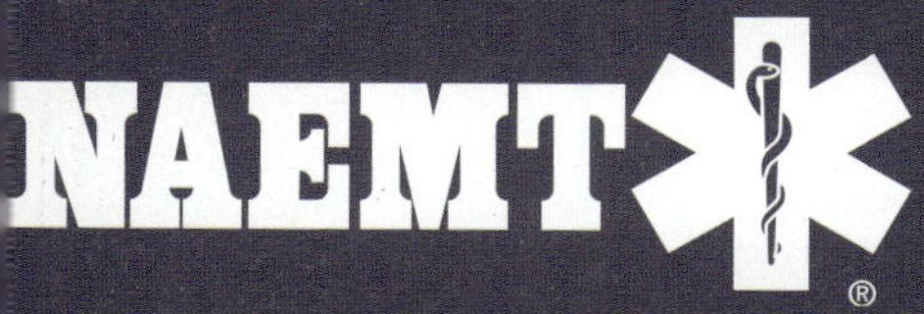

In Cooperation With

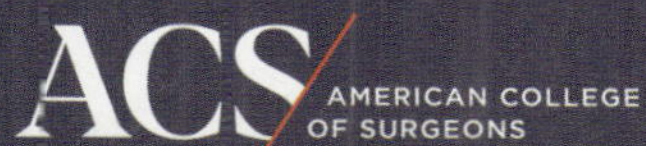

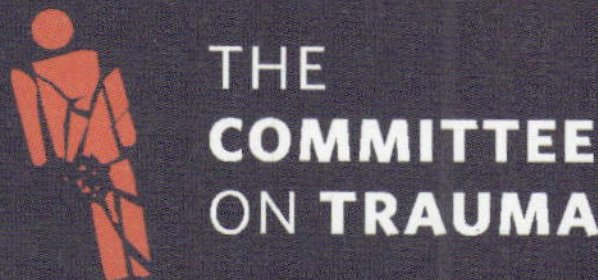

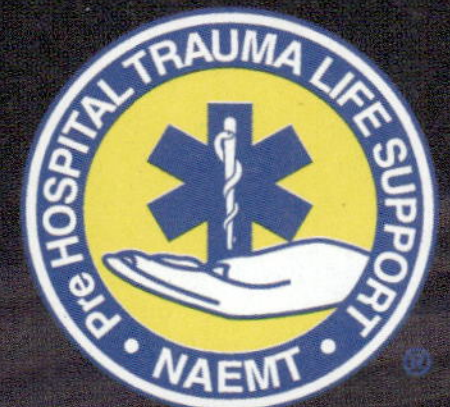

병원 전 외상 소생술

Prehospital Trauma Life Support

TENTH EDITION

지음 NAEMT | 옮김 김진우 외

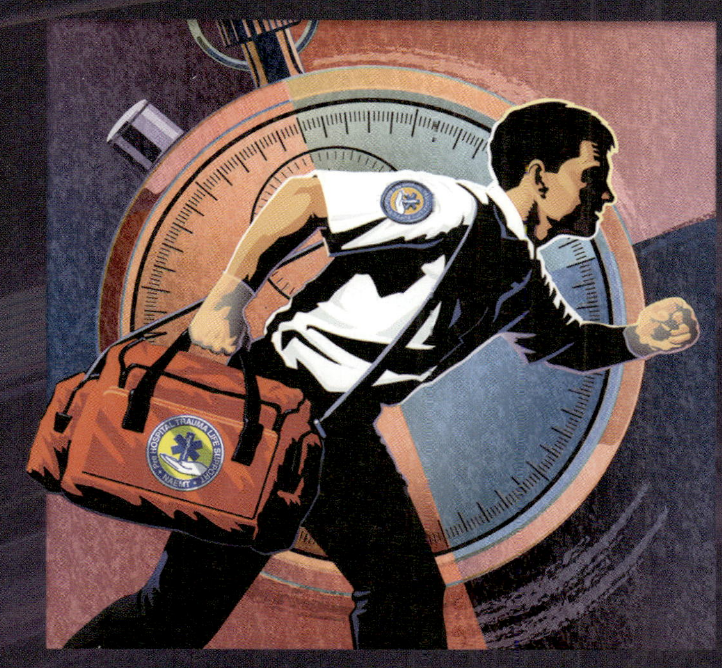

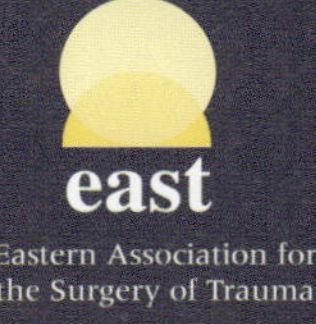

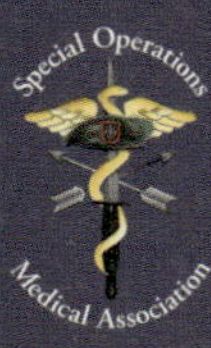

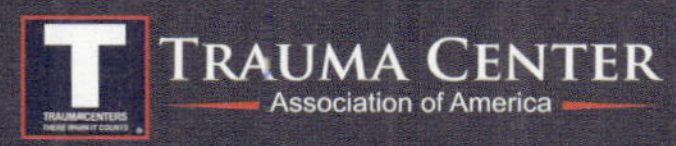

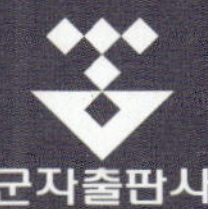

“부상자의 운명은
맨 처음 드레싱을 시행하는
바로 그 한 사람의
손에 달려있다.”

~ Nicholas Senn, MD (1844–1908)
American Surgeon (Chicago, Illinois)
Founder, Association of Military Surgeons of the United States

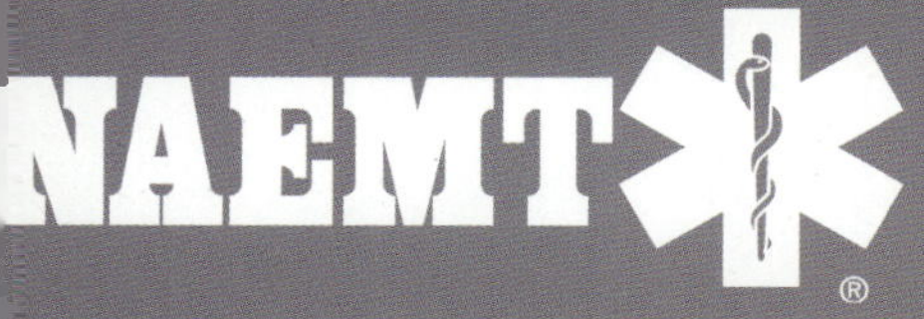
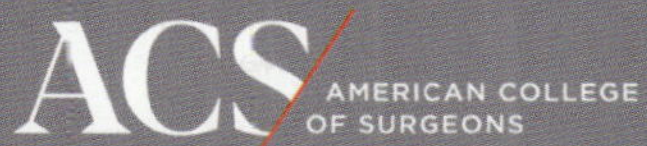
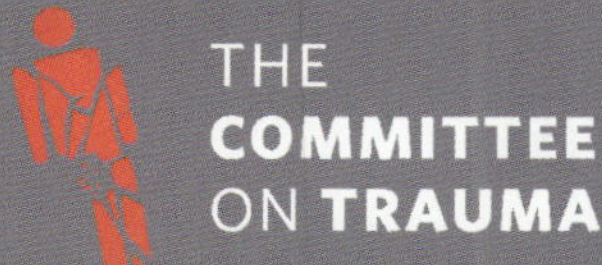

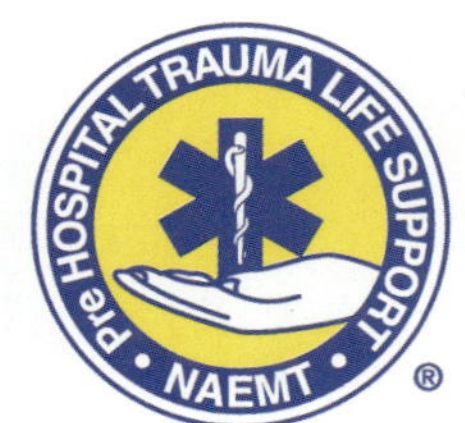

병원 전 외상 소생술
Prehospital Trauma Life Support

TENTH EDITION

지음 NAEMT | 옮김 김진우 외

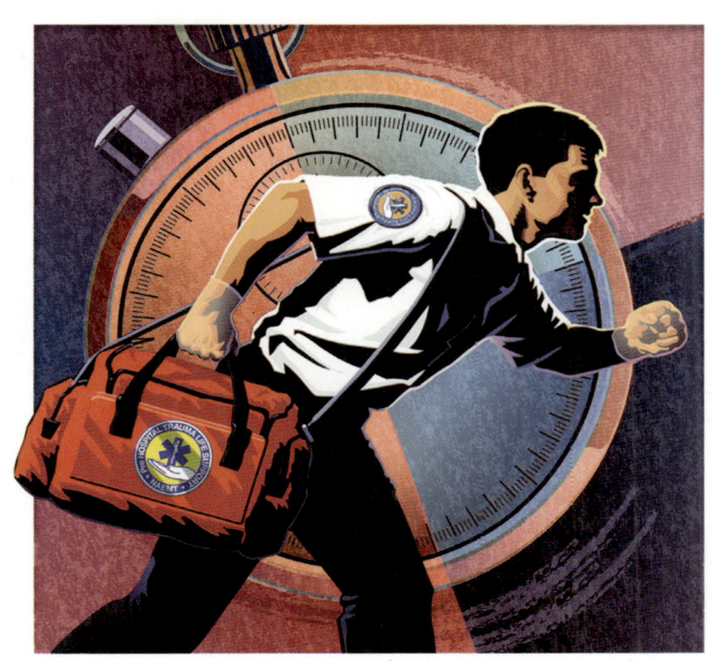

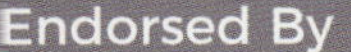
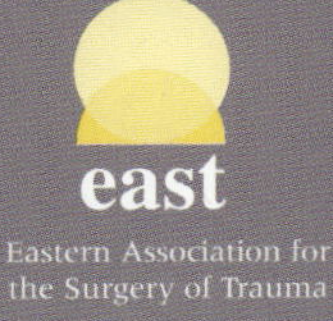
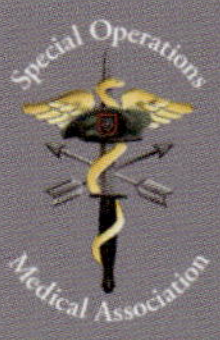
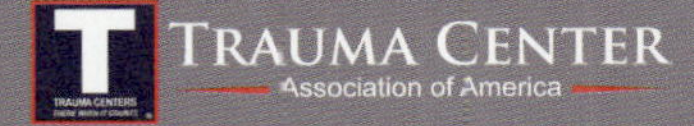
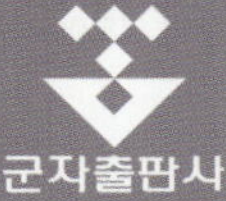

병원 전 외상 소생술 10판

첫째판 1쇄 발행 2016년 4월 15일
둘째판 1쇄 발행 2020년 4월 20일
둘째판 2쇄 발행 2021년 5월 12일
둘째판 3쇄 발행 2022년 9월   6일
열째판 1쇄 인쇄 2023년 8월 28일
열째판 1쇄 발행 2023년 9월 13일

지 은 이 National Association of Emergency Medical Technicians (NAEMT)
옮 긴 이 김진우 외
발 행 인 장주연
출 판 기 획 최준호
책 임 편 집 이다영
편 집 디 자 인 강미란
표 지 디 자 인 김재욱
발 행 처 군자출판사(주)
　　　　　　등록 제 4-139호(1991. 6. 24)
　　　　　　본사 (10881) **파주출판단지** 경기도 파주시 회동길 338(서패동 474-1)
　　　　　　전화 (031) 943-1888 팩스 (031) 955-9545
　　　　　　홈페이지 | www.koonja.co.kr

* 파본은 교환해 드립니다.
* 검인은 저자와의 합의하에 생략합니다.

ISBN 979-11-7068-047-5
정가 75,000원

목차 요약

DIVISION 1 개요 1

제1장 병원 전 외상 소생술(PHTLS): 과거, 현재 그리고 미래 3

제2장 황금 원칙, 선호 및 비판적 사고 23

DIVISION 2 평가 및 처치 45

제3장 쇼크: 삶과 죽음의 병태생리학 47

제4장 외상의 물리학 101

제5장 현장 관리 147

제6장 환자 평가 및 처치 171

제7장 기도와 환기 205

DIVISION 3 특별한 손상 261

제8장 머리와 목 외상 263

제9장 척추 외상 297

제10장 가슴 외상 343

제11장 복부 외상 375

제12장 근골격 외상 395

제13장 화상 손상 421

제14장 소아 외상 449

제15장 노인 외상 479

DIVISION 4 예방 499

제16장 손상 예방 501

DIVISION 5 다수 사상자와 테러 521

제17장 재난 관리 523

제18장 폭발과 대량살상무기 547

DIVISION 6 특별한 고려 사항 583

제19장 환경 외상 I: 더위와 추위 585

제20장 환경 외상 II: 낙뢰, 익사, 잠수 및 고도 631

제21장 야생 외상 처치 673

제22장 민간 전술적 응급의료지원 (TEMS) 709

용어 해설 727

찾아보기 743

목차

DIVISION 1　개요

제1장　병원 전 외상 소생술(PHTLS): 과거, 현재 그리고 미래　3

개요 3
응급의료서비스(EMS)에서 외상 처치의 역사 3
　고대 시대 3
　라레(Larrey) 시대(1700년대 후반부터 약 1950년대) 4
　패링턴(Farrington) 시대(약 1950~1970년) 5
　현대의 병원 전 처치 시대(약 1970년~현재) 5
병원 전 외상 소생술(PHTLS)의 철학 7
　역학 및 재정적 부담 8
외상 처치의 단계 10
　사고 전 단계 11
　사고 단계 12
　사고 후 단계 13
병원 전 외상 소생술(PHTLS): 과거, 현재 그리고 미래 16
　전문 외상 소생술(ATLS) 16
　병원 전 외상 소생술(PHTLS) 16
　군대에서의 PHTLS 17
　국제 PHTLS 17
　미래를 위한 비전 18

제2장　황금 원칙, 선호 및 비판적 사고　23

개요 24
원칙과 선호 24
　상황 25
　환자의 상태 26
　병원 전 처치 제공자의 지식 기반 27
　지역 프로토콜 27
　사용할 수 있는 장비 27

비판적 사고 28
　비판적 사고로 편견을 통제하기 30
　신속한 의사 결정에서 비판적 사고 사용하기 30
　자료 분석에서 비판적 사고 사용하기 30
　환자 처치 단계 전반에 걸쳐 비판적 사고 사용하기 ... 30
윤리 31
　윤리적 원칙 31
황금 기간: 시간에 민감한 조건 33
외상 환자가 사망하는 이유 33
병원 전 외상 처치의 황금 원칙 35
　1. 병원 전 처치 제공자와 환자의 안전 보장 35
　2. 현장 상황을 평가하여 추가 자원의 필요성 결정 ... 35
　3. 심각한 외부출혈 지혈 35
　4. 생명을 위협하는 상태를 파악하기 위해 일차평가 시행 ... 35
　5. 손상을 초래한 외상의 물리학 인식 35
　6. 척추 움직임 제한을 유지하면서 적절한 기도 관리 제공 ... 35
　7. 보조 환기 및 산소를 공급하여 산소포화도를 94% 이상으로 유지 . 37
　8. 근골격 손상을 적절히 부목으로 고정하고 정상 체온 회복 및 유지를 포함한 기본적인 쇼크 처치를 제공 ... 37
　9. 환자의 호소증상과 정신 상태를 고려하고 손상 기전을 고려하여 적절한 척추 움직임 제한 원칙을 적용 ... 38
　10. 중증외상 환자의 경우 EMS가 현장에 도착한 후 가능한 한 빨리 가장 가까운 적절한 의료기관으로 이송을 시작 ... 39
　11. 기본 관류를 회복하는 데 필요한 경우 의료기관으로 이송하는 중에 수액 소생술을 시작 ... 39
　12. 환자의 생명을 위협하는 문제가 해결되었거나 배제된 경우 병력을 확인하고 이차평가를 시행 ... 39
　13. 적절한 통증 완화 제공 40
　14. 환자 및 손상 상황에 대해 환자를 이송하는 의료기관에 상세하고 정확하게 제공 ... 40
연구 40
　EMS 문헌 읽기 40
　의료 증거 수준 40

DIVISION 2　평가 및 처치

제3장　쇼크: 삶과 죽음의 병태생리학	**47**

개요 48
쇼크의 생리학 48
　대사 48
쇼크의 정의 49
쇼크의 병태생리학 49
　대사: 인체의 운동 49
　산소공급(피크의 원리) 50
　세포 관류 및 쇼크 52
쇼크의 해부학 및 병태생리학 52
　심혈관 반응 52
　혈류역학 반응 55
　내분비 반응 55
외상성 쇼크의 분류 56
외상성 쇼크의 유형 56
　저혈량 쇼크 56
　분포(혈관성) 쇼크 59
　심장성 쇼크 59
평가 62
　일차평가 63
　이차평가 66
　근골격 손상 68
　혼동 요인 68
처치 69
　대량 출혈 70
　기도 74
　호흡 74
　순환 74
　장애 75
　노출/환경 75
　환자 이송 76
　혈관 확보 76
　수액 소생술 77
쇼크의 합병증 84
　급성신부전 84
　급성호흡곤란증후군 85
　혈액 부전 85
　간부전 85
　심각한 감염 85
　다기관부전 85
이송 지연 86

제4장　외상의 물리학	**101**

개요 102
일반적인 원칙 102

사-고 전 단계 102
사고 단계 103
사고 후 단계 103
에너지 104
　에너지와 운동의 법칙 104
　단단한 물체와 인체 사이의 에너지 교환 106
무딘 외상 109
　차량 충돌 110
　오토바이 충돌 119
　보행자 손상 121
　추락 123
　스포츠 손상 124
　무딘 외상의 국소적인 영향 125
관통성 외상 129
　관통성 외상의 물리학 129
　손상 및 에너지 수준 130
　관통성 외상의 국소적 영향 134
　산탄총 상처 136
폭발 손상 139
　폭발로 인한 손상 139
　폭발의 물리학 139
　폭발파와 신체의 상호작용 140
　폭발 관련 손상 140
　파편으로 인한 손상 140
　다발성 손상 141
외상의 물리학을 이용한 평가 142

제5장　현장 관리	**147**

개요 147
현장 평가 148
　안전 148
　상황 149
안전 관리 149
　교통안전 149
　폭력 152
상황 문제 153
　범죄 현장 153
　유해 물질 154
　대량살상무기(WMD) 155
　현장 통제 지역 156
　오염제거 157
　이차 폭발물 158
　지휘체계 158
　재난 대응계획 161
　혈액 마개 병원체 161
　환자 평가 및 분류 164

제6장　환자 평가 및 처치	**171**

개요 172
우선순위 결정 173
일차평가 173
　일반적인 인상 173
　일차평가 순서 174
　동시평가 및 처치 181
　일차평가에 유용한 장비 181
소생술 182
　이송 182
　수액 요법 182
　병원 전 처치 제공자의 자격 수준 184
이차평가 184
　활력징후 185
　SAMPLER 병력 186
　해부학적 부위 평가 186
　신경학적 검사 189
현장에서의 결정적인 처치 189
　이송 준비 190
　이송 190
　손상 환자의 현장 분류 190
　이송 기간 191
　이송 방법 193
모니터링 및 재평가(지속적인 평가) 193
의사소통 193
특별한 고려사항 194
　외상성 심장정지 194
　통증 관리 196
　학대로 인한 손상 197
이송 지연 및 의료기관 간 전원 198
　환자 문제 198
　근무자의 문제 199
　장비 문제 199

제7장　기도와 환기	**205**

개요 206

해부학 206
　상기도 206
　하기도 206
생리학 208
　환기는 어떻게 조절되는가? 210
　사강 210
　산소 공급 경로 211
병태생리학 212
　외상 환자의 기도 폐쇄 원인 및 부위 213
기도 평가 214
　기도와 환자의 자세 214
　상기도 소리 214
　기도 폐쇄 여부 평가 215
　가슴 상승 및 뒤당김(수축) 확인 215
처치 215
　기도 관리 215
　필수 술기 215
도수 기도 개방 216
　간단한 도수 조작 216
　흡인 216
보조 장비의 선택 217
단순 기도유지 장비 218
　입인두기도기 218
　코인두기도기 219
성문위기도기 219
　후두마스크기도기(LMA) 221
　삽관형 후두마스크기도기(ILMA) 221
　i-gel 장치 221
　후두튜브기도기(LTA) 221
확실한 기도유지 221
　기관내삽관 222
　외과적 기도유지 232
환기 233
　모니터링 233
　산소공급 최적화 235
　환기 최적화 235
　보조 환기 236
삽관의 지속적인 품질 개선 239
이송 지연 240

DIVISION 3　**특별한 손상**	

제8장　머리와 목 외상	**263**

개요 264

해부학 264

생리학 267
　뇌 혈류 267
　뇌정맥 배액 268
　산소와 뇌 혈류 268
　이산화탄소와 뇌 혈류 268

외상성 뇌손상의 병태생리학 269
    일차 뇌손상 269
    이차 뇌손상 272
평가 및 처치 278
    외상의 물리학 278
    일차평가 279
    이차평가 284
머리와 목의 특별한 손상 284
    두피 손상 284
    두개골 골절 285
    얼굴 손상 285
    후두 손상 288
    목의 혈관 손상 288

제9장 척추 외상   297

개요 298
해부학 및 생리학 299
    척추 해부학 299
    척수 해부학 302
병태생리학 304
    골격 손상 305
    척추 외상을 유발하는 특정 손상 기전 305
    척수 손상 306
평가 308
    신경학적 검사 308
    손상 기전을 이용한 척수 손상 평가 308
    척추 움직임 제한에 대한 적응증 309
처치 312
    일반적인 방법 314
    머리를 중립 자세로 도수 고정 314
    단단한 목뼈보호대 314
    고정판에 몸통 고정 315
    척추고정판에 대한 논의 317
    머리를 중립 자세로 유지 317
    완전한 고정 318
    척추 고정 시 가장 일반적인 실수 321
    비만 환자 321
    임신한 환자 321
    스테로이드 사용 322
이송 지연 323

제10장 가슴 외상   343

개요 344
해부학 344
생리학 345
    환기 345
    순환 347

병태생리학 347
    관통성 손상 347
    무딘 손상 348
평가 349
특정 손상에 대한 평가 및 처치 350
    갈비뼈 골절 350
    동요가슴 351
    폐 타박상 352
    기흉 352
    혈흉 357
    무딘 심장 손상 358
    심장눌림증 360
    심장 진탕 361
    외상성 대동맥 파열 362
    기관기관지 파열 363
    외상성 질식 364
    가로막 파열 365
    이송 지연 366

제11장 복부 외상   375

개요 376
해부학 376
병태생리학 378
평가 379
    운동학 379
    병력 381
    신체검사 381
    특별 검사 및 주요 지표 383
처치 385
특별한 고려 사항 386
    박힌 물체 386
    내장탈출 387
    산과 환자의 외상 387
    비뇨생식기 손상 390

제12장 근골격 외상   395

개요 396
해부학과 생리학 396
평가 398
    손상 기전 398
    일차평가 및 이차평가 399
    관련 손상 400
특정 근골격 손상 400
    출혈 400
    맥박이 촉지되지 않는 팔다리 402
    불안정성(골절 및 탈구) 404
특별한 고려 사항 408

심각한 다기관 외상 환자 408
구획증후군 408
심하게 훼손된(짓이겨진) 팔다리 408
절단 409
으깸증후군 411
뱀 412

이송 지연 413

제13장 화상 손상   421

개요 422
화상의 원인 422
화상 손상의 병태생리학 422
화상 손상의 체액 변화 422
화상 손상의 전신적 영향 423
피부의 해부학 423
화상의 특성 424
화상 깊이 424
화상 평가 427
일차평가 및 소생술 427
이차평가 429
처치 431
초기 화상 처치 431
수액 소생술 434
통증 조절 436
특별한 고려 사항 436
전기 손상 436
둘레 화상 437
연기 흡입 손상 437
아동 학대 440
방사선 화상 441
화학 화상 442

제14장 소아 외상   449

개요 450
소아 외상 환자 450
소아 외상의 인구 통계 450
외상 및 소아 외상의 물리학 451
일반적인 손상 유형 451
열 항상성 451
심리 사회적 문제 452
회복 및 재활 452
병태생리학 452
저산소증 452
출혈 453
중추신경계 손상 454
평가 454
일차평가 454

기도 455
호흡 457
순환 459
장애 459
노출/환경 461
이차평가 461
처치 461
심각한 외부출혈 지혈 462
기도 462
호흡 463
순환 465
통증 조절 466
이송 466
특별한 손상 466
외상성 뇌손상(TBI) 466
척수 외상 468
가슴 손상 468
복부 손상 469
팔다리 외상 469
화상 손상 469
자동차 손상 예방 471
아동 학대 및 방임 472
이송 지연 473

제15장 노인 외상   479

개요 480
노화의 해부학 및 생리학 480
만성 질환의 영향 480
귀, 코, 목구멍(ENT) 482
호흡계 482
심혈관계 482
신경계 483
감각 변화 484
신장계통 484
근골격 484
피부 485
영양과 면역체계 486
평가 486
외상의 물리학 486
일차평가 487
이차평가 488
처치 490
대량 출혈 490
기도 492
호흡 492
순환 492
척추 움직임 제한 492
체온 조절 493
법적 고려 사항 493

노인 학대 신고.................493
노인 학대 493
학대 유형 494
COVID-19가 노인 학대에 미치는 영향.................494

중요 사항.................494
조처 495
이송 지연 495
예방 495

DIVISION 4   예방

제16장 손상 예방　501

개요 502
손상의 개념 502
손상의 정의 502
질병으로서의 손상 502
해든 매트릭스(Haddon Matrix) 503
스위스 치즈 모형 505
손상의 분류 505
문제의 범위 505
친한 동료의 폭력 508
EMS 제공자의 손상 508

해결책으로서의 예방 509
손상 예방의 개념 509
목표 509
개입할 기회 510
잠재적 전략 510
전략 실행 510
공중 보건 접근법 513
손상 예방에서 EMS의 역할 변환 514
일대일 개입 514
지역사회 개입 515
EMS 제공자를 위한 손상 예방 515

DIVISION 5   다수 사상자와 테러

제17장 재난 관리　523

개요 523
재난 주기 524
종합적인 응급 상황 관리 525
개인 준비 525
다수 사상자 사고(MCI) 관리 527
국가 사고관리체계(NIMS) 528
재난지휘체계(ICS) 528
재난지휘체계의 구성 531
재난 발생 시 의료 대응 533
초기대응 533
수색 및 구조 534
분류 535
처치 537
이송 537
의료 지원팀 537
테러 및 대량살상무기의 위협 538
오염 제거 539
처치 구역 539
재난에 대한 심리적 반응 539
정신 건강에 영향을 미치는 재난의 특징 539

심리적 반응에 영향을 미치는 요인 539
재난으로 인한 심리적 후유증 540
중재 540
EMS 제공자 스트레스 540
재난 교육 및 훈련 541
재난 대응의 일반적인 함정 542
대비 542
통신 542
현장 안전 543
직접 파견 지원 543
공급 및 장비 자원 543
병원에 알리지 않음 543
미디어 543

제18장 폭발과 대량살상무기　547

개요 548
일반적인 고려 사항 549
현장 평가 549
재난지휘체계(ICS) 550
개인보호장비 550
통제지역 552

환자 분류 552
오염 제거의 원칙 553

폭발, 폭발물 및 소이제 554
폭발물의 종류 554
손상 기전 555
손상 유형 557
평가 및 처치 557
이송 고려 사항 558
소이제 558

화학 물질 559
화학 작용제의 물리적 특성 559
개인보호장비 559

평가 및 관리 560
이송 고려 사항 560
특정 화학 물질 선택 561

생물학적 제제 564
농축된 생물학적 작용제와 감염된 환자 565
선택된 제제 567

방사선 재난 573
방사선 재난의 의학적 영향 574
개인보호장비 577
평가 및 처치 577
이송 시 고려사항 577

DIVISION 6   특별한 고려 사항

제19장 환경 외상 I: 더위와 추위   585

개요 586
역학 586
열 관련 질환 586
저온 관련 질환 586
해부학 586
피부 586
생리학 587
체온 조절 및 체온 균형 587
항상성 589
열 질환의 위험 요인 589
비만, 체력 및 체질량 지수 589
나이 589
건강 상태 590
약물 590
탈수 590
열로 인한 손상 591
경미한 열 관련 질환 591
주요 열 관련 질환 593
열 관련 질환 예방 599
환경 600
수분공급 600
운동 602
열 순응 602
응급 사고 재활 603
한랭으로 의한 손상 603
탈수 603
경미한 한랭 관련 질환 604
주요 한랭 관련 질환 606
2020 AHA 심폐소생술 및 응급 심혈관 치료를 위한 지침 617
특수 상황에서의 심정지-우발적 저체온증 617
경증에서 중증 저체온증 처치를 위한 BLS 지침 618

저체온증 처치를 위한 ACLS 지침 618
추위와 관련된 손상 예방법 619
이송 지연 620
열 관련 질환 621
한랭과 관련된 질환 622

제20장 환경 외상 II: 낙뢰, 익사, 잠수 및 고도   631

개요 632
낙뢰 관련 손상 632
역학 632
손상 기전 632
낙뢰로 인한 손상 633
평가 635
처치 636
예방 636
익사 638
역학 639
익사의 위험 요소 639
손상 기전 640
수중 구조 642
생존의 예측 요인 642
평가 642
처치 644
익사 예방 646
레크리에이션 스쿠버 관련 손상 647
역학 648
압력의 기계적 영향 648
압력 손상 649
동맥기체색전증과 감압병 평가 654
처치 654
스쿠버 다이빙과 관련 손상 예방 655
고소병 658

역학 659
저압 저산소증 659
고소병과 관련된 요인 660
급성 고산병(AMS) 660
고지성 뇌부종(HACE) 661
고지성 폐부종(HAPE) 662
예방 663

이송 지연 665
익사 665
낙뢰 손상 665
레크리에이션 스쿠버 관련 다이빙 손상 666
고소병 666

제21장 야생 외상 처치　　673

개요 674
야생 EMS 정의 674
야생 EMS와 기존 거리 EMS 비교 675
야생 EMS 시스템 676
야생 EMS 제공자를 위한 교육 676
야생 EMS 의료 지도 677
야생 EMS 기관 677
야생 EMS 상황 677
주요 야생 EMS/수색 및 구조 원칙: 위치 파악, 접근, 처치, 구출
　　(LATE) 677
전문적인 구조의 조화 678
야생 EMS 영역 678
야생에서의 손상 유형 678
안전 679
상황에 따른 적절한 처치 679
이상적인 처치 679
야생 EMS 의사 결정: 위험과 이점의 균형 681
야생에서 외상 처치에 적용되는 TCCC 및 TECC 원칙 681
환자 이송 원칙 681
부목 적용 682
기도 유지 고려 사항 682
척추 손상 및 척추 움직임 제한 683

야생 구출 방법 684
기타 야생 EMS 환자 처치 고려 사항 685
환자 평가의 원칙 685
MARCH PAWS 685
장시간 환자 처치 시 고려 사항 686
배설(배뇨/배변) 욕구 충족 686
식량과 물 필요량 686
서스펜션 증후군(현수 증후군) 688
눈과 머리 보호 690
자외선 차단 690
야생 EMS의 특성 691
상처 관리 691
통증 관리 694
탈구 695
야생에서의 심폐소생술 695
물림 및 쏘임 696
야생의 EMS 상황 재조명 701

제22장 민간 전술적 응급의료지원 (TEMS)　709

개요 710
전술적 응급의료지원의 역사와 발전 710
민간 전술적 응급의료지원의 실습 구성 요소 ... 711
기존 EMS 이용의 장애 요인 711
작전 지역 712
처치 단계 712
교전 중 처치(CUF)/위협 상황에서의 처치(직접 위협 관리) 712
전술적 현장 처치(간접적 위협 관리) 713
전술적 후송 처치(후송 중 처치) 719
다수 사상자 사고 720
의료 정보 및 의료 지침 720

용어 해설 727
찾아보기 743

내용의 특수 술기 표

© Ralf Hiemisch/Getty Images

골내 혈관 접근 91

지혈대 적용 93

C-A-T 지혈대 팔에 적용 93

C-A-T 지혈대 다리에 적용 95

국소 지혈 드레싱 및 일반 거즈를 사용한 상처 패킹 97

이스라엘 외상 붕대를 이용한 압박 드레싱 99

특별한 기도 관리 방법 245

외상 턱밀어올리기법 245

변형된 외상 턱 밀어올리기 245

외상 턱들기법 246

입인두기도기(OPA) 247

입인두기도기: 설압자를 이용한 삽입 방법 248

코인두기도기(NPA) 249

백마스크 환기 250

성문위기도기 251

후두튜브기도기 251

I-gel 후두마스크 253

삽관형 후두마스크기도기(ILMA) 254

외상 환자의 시각화 입기관삽관 256

대면 입기관삽관 258

Airtraq 채널 비디오 후두경을 이용한 삽관 259

외과적 반지갑상연골절개 260

척추 관리 328

목뼈보호대 크기 측정 및 적용 328

통나무굴리기법(Logroll) 330

앉은 자세로 발견된 환자의 척추 움직임 제한 334

소아 고정 장비 338

헬멧 제거 339

진공부목 적용 341

가슴 외상 술기 372

바늘감압 372

넙적다리뼈 골절에 견인부목 적용 416

골반 고리 골절에 대한 골반고정대 적용 419

정맥 라인 고정 724

Contributors

Medical Editor–Tenth Edition

Andrew N. Pollak, MD, FAAOS
The James Lawrence Kernan Professor
  and Chairman
Department of Orthopaedics
University of Maryland School of
  Medicine
Chief Clinical Officer
University of Maryland Medical System
Medical Director Baltimore County Fire
  Department
Special Deputy U.S. Marshal
Baltimore, Maryland

Editor–Military Edition

Frank K. Butler Jr., MD
Capt, MC, USN (Retired)
Chairperson
Committee on Tactical Combat Casualty
  Care
Joint Trauma System
Pensacola, Florida

Chapter Editors

**Heidi Abraham, MD, EMT-B, EMT-T,
FAEMS**
Deputy Medical Director Austin/Travis
  County Office of the Chief Medical
  Officer
Austin, Texas
Medical Director New Braunfels Fire
  Department
New Braunfels, Texas

Faizan H. Arshad, MD
Section Chief, Division of EMS
EMS Medical Director—Vassar EMS part
  of NuVance Health
Asst Residency Program Director—Dept
  of Emergency Medicine
USAF-R Flight Commander—Critical
  Care Air Transport Team
Evaluations Subcommittee Chair,
  Hudson Valley REMAC, New York
Host and Producer of EMS Nation
  Podcast
Hudson Valley, New York

**Robert D. Barraco, MD, MPH,
FACS, FCCP**
Chief Academic Officer
Lehigh Valley Health Network
Associate Dean for Educational Affairs
USF Health Morsani College of
  Medicine–Lehigh Valley
Allentown, Pennsylvania

Thomas Colvin, NREMT-P
Firefighter/Paramedic
Houston Fire Department
Houston, Texas

**Alexander L. Eastman, MD, MPH,
FACS, FAEMS**
Senior Medical Officer—Operations
Medical Operations/Office of the Chief
  Medical Officer
Countering Weapons of Mass
  Destruction Office
U.S. Department of Homeland Security
Tactical Medical Director, NAEMT
  Prehospital Trauma Committee
Washington, D.C.

Emily Esposito, DO
Assistant Professor, Department of
  Emergency Medicine
University of Maryland School of Medicine
R Adams Cowley Shock Trauma Center
Baltimore, Maryland

**Samuel M. Galvagno Jr., DO, PhD,
MS, FCCM**
Professor and Executive Vice Chair
Department of Anesthesiology
University of Maryland School of
  Medicine
State Medical Director, Critical Care
  Coordination Center (C4), Maryland
  Institute for Emergency Medical
  Services Systems
Baltimore, Maryland

Mark Gestring, MD, FACS
Medical Director, Kessler Trauma Center
Chief, Acute Care Surgery Division
Professor of Surgery, Emergency
  Medicine and Pediatrics
University of Rochester School of
  Medicine
Rochester, New York

Jennifer M. Gurney, MD, FACS
COL, MC, U.S. Army
Surgeon, U.S. Army Institute of Surgical
  Research
Chief, Defense Committee on Trauma
  and Chair, Committee on Surgical
  Combat Casualty Care, Joint Trauma
  System
San Antonio, Texas

Danielle Hashmi, DO, MS
Trauma/Burn/Surgical Critical Care
Crozer Chester Medical Center
Upland, Pennsylvania

Seth C. Hawkins, MD
Associate Professor of Emergency
  Medicine, Wake Forest University
Medical Director, Western Piedmont
  Community College Emergency
  Services Programs
Medical Director, North Carolina State
  Parks
Medical Director, National Association
  for Search & Rescue
Medical Director, Landmark Learning
Chief, Appalachian Mountain Rescue
  Team
Morganton, North Carolina

Nancy Hoffmann, MSW
Senior Director, Education Publishing
National Association of Emergency
  Medical Technicians
Hopkinton, New Hampshire

Michael Holtz, MD
Clinical Assistant Professor of
  Emergency Medicine
UNLV School of Medicine
Las Vegas, Nevada

Jay Johannigman, MD, FACS
Chief Medical Officer
Knight Aerospace's
Trauma Surgeon
Brooke Army Medical Center
San Antonio, Texas

Brandon Kelly, MD
Orthopedic Surgery Resident
University of Minnesota
Minneapolis, Minnesota

Spogmai Komak, MD, FACS
Assistant Professor, Department
 of Surgery
McGovern Medical School
University of Texas Health—Houston
Houston, Texas

Matthew J. Levy, DO, MSc
Deputy Director of Special Operations
Associate EMS Fellowship Director
Associate Professor of Emergency
 Medicine
Johns Hopkins University School of
 Medicine
Baltimore, Maryland

Angel Ramon Lopez, MD
General and Trauma Surgeon
Trauma Medical Director
Yuma Regional Medical Center
Yuma, Arizona

Anthony Loria, MD
Department of Surgery, Emergency
 Medicine and Pediatrics
University of Rochester School of
 Medicine
Rochester, New York

Steven C. Ludwig, MD
Professor of Orthopaedics
Chief of the Division of Spine Surgery
Spine Surgery Fellowship Director
Department of Orthopaedics
University of Maryland Medical Center
Baltimore, Maryland

Angela Lumba-Brown, MD
Associate Professor and Associate Vice
 Chair
Department of Emergency Medicine
Stanford University School of Medicine
Co-Director, Stanford Brain Performance
 Center
Palo Alto, California

Faroukh Mehkri, DO
Assistant Professor
Division of Emergency Medical Services
Department of Emergency Medicine
University of Texas at Southwestern
 Medical Center at Dallas
Deputy Medical Director, Dallas Fire
 Rescue
Police Officer & Tactical Physician, Dallas
 SWAT
Dallas Police Department
Dallas, Texas

Vince Mosesso, MD, FACEP, FAEMS
Professor of Emergency Medicine
Associate Chief, Division of EMS
University of Pittsburgh School of Medicine
Medical Director, UPMC Prehospital Care
Medical Director, NAEMT Advanced
 Medical Life
Support Committee
Pittsburgh, Pennsylvania

Jessica A. Naiditch, MD, FACS
Trauma Medical Director
Dell Children's Medical Center of
 Central Texas
Assistant Professor of Surgery &
 Perioperative Care
Dell Medical School
University of Texas—Austin
Austin, Texas

Daniel P. Nogee, MD, MHS
Medical Toxicology Fellow
Department of Emergency Medicine
Emory University School of Medicine
Atlanta, Georgia

Jean-Cyrille Pitteloud, MD
Head of Anesthesiology, HJBE Hospital
 Bern County, Switzerland
EMS Medical Director, Jura County
 Switzerland
At-Large Member, NAEMT Prehospital
 Trauma Committee
Sion, Switzerland

Christine Ramirez, MD, FACS
Acute Care Surgeon
Associate Chief Medical Information
 Officer
St. Luke's University Health Network
Clinical Assistant Professor of Surgery
Department of Surgery, Lewis Katz School
 of Medicine at Temple University
Philadelphia, Pennsylvania

**Katherine Remick, MD, FAAP,
 FACEP, FAEMS**
Medical Director, San Marcos Hays
 County EMS System
Executive Lead, National EMS
 for Children Innovation and
 Improvement Center
Associate Professor, Departments of
 Pediatrics and Surgery, Dell Medical
 School at the University of Texas at
 Austin
EMS Director, Pediatric Emergency
 Medicine Fellowship, Dell Medical
 School
Medical Director, NAEMT Emergency
 Pediatric Care Committee
Austin, Texas

Christopher H. Renninger, MD
Orthopaedic Traumatology
Chief, Orthopaedic Trauma, Tumor and
 Foot & Ankle Surgery
Walter Reed National Military Medical
 Center
Bethesda, Maryland

Thomas Scalea, MD
Physician in Chief, R Adams Cowley
 Shock Trauma Center
Distinguished Francis X Kelly Professor
 of Trauma
University of Maryland School of
 Medicine
Baltimore, Maryland

Andrew Schmidt, MD
Chair, Department of Orthopaedic Surgery
Hennepin Healthcare
Professor, Department of Orthopaedic
 Surgery
University of Minnesota
Minneapolis, Minnesota

Justin R. Sempsrott, MD, FAAEM
Executive Director, Lifeguards Without
 Borders
Director, International Drowning
 Researchers' Alliance
Kuna, Idaho

Jesse Shriki, DO, MS, FACEP
Department of Critical Care
Vice Chair of Quality and Safety,
 Department of Medicine
Assistant Clinical Professor, Creighton
 University
Omaha, Nebraska

**R. Bryan Simon, RN, MSc,
 DiMM, FAWM**
Co-owner of Vertical Medicine Resources
Owner, Peripatetic Solutions
Director, New River Alliance of Climbers
Associate Editor, Medical Screening for
 Outdoor Activities
Fayetteville, West Virginia

**Gerard Slobogean, MD, MPH,
 FRCSC**
Associate Professor
Director of Clinical Research
Department of Orthopaedics
University of Maryland School of Medicine
R Adams Cowley Shock Trauma Center
Baltimore, Maryland

Will Smith, MD, Paramedic, FAEMS
Medical Director, Teton County
Search and Rescue, Grand Teton
National Park, Jackson Hole Fire/
EMS, USFS-BTNF
Clinical Assistant Professor, University
of Washington School of Medicine
Colonel, MC, U.S. Army Reserve—
62A (EMS and Emergency Medicine)
Emergency Medicine, St. John's Health
Jackson, Wyoming

Deborah M. Stein, MD, MPH
Professor of Surgery
University of Maryland School of
Medicine
Director for Critical Care Services
University of Maryland Medical Center
Baltimore, Maryland

Alexandra E. Thomson, MD, MPH
Spine Research Fellow
Department of Orthopaedics, Spine
Division
University of Maryland School of
Medicine
Baltimore, Maryland

John Trentini, MD, PhD, FAWM
Major, USAF, MC
United States Air Force
Las Vegas, Nevada

David Tuggle, MD, FACS, FAAP
Associate Trauma Medical Director
Dell Children's Medical Center in Texas
Former Vice-Chair of Surgery and Chief
of Pediatric Surgery, OU Medical Center
Austin, Texas

Brian H. WIlliams, MD, FACS
Professor of Trauma and Acute Care
Surgery
University of Chicago Medicine
Robert Wood Johnson Foundation
Health Policy Fellow
National Academy of Medicine
Chicago, Illinois

Kelsey Wise, MD
Orthopedic Surgery Resident
University of Minnesota
Minneapolis, Minnesota

Ivan B. Ye, MD
Spine Research Fellow
Department of Orthopaedics, Spine
Division
University of Maryland School of
Medicine
Baltimore, Maryland

National Association of Emergency Medical Technicians 2022 Board of Directors Officers

President: Bruce Evans, MPA, NRP, CFO, SPO
President-elect: Susan Bailey, MSEM, NRP
Secretary: Troy Tuke, RN, NRP
Treasurer: Christopher Way, BA, Paramedic
Immediate Past President: Matt Zavadsky, MS-HSA, NREMT

Directors:
Region I:
Robert Luckritz, NRP, Esq.
Steven Kroll, MHA, EMT
Region II:
Melissa McNally, MMSC, BCEM, PA-C, NRP
Juan Cardona, MPA, NRP
Region III:
Garrett Hedeen, MHA, Paramedic
David Edgar, MHA, CCP
Region IV:
Macara Trusty, MS, LP
Karen L. Larsen, DNP, MSN, APRN, NP-C, CEN, CFRN, CPEN, FP-C, Paramedic
At-Large:
Allison G. S. Knox, MPH, MA, EMT-B
Maria Beermann-Foat, PhD, MBA, NRP
Medical Director:
Douglas F. Kupas, MD, FAEMS, FACEP

PHTLS—Medical Directors

Warren Dorlac, MD, FACS
PHTLS Medical Director
Col (Retired), USAF, MC, FS
Medical Director, Trauma and Acute
Care Surgery
Medical Center of the Rockies
Loveland, Colorado

Margaret M. Morgan, MD, FACS
PHTLS Associate Medical Director
Medical Director, Perioperative Services
UC Health Memorial
Colorado Springs, Colorado

PHT Committee

Dennis W. Rowe, EMT-P
Chair, PHT Committee
Director of Government and Industry
Relations
Priority Ambulance
Knoxville, Tennessee

Alexander L. Eastman, MD, MPH, FACS
Tactical Medical Director
Senior Medical Officer—Operations
Medical Operations/Office of the Chief
Medical Officer
Countering Weapons of Mass
Destruction Office
U.S. Department of Homeland Security
Washington, D.C.

Frank K. Butler Jr., MD
Military Medical Advisor, PHT
Committee
CAPT, MC, USN (Retired)
Tactical Combat Casualty Care
Consultant to the Joint Trauma
System
Pensacola, Florida

Jean-Cyrille Pitteloud, MD
At-Large Member, PHT Committee
Head of Anesthesiology, HJBE Hospital
Bern County, Switzerland
EMS Medical Director, Jura County
Switzerland
Sion, Switzerland

Anthony S. Harbour, BSN, MEd, RN, NRP
Member, PHT Committee
Acute Care/EMS Educator, Center for
Trauma and Critical Care Education
Virginia Commonwealth University,
School of Medicine
Richmond, Virginia
Paramedic/Quality Assurance &
Performance Improvement
Committee
Goochland County Department of Fire-
Rescue and Emergency Services
Goochland, Virginia

Jim McKendry, BSc, MEM, ACP (Retired)
Member, PHT Committee
Winnipeg, Manitoba, Canada

Joanne Piccininni, MBA, NRP, MICP
Member, PHT Committee
Program Director, Assistant Professor
Bergen Community College Paramedic
Science Program
Lyndhurst, New Jersey

Brian Simonson, MBA, NRP, CHEC
Member, PHT Committee
SERAC Trauma Coordinator
Novant New Hanover Regional Medical
Center
Wilmington, North Carolina

Reviewers

Tenth Edition Reviewers

William Armonaitis, DHPE, MS, NRP, NCEE
University Hospital EMS
Newark, New Jersey

Ryan Batenhorst, MEd, NRP
Creighton University
Omaha, Nebraska

Shawn Bjarnson, AEMT
EMS Instructor
Retired Law Enforcement Officer
Gunnison Valley Hospital
Gunnison, Utah

Mark A. Boisclair MPA, NRP
EMS Education
Chattahoochee Valley Community
    College
Phenix City, Alabama

Dr. Susan Braithwaite
Western Carolina University
Cullowhee, North Carolina

Edward Caballero, MBA, NRP, FP-c, CCP-c
University of Hawai'i at Kapi'olani
    Community College
Honolulu, Hawaii

Bernadette Cekuta
Dutchess Community College
Poughkeepsie, New York

Joshua Chan
Flight Paramedic
Life Link III
Minneapolis, Minnesota
EMS Educator/Paramedic
Glacial Ridge Health System
Glenwood, Minnesota

Claudia Clark, MA, NRP
Anne Arundel Community College
Arnold, Maryland

Kevin Curry, AS, NRP, CCEMTP
United Training Center
Lewiston, Maine

Charles Dixon, NRP, NCEE
Nucor Steel Berkeley
Huger, South Carolina

Joel Ellzie, BS, NRP
University of South Alabama
Mobile, Alabama

Ronald Feller Sr., BSEd, MBA, NRP
Oklahoma EMS Education
Oklahoma City, Oklahoma

John A. Flora, Firefighter/ Paramedic, EMS-I
EMS Coordinator
Urbana Fire Division
Urbana, Ohio

Victoria Gallaher, FP-C, CCP
Nauvoo Fire Protection District
Nauvoo, Illinois

Jeffery D. Gilliard, PMD, NRP, CCEMTP, FPM, MEd
EMETSEEI Institute, Inc.
Rockledge, Florida

David Glendenning
Captain/Education Coordinator
New Hanover Regional EMS
Wilmington, North Carolina

James E. Gretz, MBA, NRP, CCP-C
JeffSTAT – Jefferson Health
Philadelphia, Pennsylvania

Jason D. Haag, CCEMT-P, CIC
Upstate Medical University
Syracuse, New York

Frederick A. Haas Jr., NRP, BS
Sussex County EMS
Georgetown, Delaware

Randy Hardick, MA, NREMT-P
EMS Department Chair, Paramedic
    Program Director
Saddleback College
Mission Viejo, California

Greg P. Henington, Paramedic, FP-C, BBA, MBA
Terlingua Fire & EMS
Terlingua, Texas

Melanie Jorgenson, BLS Education Specialist
Regions Hospital EMS Education
St. Paul, Minnesota

Alan F. Kicks, BSEE
EMT/BLS/PHTLS Instructor
Bergen County EMS Training Center
Paramus, New Jersey

Robert Loiselle, MA, NRP, IC
Patriot Ambulance Service
Flint, Michigan

Josh Lopez, MA, BS-EMS, NRP, I/C
University of New Mexico School of
    Medicine
Department of Emergency Medicine
    EMS Academy
Albuquerque, New Mexico

Michael McDonald, RN, NRP
Loudoun County Combined Fire and
    Rescue System
Leesburg, Virginia

Gregory S. Neiman, MS, NRP, NCEE
VCU Health System
Richmond, Virginia

Keito Ortiz, Paramedic, NYS CIC, NAEMSE Level II
Pre-Hospital Care Training Coordinator
Jamaica Hospital Medical Center
Queens, New York

Kevin Ramdayal
EMS Deputy Chief
FDNY EMS Training Academy
Queens, New York

Josh Steele, MBAHA, NRP, FP-C, CMTE
Hospital Wing
Memphis Medical Center Air
    Ambulance, Inc.
Memphis, Tennessee

Melissa Stoddard, MPH, NRP
Tacoma Community College
Tacoma, Washington

Brian Turner, CCEMT-P, RN
Genesis Medical Center
Davenport, Iowa

Jackilyn E. Williams, RN, MSN, NRP
Portland Community College Paramedic
    Program
Portland, Oregon

Rich Wisniewski, MA, NRP
South Carolina Department of Health
    and Environmental Control
Columbia, South Carolina

Karen "Keri" Wydner Krause RN, CCRN, EMT-P
Lakeshore Technical College
Cleveland, Wisconsin

Ninth Edition Reviewers

Alberto Adduci, MD, ED
Molinette Hospital
Turin, Italy

J. Adam Alford, BS, NRP
Old Dominion EMS Alliance
Bon Air, Virginia

Justin Arnone, BS, NRP, NCEE, TP-C
East Baton Rouge Parish EMS
Baton Rouge, Louisiana

Hector Arroyo
New York City Fire Department Bureau
of Training
Bayside, New York

Ryan Batenhorst, MEd, NRP
Southeast Community College
Lincoln, Nebraska

Nick Bourdeau, RN, Paramedic I/C
Huron Valley Ambulance
Ypsilanti, Michigan

**Dr. Susan Smith Braithwaite,
EdD, NRP**
Western Carolina University
Cullowhee, North Carolina

Lawrence Brewer, MPH, NRP, FP-C
Rogers State University/Tulsa
LifeFlight
Claremore, Oklahoma

Aaron R. Byington, MA, NRP
Davis Technical College
Kaysville, Utah

Bernadette Cekuta
Dutchess Community College
Wappingers Falls, New York

Ted Chialtas
Fire Captain/Paramedic, Paramedic
Program Coordinator
San Diego Fire-Rescue Department
Paramedic Program
San Diego, California

Hiram Colon
New York City Fire Department Bureau
of EMS
New York, New York

Kevin Curry, AS, NRP, CCEMT-P
United Training Center
Lewiston, Maine

Charlie Dixon, NRP, NCEE
Nucor Steel Berkeley
Huger, South Carolina

John A. Flora, FF/Paramedic, EMS-I
Urbana Fire Division
Urbana, Ohio

Fidel O. Garcia, EMT-P
Professional EMS Education
Grand Junction, Colorado

Jeff Gilliard, NRP/CCEMT-P/FPC, BS
President/CEO, Central Florida Office
Emergency Medical Education &
Technology Systems Inc.
Rockledge, Florida

David Glendenning, EMT-P
Education & Outreach Officer
New Hanover Regional EMS
Wilmington, North Carolina

Conrad M. Gonzales, Jr., NREMT-P
San Antonio Fire Department (retired)
San Antonio, Texas

David M. Gray, BS, EMTP-IC
Knoxville Fire Department
Knoxville, Tennessee

**Jamie Gray, BS, AAS, FF, NRP
(NAEMT/NAEMSE/ATOA)**
State of Alabama Office of EMS
Montgomery, Alabama

Kevin M. Gurney, MS, CCEMT-P, I/C
Delta Ambulance
Waterville, Maine

**Jason D. Haag, CCEMT-P, CIC,
Tactical Medic**
Finger Lakes Ambulance
Clifton Springs, New York
Wayne County Advanced Life
Support Services
Marion, New York
Finger Lakes Regional Emergency
Medical Services Council
Geneva, New York

Poul Anders Hansen, MD
Medical Director
EMS North Denmark Region
Chairman PHTLS Denmark

**Anthony S. Harbour, BSN, MEd,
RN, NRP**
Executive Director
Southern Virginia Emergency Medical
Services
Roanoke, Virginia

Brad Haywood, NRP, FP-C, CCP-C
Fairfax County Fire and Rescue
Academy
Fairfax, Virginia

Greg Henington
Terlingua Fire & EMS
Terlingua, Texas

Paul Hitchcock, NRP
Front Royal, Virginia

Sandra Hultz, NREMT-P
Holmes Community College
Ridgeland, Mississippi

**Joseph Hurlburt, BS, NREMT-P,
EMT-P I/C**
Instructor Coordinator/Training Officer
Rapid Response EMS
Romulus, Michigan

Melanie Jorgenson
Regions Hospital EMS
Oakdale, Minnesota

Travis L. Karicofe, NREMT-P
EMS Officer
City of Harrisonburg Fire Department
Harrisonburg, Virginia

Brian Katcher NRP, FP-C
Warrenton, Virginia

Alan F. Kicks, EMT
PHTLS Instructor
Bergen County EMS Training Center
Paramus, New Jersey

Jared Kimball, NRP
Tulane Trauma Education
New Orleans, Louisiana

Timothy M. Kimble, AAS, NRP
Education Coordinator
Carilion Clinic Life Support Training
Center
Craig County Emergency Services
New Castle, Virginia

Don Kimlicka, NRP, CCEMT-P
Executive Director
Clintonville Area Ambulance Service
Clintonville, Wisconsin

Jim Ladle, BS, FP-C, CCP-C
South Jordan City Fire Department
South Jordan, Utah

Frankie S. Lobner
Mountain Lakes Regional EMS Council
Queensbury, New York

Robert Loiselle, MA, NRP, EMSIC
Bay City, Michigan

Joshua Lopez, BS-EMS, NRP
University of New Mexico EMS
   Academy
Albuquerque, New Mexico

Kevin M. Lynch, NREMT, NYS CIC
Greenburgh Police Department: EMS
White Plains, New York

Christopher Maeder, BA, EMT-P
Chief
Fairview Fire District
Fairview, New York

Jeanette S. Mann, BSN, RN, NRP
Director of EMS Programs
Dabney S. Lancaster Community College
Clifton Forge, Virginia

Michael McDonald, RN, NRP
Loudoun County Fire Rescue
Leesburg, Virginia

Jeff McPhearson, NRP
Southside Regional Medical Center
Petersburg, Virginia

David R. Murack, NREMT-P, CCP
EMS Educator
Lakeshore Technical College
Assistant Chief of Emergency Operations
City of Two Rivers Fire/Rescue
Cleveland, Wisconsin

**Stephen Nacy, FP-C, TP-C,
CCEMT-P, NRP, DMT**
Leesburg, Virginia

**Gregory S. Neiman, MS, NRP, NCEE,
CEMA(VA)**
VCU Health System
Richmond, Virginia

Norma Pancake, BS, MEP, NREMT-P
Pierce County EMS
Tacoma, Washington

Deb Petty
St. Charles County Ambulance District
St. Peter's, Missouri

Mark Podgwaite, NECEMS I/C
Waterbury Ambulance Service
Waterbury, Vermont

Jonathan R. Powell, BS, NRP
University of South Alabama
Mobile, Alabama

Kevin Ramdayal
New York City Fire Department Bureau
   of EMS
New York, New York

**Christoph Redelsteiner, PhD, MSW,
MS, EMT-P**
Academic Director Social Work (MA)
Danube University, Krems Austria
Scientific Director
Emergency Health Services Management
   Program
University of Applied Sciences St. Pölten

Les Remington, EMT-P, I/C, FI1
EMS Educator, Trauma Course
   Coordinator Genesys EMS and
   Employee Education
Grand Blanc, Michigan

Ian T.T. Santee, MPA, MICT
City and County of Honolulu
Honolulu, Hawaii

Edward Schauster, NREMT-P
Air Idaho Rescue
Idaho Falls, Idaho

Justin Schindler, BS, NRP
Monroe Ambulance
Rochester, New York

**Kimberly Singleton, APRN, MSN,
FNP-C**
Gwinnett Medical Center
Lawrenceville, Georgia

Jennifer TeWinkel Smith, BA, AEMT
Regions Hospital Emergency Medical
   Services
Oakdale, Minnesota

**Josh Steele, MBAHA, BS, AAS, NRP,
FP-C, I/C**
Hospital Wing (Memphis Medical Center
   Air Ambulance, Inc.)
Memphis, Tennessee

Richard Stump, NRP
Central Carolina Community College
Erwin, North Carolina

William Torres, Jr., NRP
Marcus Daly Memorial Hospital
Hamilton, Montana

Brian Turner, CCEMT-P, RN
Genesis Medical Center
Davenport, Iowa

Scott Vanderkooi, BS, NRP
Department of EMS Education
University of South Alabama
Mobile, Alabama

Gary S. Walter, NRP, BA, MS
Union College
International Rescue & Relief
Lincoln, Nebraska

Mitchell R. Warren, NRP
Children's Hospital and Medical
   Center
Omaha, Nebraska

David Watson, NRP, CCEMT-P, FP-C
Pickens County EMS
Pickens, South Carolina

Jackilyn E. Williams, RN, MSN, NRP
Portland Community College Paramedic
   Program
Portland, Oregon

Earl M. Wilson, III, BIS, NREMT-P
Nunez Community College
Chalmette, Louisiana

Rich Wisniewski, BS, NRP
Columbia, South Carolina

**Karen "Keri" Wydner Krause, RN,
CCRN, EMT-P**
Lakeshore Technical College
Cleveland, Wisconsin

Dawn Young
Bossier Parish School for Technology
   and Innovative Learning
Bossier City, Louisiana

Photoshoot Acknowledgments

We would like to thank the following
people and institutions for their
collaboration on the photoshoot for
this project. Their assistance was
appreciated greatly.

Technical Consultants and Institutions

UMass Memorial Paramedics,
   Worcester EMS
Worcester, Massachusetts

Richard A. Nydam, AS, NREMT-P
Training and Education Specialist, EMS
UMass Memorial Paramedics, Worcester
   EMS
Worcester, Massachusetts

Southbridge Fire Department

Southbridge, Massachusetts

Jerry Flanagan
Account Manager
BoundTree Medical
Dublin, Ohio

추천 서문

It is an honor to recognize the significant accomplishments of the Prehospital Trauma Life Support (PHTLS) program with the launch of the 10th Edition of the PHTLS textbook. For over 40 years, PHTLS has been the gold standard for training EMS professionals in the latest strategies to minimize death and disability after severe injury. Thanks to the long-standing collaboration between the National Association of Emergency Medical Technicians (NAEMT) and the American College of Surgeons (ACS) Committee on Trauma (COT), the PHTLS course has evolved in parallel to the Advanced Trauma Life Support (ATLS) program, ensuring seamless care of patients from the prehospital to hospital environment.

This year, as the ACS Committee on Trauma celebrates our Centennial, we reflect on the history of the evolution of EMS in the United States. Optimizing the prehospital care of injured patients has been a priority of the ACS since 1922 when Transportation of the Injured was established as one of the first subcommittees of the original ACS Committee on Fractures. In the 1950s and 60s, surgeons of the COT developed standards for ambulance equipment and for the training of ambulance personnel and first responders in basic trauma care. As EMS systems began to develop, Norman E. McSwain Jr., MD, FACS, a founding member of NAEMT and Chair of the ACS COT's Subcommittee on Emergency Services Prehospital (1981–1986), saw the need for a comprehensive education program for prehospital providers comparable to the ATLS course, and so PHTLS was born.

Like ATLS, PHTLS has grown exponentially into a global program taught across the world as a uniform, evidence-based approach to care for the most critically injured. PHTLS has expanded to support both civilian and military prehospital care and has been instrumental in the implementation of the Tactical Combat Casualty Care guidelines developed during the wars in Iraq and Afghanistan. In return, lessons learned in the care of combat casualties have enhanced the care of civilian trauma patients.

This edition of PHTLS also incorporates the recently updated 2021 National Guidelines for the Field Triage of Injured Patients, which recognize the critical importance of the triage decisions of EMS clinicians in ensuring the right patient receives the right level of care in the right amount of time. EMS is the first link in the chain of survival for critically injured patients and the portal of entry into our trauma systems.

Dr. McSwain taught us, *"Trauma is a surgical disease from beginning to end. Trauma begins when the incident occurs. Trauma care begins when the first emergency medical technician or first responder arrives on the scene, not when the patient arrives at the hospital. At least half of the care provided in the golden hour is in the hands of the [paramedics and] EMTs. Trauma is a team effort and EMS is a critical part of that team."* (Scudder Oration on Trauma, 2003)

This 10th Edition of PHTLS ensures a standardized approach to the immediate care of these patients, which will save lives and support optimal outcomes for all those impacted by traumatic injury.

Eileen M. Bulger, MD, FACS
Medical Director of Trauma Programs
American College of Surgeons
Professor of Surgery & Chief of Trauma
Harborview Medical Center, University of Washington

PHTLS Textbook Development Philosophy

When we began to develop the 10th edition of this textbook, we very purposefully intended it to serve as a resource. However, we did not want it to be merely a resource that just sits on a shelf for when questions arise. We also did not want it to simply serve as the academic medicine that supports the PHTLS course. We wanted this book to be something that prehospital trauma practitioners read and then use to begin or to sustain a lifelong journey through the literature. And we wanted to provide them with a way to prepare.

When taking care of trauma victims, it is necessary to have a plan. That plan can be based on local protocols, jurisdictional algorithms, or even nationally driven standards. But as famous boxer Mike Tyson once said, *"Everyone has a plan until they get punched in the mouth."* Trauma often represents that punch in the mouth. The punch may knock your plan out from under you, but a solid foundation of knowledge and critical thinking prepares you for the unexpected.

Patients present with different challenges in different scenarios, and being prepared for the unexpected requires knowledge and reading. Being prepared requires learning from the mistakes and successes of others and requires understanding the literature written about those mistakes or successes. Whether in architecture, surgery, or prehospital trauma care, understanding the literature begins with thoroughly reading textbooks and continues with using the references in those books to delve further into the journal articles, textbook chapters, and further readings that comprise the supporting evidence.

Preparing for anything involves reading the history of what others have done before in similar situations and what they have learned. Former Marine Corps General and former Secretary of Defense James Mattis has advocated for continual preparation through reading. He argues that every problem warriors are likely to face in battle has likely been faced previously and has likely already been described in the literature. He further argues that preparing for battle by voraciously reading this literature is the solemn obligation of every warrior. You could certainly make an argument that the same is true in trauma care. Whatever constellation of injuries a patient presents with, it is highly likely that trauma victims have presented with similar injuries in the past. It is also highly likely that someone has already written about what worked and what didn't work in the care of such a patient. Gen. Mattis is famously quoted as having said, *"'Winging it' and filling body bags as we sort out what works reminds us of the moral dictates and the cost of incompetence in our profession."* While he intended for that statement to apply to performing the job of leading soldiers into battle, it certainly applies equally well to the task of caring for the injured. We cannot afford to 'wing it' when patients' lives are at stake.

In addition to serving as an important general resource for the trauma practitioner, this book is also intended to help prepare and guide students through the formal PHTLS course. While studying trauma care and the science behind it is critically important, so too is training. Prehospital trauma care practitioners must consistently and frequently practice their skills and be thoroughly prepared to perform those skills under stressful situations.

Ancient Greek poet and mercenary Archilochus wrote, *"We don't rise to the level of our expectations, we fall to the level of our training."* He, too, was referring to performance of warriors in battle, but the quote applies equally to the response of trauma care practitioners in the care of injured patients. Understanding the skills we perform and developing the muscle memory necessary to apply those skills perfectly under duress must also be part of every prehospital care practitioner's regular work of preparation.

It is the combination of planning, learning, and practicing that allows any practitioner to be as prepared as possible to care for trauma patients. This book is intended to be an important resource to allow practitioners to train effectively, to avoid 'winging it,' and to prepare to be punched in the mouth once or twice.

Why PHTLS?

Course Education Philosophy

Prehospital Trauma Life Support (PHTLS) focuses on principles, not preferences. By focusing on the principles of good trauma care, PHTLS promotes critical thinking. The PHT Committee of the National Association of Emergency Medical Technicians (NAEMT) believes that emergency medical services (EMS) practitioners make the best decisions on behalf of their patients when prepared with a sound foundation of key principles and evidence-based knowledge. Rote memorization of mnemonics without understanding their foundation is discouraged. Furthermore, there is no one 'PHTLS way' of performing a specific skill. The principle of the skill is taught, and then one acceptable method of performing the skill that meets the principle is presented. The authors realize that no one method can apply to the myriad unique situations encountered in the prehospital setting.

Up-to-Date Information

Development of the PHTLS program began in 1981, on the heels of the inception of the Advanced Trauma Life Support (ATLS) program for physicians. As the ATLS course is revised every 4 to 5 years, pertinent changes are incorporated into the next edition of PHTLS. This 10th edition of the PHTLS program has been revised based on the forthcoming 2022 ATLS course, the 10th edition of the ATLS textbook, discussions with members of the ACS-COT, and subsequent publications in the medical literature. Although aligned with ATLS principles, PHTLS is specifically designed to prepare learners to address the unique challenges encountered when caring for trauma outside of the hospital. All chapters have been revised and updated to reflect current evidence. Video clips of critical skills and an eBook are available online.

Scientific Base

The authors and editors have adopted an evidence-based approach that includes references from medical literature supporting the key principles, and additional position papers published by national organizations are cited when applicable. References have been added or updated, allowing those prehospital care practitioners with inquisitive minds to read the original scientific papers that form the evidentiary basis for our recommendations.

PHTLS—Commitment and Mission

As we continue to pursue the potential of the PHTLS course and the worldwide community of prehospital care practitioners, we must remember the goals and objectives of the PHTLS program:

- To provide a description of the physiology and kinematics of injury
- To provide an understanding of the need for and techniques of rapid assessment of the trauma patient
- To advance the participant's level of knowledge with regard to examination and diagnostic skills

- To enhance the participant's performance in the assessment and treatment of the trauma patient
- To advance the participant's level of competence in regard to specific prehospital trauma intervention skills
- To provide an overview and establish a management method for the prehospital care of the multisystem trauma patient
- To promote a common approach for the initiation and transition of care beginning with civilian first responders continuing up and through the levels of care until the patient is delivered to the definitive treatment facility

It is also fitting to reprise our mission statement, which was written during a marathon session at the NAEMT conference in 1997:

The Prehospital Trauma Life Support (PHTLS) program of the National Association of Emergency Medical Technicians (NAEMT) serves trauma victims through the global education of prehospital care providers of all levels. With medical oversight from the American College of Surgeons Committee on Trauma (ACS-COT), the PHTLS programs develop and disseminate educational materials and scientific information and promote excellence in trauma patient management by all providers involved in the delivery of prehospital care.

The PHTLS mission also enhances the achievement of the NAEMT mission. The PHTLS program is committed to quality and performance improvement. As such, PHTLS is always attentive to changes in technology and methods of delivering prehospital trauma care that may be used to enhance the value of this program.

Support for NAEMT

NAEMT provides the administrative structure for the PHTLS program. All profits from the PHTLS program are reinvested into NAEMT to support programs that are of prime importance to EMS professionals, such as educational conferences and advocacy efforts on behalf of prehospital care practitioners and their patients.

PHTLS Is a World Leader

Because of the unprecedented success of the prior editions of PHTLS, the program has continued to grow rapidly. PHTLS courses continue to proliferate across civilian and military sectors in the United States. It has also been taught worldwide in more than 80 nations, with more countries expressing interest in PHTLS to improve prehospital trauma care.

Prehospital care practitioners have the responsibility to assimilate this knowledge and these skills in order to use them for the benefit of their patients. The editors and authors of this material and the PHT Committee of NAEMT hope that you will incorporate this information into your practice and that you will rededicate yourself to the care of trauma patients.

National Association of Emergency Medical Technicians

Founded in 1975, NAEMT is the only national organization in the United States that represents and serves the professional interests of EMS practitioners, including paramedics, emergency medical technicians, emergency medical responders, and other professionals providing prehospital and out-of-hospital emergent, urgent, or preventive medical care. NAEMT members work in all sectors of EMS, including government service agencies, fire departments, hospital-based ambulance services, private companies, industrial and special operations settings, and the military.

NAEMT serves its members by advocating on issues that impact their ability to provide quality patient care, providing high-quality education that improves the knowledge and skills of practitioners, and supporting EMS research and innovation.

One of NAEMT's principal activities is EMS education. The mission of NAEMT education programs is to improve patient care through high-quality, cost-effective, evidence-based education that strengthens and enhances the knowledge and skills of EMS practitioners.

NAEMT strives to provide the highest quality education programs. All NAEMT education programs are developed by highly experienced EMS educators, clinicians, and medical directors. Course content incorporates the latest research, newest techniques, and innovative approaches in EMS learning. All NAEMT education programs promote critical thinking as the foundation for providing quality care. This is based on the belief that EMS practitioners make the best decisions on behalf of their patients when given a sound foundation of evidence-based knowledge and key principles.

Once developed, education programs are tested and refined to ensure that course materials are clear, accurate, and relevant to the needs of EMS practitioners. Finally, all education programs are reviewed and updated every 4 years or as needed to ensure that the content reflects the most up-to-date research and practices.

NAEMT provides ongoing support to its instructors and the EMS training centers that hold its courses. Over 2,500 training centers, including colleges, EMS agencies, fire departments, hospitals, and other medical training facilities located in the United States and more than 80 other countries, offer NAEMT education programs. NAEMT headquarters staff work with the network of education program faculty engaged as committee members; authors; national, regional, and state coordinators; and affiliate faculty to provide administrative and educational support.

Andrew N. Pollak, MD, FAAOS
Medical Editor, PHTLS
The James Lawrence Kernan Professor and Chairman
Department of Orthopaedics
University of Maryland School of Medicine
Chief Clinical Officer
University of Maryland Medical System
Medical Director Baltimore County Fire Department
Special Deputy U.S. Marshal

역자 소개

편집위원

김 진 우 김진우 대전보건대학교 응급구조과, NAEMT Affiliate Faculty
유 은 지 주한미8군의무사령부, NAEMT National Coordinator
양 희 범 노원을지대학교병원 응급의학과, NAEMT Medical director
이 석 원 대전소방본부 둔산소방서, NAEMT Instructor
박 세 훈 국군수도병원 응급의학과
서 상 원 을지대학교병원 응급의학과
최 강 국 가천대길병원 외상외과, NAEMT Instructor
홍 성 엽 카톨릭대학교 대전성모병원 응급의학과

역자 명단

김진우 대전보건대학교 응급구조(학)과
강신우 경기도소방본부 양평소방서
강효영 명지병원 권역응급의료센터
김경용 한국교통대학교 응급구조학과
김광석 충북보건과학대학교 응급구조과
김성주 동주대학교 응급구조(학)과
김수일 선린대학교 응급구조(학)과
김숙희 경기도소방본부
김용석 건양대학교 응급구조학과
김종호 경기도소방본부
문성모 청암대학교 응급구조과
민성기 해양경찰청
박영석 선문대학교 응급구조학과
박세훈 국군수도병원 응급의학과
박재성 동주대학교 응급구조(학)과
백승일 강원도소방본부
서상원 을지대학교병원 응급의학과
안신욱 울산소방본부

양희범 의정부을지대학교병원 응급의학과
오희석 소방청 119구급과
유은지 주한미8군의무사령부
유창환 충북보건과학대학 응급구조과
육지혜 해양경찰청
윤병길 건양대학교 응급구조학과
이남종 전주기전대학교 응급구조과
이다은 주한미8군의무사령부
이석원 대전소방본부
이재인 경기도소방학교
정수연 주한미8군의무사령부
정필중 소방청 119종합상황실
주종만 경기도소방본부
최강국 가천대길병원 외상외과
최명재 서울대학교병원 권역응급의료센터
홍성엽 가톨릭대학교 대전성모병원 응급의학과
홍영표 충청소방학교
황성훈 삼성전자 평택방재센터

역자 서문

COVID-19 발생으로 인해 전 세계적으로 수백만 명의 사망자와 수억만 명의 확진자가 발생했으며 이로 인해 우리에게도 많은 영향을 주었습니다. COVID-19의 확산으로 인해 많은 국가에서 PHTLS 교육에도 큰 영향을 주었습니다. 우리는 이런 상황에서 정부 방역 지침을 준수하면서 안전하게 교육을 진행했습니다.

PHTLS 제10판은 대한의사협회 의학용어위원회 6판을 기준으로 EMS 제공자가 쉽게 이해할 수 있도록 번역하기 위해 노력하였습니다.

병원 전 단계의 응급처치는 개인 또는 팀 단위로 변화가 되었으며 병원 전 EMS 제공자는 현장에서 부상이나 질병으로 인해 발생한 환자의 손상과 사망을 예방하고 통증을 경감시킬 수 있도록 구조와 응급처치를 효율적으로 제공해야 합니다. 그리고 예방 가능한 외상 사망률이 개선될 수 있도록 전문지식 및 술기 그리고 태도를 갖추어야 합니다. 병원 전 EMS 제공자들은 열악한 환경에서도 직업의식과 책임감을 느끼고 직무에 임해야 합니다.

병원 전 단계에서 외상 처치에 대한 국내 지침은 매우 중요합니다. 외상 환자를 처치하는 응급구조사, 응급 전문간호사, 의사에게 필수적인 요소입니다. 그리고 외상처치에 대한 표준지침과 교육과정이 확립되지 않은 병원 전 또는 병원 내 환경에서 이러한 교육 과정이 필요하며 그 외 외상 처치를 위한 관련 기관 및 관계자의 노력도 절실하게 필요합니다.

PHTLS 교육 프로그램을 잘 활용해 PHTLS의 가장 중요한 원칙인 병원 전 단계의 EMS 제공자들이 훌륭한 지식과 비판적 사고 능력을 통해 최적의 상황이 아니더라도 적절한 처치를 수행할 수 있는 술기 능력을 갖춘다면 예방 가능한 외상 환자의 사망률을 감소시킬 수 있을 것입니다. 또한 이러한 교육 프로그램의 시행은 병원 전 단계에서 외상 환자를 치료하는 EMS 제공자와 외상 환자를 처치하는 의사들에게 많은 도움이 되리라 생각합니다.

끝으로 이 책이 출판되기까지 고생하신 NAEMT Medical director 양희범 교수님, NAEMT National Coordinator 유은지 선생님, 국내 PHTLS 도입을 위해 노력하신 이석원 선생님, 그리고 군자출판사 최준호 과장님과 여러분의 노고에 감사드립니다.

역자 대표

김진우

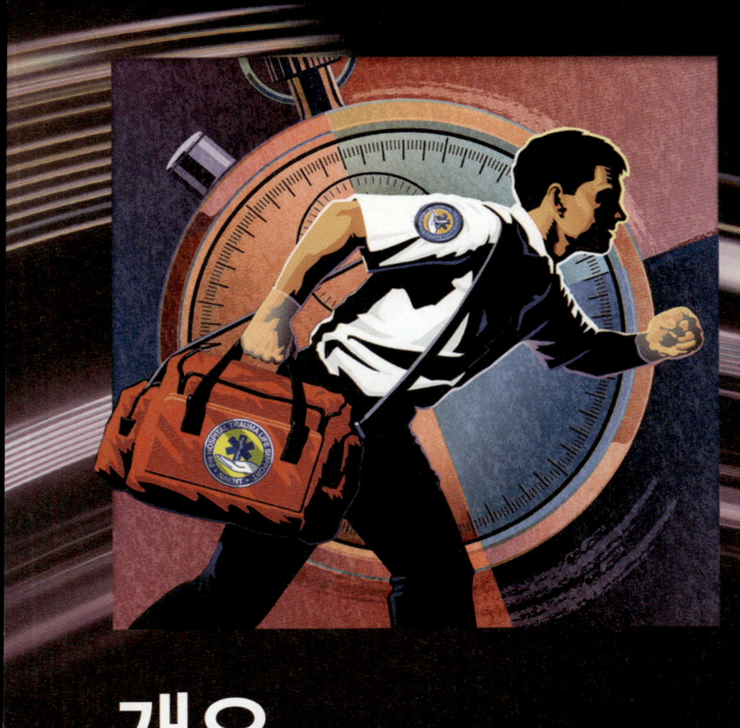

개요

제1장   병원 전 외상 소생술(PHTLS): 과거, 현재 그리고 미래

제2장   황금 원칙, 선호 및 비판적 사고

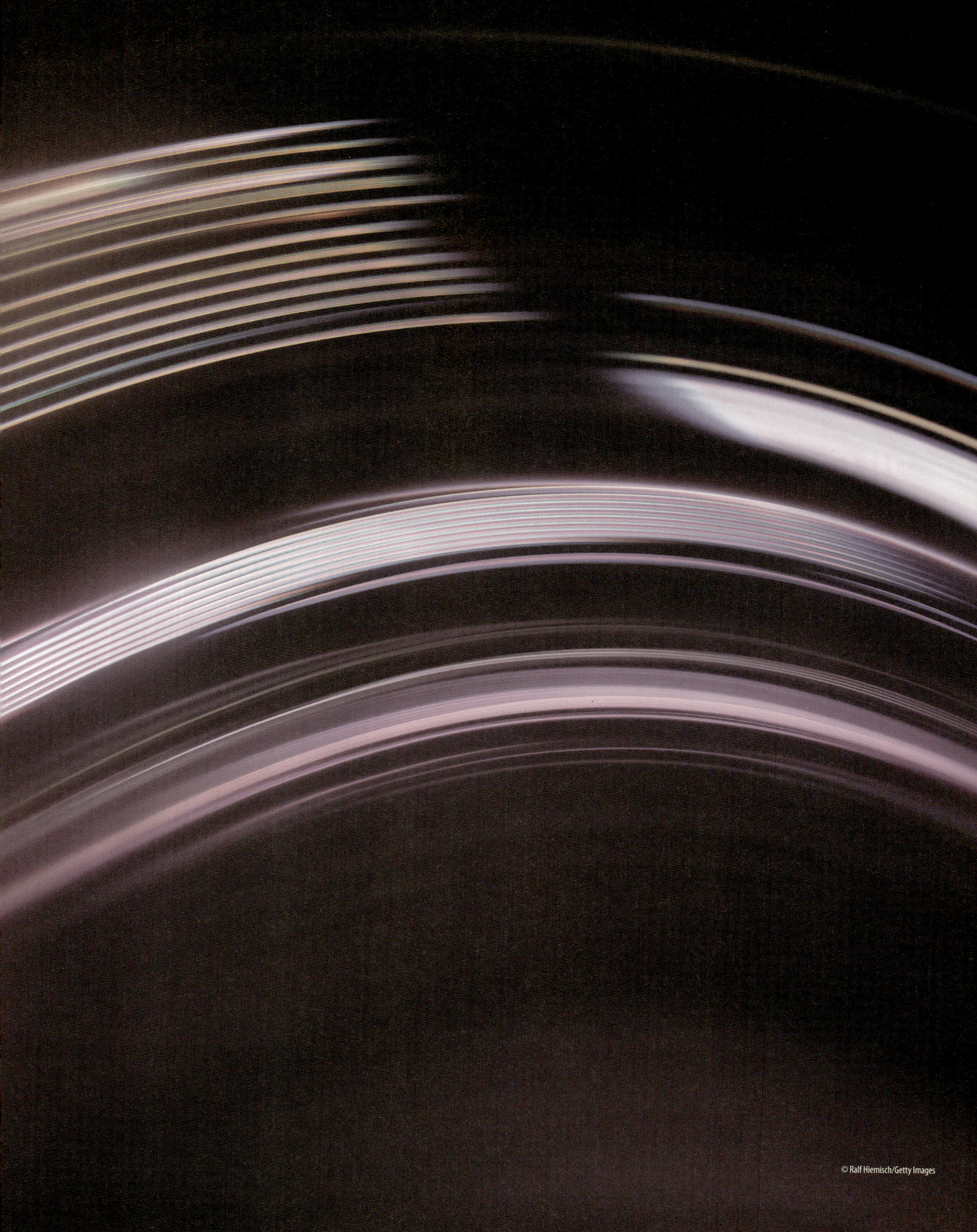
© Ralf Hiemisch/Getty Images

병원 전 외상 소생술(PHTLS): 과거, 현재 그리고 미래

Lead Editors
Andrew N. Pollak, MD, FAAOS
Nancy Hoffmann, MSW

학습 목표   이 장의 학습을 완료하면 다음과 같은 내용을 수행할 수 있다.

- 병원 전 외상 처치의 역사와 발전을 이해할 수 있다.
- 외상성 손상의 인적 및 재정적 영향의 중대성을 인식할 수 있다.
- 외상 처치의 세 가지 단계를 이해할 수 있다.

개요

환자가 우리를 선택한 것이 아니라 우리가 그들을 선택하였다. 우리는 다른 직업을 선택할 수도 있었지만, 선택하지 않았다. 우리는 우리가 피곤하거나 추울 때, 비가 내리고 어두울 때, 어떤 상황에 직면하게 될지 예측할 수 없는 최악의 상황에서 환자 처치에 대한 책임을 받아들였다. 우리는 이 책임을 받아들이거나 아니면 포기해야 한다. 우리는 공상에 잠겨 있지 말고 지속적인 장비 점검, 충분한 물품 공급 그리고 최신 지식을 가지고 우리가 할 수 있는 가장 최상의 처치를 환자에게 제공해야 한다. 우리는 최신 의료 정보가 무엇인지 알 수 없으며 매일 배우지 않는다면 환자를 처치할 준비가 되어있다고 말할 수 없다. 병원 전 외상 소생술(Prehospital Trauma Life Support; PHTLS) 과정은 병원 전 처치 제공자에게 해당 지식의 일부를 제공하지만, 더 중요한 것은 우리를 필요로 하는 모든 환자에게 도움이 된다는 것이다. 근무가 끝날 때마다 우리는 환자에게 최선을 다했다는 것을 느껴야 한다.

응급의료서비스(EMS)에서 외상 처치의 역사

외상 환자 관리의 단계와 발전은 2003년 미국 외과 대학의 스커더 연설에서 노먼 맥스웨인(Norman McSwain, MD)이 설명한 것처럼 여러 기간으로 나눌 수 있다. 이 장에서 설명하는 네 가지 시대는 1) 고대 시대, 2) 라레(Larrey) 시대, 3) 패링턴(Farrington) 시대, 4) 현대 시대이다. 이 교재와 PHTLS 교육 과정 및 외상 환자 처치는 병원 전 처치의 초기 개척자들이 개발하고 가르친 원칙을 기반으로 한다. 이러한 혁신자들은 많지만, 일부는 특별한 인정을 받을 자격이 있다.

고대 시대

이집트, 그리스, 로마, 이스라엘 사람들에 의해 그리고 나폴레옹 시대까지 이루어진 모든 의료는 전근대적 EMS로 분류된다. 대부분의 의료 서비스는 기본적인 의료시설 내에서 이루어졌으며 현장에서 병원 전 처치 제공자가 시행하는 것은 거의 없었다. 이 시대에 대한 우리의 지식에 가장 중요한 기여는 약 4,500년 전의 에드윈 스미스 파피루스(Edwin Smith Papyrus)로 일련의 사례 보고서에서 의료 서비스를 설명한 것이다.

라레(Larrey) 시대(1700년대 후반부터 약 1950년대)

1700년대 후반 나폴레옹의 수석 군의관인 도미니크 장 라레(Dominique Jean Larrey) 남작은 신속한 병원 전 처치의 필요성을 인식하였다. 1797년 그는 "구급차가 멀리 떨어져 있으므로 부상자들로부터 필요한 관심을 받지 못한다"라고 지적했으며 "날아다니는 구급차라고 부르는 마차를 만들 수 있는 권한을 부여받았다"라고 했다. 그는 전장에서 다친 전사들을 적시에 이송하기 위해 말이 끄는 "날아다니는 구급차"를 개발했고, 이러한 "날아다니는 구급차"에서 일하는 개인은 환자에게 현장 및 이송 중에 의료 서비스를 제공할 수 있도록 훈련되어야 한다는 전제를 도입했다.

1800년대 초반까지 그는 우리가 오늘날까지 계속 사용하고 있는 병원 전 처치의 기본 이론을 확립했다.

- 신속한 이송
- 의료진의 적절한 교육
- 전투 중 환자 이송 및 처치를 위해 현장으로 이동
- 현장에서 출혈 지혈
- 가까운 병원으로 이송
- 이송 중 처치 시행
- 최전선에 병원 설치
- 손상 중증도에 따른 현장 분류

그는 최전선과 가까운 병원(오늘날의 군대처럼)을 발전시켰고 환자를 전장에서 병원까지 신속한 이송을 강조했다. 라레 남작은 현재 많은 사람에게 현대 EMS의 아버지로 인정받고 있다.

하지만, 라레 남작이 개발한 치료의 유형은 미국 남북 전쟁이 시작된 60년 후에 미국의 연합군에 의해 사용되지 않았다. 1861년 8월에 제1차 불런 전투에서 3일 동안 3,000명의 부상자가 발생하였고 최대 1주일 동안 600명의 부상자가 발생하였다. 조나단 레터맨(Jonathan Letterman)이 의무 국장으로 임명되어 더 잘 조직된 의료 서비스를 제공하기 독립된 의료지원팀을 만들었다(**그림 1-1**). 13개월 후 2차 불런 전투에는 300대의 구급차와 의료 인력이 투입되었고 24시간 동안 약 1만 명의 부상자를 이송할 수 있었다.

1864년 8월에 제1차 제네바 협약에서 국제적십자사가 창설되었다.

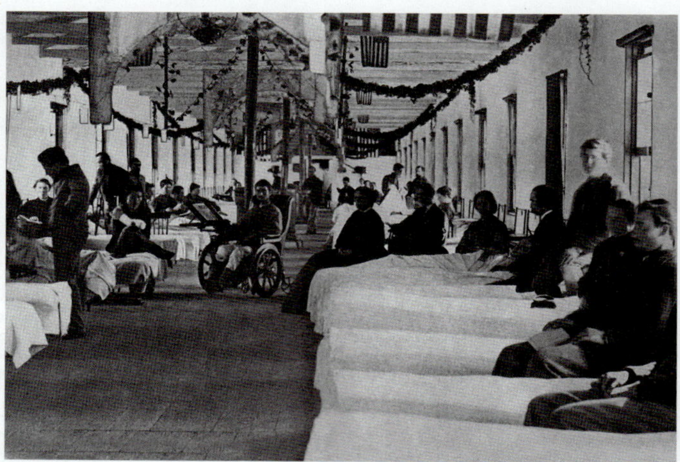

그림 1-1 미국 남북전쟁 당시 최전선 근처에 임시 병원을 짓는 것과 같이 라레(Larrey)가 개발한 군인을 위한 환자 치료 관행이 시행되었다.
© Unknown/Alamy Stock Photo

이 협약은 병원, 환자와 부상자, 관련된 모든 인원 그리고 구급차의 중립성을 인정했고 구급차와 의료인이 부상자를 이송할 수 있도록 안전한 통행을 보장했다. 또한, 환자가 어느 쪽에 있는지에 관계없이 제공되는 의료의 평등을 강조했다. 이 협약은 오늘날까지 미군이 사용하는 행동강령을 향한 첫걸음을 내디뎠다. 이 행동강령은 전술적 전투 사상자 처치(TCCC) 과정의 중요한 구성 요소이다.

병원, 군대, 영안실

1865년 미국 최초의 민간 구급차 서비스가 오하이오주에 있는 신시내티 종합병원에서 만들어졌다. 그 후 얼마 지나지 않아 여러 EMS 시스템이 미국에서 개발되었다. 1867년 뉴욕의 벨뷰 병원 구급차, 1880년대 애틀랜타 그레디 병원의 구급차 서비스(지속해 운영되는 가장 오래된 병원 기반 구급차), 1885년 외과 의사 마일스(A.B. Miles)가 만든 뉴올리언스의 자선 병원 구급차 서비스 및 수많은 기타 시설에서 운영하였다. 이러한 구급차 서비스는 1950년까지 주로 병원, 군대 또는 영안실에서 운영되었다.

1891년 군의관협회의 설립자인 니콜라스 센(Nicholas Senn) 박사는 "부상자의 운명은 첫 번째 드레싱을 시행한 사람의 손에 달려있다."라고 말했다. 센 박사가 발언했던 시기에는 병원 전 처치가 초보적인 수준이었지만, 많은 면에서 오늘날 그 말은 훨씬 더 사실이다. 외상 환자가 병원에 도착하기 훨씬 전에 이루어진 치료와 결정은 종종 다친 환자의 생존 여부를 결정한다.

제2차 세계대전이 끝날 때까지 여러 차례의 전쟁을 치르면서 의료

서비스에 약간의 변화가 있었지만, 일반적으로 군대 내 내대 지원소(Echelon II)나 민간 병원에 도착하기 전에 제공되는 시스템과 치료 유형은 1950년대 중반까지 비교적 변하지 않았다.

이 기간에 수련 병원이 있는 주요 도시의 많은 구급차에는 인턴이 근무했다. 의사가 탑승했던 마지막 구급차 서비스는 1960년대 뉴올리언스의 자선 병원이었다. 의사가 탑승했음에도 불구하고 그들이 제공할 수 있었던 외상 처치는 대부분 원시적이었다. 장비와 소모품은 미국 남북전쟁 당시 사용된 것과 크게 다르지 않았다.

패링턴(Farrington) 시대(약 1950~1970년)

J.D. 데크 패링턴(J.D. "Deke" Farrington; 1909~1982) 박사의 시대는 1950년에 시작되었다. 미국 EMS의 아버지라 불리는 패링턴 박사는 "도랑 안에서의 죽음"이라는 기사를 통해 개선된 병원 전 처치의 발전을 자극했다. 1960년대 후반 패링턴 박사와 오스카 햄튼(Oscar Hampton) 박사 그리고 커티스 아츠(Curtis Artz) 박사와 같은 다른 초기 여러 지도자는 미국을 EMS와 병원 전 처치의 현대 시대로 이끌었다. 패잉턴 박사는 구급차에서 시행하는 치료의 모든 측면에 적극적으로 참여했다. EMS의 기초를 확립하는 세 가지 초기 문서(미국 외과위원회 구급차 내 필수 장비 목록, 미 교통부의 구급차 설계 사양 및 최초의 응급구조사 기본 교육 프로그램)를 만드는 위원회의 의장으로 일하는 등 병원 전 처치의 아이디어와 개발을 촉진했다. 패링턴 박사의 노력 외에도 다른 사람이 외상 환자를 위한 병원 전 처치의 중요성을 홍보하는 데 적극적으로 도움을 주었다. 로버트 케네디(Robert Kennedy) 박사는 "아프고 다친 환자의 초기 처치"의 저자이다. 샘 뱅크스(Sam Banks) 박사는 패링턴 박사와 함께 1957년 시카고 소방서에서 최초의 병원 전 처치 교육 과정을 개설하여 가르쳤고 외상 환자의 적절한 치료에 대한 최초 반응자 교육 과정을 시작했다.

1965년 미국 외과학회 리더인 조지 커리(George J. Curry) 박사가 편집한 교과서가 출간되었는데 다음과 같이 말했다.

> 사고로 인한 손상은 인체의 모든 부분에 영향을 미친다. 경미한 찰과상과 타박상부터 여러 신체 조직을 포함하는 복합적인 손상에 이르기까지 다양하다. 이를 위해서는 이송 전에 개별적으로 효율적이고 지능적인 일차평가 및 처치가 필요하다. 훈련된 구급차 승무원의 서비스가 필수적이라는 것은 명백하다. 구급차 승무원에게 최대한의 효율성을 기대하려면 특별 교육 프로그램을 마련해야 한다.

역사적인 백서인 사고로 인한 사망과 장애: 현대 사회의 방치된 질병은 1967년에 그 과정을 더욱 가속했다. 미국 국립과학원(NAS)과 미국 국립 연구위원회(NRS)는 커리 박사가 행동을 촉구한 지 불과 2년 만에 이 논문을 발표했다.

현대의 병원 전 처치 시대(약 1970년~현재)

1970년대

병원 전 처치의 현대 시대는 1968년에 던랩(Dunlap)과 그의 동료들이 미 교통부에 EMT 구급차 훈련을 위한 교육 과정을 정의하여 보고하면서 시작되었다. 이 교육 과정은 나중에 'EMT-Basic'으로 알려지게 돼었으며 오늘날에는 'EMT'로 알려져 있다.

NREMT(The National Registry of EMTs)는 1970년에 설립되었으며 미국 국립과학원과 미국 국립연구회에서 출간한 백서에 주장한 대로 훈련된 EMS 제공자의 등록 및 시험 기준을 위한 표준을 개발했다. 로코 모란도는 15년 이상 NREMT의 집행이사였으며 패링톤 박사, 햄튼 박사, 아츠 박사와 관련이 있었다.

외상 환자에 대한 병원 전 처치 제공자의 전문적인 교육 프로그램을 만들어야 한다고 말한 커리 박사의 요청으로 개발한 교육 프로그램을 사용하여 해결되었다. 미국 도로교통안전국(NHTSA)의 EMT 교육 과정에 의해 패링턴과 뱅크스는 미국 정형외과 학회(AAOS)에서 출판한 부상자의 응급처치 및 이송과 NAEMT가 PHTLS 과정의 초기 교재 개발과 출판에 참여했다. 첫 번째 훈련 노력은 원시적이었지만, 비교적 짧은 시간 내에 크게 발전했다.

이 시대에 출판된 첫 번째 교재는 월터 호이트(Walter A. Hoyt) 박사의 아이디어로 미국 정형외과학회가 1971년에 출판했던 "부상자의 응급처치 및 이송"이고 현재 12번째 판이 출판되었다.

같은 시기에 그레이엄 티즈데일(Graham Teasdale) 박사와 브라이언 제네트(Bryan Jennett) 박사가 연구 목적으로 스코틀랜드의 글래스고 도시에서 글래스고혼수척도(Glasgow coma Scale)를 개발했다. 하워드 챔피언(Howard Champion) 박사는 환자의 지속적인 신경학적 상태를 평가하기 위한 목적으로 글래스고혼수척도를 미국으로 가져온 후 외상 환자의 처치에 통합시켰다. 글래스고혼수척도는 환자 상태의 호전 또는 악화에 대한 민감한 지표로 사용되고 있다.

1973년에는 포괄적인 EMS 시스템의 개발을 위해 연방 EMS 법률이 제정되었다. 이 법안은 통합 EMS 시스템을 갖추는 데 필요한 15개의 개별 구성 요소를 확인했다. 미국 보건복지부(DHHS)에서 근무하는 데이비드 보이드(David Boyd)박사는 이 법안의 시행을 담당하게 되었다. 이 법률에는 EMS 시스템을 구축하는 데 필요한 15가지 구성 요소가 있었는데 이 중 하나가 교육이다. 오늘날 이러한 수준의 교육을 EMT, AEMT 및 Paramedic이라고 한다. 이 교육 과정은 처음에 미국 도로교통안전국 내 교통부(DOT)에 의해 처음 정의되었으며 이후 국제 표준교육 과정 또는 미 교통부의 교육 과정으로 알려지게 되었다.

EMS 교육의 초기 선구자인 낸시 캐롤라인(Nancy Caroline) 박사는 최초의 파라메딕(Paramedic) 교육 과정 기준을 정의하였고 "현장 응급처치학"이라는 책을 집필하여 교육 과정에 사용하였다. 이 교재는 현재 9판까지 출간되었다.

생명의 별(The Blue Star of Life)로고는 원래 미국 의사협회(AMA)에서 "의료 경보"의 상징으로 디자인했으며 나중에 미국 의사협회는 이 로고를 미국 응급구조사협회(NREMT)가 공식적으로 사용했다. 당시 미국 적십자사는 "응급"을 상징하는 의미로 구급차에 "적십자" 로고를 사용하는 것에 대하여 허가하지 않았기 때문에 미국 도로교통안전국의 EMS 책임자였던 루 슈워츠(Lew Schwartz)는 NREMT 이사회 의장인 패링턴 박사에게 구급차를 상징할 수 있는 로고로 생명의 별을 사용할 수 있도록 요청하였다. NREMT에서 허가받았고 생명의 별은 이후 EMS 시스템의 국제적 상징이 되었다.

NAEMT는 NREMT의 재정적 지원으로 1975년에 설립되었다(**그림 1-2**). NAEMT는 Paramedic, AEMT, EMT, 최초반응자와 병원 전 응급의학 분야에서 일하는 기타 전문가를 포함하여 모든 EMS 종사자의 전문적 이익을 대변하는 데 전념하는 미국 내 유일한 기관이다.

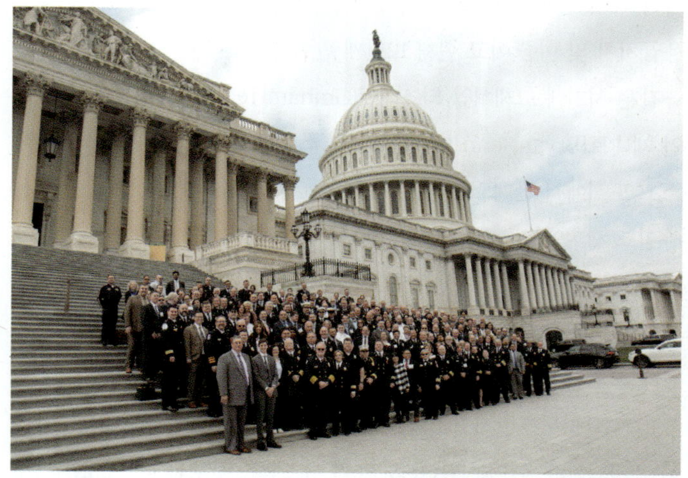

그림 1-2 1975년에 설립된 NAEMT는 파라메딕, EMT, AEMT, 응급의료대응자, 중환자 파라메딕, 항공응급구조사를 포함하여 모든 응급 및 이동 의료 종사자의 전문적 이익을 대변하는 미국 내 유일한 기관이다.

1980년대

1980년대 중반에 외상 환자는 병원 전 처치 및 교육의 관점에서 심장병 환자와 다르다는 것이 명백해졌다. 프랭크 루이스(Frank Lewis) 박사와 도널드 트런키(Donald Trunkey) 박사와 같은 외상 전문의는 이 두 그룹 사이의 주요 차이점을 인식했다. 심장질환 환자의 경우 심박출량을 회복하는 데 필요한 도구(심폐소생술, 체외 제세동기와 보조 약물)의 전부 또는 대부분을 현장에서 적절하게 훈련된 파라메딕이 사용할 수 있었다. 그러나 외상 환자의 경우 가장 중요한 물품(내부출혈의 외과적 지혈 및 혈액 보충)을 현장에서 사용할 수 없었다. 이는 적절한 의료기관으로 외상 환자를 신속하게 이송해야 한다는 중요성은 병원 전 처치 제공자뿐만 아니라 EMS 의료책임자 모두에게 명백해졌다. 잘 준비된 의료시설에는 응급의학과 의사, 외과 의사, 간호사, 수술실 관계자로 구성된 외상팀이 통합되었다. 혈액은행, 원무과, 질 향상 과정 등은 외상 환자 처치에 필요한 나머지 모든 구성요소이다. 필요한 모든 자원이 준비되어 도착하는 환자를 받을 준비가 되어있어야 하고 필요한 경우 외상팀은 환자를 직접 수술실로 데려가기 위해 대기해야 했다. 시간이 지남에 따라 이러한 기준은 켄 매톡스(Ken Mattox) 박사의 허용적 저혈압과 적혈구와 혈장의 1:1 수혈 비율과 같은 개념을 포함하도록 수정되었다. 그러나 장비가 잘 갖춰진 수술실을 신속하게 이용할 수 있어야 한다는 결론은 바뀌지 않았다.

외상 환자의 신속한 처치는 이러한 시스템에 쉽게 접근할 수 있는 '병원 전 처치 체계'에 달려있다. 이러한 접근은 단일화된 신고번호(예: 미국의 911), 구급차를 출동시키기 위한 통신 시스템 및 잘 훈련된 병원 전 처치 제공자의 도움을 받는다. 많은 사람은 신속한 신고와 심폐소생술이 심정지 환자를 살릴 수 있다고 배워왔다. 외상도 같은 방법으로 접근할 수 있다. 방금 열거한 원칙은 환자 처치를 위한 기초가 된다. 이러한 기본 원칙에 외상센터와 수술실 이외에서는 시행할 수 없는 내부출혈 지혈의 중요성이 추가되었다. 따라서 신속한 평가, 적절한 이송, 즉시 수술실을 이용할 수 있는 의료기관으로 환자를 신속하게 이송하는 것은 1980년대 중반까지 완전히 이해되거나 수용되지 않았던 추가 원칙이 되었다. 이러한 기본 원칙은 오늘날까지 EMS 처치의 기반으로 남아 있다.

지금까지 언급된 의사, 병원 전 처치 제공자 및 조직의 업적은 돋보이지만, 이 외에도 EMS의 발전에 이바지한 다른 많은 사람은 언급할 수 없을 정도로 많다. 우리는 그들 모두에게 큰 은혜를 입고 있다.

2000년대

무력 충돌 때마다 외상 처치에 큰 발전을 가져왔고 지난 20년은 예외가 아니었다. 지난 20년간의 군사 작전은 전장에서 발생한 부상자의 처치에 가장 실질적인 변화를 보여주었다. 이러한 발전을 주도하는 주요 조직 중에는 미 국방성 합동 외상 체계(JTS)와 전술적 전투 사상자 처치 위원회(CoTCCC)가 포함되었다. 미 국방성은 전투 중에 발생한 모든 부상자에게 최적의 생존 기회와 기능 회복을 위한 최대 기회를 제공하는 것을 목표로 합동 외상 체계를 구축했다. 이를 위해 미 국방성은 부상자와 그들이 받는 치료에 관한 자료와 통계를 수집하기 위해 외상 등록소(이전의 합동 외상 등록소)를 설립했다. 전술적 전투 사상자 처치 위원회는 이러한 자료와 추가적인 자원을 임상 진료 지침 개발로 이어질 수 있는 연구의 기초로 사용한다. 이러한 임상 업무 지침은 부상자의 처치와 안정화에 사용하기 위해 현장의 의료 요원에게 배포되었다.

현재도 진행 중인 이 과정의 결과로 많은 부상자의 생명을 구했다. 전투에서 부상자의 사망률은 이전의 전쟁과 비교할 때 현저하게 감소했다. 전투에서 다친 환자의 생존율은 90% 이상으로 증가했다. 일반적으로 대량 수혈이 필요한 가장 중증의 손상을 입은 환자의 경우 손상 통제 소생술(이장의 뒷부분에서 설명)을 시행하여 사망률을 40%에서 20%로 감소시켰다.

외상 처치의 이러한 발전의 이점은 군대 의료에만 국한되지 않는다. 민간 의료 환경에서는 최전선에서 멀리 떨어진 병원에서 사용하기 위해 이러한 변화를 빠르게 채택하고 있다. 한때 최후의 수단으로 여겨졌던 지혈대 사용은 현장과 응급실에서 환자의 안정화 중에 중증 출혈을 지혈하기 위한 일차적인 처치가 되었다. 지난 20년 동안 다친 군인을 치료하면서 얻은 교훈은 앞으로 수십 년 동안 민간 외상 처치의 질과 전달에 중대한 영향을 미칠 것이다.

병원 전 외상 소생술(PHTLS)의 철학

PHTLS는 해부학 및 생리학, 외상의 병태생리학, XABCDE 접근 방법을 사용한 외상 환자의 평가 및 처치 그리고 처치를 제공하는 데 필요한 술기를 이해할 수 있는 도구를 제공한다. 출혈이나 호흡이 부적절한 환자는 중증 장애를 초래하거나 치명적으로 되기까지 시간이 제한적이다(**Box 1-1**). 병원 전 처치 제공자는 비판적 사고 기술을 보유하고 적용하여 외상 환자의 생존율을 향상할 수 있는 결정을 신속하게 내리고 수행한다. PHTLS는 병원 전 처치 제공자에게 "일률적인" 접근 방법을 암기하도록 가르치지 않는다. 오히려 병원 전 처치 제공자에게 외상 환자 처치 및 비판적 사고에 대한 이해를 개발하도록 가르친다. 각 병원 전 처치 제공자의 환자 접촉에는 고유한 상황이 포함된다. 병원 전 처치 제공자가 주어진 상황에 따라 의료 서비스의 기본 원칙과 당면한 상황에서 개별 환자의 특정 요구 사항을 이해하는 경우 해당 환자의 생존 가능성을 최대화는 정확한 환자 처치 결정을 내릴 수 있다.

Box 1-1 XABCDE

ABCDE는 일차평가(기도, 호흡, 순환, 장애, 노출/환경)의 단계를 기억하는 데 사용되는 전형적인 암기 기호이다. 이러한 접근 방식은 팔다리 또는 접합부에 출혈이 있는 경우 즉시 돌이킬 수 없는 결과를 인식하여 출혈에 초점을 맞추는 것을 포함하도록 이 교과서의 마지막 판에서 수정되었다. 전형적인 "ABCDE" 암기 기호의 가장 앞에 있는 "X"는 현장 안전을 확보한 후 처치 인력이 제한되면 기도를 개방하기 전에 치명적인 출혈을 즉시 지혈해야 할 필요성을 설명한다. 중증 외부출혈 특히 동맥 출혈은 비교적 짧은 시간에 전체 혈액량에 가까운 출혈을 초래할 가능성이 있다. 출혈 속도에 따라 그 시간은 단 몇 분밖에 되지 않을 수 있다. 또한 수혈할 수 없는 병원 전 환경에서 결정질 수액을 투여하는 것은 산소를 세포로 운반할 수 있는 능력을 회복시키지 못하기 때문에 출혈 후 발생하는 문제를 해결할 수 없다. 따라서 병원 전 단계에서는 기도를 유기하기 이전에 팔다리 또는 압박할 수 있는 부위의 중증 외부출혈을 먼저 지혈하는 것이 우선이다. 기도 문제 관리하고 적절한 호흡을 제공하며 순환 상태와 장애를 평가하고 신체를 노출하여 철저한 평가를 수행한다. 미 국외과대학 ATLS 과정을 이수하고 일차평가에 대한 접근 방식의 차이에 주목할 수 있는 사람들은 이러한 차이가 초기 출혈 조절의 중요성과 관련하여 두 과정 간의 철학적 차이를 반영하지 않는다는 것을 이해하는 것이 중요하다. 초기 출혈 조절의 중요성과 관련하여 병원 전 처치와 병원 내 처치 사이의 몇 가지 차이점에 대한 인식을 나타낸다. 첫째, 대부분의 Level I 또는 Level II 외상센터에는 외상 환자가 도착할 때 팔다리 출혈을 해결하고 기도 조절을 동시에 시행할 수 있는 충분한 인력이 있다. 둘째, 서혜부의 넓적다리동맥 절단과 관련된 것과 같은 팔다리 출혈 또는 접합부 출혈은 현장에서 효과적으로 지혈되지 않는 경우 환자가 병원에 도착할 때까지 더 이상 문제가 되지 않는다. 마지막으로 환자가 서혜부의 동맥에서 혈액이 분출되는 상태로 외상 환자 처치 구역에 도착하면 즉시 해결해야 하지만, 이미 출혈된 혈액을 대체하기 위해 대규모 수혈 프로토콜을 시작하는 것도 가능하지만, 이는 대부분 병원 전 시나리오에서 실현 가능하지 않다.

PHTLS의 가장 중요한 원칙은 병원 전 처치 제공자가 충분한 지식을 바탕으로 비판적 사고를 해야 하며 최적의 상황이 아니더라도 뛰어난 환자 처치를 수행할 수 있는 적절한 술기 능력을 갖추고 있어야 한다. PHTLS는 병원 전 처치 제공자에게 특정 조치를 금지하거나 규정하지 않은 대신 병원 전 처치 제공자가 비판적 사고를 사용하여 각 환자에 대한 최상의 처치를 제공할 수 있도록 적절한 지식과 술기를 제공한다.

병원 전 처치 전문가가 환자를 도울 기회는 매우 많을 수 있다. 외상은 종종 인생에서 가장 생산적인 시기에 있는 사람들에게 영향을 미치기 때문에 병원 전 단계와 병원 내 모든 환경에서 최상의 외상 처치를 받는 외상 환자의 생존이 사회적으로 미치는 영향은 강력하다. 병원 전 처치 제공자는 외상 환자의 생명과 생산성을 연장하고 제공되는 처치를 통해 사회에 혜택을 줄 수 있다. 외상 환자에게 효과적인 처치를 제공함으로써 병원 전 처치 제공자는 사회에 상당한 긍정적인 영향을 미칠 수 있다.

역학 및 재정적 부담

손상은 사회에 막대한 영향을 미친다. 매일 전 세계적으로 약 14,000명이 손상으로 인해 사망한다. 의도하지 않은 손상은 1~45세까지의 주요 사망 원인이다. 매년 전 세계적으로 약 440만 명 이 손상으로 사망하며 전체 사망의 약 8%를 차지한다. 결핵, 말라리아, 사람면역결핍바이러스(HIV), 후천면역결핍증후군(AIDS)과 같은 질병으로 인한 총 사망자 수는 부상으로 인한 사망자 수의 절반이 조금 넘는다. 추가적인 관점에서 코로나19 범유행의 첫해 동안 약 300만 명의 사람들이 사망했다. 외상이 매년 발생하는 유행병 비율의 문제라고 보는 것은 어렵지 않지만, 외상의 원인과 이를 처치하는 가장 효과적인 방법을 이해하는 것은 그 주제에 대한 풍부한 데이터에도 불구하고 여전히 복잡하다.

미국 질병통제예방센터(CDC)는 외상으로 인한 사망을 "비의도적 손상 및 폭력 관련 손상"이라는 포괄적인 용어를 사용하고 있다. 사망 원인으로 외상을 조사하려고 시도할 때 이러한 데이터는 의도하지 않은 모든 손상이 외상이 아니라는 사실에 의해 혼란스러워진다. 비의도적 손상에는 익사, 중독, 화재, 추락 및 자동차 충돌을 포함하여 여러 가지 원인을 포함한다. 중독이 의도하지 않은 손상의 원인이라는 사실과 마약성 진통제의 과다복용으로 인한 사망이 이 범주에 포함된다는 사실을 고려한다. 이 예는 우리가 직면 한 문제를 완전히 이해하기 위해 사용할 수 있는 자료를 얼마나 신중하게 분석해야 하는지 보여준다.

중요한 맥락을 제공하기 위해서는 연령대에 걸쳐 가장 흔한 사망 원인 중 일부에 대한 추세를 평가하는 것이 도움이 된다. 이러한 접근 방식을 취하면 예방, 교육 및 공중 보건에 대한 강조 영역을 확인할 수 있다. **그림 1-3**과 **그림 1-4**에서 이러한 영역 중 몇 가지를 볼 수 있으며 익사 및 자동차 충돌이 초기에 사망의 중요한 원인임을 명확하게 보여준다. 나이가 증가함에 따라 익사로 인한 사망자 수가 감소하기 시작하고 자동차 충돌사고가 25세 전후까지 급증하여 사망의 주요 원인이 되고 중독은 의도하지 않은 손상으로 사망의 주요 원인으로 나타난다. 중독은 65~70세가 될 때까지 의도하지 않은 손상으로 인한 사망의 주요 원인이다.

이러한 방식으로 데이터를 분석하면 나이와 관계없이 자동차 충돌이 주요 사망 원인으로 지속되지만, 생애 초기 사망 원인은 익사이다. 외상성 사망으로 간주하지는 않지만, 중독은 의도하지 않은 손상으로 인한 사망의 주요 원인으로 증가하고 있으며 코로나19 팬데믹 동안 악화한 것으로 보이는 마약성 진통제 사용이 지속되면 이러한 추세는 앞으로도 지속될 가능성이 있다.

이러한 통계는 의도하지 않은 손상의 원인과 관련하여 우려할 만한 추세를 보여주고 있으며 이러한 추세가 새로운 것은 아닐 수도 있지만, 이러한 추세에 의해 가장 영향을 받는 지역은 변화하고 있다. 자동차 충돌로 인한 사망자를 줄이기 위한 노력으로 선진국에서는 지난 수십 년 동안 전반적인 감소가 이루어졌지만, 전 세계적으로 자동차 충돌로 인한 전체 사망자 수는 증가하고 있다. 매일 전 세계적으로 약 3,700명이 자동차, 자전거 또는 보행자와 관련된 충돌 사고로 사망한다. 이러한 경향은 주로 개발도상국에서 자동차 사용이 급속도로 증가한 결과로 교통량 증가로 인한 수요에 대응할 수 있는 지역 인프라와 자원(EMS 포함)의 능력을 능가한다. 낙상 관련 손상으로 인한 사망과 관련하여 향후 수십 년 동안 유사한 패턴이 예상된다. 낙상은 전 세계적으로 의도하지 않은 손상으로 인한 두 번째로 흔한 사망 원인이다. 이로 인해 매년 전 세계적으로 650,000명 이상이 사망하며 저소득 및 중간 소득 국가에서 불균형적으로 발생한다. 매년 낙상으로 인한 사망률이 증가함에 따라 선진국에서는 낙상 위험 검사, 교육 및 예방 프로그램을 시작했다. 그런데도 미국에서는 매년 300만 명의 노인들이 낙상 관련 손상으로 응급실에서 치료받고 있으며 그들 중 800,000명 이상이 결국 병원에 입원한다. 2015년에 이러한(치명적 및 비치명적) 손상에 대한 추정 총 의료비용은 500억 달러를 초과했다.

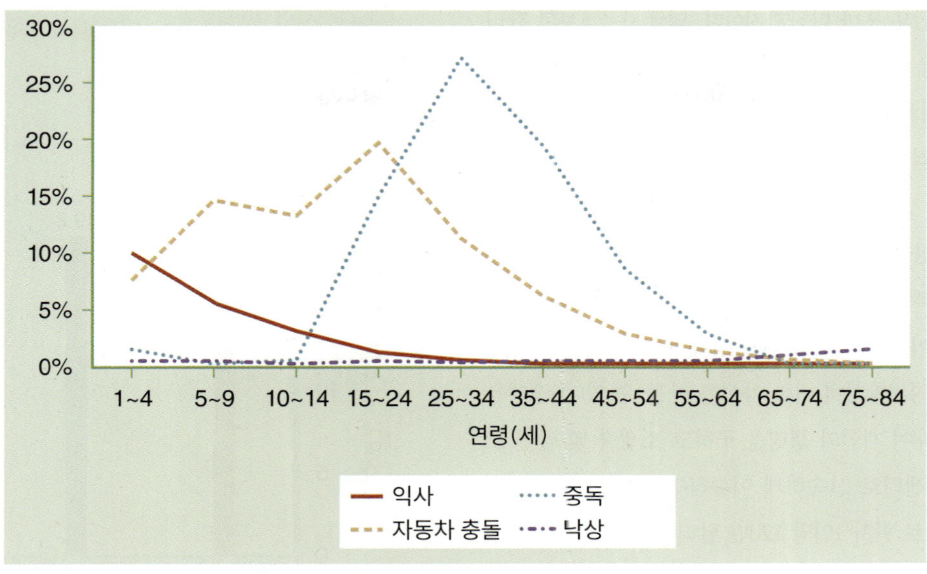

그림 1-3 나이(1~85세)에 따른 원인별 전체 사망자 비율(2019년)

Data from the National Center for Injury Prevention and Control: WISQARS. 10 leading causes of death, United States, 2019, all races, both sexes. Centers for Disease Control and Prevention. https://wisqars.cdc.gov/fatal-leading

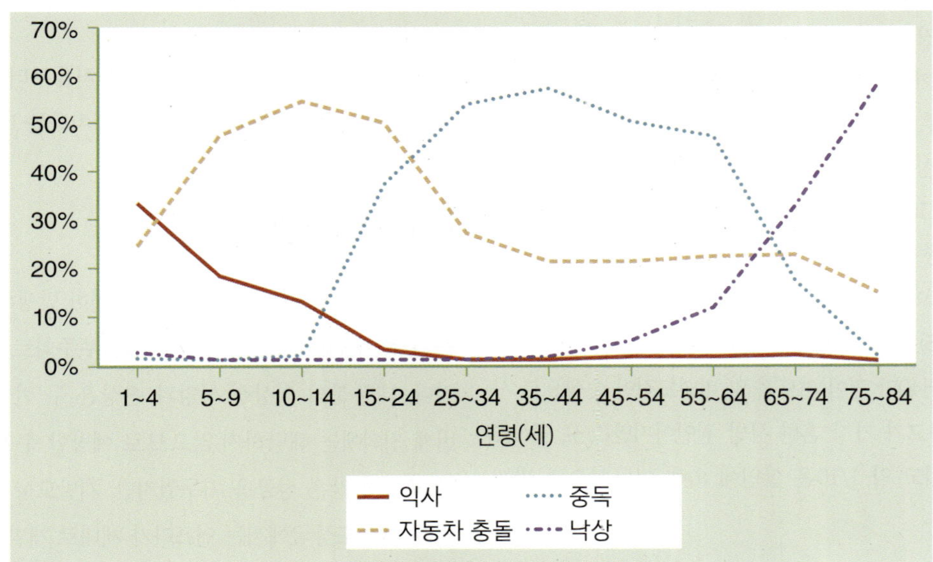

그림 1-4 비의도적인 손상으로 인한 나이(1~85세)에 따른 사망자 비율(1~85세, 2019년)

Data from the National Center for Injury Prevention and Control: WISQARS. 10 leading causes of death, United States, 2019, all races, both sexes. Centers for Disease Control and Prevention. https://wisqars.cdc.gov/fatal-leading

　낙상 및 자동차 충돌로 인한 사망을 분석하면 전 세계적으로 비의도적 손상 및 외상을 해결하려는 노력의 중요성을 알 수 있다. 2014년 보고서는 낙상과 자동차 충돌이 2030년까지 전 세계적으로 증가할 것으로 예상되는 유일한 외상성 사망 원인이라고 밝혔다. 이러한 손상의 부담은 모든 곳에서 경험되지만, 이들 국가가 전 세계 자동차의 60%에 불과하지만, 전 세계 도로 교통 사망의 93%가 저소득 및 중간 소득 국가에서 발생한다. 2014년 보고서에 이어 UN은 2021~2030년을 전 세계 교통사고 사망자를 50% 줄이는 것을 목표로 도로교통 안전을 위한 두 번째 행동 10년으로 공식적으로 결정했다.

　외상으로 인한 인명 피해도 어마어마하지만, 생존한 환자를 돌볼 때 발생하는 경제적 부담도 또한 마찬가지이다. 임금 손실, 보험 관리 비용, 재산 피해 및 고용주 비용을 제외하고 외상 환자 치료에 수십억 달러가 사용된다. 미국 국가안전보장회의(NCS)는 2019년에 발생했던 치명적 및 비치명적 외상으로 인한 경제적 영향이 미국에서 약 1조 1천억 달러에 이를 것으로 추산했다. 병원 전 처치 제공자는 외상으로 인한 사회적 비용을 줄일 기회가 있다. 예를 들어 병원 전 처치 제공자가 골절된 목뼈를 적절하게 보호하는 것은 환자가 팔다리 마비를 가지고 평생 살아가야 할지 아니면 장애가 없이 생산 활동을 유지하며 건강한 삶을 영위할지에 대한 차이를 만들 수 있다. 생명을 위협하는 출혈을 확인하여 개인의 생명을 구하고 소생술 및 출혈 조절을 위해 환자를 외상센터로 신속하게 이송하면 사회 전체에서 평생 임금 및 생산성 손실로 환자 1인당 120만 달러를 절약할 수 있다.

다음 데이터는 세계보건기구(WHO)에서 발표한 자료이다.

- 교통사고로 인한 손상은 공중 보건 문제이다. 전 세계적으로 교통사고로 인해 연간 130만 명이 사망하고 매일 평균 3,500명 이상이 사망한다. 교통사고는 5세~29세 사이의 사망 원인 중 1위이고 전 세계적으로 전체 사망자의 약 4%를 차지한다. 세계보건기구는 교통사고 예방 조치가 개선되지 않으면 2030년까지 도로 교통사고가 전 세계적으로 7대 주요 사망 원인이 될 것으로 예측했다.

- 교통사고로 인한 손상 대부분은 저소득과 중간 소득 국가 사람들에게 영향을 미치며 교통사고 사망자 4명 중 3명은 남자에게서 발생한다. 저소득 및 중간 소득 국가의 개인은 전 세계 차량의 절반만 소유하고 있지만, 이들 국가는 모든 도로 교통 사망의 90%를 차지하고 있다(**그림 1-5**).

- 전 세계적으로 매년 440만 명이 의도적 및 비의도적인 손상으로 사망한다. 도로 교통사고가 가장 흔한 사망 원인이지만(1/3), 약 1/6은 자살로 인한 것이고 약 1/10은 살인에 의해 이차적으로 발생한다.

이러한 통계가 분명히 보여주듯 외상은 세계적인 문제이다. 손상과 사망으로 이어지는 특정 사건은 국가마다 다르지만, 그 결과는 다르다.

외상이 발생하는 사회에서 일하는 우리는 손상이 발생한 환자를 처치할 뿐만 아니라 손상을 예방할 의무가 있다. EMS에 대해 자주 언급되는 이야기가 이 점을 가장 잘 보여준다. 길고 구불구불한 산악 도로는 그곳을 지나는 차량이 종종 미끄러져 30m 절벽 아래로 추락할 수 있는 커브가 있다. 지역 사회는 이러한 사고와 관련된 환자를 신속하게 처치하기 위해 절벽 아래에 구급차를 배치하기로 결정 했

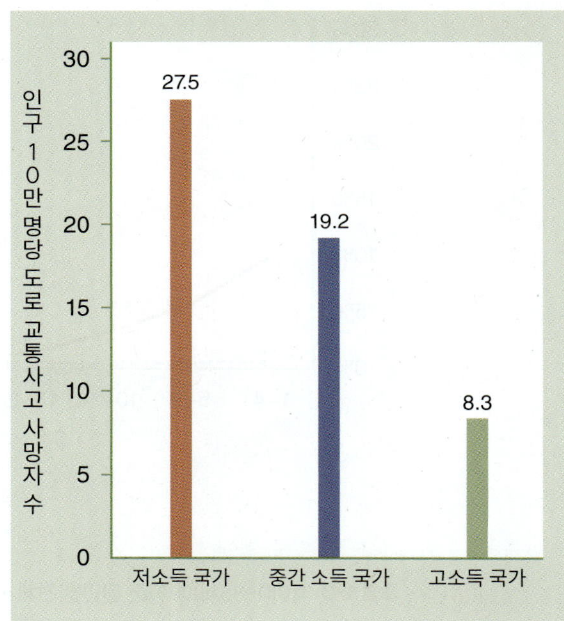

그림 1-5 인구 10만 명당 전 세계 도로 교통사고 사망자의 전세계 분포

Data from World Health Organization. Global Status Report on Road Safety 2018. World Health Organization; 2018. https://www.who.int/publications/i/item/9789241565684

다. 하지만 이것보다 더 나은 대안은 처음부터 이러한 사고가 발생하지 않도록 커브를 따라 가드레일을 설치하는 것이다.

외상 처치의 단계

외상은 흔히 사고라고 말하지만, 우연히 발생하는 것은 아니다. 사고는 종종 우연한 사고로 발생하거나 부주의로 인한 사고로 정의하고 있다. 대부분의 외상성 사망과 손상은 두 번째 정의에 부합하며 첫 번째 정의에는 해당하지 않으므로 예방할 수 있다. 선진국에서는 예방 교육이 많은 성공을 거두었지만, 개발도상국에서는 아직 갈 길이 멀다. 개발도상국에서는 인프라가 제대로 개발되지 않아 교육과 노력에 큰 장벽이 된다. 외상성 손상은 의도적인 것과 비의도적인 두 가지 범주의 손상으로 나뉜다. 의도적인 손상은 해를 입히거나 상해 또는 죽일 목적으로 의도적으로 행한 행위로 인해 발생한다. 고의적인 행동의 결과가 아니라 의도하지 않거나 우발적인 결과로 발생하는 외상성 손상은 비의도적인 것으로 간주한다.

외상 처치는 사고 전 단계, 사고 발생 단계, 사고 후 단계로 나뉜다. 외상 처치의 세 가지 단계 중 어느 단계에서든 외상성 손상의 영향을 최소화하려고 조치할 수 있으며 병원 전 처치 제공자는 단계마다 중요한 책임을 진다.

사고 전 단계

사고 전 단계는 손상으로 이어지는 상황이 포함된다. 이 단계의 노력은 주로 손상 예방에 중점을 둔다. 사고 전 단계에서 최대 효과를 달성하기 위해서는 외상성 사망과 손상을 해결하기 위한 전략은 사망률과 손상률에 가장 중요한 기여자에 초점을 맞춰야 한다. 이용 가능한 가장 최신의 자료에 따르면 비의도적 손상은 미국에서 매년 모든 연령대 전체 사망 원인 중 네 번째이다. 미국에서 손상으로 인한 사망의 거의 절반이 자동차 충돌, 추락 또는 화기로 인한 것이다(**그림 1-6**).

2011년 35%에 비해 2021년에는 미국인의 약 85%가 스마트폰을 소유하고 있다. 이러한 증가는 운전 부주의로 인한 사망자 수의 점진적인 증가와 관련이 있다. 미국 질병통제예방센터는 산만한 운전으로 인해 매년 약 3,000명이 사망하고 젊은 운전자들은 불균형적으로 더 높은 위험에 처해 있다고 추정한다. "기다릴 수 있다(It Can Wait)"와 같은 대중 인식캠페인과 관련된 예방 노력은 최근 몇 년 동안 이러한 사고 발생률의 상승 추세를 억제하기 개발되었다(**그림 1-7**). 일부 주에서는 이러한 프로그램이 자동차 운전 중 휴대전화 및 모바일 장치 사용 관련 법률과 결합하였다. 고속도로 안전에 초점을 맞춘 단체인 주지사 고속도로 안전협회(GHSA)에 따르면, 24개 주에서 운전 중 모든 개인의 휴대전화 사용을 금지하는 기본 집행법을 시행하고 있다. 운전 중 문자 메시지 사용은 48개 주에서 금지되어 있다. 초보 운전자(18세 미만)의 운전 중 휴대전화 사용은 37개 주와 컬럼비아 특별구에서 전면 금지되었다. 나이와 경력에 따른 차별화된 법적 집행은 특히 취약 계층의 교통사고 예방을 목표로 한다.

자동차 사고의 예방 가능한 또 다른 원인은 음주 운전이다. 사고 전 단계에서 이 문제를 해결하기 위해 상당한 노력을 기울였다. 만취한 것으로 간주하는 최소 혈중알코올농도에 대한 대중의 인식과 교육, 법 개정 압력이 증가한 결과 1989년 이후 치명적인 충돌 사고에 연루된 음주 운전자의 수는 지속해 감소하고 있다. 최근 몇몇 주에서 대마초의 의학적인 사용과 오락적인 사용을 모두 합법화했다. 이러한 변화가 대마초 장애 운전과 관련된 사망 및 손상에 미치는 영향에 대한 데이터는 현재 부족하다. 그러나 알코올과 대마초를 함께 복용

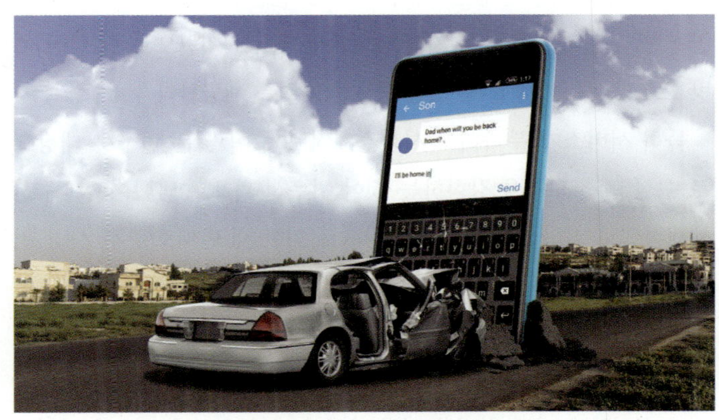

그림 1-7 점점 더 많은 대중 인식 캠페인에서 주의가 산만한 운전의 위험성을 강조한다.

© Mosab Bilto/Shutterstock

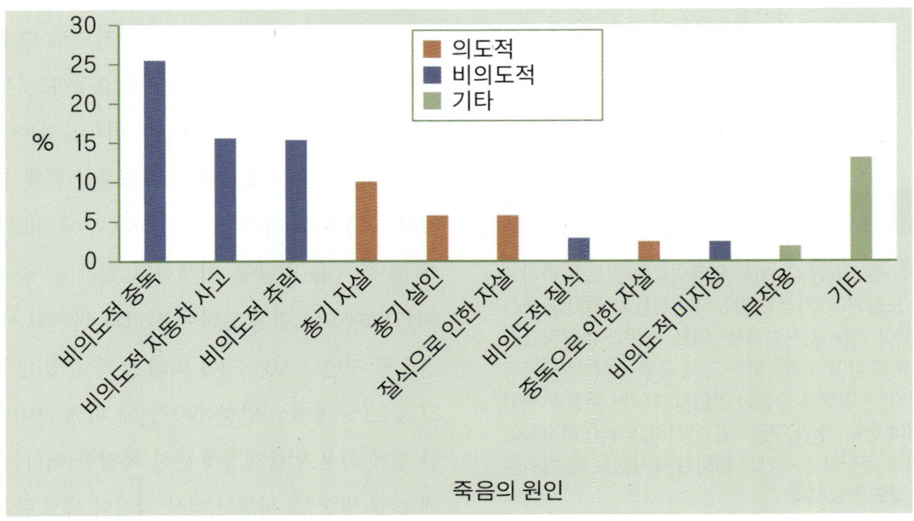

그림 1-6 자동차 외상, 추락, 총기 사고는 손상으로 인한 사망의 거의 절반을 차지한다.

한 상태에서 운전할 때 발생하는 자동차 사고의 위험이 두 가지 물질 중 하나를 단독으로 복용한 상태에서 운전할 때보다 더 크다.

낙상 위험에 처한 사람의 인식을 높이는 프로그램을 홍보하는 것도 상당한 노력이 필요한 분야이다. 미국 질병통제예방센터는 의료 제공자가 낙상의 위험이 있는 개인을 구별하고 해당 개인에 대해 수정할 수 있는 모든 위험 요소를 인식하고 낙상이 발생하기 전에 예방할 수 있는 효과적인 방법을 제공하기 위해 STEADI(노인 사고, 사망 및 손상 예방)을 개발했다. 병원 전 처치 제공자는 낙상 예방에 중요한 역할을 하는 위치에 있다. 노인들 사이에서 손상이나 사망을 초래하는 낙상에 대한 주요 위험 요소 중 하나는 이전에 겪은 낙상 사고였기 때문에 EMS 제공자는 출동 시 위험에 처한 환자를 만날 가능성이 있다. 이러한 출동은 지역 내 공공 안전부서에서 다른 의료 제공자 및 기관과 협력하여 지역 사회에서 증거를 기반으로 한 낙상 예방 프로그램을 개발할 수 있는 중요한 기회를 제공한다.

특히 서비스가 부족하고 사회경제적 수준이 낮은 인구를 대상으로 수상 안전 교육을 강화하는 것이 최우선 과제로 남아야 한다. 전 세계적으로 익사는 비의도적 손상으로 인한 세 번째로 흔한 사망 원인이다. 미국 내 도시에서 수영장 주변에 울타리를 설치해야 하는 법이 시행되었다. 또한 부모님과 수영하는 사람들에게 물 주변의 안전 수칙에 대한 지침을 제공하는 프로그램이 널리 제공된다. 공공 안전 기관의 역할과 이들에 대한 지역 사회의 신뢰 수준과 고유한 위치를 고려할 때 이러한 지원 프로그램에 대한 참여는 사건 전 단계에서 익사 문제를 완화하는 데 중요하다.

사고 전 단계의 또 다른 중요한 구성 요소는 공공 안전 인식 프로그램으로 예방할 수 없는 사고에 대한 병원 전 처지 제공자가 준비하는 것이다(**Box 1-2**).

Box 1-2 준비

준비에는 최신 의료 서비스를 제공하기 위해 업데이트된 정보를 가지고 적절하고 완전한 교육이 포함된다. 가정용 컴퓨터나 휴대용 장치를 최신 소프트웨어로 업데이트해야 하는 것처럼 최신 의료 관행과 통찰력으로 자신의 지식을 업데이트해야 한다. 또한, 모든 교대 근무 시작 시 제공자는 장비를 확인하고 누가 어떤 임무를 수행할 것인지에 대한 역할과 책임을 팀원들과 함께 검토해야 한다. 누가 구급차를 운전하고 누가 환자실에 환자와 함께 있을 것인지를 결정하는 것만큼 현장에 도착했을 때 처치를 시행할 것인지 검토하는 것도 중요하다.

© National Association of Emergency Medical Technicians (NAEMT)

비의도적 손상을 완전히 제거할 수는 없지만, 언급된 것과 같은 프로그램을 통해 중요한 비의도적 손상이 중요한 사망 원인인 것을 최소화할 수 있다. EMS 제공자는 사고 전 단계에서 예방 노력에서 중요한 임무를 수행할 것이다.

사고 단계

사고 단계는 실제로 외상이 발생하는 순간이다. 사고 단계에서 시행하는 조치는 외상성 사고로 인한 손상을 최소화하는 데 목적이 있는. 안전 장비의 사용은 외상성 사고로 인한 손상의 심각성에 상당한 영향을 미친다. 자동차 안전 제어시스템, 에어백과 오토바이 헬멧 등은 일반적으로 사고 단계에서 손상을 줄이고 예방하는 역할을 한다 (4장, 외상의 물리학 참조).

오토바이 헬멧 착용 법률을 둘러싼 역사는 특정 안전 장비의 사용을 의무화하는 법이 외상성 손상의 발생률과 심각성에 미칠 수 있는 영향을 잘 보여주고 있다. 1966년 미 의회는 오토바이 헬멧 착용을 의무화하는 법률을 통과시키지 않은 주(State)를 처벌할 수 있는 권한을 미 교통부에 부여했다. 이후 10년 동안 47개 주에서 보편적인 헬멧 착용 법률을 제정했다. 하지만 의회는 1975년에 미 교통부에서 이 권한을 철회했고 이에 따라 법률을 제정했던 주에서는 보편적인 헬멧 착용 법률을 폐지하기 시작했다. 오토바이 사고와 관련된 사망은 1980년대 초부터 꾸준히 감소했지만, 미 교통부의 처벌 권한이 해제된 지 불과 20년이 지난 1998년에는 그 비율이 증가하기 시작했다. 2021년 8월 기준으로 18개 주와 컬럼비아 특별구만이 모든 오토바이 탑승자에게 헬멧을 착용하도록 요구하는 법률을 시행하고 있으며 30개 주에서는 일부 탑승자(일반적으로 17세 이하, 특정 연령 17~25세까지)에게 헬멧을 착용하도록 요구하는 부분적인 법률을 시행하고 있다. 남은 2개 주(일리노이, 아이오와)에는 나이 또는 면허 유무에 관계없이 모든 오토바이 탑승자의 헬멧 사용을 규제하는 법률이 없다. 이것은 의회가 초기 미 교통부에 처벌 권한을 부여한 이후 현재 헬멧 착용 법률을 시행하고 있는 주 중에서 가장 적은 수이다. NHTSA에 따르면 오토바이 사고와 관련된 사망자 수는 2019년 5,014명으로 전년도 5,038명에 비해 소폭 줄었지만, 미국에서 오토바이 사고로 2,056명이 사망한 1997년에 비해 많이 증가했다. 지난 50년 동안 헬멧 착용 법률제정에 관한 복잡한 역사는 특정 안전 장비의 사용에 관한 법령 및 시행이 외상 처치의 사고 단계에서 환자의 예후를 극적으로 변화시킬 수 있는지를 보여주는 한 가지 예에 불과하다.

외상성 손상의 가능성을 최소화하는 또 다른 방법은 어린이용 안전 시트를 사용하는 것이다. 많은 외상센터, 경찰관, EMS 및 소방관은 부모에게 어린이용 안전 시트의 올바른 설치와 사용에 관한 교육을 실시한다. 어린이용 안전 시트를 올바르게 설치하여 사용한다면 외상 처치의 사고 단계에서 영아와 어린이에게 최상의 보호 기능을 제공할 수 있다.

EMS 제공자가 취한 특정 조치는 사고 단계의 결과에 큰 역할을 한다. "더 이상 해를 끼치지 말라"는 것은 좋은 환자 처치를 위한 충고이다. 개인 차량을 운전하든 응급 차량을 운전하든 병원 전 처치 제공자는 항상 자신을 보호하고 모범을 보여야 한다. 당신은 업무를 수행하는 동안 자신과 동료 그리고 환자에 대한 책임이 있다. 개인 차량을 운전할 때 자신과 다른 사람의 안전을 위해 같은 노력을 기울여야 한다. 따라서 안전하고 주의 깊게 운전하여 손상을 예방한다. 환자를 처치할 때 주의를 기울이는 것과 같은 수준의 주의가 모든 운전에 주어져야 한다. 항상 운전석에 있거나 환자 처치실에 있든, 안전띠와 같은 개인 보호 장비를 사용한다. 운전 중에는 주의가 산만해지지 않도록 한다. 운전을 시작하기 전에 자동차 또는 스마트폰용 GPS를 설정한다. 꼭 필요한 경우를 제외하고 운전 중에는 휴대전화를 사용하지 말고 핸즈프리 상태에서만 사용한다. EMS 전문가인 당신은 자기 행동이 초래하는 위험 외에도 다른 사람의 본보기라는 것을 기억한다. 만약 사람들이 당신이 안전띠를 착용하지 않고 운전하거나 문자를 주고받는 것을 본다면 그들은 당신과 같은 습관을 가질 수 있다. 마찬가지로 여러분이 세운 좋은 본보기는 다른 사람이 똑같이 하도록 자극할 수 있다. 다른 사람들은 자동차 충돌 사고와 관련된 사람을 돌본 경험이 이러한 안전 조치를 채택하게 한다면 그들이 그렇게 하는 것에 잠재적인 장점이 있다는 것을 이해한다.

사고 후 단계

사고 후 단계는 외상 사고의 결과를 다룬다. 외상 사고로 인한 최악의 결과는 환자의 사망이다. 외상 전문의 도널드 트런키(Donald Trunkey) 박사는 외상 사망의 세 단계를 설명했다. 사망의 첫 번째 단계는 사고 후 처음 몇 분 이내에 발생하고 최대 1시간 안에 발생한다. 이러한 사망은 대부분은 외상성 손상을 입은 후 즉시 또는 몇 초 이내에 발생한다. 그러나 일부는 의료진이 도착하기까지 걸리는 짧은 시간 동안 대량 출혈로 인해 발생한다. 이러한 사망을 예방할 수 있는 가장 좋은 방법은 손상 예방 전략과 공공 교육 프로그램을 이용하는 것이다. 또한 최근의 대중 인식캠페인에는 병원 전 처치 제공자

를 기다리는 동안 일반인의 지혈대 사용에 대한 교육과 공공장소 및 경찰차에 사용할 수 있는 지혈 키트를 설치하는 것이 포함된다. 이러한 노력은 첫 번째 단계에서 종종 환자의 사망으로 이어지는 압박으로 지혈할 수 있는 출혈을 지혈하는 데 도움이 될 수 있다. 사망의 두 번째 단계는 사고 발생 후 1시간에서 몇 시간 사이에 발생한다. 이러한 사망은 적절한 병원 전 처치와 병원 내 치료로 예방할 수 있다. 사망의 세 번째 단계는 사고 발생 후 며칠에서 몇 주 후에 발생한다. 이러한 사망은 일반적으로 다기관 부전으로 인해 발생한다. 연구에 따르면 이 단계는 현대의 외상과 중환자 처치의 결과로 감소하고 있다. 손상 제어 소생술은 단계적 외상 처치와 광범위한 외상 환자를 중환자실에서 안정화와 결합하여 3단계 사망을 해결하는 외상 처치의 발전 추세이다. 그 증거는 결정질 수액 소생술이 제한되고 초기 수술 개입이 짧고 출혈의 주요 원인만 다루어 환자의 결과가 개선되어 환자가 생리적으로 적절한 대사 상태로 안정화될 수 있는 외상 중환자실로 옮길 수 있음을 나타낸다. 일단 중환자실에서 안정화되면 환자의 필요에 따라 간헐적인 중환자실에서 재 안정화를 통해 추가적인 수술을 시행할 수 있다. 병원 전 환경에서 결정질 수액과 달리 혈액 및 혈액제제를 사용하여 쇼크를 조기에 적극적으로 관리하는 것은 이러한 사망을 예방하는 데 중요한 역할을 한다(**그림 1-8**). 중환자실과 외상 처치를 이용할 수 있는 지역에서 EMS의 조기 개입은 출혈의 적극적인 조절과 함께 외상센터로 신속하게 이송하고 병원에서 손상 통제 소생술을 통해 외상 환자의 결과를 개선한다.

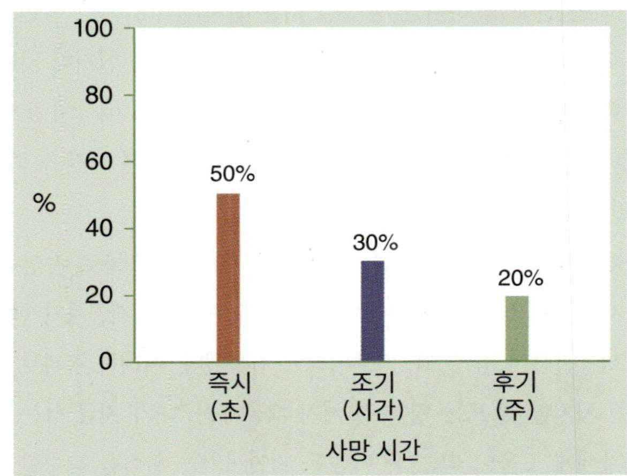

그림 1-8 즉각적인 사망은 손상 예방과 응급처치 교육으로 예방할 수 있다. 조기 사망은 적시에 적절한 병원 전 처치와 적절한 외상센터로 이송을 통해 예방할 수 있다. 후기 사망은 최신 손상 제어 기술을 통해 지혈, 혈액 및 혈액제제로 소생시키는 기술 그리고 환자의 적절한 생리적 안정화 후 단계적인 손상 치료를 진행하는 기술을 통해 예방할 수 있다.

미국 최초의 외상센터 중 하나인 메릴랜드 EMS 기관(MIEMSS) 설립자인 애덤스 카울리(R Adams Cowley) 박사는 황금 시간(Golden Hour)이라고 부르는 것을 정의했다. 자신의 연구를 바탕으로 카울리 박사는 손상 직후 결정적인 처치를 받은 환자는 처치가 지연된 환자보다 생존율이 훨씬 높다고 믿었다. 이러한 생존율 향상의 한 가지 이유는 출혈을 신속하게 처치하고 장기 기능을 유지하기 위한 신체의 에너지 생산 능력을 보존하기 때문이다. 병원 전 처치 제공자의 경우 이것은 산소공급과 관류를 유지하고 혈액과 혈장을 사용하여 소생술(손상 통제 소생술) 과정을 시행하면서 즉시 외과적 방법으로 지혈을 시행할 수 있도록 준비된 의료기관으로 신속하게 이송하는 것을 의미한다.

이 중요한 시간은 말 그대로 1시간이 아니기 때문에 황금 시간은 "황금 기간(Golden Period)"으로 생각하는 것이 좋다. 일부 환자는 치료받을 시간이 한 시간 미만이지만, 다른 환자는 더 많은 시간을 갖는다. 미국의 많은 도시에서 EMS 활성화와 구급차가 현장에 도착하는 평균 시간은 8~9분이지만, 이 시간에는 사고 발생부터 신고한 시간까지는 포함하지 않는다. 일반적으로 환자를 의료기관까지 이송하는 데 걸리는 시간은 8~9분이다. 병원 전 처치 제공자가 현장에서 10분만 보낸다고 하더라도 환자가 의료기관에 도착할 때까지 30분 이상의 시간이 이미 지났을 것이다. 현장에서 보내는 추가 시간은 환자가 피를 흘리고 있는 추가 시간이며 황금 기간 내 소중한 시간이 계속 흘러가고 있음을 의미한다.

연구 자료는 결정적인 처치를 위한 신속한 이송 개념을 뒷받침한다. 이러한 연구 중 하나는 중상을 입은 환자가 구급차가 아닌 자가용을 이용해 의료기관으로 이송되었을 때 사망률이 현저히 낮은 것으로 나타났다(자가용 17.9% vs. 구급차 28.2%). 이 예상치 못한 연구 결과는 병원 전 처치 제공자가 현장에서 너무 많은 시간을 허비한 결과일 가능성이 크다.

1980년대와 1990년대에 한 외상센터는 자동차 충돌로 손상을 입은 환자와 관통상 환자의 경우 출동한 병원 전 처치 제공자가 현장에 머무르는 시간이 평균 20~30분이라고 기록했다. 이러한 결과로 외상 환자를 처치할 때 모든 병원 전 처치 제공자는 "내가 지금 하는 행위가 환자에게 도움이 되는가? 이송을 지연시키는 위험을 감수할 정도로 이득이 있는가?"라는 질문을 스스로 해볼 필요가 있다.

병원 전 처치 제공자의 가장 중요한 책임 중 하나는 현장에서 가능한 한 적은 시간을 보내고 외상 환자의 현장 처치와 신속하게 의료기관으로 이송하는 것이다. 병원 전 처치 제공자는 현장 도착 후 첫 몇 분 동안 환자를 신속하게 평가하고 생명을 유지할 수 있는 처치를 시행하고 환자를 이송할 준비를 한다. PHTLS의 명확한 목표는 모든 제공자(소방, 경찰, EMS)가 단일화된 방법으로 수행하고 응급의료 서비스 전반에 표준 방법론을 채택하여 병원 전 현장 체류 시간을 줄기는 것이었다. 이것은 이 기간에 환자의 생존율 증가에 이바지할 것으로 기대된다. 두 번째 책임은 환자를 적절한 의료기관으로 이송하는 것이다. 외상 환자의 생존에 가장 중요한 요소는 사고 발생부터 결정적인 처치를 제공하는 데까지 걸리는 시간이다.

외상 환자를 처치할 때 손상을 입은 순간부터 적절한 외상센터에 도착할 때까지 걸린 시간은 생존에 매우 중요하다. 외상 환자에 대한 결정적인 처치는 일반적으로 지혈을 시행하고 가능한 한 전혈에 가까운 수액을 투여하여 적절한 관류를 회복시키는 것이다. 손실된 혈액을 대체하기 위해 가공된 전혈(적혈구와 혈장을 1:1 비율로 혼합)을 투여한 결과 이라크와 아프가니스탄 그리고 현재 민간 사회에서 인상적인 결과를 보여주었다. 이러한 수액은 손실된 산소운반능력, 응고인자, 혈관계의 체액 손실을 예방하기 위한 삼투압을 대체한다. 현장에서 널리 사용할 수 없으며 외상 환자를 신속하게 의료기관으로 이송해야 하는 중요한 이유이다. 의료기관으로 이송하는 중에 균형 잡힌 소생술(3장, 쇼크: 삶과 죽음의 병태생리학 참고)이 중요한 것으로 입증되었다. 지혈은 항상 현장이나 응급실에서 성공적으로 시행할 수 있는 것은 아니며, 수술실에서만, 가능할 수도 있다. 따라서 환자를 이송하기 위해 적절한 의료기관을 결정할 때 병원 전 처치 제공자는 비판적 사고방식으로 주어진 상황에서 의료기관으로의 이송 시간과 의료기관의 역량을 고려해야 한다.

환자가 의료기관에 도착하기 직전 또는 직후에 즉시 환자를 처치할 수 있는 외상 전문의, 잘 훈련되고 외상 환자에 대한 경험이 풍부한 소생팀 및 즉시 이용할 수 있는 수술팀이 있는 외상센터는 환자의 생명을 구할 수 있다. 환자 도착 후 신속하게 수술실에서 생명을 위협하는 출혈이 있는 외상 환자를 처치할 수 있으며 이는 삶과 죽음의 차이를 만들 수 있다(**Box 1-3**).

반면에 자체 수술 능력이 없는 병원은 응급실에서 수술실로 환자를 이동시키기 전에 외과 전문의와 수술팀의 도착을 기다려야 한다. 출혈이 지혈되기 전에 추가 시간이 지나 관련 사망률이 증가할 수 있다(**그림 1-9**). 만약 모든 중증 외상 환자를 필요하다면 더 가까운 의료기관으로 이송하는 것보다 직접 외상센터로 곧장 이송하면 생존율

Box 1-3 외상센터

미국 외과학회(ACS)는 손상을 입은 환자의 최적화된 처치를 위한 자원이라는 제목의 문서를 통해 외상센터에 대한 요구 사항을 정하였다. 주와 지방 관할구역은 이러한 요구 사항과 미국 외과학회 외상위원회의 외상 현장 조사 보고서를 활용하여 다양한 Level의 외상센터를 지정한다. 미국 외과학회에 따르면 Level Ⅰ 및 Level Ⅱ 외상센터에 대한 임상 요구 사항에 차이가 없어야 한다. 두 Level의 주요 차이점은 의료 교육, 연구, 전문 서비스 및 환자 수가 많고 Level Ⅰ이 더 높다는 것이다. Level Ⅰ 외상센터는 특정 지역에서 외상 처치를 조직화시키는 중추 역할을 한다. Level Ⅲ 외상센터는 일반적으로 자원이 적고 교외 또는 농촌 지역에 있다. 이들의 주요 역할은 즉각적인 처치와 안정, 전문적인 처치가 제공되는 Level Ⅰ 및 Level Ⅱ 외상센터로 신속하고 효율적으로 이송이다. Level Ⅳ 외상센터는 24시간 운영되는 응급실 외에는 거의 자원이 없으며 이들의 주요 역할은 즉각적인 처치 및 안정화이며 더 높은 Level의 외상센터로 자원이 거의 없으며 주요 역할은 즉각적인 기본 처치와 안정을 위한 안내자 역할을 하고 상위 외상센터로 신속하게 이송하는 것이다.

미국 외상학회는 외상센터로 간주하는 기관을 지정하지 않으며 단순히 병원이 특정 수준의 외상 서비스에 대해 권장 기준을 충족했는지만 확인한다. 특정 병원을 외상센터로 지정하고 해당 병원을 어떤 Level의 외상센터로 지정할 것인지에 관한 결정은 미국 외상학회의 특정 기준이 충족되었는지 확인한 후 주 및 지방 정부에서 한다.

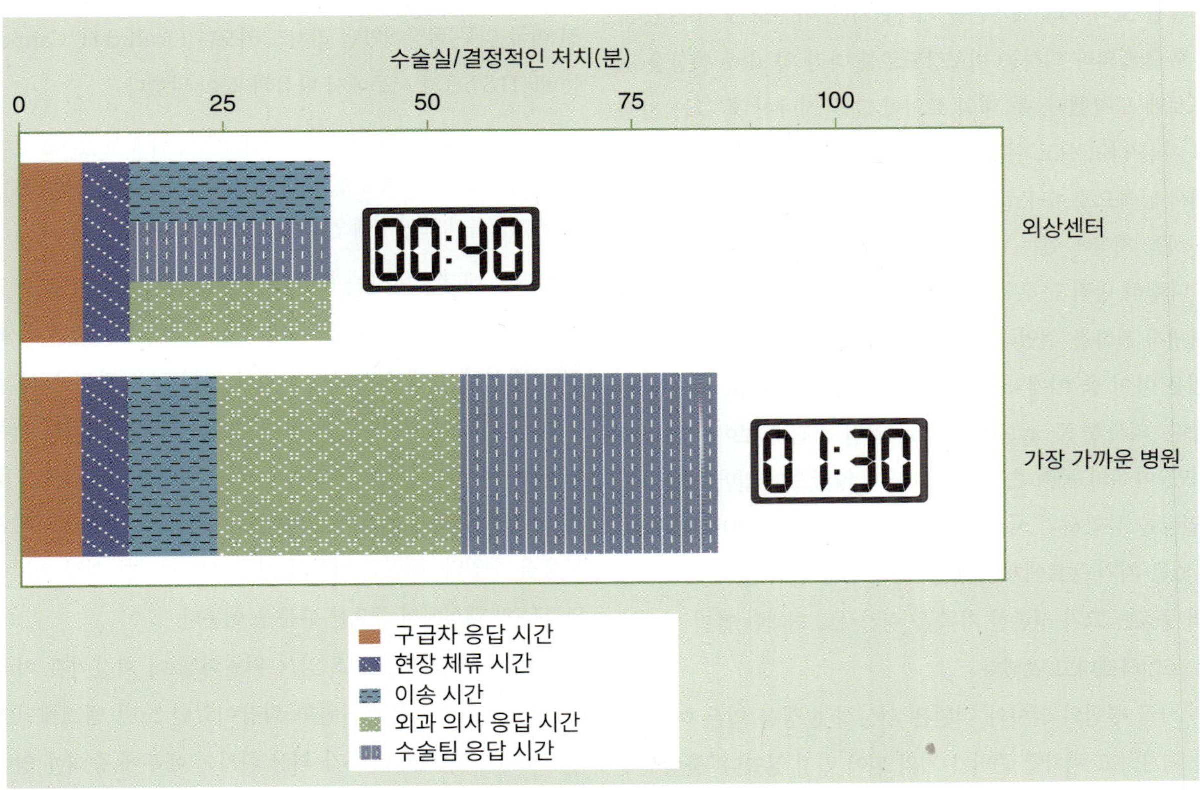

그림 1-9 외상센터를 이용할 수 있는 장소에서는 외상 환자 처치를 전문적으로 시 행할 수 없는 병원을 우회하는 것이 환자 처치를 크게 개선할 수 있다. 중증 외상을 입은 환자의 경우 결정적인 환자 처치는 종종 수술실에서 이루어진다. 환자를 병원으로 이송 중에 외과 의사 및 수술팀이 10~20분 정도를 더 보내면 수술실에서 최종 처치 받는 시간을 상당히 줄일 수 있다.

이 상당히 증가할 것이다.

수술이나 외상에 대한 조기 교육 외에도 경험이 중요하다. 연구에 따르면 분주한 외상센터에서 경험이 많은 외과 의사가 경험이 적은 외과 의사보다 더 나은 결과를 보였다.

병원 전 외상 소생술(PHTLS): 과거, 현재 그리고 미래

전문 외상 소생술(ATLS)

인생에서 자주 일어나는 일처럼 개인적인 경험은 응급처치의 변화를 가져왔고 그 결과 ATLS 교육 과정 그리고 PHTLS 교육 과정이 만들어졌다. ATLS는 미국 네브래스카의 시골 지역에서 민간 비행기가 추락한 지 2년 후인 1978년에 시작되었다. 당시 이 비행기에는 한 정형외과 의사와 아내 그리고 그의 4명의 아이가 타고 있었다. 추락 당시 아내는 현장에서 즉사했고 아이들은 중상을 입었다. 이들은 누군가가 자신들을 도와주러 오기만을 기다렸지만, 아무도 오지 않았다. 약 8시간 후 정형외과 의사는 비포장도로를 따라 약 1km 이상을 걸어 고속도로에 도착했다. 두 대의 트럭이 그를 지나친 후 그는 차를 세웠고 그 차를 타고 사고 현장으로 돌아가 아이들을 차에 태우고 사고 현장에서 남쪽으로 수 km 떨어진 가장 가까운 병원으로 갔다.

그들이 시골 지역에 있는 병원의 응급실에 도착했을 때 문은 잠겨 있었으나 다행히 당직 근무 중이던 간호사가 퇴근 후 집에 있던 2명의 일반의에게 전화를 걸었다. 아이들을 진찰한 후 의사 중 한 명이 손상을 입은 아이 중 어깨와 무릎을 다친 아이를 데리고 방사선 촬영실로 갔다. 의사는 X-ray에서 두개골 골절 소견은 보이지 않는다고 말했지만, 아이의 목뼈 손상은 고려되지 않았으며 일반의는 아이가 입은 열상을 봉합하기 시작했다. 정형외과 의사는 네브래스카주 링컨시에 있는 자기 동료에게 전화를 걸어 무슨 일이 일어났는지 말했다. 그의 동료는 그가 생존한 가족을 링컨시로 최대한 빨리 이송할 수 있도록 조치하겠다고 말했다.

이 작은 시골 병원의 의사와 직원은 외상성 손상을 입은 여러 명의 환자를 평가하고 처치할 준비가 거의 되어 있지 않았다. 불행하게도 외상성 손상에 대한 분류, 평가 및 처치에 대한 훈련과 경험이 부족했다. 이후 몇 년 동안 네브래스카 정형외과 의사와 그의 동료들은 시골 환경에서 급성 손상을 입은 환자를 처치하기 위한 외상 처치 시스템의 일반적인 부족에 대해 무언가 조치가 필요하다는 것을 인식했다. 이들은 시골의 의사들이 외상 환자 처치에 대해 체계적인 교육을 받을 필요가 있다고 결정했다. 그들은 ACLS와 유사한 형식의 ATLS이라고 부르기로 했다.

외상 처치를 위한 논리적인 접근 방식으로 교육 과정이 만들어지고 정리되었다. 외상 환자 평가와 처치의 우선순위를 결정하기 위한 ABC (기도, 호흡, 순환)뿐만 아니라 "진행과 동시에 처치"라는 방법론이 개발되었다. 1978년에 많은 외과 의사의 도움으로 네브래스카주 오번에서 ATLS 시범 교육이 시행되었고, 이 과정은 이후 네브래스카 대학교와 결국 외상에 관한 미국 외과학회 외상위원회에 소개되었다.

네브래스카주 오번에서 첫 ATLS 교육 과정을 시작한 이후로 40년 이상이 지났고 ATLS는 계속 확산하고 성장하고 있다. 원래 네브래스카 시골 지역을 위해 만들었던 교육 과정이 현재는 전 세계 모든 외상 사고 환경을 위한 과정이 되었다. PHTLS의 기초가 되는 것이 이 과정이다.

병원 전 외상 소생술(PHTLS)

전 미국 의무 국장이었던 리처드 카모나(Ricahrd H. Carmona) 박사는 PHTLS 6판의 서문에서 다음과 같이 말했다.

> 우리는 많은 명백한 성공에서 거인의 어깨 위에 서 있다고 말해져 왔고, PHTLS도 다르지 않다. 큰 비전과 열정 그리고 도전으로 소수의 리더 그룹이 25년 전에 인내하고 PHTLS를 개발했다.

1958년 패링턴 박사는 소방관이 응급 환자를 처치할 수 있도록 교육을 받아야 한다며 시카고 소방서를 설득했다. 패링턴 박사는 샘 뱅크스 박사와 함께 시카고에서 외상 처치 교육 과정을 시작했다. 무수한 사람이 이 획기적인 교육 과정에서 개발된 지침에 따라 교육을 받았다. 패링턴 박사는 현장에서 교육, 입법에 이르기까지 EMS의 모든 수준에서 계속 노력하여 EMS를 직업으로 확장하고 개선하는 데 도움을 주었다. 패링턴 박사의 연구에서 제시한 외상 처치의 원칙은 PHTLS의 핵심에서 중요한 부분을 이룬다.

미국 외과학회의 ATLS 임시 위원회 초대 회장이자 미국 외과학회 병원 전 처치 분과위원회 회장이었던 노먼 멕스웨인(Norman McSwain) 박사는 ATLS가 외상 환자의 예후에 중대한 영향을 미치리라는 것을 알고 있었다. 게다가 그는 이러한 유형의 중요한 교육을 병원 전 처치 제공자에게 제공함으로써 훨씬 더 큰 효과를 얻을 수 있다는 강한 느낌이 있었다.

NAEMT 이사회의 창립 구성원인 멕스웨인(McSwain) 박사는 협회 회장인 게리 라보(Gary LaBeau)의 지지를 얻었고 ATLS의 병원 전 단계 버전을 만들기 위한 계획을 세우기 시작했다. 라보 회장은 멕스웨인 박사와 NAEMT-P인 로버트 넬슨(Robert Nelson)에게 병원 전 처치 제공자를 위해 ATLS와 유사한 교육 과정의 실현 가능성을 결정하도록 지시했다.

루이지애나주 뉴올리언스에 있는 툴레인 의과대학 외과 교수인 맥스웨인 박사는 학교의 지원을 받아 PHTLS 교육 과정의 초안을 작성했다. 이 초안이 마련되면서 1983년에 PHTLS 위원회가 설립되었다. 이 위원회는 계속해서 교육 과정을 개선했으면 같은 해 하반기에 루이지애나주 라파에트와 뉴올리언스에서 시험 교육 과정을 실시했다. 아이오와주 수시티의 마리안 건강센터, 코네티컷주 뉴헤이븐에 있는 예일대학교 의과대학, 코네티컷주 노워크에 있는 노워크 병원에서 시범 교육을 시작했다.

리처드 보마카(Richard W. Vomacka; 1946~2001)는 초기 PHTLS 교육 과정을 개발한 특별 전문위원회의 일원이었다. PHTLS는 과정이 합쳐지면서 그의 열정이 되었고 1980년대 초에 전국을 여행하며 시범 교육과 지역 내 강사 워크숍을 진행했다. 그는 멕스웨인 박사 및 다른 팀원들과 함께 교육 과정을 수정하는 작업을 하였다. 보마카는 PHTLS와 미군 사이의 관계를 형성하는 데 중요한 역할을 했으며 그는 또는 최초의 국제 PHTLS 교육 기관에서 일했다.

PHTLS의 전국적 보급은 1984년 9월에서 1985년 2월 사이에 콜로라도주 덴버, 메릴랜드주 베데스다, 플로리다주 올랜도에서 세 번의 집중적인 워크숍에서 시작되었다. 이러한 초기 PHTLS 교육 과정을 이수한 사람들은 "지방 순회자"와 같은 역할을 하였다. 이들은 PHTLS 교수진으로 전국을 이동하면서 추가로 강사를 양성하고 PHTLS의 핵심 원칙에 대한 정보를 전파했다. NAEMT-P인 알렉스 부트만은 보마카와 함께 사비를 들여 PHTLS 교육 과정의 1판과 2판을 결실을 보기 위해 부지런히 일했다.

이러한 성장 과정 전반에 걸쳐 미국 외과학회 외상위원회를 통해 의료감독이 제공되었다. 30년 이상 동안 미국 외과학회와 NAEMT의 협력관계를 통해 PHTLS 교육 과정을 이수한 사람들은 외상 환자에게 최상의 생존할 기회를 제공할 기회를 얻을 수 있었다.

1994년부터 2001년까지 스캇프레임(Scott B. Frame; 1952~2001) 박사는 PHTLS 교육 과정의 부 의료책임자였다. 그의 주요 강조점은 PHTLS 교육 과정을 위한 시청각 자료의 개발과 국제적으로 보급하는 것이었다. 그가 사망할 때까지 PHTLS 교재 제5판에 대한 책임을 맡았다. 그가 개정한 5판에는 교재뿐만 아니라 강사 설명서와 관련 교재를 모두 개정하는 내용이 포함된다. 그는 5판이 출판되었을 때 PHTLS 교육 과정의 의료책임자로 임명되었다. PHTLS 교육 과정은 프레임 박사의 지도로 엄청나게 성장했고 그가 환자를 위하고 PHTLS를 위해 쏟은 그의 삶과 지속적인 노력에 힘입어 PHTLS는 앞으로도 계속 성장할 수 있을 것이다.

PHTLS의 지속해 성장하는 것은 앞으로도 많은 개개인의 노력에 달려있다.

군대에서의 PHTLS

1998년부터 미군은 적극적으로 PHTLS에서 의무병들을 교육하기 시작했다. 텍사스주 포드샘휴스턴에 있는 국방 의료 준비 훈련소(DMRTI)가 주관하는 PHTLS 교육 과정은 미국과 해외에 주둔한 사람들에게 가르쳤다. 2001년 미 육군의 91WB 프로그램에 PHTLS 교육 과정을 포함하여 58,000명 이상의 의무병에게 표준화된 훈련을 제공했다.

PHTLS 제4판에는 전투 관련 손상을 치료하는 군의관의 요구를 더 잘 다루기 위해 군사 챕터가 추가 되었다. PHTLS 제5판이 출판된 후 PHTLS 위원회와 새로 설립된 미 국방성 내 국방 보건위원회의 TCCC 위원회 사이에 밀접한 관계가 형성되었다. 이러한 관계에 따라 광범위하게 개정된 PHTLS의 군사 버전은 2005년 제5판 개정판으로 출판되었다. PHTLS 위원회와 TCCC 위원회 간의 협력으로 PHTLS 제6판의 군사 버전에는 여러 군사 챕터가 만들어졌다. 그리고 2010년 NAEMT는 미 국방성의 TCCC 교육 과정을 제공하기 시작했다.

국제 PHTLS

PHTLS 교육 과정에서 강조된 병원 전 외상 처치의 건전한 원칙으로 인해 미국 이외 지역의 병원 전 처치 제공자와 의사가 이 교육 과정을 자국에 도입을 요청했다. 1990년대 초부터 PHTLS 교육 과정은 처음에는 영국과 멕시코에서, 그다음에는 다른 나라에서 국제적으로 시작되었다.

2019년에는 전 세계에서 25,600명 이상의 병원 전 처치 제공자가 PHTLS 교육을 이수하였으며 본 판이 출간된 이후 전 세계 70여 개 국에서 PHTLS를 교육하고 있다. 전 세계적 COVID-19 팬데믹 동안 전 세계의 NEMT 교육 센터는 병원 전 처치 제공자가 팬데믹 환자 처치 및 예방 접종 노력에 관심을 돌렸기 때문에 더 적은 수의 PHTLS 교육 과정을 진행했다. NAEMT는 교육 및 병원 전 외상(PHT) 위원회를 통해 가상 교육에 대한 혁신적인 접근 방식을 통해 이러한 교육 센터를 지원하기 위해 노력했다. PHTLS 교수진의 글로벌 네트워크는 가상적으로나 강의실에서 이 중요한 외상 프로그램을 계속해서 가르치고 있다.

번역

점점 국제적으로 증가하는 PHTLS 교육 과정은 현재 아랍어, 네덜란드어, 영어, 프랑스어, 독일어, 그리스어, 이탈리아어, 한국어, 노르웨이어, 폴란드어, 포르투갈어, 중국어 간체자, 스페인어, 스웨덴어 및 중국어 번체자 등의 언어로 번역되었다.

미래를 위한 비전

PHTLS 교육 과정은 이 기회가 필요하고 원하는 모든 사람에게 최상의 병원 전 외상 처치 교육을 제공하는 임무를 계속할 것이다. PHTLS 교육 과정은 항상 병원 전 외상과 관련된 최신의 증거를 바탕으로 우리는 확실한 출처를 통해 이 증거를 찾기 위해 최선을 다하고 있다.

병원 전 외상 처치가 발전하고 개선됨에 따라 PHTLS 교육 과정도 발전해야 한다. 우리는 프로그램에 대한 지속적인 평가와 필요한 경우 어디서나 개선 사항을 확인하고 구현하는 데 전념하고 있다. 우리는 프로그램의 임상 및 서비스 품질을 향상하기 위해 PHTLS를 제공하기 위한 새로운 방법과 기술을 추구할 것이다.

우리는 이 프로그램이 모든 국가의 병원 전 환자의 요구를 충족할 수 있도록 노력할 것이다. 2010년부터 유럽의 PHTLS 교수진은 프로그램의 품질을 측정하는 방법을 논의하고 개선이 필요한 영역을 확인하기 위해 모임을 했다. 이 모임은 2018년에 설립된 지역 유럽 교육 위원회로 발전했다. 라틴아메리카(2019년)와 중동(2021년)에도 유사한 위원회가 설립되었다. 2012년부터 세계 외상 심포지엄이 매년 개최되어 병원 전 외상 처치에 관한 최신 근거와 동향 및 논란을 제시하고 있다. 이 프로그램은 외상 처치의 지속적인 발전을 조사하기 위해 전 세계의 실무자와 연구원들의 작업을 한데 모은다. 그들의 기여뿐만 아니라 전 세계의 PHTLS 강사, 의료 책임자, 코디네이터, 저자, 검토자로 구성된 전 세계 PHTLS 가족의 기여는 모두 삶의 수많은 시간 동안 자원봉사를 통해 PHTLS 프로그램이 계속 번창하고 성장할 수 있도록 보장할 것이다.

PHTLS 교육 과정은 PHTLS를 이수한 사람이 다음과 같은 내용을 수행할 수 있도록 보장함으로써 환자에 대한 변함없는 헌신을 유지할 것이다.

- 환자를 신속하고 정확하게 평가한다.
- 쇼크와 저산소혈증을 인지한다.
- 적절한 시기에 적절한 처치를 시작한다.
- 환자에게 적절한 처치를 적절한 시간에 시행하기 위해 적절한 의료 기관으로 신속하게 이송한다.

요약

- 오늘날 우리가 알고 있는 병원 전 처치는 1700년대 후반으로 거슬러 올라간다. 당시 나폴레옹의 수석 군의관이었던 도미니크 장 라레(Dominique Jean Larrey) 남작은 신속한 병원 전 처치의 필요성을 인식했다. 1950년경 패링턴 박사가 병원 전 처치의 발전을 촉진할 때까지 비교적 느렸다. 그 이후로 병원 전 외상 처치의 개선을 위해 꾸준하고 지속해 노력했다.

- PHTLS의 가장 중요한 원칙은 병원 전 처치 제공자들이 훌륭한 지식적 기반을 갖고 비판적으로 사고해야 하며 최적의 상황이 아니더라도 뛰어난 환자 처치를 제공할 수 있는 적절한 술기 능력을 갖추어야 한다는 것이다.

- 전 세계적으로 손상은 사망과 장애의 주요 원인이며 직접적으로 관련된 사람들뿐만 아니라 재정적인 영향을 고려할 때 사회 전체에 영향을 미친다.

- 외상 처치의 결과 개선은 사고 전 단계, 사고 단계, 사고 후 단계로 나누어진다. 이 단계 중 어느 단계에서 외상성 손상의 영향을 최소화하려고 조치할 수 있으며 병원 전 처치 제공자는 각 단계에서 중요한 책임을 진다.

- 황금 시간(Golden Hour) 또는 황금 기간(Golden Period)의 개념은 병원 전 처치를 안내한다. 연구에 따르면 결정적인 처치를 시행할 수 있는 의료기관으로 신속하게 이송하는 것이 환자 결과를 개선하는 데 핵심적인 역할을 한다.

- PHTLS 과정은 1978년에 만들어진 ATLS 교육 과정을 모델로 만든 것으로 신속한 환자 이송과 이송 중 처치를 강조했다. PHTLS 프로그램이 성장함에 따라 미국 외과학회 외상위원회를 통한 의료 감독이 제공되었다. 30년 이상 동안 미국 외과학회와 NAEMT 간의 협력관계는 PHTLS 교육 과정을 이수한 사람이 외상 환자에게 생존할 가능성을 최대한으로 제공할 수 있도록 만들었다.

References

1. McSwain NE. Prehospital care from Napoleon to Mars: the surgeon's role. *J Am Coll Surg*. 2005;200(44):487-504.

2. Larrey DJ. *Mémoires de Chirurgie Militaire, et Campagnes* [*Memoirs of Military Surgery and Campaigns of the French Armies*]. Paris, France: J. Smith and F. Buisson; 1812-1817. English translation with notes by R. W. Hall of volumes 1-3 in 2 volumes; 1814. English translation of volume 4 by J. C. Mercer; 1832.

3. Rockwood CA, Mann CM, Farrington JD, et al. History of emergency medical services in the United States. *J Trauma*. 1976;16(4):299-308.

4. Farrington JD. Death in a ditch. *Bull Am Coll Surg*. 1967;52(3):121-132.

5. Federal Specifications for Ambulance, KKK-A-1822D. United States General Services Administration, Specifications Section, November 1994.

6. Kennedy R. *Early Care of the Sick and Injured Patient*. American College of Surgeons; 1964.

7. Curry G. *Immediate Care and Transport of the Injured*. Charles C. Thomas Publisher; 1965.

8. Committee on Trauma and Committee on Shock, Division of Medical Sciences. *Accidental Death and Disability: The Neglected Disease of Modern Society*. National Academy of Sciences/National Research Council; 1966.

9. Holcomb JB, Jenkins D, Rhee P, et al. Damage control resuscitation: directly addressing the early coagulopathy of trauma. *J Trauma*. 2007;62(2):307-310.

10. Holcomb JB, Tilley BC, Baraniuk S, et al. Transfusion of plasma, platelets, and red blood cells in a 1:1:1 vs a 1:1:2 ratio and mortality in patients with severe trauma: the PROPPR randomized clinical trial. *JAMA*. 2015;313(5):471-482.

11. Borgman MA, Spinella PC, Perkins JG, et al. The ratio of blood products transfused affects mortality in patients receiving massive transfusions at a combat support hospital. *J Trauma*. 2007;63(4):805-813.

12. Holcomb JB, Wade CE, Michalek JE, et al. Increased plasma and platelet to red blood cell ratios improves outcome in 466 massively transfused civilian trauma patients. *Ann Surg*. 2008;248(3):447-458.

13. Eastridge BJ, Jenkins D, Flaherty S, et al. Trauma system development in a theater of war: experiences from Operation Iraqi Freedom and Operation Enduring Freedom. *J Trauma*. 2006;61(6):1366-1372.

14. Ling GS, Rhee P, Ecklund JM. Surgical innovations arising from the Iraq and Afghanistan wars. *Annu Rev Med*. 2010;61:457-468.

15. Borden Institute. *Emergency War Surgery 2014*. 4th ed. Office of the Surgeon General; 2014.

16. World Health Organization. Injuries and violence. Published March 19, 2021. Accessed November 11, 2021. https://www.who.int/news-room/fact-sheets/detail/injuries-and-violence

17. World Health Organization. The true death toll of COVID-19. Accessed November 11, 2021. https://www.who.int/data/stories/the-true-death-toll-of-covid-19-estimating-global-excess-mortality

18. Centers for Disease Control and Prevention. Accessed November 11, 2021. Fatal injury and violence data. https://www.cdc.gov/injury/wisqars/fatal.html

19. Centers for Disease Control and Prevention. 10 leading causes of death, United States, 2019, all races, both sexes. Accessed November 11, 2021. https://wisqars.cdc.gov/fatal-leading

20. Centers for Disease Control and Prevention. Road traffic injuries and deaths—A global problem. Last reviewed

December 14, 2020. Accessed November 11, 2021. https://www.cdc.gov/injury/features/global-road-safety/index.html

21. World Health Organization. Falls. Published April 26, 2021. Accessed November 11, 2021. https://www.who.int/news-room/fact-sheets/detail/falls

22. Centers for Disease Control and Prevention. Important facts about falls. Last reviewed February 10, 2017. Accessed November 11, 2021. https://www.cdc.gov/homeandrecreationalsafety/falls/adultfalls.html

23. World Health Organization. Injuries and violence: the facts, 2014. Published 2014. Accessed November 11, 2021. http://apps.who.int/iris/bitstream/10665/149798/1/9789241508018_eng.pdf

24. World Health Organization. Road traffic injuries. Published June 21, 2021. Accessed November 11, 2021. https://www.who.int/news-room/fact-sheets/detail/road-traffic-injuries

25. United Nations General Assembly. Improving global road safety. Resolution adopted by the General Assembly on 31 August 2020. Published September 2, 2020. Accessed November 11, 2021. https://undocs.org/en/A/RES/74/299

26. National Safety Council. *Injury facts: Societal costs.* Accessed November 11, 2021. https://injuryfacts.nsc.org/all-injuries/costs/societal-costs/

27. World Health Organization. World traffic injuries: the facts. Accessed November 11, 2021. http://www.who.int/violence_injury_prevention/road_safety_status/2015/magnitude_A4_web.pdf?ua=1

28. Centers for Disease Control and Prevention. 10 leading causes of injury deaths by age group highlighting violence-related injury deaths, United States – 2018. Accessed November 11, 2021. https://www.cdc.gov/injury/images/lc-charts/leading_causes_of_death_by_age_group_violence_2018_1100w850h.jpg

29. O'Dea S. Percentage of U.S. adults who own a smartphone from 2011 to 2021. *Statista.* Published May 12, 2021. Accessed November 11, 2021. https://www.statista.com/statistics/219865/percentage-of-us-adults-who-own-a-smartphone/

30. Centers for Disease Control and Prevention. Distracted driving. Last reviewed March 2, 2021. Accessed November 11, 2021. https://www.cdc.gov/transportationsafety/distracted_driving/index.html#problem

31. Governors Highway Safety Association. Distracted driving. Accessed August 18, 2021. https://www.ghsa.org/state-laws/issues/distracted%20driving

32. Mothers Against Drunk Driving. Accessed November 11, 2021. http://www.madd.org/

33. Sewell RA, Poling J, Sofuoglu M. The effect of cannabis compared with alcohol on driving. *Am J Addict.* 2009;18(3)185-193.

34. Centers for Disease Control and Prevention, National Center for Injury Prevention and Control. Fact sheet: risk factors for falls. Published 2017. Accessed November 11, 2021. https://www.cdc.gov/steadi/pdf/Risk_Factors_for_Falls-print.pdf

35. Centers for Disease Control and Prevention, National Center for Injury Prevention and Control. Preventing falls: a guide to implementing effective community-based fall prevention programs. Published 2015. Accessed November 11, 2021. https://www.cdc.gov/homeandrecreationalsafety/pdf/falls/fallpreventionguide-2015-a.pdf

36. American Red Cross. Red Cross launches campaign to cut drowning in half in 50 cities. Published May 20, 2014. Accessed November 11, 2021. https://www.redcross.org/about-us/news-and-events/press-release/red-cross-launches-campaign-to-cut-drowning-in-half-in-50-cities.html

37. World Health Organization. Drowning. Published April 27, 201. Accessed November 11, 2021. https://www.who.int/news-room/fact-sheets/detail/drowning#:~:text=Key%20facts,000%20annual%20drowning%20deaths%20worldwide

38. Ramos W, Beale A, Chambers P, Dalke S, Fielding R. Primary and secondary drowning interventions: The American Red Cross Circle of Drowning Prevention and Chain of Drowning Survival. *Int J Aquatic Res Educ.* 2015;9(1):89-101.

39. American Red Cross. Water safety. Accessed November 11, 2021. http://www.redcross.org/get-help/how-to-prepare-for-emergencies/types-of-emergencies/water-safety

40. Association of Aquatic Professionals. Drowning prevention education. Accessed November 11, 2021. https://aquatic-pros.org/drowning-prevention-education

41. YMCA. Water safety and swimming. Accessed November 11, 2021. https://www.ymca.org/what-we-do/healthy-living/water-safety

42. Goodwin A, Kirley B, Sandt L, et al., eds. *Countermeasures That Work: A Highway Safety Countermeasure Guide for State Highway Safety Offices.* 7th ed. National Highway Traffic Safety Administration; 2013:5-7.

43. Insurance Institute of Highway Safety. Motorcycles: motorcycle helmet use. Data updated November 2021. Accessed November 11, 2021. https://www.iihs.org/topics/motorcycles/motorcycle-helmet-laws-table

44. Edgar Synder and Associates. Motorcycle helmet laws—by state. Accessed November 11, 2021. https://www.edgarsnyder.com/motorcycle-accidents/state-helmet-laws

45. Insurance Information Institute. Facts and statistics: Motorcycle crashes. Accessed November 11, 2021. https://www.iii.org/fact-statistic/facts-statistics-motorcycle-crashes

46. Trunkey DD. Trauma. *Sci Am.* 1983;249(2):28-35.

47. U.S. Department of Homeland Security. Stop the bleed. Published June 16, 2017. Accessed November 11, 2021. https://www.dhs.gov/stopthebleed

48. Cuschieri J, Johnson JL, Sperry J, et al. Benchmarking outcomes in the critically injured trauma patient and the effect of implementing standard operating procedures. *Ann Surg.* 2012;255(5):993-999.

49. Rotondo MF, Zonies DH. The damage control sequence and underlying logic. *Surg Clin North Am.* 1997;77(4):761-777.

50. Sugrue M, D'Amours SK, Joshipura M. Damage control surgery and the abdomen. *Injury.* 2004;35(7):642-648.

51. Beldowicz BC. The evolution of damage control in concept and practice. *Clin Colon Rectal Surg.* 2018;31(1):30-35.

52. Rotondo MF, Schwab CW, McGonigal MD, et al. "Damage control": an approach for improved survival in exsanguinating penetrating abdominal injury. *J Trauma.* 1993;35(3):375-382.

53. Schreiber MA. Damage control surgery. *Crit Care Clin.* 2004;20(1):101-118.

54. Parr MJ, Alabdi T. Damage control surgery and intensive care. *Injury.* 2004;35(7):713-722.

55. University of Maryland Medical Center. Tribute to R Adams Cowley, MD. Accessed November 11, 2021. https://www.umms.org/ummc/health-services/shock-trauma/about/history

56. Demetriades D, Chan L, Cornwell EE, et al. Paramedic vs. private transportation of trauma patients: effect on outcome. *Arch Surg.* 1996;131(2):133-138.

57. Cornwell EE, Belzberg H, Hennigan K, et al. Emergency medical services (EMS) vs. non-EMS transport of

critically injured patients: a prospective evaluation. *Arch Surg.* 2000;135(3):315-319.

58. Kotwal RS, Howard JT, Oramn JA, et al. The effect of a golden hour policy on the morbidity and mortality of combat casualties. *JAMA Surg.* 2016;151(1):15-24.

59. Alarhayem AQ, Myers JG, Dent D, et al. Time is the enemy: mortality in trauma patients with hemorrhage from torso injury occurs long before the "Golden Hour." *Am J. Surg.* 2016;212(6):1101-1105.

60. American Academy of Surgeons. *Resources for Optimal Care of the Injured Patient.* 6th ed. American College of Surgeons; 2014. Accessed November 11, 2021. https://www.facs.org/quality-programs/trauma/tqp/center-programs/vrc/resources

61. Demetriades D, Martin M, Salim A, Rhee P, Brown C, Chan L. The effect of trauma center designation and trauma volume on outcome in specific severe injuries. *Ann Surg.* 2005;242(4):512-519. doi: 10.1097/01.sla.0000184169.73614.09

62. Peleg K, Aharonson-Daniel L, Stein M, et al. Increased survival among severe trauma patients: the impact of a national trauma system. *Arch Surg.* 2004;139(11):1231-1236.

63. Edwards W. Emergency medical systems significantly increase patient survival rates, Part 2. *Can Doct.* 1982;48(12):20-24.

64. Haas B, Jurkovich GJ, Wang J, et al. Survival advantage in trauma centers: expeditious intervention or experience? *J Am Coll.* 2009;208(1):28-36.

65. Scheetz LJ. Differences in survival, length of stay, and discharge disposition of older trauma patients admitted to trauma centers and nontrauma center hospitals. *J Nurs Scholarsh.* 2005;37(4):361-366.

66. Norwood S, Fernandez L, England J. The early effects of implementing American College of Surgeons level II criteria on transfer and survival rates at a rurally based community hospital. *J Trauma.* 1995;39(2):240-244; discussion 244-245.

67. Kane G, Wheeler NC, Cook S, et al. Impact of the Los Angeles county trauma system on the survival of seriously injured patients. *J Trauma.* 1992;32(5):576-583.

68. Hedges JR, Adams AL, Gunnels MD. ATLS practices and survival at rural level III trauma hospitals, 1995-1999. *Prehosp Emerg Care.* 2002;6(3):299-305.

69. Konvolinka CW, Copes WS, Sacco WJ. Institution and per-surgeon volume vs. survival outcome in Pennsylvania's trauma centers. *Am J Surg.* 1995;170(4):333-340.

70. Margulies DR, Cryer HG, McArthur DL, et al. Patient volume per surgeon does not predict survival in adult level I trauma centers. *J Trauma.* 2001;50(4):597-601; discussion 601-603.

71. McSwain NE. Judgment based on knowledge: a history of Prehospital Trauma Life Support, 1970-2013. *J Trauma Acute Care Surg.* 2013;75:1-7.

Suggested Reading

Callaham M. Quantifying the scanty science of prehospital emergency care. *Ann Emerg Med.* 1997;30:785.

Cone DC, Lewis RJ. Should this study change my practice? *Acad Emerg Med.* 2003;10:417.

Haynes RB, McKibbon KA, Fitzgerald D, et al. How to keep up with the medical literature: II. Deciding which journals to read regularly. *Ann Intern Med.* 1986;105:309.

Keim SM, Spaite DW, Maio RF, et al. Establishing the scope and methodological approach to out-of-hospital outcomes and effectiveness research. *Acad Emerg Med.* 2004;11:1067.

Lewis RJ, Bessen HA. Statistical concepts and methods for the reader of clinical studies in emergency medicine. *J Emerg Med.* 1991;9:221.

MacAvley D. Critical appraisal of medical literature: an aid to rational decision making. *Fam Pract.* 1995;12:98.

Reed JF III, Salen P, Bagher P. Methodological and statistical techniques: what do residents really need to know about statistics? *J Med Syst.* 2003;27:233.

Sackett DL. How to read clinical journals: V. To distinguish useful from useless or even harmful therapy. *Can Med Assoc J.* 1981;124:1156.

황금 원칙, 선호 및 비판적 사고

Lead Editors
Andrew N. Pollak, MD, FAAOS
Nancy Hoffmann, MSW

학습 목표

이 장의 학습을 완료하면 다음과 같은 내용을 수행할 수 있다.

- 현장에서 의사 결정과 관련하여 원칙과 선호도의 차이점을 설명할 수 있다.
- 주어진 외상 시나리오를 가지고 특수 상황에 대한 외상 처치 원칙에 대해 논의할 수 있다.
- 주어진 외상 시나리오에서 비판적 사고 기술을 사용하여 응급 외상 처치의 원칙을 달성하기 위해 선호하는 방법을 결정할 수 있다.
- 윤리적 의사결정의 네 가지 원칙을 병원 전 외상 처치완 연관시킬 수 있다.
- 주어진 외상 시나리오를 가지고 이와 관련된 윤리적 문제와 이를 해결하는 방법에 더해 논의할 수 있다.
- "황금 시간(Golden Hour)" 또는 "황금 기간(Golden Period)"의 중요성을 설명할 수 있다.
- 병원 전 외상 처치의 14가지 "황금 원칙"에 대해 토론할 수 있다.
- 병원 전 연구와 문헌의 중요성과 구성 요소를 확인할 수 있다.

시나리오

당신과 동료(paramedic과 EMT)는 두 대의 차량이 측면 충돌한 사고 현장에 도착했다. 당신 팀은 현재 출동할 수 있는 유일한 구급차이다. 픽업트럭에는 술 냄새를 심하게 풍기는 한 젊은 남성이 안전띠를 착용하지 않은 채 앉아 있었고 아래팔이 변형된 것을 확인할 수 있었다. 트럭은 승용차의 조수석 문이 심하게 들어갈 정도로 충돌한 상태였다 승용차 즈수석에는 숨을 쉬지 않는 것으로 보이는 나이 든 여성이 앉아있다. 앞 유리는 과녁 모양으로 깨져 있었다. 승용차 운전자도 손상을 입었지만, 의식은 있고 매우 불안해하고 뒷좌석에는 카시트에 고정된 두 명의 어린이가 있다. 조수석 뒤쪽에 앉은 어린이는 대략 3세 정도로 보이며 의식을 잃고 카시트에 털썩 주저앉아 있다. 운전석 뒤쪽에 어린이용 보조 의자에 고정되어 앉아 있는 5세 어린이는 울고 있지만 다친 곳은 없는 것으로 보인다.

픽업트럭의 운전자는 팔이 골절되는 손상을 입은 것이 분명하지만, 매우 적대적이고 폭언하며 처치를 거부하고 있다. 한편 승용차의 운전자는 필사적으로 자녀와 어머니 상태에 관해 묻고 있다.

- 이 다수 사상자 사고를 어떻게 처리하겠는가?
- 이 환자 중 우선순위가 높은 환자는 누구인가?
- 두 자녀의 어머니에게 그들의 상태에 대해 뭐라고 설명할 것인가?
- 다른 차량의 운전자가 술에 취한 것처럼 보이는 경우 어떻게 다룰 것인가?
- 분명히 술에 취한 운전자의 처치 거부를 허용할 것인가?

개요

걱정스럽고 좌절한 의사가 아픈 아이의 머리맡에 앉아 있는 모습을 보여주는 루크 필즈 경(Sir Luke Fildes)의 그림 이후 의학은 크게 바뀌었다(**그림 2-1**). 당시에는 항생제가 없었고 대부분 질병에 대한 최소한의 이해와 기초적인 수술만 있었으며 약물 치료는 주로 약초 요법으로 구성되었다. 수년 동안 의학은 정확한 과학이 아니라 예술 형식에 가까웠다. 이제 질병에 대한 이해, 의약품 개발 및 기술 응용 분야에서 상당한 발전이 이루어졌다. 연구를 통해 우리는 증거 기반으로 의학을 통해 더 나은 환자 치료를 제공할 수 있다. 그러나 의료 행위가 보다 과학에 기반을 두기 시작하면서 예술 형태는 줄어들었지만, 아직 예술은 여전히 남아있다.

본문 전반에서 논의된 바와 같이 병원 전 처치의 과학은 다음과 같은 실무 지식을 포함한다.

1. 해부학 — 인체의 기관, 뼈, 근육, 동맥, 신경 및 정맥
2. 생리학 — 인체의 기관과 조직이 서로 어떻게 상호작용하여 인간의 기능을 수행하는지에 대한 이해
3. 약리학 — 약물의 과학과 약물이 신체와 어떻게 상호작용하는 방식
4. 이러한 구성 요소들 사이의 관계와 구성 요소들이 서로에게 미치는 영향

이러한 요소에 대한 이해를 적용함으로써 처치 제공자는 환자가

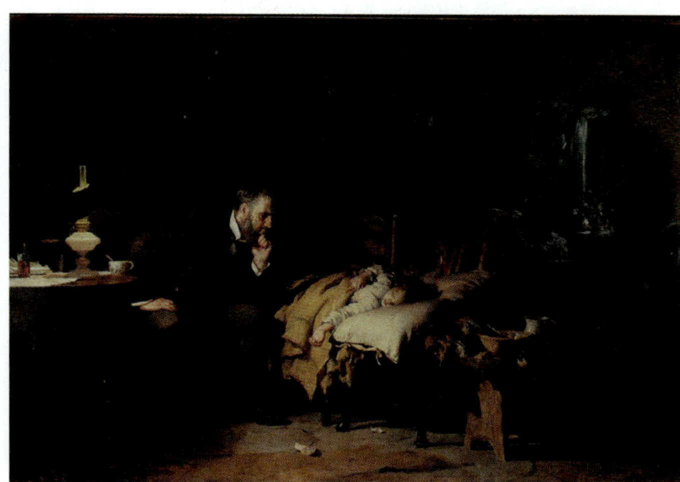

그림 2-1 루크 필즈 경(Sir Luke Fildes)의 그림 "의사"는 아픈 아이의 침대 옆에 앉아 걱정하는 의사를 보여준다. 상대적으로 원시적인 상태의 의료 서비스는 희망적인 기다림과 관찰 외에는 개입할 방법이 거의 없었다.

입은 손상과 손상의 영향을 완화하기 위해 사용하는 처치의 타당성을 이해할 수 있다.

의학의 주요 발전은 기술 및 진단 장비의 발전을 포함한다. 컴퓨터 단층활영(CT), 초음파 및 자기공명영상(MRI)의 영상 기술을 통해 환자를 평가하고 진단 및 치료하는 능력이 획기적으로 향상되었다. 임상 검사실에서는 인체에서 발견되는 거의 모든 전해질, 호르몬 또는 물질을 측정할 수 있다. 제약 산업은 지속해서 신약을 개발하고 있다. 치료는 혈관 내 및 중재적 방사선 기술을 통해 덜 침습적이고 병적이 되고 있다. EMS 통신 시스템은 획기적으로 개선되었으며 위성 항법 시스템(GPS)으로 외진 지역에서도 환자를 찾을 수 있다. 농촌 지역에서 출동 및 반응 시간이 감소했으며 기술 발전에 전반적으로 환자 처치가 개선되었다.

이러한 모든 과학적 의학 발전을 활용하기 처지 제공자는 해당 지식 기반을 개별 환자의 요구에 연결하는 기술에 능숙해야 한다. 에도 불구하고 응급 최초반응자는 환자에게 과학적인 최상의 치료를 제공함으로써 의학 기술을 제공한다. 병원 전 처치 제공자는 어떤 환자가 중상을 입었고 어느 의료기관으로 신속하게 이송해야 하는지 결정할 수 있어야 하며 어떤 처치가 환자의 결과를 악화시키지 않으면서도 환자의 처치에 도움이 될 수 있는지 균형을 맞출 수 있어야 한다. 쇼크의 경우 말초 기관까지 관류를 회복시켜야 하는 우리의 최종 목표를 달성하기 위해 사용할 수 있는 장비와 술기를 선택할 수 있는 능력이 중요하다. 이 능력은 의학의 실천인 기술을 설명한다.

의학은 다른 모든 예술적 노력과 마찬가지로 지도 원칙을 가지고 있다. 특히 이 장에서는 외상 처치의 황금 원칙에 대한 개발을 포함한다. PHTLS 프로그램의 한 가지 기본 원칙은 환자 처치가 순전히 프로토콜 중심이 아니라 지식 중심이어야 한다는 것이다. 따라서 병원 전 처치 제공자가 신속한 평가, 주요 현장 처치 및 가장 가까운 의료기관으로 외상 환자를 신속하게 이송하여 환자의 결과를 개선하는 데 도움이 되는 황금 원칙을 포함한다.

원칙과 선호

의학은 의료의 원칙(Principle)에 대한 기초를 제공한다. 간단히 말해서 원칙은 가능한 최상의 결과로 환자 생존 가능성을 극대화하기 위해 병원 전 처치 제공자가 달성해야 하는 것을 정의한다. 이러한 원칙이 환자를 가장 효율적으로 처치하기 위해 처치 제공자에 의해 구현되는 방법은 시스템과 처치 제공자가 환자 처치에 과학적 원칙을 적

용하기로 선택하는 방법을 설명하는 선호(preference)에 따라 달라진다. 이것이 환자 처치를 위해 과학과 의학 기술이 결합한 방식이다.

기도 관리와 같은 예는 원칙과 선호의 차이를 설명할 수 있다. 원칙은 산소를 포함한 공기가 개방된 기도를 통해 폐의 폐포로 이동하여 적혈구와 산소-이산화탄소 교환을 촉진하여 다른 조직으로 산소를 전달할 수 있도록 하는 것이다. 이 원칙은 모든 환자에게 적용되고 선호는 특정 환자에게 기도 관리를 수행하는 방법이다. 대부분의 경우 환자는 스스로 기도를 유지할 수 있지만, 그렇지 않은 환자의 경우 병원 전 처치 제공자가 기도 관리를 용이하게 하는 데 가장 적합한 기도유지기를 결정해야 한다. 즉 병원 전 처치 제공자는 폐로 산소를 공급하고 이차적으로 이산화탄소를 배출하기 위해 가장 좋은 기도유지 방법을 결정할 것이다. 예술 또는 선호는 병원 전 처치 제공자가 원칙을 달성하기 위해 이러한 결정을 내리고 수행하는 방법이다. 이 술기 중 일부는 고품질 무작위 임상 시험의 정보에 의해 지시된다. 이것을 근거중심의학이라고 한다. 그러나 대부분은 종종 경험과 일화에 근거한다. 처치 표준은 처치 제공자가 환자에게 처치를 제공하는 과정에서 충족해야 하는 기본적인 최소 수행 요건을 설명한다.

원칙을 달성하는 방법에 대한 선호는 상황, 환자의 상태, 사용할 수 있는 의학적 증거에 대한 처치 제공자의 지식/술기/경험, 프로토콜 및 사용할 수 있는 장비와 같은 등의 여러 요인에 따라 달라진다(Box 2-1).

PHTLS 교육의 기초는 병원 전 처치 제공자가 환자 처치에 대한 적절한 결정을 순전히 프로토콜이 아닌 지식을 기반으로 하도록 가르치는 것이다. 환자 처치의 목표는 원칙을 달성하는 것이다. 이를 달성하는 방법(즉, 처치 제공자가 환자를 처치하기 위해 내린 결정)은

Box 2-1에 설명된 현재 상황, 환자 상태, 의학적 증거, 술기, 프로토콜 및 당시 사용할 수 있는 장비를 기반으로 한 선호이다.

PHTLS 프로그램의 철학은 각각의 상황과 환자가 다르다는 것이다. PHTLS는 교육 주제에 대한 강한 이해와 적절한 처치를 수행하는 데 필요한 술기의 중요성을 가르친다. 현장에서 내리는 판단과 결정은 특정 시간과 특정 상황에서 처치하는 특정 환자의 필요에 따라 개별화되어야 한다. 프로토콜은 지침과 방향에 도움이 되지만, 현장에서 변동성이 있을 때는 충분히 융통성이 있어야 한다. 관련된 원칙을 이해하그 비판적 사고 기술을 사용하여 최종 목표를 달성하기 위해 적절한 결정을 내릴 수 있다.

선호가 병원 전 처치 제공자가 최종 목표를 달성하려는 방법이라는 점을 감안하면 원칙은 매번 같은 방법으로 달성되지 않는다. 모든 처치 제공자가 모든 술기에 숙달된 것은 아니다. 이러한 술기를 시행하는 데 사용하는 장비는 모든 응급상황에서 사용할 수 있는 것은 아니다. 한 명의 강사 또는 한 명의 의료 책임자가 한 가지 술기를 선호한다고 해서 그것이 모든 상황에서 모든 처치 제공자에게 최고의 술기라는 것을 의미하지는 않는다. 중요한 점은 원칙을 달성하는 것이다. 이를 수행하는 방법과 환자에게 처치를 제공하는 방법은 Box 2-1에 나열된 요소에 따라 다르며 이러한 요소는 다음 섹션에서 자세히 설명한다.

상황

상황은 환자에게 제공되는 처치에 영향을 미칠 수 있는 현장의 모든 요소를 포함한다. 이러한 요소에는 다음과 같은 내용이 포함되지만, 이에 국한되지는 않는다.

- 감염 우험을 포함한 현장의 위험
- 관련된 환자 수
- 환자 위치
- 차량 위치
- 오염 물질 및 위험 물질 문제
- 화재 또는 화재 가능성
- 날씨
- 경찰관에 의한 현장 통제 및 현장 안전
- 가장 가까운 병원과 가장 가까운 외상센터의 기능을 포함한 의료 기관까지의 거리 및 시간
- 현장에 있는 병원 전 처치 제공자 및 기타 지원할 수 있는 인력의 수

Box 2-1 원칙과 선호

원칙: 환자의 예후나 생존을 위한 기본적인 과학 또는 해부학 기반 원칙
선호: 병원 전 처치 제공자가 원칙을 달성하는 방법이 원칙을 달성하기 위해 사용되는 선호는 다음과 같은 몇 가지 요인에 따라 달라진다.

- 존재하는 상황
- 환자 상태
- 병원 전 처치 제공자의 지식, 술기, 경험
- 지역 내 프로토콜
- 사용할 수 있는 장비

- 목격자
- 현장에서 사용할 수 있는 이송 수단
- 원거리에 이용할 수 있는 기타 이송 수단(예; 헬기, 추가 구급차)

© National Association of Emergency Medical Technicians (NAEMT)

다른 많은 조건뿐만 아니라 이러한 모든 조건과 상황은 지속해서 변화할 수 있으며 병원 전 처치 제공자가 환자의 요구에 대응할 방법에 영향을 미칠 것이다.

예를 들어, 숲이 우거진 시골 지역의 도로에서 자동차 한 대가 가로수를 들이받았다. 날씨는 맑고 어두운 새벽 2시이며 외상센터까지 지상으로 이송하는 데 걸리는 시간은 35분이다. 현장의 병원 전 처치 제공자가 의료용 헬기를 의료 지도 의사의 승인을 받아 요청할 수 있다. 헬기가 이륙을 준비하기까지 5분이 소요되며 현장에 도착하기까지는 15분이 걸린다. 외상센터가 없는 병원은 15분 거리에 있으며 헬기 착륙장이 있다. 이러한 상황에서 당신은 외상센터까지 지상으로 이송할 것인가? 아니면 헬기 착륙장이 있는 외상센터가 없는 병원까지 지상으로 이송한 후 헬기 착륙장에서 헬기를 만날 것인가? 아니면 현장에서 의료용 헬기를 기다릴 것인가?

이러한 상황이 척추 고정과 같은 술기에 어떤 영향을 미치는지 보여주는 몇 가지 예는 다음과 같다.

상황 1

- 자동차 충돌
- 과녁 모양처럼 파손된 앞 유리
- 따뜻하고 화창한 날
- 도로에 차량 정체 없음

처치

- 차량 내에서 환자 평가 -심한 요통, 다리 쇠약이 관찰됨
- 목뼈보호대 착용
- 긴척추고정판으로 환자 구출
- 차량으로부터 구출
- 들것에 위치
- 신체 평가 완료
- 병원으로 이송한 환자

© National Association of Emergency Medical Technicians (NAEMT)

상황 2

- 연료 탱크에서 휘발유가 떨어지고 엔진에서 연기가 나며 화재 진압 장치가 현장에 없다는 점을 제외하면 상황 1과 같음
- 화재에 대한 우려

처치

- 빠른 구출 방법 사용
- 환자가 차량에서 안전한 장소로 이동
- 환자 평가 및 척추 고정을 시행의 필요성 결정
- 신체 평가 완료
- 환자를 병원으로 이송

© National Association of Emergency Medical Technicians (NAEMT)

상황 3

- 주택 화재와 관련된 환자
- 환자가 움직일 수 없음

처치

- 평가 불가능
- 환자를 화재 현장으로부터 끌어냄
- 들것 위에 환자 올려놓기
- 환자를 화재로부터 안전한 장소로 신속하게 이동
- 환자 평가 완료
- 환자의 상태에 따라 병원으로 신속하게 이송

© National Association of Emergency Medical Technicians (NAEMT)

상황 4

- 총격전을 벌이는 상황
- 경찰(또는 군인)이 무릎에 총상을 입고 심한 출혈을 보임

처치

- 거리를 두고 평가(쌍안경 이용)
- 추가 손상 평가
- 자신의 무기를 충분히 사용할 수 있는 환자
- 환자에게 스스로 지혈대를 적용할 것을 지시
- 환자에게 안전 구역까지 기어 나올 것을 지시
- 상황이 가능할 때 환자 구조

© National Association of Emergency Medical Technicians (NAEMT)

환자의 상태

의사결정 과정의 다음 구성요소는 환자의 의학적 상태와 관련이 있다. 의사결정에 영향을 미치는 주요 질문은 "이 환자가 얼마나 아픈가?"다. 이러한 결정을 쉽게 할 수 있도록 도와주는 몇 가지 주요 정보에는 환자 나이, 말초 기관 관류에 영향을 미치는 생리학적 요인(혈압, 맥박, 환기 수, 체온 등), 손상 기전, 환자 과거 병력, 복용하고 있

는 약물, 약물 및 알코올 중독이 포함된다. 이러한 요인 등은 이송 전이나 이송 중에 병원 전 처치 제공자가 수행해야 할 처치와 이송 방법을 결정하기 위한 비판적 사고력이 필요하다.

위에 언급했던 한 대의 차량이 나무에 충돌한 시나리오로 돌아가 보겠다. 환자는 분당 30회로 호흡이 곤란하며 맥박수 100회/분, 촉지에 의한 수축기 혈압 90mmHg, 환자는 명령을 따르지 않는다. 환자는 20대 중반이고 안전띠를 착용하지 않았으며 현재 에어백이 터진 핸들에 기대어 있다. 환자의 오른쪽 넓적다리 중간 부위에 변형이 발생했고 왼쪽 발목 개방 골절과 상당한 출혈이 보인다. 발목 주위 바닥에는 약 1L의 혈액이 있다.

병원 전 처치 제공자의 지식 기반

병원 전 처치 제공자의 지식은 초기 교육, 지속적인 의료 교육(CME) 과정, 지속적인 독서 및 연구, 프로토콜, 전체적인 경험과 술기 등을 포함한 여러 가지 요소에서 나온다.

다시 기도 관리를 예로 들어 보겠다. 병원 전 처치 제공자의 지식과 경험의 수준은 기도 관리와 관련된 의사 결정에 상당한 영향을 미친다. 병원 전 처치 제공자가 술기를 수행하는 숙련도는 과거에 수행된 빈도에 따라 다르다. 병원 전 처치 제공자는 다음과 같은 내용을 고려할 수 있다. 환자가 스스로 기도를 유지할 수 있는가? 그렇지 않다면 어떤 기도유지기를 사용할 수 있으며 그중에서 어떤 기도유지기를 사용하는 것이 편한가? 마지막으로 기관내삽관을 시행한 것이 언제인가? 후두경을 사용하는 것에 익숙한가? 입인두의 해부학적 구조에 대해 얼마나 알고 있는가? 살아 있는 환자나 심지어 동물 실험 모델을 대상으로 몇 번이나 반지갑상연골절개를 시행해 보았는가? 적절한 기술과 경험이 없으면 기관내삽관이나 외과적 술기와 같은 전문 처치보다는 입인두기도기나 코인두기도기와 백마스크 장비를 사용하는 것이 병원 전 처치 제공자에게 더 편안할 뿐만 아니라 환자가 생존할 가능성이 더 높다. 그런데도 고 합병증의 위험을 최소화하면서 기도를 가장 빠르게 유지하는 방법은 당신이 선택해야 한다.

단일 차량 충돌 사고 환자의 사례로 돌아가 보면 현장에 도착한 병원 전 처치 제공자는 2년 동안 함께 일했으며 둘 다 파라메딕 자격을 가지고 있다. 기관내삽관에 대한 마지막 업데이트 교육은 1년 전 있다. 한 명의 파라메딕은 2개월 전에 마지막으로 기관내삽관을 시행했고 그의 동료는 한 달 전에 배치되었다. 이들은 기관내삽관은 시행하기 위해 마비 약물을 사용할 수 있는 권한은 없지만 필요한 경우 진정제를 사용할 수 있다. 이들은 최근에 지혈대와 지혈제를 사용하여 출혈을 지혈하는 교육을 받았다. 이들이 받은 교육이 현장에서 환자를 처치하기 위해 시행할 수 있는 술기에 어떤 영향을 미칠까?

지역 프로토콜

병원 전 처치 제공자의 업무 범위는 수행할 수 있는 교육을 받고 수행 능력 인증, 자격 및 기관의 의료 책임자의 자격 증명으로 정의된다. 프로토콜은 처치 제공자가 어떤 상황에서 그들의 업무 범위를 적용해야 하는지 정의한다. 이러한 프로토콜은 모든 환자를 처치하는 방법을 요리책 형식으로 설명해서는 안 되고 설명할 수도 없지만, 모범 사례, 자원 및 교육 수준에 따라 체계적이고 일관성 있는 방식으로 환자에게 접근하는 방법을 안내하기 위한 것이다. 단일 차량 충돌 시나리오에서 진정제를 사용한 급속연속마취유도 삽관은 매우 유용할 수 있지만, 프로토콜에 포함되어 있지 않으면 병원 전 처치 제공자가 시행할 수 없다. 프로토콜은 종종 처치 제공자가 선택해야 하는 절차와 이송 의료기관을 지정한다. 예를 들어, 처치 제공자는 의료지도 의사에게 헬기를 요청하거나 환자를 특정 외상센터로 이송하도록 지시할 수 있다.

사용할 수 있는 장비

사용할 수 있는 적절한 장비가 없다면 병원 전 처치 제공자의 경험은 중요하지 않다. 병원 전 처치 제공자는 사용할 수 있는 장비 또는 소모품을 사용해야 한다. 예를 들어, 혈액은 외상 환자에게 가장 좋은 수액일 수 있다. 그러나 현장에서 혈액을 사용할 수 없는 경우가 많으므로 결정질 수액이 유일한 소생술에 사용할 수 있는 수액일 수 있다. 또 다른 고려 사항은 환자 손상의 특성을 고려할 때 허용성 저혈압이 더 나은 선택인지 여부이다. 이 특정 문제는 3장 쇼크: 삶과 죽음의 병태생리학에서 더 자세히 논의된다.

다시 한번 단일 차량 충돌 사고의 환자로 돌아가 보겠다. 완전한 구급 장비가 준비되어 있으며 교대 시작 시 확인하였다. 여기에는 기관내관, 후두경, 성문위기도기, 코인두기도기, 입인두기도기, 지혈대 및 2020년 미국 EMS 의사협회(NAEMSP)가 기본 생명 유지와 전문 생명 유지술을 시행하기 위해 권장하는 필수 장비에 대한 구급차 공동성명서에 나열된 기타 장비와 소모품이 포함된다. 파라메딕은 지혈제를 사용할 수 있고 환자는 갇혀 있지 않다. 따라서 외상센터로 가장 신속하게 이송하는 방법은 구급차를 이용하는 것이다. 환자는 스스로 기도를 유지할 수 있다. 그러나 환자의 호흡 곤란을 고려할 때 파라메딕은 보조 산소가 연결된 백마스크를 사용하여 보조 환기를 시행한다. 환자를 차량에서 구출한 발목 출혈 부위를 직접 압박으로 지혈을 시행한다. 그들은 환자의 목뼈와 척추를 고정하기 위해 목뼈 보호대와 긴척추고정판을 선택한다. 그들은 시간을 절약하기 위해 환자의 넓적다리뼈를 긴척추고정판에 고정하여 시간을 절약하고 환자를 인근 외상센터로 직접 이송한다.

원칙 대 선호의 또 따른 예는 호흡이 없는 환자를 만났을 때 기도를 개방하고 산소를 폐로 공급해야 한다는 것이다. 선택된 선호는 선호 요인(현재 상황, 환자 상태, 처치 제공자의 지식/술기/경험, 프로토콜 및 사용할 수 있는 장비)에 따라 달라진다. 심폐소생술 교육만 배운 목격자는 입 대 입 인공호흡을 시행할 수 있다. EMT는 기도유지기를 삽입하고 백마스크로 보조 환기를 시행할 수 있다. 파라메딕은 기관내삽관을 시행하거나 빠른 이송과 함께 백마스크 장비를 사용하는 것이 더 유리하다고 결정할 수 있다. 전투 중인 군인은 반지갑상연골절개를 시행하거나 적의 공격으로 인한 위험을 인지하여 아무것도 시행하지 않을 수 있다. 응급실의 의사는 마비 약물 또는 광섬유 유도를 이용해 기관내삽관을 시행할 수 있다. 주어진 환자의 특정 시점에서 잘못된 선택은 없으며 마찬가지로 항상 올바른 것은 없다.

외상 환자 처치에 있어 원칙과 선호의 개념은 군대의 전투 상황에서 가장 잘 적용된다. 이러한 이유로 전술적 전투 사상자 처치 위원회(Co-TCCC)는 PHTLS 교과서의 군사적 구성 요소를 작성했다. 군의무병의 경우 현장 상황에는 전투 중인지 아닌지, 적의 위치, 전술적 상황, 현재 사용 중인 무기와 부상자를 보호하기 위해 사용할 수 있는 보호물이 포함된다. 전투 상황에서 환자 처치와 관련된 명백한 차이가 있지만, 민간 전술적 응급의료 지원(TEMS) 제공자나 화재 현장 같은 위험한 환경에서 일하는 병원 전 처치 제공자에게도 유사한 고려 사항이 존재한다. 예를 들어, 화재에 완전히 둘러싸인 집 안에 쓰러져 있는 환자를 소방관과 구급대원이 발견한다. 이러한 상황에서 환자의 기도를 유지하고 혈역학적 평가를 시행하는 것은 안전하지 않으며 심지어 합리적이지 않다. 첫 번째 단계는 환자를 불타는 건물에서 안전한 지역으로 이동시키는 것이다. 그래야만 환자의 기도와 맥박을 평가하는 것이 적절하다.

전투에 참여할 가능성이 있는 군 의료진을 위해 전술적 전투 사상자 처치 위원회가 개발한 사상자 관리를 위한 세 가지 과정은 다음과 같다.

1. 교전 중 처치: 교전이 이루어지는 상황에서 시행하는 처치

2. 전술적 현장 처치: 교전은 종료되었지만, 여전히 위험이 남아있는 상황에서 시행하는 처치

3. 전술적 후송 처치: 상황이 종결되고 안전하다고 판단될 경우 시행하는 처치

환자 처치의 원칙은 절대 변하지 않았지만, 환자 처치가 제공되는 방식에 대한 선호는 크게 다를 수 있다. 이에 대한 세부 사항 및 자세한 논의는 22장 민간 전술적 응급의료 지원(TEMS) 또는 PHTLS 군사 버전을 참고한다(이러한 상황적 차이는 5장 현장 처치에서 자세히 설명하고 있다).

비판적 사고

특정 환자의 상태에 적용되는 원칙을 성공적으로 해결하고 그 원칙을 구현하기 위한 최선의 선호 방법을 선택하려면 비판적 사고가 중요하다. 의학에서 비판적 사고는 처치 제공자가 현재 상황, 환자 상태, 이용할 수 있는 모든 자원을 평가하는 과정이다(Box 2-2). 그런 다음 처치 제공자는 이 정보를 신속하게 분석하고 환자에게 최상의 처치를 제공할 수 있는 최적의 방법을 결정한다. 비판적 사고의 과정은 처치 제공자가 처치 계획을 수립하고 이 계획을 시행하며 환자를 평가하고 처치하는 과정이 진행됨에 따라 계획을 재평가하고 처치 단계가 완료될 때까지 환자의 상태 변화에 따라 계획을 수정해야 한다(Box 2-3). 비판적 사고는 사용과 경험을 통해 향상되는 학습된 기술이다. 병원 전 처치 제공자가 자신의 역할을 성공적으로 수행하기 위해서는 급변하는 세상에서 정보를 수집하고 처리하는 데 필요한

Box 2-2 응급의료에서 비판적 사고의 구성 요소

1. 상황을 평가한다.
2. 환자를 평가한다.
3. 사용할 수 있는 자원을 평가한다.
4. 가능한 해결 방법을 분석한다.
5. 환자와 상황을 관리하기 위한 제일 나은 방법을 결정할 때 처치 방법의 상대적 위험과 이점을 평가한다.
6. 처치 계획을 수립한다.
7. 처치 계획을 시행한다.
8. 처치에 대한 환자의 반응을 재평가한다.
9. 필요한 경우 처치 계획을 수정하거나 변경한다.
10. 이 처치 단계가 완료될 때까지 8단계와 9단계를 계속한다.

비판적 사고 기술을 갖추어야 한다.

병원 전 처치 제공자의 경우 비판적 사고는 출동 당시 제공된 초기 정보를 처리하는 것에서 시작하여 환자를 병원 의료진에게 인계할 때까지 계속된다. 사용할 수 있는 자원과 이송 시간을 고려할 필요가 있으므로 비판적 사고는 환자를 이송할 의료기관을 선택할 때도 포함된다. 이러한 모든 중요한 결정은 현재 상황, 환자 상태, 병원 전 처치 제공자의 지식 및 사용할 수 있는 장비 및 술기를 기반으로 한다.

비판적 사고 과정은 독단적이거나 기만적일 수 없으며 대신 회의적인 마음을 가지고 개방적이어야 한다. 병원 전 처치 제공자는 모든 접근 방식의 과학적 정확성에 의문을 제기해야 한다. 이것이 병원 전 처치 제공자가 적절한 결정을 내리는 데 사용할 수 있는 확실하고 근거 있는 지식을 가지고, 있어야 하는 이유이다. 그러나 이 질문이 처치를 지연시킬 정도로 받아들일 수 없다. 아리스토텔레스는 주제가 허용하는 것보다 더 많은 확실성을 요구해서는 안 된다고 제안했다. 병원 전 처치 제공자가 환자를 평가하고 처치할 때 환자의 진단에 절대적인 확실성을 확보하기 위해 행동을 보류하는 것은 어리석은 일이다. 이러한 확실성은 불가능하고 그것을 추구하는 것은 필요한 처치를 지연시킬 뿐이다. 병원 전 처치 제공자는 그 당시 이용할 수 있는 정보를 바탕으로 가능한 한 가장 정보에 입각한 최선의 평가와 결정을 내려야 한다.

PHTLS가 주장하는 적절한 의학적 처치의 기초는 "지식에 근거한 판단"이라는 비판적 사고에 의존한다. 로버트 캐롤(RobertCarroll) 박사는 비판적 사고를 엄격하고 빠른 규칙이나 단계적 절차가 아닌 개념과 원칙으로 설명했다. PHTLS 교육 전반에 걸쳐 강조되는 것은 프로토콜이 항상 비판적 사고를 위한 여지를 남겨두고 동반되어야 한다는 것이다. 환자 처치를 위한 지침과 공식적인 경로는 유연해야 하며 비판적 사고에는 유연성이 필요하다. 프로토콜은 병원 전 처치 제공자가 자신의 사고 과정을 조정하는 데 도움이 되는 지침으로 사용된다. 또한 처치 전달의 중요한 단계를 놓치지 않도록 하는 데 중요한 역할을 한다. 예를 들어, 프로토콜은 적절한 튜브 삽입을 확인하기 위해 기관내삽관 후 호기말이산화탄소 수준과 호흡음을 모두 확인하도록 요구한다. 튜브의 위치가 잘못된 것이 아니라 운항 중인 헬기의 뒤쪽에 있으므로 단순히 호흡음을 들을 수 없는 상황이라면 호기말이산화탄소에만 의존해야 할 수 있다. 또한 튜브의 위치를 확인하기 위해 가슴 X-ray 촬영을 시행할 수 있으나 이런 상황에서는 가능하지 않다.

Box 2-3 비판적 사고 평가 단계

무슨 일이 발생했는가? 무엇을 해야 하는가? 목표를 달성하는 데 필요한 자원은 무엇인가? 분석에는 다음과 같은 내용을 포함한다.

- 현장 평가
- 환자 또는 병원 전 처치 제공자에 대한 모든 위협 요소 확인
- 환자의 상태
- 문제 해결에 필요한 신속성
- 처치 장소(현장, 이송 중, 병원 도착 후)
- 현장의 환자 수
- 필요한 이송 차량 수
- 보다 신속한 이송 필요성
- 적절한 처치를 위해 환자를 이송할 의료기관

분석

이러한 각각의 조건은 개별적으로 신속하게 분석되어야 하며 병원 전 처치 제공자의 지식과 사용할 수 있는 자원이 상호 작용하여야 한다. 최상의 처치를 제공하기 위해 단계를 정의해야 한다.

계획 수립

환자에게 최상의 결과를 제공하기 위한 계획을 수립하고 비판적으로 검토한다. 잘못된 단계가 있는가? 계획된 단계를 모두 달성할 수 있는가? 빠진 단계가 있는가? 계획을 진행하는 데 사용할 수 있는 자원이 있는가? 이 모든 단계가 성공적인 결과로 이어질 가능성이 높은가? 더 좋은 계획이 있는가?

실행

수립된 계획이 실행된다. 이것은 무엇을 달성해야 하는지 또는 누가 책임자이며 누가 명령을 내리고 결정을 내리는지에 대해 혼란이 없도록 결단적이고 단호하게 시행한다. 결정이 환자의 결과에 효과적이지 않으면 병원 전 처치 제공자는 상대적인 위험과 이점을 다시 평가하고 적절하게 변경해야 한다. 변경에 대한 제안은 책임자 또는 동료가 제시할 수 있다.

재평가

현장 상황에 변화가 있는가? 실행 계획을 변경해야 할 사항이 있는가? 환자의 상태는 어떤 상태이며 개선되었는가? 처치 계획이 환자의 상태를 개선하였는가 아니면 악화시켰는가?

진행 중 변경

병원 전 처치 제공자가 확인한 모든 변경 사항은 여기서 설명된 대로 평가 및 분석되며 이게 따라 병원 전 처치 제공자가 환자에게 최상의 처치를 계속 제공할 수 있도록 변경된다. 환자의 재평가에 기초한 의사결정의 변경은 환자와 상황이 끊임없이 변화하고 계획의 변경이 요구될 수 있으므로 실패 또는 이전의 잘못된 환자 처치를 나타내는 것으로 간주해서는 안 된다. 상황에 따라 비판적으로 생각하고 역동성을 유지하는 능력을 갖추는 것은 리더의 장점을 나타내는 신호이다.

비판적 사고로 편견을 통제하기

모든 의료 종사자는 환자에 대한 비판적 사고 과정과 의사 결정에 영향을 미칠 수 있는 편견을 가지고 있다. 이러한 편견은 인식되어야 하며 환자 처치 과정에 영향을 미치지 않도록 주의해야 한다. 편견은 일반적으로 여러 근원에서 발생한다. 상당히 긍정적이거나 부정적인 영향을 미쳤던 이전의 경험이 근원이 될 수 있다. 다음 두 가지 사고 과정은 환자를 보호하는 데 도움이 된다. 1) 그렇지 않다는 것이 증명될 때까지 최악의 시나리오를 가정하고 2) "먼저 해를 끼치지 않는다"라는 원칙을 지지한다. 환자의 처치 계획은 현재 상황을 초래할 수 있는 "명백한" 상태에 대한 병원 전 처치 제공자의 의견에 상관없이 설계된다. 예를 들어, 운전자가 술에 취했다는 초기 인상은 정확할 수도 있지만, 다른 조건도 존재할 수 있다. 술에 취한 환자도 심각한 손상을 입을 수 있다. 환자가 술에 취해 장애가 있다고 해서 의식 상태의 일부 변화가 뇌손상이나 쇼크로 인한 뇌관류 감소로 인한 것이 아니라는 의미는 아니다.

종종 전체적인 그림을 초기 과정을 기반으로 이해할 수 없으므로 병원 전 처치 제공자의 비판적 사고와 대응은 최악의 상황을 가정하여 이루어져야 한다. 판단은 사용할 수 있는 최상의 정보에 기초하여 이루어져야 한다. 비판적 사고를 하는 사람은 끊임없이 "다른 정보"가 나오면 찾아보고 그에 따라 행동한다. 비판적 사고 과정은 환자, 상황 및 상태를 평가하는 동안 계속되어야 하고 병원 전 처치 제공자는 항상 몇 단계 앞을 예상하고 생각해야 한다.

신속한 의사 결정에서 비판적 사고 사용하기

EMS는 다양한 증상과 다양한 질병에 대해 적시에 결정적으로 대응할 수 있는 병원 전 처치 제공자의 타고난 능력과 신속한 조치에 의존하는 분야이다. 효율성과 정확성이 중요하며 프로토콜과 선호를 효율적으로 결합하는 것이 최적이다.

응급 상황 현장에서 비판적 사고는 신속하고 철저하며 유연하고 객관적이어야 한다. 응급 상황 현장에서 병원 전 처치 제공자는 의사 결정을 내리고 환자 처치를 시작하기 전에 상황, 환자의 상태 및 사용할 수 있는 자원을 평가하는 데 단 몇 초의 시간밖에 없다. 때때로 병원 전 처치 제공자는 어떤 상황을 생각할 수 있는 충분한 시간을 이용할 수 있지만, 그렇지 않은 경우가 많다.

자료 분석에서 비판적 사고 사용하기

정보는 시각, 후각, 촉각, 청각의 4가지 감각을 사용하여 수집된다(이것은 6장 환자 평가 및 처치에서 배울 것이다). 병원 전 처치 제공자는 일차 평가를 기반으로 이 정보 또는 수집한 데이터를 분석하고 의료 기관의 의료진에게 환자를 인계할 때까지 환자에 대한 전반적인 처치 계획을 결정한다.

일반적으로 외상 환자의 평가 과정은 XABCDE(출혈, 기도, 호흡, 순환, 장애, 노출/환경)의 일차평가로 시작하지만, 비판적 사고는 병원 전 처치 제공자를 가장 심각한 상태로 먼저 안내한다. 외부출혈로 인해 쇼크가 발생한 환자의 경우 평가 후 출혈 부위에 직접 압박을 적용하는 것이 적절한 초기 처치이다. 비판적 사고는 기도에 문제가 있는 내과 환자에게 적합한 표준 처치는 ABC 우선순위를 따르는 것이 기도를 유지할 수 있다. 그러나 현재는 출혈이 심각한 외상 환자로 이어질 수 있으므로 기도에 주의를 기울이는 대신 명백하고 심각한 출혈을 지혈하는 것이 적절한 첫 번째 처치이다. 비판적 사고는 직접 압박이 효과가 없다면 다른 처치가 필요하다는 것을 인식하는 과정이다. 비판적 사고는 상대적으로 경미한 출혈이 팔다리에서 발생하면 일차평가를 완료할 때까지 지혈을 시행하지 않는다는 것을 이해하는 것이다. 비판적 사고는 즉시 사용할 수 있는 정보를 종합하고 당시 환자의 요구, 전반적인 상황, 처치 제공자의 기식과 술기 능력 및 사용할 수 있는 장비를 기반으로 의사결정을 내리는 것이다.

비판적 사고는 판단을 내리고 임상적 결정을 내리기 위해 정보를 자세히 검토하고 차별화 및 평가하여 반영하는 것을 포함하는 광범위한 기술이다.

환자 처치 단계 전반에 걸쳐 비판적 사고 사용하기

의학의 예술과 과학, 원칙에 대한 지식, 선호의 적절한 적용은 처치가 제공되는 상황에서 환자에게 가능한 최선의 처치 예상 결과로 이어질 것이다. 급성 손상을 입은 환자의 처치 과정에는 기본적으로 네거티브 단계가 있다.

1. 병원 전 단계
2. 병원에서의 초기(소생) 단계
3. 안정화 및 최종 처치 단계
4. 환자를 기능적 상태로 되돌리기 위한 장기적인 해결 및 재활 단계

단계마다 같은 환자 처치의 원칙을 적용한다. 환자 처치 단계 전반에 걸쳐 각 처치 제공자는 비판적 사고를 사용해야 한다. 비판적 사고는 손상을 입은 시점부터 환자가 퇴원해서 집에 돌아갈 때까지 계속된다. 병원 전 처치 제공자는 초기 병원 전 처치 단계에 직접 참여하고 처치 결정의 우선순위를 확인하고 우선순위를 정하는 데 도움이 되는 중요한 비판적 사고를 사용한다. 병원 전 처치 제공자는 종종 현재 상황을 넘어 결정적인 처치 요구와 환자의 궁극적인 결과에 대해 생각해야 한다. 궁극적인 목표는 처치를 통해 환자가 손상 전과 마찬가지로 가능한 한 최고 수준의 기능으로 회복될 수 있도록 환자를 처치하는 것이다. 예를 들어, 비판적 사고는 다발성 외상 환자의 골절된 팔을 부목으로 고정하는 것이 처치의 초기 우선순위 중 하나가 아닐지라도 환자의 최종 결과와 생산적인 삶을 영위할 수 있는 능력을 고려할 때 팔의 기능을 보존하는 것을 인식하는 것을 포함한다. 환자의 병원 전 처치에서 팔다리 기능의 보존과 이송 중 추가 손상을 예방하는 것은 중요한 관심사이다.

윤리

병원 전 처치 제공자는 응급 상황과 시간에 민감한 윤리적으로 어려운 상황에 직면한다. 그러나 병원 전 상황에 맞는 특정 윤리 교육의 부족으로 인해 병원 전 처치 제공자들이 윤리적 문제에 직면했을 때 준비가 되어있지 않거나 도움을 받지 못한다고 느낄 수 있다. 비판적 사고 기술은 때때로 병원 전 처치 제공자에게 요구되는 어려운 윤리적 결정을 통해 일하는 데 도움이 되는 건전한 기반을 제공할 수 있다.

이 부문의 목표는 생명 윤리 원칙과 개념을 사용하여 윤리적 인식과 윤리적 추론 능력을 발전시키고 윤리적으로 어려운 사례를 이해하는 데 도움이 되는 공통적인 틀과 용어를 제공하는 것이다. 이 부문에서는 많은 의료 제공자에게 친숙한 기본적인 생명윤리 교육의 전통적인 요소에 의존하지만, 병원 전 상황의 사례를 사용하여 현장 환경에 적합하고 실용적인 내용을 제공할 것이다. 또한, 병원 전 처치 제공자를 일반적인 생명윤리 원칙과 개념에 노출함으로써 의료 분야와 환경 전반에 걸친 윤리적 대화를 촉진할 수 있다.

윤리적 원칙

모든 사람은 결정을 내리기 위해 어떤 가치관, 신념 또는 사회적 규칙을 사용한다. 이러한 규칙들은 일반적으로 도덕적 행동에 대해 받아들여지는 믿음이며 종종 원칙으로 언급된다. 윤리는 올바른 행동을 확인하는 데 도움을 주는 일련의 도덕적 원칙을 사용하는 것이다. 의학에서 윤리적 행동을 보장하고 임상 실습을 지도하며 윤리적 의사결정을 돕기 위해 종종 의존하는 일련의 원칙에는 자율성, 무해성, 선행 및 정의의 요소가 포함된다. 종종 원칙주의라고 불리는 이 네 가지 원칙의 사용은 일반적으로 환자의 이익을 위해 행동하기 위해 특정 환자를 처치하는 맥락 내에서 이득과 부담을 저울질하여 균형을 맞출 수 있는 틀을 제공한다.

자율성은 자신의 건강관리를 지시할 수 있는 환자의 권리로 정의된다. 무해성의 병원 전 처치 제공자가 환자에게 해를 끼칠 가능성이 있는 행동을 하지 않도록 의무화한다. 선행은 선한 일을 하는 것을 의미하며 병원 전 처치 제공자가 선행을 극대화하고 환자에 대한 위험을 최소화하는 방식으로 행동할 것을 요구한다. 정의는 외상 처치의 맥락에서 일반적으로 공정하거나 정의로운 것으로 생각되는 것으로 보통 우리가 의료 자원을 어떻게 분배하는지를 가리킨다.

외상에서 정의의 개념은 사용할 수 있는 자원이 환자 처치의 필요성에 의해 압도되는 상황에 직면했을 때 고려해야 한다. 예를 들어, 다중 사상자 사고를 분류할 때 응급 환자가 비응급 환자보다 우선순위가 높다. 따라서 가장 중증 환자는 중등이나 경미한 환자보다 처치 제공자에 의해 의료 제품과 서비스의 더 많은 부분을 제공받는다.

다수 사상자 사고에서 중증도 분류는 부분적으로 생존 확률에 기초하고 생존할 가능성이 가장 희박한 중증 환자 일부는 더 생존할 수 있는 손상을 입은 환자에게 자원이 집중될 수 있도록 지연으로 분류할 수 있다. 그러므로 특정 상황에서 자원의 가용성과 그 특정 상황에 해당 자원을 가장 공정하게 사용하고 분배하는 방법에 따라 달라질 수 있다.

이러한 윤리적 원칙을 고려하는 맥락에서 더 잘 이해되는 외상 처치 제공에는 몇 가지 중요한 문제가 있다. 예를 들어, 환자의 자율적인 의사결정 능력은 뇌손상, 쇼크 또는 화학적 중독으로 인해 손상될 수 있다. 외상 상황에서 대리인은 의사결정에 도움을 줄 수 없는 경우가 많다. 병원 전 처치 제공자는 가능한 경우 환자가 정보에 입각한 결정을 자율적으로 내릴 수 있도록 환자에게 상황을 설명하기 위해 모든 노력을 기울여야 한다. 초기 과정에서 모든 정보를 사용할 수 있는 것은 아니지만, 사용할 수 있는 정보는 환자가 자율성을 유지할 수 있도록 의식이 있고 이해할 수 있는 환자와 공유해야 한다. 마찬가지로 무해성의 원칙은 병원 전 처치 제공자가 고에너지로 인한 외상과 병적 비만으로 인한 호흡곤란이 있는 환자의 등허리 척추를 고정하도록 요구한다. 복잡한 외상 시나리오는 그러한 움직임을 제한하는 매우 수용적이고 효율적인 방법의 하나가 환자를 긴척추고정판에 고정하는 것이라고 제안한다. 선행의 원칙은 호흡을 쉽게 하기 위해 환자의 머리를 높이는 것이 옳다는 것을 시사하지만, 이는 무해성의 목표와 상충한다. 긴척추고정판을 머리 위쪽으로 30도 기울여 환자의 머리를 올리거나 들것을 역 트렌델렌버그 자세로 이동하는 해결책은 환자를 위한 두 가지 원칙을 모두 해결할 수 있다.

동의

정보에 입각한 동의는 병원 전 처치 제공자가 의사결정 능력이 있는 환자 또는 대리인(환자가 스스로 결정을 내릴 수 없는 경우 환자를 대신하여 의료결정을 내릴 수 있도록 선정된 사람)에게 의료진이 제공하려는 처치에 대한 사전 동의 또는 거부에 필요한 정보를 제공하는 절차이다. 많은 사람이 사전 동의를 법적 형식으로 생각하지만, 실제로는 형식 자체가 동의하는 대화의 기록일 뿐이다. 병원 전 처치 제공자는 환자가 자신의 가치관과 신념 및 소원에 따라 스스로 건강에 관한 결정을 내릴 수 있도록 적절한 의료 정보를 환자에게 제공해야 하는 윤리적 의무가 있다.

정보에 입각한 동의가 유효하려면 환자에게 다음과 같은 사항이 충족되어야 한다.

- 의사 결정 능력이 있어야 함
- 진단, 예후 및 처치 방법에 대해 이해하고 의사소통할 수 있는 능력이 있어야 함
- 자발적으로 동의 또는 거부할 수 있어야 함
- 적극적으로 처치를 거부하거나 동의해야 함

이러한 요소 중 하나를 평가하는 것은 통제된 임상 환경에서 충분히 어려울 수 있지만, 응급상황에서는 특히 더 어렵다. 많은 사람이 능력과 의사결정 능력이라는 용어를 번갈아 사용하지만, 능력은 개인이 스스로 좋은 결정을 내릴 수 있는 일반적인 능력을 가리키는 법적 용어이고 의사결정 능력은 특정 처치 방법이나 치료법에 관한 환자의 의사결정 능력을 의미한다.

응급 상황에서 환자의 능력을 평가하기는 특히 어렵다. 환자에 대한 기존 정보가 거의 없으며 환자가 급성 손상을 입었을 때 평가가 이루어지는 경우가 많다. 성인 환자의 의사결정 능력을 평가할 때 그들의 이해 수준을 결정하는 시도가 필요하다. 환자가 처치 방법을 이해하고 이와 관련된 위험과 이점을 평가할 수 있는가? 또한 환자는

자신의 선택에 따른 결과를 예측할 수 있을 뿐만 아니라 병원 전 처치 제공자에게 자신의 희망 사항을 표현할 수 있는 능력이 있어야 한다. 정보에 입각한 동의 절차는 환자가 스스로 결정을 내릴 수 있는 권리를 존중하지만, 다음과 같은 특정 조건의 응급 상황에서는 무시될 수 있다.

1. 환자는 의식이 없거나 심각한 인지 장애로 인해 의사 결정 능력이 부족하고 대리인이 없다.
2. 환자의 생명이나 건강을 위협할 수 있는 상태이며 처치를 받지 않을 때 돌이킬 수 없는 손상을 입을 수 있다.
3. 환자가 합리적인 사람이라면 처치에 동의할 것으로 예측되는 경우 처치 제공자는 환자 또는 대리인의 자율적인 동의 없이 처치를 시행할 수 있다.

개인 정보 보호 및 기밀 유지

의료 분야에서 개인 정보는 환자가 자기 개인 건강 정보에 접근할 수 있는 사람을 통제할 수 있는 권리를 의미한다. 기밀 유지는 환자의 처치에 관여하는 의료 종사자가 자신에게 공개된 환자 정보를 부적절하게 공유하지 않는 의무를 말한다. 환자와 의료인 관계의 상황에서 병원 전 처치 제공자가 얻은 모든 정보는 기밀로 간주해야 한다. 환자가 동의한 개인, 환자 처치에 관여하는 다른 의료 전문가와 아동 또는 노인 학대와 같이 의무적으로 보고해야 하는 담당하는 기관 이외에 개인에게 공개해서는 안 된다.

상황에 따라 병원 전 처치 제공자는 환자를 처치하는 데 필요한 정보를 얻기 위해 무능력한 환자가 아닌 다른 사람(가족, 친구 또는 이웃)에게 의존하고 상호작용해야 할 수 있다. 그러나 손상이나 사망 현장에 있을 수 있는 목격자나 뉴스 매체와 같은 의료 종사자가 아닌 사람들로부터 환자 정보를 보호하고 적절한 대리인이 있을 때까지 다른 사람에게 정보를 제공하는 데 큰 노력을 기울여야 한다.

진실을 말하기

진실을 말하는 것은 또한 윤리적인 문제를 일으킬 수 있다. 진실성은 신뢰할 수 있는 환자와 처치 제공자 사이의 관계를 구축하는 데 있어 기대이자 필수적인 부분이다. 정직한 의사소통은 환자에 대한 존중을 보여주고 진실한 정보를 바탕으로 의사결정을 가능하게 한다. 그러나 특히 병원 전 상황에서 환자에게 진실을 말하는 것은 생존자가 사망이나 중상을 입은 사랑하는 사람의 상태에 관해 물어볼 수 있는

다수 사상자 사고와 같이 환자에게 진실을 말하는 것이 큰 해를 끼칠 가능성이 있는 상황이 있다. 이러한 경우 손상의 정보와 질문하는 환자의 상태에 따라 진실을 말해야 하는 즉각적인 의무는 해를 끼치지 않아야 한다는 의무로 다소 완화될 수 있다. 환자에게 거짓말을 하는 것은 결코 용납될 수 없다. 그러나 환자에게 고통스러운 정보를 전달하는 것보다 생명을 구할 수 있는 처치를 우선시하는 맥락에서 특정 민감한 정보의 전달을 보류하거나 더 정확하게는 전달을 지연시키는 것이 때때로 필요할 수 있다.

황금 기간: 시간에 민감한 조건

1960년대 후반 애덤스 카울리(R Adams Cowley) 박사는 중증 손상을 입은 외상 환자에 대한 결정적인 처치를 시작하는 것이 중요한 시기라는 생각을 했다. 카울리 박사는 인터뷰에서 다음과 같이 말했다.

> 삶과 죽음 사이에는 "황금 시간"이 있다. 만약 당신이 중증 손상을 입는다면 생존할 수 있는 시간은 60분 미만이다. 당신은 그때 바로 사망하지 않을 수도 있고 3일 또는 2주 후에 사망할 수도 있지만, 회복 불가능한 신체적 장애가 발생할 수도 있다.

카울리 박사는 실제로 어떤 개념을 설명하고 있었고 때때로 문자 그대로 받아들여지기도 하지만, 환자가 항상 "황금 시간"을 누리는 것은 아니라는 것을 깨닫는 것이 중요하다. "시간"은 특정 기간에 대한 문자 그대로의 설명과는 반대로 비유적인 표현을 사용하기 위한 것이었다. 심장에 관통상을 입은 환자는 손상으로 인한 쇼크가 돌이킬 수 없게 되기 전에 결정적인 처치를 시행할 수 있는 시간이 몇 분밖에 없을 수 있지만, 단순 넓적다리뼈 골절로 인해 내부출혈이 서서히 진행되고 있는 환자는 결정적인 처치 또는 소생술을 받는 데 몇 시간 이상 걸릴 수 있다.

황금 시간은 엄밀히 말해 60분이라는 시간을 뜻하는 것은 아니며 손상에 따라 환자마다 다르므로 황금 기간(Golden Period)으로 생각하는 것이 좋다. 중증 손상을 입은 환자가 황금 기간 내에 지혈 및 결정적인 소생술을 받을 수 있다면 생존 가능성이 크게 향상된다. 미국 외과학회 외상위원회는 이 개념을 사용하여 외상 환자를 전문적인 외상 처치가 가능한 시설로 이송하는 것의 중요성을 강조했다.

중증외상 환자의 병원 전 외상 처치는 이러한 상황을 반영해야 한다. 그러나 다음과 같은 목표는 변하지 않는다.

1. 환자에게 접근한다.
2. 생명을 위협하는 손상을 확인하고 처치한다.
3. 신속한 평가, 신속한 환자 이송 준비, 생명을 위협하는 상태를 즉시 개선할 수 있는 현장 처치를 줄여 현장 체류 시간을 최소화한다.
4. 가장 신속한 이송 방법으로 환자를 가장 가까운 적절한 시설로 이송한다.

논의된 술기와 원칙 대부분은 새로운 것이 아니며 대부분 초기 교육 프로그램에서 가르친다. 그러나 PHTLS는 다음과 같은 점에서 다르다.

- 외상 환자를 위한 현재의 증거를 기반으로 처치 관행을 제공한다.
- 다중 손상을 입은 외상 환자에 대한 처치의 우선순위를 결정하기 위한 체계적인 접근 방식을 제공한다.
- 처치를 위한 조직적인 계획을 제공한다.

외상 환자가 사망하는 이유

외상 환자의 사망 원인을 분석한 연구는 장소와 시간에 따라 약간의 가변성을 보여준다. 1975년 러시아에서 700명 이상의 외상 사망자를 대상으로 한 연구에 따르면 부상으로 빠르게 사망한 대부분 환자는 대량 출혈(36%), 뇌와 같은 주요 장기의 중증 손상(30%), 기도 폐쇄 및 급성 환기부전(25%)의 세 가지 분류 중 하나에 속한다. 댈러스에서 2010년에 발표된 한 연구에 따르면 빠르게 사망한 환자의 76%가 머리, 대동맥, 심장에 생존할 수 없는 손상을 입어서 사망했다고 한다. 2020년 휴스턴과 칼크워프의 동료들은 외상으로 인한 사망의 17%가 출혈로 인한 것이며 이러한 사망의 45%는 조기 소생술과 출혈 조절로 예방할 수 있거나 잠재적으로 예방 가능하다고 보고했다. 2013년에 발표된 한 연구에서는 다기관부전으로 인한 사망 즉 사망의 세 번째 단계의 사망이 감소한 것으로 나타났다(1장 PHTLS: 과거, 현재, 미래 단원 참고). 이러한 사망 감소는 현장과 병원 모두에서 현대 외상 처치의 개선으로 인한 것일 수 있다.

분명히 저혈압의 중증도와 지속 기간은 외과적 출혈 조절의 속도뿐만 아니라 결과에도 영향을 미친다. 2002년 필라델피아의 클라크와 동료들은 복강 내 외상을 입은 저혈압 환자의 경우 외과적 처치 전에 응급실에 있는 시간이 길어지는 시간이 추가로 3분이 지연될 때마다 사망률이 1%씩 증가하는 독립적인 사망 위험 요소라는 사실을 입증했다. 2016년 마이애미의 메이조소와 그의 공동 연구원은 응급실 도착 후 수술까지 10분 이상 지연된 것이 저혈압을 보이는 총상 환자의 사망 위험이 3배로 증가한다고 보고했다.

그러나 세포 수준에서 이 환자에게 무슨 일이 일어나고 있는가? 인체의 대사 과정은 다른 기계와 마찬가지로 에너지에 의해 구동된다. 이에 대해서는 3장 쇼크: 삶과 죽음의 병태생리학에서 더 자세히 논의된다. 쇼크는 신체에서 산소를 전달하고 조직에서 이산화탄소를 회수하지 못해 발생하는 체내 에너지 생산 실패로 볼 수 있다. 기계와 마찬가지로 신체는 자체 에너지를 생산하지만, 그렇게 하려면 연료가 있어야 한다. 신체에 필요한 연료는 산소와 포도당이다. 신체는 포도당을 복합 탄수화물(글리코겐)과 지방으로 저장하고 나중에 사용할 수 있다. 그러나 산소는 저장할 수 없으며 신체의 세포에 지속해서 공급되어야 한다. 산소를 포함한 공기는 횡격막과 늑간근의 작용으로 폐로 유입된다. 산소는 폐포와 모세혈관벽을 가로질러 확산하여 적혈구의 헤모글로빈에 결합한 다음 순환계를 통해 신체조직으로 운반된다. 산소가 존재할 때 조직 세포는 복잡한 일련의 대사 과정(당분해, 크랩스 회로 및 전자전달계)을 통해서 포도당을 연소시켜 모든 신체 기능에 필요한 에너지를 생성한다. 이 에너지는 아데노신 삼인산(ATP)으로 저장된다. ATP 형태의 충분한 에너지가 없으면 필수적인 대사 활동이 정상적으로 일어날 수 없고 세포가 죽기 시작하며 기관부전이 발생한다.

산증, 저체온증 및 응고병증(치명적인 외상의 세 가지 요소)은 외상 환자의 쇼크와 결합하여 사망 위험을 증가시키는 요인이다. 이들 변수는 독립적인 변수가 아니다. 출혈과 쇼크는 무산소대사의 증가로 인한 산증을 유발한다. 산증은 응고를 손상한다. 출혈은 쇼크와 혈액에서 응고 인자의 손실로 이어지고 이러한 인자의 손실로 인해 손상 후 초기 몇 시간 동안 응고가 손상되며 출혈이 악화하여 쇼크 상태가 악화한다. 이후 환자에서 손상이 진행되는 과정에서 혈소판 및 응고 인자 활성화는 실제로 폐색전증 및 다기관부전 증후군과 같은 응고 관련 질환의 위험을 증가시키는 응고항진상태로 이어진다. 중증 손상을 입은 민간인의 25%와 중증 손상으로 쇼크에 빠진 군인의 1/3도 응고 장애가 있다. 마찬가지로 저체온증은 주로 차가운 공기에 노출되는 것과 관련이 있을 수 있지만, 혈액 손실과 쇼크는 차가운 온도에 반응하는 신체의 반응 능력을 감소시킨다. 저체온증은 응고병증의 독립적인 원인이므로 지속적인 출혈의 원인이 된다. 산증, 저체온증 및 응고병증은 특히 치명적이며 즉시 회복시켜야 한다.

산소 부족에 대한 세포의 민감도는 기관마다 다르다(**Box 2-4**). 산소가 부족한 기관 내의 세포는 치명적인 손상을 입을 수 있지만, 일정 기간 계속 기능할 수 있다(쇼크 발생 시 기관의 합병증은 3장 쇼크: 삶과 죽음의 병태생리학 참고). 카울리 박사가 이전에 언급했던 내용은 기관부전을 유발하는 지연된 세포 사멸은 사망을 말하는 것이다. 쇼크가 발생한 환자를 신속하게 처치하지 않으면 쇼크로 사망할 수 있다. 이러한 이유로 카울리 박사는 내부출혈을 조절하기 위해 환자를 수술이 가능한 의료기관으로 신속하게 이송해야 한다고 주장했다.

황금 시간 또는 황금 기간은 일련의 사건이 환자의 장기 생존과 전반적인 결과를 악화시킬 수 있는 중요한 간격을 나타낸다. 이 기간에 적절한 처치를 신속하게 받으면 대부분의 손상은 되돌릴 수 있다. 산소 공급을 개선하고 출혈을 조절하기 위한 적절한 처치를 시작하지 않으면 쇼크가 진행되어 결국 사망에 이르게 된다. 또한 산중, 저체온증과 응고병증의 개선이 가능한 한 빨리 일어나야 한다. 외상 환자의 생존 가능성을 높이려면 쉽게 접근할 수 있고 기능적인 응급의료 통신시스템부터 개입을 시작해야 한다. 훈련된 응급의료 전화 상담원은 지혈과 같은 도착 전 지침을 제공함으로써 현장에서 처치를 제공하는 과정을 시작할 수 있다. 현장에서의 처치는 병원 전 처치 제공자의 도착과 함께 계속되며 응급실, 수술실, 중환자실 그리고 적절한 경우 재활 시설로 진행된다. 외상은 진정한 "팀 스포츠"이다. 현장에 있는 사람들부터 외상센터에 있는 외상팀의 모든 구성원이 협력하여 개별 환자를 처치하기 위해 함께 일할 때 할 때 환자가 이긴다.

Box 2-4 쇼크

심장에 산소가 부족하면 심근 세포는 혈액을 다른 조직으로 보낼 만큼 충분한 에너지를 생산할 수 없다. 예를 들어, 환자가 대동맥에 총상을 입은 후 상당한 수의 적혈구와 혈액량을 잃었다. 심장은 몇 분 동안 계속 뛰다가 멈춘다. 심장에 너무 오랫동안 산소가 없는 상태에서 혈관을 다시 채우더라도 손상된 세포의 기능이 회복되지 않는다.

허혈은 심한 쇼크에서 볼 수 있듯이 모든 조직에 손상을 줄 수 있지만, 기관에 대한 손상은 처음에는 명백하지 않을 수 있다. 폐에서 급성 호흡곤란증후군(ARDS)은 종종 허혈 손상 후 최대 48시간 이내에 발생하는 경우가 많지만, 급성신부전과 간부전은 일반적으로 며칠 후에 발생한다. 모든 신체 조직이 산소 부족의 영향을 받지만, 일부 조직은 허혈에 더 민감하다. 예를 들면, 쇼크와 무산소증으로 인해 뇌손상을 입은 환자는 영구적인 뇌손상을 입을 수 있다. 비록 뇌세포가 기능을 멈추거나 죽더라도 신체의 나머지 부분은 몇 년 동안 생존할 수 있다.

병원 전 외상 처치의 황금 원칙

이 본문에는 특정 신체 계통에 손상을 입은 환자의 평가와 처치에 관해 설명한다. 대부분 중증 손상을 입은 환자는 두 개 이상의 신체 계통에 손상을 입기 때문에 다발성 외상 환자라는 용어를 사용한다. 병원 전 처치 제공자는 병원 전 외상 처치의 황금 원칙에 따라 다발성 손상 환자의 처치를 인식하고 우선순위를 정해야 한다. 이러한 원칙은 반드시 나열된 순서대로 시행할 필요는 없지만, 손상을 입은 환자의 결정적인 처치를 위해 모두 시행되어야 한다. 황금 원칙은 다음 논의에서 간략하게 검토된다. 각 원칙이 병원 전 외상 처치에 더 직접적으로 적용되는 특정 장에 대한 참조가 제공된다. **표 2-1**은 이러한 원칙에 대한 빠른 참조를 제공한다.

1. 병원 전 처치 제공자와 환자의 안전 보장

현장 안전은 모든 의료 지원을 요청하는 모든 현장에 도착 시 최우선 순위이다. 외상이 발생한 현장에서 도움을 요청하는 상황은 병원 전 처치 제공자가 직면하는 가장 위험한 출동 중 일부이다. 모든 현장 유형에 대한 상황 인식은 병원 전 처치 제공자가 위험을 완화하는 방법을 이해하는 데 도움이 될 수 있다(**그림 2-2**). 이러한 인식에는 환자의 안전뿐만 아니라 모든 병원 전 처치 제공자의 안전도 포함된다. 신고 접수자로부터 받은 정보를 바탕으로 현장에 도착하기 전에 잠재적인 위험을 예상할 수 있다. 더 자세한 내용은 5장 현장 관리와 16장 손상 예방을 참고한다.

2. 현장 상황을 평가하여 추가 자원의 필요성 결정

현장으로 출동하는 동안이나 현장 도착 즉시 병원 전 처치 제공자는 추가 지원 또는 전문적인 자원의 필요성을 결정하기 위해 신속한 평가를 시행해야 한다. 예로는 환자를 처치할 수 있는 추가 EMS 장비, 화재 진압 장비, 특수 구조팀, EMS 인력, 의료용 헬기 등이 포함된다. 이러한 자원의 필요성을 고려하고 가능한 한 빨리 요청해야 하며 지정된 통신 채널을 확보해야 한다. 더 자세한 내용은 5장 현장 관리를 참고한다.

3. 심각한 외부출혈 지혈

외상 환자의 경우 심각한 외부출혈은 발견 즉시 즉각적인 주의가 필요한 소견이다. 환자 처치에서 소생을 목표로 하는 조치가 즉각적인 우선순위에 있는 경우가 많지만, 심각한 외부출혈이 발생할 때 소생 술 시도는 결코 성공하지 못할 것이다. 병원 전 환경에서는 혈액을 투여할 수 있는 상황이 점점 증가하고 있음에도 불구하고 순환에 충분한 적혈구를 유지하기 위해서는 출혈 조절이 병원 전 처치 제공자에게 가장 중요한 처치이다. 출혈 조절은 이 교재 전반에 걸쳐 반복되는 주제이며 특히 3장 쇼크: 삶과 죽음의 병태생리학, 11장 복부 외상, 12장 근골격 외상, 21장 야생 외상 처치, 22장 민간 전술 응급 의료 지원에서 관련이 있다.

4. 생명을 위협하는 상태를 파악하기 위해 일차평가 시행

이 간단한 평가는 XABCDE라는 체계적인 평가를 통해 중요한 기능을 신속하게 평가하고 생명을 위협하는 상태를 확인할 수 있다(**Box 2-5**). 일차평가는 "진행과 동시에 처치"라는 철학이 포함된다. 생명을 위협하는 문제가 확인되면 가능한 한 빨리 일차평가와 동시에 처치를 시작한다. 이 원칙은 6장 환자 평가 및 처치에서 논의된다.

5. 손상을 초래한 외상의 물리학 인식

외상의 물리학을 이해하는 것은 독자에게 운동에너지가 외상 환자에게 어떻게 손상으로 이어질 수 있는지에 대한 기초를 제공한다. 자세한 내용은 4장 외상의 물리학을 참조한다. 병원 전 처치 제공자가 현장과 환자에게 접근할 때 외상의 물리학을 고려해야 한다(**그림 2-3**). 특정 손상 유형에 대한 지식은 손상을 예측하고 무엇을 찾아야 하는지 아는 데 도움이 된다. 외상의 물리학에 대한 고려는 환자 평가와 처치의 시작을 지연시키지 않아야 하지만, 전체적인 현장 평가와 환자 및 목격자에게 시행하는 질문에 포함될 수 있다. 외상의 물리학은 또한 환자를 어느 의료기관으로 이송할지 결정하는 데 중요한 역할을 할 수 있다(**Box 2-6**).

6. 척추 움직임 제한을 유지하면서 적절한 기도 관리 제공

현장 안전을 확보하고 외부출혈을 지혈한 후 중증외상 환자 처치에서 기도 관리가 최우선이다. 모든 병원 전 처치 제공자는 머리와 목 고정, 기도 내 이물질 수동 제거, 기도 개방을 위한 도수 조작(턱들기 및 턱 밀어올리기), 흡인, 입인두기도기 및 코인두기도기 사용과 같은 기도 관리의 "필수 술기"를 쉽게 수행할 수 있어야 한다. 이와 관련된 내용은 7장 기도와 환기, 8장 머리와 목 외상, 9장 척추 외상에서도 핵심적으로 고려된다.

표 2-1 14가지 황금 원칙에 대한 참조 지침

황금 원칙	관련 장
1. 병원 전 처치 제공자와 환자의 안전을 보장한다.	5장. 현장 관리 16장. 손상 예방
2. 현장 상황을 평가하여 추가 자원의 필요성을 결정한다.	5장. 현장 관리 17장. 재난 관리 18장. 폭발과 대량살상무기
3. 심각한 외부출혈을 지혈한다.	3장. 쇼크: 삶과 죽음의 병태생리학 11장. 복부 외상 12장. 근골격 외상 21장. 야생 외상 처치 22장. 민간 전술적 응급의료지원(TEMS)
4. 생명을 위협하는 상태를 파악하기 위해 일차평가를 시행한다.	6장. 환자 평가 및 처치
5. 손상을 초래한 외상의 물리학을 인식한다.	4장. 외상의 물리학
6. 척추 움직임 제한을 유지하면서 적절한 기도 관리를 제공한다.	7장. 기도와 환기 8장. 머리와 목 외상 9장. 척추 외상
7. 보조 환기 및 산소를 공급하여 산소포화도를 94% 이상으로 유지한다.	7장. 기도와 환기 8장. 머리와 목 외상
8. 근골격계 손상을 적절히 부목으로 고정하고 정상 체온 회복 및 유지를 포함한 기본적인 쇼크 처치를 제공한다.	3장. 쇼크: 삶과 죽음의 병태생리학 12장. 근골격 외상 19장. 환경 외상 I: 더위와 추위 21장. 야생 외상 처치
9. 환자의 호소증상과 정신 상태를 고려하고 손상 기전을 고려하여 적절한 척추 움직임 제한 원칙을 적용한다.	9장. 척추 외상 21장. 야생 외상 처치
10. 중증 외상 환자의 경우 EMS가 현장에 도착한 후 가능한 한 빨리 가장 가까운 적절한 의료기관으로 이송을 시작한다.	6장. 환자 평가 및 처치 8장. 머리와 목 외상 10장. 가슴 외상 13장. 화상 손상
11. 기본 관류를 회복하는 데 필요한 경우 의료기관으로 이송하는 중에 수액 소생술을 시작한다.	3장. 쇼크: 삶과 죽음의 병태생리학 13장. 화상 손상
12. 환자의 생명을 위협하는 문제가 해결되었거나 배제된 경우 병력을 확인하고 이차평가를 시행한다.	6장. 환자 평가 및 처치
13. 적절한 통증 완화를 제공한다.	6장. 환자 평가 및 처치 10장. 가슴 외상 11장. 복부 외상 12장. 근골격 외상 13장. 화상 손상 14장. 소아 외상 15장. 노인 외상
14. 환자 및 손상 상황에 대해 환자를 이송하는 의료기관에 상세하고 정확하게 제공한다.	6장. 환자 평가 및 처치

© National Association of Emergency Medical Technicians (NAEMT)

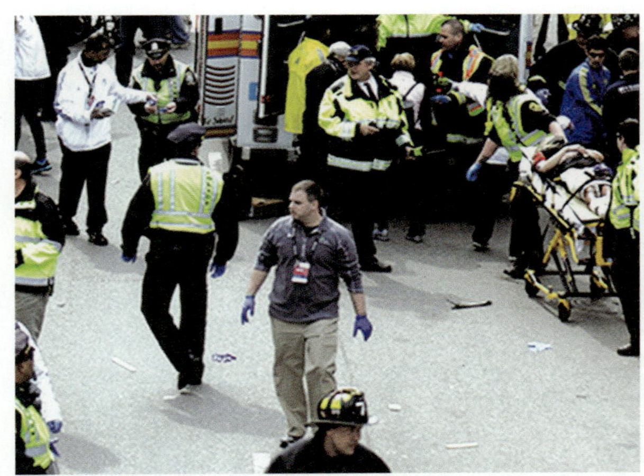

그림 2-2 현장 안전은 모든 의료 지원 요청에 대해 도착 시 최우선 순위이다. 상황 인식을 유지하는 것은 처지 제공자가 위험을 완화하는 데 도움이 되는 한 가지 방법이다.
© Charles Krupa/AP Images

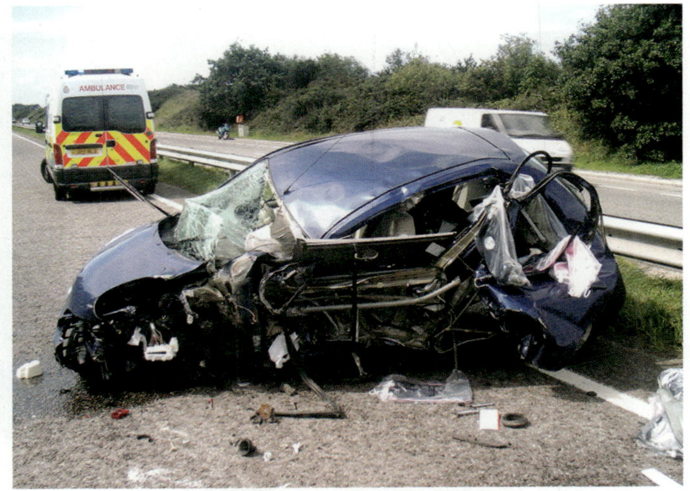

그림 2-3 손상을 초래한 외상의 물리학을 인식한다.
Courtesy of Dr. Mark Woolcock.

Box 2-5 중증이거나 잠재적으로 중증인 외상 환자: 현장 체류 시간 10분 이하

다음과 같은 생명을 위협하는 상태가 존재할 수 있다.

1. 부적절하거나 위협을 받는 기도 상태
2. 다음 중 하나에 해당하는 환기 장애가 있는 경우
   - 호흡수(RR): < 10회/분 또는 > 29회/분
   - 호흡 시 힘들어하거나 호흡 보조 필요
   - 저산소증(실내 공기에서 산소포화도 < 90%)
   - 호흡 곤란
   - 흉벽 불안정성, 변형 또는 의심되는 동요가슴
3. 지혈대 또는 상처 패킹이 필요한 활동성 출혈
4. 보상 여부와 상관없이 쇼크
5. 비정상적인 신경학적 상태
   - 명령을 따를 수 없음(GCS < 6점)
   - 발작 활동
   - 운동 기능 또는 감각 상실을 동반한 척추 손상이 의심되는 경우
6. 머리, 목, 몸통 또는 팔꿈치와 무릎 근위부의 관통상
7. 손목 또는 발목 근위부 부분 절단 또는 완전 절단

© National Association of Emergency Medical Technicians (NAEMT)

Box 2-6 외상센터로 환자를 분류하기 위한 손상 기준의 기전

- 추락
  - 모든 연령대에서 3m 이상(1층의 높이)
- 고위험 자동차 충돌(**그림 2-4**)
  - 자동차 지붕을 포함한 탑승자 공간이 30cm 이상, 그 외 공간이 50cm 이상 침범한 경우
  - 구출의 필요성(구출이 필요한 신체 부위의 물리적 걸림)
  - 차량에서 튕겨 나감(부분 또는 전체)
  - 동승자 사망
  - 차량 원격 데이터가 높은 손상 위험과 일치함
  - 보행자/자전거 탑승자가 퉁겨지거나 상당한 충격을 받음
  - 상당한 충격을 받은 수송 차량(예: 오토바이, 전지형 차량, 말 등)

Source: Adapted from *Field Triage Guidelines*. American College of Surgeons–Committee on Trauma. 2021.

Modified from the Field Triage Decision Scheme: The National Trauma Triage Protocol, U.S. Department of Health and Human Services, Centers for Disease Control and Prevention.

상 환자는 추가로 보충 산소 공급이 필요하다. 이와 관련된 내용은 7장 기도와 환기에서 자세히 논의하고 8장 머리와 목 외상에서 실행한다.

7. 보조 환기 및 산소를 공급하여 산소포화도를 94% 이상으로 유지

호흡 평가와 처치는 중상을 입은 환자 처치의 또 다른 핵심 측면이다. 병원 전 처치 제공자는 너무 느리거나(느린 호흡) 너무 빠른 호흡(빠른 호흡) 속도를 인식하고 백마스크 장비에 산소를 연결하여 호흡을 보조해야 한다. 생명을 위협하는 상태가 명백하거나 의심되는 외

8. 근골격 손상을 적절히 부목으로 고정하고 정상 체온 회복 및 유지를 포함한 기본적인 쇼크 처치를 제공

일단 심각한 외부출혈이 조절되면 병원 전 처치 제공자는 쇼크와 관련된 다른 원인과 합병증을 고려해야 한다. 예를 들어, 골절은 시각

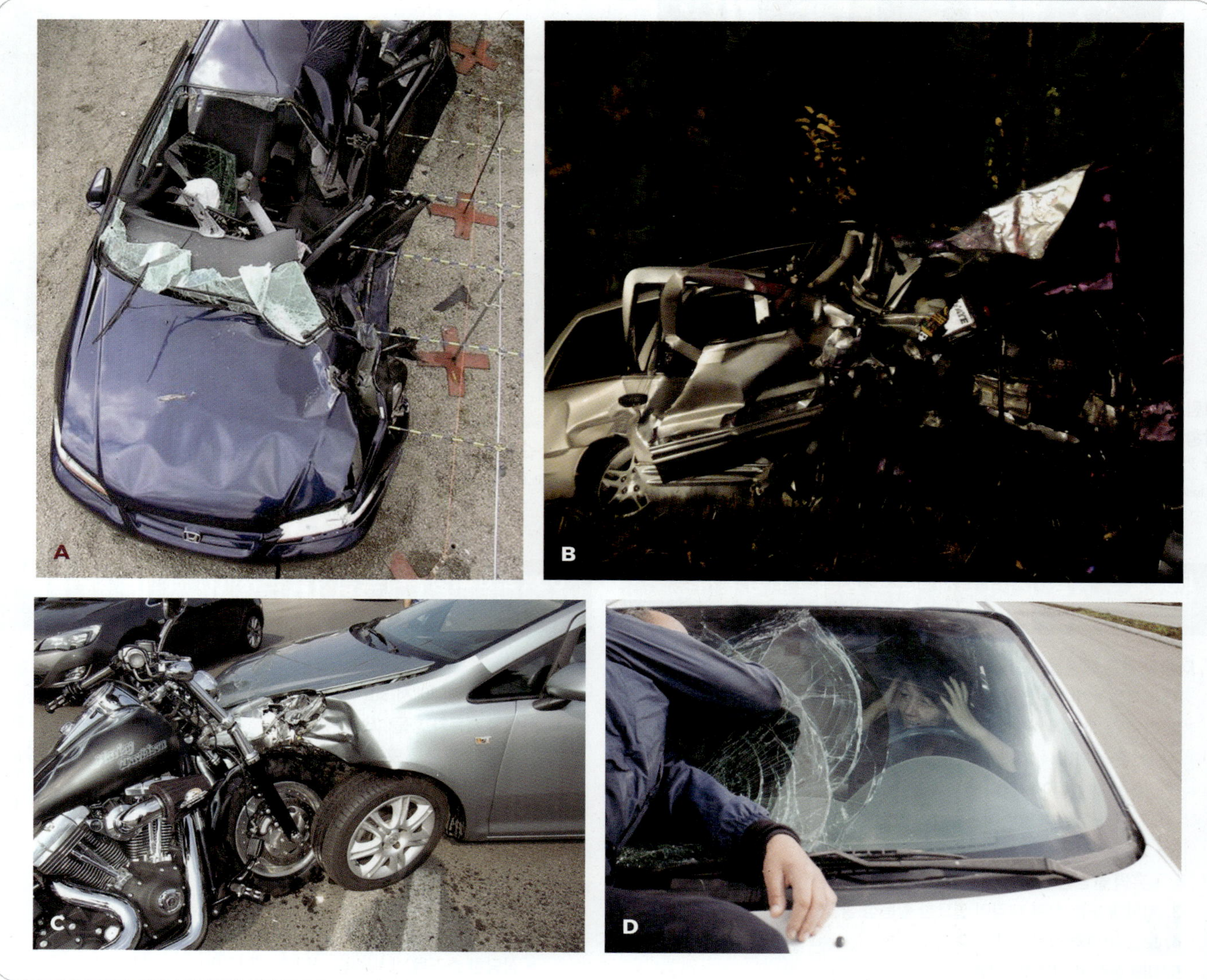

그림 2-4 고위험 자동차 충돌. **A.** 상당한 측면 충격, **B.** 엔진룸 심하게 찌그러짐, **C.** 차축 분리 충돌, **D.** 보행자가 상당한 충격을 받음
Courtesy of Stewart C. Wang, MD.

적으로 관찰할 수 없고 붕대나 압박으로 조절할 수 없는 내부출혈을 일으킬 수 있다. 골절된 팔다리를 재정렬하고 부목을 적용하는 것은 병원 전 환경에서 혈액 손실을 줄일 수 있다. 조절할 수 있는 유일한 수단일 수 있다. 환자의 체온이 유지되지 않으면 중증 저체온증이 발생할 수 있다. 저체온증은 지혈을 위한 신체의 혈액 응고 시스템 능력을 크게 손상시킨다. 그러므로 담요를 사용하고 구급차 내부를 따뜻하게 하여 체온을 유지하는 것이 중요하다. 12장 근골격 외상에서는 팔다리에 부목을 적용하는 방법에 관해 설명한다. 환자를 따뜻하게 하고 저체온증을 예방하려는 조치들이 본문 전반에 걸쳐 논의 되지만, 특히 관련된 논의는 19장 환경 외상 I: 더위와 추위, 21장 야생 외상 처치에서 찾을 수 있다.

9. 환자의 호소증상과 정신 상태를 고려하고 손상 기전을 고려하여 적절한 척추 움직임 제한 원칙을 적용

외상 환자와 접촉 시 도수로 목뼈 및 척추 움직임 제한을 시행하고 환자를 적절한 장비에 고정하거나 척추 움직임 제한의 적응증에 해당하지 않는 것으로 판단될 때까지 이송 유지해야 한다(**그림 2-5**). 척추 고정의 적응증과 방법에 대한 자세한 설명은 9장 척추 외상을 참조한다. 21장 야생 외상 처치에는 이 환경과 관련된 고유한 척추 움직

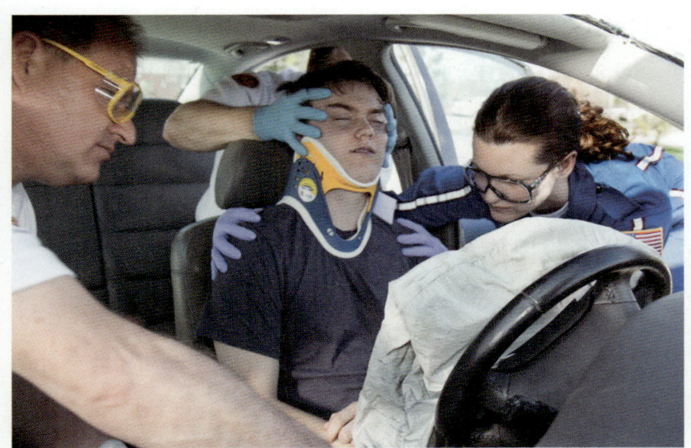

그림 2-5 이송하는 동안 척추 고정을 유지한다.
Courtesy of Rick Brady.

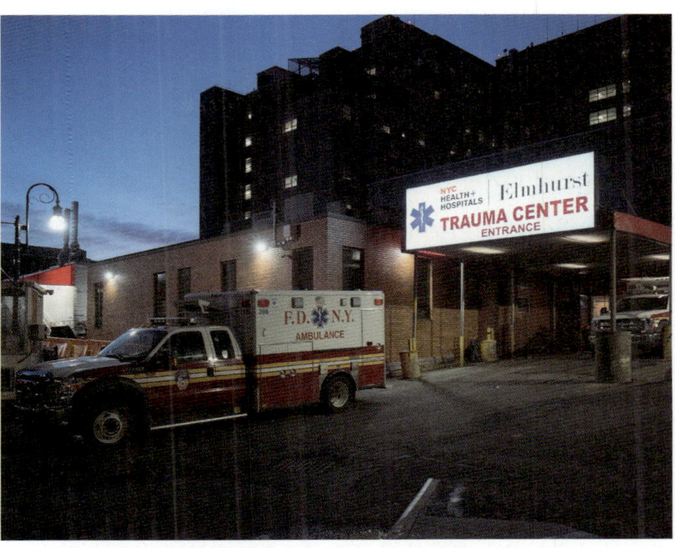

그림 2-6 중증외상 환자의 경우 현장 도착 후 10분 이내에 가장 가까운 적절한 의료기관으로 이송을 시작한다.
© Massimo Giachetti/iStock Editorial/Getty Images Plus/Getty Images

임 제한과 관련된 문제와 추가 정보가 포함되어 있다.

10. 중증외상 환자의 경우 EMS가 현장에 도착한 후 가능한 한 빨리 가장 가까운 적절한 의료기관으로 이송을 시작

중증외상 환자(**Box 2-6**)의 경우 현장에 EMS가 도착한 후 가능한 한 10분("플래티넘 10분") 이내에 이송을 시작해야 한다(**그림 2-6**). 비록 병원 전 처치 제공자가 기도 관리, 보조 환기, 수액 투여에 더 능숙해졌지만, 대부분의 중증외상 환자는 출혈 쇼크 상태에 있으며 병원 전 환경에서 제공할 수 없는 두 가지가 필요하다. 1) 산소를 운반할 혈액과, 2) 혈액 응고와 내부출혈의 조절을 제공하는 혈장이다. 병원 전 처치 제공자는 가장 가까운 병원이 다수의 외상 환자에게 가장 적절한 의료기관이 아닐 수 있다는 점을 명심해야 한다. 환자의 상태를 신중하게 고려하여 어떤 의료기관이 가장 신속하게 치료할 수 있을 것인지 결정해야 한다. 이러한 결정은 6장 환자 평가 및 처치에서 논의된다. 이 원칙은 모든 외상 상황에 적용되며 8장 머리와 목 외상, 13장 화상 손상에 잘 설명되어 있다.

11. 기본 관류를 회복하는 데 필요한 경우 의료기관으로 이송하는 중에 수액 소생술을 시작

중증 손상을 입은 외상 환자는 정맥 라인을 확보하고 수액 소생술을 시작하기 위해 이송이 지연되어서는 안 된다. 결정질 용액은 손실된 혈액량을 복원하고 관류를 개선하지만, 산소를 운반하지는 않는다. 또한 정상 혈압을 회복하는 것은 처음에 응고된 혈관에서 혈전 파괴로 인한 추가적인 출혈을 초래하여 환자의 사망률을 증가시킬 수 있다. 따라서 앞의 원칙에서 논의한 바와 같이 환자를 적절한 의료기관으로 신속하게 이송하는 것이 우선이다. 그런데도 결정질 용액을 투여(특히 락데이트 링거액)하는 것은 특정 상황에서 중요하다. 예를 들면, 외상성 뇌손상과 급성 저혈압의 증가가 있는 환자이다. 수액 투여는 거의 모든 외상 환자에게 시행할 수 있지만, 3장 쇼크: 삶과 죽음의 병태생리학과 13장 화상 손상은 이 원리를 실제로 보여준다.

12. 환자의 생명을 위협하는 문제가 해결되었거나 배제된 경우 병력을 확인하고 이차평가를 시행

일차평가에서 생명을 위협하는 상태가 발견되면 주요 처치를 시행하고 플래티넘 10분 이내에 환자를 이송해야 한다. 그러나 생명을 위협하는 상태가 확인되지 않으면 이차평가를 시행한다. 이차평가는 모든 손상을 확인하기 위해 머리부터 발끝까지 신체검사를 시행하는 것이다. 이차평가에서는 SAMPLER 병력(증상과 징후, 알레르기, 약물, 과거 병력, 마지막 식사, 손상 이전 사건, 위험 요인)도 파악한다.

초기에는 치명적인 손상이 없는 것으로 확인된 환자의 상태가 나중에 악화할 수 있으므로 활력 징후와 함께 기도, 호흡, 순환 상태는 자주 재평가해야 한다. 이 원칙은 6장 환자 평가 및 처치에서 논의된다.

13. 적절한 통증 완화 제공

중증 손상을 입은 환자는 일반적으로 심한 통증을 경험한다. 한때 통증 완화를 제공하면 환자의 증상이 가려지고 병원에 도착한 후 환자를 적절하게 평가할 수 있는 능력이 저하한다고 생각했다. 많은 연구에 따르면 실제로 이것이 사실은 그렇지 않다는 것을 보여주었다. 병원 전 처치 제공자는 금기 사항이 없는 한 통증을 완화하기 위해 진통제 투여를 고려해야 한다. 골절에 따라 부목을 고정하거나 적절하게 견인부목을 적용하는 것은 통증을 조절하는 매우 효과적인 비약물적 처치 방법이다. 통증 관리의 원리는 6장 환자 평가 및 처치에서 논의되며 이 본문의 거의 모든 장에 적용된다. 14장 소아 외상과 15장 노인 외상에서 논의한 바와 같이 통증 관리는 일부 연령대 환자에서 차이가 있지만, 환자의 나이를 기준으로 보류해서는 안 된다.

14. 환자 및 손상 상황에 대해 환자를 이송하는 의료기관에 상세하고 정확하게 제공

외상 환자와 관련된 정보를 이송할 의료기관에 제공하는 것에는 다음과 같은 세 가지 요소를 포함된다.

- 도착 전 보고
- 도착 시 구두 보고
- 환자처치기록지(PCR)와 같은 서면 문서

외상 환자를 처치하는 것은 팀의 노력이다. 중증외상 환자에 대한 처치는 병원 전 처치 제공자로부터 시작하여 병원에서 계속된다. 병원 전 상황에서 환자를 이송할 의료기관으로 정보를 전달하는 것은 환자 처치를 위해 적절한 자원과 지원을 동원하여 환자를 최적의 상태로 인계받을 수 있게 한다. 환자를 이송할 의료기관과의 효과적인 의사소통을 보장하는 방법은 6장 환자평가 및 처치에 설명되어 있으며 모든 환자 처치에 적용된다.

연구

역사적으로 병원 전 처치에 대해 의미 있는 연구가 부족했지만, 최근 몇 년 동안 변화를 하기 시작했다. 확립된 병원 전 처치 중 많은 부분이 증거 기반 연구로 인해 어려움을 겪고 있다. 예를 들어, 지혈대는 더 이상 최후의 수단으로 간주하지 않으며 전문 기도 관리는 병원 전 현장에서 점점 더 금지되고 있으며 결정질 수액 소생술은 현재 제한적이고 정의된 목표로 사용되고 있다. 일부 문헌은 논란의 여지가 있지만, 병원 전 처치는 환자에게 최선의 이익을 제공하기 위해 증거 기반 의학에 이차적으로 변화하고 있다. 이 교재를 통해 이러한 연구의 증거가 설명되고 논의하여 병원 전 처치 제공자가 지식, 교육, 술기 및 자원을 기반으로 환자를 위해 최상의 선택을 할 수 있다.

EMS 문헌 읽기

PHTLS의 주요 목표는 본 문에서 제시된 실무 권장 사항이 출판 당시 사용할 수 있는 최상의 의학적 증거를 정확하게 나타내도록 하는 것이었다. PHTLS는 이 과정을 6판부터 시작하여 후속판까지 계속하고 있다. 우리는 각 장에서 다룬 주제와 권장 사항에 대한 기본이 되는 원고, 출처 및 자료를 참고 문헌을 계속 추가한다(EMA 문헌 평가에 대한 자세한 내용은 이 장의 끝에 있는 권장 참고 자료를 참조한다). EMS 제공자를 포함한 모든 의료 종사자는 일상 업무의 구성요소에 대한 기초를 구성하는 간행물과 출처를 찾아 읽고 비판적으로 평가해야 한다.

이용할 수 있는 참고 자료를 최적으로 사용하기 위해서는 의학 논문을 구성하는 정확한 내용과 다양한 정보 출처를 해석하는 방법을 이해하는 것이 필수적이다. 대부분은 특정 주제에 대한 정보를 얻기 위해 접근하는 첫 번째 자료 출처는 의학 교재이다. 우리의 관심과 지식수준이 높아짐에 따라 해당 교재에서 전달하는 정보의 출처를 나타내는 특정 참고 문헌을 찾거나 수행 및 출판된 주요 연구가 무엇인지 찾기 위해 검색한다. 그런 다음 다양한 출처를 검토하고 분석한 후 우리의 의사 결정과 환자 처치를 안내할 증거의 품질과 강도에 관한 결정을 내릴 수 있다.

의료 증거 수준

의학적 근거의 질을 평가하고 기술하며 그 근거의 강도와 의학적 의사결정에 사용되는 방법을 이해하기 위해 다양한 시스템이 사용된다. 수년 동안 무작위 대조 실험(RCT)은 의학 문헌의 황금 표준으로 간주하였다. 여러 면에서 여전히 그렇긴 하지만, 그 디자인에도 몇 가지 제한이 있다.

어떤 연구에서든 하나의 처치 그룹, 하나의 환자 집단 또는 하나의 중재를 다른 처치 집단과 비교할 때 편향이라고 알려진 것을 도입할 위험이 있다. 예를 들어, 병원 전 처치제공자는 현장에서 긴장기흉 처치를 위한 바늘감압 시행을 양압 환기 및 신속한 이송과 비교할 수 있다. 후향적 연구 설계에서 긴장기흉이 있는 환자를 살펴보고 바늘감압을 받지 않은 환자와 그렇지 않은 환자를 비교할 것이다. 바늘감압을 시행 받은 사람들이 다른 방법으로 처치한 사람들보다 궁극적으로 사망률이 더 높다면 바늘감압이 위험하다고 결론 내릴 수 있다. 이러한 접근법의 문제는 이 모델에서 두 처치 그룹이 서로 다르다는 것이다. 바늘감압을 받은 사람들이 그렇지 않은 사람들보다 생리학적 상태 측면에서 더 나빴을 가능성이 분명히 있다. 다르게 말하면 애초에 이 환자들이 바늘감압을 받은 이유가 있었다. 즉 그들의 근본적인 상태는 더 악화하였고 받은 처치의 종류와 관계없이 사망할 가능성이 더 높았다.

그러한 연구의 대안적인 설계는 무작위 대조 실험일 것이다. 그 연구에서 병원 전 처치 제공자는 긴장기흉의 징후가 있는 환자를 제시하고 바늘감압을 시행하거나 무작위화 과정에서 환자의 위치에 따라 처치하지 않을 것이다. 이는 이전의 소급 설계와 관련된 선택 편향이 제거된다.

무작위 대조 실험은 종종 그러한 편견의 도입을 제한하기 때문에 연구를 수행하는 가장 좋은 방법이지만, 항상 실현할 수 있는 것은 아니다. 이 원칙의 좋은 예는 뉴질랜드의 영아돌연사증후군(SIDS)에 관한 역학적 인구 기반 연구이다. 해당 연구에서 조사자들은 관찰 연구 설계를 사용했다. 그들은 영사돌연사증후군으로 사망한 영아를 대조군 영아 그룹과 비교했고 엎드려 자는 자세를 위험 요인으로 확인했다. 후속 연구에서는 부모에게 영아를 엎어 재우지 않도록 교육하는 프로그램이 영아돌연사증후군의 발병률을 많이 줄인다는 사실이 입증되었다. 영아돌연사증후군의 발병률을 감소시키는 개입의 효과를 평가하기 위해 영아를 눕기 쉬운 수면 자세를 비교하기 위해 무작위 대조 실험을 수행하는 것은 명백히 실행 불가능하고 비윤리적일 것이다.

또한 무작위 대조 실험의 문제점 중 하나는 결과가 종종 일반화되지 않는다는 것이다. 바늘감압이라는 예를 사용하여 그러한 연구를 설계할 경우 연구에 포함되거나 연구에서 제외될 수 있는 환자 특성을 명확하게 정의하고자 할 것이다. 연구에 환자 수가 적은 그룹만 포함하는 경우 결과가 더 많은 환자를 포함한 그룹으로 일반화될 수 있는지가 명확하지 않다. 실용적인 연구 설계에는 종종 결과의 일반화 가능성을 높이기 위해 매우 광범위한 환자 그룹을 포함된다. 불행히도 그러한 연구는 엄격하게 설계하고 구현하기가 매우 어렵다.

이러한 모든 이유로 의학적 결정을 내릴 때 무작위 대조 실험에만 전적으로 의존하는 것은 가능하지도 바람직하지도 않다. 게다가 외상 환자를 처치할 때 EMS 제공자가 매일 내려야 하는 수많은 의학적 결정을 다루기에는 무작위 대조 실험이 충분하지 않다.

따라서 외상 환자를 처치하는 병원 전 처치 제공자는 다양한 유형의 연구를 인식하고 이해하며 제시된 증거의 장단점을 신중하게 평가할 수 있어야 한다. **표 2-2**는 일반적으로 사용되는 몇 가지 분류의 연구 설계를 설명한 것이다.

문헌에서 가장 강력한 정보는 체계적인 검토와 무작위 대조 실험, 코호트 연구, 사례 대조군 연구 및 사례 보고서의 조합에서 근거를 종합하는 요약에서 수집할 수 있다. 배경 정보와 전문가 의견은 여전히 중요한 역할을 한다. 요약하면 모든 문헌을 평가하고 해당 문헌 내에서 증거의 강도를 이해하는 것이 필요하며 순전히 완벽한 과학에 근거하여 외상 환자를 처치하는 모든 결정을 내리는 것은 불가능하다. 그렇긴 하지만, 즉 목표는 이용할 수 있는 최고 품질의 과학적 증거를 사용하고 해당 증거의 구체적인 한계를 이해하는 것이다.

표 2-2 일반적으로 사용되는 연구 설계

연구 유형	설명
체계적 검토	주제에 대한 사용 가능한 모든 연구를 수집하고 해당 결과를 검토 및 분석한다.
메타 분석	동일한 주제에 대한 여러 무작위 대조 실험의 결과를 결합한다.
무작위 대조 실험	적격한 연구 대상자를 다른 처치 또는 처치 부문에 무작위로 할당하여 선택 편향을 제거하는 연구 설계
코호트 연구	환자의 두 그룹을 종적으로 추적하고 시간 간격으로 결과를 평가하는 전향적 관찰 실험
사례 대조군 연구	일부 가정된 기본 인과적 요인을 기반으로 알려진 서로 다른 결과를 가진 두 그룹을 비교하는 관찰 연구
사례 보고서	중재 후 개별 결과 또는 유사한 환자 그룹의 결과를 설명하는 통제되지 않은 보고서
전문가 의견	특정 임상 주제 또는 질문에 대한 인정된 임상 전문가의 의견을 학술적으로 요약한 것

요 약

- 원칙(또는 의학)은 병원 전 처치 제공자가 환자의 생존과 결과를 최적화하는 데 있어 요구되는 의무를 정의한다.

- 선호(또는 의학 기술)는 원칙을 달성하는 방법이다. 방법을 선택할 때 고려해야 할 사항은 다음과 같다.
  - 현재 존재하는 상황
  - 환자의 상태
  - 지식과 경험
  - 사용할 수 있는 장비

- 의학에서 비판적 사고는 의료 종사자가 상황, 환자 및 자원을 평가하는 과정이다. 이 정보는 신속하게 분석되고 통합되어 환자에게 최상의 처치를 제공한다.

- 의학에서 네 가지 윤리적 원칙(자율성, 무해성, 유익성, 공정성)이 있다. 병원 전 처치 제공자는 병원 전 환경에서 윤리적 갈등을 해결하는 데 필요한 윤리적 추론 능력을 개발해야 한다.

- 다음은 병원 전 외상 처치의 황금 원칙이다.

  1. 병원 전 처치 제공자와 환자의 안전을 보장한다.
  2. 현장 상황을 평가하여 추가 자원의 필요성을 결정한다.
  3. 심각한 외부출혈을 지혈한다.
  4. 생명을 위협하는 상태를 파악하기 위해 일차평가를 시행한다.
  5. 손상을 초래한 외상의 물리학을 인식한다.
  6. 척추 움직임 제한을 유지하면서 적절한 기도 관리를 제공한다.
  7. 보조 환기 및 산소를 공급하여 산소포화도를 94% 이상으로 유지한다.
  8. 근골격 손상을 적절히 부목으로 고정하고 정상 체온 회복 및 유지를 포함한 기본적인 쇼크 처치를 제공한다.
  9. 환자의 호소증상과 정신 상태를 고려하고 손상 기전을 고려하여 적절한 척추 움직임 제한 원칙을 적용한다.
  10. 중증 외상 환자의 경우 EMS가 현장에 도착한 후 가능한 한 빨리 가장 가까운 적절한 의료기관으로 이송을 시작한다.
  11. 기본적인 관류를 회복시키는 데 필요한 경우 의료기관으로 이송하는 중에 수액 소생술을 시작한다.
  12. 환자의 생명을 위협하는 문제가 해결되었거나 배제된 경우 병력을 확인하고 이차평가를 시행한다.
  13. 적절한 통증 완화를 제공한다.
  14. 환자 및 손상 상황에 대해 환자를 이송하는 의료기관에 상세하고 정확하게 제공한다.

- 연구는 병원 전 처치를 포함한 모든 의료 행위에 대한 기초와 근거를 제공한다.

- 연구의 질과 결론 및 권고의 강도는 연구의 유형에 따라 다르다.

시나리오 재구성

당신과 동료(paramedic과 EMT)는 두 대의 차량이 측면 충돌한 사고 현장에 도착했다. 당신 팀은 현재 출동할 수 있는 유일한 구급차이다. 픽업트럭에는 술 냄새를 심하게 풍기는 한 젊은 남성이 안전띠를 착용하지 않은 채 앉아 있었고 아래팔이 변형된 것을 확인할 수 있었다. 트럭은 승용차의 조수석 문이 심하게 들어갈 정도로 충돌한 상태였다. 승용차 조수석에는 숨을 쉬지 않는 것으로 보이는 나이 든 여성이 앉아있다. 앞 유리는 과녁 모양으로 깨져 있었다. 승용차 운전자도 손상을 입었지만, 의식은 있고 매우 불안해하고 뒷좌석에는 카시트에 고정된 두 명의 어린이가 있다. 조수석 뒤쪽에 앉은 어린이는 대략 3세 정도로 보이며 의식을 잃고 카시트에 털썩 주저앉아 있다. 운전석 뒤쪽에 어린이용 보조 의자에 고정되어 앉아 있는 5세 어린이는 울고 있지만 다친 곳은 없는 것으로 보인다.

픽업트럭의 운전자는 팔이 골절되는 손상을 입은 것이 분명하지만, 매우 적대적이고 폭언하며 처치를 거부하고 있다. 한편 승용차의 운전자는 필사적으로 자녀와 어머니 상태에 관해 묻고 있다.

- 이 다수 사상자 사고를 어떻게 처리하겠는가?
- 이 환자 중 우선순위가 높은 환자는 누구인가?
- 두 자녀의 어머니에게 그들의 상태에 대해 뭐라고 설명할 것인가?
- 다른 차량의 운전자가 술에 취한 것처럼 보이는 경우 어떻게 다룰 것인가?
- 분명히 술에 취한 운전자의 처치 거부를 허용할 것인가?

시나리오 해결책

이 5명의 환자가 발생한 시나리오에서 추가 지원이 불가능한 상태에 놓인 당신은 병원 전 처치 제공자의 수보다 많은 환자를 분류해야 하는 상황에 직면한다. 공정성의 개념이 즉시 적용되는 것은 이러한 유형의 분류 상황이다. 두 명의 병원 전 처치 제공자와 같이 당신이 이용할 수 있는 자원은 제한되어 있고 가장 많은 수의 사람에게 가장 큰 도움이 될 수 있는 방식으로 분배되어야 한다. 이것은 누가 먼저 처치를 받고 어떤 병원 전 처치 제공자가 처치할지 결정하는 것이 포함된다. 이 시나리오에서는 나이 든 여자를 먼저 처치할지 아니면 의식이 없는 어린이를 먼저 처치할지에 대해 신속한 결정을 내려야 한다. 두 환자 모두 비슷한 외상을 입었을 때 어린이가 노인보다 생존 가능성이 더 높은 경우가 많다. 그러나 추가적인 평가와 병력은 임상 상황과 분류 결정의 적절성을 변화할 수 있다. 예를 들어, 엄마는 의식이 없는 미성년 자녀가 불치병에 걸렸다고 보고할 수 있으므로 나이만을 기준으로 분류 결정을 내리는 것은 이 경우 올바른 조치가 아닐 수 있다. 분류 프로토콜은 일반적인 상황에서 방향을 제시하고 공정성의 개념을 기반으로 하지만, 분류 지침은 마주치는 모든 고유한 상황을 설명할 수 없다. 따라서 공정성의 원칙에 대한 기본적인 이해는 "순간" 분류 결정을 내려야 하는 상황에 도움이 될 수 있다.

운전자와 그의 트럭의 모습은 병원 전 처치 제공자의 고정 관념적인 행동과 판단으로 이어질 수 있다. 고정관념은 종종 부정확하고 단순화된 일반화 또는 다른 사람들을 분류하고 그 믿음에 근거하여 처치할 수 있다는 사람들의 집단에 대한 믿음이다. 환자를 외모와 행동에 대한 선입견은 공정하고 공평한 처치를 방해할 수 있다.

비록 환자를 공정하고 일관된 방식으로 처치할 의무가 있지만, 병원 전 처치 제공자는 귀중한 자원이며 과도한 위험에 빠뜨릴 의무는 없다. 병원 전 처치 제공자는 자신을 보호할 권리뿐만 아니라 다른 사람을 처치할 수 있는 능력을 보호할 권리가 있다.

공정성의 문제 외에도 이 시나리오에 의해 제기된 자율성에 대한 몇 가지 문제가 있다. 병원 전 처치 제공자는 트럭 운전자와 승용차 운전자 모두의 의사 결정 능력을 평가해야 한다. 두 운전자 모두 손상을 입었고 정신적으로 혼란스러우며 트럭 운전자는 음주 운전 상태일 가능성이 있다. 또한 승용차 운전자는 자신을 위해 의사결정을 내리고 두 아이와 어머니를 위한 대리 의사결정자 역할을 하도록 요청받을 수도 있다. 두 운전자의 의사결정 능력을 평가한 결과 운전자 중 한 명이 무능하다고 판단한다면 병원 전 처치 제공자는 프로토콜과 환자 최선의 이익을 기반으로 응급의료서비스를 제공할 것이다.

위험과 이익의 균형은 의학적 의사 결정의 중요한 부분이다. 이 시나리오에서 승용차 운전자는 그녀의 어머니와 자녀에 대한 정보를 요청하고 있다. 환자와 병원 전 처치 제공자의 신뢰를 확립하고 운전자가 자신의 차량 탑승자에 대해 사전 동의 결정을 내리는 것을 돕기 위해 이 환자에게 진실을 이야기해야 할 의무가 있지만, 한편으로는 승용차 운전자가 손상을 입었을 가능성이 있어 올바른 결정을 내릴 능력이 없을 수 있다는 점을 명심해야 한다. 그녀의 어머니와 의식이 없는 아이의 상태에 대한 완전하고 진실한 공개는 그녀에게 더 큰 충격을 주거나 해를 끼칠 수 있다. 그러한 정보에 대한 그녀의 잠재적인 반응은 그녀의 의사결정 능력을 더욱 손상할 수 있으며 의식이 있고 이미 흥분 상태인 5세 자녀에게도 영향을 줄 수 있다. 이러면 병원 전 처치 제공자의 행동이 일으킬 수 있는 잠재적인 위해 또는 부담의 수준에 따라 무해성 및 유익성의 원칙은 환자가 더욱 안정적인 환경에 있을 때까지 완전한 공개를 연기하는 것을 고려할 것을 제안할 수 있다. 그것은 진실하게 대응할 책임을 면제하는 것은 아니다.

이 시나리오에서 분명한 것처럼 윤리는 어려운 상황에 대한 흑백 솔루션을 거의 제공하지 않는다. 오히려 윤리는 올바를 일을 하기 위해 윤리적으로 어려운 상황을 통해 고려하고 추론할 수 있는 이 장에서 논의된 자율성, 무해성, 유익성 및 공정성과 같은 네 가지 원칙과 같은 틀을 제공할 수 있다.

References

1. Lyng J, Adelgais K, Alter R, et al. Recommended essential equipment for basic life support and advanced life support ground ambulances 2020: a joint position statement. *Prehosp Emerg Care.* 2021;25(3):451-459. doi: 10.1080/10903127.2021.1886382

2. Hendricson WD, Andrieu SC, Chadwick DG, et al. Educational strategies associated with development of problem-solving, critical thinking, and self-directed learning. *J Dent Educ.* 2006;70(9):925-936.

3. Cotter AJ. Developing critical-thinking skills. *EMS Mag.* 2007;36(7):86.

4. Carroll RT. *Becoming a Critical Thinker: A Guide for the New Millennium.* 2nd ed. Pearson Custom Publishing; 2005.

5. Beauchamp TL, Childress JF. *Principles of Biomedical Ethics.* 6th ed. Oxford University Press; 2009.

6. Banning M. Measures that can be used to instill critical-thinking skills in nurse prescribers. *Nurse Educ Pract.* 2006;6(2):98-105.

7. Bamonti A, Heilicser B, Stotts K. To treat or not to treat: identifying ethical dilemmas in EMS. *JEMS.* 2001;26(3):100-107.

8. Daniels N. *Just Health Care.* Cambridge University Press; 1985.

9. Derse AR. Autonomy and informed consent. In: Iserson KV, Sanders AB, Mathieu D, eds. *Ethics in Emergency Medicine.* 2nd ed. Galen Press; 1995:99-105.

10. Post LF, Bluestein J, Dubler NN. *Handbook for Health Care Ethics Committees.* The Johns Hopkins University Press; 2007.

11. University of Maryland Medical Center. History of the Shock Trauma Center: tribute to R Adams Cowley, MD. Updated December 16, 2013. Accessed October 17, 2021. http://umm.edu/programs/shock-trauma/about/history

12. Lerner EB, Moscati RM. The Golden Hour: scientific fact or medical "urban legend"? *Acad Emerg Med.* 2001;8:758.

13. Tsybuliak GN, Pavlenko EP. Cause of death in the early post-traumatic period. *Vestn Khir Im I I Grek.* 1975;114(5):75.

14. Gunst M, Ghaemmaghami V, Gruszecki A, Urban J, Frankel H, Shafi S. Changing epidemiology of trauma deaths leads to a bimodal distribution. *Proc (Bayl Univ Med Cent).* 2010;23(4):349-354.

15. Kalkwarf KJ, Drake SA, Yang Y, et al. Bleeding to death in a big city: an analysis of all trauma deaths from hemorrhage in a metropolitan area over one year. *J Trauma Acute Care Surg.* 2020;89(4):716-722.

16. Sobrino J, Shafi S. Timing and causes of death after injuries. *Proc (Bayl Univ Med Cent).* 2013;26(2):120-123.

17. Clarke JR, Trooskin SZ, Doshi PJ, Greenwald L, Mode CJ. Time to laparotomy for intra-abdominal bleeding from trauma does affect survival for delays up to 90 minutes. *J Trauma.* 2002 Mar;52(3):420-425. doi: 10.1097/00005373-200203000-00002

18. Meizoso JP, Ray JJ, Karcutskie CA 4th, et al. Effect of time to operation on mortality for hypotensive patients with gunshot wounds to the torso: the Golden 10 Minutes. *J Trauma Acute Care Surg.* 2016 Oct;81(4):685-691. doi: 10.1097/TA.0000000000001198

19. Niles SE, McLaughlin DF, Perkins JG, et al. Increased mortality associated with the early coagulopathy of trauma in combat casualties. *J Trauma.* 2008;64(6):1459-1463; discussion 1463-1465.

20. Brohi K, Singh J, Heron M, Coats T. Acute traumatic coagulopathy. *J Trauma.* 2003;54(6):1127-1130.

21. Frieden TR. Evidence for health decision making—beyond randomized, controlled trials. *N Engl J Med.* 2017;377:465-475. doi: 10.1056/NEJMra1614394

22. Mitchell EA, Scragg R, Stewart AW, et al. Results from the first year of the New Zealand Cot Death Study. *N Z Med J.* 1991;104:71-77.

Suggested Reading

Adams JG, Arnold R, Siminoff L, Wolfson AB. Ethical conflicts in the prehospital setting. *Ann Emerg Med.* 1992;21(10):1259.

Beauchamp TL, Childress JF. *Principles of Biomedical Ethics.* 7th ed. Oxford University Press; 2013.

Buchanan AE, Brock DW. *Deciding for Others: The Ethics of Surrogate Decision Making.* Cambridge University Press; 1990.

Fitzgerald DJ, Milzman DP, Sulmasy DP. Creating a dignified option: ethical consideration in the formulation of prehospital DNR protocol. *Am J Emerg Med.* 1995;13(2):223.

Iverson KV. Foregoing prehospital care: should ambulance staff always resuscitate? *J Med Ethics.* 1991;17:19.

Iverson KV. Withholding and withdrawing medical treatment: an emergency medicine perspective. *Ann Emerg Med.* 1996;28(1):51.

Marco CA, Schears RM. Prehospital resuscitation practices: a survey of prehospital providers. *Ethics Emerg Med.* 2003;24(1):101.

Mohr M, Kettler D. Ethical aspects of prehospital CPR. *Acta Anaesthesiol Scand Suppl.* 1997;111:298-301.

Sandman L, Nordmark A. Ethical conflict in prehospital emergency care. *Nurs Ethics.* 2006;13(6):592.

Travers DA, Mears G. Physicians' experiences with prehospital do-not-resuscitate orders in North Carolina. *Prehosp Disaster Med.* 1996;11(2):91.

Van Vleet LM. Between black and white: the gray area of ethics in EMS. *JEMS.* 2006;31(10):55-56, 58-63; quiz 64-65.

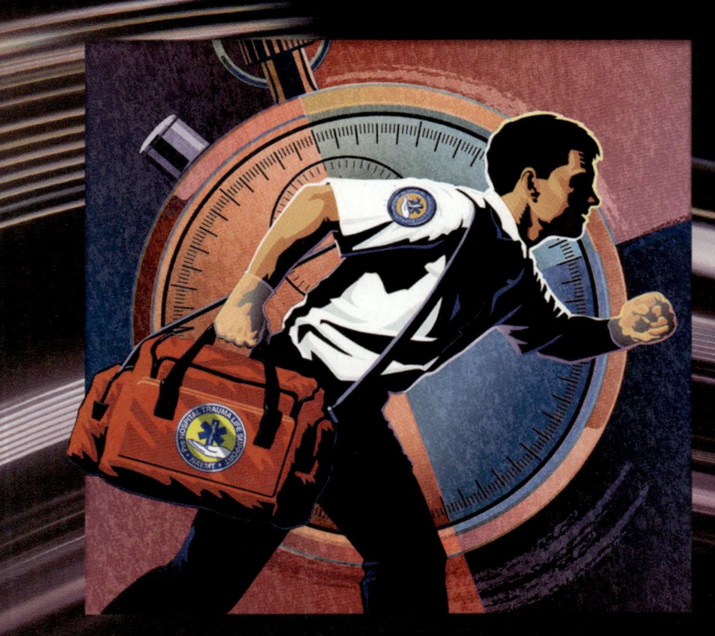

평가 및 처치

제 3 장   **쇼크: 삶과 죽음의 병태생리학**

제 4 장   **외상의 물리학**

제 5 장   **현장 관리**

제 6 장   **환자 평가 및 처치**

제 7 장   **기도와 환기**

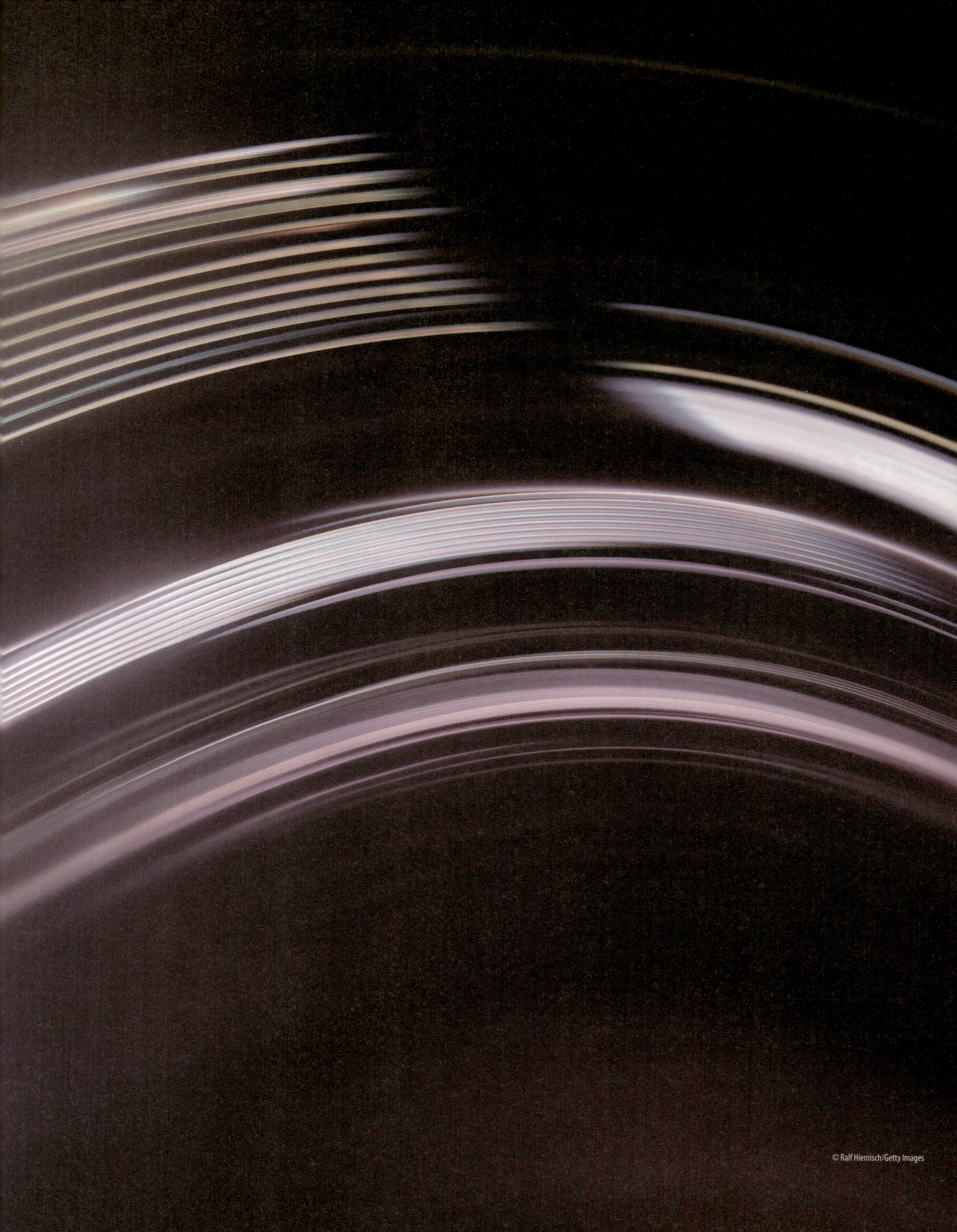
© Ralf Hiemisch/Getty Images

쇼크: 삶과 죽음의 병태생리학

Lead Editors
Samuel Galvagno, DO, PhD, FAMPA, FCCM
Jesse Shirki, DO, MS, FACEP

학습 목표

이 장의 학습을 완료하면 다음과 같은 내용을 수행할 수 있다.

- 쇼크를 정의할 수 있다.
- 전부하, 후부하 및 수축성이 심박출량에 어떻게 영향을 미치는지 설명할 수 있다.
- 원인에 따라 쇼크를 분류할 수 있다.
- 쇼크의 병태생리학과 단계별 진행 과정을 설명할 수 있다.
- 쇼크를 산-염기 상태, 에너지 생성, 원인, 예방 및 처치와 연관시킬 수 있다.
- 쇼크의 물리적 소견을 설명 설명할 수 있다.
- 쇼크를 정의하는 실질적인 평가 도구를 나열할 수 있다.
- 쇼크의 유형을 임상적으로 구분할 수 있다.
- 현장에서 쇼크 처치의 한계점에 대해 논의할 수 있다.
- 쇼크의 다양한 유형에 따라 빠른 이송과 결정적 초기 처치의 필요성을 인지할 수 있다.
- 외상 환자에게 쇼크 처치 원칙을 적용할 수 있다.
- 산소 전달에 필요한 구성 요소를 나열할 수 있다(피크 원리).
- 세포 요구를 충족시키는 무산소대사의 한계에 대해 논의할 수 있다.

시나리오

당신과 동료는 오토바이 충돌 혈장으로 출동했다. 오토바이는 도로를 벗어나 여러 번 굴러 전신주에 충돌했다. 현장에 도착하자마자 헬멧을 쓴 29세의 남성 운전자가 오토바이에서 약 15m 떨어진 곳에 바로 누워 있는 것을 발견했다. 환자는 흉부, 엉치뼈 및 왼쪽 엉덩관절 부위의 통증을 주요호소증상으로 호소한다.

환자의 신체검사 결과 피부는 창백하고 축축했으며 말초 맥박 감소, 흉부 타박상과 골반은 불안정했다. 활력징후는 맥박 110회/분, 혈압 82/56mmHg, 산소포화도는 92%, 호흡수 28회/분이며 오른쪽 호흡음이 감소했다.

- 이러한 유형의 손상 기전으로 어떤 손상이 발생할 것으로 예상하는가?
- 현장에서 이러한 손상을 어떻게 처치할 것인가?
- 이 환자에게 일어나는 주요 병리학적 과정은 무엇인가?
- 이 환자의 증상을 유발하는 병태생리학적 원인을 어떻게 교정할 것인가?
- 당신은 가장 가까운 외상센터에서 멀리 떨어진 시골 지역에서 근무하고 있다. 이 요소가 당신의 처치 계획을 어떻게 변화시키는가?

개요

프랑스어 "choc"에서 유래한 쇼크는 광범위한 산소 전달 손실과 중요한 장기의 기능 장애를 초래하는 세포로 부적절한 관류로 정의된다. 1872년 외과 의사 새무엘(Samuel Gross) 박사는 쇼크를 "생명 기계의 무례한 작동"이라고 묘사했다. 1970년대에는 외상에 따른 쇼크에 대한 추가 연구가 진행되어 조직과 세포의 부적절한 관류로 인한 사망과 병태생리학적 기전을 구분하는 데 도움이 되었다.

병원 전 응급 및 중환자 처치의 기본 목표 중 하나는 조직으로 산소공급을 촉진하는 것이다. 쇼크는 산소공급과 수요 사이의 불균형을 특징으로 하는 병리학적 상태이다. 따라서 외상으로 인한 쇼크의 신속한 진단, 소생술 및 결정적인 처치는 사망을 예방하고 환자의 결과를 최적화하는 데 필수적이다.

외상 환자의 평가와 처치는 인체 내 모든 세포로 산소를 공급하는 중요한 기능에 영향을 미치거나 방해하는 문제를 파악하고 교정하는 데 초점을 둔 일차평가에서 시작한다. 따라서 이상 징후를 확인하고 해결하기 위해서는 병원 전 처치 제공자가 사망으로 이어질 수 있는 삶의 생리학과 병태생리학에 대한 이해가 필수적이다.

병원 전 환경에서 쇼크 환자를 처치할 때 나타나는 어려움은 정교한 진단 및 처치 장비를 사용할 수 없거나 비교적 엄격하고 때로는 위험한 환경에서 이러한 환자를 평가하고 처치해야 할 필요성으로 인해 더욱 복잡해진다. 이 장에서는 외상성 쇼크의 원인에 초점을 맞추고 직접적인 처치 전략을 돕기 위해 현재 존재하는 병태생리학적 변화를 설명한다.

쇼크의 생리학

대사

인체는 1억 개가 넘는 세포로 구성되어 있으며 이 각각의 세포는 기능하기 위해 에너지가 필요하다. 세포는 아데노신삼인산(ATP) 형태의 에너지를 생산하고 사용함으로써 정상적인 대사 기능을 유지한다. 이 필요한 에너지를 생성하는 가장 효율적인 방법은 유산소대사를 통한 것이다. 세포는 산소와 포도당을 흡수하고 복잡한 생리적 대사 과정을 통해 에너지를 생산하고 부산물로 물과 이산화탄소의 부산물을 만든다. 이 과정에서 포도당은 미토콘드리아에서 피루브산으로 전환되고 아세틸조효소 A로 시트르산 회로로 들어간다.

산소 부족으로 인해 유산소대사 과정이 중단되면 피부르산이 시트

르산 회로로 들어가는 단계가 중단되고 무산소대사가 발생한다. 유산소대사와 달리 무산소대사는 산소를 사용하지 않고 일어난다. 유산소대사에서 포도당은 젖산(젖산염)으로 분해된다. 뇌, 심장, 간, 골격근과 같은 일부 기관은 일시적인 에너지원으로 젖산을 사용할 수 있지만 에너지 생산량은 포도당보다 훨씬 적다. 젖산 축적은 대사산증의 원인으로 pH 감소(혈액 내 수소 이온 증가)로 발생한다. pH가 7.20 이하로 떨어지면 심근 수축이 심하게 억제된다.

무산소대사가 빠르게 역전되지 않으면 세포가 기능을 계속할 수 없고 죽게 된다. 어느 하나의 장기에서 충분한 수의 세포가 죽으면 전체 장기의 기능이 멈춘다. 장기 사망은 환자 사망으로 진행될 수 있다.

허혈, 저산소혈증 및 저산소증의 차이를 이해하는 것이 중요하다. 허혈은 산소를 공급하기에 불충분한 혈류로 정의되며 조직으로의 혈액 공급이 중단될 때 발생한다. 허혈 후 혈액 내 산소 함량이 낮고(저산소혈증), 신체 조직 내 산소 함량이 낮으며(저산소증) 세포 사멸 간에 시간 의존적 관계가 존재한다. 산소 부족에 대한 세포의 민감도는 장기 시스템에 따라 다르다. 이 민감도는 허혈성 민감도라고 하며 뇌, 심장, 폐에서 가장 크다. 이러한 중요 장기 중 하나 이상이 회복할 수 없을 정도로 손상되기 전까지 무산소대사를 하는 데 4~6분 정도밖에 걸리지 않을 수 있다. 피부와 근육 조직은 허혈성 민감도가 4~6시간 정도로 상당히 길다. 복부 장기는 일반적으로 이 두 그룹 사이에 속하며 45~90분의 무산소대사를 견딜 수 있다(**표 3-1**).

세포의 정상적인 기능 유지는 여러 신체 계통의 중요한 관계와 상호작용에 달려있다. 환자의 기도는 개방되어 있어야 하고 호흡량과 깊이가 적절해야 한다. 심장이 정상적으로 기능하고 펌프질하고 있어야 한다. 순환계에는 인체 전체의 조직 세포에 적절한 양의 산소를 공급할 수 있는 충분한 적혈구(RBC)가 있어야 이 세포가 에너지를

표 3-1 허혈에 대한 장기의 내성	
장기	**허혈 시간**
심장, 뇌, 폐	4~6분
신장, 간, 위장관계	45~90분
근육, 뼈, 피부	4~6시간

Modified from American College of Surgeons Committee on Trauma. *Advanced Trauma Life Support: Student Course Manual.* 7th ed. American College of Surgeons; 2004.

생산할 수 있다.

외상 환자의 병원 전 평가와 처치는 무산소대사를 예방하거나 역전시켜 세포 사멸과 궁극적으로 환자 사망을 예방하는 것을 목적으로 한다. 환자의 기도가 개방되어 있고 호흡과 순환이 적절한지 확인하는 것과 같이 중요한 인체 계통이 올바르게 작동하는지 확인하는 것이 일차평가의 주요 강조 사항이다. 이러한 기능은 외상 환자에서 다음과 같은 조치를 통해 관리된다.

- 적절한 기도 유지와 환기를 유지하여 적혈구에 충분한 산소를 공급
- 보충 산소를 적절하게 사용하여 보조 환기
- 적절한 순환을 유지하여 조직 세포에 산소를 공급하는 혈액을 관류

쇼크의 정의

정상적인 생리적 기능을 방해하는 주요 합병증이 쇼크로 알려져 있다. 쇼크는 조직 세포의 저관류 상태에 따른 유산소대사에서 무산소대사로 세포 기능이 변화하는 상태이다. 결과적으로 세포 수준에서 산소공급은 신체의 대사 요구를 충족시키기에 불충분하다. 쇼크는 저혈압, 빠른맥, 차갑고 축축한 피부로 정의되지 않는다. 이것은 단순히 쇼크라고 불리는 병리학적 과정의 전신적인 징후일 뿐이다. 쇼크의 올바른 정의는 세포 수준에서 불충분한 조직 관류(산소공급)로 무산소대사와 생명을 유지하는 데 필요한 에너지 생산 손실로 이어진다. 이 정의에 따라 쇼크는 세포 관류 및 산소공급 측면에서 분류할 수 있다. 이 저관류 상태에서 발생하는 세포 변화와 내분비, 심혈관, 조직 및 말단 장기에 미치는 영향을 이해하면 처치하는 데 도움이 된다.

이 과정을 이해하는 것은 인체가 유산소대사와 에너지 생산을 회복하는 데 도움을 주는 데 중요하다. 병원 전 처치 제공자가 이 비정상적 상태를 이해하고 쇼크를 예방하거나 역전시키기 위한 처치 계획을 수립할 수 있다면 세포 수준에서 인체에 무슨 일이 일어나고 있는지 알고 이해하는 것이 중요하다. 인체가 쇼크 발생으로부터 자신을 보호하기 위해 사용하는 정상적인 생리학적 반응을 이해하고 인지하며 해석해야 한다. 그래야만 쇼크 환자의 문제를 해결하기 위한 합리적인 접근이 가능할 수 있다.

쇼크는 현장, 응급실, 수술실 또는 중환자실에서 환자를 사망에 이르게 할 수 있다. 비록 신체적 사망이 몇 시간에서 몇 주 동안 지연될 수 있지만, 가장 일반적인 사망의 원인은 쇼크로 인한 신속하고 적절한 소생술의 실패이다. 산소화된 혈액에 의한 세포의 관류 부족은 무산소대사, 에너지 생산 감소 그리고 결국 세포 사멸을 초래한다. 장기의 일부 세포가 처음에는 살아남더라도 나머지 세포가 장기의 기능을 무한정 수행할 수 없으므로 나중에 사망할 수 있다. 다음 부문에서는 이 현상을 설명한다. 이 과정을 이해하는 것은 인체가 유산소대사와 에너지 생산을 회복하는 데 도움이 된다.

쇼크의 병태생리학

대사: 인체의 운동

세포는 산소를 흡수하여 복잡한 생리학적 과정을 통해 산소를 대사하여 에너지를 생산한다. 동시에 세포의 신진대사는 에너지가 필요하며 세포는 이 과정을 수행하기 위해 연료인 포도당이 있어야 한다. 각 포도당 분자는 산소를 이용할 수 있을 때 38개의 아데노신삼인산(ATP) 분자를 생산한다. 모든 연소 과정과 마찬가지로 부산물도 생산된다. 체내에서 산소와 포도당이 대사되어 에너지를 생산하고 부산물로 물과 이산화탄소가 생성된다.

세포 대사 과정은 휘발유와 공기가 혼합되고 연소하여 에너지를 생산하고 부산물로 일산화탄소가 생성되는 자동차 엔진에서 일어나는 것과 유사하다. 자동차 엔진에서 휘발유와 공기를 혼합하여 연소시켜 생산된 에너지는 모터를 회전시켜 자동차를 움직이고 히터는 운전자를 따뜻하게 하며 생성된 전기는 헤드라이트에 사용된다.

사람의 모터도 마찬가지이다. 유산소대사는 무산소대사를 백업 시스템으로 하는 주요 구동 시스템이다. 그러나 안타깝게도 무산소대사는 강력한 백업 시스템이 아니다. 무산소대사는 유산소대사보다 훨씬 적은 에너지를 생산하며 장기간 에너지를 생산할 수 없다. 실제로 무산소대사는 에너지 생산이 19배 감소한 2개의 아데노신삼인산(ATP) 분자만을 생산한다. 그러나 병원 전 처치 제공자의 도움을 받아 인체가 스스로 회복되는 짧은 시간 동안 환자의 생존에 도움을 줄 수 있다.

무산소대사의 주요 부산물은 젖산(젖산염; **그림 3-1**)이다. 무산소대가사 빠르게 역전되지 않으면 세포는 점점 더 산성화되는 환경에서 기능을 계속할 수 없으며 적절한 에너지가 없으면 죽게 된다. 어느 장기에서든 충분한 수의 세포가 죽으면 전체 장기의 기능이 정지된다. 만약 장기에 있는 많은 수의 세포가 죽으면 전체 장기가 기능을 멈춘다. 장기의 수많은 세포가 죽으면 장기의 기능이 현저히 저하되고 해

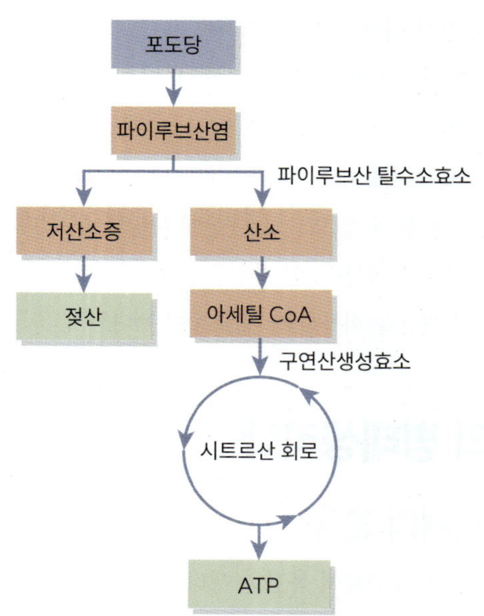

그림 3-1 저산소증 동안 젖산의 형성. 저산소증에 직면하면 피루브산은 아데노신삼인산(ATP)을 만들기 위해 시트르산 회로에 의해 처리되지 않고 젖산으로 전환된다.

© National Association of Emergency Medical Technicians (NAEMT)

당 장기의 나머지 세포는 장기 기능을 유지하기 위해 더 열심히 일해야 한다. 이러한 과로한 세포는 장기 전체의 기능을 계속해서 지원할 수도 있고 그렇지 못할 수도 있으며 장기는 여전히 죽을 수도 있다.

대표적인 예가 심장마비를 겪은 환자이다. 심근의 한 부분에 혈류와 산소가 차단되고 심장의 일부 세포가 죽는다. 이러한 세포의 손실은 심장 기능을 손상시켜 심박출량과 심장의 나머지 부분으로의 산소공급을 감소시킨다. 이는 나머지 심장 세포의 산소공급을 더욱 감소시킨다. 생존할 수 있는 세포가 너무 적거나 나머지 세포가 심장이 인체의 혈류 요구량을 충족할 수 있을 만큼 충분히 강하지 않다면 심부전이 발생할 수 있다. 심박출량이 크게 개선되지 않는 한 환자는 생존할 수 없다.

이 치명적인 과정의 또 다른 예는 신장에서 발생한다. 신장이 손상되거나 적절한 산소가 공급된 혈액이 부족하면 신장의 일부 세포가 죽기 시작하고 신장의 기능이 저하된다. 다른 세포도 손상될 수 있지만, 죽기 전에 잠깐 계속 기능할 수 있다. 결국 많은 수의 신장 세포가 죽으면 신장의 기능이 감소하여 대사 작용 시 발생하는 독성 부산물을 완전하게 제거할 수 없게 된다. 독소의 증가는 인체 전반에 걸쳐 세포 사멸을 더욱더 악화시킨다. 이러한 전신적인 악화가 계속되면 더 많은 세포와 장기가 죽고 결국 유기체(인간)가 죽는다.

초기에 관련된 장기에 따라 세포 사멸에서 유기체 사망으로의 진행은 빠르거나 지연될 수 있다. 외상 후 처음 몇 분 동안 저산소증이나 관류저하로 인한 손상이 환자의 사망을 초래하기까지 4~6분, 길게는 2~3주 걸릴 수 있다. 병원 전 단계에서 저산소증이나 관류저하를 역전시키거나 예방하기 위한 병원 전 처치 제공자의 처치에 대한 효과는 즉시 나타나지 않을 수 있다. 그러나 환자가 궁극적으로 생존하려면 이러한 소생술 처치가 필요하다. 이러한 초기 처치는 애덤스 카울리(R Adams cowley) 박사가 설명한 황금시간의 중요한 구성요소이며 현재 이 개념은 황금 기간이라고 불린다. 이는 심각한 손상을 처치하기 위한 시간의 틀이 황금시간의 비유적인 개념에 의해 전달되는 것보다 훨씬 다양하다고 알고 있기 때문이다.

산소공급(피크의 원리)

피크(Fick)의 원리는 체내 세포의 산소공급에 필요한 구성 요소에 대한 설명이다. 이 세 가지 구성 요소는 다음과 같다.

1. 폐에서 적혈구에 산소를 공급
2. 산소화된 적혈구를 조직 세포로 이동
3. 적혈구에서 조직 세포로 산소 전달

피크의 원리는 다음과 같은 공식으로 요약할 수 있다.

$$VO_2 = CO \times (CaO_2 - CvO_2)$$

VO_2는 산소 소비량[분당 소비되는 산소량(mL)]이며 인체의 활동 능력을 나타내는 지표이다. CO는 심박출량으로 심박수(분당 박동수)에 혈액의 박출량(mL)을 곱한 값이다. CaO_2는 동맥혈의 산소 농도이고 CvO_2는 정맥혈의 산소 농도이다. 동맥혈 또는 정맥혈의 산소 농도는 헤모글로빈의 양, 혈액에 용해된 산소의 양과 산소 분압에 따라 달라진다. 산소 소비량은 성별과 활동 수준에 따라 다르며 휴식 중인 남성의 정상 수치는 35~40mL/kg/분이고 휴식 중인 여성의 평균 수치는 약 27~30mL/kg/분이다. 엘리트 선수인 일부 남성은 최대 산소 소비량이 85mL/kg/분이고 엘리트 선수인 여성은 최대 77mL/kg/분을 기록했다.

기도 확보와 적절한 호흡 외에도 이 과정에서 중요한 부분은 세포가 에너지를 생산할 수 있도록 인체 전체의 조직 세포에 적절한 양의 산소를 공급할 수 있는 충분한 적혈구가 환자에게 있어야 한다는 것이다.

이 과정은 환자의 산-염기 상태에 의해 영향을 받는다. 적절한 환기와 보충 산소 공급으로 정상적인 산소포화도를 나타냄에도 불구하고 저체온증으로 인해 세포 수준에서 산소를 분리할 수 없으므로 악화하는 환자를 마주할 수 있다. 쇼크의 병원 전 처치는 무산소대사를 예방하거나 역전시켜 세포 사멸을 방지하는 것을 목표로 피크 원리의 중요한 구성요소가 유지되도록 하는 데 있다. 이러한 구성 요소는 병원 전 처치 제공자에 의해 이루어지는 일차평가에서 주요 강조사항이며 다음과 같은 처치를 통해 외상 환자를 관리할 때 구현된다.

- 대량 팔다리 출혈 조절
- 적절한 기도 유지 및 환기 유지
- 보충 산소 투여
- 환자의 체온 유지
- 적절한 순환 유지

피크 원리의 첫 번째 구성요소는 폐와 적혈구의 산소공급이다. 이에 대해서는 7장 기도와 환기에서 자세히 설명되어 있다. 두 번째 구성요소는 조직 세포에 혈액을 전달하는 관류를 포함한다. 관류를 설명하는 유용한 비유는 적혈구를 기차의 수송 차량, 폐는 산소를 공급받고 이산화탄소를 배출하는 역, 혈관을 철로, 신체 조직 세포를 기차가 정차하는 역으로 생각하면 된다. 일반적으로 건강한 사람의 경우 산소의 25%만 추출된다. 이것은 병원에서 혼합 정맥산소포화도(SvO_2; **그림 3-2**)로 측정 및 모니터링된다.

수송 열차의 수가 부족하거나 철로 주변의 장애물 또는 느린 수송 차량은 모두 산소공급 감소와 궁극적으로 조직 세포의 산소 고갈에 기여할 수 있다.

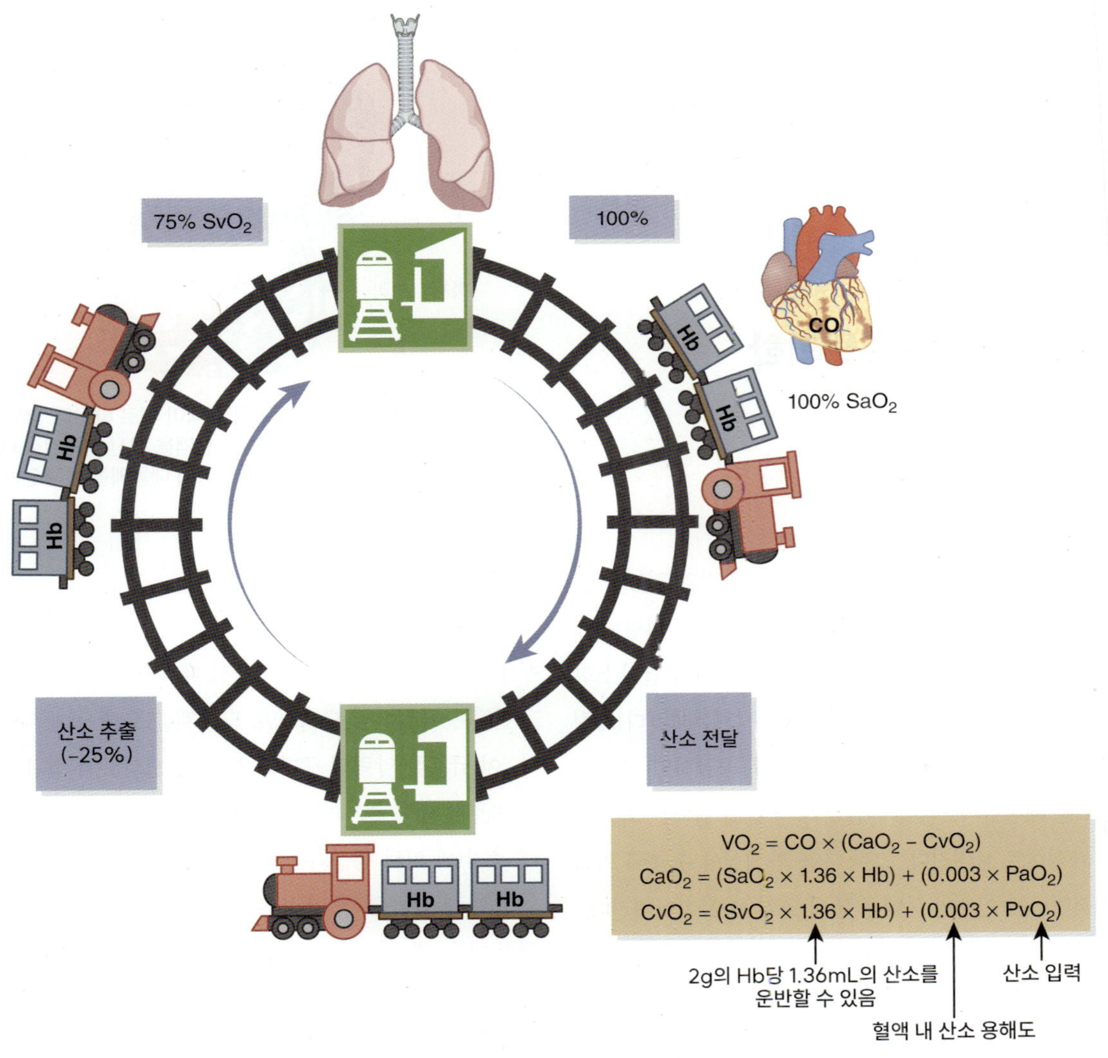

그림 3-2 혼합 정맥산소포화도(SvO_2)의 개념. 정상적인 상황에서는 산소의 25%만 사용되고 약 70~75%가 반환된다. 반환된 백분율의 척도는 혼합 정맥산소포화도이다. 낮은 혼합 정맥산소포화도는 산소 소비 증가 및 산소공급 감소를 나타낸다.

세포 관류 및 쇼크

세포 관류의 주요 결정 요인은 심장(시스템의 펌프 또는 모터 역할), 체액량(유압 유체 역할), 혈관(도관 또는 배관 역할) 그리고 마지막으로 인체의 세포이다. 이러한 관류 체계의 구성요소에 따라 쇼크는 다음과 같이 분류할 수 있다.

1. 저혈량: 주로 외상 환자에서 출혈로 인해 발생하며 순환하는 혈액 세포의 손실과 산소 운반 능력이 있는 체액량과 관련이 있다. 이것은 외상 환자에서 발생하는 쇼크의 가장 흔한 원인이다.

2. 분포(또는 혈관성): 척수 손상, 패혈증 및 급성중증과민증을 포함한 여러 가지 다른 원인으로 인해 발생하는 혈관 긴장도의 이상과 관련이 있다.

3. 심장성: 심장마비 후 종종 발생하는 심장의 펌프 활동 방해와 관련이 있다.

지금까지 외상 환자에서 쇼크의 가장 흔한 원인은 출혈로 인한 혈량 저하증이며 외상 환자에서 쇼크를 처치하는 가장 안전한 접근 방법은 쇼크의 원인이 다른 것으로 입증될 때까지 그 원인을 출혈로 간주하는 것이다.

쇼크의 해부학 및 병태생리학

심혈관 반응

심장

심장은 2개의 심방과 2개의 심실로 구성되어 있다. 심방의 기능은 심실이 빠르게 채워질 수 있도록 혈액을 축적하고 저장하여 펌핑 주기의 지연이 최소화하는 것이다. 우심방은 인체의 정맥에서 탈산소화된 혈액을 받아 우심실로 보내진다. 우심실이 수축할 때마다(**그림 3-3**) 혈액은 폐를 통해 펌핑되어 적혈구에 산소를 공급하고 날숨을 통해 이산화탄소를 배출한다. 폐에서 산소가 공급된 혈액은 좌심방으로 되돌아가 좌심실로 보내진다. 그런 다음 좌심실의 수축에 의해 산소가 공급된 적혈구는 인체의 동맥을 통해 조직 세포로 보내진다.

심장은 하나의 기관이지만, 실제로 두 개의 하위 시스템을 가지고 있다. 인체로부터 혈액을 받는 우심방과 혈액을 폐로 내보내는 우심실을 우심장이라고 한다. 폐에서 산소가 공급된 혈액을 받는 좌심방과 혈액을 내보내는 좌심실을 좌심장이라고 한다(**그림 3-4**). 이해해야 할 두 가지 중요한 개념은 전부하(심장으로 들어오는 혈액량)와

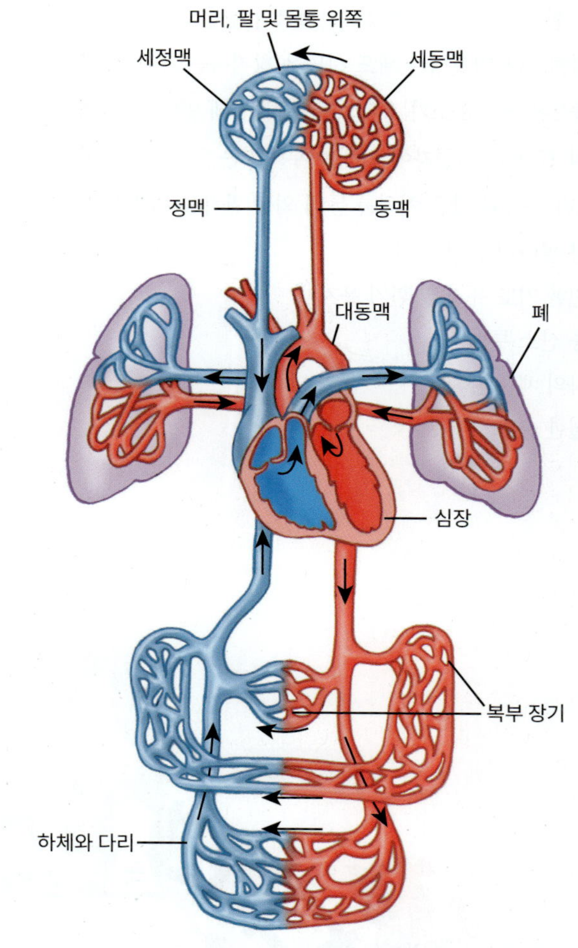

그림 3-3 우심실이 수축할 때마다 혈액이 폐로 나온다. 폐에서 나온 혈액은 심장의 왼쪽으로 들어가고 좌심실은 혈액을 전신 혈관계로 내보낸다. 폐에서 돌아온 혈액은 좌심실 수축으로 심장에서 대동맥을 통해 인체의 나머지 부분으로 내보내진다.

© National Association of Emergency Medical Technicians (NAEMT)

후부하(혈액이 좌심실에서 수축할 때 밀어내야 하는 압력)이다.

혈액은 좌심실의 수축으로 순환계를 통해 강제적으로 밀려 나간다. 이 급격한 압력의 증가는 맥파를 생성하여 혈관을 통해 혈액을 밀어낸다. 압력 증가의 정점이 수축기 혈압(SBP)이며 이는 심실 수축(수축기)에 의해 생성되는 맥박파의 힘을 나타낸다. 심실 수축 사이의 혈관에 있는 휴식 압력은 이완기 혈압(DBP)이며 이는 심실이 혈액의 다음 맥박(이완기)을 위해 다시 채워지는 동안 혈관을 통해 혈액을 계속해서 이동시키는 혈관에 남아 있는 힘을 나타낸다. 수축기 혈압과 이완기 혈압의 차이를 맥압이라고 한다. 맥압은 혈액이 순환계로 밀려 나가는 압력으로 환자의 맥박을 측정할 때 병원 전 처치 제공자의 손가락 끝에서 느껴지는 압력이다.

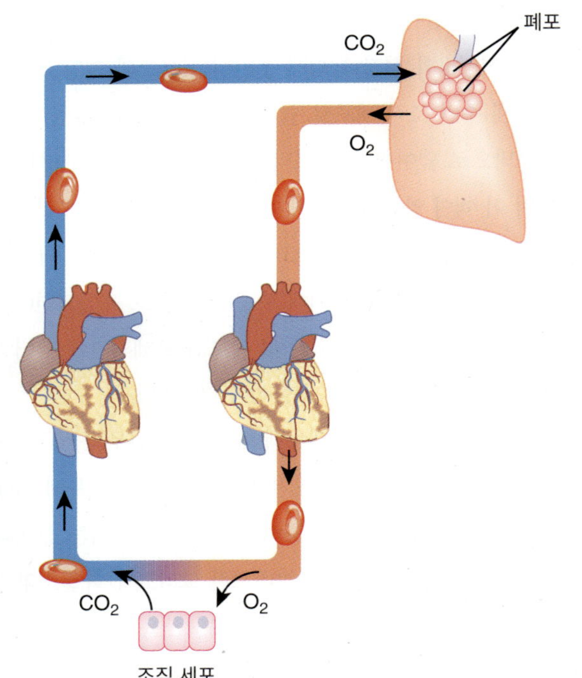

그림 3-4 심장은 하나의 기관으로 간주하지만, 두 개의 기관인 것처럼 기능한다. 탈산소화된 혈액은 위대정맥과 아래대정맥을 통해 우심장으로 유입되고 폐동맥을 통해 폐로 내보내진다. 혈액은 폐에서 산소화되고 폐정맥을 통해 심장으로 들어와 좌심실에서 배출된다.

혈압과 쇼크를 설명할 때 사용되지만, 종종 병원 전 환경에서 충분히 강조되지 않는 다른 용어는 평균 동맥압(MAP)이다. 이 수치는 수축기 압력이나 이완기 압력보다 혈류를 생성하는 전반적인 압력에 대한 더 현실적인 평가를 제공하며 사실상 말단 장기 관류의 수치적 표현을 제공한다. 평균 동맥압은 혈관계의 평균 압력이며 다음과 같이 계산한다.

$$\text{평균 동맥압(MAP)} = \text{이완기 혈압} + 1/3\ \text{맥압}$$

$$\text{또는}$$

$$\text{평균 동맥압(MAP)} = \frac{(2 \times \text{이완기 혈압}) + \text{수축기 혈압}}{3}$$

예를 들어, 혈압이 120/80mmHg인 환자의 평균 동맥압은 다음과 같이 계산한다.

$$\text{평균 동맥압} = 80 + ([120 - 80]/3)$$
$$= 80 + (40/3)$$
$$= 80 + 13.3$$
$$= 93.3\ (약\ 93)$$

많은 비침습적 자동 혈압계(NIBP)는 수축기 및 이완기 혈압 외에도 평균 동맥압을 자동으로 계산하여 나타낸다. 이것은 외상 환자에게 허용 저혈압 처치를 시행할 때 매우 유용하다. 허용할 수 있는 저혈압은 이 장의 수액 소생술 부문에서 자세히 설명한다. 정상 평균 동맥압은 70~100mmHg로 간주한다.

쇼크 지수(SI)는 쇼크 수준을 평가하는 데 자주 사용되는 또 다른 계산 방법이다. 쇼크 지수는 심박수를 수축기 혈압으로 나누어 계산한다. 심박수와 혈압은 모두 쇼크의 초기 보상 단계에서 정상적으로 나타날 수 있다. 더욱이 약물, 극단적인 연령과 같은 다른 교란 변수는 이러한 활력징후를 변화시킬 수 있다. 쇼크 지수는 출혈, 심근경색, 폐색전증 및 패혈증을 포함한 다양한 원인으로 인한 쇼크의 위험이 있거나 쇼크로 고통받는 환자를 대상으로 연구되었다. 수축기 혈압에 대한 심박수의 정상 비율은 일반적으로 < 0.7이다. 쇼크 지수 ≥ 0.9인 외상 환자는 사망률이 더 높고 치명적인 출혈 위험이 더 높은 것으로 나타났다.

심실이 수축할 때마다 순환계로 내보내지는 유체의 양을 일회박출량이라 하고 1분 동안 순환계로 내보내지는 혈액의 양을 심박출량이라고 한다. 심박출량을 구하는 공식은 다음과 같다.

$$\text{심박출량(CO)} = \text{심박수(HR)} \times \text{일회박출량(SV)}$$
$$\text{정상 심박출량} = 5{\sim}6L/분$$

심박출량은 분당 리터(L/분)로 기록한다. 심박출량은 병원 전 단계에서 측정하지 않는다. 그러나 심박출량과 일회박출량의 관계를 이해하는 것은 쇼크를 이해하는 데 중요하다. 심장이 효과적으로 작동하려면 대정맥과 폐정맥에 충분한 양의 혈액이 있어야 심실을 채울 수 있다.

스탈링의 법칙(Starling's law)은 이 관계가 어떻게 작용하는지 설명하는 데 도움이 되는 중요한 개념이다. 이 압력은 심장을 채우고(전부하) 심근 섬유를 늘린다. 심실에 혈액이 더 많이 채워질수록 심근 섬유는 더 많이 늘어나고 과도하게 늘어날 때까지 심장 수축의 강도가 커진다. 심각한 출혈이나 상대적인 혈량저하증은 심장의 전부하를 감소시켜 혈액량이 감소하고 심근 섬유가 그만큼 늘어나지 않아 수축 강도와 일회박출량이 줄어들어 혈압이 낮아진다. 체액 과부하 환자에서 발생할 수 있는 것처럼 심장의 충만 압력이 너무 높으면 심근 섬유가 과도하게 늘어나 적절한 일회박출량을 전달하지 못하고 다시 혈압이 낮아진다.

좌심실이 혈액을 동맥계로 내보내기 위해 극복해야 하는 혈류에 대한 저항을 후부하 또는 전신 혈관 저항이라 한다. 말초 동맥혈관 수축이 증가함에 따라 혈류에 대한 저항이 증가하고 심장은 혈액을 동맥계로 내보내기 위해 더 큰 힘을 생성해야 한다. 반대로 광범위한 말초 혈관의 확장은 후부하를 감소시킨다.

전신 순환은 폐순환보다 더 많은 모세혈관과 더 긴 혈관을 포함한다. 따라서 좌심장은 더 높은 압력에서 작동하며 우심장보다 더 높은 부하를 견뎌낸다. 해부학적으로 좌심실 근육은 우심실 근육보다 훨씬 두껍고 강하다.

혈관

혈관은 혈액을 포함하고 인체의 여러 부위와 세포로 혈액을 보낸다. 혈관은 생리학적 순환 과정의 "고속도로" 역할을 한다. 대동맥은 크기가 감소하는 여러 개의 작은 동맥으로 나뉘며 그중 가장 작은 것이 모세혈관이다(**그림 3-5**). 모세혈관의 너비가 하나의 세포에 불과할 수 있으므로 적혈구와 혈장에 의해 운반되는 산소와 영양소는 모세혈관벽을 통해 주변 조직 세포로 쉽게 확산할 수 있다(**그림 3-6**). 각 세포는 세포막으로 덮여 있고 세포막과 모세혈관 사이에는 사이질액이 존재하며 이 액의 양은 엄청나게 다양하다. 사이질액이 작으면 세포막과 모세혈관벽이 더 가까워지고 산소가 이 사이에서 쉽게 확산할 수 있다. 이 공간에 여분의 체액(부종)이 강제로 유입되면(결정질 수액을 과다 사용한 소생술에서 발생) 세포가 모세혈관에서 더 멀리 이동하여 산소와 영양분의 전달 효율성이 떨어진다.

혈관 용적의 크기는 동맥과 세동맥 벽에 있는 민무늬근육에 의해 조절되며 정도는 덜하지만, 정맥과 세정맥 벽에 있는 근육에 의해 조절된다. 이 근육은 교감신경계를 통해 뇌로부터 전달되는 신호와 순환 호르몬인 에피네프린과 노르에피네프린 그리고 산화질소와 같은 다른 화학물질에 반응한다. 혈관 벽에 있는 근육 섬유가 자극받아 수축하거나 이완함에 따라 혈관의 수축 또는 확장을 초래하여 심혈관계의 혈관 용적의 크기를 변화시켜 환자의 혈압에 영향을 미친다.

세 가지 체액 구획은 혈관 내액(혈관 내부의 액체), 세포 내액(세포 내부의 액체) 그리고 사이질액(세포와 혈관 사이의 액체)이다. 사이질액이 과도하게 존재하면 부종을 일으키고 손가락으로 피부를 눌렀을 때 스펀지 같은 느낌을 준다.

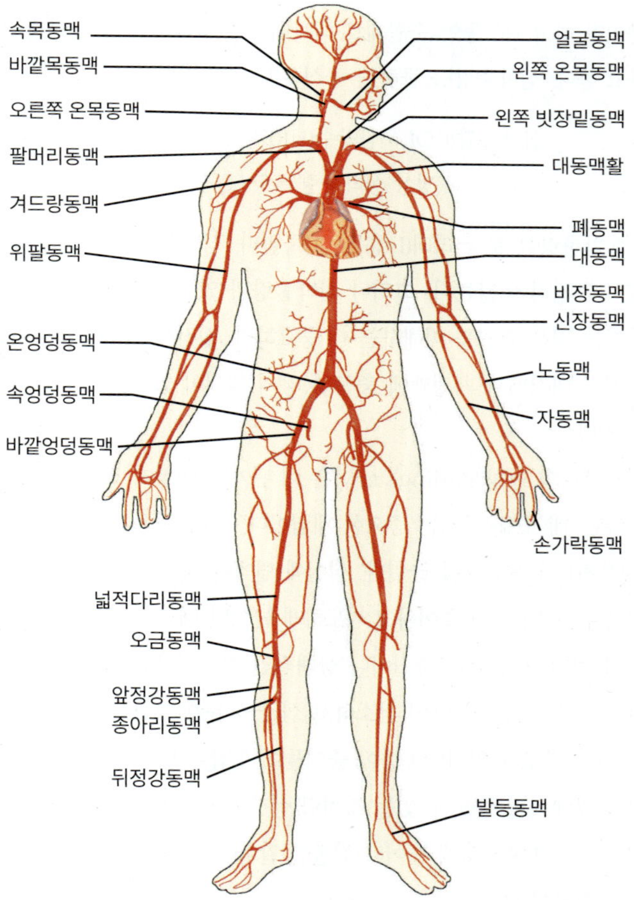

그림 3-5 인체의 주요 동맥

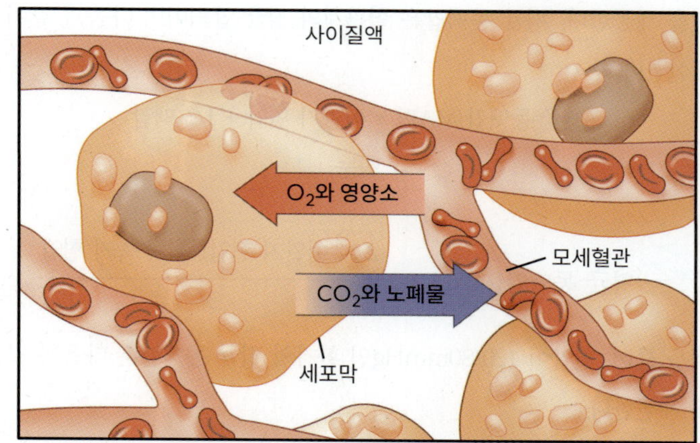

그림 3-6 적혈구에서 나온 영양소와 산소는 모세혈관벽, 사이질액, 세포막을 통해 세포 안으로 확산한다. 이산화탄소와 노폐물은 순환계를 통해 이동하여 폐에서 제거된다. 신체의 완충 시스템을 통해 이 산(acid)은 이산화탄소로 전환되어 적혈구나 혈장을 통해 폐로 이동되어 순환계에서 제거된다.

혈류역학 반응

혈액

순환계의 체액 구성 요소인 혈액에는 1) 산소를 운반하는 적혈구, 2) 감염과 싸우는 인자(백혈구 및 항체), 3) 혈관 손상 시 혈액 응고에 필수적인 혈소판 및 응고 인자, 세포 재생을 위한 단백질, 포도당과 같은 영양소 및 기타 신진대사와 생존을 위해 필요한 물질을 포함하고 있다. 다양한 단백질과 무기질은 혈관 벽을 통해 체액이 새어나가지 않도록 높은 삼투압을 제공한다. 혈관을 적절하게 채우고 관류를 유지하기 위해서 혈관계 내 체액량의 부피는 혈관의 용량과 같아야 한다. 해당 혈관의 혈액 부피와 비교하여 혈관계 용기 부피의 변화는 혈액 흐름에 긍정적 또는 부정적으로 영향을 미친다.

인체는 60%가 수분으로 모든 체액의 기초가 된다. 체중이 70kg인 사람은 약 40L의 수분을 함유하고 있다. 체수분은 세포내액과 세포외액이라는 두 가지 구성요소로 존재한다. 앞에서 언급한 바와 같이 체액의 종류에 따라 특이하고 중요한 특성이 있다(**그림 3-7**). 세포내액은 체중의 약 45%를 차지하고 세포외액은 사이질액과 혈관 내 액의 두 가지 하위 유형으로 더 분류할 수 있다. 사이질액은 조직 세포를 둘러싸고 있는 뇌척수액(뇌와 척주관에서 발견)과 윤활액(관절에서 발견)은 체중의 약 10.5%를 차지한다. 혈관에서 발견되고 혈액을 구성하는 성분과 산소 및 기타 필수 영양소를 운반하는 혈관 내 액은 체중의 약 4.5%를 차지한다.

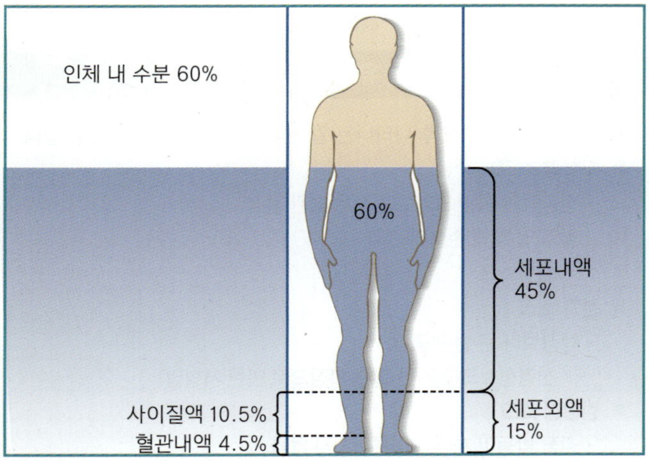

몇 가지 주요 개념을 검토하는 것은 체내에서 체액이 어떻게 움직이는지를 이해하는 데 도움이 된다. 혈관 계통을 통한 체액의 이동 외에도 1) 혈장과 사이질액 사이의 이동(모세혈관을 통해), 2) 세포내와 사이질액 구획 사이의 이동(세포막을 통해)이라는 두 가지 주요 유형의 체액 이동이 있다.

모세혈관벽을 통한 체액의 이동은 1) 모세혈관 내부(체액을 밀어내는 경향)의 정수압과 모세혈관 외부(체액을 밀어 넣는 경향)의 정수압 차이, 2) 모세혈관(체액을 유지하는) 내부의 단백질 농도와 모세혈관(체액을 끌어당기는) 외부의 삼투압 차이 그리고 3) 모세혈관의 누수 또는 투과성(**그림 3-8**)에 의해 결정된다. 정수압, 삼투압 그리고 모세혈관 투과성은 쇼크 상태뿐만 아니라 수액 소생술의 종류와 양에 영향을 받아 순환 혈액량, 혈류역학 및 조직 또는 폐부종의 변화를 초래한다.

세포 내 공간과 사이질 공간 사이의 체액 이동은 주로 세포막을 통해 이루어지며 삼투압에 의해 결정된다. 삼투란 반투막(물에 대한 투과성, 상대적으로 용질 불투과성)으로 분리된 용질이 용질의 농도에 따라 막을 통과하는 물의 이동을 제어하는 과정이다. 물은 용질 농도가 낮은 구획에서 용질 농도가 높은 구획으로 이동하여 반투막을 가로지르는 삼투 평행을 유지한다(**그림 3-9**).

내분비 반응

신경계

자율신경계는 호흡, 소화 및 심혈관 기능과 같은 인체의 비자발적 기능을 지시하고 조절한다. 그것은 교감신경계와 부교감신경계라는 두

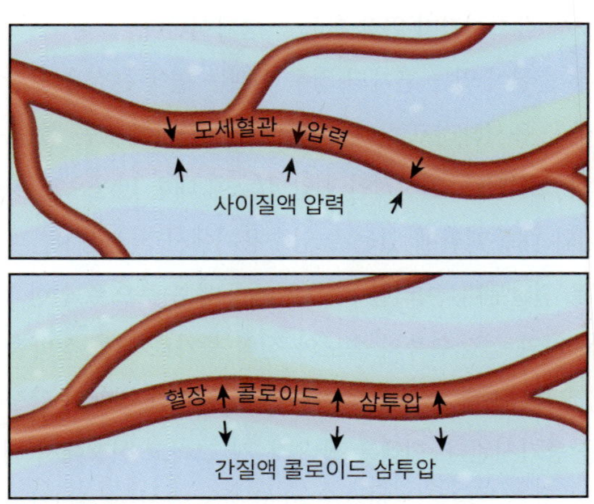

그림 3-7 인체는 약 60%가 수분으로 구성되어 있으며 이 수분은 세포내액 및 세포외액으로 나뉜다. 세포외액은 다시 사이질액과 혈관내액으로 나뉜다.

그림 3-8 모세혈관을 가로지르는 유체 흐름을 제어하는 힘

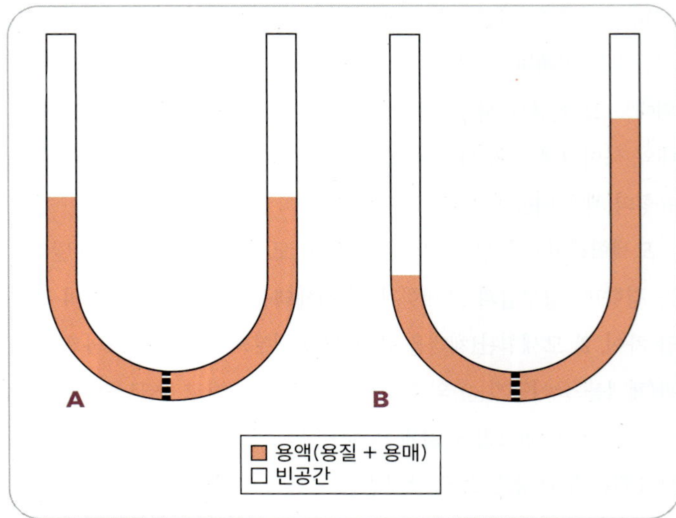

그림 3-9 **A.** 반투막에 의해 두 개로 분리되는 U 관에는 동일한 양의 물과 고체 입자가 들어 있다. **B.** 반투막을 통해 확산할 수 없는 용질이 한쪽에만 추가되고 반대쪽에는 추가되지 않으면 액체는 추가된 입자를 희석하기 위해 막을 통해 이동한다. 이 U 관에서 액체 높이의 압력 차이를 삼투압이라고 한다.

가지 하위 시스템으로 나뉘며 이 신경계는 중요한 인체 시스템의 균형을 유지할 수 있도록 서로 반대 작용을 한다.

교감신경계는 투쟁-도피 반응을 일으킨다. 이 반응은 동시에 심장은 더 빠르고 강하게 뛰게 하고 환기 속도를 증가시키며 혈관을 팽창시키고 근육으로 가는 혈류를 개선하는 동안 불필요한 장기의 혈관(피부 및 위장관)을 수축시킨다. 이 반응 시스템의 목표는 중요한 조직에 충분한 양의 산소가 공급된 혈액을 유지하여 인체가 필수적이지 않은 영역의 혈액 관류를 감소하도록 하여 응급 상황에 반응할 수 있도록 하는 것이다. 반대로 부교감신경계는 심박수를 느리게 하고 환기 속도를 감소시키며 위장 활동을 증가시킨다.

외상 후 출혈이 있는 환자의 경우 인체는 혈액 손실을 보상하고 에너지 생산을 유지하려고 한다. 심혈관계는 숨뇌에 있는 혈관 운동 중추에 의해 조절된다. 일시적인 혈압 감소에 대한 반응으로 자극은 목동맥팽대와 대동맥활에 있는 늘임수용기에서 뇌신경 9번과 10번을 통해 뇌로 전달된다. 이러한 자극은 세동맥 수축으로 인한 말초혈관 저항의 증가와 심장수축의 속도와 심의 증가로 인한 심박출량 증가와 함께 교감신경계 활동을 증가시킨다. 증가한 정맥의 탄성은 순환 혈액량을 증가시킨다. 혈액은 팔다리, 장 그리고 신장에서 더욱 중요한 부위인 심장과 뇌로 우회하며 이 부위는 강한 교감신경 자극에도 혈관이 거의 수축하지 않는다. 이러한 반응은 차갑고 청색증이 있는

팔다리, 소변 배출량 감소, 장 관류 감소를 초래한다.

좌심방의 충만압 감소, 혈압 감소, 혈장 삼투압(혈액 내 모든 화학물질의 총 농도)의 변화로 인해 뇌하수체에서 항이뇨호르몬(ADH)과 부신에서 알도스테론이 분비되어 신장에 의한 나트륨과 수분의 정체를 증가시킨다. 이 과정은 혈관 내 부피를 확장하는 데에 도움이 되지만, 이 기전이 임상적 차이를 만드는 데는 많은 시간이 필요하다.

외상성 쇼크의 분류

세포 관류의 주요 결정 요인은 심장(펌프 또는 시스템의 모터 역할), 체액량(유압 유체 역할), 혈관(도관 또는 배관 역할) 그리고 마지막으로 인체의 세포이다. 이러한 관류 체계의 구성 요소를 반으로 쇼크는 **Box 3-1**과 같이 분류할 수 있다.

외상성 쇼크의 유형

저혈량 쇼크

출혈로 인한 혈액량의 급격한 손실(혈장과 적혈구의 손실)은 체액량과 혈관 지름의 관계에 불균형을 초래한다. 혈관의 정상 지름을 유지하지만, 체액량이 감소한다. 저혈량 쇼크는 병원 전 환경에서 발생하는 쇼크의 가장 흔한 원인이고 출혈은 외상 환자에서 혈량저하증 및 쇼크의 가장 흔한 원인이다.

순환에서 혈액이 손실되면 심장이 자극되어 수축 강도와 속도를 증가시켜 심박출량을 증가시킨다. 이 자극은 부신에서 에피네프린이

Box 3-1 외상성 쇼크 유형

병원 전 환경에서 외상 후 나타나는 일반적인 쇼크의 유형은 다음과 같다.
- 저혈량 쇼크
  - 정상적인 혈관 크기보다 작은 혈관 용적
  - 혈액 및 체액 손실의 결과
    - 출혈쇼크
- 분포 쇼크
  - 정상보다 큰 혈관 공간
    - 신경성쇼크(심각한 혈관 확장으로 인한 저혈압)
- 심장성 쇼크
  - 심장 박동이 제대로 이루어지지 않음
  - 심장 손상의 결과

분비되어 발생한다. 동시에 교감신경계는 노르에피네프린을 분비하여 혈관을 수축시켜 혈관의 지름을 줄이고 남아있는 체액량에 비례하게 한다. 혈관수축은 말초 모세혈관을 폐쇄시켜 영향을 받은 세포로의 산소 전달을 감소시키고 세포 수준에서 유산소대사에서 강제로 무산소대사로 전환한다.

이러한 보상 기전은 어느 정도까지 잘 작동하며 일시적으로 환자의 활력징후를 유지하는 데 도움이 된다. 빈맥과 쇼크 지수 증가와 같은 보상 징후를 보이는 환자는 쇼크 상태가 아니라 이미 쇼크 상태이다. 보상 기전이 더 이상 손실된 혈액량을 보상할 수 없으면 환자의 혈압이 떨어진다. 이러한 혈압 감소는 보상성 쇼크에서 비보상성 쇼크로의 전환을 의미하며 이는 임박한 사망의 징후이다. 적극적인 소생술을 시행하지 않는 한 처치하지 않은 쇼크는 사망으로 이어진다.

출혈쇼크

체중이 70kg인 성인의 순환 혈액량은 약 5L이다. 출혈(출혈로 인한 저혈량 쇼크)은 출혈의 중증도에 따라 다음과 같이 4단계로 분류되며(**표 3-2**) 이 단계에 나열된 기준값과 설명은 다음과 같다. 상당히 중복되는 부분도 있으므로 출혈량의 절대적인 결정 요인으로 해석해서는 안 된다(**그림 3-10**).

1. 1단계 출혈은 성인에서 혈액량의 최대 15%(최대 750mL)까지 손실을 나타낸다. 이 단계에서는 임상 증상이 거의 없다. 빈맥은 거의 나타나지 않고 혈압, 맥압 또는 호흡수의 측정 가능한 변화가 발생하지 않는다. 이 정도의 출혈량을 유지하는 대부분의 건강한 환자는 추가 출혈이 발생하지 않는 한 상태 유지에 필요한 수액만 필요하다. 인체의 보상 기전은 혈관 내 지름-체액량 비율을 회복하고 혈압 유지를 돕는다.

2. 2단계 출혈은 성인에서 혈액량의 15~30%(750~1,500mL)의 손실을 나타낸다. 대부분 성인은 교감신경계의 활성화를 통해 혈압을 유지하여 이 정도의 출혈량을 보상할 수 있다. 임상 소견으로 호흡수 증가, 빈맥 그리고 맥압 감소 등이 있다. 이 단계에 대한 임상 단서는 빈맥, 빠른 호흡 및 정상 수축기 혈압이다. 혈압이 정상이기 때문에 이러한 반응을 보상성 쇼크라고 한다. 즉 환자는 쇼크 상태에 있지만, 당분간은 보상할 수 있다. 이 단계에서 쇼크 지수(SI)가 높아질 수 있다(>0.9). 환자는 종종 불안이나 두려움을 나타낸다. 현장에서 일반적으로 측정하지 않지만, 체액을 보존하려는 인체의 노력으로 성인의 소변 배출량은 시간당 20~30mL로 약간 감소한다. 때에 따라 이러한 환자는 병원에서 수혈이 필요할 수 있다.

3. 3단계 출혈은 성인에서 혈액량의 31~40%(1,500~2,000mL)의 손

표 3-2 출혈의 분류

	1단계	2단계	3단계	4단계
출혈량(mL)	< 750	750~1,500	1,500~2,000	> 2,000
출혈량(% 혈액량)	< 15%	15~30%	31~40%	> 40%
맥박수	↔	↔/↑	↑	↑/↑↑
혈압	↔	↔	↔/↓	↓
맥압 (mm Hg)	↔	↓	↓	↓
중추신경계/의식수준	약간 불안	약간 불안	불안, 혼란	혼란스럽고 무기력
기준초과	0 ~ -2mEq/L	-2 ~ -6mEq/L	-6 ~ -10mEq/L	-10mEq/L 이상
혈액 필요	모니터링	가능한	예	대량 수혈

↑ = 증가, ↓ = 감소, ↔ = 정상 범위

참고: 이러한 쇼크 단계에 대해 나열된 기준에 대한 추세 및 설명은 상당한 중복이 존재하므로 쇼크 등급의 절대적인 결정 요인으로 해석되어서는 안 된다.

Data from American College of Surgeons Committee on Trauma. *Advanced Trauma Life Support for Doctors: Student Course Manual*. 8th ed. American College of Surgeons; 2008.

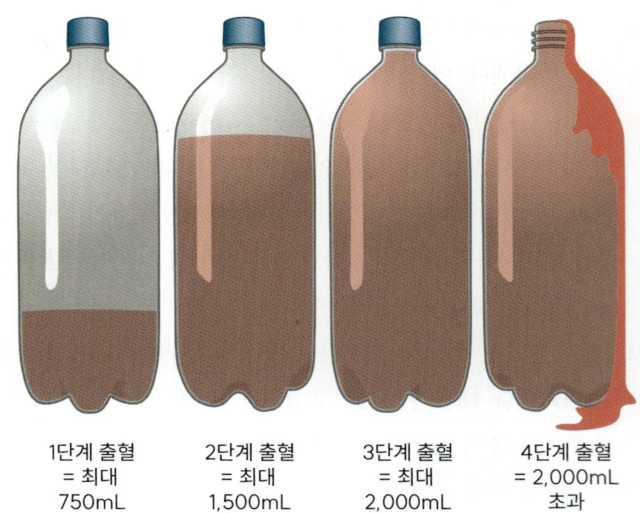

그림 3-10 출혈 단계별 대략적인 출혈량

© National Association of Emergency Medical Technicians (NAEMT)

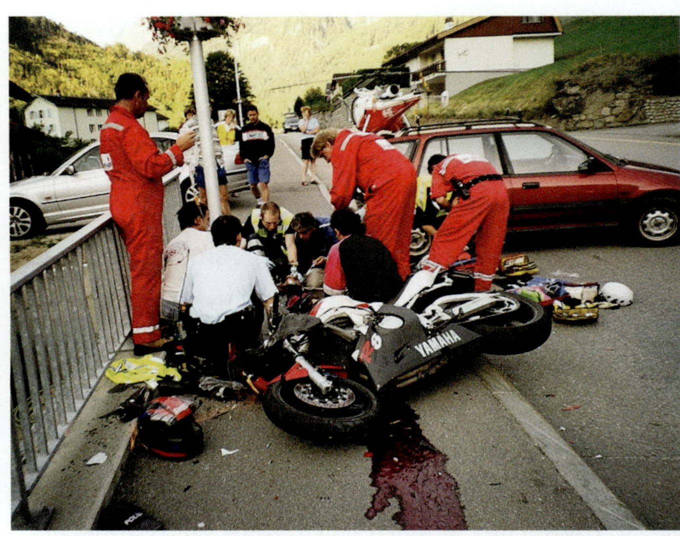

그림 3-11 이 오토바이 사고에서 환자에게 발생한 것처럼 대량 출혈은 빠르게 쇼크로 이어질 수 있다.

Photograph provided courtesy of Air Glaciers, Switzerland.

실을 나타낸다. 혈액 손실이 이 단계에 도달하면 대부분 환자는 더 이상 손실된 혈액량을 보상할 수 없으며 저혈압이 발생하고 쇼크 지수는 >1.0이다. 쇼크의 전형적인 소견이 명백하며 빈맥(심박수 120회~140회/분 이상), 빠른 호흡(호흡수 30~40회/분) 그리고 심한 불안이나 혼란이 포함되고 소변 배출량은 시간당 5~15mL로 감소한다. 이 환자 중 다수는 적절한 소생술과 출혈을 조절하기 위해 적어도 한 번의 수혈과 외과적 중재가 필요하다.

4. 4단계 출혈은 혈액량의 40% 이상(2,000mL 초과)의 손실을 나타낸다. 이 정도의 출혈은 빈맥(심박수 140회/분 초과), 빠른 호흡(호흡수 35회/분 초과), 심각한 혼란 또는 기면 그리고 수축기 혈압(일반적으로 60mmHg 범위)이 많이 감소한 것이 특징이다. 이 환자는 몇 분밖에 생존할 수 없다(**그림 3-11**). 생존은 즉각적인 출혈 조절(내부출혈을 위한 수술)과 1시간 이내에 3단위(units) 이상의 농축 적혈구(PRBC) 투여로 정의되는 대량 수혈을 포함한 혈액 및 혈액제제를 통한 적극적인 소생술 또는 24시간 이내에 10단위 이상의 농축 적혈구 투여로 정의되는 적극적인 소생술에 달려있다.

환자가 쇼크를 일으키는 속도는 혈액이 순환에서 얼마나 빨리 손실되는지에 달려 있다. 혈액이 손실된 외상 출혈이 있는 환자는 출혈의 원인을 해결해야 하며 심각한 출혈이 발생한 경우 수혈을 해야 한다. 손실된 체액은 산소 운반 능력이 있는 적혈구, 혈소판, 응고 인자

및 삼투압을 유지하는 단백질 등 다양한 구성 요소를 모두 포함하는 전혈이다.

전혈 또는 혈액제제는 일반적으로 병원 전 환경에서 사용할 수 없다. 따라서 현장에서 출혈쇼크에 빠진 외상 환자를 처치할 때 병원 전 처치 제공자는 외부출혈을 조절하고 최소 전해질 용액을 정맥 내로 투여하면서 혈장 및 응고 인자를 사용할 수 있고 출혈을 지혈할 수 있는 병원으로 신속하게 이송한다. 트라넥삼산(TXA)은 출혈을 조절하기 위해 수년 동안 사용되어 왔으며 혈전 안정제로 최근 병원 전 환경에서 사용하기 시작했다. 트라넥삼산은 플라스미노겐에 결합하여 플라스미노겐이 플라스민이 되는 것을 방지하여 혈전에서 피브린이 분해되는 것을 방지한다.

이전의 쇼크 연구에서는 손실된 혈액 1L당 3L의 전해질 용액을 투여하는 것을 권장했다. 생리식염수나 락테이트 링거액과 같은 결정질 용액을 투여하면 투여한 용액량의 1/4~1/3 정도만 투여 후 30~60분 동안 혈관 내 공간에 남아 있기 때문에 필요하다고 생각되었다.

최근의 쇼크 연구는 혈액제제 투여 전에 제한된 양의 전해질 용액을 투여하는 것이 병원으로 이송 중 올바른 처치 방법이라는 이해에 초점을 맞추고 있다. 결정질 용액을 너무 많이 투여하면 사이질액(부종)이 증가하여 남은 적혈구와 조직 세포로의 산소 전달이 잠재적으로 손상될 수 있다. 처치의 목표는 혈압을 정상 수준으로 높이는 것이 아니라 관류를 유지하고 산소화된 적혈구를 심장, 뇌, 폐로 계속

해서 공급하는 것이다. 혈압을 정상 수준으로 올리는 것은 응고 인자를 희석하고 형성된 응고를 방해하며 오히려 출혈을 증가시키는 역할만할 수 있다.

출혈쇼크를 처치하기 위해 일반적으로 선호하는 결정질 용액은 락테이트 링거액이다. 체액량 대체에 사용되는 또 다른 등장성 결정질 용액은 0.9% 생리식염수이다. 그러나 이 용액을 투여하면 고염소혈증(혈중 염화 농도 증가)을 일으켜 대량 수액 소생술이 산증을 유발할 수 있다. 노모솔(Normosol)과 플라즈마-라이트는 전해질의 혈장 농도와 더 밀접하게 일치하는 균형 잡힌 식염수의 예이지만, 비용을 증가시킬 수도 있다.

출혈이 심한 경우 최적의 대체 수액은 가능한 한 전혈에 가까운 것이 이상적이다. 첫 번째 단계는 농축 적혈구와 혈장을 1:1 또는 1:2 비율로 투여하는 것이다. 필요에 따라 혈소판, 동결침전물 또는 기타 응고인자를 추가한다. 혈장에는 작은 혈관에서 출혈을 조절하는 데 필요한 많은 응고 인자와 기타 성분이 포함되어 있다. 응고 연쇄 반응에는 13개의 확인된 인자가 있다(**그림 3-12**). 많은 양의 혈액 대체가 필요한 대량 출혈 환자의 경우 대부분의 인자가 손실되기 때문에 혈장 수혈이 신뢰할 수 있는 처치이다. 대량 출혈이 발생하면 큰 혈관의 출혈을 조절하기 위해서는 수술적 처치가 필요하거나 때에 따라 결정적인 처치를 위해 코일이나 응고용 스펀지를 혈관 내에 삽입해야 한다.

분포(혈관성) 쇼크

분포 쇼크 또는 혈관성 쇼크는 체액량이 비례적으로 증가 없이 혈관의 지름이 확장될 때 발생한다. 이 쇼크 유형은 일반적으로 급성 외상 후 척수 손상을 입은 환자에게 나타난다.

신경성 쇼크

신경성 쇼크 또는 더 적절하게는 신경성 저혈압은 척수 손상이 교감신경계 경로를 방해할 때 발생한다. 이것은 일반적으로 목뼈나 가슴 상부의 손상과 관련이 있다. 혈관 벽의 민무늬근육을 조절하는 혈관계의 교감신경 조절의 상실로 인해 손상 부위 아래의 말초혈관이 확장된다. 전신 혈관 저항의 현저한 감소는 말초혈관 확장을 유발한다. 신경성 쇼크 환자는 혈량저하가 아니다. 정상적인 혈액량은 확장된 혈관 지름을 채우기에 불충분하다.

신경성 쇼크에서 조직 산소화는 일반적으로 적절하게 유지되고 (평균 동맥압 > 65) 혈압이 낮더라도 혈류는 정상으로 유지된다(신경

성 저혈압). 또한 에너지 생산은 신경성 저혈압에서도 적절하게 유지된다.

비보상성 저혈량 쇼크와 신경성 저혈압은 모두 수축기 혈압을 감소시킨다. 그러나 그 외의 활력징후와 임상 징후는 물론 각 질환에 대한 처치 방법이 다르다(**표 3-3**). 저혈량 쇼크는 감소한 수축기 및 이완기 혈압과 좁은 맥압이 특징이다. 신경성 저혈압도 수축기와 이완기 혈압이 감소하지만, 맥압은 정상으로 유지되거나 넓어진다. 혈량저하증은 차갑고 축축하며 창백하거나 청색증인 피부와 모세혈관 재충전 시간이 지연된다. 신경성 저혈압에서 환자는 특히 손상 부위 아래가 따뜻하고 건조한 피부를 나타낸다. 저혈량 쇼크 환자의 맥박은 약하고 가늘며 빠르다. 신경성 저혈압 환자의 경우 부교감신경의 활동으로 인해 빈맥보다 일반적으로 서맥을 보이지만 맥박의 질은 약할 수 있다. 혈량저하증은 의식 수준(LOC) 감소 또는 불안이 종종 공격성을 유발한다. 외상성 뇌손상(TBI)이 없는 경우 신경성 저혈압 환자는 바로누운자세에서 일반적으로 의식이 명료하고 정상적인 지남력을 보인다(**Box 3-2**).

신경성 저혈압 환자는 종종 심각한 출혈을 일으키는 관련된 손상이 있다. 따라서 신경성 저혈압과 혈량저하증의 잠재적인 징후 또는 저혈압 이외의 쇼크 징후가 있는 환자는 먼저 출혈이 있는 것으로 간주해 처치해야 한다. 혈압상승제로 혈압을 안정화하는 것이 도움이 될 수 있지만, 출혈 원인을 해결하기 위해 적절한 수액 소생술을 확인한 후에 이를 고려해야 한다.

심장성 쇼크

심장성 쇼크 또는 혈액을 공급하는 심장의 기능 장애는 내인성(심장 자체의 직접 적인 손상 결과)과 외인성(심장 외부의 문제와 관련)으로 분류되는 원인으로 인해 발생한다.

내인성 원인

심장근육 손상

심장근육을 손상하는 모든 손상은 심박출량에 영향을 미칠 수 있다. 손상은 심장근육에 직접적인 타박상으로 인해 발생할 수 있다(심장 타박상을 유발하는 무딘 심장 손상에서와 같이). 이러한 유형의 손상에서는 반복적인 주기가 뒤따른다. 산소공급 감소는 수축력 감소를 유발하여 심탁출량 감소로 이어져 전신 관류 감소를 초래한다. 감소한 관류는 산소공급의 지속적인 감소를 초래하여 주기의 지속을 초

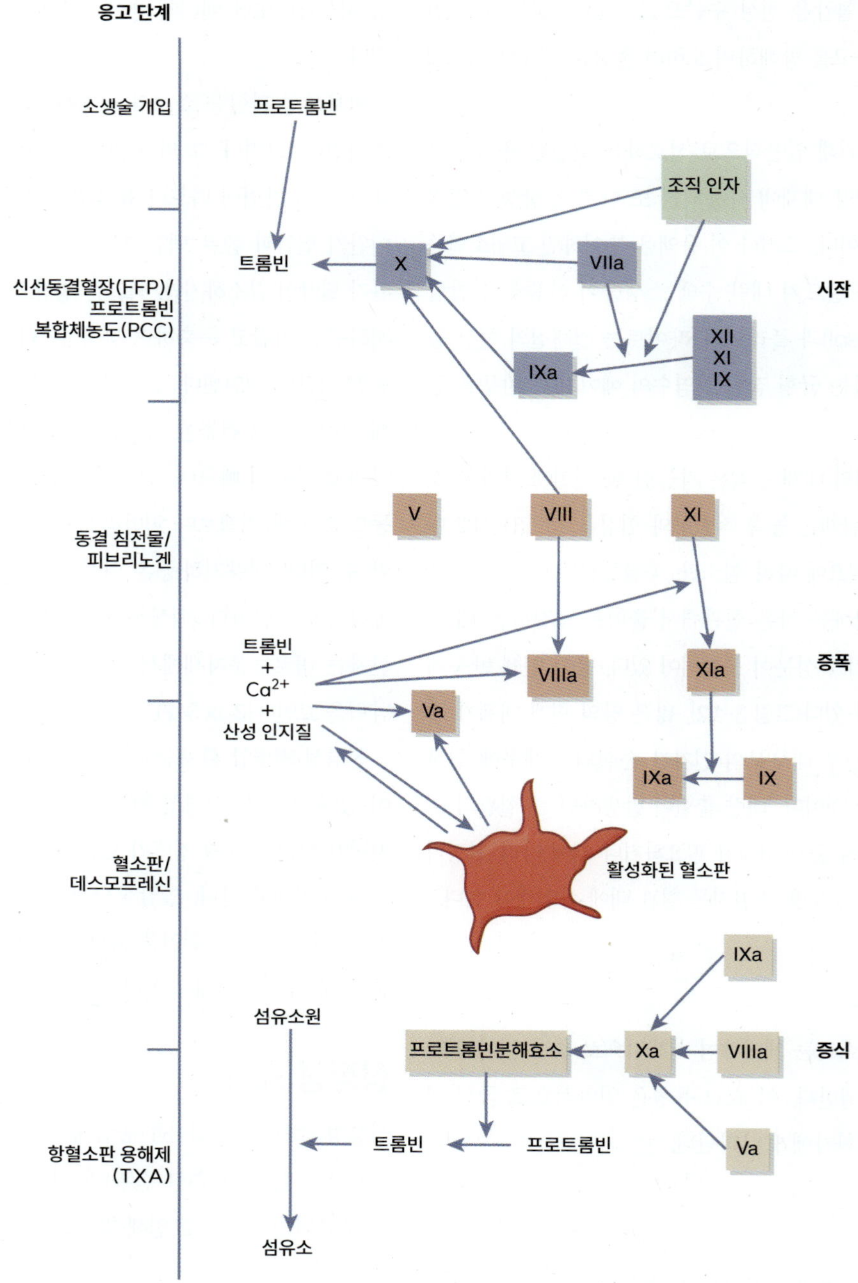

그림 3-12 응고 연쇄반응에 대한 현대적인 시각적 설명은 임상적 상관관계(소생술 처치)와 관련이 있다. 혈전은 시작, 증폭 및 전파의 세 단계를 통해 형성된다. 혈전 형성이 시작되면 다양한 응고 인자가 활성화되고 프로트롬빈이 트롬빈으로 전환된다. 혈전은 추가적인 응고 인자와 칼슘의 활성화로 증폭된다. 혈전이 전파됨에 따라 혈소판이 중심 역할을 하고 추가 응고 인자가 더 많은 트롬빈과 피브린 생성을 자극한다. 혈전은 결국 외상으로 인해 분해되고 때때로 너무 빨리 분해되어(섬유소 용해) 혈전 강도를 유지하기 위해 항섬유소 용해제(예: 트라넥삼산)가 필요하다. 응고 연쇄반응의 여러 단계에 해당하는 권장 소생술 중재술(즉 대체 혈액제제)이 나열된다.

Abbreviations: FFP, fresh frozen plasma; PCC, prothrombin complex concentrate.

표 3-3 쇼크의 유형과 관련된 징후			
활력징후	혈량저하	신경성 저혈압	심장성
피부 온도/상태	차고, 축축	따뜻하고, 건조	차고, 축축
피부색	창백, 청색증	분홍색	창백, 청색증
혈압	감소	감스	감소
의식수준	변화	명료함	변화
모세혈관 재충전 시간	느림	정상	느림

© National Association of Emergency Medical Technicians (NAEMT)

래한다. 다른 근육과 마찬가지로 심장근육도 타박상을 입거나 손상되면 효율적으로 작동하지 않는다.

판막 파열

가슴이나 복부에 갑작스럽고 강력한 압박을 가하면 심장판막이 손상될 수 있다. 심각한 판막 손상으로 인해 급성 판막 역류가 발생하여 상당량의 혈액이 심방이나 심실 내로 다시 흘러 들어간다. 이 환자들은 종종 폐부종과 심장성 쇼크로 나타나는 심부전으로 빠르게 악화한다. 새로운 심장잡음의 존재는 이 진단을 내리는 데 있어 중요한 단서이다.

외인성 원인

심장눌림증

심낭의 액체는 심장 주기의 확장기(이완) 동안 심장이 완전히 다시 채워지는 것을 방지한다. 외상의 경우 심장근육의 구멍에서 혈액이 심낭으로 유출된다. 심낭에 혈액이 축적되면서 심실 벽이 완전히 확장되는 것을 방지한다. 이는 심박출량에 두 가지 부정적인 영향을 미친다. 1) 심실이 완전히 팽창할 수 없기 때문에 매 수축에 사용할 수 있

는 혈액량이 줄어들고 2) 부적절한 충전은 심장근육의 확장을 감소시키고 심장 수축의 강도를 감소시킨다. 또한, 수축할 때마다 더 많은 혈액이 심장 손상 부위를 통해 심실 밖으로 밀려나고 심낭에 더 많은 혈액이 고여 심박출량이 더욱 감소시킨다(**그림 3-13**). 그 결과 심각한 쇼크와 사망이 빠르게 진행될 수 있다(자세한 내용은 10장 가슴 외상을 참고).

긴장기흉

가슴안의 어느 한쪽이라도 압력을 받는 공기로 채워지면 폐는 압축되어 허탈된다. 허탈된 폐는 코인두를 통해 외부로부터 공기를 다시 채울 수 없다. 이것은 적어도 네 가지 문제를 일으킨다. 1) 호흡할 때마다 일회호흡량이 감소하고 2) 허탈된 폐포가 적혈구로 산소를 전달할 수 없으며 3) 폐혈관이 허탈되어 폐와 심장으로의 혈류가 감소하고 4) 혈액이 폐혈관으로 내보내려면 더 강한 심장 수축력 필요하다(폐고혈압). 손상을 입은 가슴 내부의 공기량과 압력이 증가하게 되

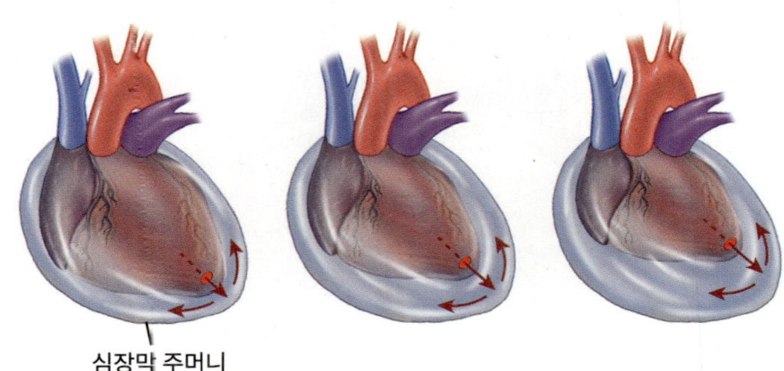

그림 3-13 심장눌림증. 심장근육의 구멍에서 심낭으로 혈액이 들어가면 심실의 확장이 제한된다. 따라서 심실을 완전히 채울 수 없다. 심낭에 더 많은 혈액이 축적되면 심실 공간이 줄어들어 심박출량이 감소한다.
© National Association of Emergency Medical Technicians (NAEMT)

면 세로칸이 손상 반대쪽으로 밀려난다. 세로칸이 이동함에 따라 반대쪽 폐는 압축되고 위대정맥과 아래대정맥의 압축 및 뒤틀림이 심장으로 들어오는 정맥혈복귀를 더욱 방해하여 전부하의 상당한 감소를 일으킨다(**그림 3-14**). 이 모든 요인은 심박출량을 감소시키고 쇼크가 빠르게 발생한다(자세한 내용은 10장 가슴 외상을 참고).

평가

쇼크의 유무에 대한 평가는 중요한 장기에 대한 혈액 관류 불량한 징후가 있는지 환자를 평가하는 것으로 시작된다. 이를 위해서는 병원 전 환경에서 즉시 접근할 수 있는 장기와 인체 계통에 대한 평가가 필요하다. 이러한 인체 계통에는 뇌와 중추신경계(CNS), 심장 및 심혈관계, 호흡계, 피부와 팔다리, 신장이 있다. 관류저하 및 에너지 생산의 감소 징후와 인체 반응은 다음과 같다.

- 의식 수준 감소, 불안, 지남력 상실, 기이한 행동(뇌 및 중추신경계)
- 빈맥, 수축기 혈압 및 맥압 감소(심장 및 심혈관계)
- 빠르고 얕은 호흡(호흡계)
- 차갑고 창백하며 축축한 피부, 발한이 있거나 모세혈관 재충전 시간 지연, 청색증 피부(피부 및 팔다리)
- 소변량 감소(신장), 병원 전 환경에서는 거의 확인하지 않지만, 도뇨

관이 적용된 환자를 이송 지연 또는 지연된 이송 상황에서 확인할 수 있음

출혈은 외상 환자에서 쇼크의 가장 흔한 원인이기 때문에 외상 환자의 저혈압은 달리 입증될 때까지 출혈로 인해 발생한 것으로 간주해야 한다. 출혈의 외부 원인을 검사하고 가능한 한 신속하고 완전하게 지혈하는 것이 최우선이다. 출혈을 조절하는 방법에는 직접 압박, 압박 드레싱, 골반 고정대, 지혈대 또는 팔다리 골절 부위 부목 고정 등이 있다.

외부출혈의 증거가 없다면 내부출혈을 의심해야 한다. 내부출혈의 적극적인 처치는 병원 전 환경에서 실용적이지 않으므로 내부출혈에 대한 원인을 확인하려면 결정적인 처치를 시행할 수 있는 의료기관으로 신속하게 이송해야 한다. 내부출혈은 가슴, 복부 또는 골반에서 발생할 수 있다. 호흡음 감소와 함께 무딘 손상이나 관통하는 가슴 손상의 증거는 가슴 손상을 시사한다. 복부, 골반(복막 내 또는 복막뒤공간)은 무딘 손상(반상출혈) 또는 관통상의 증거가 있는 출혈의 원인이 될 수 있다. 이러한 증거에는 복부 팽만 또는 압통, 골반의 불안정, 다리 길이의 차이, 움직임에 의해 악화하는 골반 부위의 통증, 회음부 반상출혈, 요도의 혈액이 포함된다. 일부 지역에서는 내부출혈의 징후를 평가하기 위해 외상 초음파 검사를 통한 확장된 집중 평가(eFAST)를 수행하기 위해 병원 전 초음파를 사용한다. 외상 초음파 검사를 통한 확장된 집중 평가는 무딘 손상 후 복막 내 체액(혈액) 또는 기흉과 일치하는 징후를 확인할 수 있다.

평가에서 출혈이 쇼크의 원인으로 확인되지 않으면 비출혈성 원인을 고려해야 한다. 여기에는 심장눌림증과 긴장기흉(두 가지 모두 목정맥 팽대가 발생하지만, 출혈쇼크에서는 목정맥 수축이 명백하게 발생) 또는 신경성 저혈압이 포함된다. 손상을 받은 가슴 쪽의 호흡음 감소, 피부밑기종, 호흡 곤란(빠른 호흡)과 기관편위(현장에서 거의 볼 수 없는 후기 소견)는 긴장기흉을 시사한다. 이러한 징후가 나타나면 손상된 가슴 쪽에 즉시 바늘감압이 필요하다는 것을 시사한다.

가슴의 무딘 손상 또는 관통상, 심장눌림증을 시사하는 심음 감소(시끄러운 병원 전 환경에서는 청진하기 어려움) 또는 부정맥과 같은 다양한 심장성 쇼크의 원인을 의심할 수 있다, 신경성 저혈압은 척추 손상, 서맥, 따뜻한 팔다리의 징후가 있는 경우 의심할 수 있다. 전부는 아니더라도 이러한 특징은 대부분은 쇼크의 원인과 현장에서 가능할 때 적절한 처치의 필요성을 결정할 수 있는 병원 전 처치 제공자에 의해 인지될 수 있다.

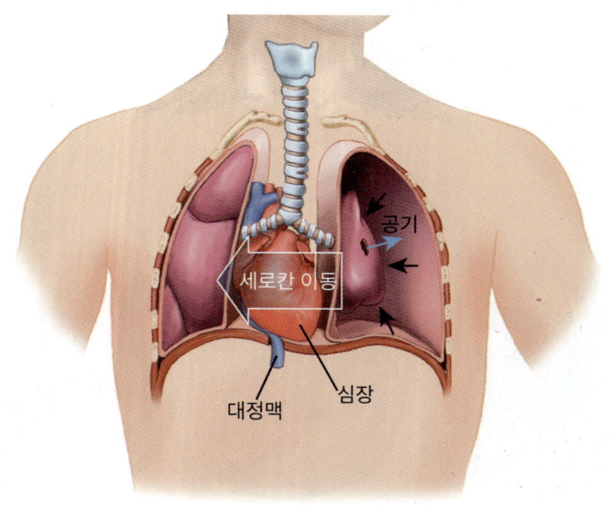

그림 3-14 긴장기흉. 가슴안에 갇힌 공기의 양이 계속 증가하면 영향을 받은 쪽의 폐가 허탈 될 뿐만 아니라 세로칸이 반대쪽으로 밀리게 된다. 세로칸이 밀려남은 대정맥을 통해 혈액이 심장으로 돌아가는 것을 방해하여 심박출량에 영향을 미치고 동시에 반대쪽 폐를 압박한다.

환자 평가 영역에는 기도 상태, 환기, 관류, 피부색 및 체온, 모세혈관 재충전 시간과 혈압이 포함된다. 각각의 내용은 일차평가와 이차평가의 내용에 별도로 제시된다. 동시 평가는 다양한 원인에서 신속하게 정보를 수집하고 처리하기 위한 환자 평가의 중요한 부분이다.

일차평가

환자 평가의 첫 번째 단계 중 하나는 환자의 상태를 가능한 한 빨리 초기 관찰하는 것이다. 다음 징후는 생명을 위협하는 상태를 의심해야 할 필요성을 나타내는 것이다.

- 경미한 불안, 혼란으로 진행 또는 의식 수준 변화
- 경미한 빠른 호흡에서 보조 호흡이 필요한 호흡으로 진행
- 경미한 빈맥에서 현저한 빈맥으로 진행
- 노동맥 약화, 노동맥이 촉지되지 않는 상태로 진행
- 창백하거나 청색증 피부색
- 모세혈관 재충전 시간 지연
- 팔다리의 맥박 소실
- 저체온증
- 갈증

일차평가를 계속하기 전에 기도, 호흡 또는 순환계의 손상이나 기능 상실을 처치해야 한다. 다음 단계는 순서대로 설명되어 있지만, 이러한 모든 평가는 거의 동시에 수행된다(**Box 3-3**, **Box 3-4**).

대량 출혈

심각한 동맥 손상으로 발생한 출혈은 몇 분 안에 환자를 사망하게 할 수 있으므로 이러한 유형의 출혈은 즉시 지혈해야 한다. 환자가 누워 있거나 옷으로 가려져 출혈의 주요 원인이 가려질 수 있다. 환자는 혈관이 밀집된 두피 열상이나 주요 혈관(빗장밑동맥, 겨드랑동맥, 위팔동맥, 노동맥, 자동맥, 목동맥, 넓적다리동맥, 오금동맥)의 손상으로 인해 많은 양의 혈액이 손실될 수 있다. 주요 혈관에서 발생한 심각한 출혈의 징후가 있는지 신속하게 확인하고 팔다리에 지혈대 적용, 두피의 압박 드레싱 또는 다른 처치가 불가능한 상처 봉합과 같은 적절한 처치를 시작한다.

기도

기도는 모든 환자에게서 신속하게 평가되어야 한다. 기도 확보는 인체의 세포에 적절한 양의 산소를 전달하는 데 필수적인 구성 요소이다. 즉각적인 기도 유지가 필요한 환자는 다음과 같다.

1. 호흡이 없는 환자
2. 명백한 기도 손상이 있는 환자

Box 3-4 MARCH

MARCH는 XABCD와 유사한 대체 환자 평가 약어로 외상 및 전술적 상황에서 근무하는 EMS 제공자가 사용한다. MARCH는 다음을 의미한다.

- **M-대량 출혈(Massive hemorrhage)**: 생명을 위협하는 출혈을 지혈대, 골반고정대, 지혈 드레싱 또는 기존의 압박 드레싱으로 지혈을 시행한다
- **A-기도(Airway)**: 기도 폐쇄 여부를 평가하고 자세 변경, 코인두기도기, 전문기도기 또는 외과적 기도 유지술을 이용하여 환자의 기도를 개방한다.
- **R-호흡(Respirations)**: 관통성 흉부 상처, 흡인성 흉부 상처 및 긴장기흉을 평가하고 처치한다.
- **C-순환(Circulation)**: 쇼크를 평가하고 처치한다. 정맥 또는 골내 경로를 확보하고 의학적으로 필요한 경우 수액 소생술을 시작한다.
- **H-머리/저체온증(Head/hypothermia)**: 저혈압, 저산소증 또는 두개내압 상승으로 인한 이차 뇌손상을 예방한다. 저체온증으로부터 환자를 보호한다. 열, 화학 물질 또는 독성 노출도 위험 요인이 될 수 있다. 주요 골절 부위에 부목을 적용하고 필요한 경우 환자에게 척추 고정을 시행한다.

MARCH 접근 방식은 EMS 제공자가 사용하는 외상 환자에 대한 환자 평가 약어인 XABCDE 접근 방식과 밀접하게 일치한다. 두 방식을 나란히 비교하면 다음과 같다.

Massive hemorrhage	e**X**sanguinating hemorrhage
Airway	**A**irway
Respirations	**B**reathing
Circulation	**C**irculation
Head/hypothermia	**D**isability
Expose/environment	

Box 3-3 XABCDE

외상 환자에 대한 일차평가는 첫 번째 단계로 생명을 위협하는 외부출혈의 지혈을 강조한다. 일차평가 단계를 순차적으로 학습하더라도 수행하더라도 추가 처치 제공자가 있는 경우 여러 단계를 동시에 수행할 수 있다. XABCDE를 사용하여 단계를 기억할 수 있다.

- **X**-중증 외부(대량)출혈 조절
- **A**-적절한 경우 기도 유지 및 목뼈 고정
- **B**-호흡(환기 및 산소공급)
- **C**-순환(관류 및 기타 출혈)
- **D**-장애
- **E**-노출/환경

3. 호흡 시 잡음이 심한 환자
4. 환기 속도가 현저하게 비정상적인 환자

호흡

감소한 세포 산소화와 관련이 있는 무산소대사는 젖산을 증가시킨다. 산중에서 생성된 수소 이온은 체내의 완충 시스템에 의해 물과 이산화탄소로 전환된다. 뇌의 감지 시스템은 이산화탄소량의 비정상적인 증가를 감지하고 호흡 중추를 자극하여 호흡 속도와 깊이를 증가시켜 이산화탄소를 제거한다. 따라서 빠른 호흡은 맥박수 증가보다 더 빠른 무산소대사와 쇼크의 초기 징후 중 하나인 경우가 많다. 일차평가에서 호흡 속도를 측정하기 위해 시간을 낭비하지 않는다. 대신 호흡은 느리거나, 정상이거나, 빠르거나 매우 빠르다고 추정해야 한다. 쇼크와 함께 느린 환기 속도는 일반적으로 환자가 심각한 쇼크 상태임을 나타내고 심정지가 발생할 수 있음을 나타낸다. 빠른 환기 속도는 문제이며 쇼크의 원인을 찾는 자극제 역할을 해야 한다. 또한 단순기흉이나 조기 심장눌림증과 같은 순전히 호흡기 문제의 징후일 수도 있다.

산소마스크를 제거하려는 환자는 특히 이러한 행동이 불안 및 혼란과 관련이 있을 때 뇌 허혈의 또 다른 징후를 보인다. 이 환자는 공기 부족을 보이며 더 많은 환기가 필요하다고 느낀다. 코와 입 위에 마스크가 있으면 환기가 제한되는 느낌이 든다. 이는 환자가 충분한 산소를 공급받지 못하고 있고 저산소혈증이라는 단서가 되어야 한다.

맥박산소측정기로 측정한 산소포화가 감소하면 저산소혈증을 확인한다. 맥박산소측정기로 측정한 산소포화도가 94% 미만인 경우 저산소혈증의 원인을 확인해야 한다. 기관내삽관과 같은 기도 처치를 받은 환자는 호기말이산화탄소분압(ETCO$_2$) 측정 및 지속적인 모니터링은 응급 환자에게 기관내삽관과 같은 방법으로 기도를 유지한 후 확인하는 일반적인 방법이다. 호기말이산화탄소분압과 동맥혈이산화탄소분압(PaCO$_2$)은 관류가 정상적일 경우 연관성이 있지만, 쇼크 상태의 환자에게서는 연관성이 낮음으로 호흡을 평가하는 데 유용성이 제한된다. 호기말이산화탄소분압을 모니터링하는 것은 관류 변화를 감지하는 데 도움이 될 수 있다.

항상 환자의 외모와 관련하여 기계의 판독값을 평가하는 것을 항상 기억하는 것이 중요하다. 환자의 외견상 저산소호혈증이 의심되는 경우 기계의 결과와 다르더라도 저산소소혈증에 대해 환자를 처치한다.

예를 들어, 환자가 비보상성 쇼크 상태라면 말초맥박산소포화도 측정값을 신뢰할 수 없다. 병원 전 환경에서는 일반적으로 중심맥박산소측정을 사용할 수 없으므로 병원 전 처치 제공자가 파형 산소측정기를 사용하여 신뢰성을 결정해야 한다. 이때 파형은 각 맥박과 일치해야 한다.

순환

순환 평가의 두 가지 구성 요소는 다음과 같다.
- 출혈 및 실혈량
- 산소화된 혈액으로 관류
  - 전신
  - 인체의 각 부위

순환 평가 중에 축적된 정보는 환자의 총혈액량과 관류 상태를 초기에 신속하게 결정하는 데 도움이 되며 이차적으로 인체의 특정 부위에 대한 유사한 평가를 시행한다. 예를 들어, 모세혈관 재충전 시간을 확인할 때 맥박, 피부색 및 다리의 체온은 관류 저하를 나타낼 수 있지만, 팔에서는 같은 징후가 정상일 수 있다. 이 불일치는 징후가 부정확하다는 것을 의미하는 것이 아니라 한 부분이 다른 부분과 다르다는 것이다. 즉시 대답해야 할 질문은 "왜?"이다. 인체의 한 부분 이상에서 다음과 같은 순환 및 관류 소견이 있는지 확인하고 전체 신체 상태의 평가가 한 부위를 기준으로 해서는 안 된다는 점을 기억하다.

출혈

관류를 회복하려는 노력은 지속해서 출혈되는 상황에서 덜 효과적이거나 완전히 비효율적이다. 중증 외부출혈은 일차평가에서 최우선으로 조절해야 한다. 병원 전 처치 제공자는 주요 출혈이 잘 조절되고 있는지 확인하고 추가 출혈의 원인을 찾기 위해 재평가해야 한다.

출혈은 적혈구의 손실과 그에 따른 산소 운반 능력의 손실을 의미한다. 따라서 출혈이 있는 환자는 환자가 가지고 있는 혈액에 산소가 포함되어 있어서 산소포화도가 정상으로 측정될 수 있지만, 전체 산소 공급은 신체의 모든 세포에 산소를 공급하기에 불충분하여 저산소중이 발생한다.

맥박

관류에 대한 다음 중요한 평가하는 맥박이다. 맥박의 초기 평가는 평가 중인 동맥에서 만져지는지를 결정한다. 일반적으로 노동맥이 촉진되지 않으면 중증 혈량저하증(또는 팔의 혈관 손상)을 의미하며, 특히 목동맥이나 넓적다리동맥과 같은 중심 동맥의 맥박이 약하고 가늘며 매우 빨리 뛰는 것은 전신 순환계 상태 저하를 나타낸다. 맥박이 촉진되면 다음과 같이 특징과 강도를 기록해야 한다.

- 맥박이 강한가? 아니면 약하고 가는가?
- 맥박수가 정상인이거나 너무 빠르거나 너무 느린가?
- 맥박이 규칙적인가? 아니면 불규칙적인가?

외상 환자 처치에서 대부분의 병원 전 처치 제공자들이 환자의 혈압에 초점을 맞추고 있지만, 일차평가에서 정확한 혈압을 측정하기 위해 귀중한 시간을 소비해서는 안 된다. 일차평가에서 혈압의 정확한 수치는 다른 쇼크의 초기 징후보다 훨씬 덜 중요하다. 중요한 정보는 맥박수와 그 특징으로 판단할 수 있다. 한 일련의 외상 환자에서 병원 전 처치 제공자가 맥박이 약하다고 평가한 것은 노동맥박은 정상으로 생각되는 맥박보다 평균 26mmHg 낮은 혈압과 관련이 있었다. 더 중요한 것은 노동맥 맥박이 약한 외상 환자는 정상 맥박을 가진 환자보다 사망할 확률이 15배 더 높다는 것이다. 일반적으로 이차평가를 시작할 때 혈압을 측정하지만, 충분한 처치 제공자가 있거나 일차평가를 완료 후 이송 중에 생명을 위협하는 문제가 해결되면 환자 평가 초기에 혈압을 촉진이나 청진으로 측정할 수 있다.

의식 수준

정신 상태는 신경학적 평가의 일부이지만, 정신 상태 변화는 관류 감소로 인한 뇌 산소 공급 장애를 나타낼 수 있다. 정신 상태 평가는 말초 장기의 관류와 기능에 대한 평가를 나타낸다. 불안하고 혼란스러운 환자는 다른 원인이 확인될 때까지 뇌 허혈과 무산소대사를 하는 것으로 가정해야 한다. 약물과 알코올 과다복용, 외상성 뇌손상은 신속하게 처치할 수 없는 상태지만, 뇌 허혈은 처치할 수 있다.

저산소혈증과 관류 감소의 존재에 대한 우려 외에도 정신 상태 변화는 외상성 뇌손상(TBI)을 시사한다. 저산소혈증이나 혈압 감소 및 외상성 뇌손상은 환자 생존에 심각한 부정적인 영향을 미친다. 13,000건이 넘는 외상성 뇌손상 사례에 관한 연구에서 저혈압 또는 저산소혈증은 사망할 확률의 증가와 관련이 있으며 두 가지 모두 존재하면 40% 이상의 사망률과 관련이 있다. 같은 연구자의 후속 연구에서 저산소혈증 및 저혈압 예방을 목표로 하는 병원 전 지침을 시행하면 중증 손상을 입은 외상성 뇌손상 환자의 생존에 도움이 된다는 것이 입증되었다. 따라서 병원 전 처치 제공자들은 외상성 뇌손상 환자의 저혈압과 저산소혈증을 예방하기 위해 노력해야 한다.

피부색

창백하거나 얼룩덜룩한 피부는 산소가 공급되지 않은 헤모글로빈과 말초에 적절한 산소 공급 부족을 나타낸다. 창백한 피부, 얼룩덜룩한 피브 또는 청색증 피부는 다음 세 가지 원인 중 하나로 인해 부적절한 혈류의 결과이다.

1. 말초혈관 수축(대부분 혈량저하증과 관련됨)
2. 적혈구 공급 감소(급성 빈혈)
3. 골절이나 혈관 손상으로 인한 인체 부위로의 혈액 공급 중단

창백한 피부는 다른 의미가 있는 국소적이거나 일반적인 소견일 수 있다. 빈맥과 같은 다른 소견은 이러한 차이를 해결하고 창백한 피부가 국소적 변화인지 전신적인 변화인지 여부를 결정해야 한다. 또한 청색증은 출혈로 인해 상당한 수의 적혈구가 소실된 저산소중 환자에게서 발생하지 않을 수 있다. 피부색이 짙은 환자의 경우 피부에서 청색증을 발견하기 어려울 수 있지만, 입술, 손바닥, 잇몸, 손발톱바닥 등에서 확인할 수 있다.

체온

신체 중요 부위에 혈액을 공급하기 위해 피부로 가는 혈액이 감소하면서 피부 온도가 낮아진다. 촉진할 때 차가운 피부는 혈관수축, 피부 관류 감소, 에너지 생산 감소, 쇼크를 나타낸다. 평가 단계에서 상당한 양의 열이 손실될 수 있으므로 환자의 체온을 유지하기 위해 조처를 해야 한다.

체온을 측정하는 환경 조건은 관류에 영향을 미칠 수 있으며 손상과 마찬가지고 결과에 영향을 미칠 수 있다. 따라서 이 평가의 결과는 전체 상황의 맥락에서 평가되어야 한다.

피부 상태

피부색과 체온 외에도 피부가 건조한지 또는 축축한지 피부 상태를 평가한다. 혈량저하증으로 인해 쇼크 상태의 외상 환자는 일반적으로 축축한 피부 상태를 나타낸다. 대조적으로 척수 손상으로 의한 저혈압 환자는 일반적으로 피부가 건조하다.

모세혈관 재충전 시간

모세혈관에서 혈액이 제거된 후 다시 혈액을 채우는 심혈관계의 능력은 중요한 지원 시스템을 나타낸다. 혈액을 제거하기 위해 모세혈관을 압축한 다음 재충전 시간을 측정하여 모세혈관의 관류를 평가할 수 있다. 일반적으로 인체는 가장 원위부의 순환을 먼저 차단하고 이 순환을 마지막에 회복시킨다. 엄지손가락이나 손발톱바닥을 평가하

면 관류저하가 발생하고 있는 조기 징후를 알 수 있다. 또한 소생술이 적절하게 진행되고 있는지를 평가할 수 있는 지표이다. 그런데도 환경적 및 생리학적 여건이 결과를 반영할 수 있다. 모세혈관 재충전 시간 측정은 피부를 재관류하는 데 필요한 시간이므로 인체의 해당 부분에 대한 실제 관류를 간접적으로 평가하는 것이다. 특정 질환이나 손상에 대한 진단검사는 아니다.

모세혈관 재충전 시간은 부정확한 쇼크 검사로 설명됐다. 그러나 이것은 쇼크 검사가 아니라 모세혈관 관류를 평가하는 검사이다. 평가의 다른 검사 및 구성 요소와 함께 사용하면 관류의 좋은 지표이며 쇼크를 암시하지만, 이는 단일 정보일 뿐이며 전반적인 상황과 환경 전체를 이해해야 한다.

쇼크는 관류 불량 및 모세혈관 재충전 지연의 원인일 수 있지만, 골절로 인한 동맥 절단, 관통상(총상 등)으로 인한 혈관 손상, 저체온증, 심지어 동맥경화와 같은 다른 원인도 있다. 모세혈관 재충전 불량의 또 다른 원인은 혈량저하증(출혈 제외)으로 인한 심박출량 감소이다.

모세혈관 재충전 시간은 소생술 또는 쇼크의 진행 상태를 모니터링하는 데 도움이 되는 진단 징후이다. 환자의 소생술이 긍정적으로 진행되고 환자의 상태가 호전되면 모세혈관 재충전 시간도 개선된다.

장애

현장에서 쉽게 평가할 수 있는 인체 시스템 중 하나가 뇌 기능이다. 다음과 같은 최소 6가지 조건이 외상 환자의 의식 수준 또는 행동(전투적이거나 공격적) 변화를 일으킬 수 있다.

1. 저산소혈증
2. 뇌졸중
3. 뇌 관류 장애를 동반한 쇼크
4. 외상성 뇌손상(TBI)
5. 알코올, 약물 또는 독극물 중독
6. 당뇨병, 발작, 자간증과 같은 대사 과정

이 6가지 상태 중에서 처치하기 가장 쉽고 처치하지 않으면 환자를 가장 빨리 사망에 이르게 하는 상태는 저산소혈증이다. 의식 수준이 변화된 환자는 뇌에 산소 공급 감소가 원인인 것처럼 처치해야 한다. 변경된 의식 수준은 일반적으로 눈에 보이는 첫 번째 쇼크 징후 중 하나이다. 외상성 뇌손상은 일차 손상(뇌 조직에 대한 직접적인 외상으로 인해 발생) 또는 이차(저산소혈증, 관류저하, 부종, 에너지 생산 손실 등의 영향으로 발생) 손상으로 간주할 수 있다. 일차 뇌손상에 대한 병원 전 환경에서 효과적인 처치는 없지만, 이차 뇌손상은 산소 공급과 관류를 유지함으로써 예방하거나 현저하게 감소시킬 수 있다.

관류 및 산소 공급이 감소하고 허혈이 발생함에 따라 뇌의 기능이 감소한다. 이 감소한 뇌 기능은 뇌의 다른 부위가 영향을 받으면서 다양한 단계를 거쳐 발달한다. 불안과 공격적인 행동이 일반적으로 첫 번째 나타나는 징후이며 사고 과정이 느려지고 인체의 운동 및 감각기능이 감소한다. 뇌 기능 수준은 중요하고 측정할 수 있는 병원 전 쇼크 징후이다. 공격적이고 전투적이며 불안한 환자 또는 의식 수준이 감소한 환자는 다른 원인이 확인될 때까지 저산소증, 뇌의 관류저하가 있는 것으로 가정해야 한다. 관류저하 및 뇌 저산소혈증은 종종 뇌손상을 동반하며 장기적인 결과를 더욱 악화시킨다. 저산소혈증과 일시적인 쇼크 과정도 원래의 뇌손상을 악화시키고 더 나쁜 결과를 초래할 수 있다.

노출/환경

환자의 신체는 덜 분명한 외부출혈 부위와 내부출혈을 나타내는 단서가 있는지 평가하기 위해 노출한다. 저체온증의 가능성도 고려한다. 이 노출은 추운 환경으로부터 환자를 보호할 수 있는 가온된 구급차의 따뜻한 환자실에서 가장 잘 수행할 수 있다.

이차평가

어떤 경우에는 쇼트의 징후가 있는 경우 현장에서 이차평가를 완료하는 데 시간을 소비하지 않는다. 시간이 허락하고 다른 문제를 해결할 필요가 없다면 의료기관으로 이송하는 중에 이차평가를 수행할 수 있다.

활력징후

활력징후의 측정은 이차평가의 첫 번째 단계 중 하나이거나 일차평가를 재평가한 후 환자를 의료기관으로 이송하는 중에 몇 분 동안 여유가 있을 때 수행할 수 있다.

환기 속도

성인의 정상 환기 속도는 분당 10~20회이다. 이 속도는 나이에 따라 달라진다(14장 소아 외상을 참고). 호흡수가 분당 20~30회인 경우는 정상과 비정상의 경계선을 나타내며 이는 쇼크의 시작과 산소 공급이 필요하다는 것을 의미한다. 분당 30회 이상의 호흡수는 쇼크의 후기 단계이며 보조 환기가 필요하다는 것을 나타낸다. 쇼크에 의한 산증은 생리적으로 호흡수를 증가시키지만, 일반적으로 일회호흡량 감소와 관련이 있다. 이러한 환기 속도는 둘 다 관류 장애의 잠재적인 원인을 찾아야 함을 나타낸다. 호기말이산화탄소분압 모니터링을 통해 정확한 환기 속도를 얻을 수 있다.

맥박

이차평가에서는 맥박수를 더 정확하게 측정한다. 성인의 정상 맥박수는 분당 60~100회이다. 운동선수를 제외하고 맥박수가 느린 것은 심장 허혈, 약물 또는 완전심장차단(CHB)과 같은 병리학적 상태를 고려해야 한다. 맥박수가 분당 100~120회인 경우 빈맥의 초기 심장 반응과 함께 조기 쇼크가 있는지 환자를 확인한다. 맥박수가 분당 120회 이상이면 통증이나 공포가 원인이 아닌 한 쇼크의 확실한 징후이며 분당 140회 이상이면 치명적인 것으로 간주한다.

혈압

혈압은 쇼크의 가장 덜 민감한 쇼크의 징후 중 하나이다. 혈압은 환자가 심각한 혈량저하 상태(실제 체액 손실이나 상대적 혈량저하증)가 될 때까지 혈압이 떨어지기 시작하지 않는다. 혈압 감소하는 것은 환자가 혈량저하증과 관류저하를 더 이상 효과적으로 보상할 수 없음을 나타낸다. 달리 건강한 환자의 경우 보상 기전이 실패하고 수축기 혈압이 90mmHg 미만으로 떨어지기 전에 혈액량의 30%를 초과하는 출혈이 발생할 수 있다. 이러한 이유로 환기 속도, 맥박 및 특징, 모세혈관 재충전 시간, 의식 수준 및 쇼크지수는 혈압보다 혈량저하증의 더 민감한 지표이다.

환자의 혈압이 감소하기 시작하면 매우 심각한 상황이 발생하므로 신속한 처치가 필요하다. 병원 전 환경에서 환자가 저혈압으로 판단되면 이미 상당한 양의 혈액을 손실했으며 지속적인 출혈이 있을 가능성이 높다. 쇼크의 첫 징후로 저혈압이 발생한다는 것은 초기 징후가 간과되었을 수 있음을 의미한다.

상황의 심각성과 적절한 처치는 상태의 원인에 따라 다르다. 예를 들어, 신경성 저혈압과 관련된 저혈압은 저혈량 쇼크로 인한 저혈압보다 치명적이지 않다. **표 3-4**는 보상성 및 비보상성 저혈량 쇼크를 평가하는 데 사용되는 징후를 보여준다.

피해야 할 중요한 위험은 수축기 혈압과 심박출량 및 조직 관류를 동일시하는 것이다. 앞에서 강조한 바와 같이 환자에게 저혈압(3단계 출혈)이 발생하기 전에 일반적으로 상당한 출혈이 발생한다. 따라서 환자는 수축기 혈압이 정상임에도 불구하고 혈액량이 15~30% 감소하면 심박출량이 감소하고 조직의 산소 공급이 저하된다. 이상적으로는 비보상성 쇼크가 발생하기 전에 초기 단계에서 쇼크를 인식하고 처치한다.

오류의 또 다른 가능한 원인은 한 번 측정한 저혈압 측정값을 신뢰하지 않는 것이다. 혈압 측정을 반복하면 보상 기전의 일부로 혈압이 정상으로 돌아올 수 있다. 또한, 비침습적 커프는 여러 번 반복적으로 혈압 측정을 시도한 후에는 정확한 판독 값을 생성할 수 없다. 이 두 가지 문제는 달리 입증될 때까지 고려해야 한다. 뇌손상은 뇌탈출이 발생하기 전까지 저혈압을 유발하지 않는다. 따라서 뇌손상과 저혈압이 있는 환자는 뇌손상이 아닌 다른 손상으로 인한 혈량저하증(일반적으로 출혈)이 있다고 가정해야 한다. 하지만 영아(6개월 미만)는 개방된 봉합선과 숫구멍으로 인해 머리 내부에 많은 양의 출혈을 수용할 수 있으므로 저혈량 쇼크를 일으킬 수 있다.

미래의 모니터링 기능

현재 연구에서는 급성 손상 환자를 처치하는 데 도움이 되는 생리학적 모니터링 기능을 확인했다. 이러한 발전은 신체 평가 능력을 대체

표 3-4 보상성 및 비보상성 저혈량 쇼크에서의 쇼크 평가

활력징후	보상성	비보상성
맥박	증가; 빈맥	매우 증가: 빈맥에서 서맥으로 진행할 수 있음
피부	창백, 차갑고 축축한	창백, 차갑고, 밀랍 같은
혈압 범위	정상	감소
의식수준	변화 없음	변화, 지남력 상실에서 혼수상태에 이르기까지 변화됨

하는 것이 아니라 능력을 향상할 것으로 예상된다. 초음파를 사용하여 체액 상태를 확인하고 조직 산소화를 모니터링, 쇼크 지수 및 보상 예비 지수를 모니터링하는 것은 미래에 병원 전 환경에서 처치 제공자의 평가 능력을 발전하는 방법이다.

보상 예비력은 혈액 손실을 보상할 수 있는 신체의 능력을 나타낸다. 보상 예비 측정(CRM) 장치는 심장이 수축할 때마다 환자의 동맥 파형을 비침습적으로 모니터링하고 임박한 보상실패를 예측할 수 있는 순환 혈액량의 지속적인 변화를 예측할 수 있다. 인간을 대상으로 한 실험실 실험에서 보상 예비 측정은 심박수, 혈압, 호흡수, 쇼크지수, 호기말이산화탄소분압, 혈중 산소포화도의 변화보다 민감도가 더 높은 것으로 나타났다. 임상 연구에서 얻은 데이터는 보상 예비 측정이 환자의 볼륨 상태에 대한 조기 경고 징후가 있는 외상 환자의 쇼크를 평가하는 정확한 방법을 제공한다는 것을 시사한다.

근골격 손상

골절 특히 다발성 골절의 경우 심각한 내부출혈이 발생할 수 있다. 넓적다리뼈와 골반 골절은 가장 큰 영향을 미친다. 골반 골절, 특히 심각한 추락이나 으깸 손상 기전으로 인한 골절은 복막뒤공간으로 대량의 내부출혈과 관련이 있다. 개방골절은 상당한 외부 및 내부출혈과 관련될 수 있지만, 주어진 골절에 대한 혈액 손실량을 뒷받침하는 데이터는 부족하다. 무딘 손상 환자는 다발성 골절과 3단계 또는 4단계 출혈이 있을 수 있지만, 외부출혈, 혈액가슴증, 복강 내 출혈, 골반 골절의 증거는 없다. 예를 들어, 성인 보행자가 차량에 치여 4개의 갈비뼈 골절과 위팔뼈 골절, 넓적다리뼈 골절, 양쪽 정강뼈와 종아리뼈 골절이 있는 경우 이를 인식하지 못하고 부적절하게 처치할 경우 환자가 쇼크로 사망할 정도로 상당한 내부출혈이 발생할 수 있다.

혼동 요인

수많은 요인이 외상 환자의 평가를 혼란스럽게 할 수 있으며 일반적인 쇼크의 징후를 모호하게 하거나 무뎌지게 할 수 있다. 이러한 요인은 부주의한 병원 전 처치 제공자가 외상 환자가 안정적이라고 잘못 생각하게 할 수 있다.

나이

삶의 극한 상황에 처한 환자(신생아)와 노인은 급성 출혈이나 쇼크 상태를 보상할 수 있는 능력이 감소한다. 건강한 성인에게는 어려움

없이 견딜 수 있는 상대적으로 경미한 손상이 이러한 개인에게는 비보상성 쇼크를 유발할 수 있다. 이와는 대조적으로 소아와 젊은 성인은 출혈을 보상할 수 있는 엄청난 능력이 있으며 신속한 검사에서 정상으로 보일 수 있다. 그들은 갑자기 비보상성 쇼크로 악화할 때까지 정상적인 것처럼 보인다. 환자를 자세히 살펴보면 경미한 빈맥, 빠른 호흡, 모세혈관 재충전 시간 지연, 창백한 피부, 불안과 같은 미묘한 쇼크의 징후가 나타날 수 있다. 강력한 보상 기전으로 인해 비보상성 쇼크 상태에서 발견된 소아는 심각한 응급 상황을 나타낸다. 노인 환자는 급성신부전과 같은 장기간 쇼크의 특정 합병증에 더 취약할 수 있다.

운동선수

컨디션이 좋은 운동선수는 종종 보상 능력이 향상된다. 대부분의 선수는 안정시 분당 40~50회의 심박수를 보인다. 심박수가 분당 100~110회 또는 저혈압은 컨디션이 좋은 운동선수에게 심각한 출혈을 나타내는 경조 징후일 수 있다. 마찬가지로 혼란스러운 것은 컨디션이 좋은 운동선수의 심박수가 분당 50회라는 것은 완전히 정상일 수도 있다는 것이다.

임신

임신 중에는 여성의 혈액량이 45~50% 증가할 수 있고 심박수와 심박출량도 증가한다. 따라서 임신부는 혈액 손실이 전체 혈액량의 30~35%를 초과할 때까지 쇼크의 징후가 나타나지 않을 수도 있다. 또한 임신부가 관류저하 징후를 보이기 훨씬 전에 태반 순환이 쇼크 상태에 대한 반응으로 분비되는 카테콜아민의 효과에 더 민감하게 반응하기 때문에 태아에게 악영향을 미칠 수 있다. 임신 3기 동안 자궁이 아래대정맥을 압박하여 심장으로의 정맥혈복귀를 많이 감소시켜 저혈압을 유발할 수 있다. 임신한 환자의 오른쪽(왼쪽 자궁 변위)을 들어 올리면 이러한 압박을 완화할 수 있다. 이 자세는 자궁을 아래대정맥으로부터 멀어지게 하여 혈액이 심장으로 돌아갈 수 있도록 한다(전부하). 이 방법을 시행한 후에도 임신부의 저혈압이 지속되면 일반적으로 생명을 위협하는 출혈이 있다는 것을 나타낸다.

기저 질환

관상동맥질환, 울혈심부전, 만성폐쇄폐질환과 같은 심각한 기저 질환이 있는 환자는 일반적으로 출혈과 쇼크를 보상할 수 있는 능력이 떨

어진다. 이러한 환자는 혈압을 유지하기 위해 심박수가 증가함에 따라 협심증을 경험할 수 있다. 박동조율기를 이식한 환자는 일반적으로 혈압을 유지하는 데 필요한 보상 작용으로 빈맥이 발생할 수 없다. 당뇨병 환자는 종종 기저 질환이 없는 환자보다 병실이나 중환자실 입원 기간이 더 길고 합병증도 더 잘 발생한다. 당뇨병 환자의 혈관은 장기간 고혈당의 영향으로 인해 순응도가 낮을 수 있으며 혈류역학적 변화에 대한 민감도와 반응 능력이 감소한다.

약물

수많은 약물이 신체의 보상 기전을 방해할 수 있다. 고혈압 치료에 사용되는 베타-아드레날린차단제 및 칼슘채널차단제는 혈압을 유지하기 위해 보상작용으로 빈맥이 발생하는 것을 예방할 수 있다. 또한, 관절염 및 근골격계 통증 치료에 사용하는 비스테로이드성 소염제(NSAID)는 혈소판 활성 및 혈액응고 장해를 유발할 수 있으며 출혈을 증가시킬 수 있다. 새로운 항응고제 약물은 며칠 동안 혈액 응고를 막을 수 있다. 항혈소판제 및 항응고제(혈액 희석제) 사용으로 인해 외상센터의 선택이 변경될 수 있다. 환자나 가족에게 약물 사용에 대한 정보를 얻을 수 있는 경우 이는 외상 팀에게 보고해야 하는 중요한 정보이다.

손상과 처치 사이의 시간

EMS 반응이 빠르면 병원 전 처치 제공자는 생명을 위협하는 내부 손상이 있지만, 쇼크를 나타낼 만큼 충분한 혈액을 손실하지 않은 환자를 만날 수 있다(3단계 출혈 또는 4단계 출혈). 대동맥, 대정맥 또는 엉덩 혈관에 관통상을 입은 환자라도 EMS 반응, 현장 체류 시간 및 이송 시간이 짧으면 정상적인 수축기 혈압으로 의료기관에 도착할 수 있다. 환자가 단지 좋아 보인다고 해서 내부출혈이 없다고 가정하는 것은 잘못된 경우가 많다. 환자는 보상된 쇼크로 인해 또는 쇼크 징후가 나타나기에 충분한 시간이 지나지 않았기 때문에 좋아 보일 수 있다. 대부분 쇼크는 보상된다는 것을 기억하는 것이 중요하다. 환자들은 아주 미세한 쇼크 징후라도 철저히 평가받아야 하며 내부출혈은 확실하게 배제될 때까지 내부출혈이 존재하는 것으로 가정해야 한다. 늦게 나타나는 내부출혈의 가능성을 평가하기 위해 외상 환자에 대한 지속적인 평가는 필수적이다.

처치

쇼크의 처치 단계는 다음과 같다.

1. 중증 외부출혈 조절
2. 산소공급 및 환기 보장(기도 관리)
3. 출혈의 원인 확인(외부출혈을 조절하고 내부출혈의 가능성을 인지)
4. 결정적인 처치를 위해 환자 이송
5. 적절한 혈액 구성 요법 시행

기도를 확보하고 산소 공급을 유지하기 위해 환기를 제공하는 것 외에드 쇼크 처치의 주요 목표는 원인을 확인하고 가능한 한 구체적으로 원인을 처치하며 순환을 지원하는 것이다. 세포로의 관류 및 산소 공급을 유지함으로써 에너지 생산이 지원되고 세포 기능이 보장된다.

병원 전 환경에서는 출혈의 외부 원인을 확인하고 즉시 직접 지혈해야 한다. 일반적으로 쇼크의 내부 원인은 병원 전 환경에서 확실하게 처치할 수 없다. 따라서 처치 방법은 가능한 최선의 방법으로 순환을 지원하면서 결정적인 처치가 가능한 의료기관으로 환자를 신속하게 이송하는 것이다. 병원 전 환경에서의 소생술은 다음이 포함된다.

- 병원 전 환경에서 가능한 한 외부출혈과 내부출혈을 모두 지혈한다. 모든 적혈구가 중요하다.
- 다음을 통해서 폐에 있는 적혈구의 산소 공급을 개선한다.
  - 적절한 기도 관리
  - 백마스크로 보조 환기를 시행하고 고농도의 보충 산소를 공급[흡입산소 농도(FiO_2) > 0.85].
- 순환을 개선하여 전신 조직에 더욱 효율적으로 산소화된 적혈구를 전달하고 세포 수준에서 산소화 및 에너지 생산을 개선한다.
  - 결정질 수액 적절하게 사용
  - 가능하고 필요한 경우 혈액제제 투여
- 저체온증을 예방한다.
- 출혈 즈절 및 소실된 적혈구, 혈장, 응고인자와 혈소판을 투여하기 위해 가능한 한 결정적인 처치를 할 수 있는 의료기관으로 신속하게 이송한다.

적절한 처치를 시행하지 않으면 환자는 사망에 이를 때까지 급속도로 악화한다. 쇼크 환자에게 제공할 처치를 결정할 때 다음과 같은 네 가지 질문을 해결해야 한다.

1. 환자에게 발생한 쇼크의 원인은?
2. 환자의 쇼크에 대한 확실한 처치는 무엇인가?
3. 환자가 결정적인 처치를 받을 수 있는 의료기관은 어디인가?
4. 결정적인 처치를 위해 환자를 이송하는 동안 환자를 지원하고 상태를 관리하기 위해 취할 수 있는 임시 조치는 무엇인가?

첫 번째 질문은 현장에서 정확하게 대답하기 어려울 수 있지만, 쇼크의 가능한 원인을 확인하면 환자의 상태에 따라 가장 적합한 의료기관과 환자의 생존 가능성을 향상하기 위해 이송 중에 필요한 조치를 결정하는 데 도움이 된다.

대량 출혈

주요 출혈은 신속하게 조절해야 한다. 팔다리 또는 접합부의 출혈에 사용할 수 있는 다양한 지혈대가 있다. 상처 패킹 그리고 응고를 촉진할 수 있는 물질도 사용할 수 있다. 생명을 위협하는 출혈은 신속하고 적극적으로 처치해야 한다.

출혈 조절

외부출혈의 현장 처치 단계는 다음과 같다.

- 손으로 직접 압박
- 가능한 경우 상처 패킹 및 지혈제가 포함된 압박 드레싱
- 지혈대
- 필요한 경우 접합부 지혈대 사용
- 불안정한 골반 골절 시 골반 고정대 적용

외부출혈의 지혈은 단계적으로 진행되어야 하며 초기 처치가 출혈 조절에 실패할 경우 단계적으로 진행해야 한다(**그림 3-15**). 일부 상황에서는 초기 출혈 조절 방법으로 지혈대 적용이 필요할 수 있다.

직접 압박

출혈 부위를 직접 손으로 압박하거나 압박 드레싱을 하는 것은 외부 출혈을 조절하기 위해 사용하는 초기 처치 방법이다. 이러한 압력 적용은 베르누이(Bernoulli's)의 원리를 기반으로 하며 다음과 같은 여러 가지 고려사항을 포함한다.

유체 누출 = 전층 압력 × 혈관 벽의 구멍 크기

전층 압력은 혈관 내부 압력과 혈관 외부 압력의 차이이다. 혈관 내 체액과 혈압 주기에 의해 혈관 벽 내부에 가해지는 압력을 혈관 내부(관내) 압력이라고 한다. 외부에서 혈관 벽에 가해지는 힘(예: 손

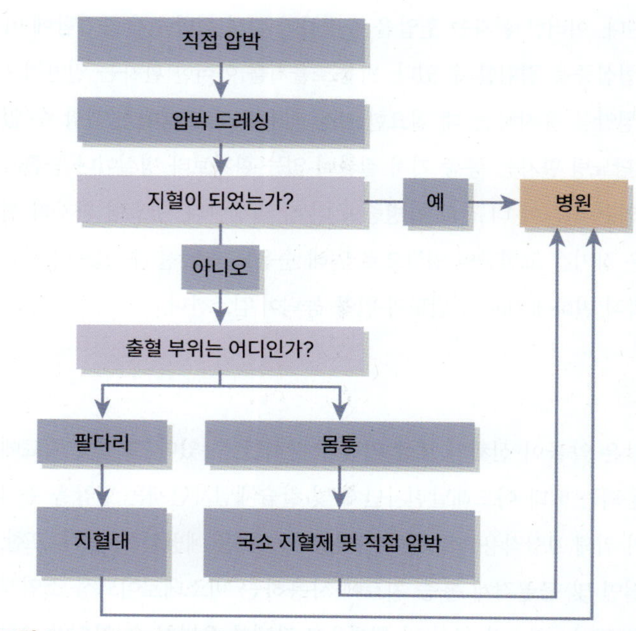

그림 3-15 현장에서의 출혈 조절
© National Association of Emergency Medical Technicians (NAEMT)

또는 드레싱)을 혈관 외부(장관 외) 압력이라고 한다. 다음 방정식은 이 관계를 설명한다.

전층 압력 = 혈관 내부 압력 − 혈관 외부 압력

혈관 내부 압력이 높을수록 혈액이 손상된 혈관 밖으로 더 빨리 빠져나간다. 병원 전 처치 제공자가 혈관 외부에 더 높은 압력을 가할수록 혈액이 더 천천히 새어 나간다. 상처 부위에 직접 압박을 가하면 외부 압력이 증가하여 누출 속도가 느려진다.

열상이 발생한 혈관의 출혈에 반응하고 조절하는 신체의 능력은 다음과 같다.

- 혈관 크기
- 혈관 내부 압력
- 응고 인자의 존재
- 손상된 혈관이 수축을 일으키고 손상 부위에서 구멍의 크기를 줄이고 혈류를 감소시키는 능력
- 손상 부위에서 혈관 주변 조직의 압력 및 병원 전 처치 제공자가 외부에서 제공하는 추가 압력

특히 동맥이 완전히 절단되면 혈관이 수축하여 연축을 일으키는 경우가 많다. 혈관이 손상되었지만, 완전히 절단되지 않은 중증 외상이 있는 팔다리보다 완전히 절단된 팔다리에서 출혈이 더 적다.

출혈 부위에 직접 압박을 가하면 혈관 외부의 압력이 증가하고 전

층의 압력이 감소하여 출혈을 느리게 하거나 멈추는 데 도움이 된다. 또한 직접 압박은 두 번째이자 중요한 기능을 수행한다. 찢어진 혈관의 측면을 압박하면 개구부의 크기(면적)가 감소하고 혈관 밖으로 누출되는 혈액이 더욱 감소한다. 출혈이 완전히 차단되지 않더라도 혈액 응고 시스템이 출혈을 멈출 수 있을 정도로 출혈이 감소할 수 있다. 이것이 바로 직접 압박이 거의 항상 출혈을 조절하는 데 성공하는 이유이다. 심장 카테터 삽입 후 넓적다리 동맥천자 부위의 출혈과 관련된 연구에서 직접 압박이 효과적인 방법이라는 것을 입증했다.

물이 새는 파이프에 비유하면 파이프에 작은 구멍이 있으면 구멍에 손가락을 대면 일시적으로 물이 새는 것을 막을 수 있다. 그런 다음 누출을 단기적으로 해결하기 위해 테이프를 파이프 주위에 감쌀 수 있다. 출혈 환자에게도 같은 개념이 적용된다. 개방 상처에 직접 압박을 가한 다음 압박 드레싱을 한다. 그러나 압박 드레싱이 가장 효과적이 되려면 혈관의 손상 부위에 직접 압박을 가해야 한다. 상처 위 피부에 적용하는 간단한 드레싱만으로는 출혈 부위 자체에 직접적인 압력을 가하지 않는다.

압박 드레싱을 가장 효과적으로 사용하려면 드레싱 재료로 상처 패킹을 시행하고 탄력 붕대로 바깥쪽을 감는 것이다. 상처 패킹의 효과는 컴뱃 거즈, 치토 거즈 또는 셀록스와 같은 지혈제를 사용하거나 일반 롤 거즈를 사용하여 수행할 수 있다. 상처 안으로 패킹 제재를 밀어 넣은 다음 출혈 부위 위에 직접 압박을 시행한 후 상처 부위 전체를 압박붕대로 감는 것이다. 상처에 지혈 거즈를 사용하는 경우 최소 3분 또는 제조업체의 지침에 따라 직접 압박을 가해야 하며 일반 거즈를 사용하는 경우 10분 동안 상처 부위에 직접 압박을 가해야 한다.

세 가지 중요 사항

직접 압박에 대한 세 가지 추가 사항이 강조되어야 한다. 첫째, 물체가 박혀있는 상처를 처치하는 경우 박혀 있는 물체 위에 압력을 가하는 것이 아니라 물체의 양쪽 옆에 압력을 가해야 한다. 박힌 물체가 혈관을 손상했을 수 있고 박혀 있는 물체 자체가 출혈을 방지할 수 있으므로 박혀 있는 물체를 현장에서 제거해서는 안 된다. 박혀 있는 물체를 제거면 조절할 수 없는 내부출혈이 발생할 수 있다.

둘째, 직접 압박으로 출혈을 조절한 후에도 일반적으로 다른 처치를 시행하거나 이송 중에는 도수로 직접 압박을 유지하는 것이 불가능하므로 압박 드레싱이 필요하다.

셋째, 출혈이 지속하는 경우 출혈 부위에 직접 압박을 가하는 것이

정맥 라인 확보 및 수액 소생술보다 우선 시행한다. 두 개의 정맥 라인을 확보하고 테이프로 고정한 상태로 외상 드레싱만 테이프로 고정한 채 출혈로 죽어가는 환자를 의료기관으로 이송하는 것은 심각한 오류가 될 수 있다.

지혈대

팔다리의 외부출혈이 직접 압박으로 즉시 조절할 수 없는 경우 지혈대를 사용하는 것이 출혈을 조절하기 위한 합리적인 다음 단계이다. 지혈대는 신경과 혈관 손상, 지혈대를 너무 오래 착용하면 팔다리를 잃을 수 있는 잠재적인 합병증에 대한 우려 때문에 선호되지 않았다. 이러한 우려 사항 중 어느 것도 입증되지 않았다. 사실 이라크와 아프가니스탄 전쟁의 데이터는 정반대임을 보여주었다. 미군이 지혈대를 적용한 결과 이러한 전쟁에서 팔다리를 잃는 사람은 없었다. 전쟁 경험에서 얻은 데이터에 따르면 지혈대를 적절하게 사용했다면 전투 사망자 100명 중 7명을 잠재적으로 예방할 수 있었다고 한다.

지혈대를 사용해서 팔다리의 외부출혈을 80% 이상 지혈할 수 있다. 또한 동맥 혈류를 차단하는 지혈대는 외과 의사들이 수술실에서 수년 동안 만족스러운 결과로 널리 사용되어 왔다. 지혈대를 적절하게 사용하면 안전할 뿐만 아니라 환자의 생명을 구할 수 있다.

이라크와 아프가니스탄에서 전쟁 중 실시한 연구에서는 지혈대를 쇼크가 발생하기 전에 적용했을 때와 혈압이 떨어진 후에 적용했을 때의 생존율에서 현저한 차이를 보였다. 환자가 쇼크 상태에 빠지기 전에 지혈대를 적용하였을 때 생존율은 96%였으며 환자가 쇼크를 일으킨 후에 지혈대를 적용한 경우 생존율은 4%였다. 대량 출혈이 발생한 상황에서 지혈대 적용을 지연시킬 이유는 없다.

장비 선택

미군은 효과적(증명된 동맥 폐색)이고 사용하기 쉬운 지혈대(특히 군인이 한쪽 팔을 다쳤을 때 다른 한 손으로도 신속하게 사용할 수 있는 지혈대)에 대한 관심으로 인해 많은 상업용 지혈대가 개발되어 판매되고 있다. 전술적 전투 사상자 처치 위원회(CoTCCC)를 통해 보건국-합동 외상 체계(Department of Health Agency-Joint Trauma System)는 다음과 같은 8개의 지혈대를 권장하는 것으로 확인했다. C-A-T 지혈대 6세대 및 7세대(Combat Application Tourniquet), EMT 지혈대(Emergency and Military Tourniquet), SOFT-W 지혈대(Special Operations Force Tactical Tourniquet - Wide), TMT 지혈대(Tactical Mechanical Tourniquet), RAM-T 지혈대(Ratcheting Medical Tourniquet-Tactical), SAT-XT 지혈대(SAM Extremity

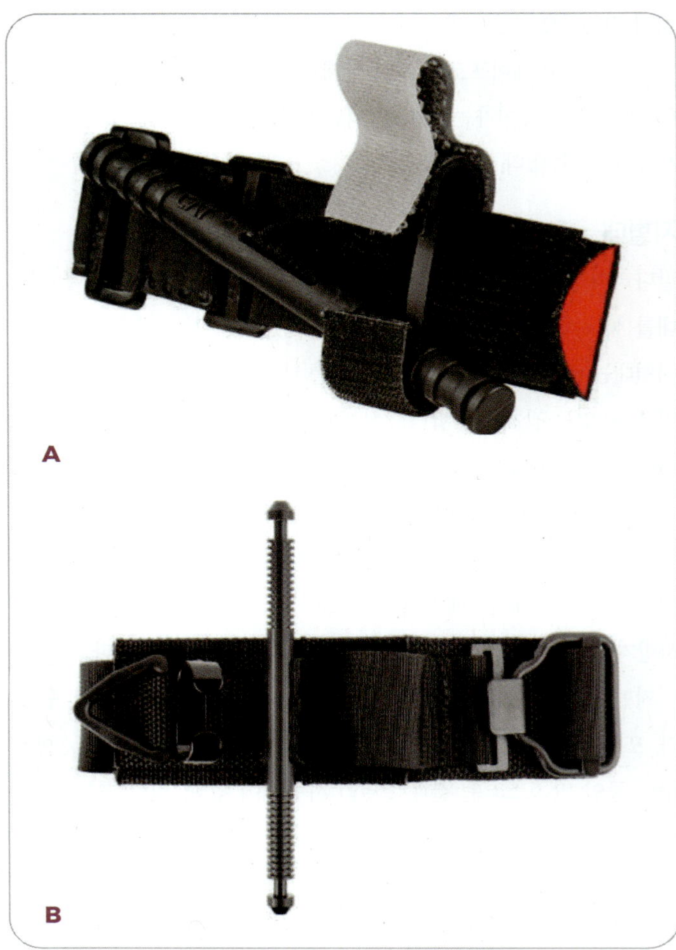

그림 3-16 **A.** C-A-T 지혈대 Gen7. **B.** SOF 지혈대 Gen4.
A. © Looka/Shutterstock **B.** Courtesy of TacMed Solutions, LCC.

Tourniquet), TPT2 지혈대(Tactical Pneumatic Tourniquet, 2-inch)이다(**그림 3-16**).

적용 부위

지혈대는 서혜부 또는 겨드랑이 부위에 사용해야 한다. 하나의 지혈대로 출혈을 완전히 조절할 수 없다면 다른 지혈대를 첫 번째 지혈대의 근위부에 추가로 적용해야 한다. 두 개의 지혈대를 나란히 적용하면 압박 면적이 두 배로 늘어나 출혈을 조절할 가능성이 높아진다. 일단 적용하면 지혈대를 적용한 부위를 노출된 상태로 유지하여 쉽게 확인하고 모니터링 할 수 있어야 한다.

이전에 일부 출처는 서혜부나 겨드랑이에 일차적으로 적용하는 것과 달리 출혈 부위에 가까운 지정된 거리에서 출혈 부위에 더 가깝게 적용할 것을 권장했다. 민간 환경에서 결정적인 처치를 시행할 수 있는 의료기관으로 이송하는 시간이 상대적으로 짧지만, 이는 다음과 같은 몇 가지 이유로 합리적이지 않다.

1. 선택적 환경에서의 수술 경험은 근위 적용이 매우 안전하고 효과적이라는 것을 강력하게 시사한다.
2. 외부출혈 부위는 내부출혈의 정도를 나타내지 않을 수 있다. 이것은 무딘 손상과 관통상 모두에 해당한다. 손상 부위는 실제로 지혈대 적용 부위보다 더 근위부로 확장되어 지혈대 조임에도 불구하고 지속적인 손상에서 출혈로 이어질 수 있다. 따라서 가능한 한 가장 근접한 적용 부위가 선호된다.
3. 적어도 이론적으로는 중요한 신경 구조가 피부밑에 있는 뼈 융기(예: 종아리뼈 목의 일반적인 종아리신경 또는 팔꿈치굴 주위의 자신경)에 가까운 부위에서 손상 위험이 더 크다. 이러한 위치에 적용하면 심각한 신경 손상이 발생할 수 있다.
4. 팔다리의 길이에 따라 특정 위치에서 뼈의 융기가 피부에 가까이 있어 연부조직이 눌리는 것을 방해해 동맥을 압박하는 것을 방해하기 때문에 출혈을 조절하기 어렵다.

지혈대 조임 강도

지혈대는 동맥의 혈류와 말초 맥박을 차단할 수 있을 만큼 충분히 조여야 한다. 팔다리의 정맥 관류만 차단할 정도로 조이면 오히려 상처에서 출혈을 증가시킨다. 출혈을 조절하는 데 필요한 압력과 팔다리의 크기 사이에는 직접적인 관계가 있다. 따라서 평균적으로 출혈을 조절하기 위해서는 팔보다 다리에 지혈대를 더 단단하게 고정해야 한다.

제한 시간

동맥에 적용한 지혈대는 선택적 팔다리 수술 중 출혈을 조절하기 위해 심한 신경이나 근육 손상 없이 수술실에서 최대 150분 동안 일반적으로 안전하게 사용되었다. 교외나 시골 지역에서도 대부분의 EMS 이송 시간은 이보다 훨씬 짧다. 일반적으로 병원 전 환경에서 적용한 지혈대는 환자를 가장 가까운 적절한 의료기관으로 이송해서 결정적인 처치를 받을 때까지 적용되어 있어야 한다. 미군에서의 사용은 적용 시간이 길어져도 크게 악화하지 않았다. 지혈대 적용이 필요한 경우 환자는 출혈을 조절하기 위해 응급 수술이 필요할 가능성이 높다. 따라서 이러한 환자에게 가장 적절한 의료기관은 외상센터 또는 최소한 즉시 수술이 가능한 비외상 전문 병원이다.

과거에는 손상된 팔다리로 약간의 혈류가 흐르도록 10~15분마다 지혈대를 느슨하게 풀어 주는 것이 팔다리를 보존하고 추가 절단을 방지하는 데 도움이 될 것으로 생각하고 권장했다. 그러나 이 방법은

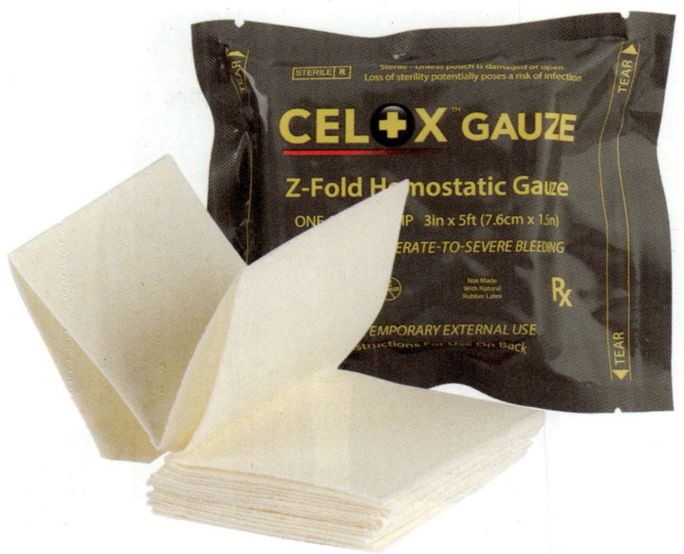

그림 3-17 지혈 거즈는 지혈대를 적용할 수 없는 신체 부위의 상처에 사용하거나 드레싱 할 수 있도록 설계되었다.

손상 부위에서 혈액 손실을 증가시키는 역할만 할 뿐 팔다리 자체에는 아무런 효과가 없는 경우가 많다. 현재 권장 사항은 지혈대가 일단 적용되면 결정적인 처치가 가능한 의료기관에서 팔다리를 평가할 수 있을 때까지 지혈대를 계속 적용하는 것이다. 지혈대는 몇 가지 제한된 상황에서 제거해야 할 수 있지만, 이는 드문 경우이며 가능하면 온라인 의료 방향의 맥락에서만 수행해야 한다.

지혈대 적용은 의식이 있는 환자가 견디기에는 고통스러울 수 있으므로 통증 관리를 고려해야 한다. **Box 3-5**는 지혈대 적용을 위한 예시 프로토콜을 제공한다.

지혈제

미 식품의약청(FDA)은 다수의 국소 지혈제 사용을 승인했다. 지혈제는 혈액 응고를 촉진하고 지혈대를 적용하기가 불가능한 신체 부위에 직접 압박만으로 출혈을 조절할 수 없는 생명을 위협하는 출혈을 조절하기 위해 상처에 패킹하거나 드레싱 할 수 있도록 설계되었다. 이러한 지혈제는 일반적으로 지혈 물질이 함유된 거즈 형태로 상처 부위에 직접 적용한다(**그림 3-17**).

복부나 서혜부와 같이 지혈대를 적용할 수 없는 부위에서 발생하는 출혈의 경우 지혈제를 사용하는 것이 합리적이다. 컴벳 거즈, 셀록스 및 치토 거즈는 상처에 단단하게 패킹할 수 있도록 설계된 지혈 드레싱이다. XStat (깊고 좁은 접합부 상처에 가장 적합)은 상처 깊숙이 주입되는 여러 개의 작은 지혈 스펀지가 들어있는 장비를 사용한다. iTClamp는 금속 침이 있는 폴리카보네이트 클램프로 압박 효과를 얻기 위해 출혈 상처를 일시적으로 봉합하는 데 사용한다. 지혈 드레싱과 지혈 스펀지는 최소 3분 동안 직접 압박을 가하는 것이 가장 좋다. 지혈 드레싱은 상처에 직접 적용해야 하며 단순히 개상 손상을 덮기 위한 드레싱으로만 사용해서는 안 된다. 이러한 드레싱은 작용 기전이 다르므로 한 종류의 드레싱이 출혈을 조절하지 못하는 경우 다른 드레싱을 적용할 수 있다. XStat 장치는 현장에서 제거할 수 없도록 설계된 고유의 제품이기 때문에 한 번 부착한 드레싱은 그대로 유지해야 한다. 필요한 경우 추가 XStat 드레싱 또는 다른 드레싱을 적용할 수 있다.

최신 지혈 드레싱 제품은 여러 대형 동물 연구에서 치명적인 손상 모델을 활용할 때 생존과 출혈 차이를 보여주었다.

접합부 출혈 조절

팔다리와 머리가 몸통과 연결되는 부위(서혜부, 겨드랑 부위, 어깨, 목)를 접합부라고 하며 이러한 접합부에서 발생한 손상은 주요 혈관이 손상되어 다량의 출혈을 일으킬 수 있다. 특히 사제폭발물(IED)로 인한 다리의 상처는 종종 지혈대를 적용할 수 없는 상처를 초래한다. 중증 출혈을 조절하기 위해 전술적 현장에서 미군에 의해 많은 장치가 사용되었다(**그림 3-18**). 전술적 상황에서 접합부에 적용할 수 있는 지혈대로는 CRoC (Combat Ready Clamp) 접합부 지혈대, JETT (Junctional Emergency Treatment Too) 접합부 지혈대, SAM 접합

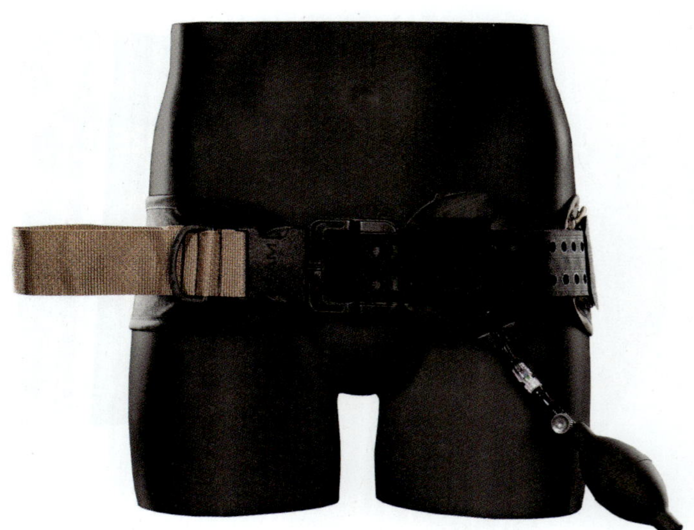

그림 3-18 SAM 접합부 지혈대
Used with permission from SAM Medical.

부 지혈대(SAM Junctional Tourniquet) 등이 있다. 민간 환경에서 이러한 장비에 대한 경험이 거의 없으며 접합부 출혈이 발생하는 대부분의 민간 상황에서 효과적일 수 있다는 최소한의 증거가 있다.

들어올리기기법(거상)과 압박점

과거에는 출혈을 조절하는 중간 단계로 팔다리의 거상과 압박점(출혈 부위 몸쪽)을 압박에 중점을 두었다. 출혈이 발생한 팔다리 말단을 들어 올리는 것이 출혈을 늦추는지에 관한 연구는 발표되지 않았다. 팔다리의 뼈가 부러진 경우 이러한 조작은 잠재적으로 내부출혈을 증가시킬 수 있다. 출혈을 조절하기 위해 압박점을 압박하는 것은 연구되지 않았으며 효과적이라도 이러한 압박을 환자를 이송하는 동안 효과적으로 유지될 가능성이 작다. 따라서 설득력 있는 데이터가 없는 상황에서 이러한 처치는 더 이상 권장되지 않는다.

기도

병원 전 환경에서는 기도를 확보하고 환기를 유지하기 위한 전문 술기가 필요할 수 있다(7장 기도와 환기를 참고). 특히 이송 시간이 짧은 경우 필수 기도 유지술의 중요성을 과소평가해서는 안 된다.

호흡

일단 기도가 확보되면 쇼크 상태에 있는 환자나 쇼크가 발생할 위험이 있는 환자(거의 모든 외상 환자)는 가능한 한 100%(FiO$_2$ 1.0)에 가

까운 농도의 산소를 공급해야 한다. 이 수준의 산소 공급은 산소 보유주머니가 부착된 장비를 산소통에 연결한 상태에서만 가능할 수 있다. 코삽입관 또는 단순얼굴마스크로는 고농도의 산소를 공급할 수 없다. 맥박산소측정기로 산소포화도를 모니터링하고 모든 외상 환자에서 환자의 상태와 상관없이 산소포화도를 94% 이상으로 유지해야 한다.

호흡하지 않거나 적절한 깊이와 호흡수를 유지하지 못하는 환자는 기도를 개방하고 코인두기도기나 입인두기도기와 같은 보조기도기를 삽입한 후 보조 환기가 필요하다. 이러한 조작에 반응이 없으면 백마스크 장치를 즉시 사용한다.

보조 환기의 품질에 세심한 주의를 기울이는 것이 중요하다. 보조 환기 중 과다환기를 시행하면 특히 외상성 뇌손상 환자나 저혈량 쇼크 환자에게서 부정적인 생리학적 반응을 일으킨다. 너무 빠르거나 너무 깊게 환기를 시행하면 환자를 알칼리성 상태로 만들 수 있다. 이 화학반응은 산소에 대한 혈색소의 친화력을 증가시켜 조직으로의 산소 전달을 감소시킨다. 또한, 과다환기는 가슴속 압력을 증가시켜 심장으로의 정맥혈복귀를 감소시키고 저혈압을 유발할 수 있다. 가슴속 압력의 증가는 많은 일회호흡량(10~12mL/kg) 또는 자동호기말양압(auto-PEEP)으로 너무 빨리 환기할 때 발생할 수 있다(부적절한 날숨은 폐에서 공기 갇히므로 이어짐). 외상성 뇌손상 환자에서 부주의한 과다환기는 뇌혈관 수축과 뇌 혈류 감소로 이어질 수 있다. 이것은 뇌에서 발생하는 이차 손상을 악화시킨다. 몇몇 연구에서 과다환기를 시행한 외상성 뇌손상 환자에서 더 나쁜 결과가 나타났다. 성인 환자의 경우 분당 10회의 환기 속도로 적절한 일회호흡량(350~500mL)을 제공하면 충분하다.

호기말이산화탄소분압 모니터링은 종종 맥박산소측정기와 같이 사용되어 충분한 산소 공급으로 정상 혈중이산화탄소 농도를 유지하는지 평가하기 위해 사용하지만, 관류가 저하된 환자의 경우 호기말이산화탄소분압과 동맥혈이산화탄소분압(PaCO$_2$)과의 상관관계가 변화될 수 있으며 환기를 정확하게 판단하려는 방법으로 신뢰할 수 없다.

순환

심각한 외부출혈이 먼저 해결되었지만, 임박한 순환부전을 해결하려면 내부출혈을 인식하고 처치하는 방법을 이해해야 한다. 기능적 순환 회복은 또한 적절한 환자의 수액 소생술을 포함할 수 있다.

내부출혈

골절 부위의 내부출혈도 고려해야 한다. 드문 경우지만 손상된 팔다리 부위를 조심해서 다루지 않으면 폐쇄골절이 개방골절로 전환될 가능성이 있다. 이러한 움직임으로 인해 골절된 뼈끝이 주변 근육 또는 혈관에 손상을 주어 내부출혈을 증가시킬 수 있다. 골절이 의심되는 팔다리의 모든 골절은 이차 손상을 최소화하기 위해 움직이지 않도록 고정해야 한다. 환자가 쇼크와 같은 생명을 위협하는 상태의 증거가 없는 경우 각 골절 부위를 부목으로 고정을 시행한다. 그러나 일차평가에서 환자의 생명을 위협하는 상태가 확인되면 환자를 적절한 장비에 신속하게 해부학적 자세로 고정하고 적절한 의료기관으로 이송한다. 골반 고정대는 골반 골절 및 골반 고리의 기타 파열을 부목 적용과 유사하게 고정하는 것으로 나타났다. 병원 전 환경에서 사용하는 경우 결과의 변화를 보여주는 연구는 수행되지 않았지만, 골반 고정대를 조기에 적절하게 사용한다면 골반 골절로 인한 출혈을 줄이고 잠재적으로인 사망을 줄일 수 있다고 믿을 만한 타당한 이유가 있다. 또한 병원 전 환경이나 다른 외부 환경에서 골반 고정대를 사용하는 것이 위험하다는 증거는 없다.

저혈압 소생술

혈관 및 환자의 관점에서 평균 동맥압(관내 압력)과 혈관을 둘러싼 조직의 압력(장관 외 압력)은 혈관의 구멍 크기뿐만 아니라 혈관으로부터의 출혈 속도를 조절하는 데 직접적인 관계가 있다. 참고로 출혈로 인해 환자의 혈압이 낮아진 경우 혈압을 다시 정상 수준으로 올리지 않은 것이 적절하다. 오히려 출혈을 멈추고 중요한 장기에 관류하기에, 충분한 수준으로 혈압을 유지해야 한다. 이 수치는 일반적으로 환자의 수축기 혈압이 80~90mmHg일 때 발생한다. 이는 환자에게 정맥 내로 수액을 과도하게 투여하는 것을 피하고 적당한 정도의 저혈압을 유지하는 것을 의미한다. 많은 양의 결정질 수액을 정맥 내로 투여하여 혈압을 정상 수준으로 회복시키면 원하는 효과와 정반대의 효과가 발생하여 혈관의 개구부에 형성된 혈전을 떨어뜨려 출혈이 증가한다.

여러 연구에서 출혈이 조절될 때까지 수액 소생술을 보류하는 것이 사망률을 증가시키지 않는다는 것이 입증되었다. 저혈압 소생술은 실행 가능하고 안전한 것으로 나타났으며 관통성 외상 환자와 같은 일부 환자군에서 생존율이 향상되는 경향이 있다. 예외는 외상성 뇌손상 또는 척수 손상 환자이다. 이러한 손상과 출혈로 인한 저혈압이 동반된 환자는 수축기 혈압을 110mmHg 이상으로 유지하기 위해 수액, 혈액제제 또는 혈압상승제를 더욱 적극적으로 사용해야 한다.

출혈을 관리하는 단계는 1) 외부 압력(손으로 직접 압박)을 증가시켜 혈관에 발생한 구멍 크기를 줄이고 내부 압력과 외부 압력의 차이를 감소시키는 것으로 두 가지 방법 모두 손상을 입은 혈관의 혈류를 감소시키는 데 기여하며, 2) 저혈압 소생술을 시행하여 혈관 내 압력이 정상보다 높게 상승하지 않도록 한다.

장애

쇼크 환자의 의식상태 변화에 대한 독특하고 구체적인 처치는 없다. 환자의 비정상적인 신경학적 상태가 뇌 저산소중과 관류저하로 발생한 것이라면 저산소중을 교정하고 관류저하를 회복시키려는 노력으로 의식상태가 호전되어야 한다. 외상성 뇌손상 후 환자의 상태를 평가할 때 초기 글래스고혼수척도(GCS) 점수는 일반적으로 적절한 소생술과 뇌 관류의 회복을 반영하는 것으로 간주한다. 쇼크 상태에서 환자의 글래스고혼수척도 점수를 평가하는 것은 지나치게 암울한 예후를 나타낼 수 있다.

노출/환경

환자의 체온을 정상 범위 내로 유지하는 것이 중요하다. 저체온증은 추운 환경에 노출되었을 때 대류나 전도 및 기타 물리적 방법(19장 환경 외상 I: 열과 한랭 손상 참조)을 통해 더 추운 환경에 노출되고 무산소대사로 인한 에너지 생산 감소로 인해 발생한다. 저체온증에 대한 가장 큰 우려는 혈액 응고에 미치는 영향이다. 체온이 감소하면 혈액 응고 장애가 발생한다. 또한, 저체온증은 응고 장애, 심근 기능 장애, 고칼륨혈증, 혈관 수축 및 환자의 생존 가능성에 부정적인 영향을 미치는 기타 많은 다른 문제를 악화시킨다. 저온은 짧은 시간 동안 조직을 보존할 수 있지만, 보존이 발생하려면 온도 강하가 매우 빠르고 매우 낮아야 한다. 이러한 급격한 변화는 외상 후 쇼크 환자에게 효과적인 것으로 입증되지 않았다.

병원 전 환경에서 저체온이 발생하면 중심 체온을 높이기가 어려울 수 있다. 따라서 정상 체온을 유지하기 위해 현장에서 취할 수 있는 모든 조치를 시작해야 한다. 환자를 노출하고 평가를 시행한 후에는 주변 환경으로부터 보호하고 체온을 유지해야 한다. 젖은 옷은 열손실을 증가시키기 때문에 피로 적신 옷을 포함하여 모든 젖은 옷은 제거하고 환자를 따뜻한 담요로 덮어준다. 환자를 따뜻하게 해주어야 하는 필요성을 예상해야 하며 구급차가 현장으로 출동하는 동난 담요를 히터의 송풍구 근처에 놓았다가 사용할 수 있다. 담요의 대안으로 두꺼운 비닐봉지와 같은 비닐 시트를 사용해 환자를 덮는 것이다. 이러한 물건은 저렴하고 보관이 쉬우며 일회용으로 효과적인 보온 장치이다. 특히 기관내삽관이 시행된 환자에게 가습된 산소를 공급하면 체온을 유지하는 데 도움이 될 수 있다.

환자를 평가한 후 쇼크 환자는 구급차를 따뜻하게 하여 환자실로 이동시킨다. 중증외상 환자를 이송할 때 이상적인 구급차의 환자실 온도는 29°C 이상으로 유지하는 것이다. 차가운 실내에서 환자의 열 손실률은 매우 높다. 모든 응급 상황에서 환자가 가장 중요한 사람이기 때문에 이 조건은 병원 전 처치 제공자가 아니라 환자에게 이상적이어야 한다. 구급차의 환자실 온도가 병원 전 처치 제공자에게 적절하다면 환자에게 너무 춥다는 것이 일반적으로 이다.

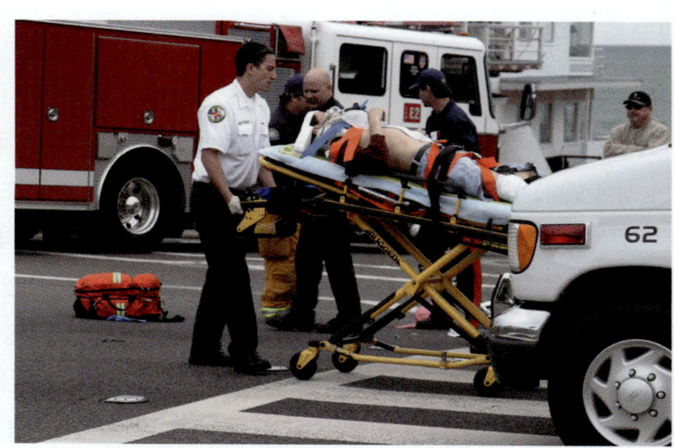

그림 3-19 주들것의 머리 부분은 들것을 기울이거나(역 트렌델렌버그 자세) 등받이 또는 진공부목을 들어 올려 주들 것 머리 부분을 발과 신체의 나머지 부분에 대해 상대적으로 들어 올린다. 등허리 척추 손상 가능성이 배제될 때까지 환자는 허리를 구부리거나 앉은 자세로 이동시켜서는 안 된다.
© Michael Ledray/Shutterstock

환자 이송

심각한 출혈성 쇼크를 효과적으로 처치하려면 병원 전 환경에서 일반적으로 사용할 수 없는 자원(수술 및 혈액제제)이 필요하기 때문에 신속한 평가와 환자를 처치할 수 있는 의료기관으로 이송하는 것이 중요하다. 병원 전 단계에서는 이러한 것을 일반적으로 사용할 수 없으므로 환자를 치료할 수 있는 의료기관으로 신속하게 이송하는 것이 중요하다. 신속한 이송은 환자 처치에서 중요한 처치 양상을 무시하거나 무시하는 구식의 "scoop and run"을 의미하지 않는다. 병원 전 처치 제공자는 출혈 조절, 기도 관리 및 호흡 보조와 같은 중요하고 잠재적으로 생명을 구할 수 있는 처치를 신속하게 시행해야 한다. 부적절한 환자 평가나 불필요한 고정으로 시간을 낭비해서는 안 된다. 중증의 외상 환자를 처치할 때 적절한 외상시설로 이송하는 동안 구급차에서 환자를 따뜻하게 하고 정맥 내로 수액 투여를 시작하며 이차평가를 수행하는 것과 같은 처치를 수행한다.

환자 자세

일반적으로 쇼크 상태에 있는 외상 환자는 바로누운자세로 고정하여 이송해야 한다. 트렌델렌버그 자세(머리 쪽을 낮게 하고 발 쪽을 올린 자세) 또는 쇼크 자세(바로누운자세에서 다리를 올린 자세)와 같은 특수한 자세는 지난 150년 동안 사용되었지만, 효과적인 것으로 입증되지 않았다. 트렌델렌버그 자세는 이미 손상된 환기 기능을 악화시킬 수 있고 흡인이나 기도 폐쇄 위험을 나타낼 수 있으며 외상성 뇌

손상 환자의 두개내압을 증가시킬 수 있다. 더 중요한 것은 중증의 저혈량 쇼크 상태에 있는 환자는 일반적으로 최대한 혈관 수축이 일어난다는 것이다. 외상성 뇌손상 환자의 경우 일반적으로 머리 쪽을 30도 올린 상태로 이송해야 한다. 이 자세는 뇌관류압 개선을 촉진하고 두개내압을 감소시킨다. 또한, 기관내삽관이 시행된 환자의 경우 흡인의 위험을 줄이기 위해 머리 쪽을 30도 올려 환기와 관련된 폐렴의 위험을 줄일 수 있는 이점이 있다. 중요한 것은 이 자세는 환자가 허리를 굽히지 않고 머리를 들어 올려서 등허리 척추 손상을 악화시킬 가능성이 있다는 것이다(**그림 3-19**).

혈관 확보

정맥 내 경로

심각한 손상을 입었거나 의심되는 외상 환자의 경우 병원 전 처치 제공자는 정맥 라인을 확보한 후 수액 소생술을 시작할 수 있다. 환자가 차량에서 구출되거나 병원 전 처치 제공자가 헬기 도착을 기다리고 있는 경우와 같은 특수한 상황을 제외하고는 환자를 가장 적절한 의료기관으로 이송하는 중에 정맥 라인을 확보해야 한다. 중증 손상을 입은 환자의 정맥 라인을 확보하기 위해 이송이 지연되어서는 안 된다.

쇼크 상태의 외상 환자에게 수액 소생술이 경험적으로 타당하지

만, 병원 전 환경에서 수액 소생술을 시작했을 때 중증외상 환자의 생존율이 개선되었다는 연구는 없다. 정맥 라인을 확보하기 위해 외상 환자의 이송이 지연되어서는 안 된다. 사실 몇몇 연구에서 출혈이 조절되기 전에 결정질 수액을 정맥으로 투여하는 이점을 입증하지 못했다.

쇼크 상태이거나 잠재적으로 심각한 손상을 입은 환자의 경우 시간이 허락한다면 1개 또는 2개의 큰 구경(18 게이지 이상), 짧은 (2.5cm) 정맥 내 카테터를 경피적으로 삽입해야 한다. 수액 투여 속도는 카테터 반경의 4제곱에 비례하고 길이에 반비례한다(짧고 지름이 큰 카테터가 길고 지름이 작은 카테터에 비해 더 많은 수액을 빠르게 투여할 수 있다). 경피적으로 정맥 라인 확보하기 위해 선호되는 부위는 아래팔 정맥이다. 정맥 라인을 확보하기 위한 대체 부위는 팔오금 안쪽 정맥, 손 및 위팔(노쪽피부정맥)이다.

골내(IO) 경로

성인의 혈관 라인을 확보하기 위한 다른 방법으로 골내(IO) 경로가 있다. 골내 경로로 수액을 투여하는 것은 새로운 것이 아니며 1941년 와터(Walter E. Lee) 박사에 의해 설명되었다. 이 혈관 확보 방법은 여러 가지 방법으로 수행할 수 있다. 가장 일반적인 부위로는 넓적다리뼈 원위부, 위팔뼈머리 또는 정강뼈 원위부 및 근위부와 같은 같은 부위에서 일반적으로 골내 경로를 확보한다. 연구에 따르면 최고의 유속으로 수액을 투여할 수 있는 부위는 위팔뼈머리와 넓적다리뼈 원위부이다. 적절하게 제작된 장비를 사용하여 복장뼈에 적용할 수도 있다(**그림 3-20, 그림 3-21** 및 **그림 3-22**). 이러한 술기는 일반적으로 병원 전 환경에서 사용되지만, 정맥 내로 수액을 투여하는 것보다 신속한 이송에 중점을 두어야 한다. 결정적인 처치를 받을 수 있는 의료기관으로 이송이 지연되거나 이송 시간이 오래 걸리는 경우 골내 경로 확보는 성인 외상 환자에게 중요한 역할을 할 수 있다. 의식 있는 환자에게 골내 경로로 수액을 투여하면 매우 심한 통증을 일으킬 수 있으며 지침에 따라 적절한 통증 조절이 필요하다.

수액 소생술

외상 환자 처치를 위해 지난 50년 동안 수액 소생술에 사용된 제품에는 일반적으로 혈액과 정맥 내 투여할 수 있는 용액으로 분류한다. 이러한 제품은 다음과 같이 더 세분화할 수 있다.

- 혈액
  - 전혈
  - 혈액제제로 재구성된 전혈
  - 농축 적혈구(PRBCs)
  - 혈장(예: 해동, 동결건조)
  - 추가 혈액 성분 요법(즉 저온 침전물)
- 정맥 내 용액
  - 결정질 용액(예: 젖산 링거액, 0.9% 생리식염수)
  - 고장액
  - 3% 생리식염수
  - 교질 용액(예: 덱스트란, 헥스텐트, 알부민)
  - 저혈압 또는 제한된 수액 전략(예: 물에 5% 포도당 희석)
  - 혈액 대체제

이러한 각 제품에는 장단점이 있다.

혈액

산소를 운반하는 능력 때문에 혈액이나 다양한 혈액제제는 중증 출

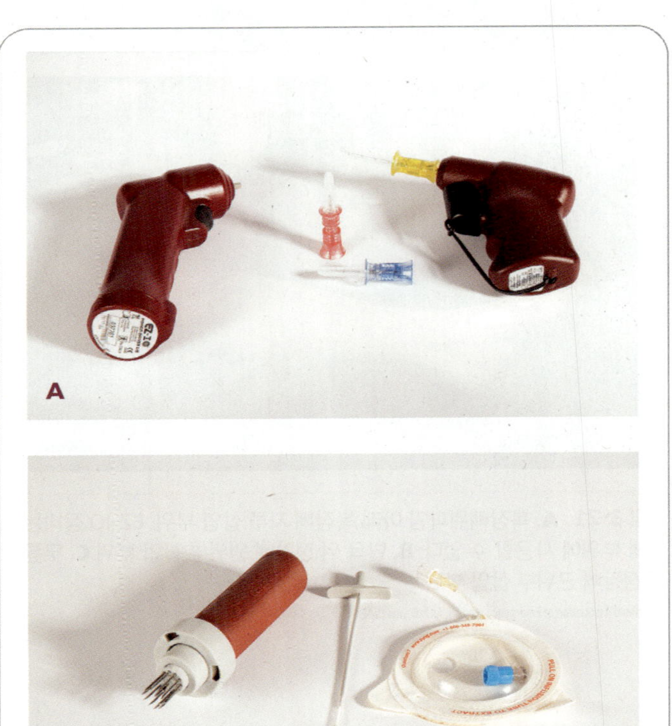

그림 3-20 A. EZ-IO 및 바늘(여러 종류). **B.** 복장뼈에 사용하는 FAST1

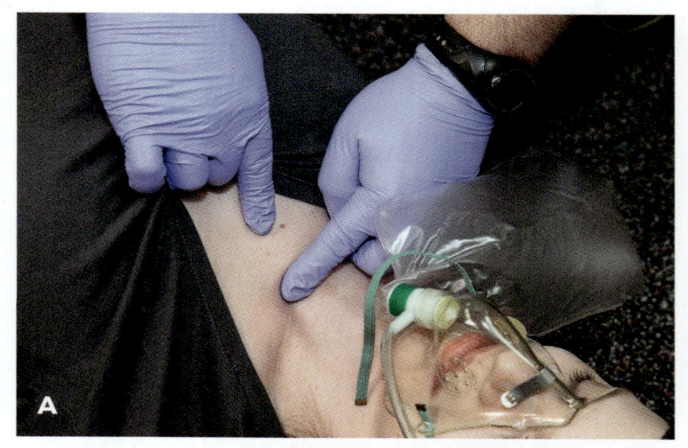

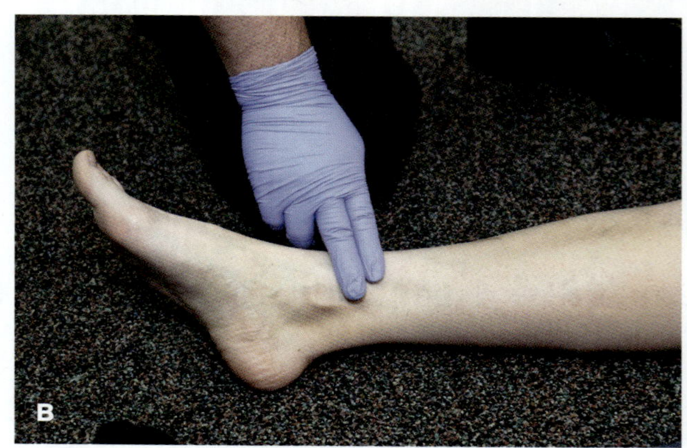

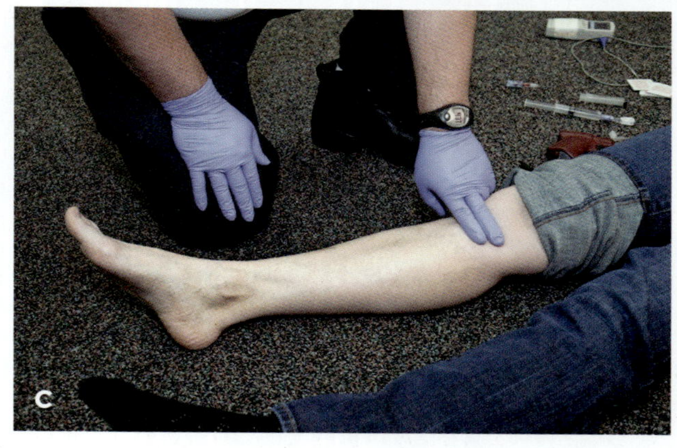

그림 3-21 **A.** 복장뼈위파임 아래 복장뼈 자루 삽입 부위. EZ-IO 장비는 복장뼈 부위에 사용할 수 없다. **B.** 발목 위 정강뼈 원위부 삽입 부위 **C.** 무릎 아래 정강뼈 근위부 삽입 부위

혈성 쇼크 환자의 소생술을 위해 선택되는 수액이다. 이라크와 아프가니스탄 전쟁의 결과로 미군이 얻은 경험은 손상을 입은 미군의 생존을 위해 전혈, 적혈구, 혈장 투여가 중요하다는 것을 보여주었다. 이 재구성된 혈액은 손실된 산소운반능력, 응고 인자 및 혈관에서 체

액 손실을 방지하기 위해 삼투압을 유지하는 데 필요한 단백질을 대체한다. 불행하게도 대부분의 경우 혈액과 혈액제제를 사용할 때까지 냉장 보관 또는 동결된 상태로 보관하지 않으면 부패하기 쉽기 때문에 현재 많은 민간 병원 전 환경에서 혈액을 사용하기가 어렵다. 그런데도 몇몇 EMS 시스템은 병원 전 수혈을 위한 프로토콜을 확립했다.

동결건조 혈장은 여러 나라의 현장에서 사용하고 있다. 동결건조 혈장은 사람의 혈장을 냉동해 건조한 것이다. 이 제품의 유통기간이 약 2년이고 냉장 보관이 필요하지 않으며 사용하기 전에 재구성해야 한다. 액체 혈장은 미국에서 일부 EMS와 항공 EMS(헬기 EMS)에서 사용하고 있으며 500명 이상의 외상 환자를 대상으로 한 연구에서 해동 혈장의 병원 전 투여는 출혈성 쇼크의 위험이 있는 환자의 30일 사망률을 크게 개선하는 것과 관련이 있었다.

정맥 내 용액

수액 소생술을 위한 대체 수액은 1) 등장성 결정질, 2) 고장성 결정질, 3) 합성(인공) 교질용액, 4) 혈액 대체재 중 하나이다.

등장성 결정질 용액

등장성 결정질은 전해질(용액에 용해될 때 전하 이온으로 분해되는 물질)로 구성된 균형 잡힌 염분 용액이다. 이 용액은 짧은 시간 동안 효과적인 부피 확장제로 작용하지만, 산소운반 능력은 없다. 결정질 용액은 투여 직후 출혈로 인해 감소한 혈관 내 공간을 채워 전부하와 심박출량을 개선한다. 젖산 링거액은 그 구성 성분이 혈장의 전해질 성분과 가장 유사하므로 쇼크 처치를 위해 사용하는 등장성 결정질 용액이다. 이 용액은 특정한 양의 칼륨, 칼슘, 나트륨, 염화물 및 젖산염 이온을 포함한다. 생리식염수(pH5.5의 0.9% 염화나트륨 용액)는 여전히 사용할 수 있는 수액이지만, 생리식염수를 다량으로 소생술을 시행하면 고염소혈증(혈액 중 염소 농도의 현저한 증가) 및 대사산증이 발생할 수 있다. 노모솔 및 플라즈마라이트는 생리식염수보다 더 균형 잡힌 산-염기 용액(pH 7.4)을 제공하기 위한 대체 수액이다. 이러한 수액은 중증 환자에게 사용할 때 신장 기능 장애가 덜한 것으로 나타났다. 포도당 용액(예: D5W)은 효과적인 부피 확장제가 아니며 외상 환자의 소생술에 사용할 수 없다.

결정질 용액을 투여한 후 30~60분 이내에 투여된 부피의 1/3~1/4 정도만이 심혈관계에 남아 있다. 용액의 수분이나 전해질이 모세혈관막을 자유롭게 통과할 수 있으므로 나머지는 사이질 공간으로 이동

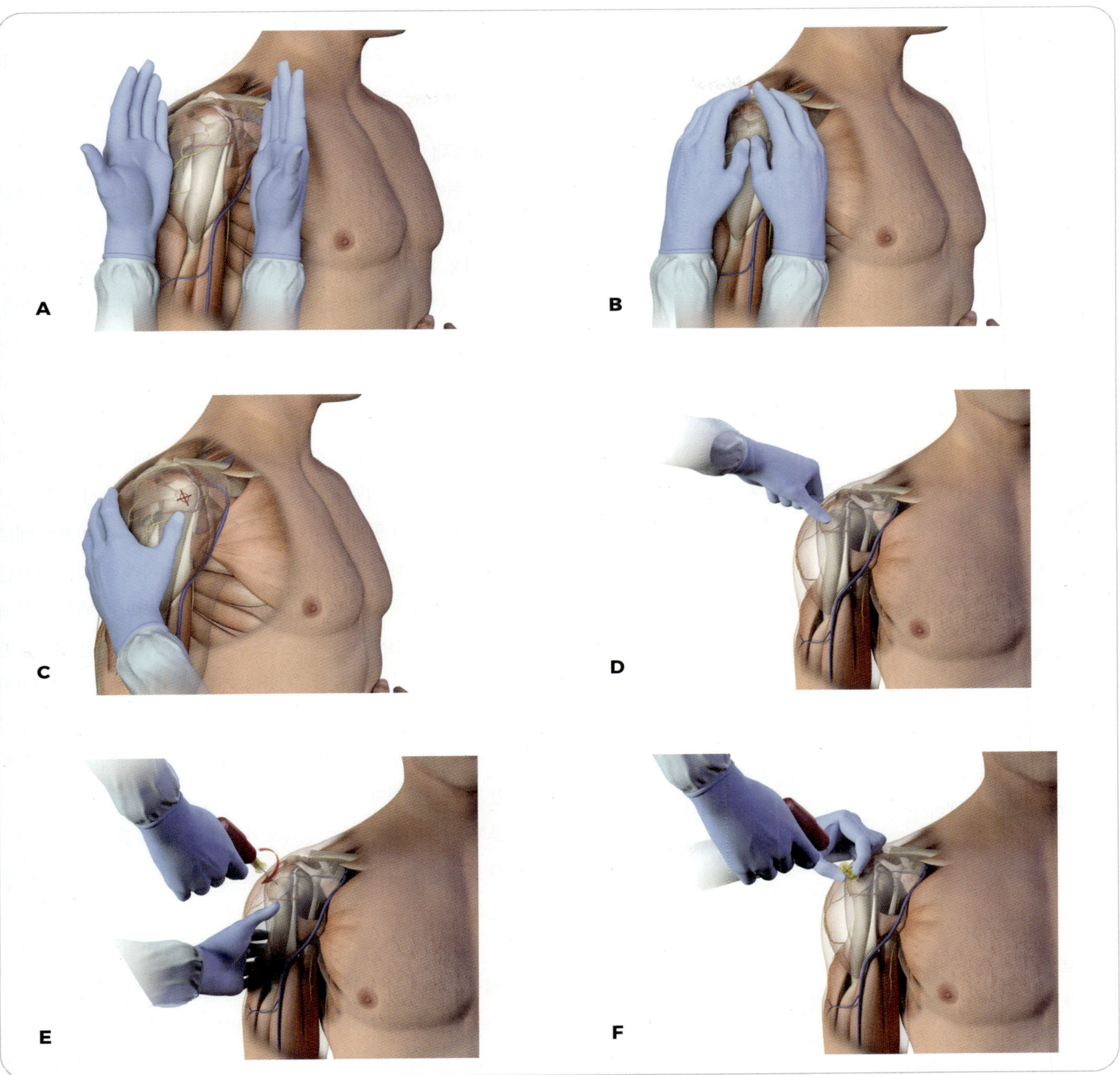

그림 3-22 EZ-IO 장치의 위팔뼈 근위 삽입 부위. **A.** 손의 자뼈 부분을 겨드랑이 위에 수직으로 위치시켜 삽입 부위를 찾는다. 다른 손의 자뼈 측면은 위팔의 정중선을 따라 측면으로 위치시킨다. **B.** 엄지손가락을 모아 팔 위에 놓는다. 이렇게 하면 위팔뼈 근위부에 수직 삽입선이 확인된다. **C.** 위팔뼈의 외과목을 촉진한다. 티 위에 골프공이 있는 것처럼 느껴져야 하며 공과 티가 만나진 지점이 외과목이다. 삽입 부위는 외과목에서 1~2cm 위에 있다. **D.** 삽입 부위를 엄지손가락으로 누른다. **E.** 다른 손으로 바늘 끝이 뼈에 닿을 때까지 피부를 통해 바늘을 누른다. 부드럽게 일정한 압력을 가하면서 방아쇠를 당긴다. **F.** 바늘을 삽입한 후 바늘의 중심부를 안정시키고 고정 장치를 적용한다. 생리식염수(성인의 경우 5~10mL, 영아나 소아의 경우 2~5mL)를 주입하여 바늘 삽입을 확인한다.

한다. 손실된 액체는 신체의 장기와 연부조직에 부종을 발생시켜 적혈구에 산소가 결합하고 분리되는 것을 어렵게 한다.

고장성 결정질 용액

고장성 결정질 용액은 혈장에 비해 전해질 농도가 매우 높다. 가장 일반적으로 사용되는 수액은 일반 생리식염수의 염화나트륨 농도보다 8배 이상인 7.5% 염화나트륨 용액인 고장식염수이다. 2%와 3%의 추가 농도의 고장식염수를 사용할 수 있으며 외상센터와 신경외과 중환자실에서 널리 사용된다. 고장식염수는 효과적인 혈장 확장제이다. 이 용액은 250mL 주입으로 2~3L의 등장성 결정질 용액을 투여하는 것과 같은 동일한 효과를 낼 수 있다. 그러나 고장식염수에 대한 여러 연구의 분석은 등장성 결정질 용액 투여에 비해 개선된 생존율을 입증하는 데 실패했다. 그런데도 고장식염수는 항감염 및 항염증 효과를 포함하여 실험 모델에서 몇 가지 추정되는 이점이 있었다. 이 용액은 미국에서 환자 치료를 위해 미 식품의약처의 승인을 얻지 못했다. 3%와 같은 상대적으로 낮은 농도의 용액은 환자 치료를 위해 승인되어 중환자실에서 사용되고 있다.

합성 교질용액

단백질은 아미노산으로 구성된 신체에서 생성되는 큰 분자이며 수많은 기능을 가지고 있다. 혈액 내 단백질의 한 형태인 알부민은 혈관 내 공간의 체액을 유지하는 데 도움을 준다. 사람의 알부민을 정맥 내 투여는 비용이 많이 들고 출혈성 쇼크 환자의 결과를 개선하는 것으로 나타나지 않았다. 출혈성 쇼크 환자에게 투여하는 경우 합성 교질용액은 사이질 및 세포 내 공간으로 체액을 끌어당겨 혈액량을 증가시킨다. 그러나 결정질 수액과 마찬가지로 교질 혈장 증가는 산소를 운반하지 못한다.

헤타스타치(Hespan, Hextend)와 덱스트란(Gentran)은 수많은 목말(아밀로펙틴) 또는 덱스트로스 분자가 알부민 분자와 크기가 비슷해질 때까지 서로 연결되어 만들어진 합성교질이다. 이러한 용액은 결정질 용액에 비해 비싸고 알레르기 반응 및 혈액형 장애와 관련이 있다. 최근 헤타스타치 사용과 관련된 두 가지 메타분석은 이러한 합성물의 투여가 급성 신장 손상의 발생률 증가와 사망률 증가에 대한 우려를 제기했다.

결정질 용액과 콜로이드의 사용은 외상 환자 처치에 있어 오랜 논쟁을 불러일으켰다. 중환자실에 입원한 약 7,000명의 환자에 대한 연구에서 콜로이드(알부민)와 일반 생리식염수로 소생술을 시행했을 때 결과에 차이가 없는 것으로 나타났다. 민간 병원 전 환경에서 이러한 합성 교질용액을 사용하는 것과 관련된 연구는 거의 발표되지 않았으며 병원에서 사용하는 결정질 수액보다 우수하다는 데이터도 없다. 이러한 제품은 병원 전 쇼크 처치에 권장되지 않는다.

혈액 대체재

수혈에는 혈액형 및 교차 일치의 필요성, 짧은 유통기간, 냉장 보관하지 않을 경우 부패 가능성, 전염병 전파 가능성, 병원 전 환경에서 사용의 어려움 등 몇몇 제한점과 바람직하지 않은 특성이 있다. 이것은 지난 20~30년 동안 혈액 대체물에 대한 집중적인 연구로 이어졌다. 미군은 냉장이 필요 없고 혈액형 검사가 필요 없는 대체혈액을 전쟁터에서 손상을 입은 군인에게 가져가 쇼크 처치를 위해 신속하게 투여할 수 있기 때문에 이번 연구에서 중심적인 역할을 해왔다.

대부분의 산소운반체(HBOC)는 인간, 소 또는 돼지의 혈액 세포에서 발견되는 것과 동일한 산소 운반 분자(헤모글로빈)를 사용한다. 산소운반체와 인간의 혈액 사이의 주요한 차이점은 산소운반체의 헤모글로빈이 세포막 내에 포함되어 있지 않다는 것이다. 이것은 헤모글로빈이 세포에서 추출될 때 항원-항체 위험이 제거되기 때문에 혈액형 및 교차 일치 검사를 수행할 필요가 없다. 또한 이러한 산소운반체 중 다수는 장기간 보관할 수 있어 다수 사상자 사고에 이상적이다. 산소운반체의 초기 문제에는 헤모글로빈의 독성이 포함되어 있었다. 현재까지 이러한 실험 용액 중 어느 것도 인간에게 안전하거나 효과적인 것으로 밝혀지지 않았다.

과불화탄소(PFCs)는 산소 용해도가 높은 합성 화합물이다. 이러한 불활성 물질은 혈장보다 약 50배나 많은 산소를 용해할 수 있다. 과불화탄소에는 적혈구나 단백질을 포함하지 않으며 어떠한 생물학적 물질을 전혀 함유하지 않기 때문에 감염의 위험이 적고 산소가 용해되어 혈장으로 전달된다. 1세대 과불화탄소는 반감기가 짧고 동시에 고농도의 산소를 공급해야 하는 등의 많은 문제점 때문에 제한된 사용을 했다. 새로운 과불화탄소는 이러한 단점이 개선되었지만, 산소를 운반하는 역할은 아직 명확하지 않다.

대부분의 헤모글로빈 기반 산소운반체는 사람, 소 또는 돼지 혈액 세포에서 발견되는 것과 같은 산소를 운반하는 헤모글로빈을 사용한다. 헤모글로빈 기반 산소운반체와 사람 혈액의 주요 차이점은 헤모글로빈 기반 산소운반체의 헤모글로빈이 세포막 내에 포함되어있지 않다는 것이다. 헤모글로빈이 세포에서 추출될 때 항원-항체의 위험이 제거되기 때문에 혈액형 및 교차 검사를 시행할 필요가 없다. 또한, 이러한 헤모글로빈 기반 산소운반체의 대부분은 장기간 보관할 수 있으므로 대량 사상자 발생 시 사용하기에 적합하다. 헤모글로빈 기반 산소운반체 용액의 초기 문제에는 헤모글로빈의 독성을 포함했다. 현재까지 이러한 실험용 용액 중 어떤 것도 사람에게 안전하거나 효과적인 것으로 밝혀진 것은 없다.

정맥 내 가온 수액 투여

쇼크 상태의 환자에게 정맥 내로 투여하는 모든 수액은 상온이나 차갑지 않고 따뜻해야 한다. 이러한 수액의 이상적인 온도는 39°C이다. 수액이 들어 있는 가방에 핫팩을 넣으면 수액을 데울 수 있다. 시중에 판매되는 수액 가온 장치를 사용하면 수액을 정확한 온도로 유지하는 쉽고 신뢰할 수 있는 수단을 제공한다. 이러한 장비는 비용이 많이 들지만, 환자를 이송 지연하거나 냉장 보관된 제품을 수혈할 때 적합하다. 외상 환자의 신속한 일반적인 이송의 경우 제한된 양의 수액 소생술과 신속한 이송에 중점을 두기 때문에 이러한 가온기는 그다지 적절하지 않다.

수액 소생술 처치

앞서 언급한 바와 같이 쇼크 상태에 있는 외상 환자에 대한 병원 전 상황에서 수액 투여를 둘러싼 상당한 논란이 있다. PHTLS가 미국에서 처음 도입되었을 때 병원 전 처치 제공자는 대부분 외상센터에서 응급의학 의사나 외과 의사가 사용하는 방식을 채택했다. 활력징후가 정상으로 돌아올 때까지 정맥 내로 결정질 용액을 투여한다(일반적으로 맥박은 분당 100회 미만, 수축기 혈압 100mmHg 이상으로 유지). 결정질 용액을 충분히 투여하여 활력징후를 정상으로 회복시키면서 환자의 관류가 개선되어야 한다. 당시 전문가들은 이러한 신속한 처치가 젖산을 제거하고 신체 세포의 에너지 생산을 회복시키며 비가역성 쇼크 및 신부전 발생 위험을 감소시킬 것이라고 믿었다. 그러나 병원 전 환경에서 외상 환자에 대한 연구에서는 정맥 내로 수액을 투여하는 것이 합병증과 사망이 감소한다는 결과가 나오지 않았다.

지난 20년 동안 PHTLS의 주요 기여는 중증 손상을 입은 외상 환자에게 정맥 라인을 확보하고 수액을 투여하기 위해 이송이 지연되어서는 안 된다는 개념적 변화를 확립하는 것이었다. 776,000명 이상의 환자를 대상으로 한 국립 외상 데이터 뱅크(NTDB)의 연구에서 병원 전 정맥 내 수액 투여는 사망 확률 증가와 관련이 있었다. 정맥 라인은 가장 가까운 적절한 의료기관으로 이송하는 중에 구급차의 환자실에서 시행할 수 있다. 쇼크 상태에 있는 중증외상 환자는 일반적으로 내부출혈을 조절하기 위해 수혈과 중재술이 필요하며 대부분은 현장에서 수행할 수 없다. 출혈을 조절할 수 있는 수술실이나 응급실로 출혈 환자의 신속한 이송을 지연시켜서는 안 된다.

병원 전 수액 소생술은 다음 논의에서 설명된 대로 임상 상황에 맞게 조정해야 한다(**그림 3-23**).

조절되지 않는 출혈

가슴, 복부, 골반에 내부출혈이 의심되는 환자의 경우 수축기 혈압을 80mmHg 이상으로 유지하거나 평균 동맥압을 60~65mmHg로 유지할 수 있도록 정맥 내로 충분한 결정질 용액(혈액 제제를 사용할 수 없는 경우)을 투여한다. 이 혈압 수치는 신장에 적절한 관류를 유지하고 내부출혈을 악화시킬 위험이 적어야 한다. 목표 혈압 범위를 초과하여 흉곽 내, 복강 내, 골반 내 출혈이 반복될 수 있으므로 대량의 수액을 덩이로 투여해서는 안 된다.

병원 전 환경 및 초기 병원에서 처치하는 동안 제한된 결정질 용액을 투여하는 현재의 처치는 허용 저혈압, 저혈압 소생술 및 균형 소생술을 포함하여 여러 이름으로 불리며 이는 투여된 수액량과 혈압 상승 사이에 균형을 이루어야 한다는 것을 의미한다. 일단 환자가 병원에 도착하면 출혈이 조절될 때까지 혈장과 혈액(1:1 비율) 또는 전혈을 투여하는 방식으로 수액 투여를 계속한다. 제한된 결정질 수액 투여와 지속적인 수혈을 통해 혈압은 정상 수치로 회복된다.

중추신경계 손상

저혈압은 외상성 뇌손상에서 사망률 증가와 관련이 있다. 외상성 뇌손상과 같은 특정한 상황에 있는 환자는 관류를 유지하고 이차 신경 손상을 줄이기 위해 더 높은 혈압이 필요하다. 뇌 외상 재단에서 발표한 지침에 따르면 외상성 뇌손상이 의심되는 환자의 경우 수축기 혈압을 110mmHg 이상으로 유지할 것을 권장한다. 급성 척추 손상 관리에 중점을 둔 합의된 지침에 따르면 저혈압(수축기 혈압 90mmHg 미만)을 피할 뿐만 아니라 척수 관류 개선을 위해 평균 동맥압을 최소 85~90mmHg로 유지할 것을 권장한다. 이 목표를 달성하기 위해 보다 적극적인 수액 소생술이 필요할 수 있지만, 관련 내부 손상으로 인한 출혈이 재발할 위험이 높아질 수 있다.

조절된 출혈

병원 전 처치 제공자가 흉곽 내, 복강 내, 골반 내 손상 및 출혈이 의심되지 않는 상황이라면 조절된 심각한 외부출혈이 있는 환자는 더욱 적극적인 수액 소생술로 처치할 수 있다. 예를 들어, 두피에 큰 열

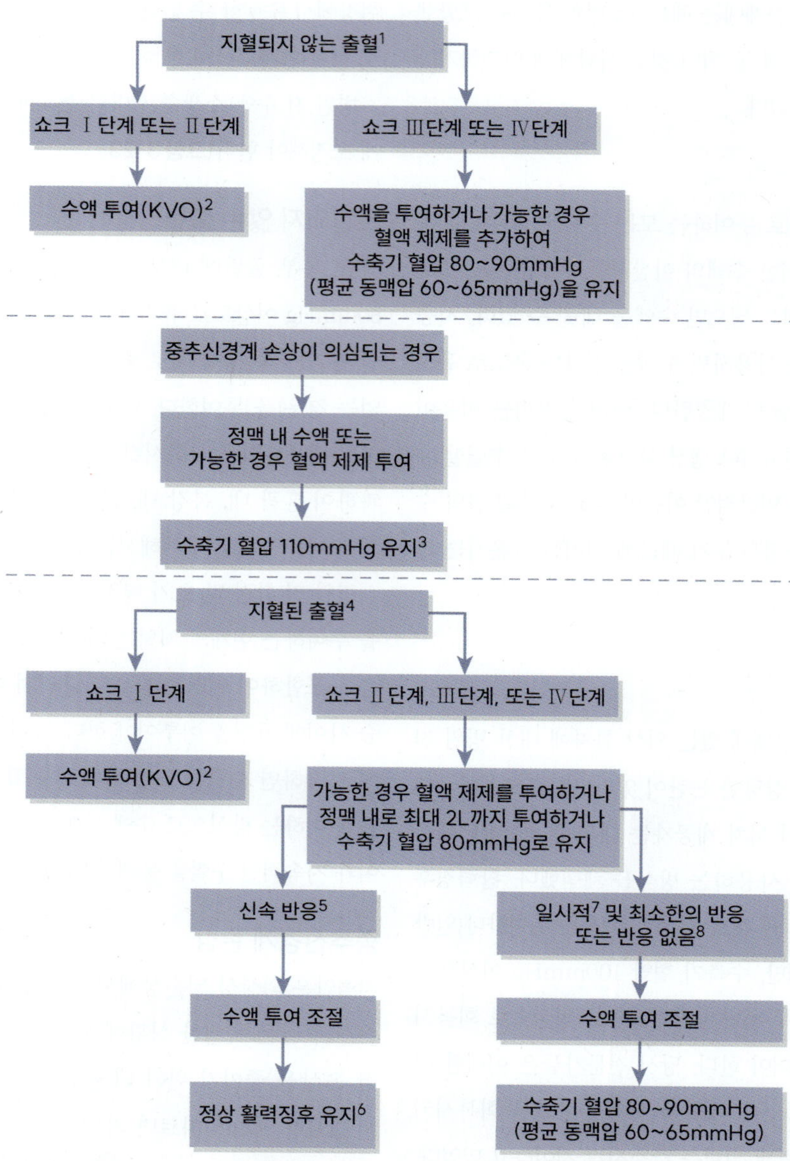

그림 3-23 **A.** 외상에서의 수액 소생술 처치 알고리즘

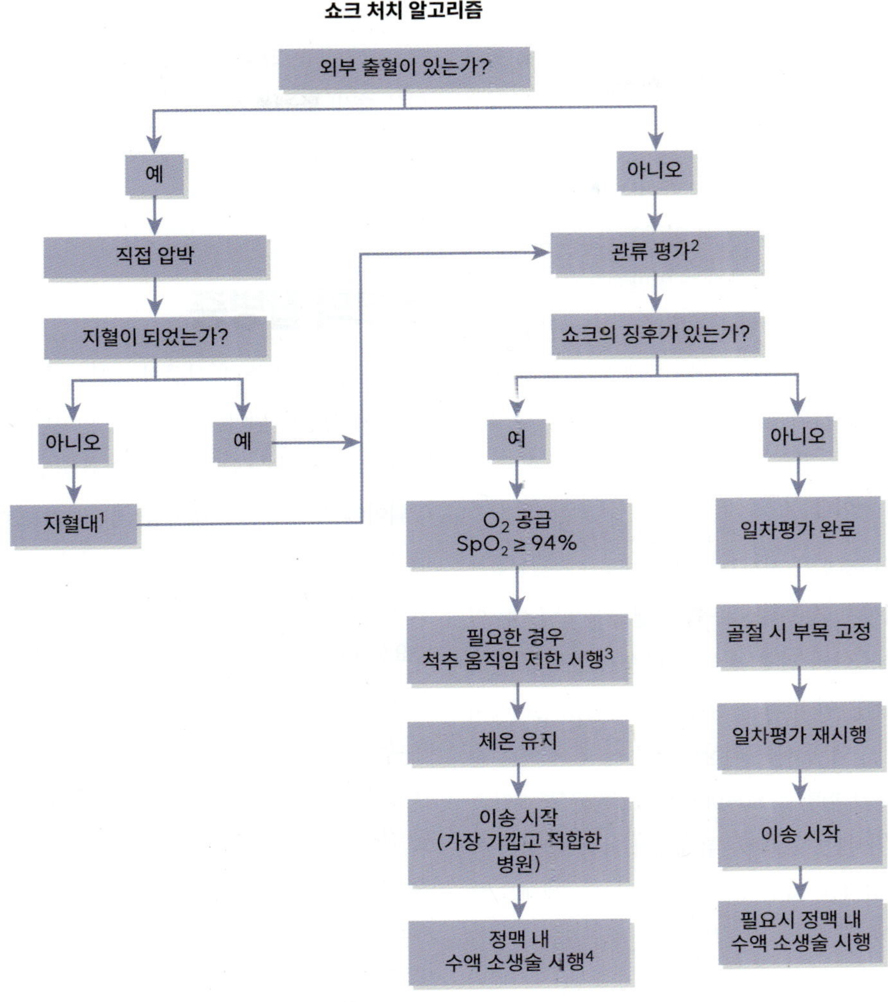

그림 3-23 (이어서) **B.** 외상에서의 쇼크 처치 알고리즘

상이 있거나 주요 혈관을 포함한 팔다리의 손상은 압박 드레싱이나 지혈대로 출혈을 조절할 수 있다. 출혈이 조절된 성인 환자 중 II, III, IV단계 출혈이 있는 경우 총 1L까지 결정질 용액을 250mL를 초기 볼루스로 반복해서 투여하거나 수축기 혈압이 90mmHg에 도달할 때까지 투여할 수 있다. 소아 환자는 가온된 결정질 용액을 20mL/kg로 볼루스로 투여한다. 앞서 언급한 바와 같이 수액 투여는 항상 가장 가까운 적절한 의료기관으로 이송하는 동안 이루어져야 한다. 초기 수액 요법에 대한 환자의 반응을 평가하기 위해 혈압, 맥박, 환기 속도를 포함한- 활력징후를 모니터링해야 한다. 대부분의 도시 환경에서 환자는 수액을 볼루스로 초기 투여가 완료되기 전에 의료기관으로 이송된다.

초기 수액을 볼루스로 투여하는 것은 다음과 같이 세 가지 반응을 보인다.

1. 신속한 반응: 활력징후가 정상으로 회복되고 유지된다. 이것은 일반적으로 환자가 혈액량이 20% 미만으로 감소하고 출혈이 멈췄음을 나타낸다.

2. 일시적인 반응: 초기에는 활력징후(맥박이 느려지고 혈압이 상승)가 개선되지만, 재평가 동안 이 환자들은 쇼크 징후가 반복되면서 악화를 보인다. 이 환자는 일반적으로 혈액량의 20~40%를 잃었고 지속적인 출혈을 경험하고 있을 수 있다.

3. 최소한의 반응 또는 무반응: 이 환자는 수액 1L를 일시에 투여한 후에도 심각한 쇼크의 징후에 거의 변화를 보이지 않는다. 이 환자들은 대량 출혈을 겪었거나 진행 중인 출혈을 겪고 있거나 둘 다일 것이다.

반응이 빠른 환자는 활력징후가 정상으로 회복되고 쇼크의 모든 임상적 지표가 해결될 때까지 지속적인 수액 소생술을 받을 수 있다. 일시적인 반응이나 최소한의 반응 또는 무반응을 보이는 환자는 내부출혈이 있을 수 있다. 이 환자는 상대적인 저혈압 상태에서 가장 잘 관리되며 정맥 내 수액 투여는 외상성 뇌손상 또는 척수 손상의 증거가 없는 한 수축기 혈압을 80~90mmHg(평균 동맥압을 60~65mmHg) 범위로 유지하는 적절하게 유지해야 한다. 일시적 반응의 개념은 덜 강조되고 있지만, 기초 생리학은 여전히 이해해야 할 중요한 과정으로 남아 있다.

트라넥삼산(TXA)

트라넥삼산은 아미노산 라이신(Lysine)의 유사체이며 심한 자궁출혈 있는 부인과 환자나, 심장 또는 정형외과 수술을 받는 환자, 혈우병 환자가 치과 치료와 같은 시술을 받는 경우 출혈을 줄이기 위해 수십 년 동안 사용됐다. 손상으로 인해 응고연쇄반응(**그림 3-12**)이 활성화되어 혈전을 형성하면 동시에 혈전 분해 과정이 시작된다. 트라넥삼산은 새로 형성된 혈전을 유지하고 안정화하기 위해 분해 과정을 방해하고 항염증 효과도 있다.

여러 연구에 따르면 트라넥삼산은 중증외상 환자의 생존율을 향상할 수 있다. 트라넥삼산은 조기 투여(즉, 손상 후 3시간 미만)와 환자가 심각한 손상(즉, 저혈압, 빈맥)을 입은 경우에 가장 효과적인 것으로 보인다. 모든 연구가 확실한 이점을 입증한 것은 아니기 때문에 외상성 뇌손상 환자에게서의 사용을 포함하여 병원 전 트라넥삼산 사용에 대한 적절한 적응증을 결정하기 위한 추가 연구가 진행 중이다. 군 및 민간 전술 EMS 공동체에서 사용하기 위한 현재의 전술 사

상자 처치 지침은 수혈이 필요할 가능성이 있는 환자(즉, 출혈성 쇼크, 젖산 상승, 하나 이상의 주요 절단, 몸통 관통상 또는 심각한 출혈의 증거) 또는 심각한 외상성 뇌손상의 징후(즉, 폭발 손상 또는 무딘 손상과 관련된 의식 수준 변화)가 있으며 손상 후 최소 3시간 이내에 나타난다.

쇼크의 합병증

저체온증, 응고병증 및 산증의 증상은 흔히 치명적인 3요소로 설명된다. 실제 사망의 원인은 아니지만, 임박한 죽음을 나타내는 발견들이다. 이것은 무산소대사와 에너지 생산 감소의 지표이며 신속하게 제공되어야 하는 무산소대사를 역전시키는 데 필요한 처치를 설명한다. 몇 가지 합병증으로 인해 지속되거나 부적절하게 소생된 쇼크 환자가 발생할 수 있으며 이는 조기 인식과 적극적으로 처치하는 것이 중요한 이유이다. 병원 전 환경에서 제공되는 처치의 질은 병원 내서 환자의 처치 과정과 결과에 영향을 미칠 수 있다. 병원 전 환경에서 쇼크를 인식하고 적절한 처치를 시작하면 환자의 입원 기간을 단축하고 생존 가능성을 높일 수 있다. 다음과 같은 쇼크의 합병증은 병원 전 환경에서는 자주 나타나지 않지만, 현장과 응급실에서 발생한 쇼크의 결과이다. 또한, 시설 간에 환자를 이송할 때 발생할 수 있다. 쇼크 과정의 결과를 알면 상태의 중증도, 신속한 출혈 조절의 중요성 및 적절한 수액 소생술을 이해하는 데에 도움이 된다.

급성신부전

신장으로의 혈액 순환이 감소하면 신장의 유산소대사가 무산소대사로 바꾼다. 감소한 에너지 생산은 신장 세포의 부종을 유발하여 신장 관류를 감소시켜 추가적인 무산소대사를 유발한다. 신세관을 구성하는 세포는 허혈에 민감하며 산소 공급이 45~60분 이상 중단되면 사망할 수 있다. 급성세관괴사(ATN) 또는 급성신부전으로 불리는 이 상태는 신세관의 여과 효율을 감소시킨다. 그 결과 신장 배출량이 감소하고 독성 물질과 전해질의 제거가 감소한다. 신장이 더는 기능하지 않으므로 과도한 체액이 배설되지 않아 용적과부하가 발생할 수 있다. 또한, 신장은 대사산과 전해질을 배출하는 능력을 잃어 대사산증과 고칼륨혈증(혈중 칼륨 증가)을 유발한다. 이러한 환자들은 종종 몇 주 또는 몇 개월 동안 투석이 필요하다. 쇼크로 인해 급성세관괴사가 발생한 대부분 환자는 결국 정상적인 신장 기능을 회복할 수 있다.

급성호흡곤란증후군

급성호흡곤란증후군(ARDS)은 폐의 폐포 세포가 손상되고 이러한 세포의 신진대사를 유지하는 데 필요한 에너지 생산 감소로 인해 발생한다. 이 손상은 소생술 중 다량의 결정질 용액 투여로 인해 발생하는 체액 과부하와 동반되어 사이질 공간과 폐포 안으로 체액이 누출되어 산소가 폐포벽을 통해 모세혈관으로 확산하여 적혈구와 결합하는 것을 훨씬 더 어렵게 만든다. 이 문제는 제2차 세계 대전 중에 처음 설명되었지만, 베트남 전쟁 중에 공식적으로 인식되어 다낭 폐(이러한 사례를 많이 본 병원 위치를 따름)라고 불렸다. 이 환자는 폐부종이 있지만, 심부전(심장성 폐부종)과 같이 심장 기능 장애의 결과는 아니다. 급성호흡곤란증후군은 비 심장성 폐부종을 나타낸다. 결정질 용액 투여를 제한하고 허용 저혈압 및 손상 통제 소생술(적혈구:혈장 비율 1:1)과 같은 소생술 과정이 변경됨에 따라 외상 기간(24~72시간)에서 급성호흡곤란증후군을 현저하게 감소시켰다.

혈액 부전

응고병증이라는 용어는 혈액의 정상적인 응고 능력의 손상을 의미한다. 이 이상은 저체온증(체온저하), 수액 투여로 인한 응고 인자 희석 또는 출혈을 조절하기 위한 노력으로 소모된 응고 물질의 결핍(소모성 응고병증)으로 인해 발생할 수 있다. 정상적인 혈액 응고 연쇄반응은 결국 혈소판을 포획하고 혈관 벽에 마개를 형성하여 지혈하는 역할을 하는 피브린 분자의 생성을 초래하는 여러 효소 및 인자를 포함한다(**그림 3-24**). 이 과정은 좁은 온도 범위(즉 거의 정상 체온) 내에서 가장 잘 효과적이다. 인체의 중심 체온이 떨어지고(단지 몇 도만) 에너지 생산이 줄어들면 혈액 응고가 손상되어 출혈이 계속된다. 혈액 응고 인자는 또한 출혈을 늦추고 조절하기 위해 혈전을 형성할 때

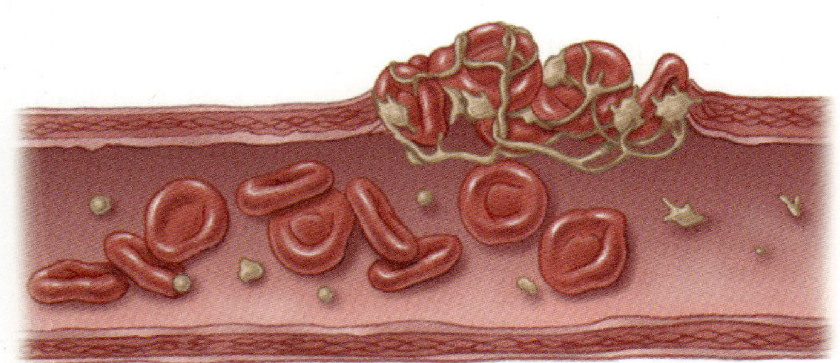

그림 3-24 혈액 응고에는 여러 가지 효소와 인자가 관여하여 결국 피브린 분자가 생성되는데 이 피브린 분자는 혈소판을 가두어 혈관 벽에 마개를 형성하여 출혈을 막는 매트리스 역할을 한다.

소모될 수 있다. 감소한 체온은 응고 문제를 악화시키고 체온을 유지하는 신체의 능력을 더욱 감소시킨다. 부적절한 소생술로 이 순환은 점점 더 악화한다.

간부전

장기간의 쇼크로 인해 덜 흔한 결과이긴 하지만, 심각한 간 손상이 발생할 수 있다. 쇼크로 인한 간 손상의 증거는 일반적으로 간 기능 검사 결과에서 간 수치가 상승한 결과가 나올 때까지 며칠 동안은 명백하지 않다. 간부전은 지속적인 저혈당증(저혈당), 지속적인 젖산 산중 및 황달로 나타난다. 간은 지혈에 필요한 많은 응고 인자를 생산하기 때문에 응고병증이 간부전을 동반할 수 있다.

심각한 감염

중증 쇼크와 관련된 감염 위험이 증가한다. 이러한 위험 증가는 다음과 같은 원인에 기인한다.

- 백혈구 수의 현저한 감소로 인해 쇼크 환자가 감염되기 쉬운 상태가 되는 것은 혈액 부전의 또 다른 증상이다.
- 쇼크 환자의 장벽 세포에서 허혈 및 에너지 생산 감소로 인해 세균이 혈루로 누출될 수 있다.
- 허혈 및 에너지 생산 손실에 직면하여 면역계의 기능이 감소한다.
- 허혈성 손상 및 순환 염증 인자로 인해 폐에 있는 모세혈관 막의 투과성이 증가하면 폐포에 액체가 축적된다. 이로 인해 호흡곤란이 발생하며 기관내삽관이 필요하다. 이러한 요인의 조합은 쇼크 환자에게 전신 패혈증을 유발할 수 있는 폐렴 증상을 유발한다.
- 가장 중요한 것은 여러 절차, 혈관 침입 및 유치 카테터 삽입으로 인해 심각한 손상을 입은 환자의 감염 위험을 증가시킨다는 것이다.

다기관부전

쇼크가 성공적으로 처치되지 않으면 처음에는 하나의 장기에서 기능 장애를 일으킬 수 있고 그다음에는 동시에 여러 장기에서 기능장애를 일으킬 수 있으며 패혈증이 동반되어 다발성 장기 기능장애 증후군(MODS)으로 이어질 수 있다.

하나의 주요 인체 계통(예: 폐, 신장, 혈액 응고 연쇄반응, 간)의 부전은 약 40%의 사망률과 관련이 있다. 심장성 쇼크와 패혈 쇼크 형태의 심혈관 부전은 때때로 회복될 수 있다. 4개의 장기 계통이 모두 망가지면 사망률은 본질적으로 100%이다.

이송 지연

쇼크 상태의 외상 환자를 장시간 이송하는 동안 중요한 장기에 대한 관류를 유지하는 것이 중요하다. 장시간 이송 전에는 기도 관리를 최적화해야 하며 기도 개방에 문제가 있는 경우 기관내삽관이나 성문외기도기 삽입과 같은 방법을 통해 기도 유지를 수행해야 한다. 환기가 부적절한 경우 적절한 일회호흡량과 환기 속도로 보조 환기를 제공하여 이미 관류가 약한 환자의 전부하 및 심박출량을 손상하지 않도록 한다. 맥박산소측은 지속해서 모니터링해야 한다. 호기말이산화탄소분압 측정은 기관내관의 위치와 환자의 관류 상태에 대한 정보를 제공한다. 호기말이산화탄소분압의 현저한 감소는 기관내관이 기도에서 이탈되었거나 환자의 관류가 현저히 감소했음을 나타낸다. 긴장기흉과 같은 추가 고려사항을 평가하고 환자에게 적절한 처치를 수행해야 한다.

이송 지연 중 심각한 외부출혈 부위를 손으로 직접 압박하는 것은 비실용적이므로 압박 드레싱으로 지혈해야 한다. 이러한 방법으로 조절되지 않으면 지혈대를 사용한다. 지혈대를 작용한 후 이송 시간이 4시간을 초과할 것으로 예상되는 상황에서는 더욱 적극적으로 국소 출혈을 지혈한 후 지혈대를 제거하는 것을 고려해야 한다. 이때 출혈의 징후가 있는지 드레싱을 관찰하면서 지혈대를 천천히 풀어야 한다. 출혈이 재발하지 않으면 지혈대를 완전히 풀고 출혈이 재발할 경우를 대비하여 그대로 둔다. 1) 출혈 3단계 또는 4단계, 2) 완전 절단, 3) 출혈의 재발에 대해 환자를 관찰할 수 없는 경우 및 4) 지혈대를 6시간 이상 적용한 경우와 같은 상황에서는 지혈대를 다시 드레싱으로 전환해서는 안 된다. 외부출혈을 조절하기 위해 모든 골절 부위를 부목으로 고정한다.

앞에서 설명한 바와 같이 정상 체온을 유지하는 술기는 이송 시간이 길어질 경우 더욱 중요하다. 구급차의 환자실을 따뜻하게 하는 것 외에도 담요나 체온을 유지할 수 있는 재료로 환자를 덮어준다. 큰 비닐봉지도 환자의 열 손실을 방지하는 데 도움이 된다. 정맥으로 수액을 투여하기 전에 수액을 따뜻하게 한다. 특히 외상 환자에게 실온의 수액을 정맥 내로 대량 투여하며 저체온증을 유발할 수 있으며 이는 환자의 혈전 형성 능력에 영향을 미칠 수 있다.

환자를 이송 지연하는 상황에서 수액 투여를 위해 정맥 라인 확보가 필요할 수 있으며 이는 두 개의 굵은 지름의 정맥 라인을 확보해야 한다. 소아와 성인에서 말초혈관을 확보하는 것이 불가능하면 앞서 설명한 바와 같이 골내 경로를 사용할 수 있다.

지속적인 출혈이 의심되는 환자의 경우 수축기 혈압을 80~90mmHg 또는 평균 동맥압 60~65mmHg 범위로 유지하면 일반적으로 내부출혈의 재발 위험을 줄이면서 중요한 장기에 대한 관류를 유지하는 목표를 달성할 수 있다. 외상성 뇌손상 또는 척수 손상이 의심되는 환자는 수축기 혈압을 110mmHg 이상으로 유지해야 한다.

활력징후를 자주 재평가하여 소생술에 대한 반응을 모니터링해야 한다. 가능한 경우 환기 속도, 맥박수, 혈압, 피부색 및 체온, 모세혈관 재충전 시간, 글래스고혼수척도, 산소포화도, 호기말이산화탄소분압 등을 간격을 두고 측정하고 기록한다.

일반적으로 빠른 이송 상황에서 요도 카테터 삽입은 필요하지 않지만, 소변 배출량을 모니터링하는 것은 이송 지연 중에 추가 수액 소생술의 필요성을 결정하는 데 도움이 되는 중요한 요소이다. 프로토콜이 허용하는 경우 요도 카테터 삽입은 소변 배출량을 모니터링하기 위해 고려해야 한다. 적절한 소변 배출량은 성인의 경우 0.5mL/kg/h, 소아 환자의 경우 1mL/kg/h, 1세 미만의 영아의 경우 2mL/kg/h이다. 이 양보다 적은 소변 배출량은 환자에게 추가 수액 투여가 필요하다는 주요 지표가 될 수 있다.

이송 지연 중에 시간과 프로토콜이 허용하는 경우 기관내삽관 환자에게 코위관 또는 입위관 삽입을 고려한다. 얼굴중간 골절이 있는 경우 입위관 삽입을 고려한다. 위 팽창은 특히 소아에서 설명할 수 없는 저혈압 및 부정맥을 유발할 수 있다. 코위관 또는 입위관 삽입하면 구토와 흡인의 위험을 감소시킬 수 있다.

요 약

- 외상 환자에서 출혈은 쇼크의 가장 흔한 원인이다.
- 인간은 포도당과 산소를 사용하여 유산소대사라는 복잡한 시스템을 통해 생명을 유지하는 데 필요한 에너지를 생산한다. 이 전체 과정은 신체의 세포에 산소를 전달할 수 있어야 하는 순환계에 적절한 양의 산소를 공급하는 호흡계에 달려있다.
- 유산소대사에 대한 백업 시스템을 무산소대사라고 한다. 무산소대사는 산소가 필요하지 않지만, 비효율적이고 소량의 에너지만 생산한다.
- 쇼크는 조직 세포의 산소 공급이 대사 요구를 충족시키기에 불충분한 조직 세포의 관류저하로 인해 유산소대사에서 무산소대사로 세포 기능의 일반화된 변화 상태이다. 그 결과 세포 에너지 생산이 감소하고 비교적 짧은 시간에 세포 기능이 손상되어 결국 세포 사멸로 이어진다.
- 쇼크는 다음과 같이 분류할 수 있다.
  - 저혈량 쇼크: 주로 외상 환자의 출혈이며 순환 혈액 세포의 손실 및 산소 운반 능력이 있는 체액량과 관련됨(외상 환자에서 쇼크의 가장 흔한 원인)
  - 분포성(또는 혈관성) 쇼크: 혈관의 긴장도 이상과 관련됨
  - 심장성 쇼크: 심장의 펌프 기능장애와 관련이 있으며 종종 심장발작 후 발생
- 쇼크 상태에 있는 환자 또는 쇼크 상태에 빠질 수 있는 환자의 처치는 쇼크와 출혈의 명백한 징후를 찾는 환자의 빠른 첫인상 평가를 시작으로 사건의 병력을 시작으로 환자를 평가하는 것으로 시작된다.
- 쇼크 처치 단계는 다음과 같다.
  1. 심한 외부출혈을 조절한다.
  2. 산소 공급 및 환지를 보장한다(기도 관리).
  3. 출혈의 원인을 확인한다.
  4. 결정적인 처치를 시행할 수 있는 의료기관으로 이송한다.
  5. 적절한 경우 혈액 성분 요법을 시행한다.
- 외부출혈은 직접 압박으로 조절한 후 압박 드레싱을 적용해야 한다. 이 방법이 신속하게 효과가 없으면 서혜부, 겨드랑 부위 말단에 지혈대를 적용해야 한다. 추가적인 출혈 조절하기 위해 국소 지혈제를 사용할 수 있다. 골반 골절이 의심되는 경우 골반 고정대 사용을 고려한다.
- 어떤 경우에는 외상 환자의 비출혈성 쇼크 원인(예: 긴장기흉)을 신속하게 교정할 수 있다.
- 쇼크 상태에 있는 모든 외상 환자는 적절한 산소 공급을 유지하는 것 외에도 쇼크의 원인을 구체적으로 확인하고 결정적인 처치를 시행할 수 있는 의료기관으로 신속하게 이송해야 한다.
- 정맥 라인을 확보하기 위해 이송이 지연되어서는 안 된다. 이러한 처치는 이송 중 구급차에서 시행한다.
- 외상 후 출혈 쇼크 환자의 추가 출혈 및 부종 형성을 최소화하기 위해 과도한 수액 투여는 피한다.

시나리오 재구성

당신과 동료는 오토바이 충돌 혈장으로 출동했다. 오토바이는 도로를 벗어나 여러 번 굴러 전신주에 충돌했다. 현장에 도착하자마자 헬멧을 쓴 29세의 남성 운전자가 오토바이에서 약 15m 떨어진 곳에 바로 누워 있는 것을 발견했다. 환자는 흉부, 엉치뼈 및 왼쪽 엉덩관절 부위의 통증을 주요호소증상으로 호소한다.

환자의 신체검사 결과 피부는 창백하고 축축했으며 말초 맥박 감소, 흉부 타박상과 골반은 불안정했다. 활력징후는 맥박 110회/분, 혈압 82/56mmHg, 산소포화도는 92%, 호흡수 20회/회이며 오른쪽 호흡음이 감소했다.

- 이러한 유형의 손상 기전으로 어떤 손상이 발생할 것으로 예상하는가?
- 현장에서 이러한 손상을 어떻게 처치할 것인가?
- 이 환자에게 일어나는 주요 병리학적 과정은 무엇인가?
- 이 환자의 증상을 유발하는 병태생리학적 원인을 어떻게 교정할 것인가?
- 당신은 가장 가까운 외상센터에서 멀리 떨어진 시골 지역에서 근무하고 있다. 이 요소가 당신의 처치 계획을 어떻게 변화시키는가?

시나리오 해결책

당신은 이 환자가 출혈 쇼크의 징후(심박수 증가, 혈압 감소 및 환기 속도 증가)를 보인다는 것을 알게 되었다. 기도, 호흡 및 순환을 평가한다. 골반 골절로 인한 내부출혈이 의심되어 척추 고정을 시행하고 골반 고정대를 적용한 후 환자는 구급차로 가장 가까운 외상센터로 이송을 시작한다.

이송 중 호기말이산화탄소분압을 확인한 후 비재호흡마스크를 통해 2L/분의 산소를 공급한다. 18게이지로 두 개의 정맥 라인을 확보하여 수축기 혈압이 90mmHg 이상으로 유지할 수 있도록 수액을 투여한다. 환자의 혈류역학 및 내부출혈의 가능성으로 인해 환자는 트라넥삼산 투여 대상자이며 가장 가까운 외상센터에서 어느 정도 떨어진 외곽 지역에 있다는 점을 고려한다. 또한, 구급차 환자실을 따뜻하게 하고 담요를 덮어주는 것과 같은 적절한 환경을 만들며 따뜻한 수액을 투여해 환자의 체온 손실을 방지한다. 외상센터로 이송하는 중에 당신은 의료 지도 의사에게 환자가 항응고제를 복용한다는 것을 보고하였고 환자는 안정적인 상태로 외상 전문의에게 인계하였다.

References

1. Janssens U, Graf J. Shock—what are the basics? *Internist (Berl)*. 2004;45(3):258-266.

2. Gross SD. *A System of Surgery: Pathological, Diagnostic, Therapeutic, and Operative*. Blanchard and Lea; 1859.

3. Knisely MH, Cowley RA, Hawthorne I, Garris D. Separation of shock types: experimental and clinical separation of hypovolemic and septic shock. *Angiology*. 1970;21(11):728-744.

4. Galvagno SM. *Emergency pathophysiology*. Teton NewMedia, 2004.

5. Cowley RA. A total emergency medical system for the state of Maryland. *Md State Med J*. 1975;45:37-45.

6. Koch E, Lovett S, Nghiem T, et al. Shock index in the emergency department: utility and limitations. *Emerg Med*. 2019;11:179-199.

7. Cannon CM, Braxton CC, Kling-Smith M, et al. Utility of the shock index in predicting mortality in traumatically injured patients. *J Trauma Acute Care Surg*. 2009;67(6):1426-1430.

8. Olaussen A, Blackburn T, Mitra B, et al. Shock index for prediction of critical bleeding post-trauma: A systematic review. *Emerg Med Austral*. 2014;26:223-228.

9. Savage SA, Sumislawski JJ, Zarzaur BL, Dutton WP, Croce MA, Fabian TC. The new metric to define large-volume hemorrhage: results of a prospective study of the critical administration threshold. *J Trauma Acute Care Surg*. 2015;78(2):224-229.

10. Meyer DE, Cotton BA, Fox EE, et al. A comparison of resuscitation intensity and critical administration threshold in predicting early mortality among bleeding patients: a multicenter validation in 680 major transfusion patients. *J Trauma Acute Care Surg*. 2018;85(4):691-696.

11. McClelland RN, Shires GT, Baxter CR, et al. Balanced salt solutions in the treatment of hemorrhagic shock. *JAMA*. 1967;199:830-834.

12. Duchesne JC, Hunt JP, Wahl G, et al. Review of current blood transfusion strategies in a mature level I trauma center: were we wrong for the last 60 years? *J Trauma*. 2008;65(2):272-276; discussion 276-278.

13. Holcomb JB, Jenkins D, Rhee P, et al. Damage control resuscitation: directly addressing the early coagulopathy of trauma. *J Trauma*. 2007;62(2):307-310.

14. Amaral CB, Ralston DC, Becker TK. Prehospital point-of-care ultrasound: a transformative technology. *SAGE Open Medicine*. 2020;8:1-6.

15. McManus J, Yershov AL, Ludwig D, Holcomb JB, Salinas J, Dubick MA, Convertino VA, Hinds D, David W, Flanagan T, Duke JH. Radial pulse character relationships to systolic blood pressure and trauma outcomes. *Prehosp Emerg Care*. 2005 Oct-Dec;9(4):423-8. doi: 10.1080/10903120500255891. PMID: 16263676.

16. Spaite DW, Hu C, Bobrow BJ, et al. The effect of combined out-of-hospital hypotension and hypoxia on mortality in major traumatic brain injury. *Ann Emerg Med*. 2017;69(1):62-72. doi: 10.1016/j.annemergmed.2016.08.00

17. Spaite DW, Bobrow BJ, Keim SM, et al. Association of statewide implementation of the prehospital traumatic brain injury treatment guidelines with patient survival following traumatic brain injury: the Excellence in Prehospital Injury Care (EPIC) study. *JAMA Surg*. 2019;154(7):e191152.

18. Convertino VA, Koons NJ, Suresh M. Physiology of human hemorrhage and compensation. *Compr Physiol*. 2021;11:1531-1574.

19. Convertino VA, Schauer SG, Weitzel EK, et al. Wearable sensors integrated with compensatory reserve monitoring in critically injured trauma patients. *Sensors*. 2020;20(22):6463.

20. Convertino VA, Johnson MC, Alarhayem A, et al. Compensatory reserve detects subclinical phases of shock with more expeditious prediction for need of life-saving interventions compared to vital signs and arterial lactate. *Transfusion*. 2021;61:S167-S173.

21. Koreny M, Riedmuller E, Nikfardjam M, et al. Arterial puncture closing devices compared with standard manual compression after cardiac catheterization: systematic review and meta-analysis. *JAMA*. 2004;291:350-357.

22. Walker SB, Cleary S, Higgins M. Comparison of the FemoStop device and manual pressure in reducing groin puncture site

complications following coronary angioplasty and coronary stent placement. *Int J Nurs Pract*. 2001;7:366-375.

23. Peng HT. Hemostatic agents for prehospital hemorrhage control: a narrative review. *Military Med Res*. 2020;7:13. doi: 10.1186/s40779-020-00241-z

24. Butler FK. The US Military Experience with Tourniquets and Hemostatic Dressings in the Afghanistan and Iraq Conflicts. *Bull Am College Surg*. 2015:100: September Supplement: 60-65.

25. Kragh JF, Walters TJ, Baer DG, et al. Survival with emergency tourniquet use to stop bleeding in major limb trauma. *Ann Surg*. 2009;249(1):1-7.doi:10.1097/SLA.0b013e31818 842ba.

26. Beekley AC, Sebesta JA, Blackbourne LH, et al. Prehospital tourniquet use in Operation Iraqi Freedom: effect on hemorrhage control and outcomes. *J Trauma*. 2008;64(2):S28-S37.

27. Kragh JF Jr, Walters TJ, Baer DG, et al. Practical use of emergency tourniquets to stop bleeding in major limb trauma. *J Trauma*. 2008;64(2):S38-S50.

28. Bellamy RF. The causes of death in conventional land warfare: implications for combat casualty care research. *Mil Med*. 1984;149:55-62.

29. Mabry RL, Holcomb JB, Baker AM, et al. United States Army Rangers in Somalia: an analysis of combat casualties on an urban battlefield. *J Trauma*. 2000;49:515-528.

30. Lakstein D, Blumenfeld A, Sokolov T, et al. Tourniquets for hemorrhage control on the battlefield: a 4-year accumulated experience. *J Trauma*. 2003;54:S221-S225.

31. Eilertsen KA, Winberg M, Jeppesen E, Hval G, Wisborg T. Prehospital tourniquets in civilians: a systematic review. *Prehosp Disaster Med*. 2021;36(1):86–94.

32. Kragh JF, Walters TJ, Baer DG, et al. Survival with emergency tourniquet use to stop bleeding in major limb trauma. *Ann Surg*. 2009;249(1):1-7.

33. Montgomery HR, Hammesfahr R, Fisher AD, et al. 2019 recommended limb tourniquets in tactical combat casualty care. *J Spec Ops Med*. 19(4);27-50.

34. Joint Trauma System. Tactical Combat Casualty Care Guidelines 2020. Accessed September 30, 2021. https://deployedmedicine.com/content/40

35. Kheirabadi BS, Scherer MR, Estep JS, Dubick MA, Holcomb JB. Determination of efficacy of new hemostatic dressings in a model of extremity arterial hemorrhage in swine. *J Trauma*. 2009 Sep;67(3):450-459; discussion 459-460. doi: 10.1097/TA.0b013e3181ac0c99

36. Kheirabadi BS, Edens JW, Terrazas IB, et al. Comparison of new hemostatic granules/powders with currently deployed hemostatic products in a lethal model of extremity arterial hemorrhage in swine. *J Trauma*. 2009 Feb;66(2):316-326; discussion 327-328. doi: 10.1097 /TA.0b013e31819634a1

37. Kunio NR, Riha GM, Watson KM, Differding JA, Schreiber MA, Watters JM. Chitosan based advanced hemostatic dressing is associated with decreased blood loss in a swine uncontrolled hemorrhage model. *Am J Surg*. 2013 May;205(5):505-510. doi: 10.1016/j .amjsurg.2013.01.014

38. Dumont TM, Visioni AJ, Rughani AI, et al. Inappropriate prehospital ventilation in severe traumatic brain injury increases in-hospital mortality. *J Neurotrauma*. 2010;27(7):1233-1241.

39. Bickell WH, Wall MJ Jr, Pepe PE, et al. Immediate versus delayed fluid resuscitation for hypotensive patients with penetrating torso injuries. *N Engl J Med*. 1994 Oct 27;331(17):1105-1109.

40. Dutton RP, Mackenzie CF, Scalea TM. Hypotensive resuscitation during active hemorrhage: impact on in-hospital mortality. *J Trauma*. 2002 Jun;52(6):1141-1146.

41. Schreiber MA, Meier EN, Tisherman SA, et al.; ROC Investigators. A controlled resuscitation strategy is feasible and safe in hypotensive trauma patients: results of a prospective randomized pilot trial. *J Trauma Acute Care Surg*. 2015 Apr;78(4):687-695; discussion 695-697.

42. Carrick MM, Morrison CA, Tapia NM, et al. Intraoperative hypotensive resuscitation for patients undergoing laparotomy or thoracotomy for trauma: early termination of a randomized prospective clinical trial. *J Trauma Acute Care Surg*. 2016 Jun;80(6):886-896.

43. Woolley T, Thompson P, Kirkman E, et al. Trauma Hemostasis and Oxygenation Research Network position paper on the role of hypotensive resuscitation as part of remote damage control resuscitation. *J Trauma Acute Care Surg*. 2018 Jun;84(6 Suppl 1):S3-S13.

44. Woodward L, Alsabri M. Permissive hypotension vs. conventional resuscitation in patients with trauma or hemorrhagic shock: a review. *Cureus*. 2021 Jul 19;13(7):e16487.

45. Carney N, Totten AM, O'Reilly C, et al. Guidelines for the management of severe traumatic brain injury, fourth edition. *Neurosurgery*. 2017 Jan 1;80(1):6-15.

46. Gentilello LM. Advances in the management of hypothermia. *Surg Clin North Am*. 1995;75(2):243-256.

47. Marino PL. *The ICU Book*. 4th ed. Lippincott Williams & Wilkins, 2014.

48. Johnson S, Henderson SO. Myth: The Trendelenburg position improves circulation in cases of shock. *Can J Emerg Med*. 2004;6:48.

49. Deboer S, Seaver M, Morissette C. Intraosseous infusion: not just for kids anymore. *J Emerg Med Serv*. 2005;34:56-63.

50. Sawyer RW, Bodai BI, Blaisdell FW, et al. The current status of intraosseous infusion. *J Am Coll Surg*. 1994; 179:353-360.

51. Macnab A, Christenson J, Findlay J, et al. A new system for sternal intraosseous infusion in adults. *Prehosp Emerg Care*. 2000;4:173.

52. Glaeser PW, Hellmich TR, Szewczuga D, et al. Five-year experience in prehospital intraosseous infusions in children and adults. *Ann Emerg Med*. 1993;22:1119.

53. Marino PL, Galvagno SM. *The Little ICU Book*. Wolters Kluwer; 2017.

54. Shand S, Curtis K, Dinh M, et al. Prehospital blood transfusion in New South Wales, Australia: a retrospective cohort study. *Prehosp Emerg Care*. 2021;25(3):404-411.

55. Roehl A, Grottke O. Prehospital administration of blood and plasma products. *Curr Opin Anaesthesiol*. 2021; 34(4):507-513.

56. Sperry JL, Guyette FX, Brown JB, et al. Prehospital plasma during air medical transport in trauma patients at risk for hemorrhagic shock. *N Engl J Med*. 2018;379(4):315-326.

57. Semler MW, Self WH, Wanderer JP, et al. Balanced crystalloids versus saline in critically ill adults. *N Engl J Med*. 2018;378:829-839.

58. Vassar MJ, Fischer RP, Obrien PE, et al. A multicenter trial of resuscitation of injured patients with 7.5% sodium chloride: the effect of added dextran 70. *Arch Surg*. 1993;128:1003-1013.

59. Vassar MJ, Ferry CA, Holcroft JW. Prehospital resuscitation of hypotensive trauma patients with 7.5% NaCl versus 7.5% NaCl with added dextran: a controlled trial. *J Trauma*. 1993;34:622-633.

60. Wade CE, Kramer GC, Grady JJ. Efficacy of hypertonic 7.5% saline and 6% dextran in treating trauma: a meta-analysis of controlled clinical trials. *Surgery.* 1997;122:609-616.

61. Galvagno SM, Mackenzie CF. New and future resuscitation fluids for trauma patients using hemoglobin and hypertonic saline. *Anesthesiol Clin.* 2013;31:1-19.

62. Zarychanski R, Abou-Setta AM, Turgeon AF, et al. Association of hydroxyethyl starch with mortality and acute kidney injury in critically ill patients requiring volume resuscitation. *JAMA.* 2013;309:678-688.

63. Lewis SR, Pritchard MW, Evans DJW, et al. Colloids versus crystalloids for fluid resuscitation in critically ill people. Cochrane Database Syst Rev. 2018;8:CD000567. doi: 10.1002/14651858.CD000567.pub7

64. Rizoli SB. Crystalloids and colloids in trauma resuscitation: a brief overview of the current debate. *J Trauma.* 2003;54:S82-S88.

65. SAFE Study Investigators. A comparison of albumin and saline for fluid resuscitation in the intensive care unit. *N Engl J Med.* 2004;350:2247-2256.

66. Haut ER, Kalish BT, Cotton BA, et al. Prehospital intravenous fluid administration is associated with higher mortality in trauma patients: a National Trauma Data Bank analysis. *Ann Surg.* 2011;253(2):371-377.

67. Jimenez JJ, Iribarren JL, Lorente L, et al.: Tranexamic acid attenuates inflammatory response in cardiopulmonary bypass surgery through blockade of fibrinolysis: a case control study followed by a randomized double-blind controlled trial. *Crit Care.* 2007;11:R117.

68. Guyette FX, Brown JB, Zenati MS, et al. Tranexamic acid during prehospital transport in patients at risk for hemorrhage after injury: a double-blind, placebo-controlled, randomized clinical trial. *JAMA Surg.* 2020;156(10):11-20.

69. The CRASH-2 Collaborators. Effects of tranexamic acid on death, vascular occlusive events, and blood transfusion in trauma patients with significant haemorrhage (CRASH-2): a randomised, placebo-controlled trial. *Lancet.* 2010;376:23-32.

70. Morrison JJ, Dubose JJ, Rasmussen TE, Midwinter MJ. Military Application of Tranexamic Acid in Trauma Emergency Resuscitation (MATTERs) study. *Arch Surg.* 2012;147:113-119.

71. Bossers SM, Loer SA, Bloemers FW, et al. Association between prehospital tranexamic acid administration and outcomes of severe traumatic brain injury. *JAMA Neurol.* 2021;78(3):338-345.

72. CRASH-3 Trial Collaborators. Effects of tranexamic acid on death, disability, vascular occlusive events and other morbidities in patients with acute traumatic brain injury (CRASH-3): a randomised, placebo-controlled trial. *Lancet.* 2019;394(10210):1713-1723.

73. Drew B, Auten J, Donham B, et al. The use of tranexamic acid in tactical combat casualty care. *J Spec Oper Med.* 2020;20(3):36-43.

74. Marshall JC, Cook DJ, Christou NV, et al. The multiple organ dysfunction score: a reliable descriptor of a complex clinical syndrome. *Crit Care Med.* 1995;23:1638-1652.

Suggested Reading

American College of Surgeons (ACS) Committee on Trauma. Shock. In: *Advanced Trauma Life Support Student Course Manual.* 10th ed. ACS; 2018.

Hemorrhage and hypovolemia. In: Marino PL, Galvagno SM. The Little ICU Book. Wolters-Kluwer, 2017.

Hypoperfusion. In: Bledsoe B, Porter RS, Cherry RA, eds. *Essentials of Paramedic Care.* 2nd ed. Brady-Pearson Education; 2011:257-265.

Revell M, Greaves I, Porter K. Endpoints for fluid resuscitation in hemorrhagic shock. *J Trauma.* 2003;54:S637.

Shock. In: Bledsoe B, Porter RS, Cherry RA, eds. *Essentials of Paramedic Care.* 2nd ed. Brady-Pearson Education; 2011:837-849.

Somand DM, Ward KR. Approach to traumatic shock. In: Tintinalli J, ed. *Emergency Medicine: A Comprehensive Study Guide.* 9th ed. McGraw-Hill; 2019:63-68.

특수 술기

골내 혈관 접근

원칙: 수액 및 약물 투여를 위한 정맥 라인 확보가 불가능할 때 골내 라인 확보 방법으로 시행한다.

이 술기는 성인과 소아 환자 모두에게 시중에서 판매되는 다양한 장비를 사용하여 시행할 수 있다.

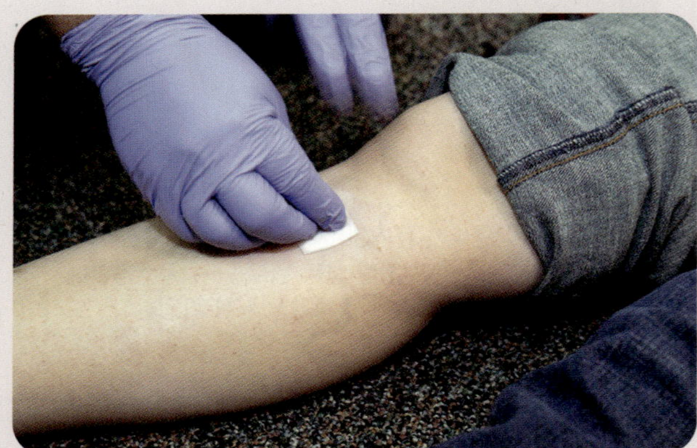

1　골내 주입 바늘, 최소 5mL의 멸균 생리식염수가 채워진 주사기, 소독제, 수액 및 수액 세트, 테이프를 포함한 장비를 확인한다. 표준 예방 조치와 적절한 신체 물질 격리를 시행하고 환자를 바로누운자세로 눕힌다.

삽입 부위는 위팔뼈머리, 넙적다리뼈 원위부, 정강뼈 또는 복장뼈가 될 수 있다. 소아 환자의 경우 정강뼈거친면 바로 아래 정강뼈 앞-내측 근위가 일반적으로 삽입하는 부위이다. 병원 전 처치 제공자는 정강뼈 삽입 부위를 확인하고 다른 처치 제공자는 다리를 움직이지 않도록 안정화한다. 삽입 부위를 소독제로 소독한다.

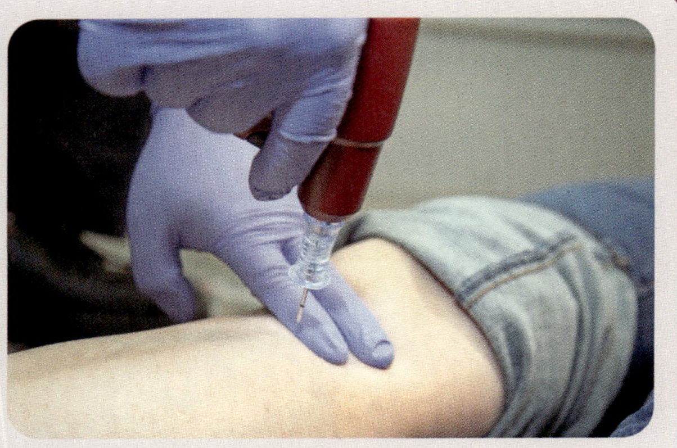

2　드릴과 바늘을 선택한 뼈에 90도 각도로 잡고 드릴을 작동시켜 회전하는 바늘을 피부를 통해 뼈 피질에 삽입한다. 뼈 피질에 들어가면 "팝"하는 소리가 난다.

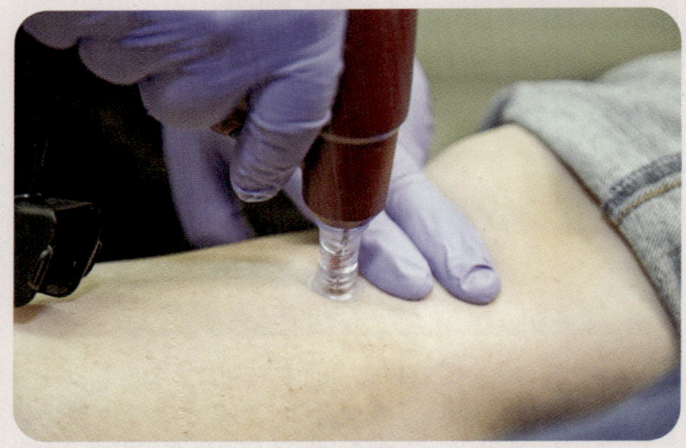

3　바늘에 대한 저항이 부족하다고 느껴지면 드릴을 더 이상 작동시키지 않는다. 바늘을 잡고 있는 동안 바늘에서 드릴을 제거한다.

(다음 페이지에 계속)

골내 혈관 접근 (이어서)

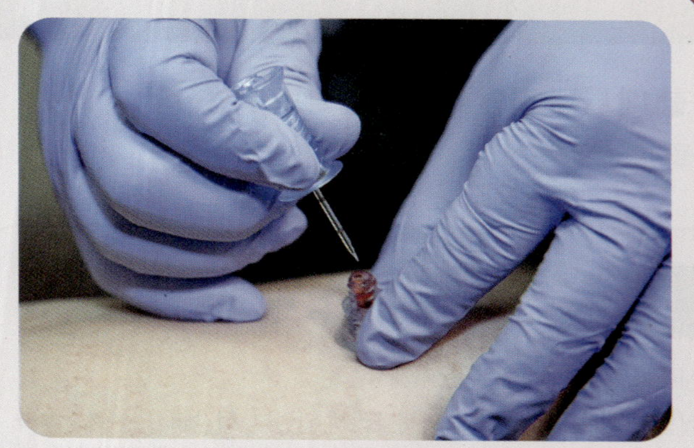

4   바늘 중앙에서 투관침을 풀어 제거한다.

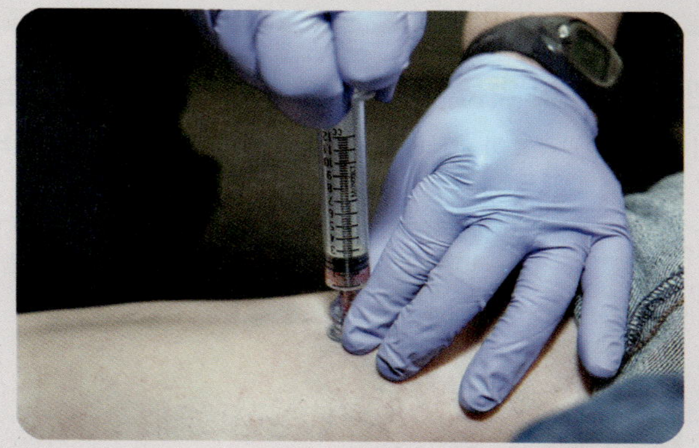

5   생리식염수가 들어있는 주사기를 바늘 허브에 연결한다. 주사기 플런저를 살짝 뒤로 당겨 골수공간에서 생리식염수와 섞이는 액체가 있는지 확인한다. "드라이" 탭은 드문 일이 아니다.

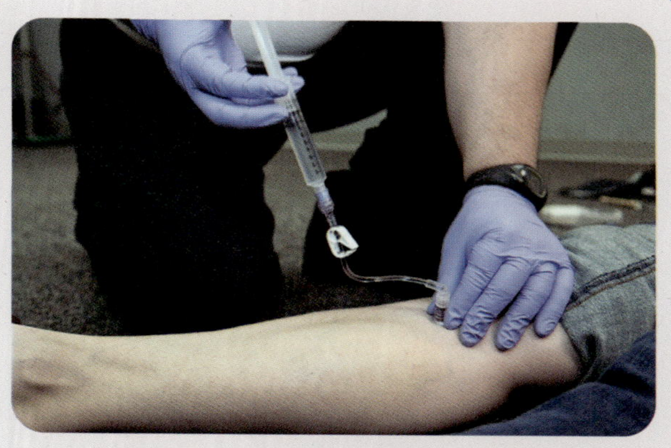

6   그런 다음 생리식염수 5mL를 주입하고 침윤 징후가 있는지 관찰한다. 침윤 징후가 없으면 바늘 허브에서 주사기를 제거하고 수액 세트를 연결한 투여량을 조절한다. 주삿바늘과 수액 세트를 고정한다.

지혈대 적용

C-A-T 지혈대 팔에 적용

이 사진에는 C-A-T 지혈대를 사용해서 지혈을 시행하는 방법이며 승인된 모든 지혈대를 사용할 수 있다.

참고: 지혈대를 사용해야 할 정도로 출혈이 심한 환자는 어지럼증과 의식 상실의 위험이 있으므로 신속하게 바로누운자세로 눕혀야 한다. 이 예시에서는 지혈대 사용 절차를 쉽게 설명하기 위해 환자를 똑바로 앉혀 놓았다.

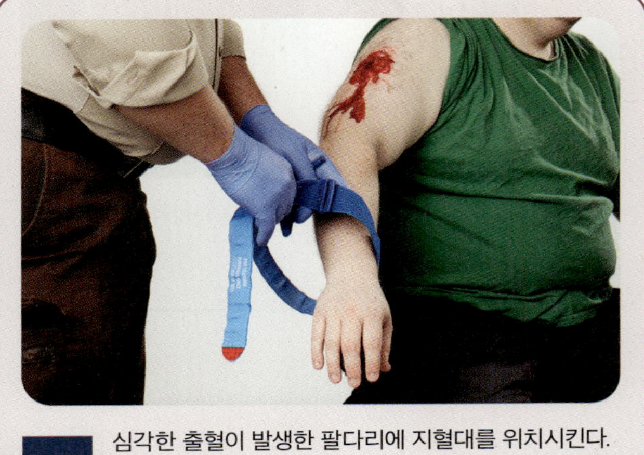

1 심각한 출혈이 발생한 팔다리에 지혈대를 위치시킨다.

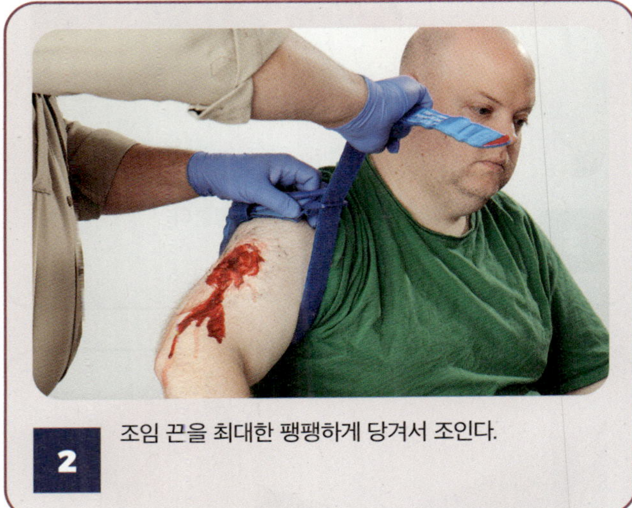

2 조임 끈을 최대한 팽팽하게 당겨서 조인다.

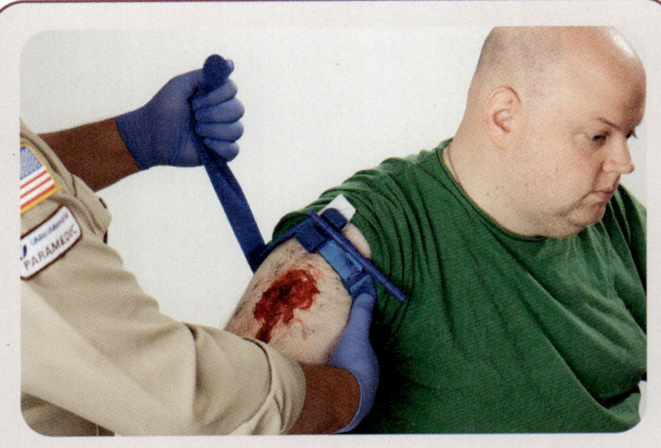

3 조임 끈을 다시 최대한 당긴 후 벨크로에 견고하게 붙인다. 조임 끈을 조임 막대를 고정하는 고정대 위에 붙이지 않는다.

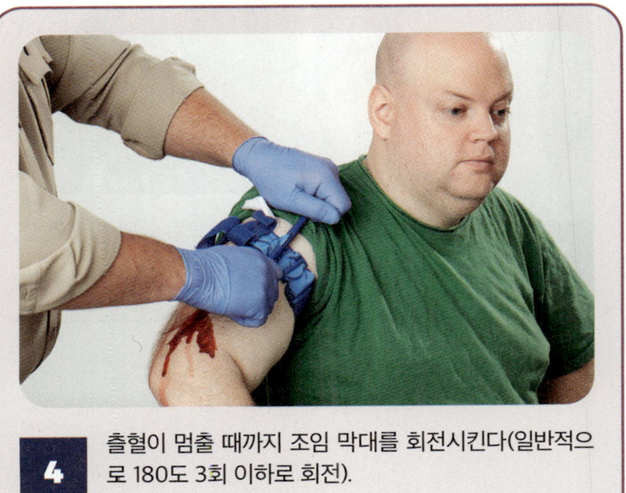

4 츨혈이 멈출 때까지 조임 막대를 회전시킨다(일반적으로 180도 3회 이하로 회전).

(다음 페이지에 계속)

지혈대 적용 (이어서)

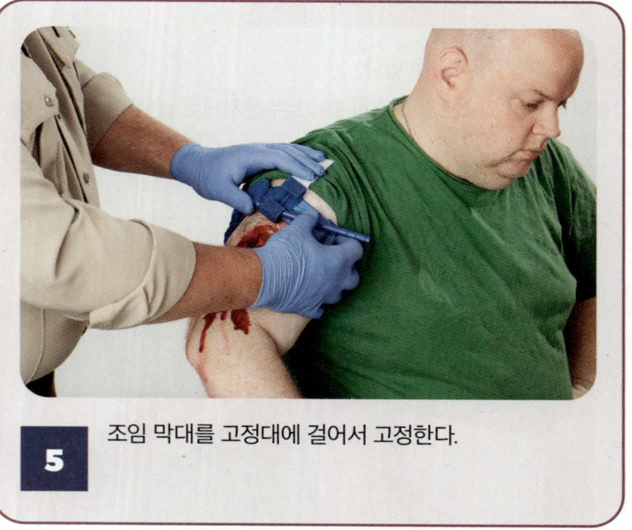

5 조임 막대를 고정대에 걸어서 고정한다.

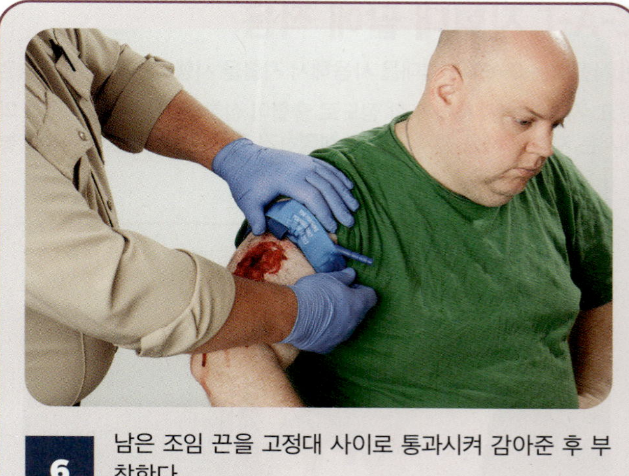

6 남은 조임 끈을 고정대 사이로 통과시켜 감아준 후 부착한다.

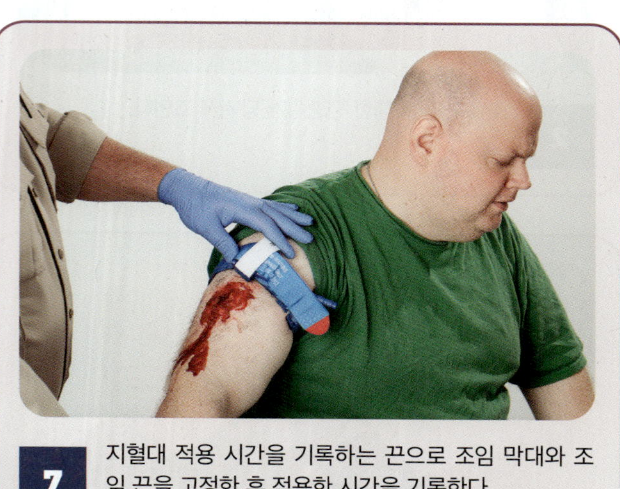

7 지혈대 적용 시간을 기록하는 끈으로 조임 막대와 조임 끈을 고정한 후 적용한 시간을 기록한다.

지혈대 적용 (이어서)

C-A-T 지혈대 다리에 적용

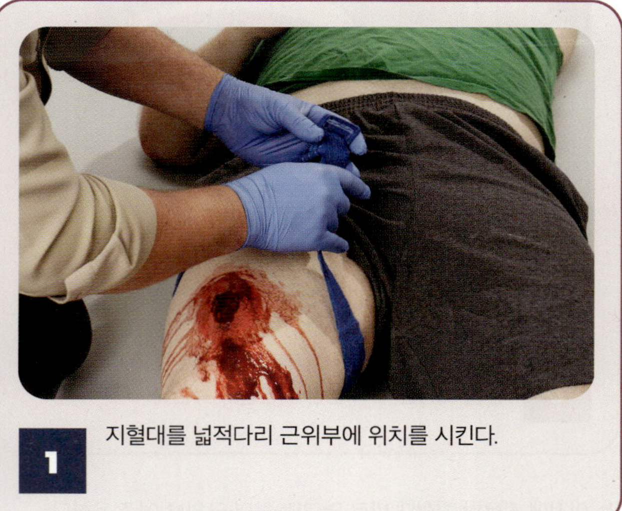

1 지혈대를 넓적다리 근위부에 위치를 시킨다.

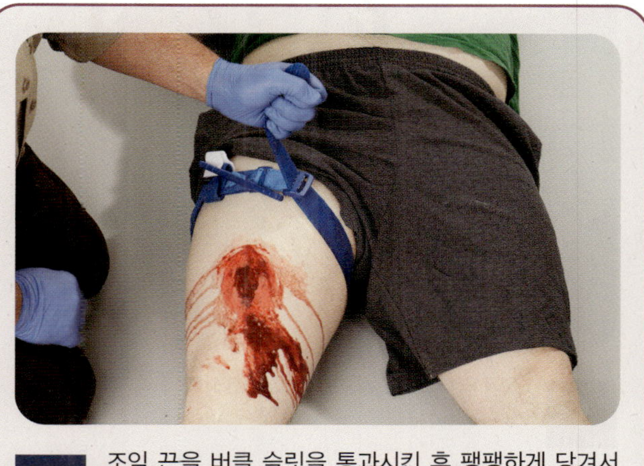

2 조임 끈을 버클 슬릿을 통과시킨 후 팽팽하게 당겨서 조인다.

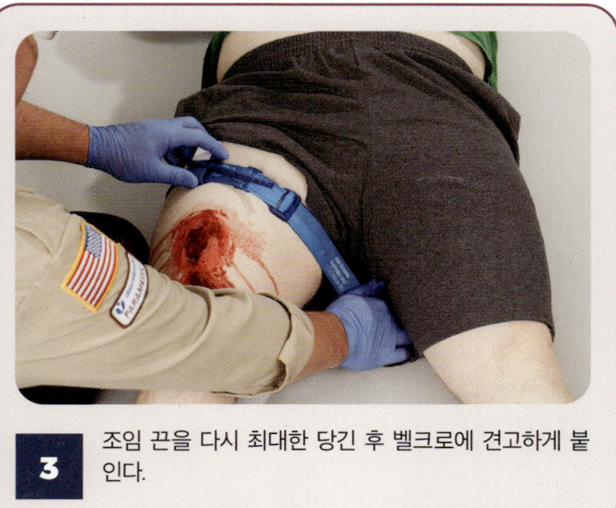

3 조임 끈을 다시 최대한 당긴 후 벨크로에 견고하게 붙인다.

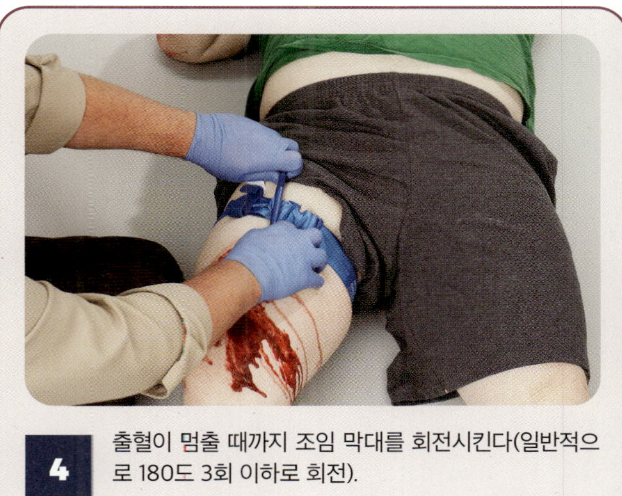

4 출혈이 멈출 때까지 조임 막대를 회전시킨다(일반적으로 180도 3회 이하로 회전).

(다음 페이지에 계속)

지혈대 적용 (이어서)

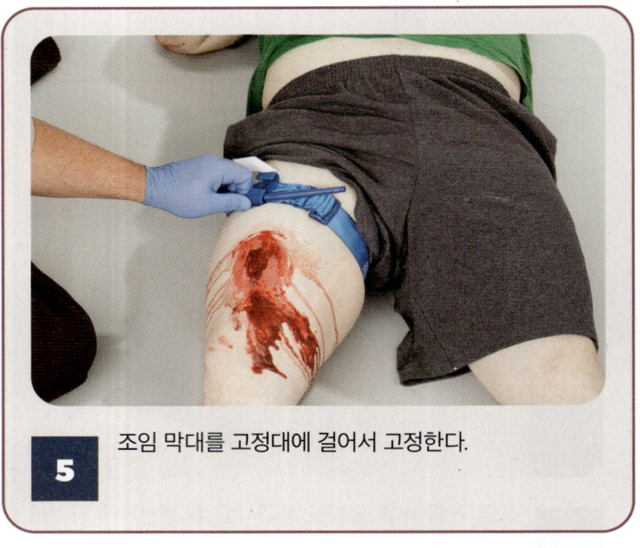

5   조임 막대를 고정대에 걸어서 고정한다.

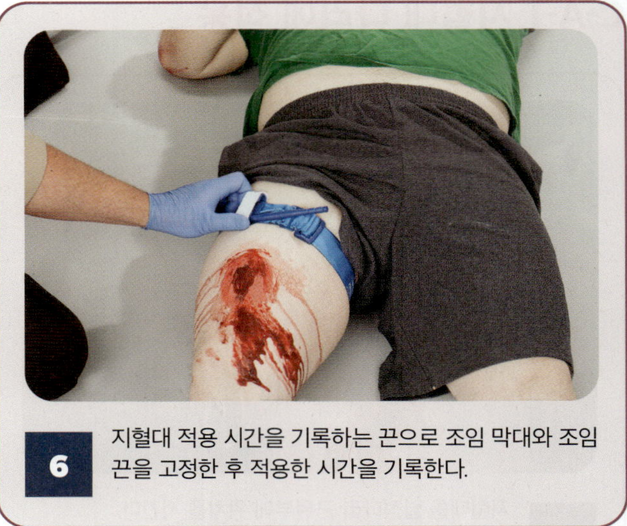

6   지혈대 적용 시간을 기록하는 끈으로 조임 막대와 조임 끈을 고정한 후 적용한 시간을 기록한다.

출혈을 조절하기 위해 여러 개의 지혈대가 필요한 경우도 있다. 추가 지혈대는 이전에 적용한 지혈대 바로 옆(가능하면 근위부)에 적용한다.

국소 지혈 드레싱 및 일반 거즈를 사용한 상처 패킹

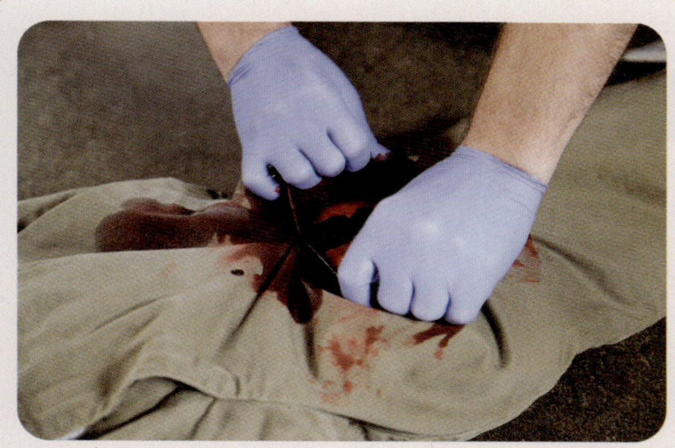

1 상처 부위를 노출한다.

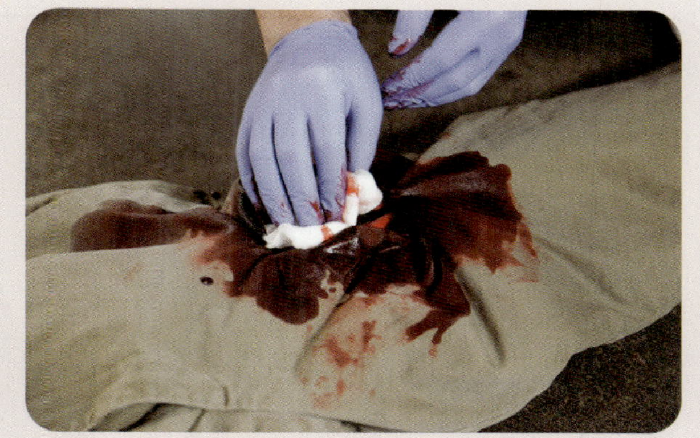

2 형성된 혈전을 보존하면서 상처 부위에 과도한 혈액을 부드럽게 제거한다. 상처에서 출혈 부위를 찾는다.

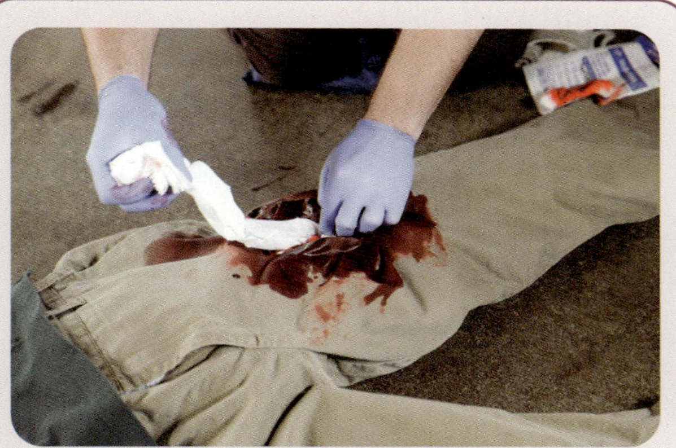

3 출혈 부위를 찾아 직접 압박을 시행하고 빈 공간을 거즈로 채워준다. 상처를 패킹하면서 지속해 압력을 유지한다.

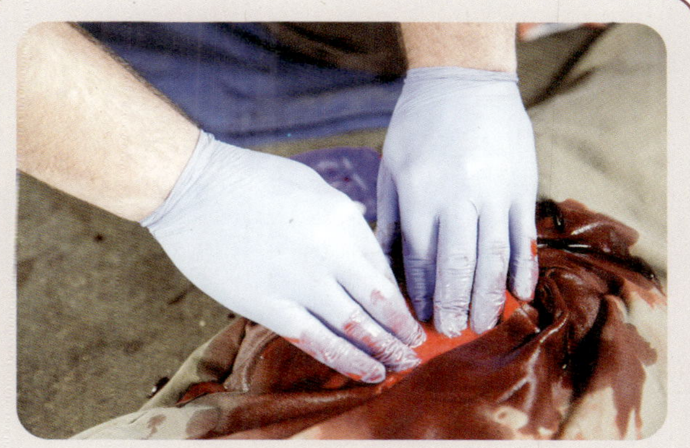

4 지혈 거즈를 사용하는 경우 최소 3분(제조업체의 지침을 따름), 일반 거즈를 사용하는 경우 10분 동안 상처 부위를 직접 압박한다.

(다음 페이지에 계속)

국소 지혈 드레싱 및 일반 거즈를 사용한 상처 패킹(이어서)

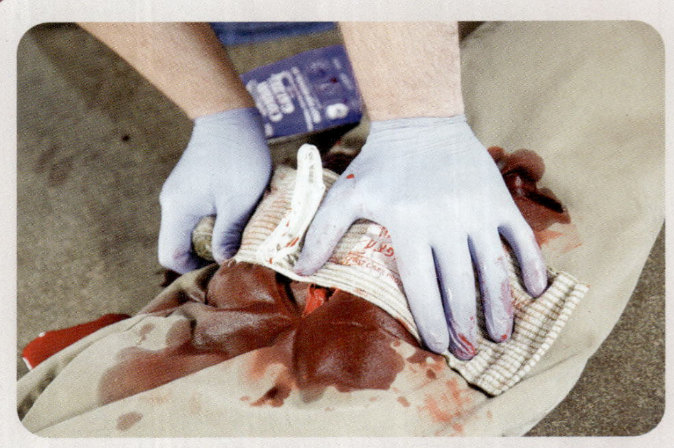

5 패킹 부위에서 출혈이 멈췄는지 재평가를 시행하고 출혈이 멈추지 않은 경우 필요하면 추가 패킹을 시행한다. 출혈이 지혈되면 패킹에 압박을 유지할 수 있도록 압박 붕대로 단단하게 고정한다.

이스라엘 외상 붕대를 이용한 압박 드레싱

원칙: 제어되지 않는 출혈을 가진 사지의 열린 상처에 기계적인 원주압과 드레싱을 제공한다.

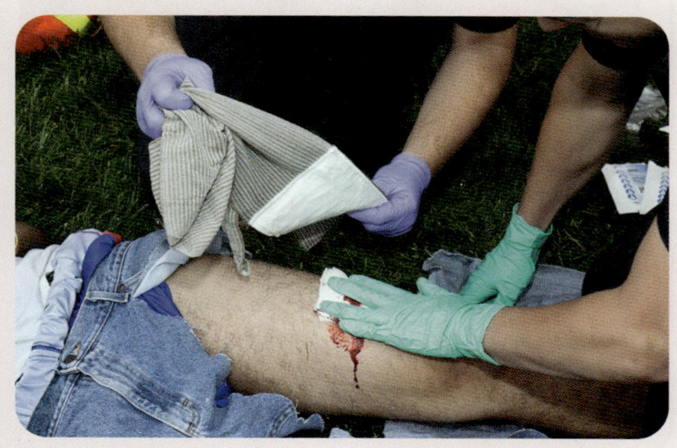
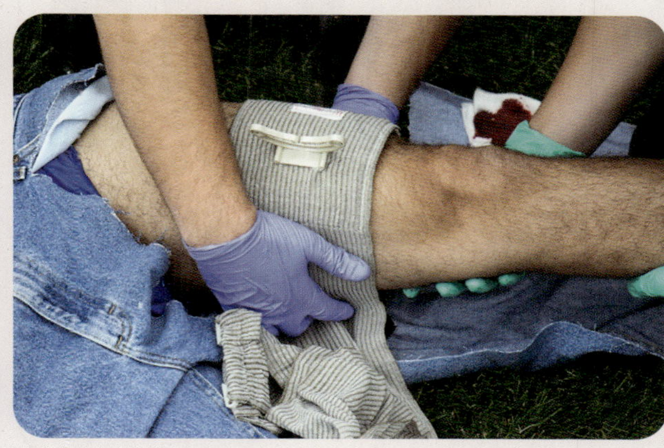

1 적절한 BSI를 시행하고 상처 위에 드레싱 패드를 올려놓는다.

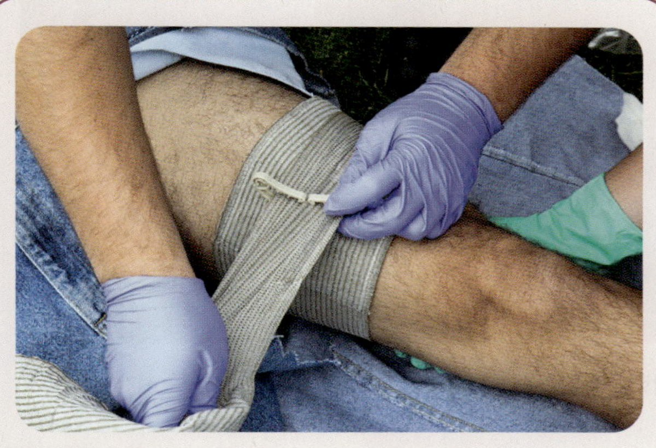

2 탄력 붕대를 팔다리에 한 번 이상 감는다.

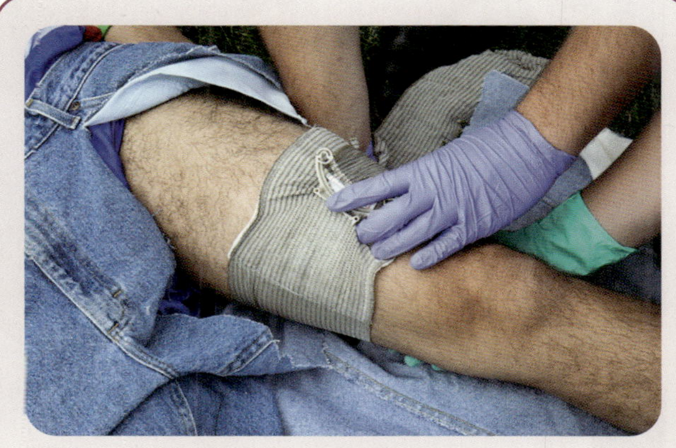

3 탄력 붕대를 바에 끼워 감는다.

(다음 페이지에 계속)

이스라엘 외상 붕대를 이용한 압박 드레싱 (이어서)

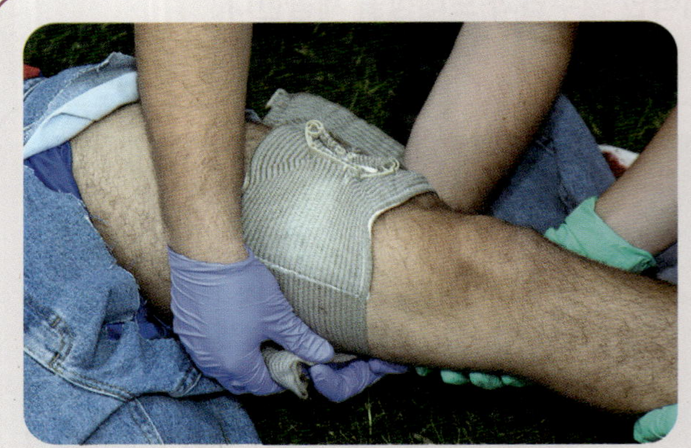

4 붕대를 상처 부위의 반대 방향으로 단단히 감아 출혈을 조절할 수 있도록 충분한 압력을 가한다.

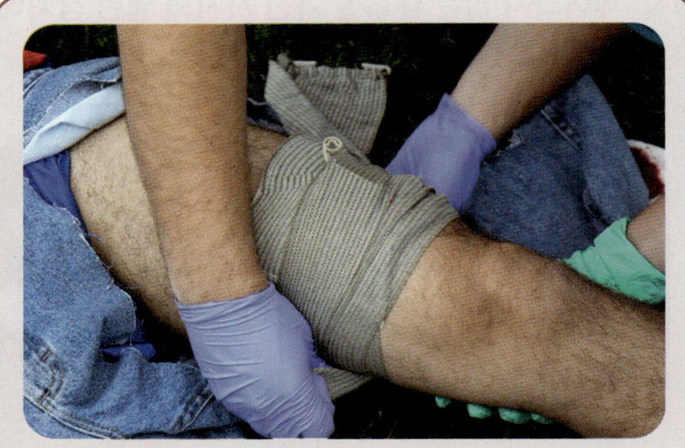

5 붕대를 팔다리에 계속 감는다.

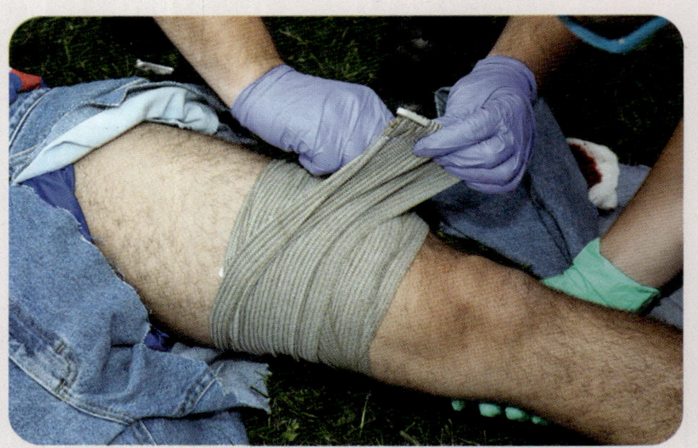

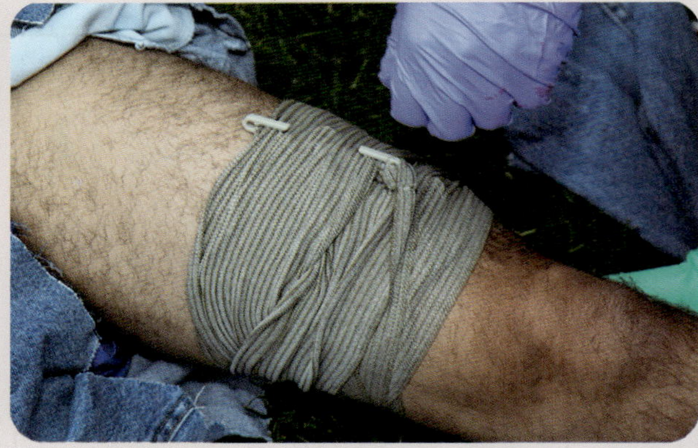

6 붕대의 원위쪽 끝을 고정하고 출혈을 조절하기 위해 지속적인 압력을 유지한다.

외상의 물리학

Lead Editors
Andrew Schmidt, MD
Kelsey Wise, MD
Brandon Kelly, MD

학습 목표
이 장의 학습을 완료하면 다음과 같은 내용을 수행할 수 있다.

- 손상을 유발하는 상황에서 에너지를 정의할 수 있다.
- 운동의 법칙, 에너지, 외상의 물리학 사이의 연관성을 설명할 수 있다.
- 속도와 에너지 교환이 손상에 미치는 관계를 설명할 수 있다.
- 에너지 교환과 공동화에 관해 설명할 수 있다.
- 차량 충돌에 대한 설명이 주어지면 외상의 물리학을 사용하여 안전띠를 매지 않은 탑승자의 손상 유형을 예측할 수 있다.
- 차량의 내부 및 외부 손상과 관련된 특정 손상 및 원인을 설명할 수 있다.
- 차량 탑승자를 위한 안전띠의 기능에 관해 설명할 수 있다.
- 운동 및 에너지 법칙을 차량 충돌 이외의 기전(예: 폭발, 추락)과 관련하여 설명할 수 있다.
- 폭발 손상의 5단계와 각 단계에서 발생하는 손상을 정의할 수 있다.
- 저에너지, 중에너지, 고에너지 무기에 의한 손상 발생 차이를 설명할 수 있다.
- 충돌하는 물체의 단면과 에너지 교환 및 손상 발생의 관계에 대해 논의할 수 있다.
- 외상의 물리학적 원리를 외상 환자 평가에 적용할 수 있다.

시나리오

추운 겨울 새벽에 당신과 동료는 단독 차량 충돌 사고 현장으로 출동하였다. 현장에 도착하자마자 당신은 시골 도로에서 가로수에 충돌한 차량 한 대를 발견하였다. 차량의 앞부분이 가로수에 충돌한 것으로 보이며 차량은 회전하면서 도로 옆 배수로에 차량의 후미 부분이 빠진 상태이다. 차량에는 운전자 한 명만 탑승했으며 에어백이 전개되었고 운전자는 여전히 안전띠를 매고 신음하고 있다. 가로수와 충돌한 차량 앞부분이 손상되었을 뿐만 아니라 회전하면서 후미 부분이 배수로에 빠져 후방 손상도 확인할 수 있었다.

- 이 사고에서 외상의 물리학에 근거하여 이 환자가 손상을 입을 가능성은 무엇인가?
- 외상의 물리학을 근거하여 환자의 상태를 어떻게 설명할 것인가?
- 어떤 손상을 입을 것으로 예상하는가?

개요

미국에서는 2019년에 36,096명이 차량 충돌 사고로 사망했다. 이는 2018년에 비해 2% 감소(739명)했지만 2015년보다 1,000명이 더 사망했다. 2019년 미국 도로에서 발생한 부상자 수는 274만 명으로 1% 조금 넘게 증가했다. 가장 최근의 세계보건기구(WHO) 보고서에 따르면 전 세계적으로 매년 135만 명이 교통사고로 사망하는 것으로 추정되며 더 나아가 교통사고로 인한 손상이 전 세계적으로 5~29세 사이의 주요 사망 원인이라고 한다. 같은 기간 동안 전 세계 도로의 차량 수가 증가했음에도 불구하고 2000년 이후 1인당 교통사고로 인한 전 세계 사망률은 거의 일정하게 유지되었다. 이러한 사망의 90% 이상이 저소득 및 중간층 국가에서 발생하며 주로 보행자, 자전거 이용자와 오토바이 운전자에게 영향을 미친다.

미국에서 총기는 주요 사망 원인으로 2019년에 39,707명이 사망했다. 총기 관련 사망의 두 가지 주요 원인은 총기 사망의 60%를 차지하는 자살과 살인이다(이 중 75%는 총기 손상으로 인해 발생). 폭발 손상은 많은 국가에서 손상의 주요 원인이지만, 칼에 의한 관통성 손상은 다른 나라에서 두드러진다.

외상 환자의 성공적인 처치는 명백한 손상과 숨겨진 손상의 확인에 데 달려 있으며 손상 기전에 대한 이해를 통해 정보를 제공하는 우수한 평가 기술을 사용해야 한다. 병원 전 환경에서 주어진 시나리오에서 발생하는 손상을 정확히 파악하기는 어렵지만, 손상 가능성과 심각한 출혈의 가능성을 이해한다면 병원 전 처치 제공자가 비판적 사고 기술을 사용하여 이러한 가능성을 인식하고 적절한 분류, 처치 및 이송 결정을 내릴 수 있다.

모든 환자의 처치(초기 소생술 후)는 환자의 손상 병력을 파악하는 것으로 시작된다. 외상에서 병력은 충격과 그 충격으로 인한 에너지 교환에 관한 이야기이다. 에너지 교환 과정에 대한 이해를 통해 병원 전 처치 제공자는 잠재적인 손상 발생 가능성을 예측할 수 있다.

외상의 물리학은 움직임을 유발하는 힘과 관계없이 물체의 움직임을 다룬다. 신체에 가해지는 힘으로 인해 발생하는 손상은 숙주와 숙주에 충격을 가하는 움직이는 물체 사이의 상호 작용과 직접적으로 관련이 있다. 병원 전 처치 제공자가 모든 처치 과정에서 외상 물리학의 원리나 관련 기전을 이해하지 못하면 손상을 놓칠 수 있다. 이러한 원칙을 이해하면 특정 기전을 고려할 때 발생할 가능성이 있는 특정 손상에 대한 의심의 수준을 높일 수 있다. 이 정보와 의심되는 손상은 현장에서 환자를 적절하게 평가하는 데 사용될 수 있으며 응급실의 의사와 간호사에게 전달될 수 있다. 현장과 이송 중에 이러한 손상이 의심되는 환자는 가장 적절한 방법으로 처치를 제공하고 더 이상 해를 끼치지 않도록 할 수 있다.

명백하지는 않지만, 여전히 심각한 손상은 현장에서 인지하지 못하고 외상센터나 적절한 의료기관에 도착해 의료진에게 전달하지 않으면 치명적일 수 있다. 어느 부위에서 손상을 찾아야 하고 어떻게 평가해야 하는지 아는 것은 손상을 발견한 후 무엇을 해야 하는지 아는 것만큼이나 중요하다. 외상 사고에 대한 완전하고 정확한 병력과 이러한 정보의 적절한 해석은 이러한 정보를 제공한다. 환자의 손상 중 상당수는 환자를 평가하기 전에 현장을 적절하게 조사하면 예측할 수 있다.

이 장에서는 외상의 물리학을 이해하기 위한 일반적인 원리에 관해 설명한다. 일반적인 원리는 에너지 교환과 에너지 교환의 일반적인 효과를 지배하는 역학의 법칙에서 시작한다. 역학적 원리는 인체와 충돌 구성 요소의 상호작용을 다룬다.

충돌은 일반적으로 에너지를 가진 단단한 물체가 다른 물체에 충돌할 때 발생하는 상호작용이다. 흔히 충돌이라는 단어를 차량 충돌과 연관시키지만, 물체가 포장도로 위로에 부딪히는 것, 총알이 신체의 외부와 내부 조직에 미치는 충격 그리고 폭발로 인한 과압과 파편 등을 의미할 수도 있다. 이러한 모든 사건은 에너지 교환을 포함하고 손상을 초래하며 잠재적으로 생명을 위협할 수 있는 상황을 초래할 수 있으므로 지식과 통찰력을 갖춘 병원 전 처치 제공자의 올바른 처치가 필요하다.

일반적인 원칙

외상 사고는 사고 전 단계, 사고 단계 그리고 사고 후 단계로 나눌 수 있다. 간단히 말해서 사고 전 단계는 예방 단계이다(**Box 4-1**). 사고 단계는 외상성 사고에서 에너지의 교환이나 외상의 물리학(에너지 역학)과 관련된 부분이다.

마지막으로 사고 후 단계는 환자 처치 단계이다. 차량 충돌, 무기, 추락, 건물 붕괴 등 손상의 원인이 무엇이든 에너지가 신체에 흡수되면 손상으로 전환된다.

사고 전 단계

사고 전 단계에는 사고 이전의 모든 사건이 포함된다. 사고가 발생하기 전에 존재하고 환자의 손상 처치에 중요한 상태는 사고 전 병력의 일부로 평가된다. 이러한 고려 사항에는 환자의 급성 또는 기존의 의

> **Box 4-1 손상 예방**
>
> 손상을 예방하는 가장 효율적이고 효과적인 방법은 처음부터 손상을 예방하는 것이다. 모든 의료 제공자는 손상 예방에 적극적인 임무를 수행하여 지역 사회 전체뿐만 아니라 자신을 위해서도 최상의 결과를 얻을 수 있다. EMS 시스템은 자체적으로 보수적인 분야에서 지역 사회 의료와 같은 측면을 포함하고 예방에 중점을 두는 더 광범위하고 효과적인 분야로 자신을 변화시키고 있다. 16장 손상 예방에서는 외상 예방을 위한 병원 전 처치 제공자의 역할에 대해 자세히 설명한다.

학적 상태 및 해당 상태를 처치하기 위한 약물, 불법 및 처방받은 약물, 알코올 등의 섭취, 환자의 정신 상태 등이다.

일반적으로 젊은 외상 환자는 만성 질환을 앓고 있지 않지만, 노인 환자의 경우 외상 사고 발생 전 기저질환이 있으면 병원 전 평가 및 환자 처치에 심각한 합병증을 유발할 수 있으며 결과에 상당한 영향을 미칠 수 있다. 예를 들어, 전봇대를 충돌한 차량의 75세 운전자는 심근경색을 나타내는 흉통이 있을 수 있다. 운전자가 전봇대를 충돌하고 심장마비를 일으켰는가? 아니면 심장마비를 일으킨 후 전봇대를 충돌했는가? 운전자가 쇼크에 반응하여 맥박이 상승하는 것을 방지하는 약물(예: 베타차단제)을 복용하고 있는가? 이러한 상태의 대부분은 평가와 처치의 전략(5장 현장 관리 및 6장 환자 평가 및 처치에서 논의)에 직접적으로 영향을 미칠 뿐 아니라 충돌 외상의 물리학적 특성에 반드시 영향을 미치지는 않더라도 전반적인 환자 처치에서 중요하다.

사고 단계

사고 단계는 하나의 움직이는 물체와 두 번째 물체 사이의 충돌 시점에 시작된다. 두 번째 물체는 움직이거나 정지해 있을 수 있으며 물체 또는 사람일 수 있다. 차량 충돌을 예로 들면 대부분의 차량 충돌 사고에서는 세 가지 충돌이 발생한다.

1. 두 물체의 충돌
2. 차량 내부와 탑승자의 충돌
3. 탑승자 내부의 중요한 장기 충돌

예를 들어 차량이 나무에 부딪히면 첫 번째 충격은 차량과 나무가 충돌하는 것이다. 두 번째 충돌은 차량 탑승자가 핸들이나 앞 유리에 부딪히는 것이다. 탑승자가 안전띠를 매고 있는 경우 탑승자와 안전띠 사이에 충격이 발생한다. 세 번째 충돌은 탑승자의 내부 장기와 흉벽, 복벽 또는 두개골 사이에서 발생한다.

앞서 언급했듯이 충돌이라는 용어는 일반적으로 자동차 사고를 떠올리게 하지만, 반드시 차량 충돌을 의미하는 것은 아니다. 차량이 보행자를 들이받거나 발사체가 복부에 부딪히거나, 건설 작업자가 아스팔트에 추락하는 것도 모두 충돌의 예이다. 추락에는 특히 첫 번째와 세 번째 유형의 충돌만 포함된다는 점에 유의한다.

모든 충돌에서 움직이는 물체와 인체 조직 사이 또는 움직이는 인체와 정지한 물체 사이에 에너지가 교환된다. 에너지 교환이 발생하는 방향과 교환되는 에너지의 양 그리고 이러한 힘이 환자에게 미치는 영향은 모두 평가를 시작할 때 중요한 고려 사항이다.

사고 후 단계

사고 후 단계에서는 충돌과 사고 전 단계에서 수집된 정보를 사용하여 환자를 평가하고 처치한다. 이 단계는 충돌로 인한 에너지가 흡수되는 즉시 시작된다. 생명을 위협하는 외상으로 인한 합병증의 발병은 현장에서 병원으로 이송되는 과정에서 제공되는 처치에 따라 느리거나 빠르게 나타날 수 있다(또는 이러한 합병증을 예방하거나 크게 줄일 수 있다). 사고 후 단계에서 외상의 물리학에 대한 이해, 손상에 대한 의심 지수, 훌륭한 평가 기술은 모두 환자 결과에 영향을 미칠 수 있는 병원 전 처치 제공자의 능력에 결정적인 역할을 한다.

인체 손상을 유발하는 힘의 영향을 이해하기 위해 병원 전 처치 제공자는 먼저 에너지 교환과 인체 해부학이라는 두 가지 요소를 이해해야 한다. 예를 들어, 차량 충돌(MCV)의 경우 현장은 어떤 모습인가? 누가 무엇을 어떤 속도로 부딪혔는가? 정지 시간은 얼마인가? 탑승자가 안전띠와 같은 적절한 구속 장치를 사용했는가? 에어백이 전개되었는가? 어린이가 유아용 카시트에 적절하게 고정되어 있었는가? 아니면 구속되지 않은 채 차량에 있었는가? 차량에서 튕겨 나온 탑승자가 있었는가? 탑승자가 어떤 물체에 부딪혔는가? 그렇다면 몇 개의 물체에 부딪혔으며 그 물체의 특성은 무엇인가? 병원 전 처치 제공자가 사고에서 발생한 에너지의 교환을 이해하고 이 정보를 손상 예측 및 적절한 환자 처치로 변환하려면 이러한 질문과 기타 많은 질문에 답해야 한다.

빈틈없는 병원 전 처치 제공자는 현장을 평가하는 과정에서 외상 물리학에 대한 지식을 사용하여 어떤 힘과 움직임이 관련되었고 그러한 힘으로 인해 어떤 손상이 발생했는지 파악한다. 외상 물리학은 물리학의 기본 원리를 기반으로 하므로 관련 물리학 법칙에 대한 이해가 필요하다.

에너지

병력을 얻기 위한 초기 단계에는 충돌 당시 발생한 사고를 평가하고 (그림 4-1) 인체와 교환된 에너지를 추정하며 그 결과로 발생한 특정 조건에 대한 대략적인 추정이 포함된다.

에너지와 운동의 법칙

뉴턴의 운동 제1 법칙에 따르면 정지한 물체는 외부의 힘이 작용하지 않는 한 정지 상태를 유지하고 운동 중인 물체는 운동 상태를 유지한다. 그림 4-2에서 스키 선수는 반대 중력에 의해 슬로프를 따라 내려갈 때까지 정지해 있었다. 일단 움직이기 시작하면 지면을 떠나더라도 무언가에 부딪히거나 지면에 착지해 멈출 때까지 움직이고 있는 상태를 유지한다.

앞서 언급했듯이 모든 충돌에서 잠재적 환자의 신체가 움직일 때 세 가지 충돌이 발생한다.

1. 이동 중이거나 정지해 있는 물체에 충돌한 차량
2. 잠재적인 환자가 차량 내부에 부딪히거나, 물체와 충돌하거나 폭발 시 발생한 에너지에 의한 충돌
3. 내부 장기가 인체 구획의 벽과 상호작용하거나 지지 구조물에서 찢어지는 경우

예를 들어 안전장치를 착용하지 않은 채 차량의 앞좌석에 앉아 있는 탑승자가 있다. 차량이 나무에 부딪혀 정지하면 안전띠를 매지 않은 탑승자는 운전대, 대시보드 및 앞 유리에 부딪힐 때까지 같은 속도로 계속 움직인다. 이러한 물체와의 충돌은 몸통이나 머리의 전진 운동을 멈추게 하지만 탑승자의 내부 장기는 흉벽, 복벽 또는 두개골 내부에 부딪혀 전진 운동이 멈출 때까지 계속 움직인다.

에너지 보존 법칙으로도 알려진 뉴턴의 운동 제2 법칙에 따르면 에너지는 생성되거나 소멸할 수 없지만, 새로운 형태로 변화할 수 있다. 차량의 움직임은 에너지의 한 형태이다. 차량을 움직이기 위해 엔진의 에너지는 일련의 기어를 통해 바퀴로 전달되고 바퀴는 회전하면서 도로를 따라 구르며 차량에 움직임을 전달한다. 차량을 정지시키려면 브레이크를 작동하거나 물체에 충돌하여 프레임을 구부리는 등 차량의 운동 에너지를 다른 형태로 바꿔야 한다. 운전자가 브레이크를 밟으면 브레이크 드럼이나 디스크의 브레이크 패드와 도로의 타이어에 의해 운동 에너지가 마찰열(열에너지)로 변환된다. 따라서 차량이 감속한다.

뉴턴의 운동 제3 법칙은 아마도 뉴턴의 세 가지 법칙 중 가장 잘 알려진 법칙일 것이다. 모든 작용이나 힘에는 반대되는 반작용이 있다고 말한다. 우리가 땅 위를 걸을 때 지구는 우리가 지구에 가하는 힘과 같은 힘을 우리에게 가하고 있다. 산탄총을 쏴본 사람은 총의 개머리판이 어깨에 전달되는 충격으로 제3 법칙을 느꼈을 것이다.

벽에 충돌하는 차량의 운동 에너지가 차량의 프레임이나 다른 부분이 구부러지면서 소멸하는 것처럼(그림 4-3) 신체 내부의 장기와 구조물의 운동 에너지도 이러한 장기가 전진 운동을 멈추면서 소멸

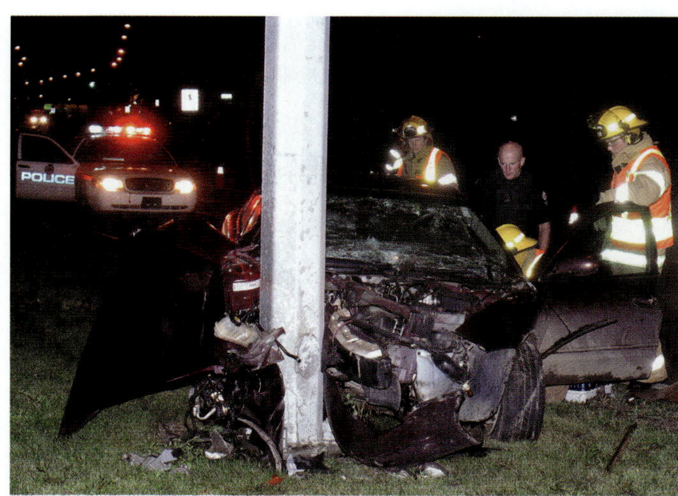

그림 4-1 사고 현장을 평가하는 것은 매우 중요하다. 충돌 방향, 탑승자 공간 침입, 에너지 교환량 등의 정보는 탑승자의 손상 가능성에 대한 통찰력을 제공한다.
© Jack Dagley Photography/Shutterstock

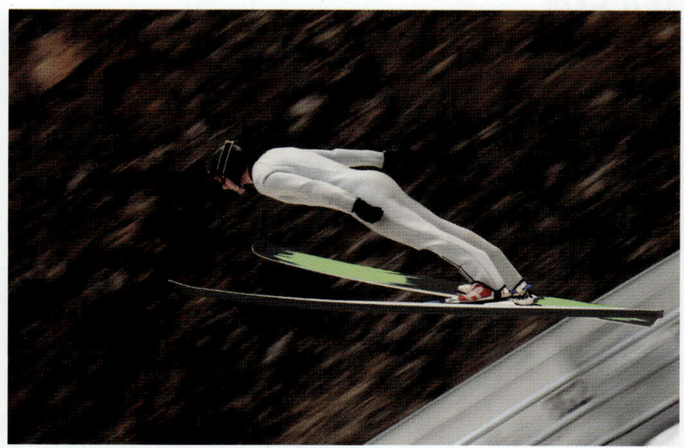

그림 4-2 스키선수는 중력 에너지가 그를 슬로프 아래로 이동할 때까지 정지해 있었다. 일단 움직이기 시작하면 지면을 떠나더라도 운동량으로 인해 무언가에 부딪히거나 지면에 돌아올 때까지 계속 움직이고 에너지 전달(마찰 또는 충돌)로 인해 정지하게 된다.
© technotr/iStock/Getty Images

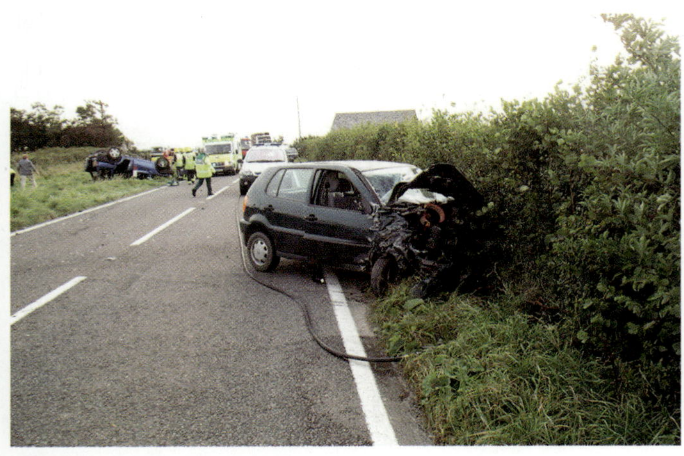

그림 4-3 차량 프레임의 변형으로 에너지가 소실된다.
© Peter Seyfferth/imageBROKER/age fotostock

하여야 한다. 같은 개념이 신체가 정지한 상태에서 칼, 총알 또는 야구 방망이와 같이 움직이는 물체와 접촉하고 상호작용할 때도 적용된다.

운동에너지는 물체의 질량과 속도의 함수이다. 기술적으로 같지는 않지만, 환자의 체중을 사용하여 질량으로 나타낼 수 있고 차량의 속도는 속도를 나타내기 위해 사용된다. 운동에너지에 영향을 미치는 무게와 속도의 관계는 다음과 같다.

$$운동에너지 = 1/2(질량 \times 속도^2)$$
$$KE = 1/2(mv^2)$$

68kg인 사람이 시속 48km를 이동할 때 운동에너지는 다음과 같이 계산한다.

$$운동에너지(KE) = 68/2 \times 48^2 = 78,336 \text{ units}$$

위의 공식에는 특정한 물리적 측정 단위(파운드, 줄)를 사용하지 않는다. 단위는 단지 이 공식에서 에너지양의 변화에 어떻게 영향을 미치는지 설명하기 위해 사용된다. 방금 설명한 것처럼 68kg인 사람이 시속 48km로 움직이는 경우 이 사람이 멈출 때 다른 형태로 변환해야 하는 에너지양은 78,336 units이다. 이러한 변화는 에너지 소실이 안전띠나 에어백과 같은 보호 장비에 전달되지 않는다면 차량 파손이나 인체 손상의 형태로 나타난다.

질량과 속도 중 어떤 변수가 발생하는 운동에너지의 양에 더 큰 영향을 미치는지 아는 것이 도움이 된다. 이를 확인하려면 앞의 예에서 시속 48km를 이동하는 68kg의 사람에 5kg을 더하여 질량을 73kg으로 증가시키면 운동에너지는 다음과 같이 계산한다.

$$운동에너지(KE) = 73/2 \times 48^2 = 84,096 \text{ units}$$

같은 속도에서 질량을 5kg 증가하면 운동에너지는 총 5,760units로 증가한다. 다음으로 체중이 68kg인 사람이 속도를 시속 64km로 증가시키면 운동에너지는 다음과 같이 계산한다.

$$운동에너지(KE) = 68/2 \times 64^2 = 139,264 \text{ units}$$

이 속도 증가로 인해 운동 에너지가 60,928 unit 증가했다.

이러한 결과는 속도를 증가시키면 질량을 증가시키는 것보다 운동에너지가 훨씬 더 증가한다는 것을 보여준다. 저속 충돌보다 고속 충돌에서 훨씬 더 많은 에너지 교환이 일어나며 따라서 탑승자, 차량 또는 둘 다에 더 심한 손상을 입힐 수 있다. 질량에 비례하고 속도의 제곱에 비례하므로 두 물체 사이에 질량 차이가 클수록 속도가 더 중요한 요소가 된다.

고속 충돌 시 발생하는 손상을 예측할 때 충돌이 시작할 때 가해지는 힘은 충돌이 끝날 때 전달되거나 소멸하는 힘과 같다는 점을 알고 있으면 도움이 될 수 있다.

$$질량 \times 가속 = 힘 = 질량 \times 감속$$

물체를 움직이려면 힘(에너지)이 필요하다. 이 힘(에너지)은 특정 속도를 생성하는 데 필요하다. 전달되는 속도는 물체의 무게에 따라 달라진다. 일단 이 에너지가 물체에 전달되어 움직이기 시작하면 물체는 에너지가 소모될 때까지 계속 움직인다(뉴턴의 운동 제1 법칙). 이러한 에너지 손실은 다른 구성 요소를 움직이게 하거나(조직 입자) 열로 손실된다(바퀴의 브레이크 디스크로 분산되면서 발생하는 열의 형태로 소모). 총상을 예로 들면, 총의 총신에는 화약이 들어 있는 탄약통이 들어 있다. 이 화약에 불이 붙으면 빠르게 연소하여 총알을 빠른 속도로 총신 밖으로 밀어내는 에너지를 생성한다. 이 속도는 총알의 무게와 화약의 연소 또는 힘으로 생성되는 에너지의 양과 같다. 뉴턴의 운동 제1 법칙에 따라 속도를 늦추려면 총알이 물체에 부딪혀 에너지를 손실시켜야 한다. 이러한 에너지 전달은 총알에 초기 속도를 줬을 때 총의 총신에서 일어난 폭발과 같은 에너지로 신체 조직 내 폭발을 일으킨다. 움직이는 차량, 건물에서 추락한 사람 또는 사제폭발물(IED)의 폭발에도 같은 현상이 발생한다.

충돌 사고의 또 다른 중요한 요소는 정지거리이다. 정지거리가 짧고 정지 속도가 빠를수록 탑승자에게 많은 에너지가 전달되어 더 많은 손상을 입힐 수 있다. 콘크리트 벽에 부딪혀 정지하는 차량과 브레이크를 밟으면 정지하는 차량을 비교하면 둘 다 다른 방식으로 같은 양의 에너지를 소모한다. 에너지 교환 속도(차체 또는 브레이크 디스크로)는 서로 다르며 서로 다른 거리와 시간에 따라 발생한다. 첫 번째로 에너지는 차량 프레임의 구부러짐에 의해 매우 짧은 거리와 시간으로 흡수된다. 두 후자의 경우 에너지는 브레이크의 열에 의해 더 긴 거리와 시간에 걸쳐 흡수된다. 차량 탑승자의 전방 운동(에너지)은 탑승자의 연부조직과 뼈에 일차적으로 흡수된다. 두 번째 사례에서 에너지는 차량의 에너지와 함께 브레이크로 분산된다.

정지거리와 손상 사이의 이러한 반비례 관계는 추락에도 적용된다. 사람들은 눈이나 깊은 물웅덩이와 같이 압축성이 있는 표면에 착지하면 추락 시 생존할 가능성이 더 높게 된다. 하지만 같은 높이에서 콘크리트와 같은 단단한 표면으로 떨어지면 더 심각한 손상을 입을 수 있다. 압축성 물질(예: 눈 또는 물)은 정지거리를 늘리고 모든 에너지가 신체에 흡수되도록 하는 것보다 최소한 일부 에너지를 흡수한다. 그 결과 신체에 대한 손상이 감소한다. 이 원칙은 다른 유형의 충돌에도 적용된다. 안전띠를 매지 않은 운전자는 안전띠를 착용한 운전자보다 더 심각한 손상을 입게 되는데, 이는 신체가 아닌 안전띠 시스템이 에너지 전달의 상당 부분을 흡수하기 때문이다.

따라서 물체가 움직이고 운동의 형태로 에너지를 가지고 있는 경우 물체가 완전히 정지하려면 에너지를 다른 형태로 변환하거나 다른 물체로 전달하여 에너지를 모두 잃어야 한다. 예를 들어, 차량이 보행자와 충돌하면 보행자는 차량에서 튕겨 나간다(**그림 4-4**). 차량이 충돌로 인해 다소 느려지지만, 차량의 더 큰 힘은 둘 사이의 무게 차이에 따라 속도의 손실보다 가벼운 보행자에게 훨씬 더 많은 가속

을 전달한다. 또한 보행자의 부드러운 신체 부위와 자동차의 단단한 부분이 충돌하면 차량보다 보행자에게 더 심한 손상을 입힐 수 있다.

단단한 물체와 인체 사이의 에너지 교환

인체가 단단한 물체와 충돌하거나 그 반대의 경우 단단한 물체에 의해 충격을 받는 신체 조직 입자의 수는 발생하는 에너지 교환의 양에 따라 결정된다. 이러한 에너지 전달은 환자에게 발생하는 손상 정도를 결정한다. 손상을 받는 신체 조직 입자 수는 1) 조직의 밀도와 2) 충격의 접촉 면적의 크기에 의해 결정된다.

밀도

조직의 밀도가 높을수록(부피당 입자로 측정) 움직이는 물체에 의해 영향을 받는 입자의 수가 많아지므로 교환되는 에너지의 비율과 총량이 커진다. 주먹으로 베개를 때렸을 때와 같은 속도로 벽돌 벽을 주먹으로 치는 것은 손에 미치는 영향이 다르다. 주먹은 밀도가 낮은 베개보다 밀도가 높은 벽돌 벽과 충돌할 때 더 많은 에너지를 흡수하므로 손에 더 심한 손상을 입힐 수 있다(**그림 4-5**).

간단히 말해서 신체는 공기 밀도(폐 대부분과 장의 일부), 수분 밀도[근육과 대부분의 고형 기간(예: 간, 비장)] 및 고형 밀도(뼈)의 세 가지 유형의 조직 밀도가 있다. 따라서 에너지 교환양(그에 따른 손상)은 영향을 받는 조직 유형에 따라 달라진다.

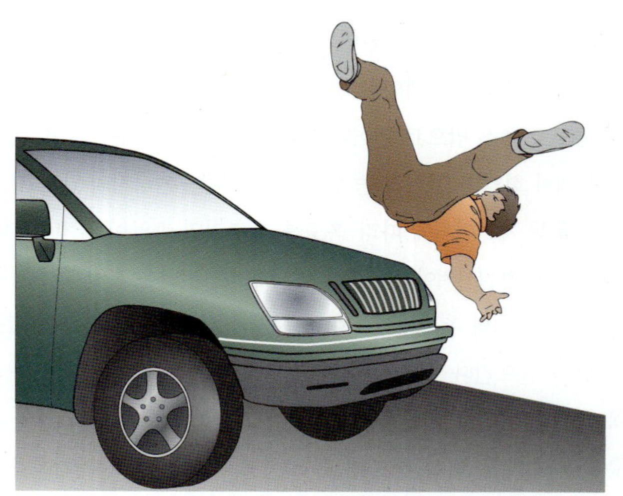

그림 4-4 움직이는 차량에서 보행자로의 에너지 교환은 보행자에게 속도와 에너지를 전달하여 조직을 부수고 차량에서 퉁겨지게 한다. 보행자가 차량에 치이거나 보행자가 바닥이나 다른 차량에 튕겨 나가면서 손상이 발생할 수 있다.

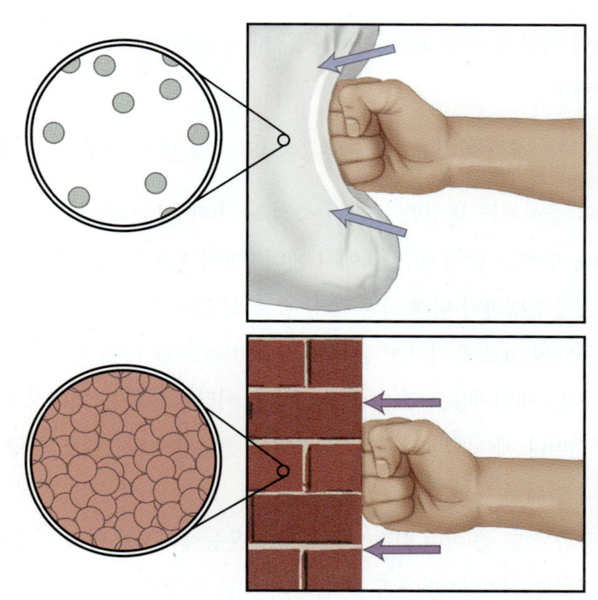

그림 4-5 사람의 주먹은 밀도가 낮은 베개보다 밀도가 높은 벽돌 벽과 충돌할 때 많은 에너지를 흡수하여 힘을 분산시킨다.

접촉 면적

달리는 차량의 창문 밖으로 손을 내밀면 바람이 손에 압력을 가한다. 손바닥이 수평이고 바람의 흐름 방향과 평행할 때 공기 입자가 손에 부딪히면서 손의 앞쪽(손가락)에 약간의 후방 압력이 가해진다. 손을 수직으로 90° 회전하면 더 넓은 표면적이 바람에 노출되므로 더 많은 공기 입자가 손에 닿아 손에 가해지는 힘의 양이 증가한다.

외상 사고의 경우 전달된 에너지와 그에 따른 손상은 충격 표면적 크기의 변화에 따라 손상이 달라질 수 있다. 인체에 미치는 이러한 영향의 예로는 자동차 전면, 야구 방망이 또는 소총의 총알이 있다. 자동차의 전면은 보행자의 많은 부분과 접촉하고 야구 방망이는 작은 부분에 닿고 총알은 아주 작은 면적에 접촉한다. 환자에게 손상을 줄 수 있는 에너지 교환의 양은 물체의 에너지와 에너지 교환 경로에 있는 조직의 밀도에 따라 다르다.

모든 충격 에너지가 작은 면적에 가해지고 이 힘이 피부의 저항을 초과하면 물체가 피부를 뚫고 나가게 된다. 망치로 나무 탁자를 치는 것과 같은 망치로 탁자 표면에 고정된 못을 치는 것의 차이를 생각해 본다. 망치로 탁자를 두드리면 망치로 탁자를 두드리는 힘이 탁자 표면과 망치 머리 전체에 퍼지면서 관통은 되지 않고 움푹 들어간 곳만 생긴다. 이와 반대로 망치로 못의 머리를 내리치면 같은 힘으로 망치의 모든 힘이 아주 작은 면적에 가해지기 때문에 못이 나무에 박히게 된다. 망치로 탁자를 내리치는 것과 같이 힘이 더 넓은 면적에 분산되어 피부를 관통하지 않는 경우의 손상을 무딘 손상으로 정의한다. 작은 면적에 힘이 가해지고 물체가 피부와 하부 조직을 관통하는 경우(망치로 탁자에 못을 박는 것과 같이)의 손상을 관통상으로 정의한다. 두 경우 모두 충격을 가한 물체의 힘으로 환자에게 공동이 생긴다.

총알과 같은 물체가 있더라도 충격 표면적은 총알 크기, 신체 내 움직임, 변형 및 파편과 같은 요소에 따라 다를 수 있다. 이러한 요소는 이 장의 뒷부분에서 설명한다.

공동화

에너지 교환의 기본 기전은 비교적 간단하다. 조직 입자에 가해지는 충격은 해당 조직 입자를 충격 지점에서 멀어지게 한다. 그러면 이러한 조직 입자는 움직이는 물체가 되어 다른 조직 입자와 충돌하여 쓰러지는 도미노 효과를 생성한다. 마찬가지로 단단한 물체가 인체에 부딪히거나 인체가 움직이다가 정지된 물체에 부딪히면 인체의 조직 입자가 정상적인 위치에서 밀려나 구멍이나 공간을 형성한다. 따라서 이 과정을 공간형성이라 한다. 공간형성을 시각적으로 설명하는 일반적인 예로 당구 게임을 들 수 있다.

큐볼은 팔 근육의 힘으로 당구대 길이만큼 움직인다. 큐볼이 당구대의 다른 쪽 끝에 있는 공에 충돌한다. 따라서 팔에서 큐볼로 전달되는 에너지는 당구대에 있는 각공으로 전달된다(**그림 4-6**). 큐볼은 다른 공에 에너지를 전달하고 에너지를 잃은 큐볼이 느려지거나 멈추는 동안 다른 공은 움직이기 시작한다. 다른 공은 이 에너지를 움

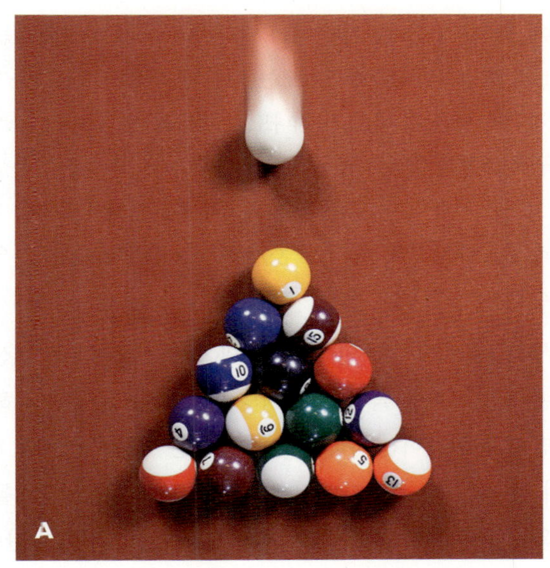

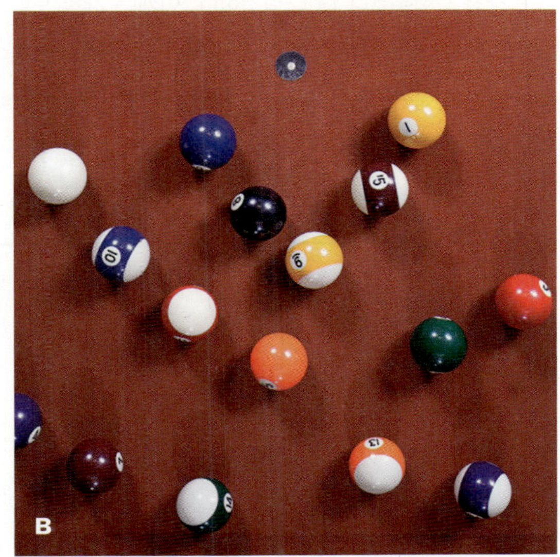

그림 4-6 **A.** 큐볼의 에너지는 각각의 다른 공으로 전달된다. **B.** 에너지 교환이 공을 서로 밀어내어 공동을 만든다.

직임으로 받아들이고 충돌 지점에서 멀어진다. 공이 놓여 있던 자리에 공간이 생성되었다. 볼링공이 레인을 따라 굴러가서 다른 쪽 끝에 있는 볼링 핀 세트를 때릴 때도 같은 종류의 에너지 교환이 발생한다. 이와 같은 유형의 에너지 교환은 둔기 및 관통상 모두에서 발생한다.

다음과 같이 두 가지 유형의 공간이 형성된다.

- 일시적 공동은 충격 발생 시 조직이 늘어나면서 발생한다. 신체 조직은 탄성력으로 인해 일시적 공동의 내용물 일부 또는 전체 내용물이 이전 위치로 돌아간다. 영구적인 손상의 일부가 되는 공동의 크기, 모양 및 부위는 조직 유형, 조직의 탄력성 그리고 조직의 반동이 얼마나 일어나는지에 따라 달라진다. 이 공동의 범위는 일반적으로 병원 전 처치 제공자 또는 병원 내 의료진이 환자를 평가할 때 충격을 받은 지 몇 초가 지나도 보이지 않는다.

- 영구적 공동은 일시적 공동이 무너진 후 남게 되며 조직 손상이 눈에 보이는 부분이다. 또한 물체가 조직에 직접적인 충격을 가하면 압궤 공동이 생긴다. 이 두 공동은 환자를 평가할 때 볼 수 있다(**그림 4-7**).

영구적 공동으로 남는 일시적 공동의 크기는 조직의 탄성(신축성)과 관련이 있다. 예를 들어, 야구 방망이로 강철 드럼통을 강하게 치면 측면에 움푹 들어간 자국이 생긴다. 같은 야구 방망이를 비슷한 크기와 모양의 고무 덩어리에 같은 힘으로 치면 야구 방망이를 제거해도 움푹 들어간 곳이 남지 않는다(**그림 4-8**). 그 차이가 탄력성이다. 고무는 강철 드럼통보다 더 탄력적이다. 인체는 강철 드럼통 보다 고무에 가깝다. 주먹으로 배를 때리면 주먹이 들어가는 느낌이 들지만, 주먹을 빼면 움푹 들어간 자국이 남지 않는다. 유사하게 야구 방망이로 가슴을 치면 가슴벽에 뚜렷한 공동이 남지는 않지만, 직접적

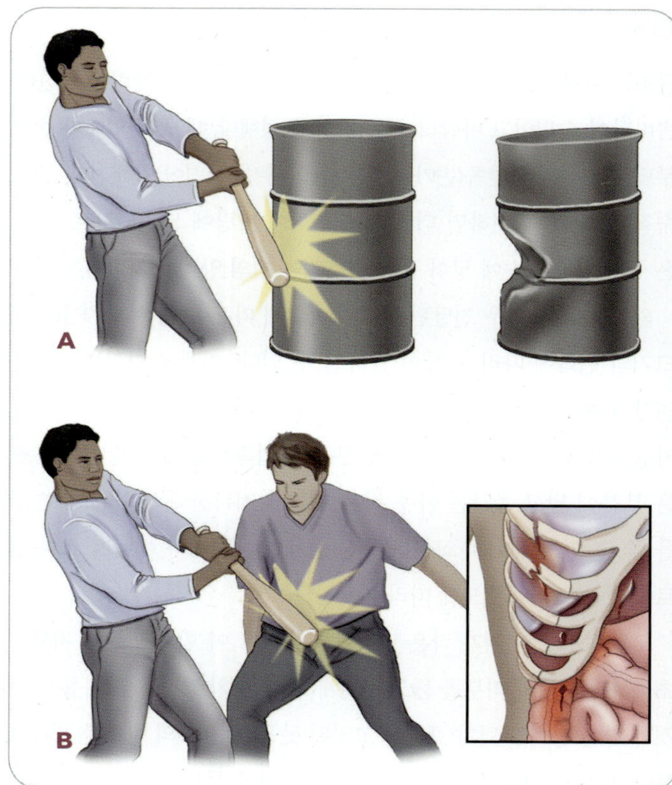

그림 4-8 **A.** 야구 방망이로 강철 드럼통을 치면 측면에 움푹 들어간 곳 즉, 공동이 생긴다. **B.** 야구 방망이로 사람을 치면 일반적으로 눈에 보이는 공동은 남지 않으며 인체의 탄력성은 손상이 발생하더라도 보통 정상적인 모양으로 돌아간다.
© National Association of Emergency Medical Technicians (NAEMT)

인 접촉과 에너지 교환에 의해 생긴 공동으로 인해 손상이 발생할 수 있다(**그림 4-8**). 사고의 이력과 에너지 전달의 해석은 충격 당시 일시적 공동의 잠재적인 크기를 결정하는 데 필요한 정보를 제공할 것이다. 관련된 장기 또는 구조는 손상을 예측할 수 있다.

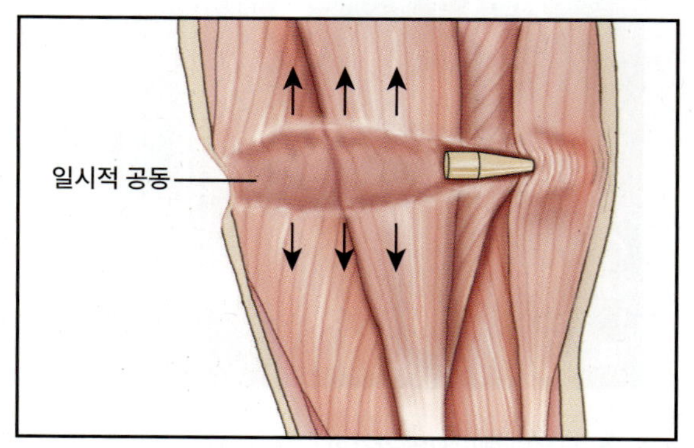

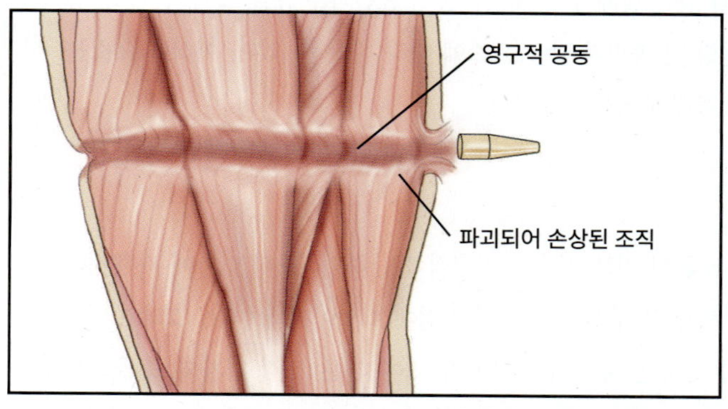

그림 4-7 조직 손상은 총상으로 인해 남아있는 영구적 공동보다 더 크다. 총알의 속도가 빠르거나 무거울수록 일시적 공동이 커지고 조직 손상 범위가 넓어진다.
© National Association of Emergency Medical Technicians (NAEMT)

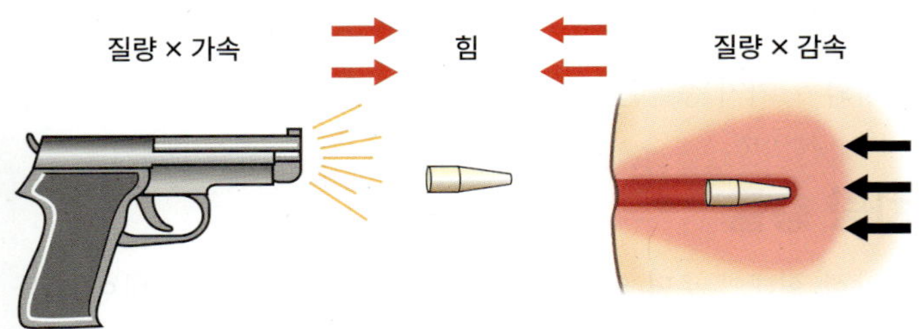

그림 4-9 총알이 조직을 관통할 때 총알의 운동에너지가 접촉하는 조직으로 전달되어 조직이 총알로부터 멀어지도록 가속한다.
© National Association of Emergency Medical Technicians (NAEMT)

장전된 총의 방아쇠를 당기면 총포의 공이가 캡을 치면서 탄약통에서 폭발이 일어난다. 이 폭발로 생성된 에너지는 총알에 가해져 총구에서 속도를 높인다. 이 총알은 에너지 즉 힘을 가지게 된다(힘 = 가속도 × 질량). 이러한 힘이 가해지면 총알은 외부의 힘으로 작용할 때까지 속도를 줄일 수 없다(뉴턴의 운동 제1 법칙). 총알이 인체 내부에서 멈추려면 총알의 에너지가 무기의 폭발에 해당하는 양(가속도 × 질량 = 힘 = 질량 × 감속도; **그림 4-9**)만큼 조직에 흡수되어야 한다. 이렇게 흡수된 에너지는 조직 입자가 정상 위치에서 벗어나게 하여 공동을 형성한다.

무딘 손상과 관통성 외상

외상은 일반적으로 무딘 손상과 관통상으로 분류된다. 그러나 두 가지 유형의 손상에서 교환되는 에너지와 발생하는 손상은 비슷하다. 공동화는 두 가지 유형 모두에서 발생하며 유형과 방향만 다를 뿐 결과적으로 피부를 관통하거나 관통하지 않을 수 있다. 물체의 전체 에너지가 피부의 한 작은 부분에 집중되면 피부는 찢어지고 물체가 몸 안으로 들어가 경로를 따라 더 집중된 에너지 교환을 일으킬 가능성이 높다. 이에 따라 한 국소 부위에 더 큰 파괴력이 발생할 수 있다. 더 큰 물체는 피부의 더 넓은 부위로 에너지가 분산되어 피부를 관통하지 못할 수 있다. 손상이 신체의 더 넓은 부위에 분산되고 손상 유형이 국소화되지 않는다. 대형트럭이 보행자에게 가하는 충격과 총에 맞은 충격의 차이를 예로 들 수 있다(**그림 4-10**).

무딘 외상으로 발생하는 공동은 일시적 공동인 경우가 많으며 충격 지점에서 멀리 떨어진 곳에 있다. 관통성 외상은 영구적 공동과 일시적 공동을 모두 생성한다. 생성된 일시적 공동은 총알의 경로에서 전방과 측면 방향으로 퍼진다.

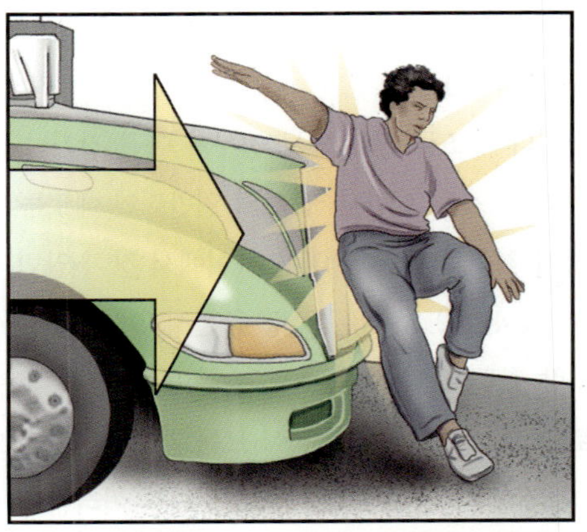

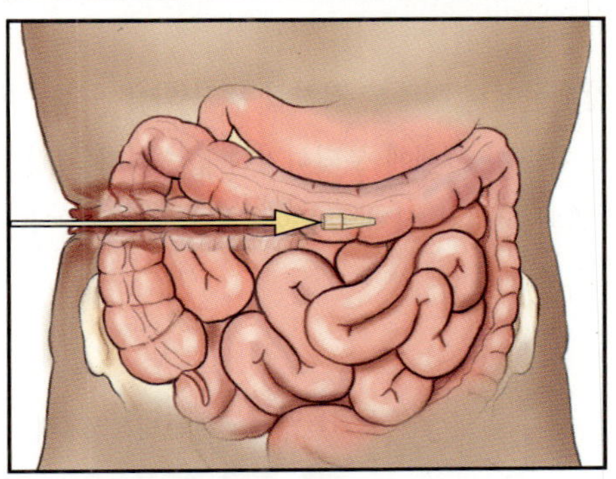

그림 4-10 차량과 사람이 충돌할 때 발생하는 힘은 일반적으로 넓은 부위에 분산되지만, 사람과 총알이 충돌할 때 발생하는 힘은 좁은 영역에 국한되어 인체와 내부 장기를 관통한다.
© National Association of Emergency Medical Technicians (NAEMT)

무딘 외상

충돌 사고로 인해 무딘 외상을 입었을 가능성이 있는 현장 평가를 통해 손상의 심각성이나 잠재적 장기 손상에 대한 단서를 얻을 수 있다. 평가 요소는 1) 충격의 방향, 2) 차량의 외부 손상(유형 및 심각도), 3) 내부 손상(예: 탑승자 공간 침입, 운전대 및 축 변형, 앞 유리 파손, 미려 손상, 대시보드-무릎 충격), 4) 차량 내 탑승자의 위치, 5) 충돌 당시 안전장치의 사용 및 작동 여부이다.

무딘 외상의 경우 두 가지 힘(전단력과 압박력)이 충격에 관여하며 이 두 힘 모두 공동을 유발할 수 있다. 전단은 하나의 장기나 구조물(또는 장기나 구조물의 일부)이 다른 장기나 구조물(또는 장기나 구조물의 일부)보다 빠르게 속도를 변화시키는 결과이다. 이러한 가속 또는 감속의 차이에 따라 장기가 구조물에 분리되고 찢어진다. 전단력의 대표적인 예는 가슴대동맥 파열이다. 오름대동맥과 대동맥활은 세로칸 내에 느슨하게 고정됐지만, 아래대동맥은 척추에 단단히 고정되어 있다. 갑작스러운 감속 사고가 발생하면 내림대동맥은 고정되어 있지만, 오름대동맥과 대동맥활은 계속 움직여 대동맥이 절단되고 파열될 수 있다(**그림 4-11**).

압박은 장기나 구조물 전체 또는 일부가 다른 장기나 구조물 사이에 직접 압박되는 것을 말한다. 압박의 일반적인 예로는 안전띠를 착용한 탑승자의 척주와 전복벽 내부 사이에서 장이 압박되는 경우를 들 수 있다(**그림 4-12**). 손상은 차량 충돌사고(차량 또는 오토바이), 보행자와 차량 충돌, 추락, 스포츠 손상, 폭발 손상과 같은 다양한 유형의 충돌로 인해 발생할 수 있다. 이 모든 기전은 개별적으로 논의되고 각 신체 부위의 특정 해부학적 구조에 대한 이러한 에너지 교환의 결과를 설명한다.

이 장의 앞부분에서 설명한 것처럼 무딘 외상에서는 세 가지 충돌이 발생한다. 차량이 물체에 부딪히거나 탑승자가 차량 내부에 부딪히거나 탑승자의 장기가 신체 공동에 부딪히는 경우이다. 이러한 충돌 중 첫 번째는 차량 충돌, 추락 및 폭발과 관련하여 논의될 것이다. 후자의 두 가지 충돌은 특정 신체 부위와 관련된 맥락에서 논의된다.

차량 충돌

다양한 형태의 무딘 외상이 발생하지만, 차량 충돌(오토바이 충돌 포함) 사고가 가장 흔하다. 2019년 미국에서는 차량 충돌 사고로 36,096명이 사망하고 약 274만 명이 손상을 입었다. 이 수치는 휴대 전화와 전자 기기를 조작할 수 있는 핸즈프리 기술의 보급이 증가했음에도 불구하고 산만한 운전이 증가한 것과 관련이 있을 수 있다. 이는 또한 이 분야에서 교육과 예방 노력을 강화할 분명한 기회이기도 하다. 대부분 부상자가 차량 탑승자였던 반면, 부상자 중 23만 명 이상이 오토바이 운전자, 46만 명 이상이 자전거 운전자 그리고 18만 명 이상이 보행자였다.

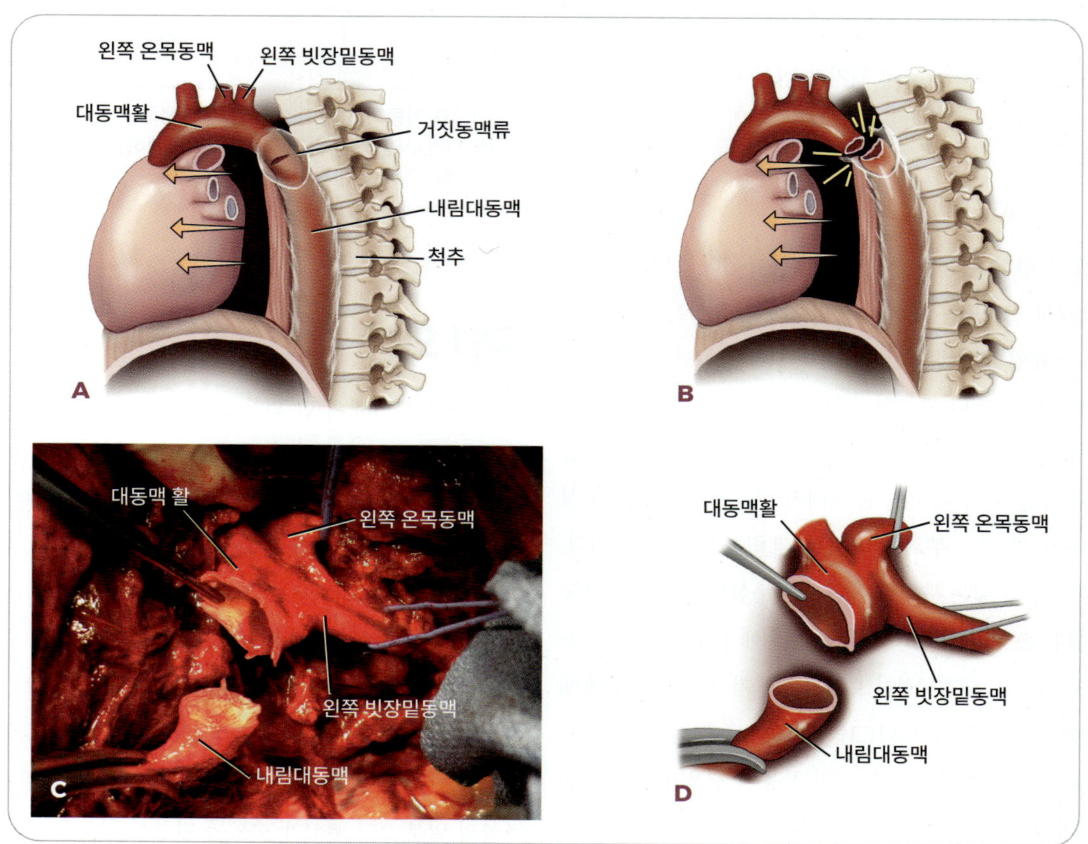

그림 4-11　**A.** 내림대동맥은 등뼈와 함께 움직이는 고정된 구조물이다. 대동맥활, 대동맥 및 심장은 자유롭게 움직임일 수 있다. 측면 충돌 시 몸통이 가속하거나 전방충돌 시 몸통이 급격히 감속하면 대동맥활-심장 복합체와 내림대동맥 사이의 운동 속도가 달라진다. 이러한 움직임으로 인해 가장 바깥쪽 층에 포함된 대동맥 내막이 찢어져 거짓동맥류(pseudo-aneurysm)가 생길 수 있다. **B.** 대동맥활과 내림대동맥의 접합부가 찢어지면 대동맥이 완전히 파열되어 가슴에 즉각적인 출혈을 일으킬 수 있다. **C.** 외상성 대동맥 파열의 수술 사진 **D.** 외상성 대동맥 파열의 그림.

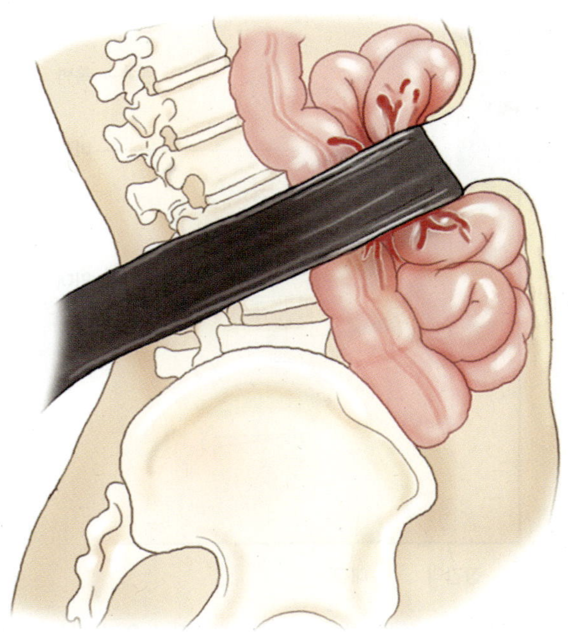

그림 4-12 안전띠가 골반 가장자리 위에 잘못 위치하면 복부 장기가 움직이는 후방 척추와 벨트 사이에 갇힐 수 있다. 췌장 및 기타 복막뒤 장기의 손상과 소장 및 결장의 파열이 발생할 수 있다.
© National Association of Emergency Medical Technicians (NAEMT)

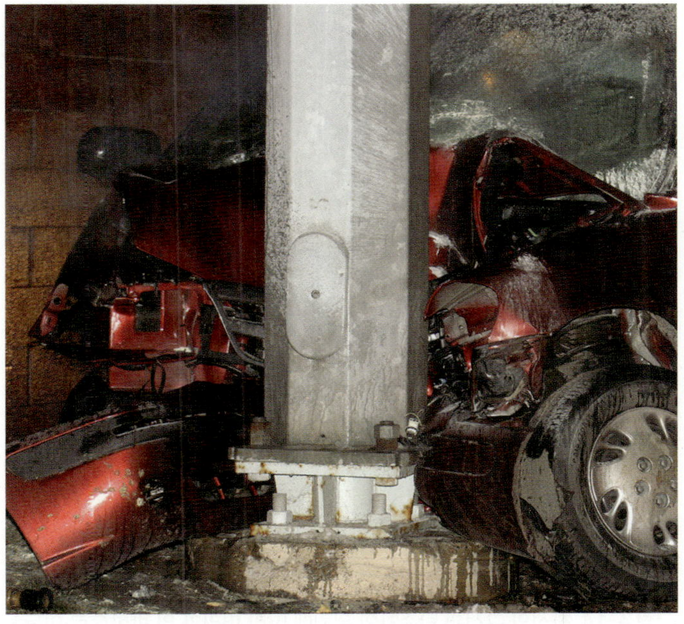

그림 4-13 차량이 전봇대에 충돌하면 차량의 앞부분은 멈추지만, 차량의 뒷부분은 계속 전진하여 차량의 변형을 일으킨다.
© Jack Dagley Photography/Shutterstock

차량 충돌은 5가지 유형으로 분류할 수 있다.

1. 전방충돌
2. 후방 추돌
3. 측면충돌
4. 회전충돌
5. 전복

각 유형에는 차이가 있지만 다섯 가지 유형을 정확하게 구분하면 다른 유사한 유형의 충돌에 대해 이해할 수 있다.

탑승자의 손상 가능성을 예측하는 한 가지 방법은 차량을 살펴보고 다섯 가지 충돌 유형 중 어떤 유형이 발생했는지, 관련된 에너지 교환 및 충돌의 방향을 파악하는 것이다. 탑승자는 차량과 같은 방향에서 차량과 같은 유형의 힘에 취약하며 잠재적인 손상을 예측할 수 있다. 그러나 탑승자와 차량이 주고받는 힘의 양은 차량의 에너지 흡수로 인해 감소한다.

전방충돌

그림 4-13에서는 차량이 차량의 중앙 부분을 전봇대에 부딪쳤다. 충돌 지점은 전진 운동을 멈추지만, 나머지 차량 부분은 차량의 변형에 의해 에너지가 흡수될 때까지 계속 전진한다. 운전자에게도 같은 유형의 운동이 발생하여 손상을 입었다. 안전한 운전대는 가슴, 아마도 복장뼈 중앙에 충격을 준다. 차량이 계속 전진하면서 차량의 전면이 크게 변형된 것처럼 운전자의 가슴도 변형되었다. 복장뼈가 운전대에 대한 전진 운동을 멈추면 뒤쪽 가슴벽은 갈비뼈의 구부러짐과 골절로 인해 에너지가 흡수될 때까지 계속된다. 이 과정에서 복장뼈와 척추, 뒤쪽 가슴벽 사이에 있는 심장이나 폐가 짓눌릴 수도 있다.

차량의 파손 정도는 충돌 당시 차량의 대략적인 속도와 관련이 있다. 차체 침입이 클수록 충돌 당시의 속도가 빨랐을 가능성이 높다. 차량의 속도가 빠를수록 에너지 교환이 커지고 탑승자가 손상을 입을 가능성이 커진다.

차량이 전방충돌 시 갑자기 전진을 멈추더라도 탑승자는 계속 이동하며 상향경로 또는 하향경로 중 하나를 따라 이동하게 된다.

안전띠를 착용하고 에어백이나 구속 시스템을 전개하면 에너지의 일부 또는 대부분을 흡수하여 피해자의 손상을 줄일 수 있다. 명확하고 간단한 설명을 위해 이 예시에서 탑승자는 안전띠를 매지 않은 것으로 가정한다.

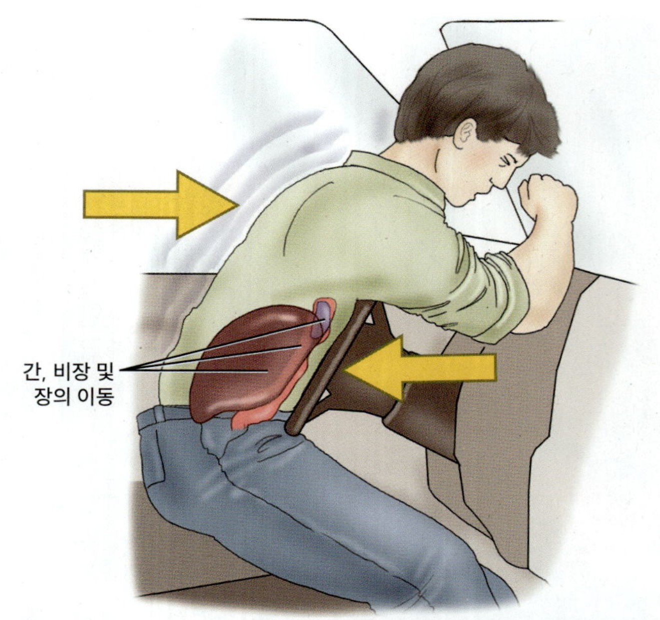

그림 4-14 좌석의 구성과 탑승자의 위치에 따라 머리가 위 방향으로 이동하는 경로를 따라 상반신에 초기 힘이 가해질 수 있다.
© National Association of Emergency Medical Technicians (NAEMT)

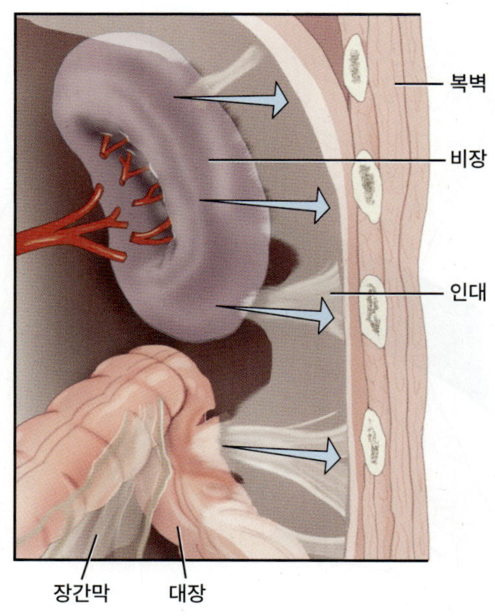

그림 4-15 장기는 복벽에 부착된 지점에서 찢어질 수 있다. 신장, 비장 및 소장은 특히 이러한 유형의 전단력에 취약하다.
© National Association of Emergency Medical Technicians (NAEMT)

상향경로

이 과정에서 신체의 전진 운동은 신체를 운전대 위로 이동하게 한다(**그림 4-14**). 일반적으로 머리가 앞 유리, 앞 유리 프레임 또는 지붕에 부딪히게 된다. 그런 다음 머리는 전진 운동을 멈추고 몸통은 척추를 따라 에너지가 흡수될 때까지 계속 움직인다. 목뼈는 척추에서 가장 덜 보호되는 부위이다. 그런 다음 몸통의 위치에 따라 가슴과 복부는 운전대와 부딪히게 된다. 가슴이 운전대와 부딪히면 가슴우리, 심장, 폐 및 대동맥 손상이 발생한다(무딘 외상의 부위별 부분 참조). 배가 운전대와 부딪히면 고형장기를 압박하고 짓눌리며 과압 손상(특히 가로막)을 일으키고 속빈 장기를 파열시킬 수 있다.

　배가 운전대에 부딪혀 갑자기 멈추면서 신장, 비장, 간도 전단 손상을 입을 수 있다. 장기가 정상적인 해부학적 구속과 지지 조직으로부터 찢어질 수 있다(**그림 4-15**). 예를 들어, 척추가 움직임을 멈춘 후에도 신장이 계속 앞으로 움직이면 혈액이 공급되는 장기의 부착 부위를 따라 전단이 발생하게 된다. 대동맥과 대정맥은 뒤쪽 배벽과 척추에 단단히 고정되어 있다. 신장의 지속적인 전진 운동은 신장 혈관이 파열 지점까지 늘어날 수 있다. 부착되지 않은 대동맥활이 단단하게 고정된 내림대동맥에 비슷하게 작용하여 가슴의 대동맥이 찢어질 수 있다(**그림 4-11** 참조).

하향 경로

하향 경로에서 탑승자는 앞쪽 아래 방향으로 좌석에서 대시보드로 이동한다(**그림 4-16**). 외상의 물리학을 이해하는 것이 얼마나 중요한지는 이 경로에서 다리에 발생하는 손상을 통해 알 수 있다. 대부분의 손상은 확인하기 어려우므로 손상의 기전을 이해하는 것이 중요하다.

　무릎을 곧게 편 채로 바닥 패널이나 브레이크 페달에 발을 올려놓

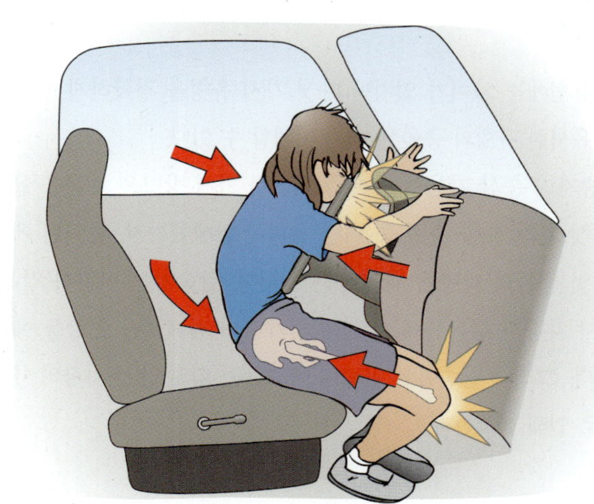

그림 4-16 탑승자와 차량은 함께 앞쪽으로 이동한다. 차량이 멈추고 안전띠 매지 않은 탑승자는 무언가에 부딪혀 움직임이 멈출 때까지 계속 전진한다.
© National Association of Emergency Medical Technicians (NAEMT)

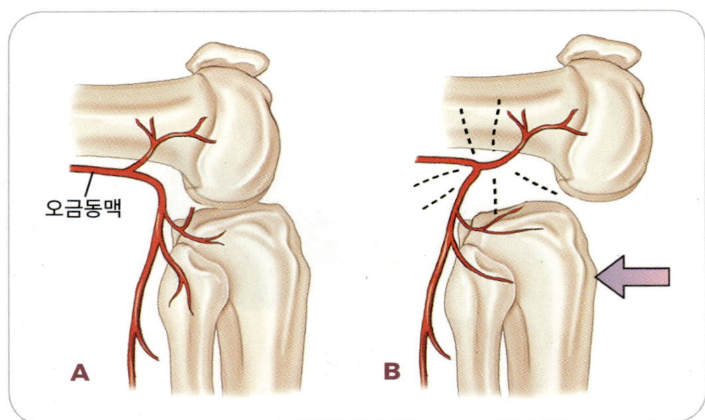

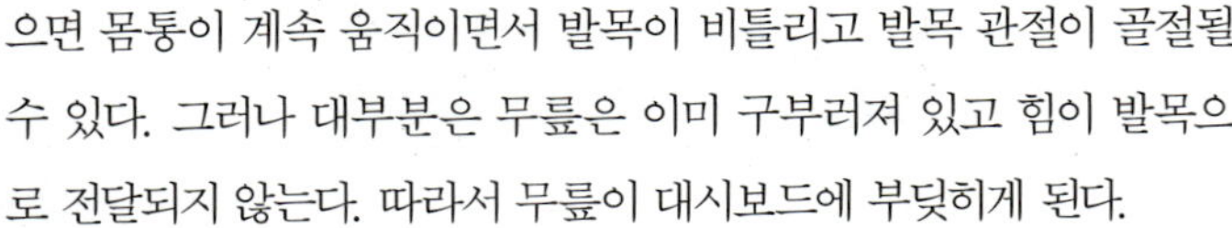

그림 4-17 **A.** 무릎은 차량 충돌 시 정강뼈와 넓적다리뼈의 두 부분에서 충격 지점이 있다. **B.** 오금동맥은 관절 가까이에 있으며 위의 넓적다리뼈와 아래의 정강뼈에 단단히 연결되어 있다. 이 두 개의 뼈가 분리되면 동맥이 늘어나거나 꼬이거나 찢어질 수 있다.

© National Association of Emergency Medical Technicians (NAEMT)

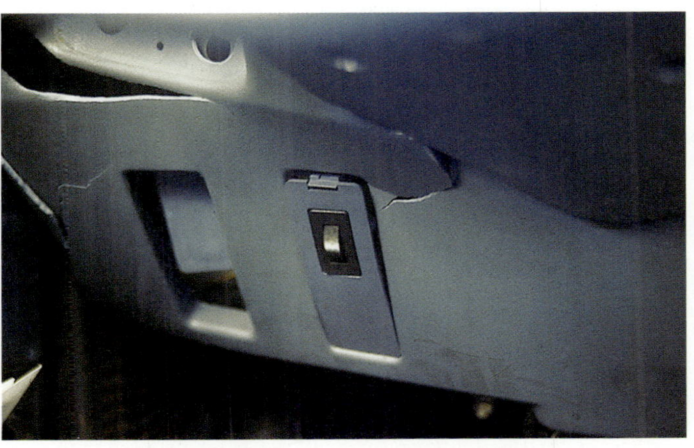

그림 4-18 무릎이 충격을 받은 대시보드의 자국은 이 관절과 인접 구조물에 상당한 에너지가 집중되었다는 것을 나타내는 중요한 지표이다.

Courtesy of Norman McSwain, MD, FACS, NREMT-P.

으면 몸통이 계속 움직이면서 발목이 비틀리고 발목 관절이 골절될 수 있다. 그러나 대부분은 무릎은 이미 구부러져 있고 힘이 발목으로 전달되지 않는다. 따라서 무릎이 대시보드에 부딪히게 된다.

무릎이 대시보드와 부딪힐 때 정강뼈와 넓적다리뼈에 충격이 가해질 수 있다(**그림 4-17A**). 정강뼈가 대시보드에 부딪혀 먼저 멈추면 넓적다리뼈는 계속 움직이면서 위로 겹치게 된다. 이에 따라 인대, 힘줄 및 기타 지지 구조가 찢어지는 무릎 탈구가 발생할 수 있다. 오금동맥은 무릎관절 부위에 위치하기 때문에 관절 탈구는 종종 이 혈관 손상과 관련이 있다. 동맥이 완전히 파열되거나 내층(내막)만 손상될 수 있다(**그림 4-17B**). 두 경우 모두 손상된 혈관에 혈전이 형성되어 무릎 아래 다리 조직으로 가는 혈류가 현저히 감소할 수 있다. 무릎 손상 및 혈관 손상의 가능성을 조기에 인지한 병원 전 처치 제공자는 응급실의 의사에게 이 부위의 혈관 평가가 필요하다는 사실을 알려야 한다.

이러한 오금동맥 손상을 조기에 확인하고 처치하면 원위부 다리의 허혈로 인한 합병증을 상당히 감소시킬 수 있다. 이 조직에 대한 관류는 약 6시간 이내에 재확립되어야 한다. 병원 전 처치 제공자가 외상의 물리학적 특성을 고려하지 않았거나 환자를 평가하는 동안 중요한 단서를 간과했기 때문에 지연이 발생할 수 있다.

이러한 환자의 대부분은 무릎 손상의 증거는 있지만 무릎과 충돌한 대시보드의 흔적은 상당한 에너지가 무릎관절과 인접한 인접 구조물에 집중되었음을 나타내는 주요 지표이다(**그림 4-18**). 가능한 손상을 더 잘 확인하기 위해 병원에서 추가 검사가 필요하다.

넓적다리뼈가 충격 지점이 되면 뼈의 축에 에너지가 흡수되어 부러질 수 있다(**그림 4-19**). 넓적다리뼈가 손상되지 않으면 골반이 넓적다리뼈 쪽으로 계속 전진하면 넓적다리 머리가 절구에서 탈구될 수 있다(**그림 4-20**).

무릎과 다리가 전진 운동을 멈춘 후 몸통이 핸들이나 대시보드 앞쪽으로 구부러진다. 그러면 안전띠를 매지 않은 탑승자는 앞서 설명한 상향경로와 같은 손상을 입을 수 있다.

이러한 잠재적인 손상을 인지하고 응급실 의사에게 정보를 전달하면 환자에게 장기적인 이점을 제공할 수 있다.

후방 추돌

후방 추돌은 서행하거나 정지한 차량을 더 빠른 속도로 움직이는 차량이 뒤에서 충돌할 때 발생한다. 이해를 돕기 위해 더 빠르게 움직이는 차량을 가해 차량이라고 하고 느리게 움직이거나 정지한 물체를 피해 차량이라고 한다. 이러한 충돌에서 충돌 순간의 가해 차량의 에너지는 피해 차량의 가속으로 변환되어 두 차량 모두에 파손이 발생한다. 두 차량의 운동량 차이가 클수록 초기 충격의 힘이 커지고 손상과 가속을 일으키는 데 사용할 수 있는 에너지가 많아진다.

후방 추돌 시 피해 차량은 앞으로 가속된다. 프레임에 고정된 모든 것이 같은 속도로 앞으로 이동한다. 여기에는 탑승자가 앉아 있는 좌석도 포함된다. 탑승자를 포함하여 차량에 부착되지 않은 물체는 프레임과 접촉한 물체가 전진 운동 에너지를 전달하기 시작한 후에야 전진 운동을 시작한다. 예를 들어, 몸통은 좌석의 스프링에 의해 일

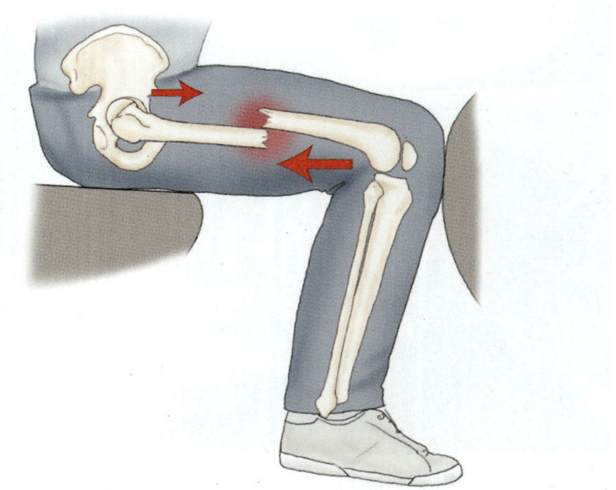

그림 4-19 넓적다리뼈가 충격 지점이 되면 에너지가 넓적다리뼈 축에 흡수되어 골절될 수 있다.
© National Association of Emergency Medical Technicians (NAEMT)

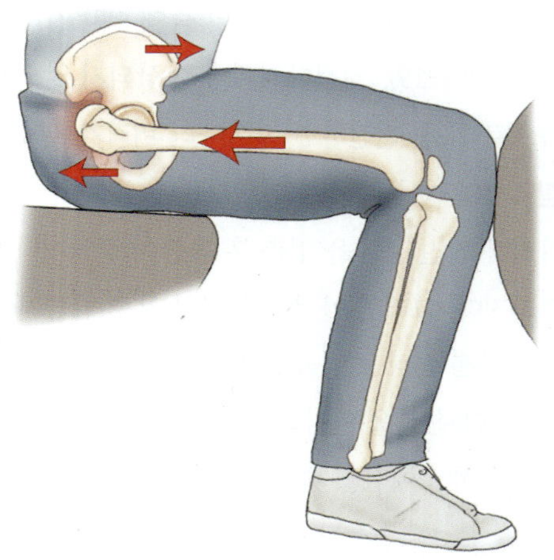

그림 4-20 넓적다리뼈에 대한 골반의 지속적인 전방 움직임은 엉덩관절의 후방탈구가 발생할 수 있다.
© National Association of Emergency Medical Technicians (NAEMT)

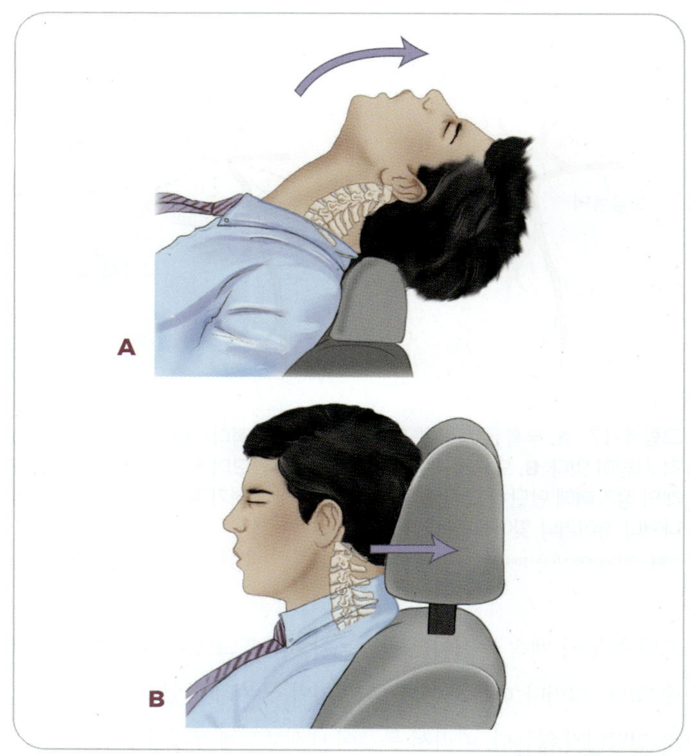

그림 4-21 **A.** 후방 충돌로 인해 몸통이 앞으로 쏠리게 된다. 헤드레스트의 위치가 부적절하면 머리가 헤드레스트 위로 과신전 된다. **B.** 헤드레스트를 올리면 머리가 몸통과 함께 움직여 목 손상을 예방하거나 줄일 수 있다.
© National Association of Emergency Medical Technicians (NAEMT)

> ### Box 4-2 헤드레스트
>
> 골다공증, 목 근육량 감소, 관절염과 같은 퇴행성 척추 질환으로 인해 노인 환자는 헤드레스트를 올바르게 사용하더라도 목 손상의 빈도가 높다.

© National Association of Emergency Medical Technicians (NAEMT)

부 에너지가 흡수된 후 좌석 등받이에 의해 가속된다. 헤드레스트가 뒤통수와 아래 부위에 부적절하게 위치하면 머리가 몸통보다 먼저 앞으로 움직이기 시작하여 목에 과신전이 발생한다. 특히 목 앞부분의 인대 및 기타 지지 구조물의 전단 및 스트레칭으로 인해 손상을 입을 수 있다(**그림 4-21A**).

헤드레스트가 적절하게 위치하면 머리는 과신전 없이 몸통과 거의 동시에 움직인다(**그림 4-21B** 및 **Box 4-2**). 피해 차량이 정지할 때까지 방해 없이 이동할 수 있다면 우주 비행사가 궤도에 진입하는 것과 유사하게 신체 움직임의 대부분이 좌석에 의해 지지가 되므로 탑승자는 심각한 손상을 입지 않을 수 있다.

그러나 차량이 다른 차량이나 물체를 들이받거나 운전자가 브레이크를 밟으며 급정거할 때 탑승자는 전방충돌의 특징적인 유형을 따라 앞으로 계속 전진하게 된다. 충돌은 후방과 정면의 두 가지 충격으로 이루어진다. 이차충돌은 손상의 가능성을 높인다.

측면충돌

측면충돌 기전은 차량이 교차로에서 충돌과 관련되거나 차량이 도로를 이탈하여 길가의 나무, 전봇대 또는 기타 장애물에 측면으로 충돌할 때 발생한다. 교차로에서 충돌한 경우 피해 차량은 가해 차량에 의해 생성된 힘에서 멀어지는 방향으로 가속된다. 부딪힌 차량의 측면이나 문이 탑승자의 측면에서 밀려난다. 탑승자는 측면으로 가속

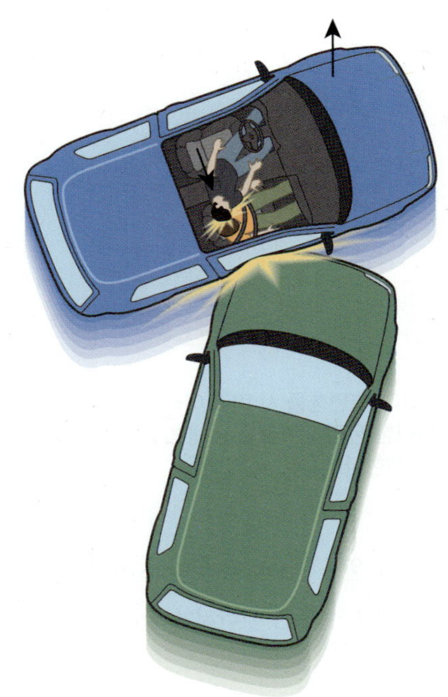

그림 4-22 차량의 측명 충돌로 인해 차량 전체가 안전띠를 매지 않은 승객쪽으로 밀려 들어간다. 안전띠를 맨 탑승자는 차량과 함께 측면으로 움직인다.
© National Association of Emergency Medical Technicians (NAEMT)

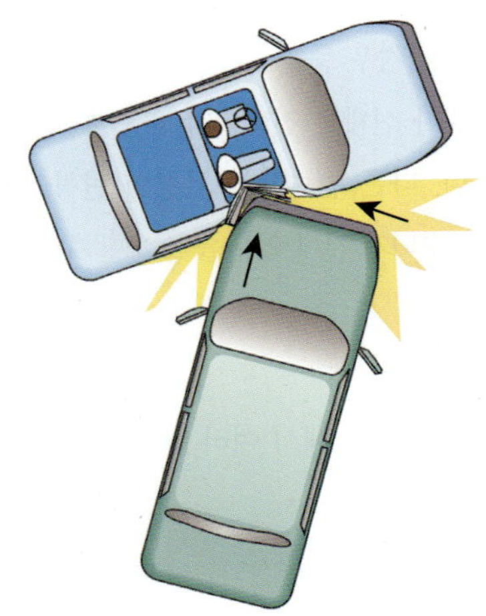

그림 4-23 차량 측면이 승객 공간으로 침입하면 또 다른 손상의 원인이 된다.
© National Association of Emergency Medical Technicians (NAEMT)

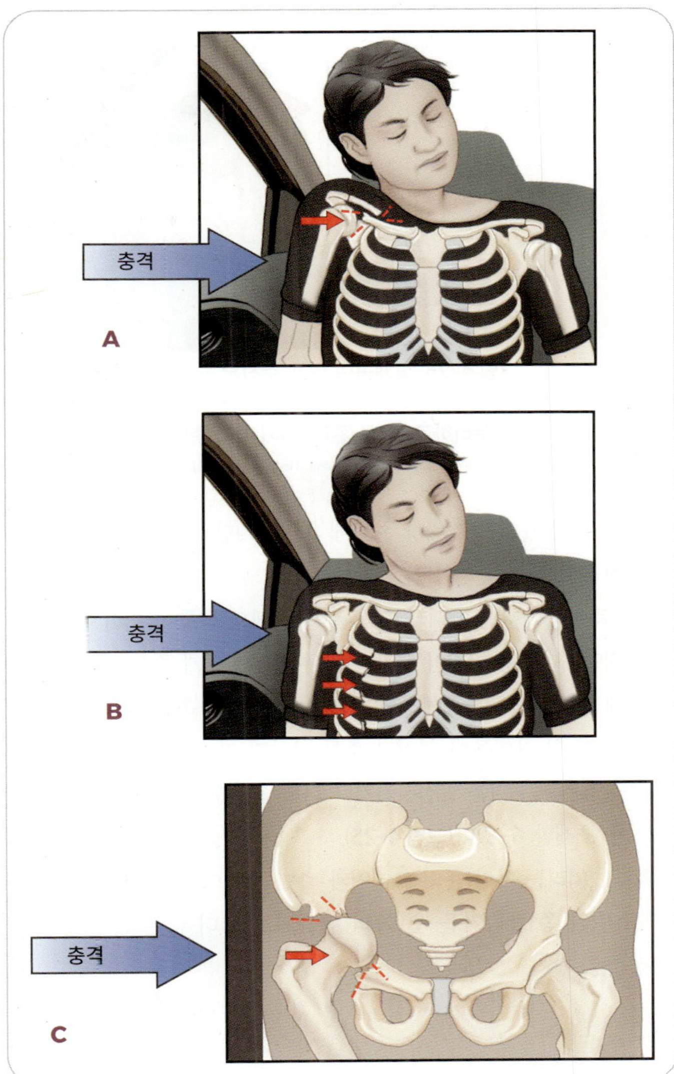

그림 4-24　**A.** 빗장뼈에 대한 어깨의 압박은 이 뼈의 중간 골절을 유발한다. **B.** 가슴 측견과 복벽에 압박을 가하면 갈비뼈가 골절되고 아래쪽 비장, 간 및 신장이 손상될 수 있다. **C.** 넓적다리뼈에 측면 충돌이 가해지면 넓적다리뼈 머리를 절구 방향으로 밀려나거나 골반이 골절될 수 있다.
© National Association of Emergency Medical Technicians (NAEMT)

되거나(**그림 4-22**) 문 돌출부에 의해 탑승자 공간이 안쪽으로 찌그러지면서 손상을 입을 수 있다(**그림 4-23**). 탑승자가 차량의 초기 움직임에 따라 움직이지 않고 고정되었으면 차량의 움직임으로 인한 손상이 덜 심각하다.

측면충돌에서는 다음과 같은 다섯 가지 신체 부위에서 손상을 입을 수 있다.

- 빗장뼈. 어깨에 힘이 가해지면 빗장뼈가 압박되어 골절될 수 있다 (**그림 4-24A**).

- 가슴. 가슴벽이 안쪽으로 압박되면 갈비뼈 골절, 폐 타박상 또는 가슴우리 아래 고형장기의 압박 손상과 과압 손상(예: 기흉)이 발생할 수 있다(**그림 4-24B**). 대동맥의 전단 손상은 측면 가속으로 인해 발생할 수 있다(대동맥 전단 손상의 25%는 측면 충돌에서 발생한다).

- 배와 골반. 함입은 골반이 압박되어 골절되고 넓적다리뼈 머리가 절구를 통해 밀려난다(**그림 4-24C**). 운전석 탑승자는 비장이 신체

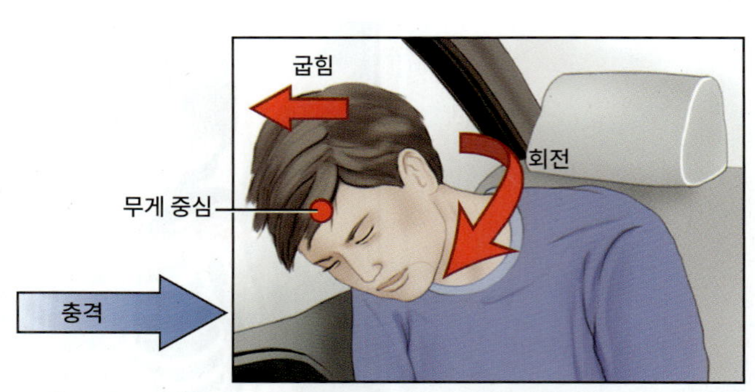

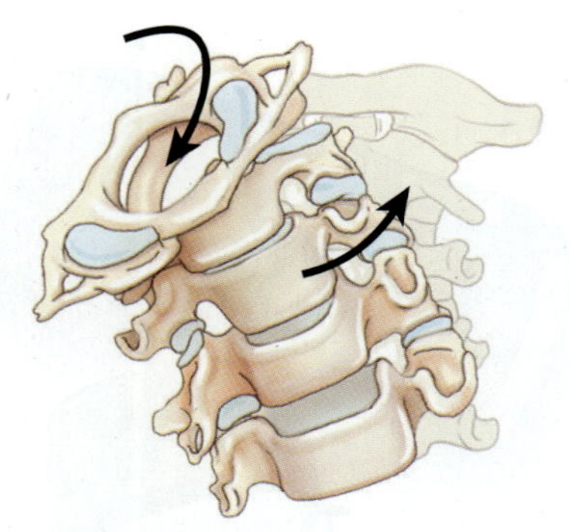

그림 4-25 두개골의 무게 중심은 두개골과 목뼈 사이의 축보다 앞쪽과 위쪽에 있다. 측면충돌 시 머리 아래에서 몸통이 급격히 가속되면 머리는 측면 및 전후방 각도에서 충격 방향을 향해 회전한다. 이러한 움직임은 충돌 반대 방향으로 척추를 분리하고 회전시킨다. 이에 따라 측면 충돌 시 인대 파열 및 측면 압박골절이 발생한다.
© National Association of Emergency Medical Technicians (NAEMT)

의 왼쪽에 있으므로 비장 손상에 취약하지만, 조수석 탑승자는 간 손상을 입을 가능성이 더 높다.

- 목. 측면충돌뿐만 아니라 후방 추돌 시에도 몸통이 머리 아래에서 움직일 수 있다. 머리의 부착 지점은 머리의 무게 중심보다 뒤쪽 아래에 있다. 따라서 목에 대한 머리의 움직임은 측면 굴곡과 회전이다. 척추의 반대쪽이 열리고 충돌 방향과 같은 쪽이 압박된다. 이 움직임은 척추뼈를 골절시키거나 척수 손상뿐만 아니라 탈구 가능성을 초래할 수 있다(**그림 4-25**).
- 머리. 머리는 차량 문의 프레임과 측면 창문에 부딪힐 수 있다. 충돌 부위 쪽 탑승자는 먼 쪽의 탑승자보다 더 많은 손상을 초래한다.

회전충돌

회전충돌은 차량의 한쪽 모서리가 움직이지 않는 물체나 다른 차량의 모서리 또는 서행하거나 반대 방향으로 움직이는 차량과 충돌할 때 발생한다. 뉴턴의 운동 제1 법칙에 따라 차량의 모서리는 정지하고 차량의 나머지 부분은 모든 에너지가 완전히 변환될 때까지 전진 운동을 계속한다.

회전충돌은 전방충돌과 측면충돌이 결합한 손상을 초래한다. 탑승자는 계속 앞으로 이동하다가 차량이 충돌 지점을 중심으로 회전하면서 측면충돌과 마찬가지로 차량 측면에 부딪히게 된다(**그림 4-26**).

탑승자가 여러 명일 경우 충돌 지점에 가장 가까운 탑승자에게 충돌 대부분의 에너지가 신체로 전달되기 때문에 가장 심각한 손상을 입을 가능성이 높다. 다른 탑승자는 차량의 변형 및 회전으로 인해 신체에 에너지가 흡수되기 전에 일부를 소모할 수 있다.

전복

전복 시 차량은 다양한 각도에서 여러 번 충격을 받을 수 있으며 안

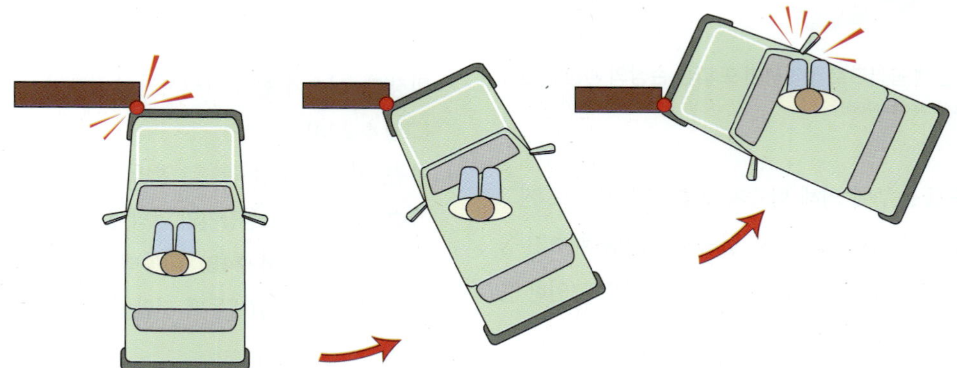

그림 4-26 회전충돌 시 탑승자는 앞쪽으로 이동한 후 차량이 충돌 지점을 중심으로 회전하면서 측면으로 이동한다.
© National Association of Emergency Medical Technicians (NAEMT)

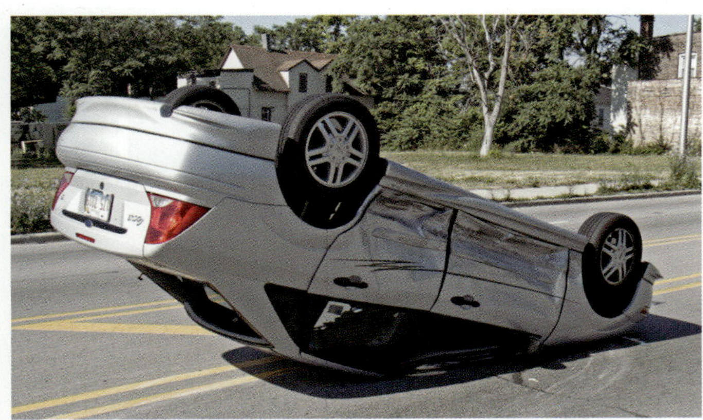

그림 4-27 전복 시 안전띠를 착용하지 않은 탑승자는 차량에서 일부 또는 완전히 튕겨 나오거나 차량 내부에서 통겨질 수 있다. 이 동작으로 인해 예측할 수 없는 다발성 손상이 발생하며 종종 심각한 손상을 입을 수 있다.
© Rechitan Sorin/Shutterstock

전띠를 매지 않은 탑승자의 신체와 내부 장기도 충격을 받을 수 있다 (**그림 4-27**). 이러한 충격으로 인해 차량 파손과 신체 손상이 발생할 수 있다. 전복 사고 시 안전띠를 매지 않은 탑승자는 구르는 차량에 의해 발생하는 상당한 힘으로 인해 전단 유형의 손상 위험이 있다. 탑승자는 안전띠를 착용하고 있더라도 내부 장기는 여전히 움직이며 연결된 조직 부위가 찢어질 수 있다. 안전띠를 매지 않으면 더 심각한 손상을 입을 수 있다. 많은 경우 탑승자는 차량이 굴러갈 때 차량에서 튕겨 나와 차량에 깔리거나 지면과의 충격으로 인해 손상을 입는다. 탑승자가 차량에서 도로로 튕겨 나오면 마주 오는 차량에 치일 수 있다. 미국 고속도로 교통안전국(NHTSA)에 따르면 2017년 사망자가 발생한 충돌 사고에서 차량에서 완전히 튕겨 나온 탑승자의 83%가 사망한 것으로 나타났다.

차량 종류에 따른 손상 차이

충돌 사고와 관련된 차량의 종류는 탑승자의 손상과 사망 가능성에 중요한 역할을 한다. 예를 들어 에어백이 없는 두 대의 차량이 측면 충돌하는 경우 피해 차량 탑승자는 가해 차량 탑승자보다 사망할 가능성이 더 높다. 충돌 차량의 탑승자에 대한 이러한 불균형한 위험은 주로 차량 측면의 상대적인 보호 장치가 상대적으로 부족하기 때문으로 설명할 수 있다. 이에 비해 탑승자 공간으로 찌그러져 들어오기 전에 차량 전면부에 많은 양의 변형이 발생할 수 있다. 측면충돌에서 피해 차량이 승용차가 아닌 스포츠 유틸리티 차량(SUV), 승합차 또는 픽업트럭일 경우 두 차량 탑승자의 사망 위험은 거의 같다. 그 이유는 SUV, 승합차 및 픽업트럭의 탑승 위치가 승용차보다 지면에서 더 높이 있어 탑승자가 측면충돌 시 직접적인 충격을 덜 받기 때문이다.

반대로 승합차, SUV, 픽업트럭이 승용차의 측면을 들이받았을 때 차량 탑승자에 더 심각한 손상과 사망 위험이 많이 증가한다는 사실이 입증되었다. 승합차와 승용차가 측면 충돌하면 측면을 부딪친 승용차의 탑승자가 승합차의 탑승자보다 사망할 확률이 더 높다. 충돌 차량이 픽업트럭이나 SUV인 경우 측면을 충돌한 차량 탑승자는 픽업트럭이나 SUV 탑승자보다 사망할 가능성이 더 높다. 이 엄청난 차이는 승합차, SUV 또는 픽업트럭의 무게중심이 높고 차량 중량이 증가하기 때문에 발생한다. 사고 시 탑승자가 어떤 차종에 탑승했는지에 대한 지식은 병원 전 처치 제공자가 심각한 손상을 의심하는 지수가 높아질 수 있다.

탑승자 보호 장치

안전띠

앞에서 설명한 손상 유형에서는 탑승자가 안전띠를 착용하지 않은 것으로 가정한 것이다. 미국 고속도로 교통안전국(NHTSA)은 2000년 이후 안전띠 착용률이 꾸준히 증가했으며 2020년에는 앞좌석 탑승자의 9.7%만이 안전띠를 착용하지 않은 것으로 보고했다. 안전띠 착용률은 여성(92.8%)보다 남성(88.4%)이 낮다. 16~24세(86.9%)에서 더 낮고 백인(90.5%)이나 다른 인종(92.8%)보다 흑인(85.2%) 탑승자가 더 낮다. 탑승자가 차량에서 튕겨 나가는 사고는 차량 사망 사고의 약 1/4을 차지한다. 승용차에서 완전히 튕겨 나간 탑승자의 83%가 사망했으며 튕겨 나온 탑승자 13명 중 1명은 척추 골절을 입었다. 차량에서 완전히 튕겨 나온 후 신체는 차량 외부의 지면 또는 다른 물체에 부딪히면서 이차 충격을 받는다. 이 이차 충격은 첫 번째 충격보다 훨씬 더 심각한 손상을 초래할 수 있다. 안전띠를 매지 않아 튕겨진 탑승자의 사망 위험은 안전띠를 착용해 차량 내부에 있는 탑승자보다 6배 더 높다. 안전띠가 생명을 구하는 것은 분명하다.

미국 고속도로 교통안전국에 따르면 미국 내 49개 주와 컬럼비아 특별구에서 성인과 미성년자 모두에 대한 안전띠 법을 시행하고 있다. 뉴햄프셔 지역만 예외적으로 미성년자에 대한 규정은 있지만, 성인에 관한 규정은 없다. 연구에 따르면 안전띠를 착용하면 앞좌석 탑승자의 치명적인 손상 위험을 45%, 심각한 손상 위험을 50% 감소시키는 것으로 나타났다. 2017년에 안전띠는 약 14,955명의 생명을 구했다. 2019년 교통사고로 사망한 승용차 탑승자는 22,215명 중 47%가 안전띠를 착용하지 않았다.

탑승자가 안전띠를 착용하면 어떤 일이 발생하는가? 안전띠를 올바르게 착용하면 충격의 압력이 골반과 가슴에 흡수되어 심각한 손상의 위험이 감소한다(**그림 4-28**). 안전장치를 올바르게 사용하면 탑승자의 신체에서 가해지는 충격의 힘이 안전띠나 안전장치로 전달된다. 안전띠를 사용하면 생명을 위협하는 손상을 입을 가능성이 크게 줄어든다.

안전띠를 올바르게 착용해야 효과적이다. 안전띠를 잘못 착용하면 충돌 시 손상을 방지하지 못할 수 있으며 심지어 손상을 입을 수도 있다. 허리 벨트를 느슨하게 착용하거나 골반 위에 매면 부드러운 배안 장기에 압박 손상이 발생할 수 있다. 부드러운 배안 장기(비장, 간, 췌장)의 손상은 안전띠와 후복벽 또는 척추 사이의 압박으로 인해 발생한다(**그림 4-12**). 배안의 압력이 증가하면 가로막 파열과 배안 장기의 탈장을 유발할 수 있다. 허리벨트는 어깨 벨트와 함께 착용해야 한다. 허리뼈 전방 골절은 몸통의 윗부분과 아랫부분이 허리벨트 위로 회전하면서 등뼈 12번, 허리뼈 1번과 2번 척추를 압박할 때 발생할 수 있다. 간혹 차량 탑승자가 대각선 안전띠를 어깨가 아닌 팔 아래에 착용하여 안전띠의 효과가 감소하는 경우가 있다.

미국에서 안전띠 착용 의무화 법안이 통과되고 시행되면서 전반적인 손상의 심각성이 감소하고 치명적인 충돌 사고가 크게 줄었다.

에어백

에어백은 차량 탑승자를 추가로 보호하는 역할(안전띠 외에)을 한다. 원래 운전석과 조수석의 에어백은 앞좌석 탑승자의 전방 움직임만 완충하도록 설계되었다. 에어백은 차체의 정지거리를 늘려 에너지를 천천히 흡수한다. 에어백은 전방충돌과 인접한 충돌의 첫 번째 충돌(전조등으로부터 30도 이내에서 발생하는 충돌의 65~70%)에서 매우 효과적이다. 그러나 에어백은 충돌 직후에 수축하므로 다중 충돌이나 후방 추돌에는 효과적이지 않다. 사고에서 부풀어 올랐다가 금방 공기가 빠지기 때문에 여러 방향의 충돌이나 충돌사고에서는 효과적이지 않다. 에어백은 0.5초 전개되고 이내에 수축한다. 최초 충돌 후 차량이 마주 오는 차량의 경로로 방향을 바꾸거나 도로를 벗어나 고정된 물체에 부딪히면 에어백의 보호 기능을 제공하지 못한다. 측면 에어백은 탑승자를 보호하는 데 도움이 된다.

에어백이 전개되면 경미하지만, 눈에 띄는 손상이 발생할 수 있으며 병원 처치 제공자가 이를 확인해야 한다(**Box 4-3**). 이러한 손상에는 팔, 가슴, 얼굴의 찰과상(**그림 4-29**), 얼굴과 눈의 이물질, 탑승자의 안경으로 인한 손상(**그림 4-30**) 등이 있다.

전개되지 않은 에어백은 여전히 환자와 병원 전 처지 제공자 모두

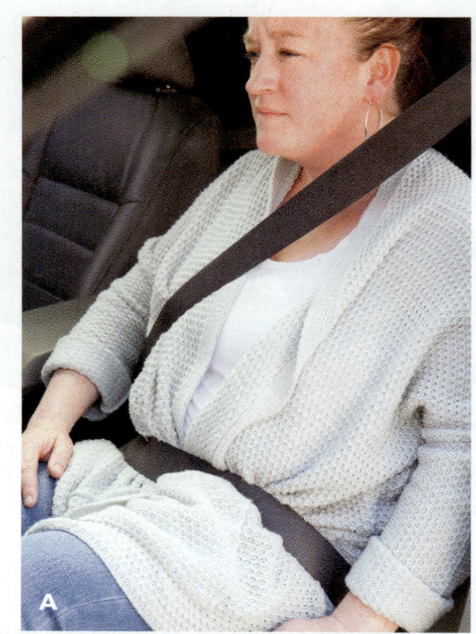

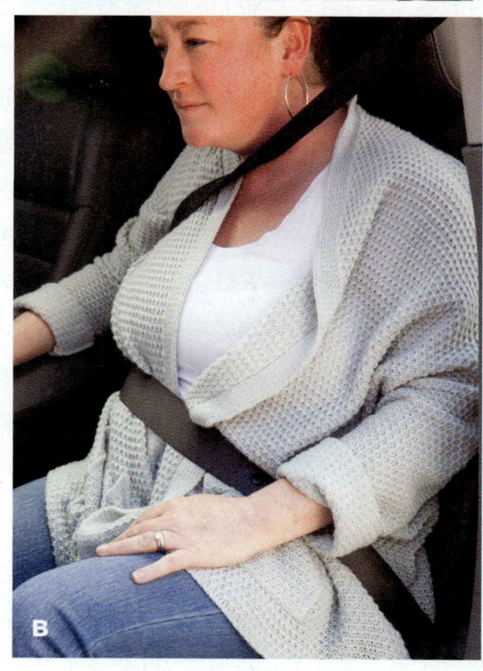

그림 4-28 **A.** 안전띠는 올바른 위치는 양쪽 넓적다리뼈 위쪽의 앞위엉덩뼈 가시에 위치하며 이 위치를 유지할 수 있도록 충분히 조여져 있어야 한다. 그릇 모양의 골반은 부드러운 배안 장기를 보호한다. **B.** 부적절하게 위치한 안전띠는 충돌 시 심각한 손상을 초래할 수 있다.
© Jones & Bartlett Learning. Photographed by Darren Stahlman.

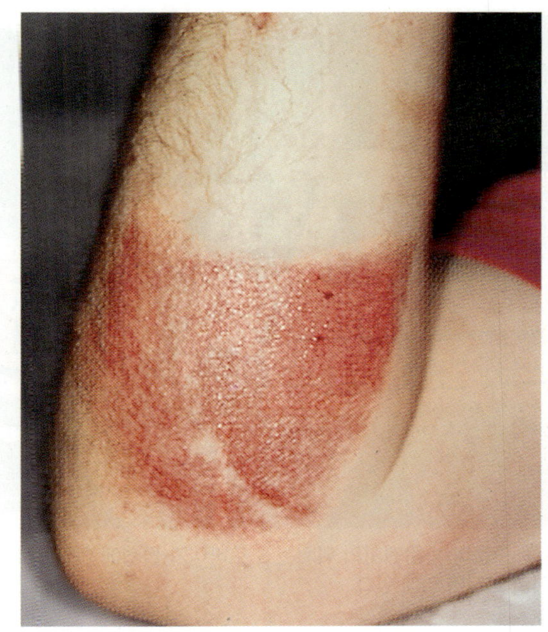

그림 4-29 아래팔 부위 찰과상은 손이 핸들에 닿았을 때 에어백이 빠르게 팽창하면서 이차적으로 발생한다.
Courtesy of Norman McSwain, MD, FACS, NREMT-P.

에게 위험할 수 있다. 에어백은 적절한 교육을 받은 구조전문가 해제할 수 있다. 이러한 비활성화로 인해 환자 처치 또는 중증 환자의 구출이 지연되어서는 안 된다.

에어백은 어린이가 안전띠를 착용하지 않았거나 조수석에 뒤쪽을 바라보도록 설치한 어린이 카시트에 앉은 영아와 어린이에게 심각한 위험을 초래할 수 있다.

오토바이 충돌

오토바이 사고는 매년 자동차 사망 사고의 상당수를 차지한다. 오토바이 충돌 사고의 물리학 법칙은 같지만, 손상 기전은 자동차나 트럭 충돌 사고와 다르다. 이러한 차이는 전방충돌, 각 충돌, 튕겨 나감과 같은 각 유형의 충돌에서 발생한다. 오토바이 사고에서 사망, 장애 및 손상을 증가시키는 또 다른 요인은 다른 자동차에 존재하는 오토바이의 구조적 프레임이 없기 때문이다.

전방충돌

단단한 물체와 전방 충돌하면 오토바이의 전진 운동이 정지한다(**그림 4-31**). 오토바이의 무게 중심은 이러한 충돌에서 종종 중심점이 되는 앞차축의 위와 뒤에 있으므로 오토바이가 앞으로 기울어지고 운전자가 핸들에 충돌할 수 있다. 운전자는 핸들이나 다른 물체와 먼저 충돌하는 신체 부위에 따라 머리, 가슴, 복부 또는 골반에 손상을 입을 수 있다. 운전자의 발이 오토바이의 발판에 고정되어 있고 허벅지가 핸들에 부딪히면 전진 운동 에너지가 넙적다리뼈 중심부에 흡수되어 때때로 양쪽 넙적다리뼈 골절이 발생할 수 있다(**그림 4-32**).

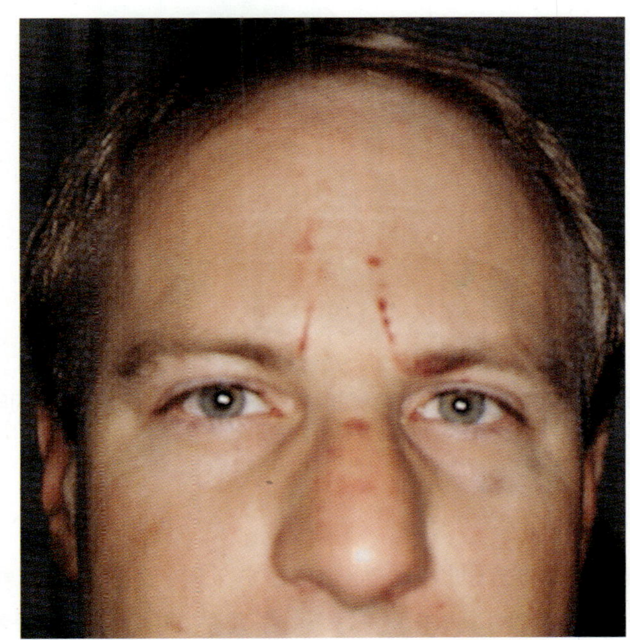

그림 4-30 안경을 낀 상태에서 에어백이 전개되면 찰과상이 발생한다.
Courtesy of Norman McSwain, MD, FACS, NREMT-P.

운전자의 골반과 핸들 사이의 상호작용은 다양한 조합의 뼈 또는 인대 손상이 발생할 수 있으며 책의 경첩처럼 후방 골반 고리가 열리는 동안 두덩결합을 방해할 수 있다("오픈북" 골반 손상). 이러한 손상은

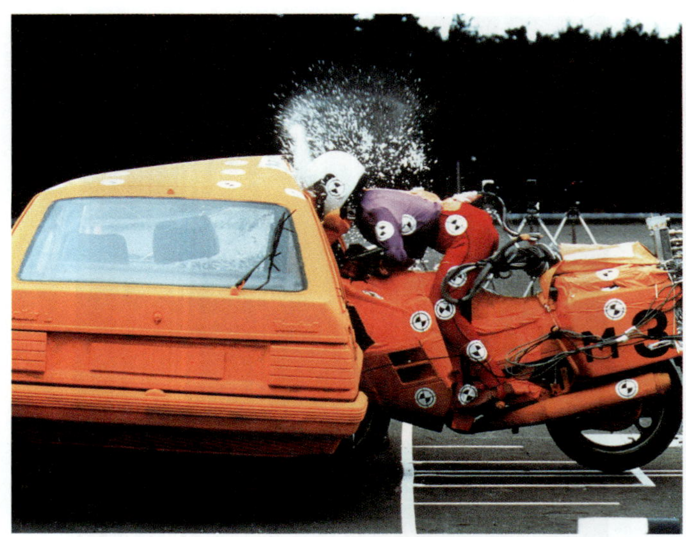

그림 4-31 오토바이 운전자의 위치는 오토바이가 물체에 전방으로 충돌할 때 앞바퀴의 회전축 위에 있다.
© TRL Ltd./Science Source

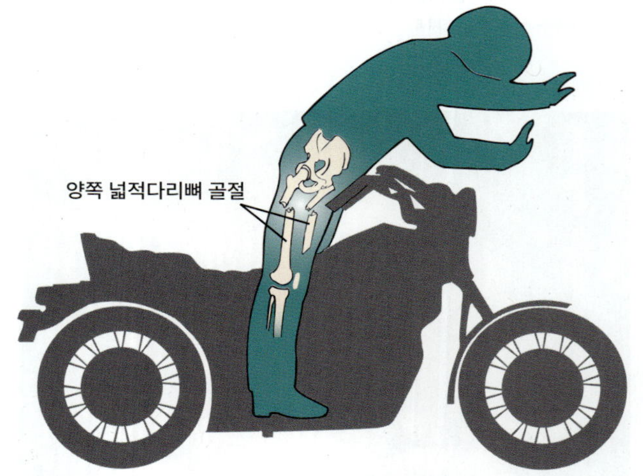

그림 4-32 운전자의 몸은 오토바이의 앞쪽과 위쪽으로 이동하며 허벅지와 넓적다리뼈가 핸들에 부딪히고 튕겨 나갈 수도 있다.
© National Association of Emergency Medical Technicians (NAEMT)

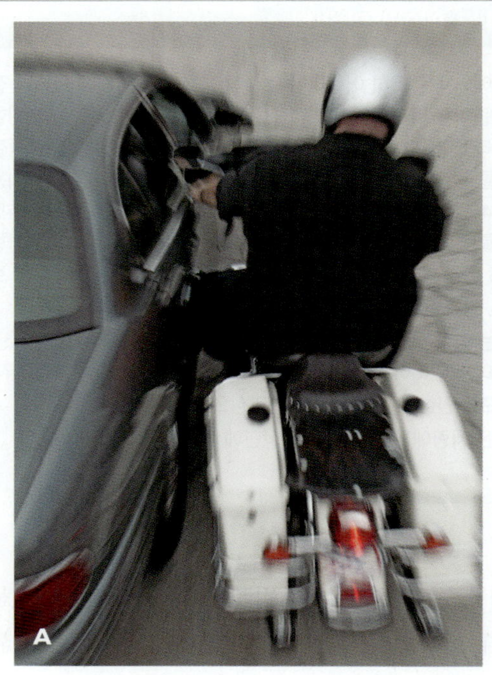

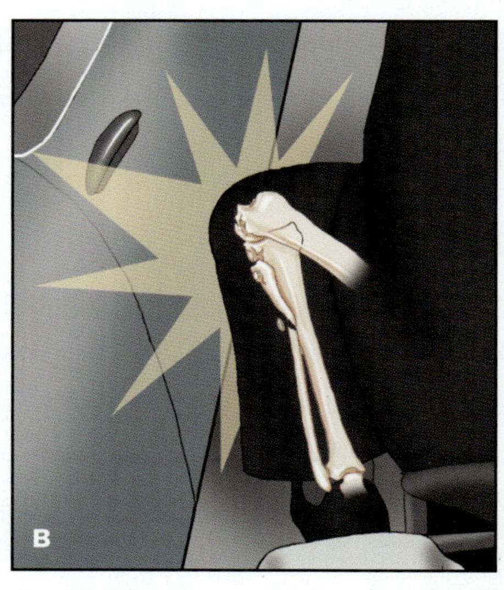

그림 4-33　**A.** 오토바이가 물체에 전방으로 부딪히지 않으면 가위처럼 쓰러진다. **B.** 이러한 충돌로 인해 오토바이 운전자의 다리가 충격을 받은 물체와 오토바이 사이에 끼이게 된다.
© National Association of Emergency Medical Technicians (NAEMT)

생명을 위협하는 골반 내 출혈을 초래할 수 있으며 골반 고정대를 즉시 적용하는 것이 생명을 구하는 처치가 될 수 있다. 이것은 운동학적 평가가 현장에서 잠재적으로 생명을 구할 수 있는 처치로 이어진 좋은 예이다.

각 충돌

각 충돌은 오토바이가 비스듬히 물체와 충돌한다. 그러면 오토바이가 넘어지면서 운전자를 덮치거나 오토바이와 충돌한 물체 사이에

끼이게 된다. 팔 또는 다리에 손상이 발생하여 골절과 광범위한 연부 조직 손상이 발생할 수 있다(**그림 4-33**). 에너지 교환의 결과로 배안의 장기에도 손상이 발생할 수도 있다.

이탈

안전장치가 없으므로 오토바이 운전자나 탑승자가 튕겨 나가기 쉽

다. 운전자는 머리, 팔, 가슴, 복부 또는 다리가 차량, 전신주 또는 도로와 같은 다른 물체에 부딪힐 때까지 날아가게 된다. 손상은 충돌 부위에서 발생하고 에너지가 흡수되면서 신체 나머지 부분으로 방출된다.

손상 예방

많은 오토바이 운전자는 적절한 보호 장비를 착용하지 않는다. 오토바이 운전자를 위한 보호 장비에는 부츠, 가죽의류, 헬멧이 포함된다. 이 세 가지 중에서 헬멧이 가장 뛰어난 보호 기능을 제공한다. 헬멧은 머리뼈와 유사하게 만들어져 외부는 튼튼하고 지지력이 뛰어나며 내부는 에너지를 흡수한다. 헬멧의 구조가 충격을 상당한 부분 흡수하여 얼굴, 머리뼈 및 뇌의 손상을 줄여준다. 헬멧은 목을 최소한으로 보호할 뿐 목 손상을 유발하지는 않는다. 헬멧 착용 의무화 법안은 운전자의 헬멧 사용을 늘리는 데 효과적이다. 오토바이 헬멧을 착용은 오토바이 충돌 사고에 연루된 운전자의 머리 손상 및 사망 위험을 줄이는 데 매우 효과적이다.

 오토바이를 눕히는 것은 운전자가 충돌이 임박한 상황에서 오토바이에서 몸을 분리하기 위해 사용하는 보호 동작이다(**그림 4-34**). 운전자는 오토바이를 옆으로 돌리고 안쪽 다리를 땅바닥에 끌게 한다. 이런 동작은 오토바이보다 운전자의 속도를 더 느리게 하여 오토바이가 운전자 위치에서 움직이도록 한다. 운전자는 아스팔트를 따라 미끄러지지만, 오토바이와 충돌하는 물체 사이에 끼이지는 않는다. 이 동작을 사용하면 운전자는 일반적으로 찰과상과 경미한 골절

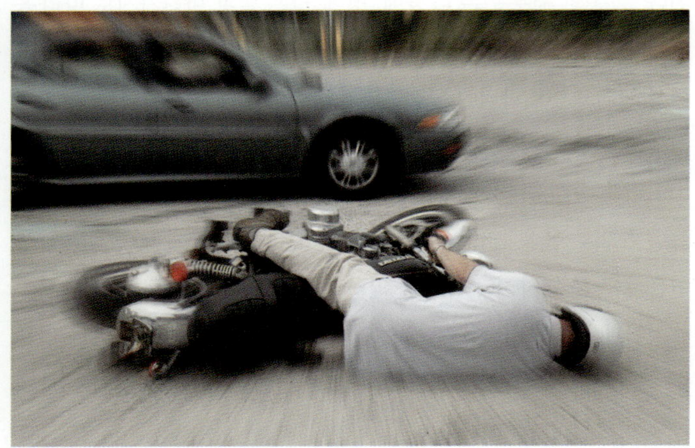

그림 4-34 오토바이와 차량 사이에 끼이는 것을 방지하기 위해 운전자는 오토바이를 눕혀 손상을 완화한다. 이 동작은 종종 아스팔트 위에서 운전자의 속도가 느려지면서 찰과상을 유발한다.
© National Association of Emergency Medical Technicians (NAEMT)

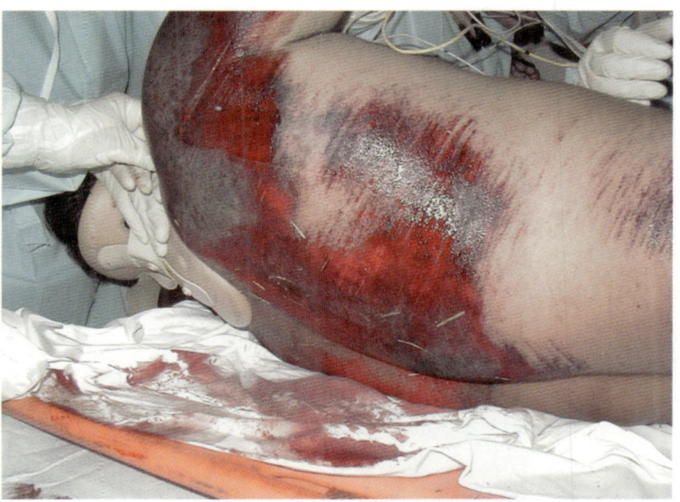

그림 4-35 보호복을 입지 않은 오토바이 운전자가 충돌 후 도로에 의한 화상을 입었다.
Courtesy of Dr. Jeffrey Guy.

을 입지만 다른 물체에 직접 부딪히지 않는 한 일반적으로 다른 유형의 충돌과 관련된 심각한 손상을 피할 수 있다(**그림 4-35**).

보행자 손상

차량이 보행자와 충돌하는 일반적인 시나리오는 다음과 같이 세 가지 단계로 나뉘며 단계마다 고유한 손상 유형이 있다. 각 고유한 손상 유형이 있는 세 가지 단계를 포함한다.

1. 초기 충격은 다리와 때로는 엉덩이 부위에 가해진다(**그림 4-36A**).
2. 몸통이 차량의 보닛 위로 굴러가면서 앞 유리에 부딪힐 수 있다(**그림 4-36B**).
3. 보행자는 차량에서 땅으로 떨어지며 일반적으로 머리부터 바닥에 떨어지고 목뼈 손상을 입을 수 있다(**그림 4-36C**).

보행자 충돌로 인한 손상은 보행자의 키와 차량의 높이에 따라 달라진다(**그림 4-37**). 차량 앞에 서 있는 소아와 성인은 차량에 부딪히는 해부학적 충돌 지점이 다르다.

성인은 일반적으로 차량의 범퍼에 다리 아래쪽을 먼저 부딪쳐서 정강뼈와 종아리뼈가 골절된다. 보행자는 차량의 보닛 앞부분에 부딪히며 보닛의 높이에 따라 배와 가슴이 보닛의 윗부분과 앞 유리에 부딪히게 된다. 두 번째 충격은 위쪽 넓적다리뼈, 골반, 갈비뼈 및 척추의 골절을 초래할 수 있으며 복강 및 가슴안에 으깸 및 전단 손상이 발생할 수 있다. 보행자의 머리가 보닛에 부딪히거나 보행자가 보닛

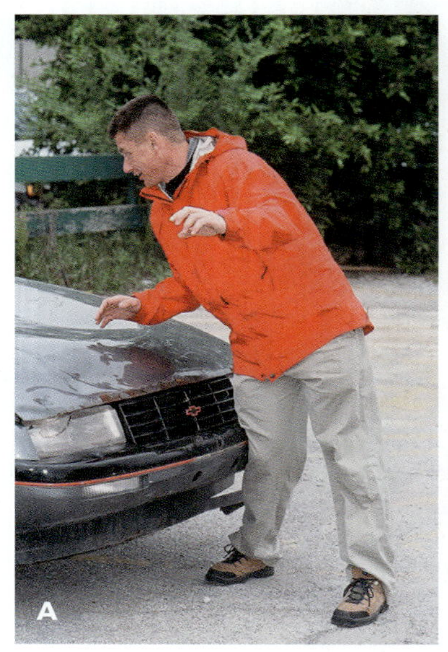

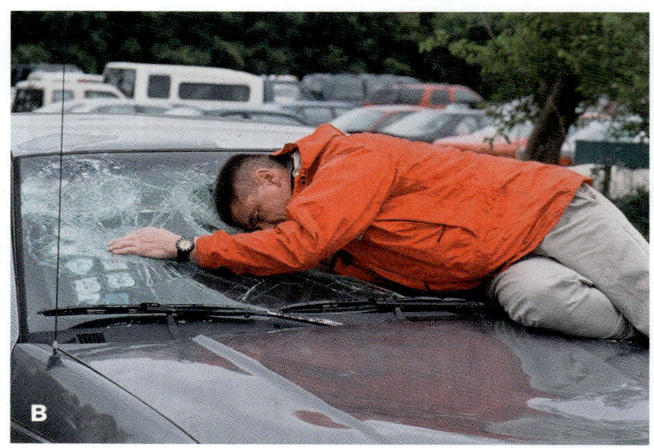

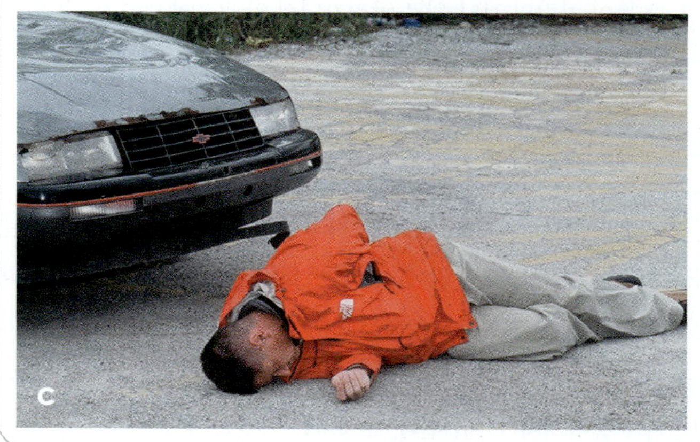

그림 4-36 차량과 보행자 충돌 단계. **A.** 1단계: 초기 충격은 보행자의 다리에 가해지고 때로는 엉덩이에 가해지는 경우도 있다. **B.** 2단계: 보행자의 몸통이 차량의 보닛 위로 굴러간다. **C.** 3단계: 보행자가 차량에서 팅겨 바닥에 부딪힌다.
© National Association of Emergency Medical Technicians (NAEMT)

위쪽으로 계속 이동할 경우 머리가 앞 유리에 부딪히면 얼굴, 머리, 목뼈 및 등뼈 손상이 발생할 수 있다. 차량의 전방 면적이 넓은 경우(예: 트럭, SUV) 보행자 몸 전체 부위가 동시에 충격을 받는다.

세 번째 충격은 보행자가 차체에서 팅겨 나와 도로에 부딪히면서 발생한다. 보행자는 신체의 한쪽에 상당한 타격을 받아 엉덩이, 어깨 및 머리에 손상을 입을 수 있다. 머리 손상은 보행자가 차량이나 도로에 부딪힐 때 주로 발생한다. 마찬가지로 세 가지 충돌 모두 몸통, 목, 머리의 갑작스러운 격렬한 움직임을 유발하기 때문에 불안정한 척추 골절이 발생할 수 있다. 땅에 떨어진 후 보행자는 다른 차량에 치일 수 있다.

키가 더 작으므로 소아는 처음에 성인보다 신체의 윗부분에 충격을 받는다(**그림 4-38A**). 첫 번째 충격은 일반적으로 범퍼에 무릎 위나 골반에 부딪혀 넓적다리뼈 또는 다리이음뼈 손상이 발생할 수 있다. 두 번째 충격은 차량이 앞으로 이동하면서 보닛의 앞부분이 소아의 가슴에 부딪히면서 거의 즉시 발생한다. 그러면 머리와 얼굴이 차량 보닛의 앞쪽이나 위쪽에 부딪힌다(**그림 4-38B**). 소아는 가볍고 키가 작으므로 일반적으로 성인과 마찬가지로 차량에서 팅겨 나가지 않을 수 있다. 대신 소아가 차량의 앞쪽 끈 부분 아래에 있는 상태에서 차량에 끌려갈 수 있다. 소아가 옆으로 넘어지면 다리도 앞바퀴에 깔릴 수 있다(**그림 4-38C**). 소아가 뒤로 넘어져 차량 밑으로 완전히 들어가면 거의 모든 손상이 발생할 수 있다(차량에 끌려가거나 돌출부에 부딪히거나 바퀴에 깔리는 경우).

충돌 시 발이 땅에 닿으면 소아는 다리 위쪽, 엉덩이 및 배에 에너지가 전달된다. 이렇게 하면 엉덩이와 배가 충격으로부터 멀어지게 된다. 몸통의 윗부분은 나중에, 땅에 닿은 발과 마찬가지로 따라올 것이다. 몸통은 움직이지만 발은 움직이지 않는 에너지 교환은 골반이 골절되고 넓적다리뼈가 전단되어 충격 지점에서 심각하게 각을 형성하여 척추 손상을 일으킬 수 있다.

이러한 손상을 더욱 복잡하게 만드는 것은 소아의 호기심 때문에 차량 쪽으로 몸을 돌리면서 앞쪽 몸과 얼굴이 손상에 노출되지만, 성인은 충돌을 피하려다 등이나 옆구리를 부딪치게 될 것이다.

성인과 마찬가지로 차량에 치인 소아도 일종의 머리 손상을 입을 수 있다. 머리, 목, 몸통에 갑작스럽고 격렬한 힘이 가해지기 때문에 목뼈 손상의 가능성이 높다.

차량과 보행자 충돌 시 다중 충돌의 단계를 파악하고 이에 따라 발생할 수 있는 여러 가지 기본적인 손상을 이해하는 것은 초기 평가를 수행하고 환자의 적절한 처치를 결정하는 데 있어 중요하다.

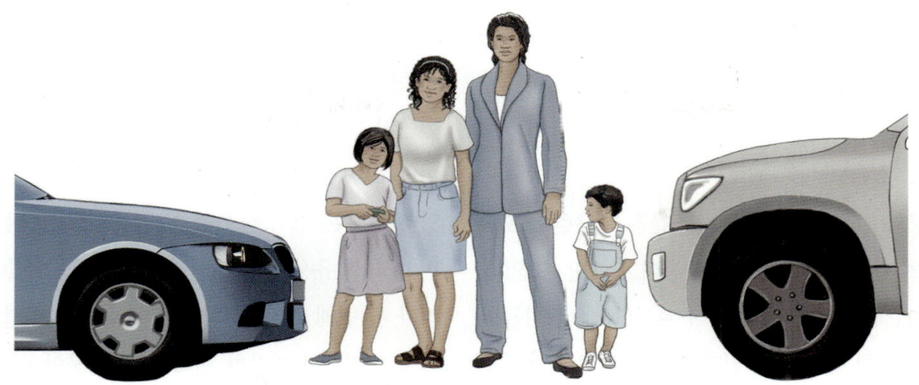

그림 4-37 차량과 보행자 충돌로 인한 손상은 보행자의 키와 차량의 높이에 따라 달라진다.
© National Association of Emergency Medical Technicians (NAEMT)

추락

추락 환자는 여러 번의 충격으로 인해 손상을 입을 수 있다. 환자가 추락한 예상 높이, 환자가 착지한 표면, 먼저 충격을 받은 신체 부위는 관련된 에너지 수준과 그에 따라 발생한 에너지 교환을 나타내므로 결정해야 할 중요한 요소이다. 더 높은 곳에서 추락하는 환자는 추락 시 속도가 증가하기 때문에 손상 발생률이 높다. 성인의 경우 6m 이상, 소아의 경우 3m 이상(소아 키의 2~3배)에서 추락하는 경우 심각한 손상을 입는 경우가 많다. 환자가 착지하는 표면의 유형과 압축성(에너지 전달 때문에 변형되는 능력)도 정지거리에 영향을 미친다. 소아의 추락에 대한 외상 물리학에 대한 정보는 14장 소아 외상에 나와 있다.

실생활에서 양쪽 발꿈치뼈 골절, 발목의 전단 및 압박 골절, 먼쪽 정강뼈 또는 종아리뼈 골절 등이 발로 착지할 때 발생한다. 발이 착지하고 움직임을 멈춘 후 다리는 에너지를 흡수하는 다음 신체 부위이다. 무릎의 정강뼈 상단 골절, 긴뼈 골절 및 엉덩관절 골절이 발생할 수 있다. 신체는 계속 움직이는 머리와 몸통의 무게로 인해 압박을 받아 등뼈와 허리뼈 부위의 척추 압박골절이 발생할 수 있다. 과굴곡은 S자형 척추의 오목한 굴곡 부위마다 발생하여 오목한 쪽은 압박 손상, 볼록한 쪽은 당김 손상을 일으킨다.

환자가 추락할 때 손을 뻗으면서 앞으로 넘어지면 한쪽 또는 양쪽 손목에 골절이 발생할 수 있다. 환자가 추락 시 발로 착지하지 않은 경우 병원 전 처치 제공자는 먼저 부딪힌 신체 부위를 평가하고 에너지 이동 경로를 평가한 후 손상 유형을 결정한다.

얕은 수심에서 다이빙하다 손상을 당한 경우처럼 몸이 거의 일직선이 된 상태에서 머리부터 떨어지면 움직이는 몸통, 골반, 다리의 전

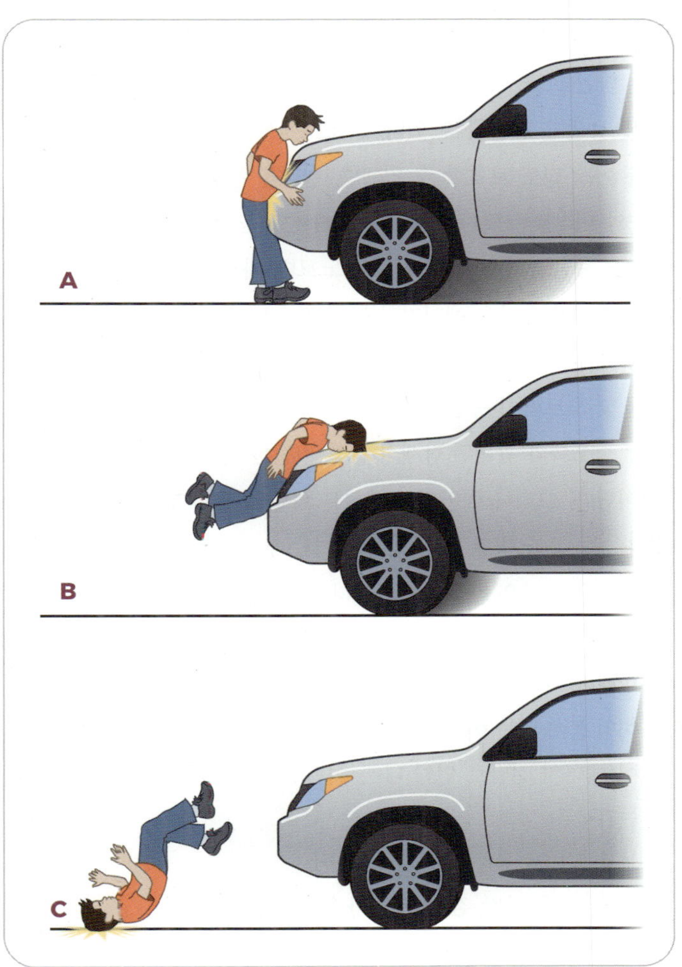

그림 4-38 **A.** 소아의 초기 충돌은 차량이 어린이의 다리 위쪽이나 골반에 부딪힐 때 발생한다. **B.** 두 번째 충격은 소아의 머리나 얼굴이 차량의 보닛 앞부분 또는 상단에 부딪힐 때 발생한다. **C.** 소아는 그림과 같이 차량에서 튕겨나갈 수도 있지만, 차량에 끌려갈 수도 있다.
© National Association of Emergency Medical Technicians (NAEMT)

체 무게와 힘이 머리와 목뼈를 압박하게 된다. 전방충돌 차량의 상향 경로와 마찬가지로 목뼈 골절이 발생할 수 있다.

스포츠 손상

스키, 다이빙, 야구, 축구와 같은 접촉 스포츠와 같은 다양한 스포츠나 레크리에이션 스포츠 활동 중에 심각한 손상이 발생할 수 있다. 이러한 스포츠 손상은 갑작스러운 감속력이나 과도한 압박, 비틀림, 과신전 또는 과굴곡으로 인해 발생할 수 있다. 최근에는 필요한 훈련과 컨디션 조절 또는 적절한 보호 장비를 갖추지 못하고 레크리에이션 스포츠를 즐기는 사람들이 다양한 스포츠 활동을 즐길 수 있게 되었다. 레크리에이션 스포츠 활동은 모든 연령대가 즐긴다. 스키, 수상스키, 자전거, 스케이트보드와 같은 스포츠는 잠재적으로 빠른 속도를 낼 수 있는 운동이다. 산악자전거, 사륜 오토바이, 스노모빌과 같은 다른 스포츠는 오토바이 충돌이나 차량 충돌과 유사한 속도 감속 및 충돌을 유발할 수 있다. 스포츠에서 착용하는 보호 장비는 신체를 어느 정도 보호할 수 있지만, 헬멧을 쓴 미식축구 선수가 다른 선수와 머리를 부딪치는 경우와 같이 손상을 초래할 수 있다.

고속 충돌 후 스케이트보드, 스노모빌, 자전거에서 튕겨 나온 환자의 잠재적인 손상은 에너지의 양이 같으므로 탑승자가 같은 속도로 자동차에서 튕겨 나올 때 입은 손상과 비슷하다(앞서 설명한 차량 충돌 및 오토바이 충돌의 특정 기전을 참조)

각 스포츠와 관련된 잠재적 손상 기전은 너무 많아 일일이 열거하기 어렵다. 그러나 일반적인 원칙은 차량 충돌과 같다. 손상 기전을 평가하는 동안 병원 전 처치 제공자는 손상을 확인하는 데 도움이 되는 다음과 같은 질문을 고려한다.

- 환자에게 어떤 힘이 어떻게 작용했는가?
- 명백한 손상은 무엇인가?
- 어떤 물체 또는 어느 신체 부위에 에너지가 전달되었는가?
- 이 에너지 전달로 인해 다른 어떤 손상이 발생했을 가능성이 있는가?
- 보호 장비를 착용하고 있었는가?
- 갑작스러운 압박, 감속 또는 가속이 있었는가?
- 어떤 손상을 유발하는 움직임(예: 과신전, 과굴곡, 압박, 과도한 측면 굴곡)이 발생했는가?

두 명의 스키어 간의 충돌 사고처럼 손상 기전이 두 사람 간의 고속 충돌과 관련되면 목격자 진술로부터 사고 상황을 재구성하기가 어려운 경우가 많다. 이러한 충돌 사고에서 한 명의 스키어가 입은 손상이 다른 스키어를 평가하는 데 지침이 되는 경우가 많다. 일반적으로 한 환자의 어느 신체 부위가 다른 환자의 어느 신체 부위와 충돌했는지 그리고 에너지 전달로 인해 어떤 손상이 발생했는지 아는 것이 중요하다. 예를 들어, 한 명의 환자가 충격으로 엉덩관절이 골절되었다면 다른 스키 선수의 신체 일부가 상당한 심으로 부딪혔을 것이며 따라서 유사한 충격 손상을 입었을 수 있다. 두 번째 스키어의 머리가 첫 번째 스키어의 엉덩이에 부딪히면 병원 전 처치 제공자는 두 번째 스키어의 심각한 머리 손상과 불안정한 척추 손상을 의심해야 한다.

장비의 파손도 손상의 중요한 지표이며 손상 기전을 평가할 때 반드시 포함해야 한다. 스포츠 헬멧이 부서졌다는 것은 그만큼 큰 힘이 가해졌다는 증이다. 스키는 내구성이 뛰어난 소재로 만들어졌기 때문에 스키가 파손되었다는 것은 손상의 기전이 인상적이지 안은 것처럼 보일지라도 극도의 국소적인 힘이 가해졌음을 나타낸다. 앞부분이 심하게 찌그러진 스노모빌은 나무에 부딪힌 힘을 나타낸다. 아이스하키 경기 후 스틱이 부러져 있으면 몸싸움으로 인해 스틱이 부러진 것인지 아니면 정상적인 하키 경기 중에 부러진 것인지에 대한 의문을 가진다.

심각한 충돌 후 환자가 통증을 호소하지 않더라도 심각한 손상이 있을 수도 있으므로 다음과 같은 단계로 철저히 평가해야 한다.

1. 생명을 위협하는 손상에 대해 환자를 평가한다.
2. 손상 기전에 대한 환자를 평가한다(무슨 일이 발생했으며 정확히 어떻게 발생했는가?)
3. 한 환자에게 손상을 유발한 힘이 다른 사람에게 어떤 영향을 미쳤는지 결정한다.
4. 보호 장비를 착용했는지 확인한다(이미 제거되었을 수도 있다.).
5. 보호 장비의 파손 정도를 평가한다(이 손상이 환자의 신체에 미치는 영향은 무엇인가?).
6. 손상이 이번 사고로 인한 발생한 것인지 아니면 기존에 있던 것이 악화하여 발생한 것인지 평가한다.
7. 가능한 관련 부상에 대해 환자를 철저하게 평가한다.

많은 접촉 스포츠에서 심각한 손상을 입지 않고 높은 곳에서 빠른 속도로 추락, 충돌은 흔한 일이다. 운동선수들이 엄청난 충돌과 추락을 경험하고도 경미한 손상만 입는 것은 대부분 충격 흡수 장비의 결과이므로 혼란스러울 수 있다. 스포츠 참가자의 손상 가능성은 간과될 수 있다. 외상 물리학의 원리와 손상의 정확한 순서와 기전을 주의 깊게 고려하면 평소보다 더 큰 힘이 가해지는 스포츠 충돌에 대한 통찰력을 제공한다. 외상의 물리학은 가능한 근본적인 손상을 확인하고 의료기관에서 추가 평가와 처치가 필요한 환자를 결정하는 데 필수적인 도구이다.

무딘 외상의 국소적인 영향

신체는 머리, 목, 가슴, 복부, 골반 및 팔다리 등 여러 부위로 나눌 수 있다. 각 신체 부위는 1) 일반적으로 피부, 뼈, 연부조직, 혈관 및 신경으로 구성된 신체의 외부 부분과 2) 일반적으로 중요한 내부 장기로 구성된 신체 내부 부분으로 세분화된다. 압박 및 전단력의 결과로 발생하는 손상은 각 구성 요소와 부위에서 잠재적인 손상에 대한 개요를 제공하는 데 사용된다.

머리

환자의 머리에 압축 및 전단 손상이 발생했다는 유일한 외부 징후는 두피의 연부조직 손상, 두피 타박상 또는 차량 앞 유리의 과녁 모양의 파손일 수 있다(**그림 4-39**).

압축

차량 전방충돌이나 머리부터 추락하는 경우처럼 머리가 앞쪽으로 향하여 몸이 앞으로 나아갈 때 머리는 충격과 에너지 교환을 가장 먼저 받는 구조물이다. 그런 다음 몸통의 지속적인 운동이 머리를 압박한다. 초기 에너지 교환은 두피와 두개골에 발생한다. 두개골이 압박되고 골절되어 두개골의 골절된 뼛조각이 뇌로 밀려들어 갈 수도

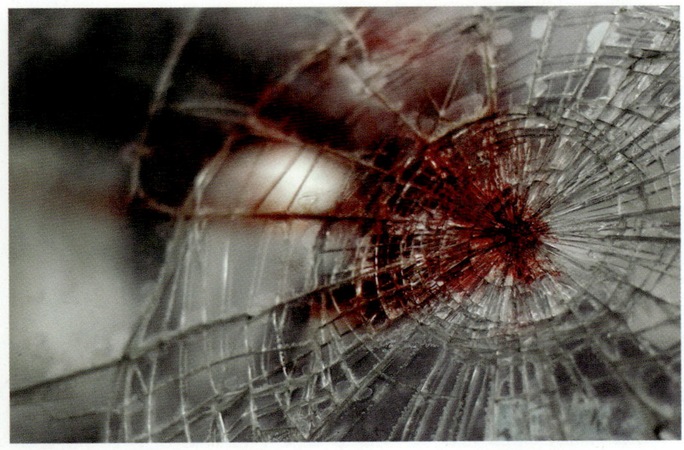

그림 4-39 차량 앞 유리의 황소 눈 모양의 파손은 머리뼈에 충격이 가해져 두개골과 목뼈에 에너지가 전달되었음을 나타내는 주요 징후이다.

© Kristin Smith/Shutterstock

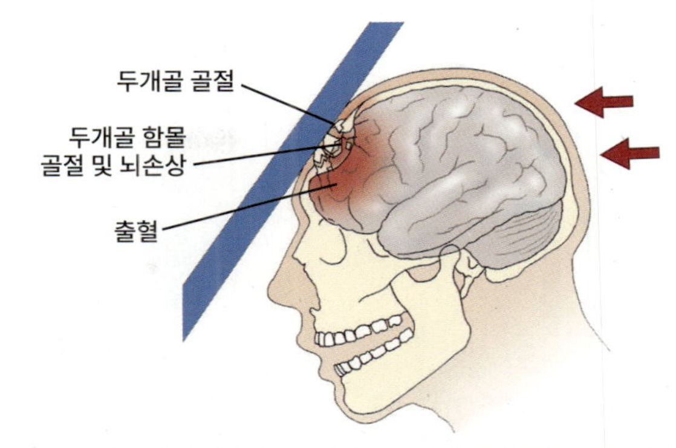

그림 4-40 두개골이 물체에 충격을 받으면 두개골이 골절되어 뇌로 밀려들어 갈 수 있다.

© National Association of Emergency Medical Technicians (NAEMT)

있다(**그림 4-40**).

전단

두개골이 전진 움직임을 멈춘 후에도 뇌는 계속 전진하면서 정상적이거나 골절된 두개골을 압박하여 뇌진탕, 타박상 또는 열상을 유발한다. 뇌는 부드럽고 압축할 수 있으므로 길이가 짧아진다. 뇌의 뒤쪽 부분은 이미 움직임을 멈춘 멀어지면서 계속 앞으로 나아갈 수 있다. 뇌가 두개골에서 분리되면 뇌 조직 자체 또는 해당 부위의 혈관이 늘어나거나 끊어지는(전단) 현상이 발생한다(**그림 4-41**). 경막외, 경막밑 또는 거미막밑 공간으로의 출혈과 뇌의 미만성 축삭 손상이 발생할 수 있다. 뇌가 척수에서 분리된다면 그것은 뇌줄기에서 발생할 가능성이 높다.

목

압축

두개골의 천장 부분은 상당히 강하고 강한 충격을 흡수할 수 있지만, 목뼈는 훨씬 더 유연하다. 두개골은 정지했지만, 몸통의 운동이 정지된 두개골을 향해 계속 압박을 가하면 목뼈에 각이 생기거나 압박이 발생한다. 이 전방으로 진행하면서 계속된 압력을 머리뼈에 가하여 목뼈에 각 형성 또는 압박이 발생한다(**그림 4-42**). 목의 과신전 또는 과굴곡은 하나 이상의 척추의 골절 또는 탈구와 척수 손상을 초래할 수 있다. 그 결과 관절면, 골절, 척수 압박 또는 연부조직(인대) 손상이 발생할 수 있다(**그림 4-43**). 직접적인 직렬식 압박은 척추몸통을 분쇄한다. 각 형성과 직렬식 압박은 척추를 불안정하게 만들 수 있다.

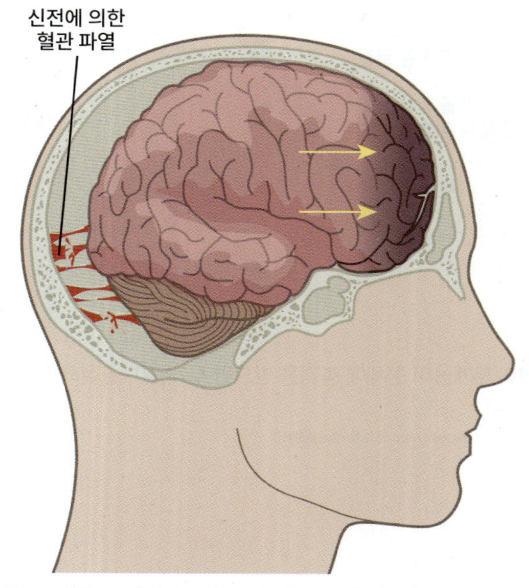

그림 4-41 두개골이 전진 운동을 멈추더라도 뇌는 계속 전진한다. 충돌지점에서 가장 가까운 뇌 부위는 충격으로 인해 압박을 받고 멍이 들며 열상을 입을 수도 있다. 충돌지점에서 가장 멀리 떨어진 부분은 두개골에서 분리되어 혈관이 찢어지고 열상을 입는다.
© National Association of Emergency Medical Technicians (NAEMT)

전단

두개골의 무게 중심은 머리뼈가 목뼈에 부착되는 지점의 앞-위쪽이다. 따라서 목이 고정되어 있지 않은 상태에서 몸통에 측면 충돌이 가해지면 목이 측면으로 꺾이고 회전한다(**그림 4-24**). 목을 과도하게 굴곡하거나 과신전하면 목의 연부조직에 스트레칭 손상을 입을 수도 있다.

가슴

압축

충돌이 가슴 앞부분에 집중되면 복장뼈가 초기 에너지 교환을 받게 된다. 복장뼈가 움직임을 멈추면 가슴 뒷부분(근육과 등뼈)과 가슴 안의 장기가 충돌하여 복장뼈에 눌릴 때까지 장기가 계속 앞으로 이동한다.

가슴 뒷부분이 계속 앞으로 움직이면 갈비뼈가 구부러진다. 갈비뼈의 인장 강도가 초과하면 갈비뼈 골절과 동요가슴이 발생할 수 있다(10장 가슴 외상, **그림 4-44**). 등허리 척추 압박 또는 파열 골절을 동반한 굽힘 손상이 발생할 수 있다. 이 손상은 차량이 흙으로 된 제방에 부딪혀 갑자기 정지할 때 발생하는 손상과 유사하다(**그림 4-3** 참고). 차량의 프레임이 구부러지면서 일부 에너지를 흡수한다. 차량

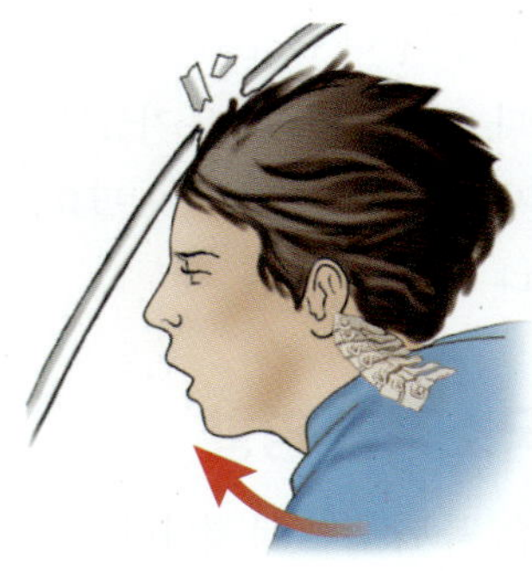

그림 4-42 두개골은 전진 운동을 자주 멈추지만, 몸통은 에너지가 흡수될 때까지 계속 앞으로 움직인다. 이 전진 운동의 가장 약한 부분은 목뼈이다.
© National Association of Emergency Medical Technicians (NAEMT)

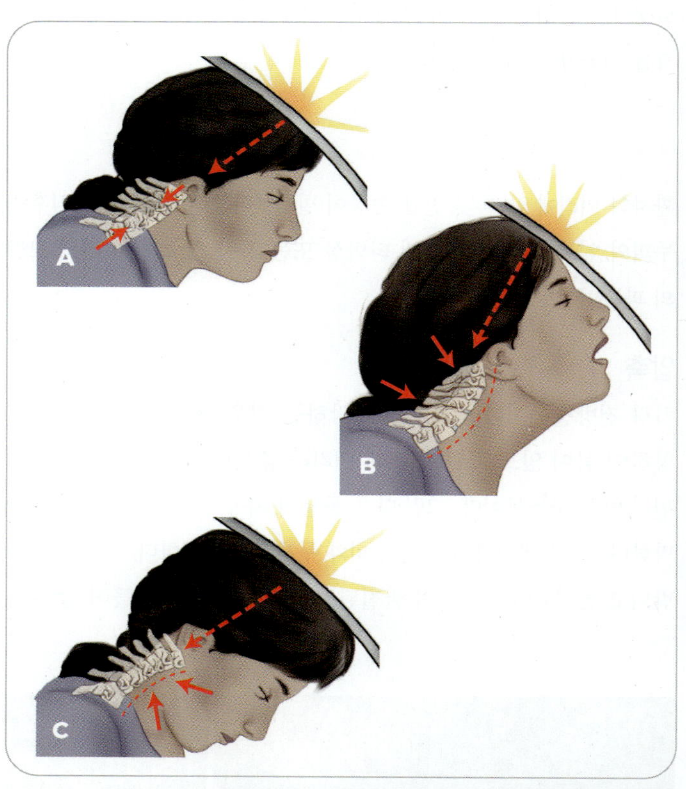

그림 4-43 목뼈는 축을 따라 **A.** 직접 압박하거나, **B.** 과신전, 또는 **C.** 과굴곡으로 각이 형성될 수 있다.
© National Association of Emergency Medical Technicians (NAEMT)

의 뒤쪽은 프레임의 변형이 모든 에너지를 흡수할 때까지 앞으로 나아간다. 같은 방식으로 가슴 뒷부분은 갈비뼈가 모든 에너지를 흡수할 때까지 계속 움직인다.

가슴벽의 압박은 전방 및 측면 충돌에서 흔히 발생하며 기흉을 유발할 수 있는 "종이 봉지 효과"라는 현상을 일으킨다. 환자는 충돌 직전에 본능적으로 심호흡을 하고 충돌 직전에 숨을 참는다. 이렇게 하

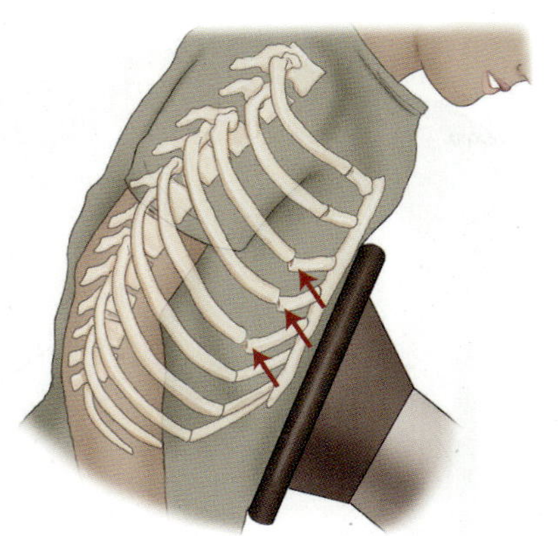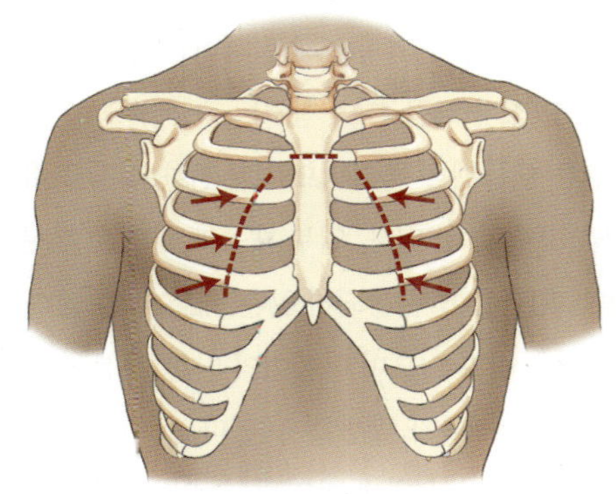

그림 4-44 외부 압박에 의해 가슴안으로 강제로 들어간 갈비뼈는 일반적으로 여러 곳에서 골절되어 때때로 동요가슴이라고 알려진 임상 증상을 유발한다.
© National Association of Emergency Medical Technicians (NAEMT)

면 성문이 닫혀 폐가 효과적으로 밀폐된다. 가슴벽에 충격과 압박이 가해질 때 상당한 에너지 교환이 일어나면 가슴벽을 압박하면 공기가 가득한 종이 봉지가 터지는 것처럼 폐가 파열될 수 있다(그림 4-45). 또한 폐가 압박되고 타박상을 입어 환기 기능이 저하될 수 있다.

　가슴 내부 구조의 압박 손상에는 복장뼈와 척추 사이에서 심장이 눌려 심각한 부정맥을 초래할 수 있는 심장 타박상이 포함될 수 있다. 더 빈번한 손상은 폐 압박으로 인한 폐 타박상일 수 있다. 임상적 결과는 시간이 지남에 따라 나타날 수 있지만, 환자는 즉시 적절한 환기 기능을 상실할 수 있다. 폐 타박상은 병원 전 처치 제공자나 병원 도착 후 소생술 중 영향을 미칠 수 있다. 긴 이송 시간이 필요한 상황에서는 이 상태가 이송 중에 영향을 미칠 수 있다.

전단

심장, 오름대동맥 및 대동맥활은 가슴안에서 상대적으로 고정되어 있지 않지만, 내림대동맥은 가슴 후벽과 척추에 단단히 부착되어 있다. 대동맥의 움직임은 청진기의 이어폰이 연결되는 딱딱한 튜브가 끝나는 부분 바로 아래의 유연한 튜브를 잡고 청진기의 소리를 듣는 부분을 좌우로 흔드는 것과 비슷하다. 충돌로 골격이 갑자기 멈추면 심장

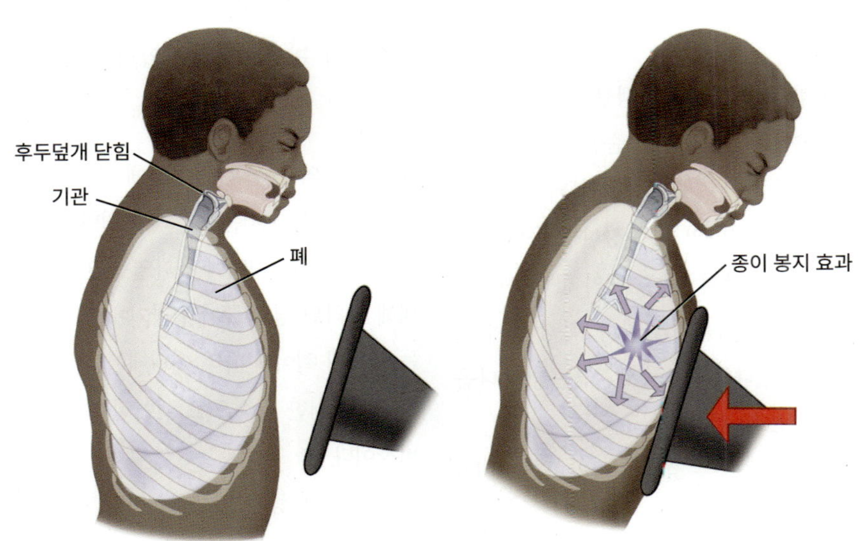

그림 4-45 앞쪽 또는 옆쪽 가슴벽에 충격이 가해지면 폐가 성문이 닫힌 상태에서 압박되면 입구가 단단히 봉해진 봉투를 압박하는 것과 비슷한 효과가 발생한다. 종이 봉투와 마찬가지로 폐가 파열된다.
© National Association of Emergency Medical Technicians (NAEMT)

과 대동맥의 시작 부분은 전진 운동을 계속한다. 이때 발생하는 전단력으로 인해 단단히 고정된 부분과 자유롭게 움직이는 부분의 접합부에서 대동맥이 찢어질 수 있다(**그림 4-14** 참고).

대동맥이 파열되면 파열은 대동맥을 즉각적으로 완전한 절단을 유발하여 빠르게 과다출혈을 초래할 수 있다. 일부 대동맥 파열은 부분 파열로 하나 이상의 대동맥 혈관층이 손상되지 않은 채로 남아 있다. 그러나 나머지 층은 큰 압력을 받고 있으며 타이어의 약한 부분에 형성되는 기포와 유사한 외상성 동맥류가 발생할 수 있다. 동맥류는 최초 손상 후 몇 분, 몇 시간 또는 며칠 내에 파열될 수 있다. 병원 전 처치 제공자는 이러한 손상의 가능성을 인지하고 이 정보를 환자를 이송하는 병원의 의료진에게 제공하는 것이 중요하다.

등허리 척추에 전단 손상이 발생하면 신경학적 손상과 관련될 수 있는 골절 및 골절-탈구가 발생할 수 있으며 환자는 추가적인 움직임으로 인해 이차적인 신경학적 손상의 위험에 처할 수 있다. 마찬가지로 등허리 척추의 어느 부위든 과도하게 신전되면 불안정한 골절이나 탈구를 유발하여 잠재적인 신경학적 손상을 초래할 수 있다.

복부

압축

전방충돌 시 척추와 핸들 또는 대시보드 사이에서 눌린 내부 장기가 파열될 수 있다. 이러한 갑작스러운 압력 증가의 효과는 내부 장기를 모루에 올려놓고 망치로 치는 것과 효과가 유사하다. 이러한 방식으로 인해 자주 손상되는 고형장기에는 비장, 췌장, 간 및 신장이 포함된다.

손상은 또한 복강 내 과도한 압력으로 인해 발생할 수 있다. 가로막은 복부 상단에 있는 5mm 두께의 근육으로 가슴안과 복강을 분리하는 역할을 한다. 가로막이 수축하면 가슴안이 확장되어 환기가 이루어진다. 전복벽은 두 개의 근막과 하나의 매우 강한 근육으로 구성되어 있다. 복벽의 측면에는 관련 근막이 있는 3개의 근육층이 있으며 허리뼈 및 관련 근육은 후복벽에 힘을 제공한다. 복강 내 압력이 증가하면 찢어지거나 파열될 수 있다(**그림 4-46**). 이 손상은 다음과 같은 네 가지 일반적인 결과를 초래한다.

- 일반적으로 가로막에 의해 생성되는 '풀무' 효과가 사라지고 환기가 손상된다.
- 복부 장기가 가슴안으로 들어가 폐가 확장할 수 있는 공간이 줄어들 수 있다.

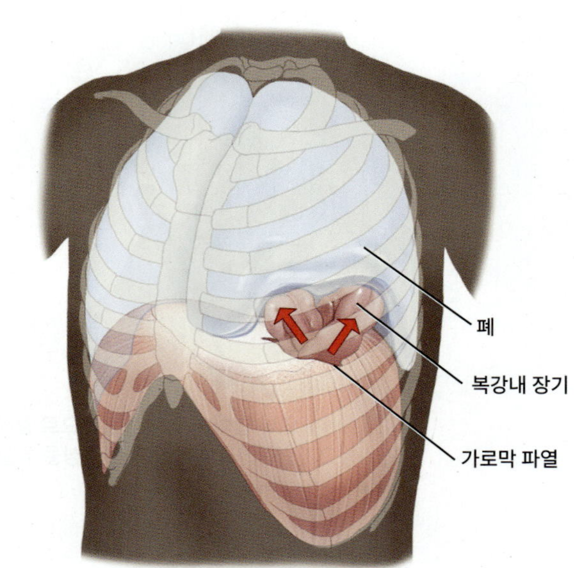

그림 4-46 복강 내 압력이 증가하면 가로막이 파열될 수 있다.
© National Association of Emergency Medical Technicians (NAEMT)

- 변위된 장기는 혈액 공급이 압박으로 인해 허혈이 발생할 수 있다.
- 복강 내 출혈이 있는 경우 혈액으로 인해 혈흉이 발생할 수도 있다.

복압 상승으로 인해 또 다른 손상은 갑작스러운 대동맥 역류로 인해 대동맥 판막을 압박하는 것이며 판막에 가해지는 이러한 힘은 판막을 파열시킬 수 있다. 이 손상은 드물지만, 핸들과의 충돌이나 다른 유형의 사고(예: 도랑 또는 터널 붕괴)로 인해 복강 내압이 급격히 상승하면 발생할 수 있다. 이러한 급격한 압력 증가는 대동맥압의 급격한 상승을 초래한다. 혈액이 대동맥 판막에 밀려(역류) 판막 첨판이 파열될 수 있는 충분한 압력을 받게 된다.

전단

복부 장기의 손상은 장간막에 부착된 지점에서 발생한다. 충돌하는 동안 신체의 전진 운동은 멈추지만, 장기는 계속 전진하여 장기가 복벽에 부착되는 지점에서 파열을 일으킨다. 장기가 줄기(조직 줄기)에 의해 부착된 경우 줄기가 장기에 부착되는 곳, 복벽에 부착되는 곳 또는 줄기의 길이에 따라 어디에서나 파열이 발생할 수 있다(**그림 4-13** 참고). 이러한 방식으로 찢어질 수 있는 장기는 신장, 소장, 대장 및 비장이다.

감속 중에 종종 발생하는 또 다른 유형의 손상은 간이 둥근인대와의 충돌로 인한 간 열상이다. 간은 가로막에 매달려 있지만, 허리뼈 근처의 후복부에 최소한으로만 부착되어 있다. 둥근인대는 배꼽

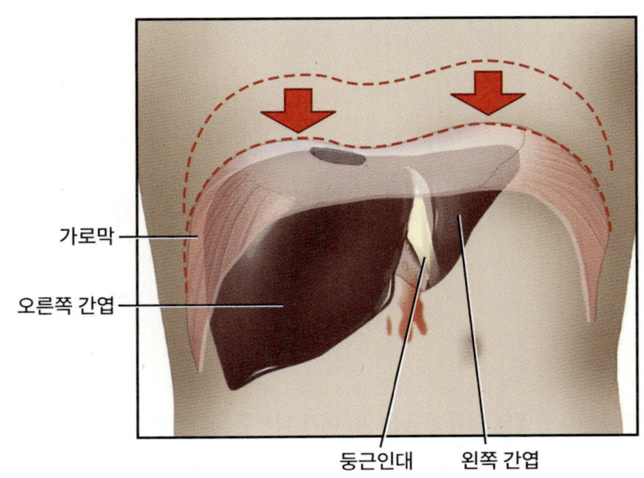

그림 4-47 간은 고정된 구조에 의해 지지되지 않는다. 간은 자유롭게 움직이는 가로막에 의해 주로 지지된다. 신체가 위아래로 움직일 때 간도 함께 움직인다. 몸통은 멈추지만, 간이 멈추지 않으면 간이 계속 둥근인대 아래쪽으로 내려가서 간이 찢어진다. 이것은 치즈 절단 와이어를 치즈 덩어리에 밀어 넣는 것과 매우 유사하다.
© National Association of Emergency Medical Technicians (NAEMT)

의 전복벽과 신체 정중선에 있는 간의 좌엽에 부착되어 있다(간 대부분은 정중선의 오른쪽에 위치). 전방충돌이나 발로 먼저 넘어질 때 간이 아래로 내려가면서 가로막을 끌어당겨 둥근인대가 있는 곳까지 내려가게 된다(**그림 4-47**). 이 경우 치즈 절단용 와이어로 치즈 덩어리를 누르는 것과 유사하게 둥근인대는 간을 파괴하거나 절단한다.

골반 골절은 외부 복부 손상의 결과이며 방광 손상이나 골반안의 혈관 열상을 유발할 수 있다. 골반 골절 환자의 4~15%는 비뇨생식기 손상도 동반한다.

일반적으로 측면 충돌로 인한 측면 압박으로 인해 발생하는 골반 골절은 두 가지 구성 요소가 있다. 하나는 근위 넓적다리뼈가 골반으로 압박되어 넓적다리뼈 머리가 절구 안으로 밀려들어 가는 것이다. 이에 따라 엉덩관절과 관련된 골절이 자주 발생한다. 넓적다리뼈와 골반의 측벽이 더 압박되면 골반 또는 두덩뼈가지에 압박골절이 발생한다. 두덩뼈가지는 일반적으로 한 곳에서만 골절될 수 없기 때문에 일반적으로 골반 고리를 따라 다른 곳에서 골반의 골절이 발생한다.

다른 유형의 압박골절은 압박력이 직접적으로 두덩결합의 앞쪽을 압박할 때 발생한다. 이 힘은 두덩뼈의 양쪽을 밀어서 부러뜨리거나 한쪽을 부러뜨려 천장관절 쪽으로 다시 밀어낸다. 이 후자의 손상 기전은 관절을 열어 소위 오픈 북 골절을 생성한다.

전단골절은 일반적으로 엉덩뼈와 엉치뼈 부위를 포함한다. 이 전단으로 인해 관절이 찢어진다. 골반과 같은 두덩뼈가지의 관절은 일반적으로 두 곳에서 골절이 발생하기 때문에 골반 고리를 따라 다른 곳에 발생하는 경우가 많다.

골반 골절에 대한 자세한 정보를 앤드루 버지스(Andrew Burgess)와 그의 공정 저자는 이러한 손상 기전에 대해 논의했다.

관통성 외상

관통성 외상의 물리학

앞에서 논의한 물리학의 원리는 관통상을 다룰 때 똑같이 중요하다. 다시 말하면 어떤 물체가 신체 조직에 전달되는 운동에너지는 다음 공식으로 나타낸다.

$$운동에너지 = 1/2(mv^2)$$

에너지는 생성되거나 파괴할 수 없지만, 변형할 수는 있다. 이 원칙은 관통성 외상을 이해하는 데 중요하다. 예를 들어, 납 총알이 폭발성 화약으로 채워진 놋쇠 탄피 안에 들어 있지만, 총알에는 힘이 없다. 그러나 뇌관이 폭발하면 화약이 연소하여 힘으로 변화되는 빠르게 팽창하는 가스를 생성한다. 그러면 총알이 총구에서 나와 목표물을 향해 이동한다.

뉴턴의 운동 제1 법칙에 따르면 이 힘이 총알에 작용한 후 총알은 외부 힘이 작용할 때까지 그 속도와 힘을 유지한다. 총알이 인체와 같은 무언가에 부딪히면 개별 조직 세포에 부딪힌다.

총알 운동 에너지(속도 및 질량)는 이러한 세포를 부수고 총알의 경로에서 멀리 이동시키는 에너지로 교환된다.

$$질량 \times 가속도 = 힘 = 질량 \times 감속도$$

정면 영역의 크기에 영향을 미치는 요인

이동하는 총알의 정면 표면적이 클수록 타격을 받는 입자의 수가 많아지므로 에너지 교환이 더 많이 일어나고 생성되는 공동이 더 커진다. 발사체의 정면 표면적은 단면 윤곽, 회전 및 파편의 세 가지 요소에 의해 영향을 받는다. 이러한 요소를 기반으로 에너지 교환 또는 잠재적 에너지 교환을 분석할 수 있다.

측면 윤곽

윤곽은 물체의 초기 크기와 충돌 시 크기가 변하는지에 관한 것이다. 얼음을 깨는 송곳의 단면 윤곽, 즉 정면 면적은 야구 방망이보다 훨씬 좁고 야구 방망이는 트럭보다 훨씬 좁다. 할로우 포인트

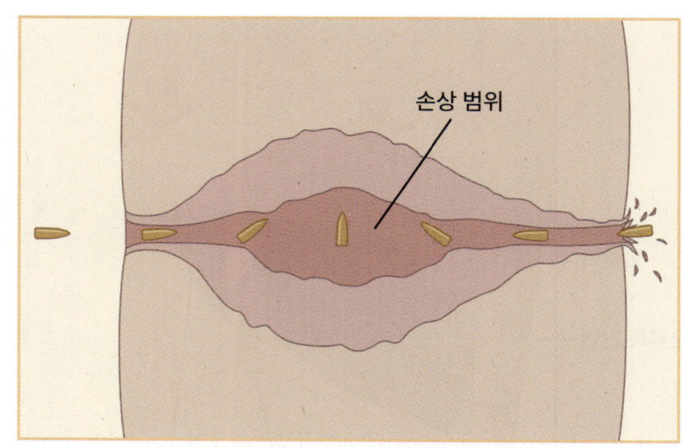

그림 4-48　총알의 텀블 운동은 90°에서 피해를 극대화한다.
© National Association of Emergency Medical Technicians (NAEMT)

(Hollow-Point) 탄은 충돌할 때 편평해지면서 퍼진다(**Box 4-4**). 이러한 변화는 정면 면적을 확대해 더 많은 조직을 파괴하고 더 큰 에너지 교환을 가져온다. 조직 입자들이 더 넓게 충돌하게 되고 큰 에너지 교환을 생성하도록 정면 영역을 확대한다. 그 결과 더 큰 공동을 형성하고 더 심한 손상을 유발한다.

　일반적으로 총알은 목표물을 향하는 동안 공기를 통해 이동하면서 공기 역학적인 상태를 유지해야 한다. 공기를 통과하는 동안 낮은 저항(공기 입자를 최대한 적게 때리는 것)을 가지는 것이 좋다. 이런 상태에서는 총알의 속도를 그대로 유지할 수 있다. 저항을 줄이기 위해 정면 면적이 원뿔 모양으로 작게 유지된다. 저항이 많은 것은 좋지 않다. 좋은 총알은 공기를 통과할 때 아주 작은 저항을 하지만 인체조직을 통과할 때는 더 큰 항력을 갖도록 디자인된 것이다. 총알이 피부를 관통할 때 변형되면 큰 영역을 포함하여 더 많은 항력을 생성하여 더 많은 에너지 교환이 발생하게 된다. 따라서 이상적인 총알은 공기 중에서는 그 모양을 유지하고 충격 시에만 변형되도록 설계된다.

텀블(TUMBLE)

텀블은 물체가 계속해서 회전하면서 신체 내부에 진입할 때 가정했던 각도와 다른 각도를 갖게 되어 공기보다 신체 내부에서 더 많은 저항력이 발생하는 상황을 설명한다. 쐐기 모양 총알의 무게 중심은 총알의 탄두보다 기저부에 더 가깝다. 탄두가 어떤 물체에 부딪히면 그것은 빠르게 느려진다. 탄환의 무게 중심이 탄환의 앞부분으로 이동하면서 운동량에 의해 총알의 기저부가 계속 앞으로 나아간다. 약간 비대칭적인 모양은 빙글빙글 도는 동작 또는 텀블을 유발한다. 총알이 텀블할 때 일반적으로 수평인 총알의 측면이 총알의 앞쪽 가장자리가 되어 총알이 공중에 떠 있을 때보다 더 많은 입자를 타격한다(**그림 4-48**). 더 많은 에너지 교환이 발생하므로 더 심각한 조직손상이 발생한다.

파편

파편화는 물체가 여러 조각 또는 잔해로 부서져 저항력을 향상하고 에너지가 더 많이 교환되는지를 나타낸다. 파편화 탄환에는 1) 무기를 떠날 때 파편화되는 경우(예: 엽총 탄알, **그림 4-49**), 2) 탄환이 신체에 들어간 후 파편화되는 경우의 두 가지 유형이 있다. 신체 내부의 파편화는 능동적이거나 수동적일 수 있다. 총알이 산산이 부서지면서 너 넓은 지역으로 퍼지나가 두 가지 결과가 발생한다. 1) 더 큰 전방 돌출부로 인해 더 많은 조직 입자가 타격을 받고 2) 더 많은 장기가 타격을 받기 때문에 손상이 신체의 더 넓은 부분에 손상이 분산된다(**그림 4-50**). 산탄총 발사로 인한 여러 개의 총알도 비슷한 결과를 초래한다. 산탄총의 상처는 파편화된 손상 유형의 훌륭한 예이다.

손상 및 에너지 수준

관통하는 물체의 에너지 용량을 알면 관통상을 예측하는 데 도움이 된다. 관통상을 유발하는 무기는 에너지 용량에 따라 저에너지, 중에너지, 고에너지 무기로 분류할 수 있다.

저에너지 무기

저에너지 무기에는 칼이나 송곳같이 손으로 사용하는 무기가 포함된다. 이러한 무기는 날카로운 끝이나 절단면으로만, 손상을 입힌다. 이것은 저속 손상이므로 일반적으로 이차 손상이 적다(공동이 적게 발생). 이러한 환자의 손상은 무기가 신체에 들어간 경로를 따라 예측

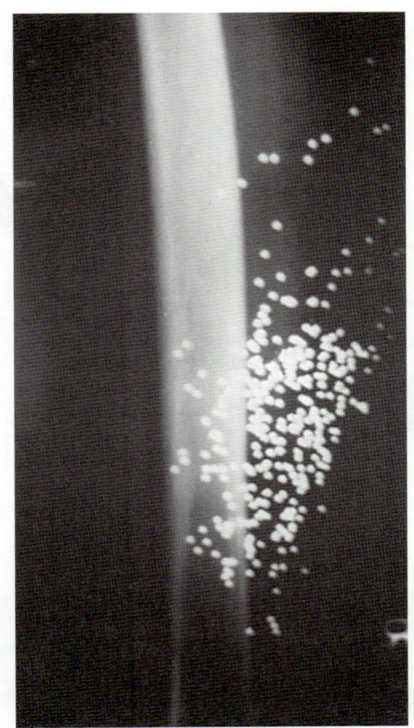

그림 4-49 산탄총 탄알은 무기에서 나올 때 분산되어 파편화된다. 파편화가 가장 적을 때 근거리에서 최대 피해를 입힌다.
© National Association of Emergency Medical Technicians (NAEMT)

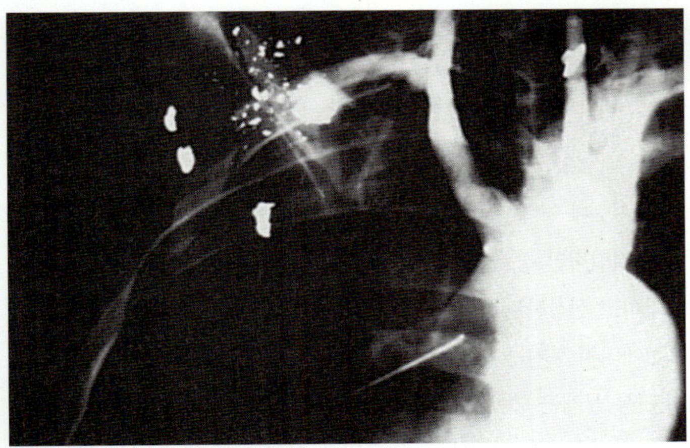

그림 4-50 충돌 시 발생하는 탄환 파편은 총알의 전방 돌출을 증가시키고 신체의 더 넓은 부분에 손상을 분산시킨다.
Courtesy of Norman McSwain, MD, FACS, NREMT-P.

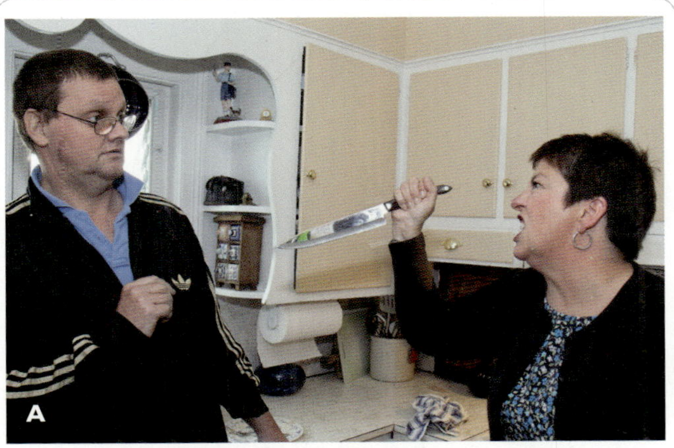

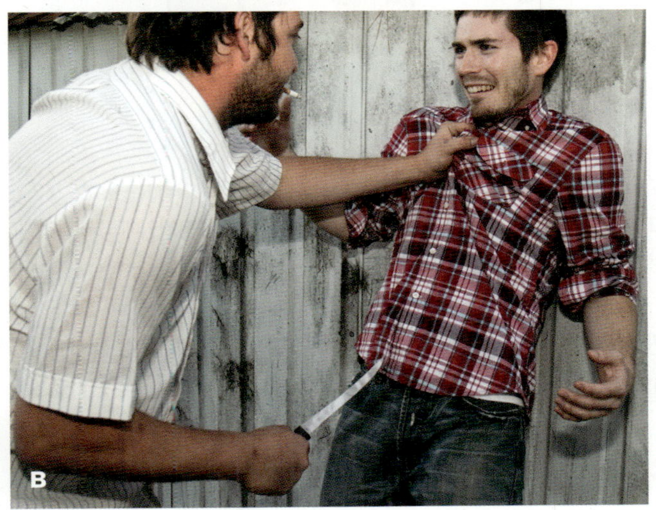

그림 4-51 칼의 궤적은 손잡이를 잡은 손의 위치에 따라 결정된다. **A.** 새끼손가락이 상단에 있으면 아래쪽으로 궤적이 생성된다. **B.** 엄지손가락이 위쪽에 있으면 궤적이 위쪽을 향한다.
© National Association of Emergency Medical Technicians (NAEMT)

할 수 있다. 무기를 제거한 경우 병원 전 처치 제공자는 시간이 허락하는 경우 사용된 무기의 종류를 파악해야 한다.

칼의 궤적은 공격자가 칼을 어떻게 잡았는지를 반영할 수 있다. 공격자가 엄지손가락이 위쪽으로 오도록 무기를 잡으면 궤적이 위쪽을 향하게 된다. 새끼손가락을 위에 있는 상태에서 잡으면 궤적이 아래쪽으로 향한다(**그림 4-51**).

공격자는 피해자를 찌른 다음 칼을 신체 내부에서 움직일 수 있다. 단순하게 보이는 사입구 상처는 안전하다고 착각하게 만들 수 있다. 사입구 상처는 작을 수 있지만, 내부 손상은 광범위할 수 있다. 삽입된 칼날이 움직일 수 있는 잠재적인 범위는 손상이 발생할 수 있는 영역이다(**그림 4-52**).

환자의 관련 손상을 평가하는 것이 중요하다. 예를 들어, 숨을 깊게 내쉴 때 가로막이 유두선까지 올라가라 수 있다. 가슴 아랫부분에 자상을 입으면 배안 및 가슴안 구조물이 손상될 수 있으며 상복부 상처는 가슴 아랫부분을 침범할 수 있다.

관통성 외상은 차량 충돌 및 추락 시 울타리 기둥이나 도로 표지

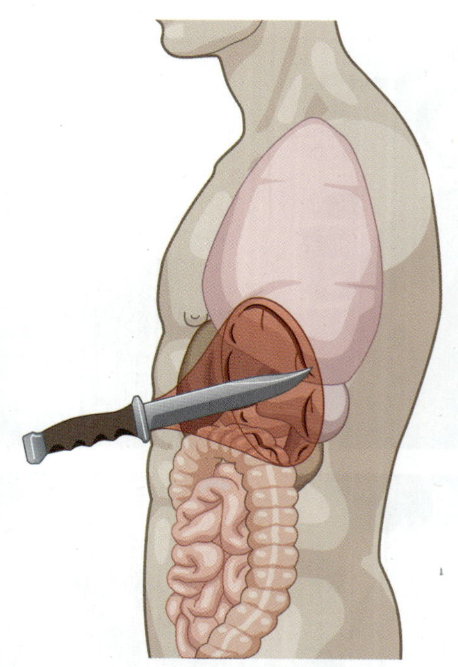

그림 4-52 칼에 의한 손상은 환자 신체 내부에서 칼날의 움직임에 따라 달라진다.
© National Association of Emergency Medical Technicians (NAEMT)

판, 스키 사고에서 스키 폴, 자전거 사고 시 핸들과 같은 물체에 찔려 발생할 수 있다.

중에너지와 고에너지 무기

총기는 중에너지와 고에너지의 두 그룹으로 나뉜다. 중에너지 무기에는 권총과 총구 속도가 초당 305m인 일부 소총이 포함된다. 이 무기에 의해 생성된 일시적 공동은 총알 구경의 3~5배에 달한다. 고에너지 무기는 총구 속도가 초당 610m를 초과하고 총구 에너지가 훨씬 더 크다. 이러한 무기는 총알 구경의 25배 이상에 달하는 일시적 공동을 만든다. 탄약통의 화약량이 증가하고 총알의 크기가 커지면 총알의 속도와 질량이 증가하고 따라서 운동에너지가 증가한다(**그림 4-53**). 총알의 질량은 중요하지만, 속도에 비해 운동 에너지 전달에 기여하는 바는 작다(운동에너지 = $1/2mv^2$).

그러나 총알의 질량을 무시해서는 안 된다. 미국 남북전쟁에서 켄터키 장총 0.55 구경 미니 총알은 현대식 M16 소총과 거의 같은 총구 에너지를 가졌다. 근거리 거리에서 12게이지 산탄총이나 급조폭발물로 인한 피해를 고려하면 총알의 질량이 더 중요해진다.

일반적으로 중에너지 및 고에너지 무기는 총알이 통과하는 경로에 있는 조직뿐만 아니라 총알의 경로 양쪽에 있는 일시적 공동에 포함된 조직도 손상한다. 총알의 윤곽, 텀블, 파편 등의 변수는 에너지 교

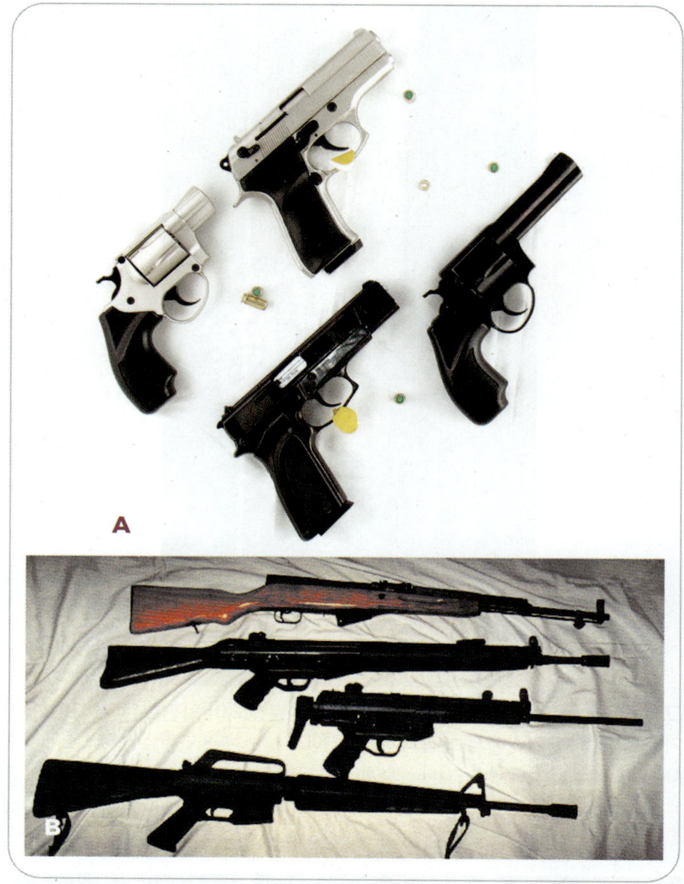

그림 4-53　**A.** 중에너지 무기는 일반적으로 총신이 짧고 탄창에 적은 화약이 들어있는 총이다. **B.** 고에너지 무기.
A. © National Association of Emergency Medical Technicians (NAEMT). **B.** Courtesy of Norman McSwain, MD, FACS, NREMT-P.

환의 속도에 영향을 미치며 손상의 정도와 방향에 영향을 미친다. 총알의 직접적인 경로를 벗어나 이동한 조직 입자의 힘은 주변 조직을 압박하고 신장시킨다(**그림 4-54**).

고에너지 무기는 빠른 속도의 총알을 발사한다(**그림 4-55**). 고에너지 관통 물체는 중에너지 관통 물체보다 조직 손상이 훨씬 더 광범위하다 조직손상을 입는다. 고속 총알에 의해 공동 내 진공이 생성되면 상처의 표면의 의류, 박테리아 및 기타 파편이 상처로 빨려 들어갈 수 있다.

총상으로 인한 손상을 예측할 때 고려해야 할 사항은 총(중에너지 또는 고에너지)이 발사되는 범위 또는 거리이다. 공기 저항은 총알 속도를 느리게 한다. 따라서 거리를 늘리면 충돌 시 에너지가 감소하고 손상이 줄어든다. 권총을 이용한 대부분의 총격은 근거리에서 이루어지므로 심각한 손상을 입을 가능성은 운동에너지의 손실보다는 관련된 해부학적 구조와 무기의 에너지와 관련이 있다.

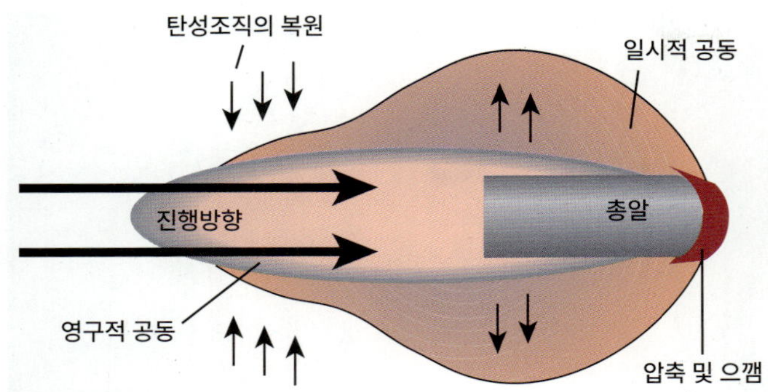

그림 4-54 총알은 총알이 지나는 경로에 있는 조직을 직접 부숴버린다. 총알이 지나간 자리에 공동이 생기며 총알의 궤적을 따라 형성된다. 분쇄된 부분은 영구적이며 일시적인 팽창은 또한 손상을 유발한다.
© National Association of Emergency Medical Technicians (NAEMT)

고에너지 무기

공동화

AK-47 소총의 특이한 손상 유형은 패클러(Fackler)와 말리노프스크(Malinowski)가 설명했다. 총알의 편심 때문에 총알이 구르며 사입구 부위와 거의 직각으로 이동한다. 이 텀블링하는 동안 총알이 계속해서 이동하여 총알이 체내에 머무르는 시간에 따라 2개 또는 3개의 공동이 생긴다. 매우 높은 에너지 교환은 공동과 심각한 손상을 일으킨다.

영구적 공동의 크기는 총알에 맞은 조직의 탄성과 관련이 있다. 예를 들어, 같은 속도의 총알이 근육이나 간을 관통하는 경우 그 결과는 매우 다르다. 근육은 훨씬 더 탄력이 있고 팽창하여 상대적으로 작은 영구적 공동을 형성한다. 그러나 간은 탄력이 거의 없기 때문에 근육에서 같은 에너지 교환으로 생성되는 것보다 골절선(fracture lines)이 생기고 훨씬 더 큰 영구적 공동이 생긴다.

파편

고에너지 무기와 파편이 결합하면 심각한 손상이 발생할 수 있다. 고에너지 총알이 신체에 충돌하여 파편화되는 경우(대부분은 그렇지 않음) 초기 관통 부위가 넓어 심각한 연부조직 손상을 초래할 수 있다. 총알이 뼈와 같은 신체의 단단한 구조물에 부딪혀 파편화되면 이 충돌 지점에서 큰 공동이 발생하고 뼈 조각 자체가 손상을 유발하는 구성요소 일부가 된다. 뼈와 주변 장기 및 혈관에 심각한 파괴가 발생할 수 있다.

19세기 후반 살았던 외과 의사 에밀 테오도르 코허(Emil Theodor Kocher)는 탄도학과 무기로 인한 피해에 대한 이해에 매우 적극적이

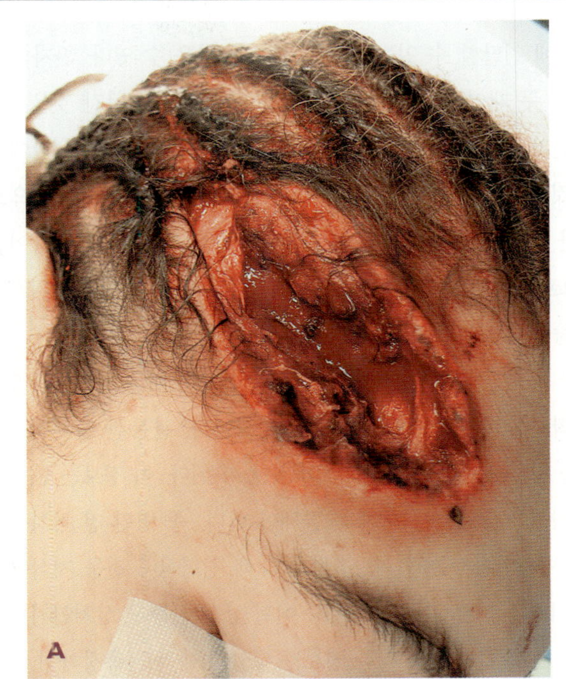

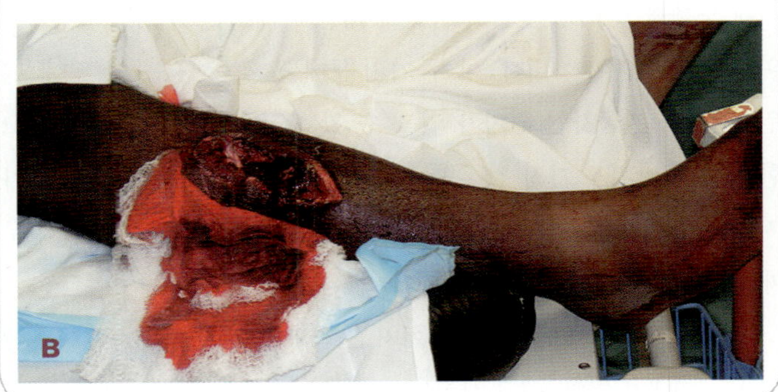

그림 4-55 A. 고속 무기의 발사체에 의해 두피에 찰과상이 생겼다. 머리뼈는 골절되지 않았다. **B.** 다리에 고속 총상을 입어 영구적인 큰 공동이 생겼음을 보여준다.
Courtesy of Norman McSwain, MD, FACS, NREMT-P.

었다. 그는 덤덤(Dum-Dum) 탄환을 사용하지 말 것을 강력히 주장했다.

입구 및 출구 상처

조직 손상은 관통 물체의 경로를 따라 신체로 총알이 진입하는 부위와 관통한 물체의 경로를 따라 신체에서 빠져나올 때 발생한다. 피해자의 위치, 공격자의 위치, 사용된 무기의 종류에 관한 정보는 손상 경로를 결정하는 데 도움이 된다. 입구 상처와 출구 상처가 관련될 수 있다면 이 경로에 있을 수 있는 해부학적 구조물을 대략적으로 추정할 수 있다.

상처 부위를 평가하는 것은 환자를 처치하거나 환자를 이송할 의료기관에 전달할 수 있는 중요한 정보를 얻을 수 있다. 환자의 복부에 있는 두 개의 구멍은 총알 한 발이 들어왔다가 나간 것을 의미하는 것인가 아니면 총알 두 발이 들어와서 두 발이 환자 몸 안에 남아 있는 것을 의미하는가? 총알이 정중선을 통과했을까?(일반적으로 더 심각한 손상을 초래함) 아니면 같은 쪽에 남아있는가? 총알이 어느 방향으로 이동했는가? 총알이 지나간 경로에 어떤 내부 장기가 있었을 가능성이 있는가?

입구 및 출구 상처는 일반적으로 항상 그런 것은 아니지만 연부조직에 확인할 수 있는 손상 유형을 형성한다. 관통한 물체의 보이는 궤적을 평가하는 것은 임상의에게 도움이 된다. 이 정보는 환자를 이송할 병원에 있는 의사에게 제공해야 한다. 즉 병원 전 처치 제공자와 대부분의 의사는 법의병리학에 대해 경험이나 전문 지식이 없으므로 어떤 상처가 입구 상처이고 어떤 상처가 출구 상처인지 평가하는 것은 불확실하다. 이러한 정보는 총알의 궤적을 측정하여 환자 처치에 도움을 주려는 것이지 사건에 대한 구체적인 사항을 결정하기 위한 법적 목적이 아니다. 이 두 가지 문제를 혼동해서는 안 된다. 병원 전 처치 제공자는 환자가 입을 수 있는 잠재적 손상을 파악하고 환자 처치 방법을 가장 잘 결정하기 위해 가능한 한 많은 정보를 가지고, 있어야 한다. 입구 및 출구 상처의 세부 사항과 관련된 법적 문제는 다른 전문가에게 맡기는 것이 가장 좋다.

총상으로 인한 입구 상처는 기저 조직에 닿아 있지만, 사출구 상처는 지지대가 없다. 입구 상처는 일반적으로 경로에 따라 원형 또는 타원형 상처이고 출구 상처는 별 모양 상처이다(**그림 4-56**). 총알이 피부에 들어갈 때 회전하기 때문에 분홍빛의 작은 찰과상(1~2mm)이 남는다(**그림 4-57** 및 **그림 4-58**). 출구 상처에는 찰과상이 없다. 발사 시 총구가 피부에 직접 닿으면 팽창하는 가스가 조직으로 들어가 촉진 시 비빔소리가 생성된다(**그림 4-59**). 총구가 피부에서 5~7cm 이내에 있으면 분출되는 뜨거운 가스에 의해 피부에 화상을 입게 되고 5~15cm 이내에 있으면 연기가 피부에 달라붙으며 25cm 이내에 있으면 연소하는 코르다이트 입자가 피부에 작은(1~2mm) 화상 부위와 문신처럼 자국이 남는다.

관통성 외상의 국소적 영향

이 부문에서는 관통성 외상 의한 신체의 다양한 부위에 입을 수 있는 손상에 관해 설명한다.

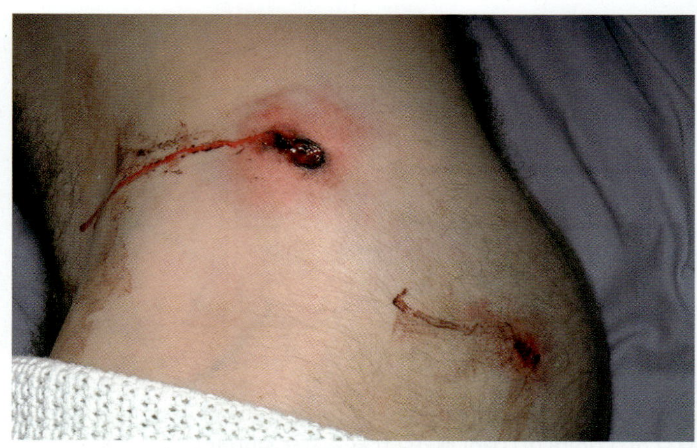

그림 4-56 입구 상처는 모양이 둥글거나 타원형이며 출구 상처는 종종 별 모양 또는 선형이다.
© Mediscan/Alamy Stock Photo

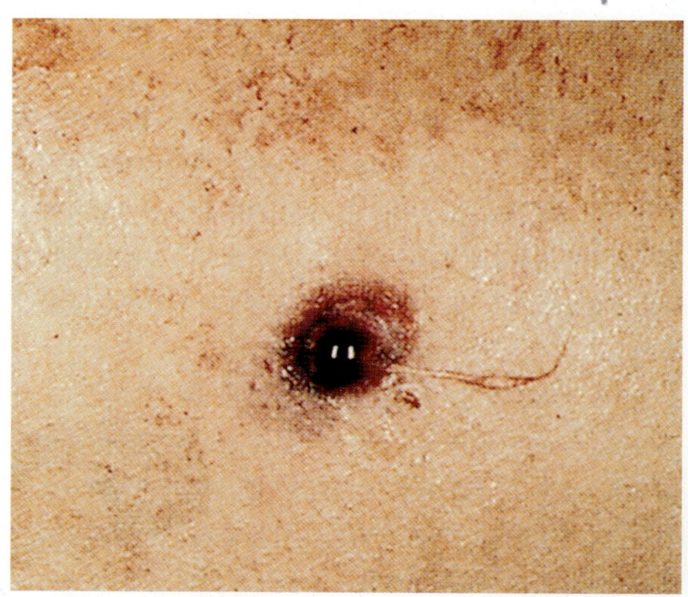

그림 4-57 가장자리에 찰과상이 생기는 것은 총알이 오른쪽 상단에서 왼쪽 하단으로 이동했음을 나타내는 것이다.
Courtesy of Norman McSwain, MD, FACS, NREMT-P.

머리

총알이 두개골을 관통한 후 그 에너지는 밀폐된 공간에 분산된다. 총알에서 가속하는 입자는 피부, 근육, 심지어 복부처럼 팽창할 수 없는 견고한 두개골에 부딪히게 된다. 따라서 뇌 조직이 두개골을 안쪽에 눌려 자유롭게 확장할 수 있을 때보다 더 많은 손상을 입게 된다. 이것은 사과에 폭죽을 넣은 다음 사과를 금속 캔에 넣는 것과 유사하다. 폭죽이 터지면 사과는 캔 벽에 부딪혀 파괴된다. 총알이 두개

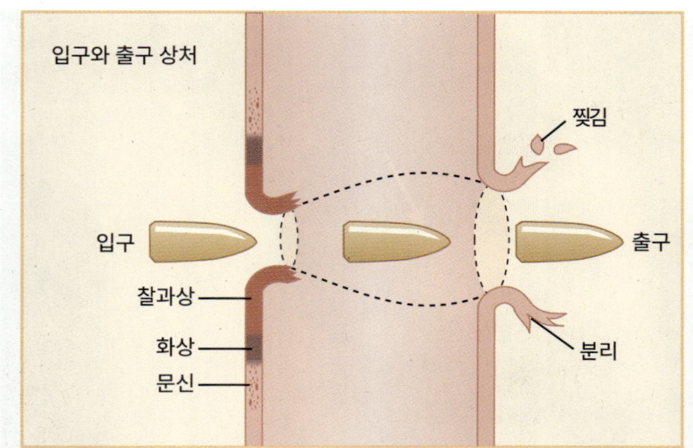

그림 4-58 입구에서 총알의 회전 및 압박은 원형 또는 타원형 구멍을 생성한다. 총알이 빠져나갈 때 상처가 눌려 벌려진다.
© National Association of Emergency Medical Technicians (NAEMT)

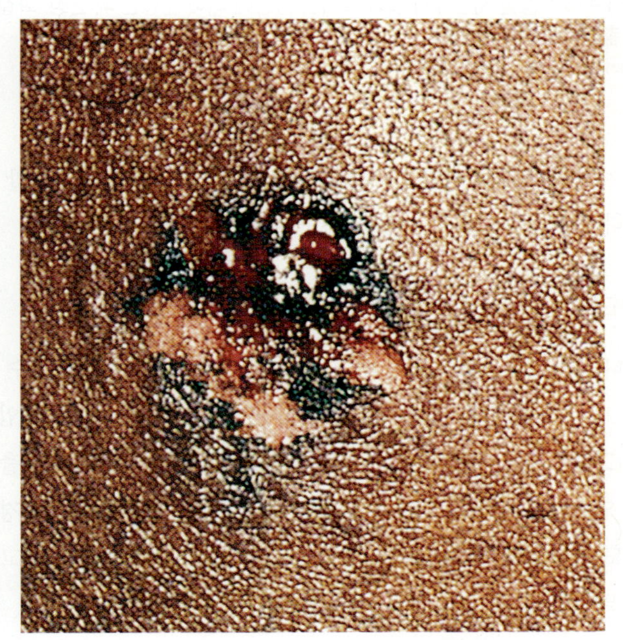

그림 4-59 피부에 근접한 총구 끝에서 나오는 뜨거운 가스는 피부에 부분층 화상과 전층 화상을 입힌다.
Courtesy of Norman McSwain, MD, FACS, NREMT-P.

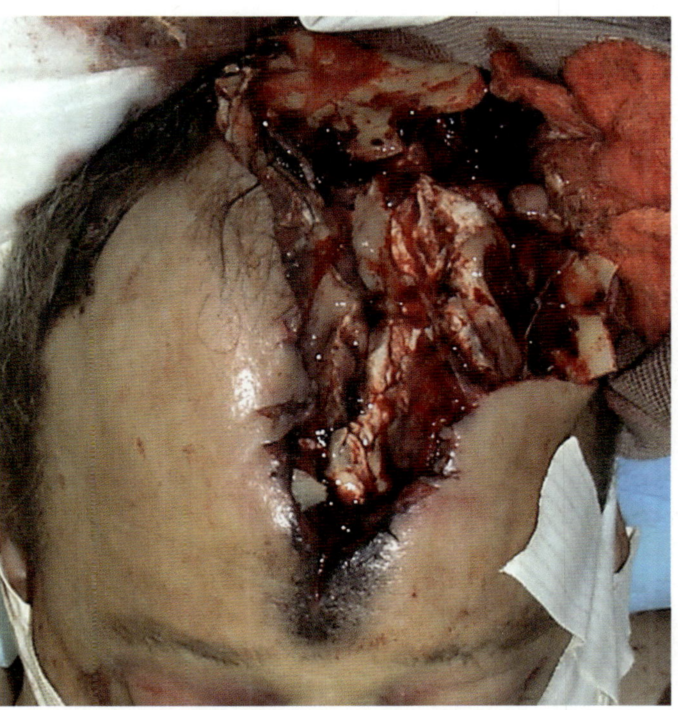

그림 4-60 총알이 두개골을 관통한 후 그 에너지는 밀폐된 공간에서 분산된다. 마치 밀폐된 용기에 폭죽을 넣는 것과 같다. 힘이 충분히 강하면 용기(두개골)가 안쪽에서 바깥쪽으로 폭발할 수 있다.
Courtesy of Norman McSwain, MD, FACS, NREMT-P.

골을 관통하는 경우 힘이 충분히 강하면 머리뼈는 안쪽에서 바깥쪽으로 폭발할 수 있다(**그림 4-60**).

총알이 비스듬히 들어와 두개골을 빠져나갈 힘이 충분하지 않으면 총알이 두개골 내부의 굴곡을 따라갈 수 있다. 이 경로는 심각한 손상을 일으킬 수 있다(**그림 4-61**). 이러한 특성 때문에 0.22 구경이나 0.25 구경 권총과 같은 소구경 중간 속도의 무기는 "암살자의 무기"로 불려 왔다. 이러한 무기는 총알이 들어가면서 모든 에너지가 뇌로 전달된다.

가슴

가슴안에는 폐, 혈관계 및 위장관의 세 가지 주요 구조물이 있다. 가슴벽과 척추와 근육은 가슴우리 구조를 구성한다. 이러한 시스템의 해부학적 구조 중 하나 이상이 관통하는 물체에 의해 손상될 수 있다.

폐

폐 조직은 혈액, 고형장기 또는 뼈보다 밀도가 낮으므로 관통하는 물체는 더 조은 입자에 부딪히고 더 적은 에너지를 교환하며 폐 조직에 더 적은 손상을 입힌다. 폐 손상은 임상적으로 중요할 수 있지만(**그림 4-62**), 수술적 치료가 필요한 환자는 15% 미만이다.

혈관계

가슴벽에 쿠착되어 있지 않은 작은 혈관은 심각한 손상 없이 옆으로 밀려날 수 있다. 그러나 대동맥 및 대정맥과 같은 큰 혈관은 척추나 심장에 부착되어 있어서 덜 움직인다. 이에 따라 쉽게 옆으로 움직일

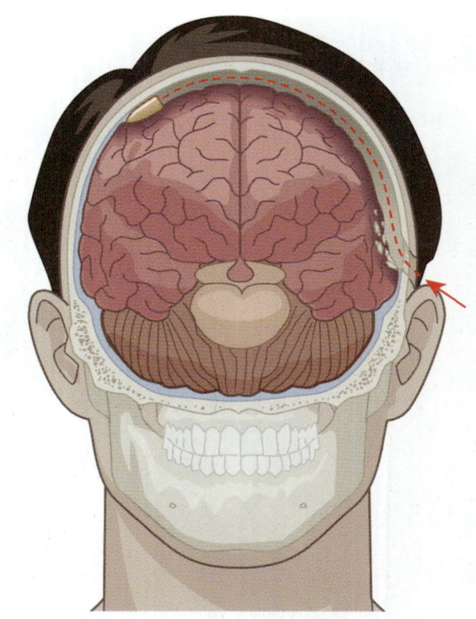

그림 4-61 총알이 두개골의 굴곡을 따라갈 수 있다.
© National Association of Emergency Medical Technicians (NAEMT)

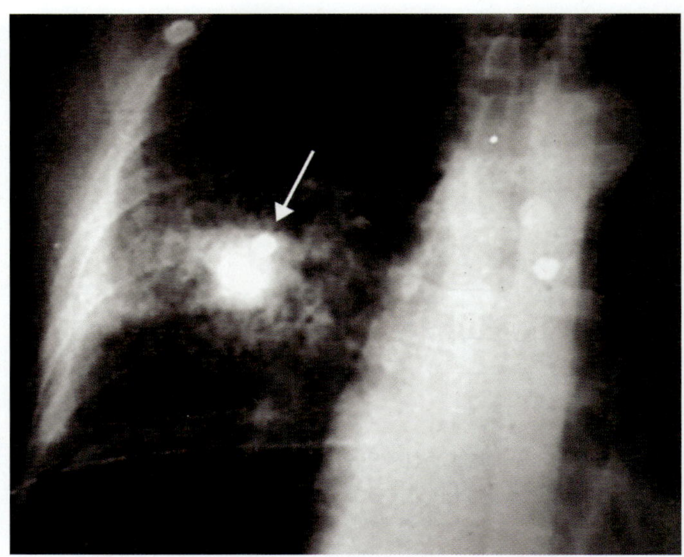

그림 4-62 충돌 지점에서 멀리 떨어진 공동에 의해 발생한 폐 손상. 화살표는 총알 파편을 나타낸다.
Courtesy of Norman McSwain, MD, FACS, NREMT-P.

수 없고 손상되기 쉽다.

심근(거의 전체 근육)은 총알이 통과하면서 늘어났다가 수축하여 더 작은 결함을 남긴다. 근육의 두께는 칼과 같은 저에너지 관통이나 0.22 구경의 작은 중간 에너지 총알로 인한 출혈을 조절할 수 있다. 이러한 폐쇄는 즉각적인 출혈을 방지하고 피해자를 적절한 의료기관으로 이송할 수 있는 시간을 확보할 수 있다.

위장관

가슴안을 가로지르는 위장관의 일부인 식도가 관통되어 내용물이 가슴안으로 누출될 수 있다. 이러한 손상의 증상과 징후는 몇 시간 또는 며칠 동안 지연될 수 있다.

복부

복부에는 속빈장기(공기가 채워진 장기), 고형장기, 뼈로 이루어진 구조의 세 가지 유형으로 구성되어 있다. 저에너지 총알에 의한 관통은 심각한 손상을 일으키지 않을 수 있으며 배안을 관통하는 칼에 의해 발생한 상처의 30%만이 수술적 치료가 필요하다. 권총과 같은 중에너지 손상은 더 심한 손상을 입히므로 85~95% 정도에서 수술적 치료가 요구된다. 중에너지 손상(권총 손상)은 더 심한 손상을 입히며 대부분 수술적 치료가 필요하다. 그러나 중에너지 총알로 인한 손상의 경우 고형장기 및 혈관구조의 손상으로 인해 즉각적인 출혈이 발생하지 않는 경우가 많다. 따라서 병원 전 처치 제공자는 효과적

인 수술적 치료를 위해 환자를 가장 적절한 의료기관으로 이송할 수 있다.

팔다리

팔다리에 관통상을 입으며 뼈, 근육, 신경 또는 혈관이 손상될 수 있다. 뼈가 맞으면 뼛조각이 이차 총알이 되어 주변 조직은 열상을 입힌다(그림 4-63). 근육은 종종 총알의 경로에서 벗어나 팽창하여 출혈을 일으킨다. 총알은 혈관을 관통하거나 아슬아슬하게 빗나간 경우에도 혈관 내벽이 손상되어 몇 분 또는 몇 시간 내에 혈관이 응고되고 막힐 수 있다.

산탄총 상처

산탄총은 고속 무기는 아니지만, 고에너지 무기이며 근거리에서는 일부 고에너지 소총보다 더 치명적일 수 있다. 권총과 소총은 총열 내부에 강선을 사용하여 목표물을 향해 비행 패턴으로 하나의 비행 패턴으로 회전시킨다. 이와는 대조적으로 대부분 산탄총은 매끄러운 원통형 튜브 총열을 사용하여 여러 발의 총알을 목표물 방향으로 발사한다. 초크와 다이버터라고 하는 장치는 산탄총 총열 끝에 부착하여 탄두를 특정 패턴(예: 원통형 또는 직사각형)으로 형성하고 모양을 만들 수 있다. 그런데도 산탄총을 발사하면 많은 수의 총알이 퍼지거나 분산되는 패턴으로 발사된다. 총알의 궤적을 조기에 넓히기 위해

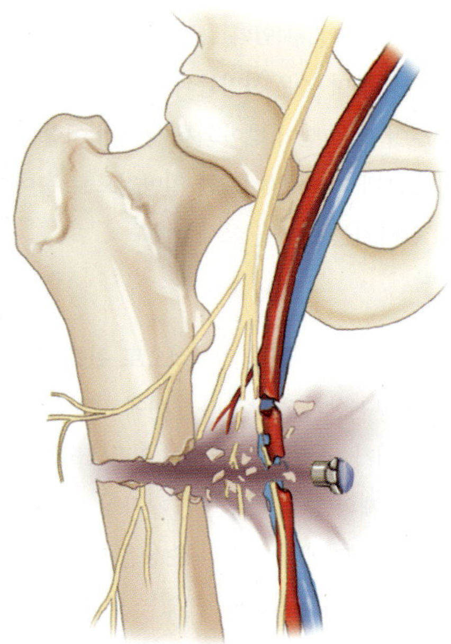

그림 4-63 뼛조각은 이차 총알이 되어 원래 관통하는 물체와 같은 기전으로 손상을 입힌다.
© National Association of Emergency Medical Technicians (NAEMT)

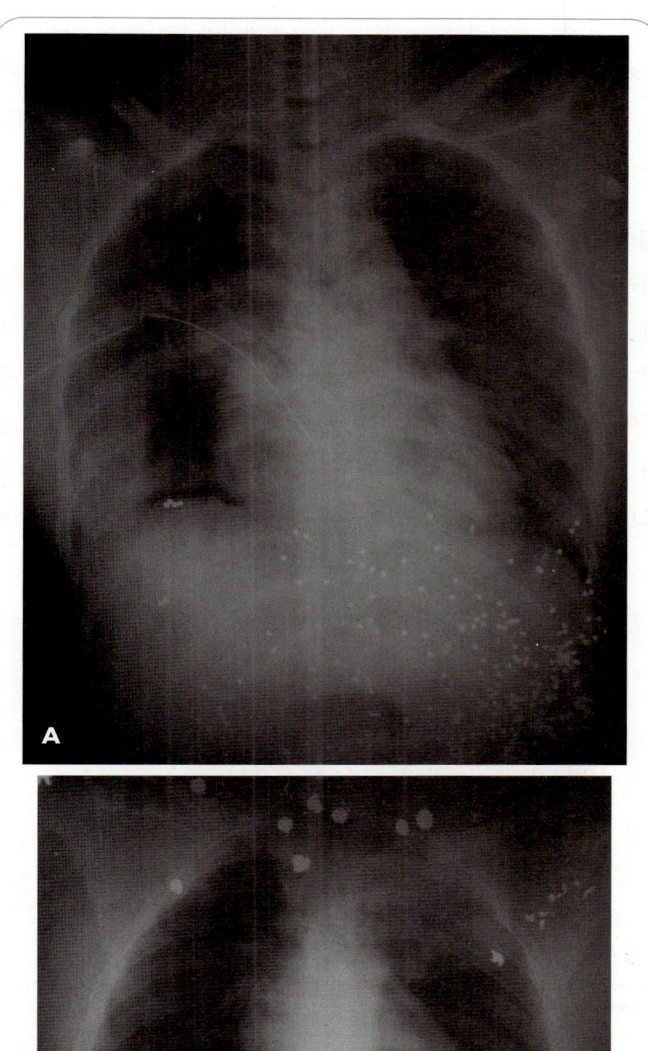

그림 4-64 A. 평균 새 사냥용 탄피에는 200~2,000개의 알갱이가 들어있을 수 있다. **B.** 벅샷 탄피에는 6~20개의 알갱이가 들어있을 수 있다.
Courtesy of Norman McSwain, MD, FACS, NREMT-P.

총열을 짧게 할 수 있다.

산탄총은 다양한 종류의 탄약을 사용할 수 있지만, 대부분 산탄총 탄피의 구조는 비슷하다. 일반적인 산탄총 탄피에는 화약, 충전재 및 발사체가 포함되어 있다. 총알이 발사되면 모든 구성 요소가 총구에서 발사되어 피해자에게 손상을 입힐 수 있다. 특정 유형의 화약은 근거리 손상의 경우 피부에 점(문신)을 남길 수 있다. 일반적으로 총알과 화약을 분리하는 데 사용되는 윤활 처리된 종이, 섬유 또는 플라스틱인 충전재는 제거하지 않으면 상처에 또 다른 감염원을 제공할 수 있다. 총알은 크기, 무게 및 구성이 다양할 수 있다. 압축 금속 분말에서 새 사냥용 산탄(작은 금속 알갱이), 벅샷(큰 금속 알갱이), 산탄(단일 금속 알갱이), 최근에는 플라스틱이나 고무 형태로도 대체된 총알에 이르기까지 다양한 총알을 사용할 수 있다. 평균적으로 탄피에는 28~43g의 샷이 장전되어 있다. 샷 내에 충전된 필러(폴리에틸렌 또는 폴리프로필렌 과립)는 피부의 표면에 박힐 수 있다.

평균적인 새 사냥용 산탄에는 200~2,000개의 알갱이를 포함할 수 있지만, 벅샷 탄피에는 6~20개의 알갱이가 들어 있을 수 있다(**그림 4-64**). 알갱이의 크기가 커질수록 유효 사거리와 에너지 전달 특성 측면에서 0.22 구경 총알의 상처 특성에 가까워진다는 점에 유의해야 한다. 더 크거나 매그넘 탄환도 사용할 수 있다. 이 탄환은 더 많은 화약이나 장약을 충전하여 총구 속도를 높일 수 있다.

산탄총 상처의 분류

사용된 탄약의 종류도 손상을 측정하는 데 중요하지만, 환자가 총에 맞은 범위(거리)는 산탄총 손상 부상자를 평가할 때 가장 중요한 변수이다(**그림 4-65**). 산탄총은 많은 수의 총알을 발사하며 그중 대부분은 원형이다. 이러한 발사체는 특히 공기 저항의 영향을 받기 쉬우며 총구를 벗어나면 속도가 빠르게 느려진다. 발사체에 대한 공기 저항의 영향은 무기의 유효 사거리를 감소시키고 무기가 생성하는 상처의 기본 특성을 변경한다. 결과적으로 산탄총 상처는 접촉 상처, 근거리 상처, 원거리 상처의 네 가지 주요 범주로 분류되었다(**그림 4-66**).

접촉 상처

접촉 상처는 무기가 발사될 때 총구가 피해자에게 닿았을 때 발생한다. 이 범위에서 총기를 발사하면 일반적으로 그을음이나 총구의 자국이 있을 수도 있고 없을 수도 있는 원형 사입구 상처가 생긴다. 총알이 총구에서 빠져나갈 때 고온과 뜨거운 가스의 팽창으로 인해 상처 가장자리가 타거나 화상을 입는 것이 일반적이다(**그림 4-59** 참조). 일부 접촉 상처는 조직에서 빠져나가는 총열의 과열된 가스로

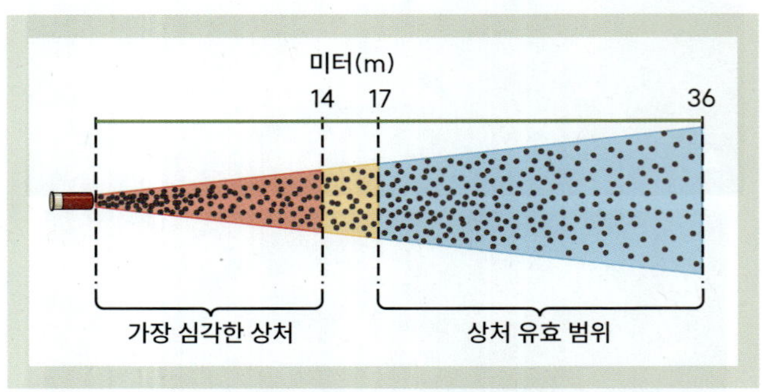

그림 4-65 사거리가 늘어날수록 샷 열의 확산 직경이 확장된다.

Data from DeMuth WE Jr. The mechanism of shotgun wounds. J Trauma. 1971;11:219–229; Sherman RT, Parrish RA. Management of shotgun injuries: a review of 152 cases. J Trauma. 1963;3:76–86.

인해 더 별 모양으로 보일 수 있다. 접촉 상처는 일반적으로 광범위한 조직 손상을 초래하며 높은 사망률과 관련이 있다. 표준 산탄총의 총신은 길이가 길어 손을 뻗어 방아쇠를 당기기 어렵기 때문에 이 무기로 자살하기 어렵다. 이러한 시도는 일반적으로 총이 뇌에 도달하지 않고 얼굴이 갈라지는 손상을 초래한다.

근거리 상처

근거리 상처(1.8m 미만)는 여전히 일반적으로 원형 입구 상처가 특징이지만, 접촉 상처보다 상처 가장자리 주변에 그을음, 화약 또는 충전재가 묻어 있는 증거가 더 많을 가능성이 있다. 또한, 총알에 의한 상처와 일치하는 충전재의 충격으로 인한 찰과상 및 자국도 발견될 수 있다. 근거리 상처는 환자에게 심각한 손상을 입히며 이 거리에서 발사된 총알은 깊은 구조물을 관통할 수 있는 충분한 에너지를 보유하고 약간 더 넓게 퍼지는 패턴을 보인다. 이 패턴은 총알이 연부조직을 관통할 때 손상 정도를 증가시킨다.

중거리 상처

중거리 상처는 중앙 입구 상처 주변의 경계에서 탄환 구멍이 나타나는 것이 특징이다. 이 패턴은 탄환의 기본 열(column)에서 개별 탄환이 퍼져나간 결과이며 일반적으로 1.8~5.5m 거리에서 발사될 때 발생한다. 이러한 손상은 깊고 관통하는 상처와 표재성 상처 및 찰과상이 혼합되어 있다. 그러나 이 손상의 깊고 관통하는 요소로 인해 복합적인 상처 패턴을 보인 피해자의 사망률은 근거리 손상과 비슷할

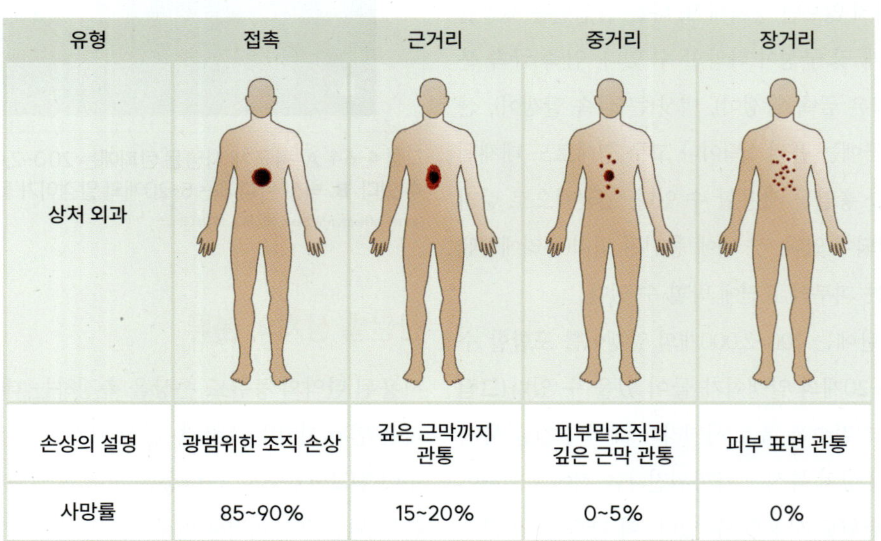

유형	접촉	근거리	중거리	장거리
상처 외과				
손상의 설명	광범위한 조직 손상	깊은 근막까지 관통	피부밑조직과 깊은 근막 관통	피부 표면 관통
사망률	85~90%	15~20%	0~5%	0%

그림 4-66 산탄총 손상의 유형

수 있다.

장거리 상처

장거리 상처는 거의 치명적이지 않다. 이러한 상처는 일반적으로 5.5m 이상의 거리에서 발생하는 전형적인 탄환 상처의 확산이 특징이다. 그러나 이렇게 느린 속도에서도 탄환은 특정 민감한 조직(예: 눈)에 심각한 손상을 입힐 수 있다. 또한 더 큰 벅샷 탄환은 충분한 속도를 유지하여 장거리에서도 깊은 구조물에 손상을 입힐 수 있다. 병원 전 처치 제공자는 민감한 조직을 중심으로 여러 개의 작은 탄환에 의한 상처와 그 부위의 누적 효과를 고려해야 한다. 외상 환자를 평가할 때 적절한 노출은 필수적이며 산탄총에 의한 손상도 예외는 아니다.

산탄총 상처 평가

산탄총 손상을 입은 환자의 손상 유형을 평가할 때는 이러한 다양한 특성을 고려해야 한다. 예를 들어, 하나의 원형 산탄총 상처는 새 사냥용 산탄이나 벅샷으로 인한 접촉 또는 근거리 손상을 나타낼 수 있다. 반대로 이것은 산탄이나 단일 총알에 의한 중거리 및 장거리 손상을 나타낼 수 있다. 상처에 대한 자세한 평가만이 이러한 손상을 구별할 수 있으며 이는 총알의 특성이 현저히 다르더라도 내부 구조물에 심각한 손상을 초래할 수 있다.

가슴의 접촉 및 근거리 상처는 크고 시각적으로 인상적인 상처가 생겨 개방성 기흉이 발생할 수 있으며 이러한 상처를 통해 장이 복부로 빠져나올 수 있다. 간혹 중거리에서 발사된 총알 하나가 장에 천공을 일으킬 정도로 깊숙이 들어가 복막염으로 이어지거나 주요 동맥을 손상해 팔다리나 장기의 혈관 손상을 일으킬 수 있다. 또는 여러 개의 작은 상처가 퍼지는 패턴을 보이는 환자는 수십 개의 사입구 상처가 있을 수 있다. 그러나 어떤 총알도 내부 구조물에 심각한 손상을 입히는 것은 고사하고 근막을 관통할 만큼 충분한 에너지를 보유하지 못했을 수 있다.

즉각적인 환자 처치가 항상 우선시되어야 하지만, 병원 전 처치 제공자는 현장에서 수집하여 환자를 이송할 의료기관에 전달할 수 있는 모든 정보(예: 탄피 형태, 총을 발사한 거리, 발사된 총알 수)는 총기 손상 환자의 적절한 진단 평가 및 처치에 도움이 될 수 있다. 또한 다양한 상처 유형에 대한 인식은 병원 전 처치 제공자가 손상의 초기 인상과 관계없이 내부 손상에 대한 높은 의심 지수를 유지하는 데 도움이 될 수 있다.

폭발 손상

폭발로 인한 손상

폭발물은 전투 및 테러리스트가 가장 빈번하게 사용하는 무기이다. 폭발 장치는 여러 기전을 통해 인체에 손상을 유발하며 그중 일부는 매우 복잡하다. 폭발 후 환자를 처치하는 의료진이 직면하는 가장 큰 어려움은 다수 사상자와 여러 관통상의 존재이다(**그림 4-67**).

폭발의 물리학

폭발은 물리적, 화학적 또는 핵반응으로 열과 빠르게 팽창하는 고도로 압축된 가스의 형태로 대량의 에너지가 거의 즉각적으로 방출되어 파편을 매우 빠른 속도로 투사할 수 있다. 폭발과 관련된 에너지는 폭발파의 운동에너지와 열에너지, 무기 상자와 주변 파편이 부서지면서 형성되는 파편의 운동에너지, 전자기 에너지 등 다양한 형태로 나타날 수 있다.

폭발파는 초당 5,000m 이상의 속도로 이동할 수 있으며 정적 및 동적 구성요소로 이루어져 있다. 정적 구성요소(폭발 과압)는 폭발 영역에 있는 물체를 둘러싸고 충격 전선 또는 충격파라고 하는 불연속적인 압력 상승으로 최대 과압까지 사방에 충격을 가한다. 충격파에 이어 과압이 주변 압력으로 떨어지고 공기가 다시 빨려 들어가면서 부분 진공이 형성되는 경우가 많다(**그림 4-68**). 동적 구성요소(동적 압력)는 방향성이 있으며 폭발풍으로 나타난다. 폭발풍의 주요 의

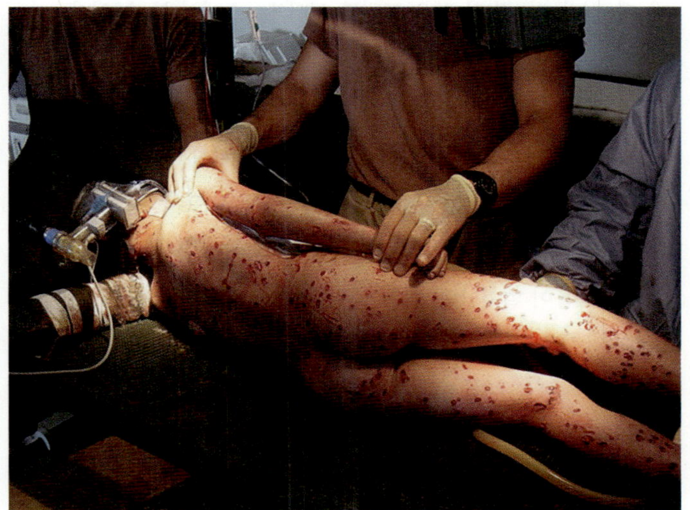

그림 4-67 폭탄 폭발로 인한 다발성 파편 손상을 입은 환자

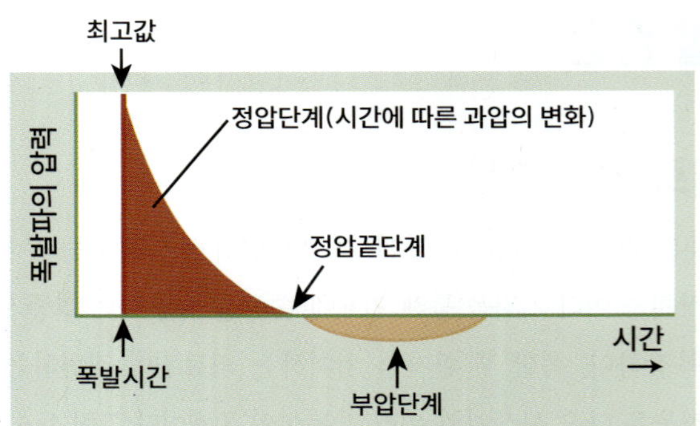

그림 4-68 폭발파의 압력과 시간의 관계. 이 그래프는 압력 감소 및 음압 단계에 따른 갑작스러운 압력 증가(폭발 과압)를 보여준다.

From Federal Emergency Management Agency. Primer to Design Safe School Projects in Case of Terrorist Attacks: Providing Protection to People and Buildings. Author; 2003:Chapter 4. https://www.fema.gov/pdf/plan/prevent/rms/428/fema428_ch4.pdf

미는 총알이나 포탄과 같은 표준 탄도 무기보다 빠른 초당 수천 미터 이상의 속도로 파편을 추진한다는 것이다. 반면에 정적 및 동적 압력의 유효 범위는 수십 미터로 측정되지만, 동적 압력에 의해 가속된 파편은 폭발파를 빠르게 앞질러 수천 미터까지 손상의 주요 원인이 될 수 있다는 것이다.

폭발파와 신체의 상호작용

폭발파는 폭발파의 에너지를 구조물에 전달하여 신체 및 기타 구조물과 상호작용한다. 이 에너지는 영향을 받는 구조물의 강도 및 고유 진동 주기에 따라 구조물이 변형되는 원인이 된다. 구조물 내의 밀도 인터페이스가 변화하면 전송된 폭발파의 복잡한 재형성, 융합 및 결합이 발생한다. 이러한 상호 작용은 특히 고형장기와 공기 및 액체(예: 폐, 심장, 간, 장)와 같은 고밀도 인터페이스에서 볼 수 있다.

폭발 관련 손상

폭발로 인한 손상은 일반적으로 미 국방성 지침 6025.21E24에 설명된 손상 분류에 따라 일차, 이차, 삼차, 사차, 오차로 분류된다(**표 4-1**). 폭발물이 폭발하면 그 경로에 있는 물체와 사람 사이에 연쇄적인 상호 작용이 일어난다. 만약 사람이 가까이 있으면 초기 폭발파는 신체의 압력을 증가시켜 특히 귀, 폐 및 드물게 장과 같이 가스로 채워진 기관에서 스트레스와 전단을 유발한다. 일차 폭발 손상과 관련된 이환율과 사망률은 폭발 위치로부터의 거리가 멀어질수록 감소하고 폭발력의 크기에 비례한다(**그림 4-69**). 이러한 일차 폭발 손상은 폭발파가 표면에서 반사되어 압력파의 파괴 잠재력을 높이기 때문에

밀폐된 공간에서 폭발이 발생할 때 더 많이 발생한다.

폐 압력 손상으로 인한 즉각적인 사망은 개방된 공간보다 밀폐된 공간에서 폭발하는 경우 더 자주 발생한다. 이라크와 아프가니스탄에서 발생한 폭발 손상의 대부분(95%)은 개방된 공간에서 발생했다.

일차 폭발 손상의 가장 흔한 형태는 고막 파열이다. 고막 파열은 제곱 인치 당 5psi의 낮은 압력에서 발생할 수 있으며 종종 경험하는 유일한 심각한 과압 손상이다. 다음으로 심한 손상은 기흉, 공기색전증, 사이질 및 피부밑기종, 세로칸공기증 등 폐 손상과 관련된 것으로 알려진 임계값인 40psi 미만에서 발생한다. 이라크 자유 작전에서 화상을 입은 군인의 데이터에 따르면 고막 파열이 폐 손상을 예측할 수 없는 것으로 확인되었다.

폭발파 충격파의 전면은 빠르게 사라지고 그 뒤에는 폭발풍으로 인해 파편이 추진하여 다발성 관통상을 일으킨다. 이러한 손상을 이차 손상이라고 부르지만, 일반적으로 가장 주된 손상이다. 또한 폭발풍은 큰 물체를 사람 쪽으로 밀어내거나 사람을 딱딱한 표면으로 밀어내어(전신 또는 부분 신체 전위) 무딘 손상(삼차 폭발)을 입힐 수도 있다. 이 손상에는 구조물 붕괴로 인한 으깸 손상도 포함된다. 폭발 시 발생하는 열, 화염, 가스 및 연기는 화상과 연료로 인한 중독, 흡입 손상 및 질식을 포함하는 사차 손상을 일으킨다. 폭발 장치에 박테리아, 화학 물질, 방사성 물질 또는 발사체가 추가되어 폭발 시 방출될 때 오차 손상이 발생한다.

파편으로 인한 손상

기존의 폭발성 무기는 파편으로 인한 손상을 극대화하도록 설계되었다. 초기 속도가 초당 수천 미터에 달하기 때문에 23kg 폭탄의 파편이 나갈 수 있는 거리는 300m를 훨씬 넘지만, 폭발 과압의 치명적인 반경은 약 15m에 불과하다. 따라서 군용 및 테러용 무기 개발자는 파편으로 인한 피해를 극대화하기 위해 자유장 폭발물의 피해 반경을 증가시킬 수 있는 무기를 개발한다.

폭발 장치가 폭발 과압만으로 손상을 일으키는 경우는 거의 없으며 심각한 일차 폭발 손상은 이차 및 삼차 손상이 대부분인 것에 비해 상대적으로 드물다. 따라서 일차 폭발 효과로 인한 손상을 입은 환자는 거의 없다. 폭발 관련된 모든 손상 전체를 폭발 손상이라고 부르는 경우가 많기 때문에 폭발 손상을 구성하는 요소와 관련하여 큰 혼란을 일으킬 수 있다.

폭발파의 에너지는 빠르게 소멸하기 때문에 대부분의 폭발 장치는

표 4-1 폭발 손상 분류

분류	정의	일반적인 손상
일차	■ 폭발 충격파가 신체에 접촉하여 발생 ■ 조직에서 압박과 비틀림파 발생 ■ 조직 밀도 경계면에서 강화/반사되는 파동 발생 ■ 공기가 차 있는 장기(폐, 장, 귀 등) 특정 위험	■ 고막 파열 ■ 폭발성 폐/폐 압력 손상 ■ 눈 손상 ■ 뇌진탕 ■ 복부 출혈
이차	■ 파편에 의한 상처 　• 일차 퍼편(폭발하는 무기의 파편) 　• 이차 파편(유리와 같은 환경 파편) ■ 파편 손상의 위협은 폭발파에 의한 손상보다 더 멀리까지 확장된다.	■ 관통성 손상 ■ 외상성 절단 ■ 열상 ■ 폐쇄성 또는 개방성 머리 손상
삼차	■ 폭발파는 사람을 표면/물체 위 또는 물체를 사람 위로 밀어내어 전신 전위를 유발한다. ■ 구조적 손상 또는 건물 붕괴로 인한 으깸손상	■ 무딘 손상 ■ 으깸증후군 ■ 구획증후군 ■ 골절
사차	■ 기타 폭발 관련 손상, 질병 또는 질환	■ 화상 ■ 유독 가스 및 기타 흡입 손상 ■ 환경 오염으로 인한 손상이나 감염
오차	■ 세균, 화학물질 및 방사선과 같은 특정 첨가물로 인한 손상("오염된 폭탄")	■ 화학 화상 ■ 세균 감염 ■ 방사선 노출

Data from Pennardt A. Blast injuries. *Medscape*. Updated August 6, 2021. Accessed October 26, 2021. https://emedicine
.medscape.com/article/822587-overview; U.S. Department of Defense, Blast Injury Research Coordinating Office. Blast
Injury 101. June 18, 2019. Accessed October 26, 2021. https://blastinjuryresearch.amedd.army.mil/index.cfm/blast
_injury_101; Department of Defense. Taxonomy of Injuries from Explosive Devices. Department of Defense Directive (DoDD) 6025.21E. Accessed October
26, 2021. https://www.esd.whs.mil/Portals/54/Documents/DD/issuances/dodd/602521p.pdf?
ver=2018-10-24-112151-983; National Association of Emergency Medical Technicians. *PHTLS: Prehospital Trauma Life Support*. Military 9th ed. Jones &
Bartlett Learning; 2021.

주로 파편으로 인한 피해를 주도록 설계되어 있다. 파편은 폭발 장치를 둘러싼 상자가 파손되어 생성되는 1차 파편이거나 주변 환경의 파편으로 인해 생성되는 2차 파편일 수 있다. 파편이 부서진 탄약 케이스, 날아다니는 파편 또는 테러리스트가 종종 사제 폭탄에 넣는 내장된 물체 등 어떤 형태로 만들어지는 파편은 폭발물의 사거리와 치사율을 기하급수적으로 증가시키며 폭발과 관련된 손상의 주요 원인이 된다.

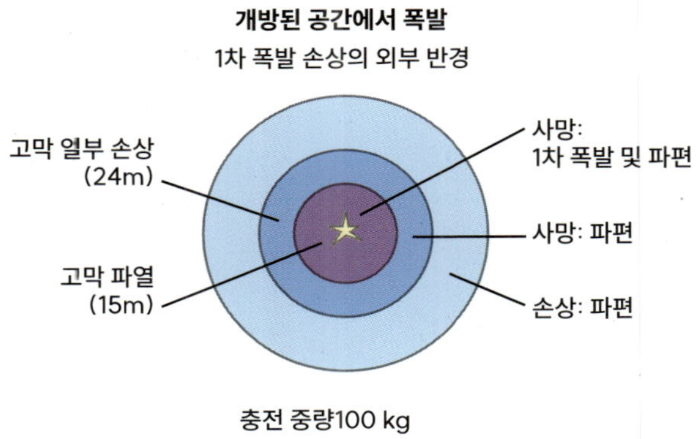

다발성 손상

폭발의 직접적인 영향 외에도 병원 전 처치 제공자는 폭발로 인한 공격으로 인한 다른 손상의 원인에 유의해야 한다. 예를 들어, 차량을 목표로 하는 급조폭발물(IED)은 차량 탑승자에게 최소한의 초기 손상을 유발할 수 있다. 그러나 차량 자체가 수직으로 변위되거나 경로

그림 4-69 100kg의 폭발물이 야외에서 폭발했을 때 거리에 따른 이환율과 사망률
© National Association of Emergency Medical Technicians (NAEMT)

를 이탈하여 충돌, 전도, 전복 등으로 인해 탑승자가 무딘 손상을 입을 수 있다. 이러한 상황에서 탑승자는 앞서 설명한 것과 같이 무딘 손상에 관해 설명한 기전에 따라 손상을 입게 된다.

군사 환경에서 차량 탑승자는 방탄복 덕분에 무딘 손상으로부터 어느 정도 보호받을 수 있다. 또한 급조폭발물 공격으로 무력화된 차량의 탑승자는 매복 공격을 받을 수 있으며 차량에서 내릴 때 총격 공격을 받을 수 있으므로 관통상을 입을 가능성이 있다.

외상의 물리학을 이용한 평가

외상 환자를 평가하려면 외상의 물리학에 대한 지식이 있어야 한다. 예를 들면, 운전자가 핸들에 부딪히면(무딘 손상) 충격 당시 가슴 전면에 큰 공동이 생기지만, 운전자가 핸들에서 튕겨 나감에 따라 가슴은 빠르게 원래 모양 또는 거의 원래 모양으로 돌아간다. 외상의 물리학을 이해하는 병원 전 처치 제공자와 그렇지 않은 병원 전 처치 제공자 두 명이 환자를 각각 평가하는 경우 외상의 물리학에 대한 지식이 없는 처치 제공자는 환자의 가슴에 보이는 타박상에만 신경을 쓰게 된다. 외상의 물리학을 이해하는 처치 제공자는 충격 당시 큰 공동이 존재했고 공동이 형성되기 위해 갈비뼈가 구부려져야 했으며 공동이 형성되면서 심장, 폐 및 대혈관이 압박되었다는 것을 인식할 것이다. 따라서 지식이 풍부한 병원 전 처치 제공자는 심장, 폐, 대혈관 및 가슴벽의 손상을 의심할 것이다. 그러다 다른 처치 제공자는 이러한 가능성을 인식하지 못할 것이다.

지식이 풍부한 병원 전 처치 제공자는 심각한 가슴안의 손상이 의심되면 경미한 폐쇄성 연부조직 손상으로 보이는 것에 대응하기보다는 이러한 잠재적 손상을 평가하고 환자를 처치하며 보다 적극적으로 이송을 시작한다. 근본적인 손상을 조기 발견, 적절한 이해 및 적절한 처치는 환자의 생존 여부에 상당한 영향을 미친다.

요 약

- 외상 환자의 평가에 외상 물리학의 원리를 통합하는 것은 중증 또는 생명을 위협하는 손상의 가능성을 발견하는 데 핵심적인 역할을 한다.
- 충돌 시 인체에서 발생하는 에너지 교환을 이해하면 대부분 손상을 예상할 수 있다. 외상의 물리학에 대한 지식은 즉각적으로 드러나지 않은 손상을 확인하고 적절하게 처치할 수 있게 해준다. 이러한 손상을 의심하지 않고 발견하지 못해 처치하지 않고 방치하면 외상으로 인한 이환율과 사망률에 영향을 준다.
- 에너지는 생기거나 파괴되지 않으며 형태만 바뀔 뿐이다. 물체의 운동에너지는 속도와 질량의 함수로 나타내며 접촉 시 다른 물체로 전달된다.
- 충격을 받은 물체나 신체 조직의 손상은 물체에 가해지는 운동에너지의 양뿐만 아니라 조직이 가해지는 힘을 견딜 수 있는 능력의 함수이기도 하다.

무딘 손상

- 충돌의 방향에 따라 전방, 측면, 후방, 회전, 전복, 각 충돌 등 손상의 유형과 가능성이 결정된다.
- 차량에서 튕겨 나가면 차량이 제공하는 충격에 대한 보호 기능이 감소한다.
- 에너지를 흡수하는 보호 장치가 중요하다. 이러한 장치에는 안전띠, 에어백, 범퍼, 충격을 흡수할 수 있는 핸들, 대시보드, 헬멧과 같은 에너지를 흡수하는 자동차 부품이 포함된다. 차량의 손상 정도와 충격 방향에 따라 어떤 탑승자가 더 심각한 손상을 입었을 가능성이 높은지 알 수 있다.
- 보행자 손상은 피해자의 키와 환자의 신체 어느 부위가 차량과 직접 접촉했는지에 따라 달라진다.

추락

- 추락 높이는 손상의 중증도에 영향을 미친다.
- 추락 지점의 에너지 흡수 능력이 손상의 중증도에 영향을 미친다.
- 추락 지점과 부딪치는 환자의 신체 부위와 환자의 신체를 통한 에너지 교환의 진행이 중요하다.

관통성 외상

- 에너지는 주요 손상 요인에 따라 다르다.
  - 저에너지: 수동식 절단기
  - 중에너지: 대부분의 권총
  - 고에너지: 고성능 소총 및 공격용 무기 등
- 환자와 가해자의 거리 및 총알이 맞았을 수 있는 물체는 신체와 충돌할 때 에너지의 양에 영향을 미치며, 따라서 신체 부위에 손상을 입히기 위해 환자에게 발사되는 가용 에너지에 영향을 미친다.
- 관통 물체의 경로에 근접한 장기는 생명을 위협할 수 있는 잠재적 상태를 결정한다.
- 관통성 외상의 경로는 입구 및 출구 상처에 따라 결정된다.

폭발

- 폭발로 인한 손상은 다섯 가지 유형이 있다.
  - 일차: 폭발 충격파
  - 이차: 발사체(가장 흔한 폭발로 인한 손상의 원인)
  - 삼차: 신체가 튕겨 나가 다른 물체와 충돌
  - 사차: 열과 화염
  - 오차: 방사선, 화학물질, 박테리아

시나리오 재구성

추운 겨울 새벽에 당신과 동료는 단독 차량 충돌 사고 현장으로 출동하였다. 현장에 도착하자마자 당신은 시골 도로에서 가로수에 충돌한 차량 한 대를 발견하였다. 차량의 앞부분이 가로수에 충돌한 것으로 보이며 차량은 회전하면서 도로 옆에 있던 배수로에 차량의 후미 부분이 빠진 상태이다. 차량에는 운전자 한 명만 탑승했으며 에어백이 전개되었고 운전자는 여전히 안전띠를 매고 신음하고 있다. 가로수와 충돌한 차량 앞부분이 손상되었을 뿐만 아니라 회전하면서 후미 부분이 배수로에 빠져 후방 손상도 확인할 수 있었다.

- 이 사고에서 외상의 물리학에 근거하여 이 환자가 손상을 입을 가능성은 무엇인가?
- 외상의 물리학을 근거하여 환자의 상태를 어떻게 설명할 것인가?
- 어떤 손상을 입을 것으로 예상하는가?

시나리오 해결책

환자에게 접근할 때 이 사고의 외상 물리학을 이해하면 머리, 목, 가슴, 복부 손상의 가능성에 대해 우려하게 된다. 환자는 반응을 보이지만 말이 어눌하고 술 냄새가 난다. 환자의 머리와 목을 도수 고정하고 손상을 평가하는 동안 콧등에 작은 열상이 있는 것을 발견했다. 그는 자신이 술을 마셨다고 인정하지만 몇 시인지 어디로 가는 중이었는지 기억이 나지 않는다고 말한다.

안전띠를 제거하는 동안 환자의 왼쪽 빗장뼈 부위에 찰과상과 압통이 있음을 확인했다. 그는 얼굴, 목, 가슴 앞쪽, 복부의 중간 부위에서 압통이 있다고 호소한다. 환자가 술을 마신 것, 어눌한 말투, 혼란스러운 상태 때문에 더 심각한 손상을 배제할 수 없으므로 환자를 차량에서 구조하기 전에 척추 고정을 시행한다.

외상센터로 이송하면서 지속적인 평가를 시행하던 중 환자가 양쪽 하복부에 심한 압통이 있다는 것을 발견하고 속빈장기가 손상이 있을 수 있다고 우려한다.

References

1. U.S. Department of Transportation, National Highway Traffic Safety Administration. 2015 motor vehicle crashes overview. Published December 2020. Accessed October 1, 2021. https://crashstats.nhtsa.dot.gov/Api/Public/ViewPublication/813060

2. World Health Organization. Global Status Report on Road Safety 2018. Published June 7, 2018. Accessed October 1, 2021. https://www.who.int/publications/i/item/9789241565684

3. Centers for Disease Control and Prevention/National Center for Health Statistics. All firearm deaths. Accessed October 1, 2021. https://www.cdc.gov/nchs/fastats/injury.htm

4. Hunt JP, Marr AB, Stuke LE. Kinematics. In: Mattox KL, Moore EE, Feliciano DV, eds. *Trauma*. 7th ed. McGraw-Hill; 2013.

5. Hollerman JJ, Fackler ML, Coldwell DM, et al. Gunshot wounds: 1. bullets, ballistics, and mechanisms of injury. *Am J Roentgenol*. 1990;155(4):685-690.

6. Centers for Disease Control and Prevention. Leading causes of death. Updated April 20, 2017. Accessed May 30, 2017. https://www.cdc.gov/injury/wisqars/index.html

7. Boyce RH, Singh K, Obremskey WT. Acute management of traumatic knee dislocations for the generalist. *J Am Acad Orthop Surg*. 2015 Dec;23(12):761-768.

8. Hernandez IA, Fyfe KR, Heo G, et al. Kinematics of head movement in simulated low velocity rear-end impacts. *Clin Biomech*. 2005;20(10):1011-1018.

9. Kumaresan S, Sances A, Carlin F, et al. Biomechanics of side-impact injuries: evaluation of seat belt restraint system, occupant kinematics, and injury potential. *Conf Proc IEEE Eng Med Biol Soc*. 2006;1:87-90.

10. Siegel JH, Yang KH, Smith JA, et al. Computer simulation and validation of the Archimedes lever hypothesis as a mechanism for aortic isthmus disruption in a case of lateral impact motor vehicle crash: a Crash Injury Research Engineering Network (CIREN) study. *J Trauma*. 2006;60(5):1072-1082.

11. Horton TG, Cohn SM, Heid MP, et al. Identification of trauma patients at risk of thoracic aortic tear by mechanism of injury. *J Trauma*. 2000;48(6):1008-1013; discussion 1013-1014.

12. Insurance Information Institute. Facts + Statistics: Highway Safety. Accessed October 1, 2021. https://www.iii.org/fact-statistic/facts-statistics-highway-safety

13. Enriquez J. Occupant restraint use in 2020: Results from the NOPUS controlled intersection study (Report No. DOT HS 813 186). National Highway Traffic Safety Administration. Published September 2021. Accessed October 1, 2021. https://crashstats.nhtsa.dot.gov/Api/Public/ViewPublication/813186

14. U.S. Department of Transportation, National Highway Traffic Safety Administration. 2011 motor vehicle crashes: overview. Published December 2012. Accessed September 29, 2017. http://www-nrd.nhtsa.dot.gov/Pubs/811701.pdf

15. Insurance Institute for Highway Safety. Seat belts. Accessed October 2, 2021. https://www.iihs.org/topics/seat-belts#laws

16. Kahane CJ. Lives saved by vehicle safety technologies and associated Federal Motor Vehicle Safety Standards, 1960 to 2012 – Passenger cars and LTVs – With reviews of 26 FMVSS and the effectiveness of their associated safety technologies in reducing fatalities, injuries, and crashes. (Report No. DOT HS 812 069). National Highway Traffic Safety Administration. Published January 2015. Accessed October 2, 2021. https://crashstats.nhtsa.dot.gov/Api/Public/ViewPublication/812069

17. National Highway Traffic Safety Administration. Seat belts. Accessed October 2, 2021. https://www.nhtsa.gov/risky-driving/seat-belts

18. U.S. Department of Transportation, National Highway Traffic Safety Administration. Lives saved in 2008 by restraint use and minimum drinking age laws. *Traffic Safety Facts*. Published May 2010. Accessed September 29, 2017. https://crashstats.nhtsa.dot.gov/Api/Public/ViewPublication/811153

19. National Center for Statistics and Analysis U.S. Department of Transportation, National Highway Traffic Safety Administration. Seat belt use in 2020: use rates in the states and territories. *Traffic Safety Facts*. Report No. DOT HS 813 109. Published April 2021. Accessed January 4, 2022. https://crashstats.nhtsa.dot.gov/Api/Public/View Publication/813109

20. Greenwell NK. *Results of the National Child Restraint Use Special Study* (Report No. DOT HS 812 142). National Highway Traffic Safety Administration; May 2015.

21. Rogers CD, Pagliarello G, McLellan BA, et al. Mechanism of injury influences the pattern of injuries sustained by patients involved in vehicular trauma. *Can J Surg*. 1991;34(3):283-286.

22. Mayrose J. The effects of a mandatory motorcycle helmet law on helmet use and injury patterns among motorcyclist fatalities. J Safety Res. 2008;39(4):429-32. Published August 6, 2008. Accessed February 25, 2022. https://pubmed.ncbi.nlm.nih.gov/18786430/

23. Centers for Disease Control and Prevention. Guidelines for field triage of injured patients: recommendations of the National Expert Panel on Field Triage. *MMWR*. 2012;61:1-20.

24. Pedersen A, Stinner DJ, McLaughlin HC, Bailey JR, Walter JR, Hsu JR. Characteristics of genitourinary injuries associated with pelvic fractures during Operation Iraqi Freedom and Operation Enduring Freedom. *Mil Med*. 2015 Mar;180(3 Suppl):64-67.

25. Burgess AR, Eastridge BJ, Young JW, et al. Pelvic ring disruptions: effective classification system and treatment protocols. *J Trauma*. 1990;30(7):848-856.

26. Fackler ML, Malinowski JA. Internal deformation of the AK-74: a possible cause for its erratic path in tissue. *J Trauma*. 1998;28(Suppl 1):S72-S75.

27. Fackler ML, Surinchak JS, Malinowski JA, et al. Wounding potential of the Russian AK-74 assault rifle. *J Trauma*. 1984;24(3):263-266.

28. Fackler ML, Surinchak JS, Malinowski JA, et al. Bullet fragmentation: a major cause of tissue disruption. *J Trauma*. 1984;24(1):35-39.

29. Fackler ML, Dougherty PJ. Theodor Kocher and the Scientific Foundation of Wound Ballistics. *Surg Gynecol Obstet*. 1991;172(2):153-160.

30. American College of Surgeons (ACS) Committee on Trauma. *Advanced Trauma Life Support Course*. ACS; 2002.

31. Wade CE, Ritenour AE, Eastridge BJ, et al. Explosion injuries treated at combat support hospitals in the Global War on Terrorism. In: Elsayed N, Atkins J, eds. *Explosion and Blast-Related Injuries*. Elsevier; 2008.

32. Department of Defense. Directive Number 6025:21E: Medical Research for Prevention, Mitigation, and Treatment of Blast Injuries. Published July 5, 2006. Accessed October 2, 2021. https://www.esd.whs.mil/Portals/54/Documents/DD/issuances/dodd/602521p.pdf?ver=2018-10-24-112151-983

33. Leibovici D, Gofrit ON, Stein M, et al. Blast injuries: bus versus open-air bombings—a comparative study of injuries in survivors of open-air versus confined-space explosions. *J Trauma*. 1996;41:1030-1035.

34. Gutierrez de Ceballos JP, Turégano-Fuentes F, Perez-Diaz D, et al. The terrorist bomb explosions in Madrid, Spain—an analysis of the logistics, injuries sustained, and clinical management of casualties treated at the closest hospital. *Crit Care Med*. 2005;9:104-111.

35. Gutierrez de Ceballos JP, Turégano Fuentes F, Perez Diaz D, et al. Casualties treated at the closest hospital in the Madrid, March 11, terrorist bombings. *Crit Care Med*. 2005;34(Suppl 1):S107-S112.

36. Avidan V, Hersch M, Armon Y, et al. Blast lung injury: clinical manifestations, treatment, and outcome. *Am J Surg*. 2005;190:927-931.

37. Ritenour AE, Blackbourne LH, Kelly JF, et al. Incidence of primary blast injury in U.S. military overseas contingency operations: a retrospective study. *Ann Surg*. 2010;251(6):1140-1144.

38. Ritenour AE, Wickley A, Ritenour JS, et al. Tympanic membrane perforation and hearing loss from blast overpressure in Operation Enduring Freedom and Operation Iraqi Freedom wounded. *J Trauma*. 2008;64:S174-S178.

39. Zalewski T. Experimentelle Untersuchungen uber die Resistenzfahigkeit des Trommelfells. *Z Ohrenheilkd*. 1906;52:109.

40. Helling ER. Otologic blast injuries due to the Kenya embassy bombing. *Mil Med*. 2004;169:872-876.

41. Nixon RG, Stewart C. When things go boom: blast injuries. *Fire Engineering*. May 1, 2004.

42. National Association of Emergency Medical Technicians. Explosions and weapons of mass destruction. In: Pollak AN, ed. *PHTLS: Prehospital Trauma Life Support*. 9th ed. Jones & Bartlett Learning; 2018.

Suggested Reading

Alderman B, Anderson A. Possible effect of air bag inflation on a standing child. In: *Proceedings of 18th American Association of Automotive Medicine*. American Association of Automotive Medicine; 1974.

American College of Surgeons (ACS) Committee on Trauma. *Advanced Trauma Life Support Course*. ACS; 2018.

Anderson PA, Henley MB, Rivara P, et al. Flexion distraction and chance injuries to the thoracolumbar spine. *J Orthop Trauma*. 1991;5(2):153.

Anderson PA, Rivara FP, Maier RV, et al. The epidemiology of seatbelt-associated injuries. *J Trauma*. 1991;31(1):60.

Bartlett CS. Gunshot wound ballistics. *Clin Orthop*. 2003;408:28.

DePalma RG, Burris DG, Champion HR, et al. Current concepts: blast injuries. *N Engl J Med*. 2005;352:1335.

Di Maio VJM. *Gunshot Wounds: Practical Aspects of Firearms, Ballistics and Forensic Techniques*. CRC Press; 1999.

Garrett JW, Braunstein PW. The seat belt syndrome. *J Trauma*. 1962;2:220.

Huelke DF, Mackay GM, Morris A. Vertebral column injuries and lap-shoulder belts. *J Trauma*. 1995;38:547.

Huelke DF, Moore JL, Ostrom M. Air bag injuries and occupant protection. *J Trauma*. 1992;33(6):894.

Hunt JP, Marr AB, Stuke LE. Kinematics. In: Mattox KL, Moore EE, Feliciano DV, eds. *Trauma*. 7th ed. McGraw-Hill; 2013.

Joksch H, Massie D, Pichler R. *Vehicle Aggressivity: Fleet Characterization Using Traffic Collision Data*. Department of Transportation; 1998.

McSwain NE Jr, Brent CR. Trauma rounds: lipstick sign. *Emerg Med*. 1998;21:46.

McSwain NE Jr, Paturas JL. *The Basic EMT: Comprehensive Prehospital Patient Care*. 2nd ed. Mosby; 2001.

Ordog GJ, Wasserberger JN, Balasubramaniam S. Shotgun wound ballistics. *J Trauma*. 1922;28:624.

Oreskovich MR, Howard JD, Compass MK, et al. Geriatric trauma: injury patterns and outcome. *J Trauma*. 1984;24:565.

Rutledge R, Thomason M, Oller D, et al. The spectrum of abdominal injuries associated with the use of seat belts. *J Trauma*. 1991;31(6):820.

States JD, Annechiarico RP, Good RG, et al. A time comparison study of the New York State Safety Belt Use Law utilizing hospital admission and police accident report information. *Accid Anal Prev*. 1990;22(6):509.

Swierzewski MJ, Feliciano DV, Lillis RP, et al. Deaths from motor vehicle crashes: patterns of injury in restrained and unrestrained victims. *J Trauma*. 1994;37(3):404.

Sykes LN, Champion HR, Fouty WJ. Dum-dums, hollowpoints, and devastators: techniques designed to increase wounding potential of bullets. *J Trauma*. 1988;28:618.

현장 관리

Lead Editor
Matthew Levy, DO

학습 목표 이 장의 학습을 완료하면 다음과 같은 내용을 수행할 수 있다.

- 모든 응급 상황에서 공통으로 발생할 수 있는 생명과 안전에 대한 잠재적 위협을 확인할 수 있다.
- 주어진 시나리오에서 발생할 수 있는 잠재적인 위험을 설명할 수 있다.
- 현장 안전, 현장 상황 및 외상의 물리학 분석을 외상 환자 평가에 통합하여 환자의 처치를 결정할 수 있다.
- 안전에 대한 위협을 완화하기 위해 취해야 할 적절한 조치를 설명할 수 있다.
- 다수 사상자 사고(MCI) 시나리오(위험 물질, 대량살상무기)가 주어지면 현장 관리에 있어 중증도 분류 방법에 대해 논의하고 평가 결과에 따라 중증도를 분류할 수 있다.

시나리오

당신과 동료는 무더운 여름 새벽 2시 45분에 부부싸움을 하는 현장으로 출동했다. 가정집에 도착하자 부부가 큰 소리로 다투는 소리와 함께 아이들이 우는 소리가 들린다. 신고를 받고 경찰이 출동했지만, 아직 현장에 도착하지 않았다.

- 현장에 대한 어떤 우려 사항이 있는가?
- 환자와 접촉하기 전에 고려해야 할 중요한 사항은 무엇인가?

개요

병원 전 처치 제공자가 출동 요청을 받고 현장에 도착할 때 고려해야 할 여러 가지 우려 사항이 있다.

1. 현장 안전에 대한 사전 평가는 응급의료상황관리자가 제공하는 도착 전 정보를 바탕으로 출동하는 동안 시작한다. 이 평가에서는 동일한 현장에 대한 이전 대응, 경찰, 추가 EMS 지원팀과 같

은 다른 공공 안전 비상대응자의 필요성 및 화재 진압 또는 특수 구조팀을 포함한 기타 자원을 고려해야 한다.

2. 사고 현장에 도착하면 가장 먼저 해야 할 일은 전반적인 평가를 수행하는 것이다. 이 평가에는 1) 즉각적으로 조치를 시행해야 할 위험이나 현장이 EMS 실무자가 진입할 수 있을 만큼 충분히 안전한지 확인하고, 2) 처치 제공자와 환자의 안전을 보장하며,

3) 현재 상황에 따라 필요한 경우 환자 처치 변경을 결정하는 것이 포함된다. 이 평가에서 확인된 문제는 환자의 평가를 시작하기 전에 해결한다. 가해자가 있거나 위험 물질에 노출과 관련된 상황과 같은 일부 상황에서는 이 평가 과정이 더욱 중요해지며 수행해야 할 환자 처치의 방법과 유형을 변경할 수 있다.

현장 평가 및 재평가는 일회성이 아닌 지속적인 과정이다. 처치 제공자자 주변에서 발생하는 환경과 상황에 지속해 주의를 기울여야 한다. 처음에 안전하다고 판단한 사고 현장은 급변할 수 있으며 대응자는 상황이 변할 경우 지속적인 안전을 보장하기 위해 적절한 조치를 할 준비가 되어 있어야 한다.

3. 전체 현장 평가는 다수의 환자가 있는지 확인하는 데 도움이 된다. 현장에 한 명 이상의 환자가 발생한 경우 해당하는 상황은 다수 사상자 사고 또는 대량 사상자 사고로 분류된다. 다수 사상자 사고는 17장 재난관리에서 자세히 설명한다. 다수 사상자 사고 발생 시 환자 수가 가용 자원을 초과하면 모든 자원을 가장 심각하게 손상을 입은 환자에게 집중하는 것에서 최대한 많은 환자를 구하는 것으로 우선순위가 바뀐다. 이 장의 마지막 부문에서 설명하는 초기 축약된 분류(이 장의 마지막 부분에서 논의됨)는 피해자가 여러 명일 때 먼저 처치할 환자를 구별하고 우선순위를 정하는 데 도움이 된다. 환자 처치의 우선순위는 즉각적으로 사망을 초래할 수 있는 상태, 팔다리를 잃을 가능성이 있는 상태 그리고 생명이나 팔다리를 위협하지 않는 그 외의 모든 상태이다.

현장 평가

현장 평가는 응급의료전화상담원이 신고자에게 질문하여 정보를 수집하고 처리하거나 이미 현장에 있는 다른 공공 안전 부서에서 제공한 정보를 얻을 때 시작된다. 그런 다음 응급의료전화상담원은 사고 및 환자에 대한 초기 정보를 출동하는 EMS 팀에 전달한다.

현장으로 이동하는 동안 시간을 내어 좋은 의사소통 기술을 준비하고 연습하는 것이 잘 관리된 현장과 혼란스러운 현장의 차이일 수 있다. 상황을 인식하고 유지하는 것이 핵심이며 이를 위해서는 관찰력, 인식 및 의사소통 기술이 필요하다.

현장 정보 수집 과정은 EMS 팀원이 사고 현장에 도착하면서 시작된다. 환자와 접촉하기 전에 병원 전 처치 제공자는 다음을 수행하여 현장을 평가한다.

1. 현장 대응팀이나 환자에 대한 즉각적인 위험이나 위협이 있는지 확인하여 현장 안전을 위한 상황에 대한 전반적인 인상을 얻는다.
2. 사고의 원인(기전)과 결과(약해진 구조, 희생자 수 등)를 확인
3. 가족 및 목격자 관찰

현장의 모습은 전반적인 평가에 영향을 미치는 인상을 만드는 데 도움을 주며 상황 인식 목적의 기초 역할을 한다. 가능한 한 많은 정보를 보고, 듣고, 분류하는 것만으로도 풍부한 정보를 수집할 수 있다.

환자의 상태가 호전되거나 악화할 수 있는 것처럼 현장 상황도 빠르게 변할 수 있으므로 현장을 지속해서 모니터링하는 것이 중요하다. 상황이 어떻게 바뀔지 재평가하지 못하면 병원 전 처치 제공자와 환자 모두에게 심각한 결과를 초래할 수 있다.

현장 평가에는 안전과 상황이라는 중요한 두 가지 주요 구성 요소로 구성된다.

안전

모든 현장에 접근할 때 가장 먼저 고려해야 할 사항은 모든 EMS 팀원의 안전이다. EMS 팀원이 피해자가 되면 더 이상 다른 환자를 도울 수 없게 되고 환자 수가 늘어난다. 환자 처치는 EMS가 과도한 위험 없이 진입할 수 있을 정도로 현장이 안전해질 때까지 기다려야 할 수도 있다. 안전에 대한 우려는 환자의 체액과 감염성 물질에 노출되는 것과 같은 일반적인 사건부터 전쟁에 사용되는 화학 무기에 노출되는 것과 같은 드문 사건에 이르기까지 다양하다. 현장의 잠재적인 위험과 위험 요소에 대한 단서에는 혼잡한 고속도로를 달리는 차량, 총소리, 혈액 및 기타 체액의 존재와 같은 명백한 것뿐만 아니라 냄새나 연기와 같은 미묘한 발견도 포함된다.

현장 안전에는 EMS 팀원의 안전과 환자의 안전이 모두 포함된다. 일반적으로 위험한 상황에 부닥친 환자는 평가와 처치를 시작하기 전에 안전한 장소로 이동해야 하며 포괄적인 평가 전에 오염 제거와 같은 개입이 필요할 수 있다. 환자나 EMS 팀원의 안전에 위협이 되는 상황에는 미끄러운 바닥, 화재, 끊어진 전선, 폭발물, 위험 물질(체액, 차량, 홍수, 무기 포함) 및 환경 조건 등이 있다. 또한 가해자가 여전히 현장에 있을 수 있으며 환자나 EMS 팀원 또는 목격자에게 위협을 가할 수 있다. 그러나 총기 난사범이 현장에 있는 상황에서는 EMS가 경찰과 협력하여 가능한 한 빨리 현장에 진입하는 것이 환자의 생존

율을 향상한다는 점에 유의한다.

상황

현장의 안전 평가를 시행한 후 상황 평가를 시행한다. 상황 평가에는 병원 전 처치 제공자가 환자를 처치하는 방법에 영향을 미칠 수 있는 문제와 환자와 직접 관련된 사건 관련 문제가 모두 포함된다. 주어진 상황에서 제기된 문제를 평가할 때 고려해야 할 질문은 다음과 같다.

- 현장에서 실제로 무슨 일이 일어났는가? 어떤 상황에서 손상을 입었는가? 의도적이었는가 아니면 의도적이지 않았는가?
- 도움을 요청한 이유는 무엇이고 누가 요청했는가?
- 손상 기전은 무엇인가?(4장 외상의 물리학 참조) 대부분의 환자 손상은 사고와 관련된 외상의 물리학을 평가하고 이해함으로써 예측할 수 있다.
- 환자는 수는 몇 명이고 연령대는 어떻게 되는가?
- 현장 관리, 환자 처치 또는 환자 이송을 위해 추가 EMS 팀이 필요한가?
- 추가 인력이나 자원(예: 경찰, 소방, 전력회사 등)이 필요한가?
- 특수 구출 및 구조 장비가 필요한가?
- 헬기 이송이 필요한가?
- 환자 분류와 현장에서 의학적 문제를 지원하기 위해 의사가 필요한가?
- 의학적 문제(예: 운전자의 심장마비나 뇌졸중으로 인한 차량 충돌 등)가 외상을 유발한 요인이 되었는가?

현장 안전 및 상황과 관련된 문제는 상당 부분 중복되며 많은 안전과 관련된 문제는 특정 상황과 관련이 있고 특정 상황은 심각한 안전 위험을 초래할 수 있다. 이러한 문제는 다음 부문에서 자세히 설명한다.

안전 관리

교통안전

매년 사망하거나 손상을 입는 EMS 팀원의 대부분은 차량 관련 사고에 연루되어 있다(**그림 5-1**). 이러한 사망 및 손상의 대부분은 대응 단계에서 직접적인 구급차 충돌과 관련이 있지만, 일부는 차량 충돌사고 현장에서 작업 중에 발생한다. 여러 가지 요인으로 인해 병원 전 처치 제공자가 차량 충돌사고 현장에서 손상을 입거나 사망할 수 있다(**그림 5-2**). 기상 조건이나 도로 설계와 같은 일부 요인은 변경할

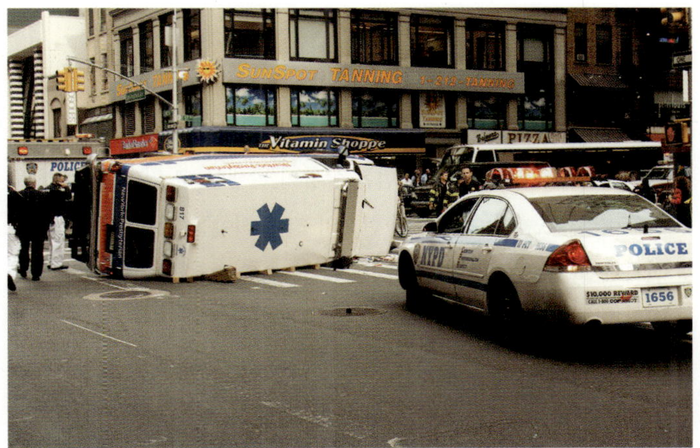

그림 5-1 매년 사망하거나 손상을 입는 EMS 팀원의 대부분은 차량 관련 사고에 연루되어 있다.
© Robert Brenner/PhotoEdit

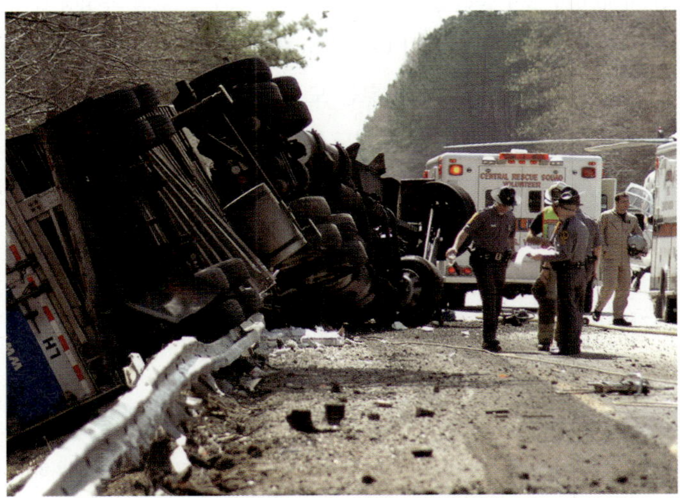

그림 5-2 손상을 입거나 사망한 병원 전 처치 제공자 중 상당수가 차량 충돌사고 현장에서 일하고 있었다.
© Jeff Thrower (We⊃ Thrower)/Shutterstock

수 없지만, EMS 팀원은 이러한 조건이 존재한다는 사실을 인지하고 이러한 상황에서 존재하는 위험을 완화하기 위해 적절하게 행동해야 한다.

날씨/빛 조건

차량 충돌사고에 대한 많은 병원 전 처치 제공자의 대응은 대부분 악천후와 야간에 이루어진다. 겨울철에 노면 결빙, 눈이 쌓이거나 안개, 폭풍우와 같은 기타 기상 조건으로 인해 마주 오는 차량이 현장에 주차된 구급차나 EMS 팀원을 피하고자 제때 멈추지 못할 수 있어 더욱 복잡해진다.

고속도로 설계

접근이 제한된 고속도로는 많은 양의 교통량을 효율적으로 이동할 수 있게 해주지만, 충돌 사고가 발생하면 교통 체증으로 인해 모든 구급대원 및 구조대원에게 위험한 상황이 발생할 수 있다. 오르막 도로와 고가도로는 마주 오는 운전자의 전방 시야를 제한할 수 있으며 운전자가 고가도로의 정점에 도달했을 때 도로에 정차한 차량과 구급대원 및 구조대원을 마주칠 수 있다. 경찰관은 접근이 제한된 고속도로를 완전히 폐쇄하는 것을 꺼릴 수 있으며 차량 흐름을 유지하기 위해 노력한다. 이러한 접근 방식은 응급 구조요원에게 추가 위험을 초래하는 것처럼 보일 수 있지만, 교통 체증으로 인한 추가 추돌 사고를 예방할 수 있다.

지방도로는 독특한 문제를 안고 있다. 교통량은 도시 도로보다 훨씬 적지만, 구불구불하고 좁고 언덕이 많은 일부 도로의 특성상 운전자는 위험할 정도로 가까이 다가가기 전까지는 차량 충돌사고 현장을 보지 못한다. 또한 시골 도로는 도시 지역 도로보다 유지 관리가 잘되지 않아 폭풍이 지나간 후에도 미끄러운 상태가 지속될 수 있으며 이에 따라 의심하지 않는 운전자가 방심할 수 있다. 차량 충돌사고를 일으켰던 눈, 노면 빙결 또는 안개 지역이 여전히 존재할 수 있으며 EMS 현장 도착을 방해할 수 있고 마주 오는 운전자에게 최적의 조건이 아닐 수 있다.

위험 완화 방안

병원 전 처치 제공자는 하루 중 언제 어떤 기상 조건에서도 대응해야 한다. 따라서 차량 충돌사고 현장에서 일하는 동안 피해자가 될 위험을 줄이려는 조치를 취해야 한다. 가장 좋은 방법은 특히 접근이 제한된 고속도로에서 출동하는 구급대원 및 구조대원의 수를 제한하는 것이다. 현장에 출동하는 인원은 당면한 작업을 수행하는 데 필요한 인원만 배치해야 한다. 예를 들어, 환자 한 명이 있는 사고 현장에 구급차 3대와 지휘 차량 1대가 있으면 구급대원이나 구조대원이 차량에 치일 위험이 많이 증가한다.

야광 의류

EMS 팀원이 마주 오는 차량에 치이는 대부분의 경우 운전자는 도로에서 EMS 팀원을 보지 못했다고 진술한다. 가시성을 높이려면 낮이든 밤이든 모든 차량 충돌사고 현장에서는 가시성이 높은 안전복(야광 의류)을 착용해야 한다. 일부 기관에서는 모든 출동 시 EMS

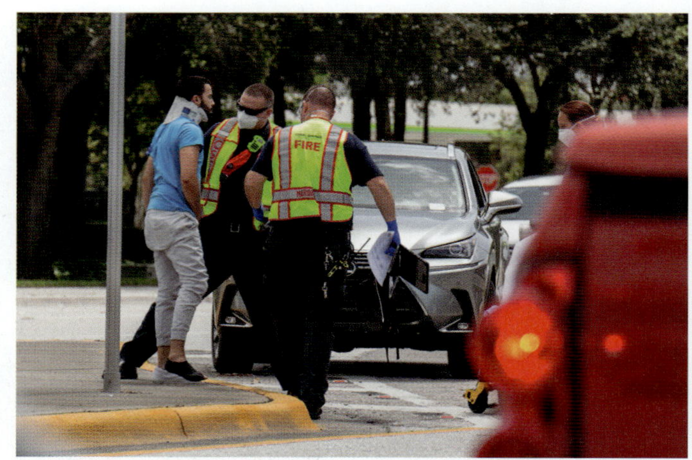

그림 5-3 미국표준협회 2등급 또는 3등급 반사 조끼는 도로에서 발상한 사고에 대응하는 사람들에게 안전성을 제공한다.
© YES Market Media/Shutterstock

팀원이 차량에서 내릴 때 눈에 잘 띄는 조끼를 착용하도록 요구하는 정책을 시행하고 있다. 미국 화재예방협회(NFPA), 산업안전보건청(OSHA), 국제 안전 장비협회는 모두 고속도로에서 작업할 때 착용해야 하는 야광 의류에 대한 표준을 가지고 있다. 미국 산업안전보건청은 고속도로에서 작업하는 근로자를 위한 3단계 보호 기준을 가지고 있으며 가장 높은 수준(3단계)은 고속도로에서 야간에 사용하도록 규정하고 있다. 미 연방고속도로국은 정부 지원금을 받는 고속도로에서 사고에 대응할 때 모든 응급 구조대원을 포함한 모든 작업자가 미국표준협회(ANSI) 2등급 또는 3등급 반사 조끼(**그림 5-3**)를 착용하도록 의무화했다. 외부 재킷에 반자 소재를 부착하거나 승인된 반사 조끼를 착용하면 미국표준협회 표준을 충족할 수 있다.

구급차 위치 및 경고 장치

구급차 내 장비의 위치도 안전에 중요한 역할을 한다. 사용하는 장비는 차도에 들어가지 않고도 수거할 수 있도록 배치해야 한다. EMS 기관에는 차량을 현장에 주차하는 방법과 위치에 관한 구체적인 정책과 절차가 있는 경우가 많다. 일부 조정된 EMS 시스템에서는 소방차와 같은 완충 차량을 사용하여 차선을 차단할 수 있다.

사고 지휘관 또는 안전 책임자는 병원 전 처치 제공자를 보호할 수 있는 최적의 위치에 대응 차량을 배치해야 한다. 사고 현장에 가장 먼저 도착한 긴급 차량이 사고 현장의 차선을 확보하는 것이 중요하다(**그림 5-4**). 구급차를 사고 현장 뒤에 배치해도 환자를 쉽게 실을 수는 없지만, 다가오는 차량으로부터 병원 전 처치 제공자와 환자를

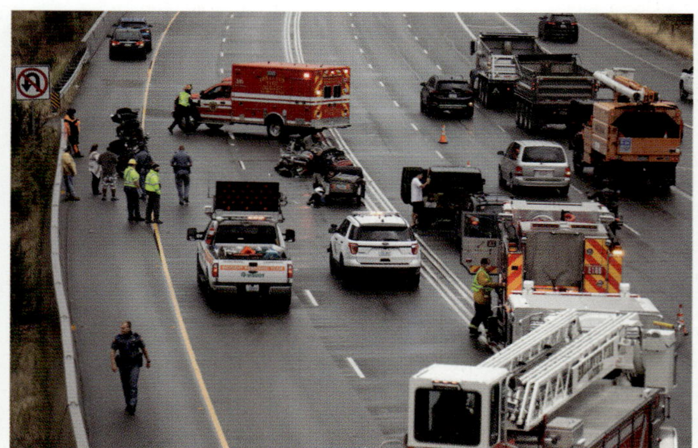

그림 5-4 긴급 차량의 올바른 위치
© VDB Photos/Shutterstock

보호할 수 있다. 긴급 차량이 추가로 도착하면 일반적으로 사고가 발생한 도로의 같은 쪽에 배치해야 한다. 이러한 차량은 사고 지점으로부터 멀리 배치하여 마주 오는 차량의 운전자에게 경고 시간을 늘려야 한다.

전조등, 특히 차량의 상향등을 깜박이는 비상 경고 시스템은 사고 현장을 비추는 데 필요한 경우가 아니라면 접근하는 운전자의 시야를 가리지 않도록 꺼야 한다. 현장에서 사용하는 경고등의 수를 확인해야 한다. 경고등이 너무 많으면 다가오는 운전자를 혼란스럽게 할 수 있다. 많은 부서에서 운전자에게 충분한 경고를 제공하기 위해 "전방에 사고가 발생했다"는 경고 표지판을 사용한다. 운전자에게 경고를 하고 차량 흐름을 유도하기 위해 야광봉이나 조명탄을 배치할 수 있지만, 건조한 환경에서는 화재를 예방하기 위해 주의해야 한다. 반사 콘은 비상 상황이 발생한 차선에서 차량 흐름을 유도하는 역할을 할 수 있다(**그림 5-5**).

실무자는 도로 작업의 모든 단계에서 안전에 대한 경계를 늦추지 말아야 한다. 여기에는 차량에서 내리기 전에 모든 방향을 확인하는 것이 포함된다. 구급차에서 내릴 때 절대로 차가 주행하는 차선을 따라 옆문을 사용하여 환자 칸에서 내리지 않는다. 부득이하게 문을 열어야 하는 경우에는 뒷문을 이용하고 문을 열기 전에 창밖을 확인한다. 긴급 차량에서 내릴 때는 사다리에서 내릴 때와 마찬가지로 항상 3개의 접촉 지점을 유지한다. 3개의 접촉 지점은 핸드레일, 문 및 계단(손 2개 + 발 1개) 차량과 접촉하는 3개의 지점이다.

차량을 통제해야 하는 경우 경찰이나 교통 통제에 대한 특수 교육을 받은 직원이 이 작업을 처리하여 EMS가 환자 처치에 집중할 수

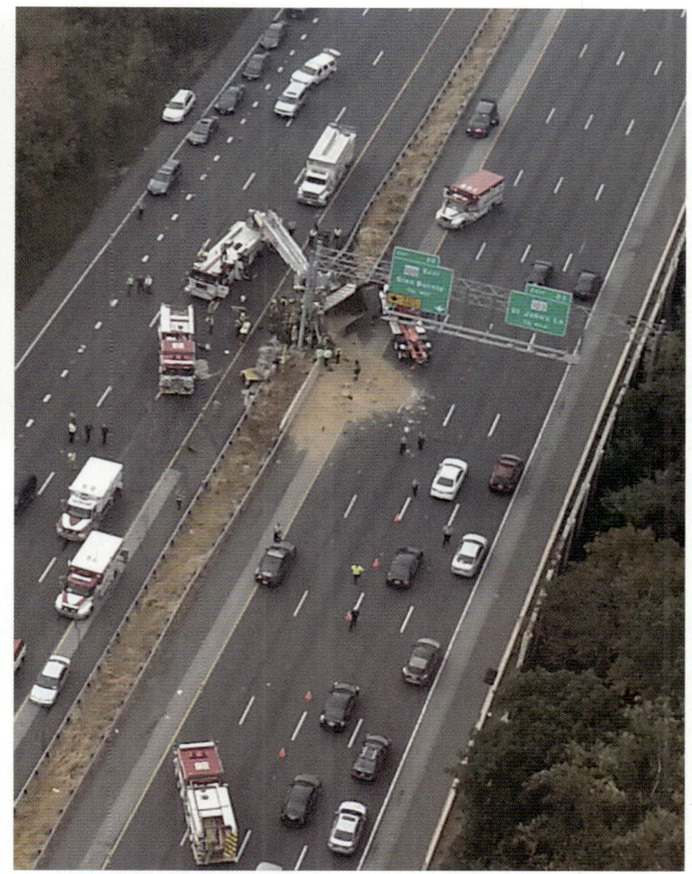

그림 5-5 교통 상황 표지판 설치
Courtesy of Andrew Pollak, MD.

있도록 해야 한다. 운전자에게 혼란스럽거나 모순되는 지침을 제공하면 추가적인 안전 위험이 발생할 수 있다. 교통이 방해받지 않고 사고 현장 주변에서 차량 흐름을 유지할 수 있을 때 최상의 상황이 만들어진다.

교통안전 교육

차량 충돌사고 현장에서 병원 전 처치 제공자에게 안전한 운전에 대해 교육하기 위해 고안된 여러 가지 교육 프로그램을 이용할 수 있다. 각 EMS 기관은 조직은 이러한 프로그램의 적용을 위해 미국 고속도로 교통안전국(NHTSA) 또는 산업보건안전청(OSHA)에 문의하여 이러한 프로그램의 현지 이용 가능 여부를 확인하고 연간 필수 교육 프로그램에 포함시킨다. NAEMT의 EMS 안전 과정은 구급대원과 구조대원들의 안전 사고 방식을 개발하고 기관 내 안전 문화를 장려할 수 있도록 준비시켜 병원 전 처치 제공자가 차량 충돌사고 현장에서 대응 및 지역사회 출동 중이거나 상관없이 모든 구조 및 구급대원을 교육한다.

폭력

출동할 때마다 병원 전 처치 제공자는 감정적으로 격양된 환경에 처할 가능성이 있다. 일부 EMS 기관에서는 병원 전 처치 제공자가 폭력 현장에 들어가기 전에 경찰의 출동을 요청하는 정책을 시행하고 있다. 위협적이지 않은 것처럼 보이는 현장도 폭력으로 악화할 가능성이 있으므로 병원 전 처치 제공자는 항상 변화하는 상황을 암시하는 미묘한 단서에 주의를 기울여야 한다. 환자나 가족, 현장에 있는 다른 사람들은 상황을 이성적으로 판단하지 못할 수 있다. 이러한 사람들은 출동 시간이 너무 길다고 생각할 수 있고 말이나 행동에 지나치게 민감할 수 있으며 환자 평가에 대해 표준화되고 체계적인 접근 방식을 오해할 수 있다. 존중과 관심을 보여주면서 자신감 있고 전문가적인 태도를 유지하는 것은 환자의 신뢰를 얻고 현장을 통제하는 데 중요하다.

EMS 팀원은 현장을 관찰할 수 있도록 스스로 훈련하는 것이 중요하다. 여기에는 현장에 도착했을 때 환자의 수와 위치, 현장을 드나드는 구경꾼의 움직임, 스트레스나 긴장의 징후, EMS의 존재에 대한 예상치 못 한 비정상적인 반응 또는 기타 직관적인 느낌을 알아차리는 방법을 배우는 것이 포함된다. 안전에 가장 큰 위험을 초래하는 것은 누군가의 손이므로 항상 환자와 구경꾼의 손을 주의 깊게 관찰한다. 누군가가 무기를 소지하고 있거나 계절에 맞지 않는 옷을 입고 있거나 무기를 쉽게 숨길 수 있는 큰 옷을 입고 있다는 징후가 있는지 살펴본다. 필요한 경우 환자의 행동을 쉽게 관찰할 수 없는 곳에 환자를 두지 말고 환자를 찾기 위해 사람들을 따라간다. 위협이 감지되면 즉시 현장을 떠날 준비를 한다. 구급차에서 평가 또는 절차를 완료해야 할 수도 있다. 병원 전 처치 제공자의 안전이 최우선이다. 가능하면 현장에서 대피할 수 있는 대체 방법을 포함하는 출구 또는 탈출 전략을 항상 마련하는 것이 중요하다.

다음과 같은 상황을 생각해 본다. 당신과 동료는 환자의 집 거실에 있다. 동료가 환자의 혈압을 측정하는 동안 술에 취한 것으로 보이는 사람이 방으로 들어온다. 그는 화가 난 것처럼 보였고 당신은 그의 허리춤에서 총 손잡이처럼 보이는 것이 튀어나온 것을 발견했다. 당신의 동료는 환자에게 집중하고 있기 때문에 이 사람이 방에 들어오는 것을 보거나 듣지 못한다. 의심스러운 사람은 당신을 의심하기 시작하고 당신의 근무복과 배지에 대해 극도로 불안해한다. 그의 손이 반복적으로 허리 쪽으로 왔다 갔다 한다. 그는 서성거리며 혼자 중얼거리기 시작했다. 당신과 동료는 이러한 상황에 어떻게 대비할 수 있는가?

폭력적인 현장 관리

당신과 동료는 폭력적인 환자나 구경꾼을 다루는 방법에 대해 논의 및 합의해야 한다. 사건 중에 해결할 수 있는 방법을 개발하려는 시도는 실패하기 쉽다. 동료는 응급상황에 대비하여서 미리 약속된 단어 및 수신호뿐만 아니라 직접 확인하는 방식을 사용할 수 있다.

- 실제 병원 전 처치 제공자의 역할은 환자 평가를 담당하고 환자에게 필요한 처치를 시행하는 것이다. 환자와 직접 접촉하지 않는 동료는 현장을 관찰하고 가족이나 목격자와 대화하고 필요한 정보를 수집하며 더 나은 출입로를 만들기 위해 노력한다. 본질적으로 환자와 접촉하지 않는 의료진은 현장을 감시하므로 동료가 환자에게만 집중할 수 있다. 병원 전 처치 제공자 모두가 환자에게만, 집중하면 현장이 빠르게 위험해질 수 있으며 초기 단서를 놓칠 수 있다. 한 명의 병원 전 처처 제공자가 환자와 상호작용하고 환자를 평가하기 시작하면 다른 병원 전 처치 제공자는 상황 인식을 유지하고 현장을 관찰하며 안전 문제가 발생할 경우 조기에 개입할 수 있다. 상황 인식을 높이면 병원 전 단계에서 병원 전 처치 제공자의 폭력적인 상황에서 대응 방법을 결정할 때 시간을 벌 수 있다.

- 미리 약속된 암호와 수신호를 사용하면 동료가 다른 사람에게 우려를 알리지 않고도 위협을 전달할 수 있다. 예를 들어 한 EMS 팀원이 환자의 동료가 무언가를 꺼내기 위해 캐비닛에 의심스럽게 손을 뻗는 것을 발견하고 암호와 수신호를 사용하여 다른 EMS 팀원에게 잠재적인 위험을 알린다. 이러한 사전 통지는 잠재적인 가해자의 의심을 불러일으키지 않으면서도 두 EMS 팀원이 모두 대응하고 도움이나 탈출을 요청할 수 있는 시간을 줄일 수 있다. 이 방법은 두 EMS 팀원이 모두 암호를 기억하고 실행 연습을 한 경우에만 효과적이다.

만약 팀원 모두가 환자에게 집중하고 있다면 현장에서 즉시 위협이 될 초기 단서를 놓칠 수 있다. 많은 상황에서 병원 전 처치 제공자가 환자를 평가하고 다른 팀원이 현장을 관찰하면 환자, 가족 그리고 목격자의 긴장 및 불안이 즉시 감소하기 시작한다.

위험해진 현장을 처리하는 방법에는 다음과 같은 다양한 방법이 있다.

1. 현장에 진입하지 않는다. 알려진 폭력적인 현장에 출동하는 경우 경찰관이 현장을 안전하게 만들고 위험이 제거될 때까지 안전한 장소에서 대기한다.

2. 후퇴한다. 현장에 접근할 때 위험이 존재하는 경우 차량으로 후퇴하여 현장을 떠나 안전한 장소에 대기하고 현장 상황을 담당

자에게 알린다.

3. 긴장 완화. 환자를 처치하는 동안 위협적인 현장 상황이 발생하면 언어적 방법을 사용하여 긴장과 공격성을 줄이면서 현장을 떠날 준비를 한다.

4. 방어한다. 최후의 수단으로 병원 전 처치 제공자는 자신을 방어해야 할 필요가 있을 수 있다. 이러한 방어 노력은 공격자와의 관계를 끊고 도망치는 것이 중요하다. 공격적인 사람을 추격하거나 제압하려고 시도하지 말고 경찰에 신고하여 협조를 요청하고 도움을 받는다.

적극적인 공격자

총기 난사범이나 가해자와 관련된 상황이 너무 빈번하게 발생하고 있다. 이러한 유형의 사고로 인해 발생한 손상으로 인한 환자 처치의 결과를 개선하기 위해 EMS 기관은 일반적으로 발생하는 것보다 훨씬 더 일찍 현장에 진입하기 위해 경찰관과 협력하는 추세가 증가하고 있다. 이럴 때 경찰관으로 구성된 대응팀이 현장에 출동하여 위협을 무력화한다. EMS 및 경찰관은 대응팀을 따라가 피해자를 신속하게 파악하고 처치를 시작한다[자세한 내용은 22장 민간 전술 응급의료 지원(TEMS)을 참조]. 이러한 프로그램에는 광범위한 계획, 교육 및 조정이 필요하다는 점에 유의해야 한다. 특별한 훈련과 훈련을 받지 않은 EMS 및 경찰관으로 구성된 즉흥적인 혼합 팀을 구성하는 것은 권장하지 않는다.

상황 문제

병원 전 처치 제공자가 환자에게 제공할 수 있는 의료서비스에 중대한 영향을 미칠 수 있는 여러 가지 상황 문제가 있다.

범죄 현장

병원 전 처치 제공자가 만나는 외상 환자는 고의적인 손상을 당했을 수 있다. 총격이나 흉기에 찔리는 것 외에도 환자들은 주먹이나 둔기로 폭행을 당하거나 목을 조르는 시도를 당했을 수 있다. 다른 경우에는 피해자가 고의로 차량에 치이거나 구조물에서 밀려나거나 움직이는 차량 밖으로 밀려나 심각한 손상을 입었을 수 있다. 차량 충돌 사고 운전자 중 한 명이 음주 또는 약물 복용, 난폭 운전, 과속 또는 운전 중 문자 메시지를 보낸 것으로 판단되는 경우 교통사고라도 범죄 현장으로 간주할 수 있다.

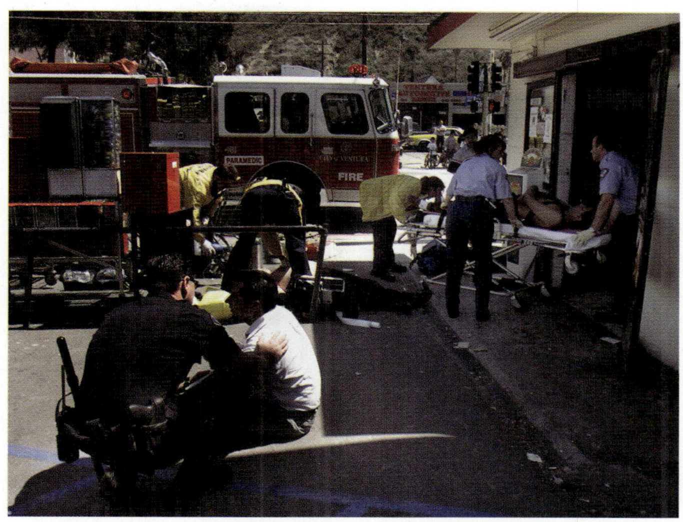

그림 5-6 병원 전 처치 제공자는 종종 범죄 현장에서 환자를 평가하고 처치를 수행하며 증거를 보존하기 위해 경찰관과 협력해야 한다. 범죄 현장의 혼란을 피하되 환자 처치 제공을 지연시켜서는 안 된다.

이러한 유형의 환자를 처치할 때 병원 전 처치 제공자는 종종 경찰관과 협조한다(**그림 5-6**). EMS와 경찰 모두 환자의 생명을 보호한다는 목표를 공유하지만, 범죄 현장에서는 때때로 두 기관의 임무가 충돌하는 경우가 있다. EMS 팀원은 피해자의 생명과 생존 가능성을 평가해야 할 필요성에 초점을 맞추지만, 경찰관은 범죄 현장에서 증거를 보존하거나 가해자를 사범 처리하는 것에 더 관심이 있다. 법 집행 및 범죄 수사가 적절한 환자 처치를 방해해서는 안 된다. 환자 평가 또는 처치를 위해 어떤 식으로든 현장을 그대로 보존하지 않는 경우 기록하고 경찰관에게 관련 내용을 전달하는 것이 필수적이다. 범죄 현장의 불필요한 방해를 최소화하기 위해 노력해야 하지만, 환자 처치를 지연시키는 방식은 절대로 해서는 안 된다.

범죄 현장에서 경찰관이 취하는 일반적인 접근 방식에 대한 인식을 키우면 병원 전 처치 제공자는 환자를 도울 수 있을 뿐만 아니라 경찰관과 더 효과적으로 협력하여 환자의 가해자를 체포할 수 있다. 주요 범죄(예: 살인, 의심스러운 사망, 강간, 교통사고 사망)가 발생한 현장에서 대부분의 경찰관은 증거를 수집하고 처리한다. 경찰관은 일반적으르 다음과 같은 업무를 수행한다.

- 현장을 조사하여 무기와 탄피를 포함한 모든 증거를 확인한다.
- 현장을 사진으로 촬영한다.
- 현장을 스케치한다.
- 현장에 출입한 모든 사람을 기록한다.

- 모든 잠재적 증거를 찾기 위해 현장 전체를 더욱 철저하게 수색한다.
- 지문이나 DNA 증거가 포함될 수 있는 물품(예: 담배꽁초, 머리카락, 섬유조직)을 찾아서 수집한다.

경찰 수사관들은 범죄 현장에 들어오는 모든 사람이 어떤 종류의 증거를 현장으로 가져오고 자신도 모르게 현장에서 일부 증거를 훼손한다고 믿는다. 범죄를 해결하기 위한 수사관의 목표는 가해자가 두고 간 증거를 확인하는 것이다. 이를 위해 수사관은 다른 경찰관, 구급 및 구조대원, 시민 및 현장에 들어갔을 수 있는 모든 사람이 남기거나 훼손한 모든 증거를 파악해야 한다. 주의를 기울이지 않는 범죄 범죄 현장에 출동한 병원 전 처치 제공자는 주의를 기울이지 않으면 중요한 증거를 방해, 파괴 또는 오염시켜 범죄 수사를 방해할 수 있다.

경우에 때라 병원 전 처치 제공자는 경찰관 보다 먼저 잠재적인 범죄 현장에 도착한다. 피해자가 사망한 것이 명백한 경우 병원 전 처치 제공자는 어떤 물건도 건드리지 말고 조심스럽게 해당 위치에서 벗어나 경찰관이 도착할 때까지 기다려야 한다. 범죄 현장이 방해받지 않기를 바라지만, 수사관들은 환자에게 접근하고 생존 가능성을 판단하기 위해 시신을 뒤집거나 범죄 현장에서 물건을 옮겨야 하는 상황도 있다는 것을 알고 있다. 병원 전 처치 제공자가 경찰관이 도착하기 전에 현장에서 환자를 이송하거나 시신 또는 기타 물체를 이동해야 하는 경우 수사관은 일반적으로 다음 사항을 확인한다.

- 현장이 언제 변경되었는가?
- 이동의 목적은 무엇이었는가?
- 누가 현장을 변경했는가?
- EMS 팀원이 환자의 사망을 확인한 시간은 언제인가?

병원 전 처치 제공자가 경찰관보다 먼저 범죄 현장에 진입한 경우 수사관은 병원 전 처치 제공자의 행동이나 관찰에 대해 면담하고 공식적인 진술을 받을 수 있다. 병원 전 처치 제공자는 이러한 요청에 놀라거나 걱정해서는 안 된다. 면담의 목적은 병원 전 처치 제공자의 행동을 비판하는 것이 아니라 수사관이 사건을 해결하는 데 도움이 될 수 있는 정보를 얻기 위한 것이다. 병원 전 처치 제공자가 장갑을 끼지 않고 범죄 현장의 물건을 만지거나 취급한 경우 수사관은 병원 전 처치 제공자에게 지문 채취를 요청할 수 있다.

환자의 의복을 적절히 처리하면 귀중한 증거를 보존할 수 있다. 환자의 옷을 제거해야 하는 경우 경찰관과 검시관은 병원 전 처치 제공자가 옷에 총알이나 칼 구멍을 자르는 행위를 하지 않는 것을 선호한다. 옷이 잘린 경우 경찰관은 옷에 어떤 변경이 있었는지, 누가 변경했는지, 변경 사유를 물어볼 수 있다. 제거한 옷은 비닐봉지가 아닌 종이봉투에 넣어 경찰관에게 제출해야 한다.

폭력 범죄 피해자와 관련된 마지막 중요한 문제 중 하나는 병원 전 처치 제공자의 처치를 받는 동안 한 진술의 가치이다. 일부 환자는 손상의 심각성을 깨닫고 손상을 입힌 사람을 병원 전 처치 제공자에게 말할 수 있다. 이 정보는 기록되어 수사관에게 전달해야 한다. 가능하면 병원 전 처치 제공자는 환자가 가해자에 관한 정보를 제공할 수 있는 경우 경찰관이 입회할 수 있도록 환자 손상의 심각성을 경찰관에게 알려야 한다. 이를 "임종시 진술"이라고 한다.

유해 물질

유해 물질에 노출될 위험은 유해 물질 노출될 가능성이 있는 환경을 인식하는 것만큼 간단하지 않다. 현대 사회에는 유해 물질이 널리 퍼져 있다. 차량, 건물 및 가정에 유해 물질이 포함된 경우가 점점 더 많아지고 있다. 유해 물질 외에도 이 논의는 대량살상무기에 대해서도 같게 적용된다. 이러한 위험은 매우 다양한 형태로 존재하므로 모든 병원 전 처치 제공자는 최소한의 위험 물질 인식 교육을 받아야 한다. 유해 물질은 종종 환경 파괴 물질(HazMat)이라고 한다.

위험 물질 교육에는 네 가지 일반적인 수준이 있다.

- **인식(Awareness)**: 이 교육은 응급의료 대응자에게 제공되는 4단계 교육 중 첫 번째 단계이며 위험 물질 사고에 대한 기본적인 지식을 제공하도록 설계되어 있다.
- **운영(Operations)**: 운영 수준 교육은 위험 물질 사건을 통제하는 데 도움이 되는 교육과 지식을 제공하므로 모든 응급의료 대응자에게 유용하다. 이 응급의료 대응자는 주변 및 안전 구역을 설정하도록 훈련되어 사고의 확산을 제한한다.
- **기술자(Technician)**: 기술자는 위험지역 내에서 작업하고 위험 물질의 방출을 막도록 훈련을 받았다.
- **전문가(Specialist)**: 전문가 수준의 응급의료 대응자가 위험 물질 사고의 관리 및 대응에 대한 전문 지식을 갖추었음을 나타낸다.

현장 평가

모든 현장에서 최우선 순위는 병원 전 처치 제공자의 안전이므로 중요한 첫 번째 단계는 위험 물질 노출 가능성이 있는지 현장을 평가하는 것이다. 출동 시 제공된 정보를 통해 위험 물질을 의심할 수 있는 높은 의심 지수를 설정할 수 있다. 호흡곤란이나 발작 등 유사한 증상을 보이는 다수의 환자와 관련된 출동은 위험 물질 노출 가능성을 제기해야 한다.

현장에 위험 물질이 있다고 판단되면 현장의 안전을 확보하고 적절한 도움을 요청하여 관련 지역을 안전하게 격리하고 노출된 환자와 개인을 구조하고 오염을 제거하는 데 초점을 맞춰야 한다. 일반적인 원칙은 현장이 안전하지 않다면 안전하게 만드는 것이다. 병원 전 처치 제공자가 현장을 안전하게 만들 수 없는 경우 도움을 요청해야 한다. 미국 교통부에서 제작한 비상대응가이드북(ERG) 또는 화학물질 비상대응서비스 기관에 연락하면 잠재적 위험을 확인하는 데 유용하다(그림 5-7). 이 가이드북(및 관련 앱)은 위험 물질의 이름이나 식별 플래카드 번호로 물질을 구별할 수 있는 간단한 시스템을 사용한다. 그런 다음 텍스트는 구급대원과 구조대원을 위한 안전거리, 생명 및 화재 위험, 환자가 호소할 수 있는 증상에 대한 기본 정보를 제공하는 페이지를 독자에게 소개한다.

쌍안경을 사용하여 멀리서 라벨을 확인한다. 쌍안경을 사용하지 않고 라벨을 읽을 수 있다면 병원 전 처치 제공자가 너무 가까이 있어 노출될 가능성이 높다. 엄지손가락을 쭉 뻗었을 때 사고 현장 전체가 가려지지 않는다면 너무 가까이 있는 것이다.

위험 물질이 노출된 현장에서는 현장의 안전이 보장되어야 한다. 아무도 들어가지 말고 아무도 나가지 않는다. 대기 지역은 바람이 불어오는 방향(바람을 안고)에 위험 요소로부터 안전한 거리에 설치해야 한다. 위험 물질 전문가가 현장에 도착할 때까지 현장 출입을 금지해야 한다. 대부분의 경우 환자 처치는 현장에서 오염을 제거한 후 병원 전 처치 제공자에게 인계하면 시작된다.

병원 전 처치 제공자가 위험 물질이 노출된 현장에서 사고 현장 현장지휘체계와 구조를 이해하는 것이 중요하다(그림 5-8). 대량살상무기나 위험 물질과 관련된 사고 현장은 일반적으로 오염지역[직접적인 위험지역(Hot Zone)], 전방통제지역(Warm Zone), 안전지대(Cold Zone)로 구분한다. 각 구역의 기능에 대한 설명은 18장 폭발 및 대량살상무기 무기를 참조한다.

규모가 크고 복합한 위험 물질 사고 현장에서 오염지역(위험지역)에 진입할 위험 물질 팀원들을 위해 응급 의료 대기 및 지원 서비스를 제공하라는 요청을 받는 경우도 종종 있다.

대량살상무기(WMD)

대량살상무기 관련 현장에 대한 대응은 앞서 설명한 바와 같이 위험 물질 관련 현장에 대한 대응과 유사한 안전 및 기타 우려 사항을 가지고 있다.

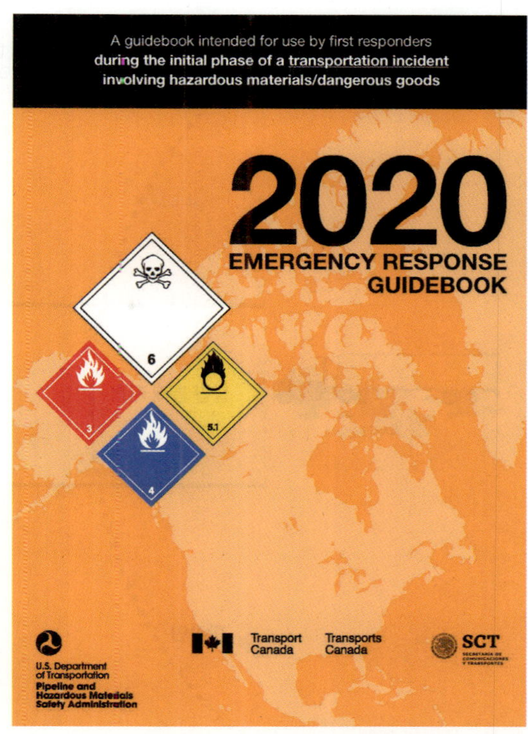

그림 5-7 미국 교통부에서 제작한 비상대응가이드북(ERG)은 잠재적 위험 물질 사고 현장에서 중요한 정보를 제공한다. 비상대응가이드북은 스마트폰용 앱으로도 제공된다.

Reproduced from J.S. Department of Transportation, Transport Canada, and Secretariat of Communications and Transport of Mexico. 2020 Emergency Response Guidebook. Pipeline and Hazardous Materials Safety Administration, U.S. Department of Transportation, 2020. https://www.phmsa.dot.gov/sites/phmsa.dot.gov/files/2021-01/ERG2020-WEB.pdf

다수의 피해자가 발생한 모든 현장, 특히 피해자들이 유사한 증상을 호소하거나 폭발로 인한 것으로 보고된 경우 1) 대량살상무기가 관련되었는가? 2) 구급대원과 구조대원에게 해를 가하기 위한 이차 장치가 있을 수 있는가?(자세한 내용은 18장 폭발 및 대량살상무기를 참조).

피해자가 되지 않으려면 병원 전 처치 제공자는 이러한 현장에서 극도로 조심스럽게 접근하고 피해자를 처치하기 위해 서두르고 싶은 충동을 억제해야 한다. 대신 병원 전 처치 제공자는 바람이 부는 방향에서 현장에 접근하여 잠시 멈춰 서서 대량살상무기의 존재 가능성을 나타내는 단서가 있는지 살펴보고 귀를 기울여야 한다. 물질의 특성이 확인될 때까지 젖은 물질이나 마른 물질, 눈에 보이는 증기 및 연기에 명백하게 유출되는 것을 피해야 한다. 밀폐된 공간이나 제한된 공간은 적절한 교육과 개인보호장비(PPE) 없이는 절대로 들어가서는 안 된다(위험 물질 및 대량살상무기 사고 발생 시 개인보호장비 착용에 대한 자세한 내용은 18장 폭발 및 대량살상무기를 참조).

대량살상무기가 가능한 원인에 포함되면 병원 전 처치 제공자는

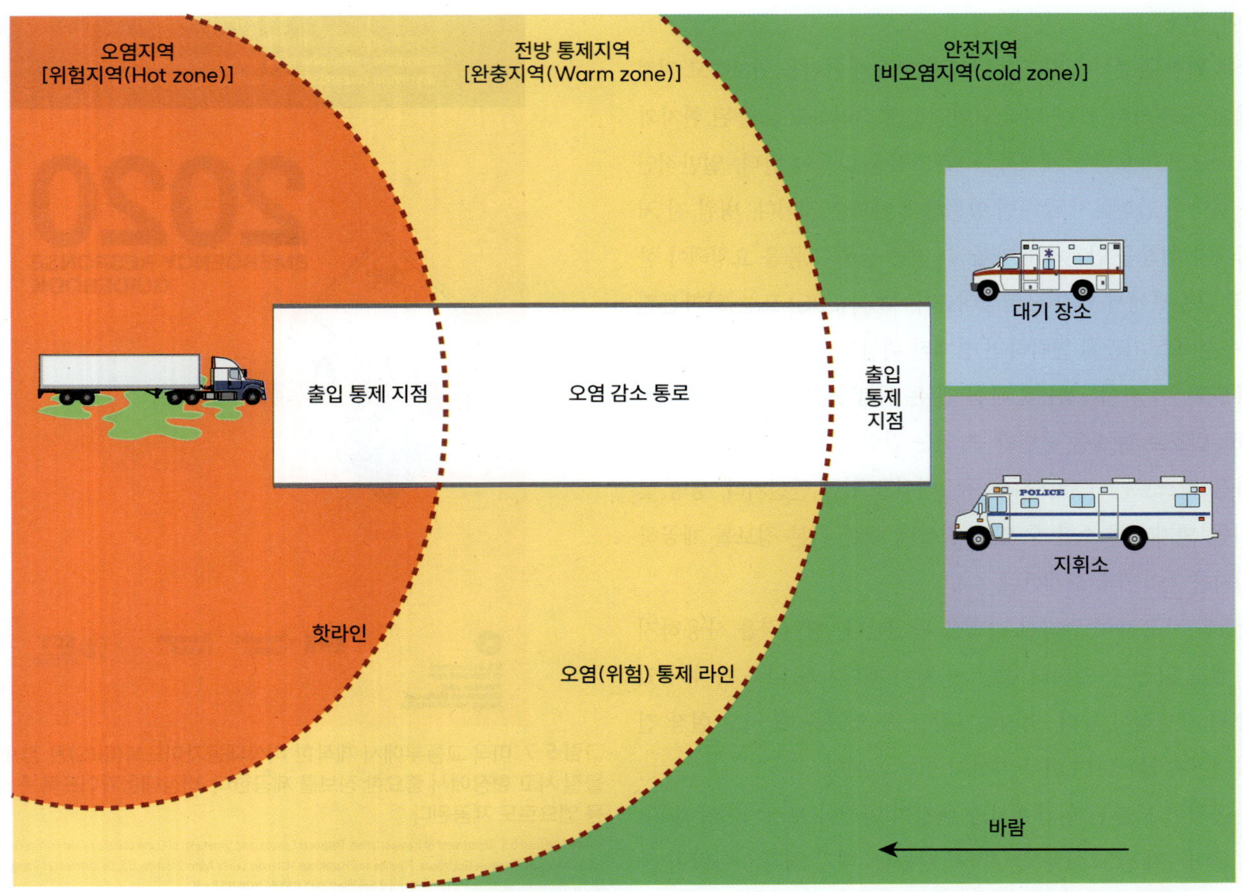

그림 5-8 대량살상무기나 위험 물질과 관련된 사고 현장은 일반적으로 오염지역[위험지역(Hot Zone)], 전방통제지역(Warm Zone), 안전지역(Cold Zone)으로 구분된다.
© National Association of Emergency Medical Technicians (NAEMT)

자기 보호와 현장에 도착하는 다른 대응자를 보호하기 위해 모든 적절한 조치를 해야 한다. 이러한 단계에는 대응자의 직무와 훈련 수준에 적합한 개인보호장비 사용이 포함된다. 예를 들어, 오염지역(hot zone)에 들어가야 하는 구급대원과 구조대원은 최고 수준의 피부 및 호흡기보호 장비를 착용해야 하며 안전지대에서는 대부분의 경우 표준 예방조치로 충분하다. 대량살상무기 사고일 수 있다는 정보는 현장에 출동하는 모든 구급대원과 구조대원에게 알릴 수 있도록 상황실에 다시 전달되어야 한다. 추가 장비, 인력, 헬기 착륙장은 바람이 불어오는 쪽에 현장으로부터 안전한 거리에 설치해야 한다.

현장 안전을 확보하고 경찰관과 협력하여 오염지역, 전방통제지역, 안전지대를 지정해야 한다. 오염 제거를 위한 장소도 설정해야 한다. 물질의 특성(화학 물질, 생물학적 물질 또는 방사성 물질)이 결정되면 해당 분야 전문가는 특정 해독제, 약물 또는 항생제를 요청할 수 있다.

현장 통제 지역

위험 물질 사고와 마찬가지로 대량살상무기 사고에서도 확산과 추가 오염을 제한하기 위한 노력으로 통제 지역을 지정하고 사용해야 한다. 이러한 원칙을 준수하면 오염 확산과 구급대원과 구조대원 및 구경꾼의 손상 가능성을 줄일 수 있다. **표 5-1**은 폭탄 위협에 대한 필수대피 거리와 선호되는 안전 대피 거리가 나와 있다.

이러한 지역은 일반적으로 3개의 동심원으로 표지되지만(**그림 5-7**), 실제로 대부분의 현장에서 이러한 지역은 지형과 바람 조건에 따라 불규칙한 모양을 띨 가능성이 있다. 위험 물질 또는 대량살상무기 사고가 발생한 현장에서 환자를 병원이나 응급치료소로 이송하는 경우 환자의 오염 제거 여부를 재평가하고 이러한 지역의 개념을 모방하는 것이 가장 현명하다.

오염제거

사고에 위험 물질이 포함되든 대량살상무기가 포함되든 노출된 개인의 오염제거가 필요한 경우가 많다. 오염제거는 해로운 화학 물질, 생화학적 물질, 방사성 물질을 줄이거나 제거하는 것을 말한다. 지속적인 노출이 의심되는 경우 최우선 순위는 개인의 안전을 보장하는 것이다. 적절한 교육을 받은 위험 물질 전문가 수준의 구급대원과 구조대원이 환자의 오염을 제거하는 것이 그다음 우선순위이다. 이렇게 하면 환자를 평가하고 처치하는 동안 병원 전 처치 제공자가 위험 물질에 노출될 위험을 최소화하고 장비와 차량의 오염을 방지할 수 있다.

미국 산업안전보건청(OSHA)은 잠재적으로 위험한 환경에서 환자에게 처치를 시행하는 동안 병원 전 처치 제공자가 사용하는 개인보호장비에 대한 규제 지침을 제공한다. 위험성이 알려지지 않은 환경에서 의료서비스를 제공하는 개인은 최소한의 적절한 교육을 받아야 하며 Level B 보호복을 착용해야 한다. Level B 보호복은 비말 방지, 내화학성 의복과 자체 호흡 장치로 구성된다. 이 수준의 개인보호장비를 사용하기 전에 사전 교육이 필요하다(위험 물질 및 대량살상무기사고에 대한 개인보호장비에 대한 자세한 내용은 18장 폭발 및 대량살상무기를 참조).

환자가 의식이 있고 도움을 줄 수 있는 경우 환자의 협조를 얻어 가능한 한 많은 오염 제거를 수행하도록 하여 병원 전 처치 제공자에게 교차 오염 가능성을 줄이는 것이 가장 좋다. 환자의 오염을 제거하거나 감독할 때 병원 전 처치 제공자는 환자로부터 위험 제품을 안전하게 제거할 뿐만 아니라 통제되어 현장을 더 이상 오염시키지 않도

표 5-1 폭탄 위협: 안전한 대피 거리

위협 설명	폭발물 용량 (TNT 용량)	필수 대피 거리	선호하는 대피 거리	위협 설명	폭발물 용량 (TNT 용량)	필수 대피 거리	선호하는 대피 거리
파이프 폭탄/압력솥	2.3kg	21.3m	365.8m	승용차	227kg	97.5m	579m
IED 자살 조끼	9.1kg	33.5m	518m	SUV/밴	454kg	122m	731.5m
서류 가방/여행 가방 폭탄	22.7kg	45.7m	564m	소형 이삿짐 밴/배송 트럭	1,814kg	195m	1,158m
				이삿짐 트럭/소형 탱크로리	4,536kg	262m	1,555m
				세미 트레일러	27,216kg	479m	2,835m

© Jones & Bartlett Learning

Data from the U.S. Department of Homeland Security.

록 해야 한다. 오염 제거 과정에 대한 자세한 검토는 13장 화상 손상을 참조한다.

이차 폭발물

모든 병원 전 처치 제공자는 이차 폭발물의 존재 가능성에 유의해야 하며 이러한 폭탄은 구급대원이나 구조대원에게 손상을 입히도록 설계되었다. 1996년 애틀랜타에서 개최된 하계 올림픽에서 폭탄 테러가 발생한 지 몇 달 만에 조지아주 애틀랜타의 대도시 지역에서 두 건의 추가 폭탄 테러가 발생했다. 유산 클리닉과 나이트클럽에서 발생한 이 폭탄 테러에는 이차 폭발물이 설치되어 있었으며 미국에서 17년 만에 처음으로 일차 폭발 현장에 출동한 구급대원이나 구조대원에게 죽이거나 다치게 하려는 목적으로 이차 폭발물을 설치한 것으로 추정된다. 안타깝게도 유산 클리닉에 설치된 이차 폭발물은 폭발 전에 발견되지 않았으며 6명의 사상자가 발생했다. 이차 폭발물은 전 세계 테러리스트들이 정기적으로 사용해 왔다.

이 사고 이후 조지아 비상 관리국은 이차 폭발물이 설치될 가능성이 있는 폭발 테러 현장에 대응하는 구급대원이나 구조대원을 위해 다음과 같은 지침을 개발했다.

1. 전자기기 사용을 자제한다. 휴대전화와 라디오에서 나오는 음파는 특히 폭탄 가까이에서 사용할 경우 이차 폭발물을 폭발시킬 수 있다. 뉴스 미디어에서 사용하는 장비도 폭발을 일으킬 수 있다.

2. 현장으로부터 충분한 안전거리를 확보한다. 오염지역은 원래 폭발 지점에서 모든 방향(수직 포함)으로 305m까지 확장해야 한다. 더 강력한 폭탄이 폭발할수록 파편이 더 멀리 날아갈 수 있다. 최초 폭탄 폭발은 가스관과 전력선 등 기반 시설을 파괴할 수 있어 구조대원의 안전을 더 위험에 빠뜨릴 수 있다. 오염지역에 대한 출입은 주의 깊게 통제해야 한다.

3. 피해자를 현장 및 오염지역에 신속하게 대피시킨다. 최초 폭발 현장에서 610~1,219m 떨어진 곳에 응급의료 현장지휘소를 설치해야 한다. 구조대원은 피해자와 구조대원이 오염지역에서 벗어날 때까지 최소한의 중재를 시행한 후 피해자를 폭발 현장에서 신속하게 대피시켜야 한다.

4. 증거 보존 및 복구에 대해 경찰관과 협력한다. 폭발 사고는 범죄 현장에 해당하므로 구급대원이나 구조대원은 피해자를 대피시키는 데 필요한 경우에만, 현장을 훼손해야 한다. 피해자에 함께

현장에서 실수로 제거된 잠재적 증거는 문서화하여 경찰관에게 넘겨 적절한 보호 체계를 확보해야 한다. 병원 전 처치 제공자는 현장에서 어디에 있었는지, 어떤 물건을 만졌는지 정확하게 기록해야 한다.

지휘체계

신고를 받고 출동하는 구급차에는 일반적으로 한 명의 병원 전 처치 제공자와 지원 역할을 보조하는 병원 전 처치 제공자 한 명이 탑승한다. 사건의 규모가 커지고 다른 팀의 구조대원이 현장에 출동함에 따라 대응을 감독하고 통제할 수 있는 공식적인 지휘체계의 필요성이 점점 더 중요해지고 있다.

재난지휘

재난지휘체계(ICS)는 대형 화재 현장에서 다중 서비스 대응을 위해 소방서에서 사용하는 계획 시스템의 결과로 수년에 걸쳐 발전해 왔다. 1987년 국제화재방지협회(NFPA)는 소방 사고지휘 관리 시스템에 관한 표준인 NFPN 표준 1561을 발표했다. NFPN 1561은 이후 응급의료서비스 사고 관리 시스템 및 지휘 안전에 관한 표준으로 개정되었다. 이 버전은 사고를 관리하는 모든 기관에서 모든 유형 또는 규모의 사건에 맞게 구현하고 조정할 수 있다. 1990년대에 단일 사고 관리 접근 방식을 더욱 개선한 국가 화재 사고관리시스템(IMS)이 만들어졌다.

재난지휘체계가 제공하는 정확한 지휘체계를 통해 크고 작은 모든 사고에 대한 대처 능력이 향상된다. 재난지휘체계의 핵심은 현장에서 중앙 집중식 지휘체계를 확립하고 이후 부서 유형별 책임을 강화하는 것이다. 가장 먼저 도착한 팀은 현장 지휘 본부를 설치하고 대응력 강화를 위한 통신을 구축한다. 재난지휘체계의 다섯 가지의 핵심 요소는 다음과 같다.

1. 명령(Command)은 사건에 대한 전반적인 통제와 사고 현장의 자원 이동과 환자 이동을 조정하는 통신을 제공한다.

2. 운영(Operations)은 사건의 전술적 요구를 처리하는 부서가 포함된다. 화재 진압, EMS, 구조가 운영 부서의 예이다.

3. 계획(Planning)은 사고의 즉각적이고 잠재적인 요구를 평가하고 대응을 계획하는 지속적인 과정이다. 사고 전반에 걸쳐 이 요소는 운영의 효율성을 평가하고 대응 및 전술적 접근 방식에 대한 변경을 제안하는 데 사용된다.

4. 물류(Logistics)는 기획 부서에서 파악한 자원을 확보하여 필요한 곳에 공급하는 업무를 담당한다. 이러한 자원에는 인력, 피난처, 차량 및 장비가 포함된다.

5. 재정(Finance)은 자금을 추적한다. 모든 관련 기관의 대응 인력은 물론 사고에 투입된 계약업체, 인력 및 공급업체를 추적하여 사고 비용을 결정하고 이 그룹에 상품, 소모품, 장비 및 서비스 비용을 지급할 수 있다.

통합지휘체계

재난지휘체계의 확장은 통합지휘체계이다. 이러한 확장은 수많은 기관(예: EMS, 소방 및 경찰)을 조정해야 할 필요성을 고려한다. 여러 지역사회, 지자체에서 자원을 지원하는 데 필요한 기술적인 측면은 이 추가 조정 구조에서 다룬다.

국가재난관리체계

2003년 2월 28일 조지 부시 대통령은 대통령령 HSPD-5를 통해 국토안보부 장관에게 국가재난관리체계(NIMS)를 만들도록 지시했다. 이 지침의 목표는 연방정부, 주 및 지방 정부가 원인, 규모 또는 복잡성과 관계없이 국내 사고에 대비, 대응 및 복구하기 위해 효과적으로 협력할 수 있는 일관되고 전국적인 접근 방식을 수립하는 것이다. 국토안보부는 2004년 3월 1일에 주 및 지방 정부 공무원, 국제응급구조사협회(NAEMT), 경찰공제조합(FOP), 소방서장협회(IAFC), 국제재난관리자협회(IAEA) 및 기타 다양한 공공안전단체의 대표로 구성된 소위원회와 협력하여 국가재난관리체계를 설립했다.

국가재난관리체계는 다음과 같은 사고관리 특성에 중점을 둔다.
- 일반적인 용어(평범한 영어로 말하는 것 포함)
- 모듈식 조직
- 목표별 관리
- 사고 실행 계획에 대한 신뢰성
- 관리할 수 있는 통제 범위
- 현장지휘소의 설치 장소 및 사전 지정된 장소
- 포괄적인 자원 관리
- 일원화된 통신
- 지휘권 이양 확립
- 지휘체계 및 지휘 일원화
- 통합지휘체계

- 자원 및 인력의 책임
- 배치
- 정보 및 정보 관리

국가재난관리체계의 주요 구성 요소는 다음과 같다.
1. 준비
2. 통신 및 정보 관리
3. 자원 관리
4. 지휘 및 관리
5. 지속적인 관리 및 유지 관리

지휘

지휘부는 재난지휘관(IC)과 지휘부 직원으로 구성된다. 모든 사고에는 대응을 감독하는 지휘관이 있어야 한다. 재난지휘관을 지원하는 지휘부 인력은 사고의 규모와 성격에 따라 적절하게 배정되며 홍보책임자, 안전 책임자, 연락 책임자 등이 포함될 수 있다. 재난지휘관이 필요하다고 판단하는 경우 다른 직책을 만들 수 있다.

앞에서 설명한 것처럼 통합지휘체계는 여러 관할구역이 관련된 상황에서 사고에 대한 지휘체계를 강화하는 것이다. 단일 지휘체계에서 재난지휘관은 사고 관리에 대한 책임을 전적으로 진다. 통합지휘체계에서 다양한 기관을 대표하는 개인이 공동으로 목표, 계획 및 우선순위를 결정한다. 통합지휘체계는 통신 및 운영 표준의 차이와 관련된 문제를 해결하고자 한다(**그림 5-9**).

통합지휘체계 및 국가재난관리체계에 추가되는 재난지휘체계에 포함되지 않은 요소 중 하나는 정보이다. 사고 규모에 따라 국가 안보와 관련된 정보 및 정보 수집에는 위험 관리 평가, 의료 정보, 기상 정보, 건물 구조 및 설계, 독성물질 억제에 대한 정보가 포함될 수 있다. 이러한 기능은 일반적으로 계획 부분에서 처리하지만, 재난지휘관은 특정 상황에서 정보 수집과 계획을 분리할 수 있다.

국가재난관리체계에서 재난지휘관은 다음과 같이 정보와 정보 수집을 할당할 수 있다.
- 지휘부 내
- 계획 부분의 한 단위로
- 운영 부문으로서
- 별도의 일반 직원 기능으로

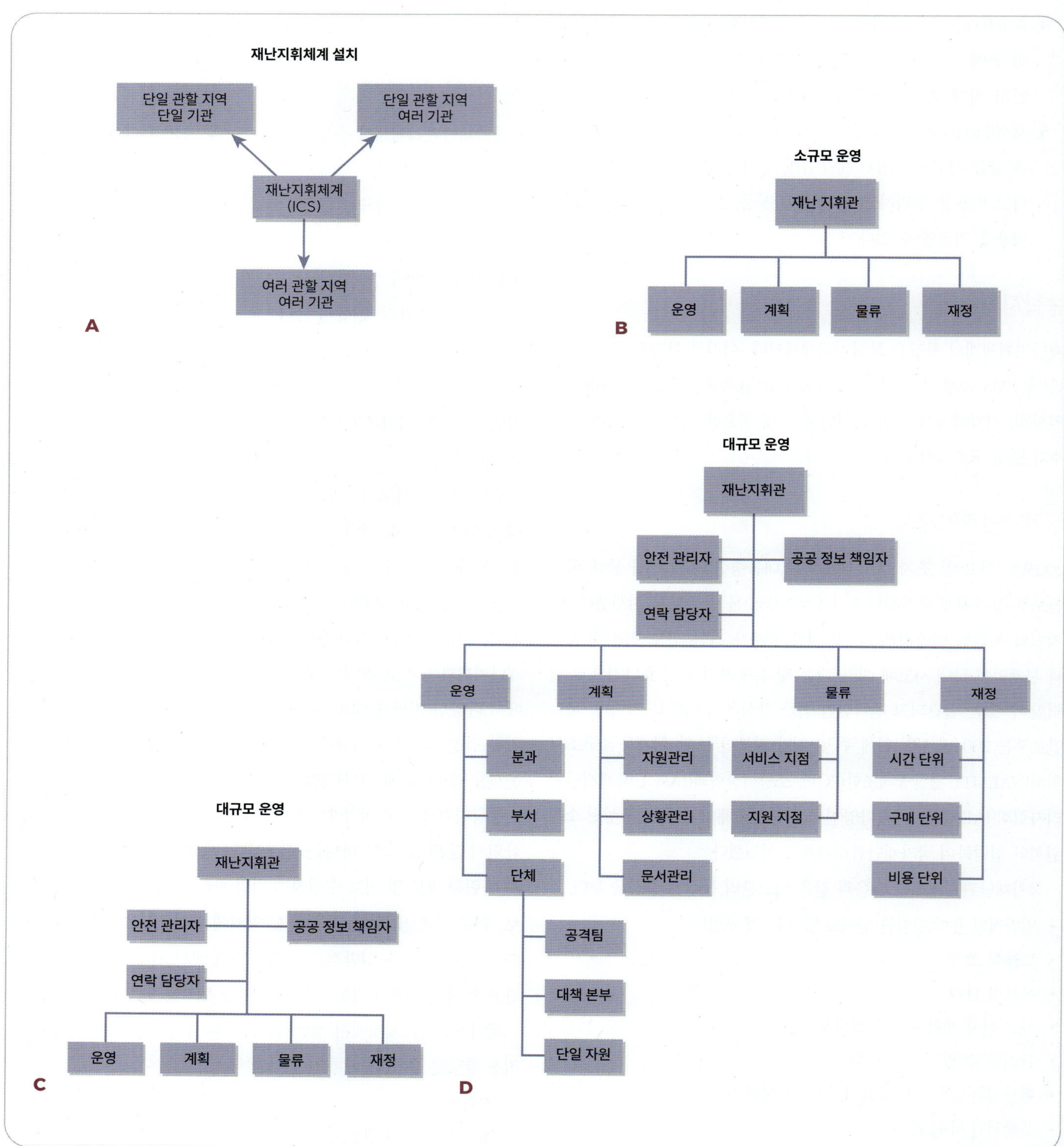

그림 5-9 재난관리체계는 환자의 수와 사고의 복잡성에 따라 확대하거나 축소할 수 있다. 재난지휘체계의 5가지 핵심 요소(지휘, 운영, 계획, 물류, 재정)로 운영된다. 사고 지휘를 담당하는 각 부문의 운영 기능은 분과로 구성된다. 의료 서비스 구역은 사고의 전술적 목표를 달성하는 데 필요한 의료서비스를 조정하고 제공하는 역할을 담당하는 운영 구성요소이다. 사고 규모에 따라 이러한 서비스는 장비, 인력, 환자 분류, 의료 시설과의 통신 및 이송을 포함하는 부서로 운영될 수 있다.

재난 대응계획

재난 대응계획(IAPs)에는 재난지휘관 또는 통합 지휘체계 구성원이 수립한 전반적인 재난 대응 목표와 전략이 포함된다. 계획부서에는 재난 대응계획을 개발하고 문서화한다. 재난 대응계획은 일반적으로 12~24시간으로 지정된 운영 기간의 전술적 목표와 지원 활동을 다룬다. 계획부서에서는 대응이 사고에서 필요한 요구 사항을 충족하는지 확인하기 위해 지속적인 비판 또는 학습된 교훈 과정을 제공한다. 대규모 사고의 경우 여러 기관에서 현장지휘소를 설치할 수 있다. 여러 현장지휘소는 조직을 관리하기 위해 지역 지휘관을 선임할 수 있다. 지역 지휘관은 운영 책임은 없지만, 다음과 같은 임무를 수행한다.

- 기관의 전반적인 사고 관련 우선순위 설정
- 설정된 우선순위에 따라 중요 자원을 할당
- 사고가 적절하게 관리되도록 보장
- 효과적인 통신 보장
- 사고 관리 목표가 충족되고 서로 또는 기관의 정책과 충돌하지 않는지 확인
- 중요한 자원 요구 사항을 파악하고 긴급상황실에 보고
- 전체 복구 작업으로 전환을 지원하기 위해 단기 비상 복구가 조정되도록 함
- 인사 책임과 안전한 운영 환경 제공

Hazardous Materials Training & Research Institute. *Emergency and Disaster Response to Chemical Releases*. January 2006. https://tools.niehs.nih.gov/wetp/public/Course_download2.cfm?tranid=6020

재난지휘체계 및 국가재난관리체계에 관한 자세한 정보 및 교육 프로그램은 연방재난관리청 웹사이트(**Box 5-1**)에서 확인할 수 있다.

혈액 매개 병원체

1980년대 초 후천면역결핍증후군(AIDS)이 알려지기 전에는 의료인, 멸균 처리 기술자, 병원 전 처치 제공자를 포함한 의료 종사자들은 체액 노출에 대해 거의 우려하지 않았다. 혈액이 특정 간염바이러스를 전염시킬 수 있다는 사실을 알고 있었음에도 의사를 비롯한 응급 의료종사자들은 환자의 혈액과 접촉하는 것을 직업적 위험이라기보다는 불편한 일로 여기는 경우가 많았다. 후천면역결핍증후군 감염으로 인한 높은 사망률과 후천면역결핍증후군의 원인인 사람면역결핍바이러스(HIV)가 혈액을 통해 전염될 수 있다는 인식으로 인해 의료 종사자들은 환자를 질병의 매개체로 생각하게 되었다. 질병통제예방센터와 산업보건안전청과 같은 정부 기관에서는 보건의료 종사

재난지휘체계 교육에 대한 연방재난관리청(FEMA) 자원에는 다음이 포함된다.

- **ICS-100.B: Introduction to Incident Command System, ICS-100** (https://training.fema.gov/is/courseoverview.aspx?code=is-100.c)
- **ICS-200.B: ICS for Single Resources and Initial Action Incidents** (https://training.fema.gov/is/courseoverview.aspx?code=IS-200.c)
- **ICS-700.A: National Incident Management System (NIMS), An Introduction** (https://training.fema.gov/is/courseoverview.aspx?code=IS-700.b)
- **ICS-800.B: National Response Framework, An Introduction** (http://training.fema.gov/EMIWeb/IS /IS800b.asp)

국가저난관리체계(NIMS) 및 연방재난관리청 교육에 대한 자세한 내용은 해당 주 비상 관리 기관 또는 비상 관리 기관 및 국립소방학교(NFA)에 문의한다. 다양한 온라인 통신 및 현장 교육 과정을 이용할 수 있다(http://training.fema.gov/IS/crslist.asp).

Data from the National Incident Management System.

자가 사람면역결핍바이러스 및 간염을 포함한 혈액 매개 병원체에 대한 노출을 최소화하기 위해 지침과 의무 사항을 개발했다. 혈액을 통해 전염되는 주요 감염원에는 B형 간염바이러스, C형 간염바이러스(HCV) 및 사람면역결핍바이러스가 있다. 이 문제는 사람면역결핍바이러스로 인해 우려의 대상이 되었지만, 간염바이러스 감염은 사람면역결핍바이러스 감염보다 훨씬 더 쉽게 발생하고 훨씬 적은 접종이 필요하다는 점에 유의하는 것이 중요하다.

역학 자료에 따르면 의료 종사자가 환자로부터 혈액 매개 질병에 걸릴 확률이 환자가 의료 종사자가로부터 질병에 걸릴 확률보다 훨씬 높다. 혈액에 대한 노출은 일반적으로 경피 또는 점막피부 노출로 특징지어진다. 경피적 노출은 바늘이나 메스 같은 오염된 날카로운 물체에 찔려 상서를 입었을 때 발생하며 전염 위험은 오염 물질과 상처로 인해 유입된 감염된 혈액의 양과 직접적으로 관련이 있다. 점막피부 노츨은 일반적으로 전염 가능성이 적으며 연부조직 상처(예: 찰과상이나 열상)나 피부 상태(예: 여드름) 또는 점막(예: 눈 결막)에 혈액이 노츨되는 것을 포함한다.

바이러스 간염

간염은 손상되지 않은 피부를 주삿바늘에 찔리거나 점막피부 노출을 통해 의료 종사자에게 전염될 수 있다. 앞에서 언급했듯이 간염

환자의 혈액에 노출된 후 감염되는 비율은 사람면역결핍바이러스에 감염되는 비율보다 훨씬 높다. 특히 B형 간염에 감염된 주삿바늘에 찔린 후 감염률은 37~62%, C형 간염 감염은 약 1.8%(50명 중 1명)이다. 다양한 감염률에 대한 가능한 설명은 감염된 혈액에서 발견되는 바이러스 입자의 상대적 농도이다. 일반적으로 B형 간염 양성 혈액에는 mL당 1억~10억 개의 바이러스 입자가 포함되어 있지만, C형 간염 양성 혈액에는 mL당 100만 개, 사람면역결핍바이러스 양성 혈액에는 mL당 100~1만 개의 바이러스 입자가 포함되어 있다.

많은 간염 바이러스가 확인되었지만, B형과 C형 간염은 혈액 노출을 경험하는 의료 종사자들에게 자장 우려되는 바이러스이다. 바이러스 간염은 간에 급성 염증을 일으킨다(**Box 5-2**). 잠복기(노출 후 증상 발현까지의 시간)는 일반적으로 60~90일이다. B형 감염자의 최대 30%는 무증상 소견을 보일 수 있다.

B형 간염 표면 항원에서 추출한 백신으로 B형 간염 바이러스 감염을 예방할 수 있다. 이 백신이 개발되기 전에는 매년 1만 명 이상의 의료 종사자가 B형 간염에 걸렸고 매년 수백 명이 중증 간염이나 만성 B형 간염 합병증으로 사망했다. 산업안전보건청은 고용주가 고위험 환경에서 일하는 의료 종사자에게 B형 간염 백신을 제공하도록 요구하고 있다. 모든 병원 전 처치 제공자는 B형 간염 예방 백신을 접종해야 한다. 3회의 예방접종을 받은 거의 모든 사람은 대부분 B형 간염 표면 항원(HBsAg)에 대한 항체가 형성되며 의료 종사자의 혈액에서 B형 간염 표면 항원의 존재 여부를 검사하여 면역 여부를 확인

할 수 있다. 의료 종사자가 면역이 형성되기 전(즉 백신 접종을 완료하기 전)에 잠재적으로 B형 간염에 걸린 환자의 혈액에 노출된 경우 B형 간염 면역글로불린(HBIG)을 투여하여 B형 간염으로부터의 수동적으로 보호받을 수 있다.

현재 의료 종사자를 C형 간염 바이러스 노출로부터 보호할 수 있는 면역글로불린이나 백신은 없으므로 표준 예방 조치의 필요성이 강조된다. 직접 작용하는 경구 약물은 C형 간염 바이러스 감염을 치료할 수 있다. 이 약물은 2011년에 미국에서 승인되었다. 치료 요법은 유전자형, 바이러스의 양 및 간경변의 정도에 따라 다르다. 이러한 새로운 약물의 비용은 보편적인 사용을 제한한다.

사람면역결핍바이러스(HIV)

감염 후 사람면역결핍바이러스는 새로운 숙주의 면역체계를 표적으로 삼는다. 시간이 지남에 따라 특정 유형의 백혈구 수가 급격히 감소하여 비정상적인 감염이나 암에 걸리기 쉽다(**Box 5-3**).

사람면역결핍바이러스 양성 혈액에 대한 주삿바늘에 노출된 경우 약 0.3%만이 감염으로 이어진다. 감염 위험은 더 많은 양의 혈액에 노출되거나 질병의 더 진행된 환자의 혈액에 노출되거나, 깊은 경피적 손상을 입거나, 혈액이 채워진 주삿바늘에 찔린 경우 더 높게 나타난다. 사람면역결핍바이러스는 주로 감염된 혈액이나 정액을 통해 감염되지만, 질 분비물과 심장막액, 복막액, 가슴막액, 양막액, 뇌척수액도 모두 감염 가능성이 있는 것으로 간주한다. 명백한 혈액이 없는 한 눈물, 소변, 땀, 대변, 침은 일반적으로 비감염성 액체로 간주한다. 고위험 노출과 관련된 상황에서 시기적절한 예방 치료는 혈청 전환 및 만성 감염의 위험을 줄일 수 있는 것으로 나타났다. 따라서 직업적 노출의 맥락에서 주삿바늘 찔림 및 감염원 노출 직통 상담 전화 또는 해당 기관의 감염관리 담당자에게 즉시 의뢰하는 것이 바람직하다.

표준 예방 지침

임상 검사로는 의료 종사자에게 잠재적 감염 위험이 되는 모든 환자를 확실하게 구별할 수 없기 때문에 의료 종사자가 환자의 체액과 직접 접촉하지 않도록 표준 예방 지침이 개발되었다. 동시에 이러한 예방 조치는 병원 전 처치 제공자가 가지고 있는 감염으로부터 환자를 보호하는 데 도움이 된다. 산업안전보건청은 고용주와 직원이 근무 중에 표준 예방 지침을 따르도록 의무화하는 규정을 개발했다. 표준

Box 5-2 간염

바이러스 간염의 임상증상은 우상복부 통증, 피로, 식욕 부진, 오심, 구토와 간 기능의 변화 등이다. 피부가 노랗게 변하는 황달은 혈액 내 빌리루빈 수치가 증가하여 발생한다. 대부분의 간염 환자는 심각한 문제 없이 회복되지만, 소수의 환자는 급성 전격성 간부전으로 발전하여 사망할 수 있다. 회복된 환자 중 상당수는 혈액이 바이러스를 전염시킬 수 있는 보균자 상태가 된다.

B형 간염과 마찬가지로 C형 간염은 경미한 무증상부터 간부전 및 사망에 이르기까지 다양할 수 있다. C형 간염의 잠복기는 6~9주로 B형 간염보다 다소 짧다. C형 간염 만성 감염은 B형 간염보다 훨씬 더 흔하며 C형 간염에 걸린 사람의 약 75%~85%는 지속해 간 기능 이상이 발생하여 간세포 암에 걸리기 쉽다. C형 간염은 주로 혈액을 통해 감염되지만, B형 간염은 혈액이나 성 접촉을 통해 감염될 수 있다. 정맥 내 약물 사용자가 C형 간염에 걸릴 위험은 정맥 내 약물 사용 기간에 따라 증가한다. 헌혈한 혈액에 대한 정기적인 B형 간염 및 C형 간염 감염 여부 검사 이전에는 수혈이 환자가 간염에 걸리는 주요 원인이었다.

Box 5-3 사람면역결핍바이러스(HIV)

두 가지 혈청형의 HIV가 확인되었다. HIV-1은 미국과 적도 아프리카의 거의 모든 AIDS를 차지하며 HIV-2는 거의 서아프리카에서만 발견된다. HIV의 초기 희생자는 남성 동성애자, 정맥주사 약물 사용자 또는 혈우병 환자였지만, 현재는 많은 청소년과 성인 이성애자 인구에서 발견되고 있으며 소수자 집단에서 가장 빠르게 증가하고 있다. HIV 선별 검사는 매우 민감하지만, 때로는 잘못된 양성 검사가 발생한다. 모든 양성 선별 검사는 더 구체적인 기술(예: 웨스턴 블롯 전기영동)로 확인해야 한다.

HIV에 걸린 후 환자가 특징적인 기회감염 또는 암 중 하나가 발생하면 HIV 양성에서 AIDS로 전환된다. 지난 10년 동안 HIV 질병의 치료, 특히 그 영향에 대처하기 위한 신약 개발에 상당한 진전이 있었다. 이러한 진전 덕분에 HIV에 걸린 많은 사람이 질병의 진행 속도가 느려져 상당히 정상적인 삶을 영위할 수 있게 되었다.

의료 종사자는 일반적으로 다양한 이유로 HIV 감염에 대해 더 우려하지만, 실제로는 B형 간염이나 C형 간염에 걸릴 위험이 더 크다.

예방 지침은 혈액 및 체액과 노출에 대한 물리적 장벽과 주삿바늘 및 기타 날카로운 도구에 관해 안전하게 취급하는 방법으로 구성되어 있다. 외상 환자는 종종 외부출혈이 있고 혈액은 매우 위험한 체액이기 때문에 병원 전 처치 제공자는 환자를 처치하거나 이송하는 동안 적절한 보호장비를 착용해야 한다.

물리적 장벽

글러브

손상된 피부, 점막 또는 혈액이나 기타 체액으로 오염된 부위를 만질 때는 글러브를 착용한다. 환자를 처치하거나 이송하는 동안 글러브가 쉽게 찢어질 수 있으므로 주기적으로 확인하고 문제가 발견되면 즉시 교체해야 한다(**그림 5-10**). 또한 다수 사상자 발생 시 각 환자와 접촉할 때마다 글러브를 교체한다.

마스크와 얼굴 보호대

마스크는 특히 비말 또는 공기 중 병원체가 알려지거나 의심되는 상황에서 감염원에 노출되지 않도록 의료진의 입과 코점막을 보호하는 역할을 한다. 마스크와 얼굴 보호대는 젖거나 더러워지면 즉시 교체한다.

외과용 마스크는 비말 매개 질병을 예방하는 데 유용하다. 비말 예방 조치가 필요한 질환의 예로는 계절성 인플루엔자, 보르데텔라백일해 등이 있다.

결핵, 수두 및 COVID-19를 유발하는 바이러스를 포함한 특정 다른 유형의 질병의 경우 공기 중 예방 조치가 필요하다. 공기 중 질병으로부터 보호하려면 N95 마스크는 또는 전동식 공기 청정기를 사

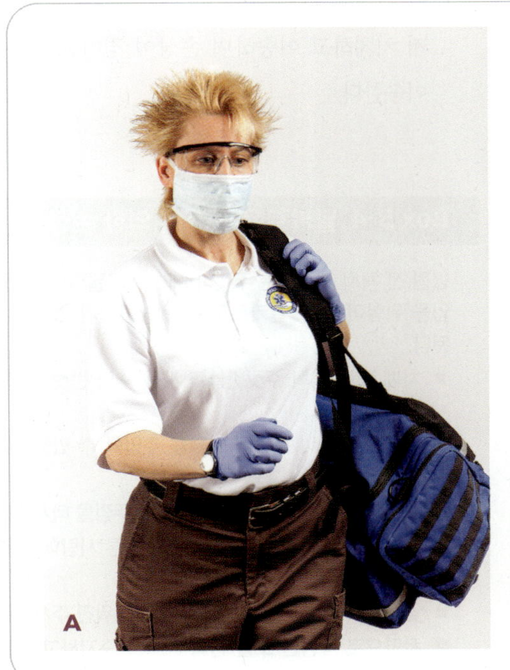
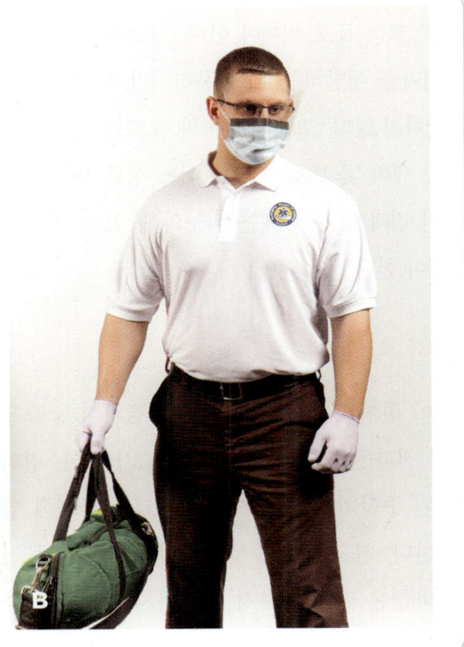

그림 5-10 병원 전 처치 제공자를 위한 개인 보호장비는 최소한 글러브, 마스크 및 보호안경으로 구성되어야 한다. **A.** 보호안경, 마스크 및 글러브 **B.** 얼굴 보호대, 얼굴 보호대 및 글러브

용해야 한다. N95 마스크는 적절한 마스크 밀착을 확인하기 위해 적합성 테스트가 필요하다.

눈 보호

EMS 팀원은 일반적으로 보호안경을 착용해야 한다. 입인두에 혈액이 있는 환자에게 기도 유지를 시행하거나 개방성 상처를 처치할 때, 얼굴 마스크를 착용하고 있을 때 등 감염 가능성이 있는 체액이나 혈액 방울이 튈 수 있는 상황에서 눈 보호 장비를 착용해야 한다.

가운

불침투성 플라스틱 라이너가 있는 일회용 가운은 최상의 보호 기능을 제공하지만, 병원 전 환경에서는 매우 불편하고 비실용적일 수 있다. 가운이나 옷에 오염이 심각하게 발생하면 즉시 갈아입는다.

소생술 장비

의료 종사자는 환자의 타액, 혈액 및 구토물에 직접 접촉하지 않도록 백마스크나 포켓마스크를 사용할 수 있어야 한다. 환자의 양압 환기에 사용되는 소생술 장비에는 일방향 바이러스 필터가 있어 의료 종사자를 추가로 보호해야 한다.

손 씻기

손 씻기는 감염 관리의 기본 원칙이다. 혈액이나 체액으로 심하게 오염된 경우 손을 비누와 흐르는 물로 씻어야 한다. 알코올 성분의 손 소독제는 많은 감염원 전파를 예방하는 데 유용하지만, 명백한 오염이 발행한 상황에는 적합하지 않다. 그러나 비누와 흐르는 물로 손을 씻을 수 없는 상황에서는 세척 및 보호 효과를 어느 정도 제공할 수 있다. 글러브를 착용하기 전과 벗은 후에는 비누와 물 또는 알코올 기반 소독제로 손을 씻어야 한다.

날카로운 물체에 의한 손상 예방

앞에서 설명한 바와 같이 환자의 혈액이나 체액의 경피적 노출은 의료 종사자에게 감염이 전파될 수 있는 중요한 경로가 된다. 경피적 노출 대부분은 오염된 주삿바늘이나 기타 날카로운 물건에 찔려 손상을 입어서 발생한다. 불필요한 주삿바늘과 날카로운 물건을 없애고 사용한 주삿바늘은 절대로 다시 사용하지 않으며 가능하면 무침 정맥주사 시스템과 같은 안전장치를 도입해야 한다(Box 5-4).

직업적 노출 관리

미국 산업안전보건청은 의료 서비스를 제공하는 모든 조직이 직원의 혈액 및 체액에 대한 직업적 노출을 관리하기 위한 통제 계획을 수립하도록 규정하고 있다. 각 노출은 손상의 유형과 예방접종을 포함하여 철저하게 문서화해야 한다. 의료 종사자가 혈액에 점막피부 또는 경피적 노출을 경험했거나 오염된 날카로운 물체에 의해 손상을 입은 경우 파상풍, B형 간염, 사람면역결핍바이러스 감염을 포함한 감염을 예방하기 위해 노력한다. C형 간염을 예방하기 위한 예방 방법은 현재 승인되었거나 이용할 수 없다. **Box 5-5**는 일반적인 혈액 및 체액 노출 지침을 설명한다.

환자 평가 및 분류

앞의 모든 문제가 해결되면 환자를 평가하고 처치하는 실제 과정을 시작할 수 있다. 가장 큰 어려움은 병원 전 처치 제공자가 다수의 환자를 마주할 때 발생한다.

　Triage는 '분류한다'를 의미하는 프랑스어 단어이다. 환자 분류는 처치 및 이송의 우선순위를 결정하는 과정이다. 병원 전 환경에서 환자 분류는 두 가지 다른 맥락에서 사용된다.

1. 모든 환자를 처치할 수 있는 충분한 자원이 확보되어 있다. 이러한 환자 분류 상황에서는 가장 심각한 손상을 입은 환자를 먼저 처치하고 이송하며 손상이 경미한 환자는 나중에 처치하고 이송한다.

> ### Box 5-4 날카로운 물체에 의한 손상 예방
>
> 병원 전 처치 제공자는 주삿바늘과 기타 날카로운 물건으로 인해 손상을 입을 위험이 크다. 날카로운 손상을 줄이기 위해 전략에는 다음이 포함된다.
> - 차폐 또는 후퇴 주삿바늘과 자동 후퇴 란셋과 같은 안전장치를 사용한다.
> - 주삿바늘 없이 포트에 약물을 주입할 수 있는 무바늘 시스템을 사용한다.
> - 주삿바늘과 기타 날카로운 물건에 뚜껑을 다시 씌우지 않는다.
> - 오염된 주삿바늘을 버리기 위해 다른 사람에게 건제지 말고 즉시 주삿바늘 폐기물통에 버린다.
> - 앰플에서 약물을 뽑기보다는 미리 채워진 주사기를 사용한다.
> - 서면으로 작성된 노출 관리 계획을 숙지하고 모든 직원이 알고 있는지 확인한다.
> - 날카로운 물체에 의한 손상을 기록한다.

2. 환자 수가 즉시 사용할 수 있는 현장 자원을 초과하는 경우이다. 이러한 환자 분류 상황의 목표는 가능한 한 많은 손상을 입은 환자의 생존을 보장하는 것이다. 환자 수가 가용 자원을 초과하기 때문에 환자를 중증도 별로 분류하고 처치를 배분해야 한다. 병원 전 처치 제공자 중 50~100명 이상의 환자가 동시에 발생하는 다수 사상자 사고를 경험한 병원 전 처치 제공자는 상대적으로 적지만, 많은 병원 전 처치 제공자가 10~20명의 환자가 발생한 사고에 관여하며 대부분의 병원 전 처치 제공자는 2~10명의 환자가 발생한 사고를 관리한 경험이 있다.

충분한 응급의료 인력과 의료 자원을 이용할 수 있는 사고는 가장 심각한 손상을 입은 환자를 먼저 처치하고 이송할 수 있다. 대규모 다수 사상자가 발생한 사고 현장에서는 제한된 자원으로 인해 생존 가능성이 가장 높은 환자를 구조하기 위해 환자 처치 및 이송에 우선순위를 두어야 한다. 이러한 환자는 처치와 이송의 우선순위가 결정되어야 한다(**그림 5-11**).

다수 사상자가 발생한 현장에서 환자 처치의 목표는 가용한 자원으로 가장 많은 환자에게 가장 큰 이익을 주는 것이다. 누굴 먼저 처치해야 하는지에 대한 결정을 내리는 것은 병원 전 처치 제공자의 책임이다. 생명을 구하는 일반적인 원칙은 다수 사상자 사고에서 다른다. 결정은 항상 가장 많은 생명을 구하는 것이다. 그러나 가용 자원이 손상을 입은 모든 환자의 요구에 충분하지 않은 경우 생존 가능성이 가장 높은 환자를 위해 자원을 사용해야 한다. 중증 외상성 뇌손상과 같은 치명적인 손상을 입은 환자와 급성 복강 내 출혈 환자 사이에서 선택해야 하는 경우 다수 사상자 사고에서 적절한 조치는 먼저 생존할 수 있는 손상을 입은 환자, 즉 복강 내 출혈이 있는 환자를 먼저 처치하는 것이다. 심각한 머리 외상을 입은 환자를 먼저 처치하면 두 환자 모두를 잃을 수 있다.

다수 사상자가 발생한 상황에서 치명적인 손상을 입은 환자는 더 많은 자원과 장비를 사용할 수 있을 때까지 처치를 연기하여 우선순위가 낮은 환자로 간주해야 할 수 있다. 이는 어려운 결정과 상황이지만, 병원 전 처치 제공자는 신속하고 적절하게 대응해야 한다. 병원 전 처치 제공자는 기도 손상이나 외부출혈로 인해 다른 환자 3명이 사망하는 동안 생존 가능성이 거의 없거나 전혀 없는 외상성 심정지 환자를 소생시키려고 노력해서는 안 된다.

그러나 환자 분류 규칙이 반드시 적용되지 않는 한 가지 독특한 시나리오는 낙뢰로 인해 다수의 사상자가 발생한 경우이다. 이 상황에서는 심정지 환자에게 집중적으로 처치를 한다(일반적으로 다수 사상자 사고에서는 그 반대). 대부분 상황에서 낙뢰를 맞은 후 의식이 있고 활력징후가 있는 사람은 즉각적인 처치 없이도 상당히 좋은 결과를 얻을 수 있기 때문이다. 반대로 대부분의 낙뢰에서 심정지의 원인은 일시적인 자율신경 마비로 인한 심정지이다. 대부분의 경우 인공호흡과 가슴압박으로 처치할 수 있다(21장 야생 외상 처치 참조).

가장 자주 사용되는 분류 체계는 처치의 필요성과 생존 가능성에

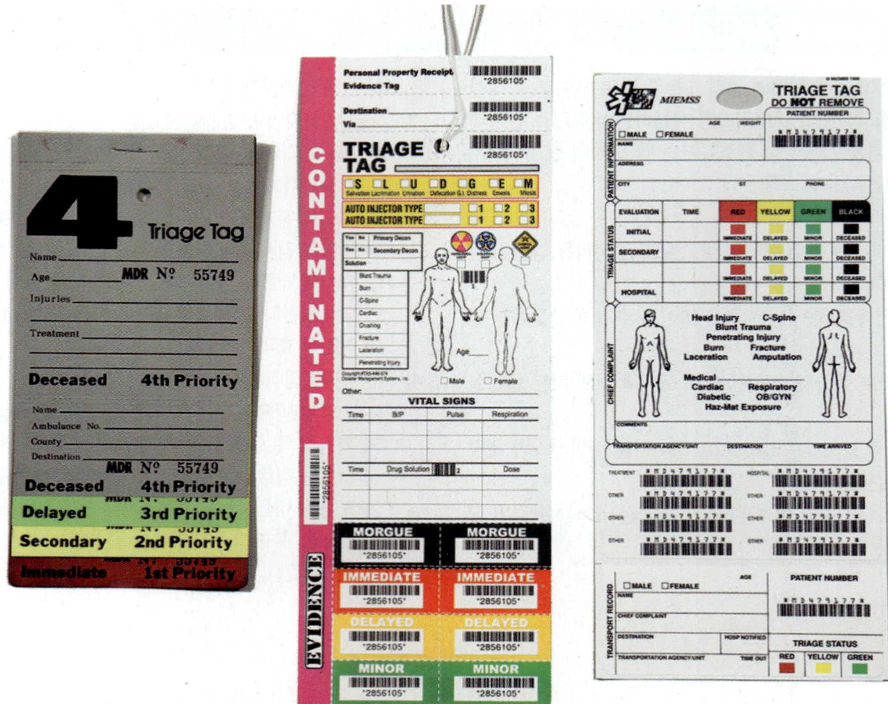

그림 5-11 환자 분류표의 예

© File of Life Foundation, Inc.

따라 환자를 다섯 가지로 구분한다.

1. **즉시(Immediate)-적색 태그:** 손상이 심각하지만, 처치하는 데 최소한의 시간이나 장비만 필요하고 생존할 가능성이 많은 환자이다. 예를 들어 기도가 손상되었거나 다량의 외부출혈이 있는 환자이다.

2. **지연(Delayed)-노란색 태그:** 손상으로 쇠약해지고 있지만, 생명이나 팔다리를 구하기 위해 즉각적인 처치가 필요하지 않은 환자이다. 예를 들어 긴뼈 골절 환자이다.

3. **경증(Minor)-녹색 태그:** 처치를 기다릴 수 있는 경미한 손상을 입거나 중간에 다른 환자 이송에 도움을 줄 수 있는 보행 부상자라고 하는 환자이다.

4. **대기(Expectant)-회색 태그:** 손상이 너무 심각해서 생존 가능성이 거의 없는 환자이다. 예를 들어 90% 전층 화상 및 열로 인한 폐 손상 환자가 있다.

5. **사망(Dead)-검은색 태그:** 무반응, 맥박 및 호흡이 없는 환자이다. 재난 상황에서 자원이 심정지 환자의 소생술을 시도하지 않는다.

Box 5-6, **그림 5-12**, **그림 5-13**은 일반적으로 사용되는 START라는 분류 체계에 관해 설명하며 이 분류 체계는 즉시, 지연, 경미, 사망의 네 가지로 분류하여 사용한다(START 분류 체계에 대한 자세한 내용은 17장 재난관리를 참조한다). 특별히 다수 사상자 사고를 염두에 두고 개발된 분류 시스템은 SALT 분류 시스템이다(**Box 5-7** 및 **그림 5-14**).

Box 5-6 START 분류 체계

1983년에 호그 메모리얼 병원의 의료진과 뉴포트 비치 소방서의 구급대원은 START 분류라는 응급의료 대응자를 위한 분류 과정을 만들었다(**그림 5-12** 참고). 이 분류 과정은 중상을 입은 환자를 쉽고 빠르게 구별하도록 설계되었다. START는 의학적 진단을 확립하지 않고 대신 신속하고 간단한 분류 과정을 제공한다. START는 세 가지 간단한 평가를 사용하여 손상으로 사망할 위험이 가장 높은 피해자를 확인한다. 일반적으로 평가는 피해자 1인당 30~60초가 걸린다. START는 도구나 특수 의료 장비 또는 특별한 지식이 필요하지 않다.

START 분류는 어떻게 시행하는가?

첫 번째 단계는 걸을 수 있는 사람을 지정된 안전한 지역으로 안내하는 것이다. 피해자가 걸을 수 있고 지시를 따를 수 있으면 경증으로 분류되며 더 많은 구조대원이 도착하면 추가로 분류하여 분류표를 붙인다. 이 초기 분류를 통해 더 심각한 손상을 입은 것으로 추정되는 피해자 그룹이 분류 대상에 남게 된다. "30-2-can do"라는 암기 기호는 START 분류 시 신속하게 사용할 수 있다(**그림 5-13** 참고). "30"은 피해자의 호흡수, "2"는 모세혈관 재충전 시간, "can do"는 피해자가 지시를 따르는 능력을 말한다. 호흡수 분당 30회 미

만이고 모세혈관 재충전 2초 미만이며, 구두 명령을 따르고 걸을 수 있는 능력이 있는 피해자는 경증(minor)으로 분류된다. 피해자가 이러한 기준을 충족하지만, 걸을 수 없는 경우 지연(delayed)으로 분류된다. 의식이 없거나 호흡이 빠른 피해자, 모세혈관 재충전 시간이 지연되거나 노동맥이 촉지되지 않는 경우 즉시(immediate)로 분류된다.

피해자의 곁에서 기도 개방과 외부출혈을 조절하는 두 가지 기본적인 인명구조 처치를 수행할 수 있다. 숨을 쉬지 않는 환자의 경우 병원 전 처치 제공자는 기도를 개방하고 호흡이 재개되면 즉시 환자로 분류한다. 심폐소생술을 시도해서는 안 된다. 피해자가 호흡을 재개하지 않으면 피해자는 사망한 것으로 분류된다. 구경꾼 또는 "걸을 수 있는 부상자"는 병원 전 처치 제공자가 기도 유지 및 출혈 조절을 유지하는 것을 도울 수 있도록 지시할 수 있다.

이송 수단 부족으로 피해자가 현장에 머무는 시간이 길어지는 경우 재분류가 필요하다. START 기준을 사용하여 심각한 손상을 입은 피해자는 지연으로 분류할 수 있다. 피해자가 처치 없이 현장에 머무는 시간이 길어질수록 상태가 악화할 가능성이 커진다. 따라서 시간이 지남에 따라 반복적인 평가와 분류가 적절하다.

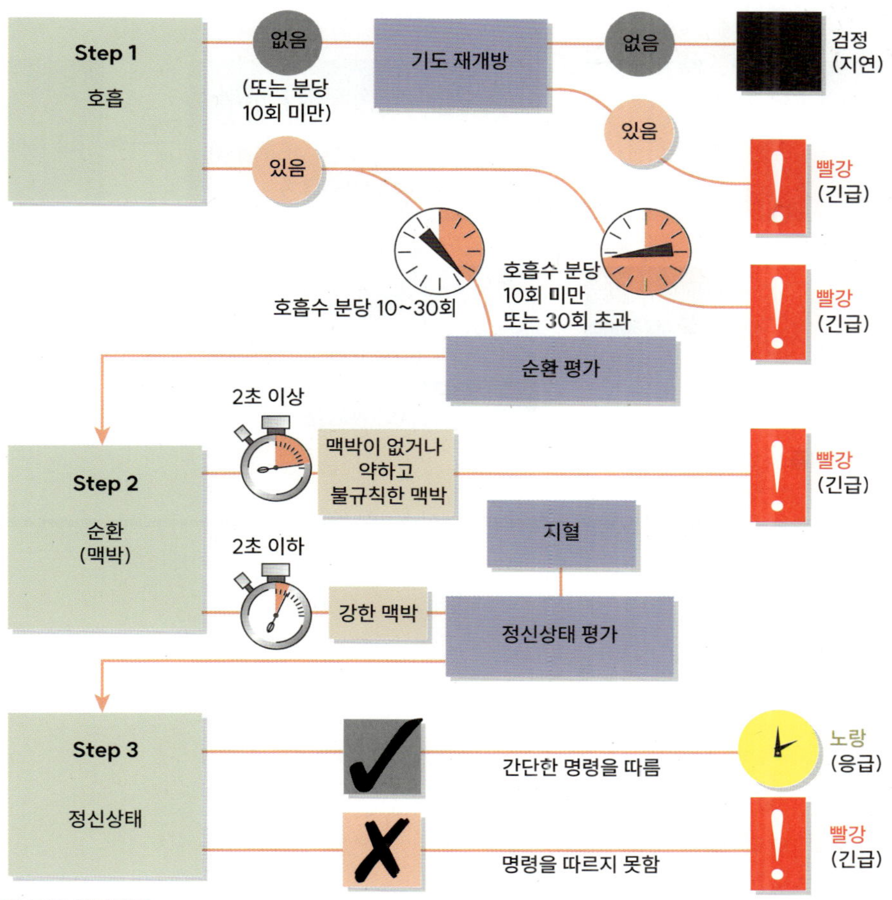

그림 5-12 START 분류 알고리즘

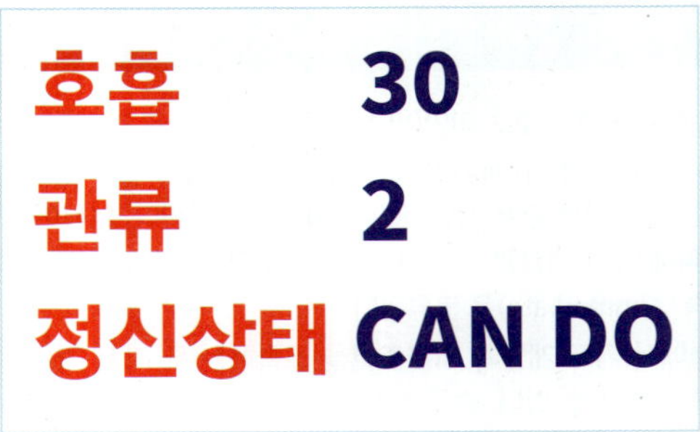

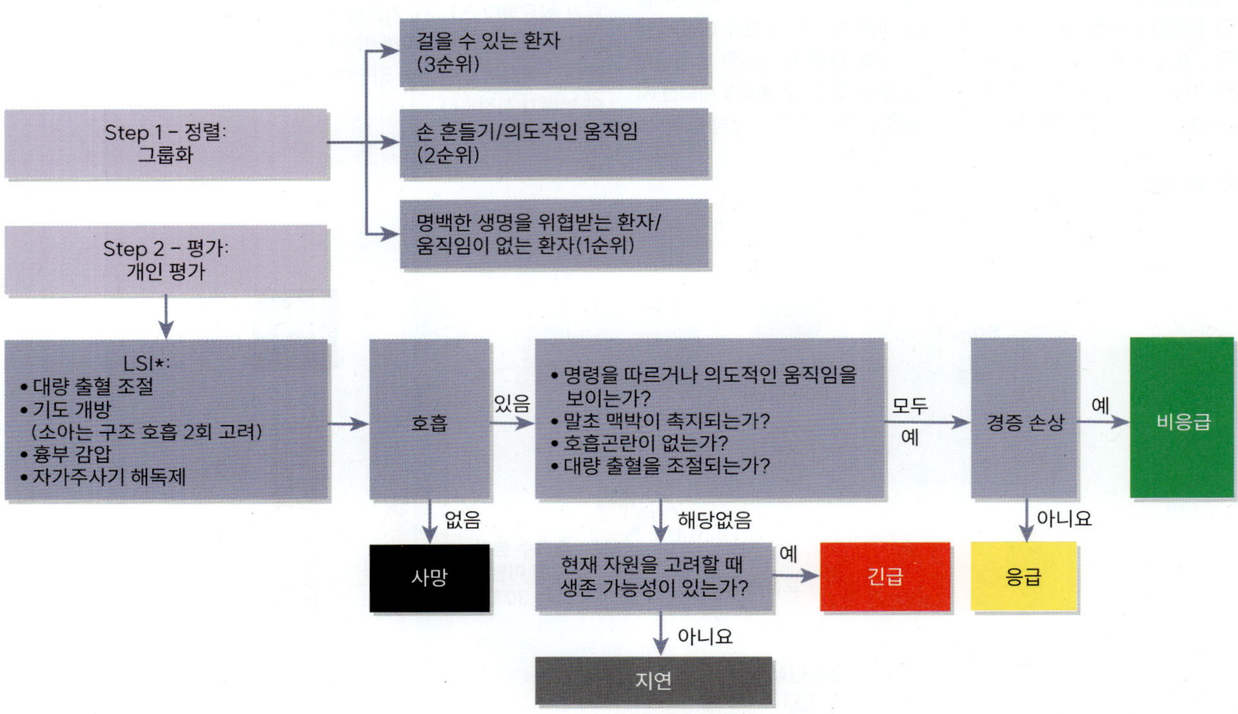

그림 5-13 START 분류 알고리즘; "30-2-can do."

Courtesy of Hoag Hospital Newport Beach and the Newport Beach Fire Department.

Box 5-7 SALT 분류체계

미국 질병통제예방센터는 많은 의료기관을 대표하는 전문가 패널과 함께 SALT 분류체계를 개발했다. 이 프로젝트의 목적은 국가적으로 합의된 분류 시스템의 기반이 될 수 있는 분류 방법을 개발하는 것이었다. 이 방법은 피해자에게 걷거나 손을 흔들도록 요청하는(명령을 따름) 전체 분류 과정을 사용하는 것으로 시작한다. 그런 다음 응급하지 않는 피해자는 생명 위협 여부를 평가한 후 즉시, 지연, 최소, 대기 또는 사망으로 분류된다(**그림 5-14** 참조).

그림 5-14 SALT 분류 알고리즘.

*Note: LSI stands for lifesaving interventions.

Modified from Chemical Hazards Emergency Medical Management, U.S. Department of Health and Human Services. SALT mass casualty triage algorithm (sort, assess, lifesaving interventions, treatment/transport). Accessed December 14, 2021. https://chemm.hhs.gov/salttriage.htm

요 약

- 현장의 안전을 평가할 때 교통 문제, 환경 문제, 폭력, 혈액 매개 병원체 및 위험 물질 등 모든 유형의 위험 요소를 평가하는 것이 중요하다.

- 현장에 대한 지속적인 평가를 통해 EMS 인력과 장비가 손상되어 다른 사람이 사용할 수 없는 상황이 발생하지 않도록 하고 다른 구조대원이 격리되거나 제거되지 않은 위험으로부터 보호받을 수 있도록 해야 한다.

- 때로는 위험을 신속하게 배제할 수 있지만, 평가하지 않으면 보이지 않는 경우도 있다.

- 병원 전 처치 제공자는 잠재적으로 위험한 현장에서 위험을 완화할 수 있는 계획을 세워야 한다. 예를 들어, 자동차 사고 현장에서는 반사 복장을 착용하고 전략적으로 주차해야 하며 적대적인 사람이 있는 현장에서는 동료가 폭력을 예방할 수 있는 계획을 세워야 한다.

- 범죄 현장이나 대량살상무기 사용 등 의도적인 행위와 같은 특정 상황은 병원 전 처치 제공자가 현장에 대응하는 방식에 영향을 미친다.

- 사고는 재난지휘체계(ICS) 구조를 사용하여 관리된다. 병원 전 처치 제공자는 재난지휘체계와 해당 시스템 내에서 자신의 역할을 알고 이해해야 한다.

- 병원 전 처치 제공자는 간염 바이러스 및 사람면역결핍바이러스와 같은 혈액 매개 병원체를 포함한 감염성 물질에 의한 감염을 피하기 위한 예방 조치를 취해야 한다. 주요 고려 사항에는 표준예방조치 사용, 물리적 장벽 사용, 손 씻기 및 날카로운 물건에 의한 손상 방지 등이 포함된다.

- 다수의 사상자를 마주하는 병원 전 처치 제공자는 환자의 상태와 가용 자원에 따라 환자를 분류할 준비가 되어 있어야 한다.

시나리오 재구성

당신과 동료는 무더운 여름 새벽 2시 45분에 부부싸움을 하는 현장으로 출동했다. 가정집에 도착하자 부부가 큰 소리로 다투는 소리와 함께 아이들이 우는 소리가 들린다. 신고를 받고 경찰이 출동했지만, 아직 현장에 도착하지 않았다.

- 현장에 대한 어떤 우려 사항이 있는가?
- 환자와 접촉하기 전에 고려해야 할 중요한 사항은 무엇인가?

시나리오 해결책

현장을 평가하면 몇 가지 잠재적인 위험이 드러난다. 가정 폭력 사건은 구급대원에게 가장 위험한 사건 중 하나이다. 이러한 사건은 종종 확대되어 구급대원의 폭행으로 이어질 수 있다. 따라서 현장에 진입하기 전에 경찰관에게 도움을 요청하는 것을 고려해야 한다. 모든 외상 사례와 마찬가지로 출혈이 있는 환자는 병원 전 처치 제공자를 혈액 매개 감염의 위험에 노출하므로 구급대원은 글러브, 마스크, 보호안경을 포함한 개인보호장비를 착용해야 한다.

이 경우 경찰관이 도착할 때까지 기다렸다가 집에 들어간다. 집에 들어가자마자 한 사람의 얼굴에 다발성 타박상을 입었고 한쪽 뺨에 작은 열상이 있는 것을 발견한다. 경찰관은 다른 한 명을 구금하고 아이들을 돌보기 위한 준비를 한다. 일차평가를 시행한 결과 생명에 위협이 없는 것으로 확인되었다. 이차평가에서도 추가 손상이 발견되지 않았다. 아무 문제 없이 환자를 가장 가까운 병원으로 이송한다.

References

1. Miller A. Emergency medical service personnel injury and fatality in the United States. *J Epidemiol Res*. 2018;4(2): 9-18.
2. Federal Emergency Management Agency, U.S. Department of Homeland Security. *National Incident Management System*. 3rd ed. October 2017. Accessed October 17, 2021. https://www.fema.gov/sites/default/files/2020-07/fema_nims_doctrine-2017.pdf
3. Kuhar DT, Henderson DK, Struble KA, et al. Updated US Public Health Service guidelines for the management of occupational exposures to human immunodeficiency virus and recommendations for postexposure prophylaxis [published correction appears in *Infect Control Hosp Epidemiol*. 2013 Nov;34(11):1238. Dosage error in article text]. *Infect Control Hosp Epidemiol*. 2013;34(9):875-892. doi:10.1086/672271
4. Chen SL, Morgan TR. The natural history of hepatitis C virus (HCV) infection. *Int J Med Sci*. 2006;3(2):47-52.
5. Bell J, Batey RG, Farrell GC, Crewe EB, Cunningham AL, Byth K. Hepatitis C virus in intravenous drug users. *Med J Aust*. 1990 Sep 3;153(5):274-276.
6. Poland GA, Jacobson RM. Prevention of hepatitis B with the hepatitis B vaccine. *N Engl J Med*. 2004;351:2832.
7. U.S. Department of Health and Human Services, Centers for Disease Control and Prevention. Exposure to blood: what healthcare personnel need to know. July 2003. Accessed October 17, 2021. https://www.cdc.gov/hai/pdfs/bbp/exp_to_blood.pdf
8. Lerner EB, Schwartz RB, Coule PL, et al. Mass casualty triage: an evaluation of the data and development of a proposed national guideline. *Disaster Med Pub Health Prep*. 2008;2:S25-S34.

Suggested Reading

Centers for Disease Control and Prevention: See website for information on standard precautions and postexposure prophylaxis, www.cdc.gov.

National Institute for Occupational Safety and Health. Workplace solutions: preventing exposure to bloodborne pathogens among paramedics. DHHS (NIOSH) Publication No. 2010-139.

Rinnert KJ. A review of infection control practices, risk reduction, and legislative regulations for blood-borne disease: applications for emergency medical services. *Prehosp Emerg Care*. 1998;2(1):70.

Rinnert KJ, O'Connor RE, Delbridge T. Risk reduction for exposure to blood-borne pathogens in EMS: National Association of EMS Physicians. *Prehosp Emerg Care*. 1998;2(1):62.

© Ralf Hiemisch/Getty Images

환자 평가 및 처치

Lead Editors
Vince Mosesso, MD, FACEP
Michael Holtz, MD

학습 목표

이 장의 학습을 완료하면 다음과 같은 내용을 수행할 수 있다.

- 외상 환자의 전반적인 처치 맥락에서 환자 평가의 중요성에 관해 설명할 수 있다.
- 신속한 일차평가를 수행하는 방법과 일차평가를 시행하는 중에 평가 및 처치가 어떻게 통합되는 설명할 수 있다.
- 이차평가의 구성 요소와 외상 환자 평가에서 사용되는 시기를 설명할 수 있다.
- 현장에서 환자 분류 결정 체계를 활용하여 외상 환자를 이송할 의료기관을 결정할 수 있다.

시나리오

11월 초 토요일 아침 날씨는 맑고 기온은 5.5℃이다. 당신이 소속된 구급팀은 2층 건물 옥상에서 추락한 사람이 있다는 신고를 받고 현장으로 출동한다. 현장에 도착하자마자 환자의 가족이 당신을 집 뒷마당으로 안내한다. 가족은 환자가 지붕에서 빗물받이의 낙엽을 빗자루로 청소하던 중 균형을 잃고 지붕에서(약 3.6m) 등부터 추락했다고 말한다. 환자는 처음에 잠시 의식을 잃었지만, 119에 신고할 때는 의식이 있었다.

환자에게 다가가 보니 약 40대의 남성이 바닥에 반듯하게 누워 있고 두 명의 가족이 그의 옆에 무릎을 꿇고 있는 것을 목격한다. 환자는 의식이 있고 가족과 이야기하고 있으며 심한 출혈의 징후는 보이지 않는다. 동료가 환자의 머리와 목을 도수로 고정할 때 당신이 환자에게 어디가 아픈지 물어본다. 환자는 등 전체가 가장 아프다고 말한다.

초기 문진은 환자의 주요호소증상을 파악하고 그의 초기 의식 수준을 결정하며 환기 노력을 평가하는 등 다양한 목적으로 수행된다. 명백한 호흡곤란이 발견되지 않으면 환자 평가를 진행한다. 환자는 당신의 질문에 적절하게 대답하며 사람, 시간, 장소에 대한 지남력은 정상이다.

- 이 사고와 관련된 외상의 물리학에 근거하여 평가하는 중에 어떤 잠재적인 손상을 발견할 것으로 예상하는가?
- 다음 우선순위는 무엇인가?
- 이 환자를 어떻게 처치할 것인가?

개요

평가는 모든 환자 처치의 초석이다. 외상 환자의 경우 다른 중증 환자와 마찬가지로 평가는 모든 처치 및 이송 결정의 기초가 된다. 환자의 상태에 대한 전반적 인상이 형성되고 호흡, 순환, 신경계 상태에 대한 기준값이 설정된다. 생명을 위협하는 상태가 확인되면 즉각적인 처치와 소생술을 시작한다. 시간과 환자 상태가 허락하는 경우 생명이나 팔다리에 위협이 되지 않는 손상에 대해 이차평가를 한다. 이차평가는 종종 환자 이송 중에 이루어진다.

이러한 모든 단계는 현장에서 소요되는 시간을 최소화하는 것을 목표로 신속하고 효율적으로 수행된다. 중증 환자는 구조가 필요하거나 신속한 이송을 방해하는 다른 문제가 없는 한 즉각적으로 생명을 위협하는 것을 처치하는 것 외에 다른 처치를 수행하기 위해 현장에 남아 있어서는 안 된다. 이 과정에서 배운 원칙을 적용하면 현장 체류 시간을 최소화고 환자를 적절한 의료기관으로 신속하게 이송할 수 있다. 성공적인 평가와 처치를 수행하기 위해서는 외상 생리학에 대한 충분한 지식을 기반으로 신속하고 효과적으로 수행할 수 있도록 잘 수립된 처치 계획이 필요하다.

외상 처치와 관련된 문헌에서는 외상 환자를 손상 발생 후 짧은 시간 내에 최종 수술 치료를 받을 수 있도록 이송해야 한다고 자주 언급한다. 이러한 긴급성은 중증외상 환자의 경우 내부출혈과 같이 병원 전 환경에서 처치할 수 없는 손상이 있을 수 있기 때문이다. 대부분의 심각한 출혈에 대한 결정적인 출혈 조절은 병원 환경, 주로 수술실에서 이루어진다.

외상 환자의 평가 및 처치에 대한 주요 관심사는 1) 대량 출혈 지혈, 2) 기도, 3) 산소 공급, 4) 환기, 5) 관류 및 6) 신경학적 기능이다. 이 순서는 신체가 산소를 공급하는 능력과 적혈구(RBC)가 조직에 산소를 전달하는 능력을 모두 보호한다.

애덤스 카울리(R Adams Cowley) 박사는 외상의 "황금 시간"이라는 개념을 개발했다. 그는 손상 발생 후 결정적인 처치까지 걸리는 시간이 매우 중요하다고 생각했다. 이 시간 동안 출혈이 조절되지 않고 관류 감소로 인해 조직으로 산소 공급이 불충분하면 신체 전체에 손상이 발생한다.

황금 시간은 정확히 1시간이 아니기 때문에 "황금 기간(Golden Period)"이라고 표현하는 것이 더 좋다. 어떤 환자는 치료를 받을 수 있는 시간이 1시간 미만이지만, 어떤 환자는 그보다 더 긴 시간이 걸릴 수 있다. 병원 전 처치 제공자는 주어진 상황의 긴급성을 인식하고 환자를 가능한 한 빨리 최종 치료를 받을 수 있는 의료기관으로

이송할 책임이 있다. 외상 환자에게 결정적인 처치를 시행할 수 있는 의료기관으로 이송하려면 환자의 생명을 위협하는 손상의 심각성을 신속하게 파악하고 현장에서 생명을 구할 수 있는 필수적인 처치만 제공하며 적절한 의료기관으로 신속하게 이송을 시작해야 한다. 많은 도시의 병원 전 시스템에서 EMS가 활성화되고 현장에 도착하기까지 평균 8~9분이 걸리며 이 시간에는 사고 발생부터 신고하는 시간은 포함되지 않는다. 일반적으로 환자를 이송하는 데 8~9분이 더 소요된다. 병원 전 처치 제공자가 현장에서 10분 미만의 시간을 보낸다면 환자가 의료기관에 도착할 때는 이미 30분 이상의 시간이 흐른 후일 것이다. 현장에서 머무는 시간이 1분 더 늘어날 때마다 환자의 출혈 시간이 늘어나는 것이며 황금 시간 또는 황금 기간에서 소중한 시간이 흘러가고 있다.

이 중요한 외상 처치 문제를 해결하기 위해서는 환자를 신속하고 효율적으로 평가하고 처치하는 것이 궁극적인 목표이다. 현장 체류 시간을 최소화해야 하며 "백금 10분"은 연구에 의해 직접적으로 뒷받침되지는 않지만, 신속한 처치를 뒷받침하는 증거가 있다. 외상으로 인한 출혈 쇼크 환자의 경우 응급실에서 수술실에 도착하는 시간이 지연되면 사망률이 증가한다는 증거가 있다. 그러므로 애초에 응급실에 도착하는 것이 지연되는 것은 해로울 수 있다는 것은 논리적이다. 출혈 조절이 출혈쇼크 처치에 필수적인 요소라는 것은 본질적으로 논리적이고 논란의 여지가 없다. 또한 현장 체류 시간이 길어지는 것이 유익하다거나 어떤 식으로든 환자 처치를 개선한다는 증거도 부족하다.

외상 환자가 현장에 오래 머물수록 출혈과 사망 가능성이 커진다. 현장 체류 시간 연장은 구출 지연, 현장 위험 및 기타 예상치 못한 현장 상황과 같은 특별한 상황에서만 발생해야 한다. 외상으로 인해 출혈이 있는 환자가 수술실로 이동하는 데 방해가 되는 것은 거의 없어야 한다.

이 장에서는 현장에서의 환자 평가 및 초기 처치의 필수 사항을 다루며 ATLS 프로그램에서 의사에게 가르치는 접근 방식을 기반으로 한다. 또한, PHTLS에서 가르치는 접근 방식은 ATLS에서 가르치는 병원 전 처치와 병원 내 처치의 차이점을 반영한다. 설명된 원칙은 때때로 다른 용어가 사용될 수 있지만, 초기 기본 또는 전문 교육 프로그램에서 배운 원칙과 같다. 예를 들어, 일차평가라는 용어는 ATLS 프로그램에서 국가 EMS 교육 표준에서 일차평가로 알려진 환자 평가 활동을 설명하기 위해 사용된다. 대부분의 경우 이 단계에서 수행되는 활동은 동일하며 다양한 과정에서 단순히 다른 용어를 사용한다.

우선순위 결정

현장에 도착하면 즉각적으로 처리해야 할 세 가지 우선순위가 있다.

1. 외상 사고에 관련된 모든 사람의 최우선 순위는 현장 평가와 현장 안전이다. 상황에 적절한 개인보호장비를 착용하고 표준 예방 조치(혈액 및 체액으로부터 보호)를 준수한다. 지역사회에 확산하는 에어로졸화된 질병 확산과 관련하여 현재 상황에 따라 적절한 경우 전염성 질병에 대한 비말 및 공기 중 예방 조치를 사용해야 한다. 5장 현장 관리에서 이 주제에 대해 자세히 설명한다.

2. 추가 자원의 필요성을 파악한다. 대응자는 다발성 환자 발생사고 및 다수 사상자 발생사고의 가능성을 인식해야 한다. 다수 사상자 발생 사고에서는 모든 자원을 가장 심각하게 손상을 입은 환자에게 집중하는 것에서 최대한 많은 환자를 구하는 것(최대 다수에게 최대 이익을 제공하는 것)으로 우선순위가 바뀐다. 환자가 여러 명일 때 환자 분류에 영향을 미칠 수 있는 요인에는 손상의 심각성과 환자 처치하는 데 사용할 수 있는 자원(인력과 장비)이 포함된다. 5장 현장 관리 및 17장 재난 관리에서도 환자 분류에 관해 설명한다.

3. 간단한 현장 평가를 수행하고 관련 요구 사항이 해결되면 개별 환자를 평가하는 데 주의를 기울일 수 있다. 평가 및 처치 과정은 자원이 허용하는 한 가장 중증인 것으로 확인된 환자에게 집중하는 것으로 시작된다. 1) 생명을 잃을 수 있는 상태, 2) 팔다리를 잃을 수 있는 상태, 3) 생명이나 팔다리를 위협하지 않는 기타 모든 상태의 순서로 강조된다. 손상의 심각성, 환자 수, 의료기관의 접근성에 따라 생명이나 팔다리를 위협하지 않는 상태는 현장에서 처치하지 않을 수 있다.

이 장의 대부분은 적절한 평가를 수행하고 결과를 해석하며 적절한 환자 처치를 위한 우선순위를 결정하는 데 필요한 비판적 사고 기술에 중점을 둔다. 이 과정을 통해 필요한 처치를 적절히 제공할 수 있다.

일차평가

중증 다발성 외상 환자에서 처치의 우선순위는 생명을 위협하는 상태를 신속하게 파악하고 처치하는 것이다(**Box 6-1**). 대부분의 외상 환자는 한 가지 계통(예: 다리 골절)에만, 손상을 입는다. 이러한 단일 계통 외상 환자의 경우 일차평가 및 이차평가를 모두 철저하게 수행

할 수 있는 경우가 더 많다. 다기관 손상이 있는 생리학적으로 불안정한 환자의 경우 병원 전 처치 제공자가 일차평가 이상의 조치를 시행하지 못할 수도 있다. 이러한 중증 환자의 경우 신속한 평가, 소생술 시작 및 적절한 의료기관으로 이송에 중점을 두어야 한다. 신속한 이송에 대한 강조는 병원 전 처치의 필요성을 배제하는 것이 아니다. 오히려 생명을 위협하는 경우 즉시 처치를 시작하고 가장 가까운 적절한 외상센터로 이송하면서 처치를 계속해야 한다.

우선순위를 빠르게 결정하고 생명을 위협하는 손상에 대한 일차평가를 신속하게 시행한다는 것을 병원 전 처치 제공자는 기억해야 한다. 따라서 일차평가 및 이차평가의 구성 요소를 기억하고 손상의 심각성과 관계없이 매번 같은 방식으로 우선순위에 따른 평가와 처치를 이해하고 수행해야 한다. 병원 전 처치 제공자는 환자의 손상과 상태의 병태생리에 대해 생각해야 한다.

외상에서 가장 흔한 생명을 위협하는 것 중 하나는 조직으로 적절한 산소 공급 부족(쇼크)으로 인해 무산소대사가 일어나는 것이다. 대사는 세포가 에너지를 생산하는 기전이다. 정상적인 대사 과정이 이루어지기 위해서는 1) 적절한 적혈구 수, 2) 폐에서 적혈구의 산소화, 3) 적혈구가 전신의 세포로 전달, 4) 이러한 세포에 산소가 공급되는 네 가지 조건이 필요하다. 일차평가에 포함된 활동은 이러한 상태의 문제를 파악하고 교정하는 데 목적이 있다. 무산소대사는 에너지 생산 효율이 떨어지고 젖산산증을 유발한다.

일반적인 인상

일차평가는 환자의 호흡기, 순환계 및 신경계 상태를 신속하게 파악하여 심각한 출혈의, 기도, 호흡, 순환 장애, 심각한 변형 등 생명이나 팔다리에 대한 명백한 위협을 파악하는 것으로 시작된다. 병원 전 처치 제공자는 처음에 환자에게 접근할 때 심각한 외부출혈이 있는

지 확인하고 환자가 효과적으로 호흡을 하는 것처럼 보이는지, 의식이 있거나 반응이 없는지, 자발적으로 움직일 수 있는지 확인한다. 병원 전 처치 제공자는 환자 곁에 도착하면 자신을 소개하고 환자의 이름을 물어본다. 합리적인 다음 단계는 환자에게 "무슨 일이 일어났나요?"라고 물어보는 것이다. 환자가 편안해 보이고 완전한 문장으로 일관성 있게 대답하면 환자의 기도는 개방되어 있고 말을 할 수 있을 만큼 호흡 기능이 충분하며 뇌관류가 적절하고 신경학적 기능이 정상이며 이 환자는 즉각적으로 생명을 위협하는 손상은 없다는 결론을 내릴 수 있다.

환자가 그러한 대답을 할 수 없거나 고통스러워 보이는 경우 생명을 위협하는 문제를 파악하기 위해 자세한 일차평가를 시작한다. 몇 초 안에 환자의 전반적인 상태에 대한 일반적인 인상을 얻을 수 있다. 일차평가는 주요 기능을 신속하게 평가하여 환자가 현재 위독한 상태인지 또는 위독한 상태가 임박 한지를 확인하는 역할을 한다.

일차평가 순서

일차평가는 신속하고 논리적인 순서로 진행되어야 한다. 병원 전 처치 제공자가 혼자인 경우 생명을 위협하는 상태가 확인되면 몇 가지 주요 처치를 수행할 수 있다. 기도를 흡인하거나 지혈대를 적용하는 것과 같이 문제를 쉽게 해결할 수 있는 경우 병원 전 처치 제공자는 다음 단계로 넘어가기 전에 문제를 해결할 수 있다. 반대로 내부출혈로 인해 쇼크가 발생한 경우와 같이 현장에서 문제를 신속하게 해결할 수 없는 경우 일차평가를 신속하게 완료한다. 두 명 이상의 병원 전 처치 제공자가 현장에 있는 경우 한 명의 병원 처치 제공자가 일차평가를 완료하는 동안 다른 병원 전 처치 제공자는 확인된 문제에 대한 처치를 시작할 수 있다. 여러 가지 심각한 상태가 확인되면 일차평가를 통해 병원 전 처치 제공자는 처치의 우선순위를 결정할 수 있다. 일반적으로 압박으로 지혈할 수 있는 외부출혈을 먼저 처치한 후 기도 문제를 호흡장애가 발생하기 전에 처치하는 등의 방식으로 처치한다.

환자의 유형과 관계없이 같은 일차평가 방법을 사용한다. 노인, 소아 또는 임신한 환자를 포함한 모든 환자를 유사한 방법으로 평가하여 평가의 모든 구성 요소를 바탕으로 중요한 병리학적 상태를 놓치지 않도록 한다.

외상 환자에 대한 일차평가는 생명을 위협하는 외부출혈의 조절하는 것을 첫 번째 단계로 강조한다. 일차평가의 단계가 차례대로 교육되고 실습하더라도 많은 단계가 동시에 수행될 수 있고 수행되어야

한다. 각 단계는 XABCDE를 사용하여 기억할 수 있다.

- **X**(**Ex**sanguinating Hemorrhage): 대량 출혈(심각한 외부출혈 지혈)
- **A**(**A**irway): 기도 관리 및 척추 움직임 제한
- **B**(**B**reathing): 호흡(환기 및 산소 공급)
- **C**(**C**irculation): 순환(관류 및 기타 출혈)
- **D**(**D**isability): 장애(신경학적 평가)
- **E**(**Ex**pose/**E**nvironment): 노출/환경

X—대량 출혈(심각한 외부출혈 지혈)

외상 환자의 일차평가에서 생명을 위협하는 외부출혈을 즉시 확인하고 지혈해야 한다. 대량의 외부출혈이 있는 경우 기도를 평가하기 전(또는 현장에 적절한 지원이 있는 경우 동시) 또는 척추고정과 같은 다른 처치를 수행하기 전에 출혈을 지혈해야 한다. 이러한 유형의 출혈은 일반적으로 팔다리의 동맥 출혈에서 발생하지만, 두피나 몸통과 팔다리가 연결되는 부분(접합부 출혈) 및 기타 부위에서 발생할 수도 있다.

팔다리에서 발생한 대량 동맥출혈은 즉시 지혈대를 가능한 한 손상된 팔다리의 근위부(즉, 서혜부 또는 겨드랑이 부위)에 적용하는 것이 가장 효과적이다. 직접 압박 및 지혈제와 같은 다른 지혈 방법도 사용할 수 있지만, 이러면 지혈대 배치를 지연시키거나 대신해서는 안 된다. 팔다리의 비동맥성 중증 출혈과 몸통 부위의 중증 출혈이 있는 경우 직접 압박과 지혈 패킹 및 드레싱을 적용한다. 때때로 원위부 동맥이나 더 작은 동맥의 출혈은 집적 압박으로 지혈할 수 있다. 그러나 이 방법은 일반적으로 지혈대를 근위부에 적용할 수 있을 때까지 일시적으로 시행하는 조치이다. 접합 부위의 심한 출혈은 가능한 경우 적절한 접합부 지혈대 또는 클램프를 사용하거나 지혈 거즈로 패킹하고 압박 드레싱을 시행하면 처치할 수 있다(**Box 6-2**).

A—기도 관리 및 척추 움직임 제한

기도

환자의 기도 상태를 신속하게 평가하여 기도가 개방되어 있고 기도 폐쇄 위험이 없는지 확인한다. 기도가 손상된 경우 처음에는 도수 방법(외상 턱들기 또는 외상 턱밀어올리기)으로 기도를 개방하고(**그림 6-2**) 필요한 경우 혈액, 분비물 및 이물질을 제거한다. 결국 장비와 더 많은 인력이 확보되면 기도 관리는 흡인 및 기계적 수단(입인두기도기, 코인두기도기, 성문위기도기, 기관내삽관 또는 기관절개술)을

Box 6-2 접합부의 심한 출혈

접합부 출혈은 목 밑부분을 포함하여 몸통과 팔다리의 접합부에서 발생하는 출혈로 정의된다. 접합부의 예로는 서혜부, 볼기 및 겨드랑이가 있다(그림 6-1). 이러한 부위에 지혈대나 압박 드레싱을 사용하는 것은 종종 비실용적이고 효과적이지 않은 경우가 많다.

접합부 출혈의 주요 처치 방법은 손상 부위 근위부에 걸쳐 있는 큰 혈관을 직접 압박하는 것이다. 병원 전 환경에서 출혈 속도를 늦추기 위해 넓적다리동맥, 엉덩동맥 또는 겨드랑동맥에 상당한 양의 직접 압박이 필요할 수 있다. 이를 위해 다양한 상용 장비를 사용할 수 있다. 이는 종종 외부에서 적용하는 지혈제와 압박 드레싱의 사용과 결합한다. 또한 무릎 위 다리의 외상성 절단 환자에게 골반 고정대를 적용하여 출혈 조절에 도움이 된다는 경험적 증거가 있다.

외부출혈 조절에 사용하는 지혈제와 압박 드레싱을 함께 수행하기도 한다. 또한, 무릎 높이 이상의 다리가 절단된 외상 환자에게 골반 고정대를 적용한 경험적 사례가 이 주장을 뒷받침한다. 이러한 외상 환자에게 가해지는 강력한 힘은 골반 및 어깨와 같이 인접한 부위에 손상을 입을 수 있기 때문에 이러한 부위의 안정화도 함께 고려해야 한다. 이러한 외상성 손상에서 발생하는 상당한 힘은 종종 골반과 팔이음뼈와 같은 인접한 구조물을 손상하므로 이러한 부위의 안정화도 고려되어야 한다.

전술적 전투 사상자 처치 위원회(CoTCCC)는 접합부 출혈 부위에 사용하기 위해 특별히 제작된 세 가지 지혈대를 권장한다. 여기에는 접합부 지혈대(CRoC, JETT, SAM)가 포함된다. 실험실 환경에서 이러한 장비를 비교한 연구에서 다양한 장단점이 확인되었으며 현장에서 장비를 사용하는 인력이 장비를 선택할 때 이러한 모든 사항을 고려해야 한다.

접합부 부위의 출혈을 조절하려고 시도할 때 고려해야 할 가장 중요한 개념은 1) 해당 부위에 걸쳐 있는 혈관에 강한 힘으로 직접 압박이 필요하다는 것과 2) 지혈제를 사용한 직접 압박 드레싱을 상처의 개방된 부위에 시행해야 한다는 점이다. 이 두 가지 처치 방법이 결합하면 치명적인 외상을 입은 상황에서 생존 가능성을 높일 수 있다. 결론은 가능한 한 빨리 손상 부위에 압박 드레싱을 하고 출혈이 있는 동맥 부위를 압박해야 한다는 것이다.

© National Association of Emergency Medical Technicians (NAEMT)

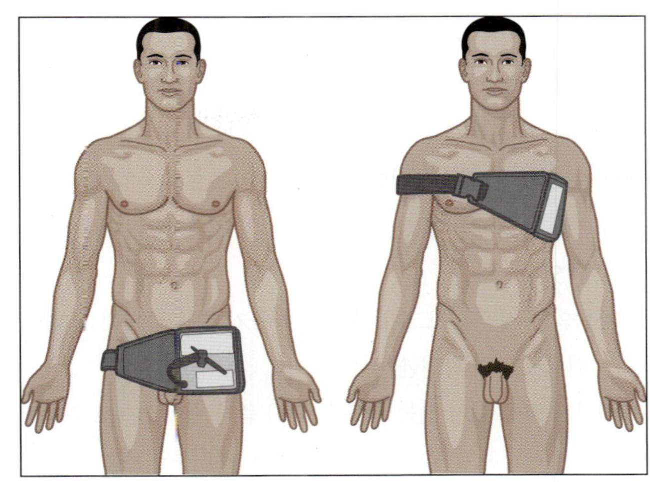

그림 6-1 겨드랑이와 서혜부의 접합 부위.
© Jones & Bartlett Learning

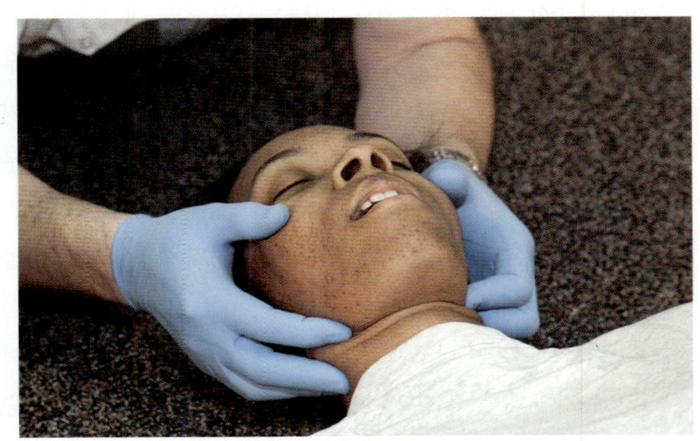

그림 6-2 기도가 손상된 것처럼 보이면 척추 고정을 유지하면서 기도를 개방해야 한다.
© National Association of Emergency Medical Technicians (NAEMT)

사용할 수 있다. 기도 유지 방법을 결정하는 데는 사용할 수 있는 장비, 병원 전 처치 제공자의 숙련도, 외상센터까지의 이송 거리 등 다양한 요인이 영향을 미친다. 후두 골절이나 불완전한 기도 가로절단과 같은 일부 기도 손상은 기관내삽관 시도로 인해 악화할 수 있다. 기도 관리는 7장 기도와 환기에서 자세히 설명한다.

척추 움직임 제한

척추 손상이 결정적으로 배제될 때까지 심각한 무딘 손상 기전이 있는 모든 외상 환자에서 척추 손상을 의심해야 한다. 특히 노인이나 만성적으로 쇠약해진 환자의 경우 경미한 손상 기전이 있더라도 척추 손상의 의심 지수를 높게 유지하는 것이 중요하다(척추 움직임 제한에 대한 적응증 9장 척추 외상을 참조). 기도를 유지하는 것이 우선이지만 목뼈 손상의 가능성을 항상 고려해야 한다. 척추 골절이 있는 경우 골절된 척추가 척수에 압박을 가할 수 있으므로 어떤 방향으로든 과도한 움직임은 신경학적 손상을 유발하거나 악화시킬 수 있다. 따라서 전체 평가 과정 특히, 기도를 유지하고 보조 환기를 시행할 때 도수 고정으로 환자의 머리와 목을 중립 자세로 유지해야 한다. 이러한 목뼈의 안정화가 필요하다고 해서 필요한 기도 유지 절차를 적용할 수 없다는 것을 의미하는 것은 아니다. 대신 환자의 척추가 불필요하게 움직이지 않도록 보호하면서 처치를 진행한다는 의미이다. 환자를 재평가하거나 필요한 처치를 수행하기 위해 적용한 척추 고정 장비를 제거해야 하는 경우 장비를 다시 적용할 수 있을 때까지 머리와 목을 도수로 고정한다. 관통성 외상만 입은 환자의 경우 척추 고정 장비가 필요하지 않다.

B—호흡(환기 및 산소 공급)

호흡은 산소를 환자의 폐로 효과적으로 전달하여 유산소 대사 과정을 유지하는 데 도움을 준다. 저산소증은 폐의 부적절한 환기로 인해 발생할 수 있으며 신체 조직의 산소 공급 부족으로 이어질 수 있다. 환자의 기도가 개방되면 환자 호흡(환기)의 질과 양을 다음과 같이 평가할 수 있다.

1. 가슴의 움직임을 보고 입과 코에서 공기 흐름을 느껴 환자가 숨을 쉬고 있는지 확인한다.

2. 환자가 숨을 쉬지 않는 경우(무호흡) 즉시 백마스크로 환자에게 환기를 시작하고 평가를 계속한다. 가능한 경우 보충 산소를 공급하고 필요한 경우 척추 움직임 제한을 유지한다.

3. 환자의 기도가 확보되었는지 확인하고 보조 환기를 계속 제공하거나 가능한 경우 입인두기도기 또는 코인두기도기(심각한 얼굴 외상이 없는 경우)를 삽입한다. 환자가 계속 반응이 없는 경우 환자 상태와 외상센터와의 접근성에 따라서 보다 더 확실한 기도유지기를 삽입해야 하는지 아닌지를 고려한다. 여기에는 성문위기도기(심각한 입인두 외상의 징후가 없는 경우), 기관내삽관(숙련된 처치 제공자)이 포함될 수 있다. 기도에서 혈액, 구토물 또는 기타 액체를 흡인할 준비를 한다.

4. 일반적으로 호흡수라고 부르지만, 환자가 얼마나 빨리 숨을 쉬고 있는지에 대한 더 정확한 용어는 환기 속도이다. 환기는 들숨과 날숨 과정을 말하지만, 호흡은 모세혈관과 폐포 사이의 가스 교환의 생리학적 과정을 가장 잘 설명한다. 환자가 호흡하는 경우 환기수와 깊이의 적절성을 평가하여 환자가 충분한 공기를 이동시키고 있는지 확인한다(분당 환기량은 호흡수 × 깊이)(7장 기도와 환기 참조).

5. 환자가 저산소증이 없고 산소포화도가 94% 이상인지 확인한다. 적절한 산소포화도를 유지하는 데 필요에 따라 보충 산소(보조 환기)를 제공해야 한다.

6. 환자가 의식이 있는 경우 환자가 어려움 없이 완전한 문장을 말할 수 있는지 확인한다.

환기율은 다음과 같이 다섯 가지로 분류할 수 있다.

1. 무호흡: 환자가 숨을 쉬지 않는다. 여기에는 공기 교환이 효과적으로 이루어지지 않는 간헐적으로 헐떡임(임종 호흡)이 포함된다.

2. 느림: 분당 10회 미만의 매우 느린 호흡(호흡 완만)은 뇌의 심각한 손상 또는 허혈(산소 공급 감소)을 나타낼 수 있다. 이러한 경우 병원 전 처치 제공자는 충분한 양의 공기 교환이 이루어지고 있는지 확인해야 한다. 백마스크로 환자의 호흡을 보조하거나 완전히 대신해야 하는 경우가 종종 있다. 백마스크를 사용한 보조 환기 또는 전체 환기를 지원하는 경우 산소포화도가 94% 이상이 되도록 보충 산소를 공급하는 것이 포함되어야 한다(**그림 6-3**).

3. 정상: 환기 속도가 분당 10~20회인 경우 병원 전 처치 제공자는 적절한 환기량과 산소포화도가 유지되는지 확인해야 한다. 필요한 경우 보충 산소를 공급한다.

4. 빠름: 호흡수가 분당 20~30회(빠른 호흡)인 경우 환자의 상태가 호전되거나 악화하는지를 주의 깊게 관찰해야 한다. 환기수를 증가시키는 원동력은 혈중 이산화탄소 축적이 증가하거나 저산소증 또는 빈혈로 인해 혈중 산소 농도 수치가 감소하는 것이다. 통증이나 불안도 환기 속도를 증가시킬 수 있다. 환자가 비정상적인 환기 속도를 보이는 경우 원인을 확인한다. 빠른 속도는 충분한 산소가 신체 조직으로 전달되지 못한다는 것을 나타낼 수 있다. 이러한 산소 부족은 무산소대사(3장 쇼크: 삶과 죽음의 병태생리학을 참조)를 시작하고 궁극적으로 혈중 이산화탄소 수치를 증가시켜 대사성산증을 유발한다. 인체의 감지 시스템은 증가한 혈중 이산화탄소 수준을 인식하고 초과한 이산화탄소를 제거하기 위해 호흡의 양과 깊이를 증가시키도록 환기

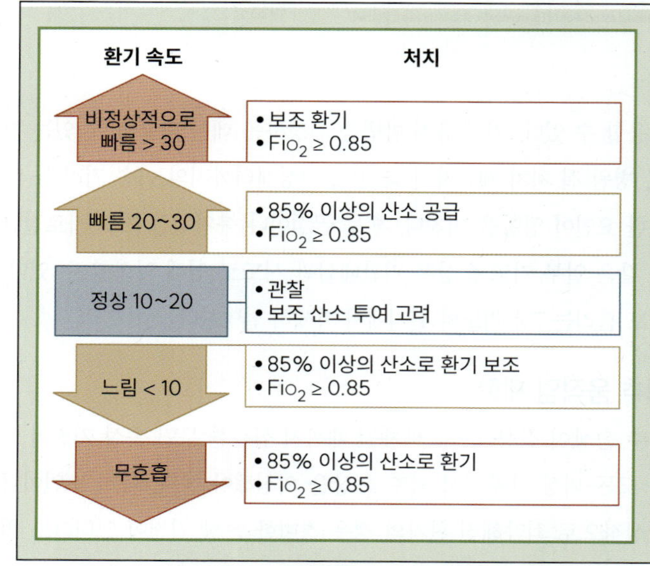

그림 6-3 자발적 환기율에 따른 기도 관리.
© Jones & Bartlett Learning

시스템에 지시한다. 따라서 환기 속도가 증가하면 환자에게 더 나은 관류나 산소 공급이 필요하거나 둘다 필요하다는 것으로 나타낼 수 있다. 산소포화도를 94% 이상으로 유지되도록 보충 산소를 공급한다. 병원 전 처치 제공자는 환자의 전반적인 상태가 악화하는지 자세히 모니터링한다.

5. **매우 빠름**: 호흡수가 분당 30회(심각하게 빠른 호흡)를 초과하면 저산소증, 무산소대사 또는 두 가지 모두를 의미하며 결과적으로 산증이 발생한다. 빠른 환기의 원인이 일차적인 환기 문제인지 아니면 부적절한 관류 또는 심각한 출혈과 같은 산소 공급 문제인지 즉시 확인해야 한다. 산소 공급 및 환기를 방해할 수 있는 손상에는 긴장기흉, 폐 타박상, 동요가슴, 대량 혈흉 및 개방 기흉이 있다. 원인이 확인되면 즉시 처치를 시행하여 문제를 해결해야 한다(10장 가슴 외상 참조). 호흡수가 분당 30회를 초과하는 환자는 산소를 공급해야 한다. 이러한 환자의 피로감이나 의식 상태 저하, 호기말이산화탄소분압 증가 또는 낮은 산소포화도와 같은 부적절한 환기의 징후가 있는지 주의 깊게 모니터링하고 필요한 경우 백마스크로 보조 환기를 시행하여 적절한 분당 환기 및 산소포화도를 유지한다.

환기가 비정상적인 환자의 경우 가슴을 노출하고 관찰하며 빠르게 촉진한다. 그런 다음 폐 청진을 통해 호흡음이 비정상적이거나 감소하거나 들리지 않는지 확인한다. 환기를 방해할 수 있는 손상에는 긴장기흉, 동요가슴, 척수 손상 및 외상성 뇌손상 등이 있다. 이러한 손상은 일차평가 중에 확인되거나 의심되는 경우 즉시 보조 환기를 시작해야 한다. 긴장기흉이 의심되는 경우 바늘감압을 즉시 실행한다.

외상 환자의 환기 상태를 평가할 때는 호흡수뿐만 아니라 깊이도 평가한다. 환자가 분당 16회의 정상적인 환기 속도로 호흡하고 있지만, 호흡 깊이가 심하게 감소할 수 있다. 반대로 환기 깊이는 정상적이지만, 환기 속도가 증가하거나 감소할 수 있다. 일회호흡량에 환기 속도를 곱하여 환자의 분당환기량을 계산한다(7장 기도와 환기 참조).

C—순환(관류 및 기타 출혈)

순환계 손상 또는 기능 상실을 평가하는 것은 외상 환자를 처치하는 다음 단계이다. 조직 세포에 전달되지 않은 적혈구의 산소 공급은 환자에게 아무런 도움이 되지 않는다. 이 과정의 첫 번째 단계에서 생명을 위협하는 출혈이 확인하고 지혈한다. 병원 전 처치 제공자는 환자의 기도와 호흡 상태를 평가한 후 환자의 심박출량과 관류 상태에 대한 전반적인 추정치를 얻어야 한다. 외부출혈 또는 내부출혈은 외상으로 인한 예방 가능한 사망의 가장 흔한 원인이다. 기도와 호흡 문제를 해결한 후 일차평가 단계에서 덜 심각한 출혈을 조절한다.

출혈 조절

중증 출혈을 가능한 한 빨리 지혈하지 않으면 환자의 사망 가능성이 급격히 증가하기 때문에 외부출혈은 일차평가에서 확인하고 지혈한다. 외부출혈의 세 가지 유형은 모세혈관, 정맥 및 동맥 출혈이며 다음과 같이 설명된다.

1. 모세혈관 출혈은 피부 표면 바로 아래에 있는 작은 모세혈관이 찰과상으로 인해 발생한다. 모세혈관 출혈은 일반적으로 생명을 위협하지 않으며 병원 전 처치 제공자가 현장에 도착하기 전에 출혈 속도가 느려지거나 지혈되었을 수도 있다.

2. 정맥 출혈은 정맥의 열상이나 기타 손상으로 인해 발생하며 이에 따라 상처에서 검붉은 혈액이 지속해서 흘러나오게 된다. 이러한 유형의 출혈은 일반적으로 직접 압박으로 지혈할 수 있다. 정맥 출혈은 출혈이 오래 지속되거나 큰 정맥이 손상되지 않는 한 일반적으로 생명을 위협하지 않는다.

3. 동맥 출혈은 동맥이 찢어지는 손상으로 인해 발생한다. 동맥 출혈은 가장 위험하며 지혈하기 가장 어려운 유형의 출혈이다. 일반적으로 밝은 선홍색 혈액이 분출하는 것이 특징이다. 그러나 동맥 출혈은 심부 동맥이 손상된 경우 상처에서 빠르게 분출되는 혈액으로 나타날 수도 있다. 심지어 작고 깊은 동맥 천자와 같은 상처라도 생명을 위협하는 출혈을 일으킬 수 있다.

동맥출혈의 신속한 지혈은 외상 환자 처치에서 중요한 목표 중 하나이다. 일차평가는 첫 번째 단계에서 출혈이 지혈되지 않으면 진행할 수 없다. 모세혈관 출혈과 정맥 출혈은 일반적으로 일차평가의 뒷부분에서 다루어진다.

출혈은 다음과 같은 방법으로 조절할 수 있다.

1. **직접 압박**: 직접 압박은 이름에서 알 수 있듯이 출혈 부위에 직접 압력을 가하는 것이다. 이는 출혈 부위(확인할 수 있는 경우) 바로 위에 드레싱(지혈 거즈 선호)을 대고 압력을 가하는 방식으로 이루어진다. 가능한 한 정확한 위치에 집중적으로 압력을 가해야 한다. 눈에 보이는 박동성 동맥 출혈은 손가락을 대는 것이 효과적이다. 지혈 거즈의 경우 최소 3분 이상 또는 제조업체 지침에 따르거나 일반거즈를 사용할 때는 10분 동안 지속해서 압력을 가해야 한다. 병원 전 처치 제공자는 그 전에 상처에

서 출혈이 계속되는지 확인하기 위해 압력을 멈추지 않는다. 직접 압박을 가하고 유지하려면 병원 전 처치 제공자는 다른 처치에 참여하지 말고 압박에 집중해야 한다. 또는 도움이 제한되는 경우 압박 드레싱을 적용할 수 있다. 여러 가지 상품화된 제품(예: 이스라엘 붕대)이나 거즈 패드와 탄력 붕대로 압박드레싱으로 사용할 수 있다. 출혈이 지혈되지 않으면 환자에게 산소나 수액을 얼마나 공급하든 상관없이 다량의 출혈이 계속되면 관류는 개선되지 않는다.

2. **지혈대**: 지혈대는 과거에 종종 최후의 수단으로 사용되는 술기로 설명되었다. 아프가니스탄과 이라크 전쟁에서의 미군 경험과 수술 시 외과 의사들에 의한 일상적이고 안전한 지혈대 사용으로 인해 이 지혈 방법이 재고되었다. 지혈대는 심각한 출혈을 지혈하는 데 효과적이며 직접 압력이나 압박 드레싱으로 팔다리에서 발생한 출혈을 즉시 지혈하지 못하거나 현장에서 다른 방법으로 출혈을 지혈할 수 있는 충분한 인력이 없는 경우 사용해야 한다(3장 쇼크: 삶과 죽음의 병태생리학 참조). 출혈 부위를 들어 올리는 방법과 선택적 동맥 압박은 효과를 뒷받침하는 데이터가 충분하지 않으므로 더 이상 권장하지 않는다. 앞에서 언급한 바와 같이 생명을 위협하거나 다량의 출혈을 유발하는 경우 다른 지혈 방법 대신 지혈대를 적용하거나 동시에 적용해야 한다(즉 이러한 유형의 출혈에 대한 첫 번째 처치). 또한 즉석에서 만드는 지혈대는 시중에서 판매하는 지혈대보다 효과가 떨어질 수 있다는 점에 유의한다. 그러나 임의로 사용하는 지혈대는 상품화된 지혈대보다 효과가 제한적일 수 있다는 점에 유의해야 한다.

관류

환자의 순환 상태는 말초 맥박을 확인하고 피부색, 체온 및 피부의 습도를 평가하고 심각한 외상성 뇌손상이 없는 경우 환자의 의식 상태를 평가하여 확인할 수 있다(**Box 6-3**). 노인이나 소아 환자, 상태가 양호하지만, 특정 약물을 복용하는 환자는 어려울 수 있다. 외상 환자의 쇼크는 대부분 출혈로 인해 발생한다(3장 쇼크: 삶과 죽음의 병태생리학 참조).

대량 내부출혈이 발생할 수 있는 잠재적 부위는 가슴(양쪽 가슴막안), 복막강, 골반, 복막뒤공간 및 팔다리(주로 넓적다리)를 포함한다. 내부출혈이 의심되면 가슴, 배, 골반 및 넓적다리를 노출해 신속하게 손상 징후가 있는지 신속하게 시진하고 촉진한다. 이러한 부위의 출

혈은 병원 전 환경에서 조절하기가 쉽지 않다. 의료 지도 의사의 지시가 있고 사용이 가능한 경우 골반고정대를 신속하게 적용하여 잠재적인 'open book' 골반 손상을 예방한다. 전반적인 목표는 수술실에서 출혈을 신속하게 조절할 수 있도록 인력과 장비를 갖춘 외상센터로 신속하게 이송하는 것이다.

맥박

맥박은 맥박의 유무, 질 및 규칙성을 평가한다. 환자의 맥박을 신속하게 확인하면 빈맥, 서맥 또는 불규칙한 리듬이 있는지 알 수 있다. 과거에는 노동맥이 촉지되면 수축기 혈압이 80mmHg 이상, 넓적다리동맥에서 촉지되면 수축기 혈압이 70mmHg 이상, 목동맥에서만 촉지되는 경우 수축기 혈압이 60mmHg 이상인 것으로 여겨져 왔다. 여러 증거에 따르면 이 이론은 부정확하고 혈압을 과대평가한다는 것으로 나타났다. 중심 맥박이 촉지되는 상태에서 말초 맥박이 촉지되지 않는다는 것은 심한 저혈압을 나타낼 가능성이 있지만, 말초 맥박이 촉지된다고 해서 환자의 혈압이 안정적이라고 판단해서는 안된다.

일차평가에서는 정확한 맥박수를 측정할 필요가 없다. 대신 대략적인 추정치를 빠르게 확인하고 실제 정확한 맥박수는 나중에 측정한다. 외상 환자의 경우 비정상적인 활력징후와 신체 소견에 따른 처치 가능한 원인을 고려하는 것이 중요하다. 예를 들어, 관류 장애와 호흡 곤란이 함께 나타나면 병원 전 처치 제공자는 긴장기흉의 유무를 고려해야 한다. 임상 징후가 나타나면 바늘감압이 생명을 구할 수 있다(10장 가슴 외상 참조).

피부

피부 검사를 통해 환자의 순환 상태에 대해 많은 것을 알 수 있다.

- 피부색: 혈액이 특정 부위에 관류되지 않으면 피부가 창백해진다. 창백한 피부색은 부적절한 관류와 관련이 있다. 푸르스름한 색은 산소 공급이 원활하지 않음을 나타낸다. 푸르스름한 색은 해당 부위에 탈산소화된 혈액이 관류되어 발생한다. 피부의 색소 침착은 종종 이러한 판단을 어렵게 만들 수 있다. 피부에 색소 침착이 심한 환자는 손발톱바닥, 손바닥, 발바닥, 점막(특히 눈꺼풀 결막)의 색을 확인하면 이러한 부위의 색소가 상대적으로 부족해 보통 눈꺼풀, 입술, 잇몸 또는 손끝에 색의 변화가 먼저 나타나기 때문에 이러한 문제를 해결할 수 있다.
- 체온: 전반적인 피부 평가와 마찬가지로 피부 온도는 환경 조건에 의해 영향을 받는다. 피부가 차가우면 원인과 관계없이 관류가 감소했음을 나타낸다. 피부 온도는 손등으로 환자의 피부를 살짝 만져보는 것으로 평가할 수 있다. 정상적인 피부 온도는 만졌을 때 따뜻하며 차갑거나 뜨겁지도 않은 상태이다.
- 피부 상태: 정상적인 상황에서는 피부가 보통 건조하다. 교감신경 자극으로 관류가 원활하지 않은 환자에게서는 차고 촉촉한 피부 상태가 나타날 수 있다(발한). 그러나 피부 상태를 평가할 때 주변 조건을 고려하는 것이 중요하다. 덥거나 습한 환경에 있는 환자는 손상의 정도와 관계없이 피부가 촉촉할 수 있다.

D—장애

폐로 산소를 전달하고 전신으로 순환시키는 데 관여하는 요인을 가능한 한 평가하고 교정한 후 일차평가의 다음 단계는 뇌의 산소 공급을 간접적으로 측정하는 뇌 기능 평가이다. 이는 환자의 의식 수준(LOC)을 결정하는 것으로 시작한다.

병원 전 처치 제공자는 혼란스럽고 호전적이며 공격적이거나 비협조적인 외상 환자는 다른 원인이 증명될 때까지 저산소증이거나 외상성 뇌손상(TBI)을 입었다고 가정한다. 대부분의 환자는 생명이 의학적으로 위협받을 때 도움을 원한다. 환자가 도움을 거부하면 그 이유를 질문해야 한다. 환자가 현장에 병원 전 처치 제공자가 있는 것에 위협을 느끼는가? 만약 그렇다면 친밀감을 형성하기 위한 추가 시도가 환자의 신뢰를 얻는 데 도움이 되는 경우가 많다. 상황이 위협적이지 않은 것 같으면 행동의 원인을 생리학적인 것으로 간주하고 가역적인 상태를 확인하고 처치해야 한다. 평가 중에 병력은 손상이 발생한 후 환자가 의식을 잃었는지 아닌지, 독성 물질이 관련되어 있는지(그리고 어떤 물질인지), 환자에게 의식 수준 감소 또는 비정상적

인 행동을 일으킬 수 있는 기존의 질환이 있는지를 결정하는 데 도움이 될 수 있다. 현장을 주의 깊게 관찰하면 이와 관련된 중요한 정보를 얻을 수 있다.

의식 수준이 감소하면 병원 전 처치 제공자에게 다음과 같은 가능성을 시사한다.

1. 뇌의 산소 공급 감소(저산소증/관류저하로 인한) 또는 심각한 저환기(이산화탄소 혼수)
2. 중추신경계 손상(예, 외상성 뇌손상)
3. 약물 또는 알코올 과다 복용 또는 독소 노출
4. 대사 장애, 특히 저혈당증(예: 당뇨병, 발작 또는 심정지로 인한)

글래스고혼수척도(GCS)를 포함한 정신 상태 변화에 대한 자세한 내용은 8장 머리와 목 외상에서 확인할 수 있다. 글래스고혼수척도는 의식 수준을 결정하는 데 사용되는 도구이며 AVPU 방법보다 선호된다(**Box 6-4**). 이는 뇌 기능을 빠르고 간단하게 판단하는 방법이며 환자의 예후, 특히 최상의 운동 반응을 예측할 수 있다. 또한, 일련의 신경학적 평가를 위한 뇌 기능의 기준을 제공한다. 글래스고혼수척도는 눈 뜨기(E), 언어 반응(V), 운동 반응(M)의 세 부분으로 나뉜다. 환자에게는 글래스고혼수척도의 각 구성 요소에 대한 최상의 반응에 따라 점수가 부여된다(**그림 6-4**). 예를 들어, 환자의 오른쪽 눈이 심하게 부어서 눈을 뜰 수 없지만, 왼쪽 눈은 자발적으로 뜬다면 환자는 최상의 안구 운동에 대해 4점을 받는다. 환자가 자발적으로 눈을 뜨지 못하는 경우 병원 전 처치 제공자는 구두 명령(예: 눈을 떠 보세요.)을 사용해야 한다. 환자가 언어적 자극에 반응하지 않으면 펜으로 손발톱바닥을 누르거나 겨드랑이 피부를 누르는 등 통증을 유발하는 자극을 가할 수 있다.

환자의 언어적 반응은 '무슨 일이 있었나요?'와 같은 질문을 통해

Box 6-4 AVPU

AVPU는 종종 환자의 의식 수준을 설명하는 데 사용된다. 이 방법에는 A는 명료, V는 언어 자극에 반응, P는 통증 자극에 대한 반응, U는 무반응을 나타낸다. 이 방법은 간단하지만, 환자가 언어 자극 또는 통증 자극에 구체적으로 어떻게 반응하는지에 대한 정보를 제공하지 못한다. 즉 환자가 구두 질문에 반응하는 경우 환자가 지남력이 있는지, 혼란스러워하는지, 이해할 수 없을 정도로 중얼거리는지 등을 알 수 없다. 마찬가지로 환자가 통증 자극에 반응할 때 환자가 통증 자극을 국소화하거나, 회피하거나 피질제거자세, 대뇌제거자세를 보이는가? 정확성이 부족하므로 AVPU의 사용은 선호도가 떨어졌다.

눈뜨기 반응	점수
자발적으로 눈 뜨기	4
명령에 따라 눈 뜨기	3
압력에 눈 뜨기	2
눈을 뜨지 않음	1
언어 반응	
적절하게 답변(지향적)	5
혼란스러운 대답	4
부적절한 단어 사용	3
알아들을 수 없는 소리를 냄	2
언어적 반응이 없음	1
운동 반응	
명령을 따름	6
통증 자극 부위를 인지	5
정상 굴곡 반응	4
비정상 굴곡 반응(겉질제거자세)	3
신전 반응(대뇌제거자세)	2
운동 반응 없음	1
합계	

그림 6-4 글래스고혼수척도(GCS).
© Jones & Bartlett Learning

확인할 수 있다. 환자의 지남력이 정상이라면 일관성 있는 답변을 한다. 그렇지 않으면 환자의 언어적 반응은 혼란스럽거나, 부적절하거나, 이해할 수 없거나, 반응이 없는 것으로 점수가 매겨진다. 환자에게 기관내삽관이 시행된 경우 글래스고혼수척도는 언어 반응이 없음을 나타내는 1점이 포함하며 눈뜨기 반응과 운동 반응을 계산하여 추가되고 언어 반응은 평가할 수 없음을 나타내는 영문자 T를 추가하여 기록한다(예: 8T).

글래스고혼수척도의 세 번째 구성요소는 운동 점수이다. 예를 들어, 환자에게 '손가락 두 개를 들어 보세요', 또는 '엄지손가락을 보여주세요.'와 같은 간단하고 명확한 명령을 내린다. 환자가 명령을 준수하면 가장 높은 점수인 6점이 부여된다. 병원 전 처치 제공자의 손가락을 쥐거나 움켜잡는 환자는 단순히 움켜쥐는 반사(grasping reflex)를 보이는 것이지 의도적으로 명령을 따르는 것이 아닐 수 있다. 환자가 명령을 따르지 않으면 앞서 언급한 대로 통증을 유발하는 자극을 주어 환자의 최고 운동 반응을 평가한다. 환자가 고통스러운 자극을 밀어내려고 시도하는 경우 국소화하는 것으로 간주한다. 통증에 대한 다른 가능한 반응으로 자극을 회피, 비정상적인 굴곡(피질제거자세), 비정상적인 신전(대뇌제거자세) 또는 운동기능의 부재가 있다.

최대 글래스고혼수척도 점수는 15점으로 장애가 없는 환자를 나타내고 가장 낮은 3점은 일반적으로 불길한 징후이다. 점수가 8점 이하는 중증 손상, 9~12점은 중등도 손상, 13~15점은 경증 손상을 의미한다. 글래스고혼수척도 점수가 8점 이하이면 환자의 적극적인 기도 관리가 필요한지 신중하게 평가해야 한다. 병원 전 처치 제공자는 점수의 개별 구성 요소를 쉽게 계산하고 관련시킬 수 있으며 환자처치보고서뿐만 아니라 환자를 이송할 의료기관에 구두로 보고할 때도 이를 포함해야 한다. 특정 변경 사항을 기록할 수 있으며 전체 점수보다는 글래스고혼수척도의 개별 구성 요소 점수를 전달하는 것이 더 바람직하다. '환자는 E4, V4, M6'라고 기록한 환자처치보고서는 환자가 혼란스러워하지만, 명령을 따른다는 것을 나타낸다.

글래스고혼수척도 점수는 외상 환자 평가에서 거의 보편적으로 사용하지만, 병원 전 환경에서 유용성을 제한할 수 있는 몇 가지 문제가 있다. 예를 들어, 평가자 간 신뢰도가 낮으므로 같은 환자에 대해 병원 전 처치 제공자가 다르게 평가해 다른 처치를 제공할 수 있다. 또한 앞서 언급한 바와 같이 기관내삽관된 환자의 경우 점수가 왜곡된다. 따라서 환자의 중증도와 결과를 예측할 수 있는 더 간단한 점수 시스템을 찾고 있다. 증거에 따르면 글래스고혼수척도의 운동 요소만으로도 전체 점수만큼 환자를 평가하는 데 유용하고 한다. 이 점수는 환자의 기관내삽관 필요성 및 퇴원까지의 생존율과 같은 결과를 정확하게 예측하는 것으로 나타났다. 한 연구에 따르면 환자가 명령을 따를 수 있는지(즉, 운동 점수 6점)에 따라 손상의 심각성과 전체 글래스고혼수척도 점수를 예측할 수 있다고 한다.

환자가 깨어 있지 않거나, 지남력이 없거나, 명령을 따를 수 없는 경우 병원 전 처치 제공자는 환자의 동공뿐만 아니라 자발적인 팔다리 움직임을 신속하게 평가할 수 있다. 양쪽 동공이 같고 둥글며 빛에 반응하는가(PERRLA)? 양쪽 동공의 크기가 같은가? 각 동공은 둥글고 정상적인 모양이며 수축하여 빛에 적절하게 반응하는가? 아니면 반응하지 않고 확장되었는가? 시선이 결합하여 있는가? 비정상적인 동공 검사와 함께 글래스고혼수척도가 14점 미만이면 생명을 위협하는 외상성 뇌손상이 있을 수 있다.

E—노출/환경

외상 환자의 노출은 모든 손상을 찾는 데 중요하기 때문에 평가 과정의 초기 단계에서 환자의 옷을 제거하는 것이다(**그림 6-5**). "노출되지 않은 신체 부위가 가장 심하게 다친 부위."라는 말이 항상 맞는 것은

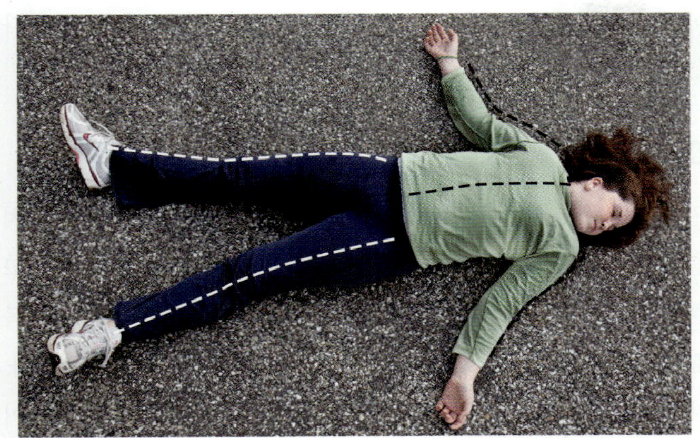

그림 6-5 점선으로 표시된 대로 옷을 자르면 빠르게 제거할 수 있다.
© National Association of Emergency Medical Technicians (NAEMT)

Box 6-5 법의학적 증거

불행하게도 일부 외상 환자는 폭력 범죄의 피해자이다. 이런 상황에서 경찰관을 위해 증거를 보존하기 위해 가능한 모든 조치를 하는 것이 중요하다. 범죄 피해자의 옷을 자를 때는 총알(발사체)이나 칼 또는 기타 물체로 인해 단들어진 귀중한 법의학적 증거를 훼손할 수 있으므로 옷의 구멍을 절단하지 않도록 주의해야 한다. 잠재적인 범죄의 피해자에게서 옷을 제거할 경우 제거한 옷을 비닐이 아닌 종이 가방에 넣어 현장에 있는 경찰관에게 인계해야 한다. 환자 평가 중에 발견된 무기, 약물 또는 개인 소지품도 경찰관에게 인계해야 한다. 환자의 상태에 따라 경찰관이 도착하기 전에 이송이 필요한 경우 이러한 물품은 환자와 함께 병원으로 가져가야 한다. 현지 경찰관에게 대상 시설을 알려야 한다. 프로토콜에 따라 환자의 소지품을 경찰관이나 병원에 인계하는 과정을 기록한다. 그러나 항상 환자 처치가 우선이라는 점에 유의한다. 진행 중인 범죄 수사라는 명목으로 평가나 처치를 지연하거나 변경해서는 안 된다.

© National Association of Emergency Medical Technicians (NAEMT)

아니지만, 전신 신체검사가 필요한 정도로 자주 해당되는 말이다. 또한 혈액이 옷에 흡수되어 눈에 띄지 않을 수도 있다. 환자의 전신을 확인한 후 병원 전 처치 제공자는 체온을 보존하기 위해 다시 환자를 덮을 수 있다.

효과적인 평가를 위해 외상 환자의 신체를 노출하는 것이 중요하지만, 체온저하는 외상 환자 처치에서 심각한 문제이다. 필요한 부분만 외부 환경에 노출해야 한다. 환자를 따뜻한 구급차의 환자 칸으로 옮긴 후에는 가능한 한 신속하게 전체 검사를 수행하고 환자를 다시 덮어준다.

평가 중에 제거해야 하는 환자의 옷은 발견된 상태나 손상에 따라 다르다. 일반적으로 의심되는 상태나 손상 유무를 판단하기 위해 필요한 만큼의 옷을 제거하는 것이 원칙이다. 환자의 정신 상태가 정상이고 외상이 있는 경우 일반적으로 손상 부위 주변만 노출하면 된다. 심각한 손상 기전이 있거나 정신 상태에 변화가 있는 환자는 손상을 평가하기 위해 완전히 노출해야 한다. 병원 전 처치 제공자는 옷을 제거하는 것이 평가와 처치를 적절히 완료할 수 있는 유일한 방법이라면 옷을 제거하는 것을 두려워할 필요가 없다. 때때로 환자는 총상을 입은 후 자동차 충돌을 경험하는 등 환자는 여러 가지 손상 기전에 의해 손상을 입을 수 있다. 환자를 부적절하게 평가하면 생명을 위협하는 손상을 놓칠 수 있다. 손상은 확인되지 않으면 처치할 수 없다.

범죄 피해자의 옷을 자르고 제거할 때는 실수로 증거를 훼손하지 않도록 특별한 주의를 기울여야 한다(**Box 6-5**).

체온을 유지하고 저체온증을 예방하기 위해 평가 및 처치 후 가능한 한 빨리 환자를 덮어준다. 추운 환경에서 병원 전 처치 제공자는 보온 담요 사용을 고려해야 한다. 환자를 구급차에 탑승시키면 병원 전 처치 제공자가 불편할 정도로 덥다고 느끼더라도 차량 히터를 조절하여 환자 칸을 적절하게 따뜻하게 해야 한다.

동시평가 및 처치

이 장의 앞부분에서 언급한 바와 같이 일차평가가 단계적으로 시행하지만, 여러 단계를 동시에 평가할 수 있다. "어디가 아프세요?"와 같은 질문을 통해 기도 개방을 평가하고 호흡 기능을 확인한다. 병원 전 처치 제공자가 노동맥을 촉지하면서 피부 온도와 피부 상태를 평가하면서 동시에 수행할 수도 있다. 환자의 의식 수준과 정신활동은 구두 반응의 적절성에 따라 결정할 수 있다. 그런 다음 병원 전 처치 제공자는 환자의 머리부터 발끝까지 빠르게 스캔하여 출혈이나 다른 손상으 징후를 찾을 수 있다. 첫 번째 병원 전 처치 제공자가 환자의 기도와 호흡을 계속 평가하는 동안 두 번째 병원 전 처치 제공자는 외부출혈 부위에 직접 압박하거나 지혈대를 적용하라는 지시받을 수 있다. 이런 방법을 사용하면 생명을 위협하는 손상을 신속하게 평가하고 처치할 수 있다. 일차평가는 특히 심각한 손상을 입은 환자에게 자주 반복해야 한다.

일차평가에 유용한 장비

환자의 상태를 모니터링하는 데 다음과 같은 몇 가지 보조 장비를 유용하게 사용할 수 있다.

- 맥박산소측정기: 맥박산소측정기는 일차평가 중 또는 가능한 한 빨리 적용해야 한다. 그런 다음 산소포화도를 94% 이상으로 유지

하도록 산소를 적절하게 공급한다. 맥박산소측정기는 병원 전 처치 제공자에게 환자의 심박수를 알려준다. 산소포화도가 감소하면 근본적인 원인을 파악하기 위해 일차평가를 반복해야 한다. 맥박산소측정은 신호가 평균화되기 때문에 실제 혈중 산소포화도와 모니터에 표시되는 수치 사이에는 일반적으로 5~30초 이상의 "지연 시간"이 발생할 수 있다는 점을 기억하는 것이 중요하다. 말초 관류가 좋지 않거나 말초혈관 수축이 있는 환자의 경우 지연 시간이 최대 120초 이상으로 상당히 길어진다. 따라서 환자는 적절한 산소 공급 없이 일시적으로 정상적인 산소포화도 측정 수치를 보일 수 있으며 그 반대의 경우도 마찬가지이다. 일산화탄소와 같은 다른 요인도 맥박산소측정기 측정값의 신뢰성에 영향을 미칠 수 있다.

- 호기말이산화탄소분압측정기(ETCO$_2$): 호기말이산화탄소분압 모니터링은 기관내관과 성문위기도기의 삽관 위치를 확인하고 환자의 동맥혈이산화탄소(PaCO$_2$) 수준을 간접적으로 측정하는 데 유용할 수 있다. 특히 다발성 외상 환자의 경우 호기말이산화탄소분압이 환자의 동맥혈이산화탄소분압과 항상 좋은 상관관계가 있는 것은 아니지만, 호기말이산화탄소분압의 측정치가 환기 속도를 알려주는 데 유용할 수 있다.

- 심전도(ECG) 모니터: 심전도 모니터링은 모니터에 조직화한 심장의 전기적 패턴이 항상 적절한 관류와 상관관계가 있는 것은 아니므로 심전도 모니터링은 맥박산소측정 모니터링보다 덜 유용하다. 관류 여부를 평가하기 위해서는 여전히 맥박 및 혈압 모니터링이 필요하다. 청각적 신호는 환자의 심박수나 리듬의 변화를 병원 전 처치 제공자에게 알릴 수 있다.

- 자동 모니터링: 일반적으로 혈압 측정은 일차평가에 포함되지 않지만, 환자의 상태가 이차평가를 허용하지 않는 중증 손상을 입은 환자의 경우 수동으로 혈압을 측정한 후 이송 중 상태 변화를 파악하기 위해 자동 혈압계를 적용하면 환자의 쇼크 정도에 관한 정보를 얻을 수 있다. 외상 환자에서 자동 혈압 측정은 수동으로 측정하는 것보다 정확도가 떨어지므로 시간이 허락할 때마다 병원 전 처치 제공자는 자동으로 혈압을 측정하는 것보다 청진으로 혈압을 측정해야 한다. 그런데도 자동으로 혈압을 측정하는 추세는 인력을 유지하면서 유용한 정보를 제공한다.

소생술

소생술은 일차평가에서 확인된 생명을 위협하는 문제를 해결하기 위해 취한 처치 단계를 설명한다. 병원 전 외상 소생술 평가는 생명에 대한 각각의 위험이 확인되거나 즉시 또는 가능한 한 가장 빠른 순간에 처치를 시작하는 "진행과 동시에 처치"라는 철학을 기반으로 한다 (**그림 6-6**).

이송

일차평가 중에 생명을 위협하는 상태가 확인되면 제한된 현장 처치를 시작한 후 신속하게 이송해야 한다. 중증외상 환자를 가장 가깝고 적절한 의료기관으로 가능한 한 빨리 이송을 시작한다(**Box 6-6**). 복잡한 상황이 아니라면 이러한 환자의 현장 체류 시간은 짧아야 한다. 제한된 현장 체류 시간과 가장 가까운 적절한 외상센터로 신속한 이송 시작은 PHTLS의 기본 요소이다.

연구에 따르면 중증외상 환자의 경우 현장 도착부터 이송 시작까지의 시간이 길수록 더 나쁜 결과가 발생했다. 이 연구 결과는 생명을 위협하는 가역적인 상태에 대한 처치만, 현장에서 실행하여 현장 체류 시간을 최대한 단축해야 한다는 개념을 더욱 뒷받침한다.

수액 요법

소생술의 또 다른 중요한 단계는 심혈관계 내의 관류량을 가능한 한 빨리 회복시키는 것이다. 이 단계는 혈압을 정상으로 회복시키는 것이 아니라 중요한 장기에 관류가 이루어질 수 있도록 충분한 수액을 공급하는 것이다. 현재 일부 지상 EMS에서는 병원 전 투여할 수 있는 혈액을 보유하고 있지만, 혈액 제제는 일반적으로 중환자실과 헬기 EMS에서만 찾을 수 있다. 병원 전 단계에서 외상 소생술에 가장 일반적으로 사용하는 수액은 젖산 링거액이나 생리식염수와 같은 결정질 용액이다. 젖산 링거액은 나트륨과 염화물 외에도 소량의 칼륨, 칼슘 및 젖산염이 포함되어 있어 생리식염수보다 산도가 낮다. 그러나 결정질 용액은 소실된 적혈구의 산소 운반 능력을 대체하거나 응고에 필요한 혈소판을 대체하지 않는다. 따라서 중증 손상을 입은 환자를 적절한 의료기관으로 신속하게 이송하는 것이 절대적으로 필요하다. 또한 과도한 결정질 수액 소생술의 위험을 고려할 때 이러한 수액은 신중하게 사용하고 특정 임상 목표에 적합해야 한다.

의료기관으로 이송하는 중에 가능하면 시간이 허락하는 한 환자의 아래팔 또는 팔오금 안쪽 정맥에 18게이지 카테터를 이용해 1개 또는 2개의 정맥 라인(IV)을 확보할 수 있다. 병원 전 처치 제공자는 움직이는 구급차에서 정맥 라인을 확보하는 경우 주삿바늘에 찔릴 수 있는 위험이 증가한다는 것을 인식하고 이러한 위험을 최소화하는 조치를 해야 한다. 정맥 라인 확보를 빠르게 성공하지 못할 경우 골내(IO) 라인 확보를 시작한다. 위팔뼈 근위부는 정강뼈 근위부보

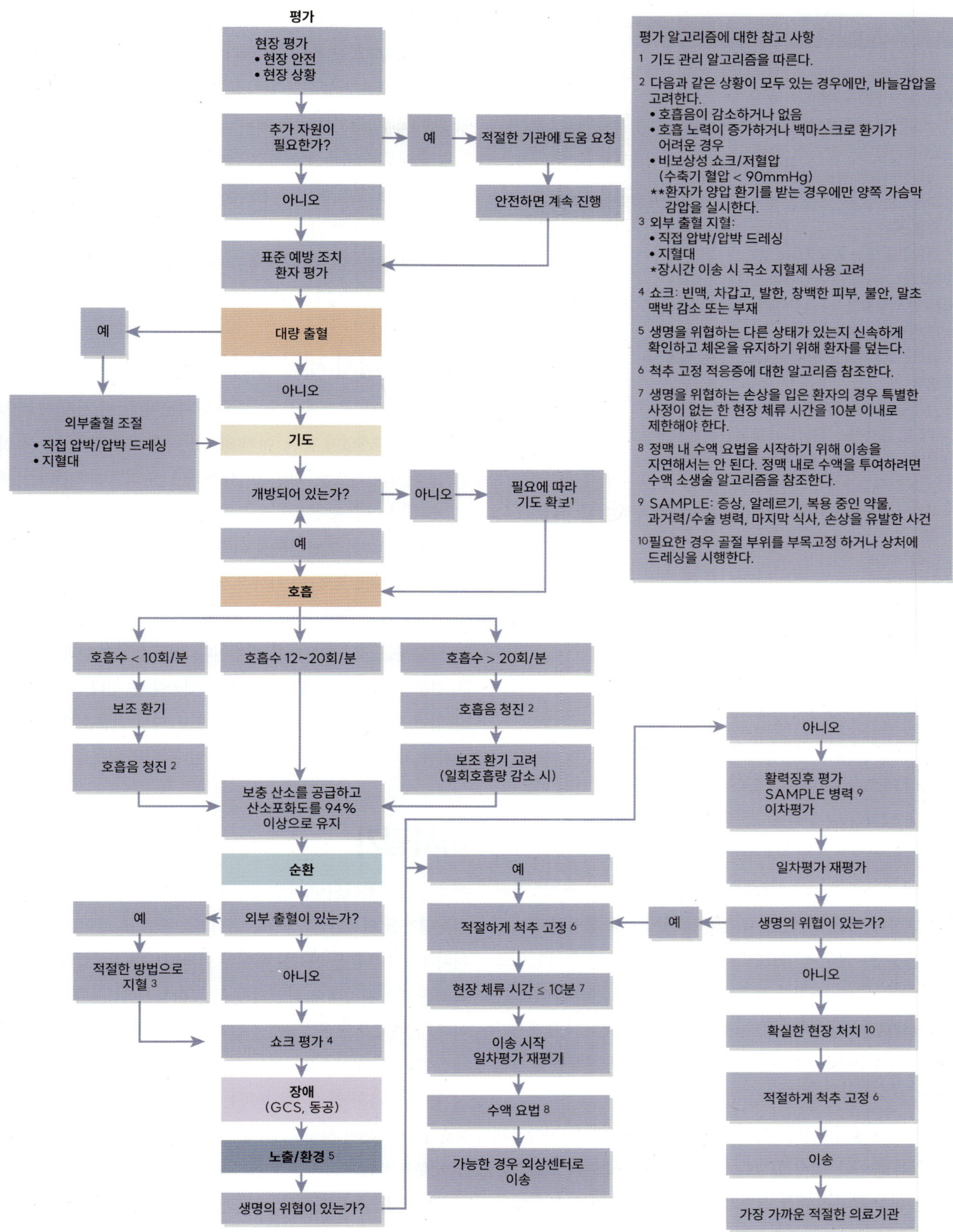

그림 6-6 평가 알고리즘

© National Association of Emergency Medical Technicians (NAEMT)

Box 6-6 중증외상 환자

다음과 같은 생명을 위협하는 상황이 있는 경우 현장 체류 시간을 가능한 한 짧게(10분 미만) 유지한다.

1. 부적절하거나 위협적인 기도 상태
2. 다음과 같은 경우 환기가 저하된다.
   - 비정상적으로 빠르거나 느린 환기 속도
   - 저산소증(보충 산소 공급에도 불구하고 산소포화도 94% 미만)
   - 호흡곤란
   - 개방기흉 또는 동요 가슴
   - 폐쇄성 기흉 또는 긴장기흉이 의심되는 경우
3. 심각한 외부출혈 또는 내부출혈이 의심되는 경우
4. 비정상적인 신경학적 상태
   - 글래스고혼수척도 점수 ≤13 또는 운동 반응 <6
   - 발작
   - 감각 또는 운동 기능 소실
5. 머리, 목, 몸통 또는 팔꿈치나 무릎 근위부 관통성 외상
6. 손가락 또는 발가락의 불완전 절단 또는 완전 절단
7. 다음과 같은 경우에 심각한 외상이 발생
   - 심각한 질환의 병력(예: 관상동맥 질환, 만성폐쇄폐질환, 출혈 장애)
   - 나이 >55세
   - 저체온증
   - 화상
   - 임신

© National Association of Emergency Medical Technicians (NAEMT)

다 수액을 더 빠르게 투여할 수 있다. 일반적으로 중심 정맥 라인(빗장뼈밑, 속목, 넓적다리)을 확보하는 것은 외상 환자의 현장 처치에서 적합하지 않다. 적절한 수액 투여량은 주로 정맥 라인으로 수액 투여를 시작할 때 환자의 출혈이 지혈되었는지 여부, 환자가 저혈압 상태인지 또는 외상성 뇌손상의 증상과 징후를 보이는 등 환자의 상태에 따라 달라진다. 한 연구에 따르면 병원 전 단계에서 정맥 라인으로 수액을 투여하는 것은 저혈압 환자에게 유익하지만, 저혈압이 없는 환자에게는 해로울 수 있다고 한다. 3장 쇼크: 삶과 죽음의 병태생리학 및 8장 머리와 목 외상에서는 수액 소생술에 대한 자세한 지침을 제공한다.

현장에서 정맥 라인 확보를 시작하면 현장 체류 시간이 길어지고 이송이 지연될 뿐이다. 앞서 설명한 바와 같이 내부출혈이나 심각한 출혈이 있는 외상 환자에 대한 결정적인 처치는 병원에서만 이루어질 수 있다. 예를 들어, 비장 손상으로 분당 50mL의 혈액이 손실되고 있는 환자는 수술실 또는 혈관 조영실에서 처치를 시작할 때까지 그 속도로 계속 출혈을 하게 된다. 조기 이송하지 않고 현장에서 정맥 라인을 확보하고 수액을 투여하기 시작하면 출혈이 증가할 뿐만 아니라 환자의 생존 가능성도 낮아질 수 있다. 환자를 즉시 이동할 수 없는 갇힌(포착) 경우와 같은 예외도 있다.

정맥 내로 수액을 투여하기 전에 외부출혈을 지혈해야 한다. 적극적인 정맥 내 수액 투여는 혈압을 상승시키고 혈소판과 응고 인자를 희석해 혈전을 터뜨려 추가 출혈을 일으킬 수 있으므로 피해야 한다. 더 중요한 것은 지속적인 수액 투여가 외부출혈에 대한 수동 조절과 내부출혈에 대한 이송 시작을 대신할 수 없다는 것이다.

병원 전 처치 제공자의 자격 수준

중증외상 환자를 소생시키는 주요 단계는 병원 전 처치 제공자의 자격 수준과 관계없이 같다. 여기에는 1) 대량 외부출혈을 즉시 지혈하고, 2) 환자의 기도를 개방하고 유지하며, 3) 적절하게 환기를 제공하고, 4) 환자 이송을 신속하게 준비하여, 5) 환자를 가장 가까운 의료기관으로 신속하고 안전하게 이송을 시작하는 것이 포함된다. 이송 시간이 길어지면 EMT는 가까운 곳에 있는 전문소생술(ALS) 팀에 도움을 요청하는 것이 적절할 수 있다. 헬기를 이용한 외상센터로 환자를 이송하는 것은 또 다른 방법이다. 전문소생술 팀과 헬기 이송팀은 전문 기도유지 및 수액 소생술을 제공할 수 있다. 항공 EMS는 또한 혈액, 신선 냉동 혈장 및 일반적으로 지상 전문소생술 팀보다 광범위한 처치를 이송 중에 시행할 수 있다.

이차평가

이차평가는 환자의 머리부터 발끝까지 더 자세히 평가하는 것이다. 일차평가를 완료한 후 생명을 위협하는 것으로 확인된 모든 손상을 처치하고 소생술을 시작한 후에만 이차평가를 수행한다. 이차평가의 목적은 일차평가에서 확인되지 않은 손상이나 문제를 파악하는 것이다. 일차평가를 완벽하게 수행하면 즉시 생명을 위협하는 모든 상태를 파악할 수 있으므로 이차평가는 정의상 덜 심각한 문제를 다루게 된다. 따라서 중증외상 환자는 일차평가 종료 후 가능한 한 빨리 이송을 시작하며 정맥 라인 확보나 이차평가를 시행하기 위해 현장에 머무르지 않는다.

이차평가는 "보고, 듣고, 느끼는" 접근 방법을 사용하여 환자를 평가한다. 병원 전 처치 제공자는 머리부터 시작하여 목, 가슴, 복부를 거쳐 팔다리까지 부위별로 손상을 파악하고 신체적 소견의 상관관계

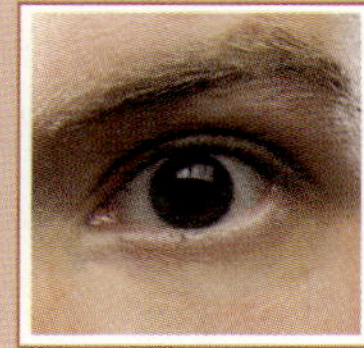
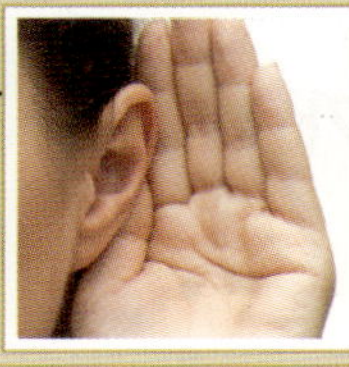
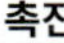
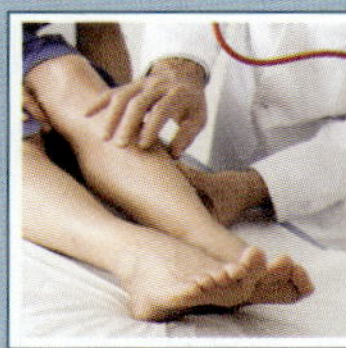

그림 6-7 외상 환자의 신체적 평가는 주의 깊은 시진, 청진 및 촉진(보고, 듣고, 느끼기)이 포함된다.

Eye photo: © REKINC1980/iStock/Getty Images; ear photo: © vvs1976/iStock/Getty Images; hands photo: © Image Point Fr/Shutterstock.

© National Association of Emergency Medical Technicians (NAEMT)

를 파악한 후 상세한 신경학적 검사로 마무리한다(**그림 6-7**). 환자를 평가하는 동안 사용할 수 있는 모든 정보를 사용하여 환자 처치 계획을 수립한다.

본다(시진).

- 각 부위의 모든 피부를 평가한다.
- 외부출혈이나 복부팽만, 팔다리의 부종 및 긴장, 혈종 확장 등 내부출혈의 징후가 있는지 주의 깊게 평가한다.
- 찰과상, 화상, 타박상, 혈종, 열상 및 찔린 상처를 포함한 연부조직 손상이 있는지 확인한다.
- 뼈의 종괴나 부종, 변형이 있는지 확인한다.
- 피부의 비정상적으로 움푹 들어간 부분과 피부색을 확인한다.
- 정상적으로 보이지 않는 모든 것을 기록한다.

듣는다(청진).

- 환자가 숨을 들이쉬거나 내쉴 때 이상한 소리가 들리는지 확인한다. 정상적인 호흡은 조용하다.
- 가슴을 청진할 때 비정상적 소리가 들리는지 확인한다.
- 양쪽 폐에서 호흡음이 같은지 청진한다(**그림 6-8**).
- 목동맥을 청진하고 혈관 손상을 나타낼 수 있는 비정상적인 소리

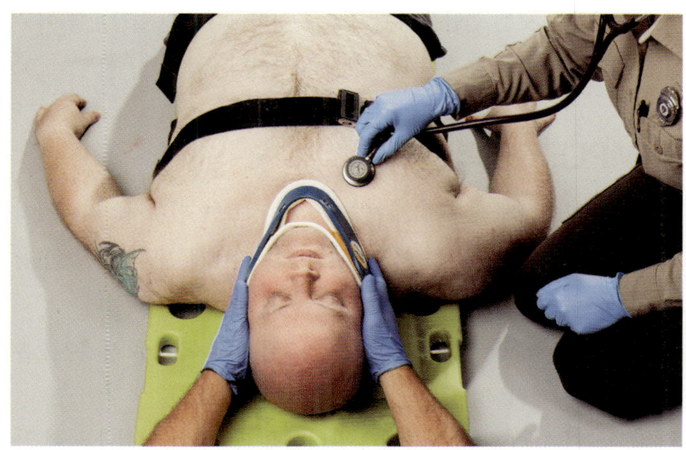

그림 6-8 모든 폐 영역에서 호흡음이 같은지 확인한다.

© Jones & Bartlett Learning. Photographed by Darren Stahlman.

(잡음)가 있는지 확인한다(흔히 외상 현장에서 현실적이지 않다).

느낌(촉진).

- 신체 모든 부위를 촉진하면서 비정상적 움직임이나 비빔소리, 피하기종, 환자가 압통을 호소하는지, 맥박이 촉지되는지 확인한다.
- 관절 부위를 조심스럽게 움직인다. 결과적으로 발생하는 비빔소리, 통증 또는 운동 범위 감소, 이완과 같은 비정상적인 움직임이 있는지 확인한다.

활력징후

이차평가의 첫 번째 단계는 활력징후를 측정하는 것이다. 맥박수와 질, 호흡수와 깊이 그리고 일차평가의 다른 구성요소는 중요한 변화가 빠르게 발생할 수 있으므로 지속해 재평가하고 이전 평가 결과와 비교한다. 상황에 따라 첫 번째 병원 전 처치 제공자가 일차평가를 완료하는 동안 두 번째 처치 제공자가 활력징후를 측정하여 추가 지연을 방지할 수 있다. 그러나 맥박수, 호흡수 및 혈압에 대한 정확한 측정은 중증 다발성 외상 환자의 초기 처치에서 중요하지 않다. 따라서 활력징후의 정확한 측정은 소생술 및 안정화의 필수 단계가 완료될 때까지 지연될 수 있다.

완전한 활력징후에는 혈압, 맥박수와 질, 호흡수와 깊이, 산소포화도(맥박산소측정기 사용), 체온이 포함된다. 중증외상 환자의 경우 가능한 한 3~5분마다 완전한 활력징후를 평가하고 기록하며 상태 변화나 의학적 문제가 발생한 시간도 기록한다. 자동화된 비침습적 혈압측정기를 사용할 수 있더라도 초기 혈압 측정은 수동으로 측정한다. 환자가 현저히 저혈압이면 자동혈압계는 부정확할 수 있으므로

이러한 환자는 모든 혈압을 수동으로 측정하거나 자동혈압계를 이용한 측정과 수동으로 측정한 측정값을 비교한다.

SAMPLER 병력

환자에 대한 병력을 신속하게 얻는다. 이 정보는 환자처치기록지에 기록하고 환자를 이송하는 의료기관의 의료진에게 전달되어야 한다. SAMPLE 약어는 주요 구성요소를 생각나게 하는 역할을 한다.

- 증상(Symptoms): 환자의 주된 호소증상은 무엇인가? 통증? 호흡곤란? 감각마비? 저림?
- 알레르기(Allergies): 환자에게 알려진 알레르기가 있거나 특히 약물에 대해 알레르기가 있는가?
- 약물(Medications): 환자가 정기적으로 복용하는 처방 약 또는 비처방약(비타민, 보충제 및 기타 비처방약 포함)은 무엇인가? 환자가 정기적으로 복용하거나 특히 오늘 어떤 기분 전환용 물질을 사용했는가?
- 과거 병력 및 수술 이력(Past medical and surgical history): 환자에게 지속해서 처치가 필요한 심각한 의학적 문제가 있는가? 환자가 이전에 수술받은 적이 있는가?
- 마지막 식사/마지막 생리 기간(Last meal and menstrual period): 환자가 마지막으로 식사를 한 지 얼마나 되었는가? 많은 외상 환자는 수술이 필요하고 최근에 먹은 음식은 마취 유도 중 흡인의 위험을 증가시킨다. 가임기 여성 환자의 경우 마지막 월경이 언제였는가? 임신 가능성이 있는가?

- 사건(Events): 손상 발생 전에 어떤 사건들이 발생했는가? 익수(익사 또는 저체온)와 위험 물질에 노출된 경우 등을 포함한다.
- 위험 요소(Risk factors): 환자가 환자 살고 있고 넘어질 위험이 더 높은가? 날씨가 기타 환경적 위험이 환자의 외상 위험을 증가시켰는가? 고려해야 할 특별한 위험 요소(예: 소아, 노인, 비만 또는 산과 환자)가 있는가?

해부학적 부위 평가

머리

머리와 얼굴을 시진으로 검사하여 타박상, 찰과상, 열상, 뼈 비대칭, 출혈, 얼굴과 머리뼈를 지지하는 뼈의 결함, 눈, 눈꺼풀, 외이, 입, 아래턱뼈의 이상을 알 수 있다. 머리 검사에는 다음과 같은 단계가 포함된다.

- 두피에 연부조직 손상이 있는지 환자의 머리카락을 샅샅이 확인한다.
- 동공 크기, 빛에 대한 동공 반사, 양측 대칭, 조절, 모양이 둥글거나 불규칙한지 확인한다.
- 얼굴과 두개골을 조심스럽게 촉진하여 국소적 압통, 비빔소리, 변형, 함몰 또는 비정상적인 움직임이 있는지 확인한다(이것은 머리 손상에 대한 비방사선 평가에서 매우 중요하다.). **그림 6-9**는 두개골의 해부학적 구조이다.
- 얼굴에 손상의 단서가 있고 의식이 없는 외상 환자의 눈을 뜨게 하

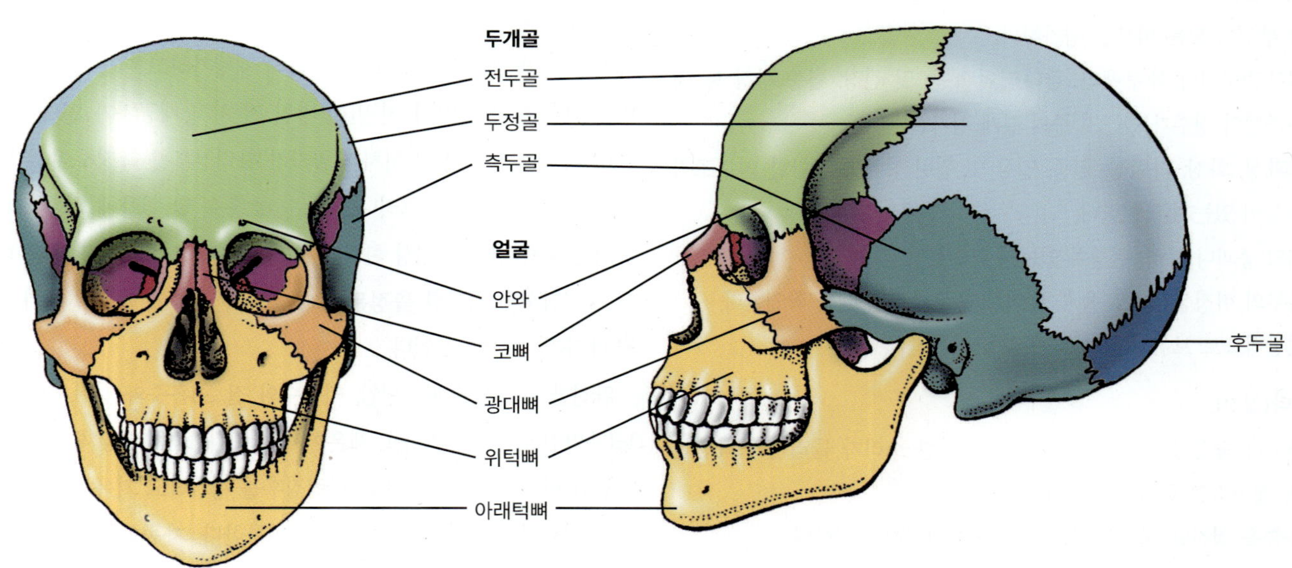

그림 6-9 얼굴과 두개골의 정상적인 해부학적 구조.

여 평가할 때 주의를 기울여야 한다. 무딘 손상 또는 관통상을 입은 눈은 소량의 압력으로도 추가 손상을 입을 수 있다.

얼굴 중간 뼈의 골절은 종종 두개골 바닥의 체판이라고 하는 부분의 골절과 관련이 있다. 환자에게 얼굴 중간에 외상(예: 윗입술과 안와 사이의 손상)이 있는 경우 위관을 삽입하는 경우 코가 아닌 입을 통해 삽입해야 한다.

목

목에 타박상, 찰과상, 열상, 혈종 및 변형이 있는지 시진으로 평가를 통해 병원 전 처치 제공자는 근본적인 손상의 가능성을 확인할 수 있다. 촉진 시 후두, 기관 또는 폐 이는 곳에서 피하기종을 확인할 수 있다. 후두의 비빔소리, 쉰 목소리, 피하기종은 후두 골절을 나타내는 전형적인 세 가지 증상이다. 목뼈에 압통이 없는 것은 목뼈 골절을 배제하는 데 도움이 될 수 있지만(엄격한 기준과 함께 사용할 경우), 압통은 종종 골절, 탈구 또는 인대 손상의 존재를 나타낼 수 있다. 이러한 촉진은 목뼈를 중립 자세로 유지하면서 조심스럽게 수행한다. 신경학적 결손이 없다고 해서 불안정한 목뼈 손상의 가능성을 배제할 수는 없다. 재평가를 통해 이전에 확인된 혈종의 확장이나 기관편위를 발견할 수 있다. **그림 6-10**은 목의 정상적인 해부학적 구조를 보여주는 것이다.

가슴

가슴은 강하고 탄성이 있고 탄력적이기 때문에 상당한 양의 충격을 흡수할 수 있다. 변형, 천자 및 관통상, 모순 운동, 타박상, 찰과상이 있는지 가슴을 주의 깊게 시진하여 잠재적인 손상을 확인해야 한다. 병원 전 처치 제공자가 주의 깊게 관찰해야 하는 다른 징후로는 환자가 가슴을 방어하거나, 가슴을 움직이려고 하지 않거나, 양쪽 가슴의 비대칭적인 움직임, 모순운동, 갈비사이, 복장위, 빗장위의 팽륜 또는 뒤당김 등이 있다.

복장뼈 위의 타박상은 잠재적인 심장 손상을 나타내는 유일한 징후일 수 있다. 관통 상처는 관통 부위에서 멀리 떨어진 신체 부위에 영향을 미칠 수 있다. 신체 표면과 가로막 및 날숨과 들숨 시 위치가 변하는 기본 장기 사이의 관계를 이해하는 것이 중요하다. 앞쪽으로 네 번째 갈비사이공간에서 측면 여섯 번째 갈비사이공간, 뒤쪽으로 여덟 번째 갈비사이공간까지 이어지는 선은 완전한 날숨 시 가로막의 상향 이동을 나타낸 것이다(**그림 6-11**). 이 선(유두 높이 정도) 아래에서 발생하거나 이선 아래를 통과할 수 있는 경로로 관통상을 입은 경우 흉강과 복강을 모두 통과한 것으로 간주해야 한다.

청진기를 이용한 청진은 가슴 평가의 필수적인 부분이다. 환자는 대부분 바로누운자세로 있어 앞쪽과 옆쪽 가슴만 청진할 수 있다. 환자가 이 자세에서 호흡음이 정상적이거나 감소한 것을 인식하는 것이 중요하다. 호흡음이 감소하거나 소실된 것은 기흉, 긴장기흉, 혈흉

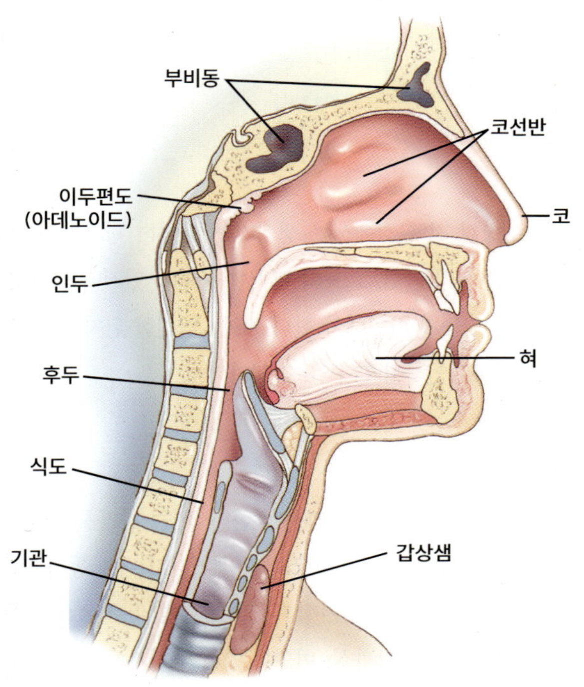

그림 6-10 목의 정상적인 해부학적 구조.
© National Association of Emergency Medical Technicians (NAEMT)

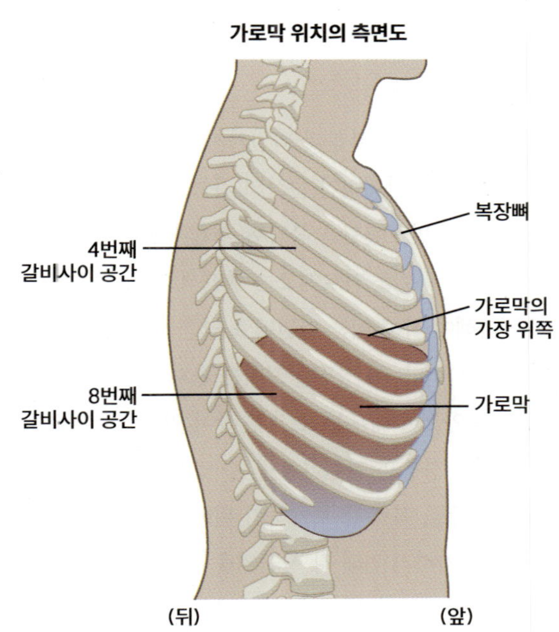

그림 6-11 최대 날숨 시 가로막 위치의 측면 모습.
© National Association of Emergency Medical Technicians (NAEMT)

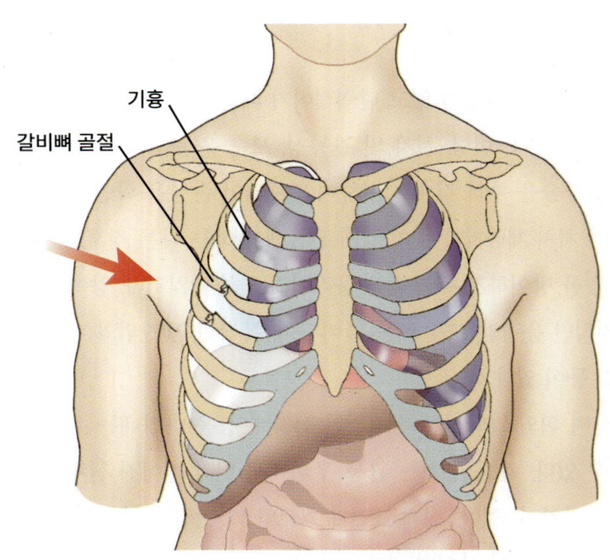

그림 6-12 가슴 압박 손상은 갈비뼈 골절 및 기흉을 유발할 수 있다.
© National Association of Emergency Medical Technicians (NAEMT)

이 있을 수 있다. 가슴 뒤쪽(환자를 통나무굴리기를 시행하는 경우)이나 측면에서 거품 소리가 들리면 폐 타박상을 의미할 수 있다. 심장눌림증은 멀리서 들리는 심음이 특징이지만, 현장에서 소란이나 이송 중 소음으로 인해 확인하기 어려울 수 있다.

갈비뼈 골절 부위가 있으면 심각한 폐 타박상을 나타낼 수 있다. 모든 유형의 가슴 압박 손상은 기흉을 유발할 수 있다(**그림 6-12**). 가슴을 촉진하여 피하기종(연부조직에 공기가 차 있는 상태)이 있는지 확인한다.

복부

복부 평가는 신체의 다른 부분과 마찬가지로 시진 평가로 시작한다. 찰과상과 반상출혈은 잠재적인 손상의 가능성을 나타내며, 특히 배꼽주위와 옆구리의 반상출혈은 복막뒤 출혈과 관련이 있다. 차량 충돌 사고의 경우 하복부를 가로지르는 빨간색 가로줄 무늬가 있는지 주의 깊게 평가해야 하며 이는 안전띠로 인한 잠재적인 손상을 입었을 수 있음을 시사한다. 이 징후를 보이는 환자의 상당수는 잠재적인 손상이 있을 수 있으며 대부분 소장 손상이 있을 것이다. 허리뼈 골절은 또한 "안전띠 징후"와 관련이 있을 수 있다.

복부 평가는 압통, 복부를 보호하기 위한 보호성 근경련 또는 덩어리가 있는지 평가하기 위해 각 사분역을 촉진한다. 촉진할 때 병원 전 처치 제공자는 복부가 부드러운지 또는 경직이나 보호성 근경련이 있는지를 평가한다. 복부 압통이나 통증을 발견한 후에도 계속 촉

진할 필요는 없다. 추가 정보는 병원 전 처치를 변경하지 않으며 복부 평가를 계속하면 환자가 더 불편해지고 이송이 지연될 뿐이다. 마찬가지로 복부 청진은 외상 환자의 평가에 사실상 아무런 도움이 되지 않는다. 복막강은 다량의 혈액을 숨길 수 있으며 종종 복부 팽창이 거의 또는 전혀 없는 경우가 많다.

외상성 뇌손상 또는 알코올이나 기타 약물 중독으로 인한 의식 상태 변화는 종종 복부 평가를 모호하게 만든다.

골반

골반은 시진과 촉진으로 평가한다. 먼저 골반에 찰과상, 타박상, 혈종, 열상, 개방골절, 확장 징후가 있는지 시진으로 평가한다. 골반 골절은 대량의 내부출혈을 일으켜 환자의 혈류역학적 상태를 급격히 악화시킬 수 있다.

병원 전 환경에서 골반을 촉진하는 것은 환자 처치에 영향을 미칠 수 있는 최소한의 정보를 제공한다. 평가 시 골반은 이차평가의 하나로 압통과 불안정성에 대해 한 번만 촉진한다. 불안정한 골반을 촉진하면 골절된 부분이 움직이고 형성된 혈전을 파괴하여 출혈을 악화시킬 수 있으므로 이 평가는 반복해서 시행하지 말고 한 번만 시행한다. 촉진은 두덩결합 부위에 팔꿈치로 앞에서 뒤쪽으로 부드럽게 압력을 가한 다음 양쪽 엉덩뼈 능선 부위를 부드럽게 안쪽으로 압력을 가하여 비정상적인 움직임이 있는지 평가한다. 불안정성의 증거가 있으면 골반을 더 이상 촉진하지 말고 가능한 경우 즉시 골반 고정대를 착용시켜야 한다.

생식기계

일반적으로 병원 전 환경에서는 생식기는 자세히 평가하지 않는다. 그러나 외부 생식기 출혈, 요도의 명백한 출혈이 있거나 남성의 경우 지속발기증이 있는지 확인해야 한다. 또한, 임신한 환자의 투명한 액체는 양막 파열로 인해서 양수일 수 있다.

등

등에 손상의 증거가 있는지 평가해야 한다. 이는 환자를 긴척추고정판이나 다른 이송 장비로 이동시키거나 제거하기 위해 통나무굴리기 방법을 시행할 때 가장 잘 평가할 수 있다. 가슴 뒤쪽에서 호흡음을 청진하고 등에 타박상, 찰과상, 변형이 있는지 평가하고 척추의 압통이 있는지 촉진한다.

팔다리

팔다리 평가는 팔의 빗장뼈와 다리의 골반에서 시작하여 각 팔다리의 가장 먼 부분으로 진행된다. 각 뼈와 관절의 변형, 혈종 또는 반상출혈이 있는지 시진으로 확인하고 촉진으로 뼈 마찰음, 통증, 압통 또는 비정상적인 움직임이 있는지 확인한다. 골절이 의심되는 부위는 모두 고정해야 한다. 각 팔다리의 원위부에서 순환, 운동, 감각신경 기능을 평가한다. 팔다리를 고정하는 경우 부목으로 고정하기 전과 후에 맥박, 움직임, 감각을 평가해야 한다.

신경학적 검사

앞서 설명한 다른 신체 부위 평가와 마찬가지로 이차평가의 신경학적 검사는 일차평가보다 훨씬 더 상세하게 수행한다. 글래스고혼수척도 점수 계산, 운동 및 감각기능 평가, 동공 반응 관찰이 모두 포함된다. 감각 능력과 운동 반응에 대한 전반적인 검사를 통해 팔다리의 쇠약 또는 감각 상실 유무를 판단하여 뇌 또는 척추 손상을 시사하고 추가 검사가 필요한 신체 부위를 파악한다. 환자의 동공을 검사할 양쪽 동공의 크기뿐만 아니라 빛에 대한 동공의 반응도 평가한다. 일부에서는 동공의 크기가 다르지만(동공부등), 정상 상태인 경우가 있다. 그러나 이러한 환자에게서도 동공은 비슷한 방식으로 빛에 반응해야 한다. 빛을 비추었을 때 서로 다른 속도로 반응하는 동공은 양쪽 동공이 같지 않은 것으로 간주한다. 의식이 없는 외상 환자에서 양쪽 동공이 서로 다른 것은 뇌부종이나 빠르게 팽창하는 두개내 혈종으로 인해 두개내압이 증가하거나 3번 뇌신경에 압박이 가해지고 있음을 나타낼 수 있다(**그림 6-13**). 직접적인 눈 손상도 동공의 불균형을 유발할 수 있다.

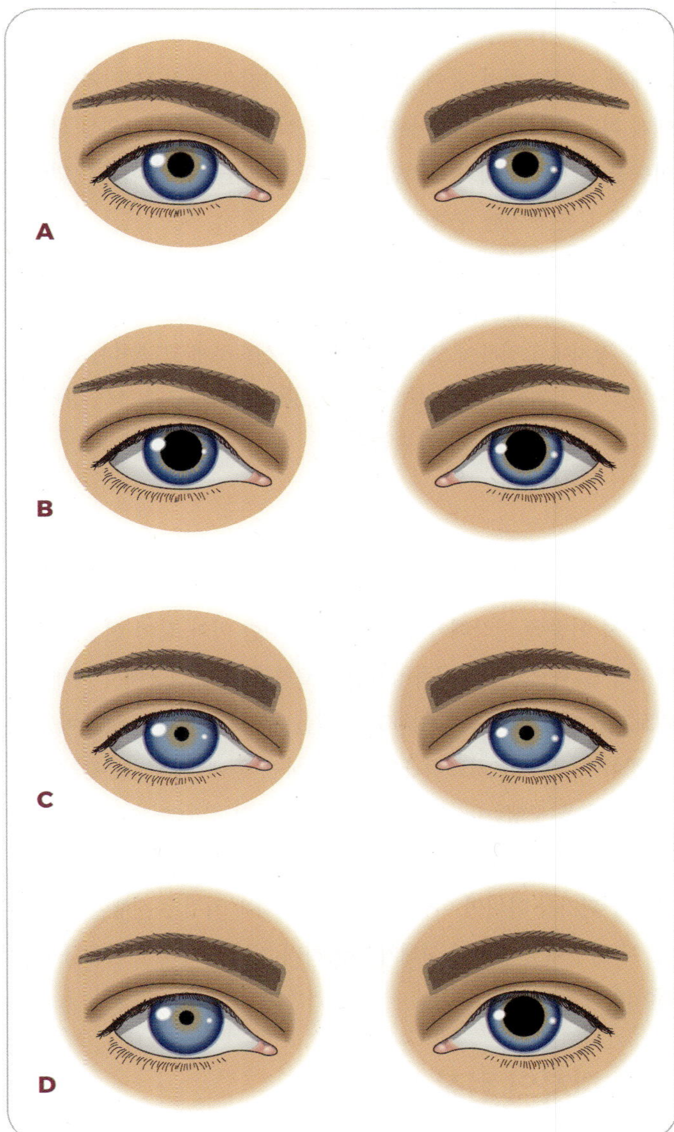

그림 6-13 **A.** 정상 동공 **B.** 동공 확장 **C.** 동공 수축 **D.** 불균등 동공.
© Jones & Bartlett Learning.

현장에서의 결정적인 처치

결정적인 처치는 환자의 특정 상태를 완전히 교정하는 처치이다. 다음은 결정적인 처치의 예이다.

- 심실세동으로 심정지가 발생한 환자의 경우 결정적인 처치는 제세동을 실시하여 자발 순환을 회복(ROSC)시키는 것이다.
- 당뇨병성 저혈당 혼수상태에 있는 환자의 경우 결정적인 처치는 포도당을 투여해 정상 혈당 수치로 회복시키는 것이다.
- 기도가 폐쇄된 환자의 경우 결정적인 처치는 턱 밀어올리기 방법으로 기도를 개방하고 보조 환기와 같은 간단한 조작으로 기도 폐쇄를 완화하는 것이다.

- 심각한 출혈이 있는 환자의 경우 결정적인 처치는 수술적 처치 또는 혈관 폐색을 통한 출혈 조절과 쇼크 소생술을 시행하는 것이다.

일반적으로 병원 전 환경에서 발생할 수 있는 일부 문제에 대한 결정적인 처치는 현장에서 제공할 수 있지만, 중증외상 환자의 경우 손상에 대한 결정적인 처치는 병원 환경에서만 제공할 수 있다. 그 결정적인 처치가 지연되면 환자의 생존 가능성이 감소한다. 또한, 현장에서 한 가지 손상이나 조건은 결정적으로 처치할 수 있지만, 대부분의 중증외상 환자는 병원에서 처치해야 하는 다른 손상이 있을 수 있다.

이송 준비

앞에서 논의한 바와 같이 심각한 손상 기전을 가진 모든 외상 환자에게 척추 손상을 의심해야 한다. 따라서 척추 안정화는 외상 환자의 이송을 준비하는 데 필수적인 구성 요소이다. 시간적 여유가 있다면 다음과 같은 조치를 수행한다.

- 특정 부목을 사용하여 팔다리 골절을 조심스럽게 고정한다.
- 환자가 위독한 상태면 환자를 긴척추고정판 또는 기타 이송용 구출 장치에 고정하여 모든 골절 부위를 신속하게 고정한다.
- 필요하고 적절한 경우 주요 상처를 붕대(출혈이 지속하는 상처, 내장 적출이 있는 상처)로 감는다.

이송

즉각적으로 생명을 위협하는 문제가 해결되면 환자를 구급차에 태우고 즉시 이송을 시작해야 한다. 앞에 설명한 바와 같이 현장에서 정맥 라인을 확보하거나 이차평가를 완료하기 위해 현장에서 지체하면 의료기관에서 혈액을 투여하고 출혈을 지혈할 수 있는 시간이 지연될 뿐이다. 환자를 의료기관으로 이송하는 중에 지속적인 평가와 추가 소생술을 수행한다. 일부 중증외상 환자의 경우 이송을 시작하는 것이 현장에서의 결정적인 처치에서 가장 중요한 부분이다.

중증 환자가 아니면 이송 전에 손상 부위에 처치를 시행할 수 있지만, 이 경우에도 숨겨진 상태가 악화하기 전에 신속하게 이송을 시작해야 한다.

손상 환자의 현장 분류

중증 환자를 이송할 수 있는 적절한 의료기관을 선택하는 것은 병원 전 환경에서 제공되는 다른 생명을 구하기 위해 처치만큼 중요할 수 있으며 이는 환자의 손상 또는 의심되는 손상에 대한 평가를 기반으로 한다(**Box 6-7**). 40년 이상 동안 의학 문헌에 발표된 수많은 논문에서 손상을 입은 환자를 처치할 준비가 되어 있는 외상센터가 더 나은 치료 결과를 보인다는 사실이 입증되었다. 2006년에 발표된 미 질병통제예방센터의 지원을 받은 연구에 따르면 환자가 비 외상센터에서 치료를 받은 경우보다 Level Ⅰ 외상센터에서 치료를 받은 경우 손상에서 생존할 가능성이 25% 더 높은 것으로 나타났다. 미국 인구의 82.1%가 외상센터에서 60분 이내에 거주하지만, 중증외상 환자의 36%를 포함하여 전체 외상 환자의 절반 이상이 지정된 외상센터에서 치료를 받지 못했다. 손상을 입은 환자를 지정된 외상센터로 이송하

면 심각한 손상으로 인한 사망률이 많이 감소한다.

병원 전 처치 제공자가 직면한 더 어려운 결정 중 하나는 어떤 손상을 입은 환자를 외상센터에서 가장 잘 치료할 수 있는지 결정하는 것이다. 외상센터로 이송할 환자를 적절히 선택하려면 "과잉 분류"와 "과소 분류" 사이의 균형을 고려해야 한다. 모든 외상 환자를 외상센터로 이송하는 것은 과잉 분류를 초래할 수 있으며 이는 상당수의 손상을 입은 환자가 외상센터에서 제공하는 전문 처치가 필요하지 않다는 것을 의미한다. 과잉 분류는 외상센터의 자원이 덜 심각한 손상을 입은 환자로 인해 과부하가 걸리기 때문에 더 심각한 손상을 입은 환자에게 더 나쁜 결과를 초래할 수 있다. 과소 분류는 심각한 손상을 입은 환자를 비외상센터로 이송하는 것이다. 과소 분류는 의료기관에서 환자를 적절히 처치할 수 있는 역량이 부족할 수 있으므로 환자의 예후가 나빠질 수 있다. 생명을 위협하는 상황을 병원 전 환경에서 파악할 수 없으므로 어느 정도의 과소 분류는 불가피해 보인다. 과소 분류를 최소화하기 위해 전문가들은 30~50%의 과잉 분류가 필요하다고 추정하는데, 이는 외상센터로 이송되는 손상을 입은 환자의 30~50%는 전문적인 처치가 필요하지 않다는 것을 의미한다.

일반적으로 중증외상 환자에 대한 정의는 손상 중증도 점수(ISS)가 16점 이상인 환자이다(**Box 6-8**). 안타깝게도 손상 중증도 점수는 고급 영상(예: 컴퓨터 단층촬영) 또는 수술을 통해 발견된 손상을 포함하여 환자의 모든 손상이 진단된 경우에만, 계산할 수 있다. 따라서 손상중증점수는 병원 전 현장에서 계산할 수 없다. 1) 응급실 또는 입원 후 24시간 이내에 사망한 외상 환자, 2) 혈액제제의 대량 수혈이 필요한 환자, 3) 중환자실 입원이 필요한 환자, 4) 손상으로 인한 긴급수술이 필요하거나 5) 중재적 혈관 조영술로 내부출혈을 조절해야 하는 환자를 포함하는 대체 정의가 제안되었다. 이러한 모든 정의는 연구 목적으로는 유용하지만, 병원 전 처치 제공자가 확인할 수

Box 6-8 손상 중증도 점수(ISS) 평가

병원 환경에서 외상성 손상을 입은 환자를 분석하고 분류하기 위해 다양한 점수 시스템이 사용된다. 점수 시스템은 외상성 손상의 중증도에 따라 환자의 예후를 예측하는 데에도 사용할 수 있다. 이러한 점수 시스템은 일반적으로 환자가 외상센터에서 완전히 평가될 때까지 계산되지 않는다. 현장에서 손상을 입은 환자의 초기 분류에 제한적으로 사용되지만, 외상 치료의 전반적인 질 개선(QA) 및 질 관리(QI) 과정에서 중요한 가치를 가지고 있다.

가장 일반적으로 논의되는 점수 시스템 중 하나는 손상 중증도 점수이다. 손상 중증도 점수는 손상을 해부학적 구분되는 6개의 신체 부위로 분류한다.

1. 머리와 목
2. 얼굴
3. 가슴
4. 복부
5. 팔다리
6. 피부

각 부위에서 가장 심각한 손상만 고려된다. 6개 부위 모두에서 가장 심각한 손상이 확인되면 간편 손상척도(AIS)를 사용하여 1에서 6까지의 값이 부여된다.

1. 경증
2. 보통
3. 심각한
4. 중증
5. 위험한
6. 생존 불가능

그런 다음 가장 높은 세 개의 값을 제곱하여 가장 높은 점수에 추가 가중치를 부여하고 가장 낮은 점수를 최소화한다. 그런 다음 이러한 값들을 합산하여 최종 손상 중증도 점수를 계산한다.

손상 중증도 점수가 높을수록 사망률, 이환율, 입원 기간 및 기타 중증도 측정과 선형적으로 관련이 있다. 손상 중증도 점수의 주요 한계는 간편 손상척도 점수 오류를 손상 중증도 점수로 계산할 때 증폭된다는 점과 신체의 특정 부위의 손상이 다른 부위의 손상보다 본질적으로 더 심각할 수 있다는 사실을 고려하지 않았다는 점이다. 외상 환자 현장 분류에 제한적으로 사용되지만, EMS 제공자가 연구 논문과 실제 업데이트된 자료를 읽을 때 손상 중증도 점수를 어떻게 계산하는 방법을 이해하는 것은 매우 중요하다.

© National Association of Emergency Medical Technicians (NAEMT)

있는 것은 없다.

외상센터로 이송하여 처치를 받으면 가장 큰 혜택을 받을 수 있는 환자를 파악하기 위해 미국 외과학회 외상위원회(ACS-COT)는 2022년 5월 손상을 입은 환자의 현장 분류를 위한 지침을 업데이트했다(**그림 6-14**). 이 문서는 EMS 제공자가 개별 외상 환자의 이송 목적지에 대해 적절한 결정을 내리는 데 도움이 되는 지침을 제공한다. 현장 분류 지침은 고려해야 할 네 가지 부분으로 구성되어 있다.

- 손상 유형. 이 부분에는 동요 가슴, 골반 골절 또는 활동성 출혈과 같이 생명을 위협하는 상태와 관련이 있을 가능성이 가장 높은 손상 유형에 관해 설명한다. 이러한 손상 유형을 보이는 환자는 가능한 최고 수준의 외상센터로 이송해야 한다.
- 의식상태 및 활력징후. 이 환자는 의식상태가 변화 및 기타 생리학적 불안정성의 증거가 있어 가능한 최고 수준의 외상센터로 이송해야 한다.
- 손상의 기전. 이러한 기준은 생리학적 장애나 명백한 외부 손상으로 나타나지 않는 잠재적인 손상이 있을 수 있는 추가 환자를 파악한다.
- EMS 판단. 이러한 기준은 항응고제 사용, 화상 또는 임신 여부와 같은 요인이 외상센터로의 이송 결정에 어떤 영향을 미칠 수 있는지를 파악한다.

손상 유형이나 의식상태 및 활력징후를 기준으로 손상 기준을 충족하는 환자는 해당 지역에서 이용할 수 있는 최고 수준의 외상치료센터로 이송해야 한다. 손상 기전 기준 또는 EMS 판단 기준을 충족하는 환자는 해당 지역에서 가장 가까운 적절한 외상센터로 이송해야 하지만, 반드시 최고 수준은 아니다. 그러나 모든 의사결정 도구와 마찬가지로 지침으로 사용해야 하며 올바른 판단을 위한 대체 수준으로 사용해서는 안 된다. 의심스러운 경우 외상센터로 이송하는 것이 좋다.

이송 기간

앞에서 논의한 바와 같이 병원 전 처치 제공자는 환자의 손상 정도에 따라 이송할 의료기관을 선택해야 한다. 간단히 말해서 환자를 가장 가까운 적절한 의료기관(즉 환자의 문제를 처치할 수 있는 가장 가까운 의료기관)으로 이송해야 한다. 환자의 손상이 심각하거나 출혈이 계속될 가능성이 있는 경우 병원 전 처치 제공자는 가능한 한 빨리 결정적 처치를 제공(가능한 경우 외상센터)할 수 있는 의료기관으로 환자를 이송해야 한다.

예를 들어, 구급대는 도움 요청을 받고 8분 만에 현장에 도착하고 현장에서 이송을 준비하고 환자를 구급차에 태우는 데 6분이 걸렸다. 지금까지 황금 기간 중 14분이 지났다. 가장 가까운 병원은 현장에서 5분 거리이고 외상센터는 14분 거리에 있다. 시나리오 1에서 환자는 외상센터로 이송된다. 의료기관에 도착하자마자 외과 의사는 응급의학과 의사, 전체 외상 팀과 함께 응급실에 있었고 수술실에 인력 배치되어 준비가 완료되었다. 응급실에서 10분 동안 소생술, 필요

손상 환자 현장 분류를 위한 대한 국제 지침

빨간색 기준
심각한 심각한 손상의 위험이 높음

손상 유형	정신 상태 & 활력징후
• 머리, 목, 몸통 및 근위 팔다리의 관통상 • 두개골 변형, 두개골 골절이 의심되는 경우 • 새로운 운동 또는 감각 상실을 동반한 척추 손상이 의심되는 경우 • 가슴벽 불안정, 변형 또는 동요가슴 의심되는 경우 • 골반 골절이 의심되는 경우 • 두 개 이상의 근위부 긴뼈 골절이 의심되는 경우 • 으깸손상, 벗겨진 손상, 짓이겨진 손상, 팔다리 맥박이 촉지되지 않는 경우 • 손목 또는 발목 근위부 절단 • 지혈대 또는 지속적인 압력을 가하는 상처 패킹이 필요한 대량 출혈	**모든 환자** • 명령을 따를 수 없음(GCS 운동 반응 < 6) • 호흡수 < 10 또는 > 29회/분 • 호흡 곤란 또는 환기 보조가 필요한 경우 • 산소포화도측정(실내 공기) < 90% **0~9세** • 수축기 혈압 < 70mmHg + (2 × 나이) **10~64세** • 수축기 혈압 < 90mmHg 또는 • 심박수 > 수축기 혈압 **65세 이상** • 수축기 혈압 < 110mmHg 또는 • 심박수 > 수축기 혈압

위의 빨간색 기준 중 하나라도 충족하는 환자는 지역 외상 시스템의 지리적 제약 내에서 이용 가능한 최고 수준의 외상센터로 이송해야 한다.

노란색 기준
심각한 손상에 대한 중간 정도의 위험

손상 기전	EMS 판단

• 고위험 차량 충돌
  – 신체의 일부 또는 전체 튕겨 나감
  – 심각한 침입(지붕 포함)
    • 탑승자 공간 >30cm
    • 차량 모든 부위 >46cm
    • 갇혀있는 관자를 구출해야 하는 경우
  – 동승자 사망
  – 어린이(0~9세) 안전띠를 매지 않았거나 고정되지 않은 어린이용 카시트에 탑승한 경우
  – 심각한 손상과 일치하는 차량 원격 측정 데이터
• 상당한 충격으로 차량에서 분리된 탑승자
  (예: 오토바이, ATV, 말 등)
• 보행자/자전거 탑승자가 퉁겨지고 부딪히거나 충격이 큰 경우
• 추락 높이 > 3m(모든 연령)
	다음과 같은 위험 요소를 고려한다.
	• 머리 충격이 심한 어린이(5세 이하) 또는 노인(65세 이상)의 낮은 수준의 낙상
	• 항응고제 사용
	• 아동 학대 의심
	• 특별하고 많은 자원이 필요한 의료서비스
	• 임신 > 20주
	• 외상과 동반된 화상
	• 소아는 먼저 소아청소년과 치료가 가능한 센터로 환자 분류
	
	우려되는 경우 외상센터로 이송

노란색 기준 중 하나에 해당하지만, 빨간색 기준을 충족하지 않는 환자는 지역 외상 시스템의 지리적 제약 내에서 가능한 경우 우선적으로 외상센터로 이송해야 한다(최고 수준의 외상센터일 필요는 없음).

그림 6-14 환자를 이송할 의료기관을 결정하는 것은 매우 중요하며 이용 가능한 기료기관의 유형과 위치, 외상센터의 지리적 제약을 고려해야 한다.

한 방사선 촬영 및 혈액 검사를 수행한 후 환자는 수술실로 이동되었다. 이제 사고 발생 후 전체 시간은 38분이 지났다. 시나리오 2에서는 환자가 외상센터보다 9분 거리에 있는 가장 가까운 병원으로 이송된다. 응급실에는 응급의학과 의사가 있지만, 외과 의사와 수술팀은 퇴근한 상태이다. 환자가 응급실에서 소생술을 위해 대기하는 10분은 외과 의사가 도착하여 환자를 검사할 때까지 45분으로 늘어날 수 있다. 외과 의사가 환자 검사하고 수술을 결정한 후 수술팀이 도착하기를 기다리는 동안 30분이 더 지날 수 있다. 시나리오 2의 사고 후 전체 시간은 94분으로 외상센터로 이송된 시나리오보다 2.5배 더 길다. 가장 가까운 병원으로 이송하는 시간을 단축하여 절약한 9분은 실제로 환자에게 56분이 소요되었으며 이 시간 동안 외상센터에서 수술 준비를 시작하고 출혈을 조절할 수 있었을 것이다.

시골 지역에서는 대기 중인 외상팀까지 이송하는 데 45~60분 또는 그 이상 소요될 수 있다. 이런 상황에서 대기 중인 외상팀이 있는 가장 가까운 병원이 환자를 이송할 적절한 의료기관이다.

또 다른 고려 사항은 비외상센터가 중증 손상을 입은 환자에게 확실한 처치를 제공하지 못하므로 이러한 환자를 외상센터로 이송한다는 것이다. 시나리오 2의 경우라면 결정적인 처치까지 지연되는 시간이 훨씬 더 길어질 수 있다.

이송 방법

환자 평가 및 이송 결정의 또 다른 측면은 이송 방법이다. 일부 체계는 항공 이송이 가능하다. 항공 의료 서비스는 중증외상 환자에게 지상 구급대보다 더 높은 수준의 처치를 제공할 수 있다. 또한 상황에 따라 항공 이송이 지상 이송보다 더 빠르고 원활할 수도 있다. 앞에서 언급한 바와 같이 지역사회에서 항공 이송이 가능하고 특정 상황에 적합한 경우 평가 과정 초기에 항공 이송을 요청하는 결정을 내릴수록 환자에게 더 큰 혜택이 돌아갈 가능성이 높다. 헬기 이송은 해당 지역에서 최고 수준의 처치를 제공하는 의료기관으로 이송하기 위한 지침 기준을 충족하는 환자에게 고려해야 한다.

모니터링 및 재평가(지속적인 평가)

일차평가 및 초치 처치가 완료된 후에는 환자를 지속해 모니터링하고 활력징후를 재평가해야 하며 이송이 지연되는 경우 현장이나 이송 중에 일차평가를 여러 번 재평가해야 한다. 일차평가의 구성요소에 대한 지속적인 재평가는 생명 기능이 악화하지 않도록 하거나 악화하면 즉시 교정하는 데 도움이 된다. 병원 전 처치 제공자는 환자의 상태에 중대한 변화에 특히 주의를 기울이고 그러한 변화가 발견되면 처치 방법을 다시 고려해야 한다. 또한 환자를 지속해서 모니터링하면 일차평가에서 간과했거나 이제야 나타난 상태나 문제를 발견하는 더 도움이 된다. 환자의 상태가 명확하지 않은 경우가 많으므로 환자를 보고, 듣는 것만으로도 많은 정보를 얻을 수 있다. 정보를 수집하는 방법은 모든 정보를 수집하는 것만큼 중요하지 않다. 재평가는 가능한 한 신속하고 철저하게 수행해야 한다. 환자를 이송 지연해야 하는 상황에서의 모니터링은 나중에 설명한다.

의사소통

병원 전 처치 제공자와 병원 의료진 사이의 의사소통은 양질의 환자 치료를 위해 매우 중요한 부분이며 병원 도착 전 보고, 병원 도착 시 의료진에게 구두 보고 및 공식적으로 작성된 환자 처치 기록지와 같은 다양한 구성 요소로 이루어져 있다. 환자를 이송할 의료기관에 가능한 한 빨리 보고가 이루어져야 한다. 조기에 연락을 취하면 의료기관에서 종종 외상 경보 시스템을 통해 환자에게 최선의 처치를 하는 데 필요한 적절한 인력과 장비를 배치할 수 있다. 이송 중에 병원 전 처치 제공자는 환자를 이송할 의료기관에 다음과 같은 정보가 포함된 간단한 환자 처치 기록지를 제공해야 한다.

- 환자의 성별 정확한 나이 또는 추정 나이
- 손상 기전
- 생명을 위협하는 손상, 확인된 상태, 손상의 해부학적 위치
- 현자 활력징후
- 수행한 처치와 처치에 대한 환자의 반응
- 예상 도착 시간(ETA)

시간이 허락하는 경우 관련 의학적 상태 및 복용 중인 약물, 기타 생명을 위협하지 않는 손상, 환자가 사용하는 보호 장비(안전띠, 헬멧 등)를 포함한 현장의 특성, 추가 환자에 대한 정보 등 추가 정보를 포함할 수 있다. 그러지 않으면 이 정보는 병원에 도착해서 제공할 수 있다.

병원 전 처치 제공자는 또한 환자를 인계받는 의료기관의 의사나 간호사에게 구두로 보고한다. 이 구두 보고는 일반적으로 무전을 이용한 보고보다는 상세하지만, 병원 전 처치 보고서보다 덜 상세하며 사고 발생과 관련된 내용, 병원 전 처치 제공자가 시행한 처치 및 이 처치에 대한 환자의 반응에 관한 내용을 제공한다. 구두 및 서면 보

고서는 모두 무선 보고 후 발생한 환자 상태에 대한 중요한 변화를 강조해야 한다. 중요한 병원 전 정보의 전달은 환자 처치에 대한 팀 개념이 더욱 강조된다.

일부 외상센터는 병원 전 처치 제공자와 병원 직원 간의 잘못된 의사소통과 오해를 피하려고 이 과정을 공식화했다. 외상 환자가 외상센터의 소생술에 도착하면 외상팀 리더는 숨을 쉬고 맥박이 있는지 확인하기 위해 신속한 일차평가를 수행한 후 잠시 멈춰서 EMS 팀 리더의 20초간 외치는 소리를 듣는다. 이 구두보고에는 다음과 같은 요소가 포함되어야 한다.

1. 나이, 성별, 손상 기전 및 사고 발생 시간
2. 수축기 혈압이 90mmHg 미만인 경우를 포함한 병원 전 단계 활력징후
3. 확인된 손상
4. 병원 전 처치
5. 환자의 상태 변화, 특히 신경학적 또는 혈류역학적인 변화
6. 환자 병력, 알레르기 및 약물 특히 혈전 용해제 복용 여부

중증외상 환자의 경우 외상팀은 20~30초를 초과하여 평가를 진행할 수 없으며 추가 정보는 환자를 직접 평가하거나 이 과정에 관여하지 않는 간호사나 다른 외상팀원에게 제공할 수 있다.

서면으로 작성한 병원 전 환자처치보고서(PCR)도 중요하다. 또한 좋은 병원 전 환자처치보고서는 다음과 같은 두 가지 이유로 가치가 있다.

1. 병원 전 처치 제공자가 떠난 후 환자가 이송된 의료기관의 의료진이 발생한 사고와 환자 상태에 대해 완전한 이해를 할 수 있게 해준다.
2. 사례검토를 가능하게 하여 병원 전 단계 시스템 전반의 품질 관리를 보장한다.

이러한 이유로 병원 전 처치 제공자는 병원 전 환자처치보고서를 정확하고 완벽하게 작성하여 환자를 이송하는 의료기관에 제공하는 것이 중요하다. 병원 전 환자처치보고서는 환자와 함께 있어야 하고 환자가 도착 후 몇 시간 또는 며칠이 지난 후에 제출하면 아무 도움도 되지 않는다. 기관에서 전자 기록 프로그램을 사용하는 경우 주요 정보의 서면 요약을 응급실의 의료진에게 할 수 있으며 전체 기록이 완료되면 병원으로 전송해야 한다.

병원 전 환자처치보고서는 환자 의무기록의 일부이다. 이것은 발견된 내용과 수행한 조치에 대한 법적 기록이며 법적 증거로 사용될 수 있다. 이 보고서는 발견된 손상과 병원 전 환경에서 수행한 조치에 대한 공식 기록이다. 따라서 이 보고서는 철저하고 정확해야 한다. 병원 전 환자처치보고서의 사본을 환자를 이송하는 의료기관에 제공하는 또 다른 중요한 이유는 대부분의 외상센터가 입원한 모든 외상 환자의 "외상 등록체계"를 유지 관리하기 때문이다. 병원 전 정보는 이 데이터베이스의 중요한 부분이며 귀중한 연구에 도움이 될 수 있다.

특별한 고려사항

외상성 심장정지

외상으로 인한 심정지는 내과적 심정지와 몇 가지 중요한 점에서 다르다. 첫째 내과적 심정지는 일반적으로 호흡기 문제(예: 이물질에 의한 기도 폐쇄) 또는 심장 부정맥의 결과이다. 이럴 때 현장에서 소생술을 시도하는 것이 가장 좋다. 외상성 심정지는 대부분 대량 출혈이나 심각한 뇌손상으로 인해 발생하는 경우가 많다. 이러한 환자는 일반적으로 현장에서 적절하게 소생시킬 수 없다. 외상성 심정지로 인한 생존율은 낮으며 전체 생존율은 4% 미만이고 양호한 신경학적 상태로 생존하는 비율은 2% 미만이다.

병원 전 환경에서 외상성 심장정지 처치와 관련된 결정은 종종 복잡하며 다양한 요소를 고려해야 한다. 미국 구급의학회(NAEMSP)와 미국 외과학회 외상위원회(ACS-COT)뿐만 아니라 유럽 소생의학회(ERC)에서 개발한 지침과 의견문은 현재 이용할 수 있는 증거에 대한 최선의 이해를 나타낸다. 그러나 새로운 연구 및 지역적 요인을 고려해야 하므로 일부 지역 프로토콜은 이러한 지침에서 벗어날 수 있다.

일반적인 원리

명백한 사망 징후(예: 뇌 조직 노출)가 즉시 나타나거나 환자가 다음 부분에 설명된 소생술 보류 기준을 명확하게 충족하지 않는 한 추가 평가를 수행하고 이송을 준비하는 동안 소생술을 시작해야 한다. 외부출혈은 즉시 지혈해야 한다. 많은 프로토콜이 외상성 심정지 환자를 처치하기 위한 알고리즘에 가슴 압박을 포함하고 있지만, 중증 외상 및 대량 출혈 상황에서 심폐소생술의 효과는 의문이다. 이러한 유보에도 불구하고 소생 가능성이 있는 환자는 외상성 심정지의 가역적 원인을 먼저 처치하면 심폐소생술을 시도하는 것이 합리적이다. 모든 심폐소생술 시도와 마찬가지로 병원 전 처치 제공자는 가슴압

박 중단을 최소화해야 한다.

전문소생술(ALS)을 제공할 수 있다면 기본소생술(BLS)을 유지하면서 전문소생술을 제공한다. 기도는 기관내삽관 또는 성문외기도기와 같은 적절한 기도유지기를 사용하여 기도를 개방한다(목뼈를 중립적 자세로 유지하면서). 호흡음을 청진하고 환기 중 호흡음이 감소하거나 부적절한 가슴의 움직임이 있다면 긴장기흉을 고려해야 한다. 환자에게 긴장기흉이 의심되는 경우 바늘감압을 시행해야 한다. 정맥 라인을 확보하고 등장성 결정질 용액을 투여한다. 심전도 모니터링을 수행하고 심장 리듬을 평가한다. 심실세동이 관찰되면 제세동을 시행해야 한다.

일반적으로 중증외상 환자는 현장 체류시간이 짧고 외상센터로 신속하게 이송하는 것이 가장 좋다. 그러나 외성성 심정지 환자의 경우 이송 시기(또는 이송 여부)를 결정하는 것이 훨씬 더 복잡하다. 항공 응급의료서비스는 수혈과 같은 전문적인 처치를 현장에서 제공할 수 있으며 지상 이동보다 의료기관에 더 일찍 도착할 수 있다. 그러나 많은 항공 응급서비스는 심정지 환자를 이송하지 않는다.

EMS 제공자가 심정지를 목격했거나 병원 전 처치 제공자가 현장에 도착하기 몇 분 이내에 심정지가 발생했다고 믿을 만한 이유가 있고 환자를 10~15분 이내에 적절한 의료기관으로 이송할 수 있는 경우 즉시 이송하고 이송 중에 추가 처치 및 소생술을 실시하는 것을 고려한다. 환자를 이 시간 내에 적절한 의료기관(외상센터)으로 이송할 수 없는 경우 병원 전 처치 제공자는 현장에서 소생술을 시행한 후 적절한 경우 소생술을 중단하는 것을 고려할 수 있다.

소생술 보류

생존 가능성이 극히 낮은 환자에게 소생술을 시도하면 병원 전 처치 제공자를 이송 중 차량 충돌로 인한 손상뿐만 아니라 혈액과 체액에 노출될 수 있는 손상을 입을 위험에 처하게 된다. 또한 소생술 시도에 실패하면 생존 가능성이 더 높은 환자에게 자원이 집중되지 못할 수도 있다. 이러한 이유로 외상성 심정지 환자에 대한 소생술 시도 여부를 결정할 때는 신중한 판단이 필요하다.

미국 구급의학회(NAEMSP)는 미국 외과학회 외상위원회(ACS-COT)와 협력하여 병원 전 환경에서 소생술을 보류하거나 중단하기 위한 지침을 개발했다. 익사, 낙뢰 또는 저체온증의 피해자와 소아 또는 임신한 환자는 소생술을 보류하거나 중단을 결정하기 전에 특별한 고려가 필요하다. 외상 사고 현장에서 심정지 상태로 발견된 환자는 내과적 문제(예: 심근경색)로 심정지가 발생했을 수 있으며, 특

히 환자가 노인이거나 손상이 경미한 경우 더욱 그렇다. 심정지의 원인이 외상보다 내과적 원인이 심정지의 원인일 가능성이 더 높은 것으로 판단되는 환자의 경우 병원 전 심정지에 대한 표준 지침을 따라서 처치를 시행한다.

심정지의 가장 큰 원인으로 추정되는 외상성 손상이 있고 다음 기준을 충족하는 환자의 경우 소생술을 보류하고 환자의 사망을 선언할 수 있다.

- 명백히 치명적인 손상(예: 목 절단, 뇌 조직 노출)이 있거나 비가역적인 증거가 있는 경우(잿빛 피부, 사후 강직, 부패 등)
- 무딘 손상 환자의 경우 병원 전 처치 제공자 도착했을 때 환자가 맥박이 없고 무호흡 상태이며 심전도 활동이 없는 경우 소생술을 보류할 수 있다.
- 관통성 환자의 경우 병원 전 처치 제공자 도착했을 때 환자가 맥박이 없고 무호흡 상태이며 다른 생명 징후(동공 반사 소실, 자발적 움직임 없음, 조직화한 심전도 활동 없음)가 없는 경우 소생술을 보류할 수 있다.

소생슬 보류 결정은 적절한 평가를 수행한 경우에만 의학적으로 정당화될 수 있으므로 사망 가능성이 있는 환자를 평가할 때는 각별한 주의를 기울여야 한다. 사망으로 잘못 추정되었던 외상 환자가 나중에 활력징후가 있는 것으로 밝혀진 사례가 매년 보고되고 있다. 이러한 환자들은 거의 모두 손상을 극복하고 회복되지만, 이러한 사건은 병원 전 처치 제공자와 해당 의료기관 모두에게 당혹스러운 일이 될 수 있다. 다수의 환자가 발생한 현장의 흥분된 상황에서 병원 전 처치 제공자는 환자의 맥박이 있는지 적절하게 평가하지 못할 수 있다. 죽어가는 외상 환자는 서맥과 저혈압이 심할 수 있으므로 임종 전 상태를 파악하기 어려울 수 있다. 명백한 사망 징후가 없는 환자에게 소생술 보류를 결정하기 전에 병원 전 처치 제공자는 맥박 확인(가능하면 여러 부위에서), 환자의 신경학적 상태 평가(예: 동공 반사, 자발적 움직임 및 통증 자극에 대한 반사) 및 심전도 모니터링 등 적절한 평가를 수행해야 한다.

외상성 심정지 환자에서 소생술 보류를 결정할 때 고려해야 할 사항은 **표 6-1**에 나와 있다.

소생술 종료

미국 구급의학회 및 미국외과학회 외상위원회는 병원 전 환경에서 소생술 종단에 대한 개정된 지침을 발표했다. 외상 환자의 소생술 중단은 가슴알박 중단을 최소화한 심폐소생술과 가역적인 심정지 원인

표 6-1 외상성 심정지 환자에서 소생술 보류 시 고려 사항

고려 사항	설명	권고
소생술을 시작하더라도 사망할 가능성이 가장 높다.	■ 환자는 맥박이 없고 무호흡 상태이며 조직화된 ECG 활동이 없고 자발적인 움직임이나 동공 반사가 없다.	소생술 보류
존재하는 손상은 생명과 양립할 수 없는 상태이다.	■ 머리제거 ■ 외상성 몸통 분리(하반신절단)	소생술 보류
장시간 심정지의 증거가 있다.	■ 사후경축 ■ 시반 ■ 부패의 증거	소생술 보류
비외상성 심정지 원인에 대한 증거가 있다.*	■ 경미한 차량 손상은 있지만, 환자가 손상을 입지 않은 것으로 보이는 경우 ■ 치명적이지 않은 높이에서 추락해 심각한 손상의 증거가 없는 경우	소생술 시작

*이들은 외상성 사건이 심정지의 원인이 아닌 심정지 이전의 결과로 의심되는 환자들이다(예: 심각한 심정지를 겪은 후 사다리에서 떨어지거나 뇌졸중을 겪은 후 차량 충돌 등).

© National Association of Emergency Medical Technicians (NAEMT)

처치를 포함한 적절한 구급대원의 처치에도 불구하고 생명 징후가 없고 자발 순환 회복이 없을 때 고려해야 한다(표 6-2). 외상성 심정지 환자에게 소생술을 중단하기 전에 고려해야 할 적절한 소생술 지속 시간은 아직 명확하지 않다. 합리적인 지침은 15분간의 소생술 시도이지만, 지역 프로토콜은 다른 시간이 정해질 수 있다. 일반적으로 이송이 시작된 후에는 소생술을 중단할 수 없다.

통증 관리

과거에는 주로 아편유사제의 부작용(환기 감소 및 혈관 확장 감소)이 저혈압 또는 저산소증을 유발하거나 악화시킬 수 있다는 우려 때문에 외상 환자 처치에서 약리학적 통증 관리의 역할이 제한적이었다. 이러한 우려로 인해 통증 관리가 필요한 일부 환자에게는 제한적이었다. 그 후 한동안 통증 관리를 목표로 아편유사 약물을 사용하는 약리학적 통증 관리가 상당히 무분별하게 시행되었다. 의학계 전반에 걸친 이러한 관행은 마약 중독 및 치명적인 과다 복용의 전국적인 유행과 관련이 있었다. 적절한 통증 관리를 사용하고 가능한 한 아편유사제 약물 사용을 피하고 비약물적 방법을 자주 사용하는 더욱 균형 잡힌 접근 방식을 사용해야 한다. 선택한 통증 관리 방법은 효과와 안전성을 기준으로 선택해야 하며 생명을 구하는 처치나 적절한 의료기관으로의 신속한 이송을 방해해서는 안 된다.

비약물적 통증 관리 방법에는 부목고정, 냉찜질 및 언어적 진정 기법 등이 있다. 아세트아미노펜, 케타민, 비스테로이드성소염진통제(NSAIDs)와 같은 비아편유사제 약물을 포함한 다양한 약리학적 통증 관리 방법을 사용할 수 있다. 펜타닐, 모르핀, 하이드로몰폰과 같은 아편유사제 약물도 사용할 수 있지만, 신중하게 사용해야 한다. 펜타닐은 작용 시간이 빠르고 작용 지속 시간이 짧으며 혈류역학에 미치는 영향이 적기 때문에 종종 1차 약물로 사용된다. 또 다른 매력적인 방법은 케타민의 해리 용량(진통제 용량)으로 적절히 투여할 때 혈류역학적 안정성과 호흡 충동을 유지하는 유리한 안전성 분석이 있기 때문이다.

표 6-2 외상성 심정지 환자에서 소생술 종료 시 고려 사항

고려 사항	설명	권고
생명의 징후가 존재한다.	■ 자발적인 호흡, 움직임, 맥박 또는 측정 가능한 혈압이 존재	소생술을 종료하지 않는다.
무맥성전기활동이 있는 ECG 가 존재	■ 좁은 QRS 이며 정상 또는 빠른 유형(생존 가능성이 높음) ■ 넓은 QRS 이며 느린 유형(생존 가능성이 낮음)	소생술을 종료하지 않는다.
환자는 응급실에서 가슴절개술을 받을 수 있다.	■ 생명의 징후가 목격된 관통성 가슴 손상 ■ ECG에서 좁은 QRS 이며 정상 또는 빠른 유형	소생술을 종료하지 않는다.
효과적인 심폐소생술에도 불구하고 환자의 ECG 활동이 좋지 않은 상태로 진행 중	■ 좁은 QRS 이며 정상 또는 빠른 유형에서 넓은 QRS 이며 느린 유형으로 역 보상	소생술 중단 고려
소생술 지속 시간은 예후가 좋지 않은 것과 일치한다.	■ 일반적으로 15분 이내로 허용한다. ■ 특정 환자에 대한 고려 사항에 따라 이 15분을 초과할 수 있다.	소생술 중단 고려

Abbreviations: CPR, cardiopulmonary resuscitation; ECG, electrocardiogram; ED, emergency department; PEA, pulseless electrical activity.

© National Association of Emergency Medical Technicians (NAEMT)

진통제를 투여하는 경우 진통 효과와 잠재적인 부작용이나 합병증에 대해 환자를 자세히 모니터링해야 한다. 모니터링에는 맥박산소측정, 심박수, 의식상태 및 빈번한 혈압측정이 포함되어야 한다. 가능한 경우 호기말이산화탄소분압 모니터링도 시행해야 한다.

학대로 인한 손상

병원 전 처치 제공자는 현장에 가장 먼저 도착하는 경우가 많으므로 학대 가능성이 있는 상황을 평가할 수 있다. 집 안에 있는 병원 전 처치 제공자는 현장을 확인한 후 현장의 세부 사항을 환자를 이송할 의료기관에 전달하여 해당 지역의 관련 기관에 학대 우려를 알릴 수 있다. 병원 전 처치 제공자는 종종 이 숨겨진 위험에 대한 정보를 의심하고 확인하여 정보를 전달할 수 있도록 의학적으로 교육을 받은 유일한 사람인 경우가 많다. 일부 지역에서는 병원 전 처치 제공자가 의료기관뿐만 아니라 관련 기관에 학대와 관련된 내용을 신고하도록 의무화하는 법률이 있다.

나이와 관계없이 누구나 잠재적인 학대의 피해자 또는 학대자가 될 수 있다. 임신부, 영아, 어린이, 청소년, 청년, 중년, 노인 모두 학대의 위험에 노출되어 있다. 신체적, 심리적(정서적), 성적, 경제적인 학대를 포함하여 여러 유형의 학대가 있다. 학대는 의도적인 행위로 인한 손상을 입히는 고의(예: 신체적 학대 또는 성적 학대), 의뢰에 의해 발생하거나 부양가족의 방치로 발생할 수 있다. 이 부분에서는 학대의 유형에 대해 논의하지 않으며 일반적인 특성을 소개하고 병원 전 처치 제공자의 학대에 대한 인식과 의심을 높인다.

잠재적인 학대자의 일반적인 특성으로는 손상과 관련 없는 사건에 대한 설명, 환자의 손상을 최소화하는 태도, 부정적인 태도, 지나치게 자신감 있는 태도, 병원 전 처치 제공자에게 폭언을 하거나 어린 환자의 경우 부모의 관심 부족 및 질문에 대답하지 않으려는 태도 등이 있다. 학대를 겪고 있는 환자의 몇 가지 일반적인 특징으로는 조용함, 사건의 세부 사항을 자세히 설명하기를 꺼리는 것, 현장에 있는 사람과 눈을 계속 마주치거나 눈을 마주치지 않는 것, 신체적 손상을 최소화하는 것, 상처가 드러날 수 있는 옷을 벗는 것을 거부하는 것 등을 들 수 있다. 학대자, 학대받는 사람은 다양한 형태를 취할 수 있으며 병원 전 처치 제공자는 현상 상황과 설명이 일치하지 않는 경우 학대 의심의 수준을 높게 유지해야 한다.

이송 지연 및 의료기관 간 전원

대부분의 도시 또는 교외 EMS 이송은 30분 이하가 걸리지만, 기상 조건, 교통 혼잡, 철도 건널목 등으로 인해 이송 시간이 길어질 수 있다. 이러한 지연은 외상센터로의 이송 시간이 지연되는 것을 설명하기 위해 환자처치보고서에 기록해야 한다. 농촌 및 교외 지역에서 근무하는 많은 병원 전 처치 제공자는 이송 중 훨씬 더 긴 시간 동안 환자를 일상적으로 처치한다. 또한 병원 전 처치 제공자는 지상 또는 항공 이송을 통해 한 의료기관에서 다른 의료기관으로 이송하는 동안 환자를 처치해야 한다. 이러한 전원에는 최대 몇 시간이 걸릴 수 있다.

병원 전 처치 제공자가 외상 환자의 이송 지연, 특히 의료기관 간 이송에 관여하는 경우 특별한 준비가 필요하다. 이러한 이송을 시작하기 전에 고려해야 하는 문제는 환자, 병원 전 처치 제공자 및 장비와 관련된 문제로 나눌 수 있다.

환자 문제

가장 중요한 것은 환자를 이송할 때 안전하고 따뜻한 환경을 제공하는 것이다. 들것은 구급차에 적절하게 고정되어야 하고 환자는 들것에 적절히 고정되어야 한다. 본문 전체에서 강조했듯이 체온저하는 외상 환자에게 치명적일 수 있는 합병증이므로 환자 칸은 아주 따뜻해야 한다. 완전히 옷을 입은 병원 전 처치 제공자가 환자 칸의 온도에 편안하다면 노출된 환자에게는 너무 추울 수 있다.

환자는 특히 손상 부위에 최대한 접근할 수 있는 위치에 환자를 고정해야 한다. 이송 전에 삽입한 기도유지기의 위치를 확인하고 구급차가 급커브를 돌거나 차량 충돌사고에 연루되었을 때 장비(예: 모니터, 산소 탱크)가 투사체가 되지 않도록 배치하고 고정해야 한다. 환자가 움직일 때 장비가 떨어질 수 있고 환자에게 불편함을 줄 수 있으며 이송 지연 시 욕창을 유발할 수 있으므로 장비를 환자 위에 올

려놓지 않는다. 이송 중에는 확보한 정맥 라인이 빠지지 않도록 카테터를 고정한다. 이송 시간이 길어질 것으로 예상되어 환자를 들것으로 옮길 때 긴척추고정판을 사용했다면, 이송 전에 적절하게 척추 움직임 제한을 유지하면서 조심스럽게 환자에게 통나무굴리기법을 시행하여 긴척추고정판을 제거하고 이송하는 것을 고려한다. 이렇게 하면 환자의 편안함을 증가시키고 딱딱한 표면에 고정하는 것과 관련된 궤양 형성의 위험을 줄일 수 있다.

환자는 일차평가와 활력징후를 주기적으로 재평가를 받아야 한다. 거의 모든 중증 환자에게 맥박산소측정과 심전도를 지속해서 모니터링하고 가능한 경우 기관내삽관이 시행된 환자는 호기말이산화탄소분압을 측정한다. 기관내삽관이 시행되지 않는 환자의 경우 코삽입관 또는 입에 삽입한 카테터를 이용해 호기말이산화탄소분압을 측정할 수 있다. 구급차에 환자와 같이 타는 병원 전 처치 제공자는 환자의 예상 요구 사항에 적합한 수준에 교육을 받아야 한다. 중증 손상을 입은 환자는 일반적으로 전문 교육을 받은 병원 전 처치 제공자가 처치해야 한다. 환자가 이송 중 수혈이 필요할 것으로 예상되는 경우 업무 범위 내에서 수혈이 가능한 처치 제공자가 동행해야 하며 미국에서는 일반적으로 중환자 처치 교육을 받은 병원 전 처치 제공자, 간호사와 의사가 동행한다.

두 가지 관리 계획을 세워야 한다. 첫 번째는 의료 계획으로 이송 중 환자에게 예상되는 문제나 예상치 못한 문제를 관리하기 위해 개발된다. 필요한 장비, 약물 및 소모품을 쉽게 사용할 수 있어야 한다. 두 번째 이송 계획은 환자를 이송할 의료기관까지 가장 신속하게 이동할 수 있는 경로를 파악하는 것이다. 기상 조건, 도로 상황(예: 공사) 및 교통 상황을 파악하고 예상해야 한다. 또한 병원 전 처치 제공자는 일차 목적지까지 이동하는 동안 현장에서 처치할 수 없는 문제가 발생한 경우를 대비하여 이송 경로에 있는 의료기관에 대해 잘 알고 있어야 한다.

이송 지연 중 또는 전원 전에 의료기관에서 수행되는 환자 처치를 위한 보조 장치는 다음과 같은 것이 포함될 수 있다.

- 위장관: 적절하게 삽입하는 방법을 교육받은 경우 코위관 또는 입위관을 환자의 위에 삽입할 수 있다. 위 내용물을 흡입하면 복부 팽만감이 감소하고 잠재적으로 구토 및 흡인의 위험을 감소시킬 수 있다.
- 도뇨관: 적절하게 삽입하도록 교육을 받았으면 환자의 방광에 도뇨관을 삽입할 수 있다. 소변 배출량은 환자의 신장 관류량을 측정하는 민감한 척도이자 환자의 체액량 상태를 나타내는 지표가 될 수 있다.

- 현장 검사 장비를 이용한 동맥 또는 정맥혈 가스 모니터링: 맥박 산소측정기는 산소헤모글로빈 포화도에 대한 유용한 정보를 제공하지만, 혈액가스 수치는 환자의 이산화탄소분압과 pH 및 쇼크의 심각성을 나타내는 염기 결핍에 대한 유용한 정보를 제공할 수 있다.

근무자의 문제

병원 전 처치 제공자의 안전은 환자의 안전만큼이나 중요하다. 병원 전 처치 제공자는 특히 장시간 이동하는 경우 충분한 휴식과 수분을 섭취해야 한다. 최근의 증거 기반 검토에 따르면 카페인이 함유된 음료, 낮잠, 24시간 이상 교대 근무 피하기 등 다양한 피로 관리 전략을 권장한다. 근무자는 운전석이나 환자 칸 모두에서 안전띠를 포함한 적절한 안전장치를 갖추고 사용해야 한다. 병원 전 처치 제공자는 표준 예방조치를 하고 체액, 혈액, 기타 가능한 노출 가능성을 방지할 수 있는 충분한 장갑과 기타 개인보호장비를 준비해야 한다.

장비 문제

이송 지연 중에 발생하는 장비 문제에는 차량, 소모품, 의약품, 모니터링 장비 및 통신 등이 포함된다. 구급차 또는 의료용 헬기는 충분한 양의 연료를 포함하여 정상으로 작동되어야 한다. 병원 전 처치 제공자는 드레싱을 수행하기 위한 거즈와 패드, 정맥 내로 투여할 수액, 산소 및 진통제 등 이송에 필요한 충분한 물품과 의약품을 충분히 사용할 수 있는지 확인해야 한다. 의약품은 예상되는 환자의 필요에 따라 준비하며 진정제, 마비제, 진통제 및 항생제 등을 포함한다. 일반적인 규칙은 상당한 이송 지연이 발생하는 경우 예상되는 필요량보다 약 50% 더 많은 소모품과 의약품을 구급차에 비축하는 것이다. 환자 처치 장비는 모니터 장비(알람 기능이 있는), 산소 조절기, 흡인기를 포함하여 모든 장비에 적절한 전원 공급이 보장되어야 한다. 또한 이송 지연의 성공은 다른 병원 전 처치 제공자와 의사소통할 수 있는 통신장비 사용을 포함한 의료 지도, 환자를 이송할 의료기관이 의사스통 능력에 달려 있을 수 있다.

이송 지연 중 특정 손상에 대한 처리는 이 본문의 해당 장에서 설명한다.

요 약

- 외상성 손상을 입은 환자의 생존 가능성은 조직 관류를 방해하는 상태를 즉시 파악하고 완화하는 데 달려 있다.
- 이러한 상태를 파악하려면 체계적이고 우선순위를 정하여 논리적으로 정보를 수집하고 그에 따라 조처하는 과정이 필요하다. 이 과정을 환자 평가라고 한다.
- 환자 평가는 현장의 안전성 평가를 포함한 현장 평가로 시작하며 환자에 대한 일반적인 인상, 일차평가 및 환자의 상태와 추가 EMS 인력의 가용성이 허용되는 경우 이차평가를 포함한다.
- 이 평가 과정을 통해 얻은 정보를 분석하여 환자 처치 및 이송 결정의 기초 자료로 사용한다.
- 외상 환자의 처치에서 놓친 문제는 잠재적으로 환자의 생존을 도울 기회를 놓친 것이다.
- 현장 안전과 상황에 대한 일반적인 인상을 동시에 결정한 후 병원 전 처치 제공자는 XABCDE 형식에 따라 일차평가를 시작한다.
  - X(Exsanguinating Hemorrhage): 대량 출혈(심각한 외부출혈 지혈)
  - A(Airway): 기도 관리 및 척추 고정
  - B(Breathing): 호흡(환기 및 산소 공급)
  - C(Circulation): 순환(관류 및 기타 출혈)
  - D(Disability): 장애
  - E(Expose and Environment): 노출/환경
- 이러한 형식의 순차적 표시에도 불구하고 일차평가는 본질적으로 동시에 빠른 순서로 이루어진다.
- 환자의 생명에 대한 즉각적인 위협은 "진행과 동시에 처치" 방식으로 신속하게 해결한다. 병원 전 처치 제공자가 출혈을 조절하고 환자의 기도와 호흡을 처치하면 현장에서 추가 처치 없이 이송을 시작한다. 외상 현장 처치의 한계로 환자를 결정적인 처치를 받을 수 있는 의료기관으로 신속하게 이송해야 한다.
- 일차평가 및 이차평가를 자주 반복하여 환자 상태의 변화와 신속한 처치가 필요한 새로운 문제를 파악해야 한다.
- 병원 전 처치 제공자가 환자에게 가장 적절한 의료기관을 선택하고 의료기관과 원활하게 의사소통하며 환자의 상태와 병원 전 환경에서 수행한 조치를 철저히 문서화하면 환자의 예후를 크게 개선할 수 있다.

시나리오 재구성

11월 초 토요일 아침 날씨는 맑고 기온은 5.5℃이다. 당신이 소속된 EMS 팀은 2층 건물 옥상에서 추락한 사람이 있다는 신고를 받고 현장으로 출동한다. 현장에 도착하자마자 환자의 가족이 당신을 집 뒷마당으로 안내한다. 가족은 환자가 지붕에서 빗물받이의 낙엽을 빗자루로 청소하던 중 균형을 잃고 지붕에서(약 3.6m) 등부터 추락했다고 말한다. 환자는 처음에 잠시 의식을 잃었지만, 119에 신고할 때는 의식이 있었다.

환자에게 다가가 보니 약 40대의 남성이 바닥에 바로누워 있고 두 명의 가족이 그의 옆에 앉아 있는 것을 목격한다. 환자는 의식이 있고 가족과 이야기하고 있으며 심한 출혈의 징후는 보이지 않는다. 동료가 환자의 머리와 목을 도수로 고정할 때 당신이 환자에게 어디가 아픈지 물어본다. 환자는 등 전체가 가장 아프다고 말한다.

초기 문진은 환자의 주요호소증상을 파악하고 그의 초기 의식 수준을 결정하며 환기 노력을 평가하는 등 다양한 목적으로 수행된다. 명백한 호흡곤란이 발견되지 않으면 환자 평가를 진행한다. 환자는 당신의 질문에 적절하게 대답하며 사람, 시간, 장소에 대한 지남력은 정상이다.

- 이 사고와 관련된 외상의 물리학에 근거하여 평가하는 중에 어떤 잠재적인 손상을 발견할 것으로 예상하는가?
- 다음 우선순위는 무엇인가?
- 이 환자를 어떻게 처치할 것인가?

시나리오 해결책

1분 동안 현장에 있었지만, 환자에 대한 추가 평가 및 처치를 안내하는 중요한 정보를 얻었다. 환자와 접촉한 처음 15초 동안 환자에 대한 일반적인 인상이 형성되어 소생술이 필요하지 않다고 판단했다. 몇 가지 간단한 조치로 일차평가의 XABCD를 평가했다. 눈에 보이는 심한 외부출혈은 없다. 환자가 어려움 없이 말을 하여 기도가 개방되어 있고 어려움 없이 숨을 쉬고 있음을 나타낸다. 동시에 손상 기전을 인지하고 목뼈를 고정했다. 동료가 노맥박을 평가하고 환자의 피부색, 피부 상태 및 체온을 확인했다. 이러한 결과는 환자의 순환 상태에 대한 즉각적인 위협이 없음을 나타낸다. 또한 환자가 깨어 있고 지남력이 있고 질문에 적절하게 대답하고 모든 팔다리를 움직일 수 있으므로 장애의 초기 증거를 동시에 발견하지 못했다. 추락에 대한 정보와 함께 이 정보는 추가 자원의 필요성, 이송 방법 및 환자를 이송할 의료기관 유형을 결정하는 데 도움이 된다.

이제 이러한 단계를 완료했으며 즉각적인 소생술이 필요하지 않다면, 평가 과정 초기에 일차평가의 E 단계를 진행한 다음 활력징후를 측정한다. 환자를 노출해 옷에 가려졌을 수 있는 추가 손상과 출혈을 확인한 다음 환자를 덮어 외부 환경으로부터 보호한다. 이 과정에서 덜 심각한 손상에 주목하여 더 자세한 검사를 수행한다.

다음 단계는 척추 전체의 움직임 제한, 팔다리의 손상 부위에 드레싱을 시행하거나 부목을 고정하고 이송한다. 이송 중 환자를 재평가하고 모니터링하며 정맥 라인을 확보한 후 수액을 투여하거나 지시에 따라 적절한 진통제를 투여하고 시간이 허락하는 대로 개방 상처에 드레싱을 시행한다. 외상의 물리학에 대한 당신의 지식과 환자의 목격된 의식 소실은 외상성 뇌손상, 다리 손상 및 척추 손상을 의심할 수 있다.

References

1. Brown JB, Rosengart MR, Forsythe RM, et al. Not all prehospital time is equal: influence of scene time on mortality. *J Trauma Acute Care Surg*. 2016;81:93-100.

2. Meizoso JP, Ray JJ, Karcutskie CA 4th, et al. Effect of time to operation on mortality for hypotensive patients with gunshot wounds to the torso: the golden 10 minutes. *J Trauma Acute Care Surg*. 201;81(4):685-691. doi: 10.1097/TA.0000000000001198

3. Clarke JR, Trooskin SZ, Doshi PJ, Greenwald L, Mode CJ. Time to laparotomy for intra-abdominal bleeding from trauma does affect survival for delays up to 90 minutes. *J Trauma*. 2002;52(3):420-425. doi: 10.1097/00005373-200203000-00002

4. Brown E, Tohira H, Bailey P, et al. Longer prehospital time was not associated with mortality in major trauma: a retrospective cohort study, *Prehosp Emerg Care*. 2019;23(4):527-537. doi: 10.1080/10903127.2018.1551451

5. Advanced Trauma Life Support (ATLS) Subcommittee, Committee on Trauma. Initial assessment and management. In: *Advanced Trauma Life Support Course for Doctors, Student Course Manual*. 10th ed. American College of Surgeons; 2018.

6. Kotwal RS, Butler FK, Gross KR, et al. Management of junctional hemorrhage in Tactical Combat Casualty Care: TCCC guidelines–proposed change 13-03. *J Spec Oper Med*. 2013;13:85-93.

7. Kragh JF Jr, Mann-Salinas EA, Kotwal RS, et al. Laboratory assessment of out-of-hospital interventions to control junctional bleeding from the groin in a manikin model. *Am J Emerg Med*. 2013;31:1276-1278.

8. Kragh JF Jr, Parsons DL, Kotwal RS, et al. Testing of junctional tourniquets by military medics to control simulated groin hemorrhage. *J Spec Oper Med*. 2014;14:58-63.

9. Kragh JF, Kotwal RS, Cap AP, et al. Performance of junctional tourniquets in normal human volunteers. *Prehosp Emerg Care*. 2015;19:391-398.

10. Chen J, Benov A, Nadler R, et al. Testing of junctional tourniquets by medics of the Israeli Defense Force in control of simulated groin hemorrhage. *J Spec Oper Med*. 2016;16:36-42.

11. Bulger EM, Snyder D, Schoelles K, et al. An evidence-based prehospital guideline for external hemorrhage control: American College of Surgeons Committee on Trauma. *Prehosp Emerg Care*. 2014;18(2):163-173.

12. Fischer PE, Perina DG, Delbridge TR, et al. Spinal motion restriction in the trauma patient: a joint position statement. *Prehosp Emerg Care*. 2018;22(6):659-661. doi: 10.1080/10903127.2018.1481476

13. Kragh JF, Littrel ML, Jones JA, et al. Battle casualty survival with emergency tourniquet use to stop limb bleeding. *J Emerg Med*. 2011;41:590-597.

14. Beekley AC, Sebesta JA, Blackbourne LH, et al. Prehospital tourniquet use in Operation Iraqi Freedom: effect on hemorrhage control and outcomes. *J Trauma*. 2008;64:S28-S37.

15. Doyle GS, Taillac PP. Tourniquets: a review of current use with proposals for expanded prehospital use. *Prehosp Emerg Care*. 2008;12:241-256.

16. First Aid Science Advisory Board. First aid. *Circulation*. 2005;112(III):115.

17. Swan KG Jr, Wright DS, Barbagiovanni SS, et al. Tourniquets revisited. *J Trauma*. 2009;66:672-675.

18. King DR, Larentzakis A, Ramly EP; Boston Trauma Collaborative. Tourniquet use at the Boston Marathon bombing: lost in translation. *J Trauma Acute Care Surg*. 2015;78(3):594-599.

19. Deakin CD, Low JL. Accuracy of the advanced trauma life support guidelines for predicting systolic blood pressure using carotid, femoral, and radial pulses: observational study. *Br Med J*. 2000;321(7262):673-674.

20. Teasdale G, Jennett B. Assessment of coma and impaired consciousness: a practical scale. *Lancet.* 1974;2:81-84. doi: 10.1016/s0140-6736(74)91639-0

21. Bledsoe B, Casey M, Feldman J, et al. Glasgow Coma Scale scoring is often inaccurate. *Prehosp Disaster Med.* 2015;30(1): 46-53.

22. Gill MR, Reiley DG, Green SM. Interrater reliability of Glasgow Coma Scale scores in the emergency department. *Ann Emerg Med.* 2004;43(2):215-223.

23. Kerby JD, Maclennan PA, Burton JN, Mcgwin G, Rue LW. Agreement between prehospital and emergency department Glasgow Coma scores. *J Trauma.* 2007;63(5):1026-1031.

24. Healey C, Osler TM, Rogers FB, et al. Improving the Glasgow Coma Scale score: motor score alone is a better predictor. *J Trauma.* 2003;54:671-678.

25. Beskind DL, Stolz U, Gross A, et al. A comparison of the prehospital motor component of the Glasgow Coma Scale (mGCS) to the prehospital total GCS (tGCS) as a prehospital risk adjustment measure for trauma patients. *Prehosp Emerg Care.* 2014;18(1):68-75.

26. Kupas DF, Melnychuk EM, Young AJ. Glasgow Coma Scale motor component ("patient does not follow commands") performs similarly to total Glasgow Coma Scale in predicting severe injury in trauma patients. *Ann Emerg Med.* 2016;68(6):744-750.

27. Aguilar SA, Davis DP. Latency of pulse oximetry signal with use of digital probes associated with inappropriate extubation during prehospital rapid sequence intubation in head injury patients: case examples. *J Emerg Med.* 2012;42(4):424-428.

28. Vithalani VD, Vlk S, Davis SQ, Richmond NJ. Unrecognized failed airway management using a supraglottic airway device. *Resuscitation.* 2017;119:1-4.

29. Davis JW, Davis IC, Bennink LD, Bilello JF, Kaups KL, Parks SN. Are automated blood pressure measurements accurate in trauma patients? *J Trauma.* 2003;55(5):860-863.

30. Brown JB, Rosengart MR, Forsythe RM, et al. Not all prehospital time is equal: influence of scene time on mortality. *J Trauma Acute Care Surg.* 2016;81:93-100.

31. Pokorney DM, Braverman MA, Edmundson PM, et al. The use of prehospital blood products in the resuscitation of trauma patients: a review of prehospital transfusion practices and a description of our regional whole blood program in San Antonio, TX. *IBST Sci Ser.* 2019;14(3):332-342.

32. Pasley J, Miller CH, Dubose JJ, et al. Intraosseous infusion rates under high pressure: a cadaveric comparison of anatomic sites. *J Trauma Acute Care Surg.* 2015;78(2):295-299.

33. Brown JB, Cohen MJ, Minei JP, et al. Goal directed resuscitation in the prehospital setting: a propensity adjusted analysis. *J Trauma Acute Care Surg.* 2013;74(5):1207-1214.

34. Biswas S, Adileh M, Almogy G, Bala M. Abdominal injury patterns in patients with seatbelt signs requiring laparotomy. *J Emerg Trauma Shock.* 2014;7(4):295-300.

35. Bansal V, Conroy C, Tominaga GT, Coimbra R. The utility of seat belt signs to predict intra-abdominal injury following motor vehicle crashes. *Traffic Inj Prev.* 2009;10(6):567-572.

36. Chandler CF, Lane JS, Waxman KS. Seatbelt sign following blunt trauma is associated with increased incidence of abdominal injury. *Am Surg.* 1997;63(10):885-888.

37. Moylan JA, Detmer DE, Rose J, Schulz R. Evaluation of the quality of hospital care for major trauma. *J Trauma.* 1976;16(7):517-523.

38. West JG, Trunkey DD, Lim RC. Systems of trauma care: a study of two counties. *Arch Surg.* 1979;114(4):455-460.

39. West JG, Cales RH, Gazzaniga AB. Impact of regionalization: the Orange County experience. *Arch Surg.* 1983;118(6):740-744.

40. Shackford SR, Hollingworth-Fridlund P, Cooper GF, Eastman AB. The effect of regionalization upon the quality of trauma care as assessed by concurrent audit before and after institution of a trauma system: a preliminary report. *J Trauma.* 1986;26(9):812-820.

41. Waddell TK, Kalman PG, Goodman SJ, Girotti MJ. Is outcome worse in a small volume Canadian trauma centre? *J Trauma.* 1991;31(7):958-961.

42. MacKenzie EJ, Rivara FP, Jurkovich GJ, et al. A national evaluation of the effect of trauma-center care on mortality. *N Engl J Med.* 2006;354(4):366-378.

43. Branas CC, MacKenzie EJ, Williams JC, et al. Access to trauma centers in the United States. *JAMA.* 2005; 293(21):2626-2633.

44. Nathens AB, Jurkovich GJ, Rivara FP, Maier RV. Effectiveness of state trauma systems in reducing injury-related mortality: a national evaluation. *J Trauma.* 2000;48(1):25-30; discussion 30-31.

45. Report Card Task Force Members, American College of Emergency Physicians (ACEP) Staff. America's emergency care environment, a state-by-state report card: 2014 edition. *Ann Emerg Med.* 2014;63(2):97-242.

46. American College of Surgeons. *COT Releases Updated National Guideline for Field Triage of Injured Patients.* Reviewed May 3, 2022. Accessed June 1, 2022. https://www.facs.org/for-medical-professionals/news-publications/news-and-articles/acs-brief/may-10-2022-issue/cot-releases-updated-national-guideline-for-field-triage-of-injured-patients/

47. American College of Surgeons. *Resources for the Optimal Care of the Injured Patient.* 6th ed. American College of Surgeons; 2014.

48. Baker SP, O'Neill B, Haddon W Jr, Long WB. The injury severity score: a method for describing patients with multiple injuries and evaluating emergency care. *J Trauma.* 1974;14(3):187-196.

49. McCoy CE, Chakravarthy B, Lotfipour S. Guidelines for field triage of injured patients: in conjunction with the *Morbidity and Mortality Weekly Report* published by the Centers for Disease Control and Prevention. *West J Emerg Med.* 2013;14(1):69-76.

50. Centers for Disease Control and Prevention. Guidelines for field triage of injured patients: recommendations of the national expert panel on field triage 2011. *Morb Mortal Wkly Rep.* 2012;61:1-21.

51. Truhlar A, Deakin CD, Soar J, et al. European Resuscitation Council Guidelines for Resuscitation 2015. Section 4: cardiac arrest in special circumstances. *Resuscitation.* 2015;95:148-201.

52. American Heart Association. 2015 guidelines for cardiopulmonary resuscitation and emergency cardiovascular care. *Circulation.* 2015;132:S313-S314.

53. National Association of EMS Physicians and American College of Surgeons Committee on Trauma. NAEMSP position statement: withholding of resuscitation for adult traumatic cardiopulmonary arrest. *Prehosp Emerg Care.* 2013;17:291.

54. The National Association of EMS Physicians (NAEMSP) and the American College of Surgeons Committee on Trauma (ACS-COT). Termination of resuscitation for adult traumatic cardiopulmonary arrest. *Prehosp Emerg Care.* 2012;16(4):571.

55. U.S. Department of Health and Human Services. *What is the U.S. opioid epidemic?* Reviewed October 27, 2021. Accessed February 11, 2022. https://www.hhs.gov/opioids/about-the-epidemic/index.html

56. Alonso-Serra HM, Wesley K. Prehospital pain management. *Prehosp Emerg Care*. 2003;7(4):482-488. doi: 10.1080/312703002260

57. Morgan MM, Perina DG, Acquisto NM, et al. Ketamine use in prehospital and hospital treatment of the acute trauma patient: a joint position statement. *Prehosp Emerg Care*. 2021;25(4):588-592, doi: 10.1080/10903127.2020.1801920

58. Patterson DP, Higgins JS, Van Dongen HPA, et al. Evidence-based guidelines for fatigue risk management in emergency medical services. *Prehosp Emerg Care*. 2018;22(1):89-101.

Suggested Reading

Merchant RM, Topjian AA, Panchal AR, et al. Part 1: executive summary: 2020 American Heart Association guidelines for cardiopulmonary resuscitation and emergency cardiovascular care. *Circulation*. 2020;142:S337-S357.

기도와 환기

Lead Editors
Jean-Cyrille Pitteloud, MD
Jay Johannigman, MD, FACS, FCCM

© Ralf Hiemisch/Getty Images

학습 목표 이 장의 학습을 완료하면 다음과 같은 내용을 수행할 수 있다.

- 환기와 가스 교환의 원리를 통합할 수 있다.
- 외상성 손상이 환기와 산소 공급의 정상적인 과정을 손상시키는 방법을 수 있다.
- 산소 공급 및 환기 장애가 관류 및 외상성 쇼크의 진행에 미치는 영향을 명확히 설명할 수 있다.
- 외상이 분당호흡량과 산소 공급에 어떤 영향을 미치는지 이해할 수 있다.
- 환기와 산소 공급의 차치를 구별할 수 있다.
- 손상을 입은 환자에게 보충 산소 및 보조 환기가 도움이 될 수 있는 기전을 설명할 수 있다.
- 외상 환자와 관련된 시나리오를 제시하고 기도 개방을 제공하는 가장 효과적인 방법을 선택할 수 있다.
- 다양한 시나리오가 주어지면 기도 관리, 산소 공급 및 환기에 대한 적절한 대응 및 처치를 개발할 수 있다.
- 현재 연구의 새로운 계획을 인식하고 다양한 침습적 처치의 위험과 이점을 이해할 수 있다.
- 외상 환자에서 호기말이산화탄소(ETCO$_2$) 모니터링의 적응증과 한계에 대해 논의할 수 있다.

시나리오

당신은 혼잡한 도로에서 오토바이 충돌 사고가 발생했다는 신고를 받고 현장으로 출동한다. 현장에 도착했을 때 심하게 파손된 오토바이에서 약 15m 떨어진 곳에 환자가 누워있는 것을 보게 된다. 환자는 헬멧을 쓰고 있는 젊은 남성이다. 환자는 움직이지 않고 멀리서 보면 빠르게 숨을 쉬고 있는 것을 알 수 있다. 환자에게 다가가면서 머리 주위에 피가 고여 있고 코를 골며 목을 울리는 소리와 함께 호흡음이 시끄럽다는 것을 알 수 있다.

당신은 외상센터에서 15분 거리에 있으며 상황실에서 기상 악화로 인해 헬기 이송은 불가능하다고 알려준다.

- 이 환자에서 분명한 기도 손상의 지표로 무엇인가?
- 목격자나 응급의료반응자(EMR)로부터 어떤 다른 정보를 확인해야 하는가?
- 현장에서 초기 신속한 평가를 시행하는 동안 찾고 관찰해야 하는 산소 공급 및 환기를 악화시키는 중요한 징후와 증상은 무엇인가?
- 이송 전과 이송 중에 환자를 처치하기 위해 취할 조치의 순서를 설명한다.

개요

병원 도착 전 가장 중요한 두 가지 술기는 기도 개방과 가스 교환을 제공하고 유지하는 것이다. 기도를 적절하게 유지하고 적절한 산소 공급 및 환기를 제공하지 못하면 주요 중기가 빠르게 손상되어 돌이킬 수 없는 손상을 입을 수 있다. 기도 손상과 부적절한 산소 공급 및 환기를 인식하는 능력은 손상의 전반적인 부담을 최소화하는 데 중요한 단계이다. 정의의 목적으로 다음 사항을 고려할 수 있다.

- 산소공급은 흡기된 분자 산소가 폐포막을 통과해 헤모글로빈과 결합하여 신체 조직에 전달되는 과정을 말한다.
- 환기는 들숨과 날숨으로 인한 기체 교환 과정을 말한다.

유산소대사는 인체에서 가장 효율적인 에너지 전환 형태이다. 이 과정에서 산소는 연료 공급원이 세포 에너지로 전환되어 생명과 관련된 기관을 유지하는 데 중요한 요소이다.

호흡기의 두 가지 주요 기능은 다음과 같다.

1. 헤모글로빈이 흡수하여 세포로 운반할 수 있도록 산소를 전달한다. 신체에는 산소가 거의 없으므로 산소가 부족하면 몇 분 안에 세포 사멸로 이어질 수 있다.
2. 체내 대사 과정에서 생성된 이산화탄소를 제거한다. 환기가 불충분하면 이산화탄소가 축적되어 산증과 혼수상태로 이어진다.

호흡계가 적절하게 작동하려면 산소 공급과 환기가 모두 이루어져야 생명을 유지할 수 있다.

해부학

호흡계는 폐를 포함한 상기도와 하기도로 구성되어 있다(**그림 7-1**). 호흡계의 각 구성 요소는 가스 교환을 보장하는 데 중요한 역할을 한다.

상기도

상기도는 코안과 입안으로 구성되어 있다(**그림 7-2**). 상기도는 음식과 수분을 섭취하고 환기하는 이중 기능을 가지고 있다. 그런 이유로 상기도는 견고하지만, 정교한 해부학적 구조와 정교한 신경 공급을 하고 있다. 코안으로 들어오는 공기는 따뜻해지고 가습되며 여과된다. 입과 코안 너머에는 인두라고 알려진 부위가 있는데, 인두는 물렁입천장에서 식도의 상단까지 이어져 있다. 인두는 점막으로 둘러싸인 근육 구조이며 코인두(상부), 입인두(중간 부분), 후두인두(인두의

하부 또는 말단부)의 세 부분으로 나뉜다. 인두의 아래에는 위와 연결되는 식도와 하기도의 시작인 기관이 있다. 하인두와 기관의 교차점에는 후두(**그림 7-3**)가 있으며 후두에는 성대와 그 기능을 조정하는 근육이 있다. 후두는 튼튼한 연골에 의해 보호되고 성대는 기도로 돌출되어 소리를 내는 주름이다. 성대는 소리를 생성하고 수정하는 운동 범위와 기도를 흡인으로부터 보호하기 위해 정중선에서 만나는 기능을 가지고 있다. 가성대 또는 안뜰주름은 성대를 통해 공기의 흐름을 유도한다. 성대를 뒤에서 지지하는 것은 모뿔연골이다. 후두 바로 위에는 후두개라는 나뭇잎 모양의 구조물이 있다. 후두개는 공기를 기관으로 고체 및 액체를 식도로 보내는 입구 또는 플래퍼 밸브 역할을 한다.

하기도

하기도는 기관, 기관지 및 폐로 구성된다. 하기도의 기능은 기관, 기관지 및 세기관지 등의 여과 기능과 폐포에서 가스 교환을 위한 통로를 제공하는 것이다. 기관의 내벽은 섬세하고 공기 이외의 다른 물질에 매우 민감하다. 들숨 시 공기는 상기도를 거쳐 하기도로 이동한 후 실제 가스 교환이 일어나는 폐포에 도달한다.

기관은 오른쪽과 왼쪽 주기관지로 나뉜다. 오른쪽 주기관지는 왼쪽보다 더 짧고 굵으며 수직 방향이다. 오른쪽 주기관지는 기관에서 약 25도 각도로 나오지만, 왼쪽 주기관지는 45도 각을 이룬다. 이러한 해부학적 차이는 기관내관의 오른쪽 주기관지로 삽입되는 기관내삽관의 흔한 합병증이 발생하는 이유이다. 각각의 주기관지는 여러 개의 일차기관지와 이차기관지로 반복적으로 나뉘며 그 후 말단 세기관지로 끝난다. 세기관지(아주 작은 기관지)는 가스를 폐포 안팎으로 운반하는 역할을 한다. 폐포는 폐의 기능적 단위이며 혈액을 함유한 모세혈관으로 둘러싸인 작은 공기주머니로 구성되어 있다. 폐포는 호흡기와 순환기가 만나는 가스 교환 장소이다.

폐 조직은 수백만 개의 작은 풍선(폐포)이 들어 있는 스펀지에 비유할 수 있으며 각 폐포는 혈관이 가득한 얇은 벽으로 이루어져 있어 공기 교환이 일어날 수 있는 넓은 표면을 제공한다. 성인의 경우 폐포의 총 표면적은 약 100m²로 피부 표면적의 50배에 달한다. 폐에는 자체 근육이 없으며 오히려 가슴우리의 탄성 반동이 지속해서 팽창하여 폐포 공간을 팽창시킨다. 이러한 가슴 공간의 고유한 반동은 정상적인 사람의 폐가 절대 완전히 붕괴하지 않는 이유를 설명하는 데 도움이 된다. 정상적인 날숨이 끝날 때 폐에 남아있는 공기의 양을 기능잔기용량(FRC)이라고 한다. 이 용량은 일반적으로 성인의 경

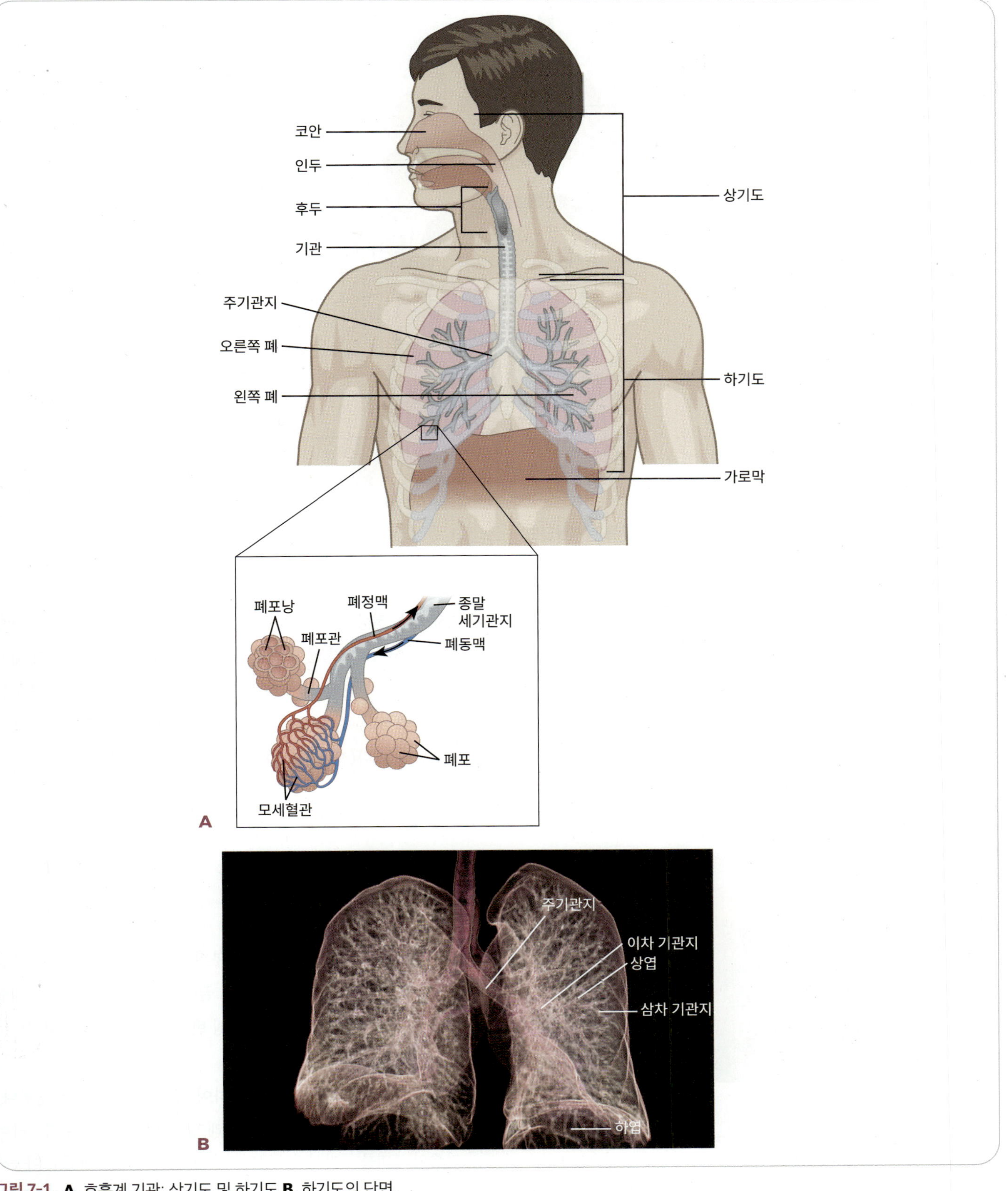

그림 7-1 **A.** 호흡계 기관: 상기도 및 하기도 **B.** 하기도의 단면.

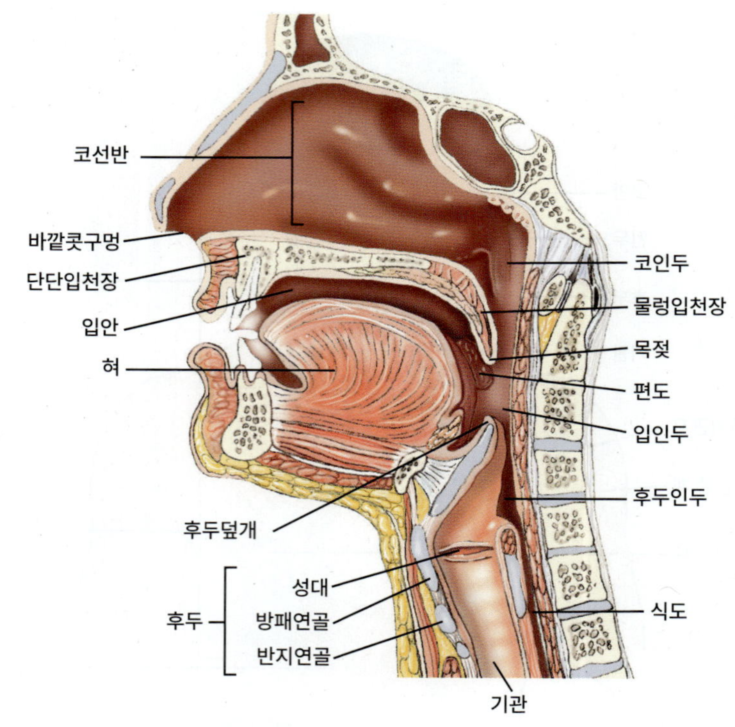

그림 7-2 코안과 인두를 통한 시상단면.
© National Association of Emergency Medical Technicians (NAEMT)

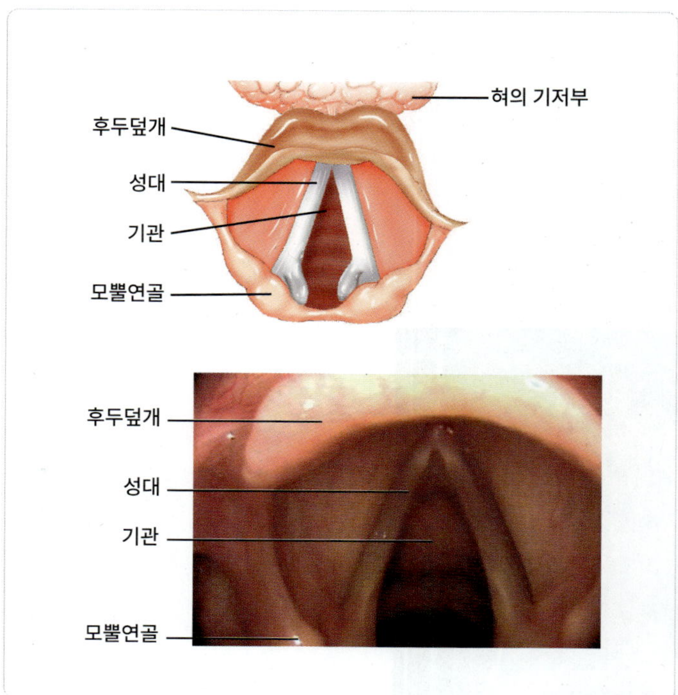

그림 7-3 위에서 본 성대는 후두와 후두개 연골의 쌍을 이루는 연골과의 관계를 보여준다. 상기도는 단단한 치아와 입안 근육으로 구성되어 있고 후두는 얇은 점막과 섬세한 연골을 포함한 더 섬세한 구조로 이루어져 있다. 후두 구조는 처치 중 손상에 더 취약하므로 이러한 탄력성의 차이가 중요하다.

A: © National Association of Emergency Medical Technicians (NAEMT); B: Courtesy of James P. Thomas, M.D., www.voicedoctor.net

우 2.5L이다. 정상적인 들숨 후에는 흉곽의 확장과 폐의 수축이 균형을 이루며 이 두 가지 균형 잡힌 구조물 사이의 가슴막 공간의 얇은 액체층의 표면 장력에 의해 억제된다. 폐에서 모든 공기를 배출하는 것은 불가능하다. 절대 강제 최대 날숨 후에도 폐에 여전히 약 1L의 공기가 남아 있다(잔기량; RV). 이 균형 잡힌 시스템은 호흡 주기 동안 산소와 이산화탄소 교환 과정을 수행할 수 있는 충분한 양의 기능적 폐포가 항상 존재하도록 보장한다.

생리학

정상적인 호흡 주기 동안 가슴안의 부피가 팽창하여 가슴안에 음압이 생성한다. 이 음압은 공기를 폐로 끌어당긴다. 반대로 숨을 내쉴 때는 가슴안의 탄성과 그에 폐의 탄성 반동이 공기가 외부 환경으로 이동하는 것을 촉진한다.

다음 세 가지 요소가 동시에 작동하여 가슴안의 부피를 확장한다.

• 가로막은 주사기의 플런저처럼 아래 방향으로 이동하여 작용하여 가슴의 부피를 증가시키고 음압차를 만들어 공기를 폐포로 이동시킨다(**그림 7-4A**). 가로막은 가로막신경(C3~C5)에 의해 활성화된다. 정상적이고 조용한 호흡 중에 가로막 움직임은 환기 작업을 수행하

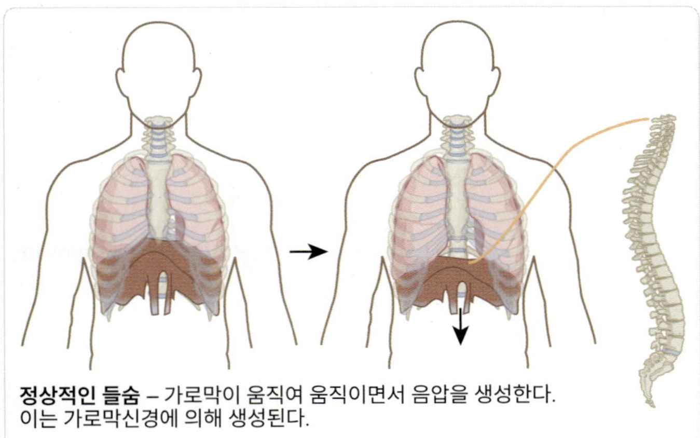

정상적인 들숨 – 가로막이 움직여 움직이면서 음압을 생성한다. 이는 가로막신경에 의해 생성된다.

A

증가한 들숨 – 갈비사이근은 갈비뼈를 바깥쪽으로 벌린다. 이는 갈비사이신경(D2~D10)에 의해 생성된다.

B

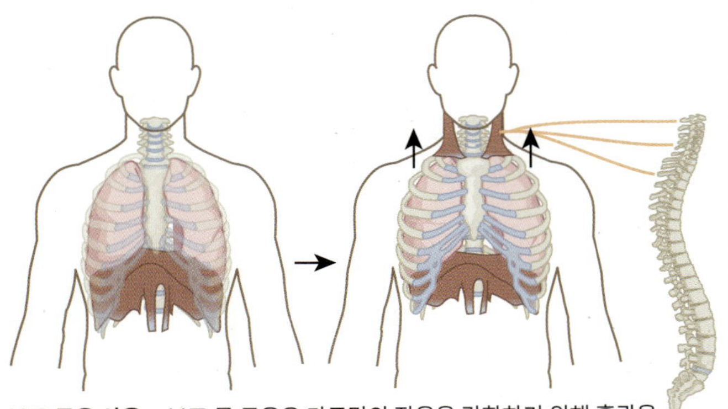

보조 근육 사용 – 보조 목 근육은 가로막의 작용을 강화하기 위해 흉곽을 위쪽으로 당긴다. 이 움직임은 목 신경근(C3~C6)에 의해 생성된다.

C

그림 7-4   **A.** 정상 들숨 **B.** 들숨 증가 **C.** 보조 근육 사육.
© National Association of Emergency Medical Technicians (NAEMT)

는 데 필요한 압력차를 생성한다.

- 산소 흡입량을 늘리거나 이산화탄소를 배출하거나 기도 저항 증가를 극복하기 위해 추가 호흡량이 필요한 경우 갈비뼈가 복장뼈 및 척추와의 관절에서 바깥쪽으로 활발하게 움직여 양동이 손잡이 모

표 7-1 호흡 역학		
	들숨	**날숨**
정상 호흡	가로막	수동적인
호흡 노력 증가	가로막 및 갈비사이근	갈비사이근
극심한 호흡 노력	가로막, 갈비사이근 그리고 보조근육	갈비사이근 복근

© National Association of Emergency Medical Technicians (NAEMT)

양을 형성하여 가슴의 부피를 확장된다(**그림 7-4B**). 이 호흡 단계에서는 가슴벽의 움직임이 더 잘 보인다.

- 추가 일회호흡량이 필요하면 목 근육(즉, 목빗근)이 작동하여 흉곽이 위쪽으로 확장되고 가슴안의 부피를 더욱 확장한다(**그림 7-4C**). 이러한 호흡 보조 근육은 목뼈 C2~C7 뿌리에 의해 신경이 분포된다.

- 정상적인 날숨은 가슴우리의 수동적인 탄성의 결과로 발생한다. 더 빠른 날숨 과정이 필요한 경우 갈비사이근과 복근을 동원하여 날숨 과정을 능동적으로 강화할 수 있다(**표 7-1**).

들숨과 날숨을 촉진하기 위한 압력 변화가 발생하려면 가슴벽이 손상되지 않아야 한다. 가슴벽이 손상되거나 손상되면 적절한 환기를 촉진하는 데 필요한 압력차를 생성하는 환자의 능력이 저하될 수 있다. 정상적으로 손상되지 않은 가슴안에 상처가 생기면 대기와 흉강 사이에 공기가 유입되는 대체 통로가 생긴다. 이 구멍이 뚫리면 공기가 가슴안으로 유입되지만, 폐포 영역 외부로 유입될 수 있다. 이러한 가슴안으로의 대체 경로는 기흉이 생성될 수 있는 기전 중 하나이다(10장 가슴 외상 참조).

폐포 내에 공기가 존재하면 모세혈관-폐포 경계면을 가로질러 혈관 공간으로 이동하여 적혈구와 헤모글로빈과 접촉하는 것이 촉진된다. 산소는 헤모글로빈 분자의 산소 결합 부위를 채운다(산소공급 전에는 산소 결합 부위 4개 중 3개[75%], 산소 공급 후에는 4개 중 4개[98~100%], **그림 7-5A**). 동시에 세포 대사의 부산물로 생성된 이산화탄소는 폐포 모세혈관 경계면으로 전달되어 반대 방향(혈류에서 폐포로)으로 이동한다. 혈장에 녹아있거나(약 10%) 단백질(주로 적혈구의 헤모글로빈[약 20%])에 결합하여 있거나 탄산수소염(약 70%) 형태로 운반되는 이산화탄소는 혈류에서 폐포모세혈관막을 통과하여 폐포로 이동하여 날숨 동안 제거된다(**그림 7-5B**). 이 가스 교환이 완료되면 산소가 공급된 적혈구와 이산화탄소 농도가 낮은 혈장은 심장

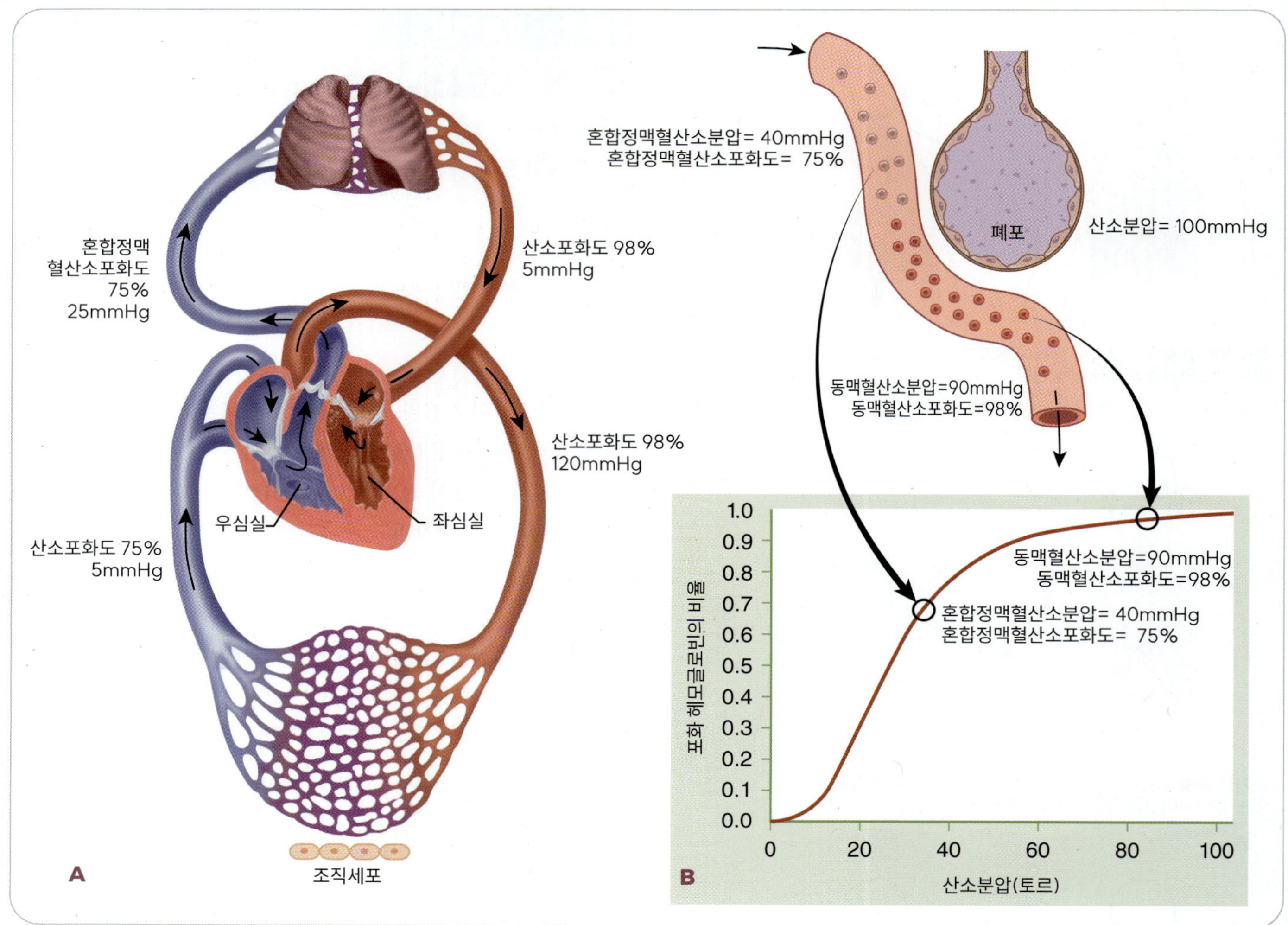

그림 7-5　**A.** 정맥혈은 저압 정맥계(심장에 들어가기 직전에 대정맥 내 5mmHg)를 통해 심장 쪽으로 끌어당겨지고 우심장에서 폐로 펌핑된다(우심실에서 나온 후 25mmHg). 산소는 폐포에서 적혈구로 흡수되고 혈장에 용해된 이산화탄소는 폐로 배출된다. 그런 다음 완전히 산소가 공급된 혈액은 고압 동맥 시스템을 통해 신체 조직으로 펌핑된다. **B.** 적혈구가 폐를 통과하면서 헤모글로빈 분자에 결합하는 산소 분자에 노출되어 헤모글로빈 분자의 산소 결합 부위가 점점 더 채워지고(산소포화도 증가) 혈액 내 산소 분압이 점차 증가하게 된다.

의 왼쪽으로 되돌아와 신체의 모든 세포로 뿜어져 나온다.

환기는 어떻게 조절되는가?

환기는 동맥혈의 pH에 따라 뇌줄기에 의해 조절된다. 산소와 포도당은 에너지와 이산화탄소를 생성한다. 이산화탄소는 약산성(pH=6.3)인 탄산수소염(HCO_3^-)으로 혈액에 용해되어 동맥혈을 더 산성으로 만든다. 혈중 이산화탄소분압이 상승하면 이산화탄소가 뇌척수액으로 확산한다. 이것은 뇌척수액에서 H^+ 이온이 방출되어 중뇌의 화학수용체 중추를 자극하여 호흡 속도와 일회호흡량을 증가시켜 더 많은 이산화탄소를 배출하게 된다. 목동맥체에 있는 말초 화학수용체도 동맥혈 이산화탄소분압에 반응하지만, 이는 환기 반응의 20% 미만을 차지한다. 혈중 pH는 산소 농도보다 호흡을 훨씬 더 강력하게 자극하며 이는 현저한 저산소혈증에 직면했을 때만 호흡을 자극하기 시작한다. 이는 처음에는 비논리적으로 보일 수 있지만, 뇌가 산소 부족에 반응하는 것이 아니라 산소 소비에 능동적으로 반응할 수 있도록 한다.

사강

폐포는 가스 교환이 일어나는 얇은 막에 의해서만 폐포 공기와 분리되는 매우 얇은 모세혈관으로 채워져 있다. 폐에 도달하기 전에 공기는 먼저 가스 교환에 관여하지 않는 입, 인두와 기관지를 통과한다. 그 결과 성인의 경우 약 150mL의 부피가 공기 교환이 일어나지 않는 사강이라고 불리는 공간으로 남게 된다. 이것은 호흡마다 마지막 150mL의 공기가 실제로 폐포에 도달하지 않는다는 것을 의미한다. 이는 정상적인 호흡 중에는 문제가 되지 않지만, 환기가 손상되면 더 심각해질 수 있다. 들숨량이 많을수록 사강 부피도 증가한다.

폐포는 적절한 양의 산소가 포함된 신선한 공기가 지속해서 공급되어야 한다. 환기라고 하는 이러한 공기 보충은 이산화탄소를 제거에도 필수적이다. 환기는 측정할 수 있다. 일회호흡량에 분당 환기수를 곱하여 분당 호흡량을 구할 수 있다.

분당 호흡량 = 일회호흡량 × 분당 환기수

정상적인 휴식 시 환기 중에는 약 500mL의 공기가 폐로 흡입된다. 앞에서 언급했듯이 이 중 일부인 150mL는 기관과 기관지의 사강으로 남아 있으며 가스 교환에 참여하지 않는다. 폐포에서 가스 교환에 사용할 수 있는 것은 350mL에 불과하다. 일회호흡량이 500mL이고 환기 속도가 분당 14회인 경우 분당 호흡량은 다음과 같이 계산할 수 있다.

분당 호흡량 = 500mL × 14회/분 = 7,000mL/분 또는 7L/분

그러나 사강을 고려하면 분당 4.9L만이 폐포와 만나 가스 교환에 참여한다는 것이 분명해진다. 즉,

500mL - 150mL = 350mL

350mL × 14회/분 = 4,900mL/분 또는 4.9L/분

이 두 번째 계산은 총 분당 환기량에서 사강 환기량을 뺀 유효환기량을 파악한다.

분당 호흡량이 증가한 수요를 충족시키지 못하면 환기가 불충분한 상태가 되는데, 이를 저환기라고 한다. 저환기는 폐포 내 산소 공급이 감소하고 폐포와 체내에 이산화탄소가 축적되는 것을 초래한다. 저환기는 머리 또는 가슴 외상으로 인해 호흡 패턴이 바뀌거나 가슴벽을 적절히 움직일 수 없을 때 흔히 발생한다.

예를 들어, 갈비뼈 골절 환자가 골절로 인한 통증으로 빠르고 얕게 호흡하는 경우 일회호흡량 200mL이고 환기 속도는 분당 30회일 수 있다. 이 환자의 분당 호흡량은 다음과 같이 계산할 수 있다.

분당 호흡량 = 200mL × 30회/분 = 6,000mL/분 또는 6L/분

손상을 입지 않은 사람이 휴식 중일 때 적절한 가스 교환을 위해 분당 7L가 필요한 경우, 신체가 충분한 산소를 흡수하고 이산화탄소를 효과적으로 제거하는 데 필요한 분당 6L보다 적으므로 폐의 산소 농도가 감소하고 이산화탄소가 축적되기 시작한다. 또한 효과적인 분당환기량을 계산하면 환자 상태의 실제 심각도를 알 수 있다.

200mL - 150mL = 50mL

50mL × 30회/분 = 1,500mL/분 또는 1.5L/분

이 단계에서는 산소가 공급된 공기가 폐포에 거의 도달하지 못하고 대부분의 공기는 기관과 기관지까지만 도달한다. 이러한 저환기를 처치하지 않고 방치하면 심각한 저산소혈증, 산증, 다발성 장기부전 그리고 궁극적으로 사망으로 이어질 수 있다(**그림 7-6**).

앞의 예에서 갈비뼈 골절 환자는 호흡수가 분당 30회인데도 저환기 상태임을 알 수 있다. 따라서 호흡수 자체만으로는 환기의 적절성을 정확하게 설명할 수 없다. 병원 전 처치 제공자는 일회호흡량을 고려해야 하며 단순히 호흡수가 정상이거나 빠르다고 해서 환기가 적절하게 이루어지고 있다고 가정해서는 안 된다.

환기 기능 평가에는 항상 환자가 조직 세포에 산소를 얼마나 잘 흡수하고 확산 및 전달하고 있는지에 대한 평가가 포함된다. 산소를 제대로 흡입하지 못하면 조직 세포에 산소를 전달하고 세포 내에서 산소를 처리하여 유산소대사와 에너지 생산을 유지하는 데 장애가 생긴다. 이를 바로잡지 않으면 세포 대사가 무산소대사로 전환된다.

산소 공급 경로

이산화탄소는 혈장 내 매우 잘 용해되지만, 혈장 내 산소 용해도는 매우 제한적이다. 그러므로 산소는 적혈구 내의 헤모글로빈에 의해 운반되어야 한다. 각 헤모글로빈 분자에는 4개의 산소 결합 부위가 있다. 헤모글로빈의 산소 친화력은 산소의 기체 분압에 따라 달라진다. 산소가 풍부한 폐의 환경에서 각 산소 결합 부위가 개별 산소 분자에 결합한다. 산소 압력이 훨씬 낮은 조직에서는 헤모글로빈 분자의 형태가 변화하여 헤모글로빈 분자로부터 조직으로 산소가 방출된다.

혈장 내에서 산소가 용해되는 능력은 매우 제한적이다. 그러므로 세포 조직으로의 산소 전달 대부분은 적혈구 내 헤모글로빈 분자의 포화도에 의해 결정된다.

산소 공급의 세 단계는 외호흡, 산소 전달 및 내호흡이다. 적절한 산소 공급은 다음 세 단계에 따라 달라진다.

1. 외호흡은 산소 분자가 공기에서 혈액으로 이동하거나 확산하는

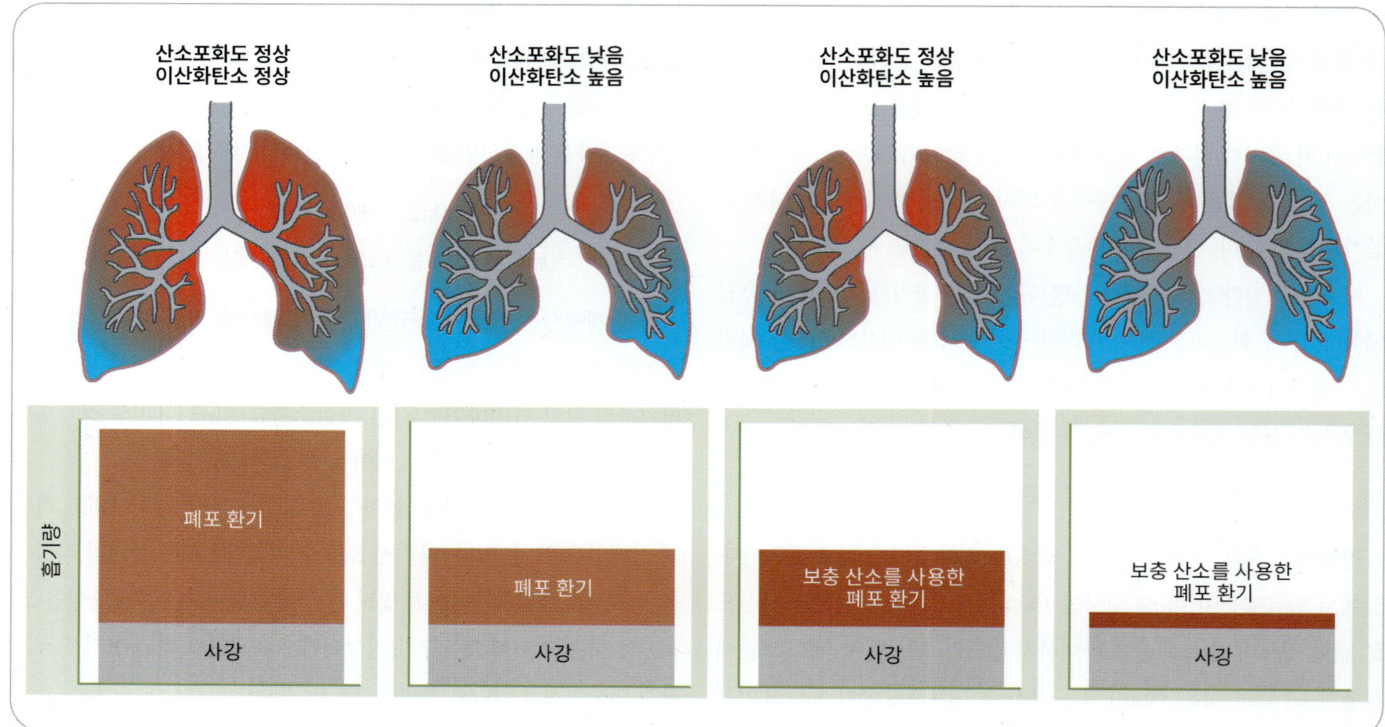

그림 7-6 흡기량이 점차 감소함에 따라 헤모글로빈 분자의 산소포화도를 충분히 유지하는 능력이 감소하고 폐에서 이산화탄소를 적절하게 제거하는 능력이 손상된다.

© National Association of Emergency Medical Technicians (NAEMT)

것을 말한다. 공기는 산소(20.95%), 질소(78.1%), 아르곤(0.93%) 및 이산화탄소(0.031%)가 포함되어 있지만, 실제로 공기의 함량은 산소 21%와 질소 79%이다. 모든 폐포 산소는 자유 기체로 존재하므로 각 산소 분자는 압력을 가한다. 흡입 공기 중 산소 비율을 높이면 폐포 산소 압력 또는 장력이 증가한다. 보충 산소를 공급하면 숨을 들이쉴 때마다 산소 비율이 증가하여 각 폐포의 산소량이 증가한다. 액체에 들어가는 가스의 양은 액체가 가하는 압력과 직접적인 관련이 있으므로 혈액으로 전달되는 기체의 양이 증가한다. 기체의 분압이 클수록 순환계의 체액(혈장) 성분으로 흡수되는 기체의 양이 많아진다.

2. 산소 전달은 산소를 최종 사용 지점(세포)에 공급하는 과정이다. 산소 전달은 심박출량, 헤모글로빈 및 산소포화도라는 세 가지 주요 구성 요소에 따라 달라진다. 산소포화도는 다음 공식으로 계산할 수 있다[$CO \times CaO_2$ ($CaO_2 = 1.31 \times Hgb \times O_2$ Sat)].

3. 내호흡은 적혈구에서 세포의 미토콘드리아로 산소가 이동하여 산소가 주요 산화제로 활용되는 것을 말한다. 세포 활동에 연료를 공급하기 위해 에너지를 방출하는 여러 가지 이화반응이 있는데 주로 해당 과정과 트라이카복실산(TCA) 회로(크렙스 회로는 시트르산 회로라고도 함)가 있다. 이러한 과정의 구체적인 세부 사항을 이해할 필요는 없지만, 에너지 생산에서 산소의 역할에 대해 전반적으로 이해하는 것이 중요하다.

병태생리학

외상은 여러 가지 방식으로 산소를 적절하게 공급하고 이산화탄소를 제거하는 호흡계의 능력에 영향을 미칠 수 있다. 임상 조건에는 저산소증의 여러 원인이 있을 수 있다. 일부 겹치는 부분이 있지만, 저산소혈증과 저산소증이라는 용어는 동의어가 아니다. 저산소혈증은 혈중 산소 분압이 감소하는 것을 말하며 저산소증은 조직의 산소화 감소로 정의된다.

저산소혈증의 원인과 외상성 원인의 예는 다음과 같다.

- 주변 환경 또는 들숨 산소 분압 감소
  - 고지대에서의 외상 또는 환자를 항공으로 이송하는 경우

- 저환기
  - 기도 폐쇄
  - 중독 또는 머리 손상과 같은 호흡 충동 감소
  - 상부 목 척수 손상과 같은 마비
  - 갈비뼈 골절 등으로 인한 통증
- 환기 관류 불일치: V/Q 불일치는 환기(V)와 관류(Q) 사이의 불균형을 의미하며 일반적으로 저산소혈증은 폐포 산소 수치 감소로 인해 V/Q 상태가 낮을 때 나타난다. 저산소혈증은 V/Q 비율이 높거나 폐가 환기되지만, 관류되지 않는 "생리학적 사강" 상황에서도 볼 수 있다. 단락은 폐에 관류는 되지만, 환기되지 않는 낮은 V/Q 불일치의 또 다른 극단적인 상황이다.
  - 낮은 V/Q 및 션트
    - 폐 타박상과 같은 폐 조직 손상
    - 흡인, 무기폐 또는 폐허탈과 같은 폐호흡 불량
  - 높은 V/Q 또는 생리학적 사강
    - 폐색전증
    - 쇼크
- 확산 이상(모세혈관-폐포막을 통과하는 가스 수송 장애)
  - 폐부종
  - 심각한 빈혈(산소 흡수 능력 감소로 인한)

조직 저산소증은 저산소혈증을 완화할 수 있는 충분한 보상적 심박출량 증가가 없는 한 모든 저산소혈증으로 인해 발생할 수 있다. 또한 저산소혈증이 없는 경우에도 세포나 조직이 정상적으로 산소를 이용할 수 없는 경우 저산소증이 발생할 수 있다.

- 시안화물 중독과 같이 이 과정을 손상하는 독소 또는 독극물로 인해 산소 이용률이 감소한다.

외상 환자의 기도 폐쇄 원인 및 부위

상기도의 기계적 폐쇄의 가장 흔한 원인은 혀가 뒤로 넘어가서 하인두를 막는 것이다(**그림 7-7A**). 혀는 상기도 보호 반사를 변화시키거나(중독이 일반적인 예) 혀가 후방으로 이동하여 하인두를 폐쇄할 수 있는 기계적 상황을 만드는 모든 과정(아래턱뼈 골절이 일반적인 예)에서 방해물이 될 수 있다. 혀가 하인두 높이에서 기도를 폐쇄하는 것은 코골이와 울려 퍼지는 소리뿐만 아니라 비정상적인 가슴 움직임이 특징적으로 나타난다. 외상 환자의 경우 이러한 폐쇄는 종종 상기도에 축적된 혈액과 분비물로 인해 더욱 복잡해진다. 외상 환자의 경우 이러한 상태를 턱밀어올리기 또는 턱들기와 같은 간단한 기

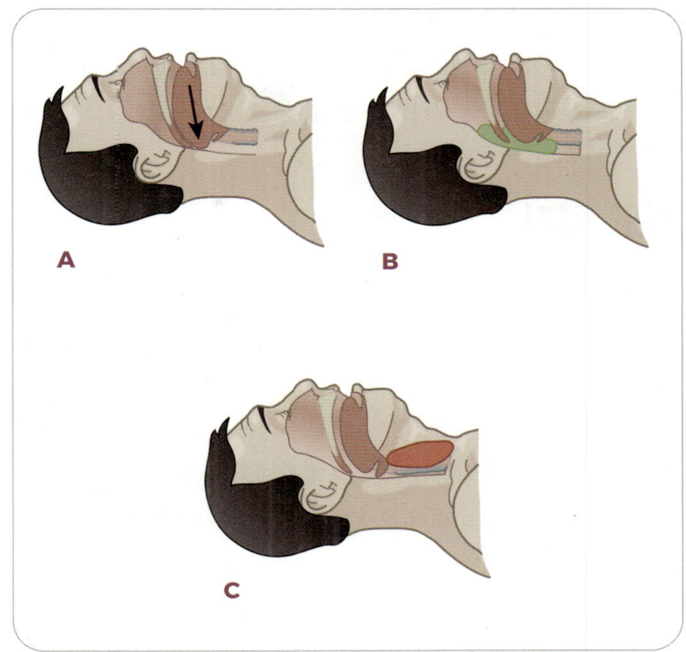

그림 7-7 상기도 폐쇄의 일반적인 원인. **A.** 혀가 기도를 막는 경우 **B.** 구토물, 혈액 또는 기타 분비물 **C.** 후두에 대한 직접적인 외상 또는 흡입 손상.
© National Association of Emergency Medical Technicians (NAEMT)

도 조작을 통해 교정할 수 있다.

상기도 폐쇄의 또 다른 일반적인 원인은 환자의 의식 수준 저하 또는 광범위한 외상으로 인해 환자가 스스로 기도를 유지할 수 없을 때마다 분비물, 혈액 및 이물질이 하인두에 축적되는 것이다(**그림 7-7B**). 그렁거리는 호흡음은 기도 내 분비물이나 이물질을 제거할 수 없다는 확실한 신호이며 다음 호흡 시 흡인 위험 및 기도 폐쇄가 발생할 수 있다. 이 상태는 환자를 옆으로 눕히거나 상기도를 흡인하여 적어도 일시적으로 교정할 수 있다.

상기도 폐쇄의 세 번째로 흔한 부위는 후두이며 후두연골에 대한 직접적인 외상이나 점막이 부어오르는 흡입 화상에 의해 폐쇄가 발생할 수 있다(**그림 7-7C**). 이 상태는 쉰 목소리와 협착음이 나타날 수 있으며 교정하기가 훨씬 더 복잡하다.

상기도가 부분적으로 막히면 저항을 극복하고 적절한 일회호흡량을 유지하기 위해 들숨 근육의 노력이 증가해야 한다. 이것은 종종 시끄러운 들숨으로 이어진다. 환자가 이러한 추가적인 노력을 제공할 수 없는 경우 일회호흡량이 감소하고 호흡이 완전히 멈추기도 한다. 이는 특히 어린이에게 흔하다. 가장 좋은 처치는 환자의 기도를 도수로 개방하고 회복 자세와 같은 보조 자세를 취하거나 환자가 앉아서 앞으로 몸을 기울이도록 하는 것이다. 가슴벽 또는 척수 손상으로

인해 들숨 노력이 제한되는 환자의 경우 기도를 개방하면 환자가 더 효율적으로 호흡하는 데 도움이 될 수 있다. 보충 산소를 공급한다고 해서 기도가 막힌 것을 보완할 수는 없다.

기도 평가

기도를 평가하는 능력은 기도를 효과적으로 관리하기 위한 전제 조건이다. 병원 전 처치 제공자는 기도 평가의 여러 측면을 자동으로 수행한다. 의식이 명료하고 정상적인 목소리로 말하는 외상 환자는 기도가 개방되어 있을 가능성이 높다. 이러한 상황에서 철저한 체계적인 평가는 여전히 임박한 기도 문제를 파악하는 데 도움이 될 수 있다(**그림 7-8**). 환자의 의식 상태가 감소하면 우선순위가 낮은 다른 손상을 평가하거나 처치하기 전에 기도를 철저히 평가하는 것이 훨씬 더 중요하다. 일차평가의 일부로 다음을 수행해야 한다.

- 기도 개방 여부를 평가한다.
- 입안에 액체나 고형물이 있는지 확인한다.
- 아래턱과 목 앞부분의 변형이나 부기가 있는지 확인한다.

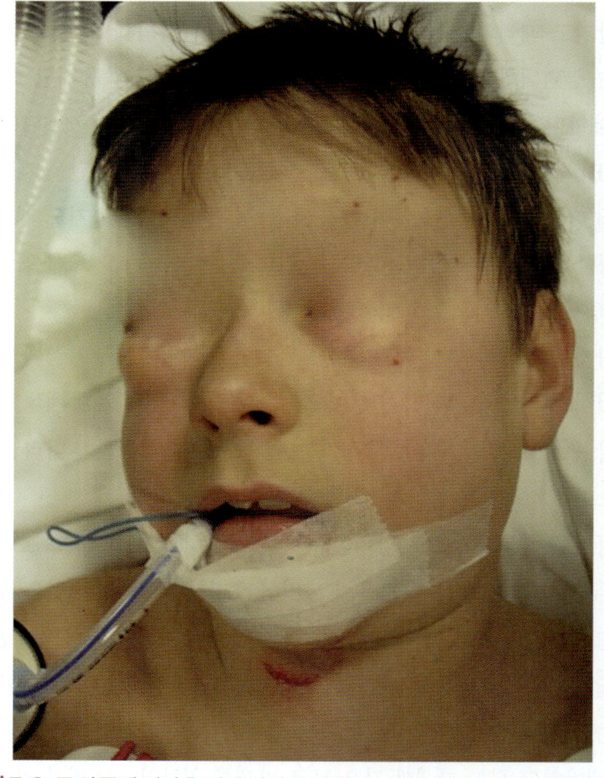

그림 7-8 목 앞쪽에 외상을 입어 기관이 파열되고 목과 얼굴에 피부밑기종이 발생한 환자이다. 목을 보지 않고 환자의 입안만 보면 중요한 정보를 놓칠 수 있다.
Courtesy of J.C. Pitteloud MD, Switzerland.

- 비정상적인 소리가 들리는지 들어본다.
- 비정상적인 가슴 움직임/뒤당김이 있는지 확인한다.

기도와 환자의 자세

환자와 시각적으로 접촉할 때 환자의 자세를 관찰하는 것이 중요하다. 의식 상태가 감소한 바로누운자세의 환자는 혀가 입안으로 밀려 들어가 기도 폐쇄의 위험이 있다. 의식 상태가 감소한 대부분의 외상 환자는 척추 움직임 제한을 위해 긴척추고정판이나 진공부목에 바로 누운자세로 고정하기 때문에 의식 상태가 감소한 징후를 보이는 모든 환자는 기도 폐쇄 여부를 지속해서 재평가해야 하며 기도 개방을 위해 보조기도기 삽입이 필요할 수 있다. 옆으로 누운 상태에서 기도가 개방된 환자는 바로누운자세로 눕힐 때 기도가 막힐 수 있다.

심한 얼굴 외상과 출혈이 심한 환자는 자세가 중요한 고려 사항이다. 이러한 환자는 스스로 기도를 유지하고 있는 경우 발견 당시의 자세를 유지해야 할 수 있다. 기도가 유지되고 있다면 환자를 똑바로 앉혀야 하는 예도 있다. 이러한 환자를 비스듬히 눕히거나 똑바로 눕히면 기도가 막히고 혈액이 흡인될 수 있다. 환자가 스스로 기도를 유지하고 있다면 환자가 생존할 수 있었던 자세를 유지하도록 하는 것이 최선의 조치일 수 있다. 필요한 경우 혈액과 분비물을 제거하기 위해 흡인을 시행할 수 있어야 한다. 또한 기도를 개방하는 데 필요한 자세로 머리를 도수로 고정하여 목뼈를 고정할 수 있다. 등허리 척추의 안정화는 바로 선 자세에서 시행하기가 더 어렵지만, 등허리 척추의 보호 강화와 바로 선 자세로 발견된 환자의 기도 개방을 유지할 수 없는 상황 중 하나를 선택해야 하는 경우 환자의 기도를 개방하고 유지하는 것을 우선시해야 한다. 이 개념은 부분적으로 바로 선 자세의 환자에게 적용된다는 점을 기억한다. 그렇다고 해서 바로누운자세로 발견된 환자를 바로 선 자세로 옮기는 것이 반드시 안전하다는 것을 의미하지는 않는다. 이렇게 하면 등허리 척추의 불안정한 골절이 변위될 위험이 있다.

상기도 소리

상기도에서 나오는 정상 이외의 비정상적인 소리는 기도 폐쇄 또는 호흡 곤란의 징후일 수 있다. 이러한 비정상적인 소리는 환자에게 다가갈 때 종종 들릴 수 있다. 일반적으로 상기도의 혀, 혈액 또는 이물질로 인한 부분적인 기도 폐쇄의 결과이다.

들리는 소리의 유형은 상기도 폐쇄의 원인과 위치에 대한 단서를 제공할 수 있다. 코골이는 혀의 기저부와 물렁입천장이 뒤로 넘어가 상기도를 막기 때문에 발생한다. 목을 울리는 소리는 인두에 혈액, 구토물 또는 분비물이 있을 때 발생하며 이는 환자가 스스로 기도를 깨끗하게 유지하거나 보호할 수 없다는 신호이다. 협착음은 성대 수준에서 좁아지는 데서 비롯된다. 이것은 숨을 들이마시거나 내쉴 때 들리는 소리이다. 협착음은 일반적으로 흡입 화상처럼 직접적인 외상, 이물질 또는 점막 부기로 인해 발생한다. 부기는 상기도의 가장 좁은 지점에서 발생하고 기도 전체가 막히는 것을 방지하기 위해 신속한 조치가 필요하므로 어려운 상황이다. 기도 폐쇄를 완화하고 기도를 개방하고 유지하는 조치를 즉시 취해야 한다.

기도 폐쇄 여부 평가

상기도는 코끝에서 복장뼈파임까지 이어져 있으므로 단순히 입안을 들여다보는 것만으로는 충분하지 않다. 입안에서 구토물, 혈액, 조직 파편 등 명백한 이물질이나 혈종, 부기와 같은 심각한 해부학적 변형이 있는지 확인한 다음 목 앞쪽을 따라 복장뼈파임까지 확인한다(그림 7-7 및 그림 7-8 참조). 특히 위험한 기도 폐쇄가 목 앞에서 발생하므로 기도에 대한 철저한 평가가 중요하다. 이물질이 발견되면 즉시 제거한다.

가슴 상승 및 뒤당김(수축) 확인

가슴이 제한적으로 상승하는 것은 기도가 막혔다는 징후일 수 있다. 가슴우리 수축, 보조 호흡근 사용 또는 호흡 노력의 향상과 같은 추가 징후가 나타나면 기도 손상을 의심해야 한다.

　환자가 부분적으로 막힌 기도를 통과하여 공기를 이동시키기 위해 열심히 노력하면 가슴 내에 더 큰 가슴 내 음압이 발생하게 된다. 그 결과 가슴벽과 갈비사이공간의 연부조직이 안쪽으로 당겨지고 들숨 노력으로 근육과 연부조직이 가슴으로 당겨지면서 갈비뼈 사이와 복장뼈파임에 뒤당김이 생긴다. 이러한 뒤당김은 특히 어린이에게서 잘 나타난다. 뒤당김이 있으면 환자가 호흡 곤란을 겪고 있음을 나타내므로 적극적으로 기도 폐쇄를 찾아 완화해야 한다.

　심한 부분 기도 폐쇄의 경우 "시소 호흡" 또는 "흔들리는 보트 호흡"이 발생할 수 있다. 환자가 폐쇄된 기도를 통해 숨을 쉬려고 하면 가로막이 아래로 내려가면서 복부가 올라가고(정상적인 들숨 시) 가슴이 내려간다(정상이 아님). 가로막이 이완되면 그 반대의 현상이 발생한다. 이러한 호흡 패턴을 관찰하는 병원 전 처치 제공자는 기도 폐쇄를 의심하고 적극적으로 이물질을 제거해야 한다.

처치

기도 관리

심각한 출혈을 조절한 후에는 기도를 확보하는 것이 외상 처치와 소생술의 다음 우선순위이다. 외상 환자의 기도는 공기가 들어올 수 있도록 개방되어 있어야 하며 부기로 인한 폐쇄와 흡인으로부터 보호되어야 하는 것이 이상적이다. 그러나 기도를 개방하고 유지하는 것이 최우선이며 대부분은 병원 전 처치 제공자의 장갑 낀 손 이외의 다른 장비 없이도 신속하게 기도를 개방할 수 있다. 기도 관리 방법과 관계없이 손상 기전이 목뼈 손상의 가능성을 시사하고 환자의 의식상태 또는 기타 요인으로 목뼈 손상의 존재를 확실히 배제할 수 없는 경우 목뼈 손상을 고려해야 한다. 위에서 설명한 기도 유지 방법을 사용하려면 환자가 완전히 고정될 때까지 목뼈를 중립 자세에서 도수로 동시에 고정해야 한다. 이 규칙에 대한 예외는 관통성 목 외상이다. 데이터에 따르면 이러한 환자에게 척추 고정이 필요하지 않으며 시간적 관점에서 해로울 수 있기 때문이다(10장 척추 외상 참조).

필수 술기

외상 환자의 기도 관리는 비교적 간단한 것부터 까다로운 것까지 다양할 수 있지만, 대부분 환자에서 초기 처치 단계에서 도수 또는 간단한 술기만으로도 충분하다. 모든 병원 전 처치 제공자는 교육 수준과 관계없이 이러한 간단하고 필수적인 도수 술기를 수행할 수 있는 능력을 유지해야 한다. 임상 상황에 따라 대부분 기도 문제는 간단한 방법으로 해결되지만, 폐쇄가 완화되지 않으면 더 복잡한 문제로 진행된다. 도수 및 간단한 술기는 시간, 인력 및 장비가 더 많이 필요하고 실패 위험이 높으며 부적절하게 사용할 때 손상을 입힐 수 있는 복잡한 술기보다 더 나은 환자의 처치 결과를 가져오는 경우가 많다. 병원 전 처치 제공자는 항상 침습적이고 복잡한 술기를 수행할 때의 위험과 이점을 비교해야 한다. 전문적인 술기는 고도의 숙련도와 의료 지도 의사의 면밀한 지도가 필요하다. 불필요하게 사용해서는 안 된다.

　기도 유지 술기는 도수, 단순, 전문 및 결정적인 처치 방법으로 나눌 수 있다. 이러한 술기의 적용, 병원 전 처치 제공자의 업무 범위에 포함되는 경우 현장 상황과 환자의 중증도에 따라 환자 중심으로 이루어져야 한다.

도수 기도 개방

기도 관리의 첫 번째 단계는 입인두 안을 빠르게 눈으로 확인하는 것이다. 외상 환자의 입안에는 이물질(예; 음식물), 부러진 치아 또는 틀니, 혈액이 있을 수 있다. 이러한 이물질은 장갑을 낀 손가락으로 입안을 쓸어내거나 흡인하여 제거해야 한다. 그런 다음 물림 보호대나 입인두기도기는 상부 기도 확보에 유용한 보도 도구가 될 수 있다. 또한 환자를 옆으로 눕히거나 척추 외상의 가능성이 없는 경우 앉은 자세를 취해주면 중력을 이용해 분비물, 혈액, 구토물을 제거할 수 있으며, 특히 양이 많은 경우 더 효과적이다. 척추 외상이 의심되는 경우 환자를 통나무굴리기법으로 측면으로 눕혀 혈액과 구토물을 제거할 수 있도록 한다.

간단한 도수 조작

반응이 없는 환자의 경우 혀가 이완되어 뒤로 떨어지면서 하인두가 막게 된다. 이것이 기도 폐쇄의 가장 흔한 원인이다. 혀가 아래턱뼈에 부착되어 앞으로 움직이기 때문에 이러한 유형의 폐쇄를 제거하는 도수 방법은 쉽게 수행할 수 있다. 아래턱뼈를 앞으로 움직이는 동작을 하면 혀가 하인두 뒤쪽에서 멀어진다.

- 외상 턱밀어올리기. 머리, 목 또는 얼굴 외상이 의심되는 환자의 경우 목뼈를 중립 자세로 유지한다. 외상 환자에게 턱밀어올리기를 시행하면 병원 전 처지 제공자는 머리와 목뼈를 거의 또는 전혀 움직이지 않고 기도를 개방할 수 있다(**그림 7-9A**). 엄지손가락을 각 광대뼈에 대고 집게손가락과 긴 손가락을 아래턱뼈에 대고 같은 각도로 아래턱뼈를 앞으로 밀면서 밀어 올린다. 이 술기는 한 명의 병원 전 처치 제공자가 환자의 머리 위쪽 또는 옆쪽에서 적용할 수 있다. 한 명의 병원 전 처치 제공자가 기도를 확보하고 목뼈를 중립 자세로 유지할 수 있으므로 일체형 술기이다.
- 외상 턱들기. 첫 번째 병원 전 처치 제공자가 머리를 잡고 목뼈의 정렬을 유지하는 동안 두 번째 병원 전 처치 제공자는 턱을 잡고 입을 벌린 다음 턱을 앞으로 당긴다(**그림 7-9B**). 외상 환자에게 턱들기 방법을 안전하게 시행하려면 두 명의 처치 제공자가 필요하다. 처치 제공자가 엄지손가락을 환자의 입에 넣는 이전 방법은 환자가 처치 제공자의 엄지손가락을 깨물 수 있으므로 위험하다.

두 술기 모두 아래턱뼈의 앞쪽(위쪽)과 약간 발 쪽으로 움직여 혀를 앞으로 당겨 기도 뒤쪽에서 멀어지게 하고 입을 벌리게 한다. 외상 턱밀어올리기 방법은 아래턱뼈를 앞으로 밀어내지만, 외상 턱들기

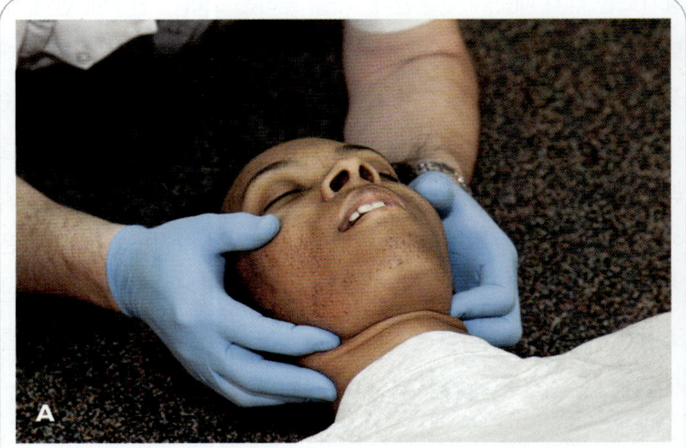

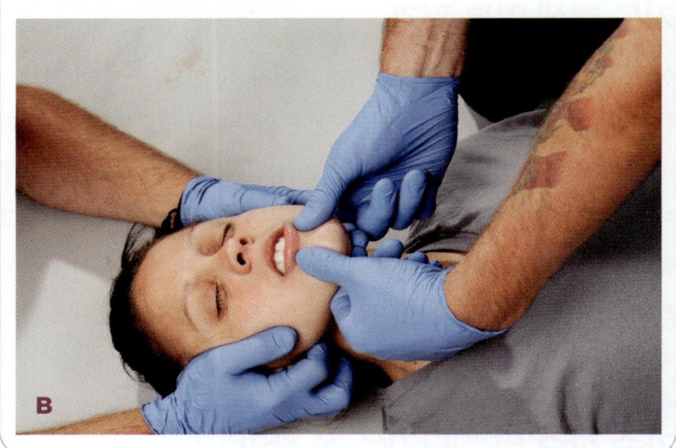

그림 7-9 A. 외상 턱밀어올리기. 엄지손가락을 각 광대뼈에 대고 집게손가락과 긴 손가락이 아래턱뼈의 각에 맞춰 놓는다. 아래턱뼈를 위쪽으로 밀어 올린다. **B.** 외상 턱들기. 턱들기는 외상 턱들어올리기와 유사한 기능을 수행한다. 아래턱뼈를 앞으로 움직여 혀를 이동시킨다.

A: © National Association of Emergency Medical Technicians (NAEMT); B: © Jones & Bartlett Learning. Photographed by Darren Stahlman.

방법은 아래턱뼈를 당긴다. 외상 턱밀어올리기 방법과 외상 턱들기 방법은 기존의 턱밀어올리기와 턱들기를 변형한 것이다. 이러한 변형은 환자의 목뼈를 보호하는 동시에 혀를 후인두에서 이동시켜 기도를 개방한다.

흡인

외상 환자가 기도 내 축적된 분비물, 구토물, 혈액 또는 이물질을 효과적으로 제거하지 못할 수 있다. 흡인을 제공하는 것은 환자의 기도를 확보화고 유지하는 데 중요한 부분이다.

기도가 아직 관리되지 않은 외상 환자는 상기도에 대한 적극적인 흡인이 필요할 수 있다. 병원 전 처치 제공자가 도착하기 전에 이미

기도에 다량의 혈액과 구토물이 축적되었을 수 있으며 이에 따라 이미 환기 및 폐포로의 산소 전달이 손상되었을 수 있다. 다량의 구토나 출혈이 있는 때 액체의 양이 간단히 흡인기로 빠르게 제거할 수 있는 양보다 많을 수 있다. 이럴 경우 목뼈 정렬을 유지하면서 통나무 굴리기 방법으로 환자를 옆 누운자세를 취해주면 중력이 기도를 확보하는 데 도움이 될 수 있다. 입인두를 흡인하기 위해서는 단단하고 흡인팁의 구멍이 큰 흡인기를 사용하는 것이 좋으며 반응이 빠른 환자가 훨씬 더 잘 견딜 수 있으므로 입안을 흡인하기 위해서는 흡인팁을 입의 중앙이 아니라 옆으로 삽입해야 한다.

장시간 흡인으로 인해 저산소증이 발생할 수 있는 것은 사실이지만, 기도가 완전히 막히면 공기 교환이 불가능하므로 기도가 부분적으로 확보될 때까지 적극적으로 흡인과 환자 자세를 유지한다. 이 시점에서 과산소화를 시행한 후 필요한 경우 흡인을 반복한다. 과산소호는 예방산소투여같이 비재호흡마스크 또는 고유량 산소가 연결된 백마스크 장치를 사용하여 수행할 수 있다. 과산소화의 목표는 짧은 시간 동안 산소포화도를 가능한 한 100%에 가깝게 유지하는 것이다.

보조 장비의 선택

일차평가에서 발견된 기도 문제는 기도를 개방하고 유지하기 위한 즉각적인 조치가 필요하다. 이러한 초기 단계는 외상 턱밀어올리기 또는 턱들기와 같은 도수 방법이다. 일단 기도가 개방되면 일반적으로 보조 장비를 사용하여 기도를 유지해야 한다. 특정 장비는 병원 전 처치 제공자의 해당 장비에 대한 교육 수준 및 숙련도와 환자와 관련된 다양한 보조 장치, 술기의 사용에 대한 위해성-유익성 분석에 따라 선택해야 한다(2장 황금 원칙, 선호 및 비판적 사고를 참조). 기도 보조 장비의 선택은 환자 중심으로 이루어져야 한다. 이 특정 상황에서 특정 환자에게 가장 적합한 기도 유지 방법은 무엇인가? 라는 질문에서 시작해야 한다(**Box 7-1**).

초기 교육과 지속적인 교육을 받는 동안 다양한 수준의 병원 전 처치 제공자는 기도를 개방하고 유지하는 데 도움이 되는 다양한 보조 장비를 접하게 된다. 훈련의 양은 장비 삽입의 어려움과 직접적으로 관련이 있다. 응급의료 제공자 수준에서 EMT는 입인두기도기 삽입에 대한 교육을 받지만, Paramedic은 전문적인 기도 유지 장비를

사용하도록 훈련을 받으며 일부 프로토콜에서는 외과적 기도유지 술기도 허용한다. 삽관이나 외과적 반지갑상연골절개와 같은 전문적인 술기의 경우 술기를 더 많은 횟수를 수행할수록 성공적인 결과를 얻을 가능성이 높아진다. 강의실에서만, 이러한 술기를 실습한 신규 구급대원은 이러한 처치를 여러 번 수행한 10년 경력의 구급대원에 비해 어려운 환자에게 성공적으로 삽관을 시행할 가능성이 적다. 절차에 단계가 많을수록 절차를 배우고 숙달하기가 더 어려워진다. 전문적인 술기는 더 다양한 지식이 필요하고 처치를 완료하는 데 더 많은 단계가 필요하므로 실패할 확률도 더 높다. 술기의 난도가 높아지면 초기 교육과 지속적인 술기 유지 관리 모두에서 교육 요구 사항도 증가한다. 일반적으로 술기의 난도가 높을수록 실패 또는 실수로 인해 환자에게 가해지는 불이익도 커진다. 이것은 기도 술기에서 특히 그렇다.

다음은 환자의 필요 또는 잠재적인 필요에 따라 선택할 수 있는 여러 유형의 기도 유지 장비이다.

- **단순 기도유지 장비**(인두 뒤쪽에서 혀를 들어 올리는 장치)
  - 입인두기도기
  - 코인두기도기
  - 환기를 시행하기 위해서는 마스크가 필요(일반적으로 백마스크 장비 사용)
- **전문 기도유지 장비**(입인두 높이에 위치하고 성대 위의 기도를 확보하기 위한 장치, 성문위기도기라고도 함)
  - 후두마스크기도기
  - 후두튜브(예: LT, LTS)
- **확실한 기도유지 장비**(폐쇄 형태로 기관을 격리하고 성대 아래 수준에서 기도를 관리할 수 있는 장비)
  - 기관내관
  - 외과적 기도유지

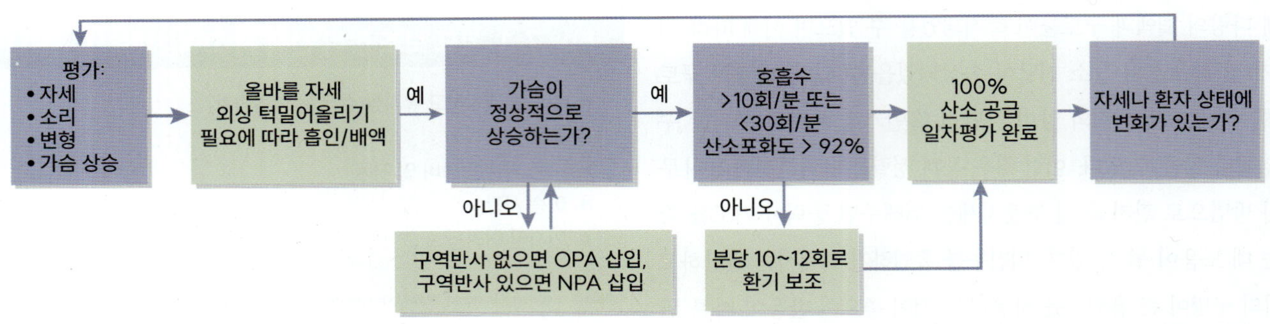

그림 7-10 기본 기도 관리 알고리즘.
© National Association of Emergency Medical Technicians (NAEMT)

단순 기도유지 장비

도수 기도유지가 실패하거나 기도 개방을 지속해 유지해야 할 경우 다음 단계는 인공기도기를 사용하는 것이다(**그림 7-10**). 단순 기도유지기를 삽입한 후 환자와 상황에 따라 전문 기도유지 장비를 삽입하는 결정이 적절할 수 있다. 다음은 단순 기도유지 장비에 대한 설명이다.

기본 생명유지술(BLS)에 사용하는 기도유지기에는 입인두기도기와 코인두기도기의 두 종류가 있다. 일반적으로 BLS 제공자는 이 장비를 삽입할 수 있는 자격을 갖추고 있으므로 BLS 장비라고 부른다. 단순히 혀의 뒷부분이 기도를 막지 않도록 하는 기본적인 장비이다. 그러나 인두에 구토물이 가득 차 있거나 후두가 부풀어 오른 경우 이러한 장비는 환자가 기도를 개방하고 유지하는 데 도움이 되지 않는다. 하지만 대부분 기도 폐쇄를 완화하는데 빠르고 유용한 장비이다.

입인두기도기

가장 자주 사용되는 인공기도기는 입인두기도기(OPA)이다(**그림 7-11A** 참조). 입인두기도기는 설압자를 이용해서 삽입하거나 90도 또는 180도 회전시켜 삽입할 수 있다.

적응증

- 혀의 기저부 후방 변위로 인해 독립적으로 기도를 유지할 수 없는 환자
- 삽관이 시행된 환자가 기관내관을 깨무는 것을 예방하기 위해

금기증

- 의식이 명료하거나 반의식이 있는 환자
- 구역 반사가 있는 환자

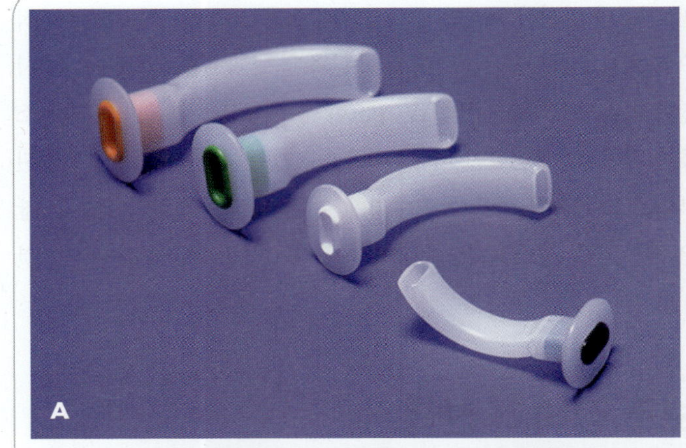

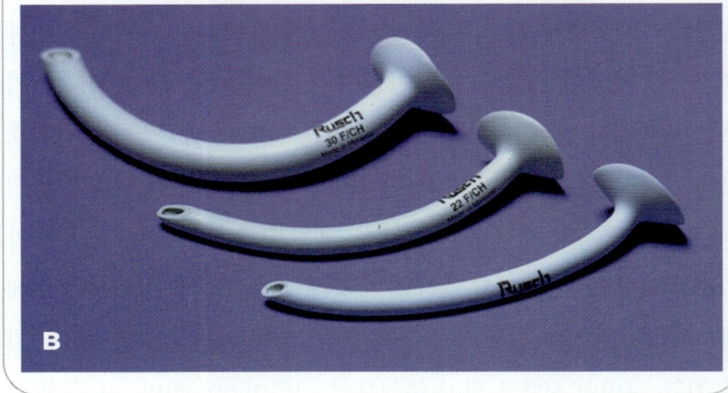

그림 7-11 A. 입인두기도기 **B.** 코인두기도기.
© Jones & Bartlett Learning. Courtesy of MIEMSS.

합병증

- 입인두기도기는 혀의 뒷부분을 누르기 때문에 이를 사용하면 의식이 있는 환자의 경우 구역, 구토 및 후두연축을 유발할 수 있다.
- 의식이 없는 환자의 경우 가장 흔한 합병증은 기도 개방을 완전하게 유지하지 못하는 것이며 이 경우 추가로 턱들기가 필요할 수 있다.

코인두기도기

코인두기도기(NPA)는 혀 뒤쪽이 상기도를 막지 않도록 한쪽 콧구멍을 통해 코인두와 입인두 후벽의 굴곡을 따라 삽입하는 부드러운 고무 재질로 만들어진 장비이다(**그림 7-11B**).

적응증

- 스스로 기도 개방을 유지할 수 없는 환자

금기증

- 코인두기도기의 두개내 삽입에 대한 일부 사례 보고가 있었지만, 얼굴/두개골기저부 골절이 코인두기도기 삽입이 필요한 경우 금기라는 주장을 뒷받침하는 증거는 없다. 그러나 두개골기저부 골절의 징후가 있는 경우 주의가 필요하다. 올바른 삽입 술기로 위험을 최소화해야 한다.

합병증

- 삽입으로 인한 출혈

성문위기도기

전문 기도기의 원리는 상기도를 개방하고 소화관과 분리된 상태로 유지하면서 단단히 밀폐하여 양압환기를 쉽게 하는 것이다. 성문위기도기(SGA)는 가장 간단한 전문 기도유지기이다. 기도 유지가 어려운 환자나 양압환기가 필요하고 마스크를 얼굴에 단단히 밀폐하기 어려운 환자에게 유용할 수 있다(**그림 7-12**).

성문위기도기의 종류에는 후두 주위를 밀봉하고 튜브 끝부분이 식도를 막는 후두마스크기도기(LMA)와 입인두를 밀봉하고 튜브 끝부분이 식도를 막는 후두튜브기도기(LTA)가 있다(**표 7-2**).

두 장비 모두 목구멍 뒤쪽을 누르기 때문에 의식이 없는 환자에게만 사용할 수 있으며 잘못 삽입하면 기도가 막힐 수 있으므로 가슴 시진, 청진 및 연속 파형 호기말이산화탄소 모니터링을 통해 튜브 위치를 확인해야 한다. LMA는 크기가 다양하며 올바른 사용을 위해 환자의 해부학적 구조와 일치해야 한다.

이 장비의 장점은 쉽고 빠른 삽입(대부분의 연구에서 20초 미만), 뛰어난 술기 유지, 환자의 위치와 관계없이 삽입할 수 있는 장점은 환자에게 접근 및 구출이 어렵거나 목뼈 손상이 의심되는 외상 환자에게 특히 중요할 수 있다. 양압환기가 필요하고 얼굴에 마스크를 단단히 밀폐하기 어려운 경우 유용하게 사용할 수 있다(**그림 7-13**).

이 장비를 사용하면 소아 환자에게도 16~26cmH$_2$O의 기도 밀폐

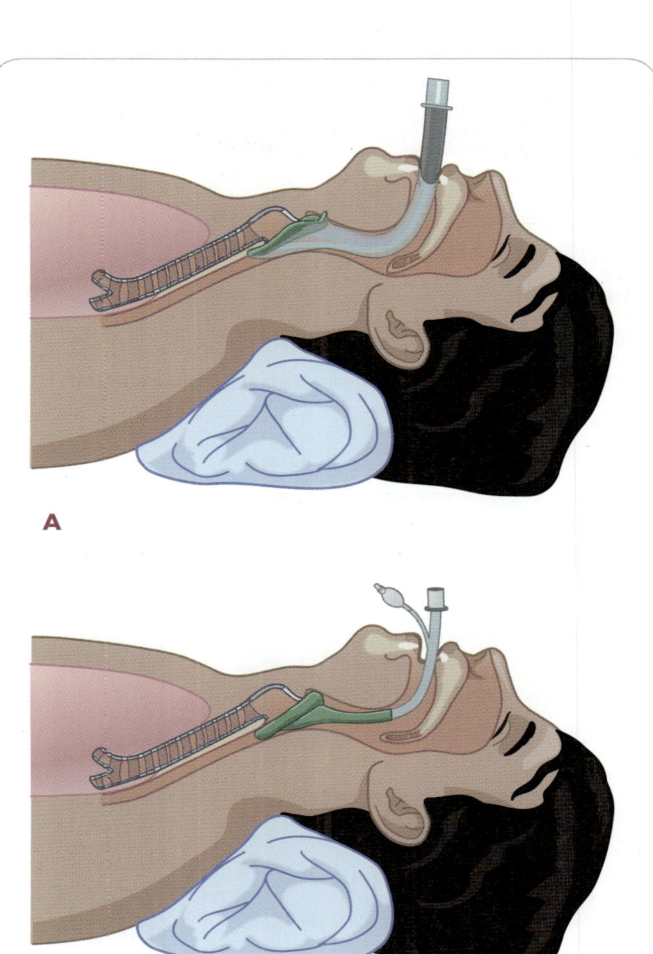

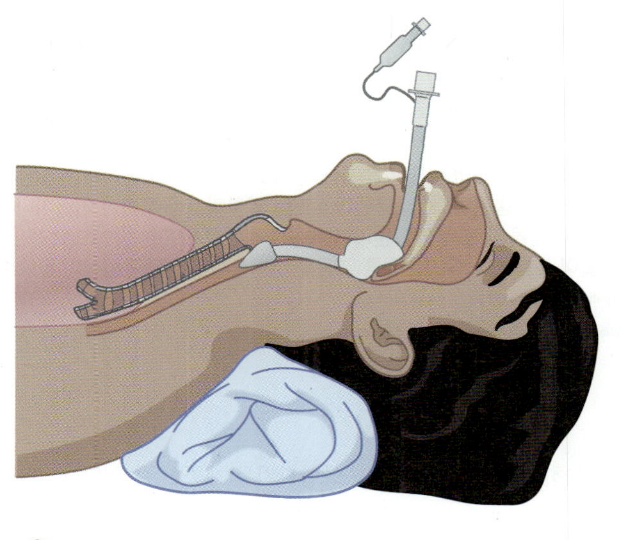

그림 7-12 **A.** i-gel은 후두 주위를 밀폐하도록 고안된 폴리머 링이다. **B.** 후두마스크에는 후두 주위를 밀폐하는 팽창식 링이 있다. **C.** 후두튜브는 후두를 향하는 개부부가 있고 근위 커프는 입인두를 밀봉한다.

표 7-2 성문위기도기

	기도 밀봉	풍선 커프	위 감압	기관내관 통과 가능성
클래식 후두마스크	후두 주변	예	아니오	예
슈프림 후두마스크 (삽관형 후두마스크)	후두 주변	예	예	No
i-gel 후두마스크	후두 주변	아니오	예	예
후두튜브	입인두	예	일부 모델	아니오

© National Association of Emergency Medical Technicians (NAEMT)

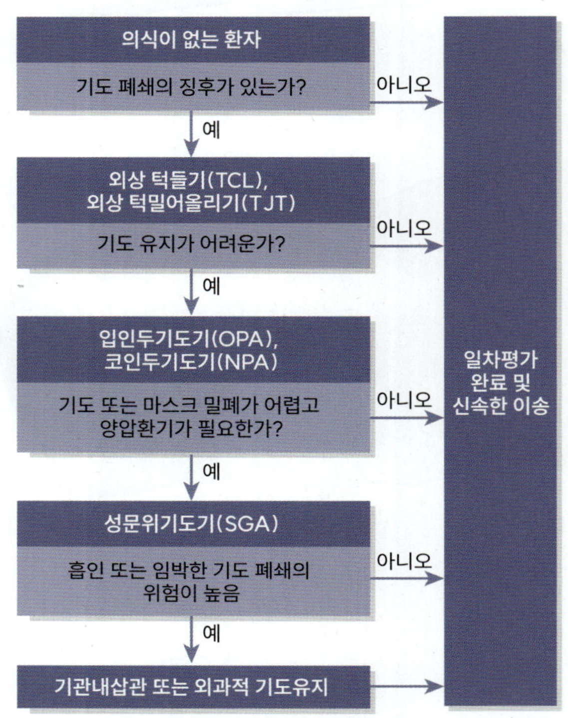

그림 7-13 의식이 없는 많은 환자에게 기도를 개방하고 유지하는 것은 기본 술기만으로도 충분하다. 얼굴에 마스크를 밀착하고 유지하기 어렵거나 흡인의 위험이 높을 때 또는 양압환기를 제공하기 위한 안전한 방법으로 전문기도유지술이 유용하다. 우선순위를 결정하려면 체계적인 접근 방식이 필요하다.

Abbreviations: TCL, trauma chin lift; TJT, trauma jaw thrust.

© National Association of Emergency Medical Technicians (NAEMT)

가 가능하므로 매우 효과적인 양압환기를 제공할 수 있다. 또한 수동적인 역류를 방지하는 데 도움이 될 수 있는 식도 밀폐(약 16cmH$_2$O)를 제공한다. 대부분 장치에는 식도를 통해 흡인 카테터를 삽입할 수 있는 내강이 있어 위를 부분적으로 감압할 수 있어 역류 위험을 더욱 줄이고 환기의 효과를 개선할 수 있다. 그러나 성인의 경우 심한 구토로 인해 최대 300cmH$_2$O의 압력이 발생할 수 있으므로 장비가 빠질 수 있다. 따라서 성문위기도기는 비교적 높은 수준의 기도 보호를 제공하지만, 완전한 기도 보호를 제공하지 않는다.

또 다른 한계는 후두 부종이 성문위기도기의 말단 끝에서 먼 쪽에서 발생하기 때문에 이러한 장비가 후두 부종을 해결하는 데 도움이 되지 않는다는 것이다.

적응증

- 성문위기도기는 병원 전 처치 제공자가 교육을 받고 승인을 받으면 구역반사가 없고 의식이 없는 외상 환자의 기도를 유지하는 데 효율적인 장비이다. 일반적으로 기관내관 삽관보다 삽입 속도가 빠르며 일차 기도 관리 도구로서 더 안정적이다. 양압환기가 가능하므로 무호흡 상태이거나 분당 10회 미만의 속도로 호흡하는 환자에게 유용하다.
- 성문위기도기는 병원 전 처치 제공자가 기관내삽관을 할 수 없고 백마스크와 입인두기도기 또는 코인두기도기로 환자에게 환기를 쉽게 할 수 없는 경우 대체 기도유지 장비로 사용하는 경우가 많다.

금기증

- 정상적인 구역반사
- 알려진 식도 질환(이 금기는 특히 후두튜브기도기와 관련이 있다. LMA는 식도로 들어가지 않기 때문에 위험이 줄어든다.)
- 최근 부식성 물질 섭취

합병증

- 구역질 및 구토(구역반사가 정상인 경우)
- 흡인
- 식도 손상
- 삽입 위치가 잘못되었을 때 저산소증 및 저환기 발생

후두마스크기도기(LMA)

후두마스크기도기는 성문위기도기 중 가장 널리 사용되는 장치이다. 이 장치는 실리콘 튜브의 원위부 끝에 대각선으로 부착된 팽창식 실리콘 링으로 구성된다(그림 7-14). 링을 삽입하면 후두 자체에 장치를 직접 삽입하지 않고도 LMA와 성문 개부부 사이에 저압 밀봉을 형성한다.

해부학적으로 구부러진 단단한 도관이 있는 일부 모델을 포함하여 다양한 브랜드와 디자인의 LMA를 사용할 수 있다. 특수 모델 중 하나는 의료용 열가소성 탄성중합체로 만든 i-gel LMA이다. 이 모델은 인두, 후두 및 후두 주위 구조물을 팽창하지 않고 해부학적으로 밀착하는 동시에 압박 외상을 방지하도록 설계되었다. 이에 따라 주사기가 필요하지 않으므로 군사적 또는 기타 전술 환경에서 특히 유용하다.

LMA의 장점은 다음과 같다.

- LMA는 맹목적 삽입용으로 설계되었으며 기관이나 성대를 직접 눈으로 확인할 필요가 없다.
- LMA는 소아와 성인 환자에게 모두 사용할 수 있도록 다양한 크기로 제공된다.

현재 유럽, 북미 및 군대의 병원 전 환경에서 LMA를 사용한 풍부한 경험이 있다. 이 장치의 더 정교한 버전은 "삽관형 LMA"이다. 이 장치는 기존 LMA와 비슷하게 삽입되지만, 유연한 기관내관을 LMA를 통해 기관으로 삽입할 수 있다.

삽관형 후두마스크기도기(ILMA)

삽관형 후두마스크기도기(ILMA) 장치는 LMA와 디자인이 유사하며 삽입 방법도 같다. 이 장치는 기관내관의 이차 삽입을 허용하고 기관내로 튜브를 유도한다. 일단 기관내관 위치가 확인되면 일반적으로 이송하는 동안 기관내관의 안정화를 돕고 백업 역할을 할 수 있도록 ILMA를 저거하지 않는 것이 일반적이다.

이 장치는 성인에게만 사용할 수 있다. 환자에게 더 잘 접근할 수 있게 되면 기관내관을 삽입하여 환자를 구출하기 전에 일시적으로 기도를 확보하는 장치로 유용할 수 있다.

i-gel 장치

i-gel 장치는 비팽창식 기전 및 맹목적 삽입 술기를 사용하여 밀봉을 생성한다. 성문 개구부 주위에 밀봉이 형성되기는 하지만, 기관내관만큼 포괄적이지 않으며 흡인은 여전히 문제로 남아 있다.

신생아부터 성인까지 사용할 수 있으며 장점으로는 기도 외상의 위험이 적그 삽입이 비교적 쉽다는 것이다.

후두튜브기도기(LTA)

후두튜브기도기는 원위부와 근위부에 커프가 있는 이중 내강 튜브이다. 일차 내강은 환기를 위한 것이고 두 번째는 위 감압을 위한 흡인 카테터 삽입을 쉽게 하기 위한 것이다. 이 장치는 기관내관보다 흡인으로부터 덜 보호하지만, 그런데도 양압환기를 시행할 수 있다.

영아부터 성인까지 사용할 수 있으며 이중 내강 디자인으로 기관 삽관을 보조하는 데 효과적일 수 있다.

확실한 기도유지

성대 아래 기관에 커프가 있는 튜브를 삽입하면 흡인에 대한 가장 효과적인 보호와 부기로 인한 기도 폐쇄를 가장 효과적으로 방지하고 양압환기를 시행할 수 있으므로 결정적 기도기라고 한다. 여기에서는 기관내관과 외과적 기도유지라는 두 종류의 결정적 기도기에 관해 설명한다.

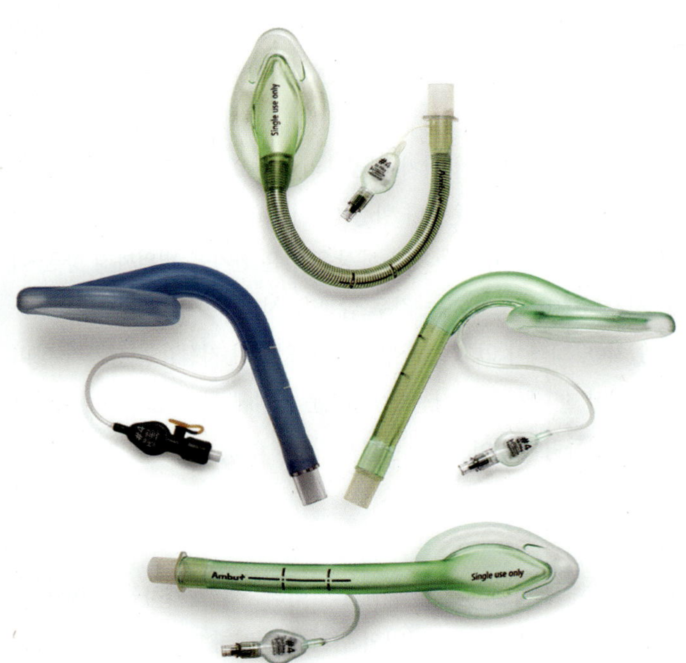

그림 7-14 후두마스크기도기

Courtesy of Ambu, Inc.

기관내삽관

전통적으로 기관내삽관(ETI)은 무호흡이거나 기도를 유지하고 보호할 수 없거나 보조 환기가 필요한 외상 환자의 기도를 유지할 수 있는 이상적인 방법이었다(**그림 7-15**). 그러나 환자의 생존 측면에서 이 술기를 사용한 결과가 다양하므로 최근 사용에 대한 논란이 커지고 있다.

합병증이 거의 발생하지 않는 안전한 수술실에서 삽관과 달리 병원 전 환경에서 중증 환자에게 시행하는 응급 삽관은 매우 위험한 술기이며 심각한 합병증과 관련이 있다. 장비와 인력이 잘 갖춰진 응급실이나 중환자실에서도 중증 환자의 응급 삽관은 40%의 심혈관 불안정, 9%의 심각한 저산소증, 최대 3%의 심정지 위험과 관련이 있었다. 이는 일부 병원 전 연구에서 삽관 성공률이 97% 이상임에도 불구하고 환자 생존에 미치는 영향이 아직 명확하지 않은 이유를 설명할 수 있다. 연구에 따르면 도시 환경에서 기관내삽관으로 중증외상 환자는 입인두기도기를 삽입한 후 백마스크 장치로 환기를 시행하면서 이송한 환자보다 예후가 더 낮은 결과를 얻지 못했다. 그 결과 기관내삽관의 역할에 대한 의문이 점점 더 커지고 있으며 현재까지 이 술기의 사용에 대한 실제 이점을 입증한 연구는 거의 없다.

그러나 술기의 적응증을 더 잘 이해하고 술기를 최적화하면 환자의 생존율에 더 긍정적인 영향을 미칠 수 있다.

장점

- 기도를 확실하고 단단하게 밀폐
- 양압환기 가능
- 기관지 흡인으로부터 최적의 보호

단점

- 시간 소요

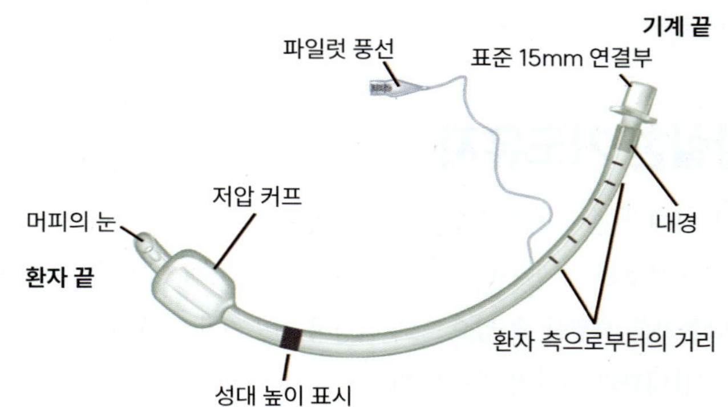

그림 7-15 기관내관의 특징

표 7-3 기관내삽관을 위한 장비 및 설명		
환기 및 산소 공급	**삽관**	**구조 계획**
백마스크 장치 산소 탱크 마스크 OPA 및 NPA	커프가 있는 기관내관 주사기 탐침 후두경 단단한 대구경 흡인 카테터	후두마스크 외과적 기도유지 세트
ECG, NIBP, SpO₂ 및 ETCO₂로 모니터링		
정맥 라인 확보 후 진정제, 근이완제 및 혈압상승제 투여		

Abbreviations: ECG, electrocardiogram; ETCO₂, end-tidal carbon dioxide; IV, intravenous; NIBP, noninvasive blood pressure; NPA, nasopharyngeal airway; OPA, oropharyngeal airway; SpO₂, peripheral oxygen saturation.

- 정맥 내 라인, 약물 및 모니터링 필요(**표 7-3**)
- 숙련되고 경험이 풍부한 시술자 필요
- 높은 합병증 발생률

기관내삽관을 수행하거나 대체 장치를 사용할지를 결정하는 것은 예상되는 어려움과 시술자의 경험 수준을 포함하여 위험과 이점을 종합적으로 평가한 후 결정해야 한다. 기관내삽관을 수행하는 데 필요한 현장 체류 시간의 증가에 따른 영향도 고려해야 한다. 한 대규모 유럽 연구에서 기관내삽관을 받는 환자의 평균 추가 현장 체류 시간은 8분이었다.

확실한 것은 병원 전 처치 제공자의 숙련도나 효율성과 관계없이 현장에서의 삽관은 병원보다 항상 더 어렵고 현장 체류 시간이 더 길어진다는 것이다. 따라서 기도 화상을 입은 환자를 병원까지 항공 이송 시간이 30분 소요되는 경우 삽관을 시행해야 하는 이유가 있을 수 있지만, 의식이 없고 얼굴에 외상이 없으며 저혈압인 환자가 장비와 인력이 잘 갖춰진 외상센터에서 5분 거리에 있는 경우에는 이러한 이유가 설득력이 떨어진다.

잠재적으로 어려운 기관내삽관의 예측

기관내삽관을 시행하기 전에 삽관의 어려움을 평가하는 것이 필수적이다. 많은 요인이 외상 환자의 삽관을 어렵게 만들 수 있다. 이 중 일부는 외상과 직접적으로 관련이 있고 다른 일부는 얼굴과 상기도의 해부학적 이상으로 인한 것이며 다른 일부는 환자의 자세로 인한

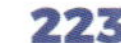

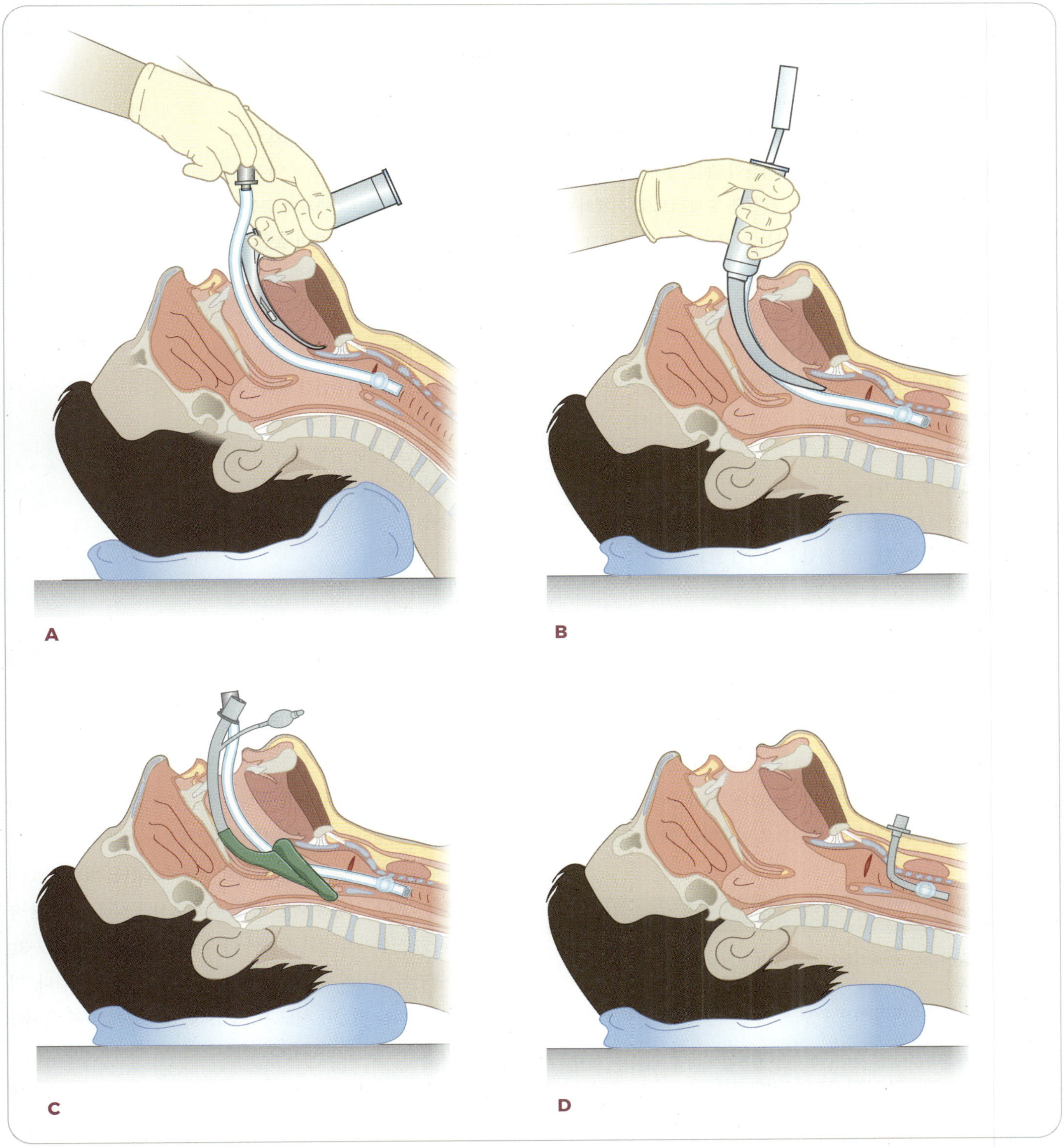

그림 7-16 확실한 기도유지는 성대 아래 기관에 커프가 달린 튜브를 삽입하는 것이다. 기관지 흡인 및 부종으로 인한 기도 폐쇄를 방지하는 확실한 보호 장치이다. 의식이 있거나 반의식 상태인 환자에게 확실한 기도유지를 확보하려면 정맥 내 라인, 진정제, 모니터링이 필요하다. **A.** 후두경으로 직접 눈으로 보면서 기관삽관. **B.** 비디오 후두경을 이용한 간접 시각화를 통한 기관삽관. **C.** 후두마스크를 이용한 삽관. **D.** 외과적 기도유지는 기본 장비와 국소 마취를 통해 신속하게 시행할 수 있지만, 광범위한 교육이 필요하다.

것이다.

HEAVEN은 기존의 병원 또는 진료실 기반 평가 방법보다 병원 전 환경에서 외상 환자에게 더 잘 적용되는 것으로 보이는 어려운 삽관을 예측하기 위한 일련의 기준이다(Box 7-2).

이송 시간도 적절한 방법을 결정할 때 고려해야 할 요소일 수 있다. 예를 들어, 외상센터로 이송하는 기간이 짧은 경우 입인두기도기를 삽입한 후 백마스크로 환자에게 환기를 효과적으로 시행하면서 이송할 수 있다. 병원 전 처치 제공자는 삽관을 시행하지 않고 간단한 기도유지 방법을 사용하여 기도를 유지하면서 이송하는 방법을 선택할 수 있다. 병원 전 처치 제공자는 전문적인 기도유지 방법을 시행하기로 할 때 위험과 이점을 평가해야 한다.

이 절차의 잠재적인 어려움에도 불구하고 기관내삽관은 다음과 같은 장점이 있으므로 여전히 선호되는 기도 관리 방법이다.

- 기도를 분리
- 100% 산소로 환기 가능
- 적절한 마스크로 얼굴에 밀봉을 유지할 필요가 없음
- 흡인(구토, 이물질, 혈액)의 위험을 현저히 감소
- 기관 깊은 곳의 흡인을 쉽게 함
- 위 흡인 방지

적응증

- 기도를 보호할 수 없는 환자, 최근 이 적응증에 대한 논란이 있지만, GCS 점수가 8점 미만인 환자
- 산소 공급에 심각한 문제가 있어 고농도 산소 투여가 필요한 환자
- 보조 환기 또는 양압환기가 필요한 심각한 환기 장애가 있는 환자
- 확실한 기도 유지가 가능한 병원으로 이송하는 데 상대적으로 긴

시간이 소요되는 경우
- 덜 침습적인 처치를 사용하여 기도유지를 적절하게 시행하고 유지할 수 없는 경우

금기증

- 술기에 대한 교육 및 교육 유지 부족
- 적절한 적응증 부족
- 환자를 이송할 의료기관과의 근접성(상대적 금기)
- 기도 확보를 실패할 확률이 높음
- 혈관 내 혈량저하증 및 출혈쇼크

합병증

- 장시간의 삽관 시도로 인한 저산소혈증
- 서맥을 유발하는 미주신경 자극
- 두개내압 증가
- 기도 외상으로 인한 출혈 및 부기 발생
- 우측 주기관지 삽관
- 식도 삽관
- 구토로 인한 흡인
- 치아가 흔들리거나 부러짐
- 성대 손상
- 신경학적 결손이 없는 목뼈 손상이 신경학적 결손이 있는 목뼈 손상으로 전환
- 단순기흉이 양압환기로 인해 긴장기흉으로 전환
- 양압환기와 함께 진정제 투여로 인한 순환계 허탈

모든 위험과 이점을 판단해야 한다. 단순히 프로토콜이 허용하기 때문에 삽관을 시행하는 것은 부적절하다. 가능한 이점과 가능한 위험을 고려하고 임상 시나리오와 환자의 신체적 소견을 바탕으로 계획을 수립해야 한다. 상황은 이송 시간, 위치(도시와 시골), 주어진 술기를 시행하는 시술자의 경험 수준에 따라 크게 달라진다(Box 7-3). 삽관 성공률만이 성공의 유일한 척도가 아니라는 점을 명심한다. 기도 확보까지 걸리는 기간과 시도 횟수는 이환율 및 사망률과 유의한 상관관계가 있는 것으로 나타났다.

2000년대 초반의 연구에서는 병원 전 삽관 중 저산소혈증의 발생률과 영향에 대한 우려가 제기되었다. 최근 발표된 논문에서는 삽관의 생리학적 측면을 강조하며 시도 횟수에 따라 합병증과 사망률이 모두 증가할 수 있다고 제안했다. 이전 접근 방법에서는 모든 단계에서 새로운 도구를 사용하여 여러 번 시도하는 것을 옹호했다. 안타깝게도 이러한 접근 방법이 결국 높은 삽관 성공률로 이어지더라도 사

Box 7-2　HEVEN 기준

- 저산소증(Hypoxemia): 초기 후두경 검사 시 산소포화도가 93% 이하인 경우
- 극단적인 크기(Extremes of size): 8세 이하의 소아 환자 또는 임상적 비만
- 해부학적 문제(Anatomic challenge): 후두경 시야를 제한하는 외상, 종괴, 부기, 이물 또는 기타 구조적 이상이 포함
- 구토물/혈액/체액(Vomit/blood/fluid): 후두경 검사 시 인두/하인두에 임상적으로 유의미한 체액이 존재
- 토혈(Exsanguination): 급속연속기관삽관 관련 무호흡 중에 불포화 반응을 가속할 수 있는 의심되는 빈혈
- 목(Neck): 목 운동 범위 제한

Reproduced from Davis D, Olvera DJ. HEAVEN criteria: derivation of a new difficult airway prediction tool. Air Med J. 2017;36(4):195-197. https://doi.org/10.1016/j.amj.2017.04.001

망률 측면에서 비참한 결과를 초래하는 경우가 많다. 그렇기 때문에 시술자는 전체 조건을 최적화하고 최상의 술기를 먼저 사용하며 중요한 매개변수를 관찰하고 실패할 경우 조기에 술기를 포기하는 것을 목표로 해야 한다(**Box 7-4**).

기관내삽관 방법

기관내삽관을 수행할 때 몇 가지 대체 방법을 사용할 수 있다. 선택 방법은 환자의 요구, 긴급성 수준, 환자 자세 또는 병원 전 처치 제공자의 훈련 및 숙련도, 업무 범위와 같은 요인에 따라 달라진다. 선택한 방법을 선택하든 술기를 시행하는 동안 환자의 머리와 목을 중립 자세로 유지하며 척추 움직임 제한 술기를 시행하는 내내 유지해야 한다. 일반적으로 두 번의 시도 후에도 삽관을 성공하지 못하면 다른 기도유지 방법을 시도해 본다. 더욱 기본적인 방법으로 시행하는 것이 제일 나은 선택이다. 저산소증이 여러 번 지속된 후 추가 뇌손상이 있는 삽관된 환자보다 기관내관 없이 산소가 잘 공급된 환자를 응급실로 이송하는 것이 더 낫다.

입기관삽관

입기관삽관은 기관내관을 입으로 기관에 삽입하는 것이다. 외상이 없는 환자는 삽관을 쉽게 하려고 '냄새 맡는 자세'를 취하는 경우가 많다. 이 자세는 목뼈 1~2번(목뼈 골절이 두 번째로 흔히 발생하는 부위)을 과신전 시키고 목뼈 5~6번(목뼈 골절이 가장 흔히 발생하는 부위)에서 목뼈를 과굴곡시키기 때문에 무딘 외상 환자에게 사용해서는 안 된다(**그림 7-17**). 그러나 수많은 연구에 따르면 비디오 후두경으로 삽관을 시행할 때 목뼈를 보호하면서 기관내삽관을 더 쉽게 시행할 수 있는 것으로 나타났다.

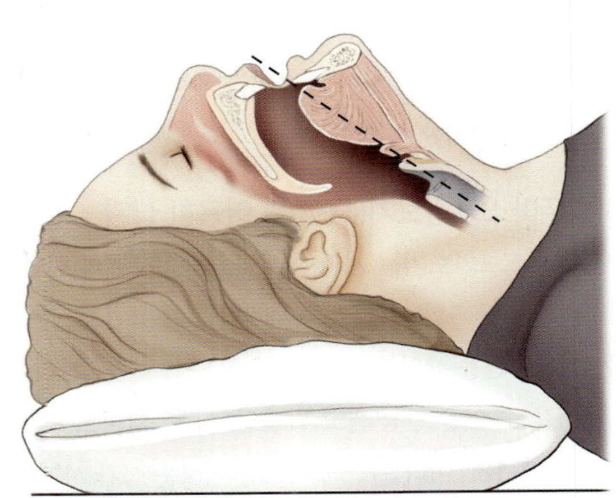

그림 7-17 환자의 머리를 냄새 맡는 자세로 위치시키면 입을 통해 후두를 이상적으로 시각화할 수 있다. 그러나 이러한 자세는 환자의 목을 C1과 C2에서 과신전시키고 C5와 C6에서 과굴곡시킨다. 이 부위가 목뼈 골절의 가장 흔한 두 지점이다.

© National Association of Emergency Medical Technicians (NAEMT)

코기관삽관

의식이 있는 외상 환자나 구역반사가 정상인 환자의 경우 기관내삽관을 수행하기 어려울 수 있다. 자발호흡이 있는 경우 이점이 위험도보다 크다면 맹목적 코기관삽관(BNTI)을 시도할 수 있다. 코기관삽관은 직접 시각화 및 입기관삽관보다 수행하기 어려운 경우가 많지만, 이 술기에 숙련된 시술자는 외상 환자에서 높은 성공률을 보인다는 보고가 있다. 맹목적 코기관삽관을 시행하는 동안 기관내관이 성대를 통과할 수 있도록 숨을 쉬고 있어야 한다. 많은 문헌에서 얼굴 중앙부 외상이나 골절이 있는 경우 맹목적 코기관삽관을 금기 사항으로 제시하고 있지만, 철저한 문헌 검색 결과 기관내관이 머리덮개뼈 들어갈 위험에 대한 증거는 드물게 발견되었다. 무호흡은 삽관을 시행하는 절차에 시간이 걸리고 그동안 환자가 효과적으로 환기할 수 없으므로 맹목적 코기관삽관의 특별한 금기 사항이다. 또한 술기 자체는 환자의 호흡으로 활성화된다. 무호흡 환자에게는 이러한 촉진 요인이 없다.

대면 삽관

대면 삽관은 병원 전 처치 제공자가 외상 환자의 머리 위쪽에서 표준 자세를 취할 수 없어 표준 외상 삽관 술기를 시행할 수 없는 경우에 사용된다. 이러한 상황에는 다음이 포함되지만, 이에 국한되지는 않는다.

- 차량에 갇힘
- 잔해물에 환자가 깔림

이 술기는 전통적으로 오른손에 곡선형 후두경을 들고 시도해 왔지만, 삽관형 후두마스크기도를 사용한 삽관이 더 쉽고 안정적이며 삽관 시도 사이에 환기할 수 있다.

삽관형 후두마스크기도기(ILMA)를 이용한 삽관

삽관형 후두마스크기도기는 기존 후두마스크기도기의 변형된 버전이며 기관내관이 통과할 수 있도록 설계되었다. 삽관형 후두마스크기도기는 기관내관을 삽입할 수 있을 만큼 넓고 기관내관의 끝이 기관으로 들어갈 수 있을 만큼 짧고 단단하며 해부학적으로 구부러진 튜브이다(**그림 7-18**). 여러 연구에 따르면 어려운 삽관 사례(즉, 직접 후두경으로 삽관에 실패한 환자)에서 높은 성공률을 보였다. 삽관을 시도하는 동안 간헐적으로 환기를 할 수 있고 삽관에 실패한 경우 대체 계획이 이미 마련되어 있다는 점 등이 삽관형 후두마스크의 추가 장점으로 꼽힌다.

비디오 후두경을 이용한 삽관

비디오 후두경은 후두를 비디오로 시각화할 수 있는 장치이다. 비디오 후두경을 이용한 삽관은 환자의 해부학적 구조(짧은 목 또는 기타 해부학적 문제)로 인해 직접적인 후두경 삽관이 어려운 상황에서 특히 유용한 것으로 보인다. 일부 연구에서는 비디오 후두경 사용이 삽관 성공률을 향상할 수 있음을 입증했다. 이는 목뼈 정렬을 유지해야 하거나 혈액과 분비물이 시술자의 시야를 가리는 외상 환자에게 특히 두드러진다. 비디오 후두경 삽관은 실외 또는 밝은 환경에서는 비디오 화면이 잘 보이지 않기 때문에 삽관이 어려울 수 있다.

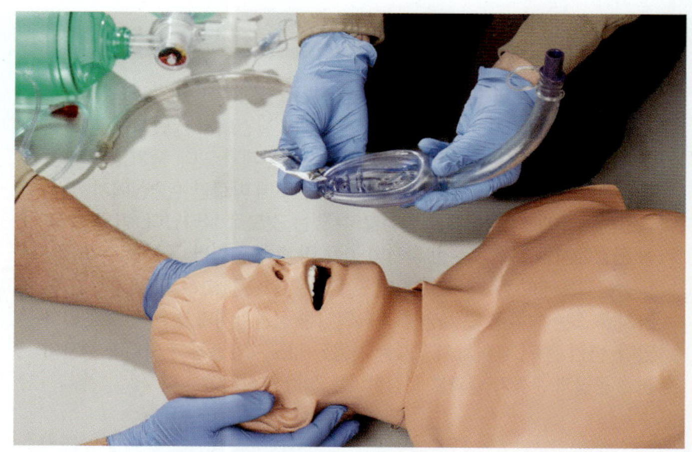

그림 7-18 삽관형 후두마스크기도기
© Jones & Bartlett Learning. Photographed by Darren Stahlman.

비디오 후두경은 기관내관을 끼울 수 있는 경로가 없거나 경로가 있다(**그림 7-19**). 경로가 없는 비디오 후두경의 경우 기관내관을 직접 자유롭게 시야로 가져와야 하지만, 경로가 있는 유형은 후두의 시야가 잘 확보되면 기관내관을 후두경 날에 삽입하고 경로를 따라 밀어 넣는다. 선명한 시야를 확보하기 위해 조직을 이동시켜야 하는 기존의 후두경과 달리 경로가 있는 비디오 후두경은 렌즈와 삽관 경로가 성대와 정렬될 때까지 연부조직 아래로 미끄러져 들어갈 수 있다.

약물 보조 삽관

여러 연구에 따르면 약물 보조 삽관(DAI) 또는 약리학적 보조 삽관이 삽관의 성공률을 높인다는 사실이 밝혀졌지만, 여기에는 비용이 따른다. 약리학적 진정 및 이완은 호흡 억제, 무호흡 및 순환계 허탈의 위험을 초래할 수 있다. 근육마비제를 사용하면 심장을 제외한 모든 근육을 차단하므로 환자에게 마비제를 투여하는 순간부터 환자의 호흡과 기도 조절은 모두 시술자의 책임이 된다. 그런데도 숙련된 시술자라면 다른 방법이 실패하거나 다른 방법을 시행할 수 없을 때 이 술기를 사용하여 효과적으로 기도유지를 시행할 수 있다. 이 절차의 효과를 극대화하고 환자의 안전을 보장하기 위해 병원 전 처치 제공자는 프로토콜, 약물 및 술기 사용 적응증을 숙지해야 한다. 현재 다양한 순서의 약물 보조 삽관이 시행되고 있으며 가장 널리 알려진 것은 급속연속기관삽관(RSI) 및 지연연속기관삽관(DSI)이다. 급속연속기관삽관은 흡인 예방에 중점을 둔 마취 기술인 반면 급속연속기관삽관은 불포화 및 저산소증 예방에 중점을 둔다. 그러나 삽관을 보조하기 위한 약물을 사용하는 경우, 특히 급속연속기관삽관은 삽관만 하는 것 이상의 위험이 있다. 약물을 사용한 삽관은 다음 세 가

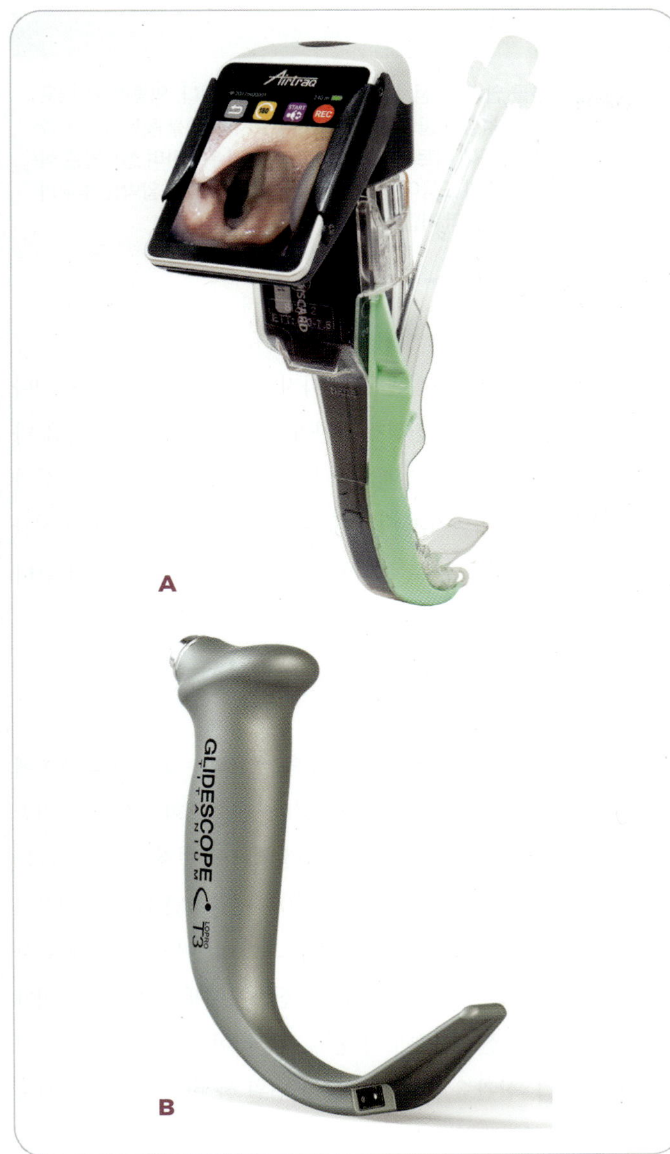

그림 7-19　**A.** 홈이 있는 비디오 후두경 **B.** 홈이 없는 후두경 날.

A: Courtesy of Airtraq LLC a subsidiary of Prodol Meditec S.A.; **B:** Courtesy of Verathon Inc.

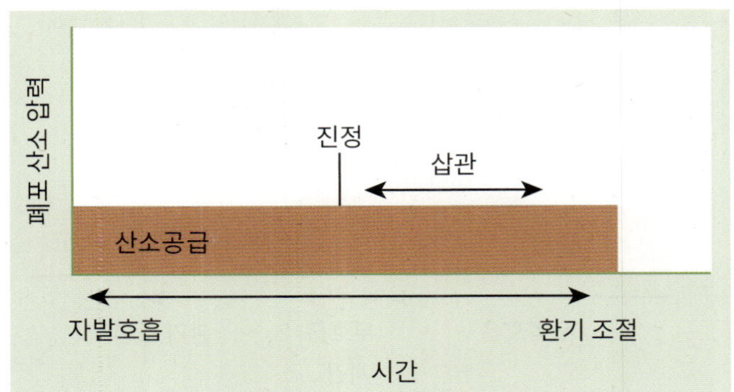

그림 7-20　약물 보조 삽관. 환자에게 진정제/마비제를 투여하여 삽관을 용이하게 한다. 환자는 삽관을 시행하는 내내 호흡을 계속하여 산소 불포화 위험을 줄인다.

© National Association of Emergency Medical Technicians (NAEMT)

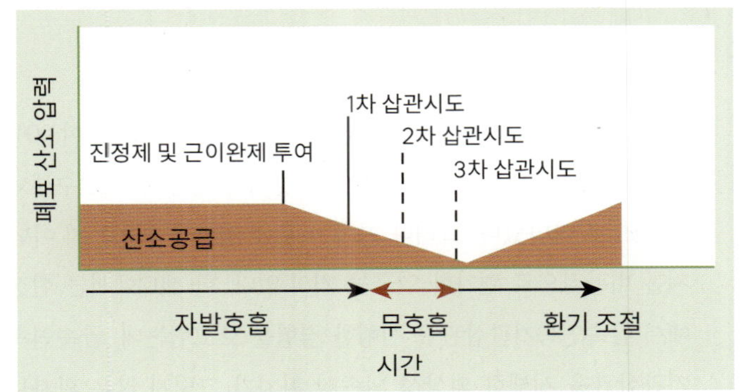

그림 7-21　급속연속기관삽관(RSI). RSI는 기관지 흡인을 예방하기 위한 술기이다. 환자에게 진정제와 속효성 근이완제를 통시에 투여한 후 삽관한다. 이 방법은 성공률이 높지만, 술기 시작 시 환자에게 산소 공급이 충분하지 않거나 삽관 시도가 길어지면 무호흡 기간 동안 저산소증 위험이 증가한다.

© National Associacion of Emergency Medical Technicians (NAEMT)

지로 분류할 수 있다.

1. 진정제나 마약류만을 사용한 삽관. 케타민, 에토미데이트 또는 프로포폴과 같은 마취제와 디아제팜, 미다졸람과 같은 바르비투르산염 또는 펜타닐이나 모르핀과 같은 마약을 단독 또는 병용하여 사용할 수 있으며, 삽관이 가능할 정도로 환자를 이완시키되 보호 반사나 호흡을 없애지 않는 것이다(**그림 7-20**). 케타민은 우수한 1차 유도제이다. 다른 유도제에 비해 순환 저하를 덜 유발하고 진통 효과가 강하다. 하지만 마비제를 사용할 때보다 성공률이 낮고 합병증이 더 자주 발생하는 것으로 보인다.

2. 마비제를 사용한 급속연속기관삽관. 급속연속기관삽관의 목적은 흡인 위험 기간을 최소화하는 것이다. 이를 위해 진정제를 먼저 투여하는 기존의 순서와 달리 진정제와 속효성 마비제를 동시에 투여한다(**그림 7-21**). 급속연속기관삽관의 목적은 환자를 부드럽고 빠르게 의식을 잃게 하고 골격근 마비를 유도하여 기관내관이 상기도를 지나 기관으로 쉽게 삽입할 수 있도록 하는 것이다. 그 결과 안정적인 뇌관류 압과 심혈관 혈류역학을 유지하면서 삽관을 쉽게 할 수 있다. 이 방법은 완전한 근육 마비를 저공하고 모든 보호 반사를 제거하며 무호흡을 유발하여 삽관을 훨씬 쉽게 만든다. 그러나 환자의 환기가 중단되는 순간부터 환자에게 효과적으로 환기를 시행할 수 없는 경우 저산소증의 위험이 분명히 존재하기 때문에 이 술기는 위험이 없는 것은

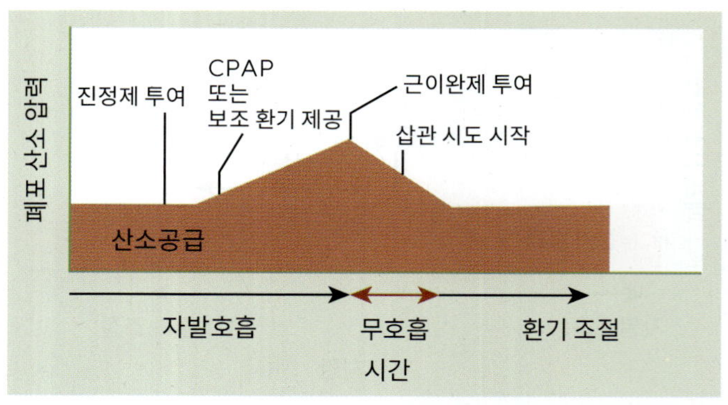

그림 7-22 지연연속기관삽관(DSI). 지연연속기관삽관은 고위험 환자의 산소포하도 저하 및 저산소증 위험을 줄이기 위해 개발된 술기이다. 환자에게 진정제를 투여하여 지속기도양압 및 보조 환기를 통한 예방산소투여가 가능하게 한 후 근이완제를 투여한다. 이 방법은 성공률이 높고 안전성이 높지만, 예방산소투여를 최적화하려면 추가 시간이 필요하다.
© National Association of Emergency Medical Technicians (NAEMT)

아니다.

　이 기도 관리 방법에 관한 연구에 따르면 삽관 성공률이 90% 중반대로 보고되는 등 현장에서 이 술기가 성공적으로 수행되는 것으로 나타났다. 그러나 환자 예후에 영향을 미치는지 아닌지를 비판적으로 평가한 연구는 거의 없다. 한 센터에서는 현장에서 급속연속기관삽관을 시행한 경험을 보고했는데, 급속연속기관삽관을 시행한 외상성 뇌손상 환자가 그렇지 않은 환자보다 예후가 더 나빴다고 기록했다. 후속 분석에 따르면 저이산화탄소혈증과 저산소증으로 이어지는 인지되지 않은 과다환기가 좋지 않은 결과의 주요 원인인 것으로 나타났다. 또 다른 연구에서는 병원에서 삽관된 환자에 비해 현장에서 삽관을 시행한 외상성 뇌손상 환자의 6개월 후 예후가 더 좋다는 결과가 나왔다. 외상 환자에서 기관내삽관과 관련된 사망률 대부분은 아니더라도 일부 특히 혈량저하 환자(즉, 출혈 쇼크 또는 외상성 쇼크)에서 기관내삽관에 수반되는 관류압(MAP 및 CPP)의 급격한 저하의 결과라는 증거가 점점 더 많아지고 있다. 따라서 병원 전 급속연속기관삽관이 장기적인 환자 예후에 긍정적인 영향을 미치는지 부정적인 영향을 미치는지에 대한 중요한 질문에 대한 최종적인 해답은 아직 이용할 수 있는 연구를 통해 밝혀지지 않았다. 확실한 것은 이 술기는 고도로 훈련된 병원 전 처치 제공자만 시행할 수 있으며 어떤 술기를 시행하든 효율적인 환기와 관류가 목표라는 점이다.

3. 지연연속기관삽관. 지속기도양압(CPAP)과 삽관 중 무호흡 산소공급을 통한 예방산소투여를 강조하는 새로운 약물 보조 삽관

© National Association of Emergency Medical Technicians (NAEMT)

술기인 지연연속기관삽관은 몇 가지 유망한 결과를 보여주었다 (**그림 7-22**). 케타민 진정제로 환자를 예방산소투여 후 다음 마비제를 투여하고 코삽입관으로 무호흡 산소를 공급하면서 삽관을 시행한다. 이 술기는 시간이 오래 걸리고 최종 치료까지 시간이 지연될 수 있으므로 이러한 위험을 평가하고 고려해야 한다 (**Box 7-5**).

삽관 중 주의해야 할 사항

저산소혈증은 단기간에 발생하더라도 외상성 뇌손상 환자의 생존에 치명적인 영향을 미치는 것으로 나타났다. 산소포화도가 90% 미만의 단일 사건은 입원실 및 중환자실 입원 기간이 현저하게 늘어나는 것으로 나타났다. 또한 산소포화도가 70% 미만이면 환자는 심장의 보상실패로 심각한 위험에 처하게 된다. 그러므로 특히 마비제를 사용하는 경우 삽관을 시도하기 전에 예방산소투여에 주의를 기울여야 한다. 일반적으로 산소포화도가 93% 이상이어야 삽관을 안전하게 시도할 수 있다. 삽관을 시도하는 동안 팀원 한 명이 모니터를 계속 주시하고 산소포화도가 93%에 가까워지면 삽관 시도를 중단하고 환자에게 환기를 다시 해야 한다. 또 다른 유용한 팁은 술기를 시행하는 동안 팀원들이 산소포화도를 명확하게 들을 수 있도록 모니터를 설정하는 것이다,

　서맥은 팀원들이 찾아야 하는 또 다른 징후이다. 뇌 저산소증은 손끝에서 발생하는 것이 아니라는 점을 기억한다. 실제로 말초 산소포화도는 뇌 산소포화도보다 훨씬 늦게 감소하는 것으로 입증되었으며 이를 맥박산소 지연이라고 한다. 따라서 병원 전 처치 제공자는 삽관 중 서맥이 발생하면 뇌 저산소혈증의 징후일 수 있으므로 이를 주의 깊게 관찰해야 한다. 이러한 사건은 처치 제공자가 인식하지 못하는 경우가 많다는 연구 결과가 입증된 만큼 인적 요인이 중요한 역할을 하는 것으로 보인다. 당신 팀에서 이런 일이 발생하지 않도록 한다(**Box 7-6**). 삽관하는 동안 산소포화도를 포함한 활력징후를 모니

Box 7-6 삽관 중 무호흡 산소 공급

새로운 개념은 아니지만, 삽관 중 무호흡 산소 공급은 최근 몇 년 동안 부활을 경험했다. 무호흡 환자의 경우 폐포는 성인의 경우 분당 약 250mL의 산소를 계속 흡수하는 동시에 약 20mL의 이산화탄소를 배출한다. 이렇게 하면 폐에 대기압 이하의 압력이 발생하여 인두에서 폐로 공기가 유입된다. 코삽입관을 통해 분당 약 15L의 산소를 공급하면 인두와 상기도가 채워져 폐로 흐르는 산소의 양이 증가한다. 이산화탄소 저류로 인해 호흡성 산증이 발생하기 시작하지만, 이 술기는 삽관 시도 중 불포화 위험을 줄이는 데 효과적인 것으로 입증되었다.

또 따른 중요한 요소는 삽관을 시도하기 전에 성대 주위에 고여 있는 입안 분비물을 제거하는 것이다. 이는 비디오 후두경을 이용한 삽관을 시행할 때 특히 유용한 것으로 보인다. 외상 환자에게 먼저 흡인을 시행하지 않고 삽관하는 것은 잼이 든 용기 안에서 시계를 고치려고 하는 것과 같다고 한다. 삽관을 여러 번 시도할수록 합병증 발생률이 높아지므로 첫 번째 성공을 목표로 한다는 점을 기억한다.

© National Association of Emergency Medical Technicians (NAEMT)

Box 7-7 기관내삽관 관련 문헌에서 확인된 문제들

- 삽관을 시도하는 동안 저산소증이 자주 발생하며 혈액순환이 좋지 않은 환자에서 산소포화도 신호가 지연되는 경우가 많으므로 인식하지 못하는 경우가 많다.
- 호기말이산화탄소 모니터링에도 불구하고 과다환기가 빈번하게 발생하며 특히 외상성 뇌손상 환자에게는 해로울 수 있다.
- 합병증은 시도 횟수에 비례한다.
- 해결책
  - 삽관을 시도하는 동안 예방산소투여 및 무호흡 산소공급을 통해 산소공급을 최적화한다.
  - 비디오 후두경을 사용하여 첫 번째 삽관 성공률을 높인다.
  - 적절한 속도와 양에 세심한 주의를 기울여 과다환기를 예방한다.

© National Association of Emergency Medical Technicians (NAEMT)

터링할 팀원을 지정한다(**Box 7-7**).

마지막으로 진정제와 양압환기가 정맥혈복귀에 영향을 미치고 혈압을 떨어뜨려 외상성 뇌손상 환자의 사망률을 많이 증가시킬 수 있다는 점을 기억한다. 그러므로 삽관 후 혈압을 포함한 활력징후를 확인하는 것이 삽관 후 처치의 중요한 부분이다. 병원 전 처치 제공자는 혈량저하 환자에게 적절한 수액 소생술을 사용하여 삽관 후 저혈압을 해결할 수 있도록 준비해야 한다.

기관에 튜브를 삽입하는 것만으로는 충분하지 않다. 환자의 생리학적 상태를 최적화하는 것이 목표여야 한다.

적응증

- 안전한 기도 유지가 필요하고 비협조적인 행동으로 인해 삽관이 어려운 환자(저산소증, 외상성 뇌손상, 저혈압 또는 중독 등)

상대적 금기증

- 대체 기도기(예: 성문위기도기)의 사용 가능 여부
- 성공적인 삽관을 방해하거나 방해할 수 있는 심각한 얼굴 외상
- 외과적 기도유지를 복잡하게 하거나 방해하는 목의 변형 또는 부기
- 지시된 약물의 사용을 방해할 수 있는 내과적 문제

절대적 금기증

- 삽관할 수 없음
- 입인두기도기 및 백마스크로 기도를 유지할 수 없음
- 지정된 약물에 대해 알려진 알레르기

합병증

- 진정제나 마비제를 사용한 환자에게 더 이상 기도를 유지하거나 자발 호흡을 할 수 없는 경우 약물을 투여한 후 삽관할 수 없는 환자는 약물이 사라질 때까지 장기간 백마스크로 환기가 필요하다.
- 장시간 삽관을 시도하는 동안 저산소증 또는 고이산화탄소혈증 발생
- 흡인
- 저혈압-거의 모든 약물은 혈압을 낮추는 부작용이 있다.

경증 또는 중증의 혈량저하이지만, 보상을 받고 있는 환자는 기관내삽관에 사용하는 약물의 정맥 내 투여와 관련하여 혈압이 급격히 떨어질 스 있다. 삽관을 위한 약물 사용을 고려할 때는 항상 주의해야 한다(**표 7-4**). 또한 용적이 고갈된 환자는 자발 호흡(활동적 들숨 중 가슴속 음압)에서 양압환기로 전환할 때 저혈압이 되는 경우가 많다.

기관내관 위치 확인

삽관 후 병원 전 처치 제공자는 기관내관이 기관의 올바른 위치에 삽입되었는지 확인하기 위해 구체적인 조처를 해야 한다. 환자에게 삽관을 하고 이완되면 환기와 산소공급이 전적으로 병원 전 처치 제공자에게 달려 있으므로 환기, 산소공급 및 활력징후를 세심하게 모니터링해야 한다. 식도에 기관내관이 의도치 않게 삽입되면 짧은 기간만 인지하지 못해도 심각한 저산소증이 발생하여 뇌손상(저산소성 뇌병증) 및 사망에 이를 수도 있다. 따라서 적절한 삽관 위치를 확인하는 것이 중요하다. 삽관을 확인하는 방법에는 임상 평가와 보조 장치의 사용이 있다. 임상 평가에는 다음이 포함된다.

표 7-4 약물 보조 삽관에서 사용되는 일반적인 약물

	용량(성인)	지속시간	효과	부작용	설명
진정제					
미다졸람	0.1~0.3mg/kg IV	1~2시간	지속성 진정제, 기억상실	호흡억제 무호흡 저혈압	전형적인 유도제, 시작이 다소 느림(최대 3분)
에토미데이트	0.2~0.3mg/kg IV	3~10분	유도 마취	무호흡 저혈압 구토	빠른 시작, 중등도의 저혈압만 유발, 부신 피질 억제
케타민	1~2mg/kg IV	10분	진정 유도 마취 진통제	빈맥 고혈압 두개내압 증가(?)	진정과 진통 효과를 모두 제공, 쇼크 환자에게 최선의 선택 수축기혈압이 정상보다 높은 경우 주의가 필요
프로포폴	1~2mg/kg IV	5~10분	진정 유도 마취	무호흡 저혈압	매우 널리 사용되는 마취제지만 심각한 저혈압 유발 숙련된 의료진이 외상 환자에게 사용
진통제					
펜타닐	2~3mcg/kg IV	20~30분	진통	호흡 억제 무호흡 저혈압	강력하고 빠르게 작용하는 RSI용 전형적인 진통제
모르핀	0.01mg/kg IV	2~3시간	진통	호흡 억제 무호흡 저혈압	매우 느리게(최대 5분) 작용하기 때문에 RSI에 적합하지 않음
케타민*	0.1~0.3mg/kg	10분		환각, 특히 0.5mg/kg 이상 용량	일체형 진통 및 마취제 저용량으로 근긴장도와 및 호흡 억제 없이 탁월한 진통 효과 제공
근이완제					
썩시니콜린	1~2mg/kg IV	3-5분	빠르고(30~60초) 단시간에 작용하는 근육 이완	고칼륨혈증 근섬유다발수축	빠르고 저렴하며 효율적 신경근 질환 환자에게 금기 사항
로큐리늄	0.6~1.2mg/kg IV	30분	빠르고 오래 지속되는 근육 이완		빠르고 효율적 해독제(슈가마덱스) 사용 가능
베큐리늄	0.1mg/kg IV	30~40분	근육 이완	느린 시작	느린 시작(최대 5분)으로 인해 RSI의 두 번째 선택

*전술 제공자를 위한 주의 사항: 환자가 무장 해제되기 전에는 절대로 케타민을 투여하지 않는다.

Abbreviations: IV, intravenous; kg, kilogram; mcg, microgram; mg, milligram; RSI, rapid-sequence intubation; SBP, systolic blood pressure.

- 성대를 통과하는 기관내관을 직접 눈으로 확인
- 양쪽 호흡음(겨드랑이 아래 측면 청진)의 존재 및 명치부위에서 공기음이 없음
- 환기 중 가슴이 오르락내리락하는지 눈으로 확인
- 날숨 시 기관내관의 김이 서림(수증기 응축)이 있음

안타깝게도 이러한 술기 중 어느 것도 적절한 기관내관 위치를 확인하는 데 100% 신뢰할 수 있는 것은 없다. 따라서 가능한 경우 이러한 모든 임상 징후를 평가하고 기록하는 것이 신중한 처치에 포함된다. 드물게 해부학적 구조가 복잡하여 성대를 통과하는 기관내관의 시각화할 수 없는 예도 있다. 움직이는 차량(지상 또는 항고 이송)에서는 엔진 소음으로 인해 호흡음 청진이 거의 불가능할 수 있다. 비만과 만성폐쇄폐질환은 환기 중 가슴 움직임을 보는 것을 방해할 수 있다.

다음과 같은 모니터링 장비를 사용할 수 있다.
- 호기말이산화탄소 모니터링(호기말이산화탄소분압측정)
- 비색이산화탄소 감지기
- 맥박산소측정기

심장 리듬이 있는 환자의 경우 호기말이산화탄소 모니터링(호기말이산화탄소분압측정)은 기관내관의 위치를 확인하기 위한 표준 역할을 한다. 이 방법은 가능하면 병원 전 환경에서 사용해야 한다. 심정지 환자는 심폐소생술이 진행 중이더라도 이산화탄소가 충분히 생성되지 않을 수 있다. 이러한 이유로 비색이산화탄소 감지기나 호기말이산화탄소분압측정은 심장 리듬이 없는 환자에게 제한적으로 사용된다.

이러한 방법 중 어느 것도 보편적으로 신뢰할 수 있는 것은 없으므로 이전에 언급한 임상 평가를 가능한 한 모두 수행해야 한다. 임상 평가 후에는 모니터링 장비 중 하나 이상 사용해야 한다. 적절한 삽관 위치를 확인하는 데 사용되는 방법 중 하나라도 기관내관이 적절하게 삽입되지 않았을 수 있다고 판단되는 경우 기관내관을 즉시 제거했다가 다시 삽입하고 위치를 다시 확인해야 한다. 기관내관 삽입 위치를 확인하는 데 사용되는 모든 방법은 환자 처치 보고서에 적절하게 기록해야 한다.

기관내관 고정

기관내삽관을 시행한 후 기관내관을 손으로 잡고 적절한 튜브 위치를 확인해야 한다. 기관내관은 앞니 중앙에 삽입된 깊이를 확인한 다음 고정하고 기록한다. 시중에 판매되는 여러 제품이 기관내관을 적절하게 고정하는 데 도움이 될 수 있다. 한 연구에 따르면 배꼽 테이프는 상업용 장치만큼 효과적으로 기관내관을 고정하는 것으로 확인되었지만 적절한 매듭과 방법을 사용하여 기관내관 주위에 테이프를 묶어야 한다. 충분한 EMS 인력이 있는 경우 기관재관이 움직이지 않도록 도수로 적절한 위치에 고정하는 작업을 누군가에게 맡기는 것이 이상적이다.

기관내삽관이 필요한 모든 환자에게 지속적인 맥박산소측정을 필수적으로 고려해야 한다. 산소포화도가 감소하거나 청색증이 발생하면 기관내관의 유치를 다시 확인해야 한다. 또한 환자가 움직이는 동안 기관내관이 빠질 수 있다. 환자를 통나무굴리기 방법으로 긴척추고정판으로 이동하거나 구급차에 싣거나 내릴 때 계단으로 이동하는 것과 같이 환자를 움직일 때마다 기관내관의 위치를 다시 확인해야 한다. 모든 환자를 움직이는 동안 팀원 한 명을 지정하여 기관내관의 위치를 유지하고 모니터링하는 것이 중요하다.

삽관된 환자 흡인

기관내관을 통해 삽관된 환자를 흡인할 때는 기관 점막의 손상을 제한하고 마찰 저항을 최소화하기 위해 시중에 판매되는 표준 기관 흡인관을 사용해야 한다. 이 튜브는 인공기도기의 끝을 통과할 수 있을 만큼 충분히 길어야 한다(50~55cm). 부드러운 카테터는 외상 환자의 인두에서 다량의 이물질이나 액체를 흡인하는데 효과적이지 않을 수 있으며 이 경우에 tonsil 팁 또는 Yankauer 팁을 선택할 수 있다. 어떤 경우에도 tonsil 팁 또는 Yankauer 팁을 기관내관 끝에 위치시켜서는 안 된다. 삽관된 환자를 흡인할 때는 무균 절차가 필수적이다. 이 술기에는 다음 단계가 포함된다.

1. 외상 환자에게 100% 산소로 예방산소투여(전산소화)를 한다.
2. 멸균 상태를 유지하면서 장비를 준비한다.
3. 흡인을 시행하지 않으면서 카테터를 삽입한 후 카테터를 빼내면서 흡인을 시작하고 최대 10초 동안 계속한다.
4. 환자에게 산소를 다시 공급하고 보조 환기를 최소 5회 실시한다.
5. 술기 사이에 재산소화가 이루어질 수 있도록 시간을 두고 필요에 따라 이 과정을 반복한다.

대체 방법

세 번의 시도 후에도 기관내삽관에 실패한 경우 앞서 설명한 도수 및

간단한 술기를 사용하여 기도유지를 고려하고 백밸브마스크 장비로 환기하는 것이 적절하다. 환자를 이송할 의료기관까지 가까운 경우, 이송 시간이 짧을 때는 이러한 방법이 기도유지를 위한 가장 신중한 선택이 될 수 있다. 가까운 적절한 의료기관이 더 먼 경우 외과적 반지갑상연골절개를 고려할 수 있다. 다시 말하지만, 저산소증이 오래 지속된 후 추가 뇌손상이 있는 삽관된 환자보다 산소가 충분히 공급된 환자를 기관내관 없이 응급실로 이송하는 것이 더 낫다. 손상된 뇌를 더 손상하는 것은 저산소증이지 기관내관이 삽관되지 않은 상태가 아니라는 점을 기억한다.

외과적 기도유지

외과적 반지갑상연골절개는 후두(갑상연골)와 반지연골 사이에 있는 반지갑상막에 외과적 개구부를 만들고 이를 통해 기관 내강으로 튜브를 삽입한다. 대부분 환자에서 이 부위의 피부가 매우 얇으므로 기도에 즉시 접근할 수 있다. 또한 추가 장비가 비교적 적게 필요하다.

그러나 튜브를 해부학적으로 정확하게 위치시키는 것은 많은 경우 어려운 것으로 입증되었으며 일부 연구에서 부정확한 튜브 위치가 40%에 달하고 합병증도 빈번하게 발생한다.

병원 전 단계에서 이 외과적 기도유지를 시행하는 것은 논란의 여지가 있다. 이 술기에서 합병증이 흔히 발생한다. 반대로 반지갑상연골절개의 성공률이 97%에 달한다는 연구 결과에 따르면 외과적 기도 유지가 최후의 수단으로 여기는 전통적인 관점에 의문이 제기되

었다. 그러나 이 연구에서 사망률은 무려 89%에 달했다. 따라서 병원 전 단계에서 이 술기의 이점과 효능에 관한 문헌은 불분명하다. 현재까지 외과적 반지갑상연골절개술이 병원 전 기도 관리에 일상적 사용에 대한 국가 표준으로 확립되어야 한다는 권고를 뒷받침할 데이터는 충분하지 않다.

이 술기가 실제 현장 상황에서 성공하려면 실제 인체 조직에 대한 훈련이 이루어져야 한다. 현재의 마네킹 및 기타 시뮬레이션 장비는 실제 인체 조직과 환자의 해부학적 느낌을 재현하지 못한다. 병원 전 처치 제공자가 실제 인체 조직에 처음 시행하는 대상이 죽어가는 환자가 되어서는 안 된다. 또한 이 술기는 다른 기도 처치보다 더 많은 연습이 필요하며 실제 응급상황에서 단 몇 초 만에 정확하게 수행하는 데 필요한 해부학적 숙련도와 술기 능력을 유지하기 위해 자주 연습해야 한다. 일반적으로 정확하게 수행할 수 있는 두 번째 기회는 없다. 숙련된 기관내삽관 술기는 대부분 환자에서 외과적 반지갑상연골절개를 고려할 필요성을 극적으로 최소화하므로 이 술기에 대한 훈련에 추가 시간을 할애하는 것의 가치와 그 시간을 기관내삽관 훈련에 사용함으로써 얻을 수 있는 잠재적 이점을 비교 검토해야 한다 (**그림 7-23**).

적응증

- 백마스크 장치를 사용할 수 없는 심한 얼굴중간 및 입안 외상이 있는 경우

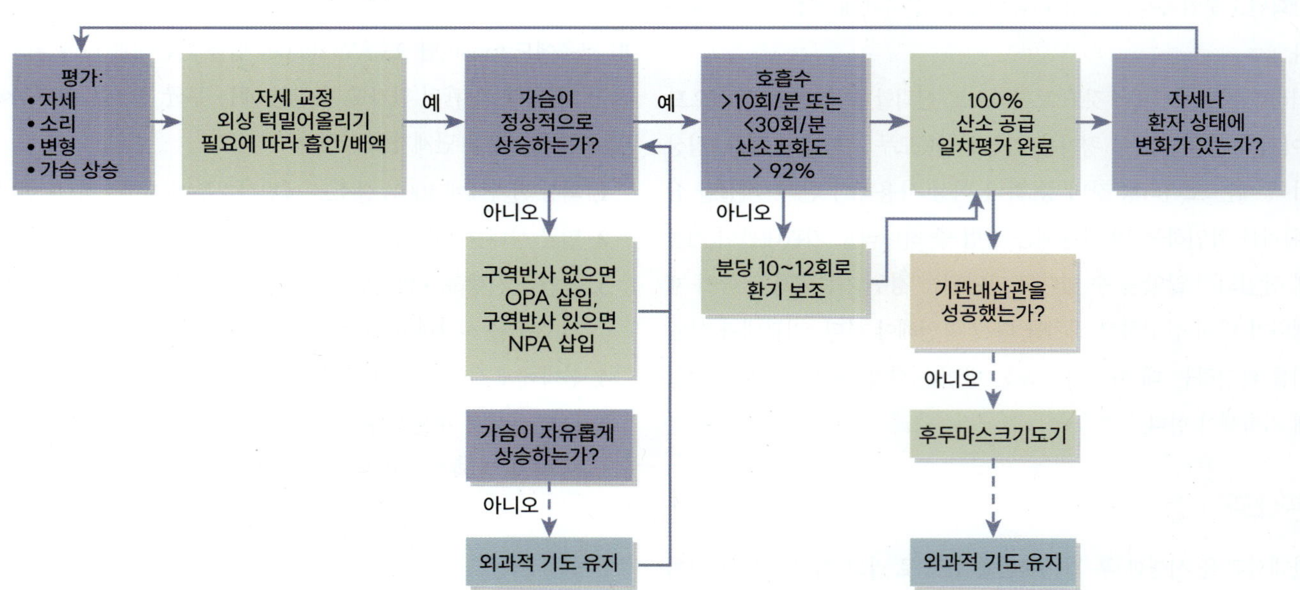

그림 7-23 외과적 기도 관리 시스템

© National Association of Emergency Medical Technicians (NAEMT)

- 덜 침습적인 조작으로 기도를 유지할 수 없는 경우

금기증

- 입 또는 코로 안전하게 삽관할 수 있는 모든 환자
- 후두기관 손상이 있는 환자
- 10세 미만의 어린이
- 외상성 또는 감염성 급성 후두 질환이 있는 환자
- 불충분한 교육

합병증

- 시술 시간 지연
- 출혈
- 흡인
- 기관내관의 잘못된 위치 또는 잘못된 삽관
- 목 구조 또는 혈관 손상
- 식도 천공

환기

기도를 확보한 후 다음 단계는 적절한 환기를 시행하는 것이다. 호흡에 필요한 네 가지 요소는 기도 개방, 정상적인 가슴우리, 기능적인 호흡근, 산소를 흡수하는 건강한 폐이다.

불안정한 가슴벽, 심각한 기흉 또는 호흡근 약화와 같은 대부분의 외상성 질환의 가장 즉각적인 영향은 일회호흡량의 급격한 감소이다. 산소 확산 감소와 같은 더 복잡한 문제는 대부분 중환자실 입원 후반에 발생하며 처치하기는 어렵지만, 병원 전 단계에서는 거의 문제가 되지 않는다. 일회호흡량의 급격한 감소는 현장에서 직면하는 일차적인 환기 문제이다.

일차평가 중에 환기를 평가하려면 다음을 확인하는 것이 중요하다.

- 일회호흡량. 가슴을 본다. 환자가 공기를 얼마나 효과적으로 이동시키고 있는가? 가슴이 어떻게 팽창하고 있는가? 환자가 의식이 있는 경우 언어의 질은 어떠한가??(예: 전체 문장을 말할 수 있는가? 아니면 한 번에 몇 단어만 말할 수 있는가?).
- 가슴우리를 평가한다. 변형이나 불안정성 또는 개방 상처가 있는가? 오른쪽과 왼쪽이 대칭적으로 확장되어 있는가? 가슴벽의 모순 운동이 있는가?
- 호흡수. 호흡수를 대략적으로 추정한다. 호흡이 정상, 빠름, 매우 빠름, 느림 중 어디에 해당하는가?

- 양쪽 가슴에서 호흡음을 청진한다. 양쪽에서 호흡음이 들리는가?
- 산소포화도. 산소포화도는 호흡 과정의 효과를 측정하는 척도이므로 모니터링한다. 동맥혈에 산소가 공급되지 않으면 성공적인 소생술이 불가능하다.

초기 평가 후에는 환자의 상태가 매우 빠르게 변화할 수 있으며 지속적인 환기 모니터링이 필수적이라는 점을 기억하는 것이 중요하다.

임상 검사 외에도 환기의 효과를 지속해서 모니터링하는 데 매우 유용한 두 가지 장비가 있는데, 바로 맥박산소측정기와 파형 호기말 이산화탄소분압측정이다.

모니터링

맥박산소측정

맥박산소측정기의 사용은 병원 전 환경에서 보편화되고 표준이 되었다. 사실 이 기술은 일반인도 사용할 수 있다. 맥박산소측정기를 적절히 사용하면 다른 신체적 징후가 나타나기 전에 폐 손상이나 심혈관 기능 저하를 조기에 발견할 수 있다. 맥박산소측정기는 높은 신뢰성, 휴대성, 적용 용이성 및 모든 연령대와 인종에 걸쳐 적용할 수 있으므로 병원 전 단계에서 특히 유용하다.

맥박산소측정기로 산소포화도와 맥박수를 측정한다. 산소포화도는 조직을 통과한 적색광과 적외선의 흡수 비율을 측정하여 결정된다. 소형 마이크로프로세서는 혈액이 혈관을 통과할 때 발생하는 광흡수 변화를 연관시켜 동맥 포화도와 맥박수를 결정한다. 정상 산소포화도는 해수면에서 94%를 초과한다. 헤모글로빈의 해리 곡선으로 인해 산소포화도가 90% 이하로 떨어지면 조직으로의 산소 전달 효율이 급격히 저하될 수 있다(**그림 7-24**). 높은 고도에서 작업할 때는 허용 가능한 산소포화도 수준이 해수면보다 낮다. 병원 전 처치 제공자는 고지대에서 처치할 경우 허용할 수 있는 산소포화도 수치가 어느 정도인지 알고 있어야 한다.

정확한 맥박산소측정값을 얻으려면 다음과 같은 일반 지침을 따라야 한다.

1. 적절한 크기와 유형의 센서를 사용한다.
2. 센서 조명이 올바르게 정렬되었는지 확인한다.
3. 광원과 광검출기가 깨끗하고 건조하며 상태가 양호한지 확인한다.
4. 심한 부종이 있는 부위에 센서를 배치하지 않는다.
5. 필요한 경우 매니큐어를 제거한다.

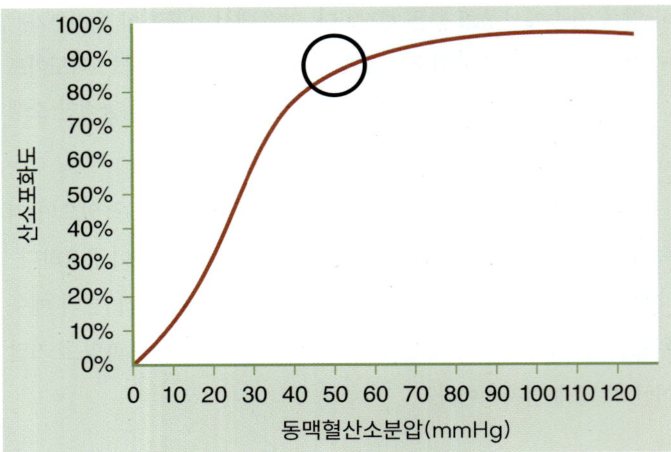

그림 7-24 맥박산소측정기. 대부분의 맥박산소측정기는 산소포화도뿐만 아니라 맥박수도 표시한다. 산소포화도 90%는 단순히 100%에서 10%를 뺀 값이 아니라는 점을 이해하는 것이 중요하다. 그보다는 불포화가 매우 빠르게 진행되는 전환점을 나타낸다.
© National Association of Emergency Medical Technicians (NAEMT)

6. 손가락과 센서를 알루미늄 포일로 감싸면 손가락 끝을 따뜻하게 하고 센서가 간섭받지 않도록 보호할 수 있다.

산소포화도 측정이 부정확해질 수 있는 일반적인 문제는 다음과 같다.

- 과도한 움직임
- 측정기 센서의 습기
- 부적절한 센서 적용 및 배치
- 저체온증/저혈량증으로 인한 환자 관류 불량 또는 혈관 수축
- 빈혈
- 일산화탄소 중독

중증외상 환자의 경우 모세혈관 관류 상태가 좋지 않고 급성 출혈과 관련된 빈혈로 인해 맥박산소측정이 정확하지 않을 수 있다. 따라서 맥박산소측정기는 외상의 병태생리학에 대한 지식과 평가 및 중재 기술이 결합한 경우에만 병원 전 처치 제공자가 추가할 수 있는 유용한 장비이다. 외상 환자를 처치하는 병원 전 처치 제공자는 팔다리에서 맥박산소측정기가 작동하지 않는 것 같으면 즉시 의문을 제기하고 문제가 맥박산소측정기인지 아니면 조직 관류(쇼크) 불량인지 고려해야 한다.

호기말이산화탄소분압

호기말이산화탄소분압 또는 호기말이산화탄소($ETCO_2$) 모니터링은 수년 동안 중환자실에서 사용됐으며 대부분의 EMS에서 일반적으로 사용하고 있다.

날숨에서 CO_2를 감지하면 환자가 대사가 활발하여 대사의 부산물로 CO_2를 생성할 수 있다는 것을 확인할 수 있다. 또한 날숨 중 CO_2가 존재한다는 것은 폐로 CO_2를 가져올 수 있는 충분한 순환이 계속되고 있으며 효과적인 폐포 환기 및 공기 교환이 일어나고 있음을 확인한다(그림 7-25).

환자에게 삽관되었거나 성문위기도기를 사용할 때 기도가 단단히 밀폐된 상황에서 $ETCO_2$를 측정할 수 있다. 이 경우 파형 호기말이산화탄소분압을 정확한 곡선으로 표시된다(그림 7-26A).

반면 기도에 밀착하지 않고 자발적으로 호흡하는 환자에서 측정하는 경우(예: 코 호기말이산화탄소분압) 곡선의 정확도가 떨어진다(그림 7-26B). 그런데도 코 호기말이산화탄소분압은 대략적인 관류 및 환기 효과를 제공할 수 있다. 또한 호흡수를 모니터링하는 데 도움이 되는 도구를 제공한다.

최근 기술의 발전으로 병원 전 단계에서 사용할 수 있는 더 작고 내구성이 뛰어난 장치를 생산할 수 있게 되었다. 호기말이산화탄소분압측정은 가스 샘플에서 이산화탄소의 비율을 측정하고, 기계는 이 비율(%)을 이산화탄소의 분압(mmHg)으로 변환한다. 말초 관류가 양호한 환자의 날숨이 끝날 때 이 샘플을 채취하면($ETCO_2$) 동맥혈이산화탄소분압($PaCO_2$)과 밀접한 상관관계가 있다. 그러나 관류가 손상된 다발성 외상 환자의 경우 $ETCO_2$와 $PaCO_2$의 상관관계는 훨씬 덜 신뢰할 수 있다.

중증 환자의 경우 $PaCO_2$은 일반적으로 $ETCO_2$보다 2~5mmHg 더 높다(정상적인 $ETCO_2$ 수치는 30~40mmHg). 이러한 수치가 환자의 $PaCO_2$를 완전히 반영하지 못할 수도 있지만, 정상 범위 내에서 수치를 유지하기 위해 노력하는 것이 일반적으로 환자에게 도움이 될 수 있다.

실용적인 관점에서 호기말이산화탄분압은 적절한 튜브 위치를 모니터링하기 위한 최고의 표준이며 기관내관의 이탈 또는 관류 감소

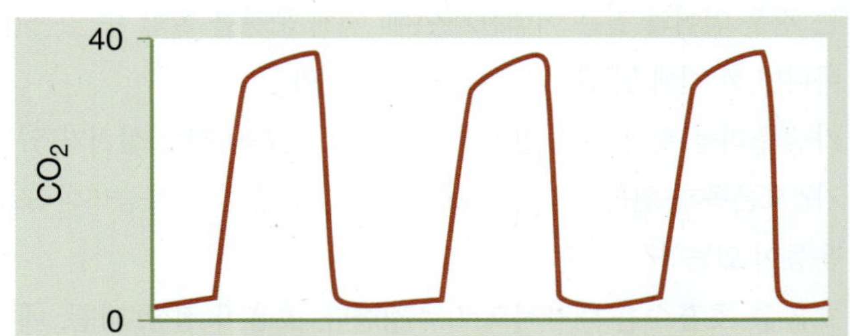

그림 7-25 정상 호기말이산화탄소분압측정 파형.
© plo/Shutterstock

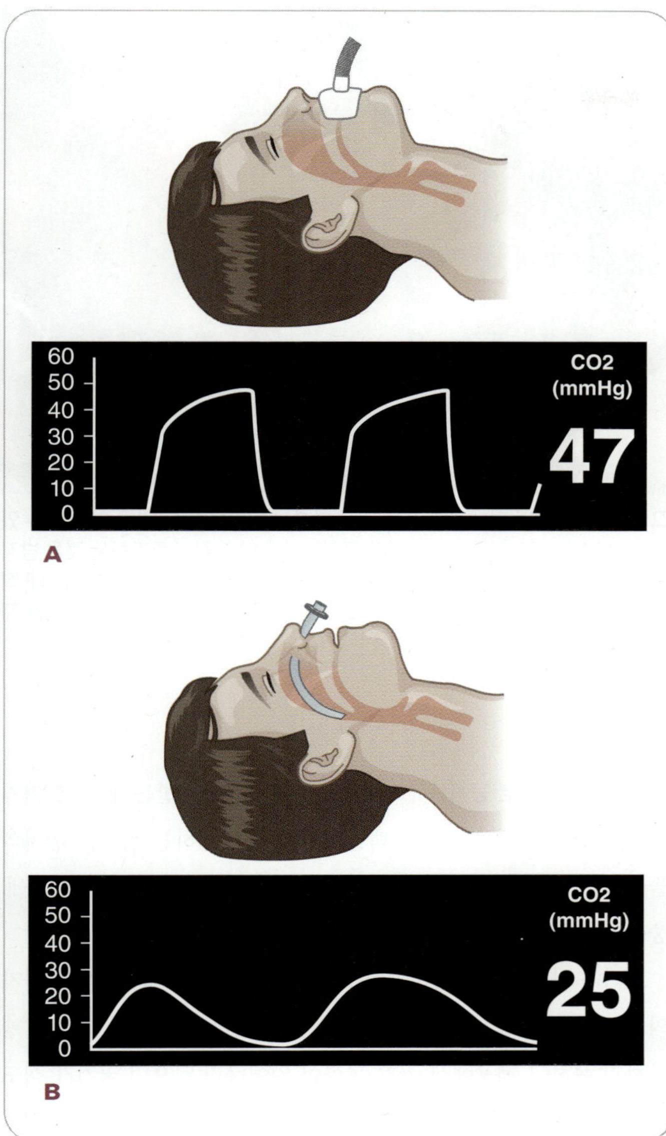

그림 7-26   A. 기도 삽관 환자와 같이 기도를 단단히 밀봉한 상태에서 호기말이산화탄소분압측정을 하면 4단계의 정밀한 곡선을 얻을 수 있다. **B.** 자발 환기 중에 코삽입관과 함께 사용하면 이산화탄소가 희석되어 곡선이 둥글어진다. 그러나 곡선의 모양을 통해 공기 교환이 일어나고 있음을 확인하고 환기 속도를 추정할 수 있다. 또한 기준선이 0으로 내려가지 않으면 산소 흐름이 불충분하여 재호흡이 발생하고 있음을 나타낼 수 있다.

© National Association of Emergency Medical Technicians (NAEMT)

로 인해 배출된 이산화탄소가 갑자기 감소하면 환자의 상태와 기관내관의 위치를 재평가해야 한다는 것을 기억한다. ETCO₂는 폐 내에서 공기 교환이 일어나고 있는지를 판단하는 궁극적인 도구이다. 전문 기도유지 술기를 시행할 때 CO₂ 모니터를 사용하는 것이 EMS의 표준 관행이다.

산소공급 최적화

폐가 실내 공기에서 충분한 산소를 공급받지 못할 때 폐의 산소 압력을 높이는 한 가지 방법은 들숨 공기의 산소 비율을 높이는 것이다. 이는 폐모세혈관막을 통과하여 혈류로 들어가 헤모글로빈 분자에 부착하는 산소 분자의 가용성을 증가시키는 효과가 있다.

환자가 흡입하는 산소의 양을 늘리기 위해 일반적으로 사용되는 장비에는 코삽입관과 비재호흡마스크(NRB)가 있다.

코삽입관

코삽입관은 콧구멍에 삽입하여 공기와 보충 산소가 혼합된 혼합물이 흐르는 두 개의 갈래가 있는 가벼운 관으로 구성된다. 일반적으로 분당 2~6L의 산소 유량을 공급하며 최대 흡입산소농도(FiO₂)는 0.4이다. 코호기말이산화탄소분압은 입으로 숨을 쉬는 환자에게 잠재적으로 이점이 적을 수 있다.

고유량 코삽입관을 사용하여 전달되는 산소의 농도를 증가시킬 수 있지만, 이는 병원 전 환경에서는 일반적으로 사용할 수 없다.

비재호흡마스크

비재호흡마스크는 산소 공급원에 연결되어 코와 입을 완전히 덮는 얼굴 마스크로 구성된다. 다양한 어댑터(예: 벤투리 어댑터)를 장착하여 더 정확한 비율로 산소를 공급할 수 있다.

비재호흡마스크는 저장주머니와 함께 사용할 수 있다. 이 경우 마스크는 고능도 산소로 채워진 플라스틱 저장주머니에 연결되며 내쉬는 공기가 산소 저장주머니로 다시 들어가는 것을 방지하는 일방향 밸브가 있다. 비재호흡마스크 자체에는 배출된 공기가 마스크에 재유입되는 것을 방지하는 밸브가 장착되어 있다. 저장주머니에 항상 산소가 채워져 있는지 확인하는 것이 중요하다. 그렇지 않으면 환자가 공기를 충분히 흡입할 수 없어 호흡 곤란이 심해질 수 있으며 환자는 더 쉽게 호흡하기 위해 마스크를 벗으려고 시도하는 경우가 종종 있다. 연구에 따르면 비재호흡마스크는 의식이 있는 환자의 보조 환기 보다 견딜 수 있지만, 산소 공급 개선 효과는 떨어진다.

환기 최적화

산소 보충의 목표는 폐 내부의 산소 비율을 증가시켜 폐포 산소화를 개선하고 산소포화도를 증가시키는 것이다. 그러나 환기가 충분하지 않으면 CO₂가 계속 축적된다. 결과적으로 PaCO₂가 증가하고 호흡수도 증가한다. 이러한 호흡수 증가는 동맥혈산소분압(PaO_2)이 개선된 상황에서도 전반적인 호흡 기능이 부적절하다는 신호이다.

저환기가 심한 경우 폐포 환기를 유지하기 위한 공기 교환이 불충분해지며 흡입 산소가 100%인 상황에서도 산소공급이 감소하기 시작한다. 흡입된 산소가 폐포까지 사강을 충분히 통과하지 못하면 이를 적절하게 보상할 수 없다. 환기 속도가 증가하면서 FiO_2가 100%인 환자의 산소포호도가 감소하는 것은 환기 허탈이 가깝다는 경고이다. 마찬가지로 호흡수가 너무 낮아(분당 10회 미만) 충분한 분당 환기를 제공하지 못하는 경우 폐포에 산소를 공급하기 위해 일회호흡량을 증가시켜야 한다. 이를 위해서는 환기를 적극적으로 보조하거나 양압환기로 완전히 전환해야 한다.

일회호흡량을 확인하는 것은 환기를 평가하는 데 중요한 부분이다. 정상적인 호흡은 눈에 띄지 않는다. 정상적으로 호흡을 하는 환자는 일반적으로 완전한 문장으로 말할 수 있지만, 완전한 문장으로 말할 수 없거나 호흡이 힘들어 보이는 환자의 경우 가슴 확장을 평가하는 것이 중요하다.

다음을 사용하여 환기를 부분적으로 교정할 수 있다.

- 자세 최적화. 앉은 자세는 호흡근을 최적으로 사용할 수 있게 해주며 운동선수들이 숨을 고르기 위해 앉는 이유가 바로 여기에 있다. 특히 과체중 환자의 경우 앉으면 가로막에 가해지는 압력을 줄일 수 있다. 저혈압이나 등허리 척추 외상의 가능성으로 인해 이 방법의 적용이 제한하기 때문에 외상 환자에게는 이 방법의 유용성이 상대적으로 제한된다. 그러나 환자를 역트렌델렌버그 자세로 눕히면 가로막의 부담을 덜어주고 호흡이 개선되는 경우가 많다.
- 개방 기흉을 인식하고 밀봉한다(10장 가슴 외상 참조).
- 긴장기흉 처치. 이것은 폐 확장을 막는 압력을 완화하기 위한 핵심적인 처치이다(10장 가슴 외상 참조)

그래도 일회호흡량이 충분하지 않으면 보조 환기가 필요하다.

보조 환기

완전히 무호흡 상태인 심정지 환자에게 환기하는 것과는 달리 외상 환자는 가슴 손상이나 뇌손상으로 인해 호흡 노력이 효과가 없는 경우에도 호흡을 계속 시도하는 경우가 많다. 환기를 완전히 조절하는 것은 일반적으로 진정된 환자나 심각한 뇌손상을 입은 환자에게만 가능하다. 대부분은 호흡이 부적절한 환자에게 환기를 보조해야 하며 이 작업은 어려울 수 있다(**그림 7-27**).

정상적인 들숨 동안 가슴 팽창은 가슴 내부의 압력을 대기압 이하

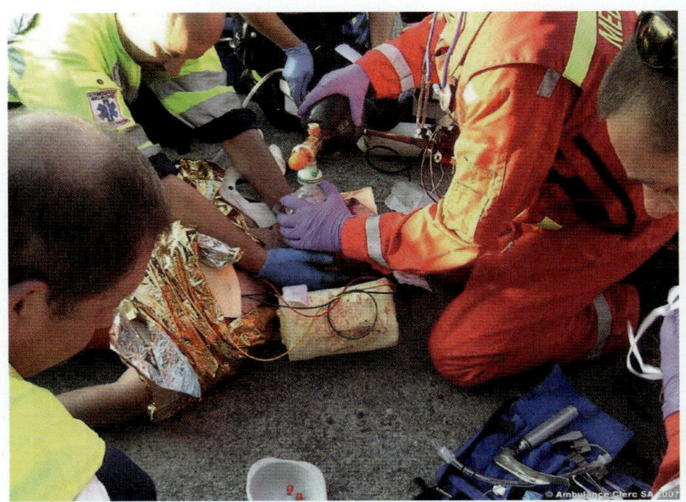

그림 7-27 부적절하게 호흡하는 외상 환자의 환기를 돕는 일은 어려울 수 있다. 구조자는 식도로 공기가 강제로 유입되어 흡인 위험이 증가하는 것을 방지하기 위해 환자의 호흡 주기에 맞춰 적절한 밀폐를 유지하고 백을 짜는 데 집중해야 한다. 환자에게 효과적으로 보조 환기를 시행하기 위해서는 술기를 지속해서 연습해야 한다.

Courtesy of J.C. Pitteloud MD, Switzerland.

로 낮추어 기도로 공기를 끌어들이는 기압 경도를 만든다. 보조 환기를 사용하면 적절한 시기에 백을 쥐어짜서 발생하는 압력이 환자의 들숨 시도로 생성되는 음압 경사도에 추가되어 폐를 팽창시키기에, 충분한 누적 압력을 생성한다.

그러나 타이밍이 정확하지 않고 백을 짜서 전달되는 압력이 환자의 숨을 내쉬려는 시도에 따른 경사도에 반하여 가해지면 폐가 팽창하지 못하고 폐포에서 공기 교환이 일어나지 않으며 공기가 식도와 위장으로 강제로 들어가 역류와 구토, 흡인으로 이어질 가능성이 있다.

따라서 환기를 성공적으로 수행하기 위해서는 타이밍과 조정이 중요한 요소이다.

백마스크 환기

앞서 설명한 세 가지 방법을 사용한 후 또는 병원 전 환경에서 환기를 최적화하기 위한 첫 번째 처치는 백마스크 장치이다. 백마스크 장치는 자체 팽창식 백과 비재호흡 밸브로 구성되어 있으며 입인두기도기나 코인두기도기를 삽입한 후 얼굴에 마스크를 밀착시켜 사용하거나 백과 마스크를 분리하여 전문기도기(LMA, 기관내, 코기관)에 백을 연결하여 사용할 수 있다. 대부분의 백마스크 장치의 용량은 1,600mL이고 90~100%의 산소 농도를 전달할 수 있다. 일부 모델

에는 비색 이산화탄소 감지기가 내장되어 있거나 마스크와 밸브 또는 튜브와 밸브 사이에 이러한 감지기를 추가할 수도 있다. 그러나 병원 전 처치 제공자 한 명이 비침습적 마스크를 충분히 밀폐한 상태에서 환자에게 환기를 시도하는 경우 효과적으로 환기를 제공하는 경우는 거의 없다. 이 술기가 효과적이고 환자가 적절한 환기 지원을 받을 수 있도록 하려면 이 술기를 지속해서 연습해야 한다.

자발적인 호흡 노력이 부족한 진정 또는 마비된 환자에게는 일반적으로 환기를 조절하는 것이 필요하다. 연구에 따르면 병원 전 처치 제공자가 가장 빈번하게 저지르는 실수는 과도한 일회호흡량과 빠른 속도로 환기를 시행하여 환자에게 과호흡하는 것이며 이는 저이산화탄소혈증, 복귀정맥혈 감소, 평균 기도 압력 상승, 삽관을 시행하지 않을 경우 위 팽창을 초래할 수 있다.

백마스크 환기를 시행하는 병원 전 처치 제공자는 신중하게 교육을 받아야 한다. 팽창량은 가슴이 눈에 띄게 상승할 수 있을 정도로 충분해야 하며 환기 속도와 호기말이산화탄소를 주의 깊게 모니터링해야 한다.

성인의 경우 분당 10~12회, 소아의 경우 분당 25회, 영아의 경우 분당 30회의 환기 속도로 시행해야 한다.

양압환기기

이송 지연 중 양압식 용적 환기기는 병원 전 단계 및 항공 의료 환경에서 오랫동안 사용됐다. 이송 시간이 짧은 대부분의 민간 환경에서는 간단하고 비교적 저렴한 용적 환기기를 사용한다. 이러한 환기기는 병원에서 사용하는 것만큼 정교할 필요가 없으며 다음 부문에서 설명된 대로 몇 가지 간단한 환기 기능만 있다.

보조 제어 환기

보조 제어(A/C) 환기는 현장에서 응급실까지 병원 전 이송 시 가장 널리 사용되는 환기 형식이다. 보조 제어 설정은 사전에 설정된 속도와 일회호흡량으로 환기를 제공한다. 환자가 스스로 호흡을 시작하면 전체 일회호흡량의 추가적인 환기가 제공되어 숨이 차고 폐가 과팽창할 수 있다.

간헐필수 환기

간헐필수 환기(IMV)는 환자에게 설정된 호흡수와 일회호흡량을 제공한다. 환자가 스스로 호흡을 시작하면 환자가 스스로 당기는 양만큼만 전달된다.

호기말양압

호기말양압(PEEP)은 호기 말기에 높은 수준의 압력을 제공하여 호기 주기가 끝날 때 폐포 허탈을 감소시킨다. 이러한 개입은 산소 공급 개선을 촉진한다. 그러나 호기말 압력을 증가시켜 전체 가슴 내 압력을 증가시킴으로써 매우 높은 수준의 PEEP은 심장으로 정맥혈 복귀를 감소시킬 수 있다. 출혈로 인해 혈량저하 상태인 환자의 경우 PEEP 수치가 높으면 혈압이 너 낮아질 수 있다. 외상성 뇌손상이 있는 환자에게서도 높은 PEEP 수치는 피해야 한다. 가슴 압력이 증가하면 두개내압의 상승을 유발할 수 있다. 반대로 외상성 뇌손상 환자는 저산소증에 특히 민감하므로 이러한 환자에게 PEEP을 신중하게 사용하는 것이 도움이 될 수 있다.

기계적 환기를 위한 초기 설정

속도

호흡이 없는 성인 환자의 경우 처음에는 분당 10~12회의 호흡 속도로 설정한다. 환자를 자세히 모니터링하여 호기말이산화탄소 수치가 정한 범위 내에 있는지 확인해야 한다.

일회호흡량

일회호흡량은 환자 표준 체중의 5~7mL/kg을 사용하여 설정한다. 표준 체중은 체질량이 아닌 환자의 성별과 키로 계산한다. 이것은 지침으로 사용되어야 하며 외상 환자에서 조정이 필요할 수도 있다.

호기말양압(PEEP)

이 방법을 사용할 때는 처음에 5cmH$_2$O로 설정해야 한다. 이 설정은 삽관 전 기도에 정상적으로 존재하는 PEEP의 양인 생리적 PEEP을 유지한다. 삽관 후에는 이론적으로 이 양의 양압이 제거된다. 외상성 손상이 악화할수록 더 많은 양의 PEEP이 필요할 수 있지만, 손상 후 처음 몇 시간 동안은 거의 발생하지 않는다. 병원 전 처치 제공자는 병원 간 이송 중에 높은 수준의 PEEP이 필요한 환자를 만날 수 있다. 이송 전 병원의 의료진은 이러한 수준의 PEEP을 설정했을 것이다. 정상적인 생리학적 PEEP 값의 범위는 5~10cmH$_2$O이다. 더 많이 PEEP을 사용할수록 부작용의 위험이 커진다. PEEP이 증가하면 다음과 같은 부작용이 발생할 수 있으므로 주의 깊은 모니터링이 필요하다.

- 정맥혈복귀 감소로 인한 혈압 감소
- 두개내압 증가
- 기흉으로 이어지는 가슴속 압력 증가 또는 긴장기흉

산소 농도

외상 환자의 산소 농도는 해수면에서 94% 이상의 포화도를 유지하도록 설정해야 한다. 100% 흡입산소농도로 시작하여 93~98% 포화도의 산소포화도를 달성하는 데 필요한 최소 농도까지 낮추는 것이 현명하다. 장기간이 고산소혈증(산소포화도 100% 및 동맥혈산소분압 150mmHg 이상)은 산화 손상을 초래할 수 있으므로 피해야 한다는 인식이 점점 더 확산하고 있다.

고압 알람/팝 오프

고압 알람 및 압력 완화 팝 오프는 환자에게 정상적으로 환기를 하는 데 필요한 압력(최대 흡기 압력)보다 10cmH2O 이상 높지 않게 설정해야 한다. 40cmH2O 이상으로 알람을 설정할 때는 주의해야 한다. 이 수치를 초과하면 압력 손상과 기흉이 발생할 가능성이 더 높아지는 것으로 나타났다. 원하는 일회호흡량을 전달하기 위해 40cmH2O 이상의 압력이 필요한 경우 기도와 사전 설정된 일회호흡량을 재평가해야 한다. 이 경우 같은 폐포의 미세한 환기를 유지하기 위해 일회호흡량을 줄이고 속도를 높이는 것이 현명한 조치일 수 있다.

다른 경보와 마찬가지로 고압 경보가 몇 번 이상 계속 활성화되면 인공호흡기에서 환자를 제거하고 인공호흡기 회로와 기관내관을 확인하는 동안 백마스크 장비를 이용해 수동으로 환기해야 한다. 또한 환자는 순응도 감소(같은 압력에 대해 더 적은 양의 공기를 이동시키는 것)에 대해 재평가해야 한다. 이러한 순응도 감소는 여러 가지 요인으로 인해 발생할 수 있다. 외상 환자의 순응도 감소의 흔한 초기 원인으로는 발생한 긴장기흉일 수 있다. 긴장기흉은 지시에 따라 바늘감압으로 처치한다. 기침을 하거나 인공호흡기와 맞서는 환자는 인공호흡기와 비동시성을 보이는 것으로 추가적인 진정제 투여 또는 인공호흡기 설정 변경이 필요할 수 있다. 다른 잠재적인 문제로는 기관내관의 변위 또는 막힘이 있다. 어떤 경우에도 병원 전 처치 제공자는 단순히 상한 압력 제한과 알람을 계속 높여서는 안 된다. 기본적인 인공호흡기 설명 목록은 **Box 7-8**에서 확인할 수 있다.

저압 경보

저압 알람은 환자와 인공호흡기 사이의 연결이 끊어지거나 인공호흡기 회로의 누출로 인해 상당한 양이 손실되거나 기도 장치가 이탈되면 병원 전 처치 제공자에게 경고한다. 대부분의 이동식 인공호흡기에서는 이 알람이 사전 설정되어 있으며 조정할 수 없다. 인공호흡기 문제 해결은 **Box 7-9**를 참조한다.

양압환기의 부정적인 영향

생리학적 조건에서 가슴 내부의 압력은 들숨 시 음압과 날숨 시 중간 또는 약간 양압 사이에서 진동한다. 환자가 삽관되어 양압환기(백 밸브 장치 또는 기계식 환기)를 하게 되면 측정된 가슴속 압력은 현저하게 양압이 된다. 병원 전 처치 제공자는 이러한 변화를 인지하고 그 결과를 이해하며 환자의 생리학적 변화에 대응할 준비를 하는 것이 매우 중요하다. 심장으로 돌아가는 정맥혈의 주요 구성 요소는 정상적인 호흡 주기 동안 가슴 내에서 발생하는 음압이다. 삽관과 양압은 이 압력 기울기를 반대 방향으로 바꾸어 정맥혈복귀와 심장 기능에 즉각적이고 현저한 영향을 미칠 수 있다. 가슴 압력의 이러한 큰 변화의 일반적인 증상은 삽관에 동반되는 저혈압이다. 폐와 가슴에 일정한 양압이 유지되는 것은 폐활량이 큰 건강한 환자에게는 잘 견딜 수 있지만, 외상이 발생하면 그렇지 않을 수 있다. 외상 환자가 출혈 또는 혈관 내 용적 변화로 인해 혈량저하 상태면 삽관 과정에서 심각한 저혈압이 발생할 수 있다. 심한 경우 혈량저하 환자의 삽관 순서는 삽관에 사용된 마비제의 부정적인 효과(부정적인 심장 수축 촉

Box 7-8　기본 환기기 설정

- 일회호흡량: 5~7mL/kg(이상 체중)
- 환기 속도: 10~12회/분
- 흡입산소농도(FiO2): 처음에는 100%, 이후 점차 줄여 산소포화도 > 94% 유지
- 최고 압력 알람: 28cmH2O
- 저압 알람: 정상 최고 압력보다 5cmH2O 낮을 때까지

Box 7-9　환기기 문제 해결: DOPE

- 먼저 환자를 확인한다. 환기 장치에서 환자를 분리하고 수동으로 환기를 시행한다. 그런 다음 DOPE 약어를 사용하여 확인한다.
  - 변위(Displacement). 튜브의 깊이를 확인, 치아 아케이드와의 거리는 튜브 길이의 3배여야 한다.
  - 폐색(Obstruction). 흡인 카테터를 튜브 끝까지 넣어 튜브가 꼬이거나 막히지 않았는지 확인한다.
  - 기흉(Pneumothorax). 양쪽 폐를 청진하여 기흉을 배제한다.
  - 장비(Equipment). 환기기를 확인하면서 환자에게 수동으로 환기한다.
- 항상 환자를 먼저 확인한다.

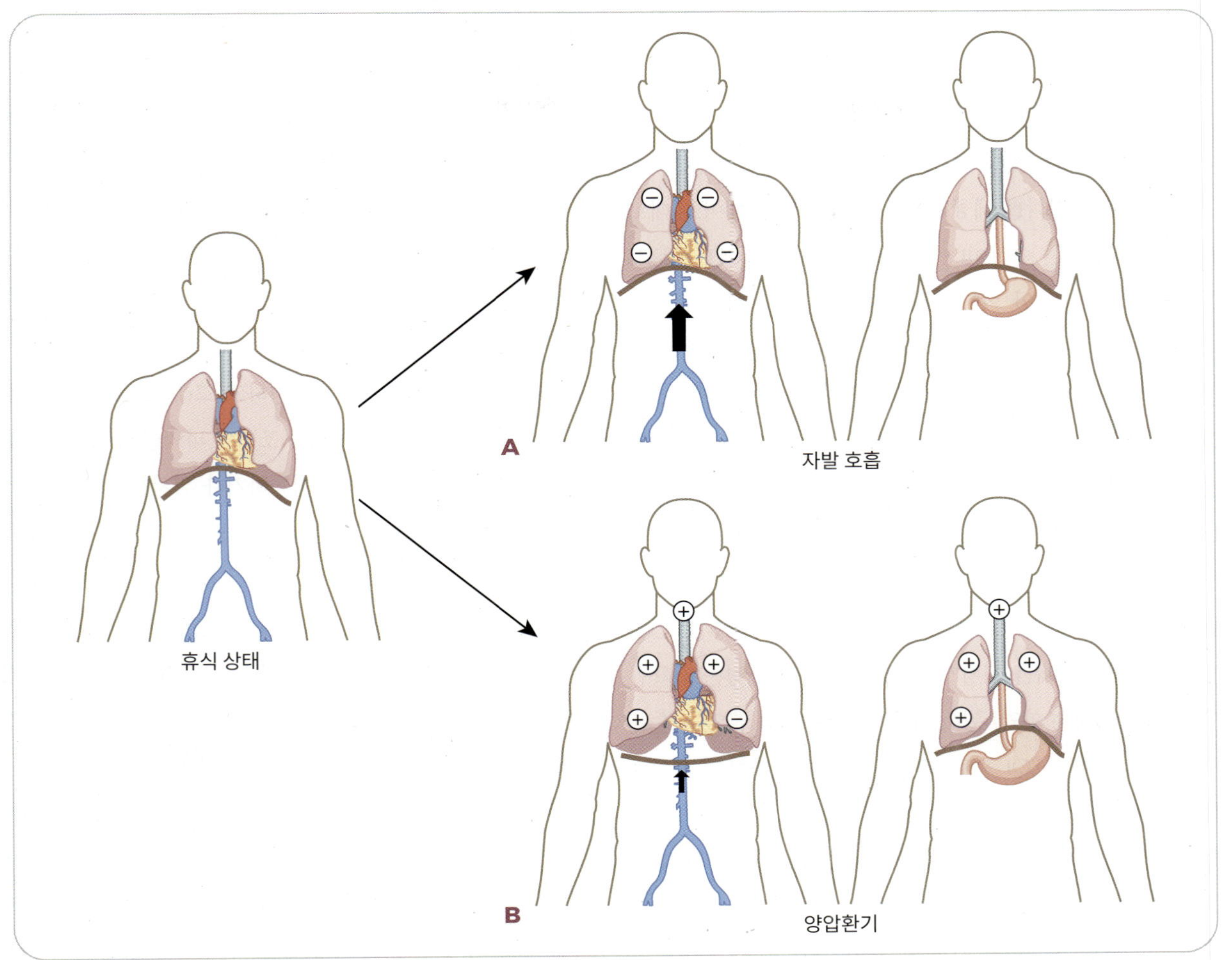

그림 7-28 음압 환기와 양압환기에 대한 생리학적 및 해부학적 반응 **A.** 정상적인 들숨 시 가로막이 내려가고 흉곽이 확장되면서 가슴 내부에 음압이 발생하여 대정맥에서 심장으로 혈액을 끌어당긴다. **B.** 양압환기를 적용하면 가슴에 양압이 생성되어 정맥혈복귀가 감소한다. 또한 공기가 위장으로 강제 유입되어 과잉팽창이 발생하고 가로막이 위쪽으로 변위될 수 있다.

© National Association of Emergency Medical Technicians (NAEMT)

진 효과)와 심장으로의 정맥혈복귀(전부하)의 현저한 감소가 결합하여 혈량저하 심정지를 초래할 수 있다(**그림 7-28**).

- 가슴에 지속적인 양압이 가해지면 심장으로의 정맥혈복귀가 감소한다. 이것은 급성 혈액 손실로 인해 혈량저하증을 겪고 있는 환자에게 특히 문제가 된다.
- 기흉이 있는 경우 폐 내부에 양압을 가하면 기흉의 크기와 심각성이 증가하고 긴장기흉이 발생할 위험이 현저히 증가한다.
- 삽관되지 않은 환자가 양압 호흡을 하는 동안 숨을 내쉬려고 하면 기도 내부의 압력이 상승하고 전달된 호흡은 저항이 가장 작은 경로를 따라 위장으로 향하게 된다.
- 관통성 가슴 외상 시 종종 발생하는 폐 열상이 있는 경우 적어도 이론적으로 기흉의 위험이 있다.

삽관의 지속적인 품질 개선

외상 환자의 병원 전 삽관의 효과에 대한 의문이 계속 제기되고 있으므로 병원 전 시스템의 관리 감독은 모든 병원 외 삽관 또는 침습적 기도유지 술기 사용과 관련된 에피소드를 지속해 검토하는 것이 중요하다. 특히 삽관 시도를 쉽게 하려고 약물을 사용하면 더욱 그렇다. 구체적인 사항은 다음과 같다.

- 프로토콜 및 절차 준수
- 삽관 시도 횟수
- 튜브 삽입 위치 확인 및 확인을 위해 사용된 절차
- 결과 및 합병증
- 유도제 사용 시 적절한 사용 적응증 확인

- 약물 투여 경로에 대한 적절한 기록 및 삽관 중 또는 삽관 후 환자 모니터링
- 삽관 전, 삽관 중, 삽관 후의 활력징후

효과적인 지속적 품질 개선(CQI) 프로그램은 환자에게 안전하고 효과적이며 가치 있는 기회를 제공하기 위해 진료 시스템이 제대로 작동하고 있는지 확인하는 수단이다. 적절하게 작동하는 CQI 프로그램은 처벌로 인식되어서는 안 되며 오히려 병원 전 처치 제공자, 행정 관리자 및 의료 책임자가 시스템이 의료 제공자에게 환자에게는 성공을 환자에게는 양질의 처치 및 결과를 제공하기 위해 작동하고 있는지 확인할 기회로 삼아야 한다. 적절하게 작동하는 CQI 프로그램의 토대는 예상치 못한 사건을 파악하는 적극적인 감시 프로그램과 결합한 표준 차트 검토 과정이다. CQI 과정을 통해 확인된 문제는 향후 새로운 교육 계획의 대상이 되며 확인된 개선 영역을 해결하기 위한 시스템 변경의 대상이 된다. 교육과 시스템 변경이 완료되면 CQI 과정의 마지막 단계는 문제를 재평가하여 수정이 이루어졌는지 확인하는 것이다. CQI 과정은 파악, 분석, 구현 및 재분석의 끝없는 순환이다. 적절하게 작동하는 CQI 프로그램은 삽관 중인 환자의 품질과 결과를 모두 향상하는 것으로 입증되었다. CQI 프로그램의 주요 대상은 시스템이다. 실무자의 개별 조치는 교육 격차가 확인될 때 발생한다. CQI 과정에서 발생하는 개별 징계 조치는 실무자가 의도적으로 프로토콜과 절차를 무시하고 환자의 안전을 위험에 빠뜨린 극히 드문 상황에만 이루어져야 한다.

이송 지연

이송 지연 전과 이송 중에 환자의 기도를 관리하려면 병원 전 처치 제공자의 복잡한 의사결정이 필요한 경우가 많다. 기도를 개방하고 유지하기 위한 처치, 특히 전문기도유지 술기의 사용에는 많은 요소를 고려해야 한다. 이러한 요소에는 환자의 손상, 실무자의 임상 술기, 사용할 수 있는 장비, 결정적인 처치를 시행할 수 있는 의료기관까지의 거리와 이송 시간 등이 포함되지만 이에 국한되지는 않는다. 최종 기도확보 결정을 내리기 전에 사용할 수 있는 모든 기도유지 방법의 위험과 이점을 고려해야 한다. 이송 거리와 예상되는 이송 시간은 이송 전에 기도를 확보할 수 있는 임계치를 낮춘다. 환자 이송에 15~20분 소요되는 경우 입인두기도기 삽입 후 백마스크 환기를 포함한 필수 술기만으로도 충분할 수 있다. 비좁고 시끄러운 환경에서는 지속적인 기도 평가 및 관리가 어렵기 때문에 항공 이송을 이용하면

기관내삽관을 시행하기 위한 임계치도 낮아진다.

이송 중 기도관리 또는 환기 지원이 필요한 환자는 이송 중 높은 수준의 지속적인 모니터링이 필요하다. 이송 중 모든 외상 환자에게 지속해서 맥박산소측정 모니터링을 사용해야 하며 모든 삽관 환자에게는 호기말이산화탄소분압측정을 필수적으로 고려해야 한다. 호기말이산화탄소 손실은 인공호흡기 서킷이 분리되었거나, 기관내관이 이탈되었거나, 환자의 관류량이 현저히 감소했음을 나타낸다. 이러한 모든 가능한 원인에는 즉각적인 조치가 필요하다.

활력징후는 지속해서 모니터링하고 그래픽으로 표시하여 병원 전 처치 제공자가 잠재적인 문제를 조기에 파악할 수 있도록 해야 한다. 앞에서 설명한 대로 환자를 이동하거나 위치를 변경할 때마다 기관내관을 확인해야 한다. 또한 모든 기도 장치의 안전성을 자주 확인하는 것이 좋다.

산소 공급을 유지하기 위해 흡입산소농도 또는 호기말양압이 필요한 환자는 신중하게 재평가해야 한다. 가능한 원인으로는 기흉의 발생이나 폐 기능 악화가 있다. 기흉이 확인되거나 의심되는 경우 긴장기흉으로 발전하는지 자세히 모니터링해야 한다. 지속적인 출혈, 혈량저하증 또는 신경성 쇼크 등 다른 원인으로 설명할 수 없는 혈류역학적 손상이 발생하면 가슴막감압술을 시행해야 한다. 환자가 양압환기를 받는 경우 이 과정에서 단순 기흉이 긴장기흉으로 전환될 수 있다. 개방 가슴 손상 부위에 폐쇄드레싱을 시행해서 과도한 가슴속 압력이 축적될 가능성이 있는 경우 드레싱을 간헐적으로 제거하여 대기 중으로 배출되도록 해야 한다.

외상 환자는 보충 산소를 투여하여 산소포화도를 94% 이상으로 유지하며 일산화탄소 중독이 확인되었거나 의심되는 환자는 100% 산소를 투여하거나 일산화탄소혈색소 포화도를 측정할 수 있는 맥박산소측정기로 모니터링해야 한다(자세한 내용은 13장 화상 손상을 참조).

환자를 이송 지연하기 전에 잠재적인 산소 요구량을 계산하고 충분한 양의 산소를 이송에 사용할 수 있도록 준비해야 한다. 환자의 산소포화도가 94%를 초과할 수 있도록 가장 낮은 흡입산소농도를 유지해야 한다. 이 전략은 의학적으로 최적이며 산소 보존을 보장한다. 일반적으로 예상되는 필요량보다 50% 더 많은 산소를 가져오는 것이 좋다(**표 7-5**).

삽관된 환자는 프로토콜에 따라 진정시켜 이송해야 한다. 인공호흡기와 환자의 호흡 부조화를 최소화하는 인공호흡기 방식을 찾아야 한다. 인공호흡기 비동기화는 환자가 인공호흡기가 적절하게 또는 적

시에 인식하지 못하는 유형으로 호흡을 시도할 때 발생한다. 인공호흡기와 싸우고 있다고 말하는 환자는 일반적으로 인공호흡기가 인식하지 못하는 유발 신호나 빠른 호흡으로 인해 인공호흡기의 유량과 양을 적절하게 공급하지 못해 어려움을 겪고 있다. 진정은 상황을 개선할 수 있지만, 근본적인 문제를 반드시 해결하지는 않는다. 선택할 수 있는 진정제는 약효가 짧고 쉽게 가역적인 것으로 프로포폴, 에토미데이트, 프리세덱스, 케타민 등이 있다. 환자가 상당히 전투적이고 기관내삽관으로 기도가 확보되어 있으며 병원 전 처치 제공자가 적절한 교육을 받고 업무 범위에 해당하는 경우 신경근 차단제 사용을 고려할 수 있다. 그러나 환자에게 적절한 진정제 투여 없이 신경근 차단제를 투여해서는 안 된다.

표 7-5 산소 탱크 크기 및 사용 시간

유량(L/분)	탱크 크기 및 사용 시간(h)				
	D	E	M	G	H/K
2	2.5	4.4	24.7	38.2	49.7
5	1	1.8	9.9	15.3	19.9
10	0.5	0.9	4.9	7.6	9.9
15	0.3	0.6	3.3	5.1	6.6

참고: 이 표는 다양한 크기의 산소 탱크와 유량에 따른 대략적인 사용 시간을 브여준다. 수치는 산소 탱크가 제곱인치당 2,100(psi)로 완전히 가득 차 있다고 가정한다.

요약

- 적절한 기도관리 및 환기를 통해 적절한 뇌 산소공급과 신체 세포 수준에서의 산소 전달은 병원 전 환자 처치에서 중요한 요소 중 하나이다.

- 병원 전 처치 제공자는 외상 환자에게 적절한 처치를 제공하기 위해 환기 및 가스 교환의 원리를 외상의 병태생리학과 통합할 수 있어야 한다.

- 유효 환기량은 총 분당 환기량에서 사강 환기량을 뺀 값으로 정의된다. 효과적인 분당 환기량이 정상 수준 이하로 떨어지기 시작하면 환기가 불충분한 상태가 될 수 있으며 이를 저환기라고 한다.

- 효과적인 환기 감소는 여러 가지 요인으로 인해 발생할 수 있다. 이 상태와 관련된 가장 흔한 병원 전 원인으로는 기계적 폐쇄(보통 혀), 의식 수준 저하 또는 효과적인 환기의 기전을 손상하는 기타 외상(동요가슴, 개방성 가슴 상처 등)이 있다.

- 상기도에서 들리는 호흡음은 부분 기도 폐쇄를 나타낼 수 있다. 부분 기도 폐쇄의 원인으로는 혀, 혈액 또는 상기도 이물에 의한 기도의 물리적 폐쇄가 있다. 병원 전 처치 제공자는 기도 폐쇄의 징후를 듣고 찾아야 한다.

- 외상 환자에서 혈량저하증(산소포화도 감소)은 피해야 한다. 특히 외상성 뇌손상을 입은 환자에게는 더욱 그렇다. 병원 전 처치 제공자는 외상 환자의 산소공급을 저해할 수 있는 모든 상태에 주의를 기울이는 것이 중요하다. 이러한 상태가 확인되면 병원 전 처치 제공자는 해당 상태를 개선하는 데 필요한 방법이나 장비를 결정해야 한다.

- 기도 보조 장비 및 절차에 대한 범주는 다음과 같다.
  - 도수 방법은 가장 간단하며 추가 장비가 필요하지 않다. 여기에는 외상 턱들기와 외상 턱 밀어올리기가 포함된다.
  - 간단한 기도관리는 단 하나의 장비만 필요한 보조 장치의 사용을 포함하여 장치를 삽입하는 술기에는 최소한의 훈련이 필요하다. 여기에는 입인두기도기 및 코인두기도기가 포함된다.
  - 성문위기도기는 전문기도기에 포함되며 추가 훈련이 필요하지만, 입인두를 더욱 완벽하게 제어할 수 있다는 이점이 있다.
  - 결정적인 기도기에는 기관내관과 외과적 기도유지가 포함된다. 이러한 방법에는 광범위한 훈련과 실습이 필요하고 시간과 자원이 많이 소요될 수 있으며 합병증 발생률이 높다. 이 술기는 또한 가장 안전한 기도유지를 제공한다.

- 기관내삽관을 실시할지 또는 대체 장치를 사용할지는 기도 평가를 통해 문제를 확인한 후에 결정해야 한다. 이는 병원 전 처치 제공자의 숙련도와 경험, 가장 가까운 외상센터까지 이송 시간 등의 요인을 고려한 위해성-유익성에 해당한다.

- 호기말이산환타소 모니터링(호기말이산화탄소분압)은 기관내관 위치를 확인하기 위한 표준 역할을 한다. 이 방법은 가능하면 병원 전 환경에서 사용해야 한다.

- 기도관리에는 위험이 없는 것은 아니다. 특정 술기와 방법을 적용할 때 위험과 해당 환자에 대한 잠재적 이득을 비교 검토해야 한다. 특정 상황에서 한 환자에게 최선의 선택일 수 있는 것이 비슷한 증상을 보이는 다른 환자에게는 그렇지 않을 수 있다.

- 외상 환자를 위한 최선의 판단을 내리기 위해서는 건전한 비판적 사고능력을 갖추어야 한다.

시나리오 재구성

당신은 혼잡한 도로에서 오토바이 충돌 사고가 발생했다는 신고를 받고 현장으로 출동한다. 현장에 도착했을 때 심하게 파손된 오토바이에서 약 15m 떨어진 곳에 환자가 누워있는 것을 보게 된다. 환자는 헬멧을 쓰고 있는 젊은 남성이다. 환자는 움직이지 않고 멀리서 보면 빠르게 숨을 쉬고 있는 것을 알 수 있다. 환자에게 다가가면서 머리 주위에 피가 고여 있고 코를 골며 목을 울리는 소리와 함께 호흡음이 시끄럽다는 것을 알 수 있다.

당신은 외상센터에서 15분 거리에 있으며 상황실에서 기상 악화로 인해 헬기 이송은 불가능하다고 알려준다.

- 이 환자에서 분명한 기도 손상의 지표로 무엇인가?
- 목격자나 응급의료반응자(EMR)로부터 어떤 다른 정보를 확인해야 하는가?
- 현장에서 초기 신속한 평가를 시행하는 동안 찾고 관찰해야 하는 산소 공급 및 환기를 악화시키는 중요한 징후와 증상은 무엇인가?
- 이송 전과 이송 중에 환자를 처치하기 위해 취할 조치의 순서를 설명한다.

시나리오 해결책

목격자들은 환자가 혼자였음을 확인하고 교통이 통제된 것을 확인하던 중 환자가 부서진 오토바이에서 15m 떨어진 곳에 누워있는 것을 목격하는데, 이는 심각한 손상 기전을 나타낸다. 환자의 호흡 양상과 머리 주위에 피가 고여 있는 것을 보면 기도 문제를 의심할 수 있다. 환자에게 다가갔을 때 코골이와 그르렁거리는 소리가 들리면 기도 문제가 확고해진다. 당신과 동료는 도수로 목뼈 고정을 유지하면서 헬멧을 제거한다. 외상 턱밀어올리기로 기도를 유지하고 흡인하면 코 고는 소리는 사라지지만, 호흡은 여전히 빠르고 얕게 유지된다. 양쪽 호흡음은 정상이지만, 산소포화도가 80%이므로 비재호흡마스크르 보충 산소를 공급한다. 이 처치는 부분적으로만 성공하고 산소포화도는 87%로 개선된다. 외상성 뇌손상이 우려되므로 산소포화도가 94%를 초과할 수 있도록 유지한다. 다음 처치는 환자의 자발 호흡에 맞춰 백마스크로 환기 보조를 시행한다. 입인두기도기 삽입으로 기도 확보를 통해 상기도를 유지하고 당신과 동료는 산소포화도를 96%까지 빠르게 개선할 수 있다. 동료가 맥박이 빠르고 가늘며 글래스고혼수척도는 편향징후 없이 7점이라고 알려준다. 헬기 이송을 사용할 수 없으므로 즉시 병원으로 이송할 준비를 한다. 구급차 안에서 환자에게 산소 공급 및 환기를 유지하기 위한 방법을 신속하게 재평가한다. 간헐적 흡인과 입인두기도기를 이용한 기도 확보로 환자는 강하고 대칭적인 호흡을 하는 것으로 보이며 산소포화도는 94% 이상으로 유지된다. 당신은 상황실에 추가 지원을 요청하여 두 명의 Paramedic 이 이송 중에 합류한다. 동료가 정맥 라인을 확보하고 모니터를 환자에게 연결하는 동안 백마스크로 환기를 계속 제공한다. 15분 후 환자를 외상팀에 인계할 때 활력징후는 산소포화도 95%, 심박수 100회/분, 혈압 110/60mmHg이었다.

References

1. Vanderlan WB, Tew BE, McSwain NE. Increased risk of death with cervical spine immobilisation in penetrating cervical trauma. *Injury*. 2009;40:880-883.

2. Barkana Y, Stein M, Scope A, et al. Prehospital stabilization of the cervical spine for penetrating injuries of the neck—is it necessary? *Injury*. 2000;31:305-309.

3. Brown JB, Bankey PE, Sangosanya AT, Cheng JD, Stassen NA, Gestring ML. Prehospital spinal immobilization does not appear to be beneficial and may complicate care following gunshot injury to the torso. *J Trauma*. 2009;67:774-778.

4. Roberts K, Whalley H, Bleetman A. The nasopharyngeal airway: dispelling myths and establishing the facts. *Emerg Med J*. 2005;22:394-396.

5. Liti A, Giusti GD, Gili A, et al. Insertion of four different types of supraglottic airway devices by emergency nurses: a mannequin-based simulation study. *Acta Biomed*. 2020 Nov 30;91(12-S):e2020016. doi: 10.23750/abm .v91i12-S.10832

6. Ruetzler K, Roessler B, Potura L, et al. Performance and skill retention of intubation by paramedics using seven different airway devices: a manikin study. *Resuscitation*. 2011 May;82(5):593-597. doi: 10.1016/j .resuscitation.2011.01.00

7. Kleine-Brueggeney M, Gottfried A, Nabecker S, Greif R, Book M, Theiler L. Pediatric supraglottic airway devices in clinical practice: a prospective observational study. *BMC Anesthesiol*. 2017 Sep 2;17(1):119. doi: 10.1186 /s12871-017-0403-6

8. Carney N, Cheney T, Totten AM, et al. *Prehospital Airway Management: A Systematic Review* [Internet]. Report No.: 21-EHC023. Agency for Healthcare Research and Quality; 2021. Accessed April 22, 2022. https://www.ncbi.nlm .nih.gov/books/NBK571440/

9. Mort TC. The incidence and risk factors for cardiac arrest during emergency tracheal intubation: a justification for incorporating the ASA Guidelines in the remote location. *J Clin Anesth*. 2004 Nov;16(7):508-516. doi: 10.1016/j .jclinane.2004.01.007

10. Stockinger ZT, McSwain NE Jr. Prehospital endotracheal intubation for trauma does not improve survival over bag-mask ventilation. *J Trauma*. 2004;56(3):531-536.

11. Davis DP, Koprowicz KM, Newgard CD, et al. The relationship between out-of-hospital airway management and outcome among trauma patients with Glasgow Coma Scale scores of 8 or less. *Prehosp Emerg Care*. 2011;15(2):184-192.

12. Gravesteijn BY, Sewalt CA, Stocchetti N, et al; CENTER-TBI collaborators. Prehospital management of traumatic brain injury across Europe: a CENTER-TBI study. *Prehosp Emerg Care*. 2021;25(5):629-643. Epub 2020 Oct 1. doi: 10.1080/10903127.2020.1817210

13. Brown CVR, Inaba K, Shatz DV, et al. Western Trauma Association critical decisions in trauma: airway management in adult trauma patient. *Trauma Surg Acute Care Open*. 2020;5:e000539.

14. Davis DP, Olvera DJ. HEAVEN criteria: derivation of a new difficult airway prediction tool. *Air Med J*. 2017;36(4):195-197.

15. American College of Surgeons (ACS) Committee on Trauma. *Advanced Trauma Life Support Course*. ACS; 2018.

16. Sakles JC, Chiu S, Mosier J, Walker C, Stolz U. The importance of first pass success when performing orotracheal intubation in the emergency department. *Acad Emerg Med*. 2013 Jan;20(1):71-78. doi: 10.1111/acem.12055

17. Garza AG, Gratton MC, Coontz D, et al. Effect of paramedic experience on orotracheal intubation success rates. *J Emerg Med*. 2003;25(3):251.

18. Buis ML, Maissan M, Hoeks SE, Klimek M, Stolker RJ. Defining the learning curve for endotracheal intubation using direct laryngoscopy: a systematic review. *Resuscitation*. February 2016;99:63-71.

19. Warner KJ, Sharar SR, Copass MK, Bulger EM. Prehospital management of a difficult airway: a prospective cohort study. *J Emerg Med*. 2008;36(3):257-265.

20. Dunford JV, Davis DP, Ochs M, Doney M, Hoyt DB. Incidence of transient hypoxia and pulse rate reactivity during paramedic rapid sequence intubation. *Ann Emerg Med.* 2003 Dec;42(6):721-728. doi: 10.1016/s0196-0644(03)00660-7

21. Walls RM, Brown CA, Bair AE, Pallin DJ. Emergency airway management: a multi-center report of 8937 emergency department intubations. *J Emerg Med.* 2011;41(4):347-354.

22. Aziz S, Foster E, Lockey DJ, Christian MD. Emergency scalpel cricothyroidotomy use in a prehospital trauma service: a 20-year review. *Emerg Med J.* 2021 May;38(5): 349-354. doi: 10.1136/emermed-2020-210305

23. Weitzel N, Kendall J, Pons P. Blind nasotracheal intubation for patients with penetrating neck trauma. *J Trauma.* 2004 May;56(5):1097-1101. doi: 10.1097/01.ta.0000071294.21893.a4

24. O'Brien DJ, Danzl DF, Hooker EA, Daniel LM, Dolan MC. Prehospital blind nasotracheal intubation by paramedics. *Ann Emerg Med.* 1989 Jun;18(6):612-617. doi: 10.1016/s0196-0644(89)80512-8

25. Marlow TJ, Goltra DD Jr, Schabel SI. Intracranial placement of a nasotracheal tube after facial fracture: a rare complication. *J Emerg Med.* 1997;15(2):187-191. doi: 10.1016/s0736-4679(96)00356-3

26. Tentillier E, Heydenreich C, Cros AM, Schmitt V, Dindart JM, Thicoïpé M. Use of the intubating laryngeal mask airway in emergency pre-hospital difficult intubation. *Resuscitation.* 2008 Apr;77(1):30-34.

27. Theiler L, Hermann K, Schoettker P, et al. SWIVIT—Swiss video-intubation trial evaluating video-laryngoscopes in a simulated difficult airway scenario: study protocol for a multicenter prospective randomized controlled trial in Switzerland. *Trials.* 2013 Apr 4;14:94. doi: 10.1186/1745-6215-14-94

28. Nabecker S, Greif R, Kotarlic M, Kleine-Brueggeney M, Riggenbach C, Theiler L. Outdoor performance of different videolaryngoscopes on a glacier: a manikin study. *Emergencias* [Spanish]. 2016;28(4):216-222.

29. Driver BE, Prekker ME, Reardon RF, et al. Success and complications of the ketamine-only intubation method in the emergency department. *J Emerg Med.* 2021 Mar;60(3): 265-272. doi: 10.1016/j.jemermed.2020.10.042

30. Wang HE, Davis DP, O'Connor RE, et al. Drug-assisted intubation in the prehospital setting. *Prehosp Emerg Care.* 2006;10(2):261-271.

31. Davis DP, Hoyt DB, Ochs M, et al. The effect of paramedic rapid sequence intubation on an outcome in patients with severe trauma brain injury. *J Trauma.* 2003;54:444-453.

32. Bernard SA, Nguyen V, Cameron P, et al. Prehospital rapid sequence intubation improves functional outcome for patients with severe traumatic brain injury: a randomized controlled trial. *Ann Surg.* 2010;252(6):959-965.

33. Galbiati G, Paola C. Effects of open and closed endotracheal suctioning on intracranial pressure and cerebral perfusion pressure in adult patients with severe brain injury: a literature review. *J Neurosci Nurs.* 2015 Aug;47(4):239-46. doi: 10.1097/JNN.0000000000000146.

34. Weingart SD, Trueger NS, Wong N, Scofi J, Singh N, Rudolph SS. Delayed sequence intubation: a prospective observational study. *Ann Emerg Med.* 2015 Apr;65(4): 349-355. doi: 10.1016/j.annemergmed.2014.09.025

35. Smith KJ, Dobranowski J, Yip G, Dauphin A, Choi PT. Cricoid pressure displaces the esophagus: an observational study using magnetic resonance imaging. *Anesthesiology.* 2003;99(1):60-64.

36. Werner SL, Smith CE, Goldstein JR, Jones RA, Cydulka RK. Pilot study to evaluate the accuracy of ultrasonography in confirming endotracheal tube placement. *Ann Emerg Med.* 2007;49(1):75-80.

37. Butler J, Sen A. Best evidence topic report: cricoid pressure in emergency rapid sequence induction. *Emerg Med J.* 2005;22(11):815-816.

38. O'Connor RE, Swor RA. Verification of endotracheal tube placement following intubation. *Prehosp Emerg Care.* 1999;3:248-250.

39. Weingart SD, Levitan RM. Preoxygenation and prevention of desaturation during emergency airway management. *Ann Emerg Med.* 2012;59(3):165-175.

40. Jeremitsky E, Omert L, Dunham CM, Protetch J, Rodriguez A. Harbingers of poor outcome the day after severe brain injury: hypothermia, hypoxia, and hypoperfusion. *J Trauma.* 2003;54:312–319.

41. Davis DP, Hwang JQ, Dunford JV. Rate of decline in oxygen saturation at various pulse oximetry values with prehospital rapid sequence intubation. *Prehosp Emerg Care.* 2008 Jan–Mar;12(1):46-51. doi: 10.1080/10903120701710470

42. Davis DP, Aguilar S, Sonnleitner C, Cohen M, Jennings M. Latency and loss of pulse oximetry signal with the use of digital probes during prehospital rapid-sequence intubation. *Prehosp Emerg Care.* 2011;15(1):18-22.

43. Cemalovic N, Scoccimarro A, Arslan A, Fraser R, Kanter M, Caputo N. Human factors in the emergency department: is physician perception of time to intubation and desaturation rate accurate? *Emerg Med Australas.* 2016 Jun;28(3):295-299. doi: 10.1111/1742-6723.12575

44. Jensen M, Barmaan B, Orndahl CM, Louka A. Impact of suction-assisted laryngoscopy and airway decontamination technique on intubation quality metrics in a helicopter emergency medical service: an educational intervention. *Air Med J.* 2020 Mar-Apr;39(2):107-110. doi: 10.1016/j.amj.2019.10.005

45. Jarvis JL, Gonzales J, Johns D, Sager L. Implementation of a clinical bundle to reduce out-of-hospital peri-intubation hypoxia. *Ann Emerg Med.* 2018 Sep;72(3):272-279.e1. doi: 10.1016/j.annemergmed.2018.01.044

46. Kupas DF, Kauffman KF, Wang HE. Effect of airway-securing method on prehospital endotracheal tube dislodgment. *Prehosp Emerg Care.* 2020;14(1):26-30. doi: 10.3109/10903120903144932

47. Moroco AE, Armen SB, Goldenberg D. Emergency cricothyrotomy: a 10-year single institution experience. *Am Surg.* 2021 Feb 10:3134821995075. doi: 10.1177/0003134821995075

48. Mabry RL, Frankfurt A. An analysis of battlefield cricothyrotomy in Iraq and Afghanistan. *J Spec Oper Med.* 2012;12(1):17-23.

49. Warner KJ, Cuschieri J, Garland B, et al. The utility of early end-tidal capnography in monitoring ventilation status after severe injury. *J Trauma.* 2009;66:26-31.

50. Groombridge CJ, Ley E, Miller M, Konig T. A prospective, randomised trial of pre-oxygenation strategies available in the pre-hospital environment. *Anaesthesia.* 2017 May;72(5):580-584. doi: 10.1111/anae.13852. Epub 2017 Mar 14.

51. Johannigman JA, Branson RD, Davis K Jr, Hurst JM. Techniques of emergency ventilation: a model to evaluate tidal volume, airway pressure, and gastric insufflation. *J Trauma.* 1991 Jan;31(1):93-8.

특수 술기

특별한 기도 관리 방법

외상 턱밀어올리기법

원리: 목뼈를 움직이지 않고 기도를 개방한다.

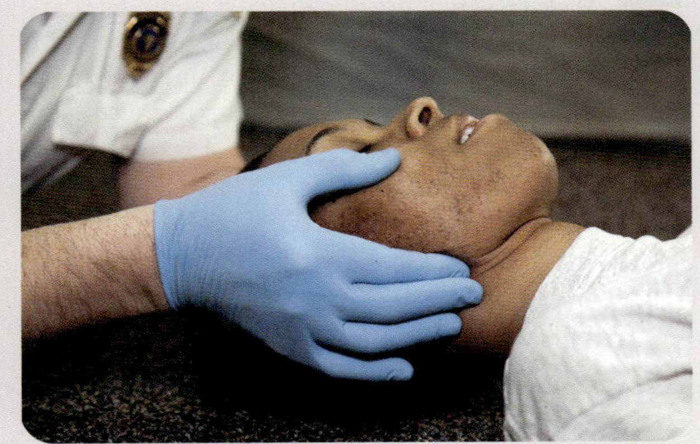

1 외상 턱 밀어올리기와 외상 턱들기 모두에서 아래턱뼈를 앞으로 이동하는 동안 머리와 목을 도수 고정으로 중립 자세를 유지한다. 이 방법은 입을 약간 벌린 상태에서 혀를 후인두에서 앞으로 이동시킨다.

병원 전 처치 제공자는 환자의 머리 위쪽에 위치해서 양손을 환자의 머리 양쪽에 놓고 손가락은 환자의 발 쪽을 향하게 하고 엄지손가락은 광대뼈예 위치시킨다. 엄지손가락이 광대뼈 위에 대고 있는 동안 반지손가락으로 가볍게 눌러 아래턱뼈를 위로 들어 올린다. 손바닥은 그 과정에서 머리를 고정한다.

변형된 외상 턱 밀어올리기

원리: 목뼈를 움직이지 않고 정면에서 기도를 개방한다.

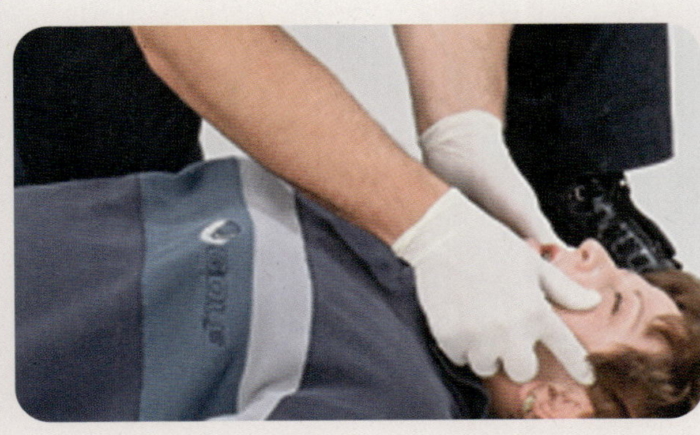

1 외상 턱 밀어올리기는 병원 전 처치 제공자가 환자 옆에서 얼굴을 마주 보면서 시행할 수도 있다. 병원 전 처치 제공자의 엄지손가락은 광대뼈에 대고 집게손가락은 아래턱뼈 각 뒤에 갈고리처럼 걸어서 앞으로 움직인다. 아래팔을 환자의 빗장뼈에 올려놓으면 안정성을 더욱 높일 수 있다. 엄지손가락으로 광대뼈를 누르고 다른 손가락으로 아래턱뼈를 안정시키는 것을 돕는 동안 반지손가락으로 아래턱뼈를 부드럽게 밀어올린다. 그런 다음 병원 전 처치 제공자는 공기 유입과 가슴 움직임을 확인한다.

외상 턱들기법

원리 : 목뼈를 움직이지 않고 기도를 개방한다.

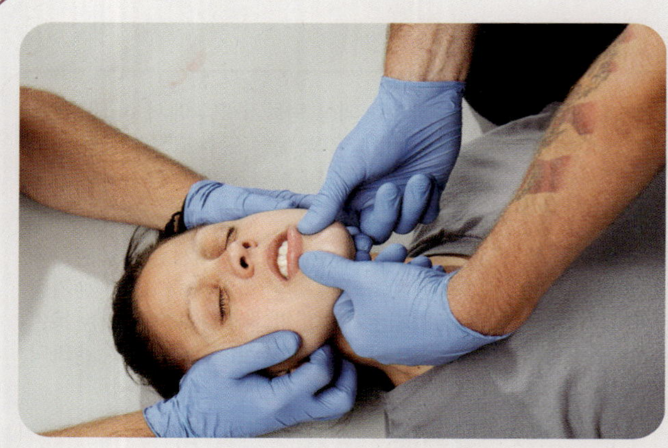

1 환자의 머리 위쪽에서 자세를 잡고 머리와 목을 도수 고정으로 유지하고 중립 자세를 유지한다. 첫 번째 병원 전 처치 제공자는 머리 위쪽에 위치하고 두 번째 병원 전 처치 제공자는 환자 옆에 무릎을 꿇고 위치한다. 첫 번째 병원 전 처치 제공자가 환자의 머리를 도수로 고정하는 동안 두 번째 병원 전 처치 제공자는 집게손가락을 환자의 턱 밑에 걸고 엄지손가락은 환자의 턱에 대고 양손으로 환자의 턱을 잡는다. 병원 전 처치 제공자는 환자의 입을 벌리고 아래턱뼈를 앞으로 당긴다. 이 과정을 성공적으로 수행하기 위해서는 먼저 환자의 입을 개방해야 한다.

이 술기는 환자가 깨물거나 발작을 일으킬 때 위험할 수 있는 엄지손가락을 환자의 입에 삽입하는 것을 방지한다.

입인두기도기(OPA)

원리: 구역반사가 없는 환자에게 기계적으로 기도 개방을 유지하기 위해 사용하는 보조기도기이다.

입인두기도기는 환자의 혀 뒷부분을 인두의 앞쪽으로 고정하도록 설계되었다. OPA는 다양한 크기로 제공된다. 기도를 개방하고 유지하려면 환자에게 맞는 적절한 크기가 필요하다. 하인두에 OPA를 삽입하는 것은 구역반사가 정상인 환자에게는 금기이다. OPA를 삽입하는 두 가지 방법이 효과적이다. 혀 턱들기 삽입 방법과 설압자를 이용한 삽입 방법이 효과적일 수 있다. 어떤 방법을 사용하든 첫 번째 병원 전 처치 제공자가 머리와 목뼈를 중립 자세로 고정하고 다른 병원 전 처치 제공자가 OPA의 길이를 측정하고 삽입한다.

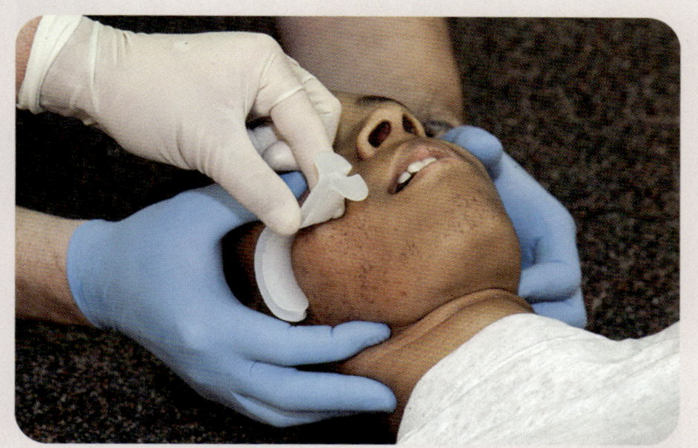

1 첫 번째 병원 전 처치 제공자가 환자의 머리와 목뼈를 중립 자세로 고정하고 턱 밀어올리기 방법으로 기도를 개방한다. 다른 병원 전 처치 제공자는 적절한 크기의 OPA를 선택하여 길이를 측정한다. OPA의 길이는 입꼬리에서 귓불까지의 거리를 측정하여 크기를 결정한다.

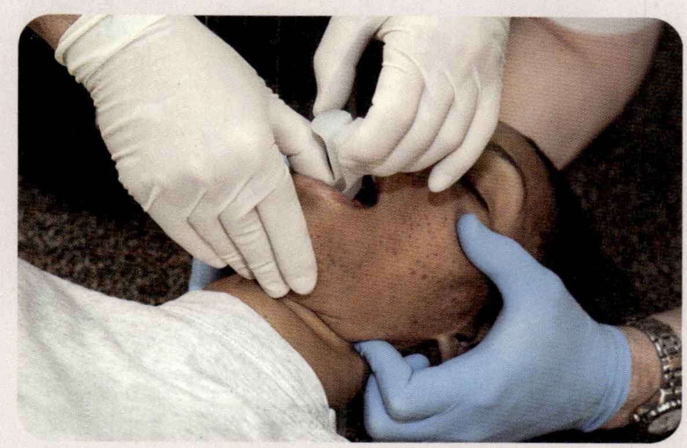

2 첫 번째 처치 제공자가 환자의 머리와 목뼈를 중립 자세로 고정하고 유지하는 동안 두 번째 병원 전 처치 제공자는 왼손으로 환자의 입을 벌리고 OPA를 삽입한다. OPA의 원위 끝이 한쪽 도는 다른 쪽을 향하도록 돌려서(플랜지 끝이 환자의 뺨을 향하도록) 환자의 입에 삽입한다. OPA의 끝이 목뒤 쪽에 도달하면 환자의 해부학적 윤곽에 맞게 회전한다.

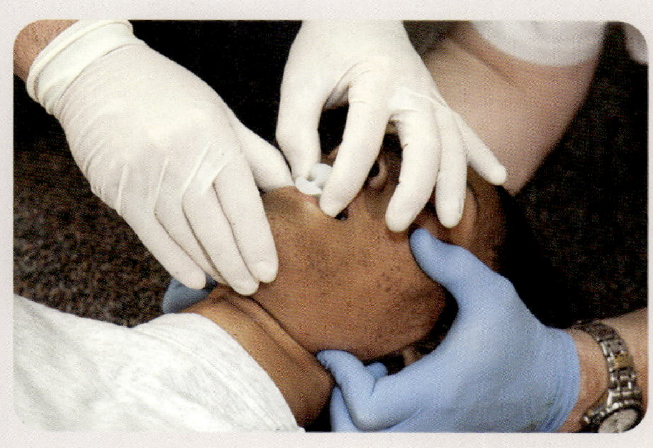

3 OPA는 안쪽 커브가 혀에 닿을 때까지 회전한다. 혀에 닿을 때까지 회전한다. OPA의 플랜지는 환자 치아의 바깥쪽에 닿아 있어야 한다. 공기 유입 및 가슴 움직임을 확인한다.

입인두기도기: 설압자를 이용한 삽입 방법

설압자를 사용하는 방법은 어느 정도의 구역 반사가 여전히 존재하는지 병원 전 처치 제공자가 설압자로 확인할 수 있으므로 아마도 혀 턱 들기보다 더 안전한 방법일 것이다. 또한 얼굴 외상의 경우 느슨해진 치아가 빠질 위험이 적다. 회전하는 기도기 끝이 물렁입천장을 손상할 수 있으므로 소아 환자에게 권장되는 술기이다.

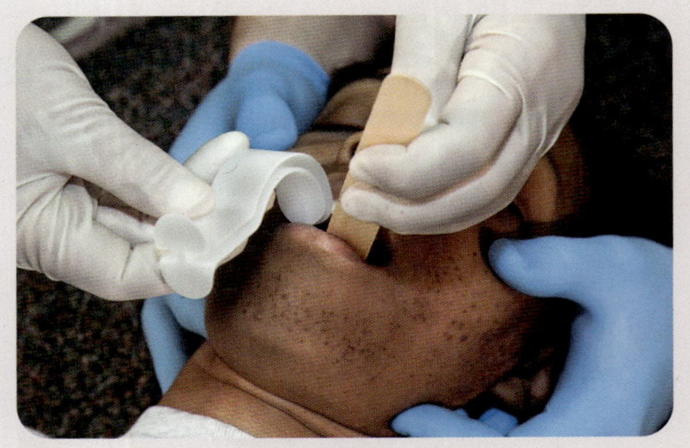

1 첫 번째 처치 제공자는 환자의 머리와 목을 중립 자세로 고정하고 유지하며 외상 턱 밀어올리기 방법으로 환자의 기도를 개방하면서 안정화를 유지한다. 두 번째 처치 제공자는 적절한 크기의 OPA를 선택하고 길이를 측정한다. 두 번째 처치 제공자가 환자의 턱을 잡아당겨 입을 벌리고 설압자를 환자의 입에 넣어 혀를 앞으로 이동시킨다. 동시에 두 번째 병원 전 처치 제공자는 구역 반사나 느슨한 구조를 확인한다.

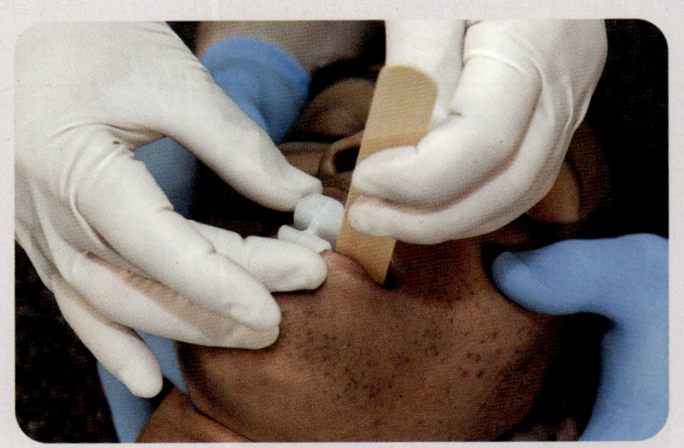

2 기도기의 굴곡을 따라 플랜지 끝부분이 환자의 발을 향하도록 하고 원위부 끝이 환자의 입을 향하도록 OPA를 삽입한다. OPA의 플랜지 끝이 환자 치아의 외부 표면에 닿을 때까지 OPA를 삽입한다. 공기 유입과 가슴 움직임을 확인하여 기도 개방의 효과를 평가한다.

코인두기도기(NPA)

원리: 구역반사가 있거나 없는 환자 또는 이를 악물고 있는 환자에서 기계적으로 기도를 유지하기 위해 사용하는 보조기도기이다.

NPA는 구역반사가 정상일 수 있는 환자의 기도를 개방하고 유지하는 효과적인 방법을 제공하는 간단한 기도 보조 장치이다. 대부분 환자는 적절한 크기의 NPA를 견딜 수 있다. NPA는 다양한 지름(내경 5~9mm)으로 제공되며 지름 크기에 따라 길이도 적절하게 달라진다. NPA는 일반적으로 유연한 고무와 같은 재질로 만들어진다.

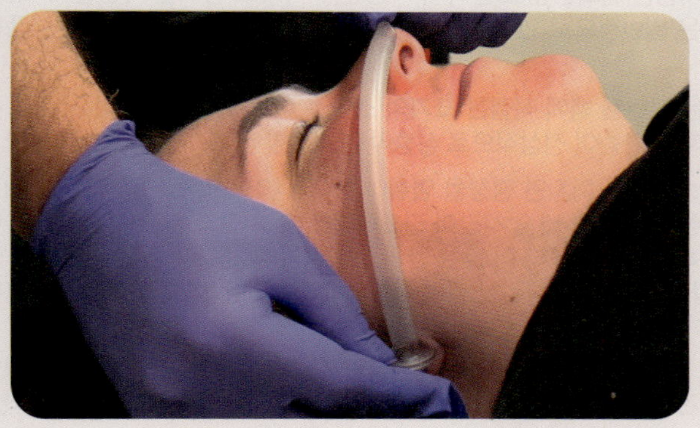

1 NPA를 삽입할 병원 전 처치 제공자는 환자의 콧구멍에 맞는 적절한 크기의 장치를 선택하는데, 이는 콧구멍 크기(대개 환자의 새끼손가락 지름)보다 지름이 약간 작은 크기를 선택한다. NPA의 길이가 중요하다. NPA는 환자의 혀와 후인두 사이에 공기 통로를 제공할 수 있을 만큼 충분히 길어야 한다. NPA의 길이는 환자의 코에서 귓불까지의 길이가 적절하다(참고: 길이를 측정할 때 NPA를 펴서는 안 된다).

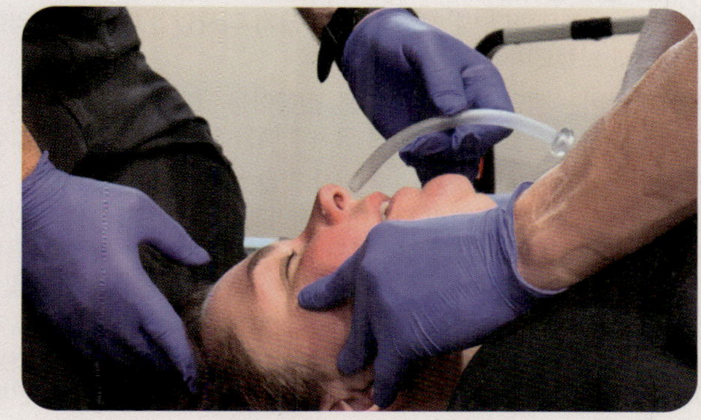

2 첫 번째 병원 전 처치 제공자는 환자의 머리와 목을 중립 자세로 고정하고 유지하며 외상 턱들어올리기 방법으로 혼자의 기도를 개방하면서 안정화를 유지한다. 두 번째 병원 전 처치 제공자는 NPA의 플랜지가 없는 끝과 외부에 수용성 젤을 바른다. 그런 다음 NPA를 선택한 콧구멍으로 천천히 삽입한다. 삽입은 코안 바닥을 따라 앞쪽에서 뒤쪽으로 삽입해야 하며 위쪽에서 아래쪽으로 삽입해서는 안 된다. NPA는 물렁입천장을 따라 들어간다. 콧구멍의 뒤쪽 끝에서 저항이 있는 경우 NPA를 부드럽게 회전시키면서 삽입하면 코안의 선반뼈를 손상 없이 통과하는 데 도움이 된다. NPA가 계속 저항에 부딪히면 NPA를 제거한 후 다시 수용성 젤을 바르고 다른 콧구멍으로 삽입해야 한다.

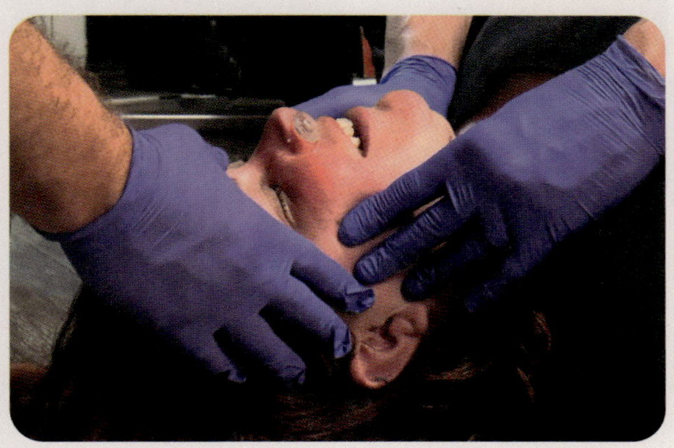

3 두 번째 병원 전 처치 제공자는 NPA의 플랜지 끝이 콧구멍의 앞쪽 가장자리에 올 때까지 또는 환자가 구토할 때까지 삽입을 계속한다. 환자가 구역질하거나 기침하면 NPA 튜브의 끝이 후두의 윗부분에 닿았기 때문에 약간 빼야 한다는 징후일 수 있다. 다시 한 번 기도 개방의 효과를 평가하기 위해 공기 유입과 가슴 움직임을 확인한다.

백마스크 환기

백마스크 장비를 사용한 환기는 병원 전 처치 제공자에게 백의 피드백을 제공하기 때문에 다른 환기 지원 시스템에 비해 이점이 있다. 긍정적인 피드백은 성공적인 환기를 보장하며 피드백의 변화는 마스크 밀착 이상, 기도 폐쇄 또는 성공적인 환기를 방해하는 가슴 문제를 나타낸다. 이러한 느낌과 조절 기능을 통해 백마스크 장비는 환기를 보조하는 데 적합하고 휴대가 간편하고 즉시 사용할 수 있어 필요할 때 즉시 환기를 제공하는 데 유용하다.

그러나 보조 산소가 없으면 백마스크 장비는 21%의 산소 농도 도는 흡입산소농(FiO_2)도 0.21을 제공할 수 있다. 시간이 허락하는 즉시 산소 보유주머니를 백마스크에 연결하고 산소 탱크에 연결한다. 산소 보유주머니를 연결하지 않고 산소만 연결하면 흡입산소농도 0.50 이하로 제한되고, 산소 보유주머니를 연결하면 흡입산소농도는 0.85 이상으로 공급할 수 있다.

환기 대상 환자가 구역반사 없고 의식이 없는 경우 백마스크 장비로 환기를 시도하기 전에 적절한 크기의 OPA를 삽입해야 한다. 환자에게 구역반사가 있는 경우 환기를 시도하기 전에 적절한 NPA를 삽입해야 한다. 비교적 저렴한 일회용을 포함하여 다양한 백마스크 장비를 사용할 수 있다. 백마스크는 브랜드마다 백, 밸브와 백의 크기 디자인이 다르다. 이러한 부품은 일반적으로 안전하게 교체할 수 없으므로 사용하는 모든 부품은 같은 모델과 브랜드여야 한다.

백마스크 장비는 성인, 소아와 영아용, 신생아용 크기가 있다. 응급상황에서는 성인용 백에 적절한 크기의 소아용 마스크를 결합하여 사용할 수 있지만, 안전한 사용을 위해 올바른 크기의 백을 사용하는 것이 좋다. 성인 환자의 가슴이 정상적으로 상승하면 적절한 환기가 이루어지고 있다.

양압 장비로 환기를 시행하는 경우 정상 일회호흡량, 즉 눈에 보이는 가슴 상승이 이루어지면 팽창을 멈춰야 한다. 백마스크 장비를 사용할 때는 가슴을 눈으로 확인하고 백의 저항이 현저하게 증가했는지 백을 만져보아야 한다. 충분한 날숨 시간이 필요하다(들숨 시간과 날숨 시간의 비율이 1:3이어야 함). 충분한 시간이 허용되지 않으면 계단식 또는 누적 호흡이 발생하여 호기량보다 더 많은 양의 흡기량을 제공한다. 계단식 호흡은 공기 교환이 제대로 이루어지지 않아 과잉팽창, 압력 증가, 식도 개방 및 위 팽창을 초래한다. 적절한 환기 속도에 주의를 기울이고 정상적인 호흡이 이루어지도록 하는 것이 매우 중요하다.

백마스크 장비로 환기를 보조하는 것은 한 명의 병원 전 처치 제공자보다 두 명 이상의 병원 전 처치 제공자가 시행하기가 더 쉽다. 첫 번째 병원 전 처치 제공자는 마스크를 적절히 밀착하는 데 집중할 수 있고 두 번째 병원 전 처치 제공자는 양손으로 백을 짜서 충분한 양을 공급할 수 있다.

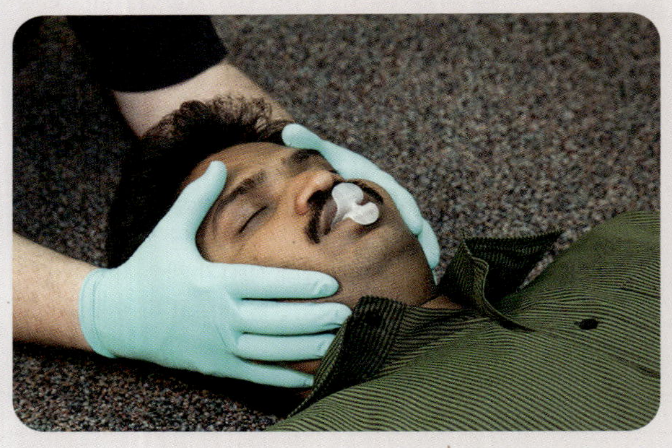

1 첫 번째 병원 전 처치 제공자는 환자의 머리 위쪽에 무릎을 꿇고 앉아 도수로 머리와 목을 중립적 자세로 고정하고 유지한다.

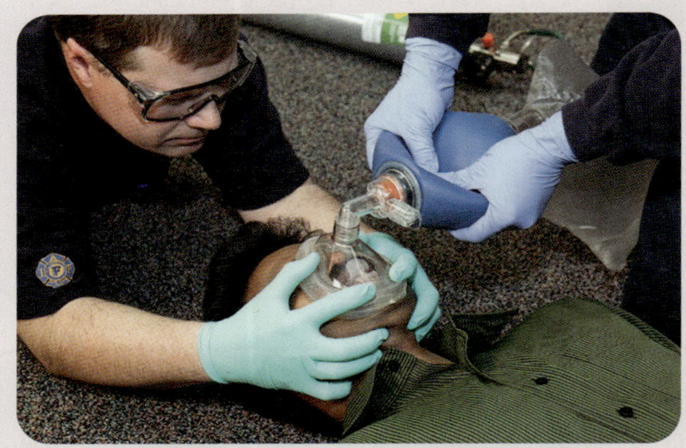

2 얼굴 마스크를 환자의 코와 입 위에 씌우고 엄지손가락으로 마스크 측면을 고정한 상태에서 아래턱뼈를 마스크 안으로 당겨서 마스크를 고정한다. 다른 손가락은 도수 고정을 유지하고 기도 개방을 유지한다. 두 번째 병원 전 처치 제공자는 환자 옆에 무릎을 꿇고 앉아 양손으로 백을 짜서 폐를 부풀리면서 적절한 환기 속도와 적절한 일회호흡량에 주의를 기울인다.

성문위기도기

기도를 개방하기 위한 첫 번째 방법으로 성문위기도기(SGA)를 사용해서는 안 된다. 성문위기도기 삽입을 시도하기 전에 환자의 산소포화도가 최소 93%(바람직하게는 100%)가 되도록 예방산소투여를 한다. 일반적으로 의식이 없는 환자가 OPA를 견딜 수 있다면 성문위기도기도 견딜 가능성이 높다.

후두튜브기도기

원리: 외상 환자에게 환기를 제공하기 위해 맹목적으로 삽입하는 이중 내강 기도기이다.

후두튜브기도기(LTA)는 원위부 및 입안(근위부) 커프가 모두 있는 이중 내강 튜브이다. 두 번째 내강은 위 감압을 위한 흡인 카테터의 삽입을 쉽게 하기 위한 것이다. 후두튜브기도기는 흡인으로부터 완전한 보호를 제공하지 않는다는 점에 유의해야 한다. 실제로 제조업체는 금식 부족과 위 내용물이 존재할 수 있는 상황(다발성 또는 대규모 손상, 급성 복부 또는 가슴 손상 등을 포함하되 이에 국한되지 않음)을 금기 사항으로 설명하고 있다. 이러한 금기 사항은 수술실 환경에도 적용되지만, 응급상황에서 후두튜브기도기는 흡인으로부터 제한적인 보호만 제공한다는 점을 상기해야 한다. 따라서 이러한 상황에서 LTA를 사용할 때 흡인을 방지하기 위해 상당한 주의를 기울여야 한다.

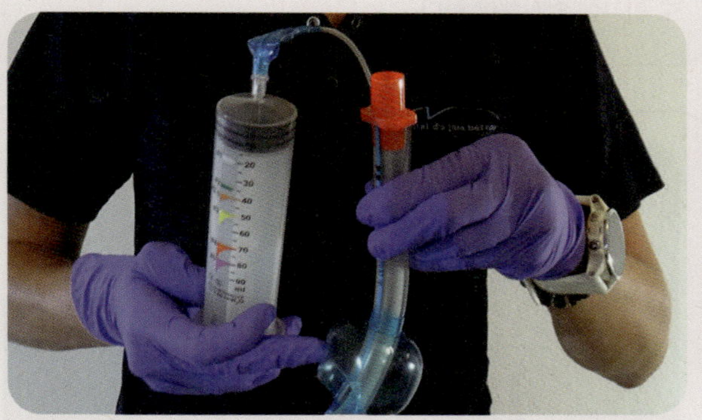

1 병원 전 처치 제공자는 환자의 키를 기준으로 올바른 후두튜브기도기 크기를 선택한다. 커프 팽창은 큰 주사기를 사용하여 커프에 최대 권장량의 공기를 주입하여 장비를 점검한다. 두 번째 병원 전 처치 제공자는 환자에게 예방산소투여를 한다.

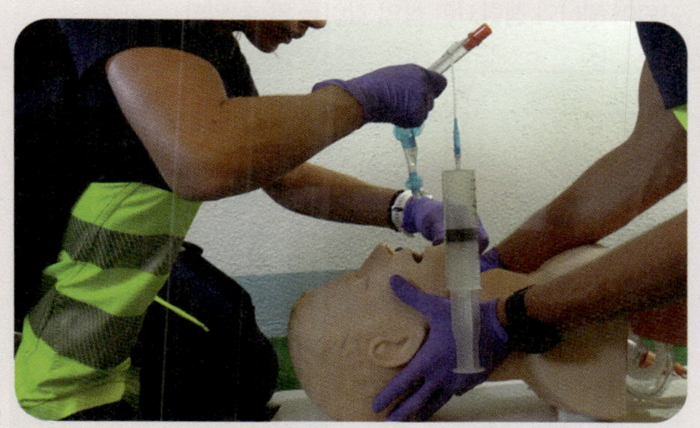

2 첫 번째 병원 전 처치 제공자는 튜브의 경사진 원위부 끝과 뒤쪽에 수용성 윤활제를 바르고 우세한 손으로 후두튜브기도기를 잡는다. 다른 손으로 수지교차법으로 환자의 입을 개방한다. 두 번째 병원 전 처치 제공자는 필요에 따라 목뼈를 안정적으로 유지한다.

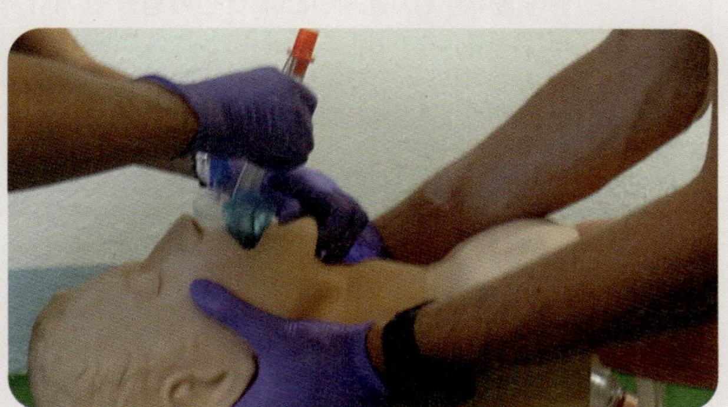

3 첫 번째 병원 전 처치 제공자는 튜브 끈을 환자의 입에 넣고 혀의 기저부 뒤쪽으로 삽입한다.

(다음 페이지에 계속)

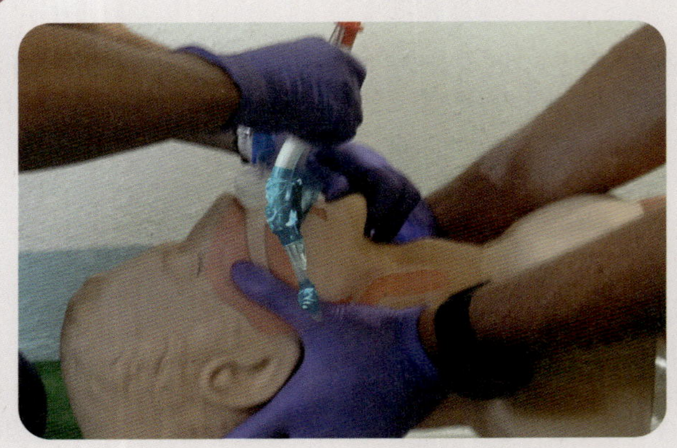

4 첫 번째 병원 전 처치 제공자는 커넥터의 밑부분이 환자의 치아와 정렬될 때까지 후두튜브기도기를 밀어 넣는다. 기준 표시는 후두튜브기도기의 근위부 끝에 제공되며 윗니와 정렬되면 삽입 깊이를 알 수 있다.

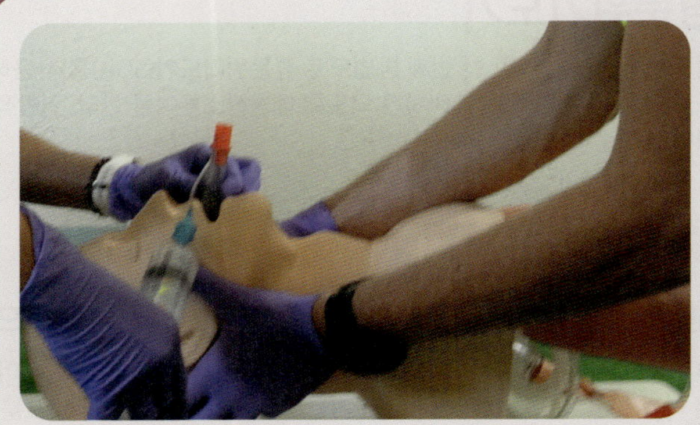

5 첫 번째 병원 전 처치 제공자는 큰 주사기로 커프를 팽창시킨다. 필요한 공기 주입량은 색상으로 구분된 주사기에 표시되어 있으며 기도를 단단히 밀봉할 수 있어야 한다. 기도 입구는 후두(흰색 원)를 향해야 하며 원위 커프는 식도 입구에 위치해야 한다.

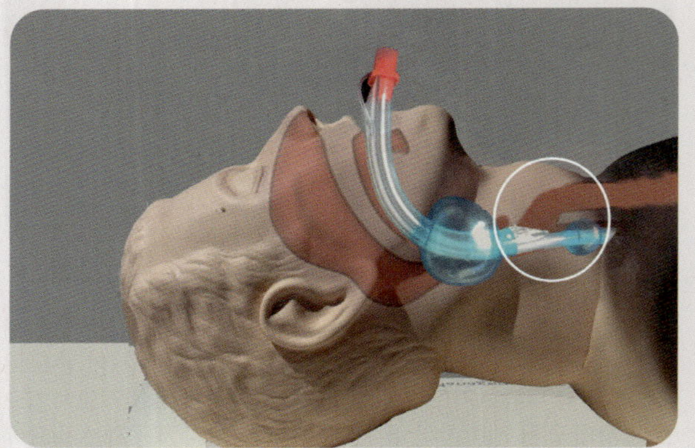

6 첫 번째 병원 전 처치 제공자는 백마스크를 후두튜브기도기에 연결한다. 환기를 평가하기 위해 환자에게 부드럽게 환기하는 동안 첫 번째 병원 전 처치 제공자는 환기가 쉽고 자유로울 때까지 기도기를 빼낸다(기도 압력을 최소화하면서 많은 일회호흡량). 이 이미지는 입인두에 큰 풍선을 부풀리고 식도에 작은 풍선을 부풀린 후 근위 내강을 식도 바로 근방에 위치시킨 LTA 장비의 이상적인 최종 위치를 보여준다.

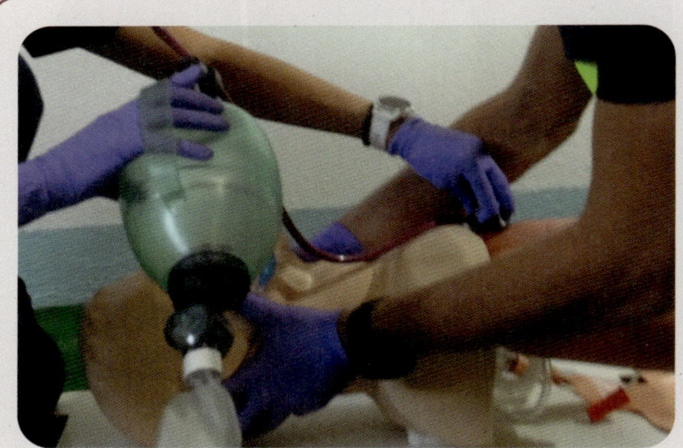

7 첫 번째 병원 전 처치 제공자는 청진, 가슴의 움직임 및 호기말이산화탄소분압측정을 통한 이산화탄소 확인을 통해 올바른 위치를 확인한다. 첫 번째 병원 전 처치 제공자는 커프 팽창을 60cmH₂O로 재조정한다. 첫 번째 병원 전 처치 제공자는 테이프 또는 기타 허용된 수단을 사용하여 환자에게 LTA를 고정한다. 원하는 경우 바이트 블록을 사용할 수도 있다.

I-gel 후두마스크

원리: 기도를 직접 눈으로 보지 않고 기도개방을 유지하는 데 사용되는 기계적 장치이다.

i-gel은 성대를 직접 눈으로 볼 필요 없이 병원 전 처치 제공자가 삽입할 수 있는 기도유지 장비이다. 이러한 맹목적 삽관 기법은 기관내삽관에 비해 초기 교육이 덜 필요하고 술기 유지가 더 쉽다는 장점이 있다.

i-gel의 목적은 압박손상을 피하면서 인두, 후두 및 기도 주위 구조물을 팽창하지 않는 밀봉을 만드는 것이다. i-gel의 한계는 성문 개구부 주위에 밀봉을 형성하지만, 기관내관 커프만큼 쇄쇄성이 높지 않다는 점이다. 흡인은 여전히 잠재적인 문제이다. 외상 환자에서 다른 기도유지기와 마찬가지로 술기를 시행하는 동안 목뼈 고정을 유지해야 한다.

i-gel LMA는 소아와 성인 환자에게 모두 사용할 수 있도록 크기가 다양하다.

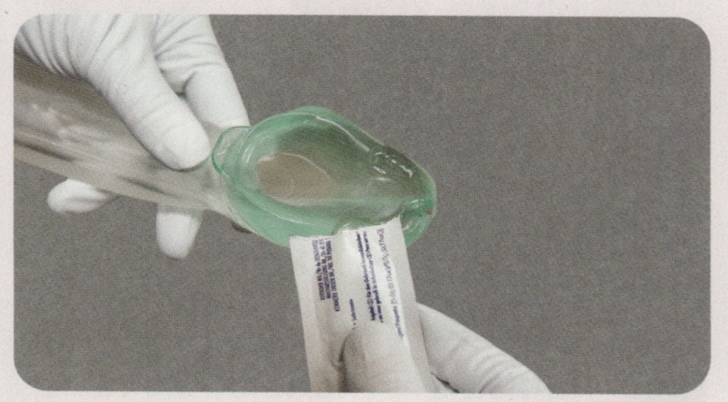

1 병원 전 처치 제공자는 보호 커버에서 꺼내서 수용성 윤활제를 후방 표면에 바른다. i-gel은 주로 사용하는 손으로 물림보호대를 따라잡는다. 두 번째 병원 전 처치 제공자는 앞쪽에서 머리를 안정시킨다.

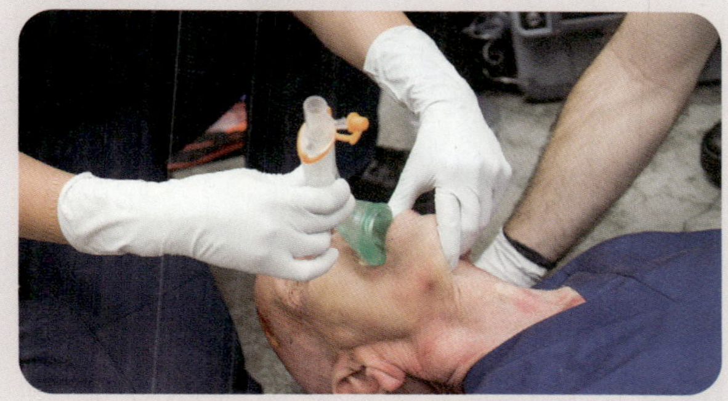

2 머리 쪽의 첫 번째 병원 전 처치 제공자는 턱을 부드럽게 누른 다음 단단입천장 쪽으로 i-gel의 부드러운 끝부분을 입안으로 삽입한다. 끝부분을 단단입천장에 대고 누르면 아래쪽으로 쉽게 삽입할 수 있다.

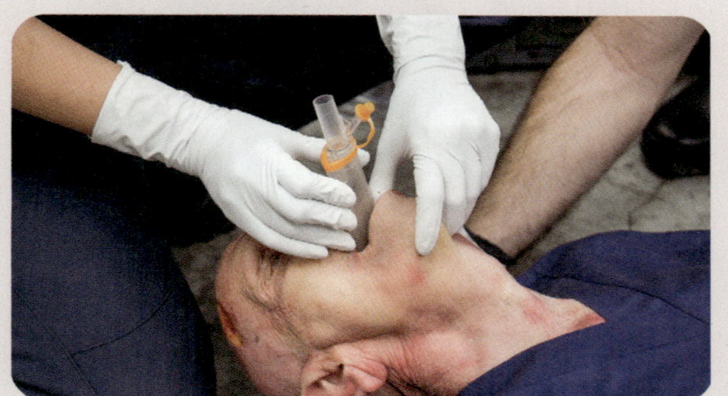

3 첫 번째 병원 전 처치 제공자는 확실한 저항이 느껴질 때까지 i-gel을 하인두로 계속 삽입한다. 이 시점에서 i-gel의 끝은 식도 상부에 위치하고 커프는 후두 주위에 있다. 앞니는 바이트 블록위에 놓여 있어야 한다.

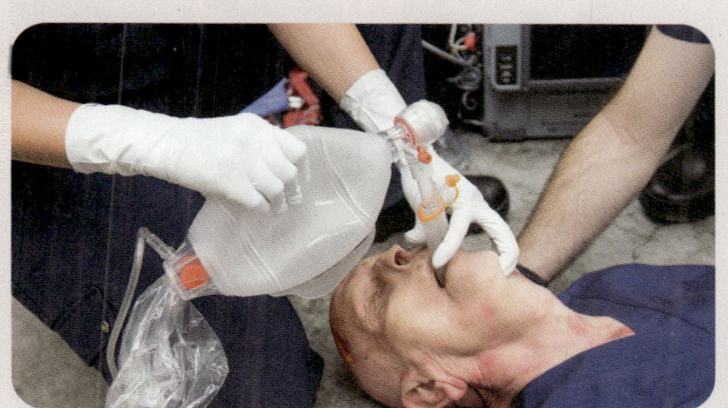

4 첫 번째 병원 전 제공자는 백마스크를 i-gel에 연결하여 환기를 시키며 두 번째 병원 전 처치 제공자는 호흡음을 확인한다. 호흡음이 확인되면 두 번째 병원 전 처치 제공자는 상업용 고정기나 테이프를 사용하여 원하는 깊이에 장치를 고정한다. 그런 다음 흡인 카테터 길이를 측정하고 흡인 포트에 삽입하여 위를 감압할 수 있다.

삽관형 후두마스크기도기(ILMA)

원리: 기도를 직접 눈으로 확인하지 않고 기도 개방을 유지하는 데 사용되는 기계 장치이다.

후두마스크는 일반적인 방법으로 삽입한다. 정상적인 가슴 상승으로 입구가 후두 앞쪽에 있고 환자에게 예방산소투여되면 기관내관을 삽관형 후두마스크(ILMA)에 삽입된 다음 기관으로 삽입한다. 후두마스크는 이송 중에 제거하지 않고 그대로 두어야 하는데 그 이유는 첫째 후두마스크가 기관내관에 대한 우수한 고정력을 제공하기 때문이고 둘째는 기관내관에 문제가 발생할 때 예비용으로 사용할 수 있기 때문이다. 외상 환자의 기도유지기와 마찬가지로 술기를 시행하는 동안 목뼈를 고정하고 유지해야 한다(명확성을 위해 사진에는 표시되지 않음).

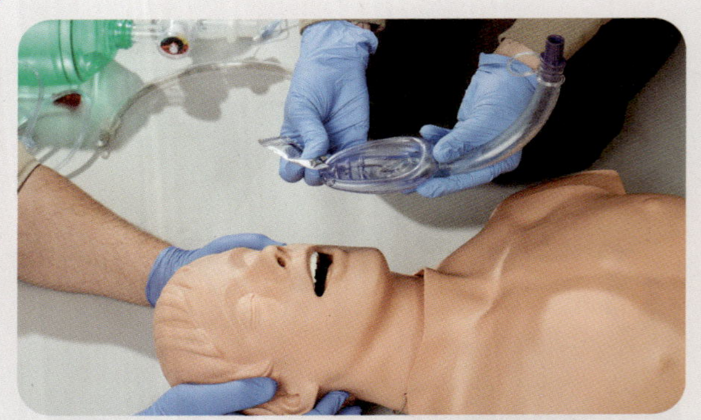

1 첫 번째 병원 전 처치 제공자는 커프의 공기를 빼고 ILMA의 후면에 수용성 윤활제를 바른다.

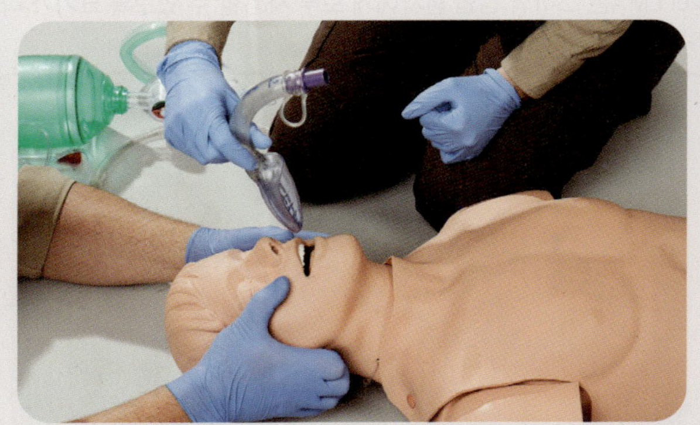

2 두 번째 병원 전 처치 제공자는 환자의 머리를 안정시키고 첫 번째 처치 제공자는 엄지와 집게손가락으로 ILMA를 잡고 커넥터가 환자의 가슴을 향해 아래쪽으로 향하도록 하고 말단 끝이 단단입천장을 향하도록 한다.

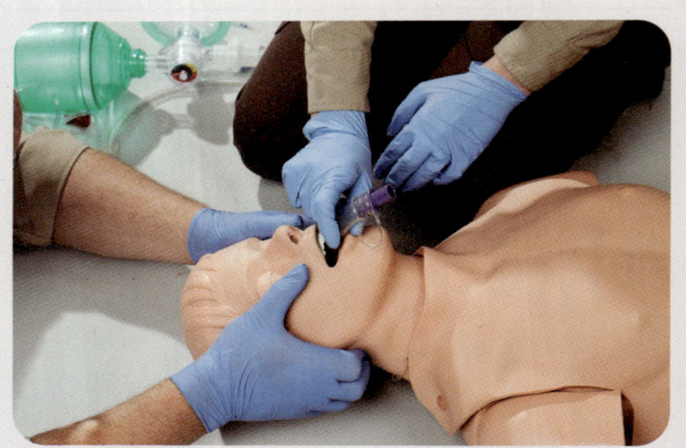

3 첫 번째 병원 전 처치 제공자는 커프 끝을 환자의 입에 넣고 압력을 유지하면서 확실한 저항이 느껴질 때까지 단단입천장을 따라 원을 그리며 아래쪽으로 계속 삽입한다.

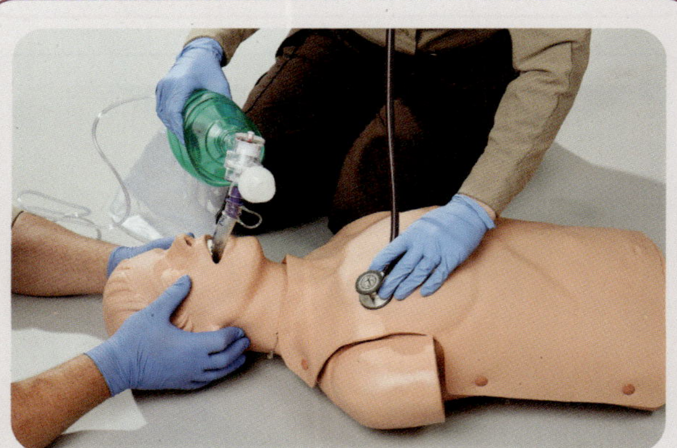

4 첫 번째 병원 전 처치 제공자는 백마스크를 후두마스크에 연결하고 환자에게 환기하면서 호흡음을 확인하고 마스크기 기관 입구 앞에 있는지 확인한다. 이 과정이 완료되고 환자가 적절하게 환기될 때까지 다음 단계로 진행하지 않는다.

(다음 페이지에 계속)

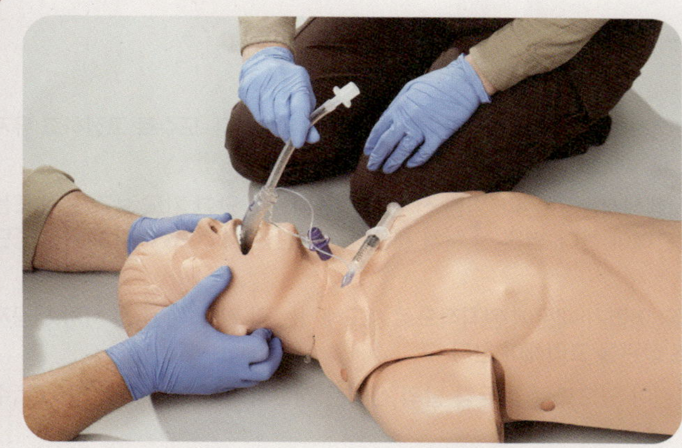

5 첫 번째 병원 전 처치 제공자는 기관낸을 ILMA의 근위 입구로 삽입한다. ILMA의 입구는 치아에서 4~5cm이다. 기관내관의 표준 삽입 깊이에 이 거리를 더해야 한다. 그런 다음 첫 번째 병원 전 처치 제공자가 커프를 팽창시킨다. 환자가 기관내관을 통해 환기되는 동안 호흡음을 청진하고 적절한 위치어 있는지 확인한다. 기관내관을 삽입할 수 없거나 이탈된 경우에도 ILMA를 사용하여 환기를 계속할 수 있다. 이러한 상황에서는 기관내관을 ILMA에 테이프로 고정하고 병원에 도착할 때까지 ILMA를 제거하지 않는다.

외상 환자의 시각화 입기관삽관

원리: 목뼈를 움직이지 않고 확실하게 기도를 확보한다.

외상이 있는 환자의 시각화된 입기관삽관은 환자의 머리와 목을 도수로 고정하여 중립 자세를 유지한 상태에서 시행한다. 도수로 고정하고 유지하는 동안 입기관삽관을 시행하려면 비외상 환자의 삽관 시 보다 추가적인 교육과 실습이 필요하다.

심정지 상태가 아닌 저산소증 외상 환자의 경우 삽관을 초기 기도 처치로 시행해서는 안 된다. 병원 전 처치 제공자는 간단한 기도 보조 장치 또는 도수 조작으로 기도를 유지하고 환자에게 고농도 산소를 공급한 후에만 삽관해야 한다. 병원 전 처치 제공자는 삽관할 때 20초 이상 환기를 중단해서는 안 된다. 어떤 이유로든 환기를 30초 이상 중단해서는 안 된다.

의식이 있는 환자나 구역 반사가 있는 환자에게는 시각적 입기관삽관이 매우 어렵기 때문에 원칙적으로 시도해서는 안 된다. 병원 전 처치 제공자는 추가 교육, 프로토콜 개발 및 의료 지도 의사의 승인을 받은 후 약물 보조 삽관을 고려해야 한다.

삽관 성공률은 종종 주어진 장비의 디자인에 대한 시술자의 편안함과 관련이 있으므로 후두경 날의 선택은 개인의 선호도에 따라 달라질 수 있다.

참고: 목뼈보호대는 아래턱뼈의 전방 움직임과 입을 완전히 벌리는 것을 제한한다. 따라서 적절한 척추 고정을 시행한 후 목뼈보호대를 제거하고 목뼈를 도수 고정을 유지하면서 기관내삽관을 시도한다. 삽관이 완료되면 목뼈보호대를 다시 착용시킨다. 삽관을 시도하기 전에 병원 전 처치 제공자는 필요한 모든 장비를 조립 및 점검하고 표준 예방 조치를 따라야 한다. 첫 번째 병원 전 처치 제공자는 환자의 머리 위쪽에 무릎을 꿇고 백마스크 장비와 고농도 산소 환기를 한다. 일반적으로 삽관을 시도하기 전에 가능하면 산소포화도가 93% 이상 유지해야 한다.

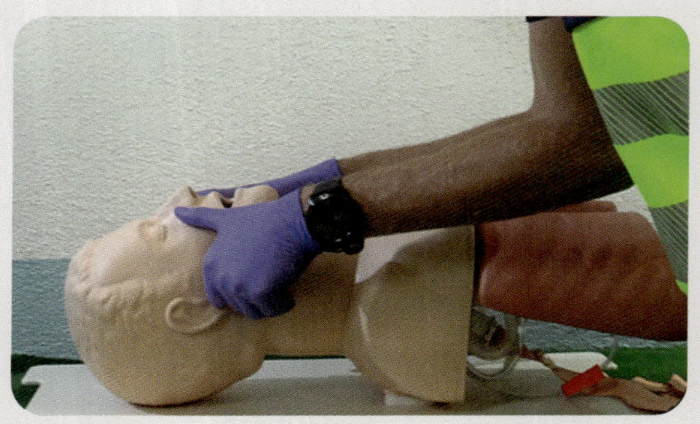

1 두 번째 병원 전 처치 제공자는 환자 옆에 무릎을 꿇고 환자의 머리와 목을 도수로 고정한다. 두 번째 병원 전 처치 제공자는 엄지손가락을 환자의 광대뼈에 대고 손가락을 머리 뒤에 위치시켜 머리를 잡는다. 손의 위치가 잘못되면 입을 막아 후두경 검사가 불가능할 수 있다. 예방산소투여 후 첫 번째 처치 제공자는 환기를 멈추고 왼손에 후두경을 잡고 오른손에 기관내관(파일럿 밸브에 주사기 연결된 상태)를 잡는다. 탐침을 사용하는 경우 장비를 확인하고 점검할 때 이미 기관내관에 삽입했어야 한다. 탐침의 원위 끝은 기관내관의 원위 입구에 약간 못 미치도록 삽입해야 한다.

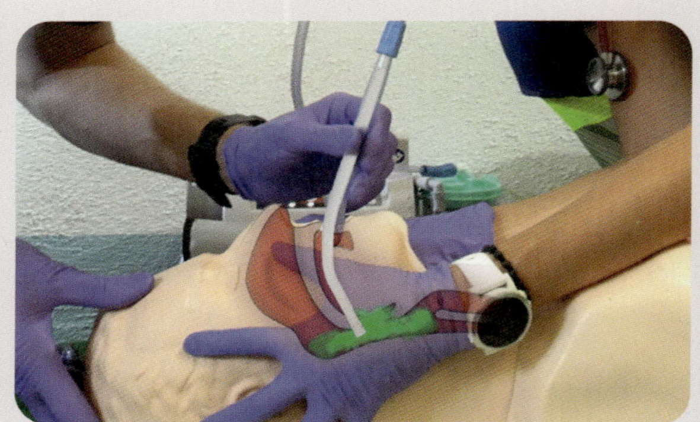

2 병원 내 삽관과 마네킹 삽관의 본질적인 차이점은 먼저 기도를 흡인하면 1차 성공률이 크게 향상되며 비디오 후두경을 사용하는 경우 더욱 그렇다. 흡인 구멍이 큰 단단한 카테터와 리버스 그립 기술을 사용하여 목구멍 뒤쪽을 깨끗이 흡인한 다음 카테터 끝을 입인두 뒤쪽에 두고 왼쪽으로 이동하여 후두경 날을 넣을 공간을 확보한다. 흡인기를 작동시키면 분비되는 분비물을 계속 제거하여 후두를 잘 볼 수 있다(듀 칸토 기법).

(다음 페이지에 계속)

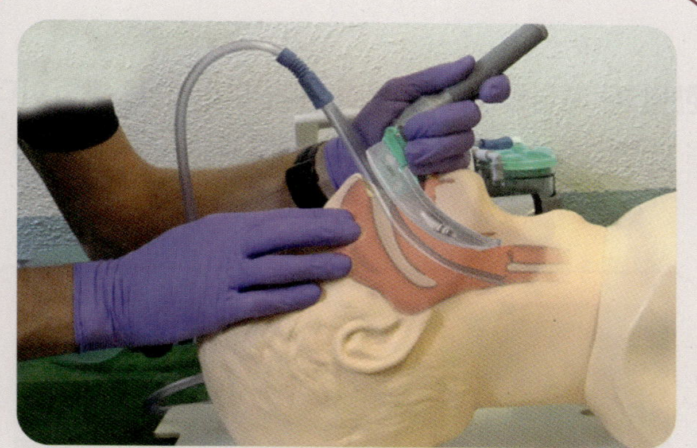

3	후두경을 왼손으로 잡고 후두경 날은 원하는 기준점을 확인하면서 기도의 중심을 향해 정확한 깊이로 환자의 기도 오른쪽으로 삽입한다.

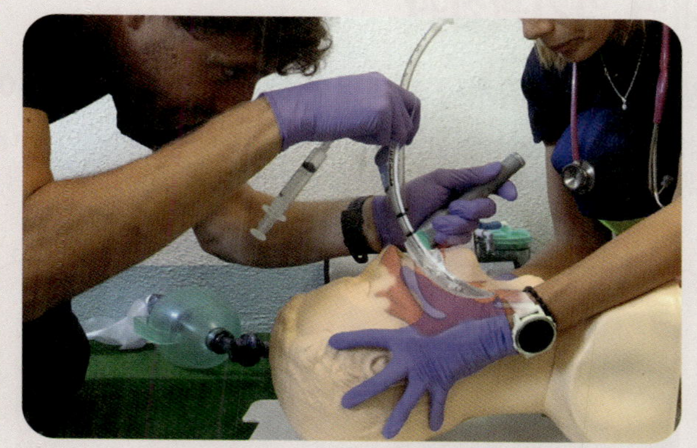

4	원하는 기준점을 확인한 후 기관내관을 환자의 성대 사이에 원하는 깊이까지 삽입한다.

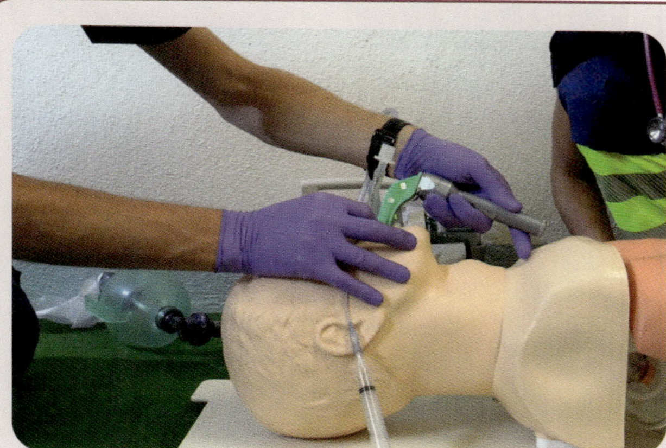

5　그런 다음 기관내관을 제자리에 고정한 상태에서 후두경을 제거하고 기관내관 측면의 깊이 표시를 확인한다. 탐침을 사용했다면 이때 탐침을 제거해야 한다. 파일럿 밸브에 환자의 기관과 기관내관의 커프 사이의 밀폐를 완료할 수 있을 만큼 충분한 공기를 주입하고(보통 5mL의 공기) 파일럿 밸브에서 주사기를 제거한다. 첫 번째 병원 전 처치 제공자는 기관내관의 근위 끝에 보유주머니가 달린 백마스크를 연결하고 호흡마다 환자의 가슴이 상승하는 것을 관찰하면서 환기를 재개한다. 환자의 머리와 목을 도수 고정으로 안정시키는 것은 과정 내내 유지해야 한다(명확성을 위해 그림에서는 표시되지 않음). 양쪽 호흡음과 상복부에서 공기음이 들리지 않는지 그리고 파형호기말이산화탄소분압측정을 포함하여 적절한 방법으로 기관내관의 위치를 확인한다(이 장의 앞부분의 기관내관 위치 확인 부분 참조). 위치가 확인되면 기관내관을 고정한다. 환자가 움직이지 않는 통제된 상황에서는 테이프나 기타 상업적으로 사용할 수 있는 장치를 사용하는 것이 적절하지만, 병원 전 상황에서 기관내관의 변위를 방지하는 가장 좋은 방법은 항상 튜브를 물리적으로 고정하는 것이다.

대면 입기관삽관

원리: 환자의 위치나 자세로 인해 기존 방법의 사용이 제한될 때 확실한 기도를 확보하기 위한 대체 방법이다.

병원 전 환경에서는 병원 전 처치 제공자가 전통적인 방법으로 기관내삽관을 시행하기 위해 환자의 머리 위쪽에 위치할 수 없는 상황이 발생할 수 있다. 삽관형 후두마스크는 이러한 상황에서 매우 효율적인 술기이다.

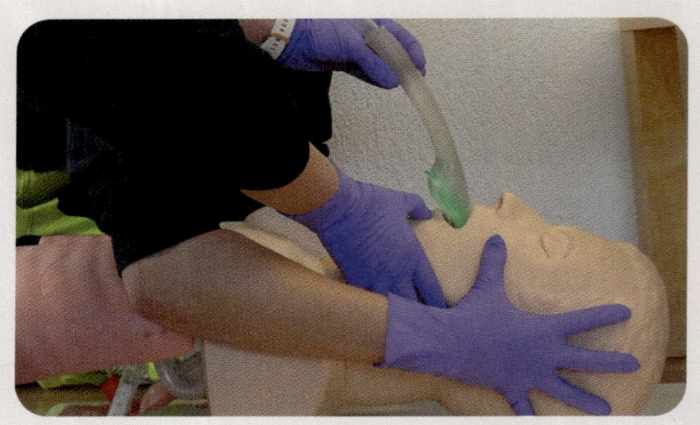

1 첫 번째 병원 전 처치 제공자는 정면에서 도수로 머리를 고정하고 두 번째 처치 제공자는 ILMA를 삽입한다. 두 번째 처치 제공자는 가슴 청진과 가능한 경우 ETCO₂를 사용하여 후두마스크의 위치를 확인한다.

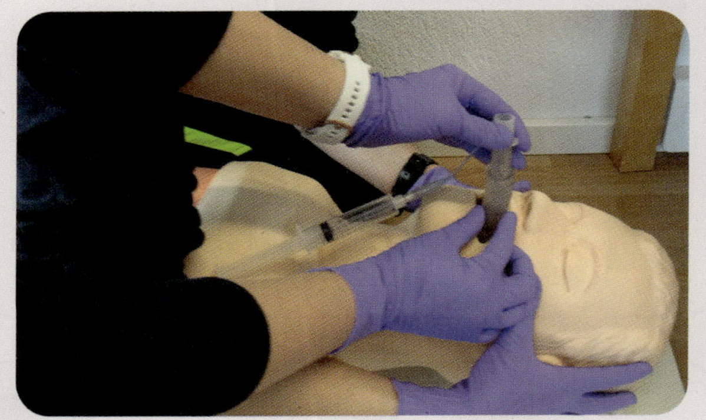

2 ILMA가 후두 입구 앞에 있는지 확인한 후 두 번째 병원 전 처치 제공자는 기관내관을 삽입한다. ILMA의 입구는 치아에서 4~5cm에 위치한다는 것을 기억한다. 따라서 이 거리를 기관내관의 표준 삽입 깊이에 더해야 한다(일반적으로 I-gal #5의 경우 4cm). 두 번째 병원 전 처치 제공자는 청진, 가슴 검사 및 ETCO₂ 파형 평가를 통해 기관내관의 삽입 위치를 주의 깊게 확인한다. 병원에 도착하기 전에 ILMA를 제거하려고 시도하지 않는다. ILMA는 기관내관에 대한 우수한 고정력을 제공하며 기관내관이 빠지거나 막히면 중요한 백업 장치이다.

Courtesy of J.C. Pitteloud MD, Switzerland.

Airtraq 채널 비디오 후두경을 이용한 삽관

원리: Airtraq 장치는 혀 주변의 성문을 시각화할 수 있으며 성대를 통해 기관내관의 방향을 쉽게 하는 경로(channel)를 포함한다(King airway는 경로가 있는 또 다른 비디오 후두경으로 매우 유사한 방식으로 작동한다).

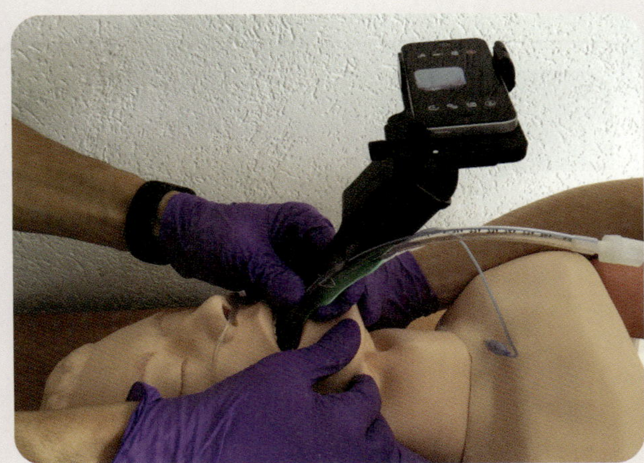

1 두 번째 병원 전 처치 제공자는 환자의 머리를 앞쪽에서 도수로 고정하고 첫 번째 병원 전 제공자는 목뼈보호대를 제거한다. 첫 번째 병원 전 처치 제공자는 비디오 후두경의 전원을 켜고 튜브를 위에서부터 Airtraq의 측면 경로로 밀어 넣어 상단을 가이드 경로의 끝에 맞춘다(경고: 튜브를 너무 깊게 삽입하면 시야를 가릴 수 있으므로 튜브 끝을 조명 뒤에 위치시킨다.). 후두경 검사 전에 기도를 흡인한다. 이는 비디오 후두경을 사용할 때 특히 필요하다. 기도를 흡인한 후 흡인 카테터 끝을 성대 아래에 그대로 두고 입의 왼쪽 모서리로 쓸어내려 후두경이 들어갈 공간을 만든다. 첫 번째 병원 전 처치 제공자는 주로 사용하지 않는 손의 엄지손가락으로 입을 벌리면서 주로 사용하는 손을 사용하여 장치를 환자의 입에 쉽게 삽입할 수 있도록 한다. Airtraq은 손바닥이 아닌 손가락으로 잡아야 하며 환자의 치아를 보호하기 위해 위에서부터 들지 않는다.

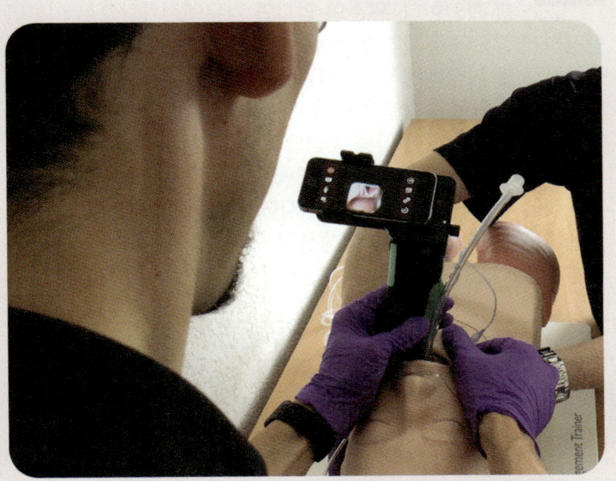

2 첫 번째 병원 전 처치 제공자는 Airtraq 끝이 혀의 뒤쪽에 닿을 때까지 윗니에 압력을 가하지 않도록 주의하면서 환자의 입 중앙선에 Airtraq를 삽입한다. Airtraq이 입인두 뒤쪽에 삽입되면 후두개, 모뿔연골 및 성대가 확인된다.

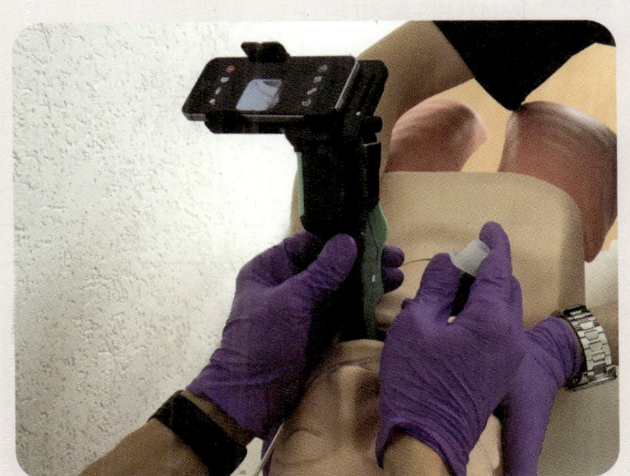

3 그런 다음 첫 번째 병원 전 처치 제공자는 튜브를 유도 경로 안에 유지하면서 앞으로 밀어서 성대 사이로 튜브를 삽입한다. 기관내관의 끝이 성대 뒤로 이동하는 경우 후두경을 1~2cm 뒤로 당기면 보통 문제가 해결된다. 첫 번째 병원 전 처치 제공자는 튜브를 고정한 상태에서 Airtraq를 옆으로 당겨서 튜브를 Airtraq에서 분리한다. 첫 번째 병원 전 처치 제공자는 청진 및 파형호기말이산화탄소분압측정 평가를 통해 튜브의 올바른 위치를 확인한다.

외과적 반지갑상연골절개

원리: 간단한 방법으로 기도 폐쇄를 완화할 수 없는 환자의 기도를 확보하는 방법이다.

시중에는 많은 장비가 있지만, 여기에 설명된 방법은 구급차에 보관된 간단하고 저렴한 장비를 사용한다. 장비에는 메스, 곡선 지혈물개, 기관 절개 튜브(또는 5.0mm~7.0mm 기관내관)가 포함된다. 표준 기관내관 튜브는 너무 길고 기관지 삽관의 위험이 있으므로 두 번째 선택이다. 이 술기는 연골이 매우 연약하여 절개가 어렵고 성문 아래의 두꺼운 점막으로 인해 내강을 찾기가 매우 어렵기 때문에 12세 미만의 소아에게는 권장되지 않는다.

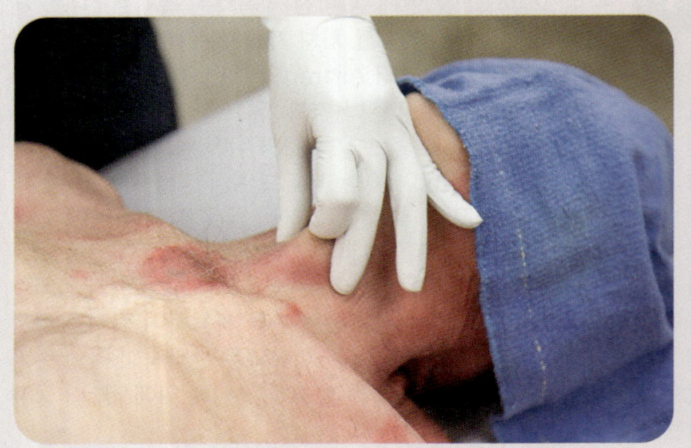

1 왼손의 엄지와 가운뎃손가락으로 후두를 고정하고 집게손가락으로 반지갑상막을 찾는다. 손바닥은 턱을 방해하지 않도록 한다.

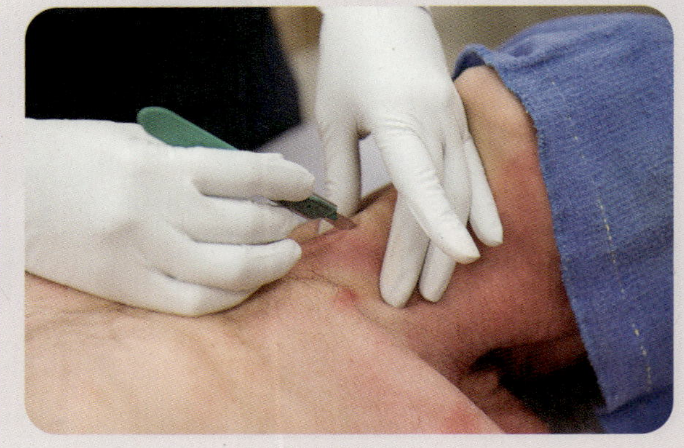

2 반지갑상연골에서 윤상돌기까지 2~3cm 수직으로 절개하고 집게손가락으로 촉진하여 반지갑상막의 위치를 확인한다. 왼손의 엄지와 가운뎃손가락으로 피부를 팽팽하게 잡으면 절개가 훨씬 쉬워진다. 메스는 오른손으로 잡고 손 뒤꿈치를 복장뼈에 단단히 얹는다. 목동맥과 목정맥이 근처에 있으므로 날카로운 칼날을 다룰 때 주의해야 한다. 반지갑상막을 찾으면 메스로 천공한 다음 수평으로 확대한다. 환자가 삼키거나 기침하는 경우 접근을 잃지 않도록 다음 단계까지 칼날을 잠시 제자리에 유지하여 살아 있는 환자에게 흔히 발생할 수 있는 상황을 방지한다. 이런 일이 발생하면 구멍을 다시 찾기가 매우 어려울 수 있다.

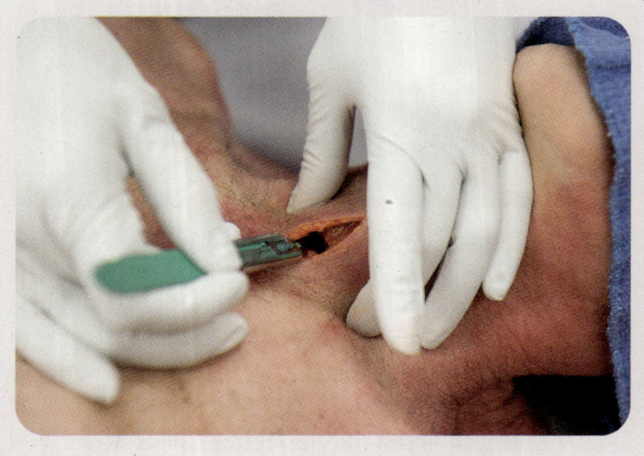

3 절개 부위에 구부러진 겸자를 삽입하고 위쪽으로 들어올려 기관을 향한 입구를 만든다. 튜브를 기관으로 삽입하고 커프를 팽창시킨다. 청진 및 파형호기말이산화탄소 분압측정 평가로 튜브의 위치를 확인한다. 외과적 기도유지에 표준 기관내관을 사용하는 경우 주의할 점은 표준 기관내관은 반지갑상연골절개 캐뉼러보다 훨씬 길기 때문에 주 기관지로 들어가기 쉽다.

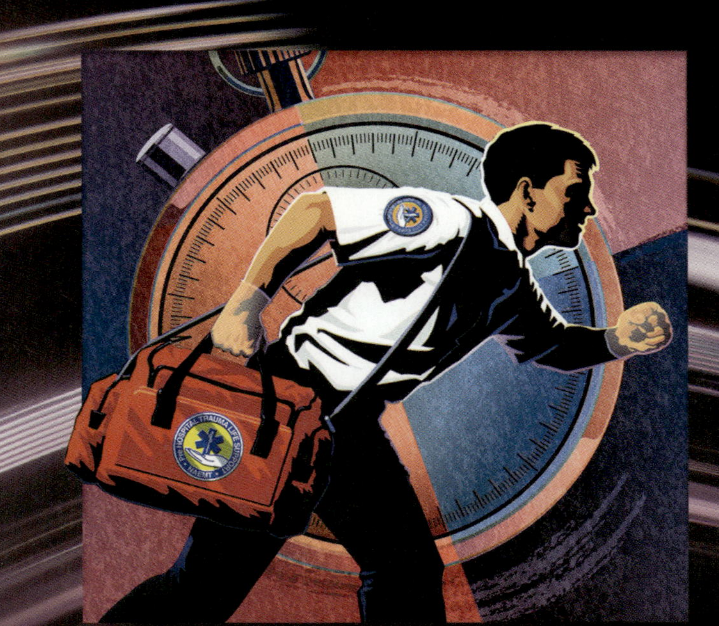

특별한 손상

제 8 장 **머리와 목 외상**

제 9 장 **척추 외상**

제 10 장 **가슴 외상**

제 11 장 **복부 외상**

제 12 장 **근골격 외상**

제 13 장 **화상 손상**

제 14 장 **소아 외상**

제 15 장 **노인 외상**

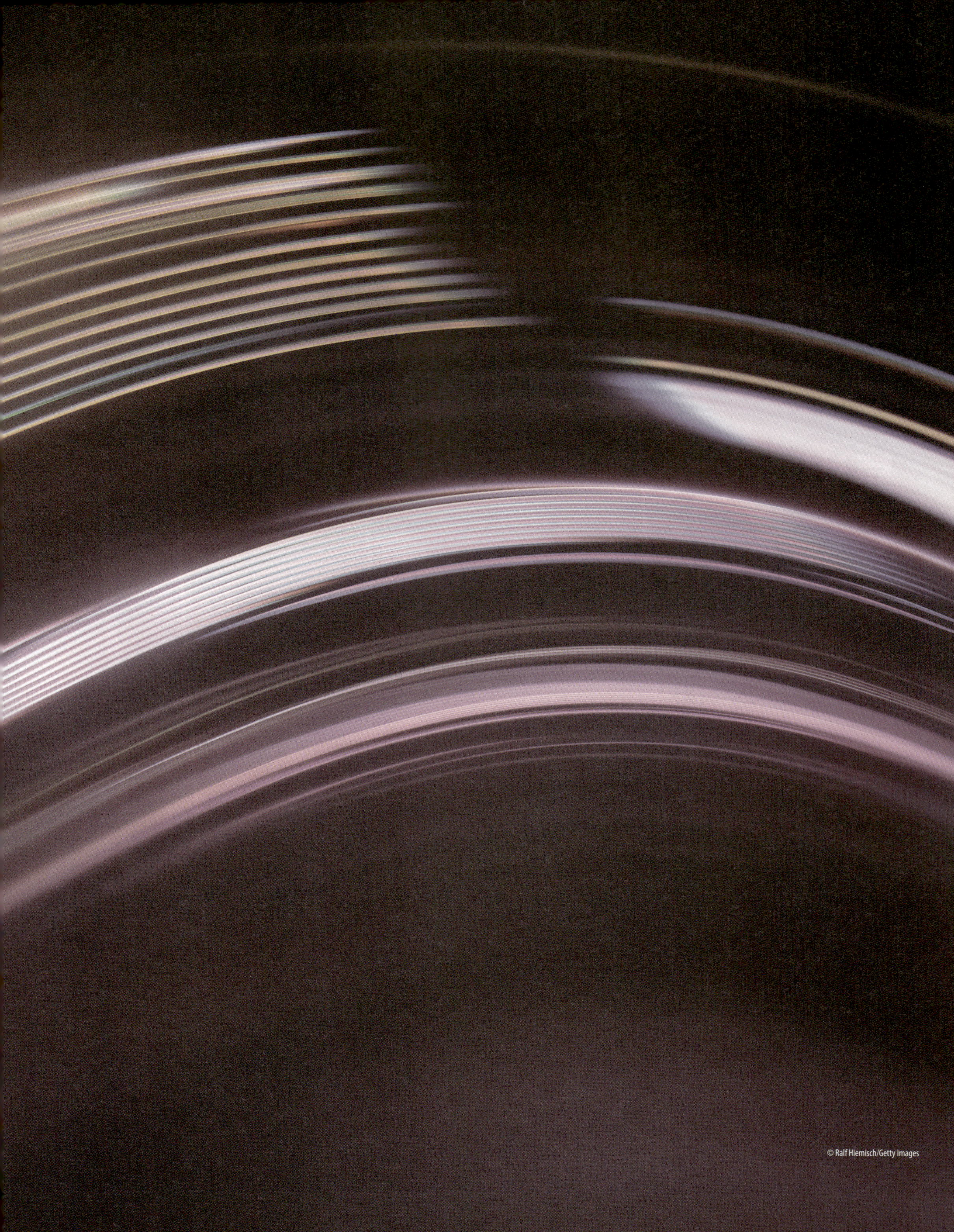
© Ralf Hiemisch/Getty Images

머리와 목 외상

Lead Editors
Christine Ramirez, MD
Angela Lumba-Brown, MD
Deborah M. Stein, MD, MPH

학습 목표   이 장의 학습을 완료하면 다음과 같은 내용을 수행할 수 있다.

- 머리 외상의 물리학을 외상성 뇌손상의 가능성과 연관시킬 수 있다.
- 머리 외상 환자의 평가를 지원하고 현장 인상을 공식화하기 위해 과거 데이터와 연관하여 외상성 뇌손상의 병태생리학적 증상을 인식할 수 있다.
- 병원 전 환경에서 글래스고혼수척도 점수를 포함한 일련의 신경학적 평가의 중요성에 대해 논의하고 환자를 이송할 의료기관에 보고할 수 있다.
- 외상성 노 손상이 의심되는 환자의 이송 시간이 짧을 때와 길어질 때를 대비하여 현장 처치 계획을 수립할 수 있다.
- 특정 유형의 일차 및 이차 TBI의 병태생리, 처치 및 잠재적인 결과를 비교하고 대조할 수 있다.
- 외상성 뇌손상이 확인되거나 의심되는 환자에 대한 적극적인 기도 관리의 중요성을 인식할 수 있다.
- 머리와 목 손상 환자의 적절한 처치에 필요한 이송, 병원 전 처치 수준, 병원 자원과 관련하여 환자 처치 결정의 기준을 파악할 수 있다.

시나리오

외부 온도가 29℃인 여름날 당신과 동료는 30세 남자가 마라톤 결승선에서 현수막을 설치하던 중 4.3m의 사다리에서 떨어졌다는 신고를 받고 사고 현장으로 출동한다. 현장에 도착했을 때 환자는 바로누워있고 반응이 없다. 목격자가 환자의 머리와 목을 일직선으로 도수 고정하고 있다.

초기 평가 시 호흡 깊이와 속도가 달라지는 불규칙한 호흡 양상이 관찰된다. 환자의 양쪽 귓구멍과 콧구멍에서 피가 섞인 액체가 나온다. 환자의 눈은 감겨 있고 당신이 말을 걸어도 반응하지 않는다.

초기 평가에서 구역 반사가 없음을 확인하고 입인두기도기를 삽입한다. 동료가 백마스크로 분당 12회의 속도로 환자에게 환기를 시행한다. 환자의 오른쪽 동공이 확장된 것을 확인하였고 노동맥박은 54회/분으로 규칙적이며 산소포화도는 96%이다. 환자의 피부는 차갑고, 건조하며 창백하다. 글래스고혼수척도(GCS)는 7점(E2, V1, M4)이다.

당신은 환자를 신속하게 이송할 준비를 하고 구급차에 환자를 태워 병원으로 이송 중에 목뼈 고정을 계속 유지하면서 이차평가를 한다. 뒤통수를 촉지하면 환자가 고통스러운 신음을 낸다. 당신은 환자의 체온을 유지하기 위해 담요로 덮어주고 혈압을 측정한 결과 184/102mmHg이었다. 심전도 검사 결과 동서맥이 관찰되며 드물게 조기심실박동이 나타난다. 오른쪽 동공은 여전히 확장된 상태이다.

(다음 페이지에 계속)

개요

외상성 뇌손상(TBI)은 손상과 관련된 사망과 장애의 주요 원인인 공중 보건 문제이다. 전 세계적으로 5,500만 명 이상의 사람들이 외상성 뇌손상 관련 장애를 겪고 있으며 그 유병률은 계속 증가하고 있다. 미국에서만 매년 최소 350만 건의 새로운 외상성 뇌손상 사례가 발생하고 있다. 미국 질병통제예방센터(CDC)에 따르면 2019년 미국에서는 약 61,000명의 외상성 뇌손상 관련 사망자가 발생했으며 이는 하루에 약 166명의 외상성 뇌손상 사망자가 발생하고 연간 약 288,000명의 입원 환자가 발생하고 있다. 또한 외상성 뇌손상은 전 세계적으로 매년 300만 명 이상의 어린이가 뇌손상을 입는 가장 흔한 사망 및 장애의 원인이다. 중등도 및 중증 뇌손상의 사망률은 각각 약 10%와 30%이다. 중등도 및 중증 뇌손상에서 살아남은 사람 중 50~99%는 어느 정도의 영구적인 신경학적 장애를 갖게 된다. 중등도 및 중증 외상성 뇌손상 환자는 이환율과 사망률이 상당히 높지만, 전체 외상성 뇌손상의 80%는 경증이며 이러한 환자의 대부분은 응급실에서 또는 일차평가 및 처치 후 집으로 퇴원한다.

외상성 뇌손상의 일반적인 원인으로는 자동차 충돌(MVCs), 의도하지 않은 추락, 관통상(예: 총기) 또는 폭행이 포함된다. 의도하지 않은 추락은 모든 TBI 관련 입원 중 연정 조정 비율과 비율(52.3%)이 가장 높으며 75세 이상의 노인에서 가장 빈번하게 발생한다. 자동차 충돌은 특히 15~54세 사이에 두 번째로 흔한 외상성 뇌손상 관련 입원(20.4%)이다. 추락과 자동차 충돌은 소아 인구에서 가장 흔한 주요 손상 기전이기도 하다.

병원 전 환경에서 외상성 뇌손상이 의심되는 환자를 처치하는 것은 여러 가지 이유로 어려운 일이다. 손상, 외상 후 발작, 동반질병, 동반된 쇼크로 인한 관류저하, 구토 등으로 인해 의식 상태가 이차적으로 변할 수 있다. 구토가 오래 지속되는 등의 외상성 뇌손상 증상은 기도 관리를 어렵게 할 수 있다. 동시에 발생하는 손상은 혈류역학적 안정성에 영향을 미치고 뇌손상이 악화하고 예후가 나빠질 위험을 증가시킬 수 있다.

병원 전 처치 제공자의 목표는 발생 가능성이 있는 외상성 뇌손상을 신속하게 파악하고 환자를 안정시켜 의료기관으로 이송하는 동안 이차 손상의 위험을 최소화하는 것이다. 외상성 뇌손상에 대한 병원 전 처치는 호흡 및 혈류역학적 안정성을 최적화하는 것을 목표로 한다.

해부학

해부학에 대한 지식은 외상성 뇌손상의 복잡한 병태생리학을 이해하고 파악하는 데 중요하다. 두피는 머리를 덮고 두개골과 뇌를 어느 정도 보호한다. 두피는 피부, 결합조직, 널힘줄(또는 머리덮개널힘줄) 및 두개골의 골막을 포함하여 여러 층으로 구성된다. 두피는 질기고 두꺼운 섬유 조직의 층으로 두피에 구조적인 지지를 제공하는 층이며 골막은 뼈에 영양을 공급한다. 두피는 혈관이 많고 상처를 입었을 때 출혈이 심할 수 있다.

두개골은 어린 시절에 하나의 구조로 융합되는 여러 개의 뼈로 구성되어 있다(**그림 6-9** 참조). 두개골 바닥을 관통하는 여러 개의 작은 구멍은 혈관과 뇌신경이 지나가는 통로를 제공한다. 큰 구멍인 대공은 두개골 바닥에 위치하며 뇌줄기에서 척수로 가는 통로 역할을 한다(**그림 8-1**). 영아의 경우 뼈와 뼈 사이에 숫구멍으로 알려진 부드러운 부분을 확인할 수 있다. 영아는 일반적으로 2세까지 뼈가 융합될 때까지 뇌의 이 부분에 대한 보호 장치가 없다. 영아의 두개골은 완전히 융합되지 않았기 때문에 두개골 내 출혈로 인해 뼈가 더 벌어져 두개골 내에 더 많은 출혈이 축적될 수 있다.

두개골은 뇌를 보호하는 중요한 역할을 한다. 두개골은 해면질 해면골 층을 둘러싸고 있는 바깥판과 속판으로 알려진 두 층의 피질 조직으로 이루어져 있다. 전두골과 같이 두개골을 구성하는 대부분의 뼈는 두껍고 튼튼하다. 그러나 두개골은 측두골과 벌집뼈 부위가 특히 얇기 때문에 이 부위에서 골절이 발생하기 쉽다. 또한 두개골기

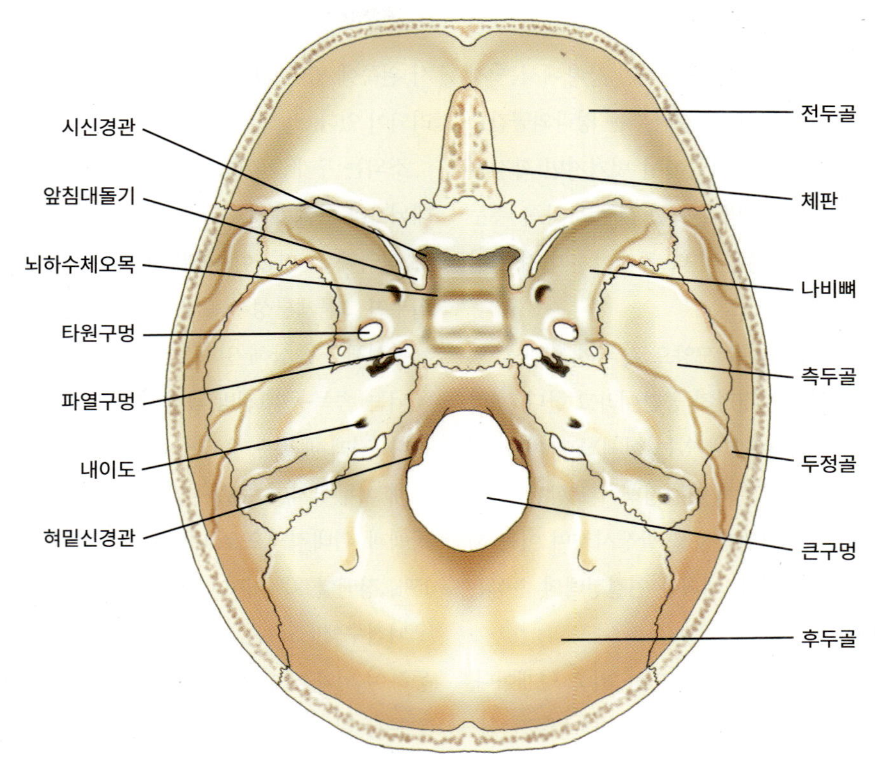

그림 8-1 두개골 바닥의 내부 모습
© National Association of Emergency Medical Technicians (NAEMT)

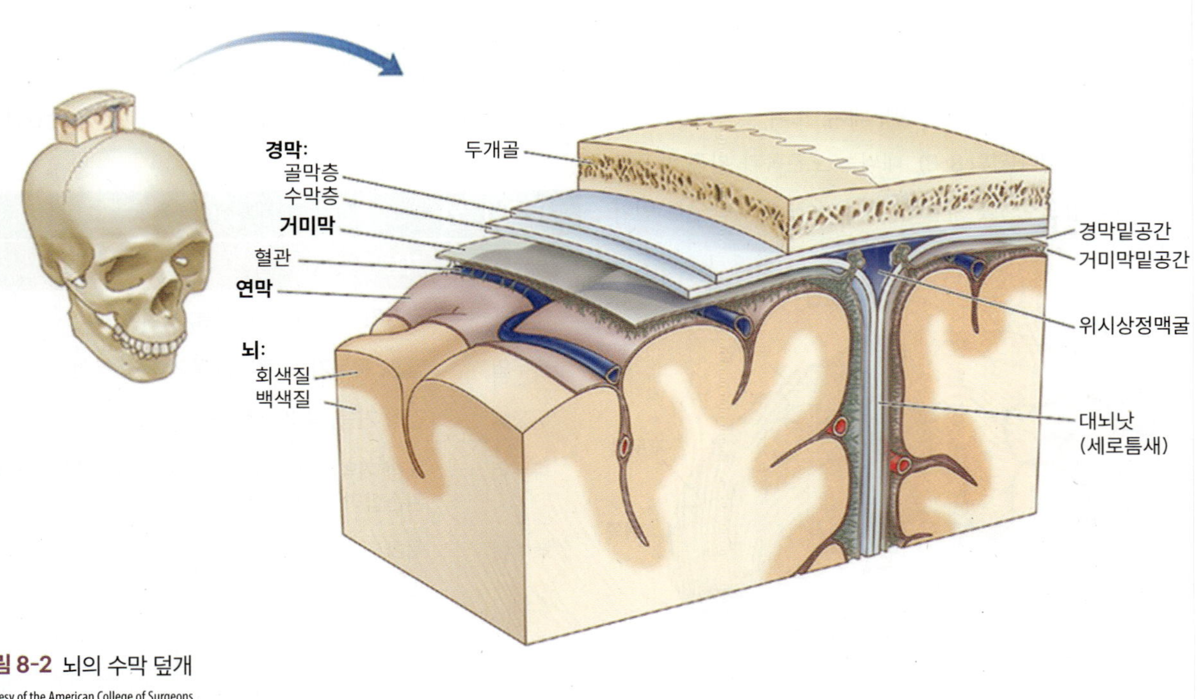

그림 8-2 뇌의 수막 덮개
Courtesy of the American College of Surgeons.

저의 내부 표면은 거칠고 불규칙하다(**그림 8-1**). 무딘 충격에 노출되면 뇌가 이러한 불규칙한 부분을 따라 미끄러지면서 뇌타박상이나 열상을 입을 수 있다.

뇌는 경막, 거미막, 연막으로 알려진 세 개의 분리된 막으로 덮여 있다(**그림 8-2**). 가장 바깥쪽 층인 경막은 단단한 섬유조직으로 구성되어 있으며 두개골의 속판을 감싸고 있다. 정상적인 상황에서는 경막과 두개골 사이에 공간이 없다. 그러나 이 접합부는 경막외공간으로 알려진 잠재적인 공간으로 경막이 두개골에서 벗겨지면 확장될 수 있다. 예를 들어, 중간 수막 동맥은 경막과 속판 사이의 양쪽 측두골의 홈에 있다. 측두골 골절로 인해 중간 수막 동맥이 찢어져 경막외혈종이 발생할 수 있다.

거미막은 경막 깊숙이 위치하며 거미줄 모양으로 뇌와 혈관을 덮고 있다. 경막과 거미막 사이의 공간은 경막하 공간이라고 한다. 경막외 공간과 달리 경막하 공간은 경막 아래에 있는 실제 공간이다. 이 공간에는 두개골과 뇌 사이 혈관의 일부인 연결정맥이 포함된다. 이러한 정맥의 외상성 파열은 종종 경막밑혈종을 발생시키며 이는 뇌 조직의 추가 손상과 관련이 있을 수 있다. 이러한 연결정맥의 손상은 경막하혈종의 이환율을 설명한다.

가장 깊은 막은 연막이다. 연막은 뇌에 붙어 있는 최종 덮개이다. 거미막과 연막 사이의 공간을 거미막밑공간이라고 하며 이 공간에는 뇌의 바닥에서 나와 뇌를 덮고 있는 뇌혈관이 있다. 일반적으로 외상이나 뇌동맥류 파열로 인해 파열되면 거미막밑공간으로 출혈이 발생하여 거미막밑혈종이 생긴다. 거미막밑혈종은 다른 심각한 뇌손상의 지표가 될 수 있다.

뇌는 머리덮개뼈의 약 80%를 차지하며 대뇌, 소뇌 및 뇌줄기의 세 가지 주요 영역으로 나뉜다(**그림 8-3**). 대뇌는 오른쪽과 왼쪽 반구로 구성되며 여러 개의 엽으로 세분화할 수 있다. 우세 대뇌반구는 언어 중추를 포함하고 있으며 오른손잡이의 대다수와 왼손잡이의 85%에서 왼쪽에 있다. 대뇌는 소뇌와 경막의 연장선인 소뇌천막에 의해 분리되어 있다.

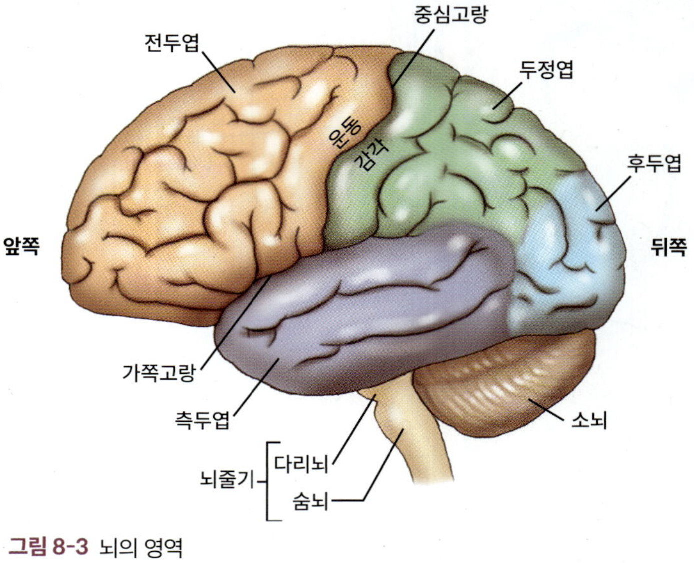

소뇌는 두개골 뒤쪽 오목, 뇌줄기 뒤, 대뇌 아래에 있다. 뇌줄기는 대뇌보다 아래쪽에, 소뇌는 대뇌보다 앞쪽에 있다. **표 8-1**은 뇌의 주요 영역과 그 기능이 나열되어 있다. 각성과 각성도를 담당하는 뇌의 일부인 그물체활성계의 대부분은 뇌줄기에도 있다. 무딘 손상은 그물체활성계를 손상해 일시적인 의식 소실로 이어질 수 있다.

뇌는 속목동맥(전방)과 척추동맥(후방)으로부터 동맥혈을 공급받는다. 정맥 배액은 주로 얕은 대뇌정맥과 깊은 대뇌정맥 네트워크를 통해 이루어지며 주로 경막정맥굴과 갈렌큰대뇌정으로 배액되고 목정맥과 위대정맥으로 배액된다. 언제든지 두개내 혈액량은 동맥혈 15%, 정맥혈 40%이며 나머지 45%는 미세순환이다.

뇌척수액(CSF)은 뇌의 뇌실계에서 생성되어 거미막밑공간으로 이동하여 뇌와 척수를 둘러싸고 있다. 뇌척수액의 주요 역할은 영양분, 호르몬 및 신경전달물질을 뇌로 전달하고 제거하는 것이다. 뇌척수액 생산량은 하루에 약 500mL이며 지속해서 생성 및 재흡수되어 총 뇌척수액 부피는 약 150mL가 된다. 이 부피는 뇌실질 및 뇌 혈류의 부피에 비해 적은 양이다.

뇌와 뇌줄기에서 유래하는 12개의 뇌신경이 있다(**그림 8-4**). 뇌신경(CN III; 눈돌림신경)은 동공 수축을 조절한다. 눈돌림신경 소뇌천

그림 8-3 뇌의 영역

표 8-1 뇌	
부위	**기능**
대뇌	감각기능, 운동기능, 지능, 기억력
전두엽	감정, 운동기능, 우세한 쪽의 언어 표현
두정엽	감각 기능, 공간 방향
측두엽	특정 기억 기능의 조절; 모든 오른손잡이와 대부분의 왼손잡이 개인의 음성 수신 및 통합
후두엽	시각
소뇌	운동
뇌줄기	뇌와 척수 사이의 신호 전달
중간뇌	그물체활성계를 통한 각성 및 각성도
다리뇌	호흡 무호흡 센터, 대뇌에서 수질 및 소뇌로 신호 전달
숨뇌	심폐 센터(호흡, 심박수)

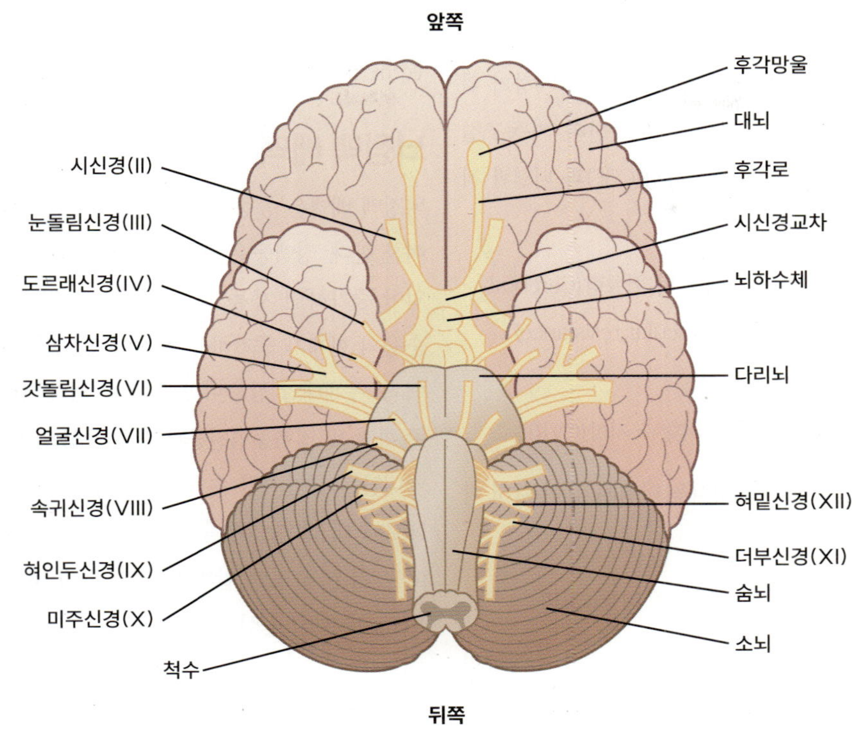

그림 8-4 뇌신경의 기원을 보여주는 뇌의 아래쪽 표면
© National Association of Emergency Medical Technicians (NAEMT)

막의 표면을 가로지르며 뇌의 아래쪽 탈출증을 유발하는 출혈이나 부종은 신경을 압박하여 기능을 손상하고 동공 확장을 유발하므로 뇌손상이 의심되는 환자를 평가하는데 중요하다.

생리학

뇌 혈류

뇌의 신경세포는 세포 활동과 생존을 위해 산소와 포도당을 공급하기 위해 지속적인 혈류가 필요하다. 뇌 혈류는 분당 약 700mL의 속도로 발생하며 이는 심박출량의 약 15%에 해당한다. 심박출량은 심장이 1분 동안 펌프질하는 혈액의 양으로 일반적으로 분당 4~8L이다. 이 일정한 뇌 혈류는 1) 뇌에 혈액이 흐르도록 하는 적절한 압력(뇌관류 압력)과 2) 관류 압력의 변화에 따라 혈류에 대한 저항을 변화시키는 조절 기전(자동조절)에 의해 유지된다. 뇌 대사율은 뇌 혈류에 영향을 미치므로 신경세포 활동이 증가하면 뇌 혈류가 증가한다. 이것은 이후 부문에서 설명할 외상성 뇌손상의 치료에서 중요하다.

뇌 관류압

뇌 관류압(CPP)은 뇌 순환을 통해 혈액을 밀어내고 뇌 혈류를 유지하는 데 사용할 수 있는 압력의 양이다. 뇌 관류압은 환자의 평균 동맥(MAP) 및 두개내압(ICP)과 직접적인 관련이 있다. 평균 동맥압은 한 번의 심장 주기 동안 동맥의 평균 압력이며 중요한 장기에 대한 관류의 지표다. 두개내압은 두개골 내에서 뇌 조직, 혈액, 뇌척수액의 결합한 압력이다.

뇌 관류압은 다음 공식으로 표현된다.

뇌 관류압(Cerebral perfusion pressure) =평균 동맥압(Mean arterial pressure) - 두개내압(Intracranial pressure)

또는

$$CPP = MAP - ICP$$

정상 평균 동맥압의 범위는 85~95mmHg이다. 성인의 두개내압은 일반적으로 15mmHg 미만이다. 소아의 경우 3~7mmHg, 영아의 경우 1.5~6mmHg이다. 따라서 뇌 관류압은 일반적으로 70~80mmHg이다. 혈압과 외상성 뇌손상 후 발생할 수 있는 혈압과 두개내압의 급격한 증가 또는 감소는 뇌 관류에 영향을 미칠 수 있다.

뇌 혈류의 자기 조절작용

뇌에 다양하게 변화하는 조건에서 뇌 혈류를 일정하게 유지하기 위해 매일 열심히 노력한다. 이 과정을 자동조절이라고 한다. 자동조절은 뇌의 정상적인 기능에 매우 중요하며 뇌 혈류량(CBF)과 뇌혈관 저항(CVR)에 따라 달라진다.

뇌 관류압(Cerebral perfusion pressure) = 뇌 혈류량(Cerebral blood flow) × 뇌혈관 저항(Cerebral vascular resistance)

또는

뇌 관류압(CPP) = 뇌 혈류량(CBF) × 뇌혈관 저항(CVR)

뇌의 주요 관심사는 뇌 혈류이므로 이 방정식을 다음과 같이 다시 작성하는 것이 유용하다.

뇌 혈류량(CBF) = 뇌 관류압(CPP)/뇌혈관 저항(CVR)

자동 조절은 혈관 확장 또는 혈관 수축을 통해 CVR을 조정하여 이루어진다. CPP가 감소하면 뇌동맥 혈관 확장이 CBF를 유지하기 위해 CVR을 감소시킨다. 마찬가지로 CPP가 증가하면 동맥 혈관 수축이 유도되어 결과적으로 CVR이 증가한다. 일반적으로 자동 조절은 50~150mmHg 사이의 CPP를 보상할 수 있다. 이 범위를 벗어나면 CBF는 CPP에 따라 선형적으로 변화한다. 따라서 뇌관류압이 50mmHg 미만이 되면 뇌 혈류가 감소하기 시작한다.

뇌 혈류 감소를 보상하는 또 다른 방법은 뇌를 통과하는 혈액에서 더 많은 산소를 추출하는 것이다. 허혈의 임상 증상과 징후(어지럼과 의식 상태 변화)는 감소한 관류가 뇌의 대사 요구를 충족시키기 위해 산소 추출을 증가시키려는 능력을 초과할 때까지 발견되지 않는다. 뇌 혈류가 감소하기 시작하면 뇌 기능이 저하되고 허혈로 인한 영구적인 뇌손상 위험이 증가한다. 손상된 뇌는 자동 조절을 활성화하고 뇌 혈류를 적절하게 유지하기 위해 정상보다 높은 뇌 관류 압력이 필요할 수 있다.

뇌 관류압은 뇌 혈류의 적절성을 평가하는 데 사용된다. 외상 시에는 CPP, 두개내압 및 MAP 사이의 관계는 중요하다. 급성 두개내출혈은 주변 조직을 압박하여 두개내압을 증가시킨다. 이것을 질량 효과라고 한다. 두개내압이 증가하면 뇌로 혈액을 보내는 데 필요한 압력도 증가한다. 이후 CPP를 유지하기 위해 MAP이 증가한다. MAP이 두개내압의 증가를 따라가지 못하거나 두개내압을 낮추기 위한 처치를 신속하게 시행하지 않으면 뇌를 통해 흐르는 혈액의 양이 감소하기 시작하여 허혈성 뇌손상과 뇌 기증 장애로 이어질 수 있다. 따라서 두개내압 모니터가 없는 경우 가장 좋은 방법은 높은 정상 MAP을 유지하는 것이다.

뇌정맥 배액

뇌정맥 배액은 종종 간과되지만, 두개내압과 자동 조절에 중요한 기여를 한다. 정맥동은 팽창과 압박에 취약하다. 예를 들어, 뇌 혈류 유입이 증가하면 자동 조절 기전으로 정맥 배수가 증가한다. 그러나 순응의 한계가 증가하는 시점이 있으며 정맥 배수가 부적절하면 정맥 및 두개내압 상승이 발생할 수 있다. 함몰두개골 골절, 두개내 혈종 확장 및 정맥동혈전증과 같은 급성 압박도 정맥 배수를 손상해 두개내압을 증가시킬 수 있다. 우성 정맥동 폐쇄는 비우성 정맥동 폐쇄보다 더 많은 영향을 미친다. 머리 굴곡이나 목뼈보호대를 꽉 조이는 경우 목정맥 압박과 같은 두개 외 원인도 정맥 배수를 거의 10mmHg까지 손상할 수 있다

산소와 뇌 혈류

뇌는 대사가 활발한 기관이므로 산소 요구량이 많다. 산소 수치가 감소하면(저산소증) 뇌 혈류를 급격히 증가시키기 위해 혈관 크게 확장된다. 이 반응은 일반적으로 동맥혈산소분압(PaO$_2$)이 50mmHg 이하로 떨어질 때까지 일어나지 않는다. 때때로 뇌 혈류량은 휴식 시 수준의 최대 400%까지 증가할 수 있다.

이산화탄소와 뇌 혈류

뇌혈관은 수축하거나 확장을 통해 동맥혈이산화탄소 수치의 변화에 반응한다. 이산화탄소의 수치가 감소하면(저이산화탄소혈증) 혈관 수축이 발생하고 수치가 높아지면(고이산화탄소혈증) 혈관 확장이 일어난다. 과다환기는 폐에서 이산화탄소가 배출되는 속도를 증가시켜 동맥혈이산화탄소분압(PaCO$_2$)을 감소시킨다. 결과적으로 저이산화탄소혈증은 뇌의 산-염기 균형을 변화시켜 혈관 수축을 일으킨다. 이 뇌혈관 수축은 뇌의 혈관 내 용적을 감소시켜 뇌 혈액 용적을 감소시키고 따라서 종종 두개내압을 감소시킨다.

과다환기로 인한 뇌혈관 수축은 CPP가 뇌 혈류를 유지하기에 적절한지 여부와 관계없이 CVR도 증가시킨다. 결과적으로 과다환기는 CBF를 감소시켜 손상된 뇌가 허혈성 손상의 위험에 더 많이 노출될 수 있다. 동맥혈이산화탄소분압이 35mmHg 미만이면 뇌 허혈의 위험이 크다. 따라서 예방적 과다환기는 외상성 뇌손상 관리에서 권장되지 않는다.

반대로, $PaCO_2$가 정상 범위인 35~45mmHg(고이산화탄소혈증) 보다 높으면 뇌 세동맥이 확장되어 뇌 혈류가 증가하면서 동시에 혈관 내 용적이 증가하여 잠재적으로 두개내압이 증가하게 된다. 과다환기를 이용한 외상성 뇌손상 관리에 대해서는 이 장의 뒷부분에서 설명한다.

외상성 뇌손상의 병태생리학

외상성 뇌손상은 일차 뇌손상과 이차 뇌손상으로 분류할 수 있다.

일차 뇌손상

일차 뇌손상은 최초 외상 당시 발생한 모든 기계적 손상을 말한다. 여기에는 뇌와 그 덮개 및 관련 혈관 구조에 대한 손상이 포함된다. 일차 뇌손상에는 뇌타박상, 출혈, 신경 및 뇌혈관 손상이 포함된다. 신경 조직이 잘 재생되지 않고 회복 가능성이 거의 없으므로 일차 손상으로 인해 손실된 구조와 기능의 회복을 기대하기는 어렵다.

경미한 외상성 뇌손상

뇌진탕을 포함한 경미한 외상성 뇌손상은 미국질병통제예방센터(CDC)에서 "머리에 부딪히거나 충격을 받거나 충격을 받아 머리와 뇌가 앞뒤로 빠르게 움직이는 외상성 뇌손상의 일종"으로 정의한다. 이 갑작스러운 움직임은 두개골에서 뇌가 튕기거나 뒤틀리게 하여 뇌에 화학적 변화를 일으키고 때로는 뇌세포가 늘어나거나 손상될 수 있다. 경미한 외상성 뇌손상에서는 신경대사 연속단계 손상이 발생하며 대게 맨눈으로 보이는 신경 손상이 없는 경우가 많다. 그러나 고도로 발전된 뇌 영상의 등장으로 미세출혈 타박상을 가시화하여 "복잡한 경증 외상성 뇌손상"를 확인할 수 있으며 이는 기존의 회복 기간인 2~4주보다 더 오래 지속되는 뇌진탕 후 증상(**표 8-2**)을 나타낼 수 있다.

두통, 어지럼, 메스꺼움은 경미한 외상성 뇌손상 후에 급성으로 발생하는 경우가 많지만, 더 심각한 손상의 초기 증상일 수도 있다. 이러한 증상이 있는 환자는 즉시 병원으로 이송하여 추가 검사를 받아야 한다. 경미한 외상성 뇌손상의 공직적인 진단은 환자를 임상적으로 평가하고 관찰한 후 뇌 영상에서 임상적으로 유의미한 두 개내 병리가 없는 것으로 확인된 후 병원에서 이루어진다. 경미한 외상성 뇌손상 환자의 최대 30%가 4주 이상 뇌진탕 후유증을 지속해 경험한다. 이러한 증상에는 두통, 균형 문제, 안구 운동 장애, 불안 및 기분

표 8-2 일반적인 뇌진탕 후 증상	
분류	**증상**
전정	불균형, 메스꺼움, 어지럼
감각	흐릿한 시야, 편두통, 이명, 사진/소리공포증
인지	집중력 저하, 건망증
감정	피로, 불면증, 과민성, 우울

Data from Quinn DK, Mayer AR, Master CL, Fann JR. Prolonged postconcussive symptoms. *Am J Psychiatry*. 2018;175(2):103-111. doi:10.1176/appi.ajp.2017.17020235

장애, 집중력 장애와 같은 인지 장애가 포함된다.

두개내출혈

두개내출혈은 경막외출혈, 경막밑출혈, 거미막밑출혈, 뇌내출혈의 4가지 일반적인 유형으로 나뉜다. 각각의 징후와 증상이 상당히 겹치기 때문에 병원 전 단계(응급실뿐만 아니라)에서의 구체적인 진단은 거의 불가능하지만, 병원 전 처치 제공자는 특정적인 임상 증상을 바탕으로 특정 유형의 출혈을 의심할 수 있다. 그렇더라도 병원에서 컴퓨터단층촬영(CT) 검사를 시행한 후에야 확실한 진단을 내릴 수 있다. 이러한 출혈은 종종 단단한 두개골 내부의 공간을 차지하기 때문에 특히 출혈량이 많은 경우 두개내압을 급격히 증가시킬 수 있다.

경막외혈종

경막외혈종은 종종 주먹이나 야구공에 의한 충격과 같이 측두골에 비교적 낮은 속도의 충격으로 인해 발생하는 경우가 많다. 이 얇은 뼈의 골절은 중간수막동맥을 손상해 두개골과 경막 사이에 동맥 출혈을 일으킨다(**그림 8-5**). 이 고압의 동맥혈은 두개골 안쪽의 경막을 절개하거나 벗겨내기 시작하여 혈액으로 가득 찬 경막외 공간을 만들 수 있다. 이러한 경막외혈종은 CT 영상에서 볼 수 있듯이 경막이 두개골의 안쪽 테이블에 혈종을 붙잡고 있으므로 특징적인 렌즈 모양을 갖는다. 뇌에 대한 주요 위협은 뇌를 대체하고 뇌출혈을 위협하는 혈액 덩어리가 팽창하는 것이다.

경막외혈종의 전형적인 병력은 환자가 잠시 의식을 잃었다가 다시 의식을 회복한 후 급격한 의식 저하를 경험하는 것이다. 의식이 있는 기간 즉 명료기간 동안 환자는 방향 감각이 없거나 무기력하고 혼란스러워하거나 두통을 호소할 수 있다. 그러나 경막외혈종 환자의 대다수는 이러한 명료기간을 경험하지 않으며 다른 유형의 두개내출

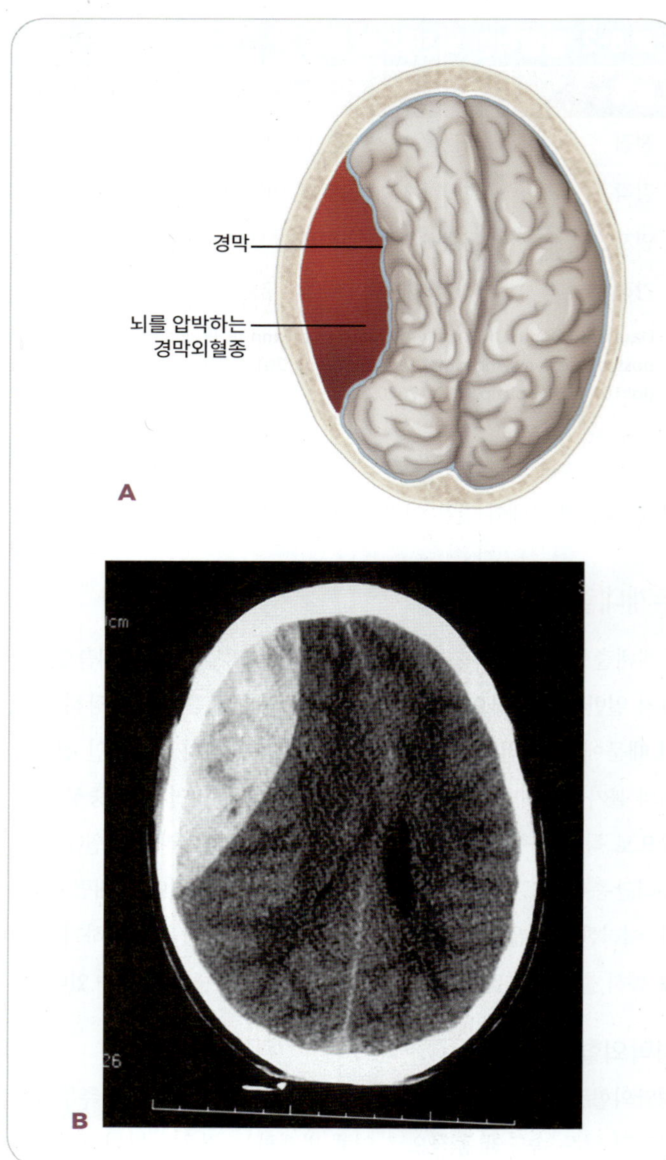

그림 8-5 **A.** 경막외혈종 **B.** 경막외혈종의 CT 영상

A. © National Association of Emergency Medical Technicians (NAEMT); **B.** Courtesy of Peter T. Pons, MD, FACEP.

한 인식과 혈종 제거가 이루어지면 사망률은 2%까지 낮아질 수 있다. 경막외혈종은 일반적으로 고립된 공간 점유 병변으로 그 아래 뇌 손상과 관련이 거의 없으므로 예후가 개선된다. 혈종을 신속하게 인식하고 제거하면 병리학적 덩이 효과가 교정되고 환자는 우수한 회복을 할 수 있다. 혈종의 신속한 제거는 사망률과 신경학적 이환율을 감소시킨다.

경막밑혈종

경막밑혈종은 연구에 따라 중증 뇌손상의 5~25%에서 발견되며 남성과 여성의 비율은 3 : 1이다. 젊은 성인의 경우 경막밑혈종은 고에너지 외상(예: 차량 충돌)과 관련이 있고 노인의 경우 경막밑혈종은 경미한 외상(예: 낙상)과 관련이 있으며 노인은 항응고제 또는 항혈소판 치료를 받고 있을 가능성이 더 높다. 이전 데이터에 따르면 경막밑혈종의 56%는 차량 충돌로 인한 것이고 12%는 낙상으로 인한 것이지만, 노인의 경우 22%는 차량 충돌로 인한 것이고 56%는 낙상으로 인한 것으로 나타났다.

경막밑혈종은 경막외혈종보다 더 흔할 뿐만 아니라 발생원인, 발생 위치 및 예후도 다르다. 동맥 출혈로 인해 발생하는 경막외혈종과 달리 경막밑혈종은 일반적으로 정맥 출혈로 인해 발생한다. 이 경우 머리 손상으로 연결정맥이 찢어진다. 경막과 그 아래 거미막 사이의 경막밑 공간에 혈액이 모인다(**그림 8-6**).

경막밑혈종은 두 가지 다른 방식으로 나타난다. 심각한 외상이 있는 환자의 경우 연결정맥의 파열로 인해 경막밑공간에 혈액이 상대적으로 빠르게 축적되어 덩이 효과가 빠르게 시작된다. 경막밑혈종 아래의 뇌실질에 대한 직접적인 손상은 정맥 파열과 동시에 발생한다. 그 결과 경막밑혈종의 덩이 효과는 손상된 뇌의 혈액 축적과 뇌부종으로 인해 발생한다. 이러한 유형의 급성 덩이 효과를 보이는 환자는 의식 상태가 급격히 저하되므로 현장에서 응급 상황을 신속하게 파악하여 CT 검사, 두개내압 모니터링 및 처리, 수술이 가능한 적절한 의료기관으로 신속하게 이송한다.

그러나 임상적으로 숨겨진 경막밑혈종은 다른 환자에게서도 발생할 수 있다. 고인이나 만성 질환과 같은 쇠약해진 환자의 경우 경막밑 공간이 뇌 위축으로 인해 이차적으로 커진다. 이러한 환자의 경우 혈액이 경막밑 공간에 축적되어도 덩이 효과를 나타내지 않으므로 증상이 나타나지 않을 수 있다. 이러한 경막밑혈종은 노인의 낙상이나 경미한 외상으로 발생할 수 있다. 와파린과 같은 항응고제나 아픽사반 또는 리바록사반과 같은 직접 경구용 항응고제를 복용하는 노인

혈에서도 발생할 수 있으므로 경막외혈종에 대해 비특이적일 수 있다. 그런데도 의식 소실 후 신경학적 기능 저하를 경험하는 환자는 두개내 진행성 과정의 위험이 있으므로 응급 검사가 필요하다.

환자의 의식이 악화함에 따라 신체검사에서 동공이 확장되고 느리거나 반응하지 않는 동공을 발견할 수 있으며 가장 일반적으로 탈출증이 발생한 쪽에서 나타난다. 운동 신경이 척수 위의 반대편으로 지나가기 때문에 일반적으로 반대쪽에서 반신불안전마비 또는 반신마비가 발생한다. 경막외혈종의 사망률은 약 20%이다. 그러나 신속

의 시작은 점진적이기 때문에 환자는 급성 경막밑혈종과 관련된 극적인 증상을 보이지 않는다. 대신 환자는 두통, 시각장애, 성격 변화, 말하기 어려움(구음장애), 서서히 진행되는 반신불완전마비나 반신마비 증상이 나타날 가능성이 더 높다. 이러한 증상 중 일부가 환자나 간병인에게 도움을 요청할 정도로 뚜렷해지면 만성 경막밑혈종이 발견된다. CT 검사에서 만성 경막밑혈종은 급성 경막밑혈종에 비해 뚜렷한 모습을 보인다. 검사와 처치를 위한 이송을 재촉하는 사건은 만성 경막밑혈종을 생성하는 가장 최근의 반복적인 경막밑출혈인 경우가 많으며 소량의 급성 혈액이 더 많은 만성 혈액에서 발견될 수 있다. 수술의 필요성과 긴급성은 환자의 증상, 덩이 효과, 환자의 전반적인 의학적 상태에 따라 결정된다.

병원 전 처치 제공자는 만성 질환자를 돌보는 시설에 출동할 때 이러한 환자를 자주 접하게 된다. 증상이 비특이적이기 때문에 현장에서 만성 경막밑혈종을 진단하는 것은 거의 불가능하며 증상이 뇌졸중, 감염, 치매 또는 환자의 전신 쇠약과 혼동될 수 있다.

이러한 환자의 경막밑혈종은 대부분 만성적이지만, 항응고제를 복용하는 환자는 겉보기에는 경미한 외상 후 경막밑혈종이 몇 시간에 걸쳐 팽창하고 응고되지 않아 탈출증으로 진행될 수 있다. 이러한 환자는 양성 증상을 보이다가 손상 후 몇 시간 후에 악화할 수 있다. 노인은 특히 경미한 낙상이 있었고 항응고제를 복용 중인 환자는 긴급하게 주의를 기울여 처치해야 한다.

거미막밑출혈

거미막밑출혈(SAH)은 뇌를 덮고 있는 경막밑공간 아래에 있는 거미막 아래에서 발생하는 출혈이다. 거미막밑공간의 혈액은 경막밑 공간으로 들어갈 수 없다. 뇌혈관 대부분은 거미막밑공간에 위치하므로 이러한 혈관에 손상을 입으면 뇌 표면의 거미막 아래에 혈액이 고이는 거미막밑출혈이 발생한다. 이 혈액층은 일반적으로 얇으며 덩이 효과를 일으키는 경우는 드물다.

거미막밑출혈은 종종 뇌동맥류의 자연 파열과 관련이 있으며 환자의 인생 최악의 두통이 갑자기 시작되는 경우가 많지만, 실제로 외상이 거미막밑출혈의 가장 흔한 원인이다. 거미막밑출혈 환자는 일반적으로 메스꺼움, 구토, 어지럼과 함께 심한 두통을 호소한다. 또한 거미막밑 공간에 혈액이 존재하면 목의 통증과 뻣뻣함, 시각적 불편감, 광 공포증과 같은 수막 징후가 나타날 수 있다. 뒤교통동맥에서 출혈이 발생하면 같은쪽의 안구 운동 신경 이상 또는 운동 상실을 유발할 수 있다. 영향을 받은 눈은 아래쪽과 바깥쪽을 바라보고 환자는

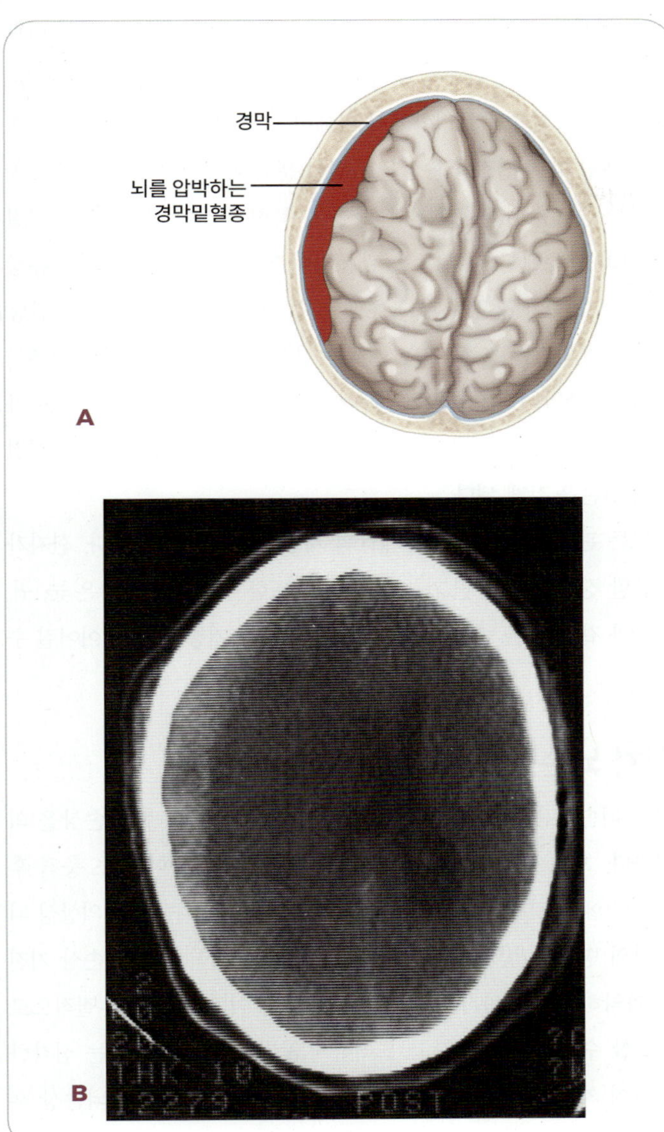

그림 8-6　**A. 경막밑혈종 B. 경막밑혈종의 CT 영상**

A. © National Association of Emergency Medical Technicians (NAEMT); **B.** Courtesy of Peter T. Pons, MD, FACEP.

환자는 낙상의 위험이 더 높다. 이러한 낙상은 경미하기 때문에 환자는 종종 검사를 받기 위해 내원하지 않는 경우가 많으며 출혈이 확인되지 않는다. 만성 경막밑혈종이 최종적으로 확인된 많은 환자는 출혈을 일으킨 외상성 사건이 너무 경미해 보였기 때문에 기억조차 하지 못한다.

숨겨진 경막밑혈종이 있는 일부 환자에게서는 경막밑혈액이 액화되지만, 경막밑공간 내에 유지된다. 시간이 지남에 따라 액체 혈종에 반복되는 작은 출혈을 포함하는 기전을 통해 만성 경막밑혈종이 확장되어 뇌에 천천히 덩이 효과를 발휘하기 시작할 수 있다. 덩이 효과

눈꺼풀을 들어 올리지 못할 수 있다. 이러한 환자는 발작이 발생할 수도 있지만, 발작 발생은 외상보다 뇌동맥류 파열이나 동정맥 기형에서 더 흔하다.

거미막밑출혈은 덩이 효과를 거의 일으키지 않기 때문에 감압을 위한 수술이 필요하지 않다. 사실, 경미한 신경학적 결손이 있는 거미막밑출혈 환자는 일반적으로 매우 호전된다. 그러나 외상성 거미막밑출혈는 다른 공간점유 병변, 두개내압 상승 및 뇌 실내 출혈의 위험을 증가시키는 잠재적 중증 뇌손상의 지표가 될 수 있다. 외상성 거미막밑출혈 환자는 뇌타박상 위험이 63~73% 증가하고 경막밑혈종이 발생할 위험이 44% 증가한다. 혈종 덩어리 두께가 1cm 이상이거나 안장위 또는 주변 부수조에 혈액이 있는 경우 나쁜 결과에 대한 예측값은 72~78%이며 외상성 거미막밑출혈은 뇌손상 환자의 사망률을 두 배로 높인다.

뇌타박상 및 뇌내출혈

뇌 자체에 손상을 입으면 뇌타박상이 발생할 수 있다. 이 손상에 뇌혈관 손상이 포함되는 경우 뇌내출혈이라고 하는 뇌내출혈이 발생할 수 있다. 뇌타박상은 중증 뇌손상을 입은 환자와 중등도 손상 환자 모두에게서 비교적 흔하게 발생한다. 일반적으로 무든 외상으로 발생하지만, 뇌에 총상을 입은 것과 같은 관통성 외상으로도 인해 발생할 수도 있다. 무딘 외상의 경우 뇌타박상은 여러 개일 수 있다. 뇌타박상은 두개골 내에서 힘이 전달되고 반사되는 복잡한 패턴으로 인해 발생한다. 예를 들어, 머리가 고정된 물체에 부딪히면 충격 부위에는 타격 손상이 발생하고 반대쪽 부위에는 뇌가 두개골의 반대쪽과 충돌하는 맞충격 손상이 발생한다. 이러한 유형의 손상을 충격-맞충격 손상이라고 한다. 결과적으로 타박상은 종종 충격 부위에서 멀리 떨어진 위치, 종종 뇌의 반대쪽에서 발생한다.

뇌타박상은 종종 CT 검사에 나타나기까지 12~24시간이 걸리는 경우가 많으며 이러한 환자는 초기 CT 검사에서 정상적일 수 있다. 뇌타박상의 존재를 알 수 있는 유일한 단서는 신경학적 검사의 저하일 수 있으며 많은 환자가 중등도의 뇌손상을 보인다. 손상 후 타박상이 진행됨에 따라 머리 CT 검사에서 타박상이 분명해지고 덩이 효과 증가와 두통이 심해질 수 있다. 특히 뇌타박상은 환자의 약 10%에서 중등도 손상이 중증 뇌손상으로 악화할 수 있다는 점이 우려된다.

관통성 머리 손상

뇌의 관통상은 가장 파괴적인 신경학적 손상 중 하나이다. 관통하는 물체는 뇌 조직을 통과할 때 뇌 조직에 직접적인 손상을 일으킬 수 있다. 발생하는 신경학적 손상의 특성은 손상된 뇌 부위에 따라 다르다. 총상은 총알과 관련된 에너지 때문에 특히 파괴적이다(이 유형의 손상은 4장 외상의 물리학에서 자세히 설명되어 있다). 총알은 조직을 통과할 때 직접적인 손상을 유발할 뿐만 아니라 관련 충격파가 공동현상 경로를 따라 조직을 손상한다. 특히 총알이 정중선을 가로질러 뇌의 한쪽에서 다른 쪽을 관통하여 뇌의 양쪽을 침범하는 총상은 예후가 좋지 않은 결과를 초래할 수 있다. 총알이 전두엽만 관통하는 경우와 같이 드물지만, 환자는 심각한 장애가 있더라도 생존할 수 있다. 총알이 뇌의 한쪽 앞쪽에서 뒤쪽으로 관통할 때도 생존 가능성도 더 높다. 그러나 이 경우에도 환자는 지속적이고 심각한 신경학적 결손을 갖게 된다.

모든 관통성 뇌손상은 두개골의 개방성 골절을 초래한다. 환자가 생존할 경우 후속 감염 가능성이 높다. 또한 두개골 관통상은 눈, 귀, 얼굴과 같은 다른 중요한 구조물을 손상시켜 기능 장애로 이어질 수 있다.

이차 뇌손상

이차 뇌손상은 최초 유발 사건 이후 구조물에 대한 추가 손상을 의미한다. 최초 손상 후 병태생리학적 과정이 발생하여 최초 충격 후 몇 시간에서 몇 주 동안 뇌에 추가 손상을 초래할 수 있다. 외상성 뇌손상의 병원 전(및 병원) 처치의 주요 초점은 이러한 이차 손상 기전을 파악하고 중단하거나 제한하는 것이다. 이차 효과는 본질적으로 방심할 수 없고 즉각적으로 드러나지 않거나 인식되지 않는 심각한 손상이 지속해서 발생할 수 있다. 이러한 영향은 외상성 뇌손상 후 사망과 장애에 중요한 역할을 한다. 이차 손상의 원인을 이해하고 이러한 손상의 발생을 예측함으로써 병원 전 처치 제공자는 이러한 합병증에 대비하고 예방하며 이를 바로잡기 위해 개입할 수 있다.

두개내 덩이 효과, 두개내압 상승 및 뇌의 기계적 이동과 관련된 병리학적 기전은 탈출증, 이환율 및 사망으로 이어질 수 있다. 임상 검사와 더불어 머리 CT 검사 및 기타 고급 영상 촬영과 두개내압 모니터링은 즉각적인 신경 외과적 수술과 같은 생명을 구하는 처치를 지원한다. 병원 전 환경에서 신속한 평가를 통해 외상 및 신경외과적 처치가 가능한 병원으로 빠르게 이송하는 것은 중증 외상성 뇌손상 및 탈출증 위험이 있는 환자를 처치하는 데 있어 매우 중요한 단계이다.

이차 손상의 다른 두 가지 중요한 원인은 저산소증과 저혈압이 이 두 가지 원인은 별도의 부문에서 자세히 설명한다. 인지하지 못하고 처치하지 않은 저산소중과 저혈압은 두개내압 상승만큼이나 손상된 뇌에 손상을 입힐 수 있다. 또한 손상된 뇌에 산소 또는 포도당 전달 장애가 발생하면 정상적인 뇌보다 더 치명적일 수 있다. 따라서 저산소중과 저혈압은 예방하고 파악하여 즉시 처치해야 한다.

이차 뇌손상의 두개내 원인

탈출증

먼로-켈리 법칙에 따르면 두개골이 온전한 환자의 경우 뇌 조직, 혈액 및 뇌척수액의 총부피가 일정하게 유지되어야 한다. 따라서 혈종, 뇌부종, 종양 등으로 인해 한 가지 구성 요소가 증가하면 다른 구성 요소 중 한두 가지가 감소해야 하며 그렇지 않으면 두개내압이 증가하게 된다(**그림 8-7**).

두개내출혈(ICH)에 대한 초기 보상 기전은 두개내 뇌척수액의 양을 감소시키는 것이다. 뇌척수액은 뇌, 뇌줄기, 척수 내부와 주변을 자연적으로 순환한다. 그러나 두개내출혈이 증가하면 뇌척수액이 머리 밖으로 강제로 배출된다. 정맥 배액도 증가하여 두개골 내 혈관내 혈액량을 줄이는 데 도움이 된다. 이 두 가지 기전은 두개내출혈의 초기 단계에서 두개내압이 상승하는 것을 방지한다. 따라서 환자는 무증상으로 보일 수 있다. 그러나 혈액 및 뇌척수액 제거의 임계치를 넘어 두개내출혈이 증가하면 두개내압이 급격히 증가하기 시작

한다. 두거내압이 증가하면 뇌가 두개골 내의 고정된 구조물을 가로질러 이동하게 되고 결국 뇌의 일부가 이러한 구조물을 통과하거나 그 주변으로 탈출하게 된다. 이에 따라 뇌의 가장 중요한 생명중추가 압박을 받아 동맥혈 공급을 위태로워진다(**그림 8-8**). 큰구멍을 통한 이러한 탈출증의 결과는 다양한 탈출증후군으로 설명된다(**그림 8-9** 및 **표 8-3**).

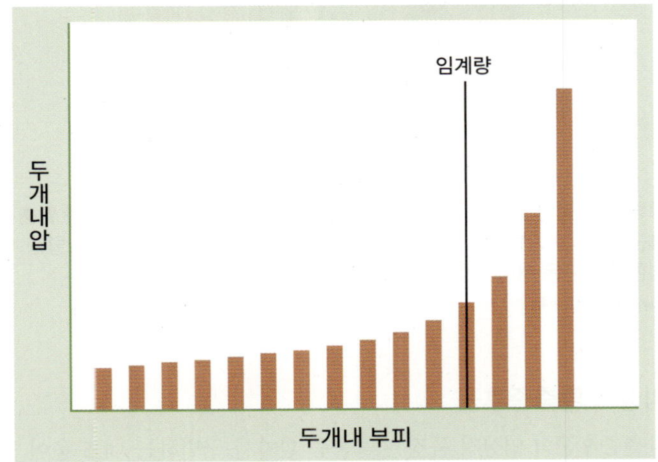

그림 8-8 이 그래프는 두개내 부피와 두개내압의 관계를 보여준다. 부피가 증가함에 다라 뇌척수액과 혈액이 강제로 배출되어 압력은 상대적으로 일정하게 유지된다. 결국 추가 보상이 일어나지 않고 두개내압이 급격히 상승하는 시점에 도달하게 된다.
© National Association of Emergency Medical Technicians (NAEMT)

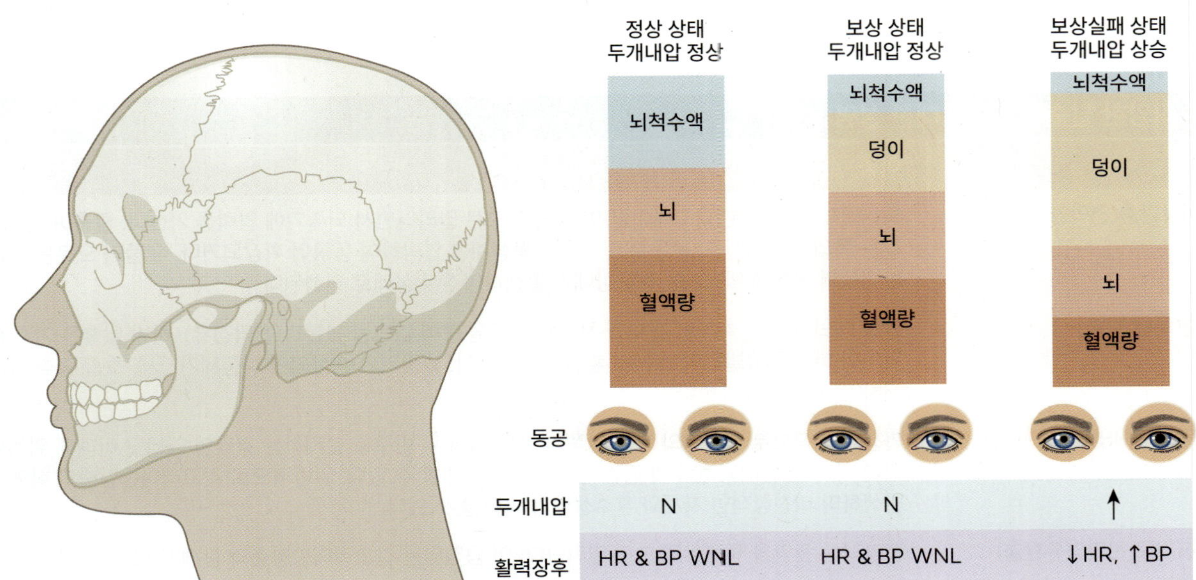

그림 8-7 먼로-켈리(Monro-Kellie) 법칙. 두개내 내용물의 부피는 일정하게 유지되어야 한다. 혈종과 같은 덩이가 추가되어 동일한 양의 뇌척수액과 혈액이 감소하면 두개내압은 정상으로 유지된다. 그러나 이 보상 기전이 소진되면 혈종의 부피가 미세하게 증가해도 두개내압이 기하급수적으로 증가한다.
© National Association of Emergency Medical Technicians (NAEMT)

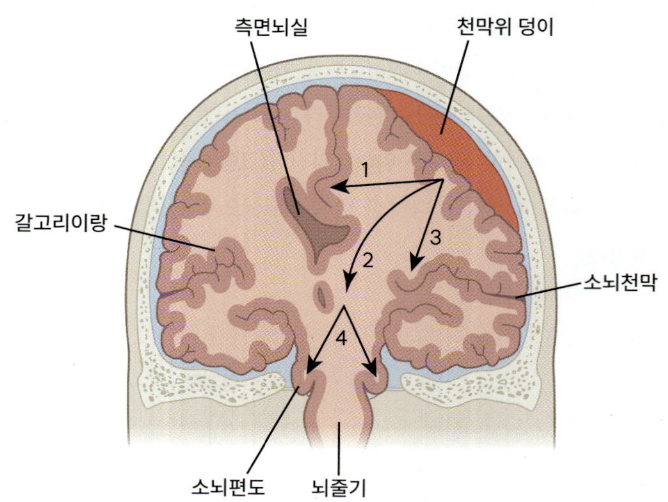

그림 8-9 덩이 효과 및 두개내압 증가로 인해 발생할 수 있는 다양한 탈출증후군. (1) 띠이랑탈출, (2) 중심탈출, (3) 갈고리이랑탈출, (4) 소뇌편도탈출. 이러한 증후군은 서로 복합적으로 발생할 수 있다.

© Jones & Bartlett Learning

임상적 탈출증후군

탈출증후군의 임상적 특징은 탈출증 환자를 구별하는 데 도움이 될 수 있다. 갈고리이랑탈출에서는 눈돌림신경(CN III)의 압박으로 인해 탈출증이 발생한 같은 쪽의 동공이 확장되거나 부푸는 현상이 발생한다. 운동로의 기능 상실은 신체의 반대쪽과 바빈스키 반사의 약화를 초래한다. 더 광범위한 탈출증은 붉은 핵 또는 안뜰핵으로 알려진 뇌줄기 구조의 파괴를 초래할 수 있다. 이에 따라 팔이 비정상적

으로 굴곡되고 다리가 경직 및 신전되는 피질제거자세가 나타날 수 있다. 더 불길한 징후로는 모든 팔다리가 신전되고 척추가 활모양으로 휘어지는 대뇌제거자세가 나타날 수 있다. 뇌줄기의 손상과 손상으로 대뇌제거자세가 발생한다(**그림 8-10**). 탈출증이 진행됨에 따라 팔다리가 이완되고 운동 활동이 없어진다.

중심탈출 및 소뇌편도탈출이 있으면 그물체활성계가 영향을 받아 비정상적인 환기 패턴 또는 무호흡이 발생하고 저산소증 및 고이산화탄소혈증이 악화한다. 체인-스톡스(Cheyne-Stokes) 호흡은 느리고 얕은 호흡이 점점 더 깊고 빨라졌다가 다시 느리고 얕은 호흡으로 돌아오는 주기를 반복하는 것이다. 호흡 주기 사이에 짧은 기간의 무호흡이 발생할 수 있다. 중추신경성 과다호흡은 지속해서 빠르고 깊은 호흡을 하는 것을 말하며 운동실조성 호흡(ataxic breathing)은 뚜렷한 패턴이 없는 불규칙한 호흡을 말한다. 자발 호흡 기능은 탈출증후군의 일반적인 최종 경로인 뇌줄기 압박으로 중단된다.

뇌 조직에 저산소증이 발생하면 뇌의 산소공급을 유지하기 위해 반사가 활성화된다. 두개내압 상승을 극복하기 위해 자율신경계가 활성화되어 정상적인 뇌관류 압력을 유지하기 위해 전신 혈압(및 MAP)을 높인다. 수축기압은 최대 250mmHg까지 증가할 수 있다. 그러나 목동맥과 대동맥활의 압력수용기가 혈압이 높게 상승한 것을 감지하면 부교감신경계를 활성화하라는 메시지가 뇌줄기로 전송된다. 그런 다음 신호는 10번 뇌신경인 미주신경을 통해 전달되어 심박수를 느리게 한다. 쿠싱 반사는 두개내압 상승과 함께 발생하는 1)

표 8-3 다양한 탈출증후군에 대한 설명	
탈출 유형	**이동**
갈고리이랑탈출(천막경유탈출)	측두엽의 내측 부분(갈고리이랑)이 천막 쪽으로 밀려나면서 뇌줄기에 압력을 가한다. 탈출이 진행되면 같은 쪽의 3번 뇌신경, 운동로 및 그물체활성계를 압박하여 동공이 확장되거나 "부풀어 오르는" 동공, 반대쪽의 운동 쇠약, 호흡 기능 장애가 발생하여 혼수상태로 진행된다.
중심탈출(하방 탈출)	양쪽 대뇌 반구의 측두엽 일부가 천막의 파임을 통해 압박을 받는다(천막경유). 하방 탈출은 기저 동맥 가지의 파열을 유발하여 소량의 출혈을 일으킨다. 뇌줄기가 손상되면 피질제거자세, 호흡 중추 기능 저하 및 사망을 초래한다.
띠이랑탈출(대뇌낫밑탈출 또는 transfalcine 탈출)	가장 일반적으로 전두엽의 가장 안쪽 부분은 뇌의 두 반구를 분리하는 경막인 대뇌낫 아래에 위치한다. 이에 따라 내측 대뇌 반구와 중간뇌에 손상이 발생할 수 있다. 일반적으로 갈고리이랑탈출과 함께 발생하며 비정상적인 자세와 혼수상태가 나타날 수 있다.
소뇌탈출(위로 천막경유탈출)	중간뇌는 천막을 통해 위쪽으로 밀려난다. 이 움직임은 갈고리이랑탈출과 함께 발생할 수 있다.
편도탈출(아래로 소뇌탈출)	소뇌편도는 큰 구멍을 통해 아래쪽으로 이동하여 소뇌와 수질 및 상부 목뼈 척수를 압박한다. 하부 수질에 손상을 입으면 심장 및 호흡 정지가 발생하며 이는 탈출증 환자에서 흔히 발생하는 최종 증상이다. 편도탈출은 "원뿔형"이라고도 한다.

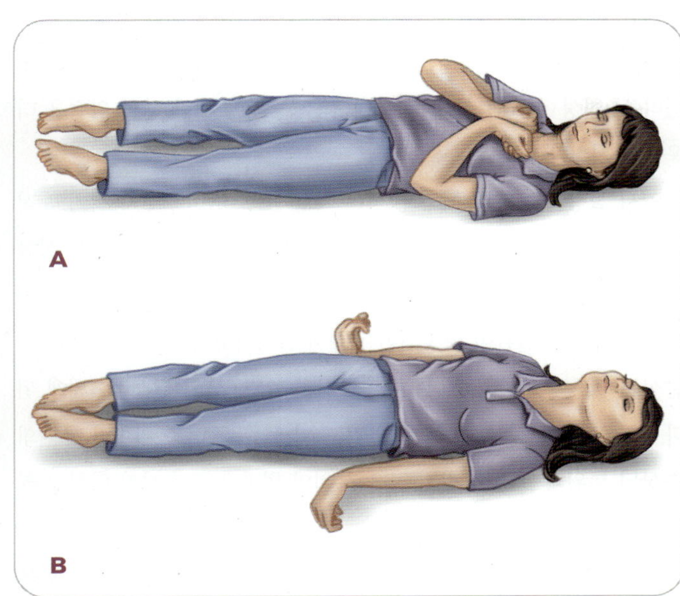

그림 8-10 **A.** 피질제거자세. **B.** 대뇌제거자세.
© Jones & Bartlett Learning

서맥, 2) 맥압 상승과 관련된 수축기 혈압 상승, 3) 체인-스톡스 호흡과 같은 불규칙한 호흡을 초래한다.

허혈 및 탈출증

탈출증후군은 두개내압이 증가하면 뇌를 압박하여 뇌손상을 유발할 수 있는지를 설명한다. 그러나 뇌부종으로 인한 두개내압 상승은 산소공급 감소와 그에 따른 뇌 허혈을 통해 뇌손상을 유발할 수도 있다. 뇌 관류압 공식(CCP=MAP-ICP)에 따르면 두개내압이 증가하면 뇌관류압이 감소하여 뇌관류가 위협받게 된다. 이것은 전신성 저혈압과 같은 다른 원인으로 인한 허혈성 손상으로 더욱 악화한다. 이러한 기계적 및 허혈성 손상은 끝없이 이어져 뇌가 더 많이 부어오르고 추가적인 기계적 및 허혈성 손상을 유발한다. 이 과정은 궁극적으로 처치하지 않으면 탈출증과 사망으로 이어진다. 이차 손상을 제한하고 이러한 이 손상 주기를 끊는 것이 외상성 뇌손상 처치의 주요 목표이다.

뇌부종

신경 세포막에 직접적인 손상을 입으면 신경세포 내에 세포내액이 고여 뇌부종이 발생할 수 있다. 또한 손상은 염증 반응을 활성화하여 신경세포와 뇌 모세혈관을 더 손상시켜 신경세포와 사이질 공간 내에 체액이 고이게 되어 뇌부종이 더욱 심해질 수 있다. 뇌부종이 진행됨에 따라 앞서 설명한 기계적 및 허혈성 손상이 발생하여 부종과

손상이 증가하는 끝없는 순환으로 이러한 과정이 악화한다.

뇌부종은 종종 두개내 혈종과 같은 일차 뇌손상 부위에서 발생하거나 뇌타박상과 같은 뇌실질에 대한 직접적인 손상의 결과로 발생하는 경우가 많다. 뇌부종은 저산소증이나 저혈압으로 인한 광범위(미만) 뇌손상의 결과일 수도 있다.

덩이 효과

외상 시 덩이 효과는 두개내 공간에 혈액이 축적되어 발생한다. 경막외, 경막밑 또는 뇌내혈종과 같은 두개내혈종은 덩이 효과의 주요 원인이다. 덩이 효과는 혈종의 크기로 인해 발생하기 때문에 이러한 혈종을 신속하게 제거하면 앞서 설명한 부종과 손상의 주기를 끊을 수 있다. 안타깝게도 혈종은 종종 뇌부종과 동반되며 손상과 부종의 순환을 멈추기 위해 혈종 제거 외에도 다른 처치가 필요하다.

정맥 폐쇄

정맥 폐쇄는 두개내 정맥 시스템의 외부 압박 또는 국소 내부 혈전증으로 인해 이차적으로 발생할 수 있다. 경막정맥동의 벽은 얇고 외부 압박을 받기 쉬우며 가장 흔하게는 함몰두개골 골절이나 확장하는 덩어리로 인해 발생한다. 외부 압박으로 경막정맥동의 얇은 벽을 국소적으로 압박하여 정맥 유출을 방지할 수 있다. 정맥 압박은 또한 정맥 혈전증을 유발하여 정맥 폐쇄를 더욱 악화시킬 것이다. 외부 정맥 압박과 정맥 혈전증은 모두 정맥 고혈압, 뇌부종 및 정맥 압박의 끝없는 주기를 시작하여 두개내압 상승을 초래한다.

가장 우려되는 손상은 대부분의 사람에게 오른쪽 가로정맥굴이 우세한 정맥굴이기 때문에 오른쪽 가로정맥굴 위의 후두 두개골 골절이다. 경막굴 혈전증과 같은 국소적인 내부 폐쇄는 드물지만, 높은 사망률과 관련이 있다. 처치에는 일반적으로 신속한 외과적 처치가 필요하다.

두개내 정맥 폐쇄 외에도 간접적으로 두개내압을 상승시킬 수 있는 두개 외 정맥 폐쇄의 원인이 있다. 정맥은 목정맥으로 흘러 들어가므로 목정맥이 압박되면 두개 내 정맥 폐쇄의 상류 효과를 유발할 수 있다. 굴곡이나 회전을 동반한 굴곡과 같이 잘못된 머리 위치는 두개내압을 크게 상승시킬 수 있다(평균 두개내압은 8.8~16.2mmHg). 후두부가 더 크고 목이 축 늘어진 어린이의 경우 이 수치는 훨씬 더 높다. 목뼈보호대는 두개내압을 4~14.5mmHg까지 증가시킬 수 있다. 가슴속 압력과 복강 내 압력이 증가하면 목 정맥압이 증가하여 뇌정맥 유출에 영향을 미칠 수 있다. 따라서 머리를 중립적인 자세로 유지하고 꽉 끼는 목뼈보호대를 피하고자 노력해야 한다.

두개내압 상승

뇌부종, 뇌 허혈, 정맥 폐쇄 및 덩이 효과와 관련된 추가 요인은 두개내압 상승을 악화시킨다. 뇌부종의 정도를 정량화하고 평가하기 위한 방법으로 두개내압을 측정된다. 의료진이 뇌부종을 정량화하고 탈출증 위험을 평가하고 뇌부종 처치의 효과를 모니터링할 수 있도록 병원에 두개내압 모니터를 배치한다. 두개내압 상승은 뇌부종의 생물표지자가 될 수 있다. 병원 전 환경에서 두개내압 모니터링을 일상적으로 사용할 수 있는 것은 아니지만, 병태생리학을 이해하면 병원 전 처치 제공자가 최상의 처치를 실천할 수 있다.

이차 뇌손상의 두개 외 원인

저혈압

뇌 허혈은 중증 뇌손상에서 매우 흔하다. 연구에 따르면 외상성 뇌손상으로 사망한 환자의 90%와 많은 생존자에게서 뇌 허혈이 확인되었다. 따라서 낮은 뇌 혈류가 외상성 뇌손상 결과에 미치는 영향은 외상성 뇌손상 후 이차 손상을 제한하기 위한 주요 초점이 되었다.

국가 외상성 뇌손상 데이터베이스에서 외상성 뇌손상으로 인한 예후 악화를 예측할 수 있는 가장 중요한 두 가지 요인은 두개내압이 20mmHg 이상인 기간과 수축기 혈압이 90mmHg 미만인 기간이다. 실제로 수축기 혈압이 90mmHg 미만인 상태가 한 번이라도 발생하면 예후가 더 나빠질 수 있다. 여러 연구에서 낮은 수축기 혈압이 외상성 뇌손상 후 결과에 미치는 심각한 영향을 확인했다.

많은 외상성 뇌손상 환자들은 출혈과 그로 인한 저혈압을 동반하는 다른 손상을 입을 수 있다. 저혈압을 예방하기 위해 수액 소생술과 이러한 손상에 대한 신속한 결정적인 처치는 이차 손상의 위험을 완화하는 데 중요하다. 병원 전 단계 또는 응급실 환경에서 모든 환자에게 일반화할 수 있는 특정 혈압 소생술 목표를 권장할 수 있는 데이터는 충분하지 않다. PHTLS와 ATLS은 모두 출혈을 조절하고 관류 징후에 대한 소생술에 중점을 두며 가능한 경우 결정질 사용을 최소화하는 것을 강조한다. 그러나 중등도 또는 중증 외상성 뇌손상이 의심되는 상황에서는 수축기 혈압을 110mmHg로 유지하는 것이 적절한 목표라는 증거가 있다.

출혈 외에도 뇌 혈류 자동 조절 기능 장애로 인해 이차 손상이 발생할 수 있다. 정상적인 피질의 뇌 혈류는 분당 뇌 조직 100g당 50mL (또는 50mL/100g/분)이다. 심각한 외상성 뇌손상 후 이 값은 30mL까지 떨어지거나 심지어 20mL/100g/분까지 낮아질 수 있다.

이러한 뇌 혈류 감소의 원인은 불명하지만, 손상에 대한 반응으로 뇌를 하향 조절하는 보호 기전 또는 자동 조절의 상실로 인한 것일 수 있다. 출혈성 쇼크와 함께 뇌 혈류 감소는 뇌에 대한 허혈 위협을 더욱 증가시킨다.

앞서 설명한 바와 같이 뇌손상은 자동 조절 기전을 손상시키고 적절한 뇌 혈류를 유지하려면 더 높은 뇌관류 압력이 필요하다. 심하게 손상된 뇌 부위는 거의 모든 자동 조절 기능을 잃을 수 있다. 이러한 부위에서는 혈관이 확장되어 충혈이 발생하고 혈액이 가장 심하게 손상된 뇌 부위와 적절한 관류로 살릴 수 있는 부위에서 멀어지게 된다. 마지막으로 적극적인 과다환기는 뇌 혈류를 더욱 위협하고 뇌의 손상된 부위와 영향을 받지 않은 부위의 혈관을 수축시켜 허혈성 위협을 더욱 악화시킬 수 있다.

이러한 생리학적 하향조절, 션트 및 출혈 쇼크의 조합은 뇌의 회복 가능한 부위에 여러 허혈성 위협을 초래하므로 적극적으로 처치하는 것이 외상성 뇌손상 처치의 필수적인 부분이다. 따라서 뇌손상 환자의 이차 손상을 제한하기 위해서는 수축기 혈압을 110mmHg 이상으로 유지하는 것을 목표로 하는 병원 전 수액 소생술과 함께 병원 전 환경에서 적극적인 처치가 필수적이다.

저산소증과 고산소혈증

혈액순환을 통해 손상된 뇌에 전달되는 가장 중요한 기질 중 하나는 산소다. 뇌 무산소증은 4분~6분만 지속되어도 돌이킬 수 없는 뇌손상이 발생할 수 있다. 연구에 따르면 외상성 뇌손상 환자의 산소포화도가 90% 미만이면 심각한 영향을 미치는 것으로 나타났다. 상당수의 외상성 뇌손상 환자는 산소포화도가 낮거나 불충분하며 이는 맥박산소측정기로 측정하지 않으면 쉽게 놓칠 수 있다. 뇌손상 환자의 병원 전 기도 관리와 산소 공급에 대한 강조는 부분적으로 이러한 연구의 결과이다. 적절한 환기와 혈류는 뇌에 적절한 산소 공급을 유지하는 데 매우 중요하다. 중증 외상성 뇌손상 환자를 대상으로 한 연구에 따르면 저산소혈증과 저혈압이 모두 발생하지 않은 경우 사망률이 26.9%, 저산소혈증만 발생한 경우 28%, 두 가지 모두 발생한 경우 57.2%로 나타났다. 따라서 병원 전 치료 제공자는 출혈을 최소화하여 혈액 순환을 원활하게 하고 기도 확보와 적절한 환기를 유지하여 적절하게 산소를 공급해야 한다.

지나치게 농축된 산소 공급 또는 고산소증도 더 나쁜 결과와 관련이 있다는 점에 유의하는 것이 중요하다. 100% 산소를 투여하면 뇌 혈관 수축을 유발하여 뇌 대사를 변화시킬 수 있다. 높은 수준의 흡입산소농도(FiO₂)와 높은 동맥혈산소분압(PaO₂)의 영향을 평가한 몇 안 되는 연구에서 기능적 결과가 나빠지고 사망률이 높아지는 것으로 나타났다. 이러한 연구에 따르면 외상성 뇌손상 후 동맥혈산소분압 수치에 대한 이상적인 치료 범위는 100~200mmHg 사이일 가능성이 높다. 그러나 정상 범위를 벗어난 고산소증과 저산소증 모두 해로울 수 있지만, 저산소증은 일시적이라도 더 위험한 것으로 간주하므로 가능한 한 예방해야 한다.

빈혈

혈액의 산소 운반 능력은 혈액에 포함된 헤모글로빈의 양에 따라 결정되므로 빈혈이 있으면 헤모글로빈 수치가 낮아져 뇌로의 산소 전달에 영향을 미친다. 헤모글로빈이 50% 감소하면 동맥혈산소분압이 50%로 감소하는 것보다 뇌로의 산소 전달에 훨씬 더 큰 영향을 미친다. 이러한 이유로 출혈로 인한 빈혈은 외상성 뇌손상에 직접적인 영향을 미친다.

응고병증

외상 및 외상성 뇌손상 자체는 혈소판 기능 장애와 피브리노겐 및 응고 인자의 변화를 포함하는 응고병증의 유발과 관련이 있으며 이는 혈전 형성 장애를 초래한다. 이러한 지혈 변화는 외상성 뇌손상의 출혈 진행에 기여하며 비응고병증 외상성 뇌손상 환자에 비해 높은 이환율 및 사망률과 관련이 있다.

　응고병증 악화의 주요 위험 요인으로는 손상 전 항응고제 또는 항혈소판 요법의 사용이 있으며 노인 인구에서 여러 적응증에 대해 점점 더 많이 처방되고 있다. 노인 인구에서 낙상으로 인한 외상성 뇌손상 발생률이 가장 높으며 현재 항응고제를 복용 중인 노인 환자는 손상 전 항응고제 또는 항혈소판 요법을 받지 않은 환자에 비해 사망률이 3배 더 높고 6개월 동안 좋지 않은 결과를 초래하는 빈도가 높다. 한 연구에 따르면 항응고 치료를 받은 환자의 사망률은 35.2%지만, 항응고 치료를 받지 않은 환자의 사망률은 11.6%에 달했다. 따라서 환자가 손상 전 항응고제 또는 항혈소판 요법을 받고 있는지 확인하여 응고병증을 가능한 한 빨리 해결하여 출혈의 진행을 제한하는 것이 매우 중요하다(**표 8-4**). 프로트롬빈 복합체 농축액은 항응고제를 빠르게 역전시키기 위해 가장 일반적으로 사용되며 데스모프레신은 항혈소판제를 역전시키는 데 사용된다.

　여러 연구에서 트라넥삼산(TXA)이 외상성 뇌손상 환자에게 미치는 영향을 평가했다. TXA은 피브린 응고 분해를 방지하고 출혈을 줄이는 데 자주 사용된다. TXA은 10분에 걸쳐 1g을 부하용량으로 투

표 8-4 일반적인 항응고제

약물 등급	예	길항제
비타민 K 길항제	Warfarin	비타민 K 프로트롬빈 복합체 농축제제 (PCC)
간접 트롬빈 억제제	Heparin 저분자량 헤파린 (LMWH)	프로타민황산염
간접 인자 Xa 억제제	Fondaparinux	N/A
직접 작용하는 경구용 항응고제 (DOAC)		PCC
직접 트롬빈 억제제	Argatroban Bivalirudin Dabigatran	Idarucizumab
인자 Xa 억제제	Apixaban Rivaroxaban	Andexanet
항혈소판제	Aspirin Clopidogrel Prasugrel	Desmopressin

Data from Yee J, Kaide CG. Emergency reversal of anticoagulation. *West J Emerg Med*. 2019;20(5):770-783. doi:10.5811/westjem.2018.5.38235

여한 후 8시간에 걸쳐 1g을 주입한다. CRASH-2 시험에 따르면 출혈성 외상 환자에게 TXA을 조기에 투여하면 출혈로 인한 사망률이 약 30%, 모든 원인으로 인한 사망률이 약 20% 감소하는 것으로 나타났다. CRASH-2 임상시험의 하위 그룹 분석 결과 두개내혈종 확장, 새로운 두개내출혈, 새로운 국소 허혈성 병변이 더 적었으며 통계적으로 유의하지는 않았지만, 외상성 뇌손상을 동반한 출혈 환자에서 TXA 투여 시 사망률이 개선되는 경향을 보였다.

　2019년의 후속 CRASH-3 임상시험에서는 특히 외상성 뇌손상 환자를 대상으로 조사한 결과 병원에서 신속한 TXA 투여(손상 후 3시간 이내)가 경증에서 중등도의 외상성 뇌손상 환자의 머리 손상 사망률을 감소시키는 것으로 나타났다. 그러나 중증 외상성 뇌손상에는 효과가 없었다. 더욱 최근의 다기관 코호트 연구(비무작위)에서는 병원 전 TXA를 투여받은 환자의 결과를 평가했으며 병원 전 TXA를 받은 환자에서 30일 사망률이 통계적으로 유의하게 높은 것으로 나

타났다. 병원 전 TXA 사용과 관련하여 논란의 여지가 있고 데이터가 제한적이기 때문에 현재 병원 전 TXA는 장시간 결정적 치료를 받을 수 없는 병원 전 이송 시간이 긴 경우를 제외하고는 병원 전 환경에서 사용을 권장하지 않는다.

저이산화탄소혈증과 고이산화탄소혈증

이 장의 앞부분에서 설명한 바와 같이 저이산화탄소혈증(PaCO₂ 감소)과 고이산화탄소혈증(PaCO₂ 증가)은 모두 뇌손상을 악화시킬 수 있다. 심각한 저이산화탄소혈증으로 인해 뇌혈관이 수축하면 뇌 혈류가 손상되어 뇌로의 산소 공급이 감소한다. 고이산화탄소혈증은 약물, 알코올 중독, 발작 및 두개내압 증가 환자에서 나타나는 비정상적인 호흡 패턴을 포함하여 다양한 원인으로 인한 저환기로 인해 발생할 수 있다. 고이산화탄소혈증은 뇌혈관 확장을 유발하여 두개내압 상승을 더욱 증가시킬 수 있다.

저이산화탄소혈증은 과다환기의 결과로 발생하며 일반적으로 기계식 환기를 받는 환자에게서 발생한다. 저이산화탄소혈증은 뇌혈관 수축을 유발하여 뇌 혈류량과 두개내압을 감소시킨다. 그러나 뇌혈관 저항을 증가시켜 뇌 혈류를 감소시키고 뇌의 허혈을 더 유발할 수 있다. 뇌 외상 재단 지침에서는 예방적 과다환기(PaCO₂가 25mmHg 이하인 경우)를 권장하지 않는다. 이상적으로는 저이산화탄소혈증과 고이산화탄소혈증의 해로운 영향을 방지하기 위해 정상 저이산화탄소혈증을 유지하는 것이다.

저혈당과 고혈당

뇌 혈류가 감소하면 산소 공급이 감소할 뿐만 아니라 포도당 및 기타 필요한 뇌 대사산물의 공급도 감소한다. 포도당은 성인 뇌의 주요 에너지 공급원이며 뇌 포도당 대사의 변화는 외상성 뇌손상에 대한 특징적인 반응이다. 영상 연구에 따르면 손상 직후 포도당 섭취가 일시적으로 급격히 증가한 후 장기간 포도당 대사가 저하되는 것으로 나타났다. 포도당 대사 억제는 중증 외상성 뇌손상 환자에서 더 심하고 이러한 억제 지속 기간은 나이가 들수록 길어진다. 시상, 뇌줄기, 소뇌의 대사율이 높을수록 의식 수준과 유의미한 양의 상관관계가 있으므로 대사가 저하되는 위치가 중요하다.

혈당 상승(고혈당)과 감소(저혈당)는 모두 허혈성 뇌 조직을 위험에 빠뜨릴 수 있다. 심각한 저혈당이 신경계에 미치는 비참한 영향은 손상을 입었을 때나 다른 때에도 잘 알려져 있다. 신경세포는 포도당을 저장할 수 없으므로 세포 대사를 수행하기 위해 지속해서 포도당을 공급해야 한다. 포도당이 공급되지 않으면 허혈성 신경세포는 영구적으로 손상될 수 있다. 그러나 혈장 포도당 수치가 150mg/dL를 초과하거나 200mg/dL를 초과하는 상태가 장기간 지속되면 손상된 뇌에 해로울 수 있다는 것도 사실이다. 혈당 수치가 상승하면 신경학적 결과가 나빠지는 것과 관련이 있으므로 혈당 수치가 높아지는 것을 피해야 한다.

병원 전 환경에서는 저혈당으로 인한 생리적 위협이 혈청 포도당 상승으로 인한 위험보다 훨씬 더 즉각적이기 때문에 저혈당 여부를 즉시 평가하고 처치한다. 의식 상태가 변화된 모든 환자의 혈당을 현장에서 측정하고 정상 수치보다 낮은 것으로 확인되면 정맥 내 또는 근육 내 포도당 투여로 처치한다. 또한 유발된 고혈당은 일시적일 가능성이 높으므로 이러한 환자를 적절히 처치하는 데 필요한 엄격한 혈당 조절은 병원 입원 시 확립되어야 한다.

발작

급성 외상성 뇌손상 환자는 발작의 위험이 있다. 환기 장애, 저혈당 및 전해질 이상으로 인한 저산소증으로 외상성 뇌손상 환자에게 전신 발작이 유발될 수 있다. 또한, 허혈성 또는 손상된 뇌 조직은 부분 또는 전신 발작 및 뇌전증 지속상태를 유발하는 과민성 초점으로 작용할 수 있다. 발작은 호흡 기능 장애로 인한 기존의 저산소증을 악화시킬 수 있다. 전신발작과 관련된 대규모 신경 활동은 산소와 포도당 수치를 빠르게 감소시켜 뇌 허혈을 더욱 악화시킨다.

평가 및 처치

손상을 일으킨 외상의 물리학에 대한 빠른 일차평가 및 이후의 이차평가는 외상성 뇌손상이 의심되는 환자의 잠재적인 생명을 위협하는 문제를 파악하는 데 도움이 된다. 또한 외상성 뇌손상의 병태생리학은 역동적인 과정이기 때문에 이러한 환자를 평소보다 더 자주 지속해서 재평가하는 것이 중요하다. 평가 결과는 시간이 지남에 때라 환자의 상태가 변화함에 따라 크게 변동할 수 있다.

외상의 물리학

손상 기전에 대한 지식은 특히 외상성 뇌손상에서 특정 손상 유형을 식별하는 데 도움이 될 수 있으므로 모든 외상 환자에게 중요하다. 외상의 물리학에 대한 주요 데이터는 종종 현장을 관찰하거나 목격자로부터 얻을 수 있다. 환자 차량 앞 유리에 거미줄 모양의 패턴이 있어 환자의 머리에 충격이 가해졌음을 암시하거나 폭행 중에 무리로 사용된 피 묻은 물체가 있을 수 있다. 머리 측면에 충격이 가해지면 측두골 골절을 유발하고 기저 중간수막동맥이 손상되어 경막외혈종이 발생할 수 있다. 고속 차량 충돌과 같이 충격이 크거나 급가속-급감속 손상으로 이어질 수 있으며 충격-맞충격 손상을 초래할 수 있다. 이 중요한 정보는 뇌손상 가능성뿐만 아니라 다른 손상과 관련이 있으므로 환자의 적절한 진단 및 처치에 필수적일 수 있으므로 의료기관의 의료진에게 보고해야 한다.

일차평가

외상성 뇌손상 환자의 효과적인 처치는 일차평가에서 확인된 생명을 위협하는 문제를 처치하는 데 초점을 맞춘 질서 있는 개입으로 시작된다. 기도, 호흡, 순환은 일차평가에서 가장 먼저 평가해야 하는 부분이다. 이러한 문제가 해결되면 환자를 신속하게 외상성 뇌손상을 처치할 수 있는 가장 가까운 의료기관으로 이송해야 한다(Box 8-1).

대량 출혈

일차평가는 외상성 뇌손상 환자를 포함하여 모든 외상 환자에 대한 첫 번째 평가이다. 질서정연하고 구조화된 접근 방식은 모든 외상 환자에게 동일하게 적용되며 출혈을 확인하고 지혈하는 것부터 시작된다. 기도 및 호흡은 대량 출혈을 조절하는 것을 지체하지 않고 현장에서 충분한 자원을 확보할 수 있는 경우 그다음 또는 동시에 처리한

다. 외부출혈이 있으면 직접 압박하거나 압박 드레싱을 적용해야 한다. 복잡한 두피 상처는 상당한 외부출혈을 일으킬 수 있다. 압박 붕대와 거즈로 압박 드레싱을 시행하여 효과적으로 출혈을 조절할 수 있다. 이 방법으로 출혈을 조절하지 못하는 경우 상처 가장자리를 따라 직접 압력을 가하여 피부와 연부조직 사이의 두피 혈관을 압박함으로써 출혈을 조절할 수 있다. 압박 드레싱은 뇌손상을 악화시키고 두개내압을 증가시킬 수 있으므로 심각한 출혈이 없는 한 함몰 또는 개방 두개골 골절에 적용해서는 안 된다. 직접적으로 부드럽게 압박하면 두개 외(두피) 혈종의 크기를 제한할 수도 있다.

기도

환자의 기도 개방 여부를 즉시 평가하고 확인한다. 의식 수준이 저하된 환자는 기도를 보호하지 못할 수 있다. 손상된 뇌에 적절한 산소를 공급하는 것은 이차 손상을 예방하는 데 매우 중요하다. 턱 밀어올리기 술기와 같은 도수 방법 및 간단한 기도 술기는 적절한 초기 기도 처치이다(7장 기도와 환기 참조). 의식이 없는 사람의 경우 혀가 기도를 완전히 폐쇄할 수 있다. 소음이 심한 환기는 혀나 이물질에 의해 기도가 부분적으로 막혔음을 나타낸다. 구토, 출혈, 혈종, 얼굴 외상으로 인한 부종은 외상성 뇌손상 환자에서 기도 손상의 흔한 원인이며 간헐적인 흡인이 필요할 수 있다.

얼굴 골절과 후두 또는 기타 목 손상을 입은 환자는 일반적으로 기도가 유지되는 자세를 취한다. 환자가 자세에 따른 기도 손상으로 저산소 상태가 되면 환자를 반듯이 눕히거나 목뼈보호대를 착용하려는 시도는 극도의 전투적 상황에 직면할 수 있다. 이러한 상황에서는 기도 개방이 척추 움직임 제한보다 우선하며 환자를 부분적으로 바로 선 자세로 이송할 수 있다. 척추를 도수로 여전히 고정해야 하지만, 기도를 손상할 수 있다고 생각되는 경우 목뼈보호대 착용을 미룰 수도 있다. 의식이 있는 환자는 필요할 때 스스로 흡인하여 기도를 관리하는 데 도움을 줄 수 있다. 총상으로 인한 손상을 포함한 얼굴 외상은 기관내삽관에 대한 금기 사항이 아니지만, 때에 따라서는 반지갑상연골절개술을 사용하여 환자를 처치해야 할 수도 있다.

기도를 관리하는 것은 대량 출혈을 조절한 후 첫 번째 처치 우선순위로 간주하며 의식 상태가 심하게 저하되어 기도를 유지할 수 없는 환자에게는 일반적으로 병원 전 기관내삽관이 권장된다. 그러나 이러한 병원 전 처치는 논란의 여지가 있다. 일부 연구에서는 현장에서 삽관한 환자의 기능적 결과가 개선되었다는 것을 뒷받침한다. 그러나 다른 연구에서는 병원 전 기관내삽관이 사망률 증가와 관련이 있

Box 8-1 알코올 사용과 외상성 뇌손상

알코올 중독은 외상성 뇌손상, 특히 경막밑혈종의 위험 요인으로 알려져 있다. 여러 요인이 이러한 위험 증가에 기여한다. 뇌의 물리적 수축(대뇌위축)은 장기간에 걸쳐 중등도 또는 과량의 알코올을 만성적으로 섭취하는 환자에게서 흔히 볼 수 있다. 뇌의 부피가 감소함에 따라 현수교의 케이블이 다리를 제자리에 고정하는 것과 유사하게 연결정맥에 가해지는 긴장이 증가한다. 이 긴장이 증가하면 손상을 일으키는 데 필요한 전단력이 줄어든다. 또한 과도한 알코올 섭취는 간에서 응고 인자를 효과적으로 생성하는 능력을 방해하여 응고 능력을 감소시키는 것으로 알려져 있다.

알코올 남용 병력이 있거나 급성 중독 환자는 손상의 정도를 완전히 표현하는 능력이 부족할 수 있다. 이는 신체 평가 결과가 혼동되고 신뢰성이 떨어질 수 있으며 심각한 머리 손상의 증상을 모호하게 만들 수도 있다.

알코올 남용 또는 급성 알코올 중독의 병력이 있는 환자에서 이러한 요인이 복합적으로 영향을 미치면 이러한 환자에서 심각한 외상성 뇌손상을 의심하는 기준을 낮춰야 한다. 이러한 환자에게 심각한 손상을 유발하는 데 필요한 힘은 알코올 남용 병력이 없는 개인에게 손상을 입히는 데 필요한 힘보다 훨씬 낮을 수 있다. 상대적으로 경미한 머리 외상을 입은 환자라도 충분한 평가를 받아야 하며 전문적인 의학적 평가를 위해 병원으로 이송할 것을 강력히 권장해야 한다.

을 수 있다고 제안했다. 2015년 메타 분석에 따르면 경험이 부족한 의사가 병원에서 삽관할 경우 사망 확률이 2배 증가했지만, 숙련된 의사가 삽관할 경우 사망률에 차이가 없는 것으로 나타났다. 경험이 없는 의사와 관련된 사망률이 높은 데에는 저산소증 및 저혈압의 인지되지 않은 에피소드를 포함하여 몇 가지 요인이 영향을 미치는 것으로 보인다. 장기간 또는 실패한 삽관 시도는 저산소증을 초래하고 삽관을 쉽게 하려고 사용되는 약물은 저혈압을 포함한 혈류역학적인 영향을 미친다. 삽관 성공 후 의도하지 않은 과다환기를 포함한 부적절한 환기는 뇌혈관 수축을 유발하여 환자의 경과를 더욱 복잡하게 만들 수 있다. 삽관을 잘못 수행하거나 삽관 후 환기를 제대로 관리하지 않으면 삽관을 전혀 하지 않는 것보다 더 해로운 것으로 보인다.

또한 병원에 도착하여 결정적인 외과적 처치가 지연되면 결과가 더 나빠지는 것과 관련이 있다. 도시 환경에서는 이송 시간이 짧으면 대체 술기를 사용하여 환자를 처치하고 보다 통제된 환경에서 기도를 확실히 관리할 수 있는 응급실로 신속하게 이송할 수 있다. 반대로 이송 시간이 더 긴 시스템에서는 경험이 적은 병원 전 처치 제공자가 삽관을 시행하더라도 삽관을 전혀 하지 않는 것보다 더 유익할 수 있다. 모든 연구가 전반적인 결과에서 의료진의 경험이 중요하다는 것이 입증되었다는 점에 유의하는 것이 중요하다. 숙련된 의사에 의한 삽관은 현장 체류시간이나 총 병원 입원 기간이 늘어나지 않으며 사망률이 현저히 낮아지는 것으로 나타났다. 따라서 환자의 기관내삽관 여부는 이송 시간과 병원 전 처치 의료진의 경험에 따라 달라진다.

이러한 조건을 염두에 두고 병원 전 의료진은 의식 상태의 심각한 저하로 인해 기도를 보호할 수 없는 모든 환자에 대해 적극적인 기도 관리를 고려해야 한다. 이러한 관리는 환자의 전투력, 입벌림 장애, 구토, 목뼈 고정을 유지해야 하는 필요성으로 인해 매우 어려울 수 있다. 따라서 삽관을 기도 관리 방법으로 선택한 경우 가장 숙련된 의료진이 수행해야 한다. 환자의 산소포화도를 지속해서 모니터링하고 저산소증(산소포화도 90% 미만)을 피하는 것이 중요하다. 맹목적코기관삽관이 대체 술기로 사용될 수 있지만, 얼굴중간에 외상이 있는 환자의 경우 맹목적코기관삽관으로 의도치 않게 두개골과 뇌를 관통할 가능성으로 인해 상대적 금기 사항이다. 그러나 이 합병증은 드물고 머리 외상 환자에서 두 번만 보고되었다.

급속연속기관삽관(RSI) 프로토콜 일부로 신경근 차단제를 사용하면 성공적인 삽관을 촉진할 수 있다. 그러나 병원 전 환경에서 급속연속기관삽관의 안전성과 유효성은 아직 결정되지 않았다. 리도카인,

펜타닐 및 에스몰롤을 사전 약물로 사용하는 급속연속기관삽관은 이환율이나 사망률을 감소시키는 것으로 입증되지 않았다. 그러나 일부 연구에서는 급속연속기관삽관이 삽관 성공률을 향상하더라도 더 나쁜 결과를 초래할 수 있다고 한다. 따라서 자발 호흡을 하고 보충 산소로 산소포화도를 90% 이상으로 유지하는 환자에게 일상적으로 마비제를 사용하는 것은 권장되지 않는다.

다른 어떤 것보다 선호되는 이상적인 기도 관리 술기는 하나도 없다. 대신, 도수 및 간단한 기도 술기를 초기 처치로 사용하고 복잡한 기도 처치는 덜 침습적인 방법으로 기도를 유지할 수 없는 경우에만 수행해야 한다. 대부분은 코인두기도기 또는 입인두기도기를 이용한 백마스크를 이용해 환자에게 산소를 공급하고 환기할 수 있다. 흡인기는 즉시 사용할 수 있어야 한다. 기도 관리 중재와 외상성 뇌손상은 종종 구토를 유발한다. 특히 이송 시간이 짧은 경우 복잡한 기도 처치를 장시간 시도하는 것은 피해야 한다.

호흡

호흡 기능 평가에는 호흡의 속도, 깊이, 적절성에 대한 평가가 포함된다. 앞서 언급했듯이 심각한 뇌손상으로 인해 발생한 발작은 호흡 조절 장애를 포함하여 여러 가지 호흡 패턴이 발생할 수 있다. 다계통 외상 환자의 경우 가슴 손상으로 인해 산소 공급과 환기를 더욱 손상할 수 있다. 목뼈 골절은 외상성 뇌손상 환자의 약 2~5%에서 발생하며 척수 손상을 초래하여 환기를 심하게 방해할 수 있다. 이전에 기도 부분에서 설명한 보조기도기를 사용하여 삽관 및 환기와 같이 호흡을 보조하기 위해 확실하게 기도를 확보하거나 필요에 따라 백마스크를 사용하여 환기를 지원할 수 있다.

이차적인 뇌손상을 최소화하려면 손상된 뇌에 적절하게 산소를 공급하는 것이 필수적이다. 산소포화도를 90% 이상으로 유지하는 것이 중요하며 그렇게 하지 않으면 뇌손상 환자의 예후가 나빠진다. 저산소증은 다른 방법으로는 임상적으로 감지하기 어려운 경우가 많으므로 모든 환자는 지속해서 맥박산소측정기로 모니터링해야 한다. 산소 농도는 맥박산소측정기로 측정하고 산소포화도를 90% 이상으로 유지하는 것을 목표로 하지만, 94% 이상이 가장 좋다. 산소 치료에도 불구하고 저산소증이 지속되면 병원 전 처치 제공자는 흡인 및 긴장기흉을 포함하여 가능한 모든 원인을 파악하고 처치해야 한다. 가능한 경우 산소 공급을 개선하기 위해 호기말양압(PEEP)을 사용하는 것을 고려할 수 있다. 그러나 15cmH_2O 이상의 호기말양압은 두개내압을 증가시킬 수 있다.

저이산화탄소혈증 및 고이산화탄소혈증 모두 외상성 뇌손상을 악화시킬 수 있으므로 환기 속도를 조절하는 것이 가장 중요하다. 병원 내에서는 동맥혈가스(ABGs) 측정을 이용하여 동맥혈이산화탄소분압($PaCO_2$)을 직접 측정하여 35~40mmHg로 유지할 수 있다. 그러나 병원 전 환경에서는 ABG와 $PaCO_2$ 일상적으로 사용할 수 없다. 호기말이산화탄소분압측정은 ABG를 사용할 수 없을 때 병원 전 환경에서 사용할 수 있는 유용한 대안이다. 이 측정기는 날숨이 끝날 때 얻은 이산화탄소의 최대 분압인 $ETCO_2$를 측정한다. 연구에 따르면 특히 건강하고 혈류역학적으로 안정된 환자에서 $ETCO_2$는 $PaCO_2$ 밀접한 관련이 있는 것으로 나타났다. 중증외상 환자의 경우 폐 관류, 심박출량, 환자 체온의 잠재적 불안정성으로 인해 $ETCO_2$와 $PaCO_2$ 사이에 불일치가 발생할 수 있으며 이에 따라 $PaCO_2$에 비해 $ETCO_2$가 더 낮게 측정될 수 있다. 그러나 외상성 뇌손상에서 $ETCO_2$의 사용을 평가한 연구에서는 $ETCO_2$가 여전히 $PaCO_2$를 신뢰할 수 있지만, 특히 ABG를 사용할 수 없는 경우 병원 전 환경에서 환기를 유도하고 저이산화탄소혈증과 고이산화탄소혈증을 모두 예방하기 위해 사용해야 한다는 것이 입증되었다.

외상성 뇌손상 환자의 환기를 보조할 때 성인의 경우 10회/분, 소아의 경우 20회/분, 영아의 경우 25회/분의 정상적인 환기 속도로 환기를 시행한다. 지나치게 빠른 환기 속도와 그에 따른 저이산화탄소혈증은 뇌혈관 수축을 일으켜 뇌 산소 공급을 감소시킨다. 일상적인 예방적 과다환기는 신경학적 결과를 악화시키는 것으로 나타났으므로 사용해서는 안 된다. 병원 전 환경에서 과다환기와 중증 저산소증은 모두 사망률 증가와 관련이 있다. 성인 환자의 경우 분당 10회의 호흡 속도로 350~500mL의 일회호흡량으로 환기를 시행하면 저이산화탄소혈증을 유발하지 않으면서 적절한 산소 공급을 유지할 수 있다.

앞서 설명한 탈출증 징후가 있는 특정 상황에서는 환자의 과다환기를 통제된 방식으로 고려할 수 있다. 이러한 징후에는 비대칭 동공, 동공 확장 및 무반응, 신전 자세 또는 운동 검사 시 무반응, 점진적인 신경학적 악화, 쿠싱 반사의 발생 등이 있다. 이러면 병원 전 처치 현장에서 경미하고 조절된 과다환기를 수행할 수 있다. 경미한 과다환기는 호기말이산화탄소분압측정 또는 환기 속도(성인의 경우 20회/분, 소아의 경우 25회/분, 1세 미만 영아의 경우 30회/분)를 주의 깊게 조절하여 $ETCO_2$를 30~35mmHg로 유지하는 것을 말한다.

순환

저혈압을 초래하는 출혈은 이차 뇌손상의 중요한 원인이므로 이러한 상태를 예방하거나 처치하기 위해 노력해야 한다. 이차 뇌손상을 예방하려면 수축기 혈압을 110mmHg 이상으로 유지하는 것이 중요하다. 이 상황에서는 수축기 혈압을 110mmHg 이상으로 유지하는 것이 바람직하지만, 과도한 결정질 투여 및 비압박성 원인으로 인한 출혈 증가의 위험과 비교해야 하므로 프로토콜을 이해하는 것이 중요하다. 단일 외상성 뇌손상에서 성인의 수축기 혈압을 110mmHg 이상으로 유지하는 것이 개선과 예후와 관련이 있다.

과거에는 소아 환자의 수축기 혈압의 기준점은 다음 공식을 사용하여 계산했다(수축기 혈압 = 70 + (2×나이)). 그러나 이러한 계산된 기준점은 75%보다 낮으며 75%보다 낮은 수축기 혈압은 단일 중증 외상성 뇌손상에서 병원 내 사망 위험이 더 높은 것과 관련이 있다. **표 8-5**는 계산된 공식을 기반으로 수축기 혈압의 기준점을 비교한 것이다. 따라서 소아 집단에서 단일 외상성 뇌손상이 발생한 경우 수축기 혈압은 연령에 따라 75% 이상으로 유지해야 한다.

저혈압 예방 및 최소화하기 위해 외부출혈이 발생하면 즉시 지혈해야 한다. 두피 손상으로 인해 조절되지 않은 출혈은 출혈쇼크의 원인이 될 수 있으므로 직접 압박을 가하거나 압박 드레싱으로 처치해야 한다. 가능하면 병원 전 처지 제공자는 외부출혈의 증거를 기록하고, 정량화해야 하며 이 정보를 환자를 이송할 의료기관에 제공해야 한다. 심각한 외부출혈이 없는 경우 무딘 외상 환자의 약하고 빠른 맥박은 가슴막 안, 복막, 복막뒤공간 또는 긴뼈 골절을 둘러싼 연부조직에서 생명을 위협하는 내부출혈이 있음을 시사한다. 숫구멍이 열려 있는 영아의 경우 두개골 내부에서 충분한 출혈이 발생하여 저혈량 쇼크가 발생할 수 있다.

저혈압은 뇌 허혈을 더욱 악화시키므로 쇼크에 대처하기 위해 표준 조치를 취해야 한다. 외상성 뇌손상 환자의 경우 저산소증과 저혈압의 조합은 높은 사망률과 관련이 있다. 쇼크가 발생하고 내부출혈이 의심되는 경우 다른 처치보다 외상센터로 신속하게 이송하는 것이 우선이다. 뇌 관류를 유지하려면 수축기 혈압을 110mmHg 이상으로 유지하기 위해 충분한 수액을 투여해야 한다. 그러나 정맥 라인을 확보하기 위해 이송이 지연되어서는 안 된다.

중증 외상성 뇌손상 환자를 대상으로 한 무작위 실험에서 고장식 염수로 병원 전 수액 소생술을 받은 환자는 결정질로 수액 소생술을 받은 환자와 비교했을 때 손상 6개월 후 거의 같은 신경학적 기능을

표 8-5 연령별 소아 수축기 혈압의 기준점

나이(년)	ATLS 정의: 70 + (2 × 나이) (mmHg)	수축기 혈압 75%(mmHg)	
		소년	소녀
0	70	92	84
1	72	92	85
2	74	95	86
3	76	98	89
4	78	100	90
5	80	102	92
6	82	103	94
7	84	104	96
8	86	106	97
9	88	107	99
10	90	109	101
11	90	111	103
12	90	113	105
13	90	115	107
14	90	118	108
15	90	120	109
16	90	123	109
17	90	125	109

연령대	수축기 혈압 75%(mmHg)	
	소년	소녀
영아(0~12개월)	92	84
유아(1~2세)	92-95	85-86
취학 전(3~5세)	98-102	89-92
취학 연령(6~12세)	103-113	94-105
청소년(13세 이상)	115-125	107-109

© National Association of Emergency Medical Technicians (NAEMT)

보였다. 생리식염수나 락테이티드 링거액(lactated Ringer solution)에 비해 비용이 증가하고 이점이 부족하므로 고장식염수는 일상적인 병원 전 수액 소생술로 권장되지 않는다.

두개내압이 증가한 상태에서 뇌 관류압을 유지하기 위한 자동 조절 기전은 주로 혈압 증가로 나타나는 일련의 심혈관 변화를 초래할 수 있다. 고혈압을 처치하려는 시도는 높은 두개내압 환경에서 뇌 관류압을 감소시켜 이차 뇌손상을 유발할 수 있으므로 피해야 한다. 앞서 설명한 바와 같이 쿠싱 현상은 서맥, 맥압 증가와 관련된 혈압 상승, 체인-스톡스 호흡과 같은 불규칙한 호흡이 복합적으로 나타나는 중중 두개내압 상승에서 나타날 수 있다. 이러한 소견은 임박한 탈출증을 나타낼 수 있다. 잠재적으로 생명을 위협하는 손상이 있는 환자의 경우 혈압 측정을 위해 이송이 지연되어서는 안 되며 시간이 허락하는 대로 이송 중에 혈압 측정을 수행해야 한다.

장애

일차평가에서 확인된 문제를 처치하기 위한 적절한 조처를 한 후에는 신속한 신경학적 검사를 해야 한다. 여기에는 기준 글래스고혼수척도(GCS)와 동공 평가가 포함된다. GCS는 환자의 눈, 언어 반응 및 운동 반응 상태를 평가할 때 나타난 가장 좋은 반응을 사용하여 계산한다. 점수의 각 구성 요소는 총계만 제공하는 것이 아니라 개별적으로 기록하여 시간이 지남에 따른 특정 변화를 확인할 수 있도록 기록해야 한다(**표 8-6**). 환자의 GCS를 결정하는 방법은 6장 환자 평가 및 처치에서 자세히 다룬다.

　GCS는 환자의 상태를 평가하는 데 도움이 되며 이송 및 분류 결정에 영향을 미칠 수 있다. 이 점수는 외상성 뇌손상의 중증도를 분류하고 외상성 뇌손상이 발생한 환경에서 환자의 기도가 확보되고 안정적인지 여부를 판단하는 데 도움이 될 수 있다. 최저 총 GCS 점수는 3점이고 최고 총 GCS 점수는 15점이다. 총 GCS 점수가 13~15점인 경우 경미한 외상성 뇌손상을 나타내고 9~12점인 경우 중등도 외상성 뇌손상을 나타내며 GCS 점수가 3~8점인 경우 중증 외상성 뇌손상을 나타낸다. 표준 지침에서는 GCS 점수가 8점 이하인 경우 삽관을 권장한다. 중독이나 기타 약물 복용을 포함하여 다른 많은 요인도 GCS 점수에 영향을 미칠 수 있다.

　GCS 점수에서 가장 중요한 부분은 운동 점수이다. 연구에 따르면 신경학적 평가와 예후에 대한 운동 점수와 총 GCS 점수 사이에 민감도와 특이성이 같은 것으로 나타났다. 병원 전 환경에서 운동 점수를 얻는 것은 현장에서 병원으로 이동하는 동안 종종 악화하는 동적인 점수이므로 특히 중요하다. 삽관, 마비 및 진정으로 인해 병원 내에서 측정한 수치와 현장에서 측정한 수치가 다른 경우가 많으므로 전체 GCS 점수의 신뢰도가 떨어진다. 연구에 따르면 현장에서 측정한 GCS 운동 점수가 병원 내에서 측정한 운동 점수보다 6개월 사망률을 더 잘 예측하는 것으로 나타났다. 이러한 연구 결과와 운동 점수 결정의 단순성을 고려할 때 병원 전 분류 환경에서는 운동 점수만 사용하는 것이 권장되고 있다.

표 8-6 글래스고혼수척도(GCS)		
하위 범주	분류	점수
눈 뜨기 반응	자발적으로	4
	소리에 반응	3
	압력에 반응	2
	눈뜨지 않음	1
언어 반응	지남력 있음	5
	혼란스러운 대화	4
	부적절한 단어 사용	3
	이해불가능한 소리	2
	반응 없음	1
운동 반응	명령을 따름	6
	통증부위 인식가능	5
	정상 굴곡	4
	비정상적인 굴곡	3
	팔다리 신전 반응	2
	전혀 움직이지 않음	1

© National Association of Emergency Medical Technicians (NAEMT)

GCS 점수를 결정하는 것 외에도 동공의 대칭과 빛에 대한 반응을 신속하게 검사한다. 성인의 안정 시 동공 지름은 일반적으로 3~5mm이다. 동공 크기가 1mm 이상 차이가 나면 비정상으로 간주한다. 고정 동공은 밝은 빛에 대한 반응으로 동공의 크기가 1mm 미만으로 수축한 동공으로 정의된다. 운동 GCS 점수와 응급실에서 검사한 동공 반응성의 조합은 외상성 뇌손상 결과를 정확하게 평가하고 예측하는 것으르 입증되었다(**Box 8-2**). 급성 동공 확장은 신경학적 응급상황을 나타내며 뇌줄기 허혈 및 갈고리이랑탈출을 시사할 수 있다.

　뇌부종이나 덩이 효과로 인한 갈고리이랑탈툴은 눈돌립신경(CN III)을 압박하여 동공 확장을 유발할 수 있습니다. 뇌줄기로의 혈류 감소와 뇌줄기 허혈도 동공 확장을 유발한다. 참고로 인구의 일부는 선천적이거나 눈 외상으로 인해 후천적으로 동공이 같지 않은 동공부등을 가지고 있다. 그러나 현장에서 외상으로 인한 동공 불균등과 선천적 또는 외상 후 기존 동공부등을 구별하는 것이 항상 가능한 것은 아니다. 따라서 동공이 같지 않은 것은 적절한 검사를 통해 뇌부종이나 운동 또는 눈 신경 손상이 배제될 때까지 항상 급성 외상에 의한 이차적인 것으로 간주해야 한다.

Box 8-2 치료 거부

EMS 전문가는 치료 및 이송을 거부하는 환자를 자주 접하게 된다. EMS 전문가는 병원으로 이송하여 평가하는 것이 환자에게 최선의 이익이라고 생각하지만, 환자가 거부하고 평가 당시 신경학적 손상이나 결손의 징후가 보이지 않을 때 이러한 상황은 더욱 복잡해진다. 심각한 손상 기전을 가진 외상성 뇌손상 환자는 종종 몇 시간 또는 며칠이 지나야 손상의 심각성을 완전히 경험하지 못할 수 있다. 경막외출혈이 있는 환자의 경우 환자가 몇 시간 후 출혈로 인한 치명적인 영향을 받기 전에 종종 의식 명료 기간이 있으며 그동안 환자의 의식은 명료하다.

　　머리 손상 가능성이 있는 환자는 의사 결정 능력에 특히 주의를 기울이면서 충분히 평가해야 한다. 또한 다음과 같은 증상과 징후는 추가적인 처치가 필요하다는 것을 나타내므로 환자에게 이를 설명해야 한다.

- 비대칭 동공
- 두통 악화
- 메스꺼움 및 구토
- 졸음 또는 잠에서 깨기 어려움
- 말이 어눌해짐
- 혼동 또는 행동 변화
- 의식 소실
- 발작
- 마비(무감각)

- 협응력 저하
- 사람이나 장소를 인식하는 데 어려움

　　EMS 제공자가 추가 평가를 위해 병원으로 이송하는 것이 환자에게 최선의 이익이라고 판단하고 의사 결정 능력이 있는 환자가 이송을 거부하는 경우 이송 거부의 위험과 치료의 이점을 명확하게 설명하기 위해 모든 노력을 기울여야 한다. 여기에는 적절한 경우 치료 지연으로 인해 발생할 수 있는 사망 및 영구 장애의 가능성에 대해 매우 직접적인 경고가 포함된다. 이러면 환자가 의사의 조언에 더 기꺼이 들을 수 있으므로 이러한 상황에서 의료 지도 의사에게 빨리 연락하는 것이 도움이 될 수 있다. 환자가 여전히 이송 및 추가 치료를 거부하는 경우 언제든지 마음을 바꿀 수 있으며 EMS가 다시 출동해서 환자를 평가할 수 있다는 점을 분명히 알려야 한다.

　　환자가 완전한 의사 결정 능력을 갖추고 있지 않은 경우 의료 지도 및 경찰관은 환자에게 최선의 이익인 추가 평가를 위해 환자를 이송하는 데 필요한 범위까지 참여해야 한다.

　　치료 결정을 내릴 때는 항상 프로토콜, 의료 지침, 업무 범위를 따라야 한다. 여기서 논의한 것과 유사한 시나리오에서 취해야 할 적절한 조치에 관한 논의는 사고가 발생하기 전에 하는 것이 가장 잘 이루어지며 지속적인 교육과 초기 직원 교육에 일상적으로 포함해야 한다. "먼저 해를 끼치지 않는다"는 원칙은 EMS 전문가가 마주치는 모든 환자를 치료하는 접근 방식에서 기본이 되어야 한다.

목뼈 골절의 발생률이 높으므로 무딘 외상으로 인해 외상성 뇌손상이 의심되는 환자에게는 척추 움직임 제한을 시행한다. 외상성 뇌손상 환자에게 목뼈보호대를 착용할 때는 머리의 정맥 배액을 방해하여 두개내압을 증가시킬 수 있으므로 주의를 기울여야 한다. 머리와 목의 움직임이 충분히 제한되는 한 목뼈보호대 착용은 필수가 아니다. 머리에 총상을 입은 환자에게는 척추 고정을 권장하지 않는다.

노출과 환경

외상성 뇌손상을 입은 환자는 뇌뿐만 아니라 생명과 팔다리를 위협하는 다른 손상을 입는 경우가 종종 있다. 이러한 모든 손상을 확인한다. 잠재적으로 생명을 위협할 수 있는 다른 문제가 있는지 전신을 검사해야 한다.

이차평가

생명을 위협하는 손상을 확인하고 처치를 시행한 후에 시간이 허락하는 경우 이차평가를 완료해야 한다. 환자의 머리와 얼굴에 상처, 함몰 및 비빔소리가 있는지 주의 깊게 촉지해야 한다. 이때 동공 크기와 반응을 다시 확인한다. 앞서 언급한 바와 같이 외상성 뇌손상 환자의 경우 목뼈 골절이 발생할 수 있으므로 목에 압통과 변형이 있는지 검사해야 한다. 코나 이관에서 맑은 액체가 흘러나오면 뇌척수액일 수 있다. 그러나 대부분의 경우 뇌척수액은 혈액과 섞여 있어 이를 공식적으로 발견하기 어렵다. 구체적인 머리 및 목 손상은 다음에 설명한다.

협조적인 환자의 경우보다 철저한 신경학적 검사를 실시할 수도 있다. 여기에는 모든 팔다리의 뇌신경, 감각 및 운동 기능에 대한 평가가 포함된다. 기능의 비대칭뿐만 아니라 전체 또는 부분적인 결손을 찾으면 신경학적 손상 가능성에 대한 중요한 단서를 발견할 수 있다. 신체의 한쪽에만 나타나는 반신불완전마비(쇠약) 또는 반신마비(마비)와 같은 소견은 "편향 징후"로 간주하며 일반적으로 외상성 뇌손상을 나타낸다.

머리와 목의 특별한 손상

두피 손상

해부학 부문에서 언급했듯이 두피는 여러 층의 조직으로 구성되어 있으며 혈관이 매우 많다. 손상은 단순한 작은 열상에서부터 두피의

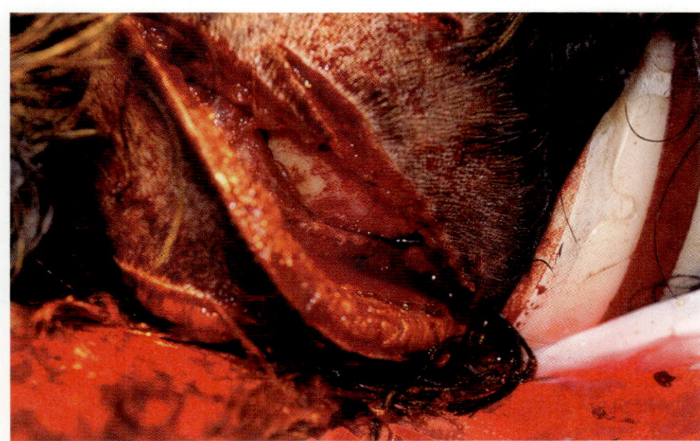

그림 8-11 광범위한 두피 손상은 대량 외부출혈을 초래할 수 있다.
Courtesy of Peter T. Pons, MD, FACEP.

넓은 부위가 두개골에서 뒤로 찢어지는 벗겨진 손상과 같은 복잡한 손상에 이르기까지 다양하다. 이러한 손상으로 인한 출혈을 지혈하지 않으면 저혈량쇼크와 대량 출혈을 초래할 수 있다(**그림 8-11**). 이러한 유형의 손상은 종종 안전띠를 착용하지 않은 차량 앞좌석 탑승자가 앞 유리에 머리를 부딪치거나 긴 머리카락이 기계에 걸리는 작업자에게 종종 발생한다. 머리에 심각한 타격을 가하면 두피 혈종이 형성될 수 있으며 이는 두피를 촉진할 때 함몰두개골 골절과 혼동될 수 있다. 두피 혈종은 근본적인 두개내 손상이 동반되어 있음을 나타낼 수 있다.

두개골 골절

두개골 골절은 무딘 손상 또는 관통성 외상으로 인해 발생할 수 있다. 선 골절은 일반적으로 무딘 외상으로 인해 발생한다. 그러나 강력한 충격으로 인해 뼛조각이 기저 뇌 조직을 향하거나 뇌 조직으로 들어가는 함몰두개골 골절이 발생할 수 있다(**그림 8-12**). 단순 선골절은 방사선 검사로만 진단할 수 있지만, 함몰두개골 골절은 주의 깊은 신체검사 중에 촉진할 수 있다. 함몰되지 않은 폐쇄 두개골 골절은 그 자체로 임상적 의미가 거의 없지만, 두개내 혈종 발생 위험을 증가시킨다. 폐쇄 함몰두개골 골절은 골절로 인한 두개내 공간을 감소시켜 두개내압이 증가하므로 신경 외과적 처치가 필요할 수 있다. 앞서 논의한 바와 같이 두개골 골절은 경막정맥동의 외부 압박을 유발하여 정맥 폐쇄를 초래하고 결과적으로 두개내압을 증가시킬 수 있다. 개방 두개골 골절은 특히 강한 충격이나 총상으로부터 발생할 수 있으며 세균이 유입되어 환자가 수막염에 걸리기 쉽다. 경막이 찢어지면 개방 두개골 골절로 인해 뇌 조직이나 뇌척수액이 누출될 수

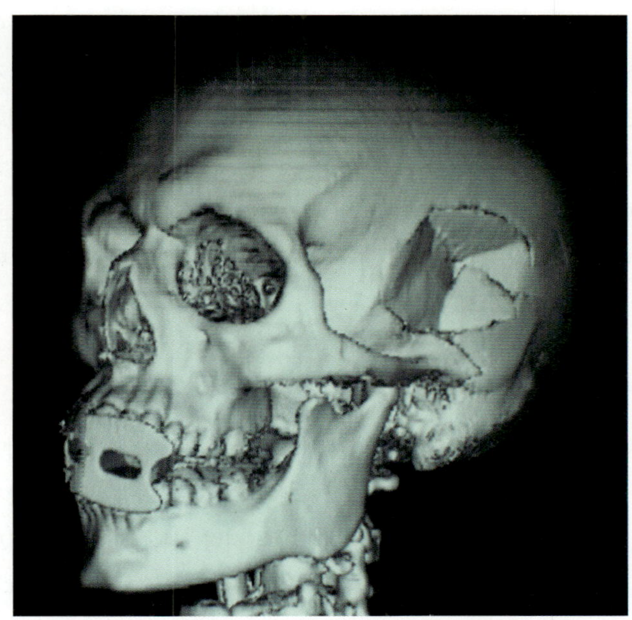

그림 8-12 폭행 후 발생한 함몰두개골 골절을 3차원으로 재구성한 모습이다.
Courtesy of Peter T. Pons, MD, FACEP.

있다. 수막염의 위험 때문에 이러한 상처는 즉각적인 신경 외과적 평가가 필요하다.

두개골 바닥 골절은 두개골 바닥의 골절로 측두골 골절이 가장 흔하다. 이러한 골절로 인해 막이 찢어져 뇌척수액이 누출될 수 있다. 두개골 바닥 골절의 약 12~30%에서 뇌척수액이 천공된 고막을 통해 귀(귓물) 또는 콧구멍(콧물)에서 통해 누출될 수 있다. 눈 주위 반상출혈(너구리 눈)과 귀 뒤쪽의 꼭지돌기 부위에 반상출혈(배틀 징후)은 두개골 바닥 골절에서 발생할 수 있지만, 손상 후 몇 시간이 지나야 뚜렷하게 나타날 수 있다. 허용되는 경우 이경으로 고막을 검사하면 고막 뒤쪽에 혈액이 보이면 이는 두개골 바닥 골절을 시사할 수 있다.

얼굴 손상

얼굴 손상은 경미한 연부조직 손상에서 기도 손상 또는 저혈량쇼크와 관련된 중증 손상까지 다양하다. 기도는 1) 구조적 손상, 2) 해부학적 변형 및 부은 조직 또는 3) 기도 내 액체나 기타 물질에 의한 폐쇄로 손상될 수 있다. 기도는 얼굴부터 기관기관지 용골까지를 포함하며 기도의 어느 곳에서나 손상이 발생할 수 있다는 점에 유의하는 것이 중요하다. 구조적인 변화는 얼굴뼈 골절로 인한 변형 또는 조직에서 발생한 혈종이 포함될 수 있다. 머리는 혈관이 밀집되어 있기 때문에 이 부위에 손상을 입으면 종종 심각한 출혈이 발생한다. 심각한

얼굴 골절은 종종 고통스럽고 덜 효과적으로 삼키므로 인해 인두에 혈액과 분비물이 고이는 것과 관련이 있다. 기도 내에서 가장 흔하게 기도를 막는 물질은 혈액과 구토물이다. 얼굴 손상은 종종 의식 변화와 잠재적으로 중증 뇌 외상과 관련이 있다. 얼굴 손상으로 인해 골절이 발생하거나 치아가 기도 안으로 변위될 수 있다. 얼굴 손상으로 인한 외상성 뇌손상과 삼킨 혈액은 구토를 일으킬 수 있으며 이에 따라 기도 폐쇄가 발생할 수 있다.

눈과 안와 외상

눈과 안와의 구조에 대한 손상은 흔하며 종종 얼굴에 대한 직접적인 외상으로 인해 발생한다. 눈(안구) 자체의 손상은 자주 발생하지 않지만, 안와 손상을 적절히 처치하면 환자의 시력 회복률을 증가시키므로 얼굴 및 안와에 외상이 확인될 때마다 안구 손상을 고려해야 한다.

눈꺼풀 열상은 안와 위에 부착된 단단한 보호대(압박 패치가 아님)로 눈을 덮어 처치한다. 보호대 아래에는 어떤 것도 부착해서는 안 된다. 눈꺼풀 열상은 기저 눈 손상과 관련이 있을 수 있다. 따라서 주요 고려 사항은 각막이나 공막 열상을 통해 안구 내 내용물이 강제로 배출되어 추가적인 손상을 입힐 수 있는 눈에 대한 압박을 피하는 것이다.

각막 찰과상은 각막을 덮고 있는 보호 상피가 손상된 것이다. 이러한 찰과상은 결함이 치유될 때까지(보통 2~3일) 극심한 통증, 눈물, 빛에 대한 민감성(눈부심), 감염 증가를 초래한다. 일반적으로 이전에 외상을 입었거나 콘택트렌즈를 사용한 병력이 있는 경우가 많다. 이 손상에 대한 병원 전 처치 방법은 빛에 대한 민감성으로 인한 불편함을 줄이기 위해 안대, 보호대 또는 선글라스로 눈을 가리는 것이다.

눈의 공막 위의 결막밑출혈은 결막과 공막 사이의 출혈로 인해 발생한다(**그림 8-13**). 진단 장비를 사용하지 않고도 쉽게 확인할 수 있다. 이 손상은 해가 없으며 처치 없이 며칠에서 몇 주에 걸쳐 저절로 회복된다. 선행된 외상이 있는 경우 더 심각한 다른 손상에 주의해야 한다. 예를 들어, 출혈로 인해 결막이 심하게 부어오르면 결막부종으로 알려진 잠복성 안구 파열을 의심한다. 이 손상의 병원 전 처치는 진단을 확인하고 다른 관련 손상을 배제할 수 있도록 환자를 병원으로 이송하는 것이다.

앞방출혈은 홍채와 각막 사이의 안구 앞방에 있는 혈액을 말한다. 이 상태는 일반적으로 눈에 직접적인 타격을 입은 급성 외상 상황에서 나타난다. 눈은 환자가 똑바로 앉은 상태에서 검사를 한다. 충분한 혈액이 존재하면 혈액이 앞방 바닥에 모여 눈의 앞방에 혈액이 모이게 되고 층을 이룬 앞방출혈로 보인다(**그림 8-14**). 환자가 바로누운자세로 검사를 받거나 혈액의 양이 매우 적은 경우 이 혈액을 확인하지 못할 수 있다. 눈 위에 보호대를 적용하고 안구 앞과 뒤를 더 잘 검사할 수 있게 하려고 환자를 앉은 자세로 병원으로 이송한다(다른 금기 사항이 없는 경우).

개방 안구 손상은 각막이나 공막을 통해 안구 내부로 들어가는 상처를 말한다. 이 상처가 확인되면 나머지 눈 검사를 중단하고 추가 손상으로부터 보호하기 위해 눈 위의 안와에 보호대를 적용해야 한다. 압박 드레싱을 적용하거나 국소 약물을 주입하지 않는다.

개방 안구 손상의 처치에는 두 가지 주요 관심사가 있다. 첫 번째는 안압을 상승시키고 각막 또는 공막 결손을 통해 안구 내 내용물

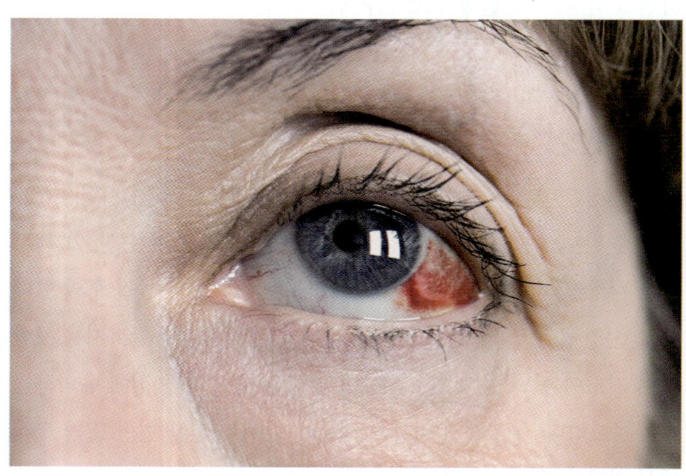

그림 8-13 결막밑 출혈

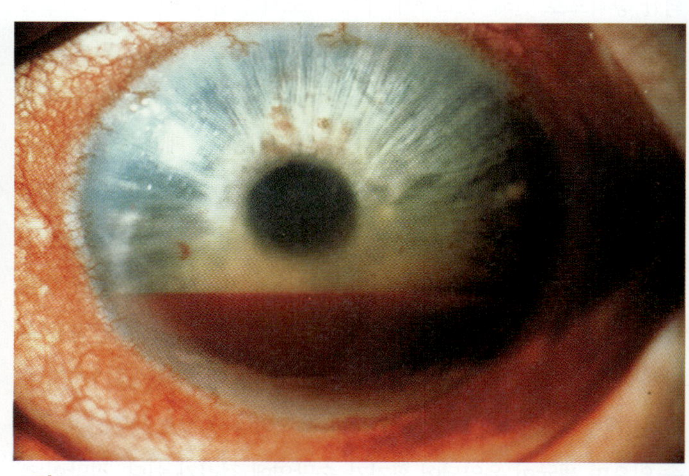

그림 8-14 앞방출혈

이 배출될 수 있는 눈의 조작이나 추가적인 외상을 최소화하는 것이다. 두 번째는 눈 안쪽의 감염인 외상 후 안구내염 발생을 예방하는 것이다. 이것은 일반적으로 시력에 치명적인 결과를 초래할 수 있다. 안과적 평가와 외과적 처치를 위해 병원으로 신속히 이송한다.

눈에 관통상을 입거나 안구 파열이 항상 분명한 것은 아니다. 잠재적인 안구 파열에 대한 단서는 손상 기전(예: 금속을 망치로 치거나 잡초 제거 도구로 인한 눈 손상)뿐만 아니라 결막 부종이 동반된 대량의 결막밑출혈, 각막과 공막의 접합부에 있거나 공막을 통해 튀어나온 어두운 포도막 조직(색깔 홍채), 왜곡된 동공(눈물방울 모양), 각막 열상 또는 천공 상처에서 누출 또는 시력 저하 등의 임상 소견이 있다. 잠재적으로 안구 파열이 의심되는 경우 명백한 개방 안구에 대해 앞서 설명한 대로 환자를 처치한다. 손상의 정도가 상대적으로 덜 심각하다고 해서 압력(외부 압력을 받는 경우)이나 안구내염으로 인한 눈의 추가 손상 위협이 사라지는 것은 아니므로 눈을 즉시 보호하고 병원으로 신속하게 이송하는 것이 여전히 필수적이다.

코 골절

코뼈 골절은 얼굴에서 가장 흔한 골절이다. 코 골절을 의심할 수 있는 증후로는 반상출혈, 부종, 코 변형, 코 출혈 등이 있다. 촉진 시 뼈 비빔소리가 나타날 수 있다.

강한 힘으로 발생한 얼굴중간 외상은 코뼈 골절뿐만 아니라 체판(두개골에서 1번 뇌신경(후각신경)이 통과하는 얇고 수평인 뼈)의 골절을 유발할 수 있다. 얼굴중간에 강한 힘을 가한 후 콧물(뇌척수액 누출)이 발생하면 체판 골절 가능성이 높다.

얼굴중간 골절

얼굴중간 골절은 르포(Le Fort) 분류에 따라 분류할 수 있다(**그림 8-15** 참조).

- 르포(Le Fort) I 형 골절은 코 바닥에서 위턱뼈까지 수평으로 분리되는 골절이다. 콧구멍을 통한 공기 통과에는 영향을 미치지 않지만, 입인두는 물렁입천장의 부종이나 혈전으로 인해 손상될 수 있다.
- 피라미드형 골절로도 알려진 르포(Le Fort) II 형 골절은 왼쪽 및 오른쪽 위턱뼈, 안와 바닥의 내측부분 및 코뼈를 포함한다. 부비동은 혈관이 잘 발달하여 있으므로 이 골절은 심각한 출혈로 인한 기도 손상과 관련이 있을 수 있다.
- 르포(Le Fort) III 형 골절은 두개골에서 얼굴뼈를 완전히 분리(머리얼굴분리)하는 골절이다. 이 손상은 강한 힘으로 인해 기도 손상, 외상성 뇌손상, 눈물관 손상, 치아의 맞물림 장애 및 코에서 뇌척수액 누출과 관련이 있을 수 있다.

얼굴중간 골절 환자는 일반적으로 정상적인 얼굴 대칭이 상실된다. 얼굴이 평평하게 보일 수 있으며 환자는 턱이나 치아를 다물지 못

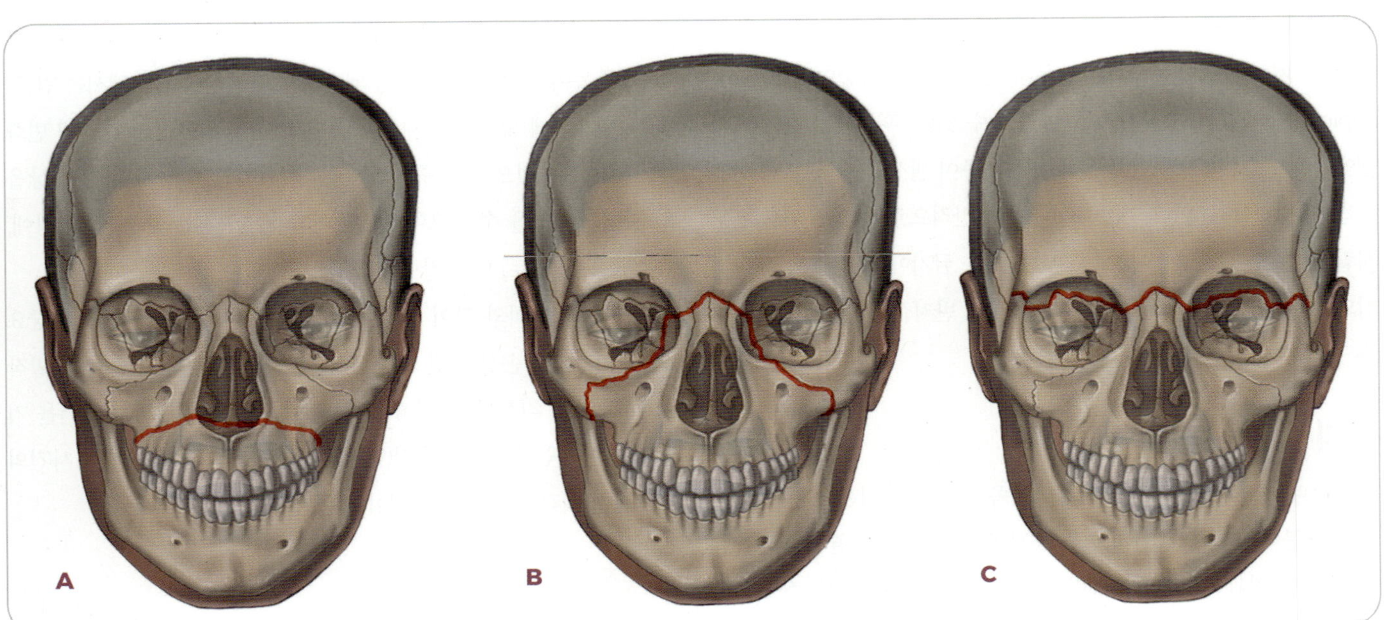

그림 8-15 얼굴중간의 Le Fort 골절 유형.　**A.** Le Fort I 골절　**B.** Le Fort II 골절　**C.** Le Fort III 골절

할 수도 있다. 의식이 있는 경우 환자는 얼굴 통증과 무감각을 호소할 수 있다. 촉진 시 골절 부위에서 비빔소리가 나타날 수 있다. 전이된 얼굴중간 골절은 때때로 기도 폐쇄를 유발할 수 있다. 얼굴 골격의 연약한 중간 1/3에 높은 에너지가 가해지면 골절 조각이 발생하여 앞뒤로 무너져 물렁입천장을 포함한 후방 구조물에 영향을 미칠 수 있다. 이에 따라 인두가 부어 기도 폐쇄를 일으킬 수 있다. 아래턱과 중간 1/3 얼굴 골절이 복합적으로 발생하면 관련된 뇌손상 및 목뼈 손상을 포함한 심각한 기저 손상을 나타낸다.

아래턱 골절

코뼈 골절에 이어 아래턱 골절은 두 번째로 흔한 얼굴 골절 유형이다. 종종 아래턱(턱뼈)은 두 곳 이상에서 부러지는 경우가 많다. 아래턱 골절 환자의 가장 흔한 호소증상은 통증 외에도 윗니와 아랫니가 더 이상 정상적인 배열에서 만나지 않는 맞물림 장애이다. 시진에서 치아의 변형이나 정렬 불량을 확인할 수 있으며 촉진 시 변형과 비빔소리가 나타날 수 있다. 아래턱 골절이 있는 바로누워 있는 환자의 경우 혀의 뼈지지 구조가 더 이상 온전하지 않기 때문에 혀가 기도를 폐쇄할 수 있다.

후두 손상

후두 골절은 일반적으로 오토바이나 자전거 운전자의 목 앞쪽이 물체에 부딪히는 것과 같이 목 앞쪽에 무딘 충격으로 인해 발생한다. 환자는 목소리(일반적으로 톤이 낮아짐)의 변화를 호소할 수 있다. 병원 전 처치 제공자는 검사 시 목의 타박상이나 갑상연골(Adam's apple)의 돌출부가 소실된 것을 발견할 수 있다. 후두 골절은 환자가 혈액이 섞인 기침(객혈)이나 목에 피하기종이 발생할 수 있으며 이는 촉진 시 발견할 수 있다. 기관내삽관은 일반적으로 골절 부위를 전위시킬 수 있어 후두 골절이 있는 환자에게는 금기이다. 후두 골절이 의심되는 환자의 기도가 손상된 경우 외과적 반지갑상연골절개로 생명을 구할 수 있다.

목의 혈관 손상

목동맥과 속목정맥은 기관 양쪽의 앞쪽 목을 가로지른다. 목동맥은 뇌 대부분에 혈액을 공급하고 속목정맥은 이 부위의 혈액을 배출한다. 이러한 혈관 중 하나에 개방 손상이 발생하면 심각한 출혈이 발생할 수 있다. 속목정맥 손상으로 인한 또 다른 위험은 공기색전증이다. 환자가 앉아 있거나 머리를 올리면 들숨 시 정맥압이 대기압보다 낮아져 공기가 정맥으로 유입될 수 있다. 큰 공기색전증은 심장 기능과 뇌 관류를 모두 방해할 수 있으므로 치명적일 수 있다. 목 혈관 외상의 또 다른 우려는 기도의 정상 해부학적 구조에 영향을 미치고 변형되어 기도 손상을 초래할 수 있는 확장하는 혈종이 발생할 수 있다는 것이다. 또한, 목정맥 압박을 유발하여 뇌정맥 유출을 막고 간접적으로 두개내압을 증가시킬 수 있다.

목에 대한 무딘 손상은 또한 뇌혈관 손상도 발생할 수 있다. 이러한 손상은 속목동맥, 온목동맥 또는 척추동맥에 발생할 수 있다. 척추동맥 손상은 거의 항상 목뼈 손상과 관련이 있다. 목동맥 손상은 중증 외상성 뇌손상, 주요 얼굴 골절, 두개골 바닥 골절 및 주요 가슴 손상 등 여러 다른 손상과 관련이 있다. 고속 차량 충돌, 목에 대한 직접적인 타격, 빨랫줄 유형의 손상, 교수형 등은 환자를 이러한 손상의 위험에 처하게 한다. 이러한 손상은 뇌졸중 위험으로 인해 심각한 병적 상태를 초래할 수 있다. 종종 이러한 환자는 현장에서 뇌졸중 징후를 나타낼 수 있으며 설명할 수 없는 신경학적 결손이 나타나면 이러한 손상에 대한 평가를 신속히 시행해야 한다.

병력

시간과 상황이 허락하는 경우 환자, 가족 또는 목격자로부터 SAMPLER 병력(증상, 알레르기, 약물, 과거 병력, 마지막 식사, 손상 전 사건, 위험 요인)을 얻어야 한다. 당뇨병, 발작 장애, 약물 또는 알코올 중독은 외상성 뇌손상을 모방하거나 외상성 뇌손상 평가를 혼란스럽게 할 수 있다. 약물 사용 또는 과다 복용의 모든 증거에 주목해야 하지만, 중독이 있는 경우 외상성 뇌손상의 가능성을 간과해서는 안 된다. 항혈소판제 및 항응고제의 사용은 외상성 뇌손상의 관리에 변화를 가져올 수 있으므로 주의해야 한다. 환자는 이전에 머리 손상을 입은 병력이 있을 수 있으며 지속적이거나 반복되는 두통, 시각 장애, 메스꺼움 및 구토, 언어 장애를 호소할 수 있다.

앞서 설명한 바와 같이 외상을 둘러싼 사건에 주목하는 것이 중요하다. 여기에는 손상 기전, 의식 상실 여부, 무반응 기간, 목격된 발작 활동 및 후속 각성 수준(발작 후 상태)이 포함된다. 환자가 사건을 기억하지 못하는 경우 외상 전(역행성) 또는 외상 후(앞 방향) 사건의 기억상실 기간을 파악하는 것이 도움이 될 수 있다.

지속적인 검사

GCS 점수를 재평가하고 시간이 지남에 따라 어떤 변화가 일어나고 있는지 파악하는 것이 중요하다. 처음에 GCS 점수가 감소하고 있는 환자는 GCS 점수가 개선된 환자보다 심각한 외상성 뇌손상에 대한 우려가 훨씬 더 높다. 경미한 뇌손상(GCS 점수 14점 또는 15점)이 있는 소수의 환자도 예상치 못한 정신 활동 변화를 경험할 수 있다. 이송 중에는 일차평가와 GCS 점수를 자주 재평가해야 한다. 이송 중 GCS 점수가 2점 이상 감소한 환자는 병리학적 과정이 진행될 수 있는 위험이 특히 높다. 이러한 환자는 적절한 의료기관으로 신속하게 이송해야 한다. 환자를 인계받는 의료기관에서는 환자의 초기 처치에 이송 중 GCS 점수 추이를 활용한다. GCS 점수 또는 활력징후의 변화는 환자를 이송할 의료기관에 보고하고 환자 처치보고서에 기록하고 환자 처치에 대한 반응도 기록해야 한다.

이송

최상의 결과를 얻으려면 중등도 및 중증 외상성 뇌손상 환자는 CT 촬영을 수행하고 신속한 신경 외과적 진료 및 처치(필요한 경우 두개내압 모니터링 포함)를 제공할 수 있는 외상센터로 즉시 이송해야 한다. 이러한 시설을 이용할 수 없는 경우 현장에서 적절한 외상센터로 항공 이송을 고려해야 한다.

이송 중 5~10분마다 환자의 맥박, 혈압, 산소포화도, 가능한 경우 호기말이산화탄소, GCS 점수를 재평가하고 기록해야 한다. 저산소증이 15cmH$_2$O 수준까지 지속되는 경우 호기말양압 밸브를 주의해서 사용할 수 있으며 15cmH$_2$O보다 큰 호기말양압은 두개내압을 증가시킬 수 있다. 이송 중에는 정상 체온을 유지해야 한다. 일반적으로 외상성 뇌손상 환자는 다른 손상이 있을 수 있으므로 바로누운자세로 이송한다. 구급차 들것이나 역트렌델렌버그 자세는 두개내압을 감소시킬 수 있지만, 특히 머리를 30도 이상으로 높이면 뇌관류압도 위험할 수 있다.

환자가 의료기관에 도착하기 전에 적절한 준비가 이루어질 수 있도록 가능한 한 빨리 환자를 이송하는 의료기관에 보고해야 한다. 무전 보고에는 손상 기전, 초기 GCS 점수 및 이송 중 변화, 국소 징후(예: 운동 검사 비대칭, 한쪽 또는 양쪽 동공 확장) 및 활력 징후, 기타 심각한 손상 및 처치에 대한 반응에 관한 정보도 포함되어야 한다.

이송 지연

이송 시간이 길어지면 전문 기도 유지를 수행하기 위한 기준이 낮아질 수 있다. 특히 항공 이송이 고려되는 경우 헬기 내에서 전투적인 환자는 탑승한 모든 사람의 안전을 위협할 수 있으므로 이러한 환경에서 급속연속기관삽관을 시행할 수 있다. 목뼈 고정을 적용하는 동안 기도를 확보하기 위한 노력이 수행되어야 한다. 적절한 산소포화도를 유지하기 위해 산소를 공급해야 한다. 딱딱한 긴척추고정판에 장시간 누워 있으면 압박으로 인한 궤양이 발생할 위험이 있으므로 특히 예상 이송 시간이 긴 경우 환자 이송에 긴척추고정판을 사용할 때는 적절한 패딩을 사용해야 한다. 환자에게 맥박산소측정기를 부착하고 환기, 맥박, 혈압, GCS 점수를 포함한 일련의 활력징후를 측정해야 한다. 빛에 대한 동공의 반응과 대칭성을 주기적으로 확인한다.

이송이 지연되거나 적절한 의료기관으로 이송하는 데 시간이 오래 걸리는 경우 추가 처치 방법을 고려할 수 있다. GCS 점수가 비정상인 환자의 경우 혈당 수치를 확인한다. 환자가 저혈당이면 혈당이 정상 수준으로 회복될 때까지 50% 포도당 용액을 정맥 내로 투여할 수 있다. 재발성 또는 장기간 발작이 발생하는 경우 벤조다이아제핀을 정맥 내로 투여할 수 있다.

외부출혈을 조절하고 쇼크 징후가 명백한 경우 결정질 수액을 투여해야 한다. 외상성 뇌손상이 의심되는 환자의 수축기 혈압을 110mmHg 이상으로 유지하기 위해 수액 소생술을 시작한다. 관련 손상은 환자를 의료기관으로 이송하는 중에 처치를 한다. 골절은 내부출혈과 통증을 조절하기 위해 적절하게 부목으로 고정해야 한다. 트라넥삼산(TXA)은 이송 시간이 길어지는 경우에만 출혈 및 외상성 뇌손상이 의심될 때 투여를 고려할 수 있다.

환자가 전원 중이고 이미 두개내압 모니터나 뇌실창냄술을 시행하지 않는 한 병원 전 현장에서 두개내압을 적절히 처치하기는 매우 어렵다. GCS 점수가 감소하는 것은 두개내압이 증가하는 것을 의미할 수도 있지만, 저혈량 쇼크로 인한 뇌관류 악화의 결과일 수도 있다. 두개내압 증가 및 탈출증 가능성에 대한 경고 징후는 다음과 같다.

- GCS 점수가 2점 이상 감소한 경우
- 동공 반응 속도가 느리거나 반응이 없는 경우
- 반신마비 또는 반신불완전마비 발생한 경우
- 쿠싱 반사

두개내압 증가에 대한 개입 및 처치 결정은 프로토콜을 기반으로 하거나 의료 지도의사의 지도를 받아 결정한다. 가능한 일시적 처치 방법에는 진정제, 화학적 마비, 만니톨과 같은 삼투성 활성제 사용, 과다환기 조절 등이 있다(**그림 8-16**). 소량의 벤조다이아제핀 진정제는 저혈압과 환기 저하라는 잠재적 부작용이 있으므로 신중하게 사용해야 한다. 환자가 삽관되었으면 베쿠로뉴과 같은 지속성 신경근

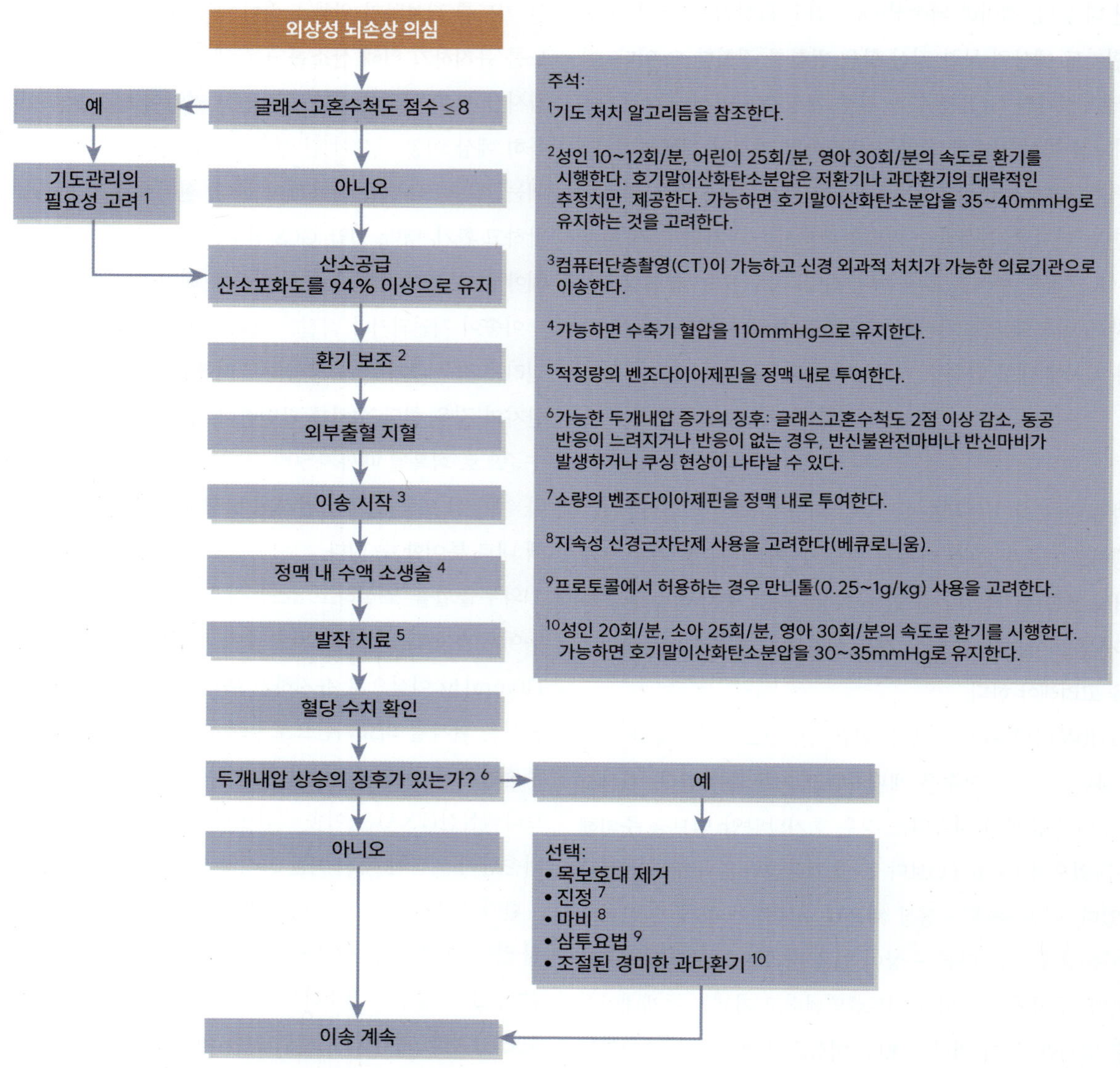

그림 8-16 외상성 뇌손상이 의심되는 환자 처치

차단제의 사용을 고려할 수 있다. 목뼈호호대가 너무 꽉 조이면 다른 방법으로 머리와 목을 적절하게 고정할 수 있느 경우 약간 느슨하게 하거나 제거할 수 있다. 가능하면 환자의 머리를 신체의 다른 부위보다 높게(역트렌델렌버그 자세)하여 뇌정맥 배액을 쉽게 해야 한다.

고장식염수(3%) 또는 만니톨(0.25~1.0g/kg)을 사용하는 것과 같은 고삼투압 요법을 사용하여 두개내압을 낮출 수 있다. 두 약물 모두 정맥 내로 투여한다. 현재 병원 전 환경에서 일상적으로 사용하는 것을 뒷받침하는 좋은 증거는 없다. 만니톨은 매우 효과적인 삼투성 이뇨제로 전신 소생술을 받지 않은 환자에게 혈량저하증을 유발할 수 있으며 이에 따라 저혈압이 발생하여 뇌 관류가 악화할 수 있다. 따라서 수축기 혈압이 90mmHg 미만인 환자에게는 사용해서는 안 된다. 만니톨은 탈출증 징후가 있는 환자에게만 제한적으로 사용해야 하며 매우 주의해서 사용한다. 또한 이송 시간이 매우 길어질 경우 폴리 카테터를 삽입하여 소변 배출량을 모니터링해야 한다.

탈출증의 명백한 징후가 있는 경우 호기말이산화탄소를 30~35mmHg로 유지하기 위해 환기 속도를 높이는 것(조절된 경도의 치료적 과다환기)을 고려할 수 있다. 성인의 경우 20회/분, 어린이의 경우 25회/분, 영의 경우 30회/분의 환기 속도로 환기를 시행한다.

앞서 언급한 바와 같이 예방적 과다환기는 외상성 뇌손상에 아무런 도움이 되지 않으며 치료적 과다환기를 시행하는 경우 두개내압 상승의 징후가 해결되면 중단한다. 스테로이드는 외상성 뇌손상 환자의 예후를 개선하는 것으로 입증되지 않았으므로 투여해서는 안 된다.

발작이 의심되는 경우 특히 장기간 또는 여러 번 목격되는 경우 디아제팜, 로라제팜 또는 미다졸람과 같은 벤조다이아제핀계 약물을 정맥 내로 투여하여 처치할 수 있다. 그러나 이러한 약물은 저혈압과 환기 저하가 발생할 수 있으므로 신중하게 투여한다.

이송 지연 중이거나 열악한 환경에 있는 외상성 뇌손상 환자에게 가장 중점을 두어야 하는 것은 뇌 산소 공급과 관류를 최대한 유지하고 뇌부종을 조절하기 위해 최대한 노력하는 것이다.

요 약

- 머리와 뇌 해부학에 대한 지식은 외상성 뇌손상의 병태생리학을 이해하는 데 필수적이다.

- 병원 전 처치 제공자는 외상 후 감소한 뇌 혈류를 뇌가 보상하는 기전을 이해해야 한다.

- 일차 뇌손상은 최초 손상 당시 발생하며 초기 외상으로 발생하는 모든 손상을 말한다.

- 이차 뇌손상은 일차 손상으로 손상되지 않은 구조물에 대한 추가 손상을 말한다. 병원 전 환경에서 덩이 효과에 의한 탈출증, 저산소증, 저혈압 등 이차 손상을 나타내는 병태생리학 과정을 인지하고 신속하게 이송하는 것이 우선순위이다.

- 손상의 기전을 알면 병원 전 처치 제공자는 특정 손상 유형을 예상할 수 있으며 이는 뇌손상과 관련된 상태가 급격히 악화하는 것을 파악하는 데 매우 중요하다.

- 외상성 뇌손상의 중증도는 즉각적으로 나타나지 않을 수 있으므로 환자의 상태 변화를 인식하기 위해서는 GCS 점수 특히 운동 점수 및 동공 반응을 포함한 환자의 신경학적 평가를 지속해서 시행해야 한다.

- 외상성 뇌손상 환자의 병원 전 단계 처치는 다른 손상으로 인한 출혈을 조절하고 수축기혈압을 110mmHg 이상으로 유지하며 산소포화도를 90% 이상으로 유지할 수 있도록 산소를 공급한다.

- 병원 전 처치 제공자는 중증 외상성 뇌손상(GCS 점수 8점 이하)이 있는 모든 환자에게 적극적인 기도 유지를 고려해야 한다. 삽관을 선택한 경우 가장 숙련된 병원 전 처치가 시행해야 한다.

시나리오 재구성

외부 온도가 29℃인 여름날 당신과 동료는 30세 남자가 마라톤 결승선에서 현수막을 설치하던 중 4.3m의 사다리에서 떨어졌다는 신고를 받고 사고 현장으로 출동한다. 현장에 도착했을 때 환자는 바로누워있고 반응이 없다. 목격자가 환자의 머리와 목을 일직선으로 도수 고정하고 있다.

초기 평가 시 호흡 깊이와 속도가 달라지는 불규칙한 호흡 양상이 관찰된다. 환자의 양쪽 귓구멍과 콧구멍에서 피가 섞인 액체가 나온다. 환자의 눈은 감겨 있고 당신이 말을 걸어도 반응하지 않는다.

초기 평가에서 구역 반사가 없음을 확인하고 입인두기도기를 삽입한다. 동료가 백마스크 장치로 분당 12회의 속도로 환자에게 환기를 시행한다. 환자의 오른쪽 동공이 확장된 것을 확인하였고 노동맥박은 54회/분으로 규칙적이며 산소포화도는 96%이다. 환자의 피부는 차갑고, 건조하며 창백하다. 글래스고혼수척도(GCS)는 7점(E2, V1, M4)이다.

당신은 환자를 신속하게 이송할 준비를 하고 구급차에 환자를 태워 병원으로 이송 중에 목뼈 고정을 계속 유지하면서 이차평가를 한다. 뒤통수를 촉지하면 환자가 고통스러운 신음을 낸다. 당신은 환자의 체온을 유지하기 위해 담요로 덮어주고 혈압을 측정한 결과 184/102mmHg이었다. 심전도는 검사 결과 동성 서맥과 드물게 심실조기박동 나타난다. 오른쪽 동공은 여전히 확장된 상태이다.

- 환자의 징후를 고려할 때 가장 가능성이 높은 손상은 무엇인가?
- 이 시점에서 처치의 우선순위는 무엇인가?
- 두개내압 증가를 해결하고 이송 지연 중 뇌 관류를 유지하기 위해 어떤 조치를 해야 할 수 있는가? 뇌 관류를 유지하기 위해 어떤 조치를 해야 하는가?

시나리오 해결책

병원으로 이송하는 중에 환자의 양손 손바닥 굴곡을 보이기 시작한다. 탈출증이 임박했다는 징후이므로 들것의 머리 부분을 들어 정맥 배액을 지원하고 일시적으로 환기 속도를 분당 16~20회로 시행하여 호기말이산화탄소를 30~35mmHg로 유지하는 것을 목표로 한다. 환자의 여전히 의식이 없다. 전문 기도유지술을 고려하지만, 산소포화도가 96%이고 외상센터까지 이송 시간이 몇 분밖에 걸리지 않으므로 입인두기도기를 삽입한 후 백마스크 장치에 100% 산소를 연결하여 환기를 보조하기로 했다.

References

1. Global Burden of Disease 2016 Traumatic Brain Injury and Spinal Cord Injury Collaborators. Global, regional, and national burden of traumatic brain injury and spinal cord injury, 1990-2016: a systematic analysis for the Global Burden of Disease Study 2016. *Lancet Neurol.* 2019;18(1):56-87.
2. Maas AIR, Menon DK, Adelson PD, Andelic N, Bell MJ, Belli A. Traumatic brain injury: integrated approaches to improve prevention, clinical care and research. *Lancet Neurol.* 2017;16(12):987-1048.
3. Centers for Disease Control and Prevention. Traumatic Brain Injury and Concussion. Accessed July 15, 2021. https://www.cdc.gov/traumaticbraininjury/
4. Dewan MC, Mummareddy N, Wellons III JC, Bonfield CM. Epidemiology of global pediatric traumatic brain injury: qualitative review. *World Neurosurg.* 2016;91:497-509.
5. Hyder AA, Wunderlich CA, Puvanachandra P, et al. The impact of traumatic brain injuries: a global perspective. *Neuro Rehabilitation.* 2007;22:341-353.
6. Cipolla MJ. *The Cerebral Circulation.* Morgan & Claypool Life Sciences; 2009.
7. Mtui E, Gruener G, Dockery P. *Fitzgerald's Clinical Neuroanatomy and Neuroscience.* 8th ed. Elsevier Saunders; 2021.
8. Chesnut RM, Marshall LF, Klauber MR, et al. The role of secondary brain injury in determining outcome from severe head injury. *J Trauma.* 1993;34:216-222.
9. Fearnside MR, Cook RJ, McDougall P, et al. The Westmead Head Injury Project outcome in severe head injury: a comparative analysis of prehospital, clinical, and CT variables. *Br J Neurosurg.* 1993;7:267-279.
10. Gentleman D. Causes and effects of systemic complications among severely head-injured patients transferred to a neurosurgical unit. *Int Surg.* 1992;77:297-302.
11. Marmarou A, Anderson RL, Ward JL, et al. Impact of ICP instability and hypotension on outcome in patients with severe head trauma. *J Neurosurg.* 1991;75:S59-S64.
12. Miller JD, Becker DP. Secondary insults to the injured brain. *J R Coll Surg Edinb.* 1982;27:292-298.
13. Berry C, Ley EJ, Bukur M, et al. Redefining hypotension in traumatic brain injury. *Injury.* 2012;43(11):1833-1837.
14. Brenner M, Stein DM, Hu PF, Aarabi B, Sheth K, Scalea TM. Traditional systolic blood pressure targets underestimate hypotension-induced secondary brain injury. *J Trauma Acute Care Surg.* 2012;72(5):1135-1139.
15. Carney N, Totten AM, O'Reilly C, et al. Guidelines for the management of severe traumatic brain injury, fourth edition. *Neurosurgery.* 2017;80(1):6-15.
16. Wilson MH. Monro-Kellie 2.0: the dynamic vascular and venous pathophysiological components of intracranial pressure. *J Cereb Blood Flow Metab.* 2016;36(8):1338-1350.
17. Mavrocordatos P, Bissonnette B, Ravussin P. Effects of neck position and head elevation on intracranial pressure in anaesthetized neurosurgical patients: preliminary results. *J Neurosurg Anesthesiol.* 2000;12:10-14.
18. Sundstrøm T, Asbjørnsen H, Habiba S, et al. Prehospital use of cervical collars in trauma patients: a critical review. *J Neurotrauma.* 2014;31:531-540.
19. Obrist WD, Gennarelli TA, Segawa H, et al. Relation of cerebral blood flow to neurological status and outcome in head injured patients. *J Neurosurg.* 1979;51:292-300.
20. Obrist WD, Langfitt TW, Jaggi JL, et al. Cerebral blood flow and metabolism in comatose patients with acute head injury. *J Neurosurg.* 1984;61:241-253.
21. Coles JP, Minhas PS, Fryer TD, et al. Effect of hyperventilation on cerebral blood flow in traumatic head injury: clinical relevance and monitoring correlates. *Crit Care Med.* 2002;30(9):1950-1959.
22. Imberti R, Bellinzona G, Langer M. Cerebral tissue PO_2 and $SjvO_2$ changes during moderate hyperventilation in patients with severe traumatic brain injury. *J Neurosurg.* 2002;96(1):97-102.
23. Stocchetti N, Maas AI, Chieregato A, van der Plas AA. Hyperventilation in head injury: a review. *Chest.* 2005;127(5): 1812-1827.
24. Centers for Disease Control and Prevention. What is a concussion? n.d. https://www.cdc.gov/headsup/basics/concussion_whatis.html
25. Quinn DK, Mayer AR, Master CL, Fann JR. Prolonged postconcussive symptoms. *Am J Psychiatry.* 2018;175(2):103-111.
26. Babcock L, Byczkowski T, Wade SL, et al. Predicting postconcussion syndrome after mild traumatic brain injury in children and adolescents who present to the emergency department. *JAMA Pediatr.* 2013;167(2):156-161.
27. Barlow M, Schlabach D, Peiffer J, Cook C. Differences in change scores and the predictive validity of three commonly used measures following concussion in the middle school and high school aged population. *Int J Sports Phys Ther.* 2011;6(3):150-157.
28. Broglio SP, McAllister T, Katz BP, et al. The natural history of sport-related concussion in collegiate athletes: findings from the NCAA-DoD CARE Consortium. *Sports Med.* 2021;52:403-415. doi: 10.1007/s40279-021-01541-7
29. Hume CH, Wright BJ, Kinsella GJ. Systematic review and meta-analysis of outcome after mild traumatic brain injury in older people. *Int Neuropsychol Soc.* 2021;1-20.
30. Meagher RL, Young WF. Subdural hematoma. eMedicine, Medscape. Updated July 26, 2018. Accessed January 3, 2022. http://emedicine.medscape.com/article/1137207-overview
31. Lucke-Wold BP, Turner RC, Josiah D, Knotts C, Bhatia S. Do age and anticoagulants affect the natural history of acute subdural hematomas? *Arch Emerg Med Crit Care.* 2016;1(2):1010.
32. Coughlin RF, Moser RP. Subdural hematoma. In: Domino FJ, ed. *The 5-Minute Clinical Consult 2013.* 21st ed. Wolters Kluwer Health/Lippincott Williams & Wilkins; 2013:1246-1247.
33. Quigley MR, Chew BG, Swartz CE, Wilberger JE. The clinical significance of isolated traumatic subarachnoid hemorrhage. *J Trauma Acute Care Surg.* 2013;74:581-584.
34. Brain Trauma Foundation. CT scan features. In: Bullock MR, Chesnut RM, Clifton GL, et al. *Management and Prognosis of Severe Traumatic Brain Injury.* 2nd ed. Brain Trauma Foundation; 2000.
35. Kihtir T, Ivatury RR, Simon RJ, et al. Early management of civilian gunshot wounds to the face. *J Trauma.* 1993;35:569-575.
36. Rimel RW, Giordani B, Barth JT. Moderate head injury: completing the clinical spectrum of brain trauma. *Neurosurgery.* 1982;11:344-351.
37. Miller JD, Sweet RC, Narayan RK, et al. Early insults to the injured brain. *JAMA.* 1978;240:439-442.
38. Silverston P. Pulse oximetry at the roadside: a study of pulse oximetry in immediate care. *BMJ.* 1989;298:711-713.
39. Stochetti N, Furlan A, Volta F. Hypoxemia and arterial hypotension at the accident scene in head injury. *J Trauma.* 1996;40:764-767.

40. Plum F. *The Diagnosis of Stupor and Coma*. 3rd ed. Oxford University Press; 1982.

41. Langfitt TW, Weinstein JD, Kassell NF, et al. Transmission of increased intracranial pressure. I. Within the craniospinal axis. *J Neurosurg*. 1964;21:989-997.

42. Langfitt TW. Increased intracranial pressure. *Clin Neurosurg*. 1969;16:436-471.

43. Ayling J. Managing head injuries. *Emerg Med Serv*. 2002;31(8):42.

44. Graham DI, Ford I, Adams JH, et al. Ischaemic brain damage is still common in fatal non-missile head injury. *J Neurol Neurosurg Psychiatry*. 1989;52:346-350.

45. Obrist WD, Wilkinson WE. Regional cerebral blood flow measurement in humans by xenon-133 clearance. *Cerebrovasc Brain Metab Rev*. 1990;2:283-327.

46. Darby JM, Yonas H, Marion DW, et al. Local "inverse steal" induced by hyperventilation in head injury. *Neurosurgery*. 1988;23:84-88.

47. Marion DW, Darby J, Yonas H. Acute regional cerebral blood flow changes caused by severe head injuries. *J Neurosurg*. 1991;74:407-414.

48. Badjatia N, Carney N, Crocco TJ, et al. Guidelines for prehospital management of traumatic brain injury: 2nd edition. *Prehosp Emerg Care*. 2007;12(1):S1-S52.

49. Bostek CC. Oxygen toxicity: an introduction. *AANA J*. 1989;57(3):231-237.

50. Brenner M, Stein D, Hu P, et al. Association between early hyperoxia and worse outcomes after traumatic brain injury. *Arch Surg*. 2012;147(11):1042-1046.

51. Tolias CM, Reinert M, Seiler R, Gilman C, Scharf A, Bullock MR. Normobaric hyperoxia-induced improvement in cerebral metabolism and reduction in intracranial pressure in patients with severe head injury: a prospective historical cohort matched study. *J Neurosurg*. 2004;101(3):435-444.

52. Hare GMT, Mazer CD, Hutchison JS, et al. Severe hemodilutional anemia increases cerebral tissue injury following acute neurotrauma. *J Appl Physiol*. 2007;103:1021-1029.

53. Cucher D, Harmon D, Myer B, et al. Critical traumatic brain injury is associated with worse coagulopathy. *J Trauma*. 2021;91(2):331-335.

54. Bohm JK, Guting H, Thorn S, et al. Global characterization of coagulopathy in isolated traumatic brain injury (iTBI): a CENTER-TBI analysis. *Neurocrit Care*. 2021;35:184-196.

55. Yee J, Kaide CG. Emergency reversal of anticoagulation. *West J Emerg Med*. 2019;20(5):770-783.

56. CRASH-2 trial collaborators. Effects of tranexamic acid on death, vascular occlusive events, and blood transfusion in trauma patients with significant hemorrhage (CRASH-2): a randomized, placebo-controlled trial. *Lancet*. 2010;376(9734):23-32.

57. Perel P, Al-Shahi Salman R, Kawahara T, et al. CRASH-2 (Clinical randomization of an antifibrinolytic in significant haemorrhage) intracranial bleeding study: the effect of tranexamic acid in traumatic brain injury—a nested randomized, placebo-controlled trial. *Health Technol Assess*. 2012;16(13):iii-xii;1-54.

58. CRASH-3 trial collaborators. Effects of tranexamic acid on death, disability, vascular occlusive events and other morbidities in patients with acute traumatic brain injury (CRASH-3): a randomized, placebo-controlled trial. *Lancet*. 2019;394(10210):1713-1723.

59. CRASH-3 Intracranial Bleeding Mechanistic Study Collaborators. Tranexamic acid in traumatic brain injury: an explanatory study nested within the CRASH-3 trial. *Eur J Trauma Emerg Surg*. 2021;47:261-268.

60. Bossers SM, Loer SA, Bloemers FW, et al. Association between prehospital tranexamic acid administration and outcomes of severe traumatic brain injury. *JAMA Neurol*. 2021;78(3):338-345.

61. Caron MJ, Hovda DA, Mazziotta JC, et al. The structural and metabolic anatomy of traumatic brain injury in humans: a computerized tomography and positron emission tomography analysis. *J Neurotrauma*. 1993;10(suppl 1):S58.

62. Caron MJ, Mazziotta JC, Hovda DA, et al. Quantification of cerebral glucose metabolism in brain-injured humans utilizing positron emission tomography. *J Cereb Blood Flow Metab*. 1993;13(suppl 1):S379.

63. Caron MJ. PET/SPECT imaging in head injury. In: Narayan RK, Wilberger JE, Povlishock JT, eds. *Neurotrauma*. McGraw-Hill; 1996.

64. Jalloh I, Carpenter KLH, Helmy A, et al. Glucose metabolism following human traumatic brain injury: methods of assessment and pathophysiologic findings. *Metab Brain Dis*. 2015;30:615-632.

65. Lam AM, Winn HR, Cullen BF, et al. Hyperglycemia and neurological outcome in patients with head injury. *J Neurosurg*. 1991;75:545-551.

66. Young B, Ott L, Dempsey R, et al. Relationship between admission hyperglycemia and neurologic outcome of severely brain-injured patients. *Ann Surg*. 1989;210:466-472.

67. Mechtcheriakov S, Brenneis C, Egger K, Koppelstaetter F, Schocke M, Marksteiner J. A widespread distinct pattern of cerebral atrophy in patients with alcohol addiction revealed by voxel-based morphometry. *J Neurol Neurosurg Psychiatry*. 2007;78(6):610-614.

68. Mayer S, Rowland L. Head injury. In: Rowland L, ed. *Merritt's Neurology*. Lippincott Williams & Wilkins; 2000:401.

69. Dimmitt SB, Rakic V, Puddey IB, et al. The effects of alcohol on coagulation and fibrinolytic factors: a controlled trial. *Blood Coagul Fibrinolysis*. 1998;9(1):39-45.

70. Perry M, Dancey A, Mireskandari K, Oakley P, Davies S, Cameron M. Emergency care in facial trauma—a maxillofacial and ophthalmic perspective. *Injury*. 2005;36(8):875-896.

71. Davis DP, Hoyt DB, Ochs M, et al. The effect of paramedic rapid sequence intubation on outcome in patients with severe traumatic brain injury. *J Trauma Injury Infect Crit Care*. 2003;54:444-453.

72. Bochicchio GV, Ilahi O, Joshi M, et al. Endotracheal intubation in the field does not improve outcome in trauma patients who present without an acutely lethal traumatic brain injury. *J Trauma Injury Infect Crit Care*. 2003;54:307-311.

73. Davis DP, Peay J, Sise MJ, et al. The impact of prehospital endotracheal intubation in moderate to severe traumatic brain injury. *J Trauma*. 2005;58:933-939.

74. Bulger EM, Copass MK, Sabath DR, et al. The use of neuromuscular blocking agents to facilitate prehospital intubation does not impair outcome after traumatic brain injury. *J Trauma*. 2005;58:718-723.

75. Wang HE, Peitzman AB, Cassidy LD, et al. Out-of-hospital endotracheal intubation and outcome after traumatic brain injury. *Ann Emerg Med*. 2004;44:439-450.

76. Chi JH, Knudson MM, Vassar MJ, et al. Prehospital hypoxia affects outcome in patients with traumatic brain injury: a prospective multi-center study. *J Trauma*. 2006;61:1134-1141.

77. Mayglothling J, Duane TM, Gibbs M, et al. Emergency tracheal intubation immediately following traumatic injury: an Eastern Association for the Surgery of Trauma practice management guideline. *J Trauma Acute Care Surg*. 2012;73:5(S4).

78. Bossers SM, Schwarte LA, Loer SA, et al. Experience in prehospital endotracheal intubation significantly influences mortality of patients with severe traumatic brain

injury: a systematic review and meta-analysis. *PLoS One.* 2015;10(10):1-26.

79. Meizoso JP, Valle EJ, Allen CJ, et al. Decreased mortality after prehospital interventions in severely injured trauma patients. *J Trauma Acute Care Surg.* 2015;79:227-231.

80. Marlow TJ, Goltra DD, Schabel SI. Intracranial placement of a nasotracheal tube after facial fracture: a rare complication. *J Emerg Med.* 1997;15:187-191.

81. Horellou MD, Mathe D, Feiss P. A hazard of nasotracheal intubation. *Anaesthesia.* 1978;22:78.

82. Davis DP, Ochs M, Hoyt DB, et al. Paramedic-administered neuromuscular blockade improves prehospital intubation success in severely head-injured patients. *J Trauma Injury Infect Crit Care.* 2003;55:713-719.

83. Cooper KR, Boswell PA, Choi SC. Safe use of PEEP in patients with severe brain injury. *J Neurosurg.* 1985;63:552-555.

84. McGuire G, Crossley D, Richards J, et al. Effects of varying levels of positive end-expiratory pressure on intracranial pressure and cerebral perfusion pressure. *Crit Care Med.* 1997;25:1059-1062.

85. Warner KJ, Cuschieri J, Copass MK, et al. The impact of prehospital ventilation on outcome after severe traumatic brain injury. *J Trauma.* 2007;62:1330-1336.

86. Godoy DA, Badenes R, Robba C, Cabezas FM. Hyperventilation in severe traumatic brain injury has something changed in the last decade or uncertainty continues? A brief review. *Front. Neurol.* 2021;12:573237.

87. Christensen MA, Bloom J, Sutton KR. Comparing arterial and end-tidal carbon dioxide values in hyperventilated neurosurgical patients. *Am J Crit Care.* 1995;4:116-121.

88. Grenier B, Dubreuil M. Noninvasive monitoring of carbon dioxide: end-tidal versus transcutaneous carbon dioxide. *Anesth Analg.* 1998;86:675-676.

89. Isert P. Control of carbon dioxide levels during neuroanaesthesia: current practice and an appraisal of our reliance upon capnography. *Anaesth Intensive Care.* 1994;22:435-441.

90. Kerr ME, Zempsky J, Sereika S, et al. Relationship between arterial carbon dioxide and end-tidal carbon dioxide in mechanically ventilated adults with severe head trauma. *Crit Care Med.* 1996;24:785-790.

91. Mackersie RC, Karagianes TG. Use of end-tidal carbon dioxide tension for monitoring induced hypocapnia in head-injured patients. *Crit Care Med.* 1990;18:764-765.

92. Russell GB, Graybeal JM. Reliability of the arterial to end-tidal carbon dioxide gradient in mechanically ventilated patients with multisystem trauma. *J Trauma Injury Infect Crit Care.* 1994;36:317-322.

93. Warner KJ, Cuschieri J, Garland B, et al. The utility of early end-tidal capnography in monitoring ventilation status after severe trauma. *J Trauma.* 2009;66:26-31.

94. Davis DP, Dunford JV, Poste JC, et al. The impact of hypoxia and hyperventilation on outcome after paramedic rapid sequence intubation of severely head injured patients. *J Trauma.* 2004;57:1-10.

95. Nagler J, Krauss B. Capnography: a valuable tool for airway management. *Emerg Med Clin N Am.* 2008;26(4):881-897.

96. Childress K, Arnold K, Hunter C, Ralls G, Papa L, Silvestri S. Prehospital end-tidal carbon dioxide predicts mortality in trauma patients. *Prehosp Emerg Care.* 2017;22(2):170-174.

97. Howard MB, McCollum N, Alberto EC, et al. Association of ventilation during initial trauma resuscitation for traumatic brain injury and post-traumatic outcomes: a systematic review. *Prehosp Disaster Med.* 2021;36(4):460-465.

98. American College of Surgeons Committee on Trauma. Head trauma. In: *Advanced Trauma Life Support for Doctors, Student Course Manual.* 10th ed. American College of Surgeons; 2017.

99. Suttipongkaset P, Chaikittisilpa N, Vavilala MS, et al. Blood pressure thresholds and mortality in pediatric traumatic brain injury. *Pediatrics.* 2018;142(2):e20180594. doi: 10.1542/peds.2018-0594

100. Cooper DJ, Myles PS, McDermott FT, et al. Prehospital hypertonic saline resuscitation of patients with hypotension and severe traumatic brain injury: a randomized controlled trial *JAMA.* 2004;291:1350-1357.

101. The Glasgow structured approach to assessment of the Glasgow Coma Scale. Accessed February 8, 2022. http://www.glasgowcomascale.org

102. Teasdale G, Allen D, Brennan P, et al. The Glasgow Coma Scale: an update after 40 years. *Nurs Times.* 2014;110:12-16.

103. Majdan M, Steyerberg EW, Nieboer D, et al. Glasgow Coma Scale motor score and pupillary reaction to predict six-month mortality in patients with traumatic brain injury: comparison of field and admission assessment. *J Neurotrauma.* 2015;32(2):101-108.

104. Ross SE, Leipold C, Terregino C, et al. Efficacy of the motor component of the Glasgow Coma Scale in trauma triage. *J Trauma.* 1998;45(1):42-44.

105. Jarvis C, ed. Physical Examination and Health Assessment. 6th ed. Elsevier Publishers; 2012:71.

106. Brain Trauma Foundation. Glasgow coma score. In: Gabriel EJ, Ghajar J, Jagoda A, et al. Guidelines for Prehospital Management *of Traumatic Brain Injury*. Brain Trauma Foundation; 2000.

107. Prosser JD, Vender JR, Solares CA. Traumatic cerebrospinal fluid leaks. *Otolaryngol Clin N Am.* 2011;44:857-873.

108. Biffl WL, Cothren CC, Moore EE, et al. Western Trauma Association critical decisions in trauma: screening for and treatment of blunt cerebrovascular injuries. *J Trauma Acute Care Surg.* 2009;67(6):1150-1153.

109. Servadei F, Nasi MT, Cremonini AM. Importance of a reliable admission Glasgow Coma Scale score for determining the need for evacuation of posttraumatic subdural hematomas: a prospective study of 65 patients. *J Trauma.* 1998:44:868-873.

110. Winkler JV, Rosen P, Alfrey EJ. Prehospital use of the Glasgow Coma Scale in severe head injury. *J Emerg Med.* 1984:2:1-6.

111. Brain Trauma Foundation. Hospital transport decisions. In: Gabriel EJ, Ghajar J, Jagoda A, et al. *Guidelines for Prehospital Management of Traumatic Brain Injury*. Brain Trauma Foundation; 2000.

112. Feldman Z, Kanter MJ, Robertson CS. Effect of head elevation on intracranial pressure, cerebral perfusion pressure and cerebral blood flow in head-injured patients. *J Neurosurg.* 1992;76:207-211.

113. Schott JM, Rossor MN. The grasp and other primitive reflexes. *J Neurol Neurosurg Psychiatry.* 2003;74:558-560.

114. Lumba-Brown A, Totten A, Kochanek PM. Emergency department implementation of the Brain Trauma Foundation's Pediatric Severe Brain Injury Guideline Recommendations. *Pediatr Emerg Care.* 2020;36(4):e239-e241.

Suggested Reading

American College of Surgeons Committee on Trauma. Head trauma. In: *Advanced Trauma Life Support, Student Course Manual*. 10th ed. American College of Surgeons; 2017.

Badjatia N, Carney N, Crocco TJ, et al. Guidelines for prehospital management of traumatic brain injury: 2nd edition. *Prehosp Emerg Care*. 2007;12(1):S1-S52.

Carney N, Totten AM, O'Reilly C, et al. Guidelines for the management of severe traumatic brain injury: fourth edition. *Neurosurgery*. 2017;80(1):6-15.

© Ralf Hiemisch/Getty Images

척추 외상

Lead Editors
Steven C. Ludwig, MD
Alexandra E. Thomson, MD, MPH
Ivan Ye, BA

학습 목표

이 장의 학습을 완료하면 다음과 같은 내용을 수행할 수 있다.

- 척추 손상의 역학을 설명할 수 있다.
- 성인과 소아에서 척추 손상을 일으키는 가장 흔한 기전을 비교하고 대조할 수 있다.
- 척추 외상의 가능성이 있는 환자를 인식할 수 있다.
- 척추 손상 및 신경성 쇼크의 증상과 징후를 근본적인 병태생리학과 관련지어 설명할 수 있다.
- 해부학 및 병태생리학의 원리를 평가 자료 및 외상 처치 원칙과 통합하여 명백하거나 잠재적인 척추 손상이 있는 환자의 처치 계획을 수립할 수 있다.
- 특정 환자에게 척추 움직임 제한이 적절한지 아닌지를 결정하는 데 필요한 다각적인 의사 결정 과정을 설명할 수 있다.
- 척추 손상의 이환율과 사망률에 영향을 미칠 수 있는 병원 전 소견 및 처치와 관련된 요인에 대해 논의할 수 있다.
- 선택적 척추 고정 원칙과 환자의 상황에 따라 이러한 원칙 적용이 어떻게 달라질 수 있는지 이해한다.
- 척수 손상에 대한 스테로이드 투여를 둘러싼 논란을 이해하고 현재 연구 중인 새로운 치료법을 이해한다.

시나리오

당신은 도로에 자전거를 타다 넘어져 손상을 입은 환자가 있다는 신고를 받고 현장으로 출동했다. 현장에 도착했을 때 경찰관이 교통을 통제하고 있었고 현장은 안전하다. 젊은 여성인 환자는 길가에 누워있다. 경찰관이 그녀 옆에 무릎을 꿇고 대화를 시도하고 있지만, 환자는 아무런 반응이 없다.

일차평가를 시작할 때 자전거를 타다가 넘어지게 된 구체적인 원인을 확인할 수 없었다. 여성이 도로를 달리던 중 넘어진 것으로 보이지만, 자동차에 치였는지는 알 수 없다. 경찰관에 따르면 목격자는 없다. 환자는 헬멧과 장갑을 포함한 안전 장비를 착용하고 있다. 이마에 찰과상이 있고 오른쪽 손목에 명백한 변형이 있다. 기도는 개방되어 있고 규칙적으로 호흡을 하고 있다. 외부출혈의 명백한 징후는 보이지 않는다. 피부는 건조하고 따뜻하며 정상적인 색을 띠고 있었다. 일차평가를 시행하는 동안 환자는 깨어났지만, 무슨 일이 있었는지 혼란스러워한다.

- 환자의 증상을 설명할 수 있는 병리학적 과정은 무엇인가?
- 어떤 즉각적인 처치와 추가 평가가 필요한가?
- 이 환자의 처치 목표는 무엇인가?

개요

외상성 척추 손상(TSI)은 잠재적으로 생명을 위협할 수 있으며 중증도는 손상된 척추 부위와 척수와 같은 주변 구조물을 손상 여부에 따라 크게 달라진다. 손상은 대부분 고에너지 힘으로 발생하지만, 노인과 같이 취약한 인구에서는 낮은 에너지의 손상 기전으로 발생할 수 있다. 척추의 골격 구성 요소에 손상을 입어도 척수 손상이 발생하지 않을 수 있으며 때에 따라 척추의 골절이나 탈구 없이 척수, 혈관 및 신경이 손상될 수 있다. 뼈 구조와 지지 인대가 손상되면 척추의 구조적 불안정성을 초래하여 척추 움직임 제한을 적절하게 시행하지 않으면 척추 및 기타 주변 구조물이 손상되기 쉽다. 심각한 손상은 척수를 회복할 수 없을 정도로 손상시켜 환자에게 평생 신경학적 장애를 남길 수 있다. 즉각적인 척수 손상은 외상이나 일차 손상의 결과로 발생한다. 이차 손상은 일차 손상에 이어 신경학적 결손을 악화시킬 수 있다. 이 이차 손상은 손상된 척추의 병리학적 움직임에 의해 유발되거나 악화할 수 있다. 척추 손상 가능성이 있는 환자를 의심하고 적절하게 평가하며 안정시키지 않으면 좋지 않은 결과를 초래할 수 있다. 이러한 손상을 신속하게 인지하고 병원 전 처치는 중상을 입은 환자를 적시에 안정시키는 데 중요하며 향후 진단 및 처치 결정을 내리는 데 도움이 될 수 있고 이차 손상의 위험을 줄일 수 있다.

신체에 갑작스럽게 강한 힘이 가해지면 척추의 골격과 인대 구조에 정상적인 운동 한계를 넘어 스트레스를 받을 수 있다. 다음 네 가지 개념은 손상 가능성을 평가할 때 에너지가 척추에 미칠 수 있는 영향을 명확히 하는 데 도움이 된다.

1. 움직이는 물체는 계속 움직이려는 경향이 있고 정지한 물체는 정지한 상태로 유지되는 경향이 있다(뉴턴의 제1 법칙).

2. 머리는 목 위에 얹혀 있는 볼링공과 비슷하며 그 질량은 종종 몸통과 다른 방향으로 이동하여 목(목뼈, 척수)에 강한 힘이 가해지는 결과를 초래한다.

3. 다리 윗부분의 갑작스럽거나 격렬한 움직임은 골반을 이동시켜 아래쪽 척추가 무리하게 움직인다. 머리와 몸통의 무게와 관성으로 인해 상부 척추에 반대 방향의 힘이 가해진다.

4. 신경학적 결손이 없다고 해서 척추의 뼈나 인대 손상 또는 척수가 견딜 수 있는 한계까지 스트레스를 받은 상태를 배제할 수는 없다.

미국에서는 매년 인구 100만 명당 약 54명(대략 17,900명)이 척수 손상(SCI)을 입고 있으며 약 252,000명에서 373,000명이 이로 인한 장애를 안고 살아가고 있다. 척수 손상은 모든 연령대에서 발생할 수 있지만, 미국의 고령화 추세에 따라 65세 이상의 인구에서 척수 손상 발생률이 증가하고 있다. 1997년~2012년 사이에 낙상으로 인한 척수 손상의 비율이 많이 증가했다. 2012년 미국에서는 의도하지 않은 낙상이 급성 외상성 척수 손상의 40%를 차지했다. 이러한 경향은 미국 인구의 평균 연령이 증가함에 따라 예측할 수 있는 결과이다. 남성이 여성보다 압도적으로 많으며 척수 손상의 78% 이상을 차지한다. 일반적인 원인은 자동차 충돌(39%), 낙상(32%), 관통상(14%), 스포츠 손상(8%) 및 기타 손상(7%)이다. 노년층에서 낙상은 척수 손상의 주요 원인으로 자동차 충돌보다 더 많다.

척수 손상은 신체 기능, 생활양식 및 재정 상황에 중대한 영향을 미칠 수 있다. 또한 일반 인구와 비교했을 때 초기 척수 손상에서 살아남은 사람들은 일반적으로 기대 수명이 짧다. 척수는 모든 수준에서 손상될 수 있으며 척수 손상의 두 가지 주요 범주에는 완전 손상과 불완전한 손상이 포함된다. 완전한 척수 손상은 신체의 양쪽에 영향을 미치며 손상 수준 이하의 움직임과 감각을 포함한 모든 기능을 완전히 상실하게 된다. 불완전 손상은 신경학적 기능의 완전한 손실 없는 모든 척수 손상을 말한다. 운동, 감각 또는 둘 다 보존되지만, 불안전한 척수 손상을 입은 환자의 경우 비대칭적일 수 있다. 일반적으로 생리학적 기능 장애와 장기적인 장애는 상부 목뼈에 손상이 발생했을 때 가장 치명적이며 손상 수준이 낮아질수록 점차 감소한다. 목뼈에서 가장 높은 수준의 완전한 손상은 치명적이며 병원 전 처치 제공자가 현장에 도착하기 전에 종종 사망할 수 있다. 척수 손상 후 운동 및 감각 기능의 상실은 경미한 쇠약감에서부터 휠체어나 인공호흡기가 필요한 경우까지 다양하다.

심각한 손상을 입은 환자는 일상 활동 수준과 독립성에 심각한 변화를 경험할 수 있다. 척수 손상은 또한 환자뿐만 아니라 일반 인구의 재정 상황에도 영향을 미친다. 이러한 손상을 입은 환자는 급성 및 장기 치료가 모두 필요하다. 이러한 처치의 평생 비용은 영구적인 척수 손상을 입은 환자 1인당 120만 달러에서 520만 달러로 추정되며 손상 정도와 손상 당시 나이에 따라 비용이 증가한다.

신경학적 결손은 다양한 중추 및 말초 신경계 구조에 대한 외상으로 발생하거나 뇌 또는 척수에 대한 산소 공급 또는 관류가 불충분한 결과로 발생할 수 있다. 환자는 말초 신경 손상 외에도 여러 장기 시스템에 손상을 입을 수 있으며 이는 결손으로 나타날 수 있다. 예를 들어, 다발성 손상을 입은 환자는 머리에 직접적인 타격을 받아 직접적인 신경 손상을 입었을 수 있고 심각한 혈관 손상으로 쇼크와 불충분한 관류가 발생하여 신경 구조에 무산소성 손상을 입었을 수 있으며 말초 신경을 직접 손상시키는 팔다리 손상을 입었을 수도 있다. 이러한 손상으로부터의 회복은 다양하며 때에 따라 영구적일 수도 있지만, 회복 가능성이 있으므로 환자의 초기 처치에 집중해야 한다. 이러한 환자의 증상은 복잡할 수 있지만, 다음과 같은 기전에서 척추 손상을 고려해야 한다.

- 머리, 목, 몸통 또는 골반에 강한 충격을 가한 무딘 손상 기전
- 목이나 몸통에 갑작스러운 가속, 감속 또는 측면 굽힘을 발생시키는 사고
- 특히 노인의 경우 높은 곳에서 추락한 경우
- 차량 또는 기타 동력 운송 장치에서 튕겨 나가거나 떨어지는 것
- 얕은 물에서 다이빙 사고

기존의 단단한 긴척추고정판을 사용한 병원 전 척추 고정은 1960년대에 처음 지지를 얻은 이후 크게 발전해 왔다. 척추 고정을 시행할지 여부는 손상 기전, 동반 질환 및 고유한 위험 요인, 환자의 신체검사 등을 신중하게 고려한 후 결정한다. 이 처치의 한계와 잠재적 합병증을 이해하는 것은 임상 의사 결정에서 똑같이 중요하다.

최근에는 단단한 긴척추고정판을 사용하는 고정의 안전성과 효능에 대한 연구자들의 도전을 받고 있으며 기존의 고정 관행에서 벗어나 패러다임 전환이 이루어지고 있다. 척추 외상에 대한 병원 전 처치가 발전함에 따라 척추 손상 환자의 척추 움직임을 효과적으로 제한하면서 단단한 고정판을 사용한 고정과 관련하여 널리 알려진 합병증을 줄이는 척추 고정 및 급성 척수 외상 처치를 위한 증거 기반 프로토콜이 광범위하게 채택되었다. 척추 외상이 의심되는 환자는 지속적인 척추 움직임 제한의 필요성을 평가할 때까지 중립 자세에서 도수 고정으로 안정시켜야 한다. 척추 외상이 의심되는 환자의 초기 처치에는 신경 조직의 관류가 중단되지 않도록 적극적인 소생술과 이차 손상 및 신경학적 기능 악화를 방지하기 위한 척추 움직임 제한이 포함되어야 한다.

해부학 및 생리학

척추 해부학

척추는 주로 세 평면 모두에서 움직임을 가능하게 하고 머리와 몸통의 하중을 골반으로 분산하는 동시에 척수의 약한 신경 조직을 보호하는 기능을 하는 복잡한 구조이다. 척주는 척추뼈라고 불리는 33개의 뼈로 구성되어 있으며 이 뼈들은 서로 겹겹이 쌓여 있다. 첫 번째 목뼈인 고리뼈(C1)와 두 번째 목뼈인 중쇠뼈(C2)와 하부 척추가 융합된 엉치뼈와 꼬리뼈를 제외한 모든 척추뼈는 형태, 구조 및 움직임이 유사하다(**그림 9-1**). 척추뼈 몸통은 앞쪽에 위치하며 각 척추뼈에서 가장 큰 부분을 차지한다. 각 척추뼈 몸통은 그 위에 있는 척주와 몸통의 무게 대부분을 지탱한다. 신경활이라 불리는 두 개의 구부러진 면은 몸에서 뒤쪽으로 돌출된 판에 의해 형성된다. 가시돌기는 근육과 인대를 부착하는 역할을 하는 판의 후방에 있는 정중선상의 뼈돌기이다. 목뼈 5번 이하에서는 가시돌기가 바로 뒤쪽을 향하고 등뼈와 허리뼈에서는 꼬리 방향(발 쪽)으로 약간 아래쪽을 향한다. 각 척추에는 뒤쪽 측면에 한 쌍의 돌기사이 관절이 있다. 이 관절은 연골로 덮여있어 척추가 서로 연결될 수 있다.

척추뼈 몸통의 측면으로 발생하는 가로돌기라고 하는 추가적인 뼈 구조물은 척추곁 근육의 부착을 위한 추가 지점 역할을 한다. 각 척추 신경의 뿌리, 척추 동맥 및 뒤뿌리신경절을 포함한 여러 신경 및 혈관 구조는 모든 척추 사이에 존재하는 추간공(신경공이라고도 함)이라고 하는 구멍을 통과한다. 신경활과 각 척추뼈 몸통의 뒤쪽부분은 척추공(척주관)이라고 하는 중앙에 구멍이 있는 거의 원형에 가까운 모양을 형성한다. 뇌척수액이 들어있는 수막으로 둘러싸인 척수가 이 공간을 통과한다. 척수는 척추에 의해 손상으로부터 어느 정도 보호되지만, 후궁간 공간을 통한 직접적인 관통상에는 여전히 취약하다. 각 척추공은 위쪽 척추와 아래쪽 척추와 나란히 정렬되어 척수가 통과하는 속이빈 척주관을 형성한다. 척추공의 구멍 크기는 병리학적 과정(예: 관절염 변화, 종양 및 척추 디스크 탈출증), 척추 하중 및 자세로 인해 달라질 수 있다. 척추공이 좁아지면 이 구멍을 통과하는 신경 혈관 구조가 손상될 위험이 증가할 수 있다.

척주

각각의 척추는 S자 모양의 기둥으로 쌓여 있다(**그림 9-2**). 이 구조는 최대한의 힘을 부여하면서 광범위한 다양한 움직임을 허용한다. 척주는 참조하기 위해 5개의 개별 영역으로 나뉜다. 척주의 위쪽에서 시작하여 아래쪽으로 내려가는 이 영역은 목뼈, 등뼈, 허리뼈, 엉치뼈 및 꼬리뼈가 있다. 척추는 위치한 부위의 첫 영문 글자와 해당 부위의 위쪽부터 순서로 구분된다. 첫 번째 목뼈는 C1, 세 번째 등뼈는 T3, 다섯 번째 허리뼈는 L5 등으로 부르며 척추 전체를 통틀어 척주라고 부른다. 각 척추는 척추를 따라 내려갈수록 증가하는 체중을 지탱한다. 증가하는 체중과 작업량을 수용하기 위해 C3에서 L5까지

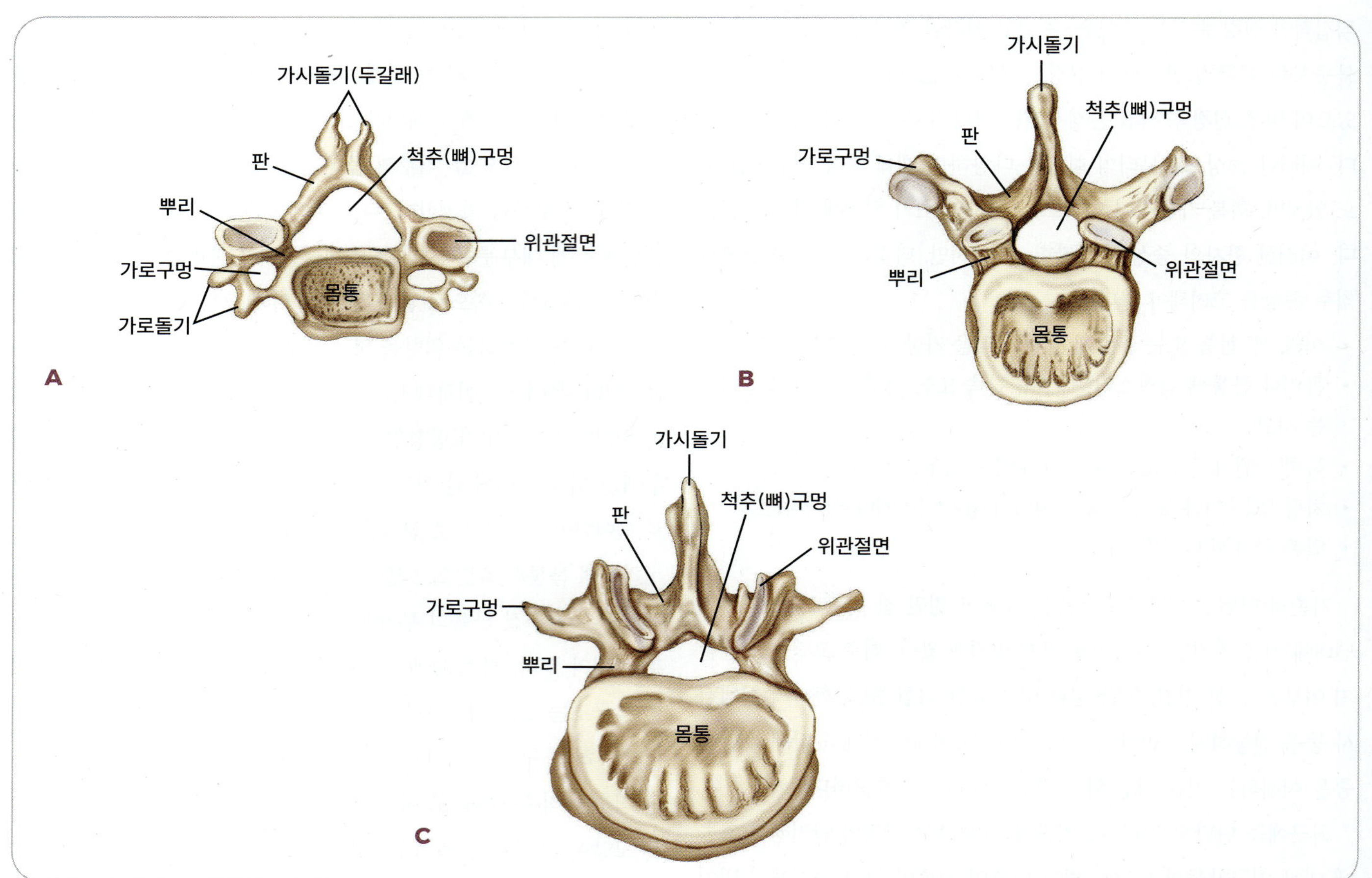

그림 9-1 각 척추의 몸통(앞 부분)은 골반에 가까워질수록 증가하는 질량을 지탱해야 하므로 아래쪽 척추에서 더 크고 강해진다. **A.** 다섯 번째 목뼈 **B.** 등뼈 **C.** 허리뼈

척추는 점차 커진다(**그림 9-1**).

머리 쪽에 있는 척주는 머리를 지탱하고 목의 골격을 구성하는 7개의 목뼈가 있다. 목뼈 부위는 유연하여 머리 전체를 움직일 수 있다. 뇌의 뒤쪽 측면에 혈액을 공급하는 척추동맥은 목뼈에 있는 별도의 구멍을 통해 흐르며 보통 C6로 들어간다. 심각한 변위나 골절이 발생하면 이 동맥이 손상되어 뇌관류가 감소하고 뇌졸중과 유사한 증상이 나타날 수 있다. 목뼈는 척추의 아래쪽 부위에 비해 상대적으로 움직임에 제한이 없으며 가장 흔하게 손상을 입는 부위이다. 다음은 12개의 등뼈이다. 각 갈비뼈 쌍은 갈비척추관절에서 등뼈 중 하나의 뒤쪽으로 연결된다. 등뼈는 목뼈보다 더 단단하고 움직임이 더 적다. 등뼈와 복장뼈 사이에 연장된 갈비뼈가 제공하는 안정성 증가는 건강한 성인 환자의 등뼈 손상이 일반적으로 고에너지 손상 기전의 상당한 물리적 힘이 있어야 하는 주요 이유이다. 그러나 등뼈 손상의 발생률은 노인 인구와 등뼈의 상대 강도를 감소시키는 요인이

있는 사람에게서 더 높다. 등뼈 아래에는 5개의 허리뼈가 있다. 허리뼈는 유연하여 여러 방향으로 움직일 수 있다. 성인이 되면 5개의 엉치뼈가 융합하여 엉치뼈라는 하나의 뼈 구조를 형성한다. 마찬가지로 4개의 꼬리뼈가 융합되어 꼬리뼈를 형성한다. 외상성 척추 골절의 발생률은 등뼈와 허리뼈에서 가장 높으며(75~90%) 대부분 등허리 접합부에 국한되어 있다. 반대로 척수 손상과 외상성 척추 손상의 전체 발병률(골절이 없는 손상 포함)은 목뼈 부위에서 가장 빈번하게 발생한다.

각 척추는 추간판에 의해 위와 아래의 척추와 분리된다(**그림 9-3**). 이 디스크는 속질핵이라고 하는 젤라틴으로 내부가 채워진 섬유질 고리로 구성되어 있다. 디스크는 척추를 여러 방향으로 구부러질 수 있는 부드러운 쿠션 역할을 한다. 또한 척추의 중력 및 기계적 축 방향 하중을 감소시켜 충격 흡수 장치 역할을 한다. 추간판이 손상되면 추간판이 척주관으로 돌출되어 추간공을 통해 나오는 척수나 신

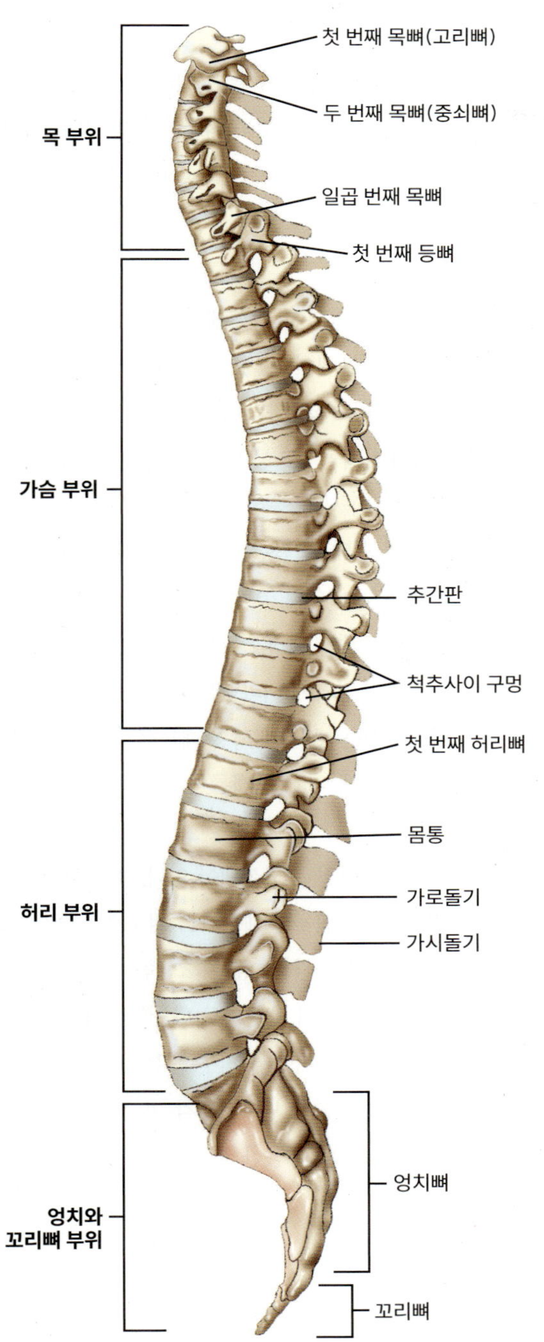

그림 9-2 척추는 곧은 막대가 아니라 여러 번 구부러질 수 있도록 쌓인 일련의 블록이다. 각 곡선마다 척추가 골절에 더 취약하기 때문에 "넘어지면 S가 부러진다"는 말이 유래되었다.
© National Association of Emergency Medical Technicians (NAEMT)

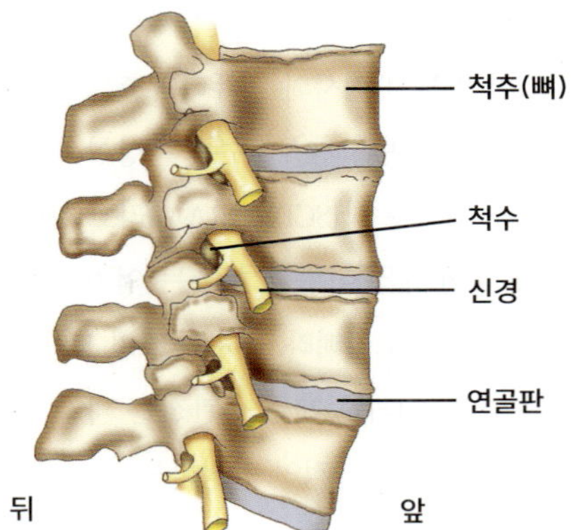

그림 9-3 인접한 척추(뼈)몸통 사이의 연골을 추간판이라고 한다.
© National Association of Emergency Medical Technicians (NAEMT)

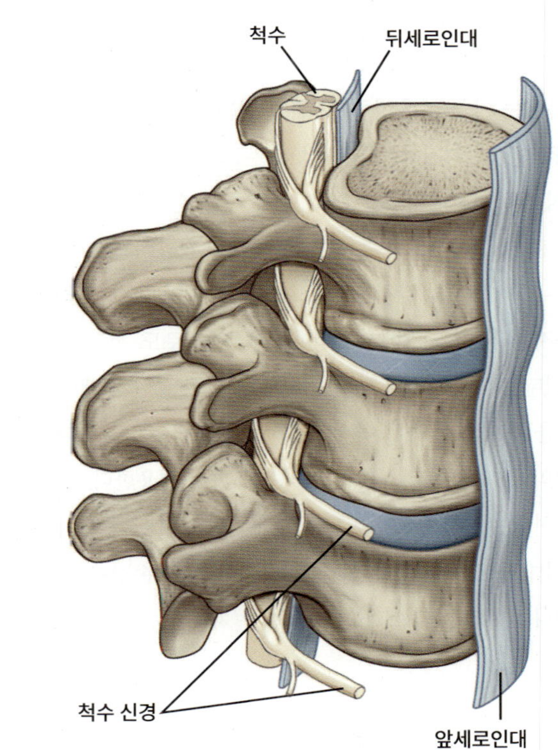

그림 9-4 척주의 앞 및 뒤 세로인대.
© National Association of Emergency Medical Technicians (NAEMT)

경을 압박할 수 있다. 인대와 근육이 두개골 바닥에서 골반까지 척추를 연결한다. 이 인대와 근육은 척주의 전체 뼈 부분을 감싸고 정상적인 정렬 상태를 유지하고 안정성을 제공하며 움직일 수 있도록 한다. 전방 및 후방 세로 인대는 척추뼈 몸통의 앞쪽과 척주관 내부를 연결한다. 가시돌기 사이의 인대는 굴곡과 신전 운동(앞뒤)을 위한 지지하고 층 사이의 인대는 측면 굴곡(측면 굽힘)을 지지한다(**그림 9-4**). 척추를 안정시키는 연부조직 구조가 찢어지면 한 척추가 다른 척추에 비해 과도하게 움직일 수 있다. 이 과도한 움직임은 척추의 탈구를 초래할 수 있으며 척수가 지나가는 공간인 척수관이 좁아져 척수 손상을 유발할 수 있다. 소아의 경우 인대 이완이 더 많이 존재한다는 점에 유의하는 것이 중요하다. 성인 척추와는 달리 소아 척추의 이완이 증가하면 일반 방사선 검사와 컴퓨터단층촬영에서 척수의 방사선학적 증거 없이 척수가 변위되어 척수를 손상할 수 있다. 이를 방사선학적 이상이 없는 척주 손상(SCIWORA)이라고 한다.

　머리는 척추 위에서 균형을 이루고 척추는 엉치엉덩관절을 통해 골반과 연결된다. 두개골은 고리뼈라고 하는 고리 모양의 첫 번째 목뼈(C1)에 자리 잡고 있다. C1과 두개골의 관절은 뼈의 안전성을 거의 제공하지 않으며 이 관절의 일차적인 안정화는 강한 머리목 인대를 통해 이루어진다. 축인 중쇠뼈(C2)는 치아처럼 위쪽으로 튀어나온 치돌기라는 못 모양의 구조로 되어있다. 이것은 고리뼈의 앞쪽 아치 바로 뒤에 위치하며 회전 관절을 형성한다(**그림 9-5**). C1과 C2 사이의 관절은 목뼈 회전 운동의 50%를 담당한다.

　사람의 머리 무게는 7~10kg으로 볼링공의 평균 무게보다 약간 더 무겁다. 목뼈는 가늘고 유연한 목 위에 있는 머리 위치, 머리에 작용하는 정상적인 힘, 지지하는 근육의 작은 크기, 보호하는 뼈 구조(갈비뼈 등)의 부족 등 여러 요인으로 인해 특히 손상을 입기 쉽다. 목뼈의 척주관은 C1과 C2 수준 이후 좁아지고 결과적으로 척수는 척수와 척주관 벽 사이의 간격을 최소화하면서 사용할 수 있는 공간의 95%를 차지한다. 이 지점에서 경미한 탈구만으로도 척수 압박을 유발할 수 있다. 반면 척수는 상부 허리 부위에서 끝나기 때문에 척수의 65%만을 차지한다. 목뒤 쪽의 근육은 강해 척수가 늘어나지 않고 굴곡 범위의 60%와 머리 신전 범위의 70%까지 허용한다. 그러나 신체에 급격한 가속, 감속 또는 측면 힘이 가해지면 운동량이 목뼈의 골격 및 인대 구조의 안정화 힘을 초과하여 척수 손상을 초래한다. 이러한 시나리오의 예로는 머리 받침대를 제대로 조정하지 않은 후

방 추돌 사고가 있다.

　엉치뼈는 척주의 기초이며 척주가 놓여 있는 플랫폼이다. 엉덩뼈는 체중의 70~80%를 지탱한다. 엉덩뼈는 척주와 골반 일부분이며 움직일 수 없는 엉치엉덩관절에 의해서 골반의 나머지 부분과 연결된다.

척수 해부학

척수는 뇌와 신체의 나머지 부분 사이에서 나가고 들어오는 신호를 전달하는 신경세포의 집합체이다. 척수는 뇌와 연속적이며 숨뇌의 끝에서 시작하여 큰구멍(두개골 바닥에 있는 구멍)과 척주관을 통해 각각의 척추를 통과하여 두 번째 등뼈(L2) 수준까지 이어진다. 혈액은 앞척수동맥 및 뒤척수동맥을 통해 척수로 공급된다.

　척수는 가장 안쪽에 연막, 중간은 거미막, 가장 바깥쪽 경막으로 알려진 세 개의 막으로 덮여 있다. 이 수막 덮개는 두 번째 엉치뼈 척추까지 이어져 주머니 모양의 저장소에서 끝난다. 연막과 거미막 사이의 공간에는 뇌에서 생성되어 뇌와 척수를 감싸고 있는 뇌척수액(CSF)이 들어 있다. 뇌척수액은 뇌에서 노폐물을 제거할 뿐만 아니라 급격한 가속도 변화로 인해 뇌가 두개골에 밀리는 손상으로부터 뇌를 보한다.

　척수 자체는 회색질과 백질로 구성되어 있다. 회색질은 주로 신경세포 세포체로 구성된다. 백질에는 해부학적 척수로를 구성하고 신경 자극이 전달되는 경로 역할을 하는 긴 수초 축삭이 포함되어 있다. 척수로는 상행과 하행의 두 가지 유형으로 나뉜다(**그림 9-6**).

　상행신경로는 말단 신체 부위에서 척수를 통해 뇌까지 감각 자극을 전달한다. 상행신경로는 통증, 온도, 촉각 및 압력 그리고 움직임, 진동, 자세 및 가벼운 접촉 등 다양한 감각 자극을 전달하는 신경로

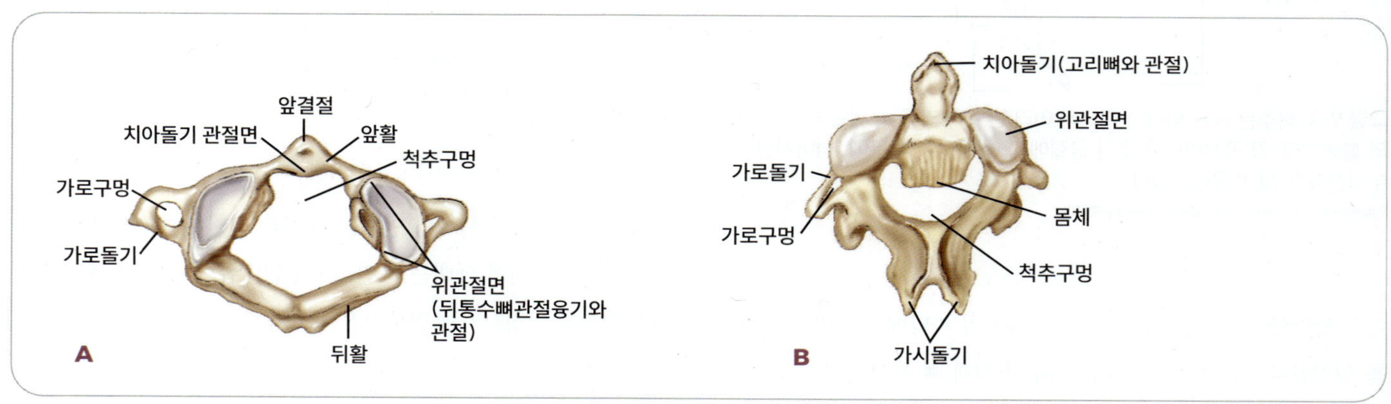

그림 9-5 첫 번째와 두 번째 목뼈의 독특한 모양이다. **A.** 고리뼈(C1) **B.** 중쇠뼈(C2)

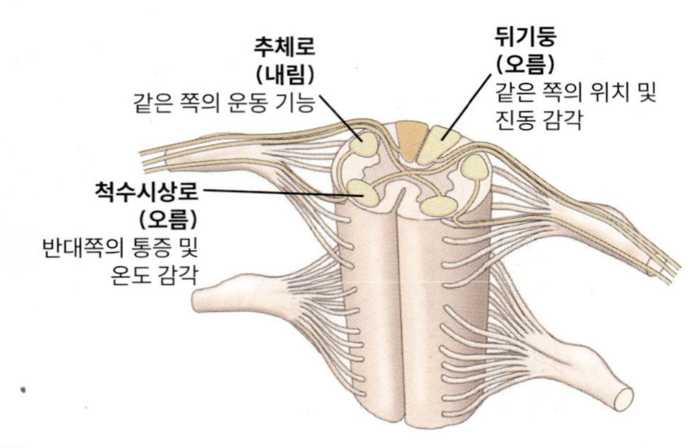

그림 9-6 척수로
© National Association of Emergency Medical Technicians (NAEMT)

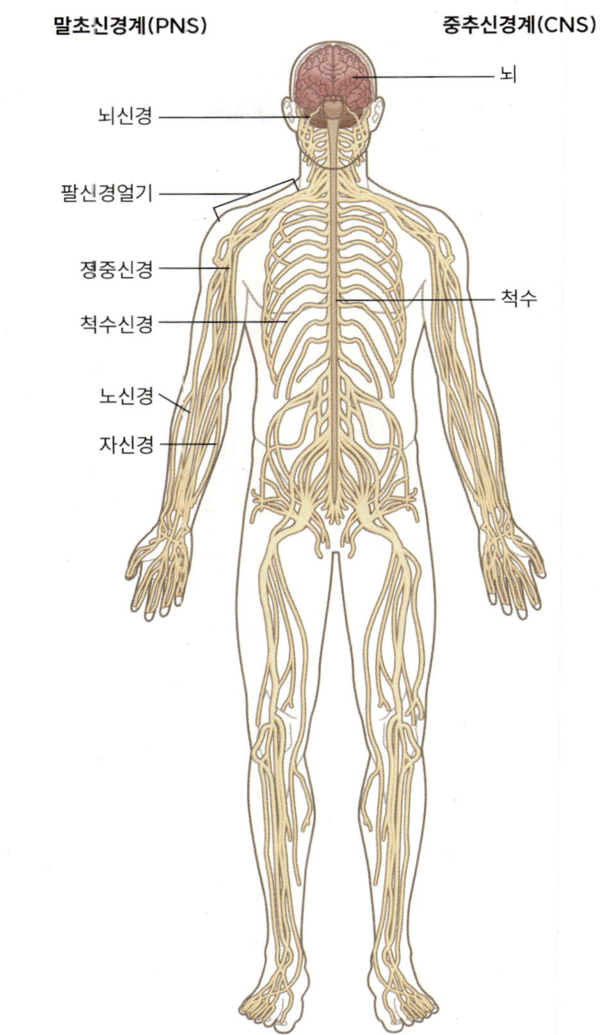

그림 9-7 중추신경계(CNS) 및 말초신경계(PNS).
© National Association of Emergency Medical Technicians (NAEMT)

로 더 나눌 수 있다. 통증과 온도 감각을 전달하는 신경로는 척수 자체에서 교차하는데 이는 신체의 오른쪽에서 정보를 전달하는 신경로가 척수의 왼쪽으로 건너가 뇌로 이동하는 것을 의미한다. 반면에 위치, 진동, 및 가벼운 접촉에 대한 감각 정보를 전달하는 신경로는 척수에서 교차하지 않고 속질 수준에서 교차한다. 따라서 감각 정보는 척수에서 신경뿌리와 같은 쪽에 있는 뇌로 전달된다.

하행신경로는 뇌에서 척수를 통해 신체로 운동 자극을 전달하는 역할을 하며 모든 근육의 움직임과 근긴장도를 조절한다. 이 하행신경로는 척수에서 교차하지 않는다. 따라서 척수의 오른쪽에 있는 운동로는 신체의 오른쪽 운동 기능을 조절한다. 그러나 이러한 운동로는 뇌줄기에서 교차하므로 뇌의 왼쪽이 신체의 오른쪽 운동 기능을 조절하고 그 반대의 경우도 마찬가지이다.

척수가 계속 내려오면서 신경 쌍이 각 척추의 척수에서 분기되어 신체의 여러 부분으로 뻗어 나간다(**그림 9-7**). 척수에는 31쌍의 척수신경이 있으며 신경이 발생하는 부위에 따라 이름이 붙여진다. 각 신경은 양쪽에 두 개의 뿌리(등 쪽과 배 쪽)가 있다.

뒤뿌리(후근)는 감각 자극에 대한 정보를 전달하고 앞뿌리(전근)는 운동 자극 정보를 전달한다. 신경 자극은 척수와 각각의 신경 쌍을 통해 뇌와 신체의 각 부분 사이를 통과한다. 척수에서 분지할 때 이 신경은 추간공이라고 하는 척추뼈 몸통의 뒤쪽의 척추의 아래쪽 측면에 있는 파임을 통과한다.

피부 분절은 하나의 뒤뿌리에 의해 신경이 지배하는 신체 피부 표면의 감각 영역이다. 피부 분절을 종합하면 각 척추 레벨에 대하여 신체 부위를 지도화할 수 있다(**그림 9-8**). 피부 분절은 척수 손상의 수준을 결정하는 데 도움이 된다. 기억해야 할 세 가지 랜드마크는 C4~5 피부 분절은 빗장뼈 수준이고 T4 피부 분절은 유두 수준이며 T10 피부 분절은 배꼽 수준이다. 이 세 가지 피부 분절을 기억하면 척수 손상의 위치를 빠르게 찾는 데 도움이 될 수 있다.

들숨과 날숨의 과정은 가슴의 움직임과 가로막 모양에 적절한 변화가 모두 필요하다. 갈비사이근과 등세모근과 같은 보조 호흡근도 호흡에 기여한다. 가로막은 C3~C5 수준 사이의 척수에서 발생하는 신경에서 비롯된 왼쪽과 오른쪽 가로막 신경에 의해 자극을 받는다. 척수가 C3 수준 이상에서 손상되거나 가로막 신경이 절단되면 환자는 자발 호흡 기능을 잃게 된다. 이런 손상을 입은 환자는 목격자가 구조 호흡을 시작하지 않으면 병원 전 처치 제공자가 도착하기 전에 질식할 수 있다. 따라서 척수 손상이 의심되는 환자의 기도를 유지하는 것이 중요하다. 이송 중에 양압 환기를 계속 시행해야 할 수도 있다.

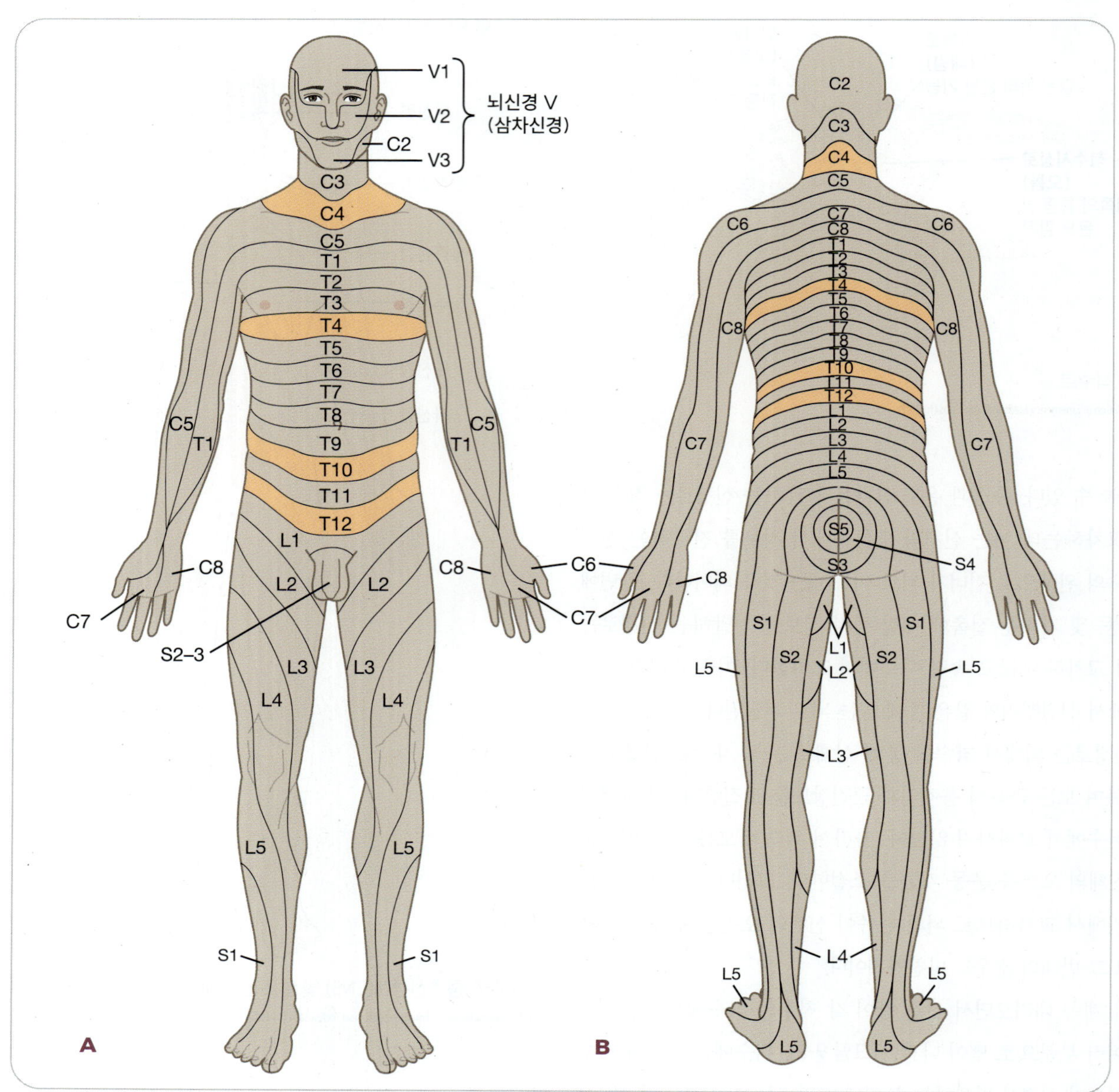

그림 9-8 피부 분절 지도는 피부의 촉각 부위와 해당 부위에 해당하는 척수 신경 사이의 관계를 보여준다. 특정 부위의 감각 상실을 나타낼 수 있다. **A.** 정면 **B.** 뒷면.

© National Association of Emergency Medical Technicians (NAEMT)

병태생리학

뼈로 된 척추는 일반적으로 최대 1,360J의 에너지를 견딜 수 있다. 고속 이동과 접촉성 스포츠는 일반적으로 척추에 이 이상을 초과하는 힘을 척추에 가할 수 있다. 저속에서 중간 속도의 차량 충돌 시에도 고정되지 않은 68kg인 사람이 앞 유리나 지붕에 머리를 갑자기 부딪치면 척추에 4,080~5,440J의 힘이 쉽게 가해질 수 있다. 오토바이 운전자가 앞쪽으로 퉁겨지거나 빠른 속도로 내려오던 스키 선수가 나

무와 충돌할 때도 비슷한 힘이 발생할 수 있다. 척추의 압박 강도는 척추 크기, 모양 및 다양한 척추 수준에서 골밀도(BMD)의 차이를 반영하여 꼬리 쪽으로 증가한다. 외상성 척추 손상을 유발하는 데 필요한 큰 힘은 종종 내장, 혈관 및 폐 구조와 관련된 손상을 초래하여 환자 처치를 더욱 복잡하게 만든다. 목뼈 손상은 척추 이외의 다른 구조물에 손상을 입힐 위험이 가장 높으며(65%), 허리뼈(52%) 및 등뼈(50%)의 손상이 그 뒤를 따른다. 등뼈 외상은 폐, 가로막, 갈비뼈 및 복장뼈와 연관된 손상을 특히 의심해야 한다. 척추 손상 부위 외

에도 척추 골절 또는 손상된 척추 부위의 수가 증가함에 따라 관련 손상의 위험이 증가한다.

골격 손상

척추에는 다음과 같은 다양한 유형의 손상이 발생할 수 있다.

- 압박골절은 척추 몸통이 쐐기형 압박되거나 완전히 납작해지는 골절
- 파열 골절은 후방 척추 벽을 침범할 수 있으며 척수 근처의 척주관에 있을 수 있는 작은 뼛조각을 생성할 수 있음
- 불완전탈구 척주의 정상적인 정렬에서 척추가 부분적으로 탈구된 것
- 인대와 근육이 과도하게 늘어나거나 찢어져 뼈의 손상 유무에 관계없이 척추 사이의 불안정성을 유발하는 추간판 손상

단순 압박 골절은 일반적으로 안정된 손상이지만, 이러한 손상은 즉시 심각한 압박이나 척수의 절단(흔하지 않지만)을 초래하여 돌이킬 수 없는 손상을 초래할 수 있다. 그러나 일부 환자에게서는 척추나 인대 손상으로 인해 불안정한 척추의 손상을 초래하지만, 즉각적인 척수 손상을 일으키지는 않는다. 불안정한 척추의 뼛조각이 움직이면 이차적으로 척수를 손상시킬 수 있다. 또한, 하나의 척추 골절이 있는 환자는 다른 비연속성 척추 손상이 발생할 확률이 10~20%에 달한다. 따라서 특정 척추 부위의 손상이 의심되는 환자에게 척추 고정의 필요성을 결정할 때 척추 전체를 고려해야 한다.

신경학적 결손이 없다고 해서 골절이나 척추가 불안정한 척추를 배제할 수는 없다. 팔다리의 운동 및 감각 반응이 양호하다는 것은 척수가 현재 손상되지 않았다는 것을 의미하지만, 그것이 척추 또는 관련 뼈, 인대 및 연부조직의 손상을 배제하지는 않는다. 척추 골절 환자의 대부분은 신경학적 결손이 없다. 척추 고정의 필요성을 결정하려면 전체 평가가 필요하다.

척추 외상을 유발하는 특정 손상 기전

척추의 축 방향 하중은 여러 가지 방식으로 발생할 수 있다. 대부분 척추 압박은 안전띠를 매지 않은 탑승자의 머리가 자동차의 앞 유리에 부딪히거나 수심이 얕은 곳에서 다이빙하다가 머리가 물체에 부딪히는 경우와 같이 머리가 물체에 부딪히고 정지한 머리에 여전히 움직이는 신체의 체중이 가해졌을 때 발생한다. 압박과 축 방향 하중은 환자가 상당한 높이에서 추락 후 지면에 서 있는 자세로 착지할 때도 발생한다. 이러한 유형의 손상은 엉치뼈가 정지된 상태에서 머리

와 가슴의 무게가 허리뼈를 압박하게 된다. 4.6m 이상의 높이에서 추락하면 약 20%에서 허리뼈 골절이 동반되지만, 특정 환자 집단, 특히 노인의 경우 4.6m보다 훨씬 낮은 높이에서 추락한 후 척추 골절 발생률이 훨씬 더 높다는 사실을 인식하는 것이 중요하다. 이러한 극단적인 에너지 교환 중에 척주는 정상적인 굴곡을 과장하는 경향이 있으며 이러한 부위에서 골절 및 압박이 발생한다. 축 방향 하중으로 인한 압박 골절 또는 파열 골절은 요추전만증 또는 흉추후만증의 정점에서 많이 발생한다.

과도한 굴곡(과다굽힘), 과도한 신전(과신전), 과도한 회전(과회전)은 뼈 또는 인대 손상을 유발하여 척수에 충돌하거나 늘어나게 할 수 있다.

갑작스럽거나 과도한 측면 굴곡은 이 방향으로의 움직임은 처음부터 제한되기 때문에 척추의 인장 또는 압박 장애가 발생하기 전에 굴곡이나 신전보다 훨씬 적인 움직임이 필요하다. 측면 충돌이 발생하면 몸통과 등뼈가 측면으로 움직인다. 머리는 목뼈 부착물에 의해 당겨질 때까지 제자리에 유지되는 경향이 있다. 머리의 무게 중심은 목뼈 결합부의 앞쪽과 위쪽에 있기 때문에 머리가 옆으로 굴러가는 경향이 있다. 이러한 움직임은 종종 탈구와 골절을 초래한다.

떼어당김(척추가 과도하게 늘어남)은 척추의 한 부분이 안정되어 있고 나머지 부분이 세로 방향으로 움직일 때 발생한다. 이렇게 척추가 분리되면 척수가 쉽게 늘어나거나 찢어질 수 있다. 떼어당김 유형의 척추 손상은 소아의 놀이터 손상, 교수형 및 특정 유형의 차량 충돌 사고에서 흔히 발생하는 손상 기전이다.

척수 손상 기전은 여러 가지가 알려졌지만, 대부분 다음과 같은 네 가지 주요 원인으로 인해 발생한다.

- 차량 충돌
- 추락
- 폭력 행위
- 얕은 물에서 다이빙을 포함한 스포츠 관련 활동

소아 환자에서 외상성 척추 손상과 척수 손상의 주요 원인은 나이와 인종에 따라 크게 다르다. 2세 미만 환자의 척추 손상의 상당 부분(17.5%)은 폭력적인 신체적 학대로 인해 발생하며 차량 충돌과 낙상은 혼자 나이와 관계없이 여전히 일반적인 원인이다. 2005년 이후 낙상과 관련된 청소년은 소아나 성인보다 스포츠 관련 활동 중에 손상을 입을 가능성이 더 높다. 총기 관련 손상은 미국 흑인 청소년의 전체 척수 손상의 1/4을 차지한다.

실제로 손상 기전이 복잡한 힘 패턴을 일으킬 수 있으므로 척추

의 정확한 손상을 결정하기는 어렵다. 추가적인 임상 및 방사선 검사를 통해 손상이 입증될 때까지 골절이나 신경학적 손상을 유발할 정도로 심각한 손상이 척추의 불안정성을 유발했다고 항상 가정해야 한다.

척수 손상

일차 손상은 충격이나 힘이 가해질 때 발생하며 척수 압박, 직접적인 척수 손상(일반적으로 날카롭고 불안정한 뼛조각이나 파편에 의한 것) 및 척수의 혈액 공급을 방해할 수 있다. 이차 손상은 일차 손상 후에 부기, 허혈 또는 뼛조각의 움직임으로 인해 발생한다.

척수 진탕은 손상 원위부의 척수 기능이 일시적 장애로 인해 발생한다. 척수 타박상은 척수 조직이 멍이 들거나 출혈을 동반하며 이로 인해 손상 원위부 척수 기능의 일시적(때로는 영구적)인 손실(척수 쇼크)을 초래할 수 있다. 척수 쇼크는 척수 손상 후 다양한 시간(보통 48시간 미만) 동안 발생하는 신경학적 현상으로 일시적인 감각 및 운동기능 상실, 근육 이완 및 마비, 척수 손상 부위 이하의 반사 상실을 초래한다. 척수 타박상은 종종 관통상 유형의 손상이나 척수에 대한 뼛조각의 움직임으로 인해 발생한다. 타박상으로 인한 손상의 심각성은 척수 조직으로의 출혈량과 관련이 있다. 척수의 혈액 공급이 손상이나 중단되면 국소적 척수 조직의 허혈이 발생할 수 있다.

척수 압박은 국소 조직의 부종으로 인한 척수 압박이지만, 외상으로 인한 디스크 파열이나 뼛조각, 압박성 혈종 발생으로 인해 발생할 수도 있다. 척수 압박은 국소 조직의 부종으로 인한 척수에 가해지는 압력이지만, 외상성 디스크 파열, 뼛조각 또는 압박성 혈종의 발병으로 인해 발생할 수도 있다. 척추 압박은 조직 허혈을 유발할 수 있으며 경우에 따라 영구적인 기능 상실을 방지하기 위해 외과적 감압이 필요할 수 있으므로 방사선학적 검사와 최종 평가를 위해 신속하게 이송하는 것이 중요하다. 척수 열상은 척수 조직이 찢어지거나 절단될 때 발생한다. 이러한 유형의 손상은 일반적으로 돌이킬 수 없는 신경학적 손상을 초래한다.

척수 절단은 완전 또는 불완전 절단으로 분류할 수 있다. 완전 척수 절단의 경우 모든 척수가 절단되고 절단된 부위 원위부의 모든 척수 기능이 상실된다. 부기로 인한 추가적인 영향 때문에 손상 후 24시간이 지나야 기능 상실 정도를 정확하게 파악할 수 있다. 대부분의 완전한 척수 절단은 손상 정도에 따라 하반신 마비나 팔다리 마비를 초래한다. 불완전한 절단의 경우 일부 척수로와 운동/감각 기능은 그대로 유지된다. 이러면 완전한 절단보다 회복에 대한 예후가 더 좋다.

병원 전 환경에서는 신경학적 결손이 척수 타박상, 척수 쇼크 또는 더 심하게 손상된 척수 때문인지 구분하는 것이 불가능하다. 따라서 척수 손상이 의심되는 모든 환자는 이러한 구분을 고려하지 않고 평가 및 처치를 한다.

불완전 척수 손상의 유형은 다음과 같다.

- 전척수증후군(Anterior cord syndrome)은 일반적으로 척수의 앞쪽 동맥에 뼛조각이나 압력이 가해져 척수의 앞쪽이 경색되거나 손상된 결과이다(**그림 9-9**). 증상으로는 운동 기능 상실, 통증, 체온, 가벼운 접촉 감각 등이 있다. 그러나 약간의 가벼운 접촉, 움직임, 위치 및 진동 감각은 손상되지 않은 뒤기둥을 통해 유지된다.
- 중심척수증후군(Central cord syndrome)은 일반적으로 목뼈 부위의 과신전으로 발생하며 특히 퇴행성 또는 선천성 원인으로 인한 협착증이 있는 환자에서 발생한다(**그림 9-10**). 증상으로는 팔의 쇠약이나 감각 이상이 있지만, 다리의 힘과 감각은 덜 하다. 이 증후군은 다양한 정도의 방광기능 장애를 유발한다.
- 브라운-시쿼드증후군(Brown-Sequard syndrome)은 관통상으로 인해 발생하며 척수의 한쪽만 손상되는 척수 반절단을 포함한다(**그림 9-11**). 증상으로는 완전한 척수 손상된 쪽의 기능 상실(운동,

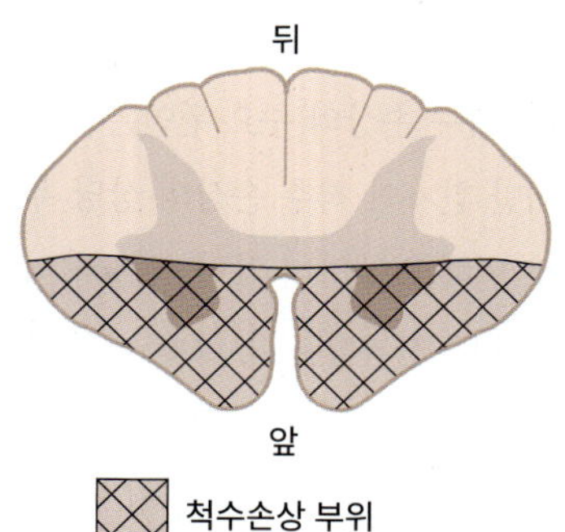

그림 9-9 전척수증후군.

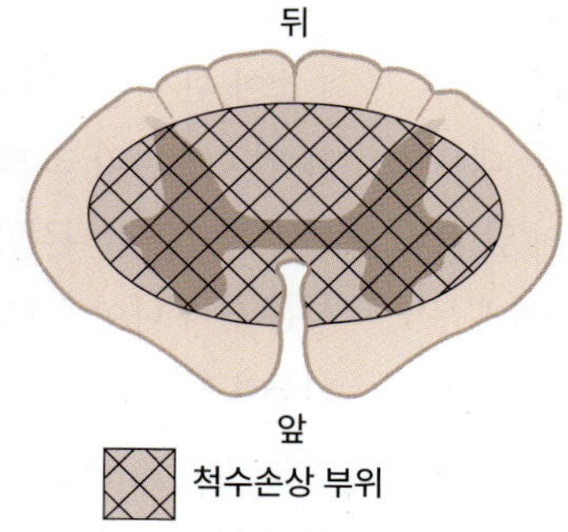

그림 9-10 중심척수증후군.

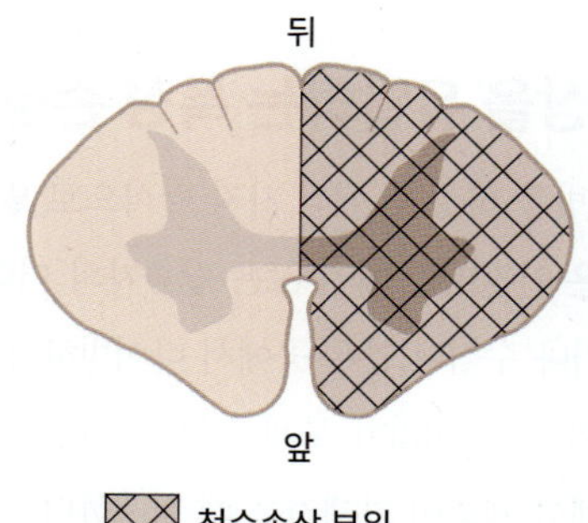

그림 9-11 브라운-시쿼드(Brown-Séquard)증후군.

진동, 동작, 자세), 손상된 반대쪽의 통증 및 온도 감각 상실 등이 있다.

척수 쇼크는 손상으로 인해 이차적으로 척수에서 운동 및 감각 신호 전달이 상실되는 것을 의미하지만, 이는 심장과 말초 혈관으로의 교감 신경 유출이 상실되어 병태생리학적 징후가 나타나는 일종의 분포성 쇼크인 신경성 쇼크와 구별해야 한다. 적절한 교감신경 자극이 없으면 부교감신경 전달이 이루어지지 않아 서맥이 발생하고 말초동맥과 정맥이 확장된다. 동맥 확장은 말초 전신 혈관 저항의 손실을 초래하고 정맥 확장은 정맥 저류를 초래한다. 이러한 결과는 정맥이 심장의 오른쪽으로 되돌아오는 심장의 전부하를 감소시킨다. 서맥과 함께 심각한 심박출량 감소가 발생할 수 있다. 저혈량 쇼크 환자는 저혈압에 반응하여 빈맥이 나타나고 말초혈관이 수축하여 혈압을 유지하기 위해 중요한 기관으로 혈액량을 순환시키기 때문에 피부가 차갑고 축축하다. 반대로 척수 쇼크와 관련된 생리학적 소견은 저혈압성 서맥이 나타나고 이를 해결하기 위해서는 적극적인 소생술과 더불어 아트로핀(또는 기타 부교감신경 차단제)으로 처치해야 할 수 있다. 부교감신경이 항진되지 않은 상태와 관련된 다른 소견으로는 혈관 확장으로 인해 피부가 따뜻하고 붉어지며 지속발기증이 나타난다. 실제로 척수 손상과 척수 쇼크 환자는 신경성 쇼크 외에도 저혈량 쇼크를 유발할 수 있는 다른 손상을 입은 경우가 많으므로 평가 및 처치가 더욱 어려워진다.

척수 관류

척수 혈류는 부분적으로 척수 관류압(SCPP)에 의해 결정된다.

척수 관류압(SCPP) = 평균 동맥압(MAP) − 외부 압력

척수 관류와 산소 공급 및 척수에 가해지는 외부 압력에 영향을 미치는 요인은 여러 가지가 있다.

1. 평균 동맥압(MAP). 평균 동맥압은 주로 척수 관류를 결정한다. 척수 관류압을 유지하려면 수액 투여와 약물 투여를 통해 평균 동맥압을 90mmHg로 적절하게 유지하는 것이 중요하다. 척수 손상 후 어느 시점에서든 전신적인 저혈압(수축기 혈압이 90mmHg 미만인 것으로 정의)은 악화한 신경학적 결과와 관련이 있다.

2. 척수 정맥 울혈. 이는 정맥 혈전증의 영향이거나 척추 정맥의 외부 압박으로 인해 혈액 유출이 불충분한 결과일 수 있다. 미세 혈관 수준에서 척수 정맥 울혈이 있는 경우 적절한 산소 교환을 위해 정맥 울혈 부위를 통해 혈액을 밀어내려면 평균 동맥압이 더 높아야 한다.

3. 저산소증. 외상 환자는 폐에 문제가 있는 경우가 많아 폐의 산소 교환이 감소하여 혈액 내 동맥혈 산소분압이 낮아질 수 있다. 척수로 가는 혈류를 적절하게 유지하려면 보충 산소를 투여하고 기도를 개방하고 유지하는 것이 중요하다.

4. 약물. 모르핀 및 기타 아편유사제를 포함한 많은 일반적인 마취제는 심근에 대한 부정적인 근육 수축 효과로 인해 심박출량을 감소시킬 수 있다. 외상 환자의 통증 조절이 중요하지만, 이러한 약물은 적절한 척수 관류 및 산소 공급을 위해 신중하게 사용해야 한다.

초기 소생술

적극적인 소생술은 척수 손상 관련 쇼크의 병원 전 처치와 신경학적 결손을 줄이고 이차 신경학적 손상을 예방하는 데 중요한 역할을 한다. 이차 신경학적 손상의 원인은 자가 조절 기능의 상실로 인해 척추 미세 순환의 손실되어 추가적인 허혈성 손상을 초래하는 데서 비롯된다. 조기에 적극적으로 혈류량과 혈압을 증가시키면 이러한 미세 순환을 개선하고 척수에 대한 이차 손상의 위험을 줄일 수 있다. 또한, 척수 손상 환자 중 최대 30%는 다발성 외상 및 중증 출혈과 관련이 있다. 이는 척수 손상 환자의 병원 입원 전 사망률이 20%에 달한다는 점과 현장에서 적절한 소생술이 얼마나 중요한지를 반영하는 결과이다.

이상적으로는 척수 손상 환자의 초기 소생술은 손상 후 7일 동안 목표 평균 동맥압을 90mmHg로 유지하는 조치가 포함되어야 한다. 이는 종종 적절한 정맥 내로 결정질 용액, 콜로이드 또는 혈액 제제를 투여하여 가능한 한 많은 신경학적 혈류를 회복하는 방식으로 이루어진다. 다발성 외상 척수 손상 환자의 경우 병원 전 처치 제공자는 허용할 수 있는 저혈압의 잠재적 위험과 이점을 평가하는 것이 중요하다. 일시적인 저관류 상태로 인해 척수 손상의 중증도가 악화할 수 있는 위험이 있으므로 일반적으로 척수 손상이 의심될 때마다 허용 저혈압을 피해야 한다.

수액 소생술에서 포도당이 함유된 것을 투여하는 것은 다음과 같은 두 가지 이유로 피해야 한다. 첫째, 포도당은 빠르게 대사되어 과량의 유리수가 남아 부종 형성을 더 쉽게 발생시킬 수 있다. 둘째, 포도당을 너무 많이 투여하면 고혈당증이 발생하여 무산소대사를 증가시켜 젖산 증가, 전신 pH를 감소시켜 예후가 나빠질 수 있다.

또한, 척수 손상 부위가 높을수록(C5 이상) 혈압상승제 및 박동조율기와 같은 심혈관 처치가 필요할 가능성이 더 높다는 점을 기억하는 것이 중요하다. 혈관운동성 교감신경 섬유는 첫 번째와 네 번째 등뼈 수준 사이에서 척수를 빠져나와 목뼈 손상이 심할 경우 절단될 수 있으며 부교감신경 섬유는 척수 외부의 미주신경을 따라 가슴으로 이동한다. 연구에 따르면 완전한 목뼈 손상 환자의 평균 동맥압은 중환자실에 도착했을 때 66mmHg에 불과하며 척수의 적절한 관류를 유지하는 데 필요한 목표 평균 동맥압인 90mmHg보다 훨씬 낮다. 한 연구에 따르면 완전한 목뼈 손상 환자의 40%가 신경성 쇼크 징후를 보였으며 즉시 승압제 사용이 필요한 것으로 나타났다. 병원 전 처치 제공자는 모든 척수 손상에 대한 소생술에 주의를 기울여야 하지만, 특히 목뼈 손상 환자에게 최상의 신경학적 결과를 도출하기 위해 특히 강조해야 한다.

평가

척추 손상은 다른 손상과 마찬가지로 동반된 손상 및 현재 상태의 맥락에서 평가해야 한다. 병원 전 처치 제공자와 현장의 안전을 확인한 후 일차평가가 최우선 순위이다. 신속한 현장 평가와 병력 청취를 통해 척수 손상의 가능성이 있는지를 확인하고 외부 고정으로 척추를 보호해야 할 필요가 있는지 결정해야 한다. 환자의 머리는 금기증이 없는 한 중립 자세로 위치시켜야 한다(이 장 뒷부분의 머리 도수 고정 부분 참조). 평가 결과 고정이 필요하지 않다고 판단될 때까지 머리를 중립 자세를 유지하거나 척추고정판을 포함한 목뼈보호대, 진공부목(진공매트리스) 또는 조끼형 장비와 같은 척추 고정 장비를 사용하여 고정할 때까지 도수 고정을 유지한다. 손상 기전이 불분명하고 현장 평가를 적절하게 시행할 수 없으며 신뢰할 수 없는 경우 척추 손상이 있는 것으로 가정하고 보다 철저한 평가를 시행할 때까지 외부 고정을 유지해야 한다.

신경학적 검사

현장에서는 신속한 신경학적 검사를 하여 척수 손상과 관련이 있을 수 있는 명백한 결손을 확인해야 한다. 환자에게 손, 팔, 다리를 움직이도록 요청하고 움직일 수 없는 경우 이를 기록한다. 그런 다음 환자는 어깨에서 시작하여 몸통에서 발로 내려가면서 감각의 유무를 확인한다. 완전한 신경학적 검사는 필요한 병원 전 처치 결정에 영향을 미치는 추가 정보를 제공하지 않고 현장에서 귀중한 시간을 소비

하고 이송을 지연시키는 역할을 할 뿐이므로 병원 전 단계에서 수행할 필요가 없다.

신속한 신경학적 검사는 환자를 고정한 후 환자를 움직일 때마다 그리고 의료기관에 도착하자마자 반복해야 한다. 이를 통해 일차평가 이후에 발생할 수 있는 환자의 상태의 변화를 파악하는 데 도움이 된다.

손상 기전을 이용한 척수 손상 평가

전통적으로 병원 전 처치 제공자는 척수 손상을 의심할 때는 손상 기전만을 기준으로 하며 손상 기전이 의심되는 환자에게는 척추 고정이 필요하다고 배웠다. 최근까지 이러한 일반화로 인해 척추 손상 평가에 대한 명확한 임상 지침이 부족했다. 손상 기전은 척추 움직임 제한이 필요한지 아닌지를 결정하는 다각적인 의사 결정 과정에서 한 가지 요소에 불과하므로 척추 움직임 제한의 필요성을 결정하는 유일한 수단이 되어서는 안 된다. 척추 고정을 위한 목과 척추의 평가에는 운동 및 감각 기능, 통증 또는 압통 유무, 척추 손상의 예측 인자로서의 환자 신뢰도에 대한 평가도 포함되어야 한다. 또한 환자는 넓적다리뼈 골절과 같이 주의를 산만하고 고통스러운 손상과 관련된 통증으로 인해 척추 통증을 호소하지 않을 수도 있다. 주의를 산만하게 하는 손상을 구성하는 요소에 대한 정의는 여전히 논란의 여지가 있다. 그러나 병원 전 처치 제공자는 환자의 잠재적인 외상성 척추 손상을 평가할 때 관련 손상을 고려해야 하며 주의를 산만하게 하는 손상이 있을 수 있는 경우 척추 움직임 제한을 적용하는 기준을 낮출 수 있다. 외상성 뇌손상이나 환자가 알코올이나 약물을 복용했을 경우 환자의 통증 인식을 둔화시키고 심각한 손상을 가릴 수 있다. 척추 운동 제한은 신뢰할 수 있는 검사 결과, 신경학적 결손이 없고 목이나 허리 통증이 없으며 주의를 산만하게 하는 심각한 손상이 없는 의식이 있는 환자에게는 척추 움직임 제한이 필요하지 않을 가능성이 높다. 검사에서 이러한 요인 중 하나라도 양성이거나 신뢰할 수 있는 검사를 제공할 수 없는 환자의 경우 척추 움직임 제한을 계속 시행해야 한다.

무딘 외상

무딘 외상은 외상성 척추 손상의 일반적인 손상 기전이며 병원 전 처치 제공자의 신중한 평가가 필요하다. 차량 충돌과 낙상은 무딘 외상과 관련된 모든 척추 골절의 절반 이상을 차지한다. 50만 명 이상의 환자를 대상으로 한 대규모 메타 분석에서 모든 무딘 외상에서 등허

리 골절의 비율이 약 7%이며 이 중 1/4 이상이 척수 손상을 유발할 정도로 심각한 것으로 나타났다. 목뼈 손상은 등뼈 또는 허리뼈 손상에 비해 척수 손상 및 그로 인한 신경학적 손상의 위험이 더 높다. 비슷한 수의 환자를 대상으로 한 연구에서 무딘 외상 환자의 6% 이상에서 목뼈가 손상되었으며 의식이 없거나 머리에 손상을 입은 환자의 경우 훨씬 더 많은 수가 발생했다. 무딘 외상으로 인한 목뼈 손상의 거의 절반이 불안정하다. 따라서 이차 손상을 예방하기 위한 병원 전 처치를 위한 중요한 기회이다.

일반적인 지침으로 척수 손상 및 잠재적으로 불안정한 척추의 존재를 추정하고 즉시 목뼈의 도수 고정을 수행하며 다음과 같은 상황에서 척추 고정의 필요성을 결정하기 위해 척추 평가를 수행해야 한다.

- 머리, 목, 몸통 또는 골반에 강한 충격을 주는 무딘 손상 기전(예: 폭행, 구조물 붕괴로 인한 끼임)
- 목이나 몸통에 갑작스러운 가속, 감속 또는 측면 굴곡을 유발하는 사고(예: 중간 속도 또는 고속의 차량 충돌, 보행자가 차량에 충돌, 폭발 사고)
- 모든 낙상, 특히 노인의 경우
- 차량 또는 기타 동력 운송 장치(예: 스쿠터, 스케이트보드, 자전거, 차량, 오토바이, 레저용 차량)에서 떨어지거나 추락
- 얕은 물에서 사고(예: 다이빙, 서핑)

척추 손상과 관련된 다른 상황은 다음과 같다.
- 의식 수준의 변화를 동반한 머리 손상
- 심각한 헬멧 파손
- 몸통에 심각한 무딘 손상
- 다리나 엉덩관절의 충격 또는 기타 감속 골절
- 척주 부위의 심각한 국소적인 손상

이러한 손상 기전에 따라 환자의 척추 움직임 제한이 필요한 징후가 있는지 확인하기 위해 철저하고 완벽하게 검사를 시행해야 한다. 징후가 발견되지 않으면 목뼈의 도수 고정을 중단할 수 있다.

적절하게 안전띠를 사용하면 생명을 구할 수 있고 머리, 얼굴 및 가슴 손상을 줄일 수 있는 것으로 입증되었다. 그러나 적절하게 안전띠를 착용했다고 해서 척추 손상의 가능성이 완전히 배제할 수는 없다. 급격한 감속이 발생하는 심각한 전면 충돌 시 안전띠를 착용한 경우 고정된 몸통은 갑자기 멈추지만, 고정되지 않은 머리는 계속 앞으로 움직일 수 있다. 감속력이 충분히 강하면 머리는 턱이 가슴벽에 부딪힐 때까지 아래쪽으로 움직이며 어깨 벨트의 대각선 끈을 따

<table>
<tr><td>Box 9-1 관통상</td></tr>
<tr><td>관통상은 그 자체로 척추 움직임 제한의 적응증이 아니다.</td></tr>
</table>

라 자주 회전한다. 이러한 빠르고 강력한 목의 과굴곡과 회전은 목뼈의 압박골절, 관절돌기의 탈구, 척수 신전을 초래할 수 있다. 후방 또는 측면 충돌로 인해 안전띠를 착용한 탑승자에게 다른 손상 기전으로 인해 척추 외상이 발생할 수 있다. 차량의 파손 정도와 환자의 다른 손상은 환자를 고정해야 하는지를 결정하는 데 중요한 요소이다.

관통성 외상

관통상은 척추 외상의 가능성과 관련하여 특별히 고려해야 할 사항이다. 일반적으로 관통성 외상이 발생한 시점에 환자가 명확한 신경 손상을 입지 않았다면 이후 척수 손상 발생에 대한 우려는 거의 없다 (**Box 9-1**). 이는 손상 기전과 관련된 힘과 관련된 운동학 때문이다. 관통상은 무딘 외상과 달리 불안정한 인대 또는 뼈 손상을 일으킬 위험이 최소화되기 때문에 불안정한 척추 골절을 일으키지 않는다. 관통하는 물체는 관통 경로를 따라 손상을 유발한다. 총상은 척수 타박상의 일반적인 원인이다. 총알이 척수를 관통하여 돌이킬 수 없는 손상을 입힐 수 있지만, 총알이 척수 가까이 지나가는 탄도 충격으로 인해 척수 타박상을 입는 경우가 더 많으며 이는 회복할 수 있다. 칼에 의한 손상이 척수 손상으로 이어지는 경우는 드물지만, 손상은 여전히 발생할 수 있다. 칼로 인한 손상은 신경 구조에 열상을 입히는 것 외에도 국소 조직 부종을 유발하여 척수 타박상을 초래할 수 있다.

척추 움직임 제한에 대한 적응증

손상 기전은 척추 움직임 제한의 적응증의 필요성을 결정하는 데 도움이 될 수 있지만, 이것이 유일한 결정 요소는 아니다(**그림 9-12**). 중요한 점은 올바른 임상적 판단과 함께 완전한 신체적 평가가 의사 결정을 내리는 데 도움이 된다는 것이다.

2018년 미국 외상학회 외상위원회, 미국 EMS 의사협회, 미국 응급의학회는 척추 움직임 제한에 관한 권장 사항을 업데이트했다. 이러한 권장 사항과 최신 문헌을 기반으로 **Box 9-2**에 나열된 적응증 중 하나라도 해당하는 무딘 손상 기전이 있는 경우 척추 고정을 고려해야 한다.

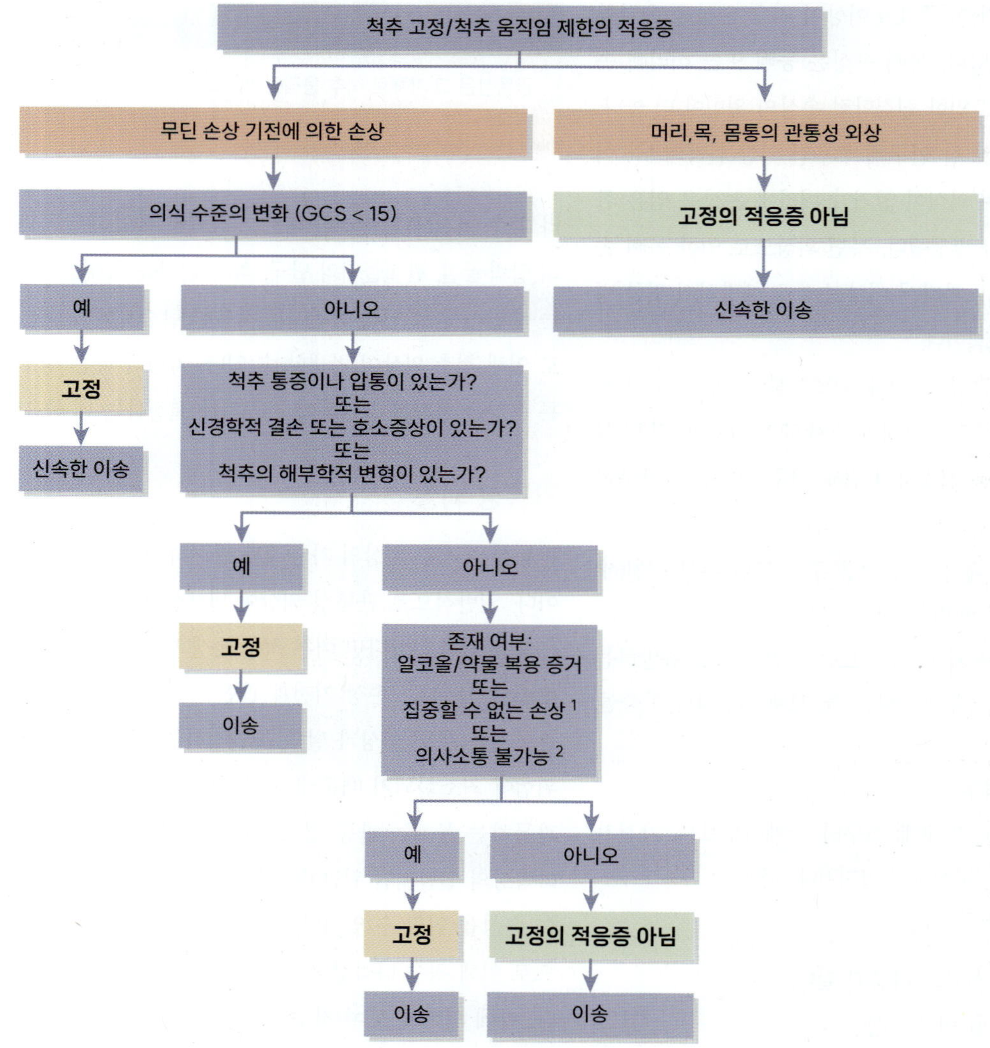

주석:
[1] 집중할 수 없는 손상
환자가 다른 송상을 인식하는 능력을 손상시킬 수 있는 모든 손상으로 예를 들면 다음과 같다.
a) 긴뼈 골절, b) 외과적 수술이 필요한 내부 손상, c) 큰 열상, 벗겨진 손상 또는 으깸 손상, d) 넓은 화상, e) 급성 기능장애를 유발하는 기타 모든 손상.
(Adapted from Hoffman JR, Wolfson AB, Todd K, Mower WR: Selective cervical spine radiography in blunt trauma: methodology of the National Emergency X-Radiography Utilization Study [NEXUS], *Ann Emerg Med.* 1998;461.)

[2] 의사소통 불가능
위의 명시되지 않은 이유로 환자의 평가에 적극적으로 참여할 수 있도록 명확하게 의사소통할 수 없는 환자이며 예를 들면,언어 또는 청각 장애, 외국어만 사용하는 사람 및 어린이

그림 9-12 척추 고정의 적응증

심각한 척추 외상과 관련된 몇 가지 중요한 징후와 증상이 있다 (**Box 9-3**). 그러나 이러한 징후가 없다고 해서 척추 손상을 완전히 배제할 수는 없다.

특히 단단한 긴척추고정판을 이용한 척추 움직임 제한의 불필요한 사용을 줄이기 위해 이러한 전문 기관에서는 환자가 **Box 9-4**에 나열된 모든 기준을 충족하는 경우 긴척추고정판에 고정할 필요가 없다고 권장한다.

머리, 목 또는 몸통에 관통상(예: 총상 또는 자상)이 있고 신경학적 징후 또는 증상(예: 무감각, 저림, 운동, 감각 기능 상실 또는 의식 상실)과 같은 척추 손상의 증거가 있는 환자는 움직이지 않아야 한다. 많은 연구에 따르면 머리, 목, 몸통의 관통성 외상으로 인해 불안정한 척수 손상이 발생하는 경우는 드물며 단독 관통상은 고정의 적

Box 9-2 척추 고정/척추 움직임 제한에 대한 적응증

- 정중선 목 또는 척추 통증 및 압통. 여기에는 주관적인 통증이나 움직임에 따른 통증, 압통 또는 척추 정중선 부위의 압통 또는 경직이 포함된다.
- 의식 수준 변화 또는 임상적 중독(예: 알코올 또는 중독성 물질의 영향으로 인한 외상성 뇌손상, GCS 점수 15점 미만).
- 마비 또는 국소 신경학적 증상(예: 무감각, 저림 및 운동 쇠약) 및 징후. 여기에는 양측 마비, 부분 마비, 불완전마비(쇠약), 무감각, 따끔거림 또는 손상 수준 이하의 신경성 쇼크가 포함된다. 남성의 경우 음경 지속발기증이 척수 손상의 추가 징후일 수 있다.
- 척추의 해부학적 변형. 여기에는 환자의 신체검사에서 발견된 척추의 변형이 포함된다.
- 주의를 산만하게 하는 손상의 존재. 여기에는 척추에 통증이 없다는 환자의 이야기를 신뢰할 수 없을 정도로 심각한 손상이 포함된다(예: 긴뼈 골절, 벗겨진 손상).
- 의사소통 불가능

© National Association of Emergency Medical Technicians (NAEMT)

Box 9-3 척추 외상의 증상과 징후

- 목이나 등의 통증
- 목이나 등을 움직일 때 통증
- 목뒤 쪽이나 정중선을 따라 등을 촉진 시 통증
- 척추의 변형
- 목 또는 등 보호대 착용 또는 고정
- 사고 후 언제라도 팔이나 다리의 마비, 무감각, 저림, 따끔거림이 나타남
- 신경성 쇼크의 증상 및 징후
- 지속발기증

© National Association of Emergency Medical Technicians (NAEMT)

Box 9-4 척추 움직임 제한이 불필요한 경우를 판단하는 기준

- 의식 수준 정상(GCS 점수 15점)
- 척추 압통 및 해부학적 이상 없음
- 주의를 산만하게 하는 손상 없음
- 중독 없음
- 신경학적 소견 또는 호소증상 없음

© National Association of Emergency Medical Technicians (NAEMT)

응증이 되지 않는다고 한다. 불안정한 척수 손상의 위험이 매우 낮고 관통성 외상으로 인한 다른 손상을 더 먼저 처치해야 하는 경우가 많으므로 관통상을 입은 환자는 척추 움직임 제한을 시행하지 않아야 한다. 실제로 국립외상 데이터 뱅크(National Trauma Data Bank)를 이용한 후향적 연구에 따르면 현장에서 척추 고정을 받은 관통성 외상 환자가 그렇지 않은 환자보다 전체 사망률이 더 높았다.

관통상은 그 자체로 척추 움직임 제한의 적응증이 아니다. 이차 손상 기전이나 척추 손상의 증거가 없는 한 관통상을 입은 환자에게 척추 움직임 제한을 일상적으로 수행해서는 안 된다.

병원 전 처치의 주요 초점은 척추를 움직이려고 시도하는 것보다 척추 움직임 제한의 적응증을 인식하는 것이다. 많은 환자에게 척수 손상이 없으므로 특히 척추 움직임 제한이 호흡 노력 향상, 피부 허혈 및 통증 증가를 포함하여 건강한 환자에게 부작용을 유발하는 것으로 나타났으므로 척추 움직임 제한에 대한 선택적 접근 방식이 적절하다. 척추 움직임 제한에 대한 이러한 선택적 접근 방식은 피부 손상에 더 취약하고 기저 폐 질환이 있는 노인에게 더 중요하다. 병원 전 처치 제공자는 척추 움직임 제한을 수행하기 위한 적절한 적응증에 초점을 맞춰야 하지만, 관련 합병증을 예방하기 위해 지시된 경우에만 고정을 시행해야 한다. 주의 깊고 철저한 검사 후 적응증이 없으면 척추 움직임 제한이 필요하지 않을 수 있다. 적절한 척추 처치의 초석은 모든 외상 처치와 같이 적절한 평가를 통해 적시에 처치를 시행한다.

방금 열거한 조건이 없는데도 환자에게 우려되는 손상 기전이 있는 경우 환자의 신뢰성을 평가해야 한다. 신뢰할 수 있는 환자는 침착하고 협조적이며 의식 상태가 완전히 정상이다.
신뢰할 수 없는 환자는 다음 중 어느 하나에 해당할 수 있다.

- 정신 상태 변화. 의식 상태에 변화를 초래하는 외상성 뇌손상을 입은 환자는 적절하게 평가를 시행할 수 없으므로 고정해야 한다. 마찬가지로 약물이나 알코올의 영향을 받는 환자는 침착하고 협조적이며 술에 취하지 않고 신체검사 소견이 정상일 때까지 척추 손상을 입은 것처럼 고정하고 처치한다.
- 주의를 산만하게 하는 고통스러운 손상. 심한 통증이 있는 손상은 환자의 주의를 덜 아픈 다른 손상으로부터 분산시켜 평가 중에 신뢰할 수 있는 답변을 제공하는 데 방해가 될 수 있다. 넓적다리뼈 골절이나 심한 화상을 예로 들 수 있다(**그림 9-12**).
- 의사소통 장애. 언어 장애가 있거나, 청력장애가 있거나, 언어를 구사하지 못하거나, 아주 어리거나 어떤 이유로든 효과적으로 의사소통을 할 수 없는 환자에게서 의사소통 문제가 발생할 수 있다.

평가의 모든 단계에서 환자를 신뢰할 수 있는지를 지속해서 재확인해야 한다. 환자에게 이러한 징후나 증상이 나타나거나 검사의 신뢰성에 문제가 있는 경우 환자에게 척추 손상이 있다고 가정하고 완

전한 고정을 시행해야 한다.

　많은 상황에서 손상 기전이 목 손상을 암시하지 않는 경우가 있다[예: 팔을 뻗은 상태에서 넘어져 콜레스 골절(원위 노뼈 및 자뼈 골절)이 발생한 경우]. 이러한 환자의 경우 정상적인 검사와 적절한 평가를 시행했다면 척추 고정은 필요하지 않다.

처치

외상성 척추 손상이 의심되고 척추 움직임 제한이 적절한 경우 병원 전 처치 제공자는 척추 움직임 제한을 안전하게 시행하여 환자를 이송할 수 있도록 준비해야 한다. 척추 움직임 제한의 목적은 척주 손상으로 불안정한 척추가 과도한 움직임으로 인해 이차 신경학적 손상을 초래할 수 있는 환자의 척추 움직임을 제한하는 것이다. 현재로서는 논란의 여지가 있지만, 일부 의사들은 조심스럽게 통나무굴리기법으로 움직이고 시트나 슬라이딩 보드를 사용하여 환자를 옮기고 구급차 주들것이나 침대에서 환자를 평평하게 유지함으로써 이러한 움직임 제한을 수행할 수 있다고 생각한다. 이러한 방법이 병원 내 환경에서 척추를 보호하는 표준 방법이지만, 병원 전 환경에서 불안정한 척추 부분의 변위 위험을 줄이기 위해 긴척추고정판, 분리형들것, 진공부목과 같은 장비를 사용하는 것이 더 안전하다고 생각하는 사람들도 있다. 병원 전 처치 제공자는 일부 환자에게 이차 신경학적 손상의 위험이 있으며 이러한 위험을 줄이기 위해 사용하는 모든 방법이 불필요한 신경학적 장애를 방지하기 위해 효과적이어야 한다는 점을 이해해야 한다. 이 텍스트에 포함된 일반적인 권장 사항에 대한 공감대가 형성되었지만, 척추 고정에 대한 현재의 과학적 연구와 이해는 아직 불완전하고 불안전하다는 점을 인정한다. 증거가 증가하고 권장 사항이 계속 발전함에 따라 임상 처치는 궁극적으로 프로토콜과 의료 지도의사가 승인한 장비 활용의 맥락에서 각 병원 전 처치 제공자의 책임이다.

　척추 고정은 몇 가지 방법으로 수행할 수 있다. 딱딱한 긴척추고정판은 짧은 시간 동안 사용하는 경우 효과적이고 적절하지만, 이 장비는 장기간 이송 시 불편하고 압박궤양 및 호흡 제한 등의 합병증을 유발할 수 있으므로 가능하면 피하는 것이 좋다. 분리형들것이나 진공부목이 딱딱한 긴척추고정판의 대안으로 사용할 수 있다. 이러한 장비는 적용하기 쉽고 더 편안할 수 있다(**Box 9-5**). 머리, 목, 몸통 및 골반을 각각 중립 자세로 고정하여 척수 손상을 초래할 수 있는 불안정한 척추가 더 이상 움직이지 않도록 해야 한다. 척추 움직임 제

분리형들것은 1943년 메인주 포틀랜드의 Wallace W. Robertson이 발명했으며 1947년 특허를 받았다. 이 들것의 발 끝부분에 하나의 개방형 조인트만 사용했다. 오늘날 우리가 알고 있는 두 개의 개방형 조인트가 있는 형태는 1970년 Ferno에 의해 특허를 받았다.

　분리형들것(그림 9-13)은 전통적으로 금속(알루미늄 또는 기타 경량 금속)으로 만들어졌지만, 최근에는 플라스틱이 더 일반적으로 사용되고 있다. 이 들것은 두 부분으로 구성된 장비로 분리된 반쪽을 과도한 조작 없이 환자의 양쪽 아래에 놓을 수 있다. 양쪽 부분을 함께 고정한 후 환자를 들어 올려 구급차 주들것이나 진공부목으로 옮길 수 있다.

　분리형들것은 접은 상태에서 길이는 약 1.6m, 너비 40cm, 환자의 키에 맞게 약 2.0m까지 길이를 조절할 수 있다. 분리형들것의 무게는 긴척추고정판과 비슷하다. 허용되는 환자의 체중 제한은 제조업체의 사양에 따라 다르다(일반적으로 160~300kg). 환자를 고정 끈으로 적절하게 고정하면 분리형들것은 환자를 장거리로 이송하는 장비를 사용할 수 있다. 분리형들것은 딱딱한 긴척추고정판보다 불편함이 적고 장비를 사용하는 동안 척추 움직임이 적을 수 있다는 증거가 일부 있다.

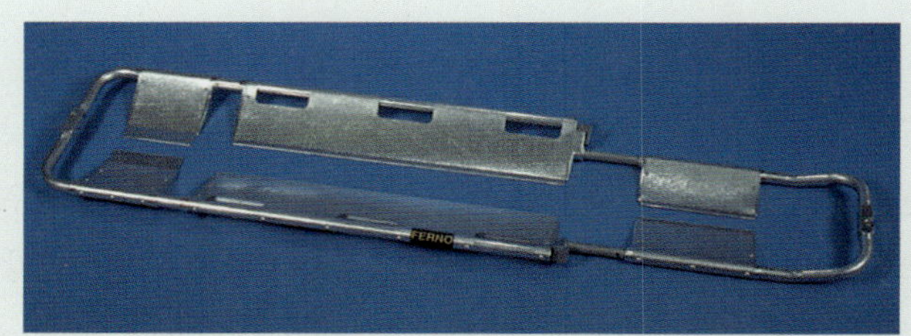

그림 9-13 분리형들것
© Jones & Bartlett Learning. Courtesy of MIEMSS.

© National Association of Emergency Medical Technicians (NAEMT)

한은 골절 처치의 일반적인 원칙인 손상 부위의 위쪽 관절과 아래쪽 관절을 고정한다. 척수의 해부학적 구조로 인해 이 고정 원칙은 척수 손상이 의심되는 관절의 위와 아래의 관절 이상으로 고정해야 한다. 척추의 위쪽 관절은 머리를 의미하고 아래쪽 관절은 골반을 의미한다.

　진공부목은 프랑스의 로드와 헤데렐레가 발명했다(**Box 9-6**). 다른 자료에서는 1960년대 후반 스웨덴 출신인 에릭 루네렐트가 진공 포장된 원두커피 패키지를 보고 아이디어를 얻었다고 한다.

　대부분의 의료 장비와 마찬가지로 진공부목은 다양한 제조사가 있으므로 병원 전 처치 제공자는 자신이 사용하는 장비에 대해 잘 알고 있어야 하며 자주 교육에 참여해야 한다.

　여러 연구에 따르면 진공부목은 딱딱한 긴척추고정판에 비해 환자에게 훨씬 더 높은 수준의 편안함을 제공하는 것으로 나타났다. 특히 진공부목은 대부분의 긴척추고정판과 마찬가지로 X-ray의 투과가 가능하기 때문에 응급실에서 환자가 검사받는 동안 제거할 필요가

© National Association of Emergency Medical Technicians (NAEMT)

없다.

긴척추고정판에 환자를 고정하면 머리를 쉽게 올릴 수 있다는 중요한 이점이 있다. 두개내압이 상승한 증거가 있고 외상성 뇌손상이 있는 특정 환자는 머리를 높이면 도움이 될 수 있다. 기도 폐쇄, 가슴 손상 또는 호흡 곤란이 있는 일부 환자는 머리를 높이면 기도 유지가 쉽고 환자가 바로 누워 있을 때보다 독립적으로 더 나은 호흡을 계속할 수 있다. 등허리 척추의 손상 가능성을 완전히 배제할 수 없는 상황에서는 일반적으로 단단한 장비를 사용하지 않는 환자의 머리를 안전하게 들어 올릴 수 있다. 바로누운자세의 환자를 위해 들것의 머리를 단순히 들어 올리면 환자가 반 앉은 자세로 이동하게 되어 불안정한 등허리 척추 손상이 있는 환자의 움직임, 정렬 불량 및 잠재적인 변위를 유발할 수 있다. 반대로 긴척추고정판에 누워 있는 환자의 머리를 들어올리기 위해 고정판 아래에 무언가를 놓거나 단단한 물

체를 사용하면 등허리, 척추의 굴곡 변형 없이 머리를 들어 올릴 수 있다. 진공부목이나 분리형들 것을 사용해도 같은 결과를 얻을 수 있다.

척추의 한 부위 골절은 종종 척추의 다른 부위 골절과 관련이 있다. 따라서 체중을 지탱하는 척추(목뼈, 등뼈, 허리뼈, 엉치뼈) 전체를 하나의 뼈로 간주하고 기저 손상이 의심되는 경우 적절한 고정을 시행하기 위해 척추 전체를 고정해야 한다는 것이 전통적인 교육이었다.

이 일반적인 규칙의 예외는 현장에서 걸을 수 있지만, 목의 통증만, 호소하는 환자에게서 발생한다. 환자의 의식 상태가 명료하고 신뢰할 수 있으며(GCS 정상, 약물 또는 알코올 사용 증거 없음) 요통이 없고 등에 압통이 없고, 원위부 신경 기능이 정상인 경우 등허리 척추의 안정화를 위해 척추 움직임 제한을 적용하는 것은 피할 수 있다. 경미한 목 통증의 경우 목을 안정시키기 위해 목뼈보호대만 착용하는 것만으로도 충분할 수 있다. 프로토콜에는 다양성이 있으며 의료 지도 의사가 이러한 환자에게 다른 고정 방법을 권장할 수 있다는 점을 이해한다.

환자는 일반적으로 앉은 자세, 옆 누운자세, 바로누운자세 또는 서 있는 자세 중 하나를 취한다. 척주 손상이 의심되는 경우 환자가 발견된 시점부터 기계적으로 고정될 때까지 환자의 척추를 즉각적이고 지속해서 브호하고 안정시켜야 한다. 도수 고정, 짧은 척추고정판, 고정 조끼, 분리형들것, 적절한 통나무굴리기법 및 완전한 도수 고정을 통한 신속 구출과 같은 술기와 장비는 환자의 척추를 보호하기 위해 사용되는 일시적인 방법이다. 이러한 술기를 사용하면 환자를 발견한 자세에서 결정적인 처치를 시행할 수 있는 의료기관에 도착할 때까지 안전하기 이동할 수 있다.

어떤 경우에는 앞서 언급한 장비 중 하나를 사용하여 척추 움직임을 완전히 제한하는 대신 척추 손상 예방조치를 취하는 것이 환자에게 도움이 될 수 있다. 척수 손상 예방 조치는 단단한 목뼈보호대를 적용하고 환자를 들것에 확실하게 고정하여 수행할 수 있다. 이 방법은 다음과 같은 상황에서 더 적절할 수 있다.

- 현장에서 보행이 가능한 환자

- 경중에서 중등도의 목 통증이 있고 신뢰할 수 있으며 신경학적 결손이나 불만이 없고 등이나 기타 등허리에 통증이 없는 환자

- 주의를 산만하게 하는 손상이 없고, 의식 수준이 정상이며 중독의 증거가 없어 긴척추고정판 또는 기타 척추 고정 장치의 적응증이 되지 않는 환자

척추 움직임 제한의 원리와 이러한 원리를 개별 환자의 필요에 맞게 수정하는 방법에 대한 이해 없이 특정 고정 장비에 지나치게 집중하는 경우가 많다. 특정 장비와 고정 방법은 모든 방법과 장비에 공통으로 적용되는 해부학적 원리를 이해해야만 안전하게 사용할 수 있다. 유연하지 않고 세부적인 장비 사용 방법은 현장에서 발견되는 다양한 조건을 충족하지 못한다. 사용하는 특정 장비나 방법과 관계없이 척추가 불안정한 환자의 처치는 다음 부문에 설명된 일반적인 단계를 따라야 한다.

일반적인 방법

외상 환자를 고정하기로 결정하면 다음과 같은 원칙을 따른다.

1. 환자의 머리를 적절한 중립 자세로 이동한다(금기 사항이 아닌 경우, 다음 부문 참조). 도수 고정과 중립 자세를 지속해서 유지한다.
2. 일차평가를 수행하여 환자를 평가하고 즉시 필요한 처치를 제공한다.
3. 환자의 상태가 허락하는 경우 팔다리에서 운동기능, 감각기능 및 순환 상태를 확인한다.
4. 환자의 목을 검사하고 적절한 크기의 목뼈보호대를 착용시킨다.
5. 척추의 불필요한 움직임 없이 조심스럽게 환자를 적절한 고정 장비로 옮긴다.
6. 환자의 몸통이 상하좌우로 움직이지 않도록 장비에 고정한다.
7. 필요에 따라 성인 환자의 머리 또는 소아 환자의 가슴 뒤쪽을 평가하고 패딩을 대어준다.
8. 환자의 머리를 중립적 자세로 유지하면서 장비에 고정한다.
9. 일차평가를 재평가하고 환자의 상태가 허락하는 경우 팔다리의 운동기능, 감각기능 및 순환 상태를 재평가한다.

머리를 중립 자세로 도수 고정

손상 기전을 통해 척추 손상이 있을 수 있다고 판단되면 첫 번째 단계는 도수 고정으로 머리의 안정화를 제공하는 것이다. 금기증이 없는 한 환자의 머리를 잡고 조심스럽게 중립 자세로 이동한다(다음 설명 참조). 적절한 중립 자세는 머리와 목에 큰 견인력 없이 유지된다. 머리와 몸통의 기계적 고정이 완료되거나 감사 결과 척추 고정이 필요하지 않은 것으로 확인될 때까지 머리는 도수 고정으로 중립 자세를 지속해서 유지해야 한다. 이러한 방식으로 환자의 머리와 목을 즉시 고정하고 필요한 경우 병원에서 검사가 끝날 때까지 고정 상태를 유지한다. 머리를 중립 위치로 이동하면 머리를 각진 상태로 환자를 고정하고 이송할 때보다 위험이 줄어든다. 또한 환자의 머리가 중립 위치에 있으면 환자의 고정과 이송이 훨씬 더 간단해진다.

금기증

환자의 머리를 중립 자세로 이동하는 것은 몇 가지 경우에 금기이다. 환자의 머리와 목을 중립 위치로 조심스럽게 움직일 때 다음 중 하나라도 발생하면 움직임을 중지해야 한다.

- 움직임에 대한 저항이 발생한 경우
- 목 근육 경련
- 통증 증가
- 무감각, 저리거나 운동 기능 상실과 같은 신경학적 결손이 발생하거나 증가
- 기도나 호흡에 문제가 발생한 경우

환자의 손상이 너무 심해서 머리가 어깨의 정중선에서 더 이상 벗어나지 않을 정도로 정렬이 잘못된 경우 중립 자세로 움직이려고 시도해서는 안 된다. 이러한 상황에서 환자의 머리는 처음에 발견된 자세로 움직이지 않도록 고정해야 한다. 다행히도 이러한 경우는 드물다.

단단한 목뼈보호대

단단한 목뼈보호대만으로는 완전한 고정을 제공할 수 없으며 단순히 목을 지지하는 데 도움을 준다. 환자를 이동하거나 이송 중 척추 움직임을 효과적으로 제한하려면 척추 움직임 제한 장비 또는 구급차 주들것에 환자를 고정해야 한다.

병원 전 척추 움직임 제한 방법은 이러한 장비가 환자를 외부적으로만 고정하고 피부와 근육 조직은 환자가 매우 잘 고정된 경우에도 골격에서 약간 움직이기 때문에 여전히 환자와 척추의 움직임이 어느 정도 허용되어야 한다. 대부분의 구조 상황에서 환자를 구출, 운반 및 환자를 구급차에 태우는 상황에서 어느 정도의 척추 움직임이 발생한다. 이러한 유형의 움직임은 구급차가 정상적인 주행 조건에서 가속 및 감속할 때도 발생한다.

효과적인 목뼈보호대는 가슴, 등뼈의 뒤쪽과 빗장뼈, 등세모근에 위치해서 조직의 움직임을 최소화한다. C6, C7 및 T1의 움직임은 여전히 허용하지만, 척추의 압박을 제한하는 데 도움이 된다. 머리는 아래턱뼈 각 부분과 두개골의 후두에 고정된다. 단단한 목뼈보호대

는 머리와 몸통 사이의 피할 수 없는 하중이 목뼈에서 목뼈보호대로 전달하여 목뼈의 압박이 발생할 수 있는 상황을 제한한다.

목뼈보호대는 척추와 머리를 완전히 고정하지는 못하지만, 머리의 움직임을 제한하는 데 도움이 된다. 목뼈보호대 앞쪽의 단단한 부분은 환자를 긴척추고정판에 고정 후 머리고정대로 고정할 때 앞쪽 목뼈보호대를 가로지르는 아래쪽 머리 고정끈이 안전하게 통과할 수 있는 경로를 제공한다.

목뼈보호대는 환자에게 맞는 크기를 사용해야 한다. 너무 짧은 목뼈보호대는 효과가 없으며 축 방향 하중으로 인해 척추의 과굴곡이나 압박을 유발할 수 있으며 너무 큰 목뼈보호대는 턱이 안으로 미끄러져 들어가 척추의 과신전 또는 목 전체의 움직임이 발생할 수 있다. 목뼈보호대를 너무 느슨하게 착용하면 머리를 고정하는 효과가 없고 실수로 앞쪽 턱, 입 및 코를 덮어 환자의 기도를 막을 수 있으며 너무 꽉 조이면 목정맥을 압박하여 두개내압을 증가시킬 수 있다.

다양한 종류의 단단한 목뼈보호대를 사용할 수 있다. 올바른 크기를 결정하는 방법과 장비의 적용은 제조업체의 권장 사항에 따라 적용해야 한다. 잘 맞지 않고 크기가 부적합한 목뼈보호대는 환자에게 도움이 되지 않으며 척추가 불안정한 경우 오히려 해로울 수 있다(**Box 9-7**).

목뼈보호대는 환자의 머리를 중립 자세로 유지한 후에 적용한다. 머리를 중립 자세로 유지할 수 없는 경우 목뼈보호대를 적용하지 않는다. 이 경우 담요나 수건 등을 말아 즉석에서 사용하면 고정에 도움을 줄 수 있다. 척추의 움직임 없이 아래턱뼈가 아래로 움직이지 않고 입이 벌어지지 않게 목뼈보호대를 착용하는 것은 환자가 구토할 때 위 내용물이 폐로 흡인될 수 있으므로 사용해서는 안 된다. 목뼈보호대를 사용할 수 없는 경우 환자를 고정하는 대체 방법으로 담요, 수건과 테이프 등을 사용할 수 있다. 병원 전 환경에서 이러한 유형의 환자를 접할 때 병원 전 처치 제공자는 창의력을 발휘해야 할 수 있다. 어떤 방법을 사용하든 척추 움직임 제한의 기본 개념을 따라야 한다(**Box 9-8**).

외상성 뇌손상 환자의 목뼈보호대 사용과 관련하여 두개내압이 증가했다는 보고가 있었다. 외상성 뇌손상이 의심되는 환자가 두개내압 증가의 명백한 징후를 보이면 목뼈보호대를 약간 느슨하게 풀어 주는 것을 고려한다.

고정판에 몸통 고정

사용하는 특정 장비와 관계없이 불안정한 척추 손상이 의심되는 환자는 몸통이 상하좌우로 움직이지 않도록 고정해야 한다. 이 장비는 환자의 몸통에 고정되어 머리와 목을 지지하고 고정할 수 있다. 환자의 몸통과 골반이 고정판에 고정되어 등뼈, 허리뼈 및 엉치뼈 부분이 지지되고 움직이지 않도록 한다. 머리를 고정하기 전에 몸통을 고정판에 고정해야 한다. 이렇게 하면 몸통을 고정 끈으로 고정할 때 발생할 수 있는 장비의 움직임으로 인해 목뼈가 움직이는 것을 방지할 수 있다.

고정판에 몸통을 고정하는 방법에는 여러 가지가 있다. 상반신(어깨 및 가슴)과 하반신(골반)을 상하좌우 어느 방향으로든 움직이지 않도록 하여 상체 척추의 압박과 측면 움직임을 방지할 수 있다. 상반신의 고정은 몇 가지 구체적인 방법으로 시행할 수 있으며 각 방법에 공통으로 적용되는 기본적인 해부학적 원리를 이해한다. 상반신이 머리 쪽으로 움직이는 것은 양쪽 어깨의 위쪽 가장자리보다 아래쪽 고정판에 그정하는 고정 끈을 사용하여 고정한 다음 어깨 위를 아랫부분에 고정한다(**그림 9-15**). 아래쪽으로의 움직임은 골반과 다리를 고정 끈으로 고정하여 움직임을 제한할 수 있다(**그림 9-16**).

한 가지 방법은 두 개의 고정 끈을 사용하여 상반신을 X자 모양으로 고정하는 것이다. 척추고정판 양쪽에서 시작한 고정 끈을 어깨 너머로 이동한 다음 가슴을 가로질러 반대쪽 겨드랑이를 통과하여 겨드랑이 부위의 고정판에 고정한다. 이 방법은 상반신의 위, 아래, 왼쪽 또는 오른쪽 움직임을 제한한다(**그림 9-17**).

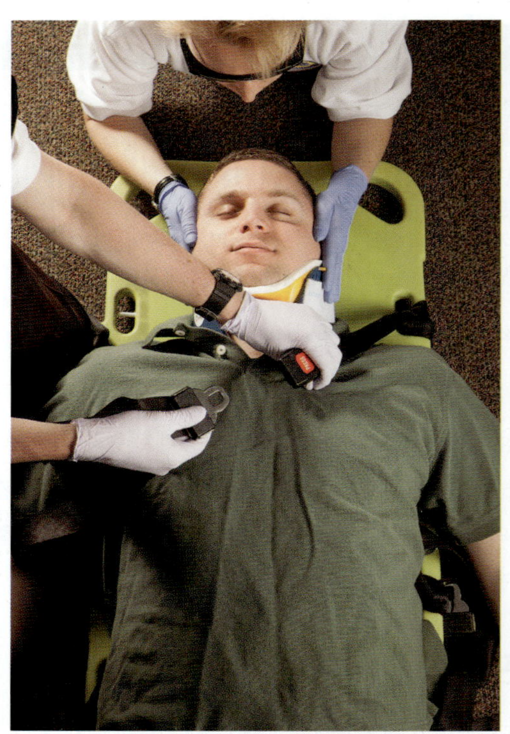

그림 9-15 상반신의 머리 쪽으로 움직이는 것은 양쪽의 고정 끈을 이용하여 X자 형태로 고정할 수 있다.

© Jones & Bartlett Learning. Photographed by Darren Stahlman.

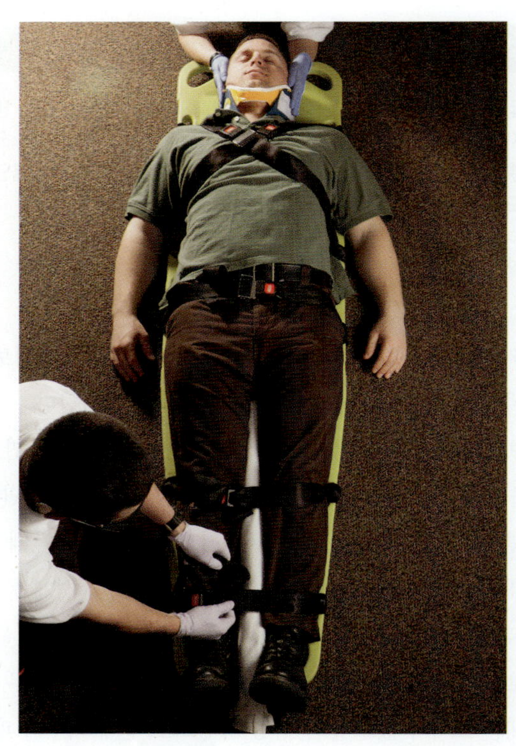

그림 9-16 골반과 다리를 고정할 수 있는 고정 끈을 사용하면 몸통의 움직임을 제한할 수 있다.

© Jones & Bartlett Learning. Photographed by Darren Stahlman.

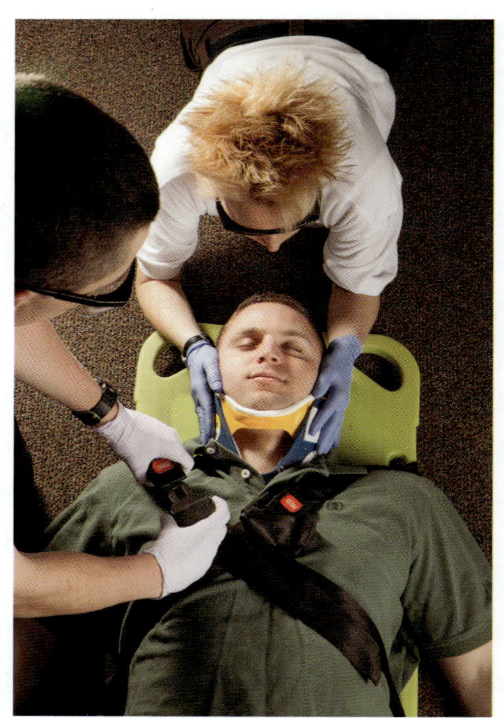

그림 9-17 두 개의 고정 끈을 사용하여 가슴 위쪽을 가로지르는 X자 모양을 만들면 상반신의 상하좌우 움직임을 막는 데 도움이 된다.

© Jones & Bartlett Learning. Photographed by Darren Stahlman.

하나의 고정을 고정판에 고정하고 한쪽 겨드랑이를 통과시킨 다음 가슴 위쪽을 가로질러 반대쪽 겨드랑이를 통과시켜 고정판의 다른 쪽에 고정한다. 그런 다음 고정 끈이나 삼각건을 양쪽에 추가하고 어깨 너머로 통과시켜 한 쌍의 멜빵과 비슷하게 겨드랑이 끈에 고정한다.

빗장뼈 골절 환자의 상반신 고정은 겨드랑이를 통해 각 어깨 주위에 배낭형 고리를 배치하고 각 고리의 끝을 같은 손잡이에 고정하여 이루어진다. 고정 끈은 상반신의 측면 가장자리 근처에 유지되며 빗장뼈를 가로지르지 않는다. 이러한 방법을 사용하면 고정 끈이 가슴의 위쪽 1/3 위에 있으며 일반적으로 가슴 아래에 꽉 조이는 고정 끈으로 인해 발생하는 환기 손상 없이 단단히 고정할 수 있다.

하체의 고정은 엉덩뼈능선에서 골반 위에 단단히 고정된 하나의 고정 끈을 사용하여 고정할 수 있다. 긴척추고정판을 위로 올리거나 계단이나 먼 거리를 이동해야 하는 경우 한 쌍의 서혜부 고정이 엉덩뼈능선을 가로지르는 단일 고정 끈보다 더 강력한 고정을 제공한다.

몸통 중앙에 고정 장비에서 멀어지는 측면 움직임이나 전방 움직임은 몸통 중앙에 추가 고정 끈을 사용하여 고정할 수 있다. 상부 가슴과 엉덩뼈능선 사이의 몸통을 고정하는 고정 끈은 환기 기능을 손상하거나 복강 내 압력을 많이 증가시킬 정도로 꽉 조이지 않아야 한다. 어떤 고정 장비나 기술을 사용하든 몸통과 머리를 고정판에 고정하는 것이 원칙이다. 선택되는 특정 장비와 기법은 병원 전 처치 제공자의 판단과 주어진 상황에 따라 달라진다.

척추고정판에 대한 논의

척추고정판은 전체 척추의 움직임 제한을 제공하지만, 척추고정판 자체에 대한 몇 가지 사실을 이해하는 것이 중요하다. 딱딱한 척추고정판에 누워 있는 환자에게는 매우 불편한 경험이다. 패딩이 없는 딱딱한 척추고정판에서 비교적 짧은 이송 시간에도 등에 대한 불편함을 호소할 수 있다. 또한 딱딱한 척추고정판에 고정되면 척추고정판과 접촉하는 뼈 돌출부에 상당한 압력이 가해진다. 일반적으로 가장 많이 영향을 받는 부위는 두피의 후두부, 어깨뼈, 궁둥뼈, 꼬리뼈와 발꿈치이다. 시간이 지남에 따라 이러한 부위의 순환이 손상되어 피부 허혈, 괴사 및 욕창 궤양으로 이어질 수 있다. 이러한 모든 요소는 병원 전 처치 제공자가 환자 아래에 패딩을 대어주고 환자가 척추고정판에 고정된 시간을 최소화해야 한다.

특히 비만 환자는 척추고정판에 바로누운자세로 고정하면 호흡기 손상을 경험할 수 있다.

이러한 모든 우려로 인해 척추고정판의 사용을 줄이려는 움직임이 증가하고 있다. 손상 기전에만 근거하여 너무 많은 환자를 불필요하게 고정하는 것은 분명하지만, 척추고정판을 둘러싼 개념적 틀은 무시할 수는 없다. 다른 처치와 마찬가지로 이러한 관리 전략의 적용은 신중하게 고려해야 한다. 또한, 잠재적인 합병증을 인식하여 척추 고정을 시행할 수 있는 유일한 방법은 아니지만, 척추고정판은 짧은 이송과 같은 일부 상황에서 유용하다.

목뼈보호대를 착용하고 바로누운자세로 구급차 주들것에 환자를 눕히는 것만으로도 척추 정렬을 유지하고 움직임을 제한할 수 있다. 이는 불안정한 목뼈 또는 등허리 손상이 공식적으로 진단된 후에도 병원에서 환자를 고정하는 데 사용되는 술기이다. 그러나 등허리 손상을 배제할 수 없는 경우 들것의 머리 부분을 들어 올려 환자를 앉게 하는 것은 안전하지 않다. 기도 보호를 강화하기 위해 머리를 높여야 하는 경우 역트렌델렌버그 자세로 해서 척추 전체가 수직으로 정렬되도록 한다. 그러나 병원에서는 여러 명이 시트를 사용하여 환자를 안전하게 움직일 수 있고 압력 궤양을 방지하기 위해 통나무굴리기법으로 환자의 위치를 변경할 수 있지만, 일반적으로 현장에서 수직으로 이동하거나 지형이 고르지 않은 장소로 이동할 필요가 없다.

또한 차량으로 과속방지턱을 지나 환자를 이송할 필요가 없으므로 병원에서는 척추 고정의 필요성이 현장만큼 중요하지는 않다.

또한, 미국 내 대부분의 EMS 이송 시간이 비교적 짧고 병원에서 환자가 척추 고정이나 고정을 유지해야 하는 시간이 상대적으로 기므로 병원에서 긴척추고정판 사용과 관련된 불편함의 정도는 병원 전 환경보다 훨씬 크며 이차 척추 변위와 그에 따른 이차 신경학적 손상의 위험은 상대적으로 적다. 그러므로 병원이나 외상센터에 도착한 직후 환자를 척추고정판이나 다른 고정 장비를 환자로부터 제거해야 하는 이유이다.

또한, 짧은 척추고정판 및 슬라이딩 보드와 같은 임시 장비를 사용하여 차량에서 환자를 안전하게 구출하고 긴척추고정판을 사용하지 않고 즉시 구급차 주들것으로 환자를 이동시킬 수 있다. 이 방법을 사용하려면 환자를 이송하는 동안 세부 사항에 더 많은 주의를 기울여야 하며 이송과 관련된 모든 인원이 이송 중에 척추 예방 조치를 유지해야 할 필요성에 대한 높은 수준의 인식이 필요하다. 병원 전 환경에서는 이러한 이송을 실행할 때 비교적 교육을 받지 않은 동료의 도움을 받는 경우가 드문 일이 아니기 때문에 이러한 수준의 통제를 유지하기가 어려울 수 있다. 그런데도 이 방법은 환자의 편안함을 높이고 생리학적으로 불안정한 환자의 현장 체류시간을 단축할 수 있다는 장점이 있다.

미국과 유럽에서는 병원 전 환경에서 긴척추고정판의 사용을 제한하려는 사례가 점점 더 빈번하게 증가하고 있지만, 현재까지 문헌에 따르면 치명적인 이차 신경학적 손상 발생률이 증가한다는 증거는 없다. 미국의 일부 EMS 기관에서는 긴척추고정판 사용을 중단했지만, 다른 기관에서는 환자를 이차적으로 치명적인 손상의 잠재적 위험에 노출하기보다 불편함을 줄이기 위해 척추고정판 사용을 수정하기로 했다. EMS 제공자는 시스템의 변화를 인지하고 최신 증거와 프로토콜 변경 사항에 대한 최신 정보를 파악하고 유지해야 한다.

머리를 중립 자세로 유지

많은 환자에서 머리를 중립 자세로 위치시킬 때 머리 뒤쪽 후두부의 가장 뒤쪽 부분이 가슴 뒤쪽 벽에서 1.3~8.9cm 앞쪽에 있다(**그림 9-18A**). 따라서 대부분 인에서 머리를 중립 자세로 유지하고 있을 때 머리 뒤쪽과 척추고정판 사이에 공간이 존재한다. 따라서 환자의 머리를 척추고정판에 고정하기 전에 적절하게 패딩을 대주어야 한다(**그림 9-18B**). 이 패딩을 효과적으로 사용하려면 쉽게 압축되지 않는 재질로 만들어야 한다. 이러한 용도로 만들어진 견고한 반 경성

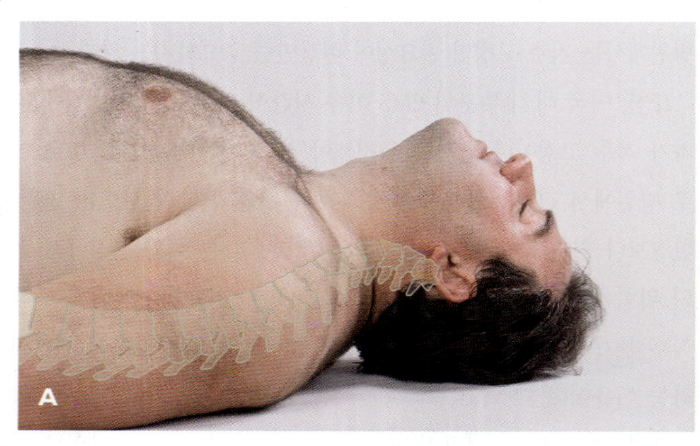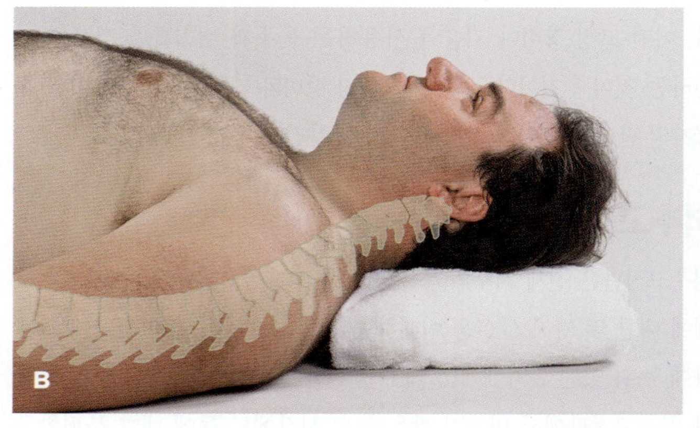

그림 9-18　**A.** 일부 환자의 경우 두개골이 척추고정판 높이까지 내려오도록 허용하면 척추가 심하게 과신전 될 수 있다. **B.** 이러한 환자의 경우 과신전을 방지하기 위해 머리 뒤쪽과 척추고정판 사이에 패딩을 대어준다.
© National Association of Emergency Medical Technicians (NAEMT)

패딩이나 접은 수건을 사용할 수 있다. 필요한 패딩의 양은 환자마다 개별적으로 결정해야 하며 일부 환자는 필요하지 않을 수도 있다. 패딩을 너무 적게 적용하거나 패딩으로 부적절한 스펀지 재질의 패딩을 사용하면 머리 고정 끈을 적용할 때 머리가 과신전 된다. 너무 많은 패딩을 적용하면 머리가 굴곡 된다. 머리의 과신전과 굴곡은 모두 척수 손상을 증가시킬 수 있으므로 피한다.

머리와 등 사이의 해부학적 관계는 대부분 사람이 바닥에 누워 있거나 척추고정판에 누워 있을 때도 같게 적용된다. 대부분 성인은 바로누운자세에서 머리가 뒤로 젖혀져 과신전이 된다. 현장에 도착하면 즉시 머리를 중립 자세로 이동하여 도수 고정으로 그 자세를 유지해야 하는데 이때 대부분 성인의 경우 머리를 지면에서 들어올려야 한다. 환자를 긴척추고정판에 눕히고 머리를 고정판에 고정하려는 경우 머리 뒤쪽과 고정판 사이에 적절하게 패딩을 삽입하여 중립 자세를 유지해야 한다. 이러한 원칙은 어깨 보호대를 착용한 운동선수와 심한 척주후만증 환자와 같이 척추가 비정상적으로 만곡된 환자를 포함한 모든 환자에게 적용한다.

일반적으로 7세 이하의 신체 크기를 가진 어린이의 경우 성인보다 머리의 크기가 신체의 나머지 부분에 비해 훨씬 크고 등 근육이 덜 발달되어 있다. 어린이의 머리가 중립 자세를 유지하고 있을 때 머리 뒤쪽은 일반적으로 등 뒤쪽 면보다 2.5~5cm까지 연장된다. 따라서 작은 소아를 딱딱한 표면에 직접 올려놓으면 머리가 굴곡된 위치로 움직이게 된다(**그림 9-19A**).

작은 소아를 표준형 긴척추고정판에 배치하면 머리와 목이 원치 않게 굴곡될 수 있다. 긴척추고정판은 후두부가 들어갈 수 있도록 고정판에 홈을 만들거나 몸통 아래에 패딩을 삽입하여 머리를 중립 자세로 유지하도록 만들어야 한다(**그림 9-19B**). 몸통 아래에 놓인 패딩은 머리가 중립 위치에서 고정판에 놓일 수 있도록 적절한 두께여야 하며 너무 두꺼우면 머리가 신전되고 너무 적으면 굴곡될 수 있다. 몸통 아래의 패딩은 단단하고 균일한 모양이어야 한다. 모양이 불규칙하거나 부적절한 패딩을 사용해서 어깨 아래에만 패딩을 넣으면 척추가 움직이거나 정렬이 틀어질 수 있다.

보호 장비를 착용한 선수가 손상을 입은 상황에서 척추고정판이나 기타 이송 장비에 위치하여 발생하는 바람직하지 않은 변형 문제는 특히 두드러진다. 보호 장비를 착용한 고에너지 운동선수의 척수 및 척추 외상은 추가 패딩을 포함한 안정화 방법을 신중하게 고려하고 잠재적으로 수정한다(**Box 9-9**).

완전한 고정

머리

환자의 몸통을 선택한 딱딱한 고정 장비에 고정하고 필요에 따라 머리 뒤쪽에 적절하게 패딩을 삽입한 후 머리를 장치에 고정한다. 머리는 둥근 모양이기 때문에 고정 끈이나 테이프만으로는 평평한 표면에 고정할 수 없다. 이것만 사용하면 머리가 옆으로 움직이거나 회전할 수 있다. 또한, 이마의 각도와 유분기가 많고 촉촉한 피부와 머리카락의 미끄러운 특성으로 인해 이마 위의 단순한 고정 끈은 안정적

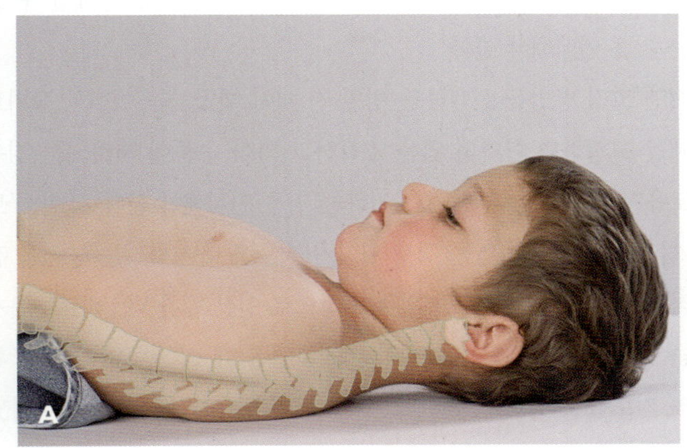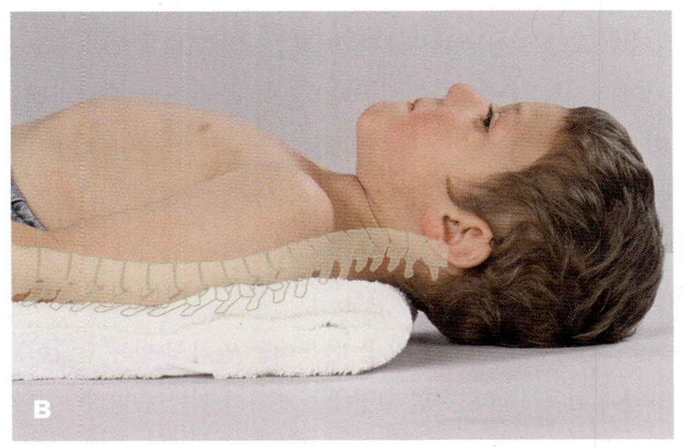

그림 9-19　**A.** 신체 크기에 비해 어린이의 머리 크기가 크고 등 쪽 가슴 근육이 발달이 감소하면 어린이를 척추고정판에 눕힐 때 머리가 과굴곡된다. **B.** 어깨와 몸통 아래에 패딩을 덧대면 이러한 과굴곡을 방지할 수 있다.

© National Association of Emergency Medical Technicians (NAEMT)

Box 9-9　운동선수 평가 및 운동 장비 제거

비교적 드물기는 하지만, 운동선수의 척추 외상은 잠재적으로 선수 생활의 종료와 인생을 바꿀 수 있는 사건이다. 스포츠 활동 중 외상은 미국 내 모든 외상성 척수 손상의 약 15%, 모든 척수 손상의 10% 그리고 모든 스포츠 관련 입원 환자의 2~3%를 차지한다. 손상이 발생하는 기전은 활동에 따라 다르다. 마찬가지로 특정 스포츠 활동은 다른 스포츠 활동보다 척수 손상 위험성이 더 높다. 레슬링, 체조 및 축구에 참여하는 미국의 운동선수들은 목 부위 척수 손상의 상당 부분을 차지한다. 고등학교 축구 선수들은 이 스포츠에 참가하는 다른 연령대보다 더 심각한 목 부위 척수 손상을 더 많이 겪고 있다. 하키는 척추 손상 위험이 상대적으로 높은 스포츠로 미국에서 하키의 인기가 계속 높아지면서 스포츠 관련 외상성 척추 손상이 더 많이 발생할 가능성이 높다. 병원 전 처치 제공자는 운동선수를 처치할 때 직면하는 고유한 문제(예: 헬멧 및 얼굴 마스크 등 보호 장비)를 인식하여 외상성 척추 손상이 의심되는 환자를 적절하게 평가하고 처치할 수 있도록 하는 것이 중요하다. 마찬가지로 EMS 시스템은 팀의 운동 트레이너 및 레크리에이션 스포츠 프로그램과 협력하여 모든 이해 관계자가 손상을 입은 운동선수의 안전하고 효과적인 병원 전 처치에 필요한 장비를 갖추고 교육을 받도록 해야 한다.

스포츠 관련 외상성 척추 손상의 평가와 처치는 환자를 현장에서 더욱 통제된 환경으로 이동하기 전에 주의를 기울여 환자가 발생한 모든 곳에서 시작해야 한다. 운동선수가 외상성 손상 기전에 노출되어 척추의 정중선 통증이나 압통, 운동 범위 감소 및 신경 학적 증상과 징후를 호소하는 경우 신중한 신체검사와 함께 도수로 척추 고정을 시행해야 한다. 지속적인 척추 움직임 제한이 적절한 경우(이 장의 앞부분에서 설명한 기준 참조) 병원 전 처치 제공자는 추가 평가를 위해 환자를 적절한 의료기관으로 이송할 수 있도록 주의 깊게 준비한다. 또한, 외상성 손상 후 의식이 없는 상태로 발견된 운동선수는 추가 평가를 통해 외상성 손상을 배제할 수 있을 때까지 외상성 척추 손상이 발생한 것으로 간주하여 처치한다. 이러한 결정을 뒷받침할 수 있는 증거는 제한적이지만, 현재로서는 지속적인 신경 학적 호소증상, 통증 또는 척추 운동 범위 감소가 있는 경우 운동선수의 경기 복귀를 허용해서는 안 된다고 권고하고 있다.

헬멧을 쓴 운동선수에게는 특별한 주의가 필요하지만, PHTLS 과정에서 가르치는 척추 고정의 일반적인 원칙이 적절하며 이를 따라야 한다. 보호대, 헬멧 또는 얼굴마스크와 같은 보호 장비를 착용하지 않은 환자는 척추 움직임 제한이 적용되는 다른 환자와 같은 방식으로 처치한다. 최근 미국 운동 트레이너협회(NATA)와 국제 EMS 관계자협회(NAEMSO)와 같은 전문기관에서 보호 장비 제거에 관한 권장 사항이 변경되었다. 선수와 발견했을 때 얼굴마스크가 장착된 헬멧을 착용하고 있는 경우 기도를 효과적으로 관리할 수 있는 충분한 접근이 가능하도록 얼굴마스크를 조심스럽게 제거해야 한다. 헬멧은 현장이나 응급실에서 벗을 수 있지만, 숙련된 인력이 충분히 지원할 수 있는 경우에만, 벗어야 한다. 헬멧과 어깨 패드를 일체형으로 벗는 것이 가장 이상적이다. 그러나 헬멧만 제거해도 목뼈의 과신전을 유발하지 않고 긴척추고정판 위에 선수를 고정할 수 있다. 어깨 패드를 제거하지 않으면 머리 뒤쪽에 패딩을 적절히 사용하여 머리를 나머지 척추와 중립 자세로 유지한다.

병원 전 처치 제공자는 손상을 입은 선수에게 필요한 의학적 요구 사항을 결정하고 이러한 요구 사항을 충족하기 위해 적절한 조치를 해야 하며 여기에는 종종 운동 장비를 즉시 제거하는 것이 포함될 수 있다. 어떤 결정을 내리든 척추 고정 방법은 보호용 운동 장비가 척추의 중립 자세 유지 능력에 어떤 영향을 미칠 수 있는지, 이송 및 이송 중에 과도한 척추 움직임을 방지할 수 있는지, 장비가 병원 전 환경에서 환자를 평가하거나 처치하는 데 제한이 되는지 등을 신중하게 고려하여 결정해야 한다. 운동 장비는 스포츠 장비 제거에 대해 훈련을 받고 경험이 있는 사람이 제거한다. 현장에서 장비를 제거하지 않기로 한 경우 스포츠 장비 제거에 대한 지식이 있는 사람이 환자와 함께 병원에 동행해야 한다.

이지 않고 쉽게 미끄러질 수 있다. 사람의 머리는 볼링공과 무게가 비슷하지만, 모양은 상당히 다르다. 머리는 난형으로 폭보다 길고 옆면이 거의 완전히 평평하며 볼링공과의 좌우를 약 5cm씩 잘라낸 모양과 비슷하다. 방법이나 장비와 관계없이 이 평평한 면에 패딩이나 말아 놓은 담요를 놓고 고정 끈이나 테이프로 고정하면 머리를 적절히 외부에서 고정할 수 있다. 조끼 형태의 장비면 조끼의 일부분인 옆 덮개를 이용하여 고정을 시행한다.

측면 고정대는 미리 성형된 폼 블록이든 말아서 만든 담요이든 머리 양옆에 위치시킨다. 측면 고정대는 환자의 귀만큼 넓거나 그 이상이어야 하며 환자가 누운 상태에서 적어도 환자의 눈높이만큼 높아야 한다. 머리고정대를 두 개의 고정 끈이나 테이프로 양옆을 서로 당겨 고정한다. 머리고정대나 담요 사이에 맞추어지면 머리는 이제 평편한 뒷면이 평평한 긴척추고정판에 고정된다. 이마 위쪽 부분의 고정 끈은 머리의 전방 움직임을 방지하기 위해 안와위 능선을 지나 이마의 아래쪽 전면에 걸쳐 고정한다. 테이프를 사용하는 경우 눈썹에 직접 붙이지 않도록 주의한다. 이 고정 끈은 머리고정대나 담요가 움푹 들어가도록 충분히 당겨 이마에 단단하게 고정해야 한다.

유형과 관계없이 머리를 고정하는 장비에는 측면을 머리 아래쪽에 단단히 밀착시키고 장비를 더 고정하고 머리와 목의 앞쪽 움직임을 방지하기 위해 아래쪽 고정 끈이 필요하다. 아래쪽 고정 끈은 측면부를 감싸고 목뼈보호대의 앞쪽 단단한 부분을 가로질러 통과한다. 이 고정 끈은 기도를 압박하거나 정맥 환류 문제를 일으킬 수 있는 목뼈보호대 앞쪽에 너무 많은 압력이 가해지지 않도록 고정한다.

고정된 환자를 옆으로 돌릴 때 머리나 목에 가해질 수 있는 무게 때문에 모래주머니는 측면 고정대로 사용하지 않는 것이 좋다. 긴척추고정판에 머리나 목의 측면을 고정하기 위해 모래주머니를 사용하는 것은 위험한 방법이다. 환자를 얼마나 잘 고정했는지에 관계없이 이러한 무거운 물체는 흔들리고 움직일 수 있다. 환자가 구토할 때와 같이 환자와 척추고정판을 옆으로 돌려야 하는 경우 모래주머니의 무게로 인해 머리와 목에 국소적인 측면 압력이 발생하여 움직일 수 있다. 환자를 이동하거나 구급차에 태우는 동안 척추고정판의 머리 부분을 올리거나 내리거나 구급차가 갑자기 가속이나 감속하면 모래 주머니가 흔들리고 머리와 목이 움직일 수 있다.

턱을 감싸는 턱받이나 고정 끈은 구토 시 입을 벌리는 것을 방해할 수 있으므로 이러한 장치를 사용해서는 안 된다.

어떤 안정화 방법을 선택하든지 처치 제공자는 이러한 장치로 목뼈의 고정이 환자의 입을 벌릴 수 있는 능력을 방해하고 의식 수준이 저하될 경우 기도유지를 위하여 기도에 접근하는 것을 방해할 수 있다는 것을 인식해야 한다.

어떤 고정 방법을 선택하든 병원 전 처치 제공자는 이러한 장비로 목뼈를 고정하면 환자의 입을 조작하고 의식 수준이 저하되는 경우 기도유지를 시행할 때 방해가 된다는 점을 인식해야 한다. 또한 구토나 입인두에 출혈이 있는 경우 환자가 기도를 유지하려는 능력을 잠재적으로 감소시킨다. 또한 척추 고정으로 인한 제한적인 바로누운자세는 측면으로 누워있는 자세와 비교하였을 때 의식이 없는 외상 환자의 기도를 개방하고 유지하는 능력을 감소시키는 것으로 나타났다. 이로 인해 기도 손상 위험이 증가한다.

턱 밀어올리기법은 다른 기도유지 방법에 비해 불안정한 목뼈 손상이 있는 경우 목의 움직임이 적다. 기도 유지가 필요한 경우 다른 병원 전 처치 제공자가 목뼈를 중립 자세로 고정한 상태에서 턱 밀어올리기를 수행하는 것이 좋다. 목뼈가 불안정한 상태에서 직접 후두경을 사용하여 기관내삽관을 시행하더라도 이러한 환자에서 이차적으로 치명적인 신경학적 손상의 위험은 나타나는 증상이나 징후 및 기전과 관계없이 적다는 점을 기억하는 것이 중요하다. 또한 구토하거나 입인두에 출혈이 있는 의식이 저하된 환자의 기도 손상 및 흡인의 위험은 실제적이고 잠재적으로 치명적일 수 있다는 점을 기억하는 것도 중요하다. 목뼈를 고정하는 과정에서 환자의 기도를 개방하고 유지하려는 능력이 손상되지 않도록 한다.

다리

발을 함께 묶으면 골반 골절이나 엉덩관절 골절로 인해 발생할 수 있는 다리의 심한 바깥쪽 회전을 방지할 수 있다. 다리 사이에 말은 담요나 패딩을 대어 주면 환자의 편안함을 높일 수 있다.

환자의 다리는 두 개 이상의 고정 끈으로 긴척추고정판에 고정한다. 하나의 고정 끈은 넓적다리 중간 정도에서 무릎의 근위부에 고정하고 다른 하나는 무릎의 원위부에 고정한다. 평균적인 성인의 경우 엉덩이의 한쪽에서 다른 쪽까지 35~50cm이고 한쪽 발목에서 다른 쪽 발목까지 15~23cm에 불과하다. 발을 모으면 엉덩이에서 발목까지 V자 모양이 형성된다. 발목은 긴척추고정판보다 상당히 좁으므로 다리 아래쪽을 고정 끈으로 고정하면 앞쪽으로의 움직임을 방지할 수 있지만, 긴척추고정판 양쪽 옆으로의 측면 움직임은 방지할 수 없다. 긴척추고정판이 기울어지거나 회전되면 다리가 긴척추고정판의 아래쪽 경계면으로 움직이게 되면서 골반이 움직이게 되고 척추가 움직임 수 있다.

환자의 다리를 효과적으로 고정할 수 있는 한 가지 방법은 긴척추고정판에 위치시키기 전에 끈으로 몇 번 감아 주는 것이다. 고정 끈을 묶기 전에 다리와 긴척추고정판의 가장자리 사이에 말은 담요를 대여 주어 척추고정판 중앙에 고정할 수 있다. 고정 끈을 너무 꽉 조여 말초 혈액순환을 방해하지 않도록 하는 것이 중요하다.

팔

안전을 위해서 환자를 이동하기 전에 환자의 팔을 척추고정판이나 몸통에 고정할 수 있다. 이를 위한 한 가지 방법은 손바닥을 안쪽으로 해서 척추고정판 양쪽에 팔을 위치시키고 아래팔과 몸통을 가로질러 고정 끈으로 고정하는 것이다. 말초 혈액순환을 방해할 정도로 고정 끈을 꽉 조이지 않도록 한다.

환자의 팔은 엉덩뼈능선이나 서혜부 고정 끈으로 같이 고정해서는 안 된다. 고정 끈으로 하반신을 적절히 고정할 수 있을 만큼 충분히 조이면 손의 순환을 방해할 수 있다. 고정 끈이 느슨하면 몸통이나 팔을 적절하게 고정하지 못한다. 팔을 고정하는 추가 고정 끈을 사용하면 환자가 구급차에 탑승한 후 혈압을 측정하거나 정맥 라인을 확보하기 위해 고정 끈을 풀어도 고정의 안전성 지장을 주지 않고 사용할 수 있다. 팔을 고정하는 끈으로 몸통을 같이 고정하면 팔을 풀어주면 몸통 고정도 함께 풀리는 부작용이 있다.

척추 고정 시 가장 일반적인 실수

다음은 척추 고정 시 가장 일반적인 실수이다.

1. 몸통이 척추고정판에서 위아래로 심하게 움직일 수 있거나 머리가 여전히 과도하게 움직일 수 있도록 척추 움직임 제한을 적절하게 제공하지 않는 경우
2. 목뼈보호대의 크기가 부적절하거나 부적절하게 적용한 경우
3. 머리를 과신전한 상태에서 환자를 고정한 경우이며 가장 흔한 원인은 머리 뒤에 적절한 패딩이 부족하기 때문이다.
4. 몸통보다 먼저 머리를 고정하거나 머리를 고정한 후 몸통 고정 끈을 재조정한다. 이렇게 하면 몸통에 대한 척추고정판의 움직임이 발생하여 머리와 목뼈가 움직일 수 있다.
5. 부적절하게 패딩을 사용한 경우이다. 바로누워 있는 환자와 척추고정판 사이의 공간을 채우지 않으면 척추가 의도치 않게 움직여 추가 손상을 초래할 수 있을 뿐만 아니라 환자의 불편함을 증가시킬 수 있다.
6. 척추 고정의 적응증에 해당하지 않는 환자에게 척추 고정을 시행한다.
7. 생리학적으로 불안정하거나 잠재적으로 불안정할 수 있는 환자에게 고정하는 데 과도한 기간을 사용하는 경우
8. 기도를 개방하고 유지하는 데 우선순위를 두지 않고 지나치게 적극적으로 고정을 시행한다.

완전한 척추 움직임 제한은 일반적으로 환자에게 편안한 경험이 아니다. 고정의 정도와 질이 높아질수록 환자의 편안함은 감소한다. 척추 고정은 척추를 완벽히 보호하고 고정해야 할 필요성, 기도를 유지하고 브로호해야 하는 필요성, 신속하게 이송을 시작해야 할 필요성과 환자가 견딜 수 있도록 해야 할 필요성 사이의 균형을 맞추는 것이 중요하다. 척추 고정의 필요성에 대한 적절한 평가가 필수적이다 (**Box 9-10**).

비만 환자

비만이 증가함에 따라 비만 환자의 처치가 더 빈번해지고 있다. 182kg의 환자를 이송하는 일은 매우 흔한 일이 되어가고 있으며 이를 위해 특수 비만 환자용 이송용 침대가 개발되었다. 그러나 미만 환자를 위해 특별히 설계되지 않은 들것 및 구출 장비를 사용할 때 안전한 작동 한계를 초과하지 않도록 각별한 주의가 필요하다. 또한 환자나 병원 전 처치 제공자에게 추가 손상을 유발하지 않도록 비만 환자를 들어 올리고 이동하기 위해 추가 인력이 있어야 한다. 이러한 외상 환자를 안전하게 고정하고 이송하면서 일반적으로 중증외상 환자에게 권장되는 현장 체류 시간을 최소화하는 것은 균형을 이루기가 매우 힘들다.

일부 비만 환자는 척추고정판에 바로누운자세로 위치하면 호흡부전으로 이어질 정도로 호흡량이 증가할 수 있다. 이러한 현상은 복부의 지방 조직에 의해 가로막에 가해지는 압력이 증가하기 때문에 이차적으로 발생한다. 이러한 경우에도 척추 움직임 제한의 원칙을 따라야 하지만, 관행을 변경해야 할 수도 있다. 잠재적인 목뼈 손상이 의심되는 비만 환자가 이송 중 들것에 앉은 채로 있는 동안 병원 전 처치 제공자가 도수 고정을 유지하고 목뼈보호대로 고정을 시행할 수 있다. 이 방법은 호흡 곤란을 증가시키지 않으면서 목뼈 고정을 시행할 수 있다.

임신한 환자

때때로 임신한 환자에게 척추 고정이 필요할 수 있다. 임신 주수에 따라서 환자를 완전히 바로누운자세를 취하는 경우 자궁에 의해 아

Box 9-10 척추 고정 술기 평가 기준

병원 전 처치 제공자는 실제 환자에게 사용하기 전에 모의 환자에게 고정 술기를 연습해야 한다. 새로운 방법이나 장비를 연습하거나 평가할 때 다음 기준은 처치가 척추 움직임 제한이 얼마나 효과적인지 측정하는 데 좋은 도구 역할을 한다.

1. 즉시 도수 고정으로 안정화를 유지하고 장비를 사용해서 고정할 때까지 유지한다.
2. 원위부에서 신경학적 기능을 확인한다.
3. 적절한 크기의 목뼈보호대를 적용한다.
4. 머리보다 몸통을 먼저 고정한다.
5. 몸통이 척추고정판 위아래로 움직이지 않도록 한다.
6. 고정 장비에 상반신과 하반신이 좌우로 움직이지 않도록 한다.
7. 가슴을 가로지르는 고정 끈이 가슴우리의 움직임을 방해하거나 환기 장애를 일으키지 않도록 한다.
8. 머리가 어떤 방향으로도 움직이지 않도록 효과적으로 고정한다.
9. 필요한 경우 머리 뒤에 패딩을 적용한다.
10. 머리를 중립 자세로 유지한다.
11. 입이 열리는 것을 방해하거나 방해하는 것이 없는지 기도를 개방하고 유지할 수 있도록 충분한 접근이 가능한지 확인한다.
12. 척추고정판과 환자를 옆으로 돌리더라도 다리가 앞, 뒤, 왼쪽, 오른쪽으로 움직이지 않도록 고정한다.
13. 골반과 다리를 중립 자세로 유지한다.
14. 팔이 척추고정판이나 몸통에 적절하게 고정되어 있는지 확인한다.
15. 고정 끈이 팔다리의 순환을 방해하지 않는지 확인한다.
16. 장비를 적용하는 동안 불안정한 척추를 손상할 수 있는 방식으로 환자에게 부딪히거나 움직이면 환자를 재평가한다.
17. 적절한 시간 내에 술기를 완료한다.
18. 원위부의 신경학적 기능을 재평가한다.

많은 방법과 변형이 이러한 목표를 달성할 수 있다. 특정 방법과 특정 장비의 선택은 현장 상황, 환자의 상태 및 사용할 수 있는 자원에 따라 결정해야 한다.

래대정맥이 압박되어 심장으로 돌아가는 정맥혈이 감소하여 임신한 환자의 혈압이 낮아질 수 있다. 이러한 상황에서 표준 방법으로 환자를 긴척추고정판에 고정해야 한다. 일단 고정이 완료되면 긴척추고정판을 비스듬히 기울여 환자를 상대적으로 왼쪽으로 기울인 자세로 해준다(환자의 오른쪽 아래에 담요나 패딩을 대어 주어 왼쪽이 아래로 향하게 하여 이 자세를 지탱할 수 있도록 한다). 이 자세를 취하면 자궁이 아래대정맥을 누르지 않아 혈압이 회복된다(**그림 9-20**).

스테로이드 사용

척수 손상 처치에 스테로이드를 사용하는 것은 논란의 여지가 있다. 국가 급성 척수 손상 연구(NASCIS) 연구는 급성 척수 손상에서 스테로이드 사용의 이점을 평가하기 위해 1984년, 1990년, 1997년에 수행된 다기관, 이중 맹검, 무작위 대조군 시험이다. 국가 급성 척수 손상 연구 I에서는 손상 후 8시간 이내에 고용량의 메틸프레드니솔론을 투여하면 무딘 외상으로 인한 급성 척추 손상 환자의 신경학적 결과를 개선할 수 있다고 제안했지만, 국가 급성 척수 손상 연구 II와 III에서는 이점을 발견하지 못했다. 2019년 미국 신경외과학회의 현재 국가 지침에서는 증거가 불충분하다는 이유로 척수 손상에 메틸프레드니솔론의 일상적인 사용을 권장하지 않는다. 스테로이드는 신경학적 결손이 있더라도 관통성 외상으로 인한 척수 손상에 대한 적응증도 없다.

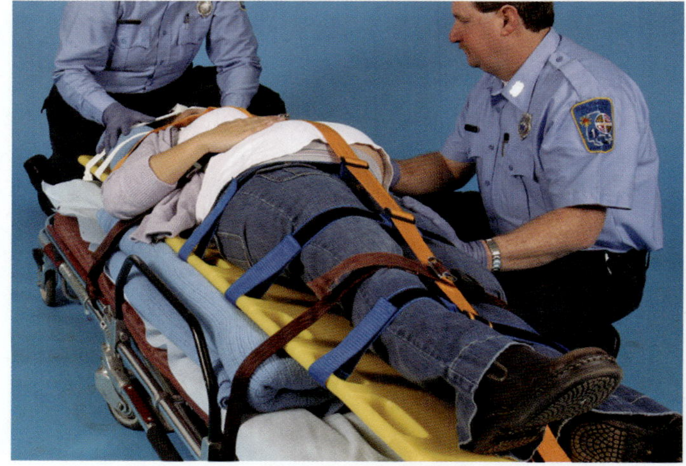

그림 9-20 임신한 환자를 왼쪽으로 기울이면 자궁이 아래대정맥을 누르는 것을 이동시켜 심장으로의 혈액 순환을 개선하여 혈압을 회복하는 데 도움이 된다.
© Jones & Bartlett Learning. Courtesy of MIEMSS.

스테로이드 사용은 부신 및 면역체계 억제를 포함한 수많은 부작용과 관련이 있다. 따라서 스테로이드 투여와 관련된 합병증의 위험은 스테로이드가 가져올 수 있는 이점보다 훨씬 더 클 수 있다. 수많은 출판물에서 더 이상 현장이나 병원에서 척수 손상에 대한 스테로이드 사용을 권장하지 않는다. 요약하면 현재 의학 문헌은 병원이나 병원 전 환경에서 척수 손상 환자에게 스테로이드를 투여하는 역할을 지지하지 않는다.

이송 지연

다른 손상과 마찬가지로 척추 및 척수 손상이 의심되거나 확인된 환자를 이송 지연할 때는 특별한 고려 사항이 필요하다. 긴척추고정판은 짧은 거리 또는 짧은 시간 이송하는 데 유용할 수 있지만 30분을 초과하는 기간 고정 장치로 사용해서는 안 된다. 이러한 노력은 척수 손상 환자의 압력 궤양 발생 위험을 줄이는 데 도움이 된다. 환자의 신체에 압력이 가해질 수 있는 모든 부위, 특히 뼈 돌출부위는 적절하게 패딩을 덧대야 한다. 환자 이송에 30분 이상 소요되는 경우 분리형들것을 사용하여 환자를 조심스럽게 들어 올리고 긴척추고정판을 제거한 다음 환자를 구급차 주들것에 눕히는 것을 고려해야 한다.

바로누운자세로 고정된 환자는 구토할 때 흡인의 위험이 있다. 환자가 구토를 시작하면 즉시 긴척추고정판과 환자를 즉시 옆으로 기울여야 한다. 흡인기는 구토가 발생하면 쉽게 사용할 수 있도록 환자의 머리 근처에 두어야 한다. 허용되는 경우 위관(코 위관, 입 위관)을 삽입하고 항구토제를 적절하게 사용하면 이러한 위험을 줄이는 데 도움이 될 수 있다.

상부 척수 손상은 가로막과 보조호흡근(예: 갈비 사이근)의 손상이 동반되어 호흡부전으로 이어질 수 있다. 임박한 호흡부전은 척추 고정을 위해 몸통을 고정한 고정 끈으로 인해 악화하고 호흡을 더욱 제한할 수 있다. 이송 지연을 시작하기 전에 병원 전 처치 제공자는 환자의 어깨와 골반, 몸통이 고정되어 있고 고정 끈이 호흡을 방해하지 않는지 다시 확인한다.

앞서 설명한 바와 같이 위쪽 척수 손상 환자는 신경성 쇼크로 인해 저혈압이 발생할 수 있다. 이러한 환자는 조직에 광범위한 저관류가 발생하는 경우는 드물지만, 일반적으로 결정질 수액만으로도 혈압을 정상적으로 회복할 수 있다. 신경성 쇼크를 처치하기 위해 혈압 상승제가 필요한 경우는 거의 없다. 목뼈 손상의 또 다른 특징은 서맥이다. 심각한 저혈압이 동반되면 서맥은 아트로핀 1.0mg을 간헐적으로 정맥 내로 투여하여 처치할 수 있다.

저혈압이 동반된 빈맥이 있으면 신경성 쇼크보다 저혈량 쇼크(출혈성 쇼크)를 의심해야 한다. 복강 내 출혈이나 골반 골절의 가능성이 가장 높지만, 주의 깊게 평가하면 출혈의 원인을 정확히 찾아낼 수 있다. 도뇨관을 삽입하면 소변 배출량을 측정하여 조직 관류의 또 다른 지침으로 사용할 수 있다. 성인의 경우 소변 배출량이 시간당 30~50mL 이상이면 일반적으로 말초 장기에 대한 충분한 혈액 관류를 의미한다. 척수 손상에 동반된 감각 상실은 의식이 있는 환자에서 감각이 없는 수준 이하의 복막염이나 다른 손상을 인지하지 못하게 할 수 있다.

척수 손상을 입은 환자는 심각한 등 통증이나 관련 골절로 인한 통증이 있을 수 있다. 통증이 완화될 때까지 소량의 마약성 진통제를 정맥 내로 투여하여 통증을 관리할 수 있다(자세한 내용은 12장 근골격 외상을 참조). 마약성 진통제는 척수 손상과 관련된 신경성 저혈압을 더 심하게 할 수 있다.

척추 손상 환자는 체온 조절 능력을 어느 정소 상실하며 이 영향은 척수의 높은 부위에서 손상을 입었을 때 더 두드러진다. 따라서 이러한 환자는 특히 추운 환경에 있을 때 저체온증 발병에 민감하다.

척추와 척수 손상은 정형외과 또는 신경외과 전문의가 있고 이러한 손상 처치에 대한 경험이 풍부한 의료기관에서 가장 잘 처치할 수 있다. 모든 Level I 및 Level II 외상센터는 척수 손상 및 모든 관련 손상을 처치할 수 있어야 한다. 척추 및 척수 손상을 전문적으로 처치하는 일부 전문 의료기관에서는 척수 손상만 입은 환자(예: 흡인의 증거가 없는 얕은 수중 다이빙 손상)를 입원시켜 치료할 수 있다.

요 약

- 척주는 24개의 분리된 척추와 엉치뼈, 꼬리뼈가 서로 겹쳐 있는 구조로 이루어져 있다.

- 척추의 주요 기능은 몸의 무게를 지탱하고 움직일 수 있게 하는 것이다.

- 척수는 척추 내에 둘러싸여 있으며 비정상적인 움직임과 자세로 인해 손상되기 쉽다. 척추 또는 척주를 제자리에 고정하는 근육 및 인대의 손상으로 인해 척주를 지지하는 기능이 손실되면 척수 손상이 발생할 수 있다.

- 병원 전 처치 제공자와 현장의 안전을 확인한 후 일차평가를 최우선으로 시행한다. 신속한 현장 평가와 손상 기전을 통해 척추 손상 가능성이 있는지를 결정해야 한다.

- 손상 기전은 척추 움직임 제한이 적절한지 아닌지를 결정하는 다양한 의사결정 과정에서 한 가지 효소에 불과하므로 척추 움직임 제한의 필요성을 결정하는 유일한 수단이 되어서는 안 된다. 척추 움직임 제한을 위한 목과 척추 평가에는 운동 및 감각 기능, 통증 또는 압통의 유무 그리고 척추 손상 위험의 예측 인자로 환자의 신뢰성도 함께 평가되어야 한다.

- 병원 전 처치 제공자는 척추 움직임 제한에 사용하는 장비(예를 들면, 분리형들것, 진공부목, 단단한 목뼈보호대)와 방법(예를 들면, 도수 고정, 머리 중립적 자세 유지)을 숙지하고 있어야 한다. 그리고 교육에 참여해 지침이나 최신 정보를 유지해야 한다.

- 비만 또는 임신한 환자를 포함한 특수 환자를 이송 지연하는 경우 표준 고정 관행을 수정해야 할 수 있다.

- 선택한 장비는 움직임을 유발하거나 허용하지 않고 머리, 가슴 및 골반 부위를 중립 자세로 고정해야 한다.

- 환자, 환자의 손상 정도 및 장비의 가용성에 따라 선택한 방법은 EMS 의료 지침에 따라 병원 전 처치 제공자의 판단에 따라 결정되어야 한다.

- 외상 환자의 성공적인 고정을 위해서는 장비를 적절하게 적용하고 고정하는 것이 가장 중요하다.

시나리오 재구성

당신은 도로에 자전거를 타다 넘어져 손상을 입은 환자가 있다는 신고를 받고 현장으로 출동했다. 현장에 도착했을 때 경찰관이 교통을 통제하고 있었고 현장은 안전하다. 젊은 여성인 환자는 길가에 누워있다. 경찰관이 그녀 옆에 무릎을 꿇고 대화를 시도하고 있지만, 환자는 아무런 반응이 없다.

일차평가를 시작할 때 자전거를 타다가 넘어지게 된 구체적인 원인을 확인할 수 없었다. 여성이 도로를 달리던 중 넘어진 것으로 보이지만, 자동차에 치였는지는 알 수 없다. 경찰관에 따르면 목격자는 없다. 환자는 헬멧과 장갑을 포함한 안전 장비를 착용하고 있다. 이마에 찰과상이 있고 오른쪽 손목에 명백한 변형이 있다. 기도는 개방되어 있고 규칙적으로 호흡을 하고 있다. 외부출혈의 명백한 징후는 보이지 않는다. 피부는 건조하고 따뜻하며 정상적인 색을 띠고 있었다. 일차평가를 시행하는 동안 환자는 깨어났지만, 무슨 일이 있었는지 혼란스러워한다.

- 환자의 증상을 설명할 수 있는 병리학적 과정은 무엇인가?
- 어떤 즉각적인 처치와 추가 평가가 필요한가?
- 이 환자의 처치 목표는 무엇인가?

시나리오 해결책

환자의 활력징후는 다음과 같다. 맥박 66회/분, 호흡 14회/분, 혈압 96/70mmHg이다. 당신은 신체검사를 계속하면서 환자가 팔이나 다리를 움직이지 못한다는 것을 확인한다. 활력징후와 신체검사 소견은 신경성 저혈압을 암시한다. 교감신경계의 차단과 척추 손상 부위 아래의 혈관계에 대한 부교감신경계의 영향으로 혈관 용적이 증가하고 상대적인 저혈량증을 초래한다. 척수 손상에 대한 환자의 반응은 저혈압과 서맥이다.

처치의 첫 번째 우선순위는 기도 유지와 산소 공급을 계속 유지하고 필요한 경우 환기를 보조하여 적절한 분당 호흡량을 확보하는 동시에 목뼈를 도수로 고정하는 것이다. 환자를 효과적이고 효율적으로 긴척추고정판에 고정하고 9분 거리에 있는 적절한 의료기관으로

(다음 페이지에 계속)

시나리오 해결책 (이어서)

환자를 이송한다. 척수 손상으로 인한 신경성 저혈압을 정맥 라인을 확보하여 두 차례에 걸쳐 250mL의 수액을 투여한다. 이송하는 동안 골절된 팔은 부목으로 고정한다.

이 환자의 병원 전 처치 목표는 추가적인 척수 손상을 예방하고 조직 관류를 유지하며 이송 중 팔다리의 외상을 처치하고 최종 처치를 위해 적절한 의료기관으로 신속하게 이송하는 것이다.

References

1. Jain NB, Ayers GD, Peterson EN, et al. Traumatic spinal cord injury in the United States, 1993–2012. *JAMA*. 2015;313(22):2236-2243. doi: 10.1001/jama.2015.6250

2. *Spinal Cord Injury: Facts and Figures at a Glance* [SCI data sheet]. National SCI Statistical Center; 2021.

3. Singh A, Tetreault L, Kalsi-Ryan S, Nouri A, Fehlings MG. Global prevalence and incidence of traumatic spinal cord injury. *Clin Epidemiol*. 2014;6:309-331.

4. DeVivo M, Chen Y, Mennemeyer S, Deutsch A. Costs of care following spinal cord injury. *Top Spinal Cord Inj Rehab*. 2011;16(4):1-9.

5. Meldon SW, Moettus LN. Thoracolumbar spine fractures: clinical presentation and the effect of altered sensorium and major injury. *J Trauma*. 1995;38:1110-1114.

6. Ross SE, O'Malley KF, DeLong WG, et al. Clinical predictors of unstable cervical spine injury in multiply-injured patients. *Injury*. 1992;23:317-319.

7. Greenbaum J, Walters N, Levy PD. An evidence-based approach to radiographic assessment of cervical spine injuries in the emergency department. *J Emerg Med*. 2009;36(1):64-71.

8. Stein DM, Knight WA IV. Emergency neurological life support: traumatic spine injury. *Neurocrit Care Soc*. 2017;27:S170-S180.

9. Hu R, Mustard CA, Burns B. Epidemiology of incident spinal fracture in a complete population. *Spine*. 1996;21(4):492-499.

10. Wood KB, Buttermann GR, Phukan R, et al. Operative compared with nonoperative treatment of a thoracolumbar burst fracture without neurological deficit: a prospective randomized study with follow-up at 16 and 22 years. *J Bone Joint Surg Am*. 2015;97:3-9.

11. Wood KB, Buttermann GR, Mehob A, Garvey T, Jhanjee R, Sechriest V. Operative compared with nonoperative treatment of a thoracolumbar burst fracture without neurological deficit: a prospective, randomized study. *J Bone Joint Surg Am*. 2003;85(5):773-781.

12. Adams MA, Dolan P. Spine biomechanics. *J Biomech*. 2005;38(10):1972-1983.

13. Izzo R, Guarnieri G, Guglielmi G, Muto M. Biomechanics of the spine. Part 1: spinal stability. *Eur J Radiol*. 2013;82:118-126.

14. Dreischarf M, Shirazi-Adl A, Arjmand N, Rohlmann A, Schmidt H. Estimation of loads on human lumbar spine: a review of *in vivo* and computational model studies. *J Biomech*. 2016;49:833-845.

15. Oxland TR. Fundamental biomechanics of the spine: what we have learned in the past 25 years and future directions. *J Biomechan*. 2016;49:817-832.

16. Leucht P, Fischer K, Muhr G, Mueller EJ. Epidemiology of traumatic spine fractures. *Injury*. 2009;40:166-172.

17. Lindsey RW, Gugala Z, Pneumaticos SG. Injury to the vertebrae and spinal cord. In: Feliciano DV, Mattox KL, Moore EE, eds. *Trauma*. McGraw Hill; 2008:479-510.

18. Jawa RS, Singer AJ, Rutigliano DN, et al. Spinal fractures in older adult patients admitted after low-level falls: 10-year incidence and outcomes. *J Am Geriatr Soc*. 2017;65(5):909-915.

19. Katsuura Y, Osborn JM, Cason GW. The epidemiology of thoracolumbar trauma: a meta-analysis. *J Orthop*. 2016;13:383-388.

20. Shin JI, Lee NJ, Cho SK. Pediatric cervical spine and spinal cord injury: a national database study. *Spine*. 2016;41(4):283-292.

21. Mohseni S, Talving P, Castelo Branco B, et al. Effect of age on cervical spine injury in pediatric population: a National Trauma Data Bank review. *J Pediatr Surg*. 2011;46:1771-1776.

22. Easter JS, Barkin R, Rosen CL, Ban K. Cervical spine injuries in children, part 1: mechanism of injury, clinical presentation, and imaging. *J Emerg Med*. 2011;41(2):142-150.

23. Patel JC, Tepas JJ III, Mollitt DL, Pieper P. Pediatric cervical spine injuries: defining the disease. *J Pediatr Surg*. 2001;36(2):373-376.

24. Parent S, Mac-Thiong J-M, Roy-Beaudry M, Sosa JF, Labelle H. Spinal cord injury in the pediatric population: a systematic review of the literature. *J Neurotrauma*. 2011;28:1515-1524.

25. Piatt JH Jr. Pediatric spinal injury in the US: epidemiology and disparities. *J Neurosurg Pediatr*. 2015;16:463-471.

26. Tator CH, Fehlings MG. Review of the secondary injury theory of acute spinal cord trauma with special emphasis on vascular mechanisms. *J Neurosurg*. 1991;75:15-26.

27. Tator CH. Spinal cord syndromes: physiologic and anatomic correlations. In: Menezes AH, Sonntag VKH, eds. *Principles of Spinal Surgery*. McGraw-Hill; 1995.

28. Ahuja CS, Martin AR, Fehlings M. Recent advances in managing a spinal cord injury secondary to trauma. *F1000Res*. 2016;5:ii.

29. Wu C, Fry CH, Henry J. The mode of action of several opioids on cardiac muscle. *Exp Physiol*. 1997;82:261-272.

30. Vale FL, Burns J, Jackson AB, Hadley MN. Combined medical and surgical treatment after acute spinal cord injury: results of a prospective pilot study to assess the merits of aggressive medical resuscitation and blood pressure management. *J Neurosurg*. 1997;87:239-246.

31. Bernhard M, Gries A, Kremer P, Bottiger BW. Spinal cord injury (SCI)—prehospital management. *Resuscitation*. 2005;66:127-139.

32. Dhall SS, Dailey AT, Anderson PA, et al. Congress of Neurological Surgeons systematic review and evidence-based guidelines on the evaluation and treatment of patients with thoracolumbar spine trauma: hemodynamic management. *Neurosurgery*. 2019;84(1):E43-E45.

33. Catapano JS, Hawryluk GWJ, Whetstone W, et al. Higher mean arterial pressure values correlate with neurologic improvement in patients with initially complete spinal cord injuries. *World Neurosurg*. 2016;96:72-79.

34. Carrick MM, Leonard J, Slone DS, Mains CW, Bar-Or D. Hypotensive resuscitation among trauma patients. *Biomed Res Int*. 2016;2016:8901938.

35. Ryken TC, Hurlbert RJ, Hadley MN, et al. The acute cardiopulmonary management of patients with cervical spinal cord injuries. *Neurosurgery*. 2013;72:84-92.

36. Bilello JP, Davis JW, Cunningham MA, et al. Cervical spinal cord injury and the need for cardiovascular intervention. *Arch Surg*. 2003;138:1127-1129.

37. Heffernan DS, Schermer CR, Lu SW. What defines a distracting injury in cervical spine assessment? *J Trauma Inj Infect Crit Care*. 2005;59(6):1396-1399.

38. Cason B, Rostas J, Simmons J, Frotan MA, Brevard SB, Gonzalez RP. Thoracolumbar spine clearance: clinical examination for patients with distracting injuries. *J Trauma Acute Care Surg*. 2015;80(1):125-130.

39. Konstantinidis A, Plurad D, Barmparas G, et al. The presence of nonthoracic distracting injuries does not affect the initial clinical examination of the cervical spine in evaluable blunt trauma patients: a prospective observational study. *J Trauma Inj Infect Crit Care*. 2011;71(3):528-532.

40. Lindborg R, Jambhekar A, Chan V, Laskey D, Rucinski A, Fahoum B. Distracting injury defined: does an isolated hip fracture constitute a distracting injury for clearance of the cervical spine? *Emerg Radiol*. 2018 Feb;25(1):35-39.

41. Young AJ, Wolfe L, Tinkoff G, Duane TM. Assessing incidence and risk factors of cervical spine injury in blunt trauma patients using the National Trauma Data Bank. *Am Surg*. 2015;81:879-883.

42. Hills MW, Deane SA. Head injury and facial injury: is there an increased risk of cervical spine injury. *J Trauma*. 1993;34(4):549-553.

43. Shekhar H, Kahn S. Cervical spine injuries. *Orthopaed Trauma*. 2016;30(5):390-401.

44. Connell RA, Graham CA, Munro PT. Is spinal immobilization necessary for all patients sustaining isolated penetrating trauma? *Injury*. 2003;34:912-914.

45. Fischer PE, Perina DG, Delbridge TR, et al. Spinal motion restriction in the trauma patient: a joint position statement. *Prehosp Emerg Care*. 2018;22(6):659-661. doi: 10.1080/10903127.2018.1481476

46. National Association of EMS Physicians and American College of Surgeons Committee on Trauma. EMS spinal precautions and the use of the long backboard. *Prehosp Emerg Care*. 2013;17(3):392-393.

47. Stuke LE, Pons PT, Guy JS, Chapleau WP, Butler FK, McSwain NE. Prehospital spine immobilization for penetrating trauma: review and recommendations from the Prehospital Trauma Life Support Executive Committee. *J Trauma Inj Infect Crit Care*. 2011;71(3):763-770.

48. Haut ER, Kalish BT, Efron DT, et al. Spine immobilization in penetrating trauma: more harm than good? *J Trauma Inj Infect Crit Care*. 2010;68(1):115-121.

49. Abram S, Bulstrode C. Routine spinal immobilization in trauma patients: what are the advantages and disadvantages? *Surgeon*. 2010;8:218-222.

50. Kennedy FR, Gonzales P, Beitler A, et al. Incidence of cervical spine injuries in patients with gunshot wounds to the head. *Southern Med J*. 1994;87:621-623.

51. Chong CL, Ware DN, Harris JH. Is cervical spine imaging indicated in gunshot wounds to the cranium? *J Trauma*. 1998;44:501-502.

52. Kaups KL, Davis JW. Patients with gunshot wounds to the head do not require cervical spine immobilization and evaluation. *J Trauma*. 1998;44:865-867.

53. Lanoix R, Gupta R, Leak L, Pierre J. C-spine injury associated with gunshot wounds to the head: retrospective study and literature review. *J Trauma*. 2000;49:860-863.

54. Barkana Y, Stein M, Scope A, et al. Prehospital stabilization of the cervical spine for penetrating injuries of the neck: is it necessary? *Injury*. 2003;34:912.

55. Cornwell EE, Chang, DC, Boner JP, et al. Thoracolumbar immobilization for trauma patients with torso gunshot wounds—is it necessary? *Arch Surg*. 2001;136:324-327.

56. American College of Surgeons Committee on Trauma. *Advanced Trauma Life Support for Doctors*. 9th ed. American College of Surgeons; 2012.

57. Ullrich A, Hendey GW, Geiderman J, et al. Distracting painful injuries associated with cervical spinal injuries in blunt trauma. *Acad Emerg Med*. 2001;8:25-29.

58. Domeier RM, Evans RW, Swor RA, et al. Prospective validation of out-of-hospital spinal clearance criteria: a preliminary report. *Acad Emerg Med*. 1997;4:643-646.

59. Domeier RM, Swor RA, Evans RW, et al. Multicenter prospective validation of prehospital clinical spinal clearance criteria. *J Trauma*. 2002;53:744-750.

60. Hankins DG, Rivera-Rivera EJ, Ornato JP, et al. Spinal immobilization in the field: clinical clearance criteria and implementation. *Prehosp Emerg Care*. 2001;5:88-93.

61. Stroh G, Braude D. Can an out-of-hospital cervical spine clearance protocol identify all patients with injuries? An argument for selective immobilization. *Ann Emerg Med*. 2001;37:609-615.

62. Dunn TM, Dalton A, Dorfman T, et al. Are emergency medical technician-basics able to use a selective immobilization of the cervical spine protocol? A preliminary report. *Prehosp Emerg Care*. 2004;8:207-211.

63. Domeier RM, Frederiksen SM, Welch K. Prospective performance assessment of an out-of-hospital protocol for selective spine immobilization using clinical spine clearance criteria. *Ann Emerg Med*. 2005;46:123-131.

64. Domeier RM, National Association of EMS Physicians Standards and Practice Committee. Indications for prehospital spinal immobilization. *Prehosp Emerg Care*. 1997;3:251-253.

65. Kwan I, Bunn F. Effects of prehospital spinal immobilization: a systematic review of randomized trials on healthy subjects. *Prehosp Disast Med*. 2005;20:47-53.

66. Akkuş Ş, Çorbacıoğlu ŞK, Çevik Y, Akıncı E, Uzunosmanoğlu H. Effects of spinal immobilization at 20° on respiratory functions. *Am J Emerg Med*. 2016;34:1959-1962.

67. Ham WHW, Shoonhoven L, Schuurmans MJ, Leenen LPH. Pressure ulcer development in trauma patients with suspected spinal injury: the influence of risk factors present in the emergency department. *Int Emerg Nurs*. 2017;30:13-19.

68. Ham WHW, Shoonhoven L, Schuurmans MJ, Leenen LPH. Pressure ulcers, indentation marks and pain from cervical spine immobilization with extrication collars and headblocks: an observational study. *Injury*. 2016;47:1924-1931.

69. Robinson WW, inventor. Scoop stretcher. U.S. patent 2417378. December 28, 1943.

70. Krell JM, McCoy MS, Sparto PJ, Fisher GL, Stoy WA, Hostler DP. Comparison of the Ferno scoop stretcher with the long backboard for spinal immobilization. *Prehosp Emerg Care*. 2006;10(1):46-51.

71. Lovell ME, Evans JH. A comparison of the spinal board and the vacuum stretcher, spinal stability and interface pressure. *Injury*. 1994;25(3):179-180.

72. Chan D, Goldberg RM, Mason J, Chan L. Backboard versus mattress splint immobilization: a comparison of symptoms generated. *J Emerg Med*. 1996;14(3):293-298.

73. Johnson DR, Hauswald M, Stockhoff C. Comparison of a vacuum splint device to a rigid backboard for spinal immobilization. *Am J Emerg Med*. 1996;14(4):369-372.

74. Hamilton RS, Pons PT. The efficacy and comfort of full-body vacuum splints for cervical-spine immobilization. *J Emerg Med*. 1996;14(5):553-559.

75. Cross DA, Baskerville J. Comparison of perceived pain with different immobilization techniques. *Prehosp Emerg Care*. 2001;5(3):270-274.

76. Luscombe MD, Williams JL. Comparison of a long spinal board and vacuum mattress for spinal immobilisation. *Emerg Med J*. 2003;20(5):476-478.

77. Ben-Galim P, Dreiangel N, Mattox KL, Reitman CA, Kalantar SB, Hipp JA. Extrication collars can result in abnormal separation between vertebrae in the presence of a dissociative injury. *J Trauma*. 2010;69(2):447-450.

78. Ho AMH, Fung KY, Joynt GM, Karmakar KM, Peng Z. Rigid cervical collar and intracranial pressure of patients with severe head injury. *J Trauma*. 2002;53:1185-1188.

79. Mobbs RJ, Stoodley MA, Fuller JF. Effect of cervical hard collar on intracranial pressure after head injury. *Anz J Surg*. 2002;72:389-391.

80. DeBoer SL, Seaver M. Big head, little body syndrome: what EMS providers need to know. *Emerg Med Serv*. 2004;33:47-52.

81. Nalliah RP, Anderson IM, Lee MK, Rampa S, Allareddy V, Allareddy V. Epidemiology of hospital-based emergency department visits due to sports injuries. *Pediatr Emerg Care*. 2014;30(8):511-515.

82. UAB Spinal Cord Injury Model System Information Network. The UAB-SCIMS information network. University of Alabama School of Medicine website. Accessed February 4, 2018. www.spinalcord.uab.edu

83. Puvanesurajah V, Qureshi R, Cancienne JM, Hassanzadeh H. Traumatic sports-related cervical spine injuries. *Trauma Spine Inj*. 2017;30(2):50-56.

84. Banerjee R, Palumbo MA, Fadale PD. Catastrophic cervical spine injuries in the collision sport athlete, part 1: epidemiology, functional anatomy, and diagnosis. *Am J Sports Med*. 2004;32(4):1077-1087.

85. Appropriate Care of the Spine Injured Athlete. National Athletic Trainers' Association. Updated August 5, 2015. Accessed February 4, 2018. https://www.nata.org/sites/default/files/Executive-Summary-Spine-Injury-updated.pdf

86. Schroeder GD, Vaccaro AR. Cervical spine injuries in the athlete. *J Am Acad Orthop Surg*. 2016;24(9):e122-e133.

87. Response to the National Athletic Trainers Association: appropriate care of the spine injured athlete; inter-association consensus statement. National Association of State EMS Officials. Published October 27, 2015. Accessed March 4, 2018. https://www.nasemso.org/Councils/MedicalDirectors/documents/NASEMSO-Response-to-NATA-Care-of-Spine-Injured-Athlete.pdf

88. Nesathurai S. Steroids and spinal cord injury: revisiting the NASCIS 2 and NASCIS 3 trials. *J Trauma*. 1998;45:1088-1093.

89. Hyldmo PK, Vist GE, Feyling AC, et al. Is the supine position associated with loss of airway patency in unconscious trauma patients? A systematic review and meta-analysis. *Scan J Trauma Resusc Emerg Med*. 2013;23:50.

90. Prasarn ML, Horodyski EB, Scott NE, Konopka G, Conrad B, Rechtine GR. Motion generated in the unstable upper cervical spine during head tilt–chin lift and jaw thrust maneuvers. *Spine J*. 2014;14:609-614.

91. Hindman BJ, From RP, Fontes RB, et al. Intubation biomechanics: laryngoscope force and cervical spine motion during intubation in cadavers—cadavers vs. patients, the effect of repeated intubations, and the effect of type II odontoid fracture on C1-C2 motion. *Anesthesiology*. 2015;123(5):1042-1058.

92. Bracken MB, Collins WF, Freeman DF, et al. Efficacy of methylprednisolone in acute spinal cord injury. *JAMA*. 1984;251(1):45-52.

93. Bracken MB, Shepard MJ, Collins WF, et al. A randomized, controlled trial of methylprednisolone or naloxone in the treatment of acute spinal-cord injury: results of the Second National Acute Spinal Cord Injury Study. *N Engl J Med*. 1990;322(20):1405-1411. doi: 10.1056/NEJM199005173222001

94. Bracken MB, Shepard MJ, Holford TR, et al. Administration of methylprednisolone for 24 or 48 hours or tirilazad mesylate for 48 hours in the treatment of acute spinal cord injury: results of the Third National Acute Spinal Cord Injury Randomized Controlled Trial National Acute Spinal Cord Injury Study. *JAMA*. 1997;277(20):1597-1604.

95. Arnold PM, Anderson PA, Chi JH, et al. Congress of Neurological Surgeons systematic review and evidence-based guidelines on the evaluation and treatment of patients with thoracolumbar spine trauma: pharmacological treatment. *Neurosurgery*. 2019;84(1):E36-E38. doi: 10.1093/neuros/nyy371

96. Bledsoe BE, Wesley AK, Salomone JP. High-dose steroids for acute spinal cord injury in emergency medical services. *Prehosp Emerg Care*. 2004;8:313-316.

97. American College of Surgeons Committee on Trauma. Spine and spinal cord trauma. In: *Advanced Trauma Life Support for Doctors*. 8th ed. Chicago, IL: American College of Surgeons; 2008.

98. Short DJ, El Masry WS, Jones PW. High dose methylprednisolone in the management of acute spinal cord injury: a systematic review from the clinical perspective. *Spinal Cord*. 2000;38:273-286.

99. Coleman WP, Benzel D, Cahill DW, et al. A critical appraisal of the reporting of the National Acute Spinal Cord Injury Studies (II and III) of methylprednisolone in acute spinal cord injury. *J Spinal Disord*. 2000;13:185-199.

100. Hurlbert RJ. The role of steroids in acute spinal cord injury: an evidence-based analysis. *Spine*. 2001;26:S39-S46.

101. Bracken MB. Steroids for acute spinal cord injury (review). *Cochrane Database Syst Rev*. 2012 Jan 18;1(1):CD001046.

102. Evaniew N, Noonan VK, Fallah N, et al. Methylprednisolone for the treatment of patients with acute spinal cord injuries: a propensity score-matched cohort study from a Canadian multi-center spinal cord injury registry. *J Neurotrauma*. 2015;32(21):1674-1683.

Suggested Reading

American College of Surgeons Committee on Trauma. *Advanced Trauma Life Support for Doctors, Student Course Manual*. 9th ed. American College of Surgeons; 2012.

Pennardt AM, Zehner WJ. Paramedic documentation of indicators for cervical spine injury. *Prehosp Disaster Med*. 1994;9:40-43.

White CC, Domeier RM, Millin MG; Standards and Clinical Practice Committee, National Association of EMS Physicians. EMS spinal precautions and the use of long backboard—resource document to the position statement of the National Association of EMS Physicians and the American College of Surgeons Committee on Trauma. *Prehosp Emerg Care*. 2014;18(2):306-314.

척추 관리

이러한 술기는 척추 움직임 제한 원칙을 설명하기 위한 것이다. 사용하는 특정 장비에 대한 선호도는 각 기관, 의료 지도, 프로토콜에 따라 결정된다.

목뼈보호대 크기 측정 및 적용

원칙: 환자의 머리와 목을 중립 자세로 정렬하고 고정하는 데 도움이 되는 적절한 크기의 목뼈보호대를 선택하여 적용한다.

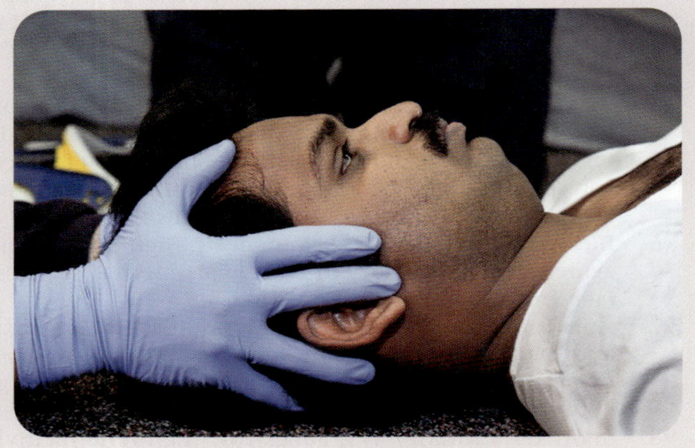

1 첫 번째 병원 전 처치 제공자가 환자의 머리와 목을 도수 고정으로 중립 자세로 유지한다.

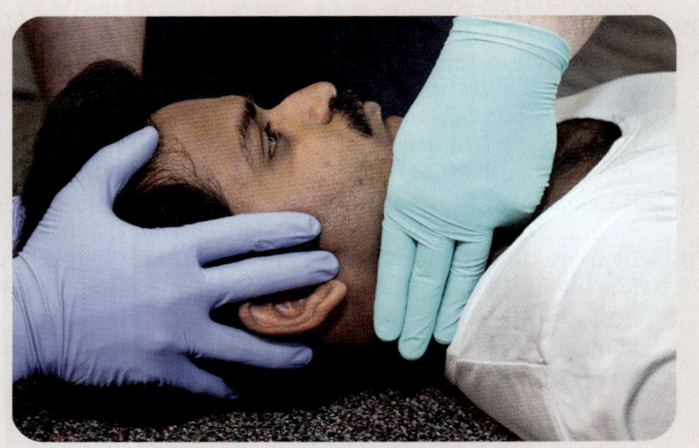

2 두 번째 병원 전 처치 제공자는 손가락을 사용하여 환자의 아래턱과 어깨 사이의 목의 길이를 측정한다.

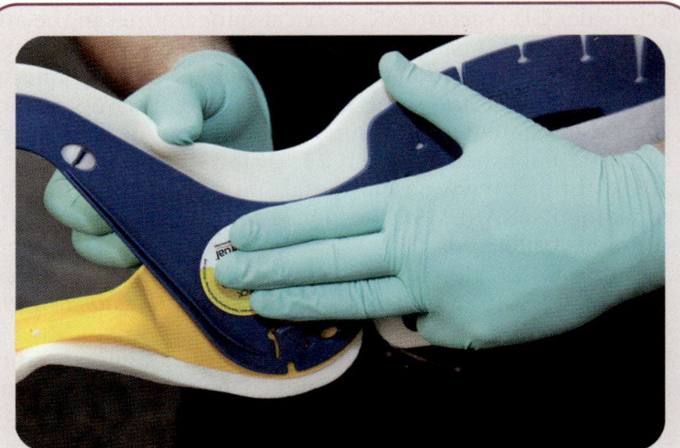

3 두 번째 병원 전 처치 제공자는 이 측정한 길이에 맞는 적절한 크기의 목뼈보호대를 선택하거나 길이 조절

(다음 페이지에 계속)

척추 관리 (이어서)

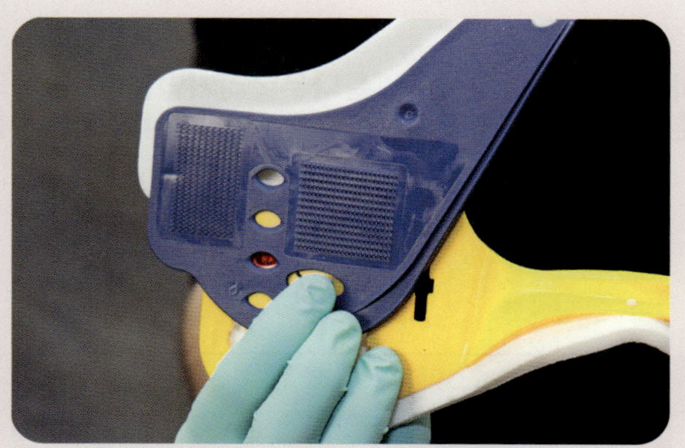

4 이 가능한 목뼈보호대라면 길이를 올바른 크기로 조절한다.

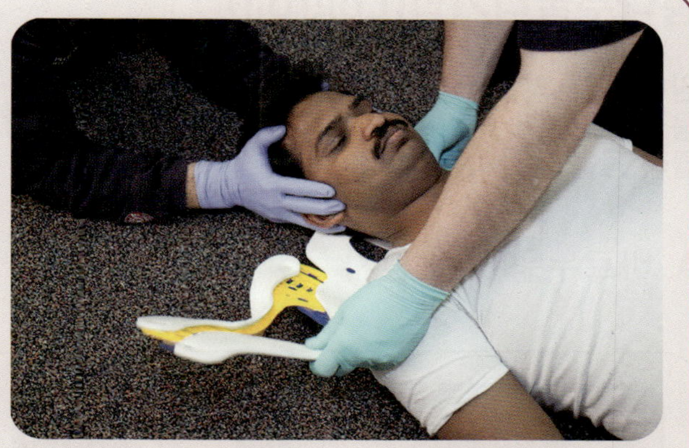

5 조절할 수 있는 목뼈보호대를 사용하는 경우 목뼈보호대를 적절한 크기로 조절하여 고정되어 있는지 확인한다.

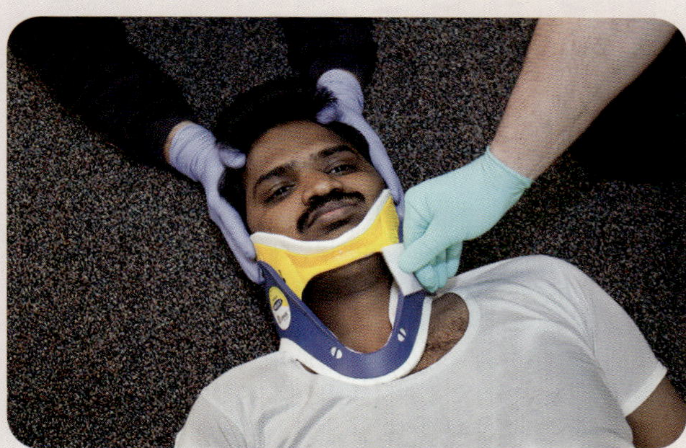

6 첫 번째 병원 전 처치 제공자가 환자의 머리와 목을 중립 자세로 계속 유지하는 동안 두 번째 병원 전 처치 제공자가 환자에게 목뼈보호대를 적용한다.

목뼈보호대를 적용하고 고정한 후 환자가 적절한 장비에 고정할 때까지 머리와 목의 도수 고정을 유지한다.

(다음 페이지에 계속)

척추 관리 (이어서)

통나무굴리기법(Logroll)

원칙: 척추의 움직임을 최소화하면서 도수 고정을 유지하면서 환자를 돌린다. 통나무굴리기법은 1) 환자의 움직임을 쉽게 하기 위해 긴척추고정판이나 다른 장비에 환자를 위치시키고, 2) 척추 외상이 의심되는 환자를 돌려 등을 검사하는 데 사용된다.

A. 바로누워 있는 환자

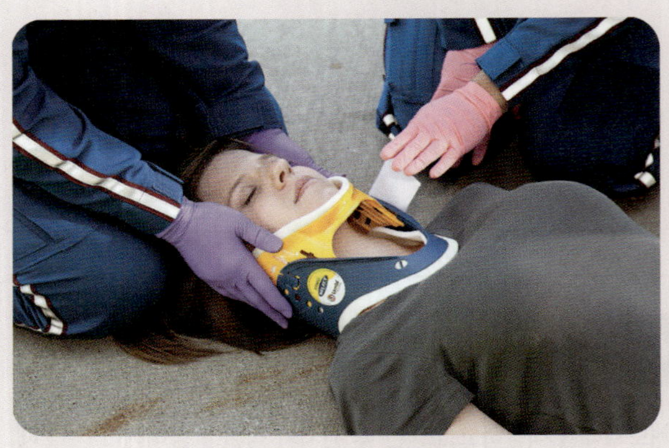

1 첫 번째 병원 전 처치 제공자가 환자의 머리와 목을 도수 고정으로 중립 자세를 유지하는 동안 두 번째 병원 전 처치 제공자는 적절한 크기의 목뼈보호대를 적용한다.

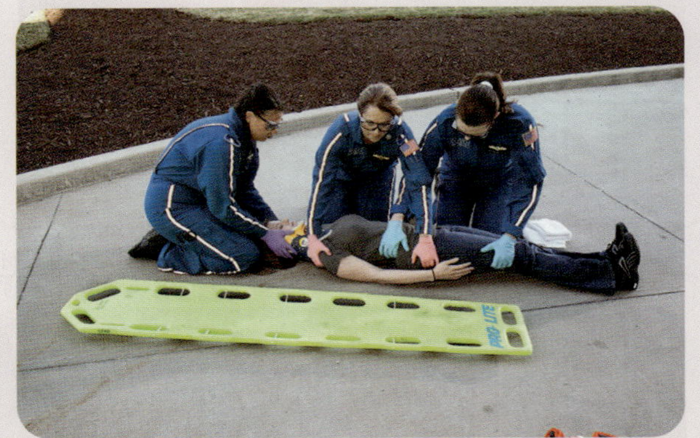

2 첫 번째 병원 전 처치 제공자가 환자의 머리와 목을 중립 자세로 유지하는 동안 두 번째 병원 전 처치 제공자는 환자의 가슴 중앙 부위에 무릎을 꿇고, 세 번째 병원 전 처치 제공자는 환자의 무릎 부위에 무릎을 꿇는다. 환자의 팔을 곧게 펴고 손바닥을 몸통 옆에 대고 환자의 다리를 중립 자세로 정렬한다. 환자의 어깨와 엉덩이를 잡고 다리를 중립 자세로 유지하는 방법으로 환자를 잡는다. 환자를 서서히 측면으로 통나무굴리기법을 시행한다.

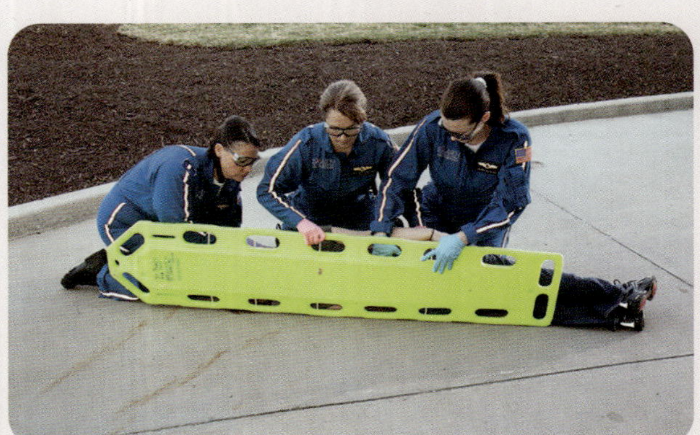

3 긴척추고정판은 또는 기타 장비는 고정판의 발 끈이 환자의 무릎과 발목 사이에 위치하도록 배치한다(고정판의 머리 부분은 환자의 머리를 지나가게 위치한다.). 긴척추고정판을 환자의 등에 대고 환자를 긴척추고정판에 다시 눕힌 다음 환자와 함께 긴척추고정판을 바닥에 내려놓는다.

(다음 페이지에 계속)

척추 관리 (이어서)

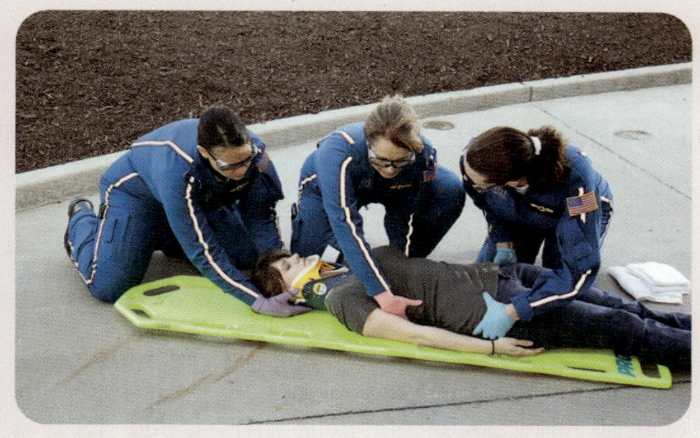

4 바닥에 내려놓은 환자의 어깨, 골반 및 다리를 단단히 잡는다.

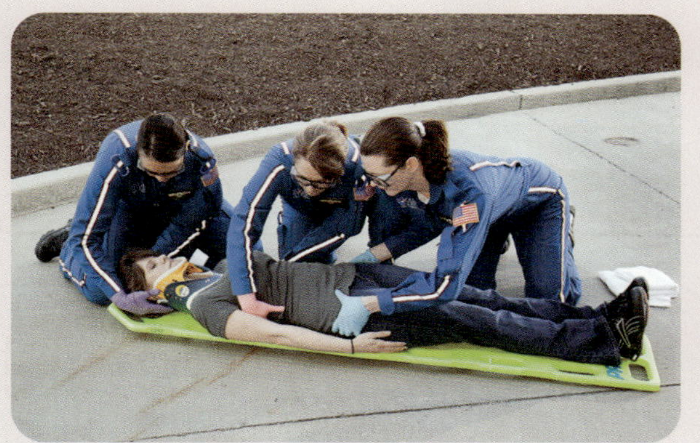

5 환자의 머리와 목을 당기지 않고 도수 고정으로 중립 자세를 유지하면서 환자를 긴척추고정판 위쪽과 옆으로 이동시킨다.

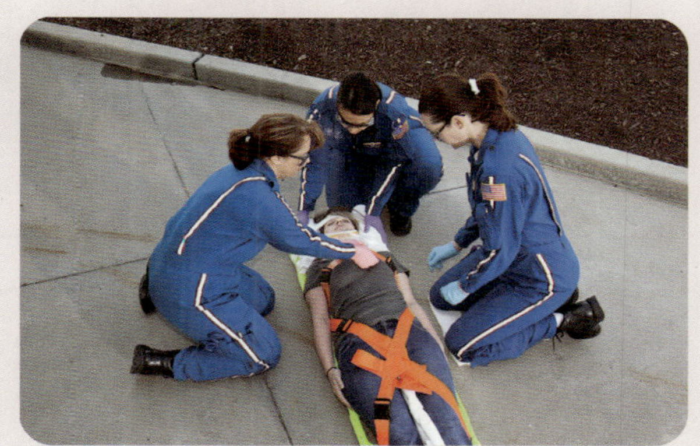

6 환자는 긴척추고정판 위에서 환자의 신체를 중앙에 위치시켜 고정한 후 머리고정대로 머리를 고정한다. 불편함이 심해지거나 이송 지연 시 환자가 바로누운자세로 구급차 주들것으로 안전하게 옮겨진 후 환자를 통나무굴리기법을 이용하여 긴척추고정판을 제거할 수 있다.

(다음 페이지에 계속)

척추 관리 (이어서)

B. 엎드린 자세 또는 반 엎드린 자세 환자

환자가 엎드린 자세나 반 엎드린 자세로 있다면 바로 누워 있는 환자에게 사용되는 것과 유사한 고정 방법을 사용할 수 있다. 이 방법은 환자의 팔다리를 중립 자세로 유지하고 병원 전 처치 제공자의 같은 위치 및 손 위치, 중립 자세를 유지하기 위한 같은 능력이 포함된다.

환자의 팔은 완전한 회전을 예상하여 위치시킨다. 반 엎드린 자세에서 통나무굴리기법을 시행하는 경우 환자를 긴척추고정판에 바로누운자세로 위치시킨 후 목뼈보호대를 적용할 수 있으며 그전에는 사용하지 않는다.

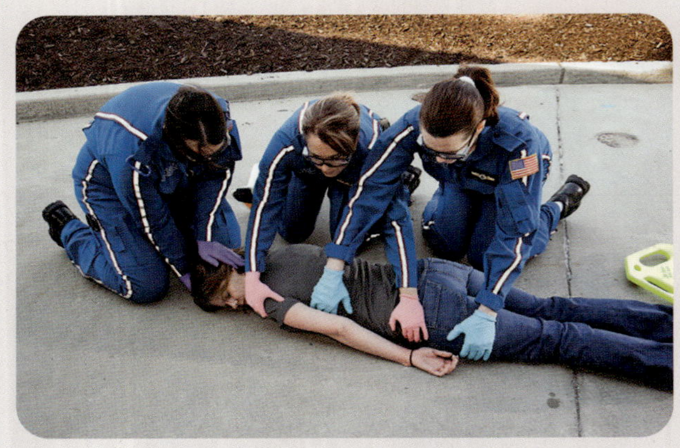

1 가능하면 항상 환자의 얼굴이 처음에 향하는 방향에서 통나무굴리기법을 시행한다. 병원 전 처치 제공자 한 명이 환자의 머리와 목을 중립 자세로 도수 고정하고 유지한다. 다른 병원 전 처치 제공자는 환자의 가슴 부위에 무릎을 꿇고 환자의 반대쪽 어깨와 손목 및 골반 부위를 잡는다. 세 번째 병원 전 처치 제공자는 환자의 무릎 부위에 무릎을 꿇고 환자의 손목과 골반 부위 및 다리 부분을 잡는다.

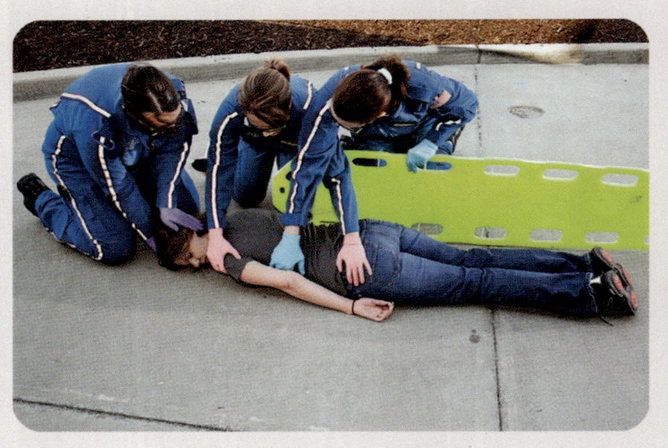

2 긴척추고정판 또는 기타 장비를 측면 가장자리에 위치시키고 환자와 병원 전 처치 제공자 사이에 위치시킨다.

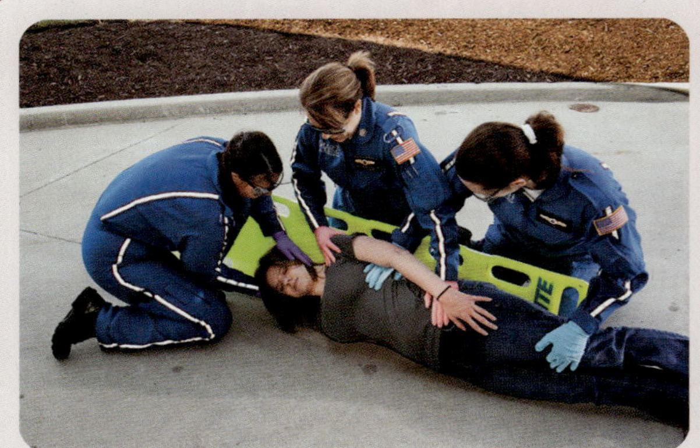

3 긴척추고정판은 발쪽 끝부분이 환자의 무릎과 발목 사이에 오도록 고정판을 위치시키고 환자를 통나무굴리기법으로 옆으로 돌린다. 환자의 머리는 몸통보다 덜 회전하므로 환자가 옆으로(지면에 수직) 누워있을 때(지면과 수직) 머리와 몸통이 적절한 중립 자세로 유지된다.

(다음 페이지에 계속)

척추 관리 (이어서)

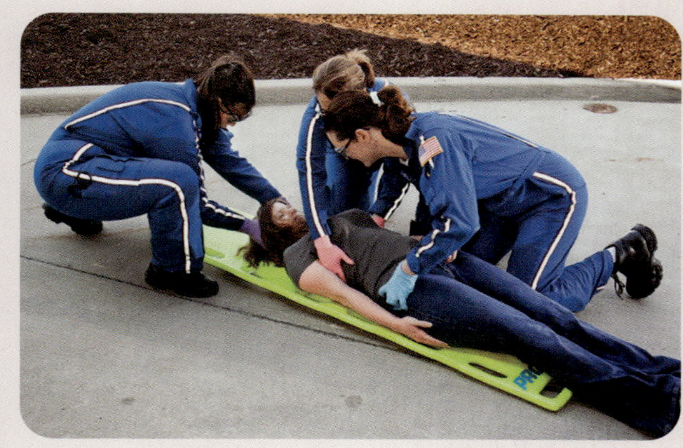

4 환자가 긴척추고정판에 바로누운 자세로 위치하면 환자를 우 쪽으로 움직여 긴척추고정판의 중앙에 위치하도록 이동시킨다. 병원 전 처치 제공자는 머리와 목을 잡아당기지 않고 중직 자세를 유지하도록 주의를 기울여야 한다. 환자가 긴척추고정판에 을바르게 위치하면 적절한 크기의 목뼈보호대를 적용하고 환자를 긴척추고정판에 고정할 수 있다. 환자가 상당히 불편해하거나 이송 시간이 길어질 때 환자가 바로누운자세로 구급차 주들것으로 안전하게 옮겨진 후 환자를 통나무굴리기법을 이용하여 긴척추고정판을 제거할 수 있다.

(다음 페이지에 계속)

척추 관리 (이어서)

앉은 자세로 발견된 환자의 척추 움직임 제한

원칙: 앉은 자세에서 이동하기 전과 이동하는 동한 환자를 도수로 고정한다.

A. 3명 이상의 병원 전 처치 제공자

척추 움직임 제한 적응증이 있는 앉아있는 환자(**그림 9-12** 참조)는 안전하게 구조할 수 있다.

다음과 같은 상황에서는 신속한 구조가 필요하다.

- 일차평가 중에 환자를 발견된 장소에서 처치할 수 없는 생명을 위협하는 상태가 확인된 경우
- 현장이 안전하지 않고 병원 전 처치 제공자와 환자에게 명백한 위험이 존재하여 안전한 장소로 신속히 이송해야 하는 경우
- 더 심각한 손상을 입은 다른 환자에게 접근하기 위해 환자를 신속하게 이동시켜야 하는 경우

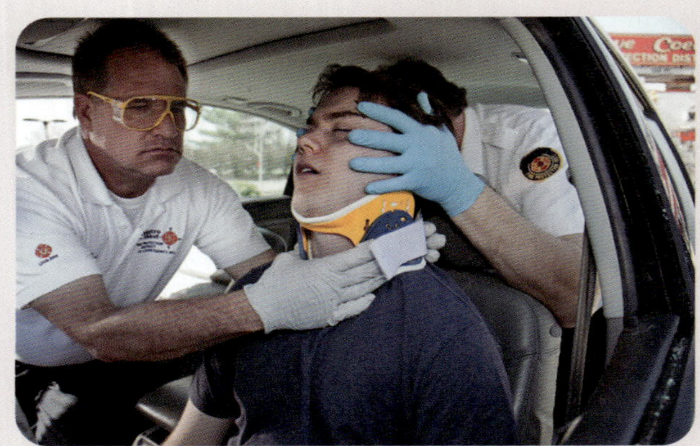

1 환자를 구출하기 전에 척추 움직임 제한을 시행하기로 하면 환자의 머리와 목을 중립 자세로 도수 고정하고 유지한다. 이것은 환자의 뒤에서 수행하는 것이 가장 좋다. 병원 전 처치 제공자가 환자 뒤로 갈 수 없는 경우 옆에서 도수 고정을 시행할 수 있다. 환자의 뒤에서든 옆에서든 환자의 머리와 목을 중립 자세로 정렬하고 환자를 신속하게 평가한 후 적절한 크기의 목뼈보호대를 착용시킨다.

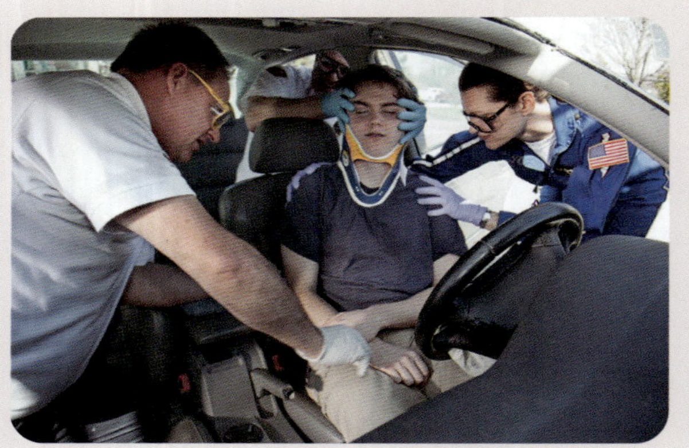

2 도수 고정을 유지하는 동안 환자의 몸통 위쪽과 아래쪽 및 다리를 제어한다. 환자는 일련의 짧고 제어된 움직임으로 회전한다.

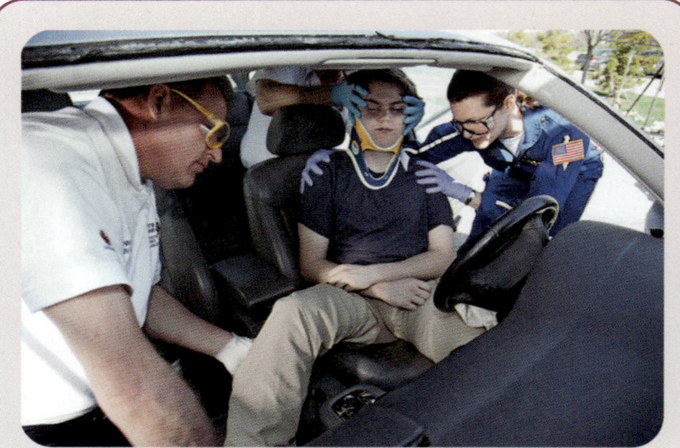

3 차량에 센터 콘솔이 있는 경우 환자의 다리를 콘솔 위로 한 번에 하나씩 이동시킨다.

(다음 페이지에 계속)

척추 관리 (이어서)

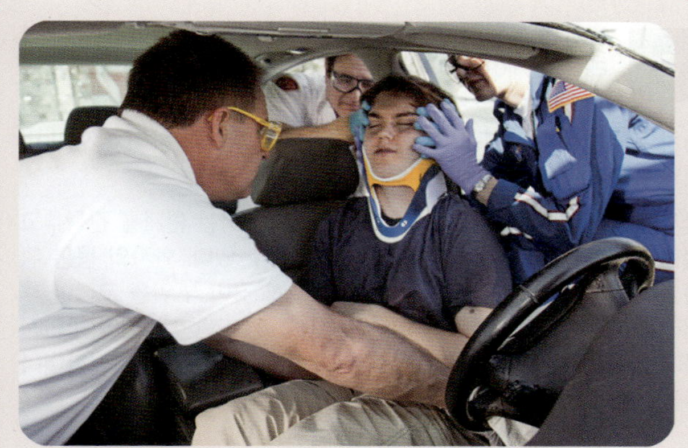

4 병원 전 처치 제공자는 차량 뒤쪽과 내부에서 도수 고정을 더 이상 유지할 수 없을 때까지 짧고 통제된 움직임으로 환자를 계속 회전시킨다. 두 번째 병원 전 처치 제공자는 차량 외부에서 서서 첫 번째 병원 전 처치 제공자로부터 도수 고정을 인계받는다.

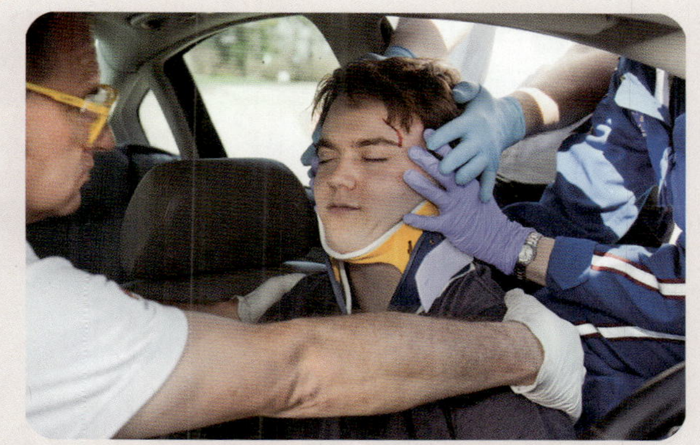

5 첫 번째 병원 전 처치 제공자는 차량 밖으로 이동하여 두 번째 병원 전 처치 제공자로부터 도수 고정을 다시 인계받는다.

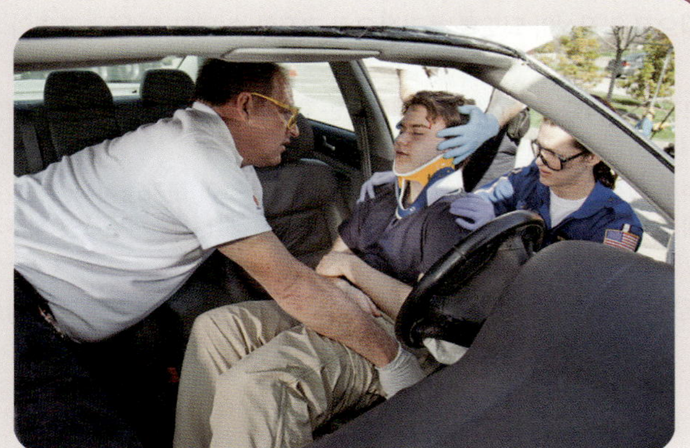

6 차량 문밖에서 환자가 앉아 있는 좌석에 긴척추고정판을 대고 위로 내릴 수 있을 때까지 환자를 계속 회전시킨다.

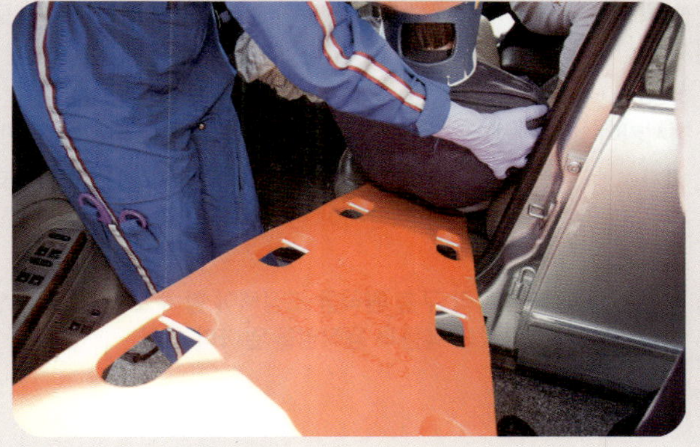

7 긴척추고정판 또는 기타 척추 고정 장비는 고정판의 발끝을 차량 좌석에 머리끝을 구급차의 주들 것에 놓는다. 주들 것을 차량 옆에 놓을 수 없는 경우 다른 병원 전 처치 제공자가 긴척추고정판을 잡고 환자를 그 위로 내릴 수 있다.

(다음 페이지에 계속)

척추 관리 (이어서)

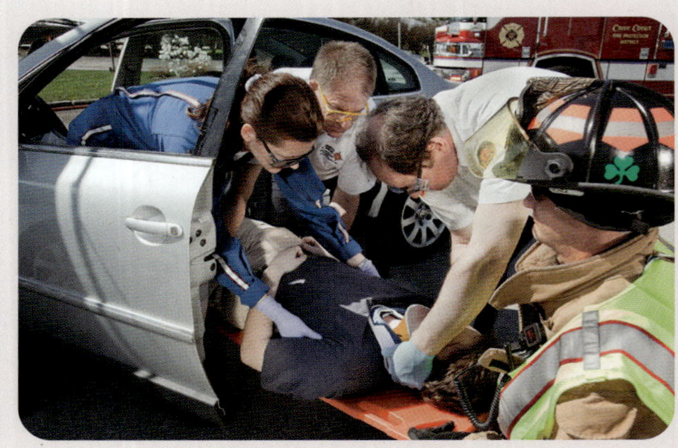

8 환자의 몸통이 고정판에 내려오면 환자의 골반과 다리 아래쪽이 제어되는 동안 환자의 가슴 무게가 제어된다. 환자를 장비 위로 이동시킨다. 도수 고정을 유지하는 병원 전 처치 제공자는 환자를 잡아당기지 않도록 주의해야 하며 환자의 머리와 목을 계속 지지해야 한다.

환자를 장비에 위치시킨 후 병원 전 처치 제공자는 환자를 긴척추고정판에 고정하고 구급차 주들것에 고정할 수 있다. 환자의 몸통 위쪽을 먼저 고정하고 그다음 몸통 아래쪽과 골반 부위를 고정한 후 머리를 고정한다. 환자의 다리는 마지막으로 고정한다. 현장이 안전하지 않으면 환자를 안전한 장소로 이동시킨 후 긴척추고정판이나 주들것에 고정해야 한다.

참고: 이 절차는 앉은 자세로 발견된 환자를 구출하는 한 가지 예시일 뿐이다. 이상적인 현장 상황은 거의 없으므로 병원 전 처치 제공자는 특정 환자와 상황에 맞게 구출 단계를 수정해야 할 수 있다. 구출 원칙은 상황과 관계없이 같게 유지되어야 한다. 구출 고정 전반에 걸쳐 중단 없이 도수 고정을 유지하고 척추 전체가 움직임 없이 일직선 자세를 유지해야 한다. 병원 전 처치 제공자는 어떤 자세를 취하든 성공할 수 있다. 그러나 수시로 자세를 바꾸고 손을 바꿔 잡는 것은 도수 고정의 실패를 초래할 수 있으므로 피해야 한다.

구출 방법은 환자를 차량에서 꺼내는 동안 환자의 머리, 목, 몸통을 도수 고정으로 일직선이 되도록 효과적으로 고정할 수 있다. 다음은 구출의 세 가지 핵심 사항이다.

1. 한 명의 병원 전 처치 제공자는 환자의 머리와 목을 도수 고정으로 항상 고정하고 다른 병원 전 처치 제공자는 환자의 몸통 위쪽을 회전시켜 안정시키며 세 번째 병원 전 처치 제공자는 환자의 몸통 아래쪽, 골반 및 다리를 움직이고 제어한다.

2. 환자를 한 번에 연속 동작으로 움직이려고 하면 환자의 머리와 목을 도수로 일직선을 유지하면서 고정을 유지하는 것이 불가능하다. 병원 전 처치 제공자는 각 동작을 제한해야 한다. 움직임을 제한하고 멈춰서 자세를 바꾸고 다음 움직임을 준비해야 한다. 지나치게 서두르면 척추가 움직일 수 있다.

3. 각 상황과 환자에 따라 구출 원칙을 조정해야 할 수도 있다. 이는 연습한 경우에만, 효과적으로 작동할 수 있다. 각 병원 전 처치 제공자는 다른 병원 전 처치 제공자의 행동과 움직임을 알아야 한다.

척추 관리 (이어서)

B. 2명 이상의 병원 전 처치 제공자

일부 상황에서는 중증 환자를 신속하게 구출할 수 있는 적절한 수의 병원 전 처치 제공자가 없을 수 있다. 이러한 상황에서는 두 명의 병원 전 처치 제공자가 환자를 구출하는 방법이 유용할 수 있다.

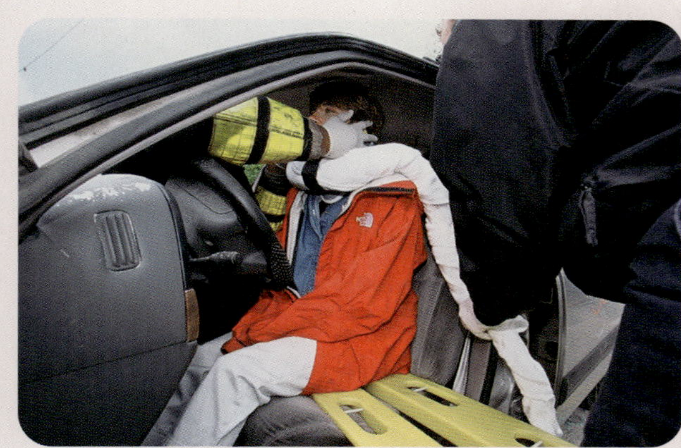

1 첫 번째 병원 전 처치 제공자가 환자의 머리와 목을 도수 고정으로 일직선이 되도록 유지한다. 두 번째 병원 전 처치 제공자는 환자에게 적절한 크기의 목뼈보호대를 착용시키고 미리 말아 놓은 담요를 환자 주위에 준비해 놓는다. 말아 놓은 담요의 중앙을 단단한 목뼈보호대에 앞쪽의 환자 정중선에 위치시킨다.

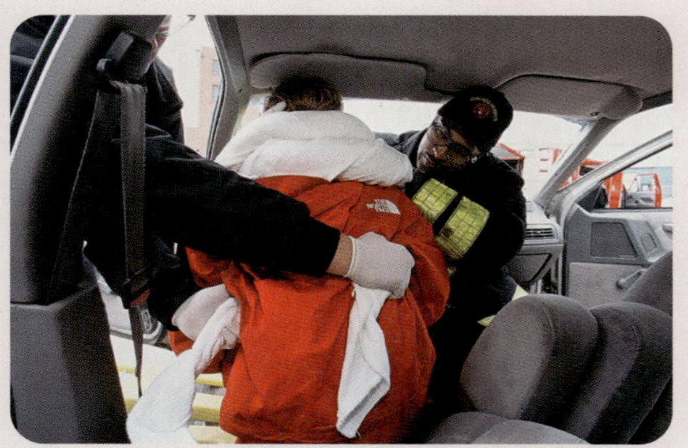

2 말은 담요 끝은 목뼈보호대를 감싸 환자의 겨드랑이에 위치시킨다.

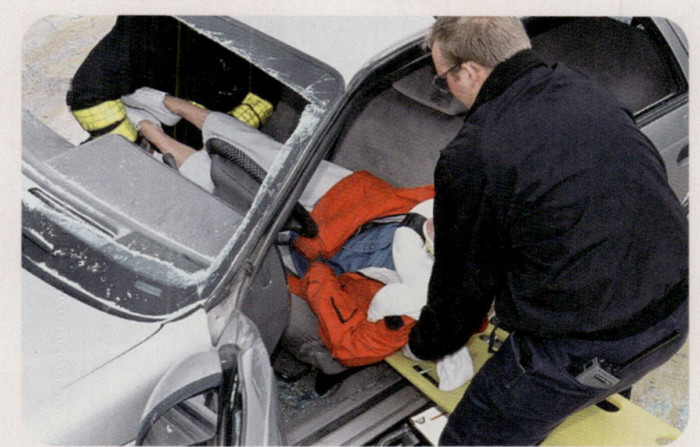

3 말은 담요 끝을 사용하여 환자의 등이 자동차 문 중앙으로 올 때까지 환자를 돌린다. 첫 번째 병원 전 처치 제공자가 담요 끝을 환자의 겨드랑이 쪽으로 담요를 당겨 환자를 이동시키는 동안 두 번째 병원 전 처치 제공자는 환자의 몸통 아래, 골반, 다리를 움직이고 제어한다.

(다음 페이지에 계속)

척추 관리 (이어서)

소아 고정 장비

원칙: 척추 손상이 의심되는 어린이에게 척추 움직임 제한을 제공한다.

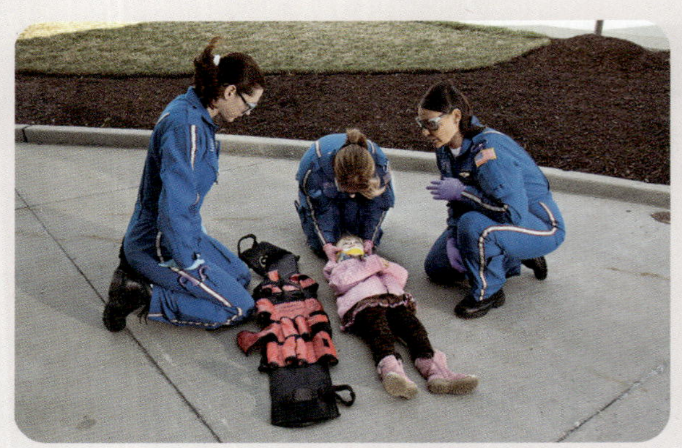

1 첫 번째 병원 전 처치 제공자가 환자의 머리 위에 무릎을 꿇고 머리와 목을 도수 고정으로 중립 자세를 유지한다. 두 번째 병원 전 처치 제공자는 첫 번째 병원 전 처치 제공자가 도수 고정을 유지하는 동안 적절한 크기의 목뼈 보호대를 적용한다. 두 번째 병원 전 처치 제공자는 필요할 경우 환자의 팔과 다리를 곧게 펴준다.

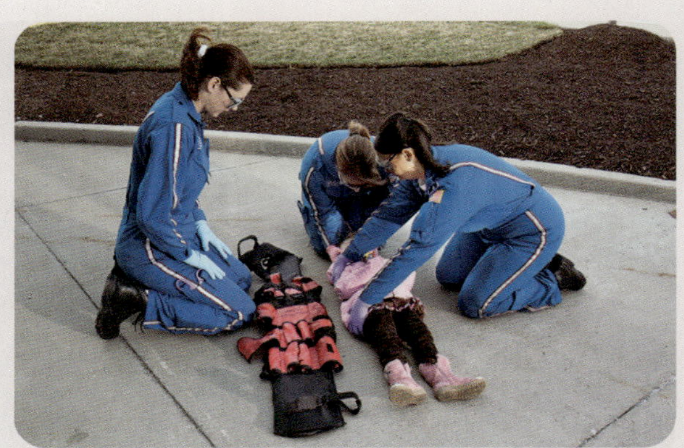

2 두 번째 병원 전 처치 제공자는 환자의 옆에서 어깨와 무릎 사이에 무릎을 꿇고 앉는다. 두 번째 병원 전 처치 제공자는 다리의 중립 자세를 유지하는 방식으로 환자의 어깨와 엉덩이를 잡는다. 첫 번째 병원 전 처치 제공자의 지시에 따라 통나무굴리기법으로 환자를 돌린다.

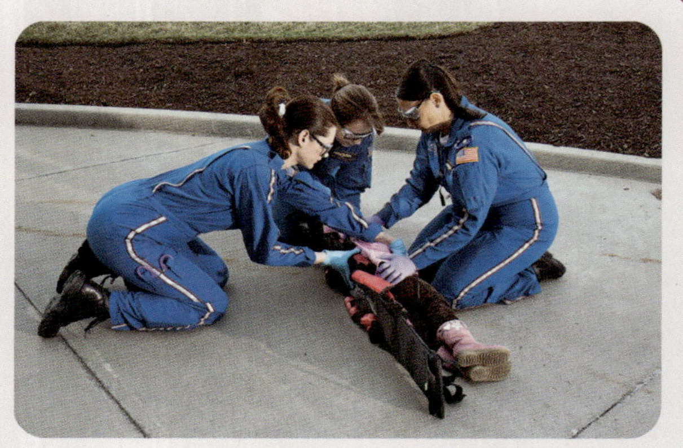

3 세 번째 병원 전 처치 제공자는 환자 등에 고정 장비를 위치시키고 유지한다.

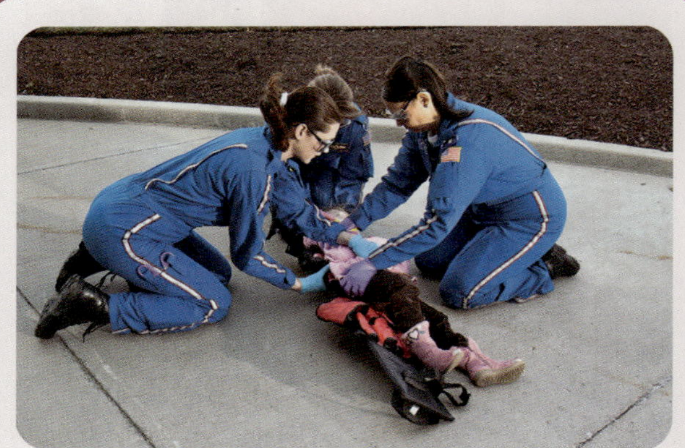

4 장비를 환자의 등에 대고 환자를 장비 위로 통나무굴리기법을 이용하여 환자와 함께 바닥으로 내려놓는다.

(다음 페이지에 계속)

척추 관리 (이어서)

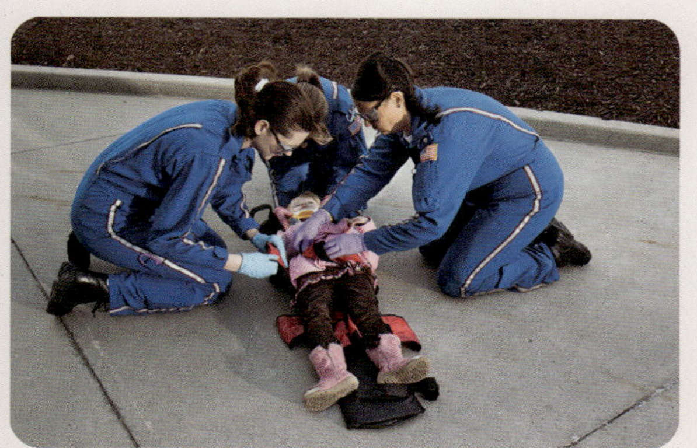

5 첫 번째 병원 전 처치 제공자가 환자의 머리와 목의 도수 고정을 유지하는 동안 두 번째 및 세 번째 병원 전 처치 제공자가 고정 장비에 환자를 고정한다.

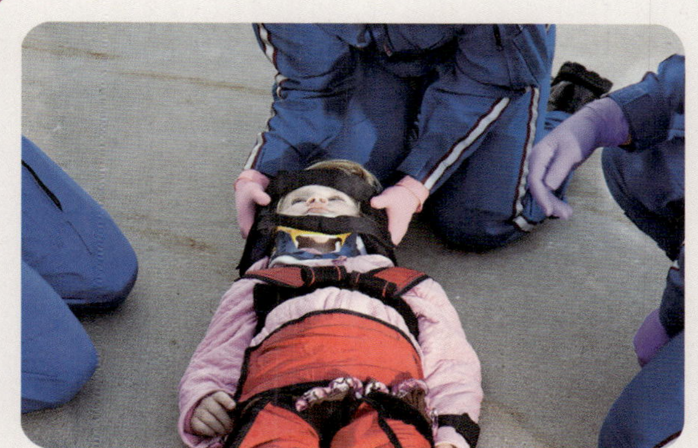

6 환자의 몸통과 다리를 장비에 고정한 후 환자의 머리를 장비에 고정한다.

© National Association of Emergency Medical Technicians (NAEMT)

헬멧 제거

원칙: 추가 손상의 위험을 최소화하면서 헬멧을 제거한다.

얼굴을 완전히 가리는 헬멧을 착용한 환자는 평가 과정 초기에 헬멧을 제거해야 한다. 이를 통해 병원 전 처치 제공자가 환자의 기도 및 환기 상태를 평가하고 처치할 수 있는 즉각적인 접근이 가능하다. 헬멧을 제거하면 숨겨진 출혈을 확인할 수 있고 환자의 머리를(큰 헬멧으로 인한 굴곡된 위치에서) 중립 자세로 이동할 수 있다. 또한, 이차평가에서 머리와 목을 완전히 평가할 수 있으며 필요한 경우 척추 고정을 쉽게 해준다(**그림 9-12**). 병원 전 처치 제공자는 환자에게 무엇을 할 것인지 설명한다. 환자가 헬멧을 제거해서는 안 된다고 말하면 병원 전 처치 제공자는 적절한 교육을 받은 인력이 환자의 척추를 보호하면서 안전모를 제거할 수 있다고 설명한다. 이 술기를 시행하기 위해서는 2명의 병원 전 처치 제공자가 필요하다.

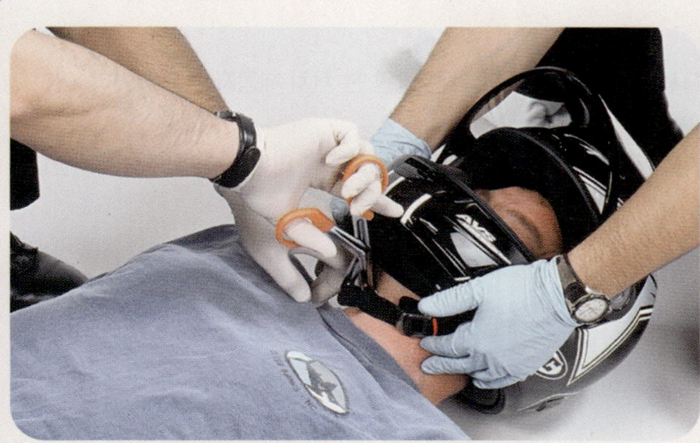

1 첫 번째 병원 전 처치 제공자가 환자의 머리 위쪽에서 위치한다. 손바닥으로 헬멧의 측면을 누르고 손가락 끝은 아래쪽 경계 부위를 잡고 헬멧이 허용하는 한 중립 자세에 가깝게 헬멧, 머리 및 목을 고정한다. 두 번째 병원 전 처치 제공자는 환자 옆에 무릎을 꿇고 필요한 경우 얼굴 보호대를 열거나 제거하고 안경을 쓰고 있는 경우 안경을 벗고 턱끈을 풀거나 자른다.

(다음 페이지에 계속)

척추 관리 (이어서)

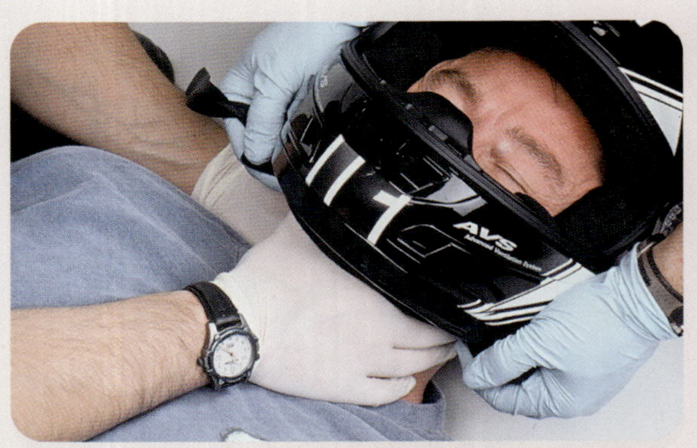

2　환자의 아래턱각 부분에서 엄지와 두 손가락 사이로 잡는다. 다른 한 손은 환자의 두개골 후두부 아랫부분에 다른 한 손을 위치시켜 도수 고정을 유지한다. 병원 전 처지 제공자는 아래팔을 바닥에 대거나 자기 넓적다리에 대고 추가적인 지지력을 확보한다.

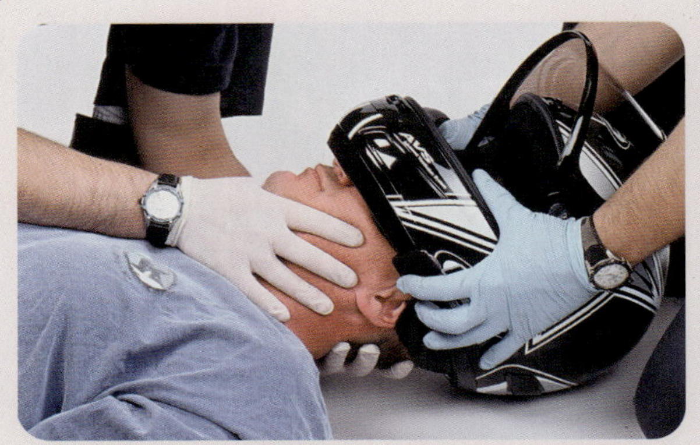

3　첫 번째 병원 전 처치 제공자는 헬멧의 측면을 환자의 머리에서 약간 떨어뜨린 후 조심스럽게 위아래로 움직이거나 돌리면서 환자의 머리에서 헬멧을 빼낸다. 헬멧을 천천히 그리고 신중하게 움직인다. 병원 전 처치 제공자는 환자의 코 부분에서 주의하면서 헬멧을 제거해야 한다.

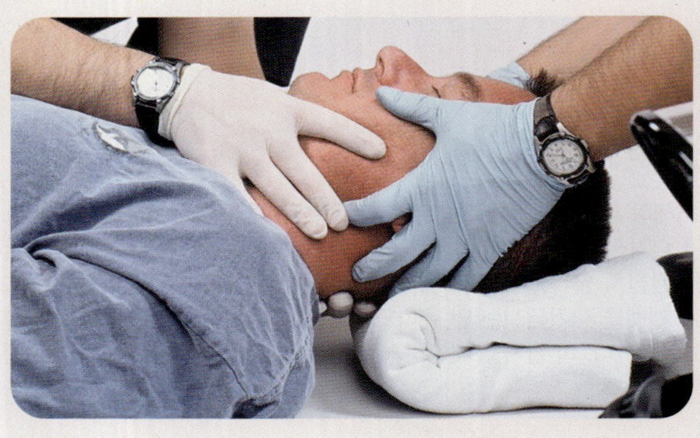

4　헬멧을 제거한 후에는 환자의 머리 뒤에 패딩을 넣어 중립 자세를 유지한다. 도수 고정을 유지하면서 적절한 크기의 목뼈보호대를 환자에게 착용시킨다.

참고: 헬멧 제거에는 다음과 같은 두 가지 핵심 요소가 관련된다.

1. 병원 전 처치 제공자가 한 명이 환자의 머리와 목을 도수 고정으로 중립 자세를 유지하는 동안 다른 병원 전 처치 제공자는 움직인다. 어떤 경우에도 두 명의 병원 전 처치제공자가 모두 손을 움직여서는 안 된다.

2. 병원 전 처치 제공자가 헬멧을 다른 방향으로 돌려서 먼저 환자의 코 부위를 제거한 후 환자의 머리 뒤쪽으로 주의하면서 헬멧을 제거한다.

척추 관리 (이어서)

진공부목 적용

진공부목을 사용할 때는 적절한 주의를 기울이는 것이 중요하다. 바닥이나 환자 옷에 있는 날카로운 물체가 부목에 구멍을 내어 사용할 수 없게 만들 수 있다.

진공부목을 적용하는 단계는 사용할 수 있는 특정 진공부목에 따라 다음 단계와 다를 수 있다. 병원 전 처치 제공자는 자신이 근무하는 기관에서 사용하는 특정 장비의 사용 방법에 익숙해져야 한다.

병원 전 처치 제공자는 진공부목을 높이를 조절할 수 있는 들것에 올려놓는다. 진공부목의 밸브가 머리 쪽에 위치하도록 한다. 진공부목 내부의 플라스틱 볼이 비교적 평평한 표면을 형성할 수 있도록 고르게 펴야 한다.

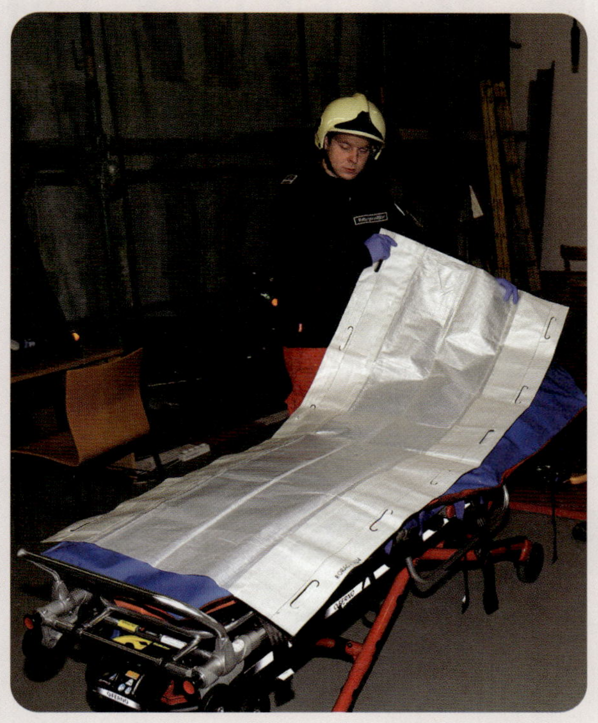

1 병원 전 처치 제공자 한 명이 주들것 위에 진공부목을 놓는다. 진공부목의 밸브가 머리 쪽에 위치하도록 한 후 내부의 플라스틱 볼이 비교적 평평한 표면을 형성할 수 있도록 고르게 편다. 그런 다음 병원 전 처치 제공자는 진공부목 위에 시트를 깔아준다.

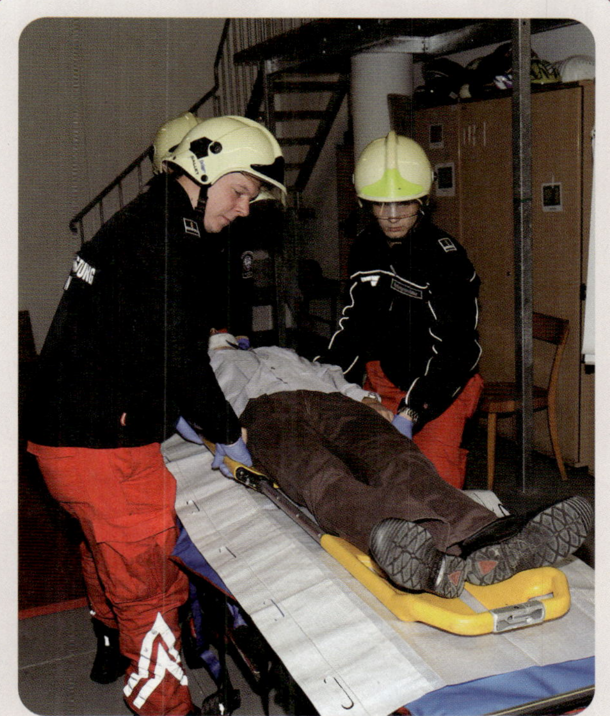

2 분리형 들것으로 환자를 진공부목으로 옮긴다.

(다음 페이지에 계속)

척추 관리 (이어서)

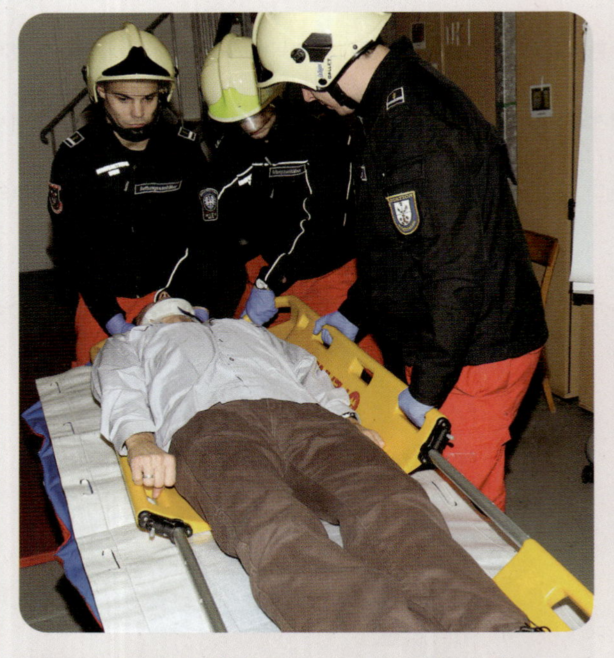

3 분리형 들것을 환자에게서 조심스럽게 제거한다.

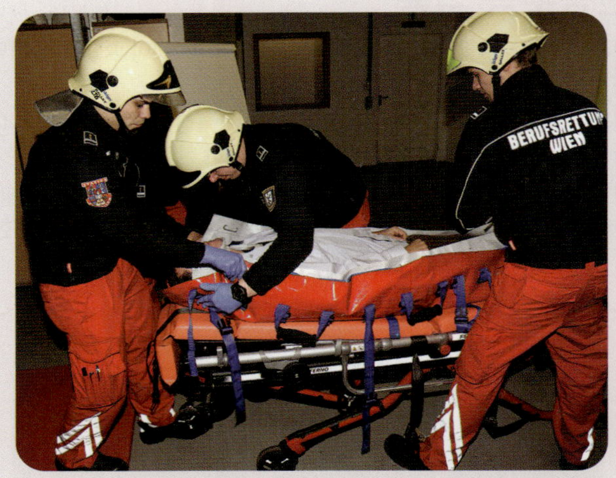

4 진공부목을 환자의 신체 윤곽에 맞게 맞추어지는 동안 병원 전 처치 제공자 한 명이 환자의 머리를 도수 고정으로 일직선을 유지한다. 진공부목이 환자의 신체 윤곽에 맞추어지면 진공부목에 부착된 고정 끈을 연결한 후 진공부목의 밸브에 공기 제거용 펌프를 연결하여 공기를 제거한다.

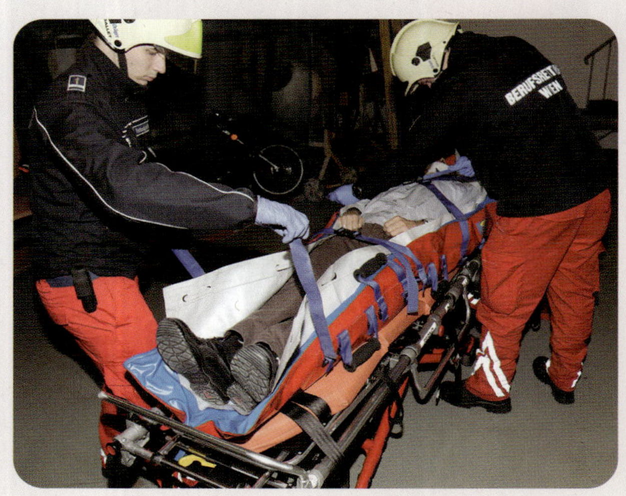

5 그런 다음 진공부목의 공기 제거가 완료되면 펌프를 제거하고 밸브의 안전 마개를 닫고 환자를 고정하고 있는 고정 끈을 다시 조절한다. 시트나 담요로 환자를 덮어준다.

제 **10** 장

가슴 외상

Lead Editors
Anthony Loria, MD
Mark Gestring, MD, FACS

학습 목표   이 장의 학습을 완료하면 다음과 같은 내용을 수행할 수 있다.

- 가슴 장기의 해부학과 생리학을 설명할 수 있다.
- 가슴 손상으로 인한 해부학 및 생리학의 변화를 설명할 수 있다.
- 가슴 외상의 기전, 해부학 및 생리학 그리고 여기에 나열된 손상과 일치하는 다양한 평가 결과 사이의 관계에 대해 토론할 수 있다.
- 신속한 안정화 및 이송이 필요한 환자와 추가 현장 평가 및 처치가 필요한 환자를 구별할 수 있다.

- 다음 손상의 증상, 징후, 병태생리학 및 처치를 설명할 수 있다.
  - 갈비뼈 골절
  - 동요가슴
  - 폐 타박상
  - 기흉(단순, 개방, 긴장)
  - 혈흉
  - 무딘 심장 손상
  - 심장눌림증
  - 심장 진탕
  - 외상성 대동맥 파열
  - 기관기관지 파열
  - 외상 질식
  - 가로막 파열

시나리오

당신과 동료는 건설 현장에서 쇠 파이프에 부딪혀 환자가 발생한 사고 현장으로 출동했다. 현장에 도착하자마자 현장 안전 관리자가 당신을 사고 발생 현장으로 안내한다. 현장 안전 관리자는 쇠 파이프를 이용해서 안전시설을 설치하던 중에 사고가 일어났다고 말했다. 환자의 동료가 말하기를 환자가 다른 쇠 파이프 기둥을 붙잡으려고 몸을 돌리다가 쇠 파이프 끝에 부딪혀 환자의 가슴에 관통했다고 하였다.

30대의 남성이 앞으로 몸을 숙이고 오른쪽 가슴을 부위에 수건을 대고 똑바로 앉아 있는 것을 발견했다. 당신은 환자에게 무슨 일이 일어났는지 물었고 환자는 당신에게 말을 하려고 하지만, 호흡하기 위해 5~6단어 후에 말을 멈춘다. 당신은 수건과 찢어진 옷을 제거한 후 약 5cm의 열상과 소량의 거품 섞인 혈액을 확인했다. 환자평가 결과 환자는 발한이 있고 노맥박은 빠르며 청진시 오른쪽의 호흡음이 감소했다. 다른 비정상적인 신체 소견은 없었다.

- 이 환자는 호흡곤란이 있는가?
- 환자에게 생명을 위협하는 손상이 있는가?
- 현장에서 어떤 처치를 수행해야 하는가?
- 이 환자를 이송하기 위해 어떤 방법을 사용해야 하는가?
- 예를 들어 농촌에서 장시간 환자를 이송하는 것은 처치 계획에 어떤 영향을 미치는가?
- 어떤 다른 손상이 의심되는가?

개요

다른 형태의 손상과 마찬가지로 가슴 외상은 무딘 손상이나 관통상 또는 폭발 기전으로 인해 발생할 수 있다. 가슴안에 무딘 힘이 가해지면 가슴 장기의 정상적인 해부학적 구조와 생리학적 기능을 방해할 수 있다. 마찬가지로 총기, 칼 또는 기타 형태의 찔림으로 인한 관통상은 가슴과 그 내용물을 손상시킬 수 있다. 폭발로 인한 가슴 손상은 심한 폐 압력 손상(타박상, 출혈, 열상, 기흉 또는 공기색전증)을 유발할 수 있다. 대부분의 가슴 손상은 가슴 절개(가슴안의 수술적 개방)가 필요하지 않다. 실제로 무딘 가슴 손상의 10% 미만과 관통에 의한 가슴 손상의 15~30% 만이 가슴 절개가 필요하다. 나머지 손상은 필요에 따라 산소공급, 호흡 보조, 진통제 또는 가슴관 삽입(흉관삽관)과 같은 비교적 간단한 처치로 잘 관리된다.

가슴 장기는 산소 공급, 환기, 관류 및 산소 전달을 유지하는 데 밀접한 관련이 있다. 따라서 가슴 손상은 특히 즉시 인지하고 적절하게 처치하지 않으면 이환율과 사망률로 이어질 수 있다. 가슴 손상을 부적절하거나 시기적절하게 처치하지 않으면 저산소혈증(혈액 내 산소 부족), 저산소증(신체 조직 내 산소 부족), 고이산화탄소혈증(혈액 내 과도한 이산화탄소), 산증(혈액 내 산 과다) 및 쇼크(순환계 이상으로 장기 관류 및 조직 산호 공급이 불충분한 상태)가 발생할 수 있다. 가슴 손상으로 인한 이러한 생리학적 이상은 또한 가슴 외상으로 인한 외상 사망의 25%를 차지하는 다기관 장기부전과 같은 후기 합병증의 원인이 될 수 있다.

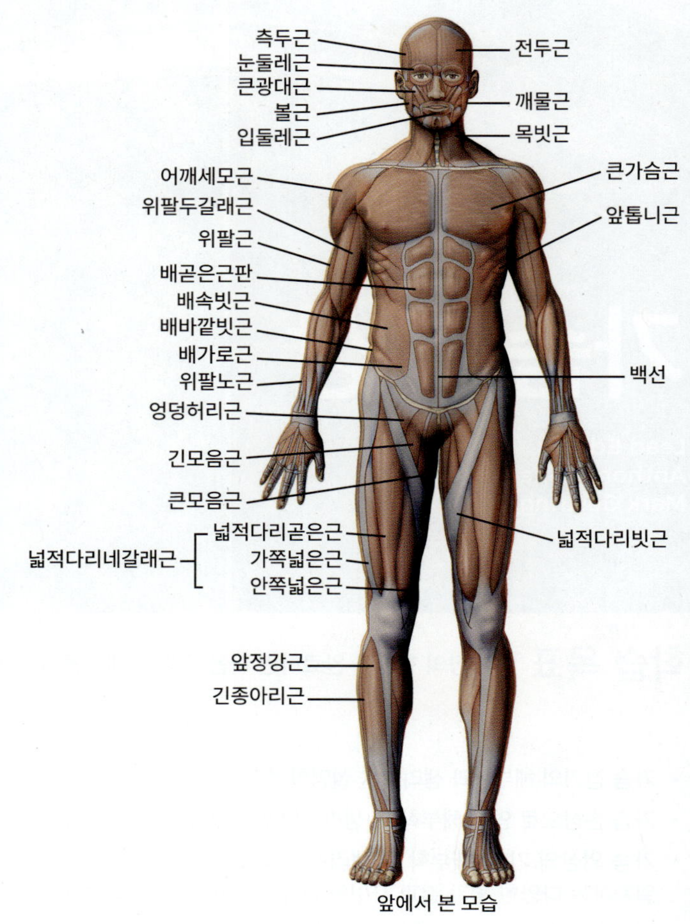

그림 10-1 근육계통
© National Association of Emergency Medical Technicians (NAEMT)

해부학

간단히 말해서 가슴 또는 가슴안은 뼈와 근육 구조로 형성된 속이 빈 원통이다. 12쌍의 갈비뼈 중 위쪽 10쌍은 척추의 뒤쪽에 부착되고 앞쪽은 갈비뼈 또는 복장뼈에 부착된다. 아래쪽 두 쌍의 갈비뼈는 척추의 뒤쪽에만 부착되어 있어 부유늑골이라고 한다. 이 뼈 구조는 가슴안과 상복부의 내부 장기(특히 비장과 간)를 보호하는 데 큰 역할을 한다. 이 갈비뼈의 구조는 갈비뼈와 갈비뼈 사이에 있는 갈비사이근에 의해 강화되며 갈비사이근은 갈비뼈와 갈비뼈를 서로 연결한다.

등의 다양한 근육과 함께 큰가슴근, 작은가슴근, 앞톱니근, 뒤톱니근, 넓은등근을 포함한 다수의 근육이 팔을 움직이고 가슴벽을 구성한다(**그림 10-1**). 이 모든 구조물은 내부 장기를 손상하는 데 상당한 힘이 필요하다는 것을 의미한다.

가슴에는 갈비사이근, 가슴 아래쪽에 부착된 돔 모양의 가로막, 위쪽 갈비뼈에 부착된 목 근육 등 호흡(환기)에 관여하는 근육이 포함되어 있다. 신경, 동맥 및 정맥은 각 갈비뼈의 아래쪽 가장자리를 따라 갈비사이근에 혈액과 감각을 제공한다.

이러한 구조에 의해 형성된 공간의 내부를 감싸는 것은 벽가슴막이라는 얇은 막이 있다. 해당 막은 내장가슴막이라고 하는 가슴안 내 두 개의 폐를 덮고 있다. 유리 사이의 매우 얇은 두께의 층을 물이 서로를 붙게 하듯이 소량의 액체가 두 개의 막 사이를 유지한다. 이 가슴막삼출액은 폐의 탄성 특성과 반대되는 펴면 장력을 생성하여 폐의 자연적으로 허탈이 발생하는 것을 방지한다. 일반적으로 이 두 막 사이에는 공간이 없다.

폐는 가슴안의 오른쪽과 왼쪽을 차지한다(**그림 10-2**). 양쪽 폐 사이에는 세로칸이라고 하는 공간이 있으며 이 공간에는 기관, 주기관지, 심장, 심장의 주요 동맥과 정맥, 식도가 있다.

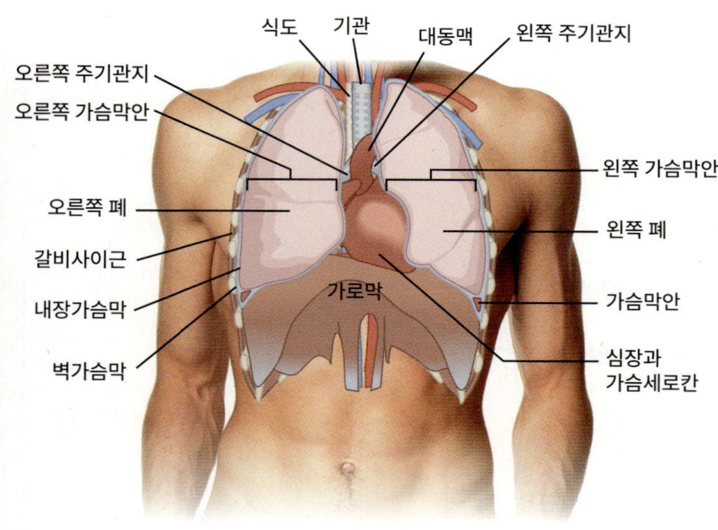

그림 10-2 갈비뼈, 갈비사이근, 가로막, 세로칸, 폐, 심장, 대혈관, 기관지, 기관 및 식도를 포함하는 가슴안
© MariyaL/Shutterstock

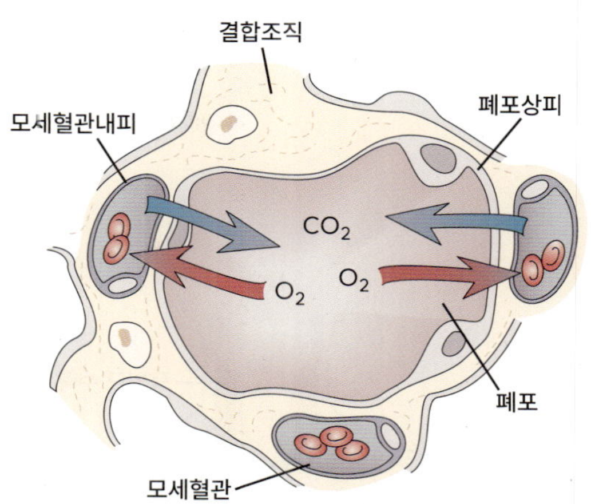

그림 10-3 모세혈관과 폐포는 서로 가까이 있으므로 폐포의 산소는 폐포, 모세혈관 및 적혈구 벽을 통해 쉽게 확산할 수 있다. 이산화탄소는 반대 방향으로 확산할 수 있다.
© National Association of Emergency Medical Technicians (NAEMT)

생리학

호흡과 순환은 가슴 손상의 영향을 가장 많이 받는 생리학의 두 가지 구성 요소이다. 산소가 장기에 도달하고 이산화탄소가 배출되려면 두 과정이 모두 적절하게 작동하고 서로 연계되어 있어야 한다. 이러한 과정을 이해하면 손상이 신체의 생리를 어떻게 변화시키는지 파악하고 손상을 처치하는 데 필요한 단계를 명확히 알 수 있다.

환기

호흡(breathing)과 호흡(respiration)은 생리적 환기(ventilation) 과정을 의미한다. 환기는 입과 코를 통해 공기를 기관과 기관지로 끌어들인 다음 폐로 들어가 폐포라고 하는 작은 공기주머니에 도달하는 기계적 과정이다. 호흡은 환기를 통해 세포에 산소를 전달하는 것이다. 공기를 들이마시는 과정을 흡입이라 한다. 흡입된 공기의 산소는 폐포의 내막을 통과하여 모세혈관이라는 인접한 작은 혈관으로 이동된다. 여기서 산소는 산소공급(산소화)이라는 과정을 통해 적혈구의 헤모글로빈에 부착되어 신체의 나머지 부분으로 운반된다. 동시에 혈액에 용해된 이산화탄소는 날숨 과정에서 폐포 내에서 공기 중으로 확산하여 배출된다(**그림 10-3**). 세포 호흡은 에너지를 생산하기 위해 세포가 산소를 사용하는 것이다(3장, 쇼크; 삶과 죽음의 병태생리학 및 7장, 기도 및 환기 참조).

흡입은 호흡근(주로 갈비사이근과 가로막)의 수축으로 발생한다. 이 근육이 수축하면 가로막이 아래쪽으로 움직이면서 갈비뼈를 들어 올리고 분리된다. 이렇게 하면 가슴안의 크기를 증가시켜 신체 외부의 기압에 비해 가슴 내부에 음압이 생성되고 그 결과 공기가 폐로 유입된다(**그림 10-4, 그림 10-5**). 숨을 내쉴 때는 갈비사이근과 가로막이 이완되어 갈비뼈와 가로막이 휴식 시 위치로 돌아오게 된다. 이렇게 하면 가슴 내부의 압력이 신체 외부의 압력을 초과하고 폐의 공기가 강제로 배출된다.

환기는 주로 뇌줄기의 호흡 중추에 의해 조절되며 중추화학수용체라고 하는 특수 세포가 동맥이산화탄소분압($PaCO_2$)과 동맥혈산소분압(PaO_2)을 모니터링하여 환기를 조절한다. 중추화학수용체가 동맥이산화탄소분압 증가를 감지하면 호흡 중추를 자극하여 호흡의 깊이와 빈도를 증가시켜 더 많은 이산화탄소를 제거하고 동맥이산화탄소분압을 정상으로 되돌린다(**그림 10-6**). 이 과정을 통해 분당 폐로 들어오고 나가는 공기의 양을 10배 증가시킬 수 있다. 기도, 폐 및 가슴벽에서 발견되는 기계 수용체는 이러한 구조물이 늘어나는 정도를 측정하고 폐 부피에 관한 피드백을 뇌줄기에 제공한다.

만성폐쇄폐질환(COPD) 환자의 경우 폐가 이산화탄소를 효율적으로 제거할 수 없다. 이에 따라 혈중 이산화탄소 수치가 만성적으로 상승하여 중추화학수용체가 동맥혈이산화탄소분압의 변화에 둔감해진다. 그 결과 말초 화학수용체(대동맥과 목동맥에 있음)가 동맥혈산소분압 감소에 반응하여 호흡을 자극한다. 중추화학수용체가 동맥혈이산화탄소분압 증가를 감지하고 호흡을 증가시켜 이산화탄소 수준

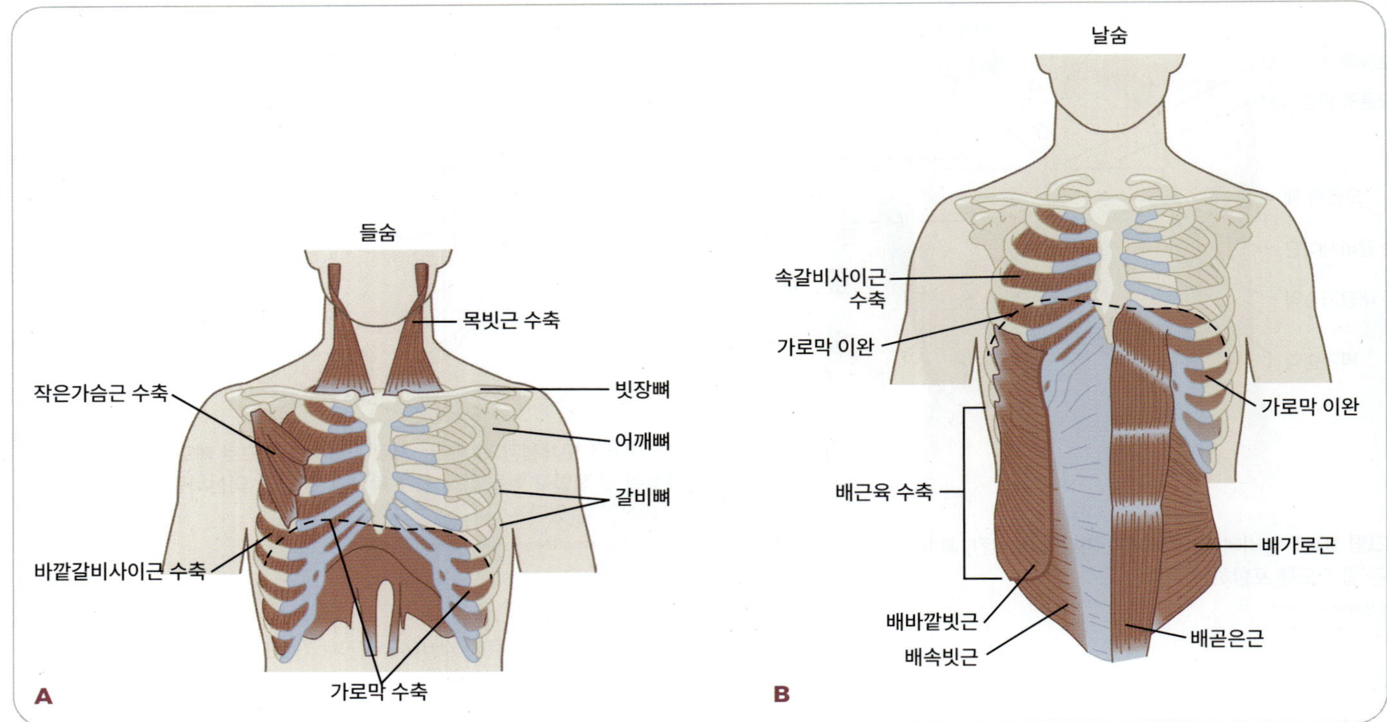

그림 10-4 A. 들숨 시 가로막이 수축하고 평평해진다. 바깥갈비사이근, 작은가슴근, 목빗근과 같은 들숨 보조근은 갈비뼈와 복장뼈를 들어 올린다. 이렇게 하면 가슴안의 부피가 증가하여 신체 외부에 비해 가슴의 압력을 감소시켜 공기가 폐로 들어간다. **B.** 안정적인 호흡 시 날숨은 가슴안의 탄성으로 인해 가로막과 갈비뼈를 본래의 위치로 돌아가게 하여 가슴안이 부피가 감소한다. 힘들게 호흡하는 동안 숨을 내쉴 때는 갈비사이근 및 복근과 같은 날숨 근육이 수축하여 가슴안의 부피가 더 빠르게 감소한다.

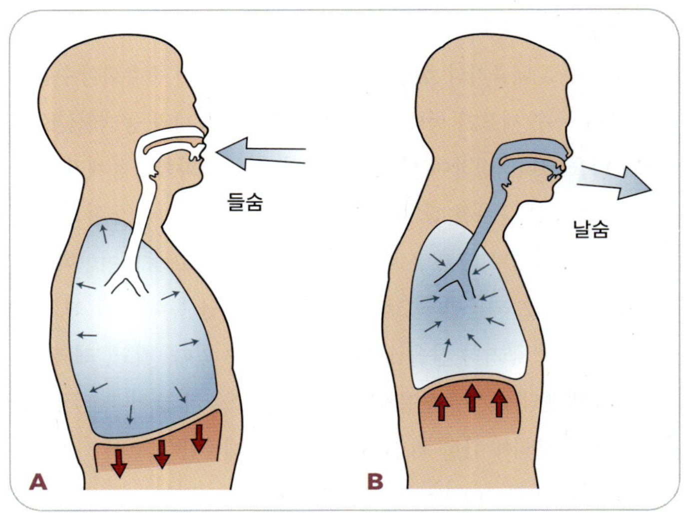

그림 10-5 들숨 중에 가슴안이 확장되면 가슴안 내 압력이 감소하고 공기가 폐로 들어간다. 가로막이 이완되고 가슴이 원래의 위치로 돌아오면 가슴안 내 압력이 증가하여 공기가 배출된다. 가로막이 이완되고 성문이 열리면 폐 안팎으로 압력이 같아진다. **A.** 들숨, **B.** 날숨

을 낮추는 것과 유사하게 말초 화학수용체는 변화하는 동맥혈산소분압을 감지하여 호흡 중추에 피드백을 보내 호흡근이 더 활동적이 되도록 자극하여 호흡 속도와 깊이를 증가시켜 동맥혈산소분압을 정상적인 값으로 높인다(**그림 10-7**). 이 기전은 혈중 산소 수치 저하와 관련이 있기 때문에 종종 "저산소 구동"이라고 한다.

저산소 구동의 개념으로 인해 호흡 자극을 억제할 수 있다는 우려 때문에 만성폐쇄폐질환 환자에게 산소 공급량을 제한하는 것이 권장되고 있다. 그러나 저산소증이 있는 외상 환자에게 병원 전 환경에서 보충 산소를 공급하지 않으면 안 된다. 저산소 구동의 실제 존재 여부는 여전히 논란의 여지가 있다. 저산소증이 존재하더라도 급성 상황에서는 나타나지 않으며 가슴 손상이 있는 환자에게 부적절한 산소 공급으로 인한 잠재적인 부작용은 능동적으로 모니터링되는 환자의 저산소 구동을 일시적으로 억제할 때 발생할 수 있는 부작용보다 훨씬 더 심각하다.

Box 10-1은 폐 생리학을 이해하는 데 중요한 용어를 정의하였다.

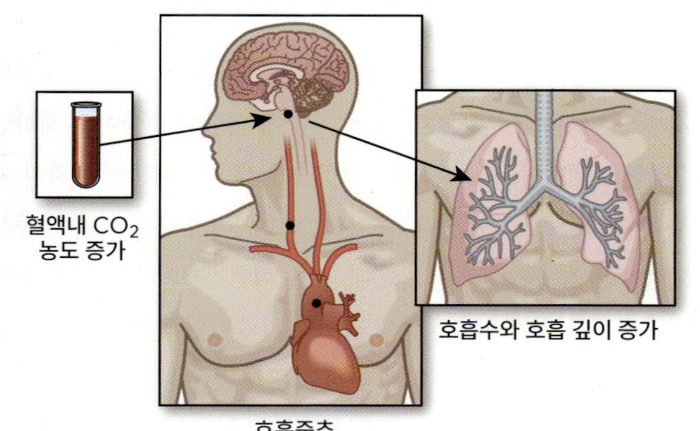

그림 10-6 이산화탄소 수치가 증가하면 이러한 변화에 민감한 신경세포가 이를 감지하여 폐를 자극하여 호흡 깊이와 호흡 속도를 모두 증가시킨다.
© National Association of Emergency Medical Technicians (NAEMT)

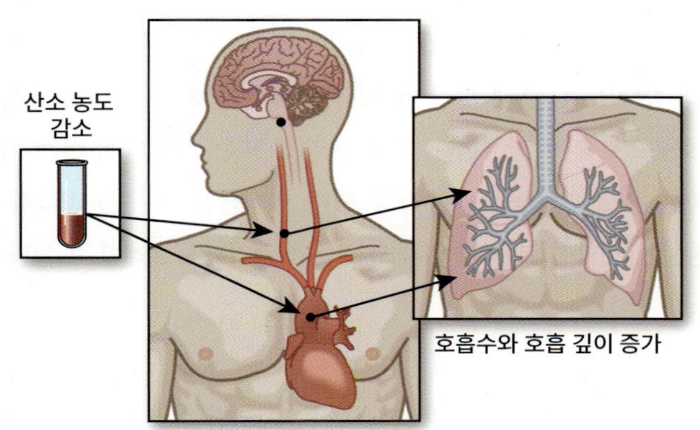

그림 10-7 대동맥과 목동맥에 있는 수용체는 혈액의 산소 수준에 민감하게 반응하여 폐를 자극하여 폐포 안팎으로 공기 이동을 증가시킨다.
© National Association of Emergency Medical Technicians (NAEMT)

순환

가슴 손상 후 영향을 받을 수 있는 또 다른 주요 생리적 과정이 순환이다. 다음 논의는 가슴 손상의 병태생리학의 단계를 설명한다. 3장 쇼크; 삶과 죽음의 병태생리학에서 이 주제를 더욱 광범위하게 다룬다.

세로칸 내 가슴 중앙에 있는 심장은 생물학적 펌프 역할을 한다. 펌프가 작동하려면 액체로 채워져 있어야 하고 액체의 수준이 유지되어야 한다. 심장의 경우 2개의 큰 정맥인 아래대정맥과 위대정맥을 통해 혈액이 되돌아온다. 심장은 일반적으로 분당 70~80회(정상 범위 60~100회/분) 수축하며 수축할 때마다 대동맥을 통해 약 70mL의 혈액을 전신으로 배출한다.

<table>
<tr><td>

Box 10-1 주요 정의

- 사강(Dead space): 가스 교환에 관여하지 않는 기도 부분의 공기량 (예: 기관 및 주기관지의 공기)
- 분당 환기량(Minute ventilation): 1분 동안 폐로 들어오고 나가는 공기의 총량
- 일회 호흡량(Tical volume): 정상적인 호흡 중에 들이마셨다가 내뱉는 공기의 양(정상=0.5L 또는 7mL/kg)
- 총 폐용량(Total lung capacity, TLC): 폐를 최대로 부풀렸을 때 폐에 들어 있는 공기의 총부피. 이 용량은 젊은 성인의 경우 6L에서 노인의 경우 4L로 나이가 들면서 감소한다.
- 호흡 노력(Work of breathing): 호흡하기 위해 가슴벽과 가로막을 움직일 때 수행되는 신체적 노력. 이런 노력은 빠른 호흡, 분당 호흡량 증가 그리고 폐 또는 가슴벽이 비정상적으로 딱딱해지면 증가한다.

</td></tr>
</table>

© National Association of Emergency Medical Technicians (NAEMT)

심장으로 혈액이 되돌아가는 것을 방해하는 과정(예: 출혈로 인한 혈액 손실, 긴장기흉으로 인한 가슴안 압력 증가)은 심장의 박출량을 감소시켜 혈압을 떨어뜨린다. 마찬가지로 심장 자체를 손상하는 과정(예: 무딘 심장 손상)은 심장의 펌프 효율을 떨어뜨려 같은 생리학적 이상을 유발할 수 있다. 화학수용체가 이산화탄소 또는 산소 수준의 변화를 인식하는 것처럼 대동맥활과 목동맥의 목동맥굴에 있는 압력수용체는 혈압의 변화를 인식하고 심장이 박동 속도와 강도를 변화하여 혈압을 정상으로 되돌리도록 지시한다.

병태생리학

앞서 언급했듯이 무딘 손상, 관통상 및 폭발 기전은 방금 설명한 생리적 과정을 방해할 수 있다. 이러한 기전에 의해 발생하는 장애에는 몇 가지 공통 요소가 있다.

관통성 손상

관통상은 다양한 크기와 유형의 물체가 가슴벽을 통과하여 가슴안으로 들어가 가슴 내 장기에 손상을 입힐 수 있다. 일반적으로 가슴막 사이에는 공간이 존재하지 않는다. 그러나 관통상으로 인해 가슴안과 외부 사이에 통로가 생성되면 가슴막 공간으로 공기가 들어갈 수 있다. 숨을 들이쉬는 동안 가슴의 압력이 가슴 외부보다 낮으면 상처를 통해 공기가 유입되어 가슴막의 부착을 방해하여 기흉이 발생한다. 상처를 통한 공기 흐름에 대한 저항이 기도를 통한 공기 흐름에 대한 저항보다 낮으면 공기가 가슴막 공간으로 더 많이 유입될

수 있다. 이러한 과정이 함께 일어나면 폐가 허탈되어 효과적인 환기를 방해한다. 관통상은 가슴벽 결손의 크기가 충분히 커서 들숨 및 날숨 중에 상처를 효과적으로 폐쇄하지 못하는 경우에만 개방성 기흉을 초래한다. 관통하는 물체로 인한 기도 또는 폐 조직에 상처를 입으면 공기가 폐에서 가슴막안으로 빠져나가 폐허탈을 초래할 수도 있다.

두 경우 모두 환자는 숨이 가빠지게 된다. 손실된 환기 능력을 보상하기 위해 호흡 중추는 빠른 호흡을 자극하여 호흡 노력을 증가시킨다. 환자는 한동안 증가한 호흡 노력을 견딜 수 있지만, 이를 인식하고 처치하지 않으면 혈중이산화탄소 수치가 상승하고 산소 수치가 떨어지면서 호흡곤란이 증가하여 호흡 부전의 위험에 처하게 된다.

공기가 빠져나가지 않고 가슴안으로 공기가 계속 유입되면 압력이 증가하여 긴장기흉이 발생한다(**그림 10-8**). 이 상태는 지속해서 증가하는 가슴안 압력으로 인해 심장으로의 정맥혈복귀가 점차 감소하여 환자의 적절한 환기 능력을 더욱 방해하고 잠재적으로 쇼크를 유발할 수 있다. 극단적인 경우 세로칸 구조(양쪽 폐 사이의 가슴 중앙에 위치한 장기와 혈관)가 영향을 받지 않은 쪽 가슴으로 이동하여 정맥혈복귀의 기계적 손상을 유발한다. 이로 인해 혈압이 감소하고 목정맥 확장이 증가하며 전형적이지만, 후기 소견인 정중선에 있는 기관이 손상되지 않은 가슴 쪽으로 기관편위가 발생할 수 있다.

가슴에 관통상을 입으면 가슴벽 근육, 갈비사이 혈관 및 폐 조직에서 가슴막안으로 출혈(혈흉)을 일으킬 수 있다(**그림 10-9**). 가슴의 주요 혈관을 관통하는 손상은 각 가슴막안에 2,500mL~3,000mL의 혈액을 수용할 수 있으므로 치명적인 출혈을 초래할 수 있다. 특히 가슴막안으로 출혈은 겉으로 쉽게 드러나지 않을 수 있지만, 쇼크 상태를 유발할 만한 양일 수 있다. 가슴막안에 대량의 혈액이 존재하면 가슴막안의 혈액이 해당 쪽 폐의 확장을 방해하기 때문에 환자의 호흡 능력에 지장을 줄 수 있다. 폐 손상으로 인해 혈흉과 기흉이 동시에 발생하는 경우는 드물지 않은데, 이를 혈액기흉이라고 한다. 혈액기흉이 발생하면 가슴막 공간의 공기와 가슴막안의 공기와 가슴안 내 혈액이 축적되어 폐가 허탈과 환기 장애가 발생한다.

폐에 상처가 생기면 폐 조직 자체에 출혈이 발생할 수도 있다. 이 혈액은 폐포로 들어가 공기로 채워지는 것을 방해하고 혈액으로 가득 찬 폐포는 가스 교환에 참여할 수 없다. 더 많은 폐포에 혈액이 많을수록 환자의 환기와 산소 공급이 더 많이 저하될 수 있다.

폐나 기도에 상처가 생기면 공기색전증이 발생할 수도 있다. 흔하지는 않지만, 치명적일 수 있다. 공기색전증은 공기 공급원(일반적으로 더 큰 기도 손상)과 혈관계(일반적으로 정맥 손상) 사이의 직접적인 소통으로 인해 발생한다. 양압 환기(백 또는 기계적 환기)는 이러한 현상의 발생 가능성을 높일 수 있다. 공기색전증은 혈류역학적 불안정성, 신경학적 결손(동맥일 때) 또는 심정지까지 초래할 수 있다.

무딘 손상

가슴벽에 가해진 무딘 힘은 가슴 내 장기로 전달된다. 이 에너지의 파동은 폐 조직을 찢어 폐포에 출혈을 일으킬 수 있다. 이러한 형태의 손상을 폐 타박상이라고 한다(**그림 10-10**). 폐 타박상은 본질적

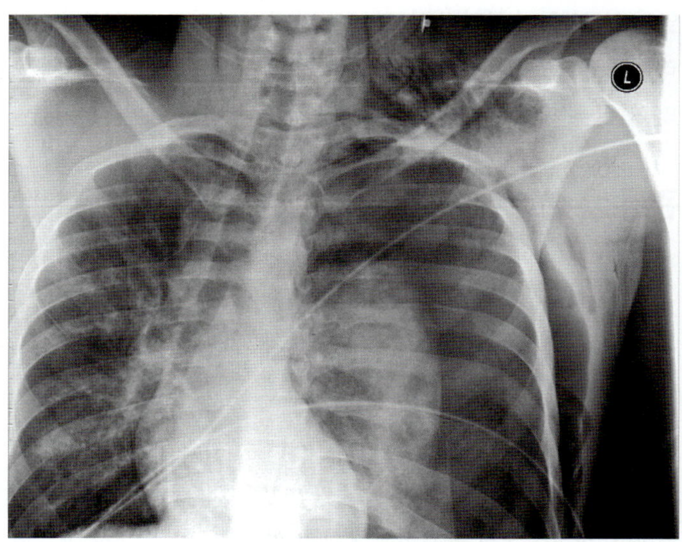

그림 10-8 왼쪽 긴장기흉을 보여주는 X-ray.

Courtesy of Dr. Mark Gestring, MD, FACS.

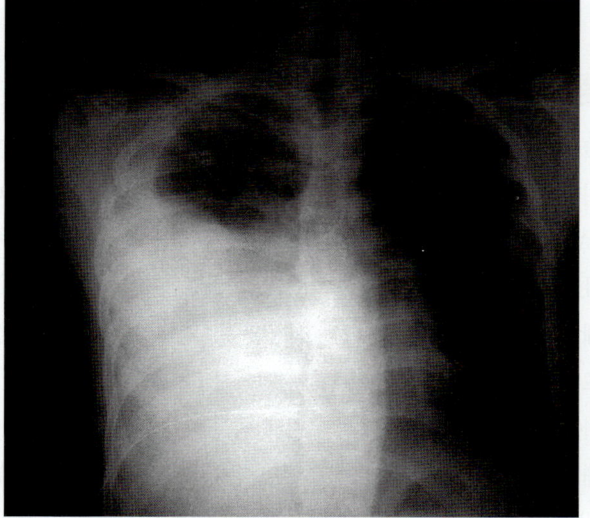

그림 10-9 오른쪽 가슴에 대량 혈흉을 보여주는 X-ray.

© Medicshots/Alamy Stock Photo

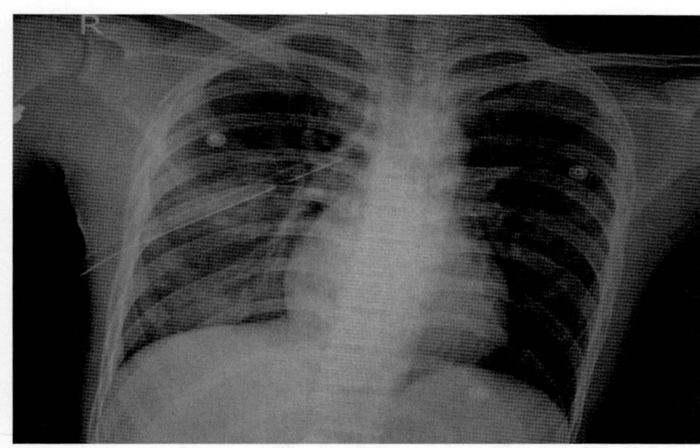

그림 10-10 오른쪽 폐 타박상을 보여주는 X-ray.
© Richman Photo/Shutterstock

으로 폐에 타박상을 입는 것으로 적극적인 수액 소생술로 인해 악화할 수 있다. 산소 공급 및 환기에 미치는 영향은 관통상과 같다. 폐 조직에 가해지는 힘으로 인해 내장가슴막이 찢어지면 공기가 폐에서 가슴막안으로 빠져나와 기흉이 발생하고 앞서 설명한 것처럼 긴장기흉이 발생할 가능성이 있다.

무딘 외상은 또한 갈비뼈를 부러뜨려 폐에 열상을 입혀 기흉과 혈흉(부러진 갈비뼈와 찢어진 폐 및 갈비사이근에서 출혈로 인해 발행)을 유발할 수 있다. 일반적으로 갑작스러운 감속 사고와 관련된 무딘 손상은 가슴의 주요 혈관 특히 대동맥 전단 또는 파열을 일으켜 치명적인 출혈로 이어질 수 있다. 마지막으로 경우에 따라 무딘 힘으로 인해 가슴벽이 손상되어 가슴벽이 불안정해지고 가슴 내 압력의 변화를 손상해 환기 장애가 발생할 수 있다.

평가

의학적 처치의 모든 측면과 마찬가지로 평가에는 병력 청취와 신체검사 시행이 포함된다. 외상이 발생한 상황에서 환자의 증상, 알레르기, 복용 중인 약물, 과거 병력, 마지막 식사 시간 및 손상과 관련된 사건 및 위험 요인을 파악할 수 있는 SAMPLE 병력을 말한다(6장 환자 평가 및 관리 참조).

가슴 외상이 있는 환자는 날카롭거나 찌르는 듯한 가슴 통증, 조이는 듯한 가슴 통증을 경험할 가능성이 높다. 종종 호흡하거나 움직임일 때 통증이 더 심해지는 경우가 많다. 환자는 숨이 가쁘거나 숨을 충분히 들이마실 수 없는 느낌을 호소할 수 있다. 쇼크가 진행 중이면 환자는 불안해하거나 어지러움을 느낄 수 있다. 증상이 없다고

해서 손상이 없는 것과 같지 않다는 것을 기억하는 것이 중요하다.

평가의 다음 단계는 신체검사를 시행하는 것이다. 신체검사는 관찰(시진), 촉진, 타진, 청진으로 구성된다.

- 관찰(Observation): 환자의 피부가 창백하고 땀을 흘리는지 관찰하며 이는 쇼크의 존재를 나타낼 수 있다. 환자는 불안해 보일 수 있다. 청색증(특히 입과 입술 주위 피부가 푸르스름하게 변색하는 증상)은 늦게 발견되며 저산소증이 진행되면 분명하게 나타날 수 있다. 호흡 속도와 환자가 호흡곤란(헐떡거림, 목의 보조 호흡근 수축, 코 벌렁거림)에 주목해야 한다. 기관이 정중선에 자리 잡고 있는가? 아니면 다른 쪽으로 치우쳐 있는가? 목정맥이 확장되어 있는가? 가슴에 타박상, 찰과상, 열상 및 가슴벽이 호흡할 때 대칭적으로 확장되는지를 검사한다. 호흡 시 가슴벽의 일부가 호흡에 따라 반대로 움직이는 부분이 있는가? 상처가 확인되면 환자가 숨을 들이쉬고 내쉴 때 상처에 공기 방울이 발생하는지 주의 깊게 확인한다.

- 청진(Auscultation): 가슴 전체를 평가한다. 한쪽의 호흡음이 다른 쪽에 비해 감소하면 평가한 쪽에 기흉이나 혈흉이 있을 수 있다. 폐 타박상은 비정상적인 호흡음(수포음)을 유발할 수 있다. 현장에서는 구분하기 어려운 경우가 많지만, 심음 청진시 심장 주위에 혈액이 고여서 들리는 심잡음과 판막 손상으로 인한 잡음도 나타날 수 있다.

- 촉진(Palpation): 손과 손가락으로 가슴벽을 부드럽게 누르면서 압통, 티빔소리(뼈, 피부밑기종), 가슴벽의 뼈 불안정성이 있는지 평가한다

- 타진(Percussion): 이 신체검사 방법은 시끄러운 환경으로 인해 현장에서 평가하기 어려운 경우가 많으므로 현장에서 수행하기 어렵다. 또한, 타진을 통해 병원 전 처치에 변화를 가져올 수 있는 얻을 수 있는 추가 정보가 거의 없다.

평가에는 활력징후에 관한 판단도 포함되어야 한다. 동맥혈산소포화도를 평가하기 위해 맥박산소측정기를 환자에게 부착하는 것은 손상 환자를 평가하는 데 유용한 보조 수단이다.

- 맥박산소측정기(Pulse oximetry): 헤모글로빈에 결합한 산소 수준을 평가하고 모니터링하여 환자의 상태 변화와 처치에 대한 반응을 감지해야 한다. 산소포화도는 94% 이상으로 유지한다. 급성 외상 및 잠재적인 쇼크 상황에서 신뢰할 수 있는 맥박산소측정 수치를 얻는 것이 어렵기 때문에 일반적으로 저산소증이 존재하는 것으로 가정하고 적절한 산고 공급에 대한 압도적인 증거가 없는 한 기본적으로 산소를 투여한다.

- 파형 호기말이산화탄소분압측정(Waveform capnography): 호기말이산화탄소분압측정은 호기말이산화탄수 수준을 평가하는 데 사용할 수 있으며 환자의 상태 변화와 처치에 대한 반응을 감지하기 위해 모니터링한다. 인라인샘플인(In-line sampling)은 직접 이산화탄소를 측정하는 반면, 사이드 스트림 평가(sidestream assessment)는 호기말 공기 샘플을 채취하여 샘플링 지점에서 멀리 떨어진 모니터 위치에서 이산화탄소 측정을 수행한다.
- 외상 초음파 검사를 통한 확장된 집중 평가(eFAST): 현장 초음파(POCUS)는 병원 전 환경에서 활발히 연구되고 있는 새로운 기술이다. 추가 교육과 경험이 필요하지만, 항공 또는 지상 이송 중에도 가능하며 신체검사에 유용한 보도 도구가 될 수 있다. 가슴 외상의 맥락에서 집중평가의 주요 역할은 기흉과 심낭삼출액을 식별하는 것이다(**Box 10-2**). 적절한 교육을 통해 병원 전 처치 제공자가 외상성 가슴 병리학을 정확하게 식별할 수 있다는 증거가 점점 늘어나고 있다. 병원 전 환경에서 이러한 기술을 사용하면 환자 생존율이 향상된다는 증거는 아직 없다. 한 가지 중요한 우려는 이러한 기술을 현장에 도입하면 현장 체류 시간이 길어지고 이송이 지연되어 환자 사망률이 높아질 수 있다는 점이다.

환자 재평가 시 호흡 속도를 반복적으로 측정하는 것은 환자의 상태가 악화하고 있음을 인식하는 가장 중요한 평가 도구가 될 수 있다. 환자가 저산소증에 빠지고 상태가 악화하면 환기 속도가 점진적으로 증가하는 것이 이러한 변화에 대한 초기 단서이다.

Box 10-2 가슴 외상에서 외상 초음파 검사를 통한 확장된 집중 평가(eFAST)의 역할

- 폐 초음파 징후(Lung sliding sign). 호흡하는 동안 내장가슴막과 벽가슴막이 서로 미끄러진다. eFAST에서 이러한 막의 접합부는 희미하게 빛나는(고에코) 흰색 선으로 나타난다. 정상적인 호흡 중에 가슴막의 앞뒤로 희미하게 움직이는 것이 폐 초음파를 정의한다. 기흉이 있으면 공기가 가슴막안을 방해하여 이 희미하게 빛나는 선이 중단되어 확인할 수 없다. 다른 질환이 폐초음파 징후를 방해할 수 있으므로 기흉을 진단하려면 이 징후를 임상적 특징과 결합해야 한다. 이 징후는 움직이는 이미지 없이는 적절하게 설명할 수 없다. eFAST 교육을 받은 병원 전 실무자는 술기를 유지하기 위해 교육과 실습을 계속해야 한다.
- 폐 초음파의 음성 예측값은 거의 100%에 가깝다. 즉 폐 초음파로 확인하면 기흉은 본직적으로 제외된다. 실제로 기흉이 임상적으로 의심되는 환자에게 초음파를 통해 불필요한 바늘감압으로 인한 피해를 예방할 수 있다는 증거가 있다. 그러나 이러한 데이터는 아직 병원 전 환경에서 검증되지 않았다.
- 폐 초음파의 양성 예측값은 90%를 초과한다. 이는 폐 초음파에서 확인되지 않으면 기흉이 있을 가능성이 높다는 의미이다. 그러나 다른 요인(예: 검사자 경험, 장치의 모드 설정, 매우 낮은 일회호흡량, 심한 유착 및 이전 폐절제술)이 기흉 확인을 더 어렵게 만들 수 있기 때문에 양성 예측값은 더 낮다. 다시 말하지만, 병원 전 환경에서의 양성 예측값이 병원 내 환경에서의 예측값과 어느 정도 일치하는지는 알 수 없다.
- 심장막 삼출액. 심장맥 삼출액은 일반적으로 외상 상황에서 혈액과 같은 체액이 심장막에 축적되는 것을 말한다. 칼돌기밑 심장 뷰를 이용한 초음파 검사로 심장막 삼출액을 확인할 수 있다. 이 혈액은 축적되어 혈류역학적 불안정성을 초래할 수 있다(이 장의 뒷부분의 심장눌림증 부분 참조).

특정 손상에 대한 평가 및 처치

갈비뼈 골절

갈비뼈 골절은 흔하며 무딘 외상 환자의 약 10%에서 발생한다. 갈비뼈 골절 환자의 이환율과 사망률에는 골절된 갈비뼈의 총개수, 양측 골절 유무, 65세 이상의 나이 등 여러 가지 요인이 영향을 미친다. 나이와 관계없이 갈비뼈 골절이 많을수록 사망률이 증가한다. 단일 갈비뼈 골절의 사망률은 5.8%이며 갈비뼈 5개가 골절되면 사망률은 10%, 갈비뼈 8개가 골절된 환자의 경우 사망률은 34%까지 증가한다. 노인은 특히 갈비뼈 골절에 취약하며 이는 피질 골량의 손실(골다공증)로 인해 갈비뼈가 적은 힘을 견디고도 골절될 수 있기 때문일 가능성이 높다.

위쪽 갈비뼈는 넓고 두껍고 어깨이음뼈와 근육으로 잘 보호된다. 위쪽 갈비뼈 골절에는 큰 에너지가 필요하므로 위쪽 갈비뼈 골절 환자는 외상성 대동맥 파열과 같은 다른 심각한 손상의 위험이 있다. 갈비뼈의 부러진 끝이 근육, 폐 및 혈관을 찢어 폐 타박상, 기흉, 혈흉의 가능성이 있다. 기저 폐 타박상은 다발성 갈비뼈 골절과 가장 흔하게 연관된 손상이다. 또한 폐 압박으로 인해 폐포가 파열되어 기흉이 발생할 수 있다. 아래 갈비뼈 골절은 비장 및 간 손상과 연관될 수 있으며 다른 복강 내 손상의 가능성을 나타낼 수 있다. 이러한 손상은 출혈 또는 쇼크 징후를 나타낼 수 있다.

평가

단순 갈비뼈 골절 환자는 대부분 호흡곤란과 숨을 들이마시거나 움직일 때 가슴 통증을 호소한다. 호흡곤란이 있을 수도 있다. 가슴벽을 주의 깊게 촉진하면 일반적으로 갈비뼈 골절 부위 바로 위에 압통점이 발견되며 갈비뼈의 부러진 끝이 서로 부딪히면서 마찰음이 느껴질 수 있다. 병원 전 처치 제공자는 환기 속도와 호흡 깊이에 특히 주의하면서 활력징후를 평가한다. 모니터링에는 필요하거나 환자의 산소 공급 상태가 불확실한 경우 추가 산소 투여와 함께 맥박산소측정을 시행해야 한다.

처치

갈비뼈 골절 환자의 초기 처치는 적절한 산소 공급, 환기 및 통증을 완화하는 것이다. 적절한 산소 공급을 위해 보충 산소를 투여하고 환기를 보조할 수 있다. 적절한 통증 조절을 위해서는 불안감을 줄이기 위해 안심시키고 환자의 팔을 편안한 위치에 두는 것이 필요할 수 있다. 환기 상태가 악화하고 쇼크가 발생할 가능성을 염두에 두고 환자를 안심시키며 지속해서 재평가하는 것이 중요하다. 환자의 상태와 예상되는 이송 시간에 따라 정맥 라인 확보를 고려한다. 정맥 내로 진통제 투여는 적절한 프로토콜이나 의료 지도를 받을 수 있는 경우 갈비뼈 골절로 인한 통증이 환자의 효과적인 호흡 능력을 방해하는 상황에서 투여하는 것이 적절할 수 있다. 환자에게 폐포의 허탈(무기폐) 및 폐렴이나 기타 합병증의 가능성을 예방하기 위해 심호흡과 기침하도록 권장한다. 테이프 또는 보호장치로 가슴우리를 단단히 고정하는 것은 무기폐와 폐렴을 유발할 수 있으므로 피해야 한다.

동요가슴

동요가슴은 인접한 2개 이상의 갈비뼈가 길이를 따라 한 곳 이상에서 골절되었을 때 발생한다. 그 결과 가슴벽의 한 부분이 연속성이 더는 유지되지 않고 갈비뼈가 들숨 중에 바깥쪽과 위쪽으로 움직여야 할 때 영향을 받은 갈비뼈가 역설적으로 안쪽으로 움직일 수 있다(**그림 10-11**). 마찬가지로 날숨 중에는 가슴 내부의 압력이 증가함에 따라 갈비뼈가 바깥쪽으로 움직일 수 있다. 분절 부위의 이러한 모순운동이 발생하면 환기 효율을 떨어뜨린다. 비효율적인 환기의 정도는 분절 부위 크기와 직접적인 관련이 있다.

　이러한 손상을 일으키는 데 필요한 상당한 힘은 일반적으로 폐로 전달되어 폐 타박상을 유발한다. 따라서 환자의 환기 및 가스 교환은 분절 부위와 폐 타박상(환기를 방해할 때 더 큰 문제)에 의해 손상된다. 앞서 설명한 바와 같이 폐 타박상은 폐포에 혈액이 충만하여 손상된 폐의 타박상 부위에서 가스 교환이 이루어지지 않는다.

평가

단순 갈비뼈 골절과 마찬가지로 동요가슴을 평가하면 통증이 있는

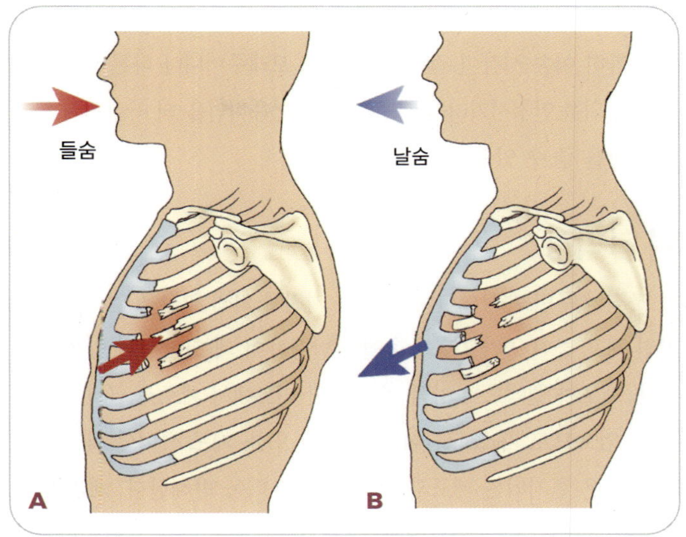

그림 10-11 모순운동. **A.** 인접한 갈비뼈가 두 군데 이상 골절되어 가슴벽의 안정성이 상실되면 들숨 시 가슴 내 압력이 감소함에 따라 외부 공기압에 의해 가슴벽이 안쪽으로 밀려나게 된다. **B.** 날숨 시 가슴 내 압력이 증가하면 가슴벽이 바깥쪽으로 밀려난다.
© National Association of Emergency Medical Technicians (NAEMT)

환자를 발견할 수 있다. 그러나 통증은 일반적으로 더 심하며 환자는 대부분 고통스러워 보인다. 환기 속도가 빨라지고 환자는 통증으로 인해 심호흡을 하지 않는다. 맥박산소측정이나 청색증으로 알 수 있듯이 저산소증이 있을 수 있다. 모순운동은 분명하거나 쉽게 인식되지 않을 수도 있다. 처음에는 갈비사이근이 경련을 일으키고 분절 부위를 안정화하는 경향이 있다. 시간이 지남에 따라 이러한 근육이 피로해지면 모순운동이 점점 더 분명해진다. 환자는 손상된 부위에 압통과 잠재적으로 뼈의 비빔소리를 들을 수 있다. 분절 부위의 불안정성은 촉진으로도 확인할 수 있다.

처치

동요가슴의 처치는 통증 완화, 보조 환기를 시행하고 환자 상태가 악화하는지 모니터링하는 것이다. 환기 속도와 일회호흡량이 가장 중요한 매개변수가 될 수 있다. 폐 타박상과 호흡기 손상이 발생한 환자는 시간이 지남에 따라 호흡 속도가 증가한다. 가능한 경우 맥박산소측정은 저산소증을 감지하는 데 유용하다. 산소포화도가 94% 이상 되도록 산소를 투여한다.

　이송 시간이 짧은 경우를 제외하고는 정맥 라인을 확보한다. 통증 완화를 위해 마약성 진통제를 신중하게 투여할 수 있다.

　적절한 산소 공급을 유지하는 데 어려이 있는 환자는 백마스크,

지속적기도양압기(CPAP) 또는 기관내삽관 및 양압 환기가 필요할 수 있다(특히 이송 시간이 길어지는 경우). 모래주머니나 다른 방법으로 분절 부위를 안정시키려는 시도는 가슴벽 움직임을 더 악화시켜 환기에 지장을 줄 수 있으므로 금기이다.

폐 타박상

폐 조직이 무딘 손상이나 관통하는 기전에 의해 열상을 입거나 찢어지면 폐포 공기 공간으로의 출혈이 발생하여 폐 타박상이 발생할 수 있다. 폐포가 혈액으로 가득 차면 말단 기도에서 폐포로 공기가 들어갈 수 없으므로 가스 교환이 손상된다. 또한, 폐포 사이의 혈액과 조직 부종은 환기되는 폐포의 가스 교환을 더욱 방해한다. 폐 타박상은 분절 부위기 있는 환자에게서 나타나며 가슴 외상의 흔하고 치명적일 수 있는 합병증이다. 손상 후 처음 24시간 이내 호흡부전으로 악화할 수 있다.

평가

환자 평가 소견은 타박상의 중증도(손상된 폐의 범위)에 따라 달라질 수 있다. 초기 평가에서는 일반적으로 호흡기 손상이 나타나지 않는다. 타박상이 진행됨에 따라 환기 속도가 빨라지고 청진시 거품소리가 들릴 수 있다. 실제로 환기 속도의 증가는 종종 폐 타박상으로 인한 환자의 상태가 악화하고 있다는 가장 빠른 단서인 경우가 많다. 특히 분절 부분이 있는 경우 높은 의심 지수가 필요하다.

처치

환자의 처치는 보조 환기를 시행하는 방향으로 이루어져야 한다. 병원 전 처치 제공자는 환기 속도와 호흡곤란 징후를 반복적으로 재평가한다. 가능한 경우에 맥박산소측정기를 활용한다. 폐 타박상이 의심되는 모든 환자에게 산소포화도를 정상 범위(≥94%)로 유지하는 것을 목표로 산소 보충을 제공한다. 지속적기도양압환기는 보조 산소 공급만으로 허용할 수 있는 산소포화도 수준을 유지하는 데 부적합한 환자의 산소 공급을 개선하기 위해 사용할 수 있다. 백마스크 장비로 환기를 기원하거나 성문위기도기 또는 기관내삽관을 통한 양압 환기가 필요할 수 있다.

적극적인 수액 소생술은 부종을 더욱 증가시키고 환기 및 산소공급을 악화시킬 수 있으므로 피해야 한다. 대신 혈압을 80~90mmHg로 유지하는 데 필요한 만큼만 정맥 내로 수액을 신중하게 투여한다.

폐 타박상은 수액 소생술이 결과를 악화시킬 수 있는 손상의 중요한 예이므로 환자의 혈압을 최소 80mmHg로 유지해야 하는 필요성과 균형을 맞춰야 한다(3장 쇼크: 삶과 죽음의 병태생리학 참조).

기흉

기흉은 심각한 가슴 손상의 최대 20%에서 발생한다. 기흉은 단순 기흉, 개방 기흉, 긴장기흉으로 분류할 수 있다.

단순 기흉은 가슴막안에 공기가 존재하는 것이다. 가슴막안 공기의 양이 증가하면 그쪽이 허탈 된다(**그림 10-12**). 개방 기흉(흡인 가슴 상처)은 가슴벽의 손상과 관련된 기흉으로 환기를 통해 외부에서 가슴막안으로 공기가 들어오고 나갈 수 있도록 허용하는 기흉이다. 긴장기흉은 가슴막 내 압력이 점진적으로 증가하면서 공기가 계속 유입되어 가슴막안에서 공기가 빠져나가지 못할 때 발생한다. 이로 인해 세로칸이 이동하여 심장으로 돌아오는 정맥혈이 감소하고 순환 기능이 손상된다.

단순 기흉

평가

단순 기흉에 대한 평가는 갈비뼈 골절 환자와 유사한 소견을 보일 가능성이 높다. 환자는 가슴막염 통증(호흡 시 악화하는 통증)과 경증에서 중증까지 다양한 호흡 곤란을 호소하는 경우가 많다. 전형적인 소견은 손상 부위의 호흡음이 감소하는 것이다. 호흡곤란과 호흡음 감소가 있는 환자는 기흉이 있는 것으로 간주한다.

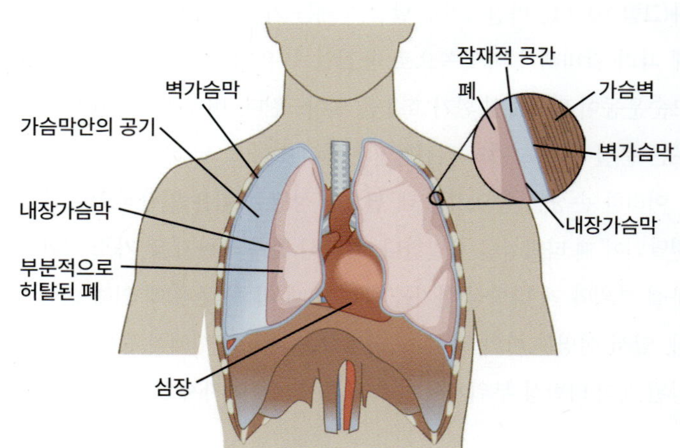

그림 10-12 가슴막안의 공기는 폐를 안쪽으로 밀어 환기할 수 있는 폐 조직의 양을 감소시켜 폐에서 나가는 혈액의 산소 수준을 감소시킨다.
© National Association of Emergency Medical Technicians (NAEMT)

처치

병원 전 처치 제공자는 보충 산소를 투여하고 정맥 라인을 확보하며 쇼크가 발생하면 처치할 준비를 한다. 호흡 약화의 조기 징후를 감지하기 위해 맥박산소측정, 파형 호기말이산화탄소분압측정 모니터링하는 것이 필수적이다. 척추 움직임 제한이 필요하지 않은 경우 환자는 반 앉은 자세를 취해주고 신속하게 이송한다. 병원 처치 제공자가 기본적인 수준의 처치만 시행할 수 있고 이송 시간이 지연된다면 전문소생술 팀과 약속된 장소에서 만나 환자를 인계하는 것을 고려한다.

처치의 핵심은 단순 기흉이 긴장기흉으로 빠르게 발전할 수 있다는 점을 인지하는 것이다. 순환이 심각하게 손상되기 전에 즉시 처치할 수 있도록 환자를 지속해서 모니터링하여 긴장기흉의 발생 여부를 확인한다.

개방 기흉

개방 기흉은 단순 기흉과 마찬가지로 가슴막안으로 공기가 유입되어 폐허탈이 발생한다. 가슴벽 손상으로 외부 공기와 가슴막안 사이에 연결 통로가 발생하는 것이 개방 기흉의 특징이다. 개방 기흉을 유발하는 기전에는 총상, 산탄총, 폭발, 관통상, 찔림 그리고 드물게 무딘 외상 등이 있다. 환자가 숨을 들이마시려고 하면 호흡근이 수축하면서 가슴안에 음압이 발생하기 때문에 공기가 개방 상처를 통해 가슴막안으로 들어간다. 더 큰 상처에서는 서로 다른 호흡 단계에 따라 가슴막안과 밖으로 공기가 자유롭게 들어오고 나갈 수 있다(**그림 10-13**). 가슴벽의 구멍을 통해 공기가 들어오고 나갈 때 가청 소음이 발생하는 경우가 많으며 이 상처를 '흡인 가슴 상처'라고 한다.

공기 흐름은 저항이 가장 적은 경로를 따르기 때문에 가슴벽을 통한 이러한 비정상적인 공기 흐름은 특히 개방 상처가 하부기도의 성문 개구부와 비슷하거나 더 큰 경우 상기도 및 기관을 통해 폐로 유입되는 정상적인 흐름보다 먼저 발생할 수 있다. 상처를 통한 공기 흐름에 대한 저항은 상처 부위가 커질수록 감소한다. 그런 다음 손상된 쪽의 폐가 허탈되고 기관을 통해 폐포가 아닌 상처를 통해 가슴막안으로 공기가 먼저 흐르기 때문에 효과적인 환기가 억제된다. 환자가 숨을 쉬고 있지만, 산소가 순환계로 유입되지 못한다.

평가

개방 기흉 환자를 평가하면 일반적으로 명백한 호흡 곤란이 나타낸다. 환자는 일반적으로 불안해하고 빠른 호흡을 보이며 맥박이 빨라

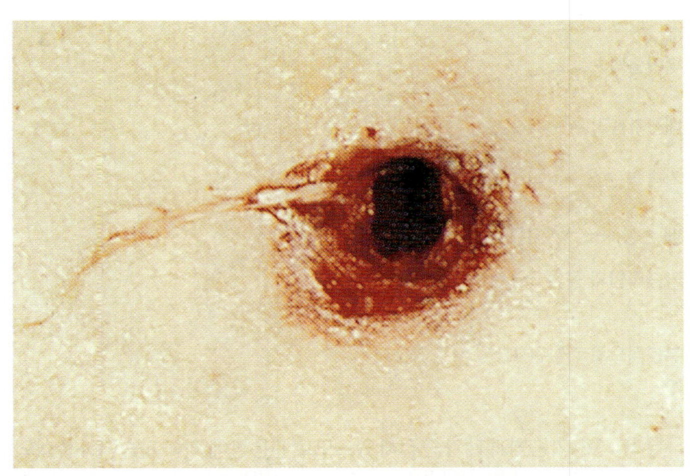

그림 10-13 가슴에 총상을 입거나 자상을 입으면 가슴벽에 구멍이 생겨 공기가 가슴막안으로 유입되거나 유출될 수 있다.
Courtesy of Norman McSwain, MD, FACS, NREMT-P.

지고 잠재적으로 가늘어질(촉진하기 어려움) 수 있다. 가슴벽을 검사하면 상처를 확인할 수 있고 들숨 시 빨아들이는 소리가 들리고 날숨 시 거품이 생길 수 있다.

처치

개방 기흉의 초기 처치에는 가슴벽 손상 부위를 밀봉하고 보충 산소를 투여하는 것이다. 상처를 통해 가슴막안으로 공기가 유입되는 것을 막기 위해 폐쇄드레싱을 적용하거나 시중에 판매하는 체스트 씰을 사용할 수 있으며 또는 알루미늄 포일이나 비닐 랩을 사용한다. 시중에 판매하는 제품을 사용할 수 없는 경우 바셀린 거즈는 제세동기 패드를 사용할 수 있다.

개방 기흉 환자는 거의 항상 폐에 손상을 입기 때문에 두 가지 원인으로 인해 공기가 누출된다. 첫 번째는 가슴벽의 구멍이고 두 번째는 폐의 구멍이다. 가슴벽 손상을 폐쇄드레싱으로 밀봉하더라도 손상된 폐에서 가슴막안으로 공기가 계속 누출되어 긴장기흉이 발생할 수 있다(**그림 10-14**).

개방 기흉을 처치할 때 폐쇄드레싱의 3면을 고정한다. 이렇게 하면 들숨 시 가슴안으로 공기가 유입되는 것을 방지하는 동시에 날숨 시 공기가 드레싱의 밀봉하지 않은 면을 통해 빠져나가 긴장기흉이 발생하는 것을 예방할 수 있다. 반대로 폐쇄드레싱의 네 면을 모두 테이프로 부착하면 긴장기흉이 발생할 위험이 있다. 개방 상처를 밀봉한 후에도 들숨과 함께 공기가 가슴막안으로 계속 이동할 수 있도록 하는 폐 조직에 근본적인 누출이 있어 기흉의 크기가 커지면 긴장기흉으로 변할 수 있다. 상처를 3면으로 밀봉하는 것이 효과적이면서 동

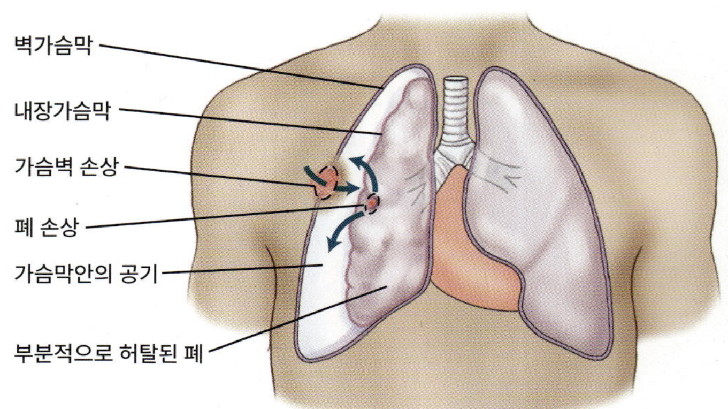

그림 10-14 가슴벽과 폐가 근접해 있으므로 관통상에 의해 가슴벽이 손상되고 폐가 손상되지 않는 것은 매우 어렵다. 가슴벽의 구멍을 막는다고 해서 폐에서 가슴막안으로 공기가 누출되는 것을 막을 수는 없다.
© National Association of Emergency Medical Technicians (NAEMT)

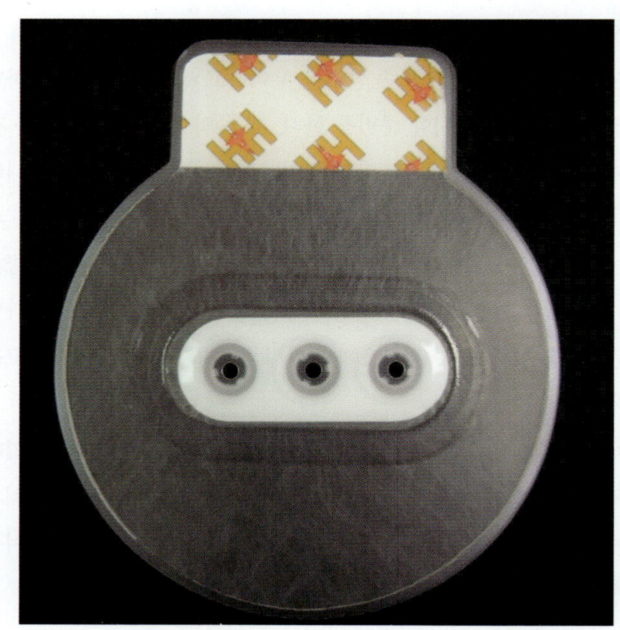

그림 10-15 개방 가슴 상처에 통기성 체스트 씰을 적용한 후 긴장기흉이 발생하는 것을 예방하는 것으로 나타났다.
Courtesy of H & H Medical Corporation.

시에 시간이 지남에 따라 가슴막안에서 공기가 방출되도록 하여 긴장기흉의 합병증을 피할 수 있다.

동물을 대상으로 한 연구에서는 통기성 체스트 씰을 사용한 동물과 비통기성 체스트 씰을 사용한 동물을 비교하여 개방 기흉 모델의 생리학적 반응을 평가했다. 이 연구에 따르면 두 가지 체스트 씰 모두 개방 기흉과 관련된 호흡 생리학을 개선했지만, 통기성 체스트 씰로 밀봉하면 긴장기흉의 발생을 예방했지만, 비통기성 체스트 씰로 밀봉하면 그렇지 않았다(**그림 10-15**). 이러한 발견으로 인해 군의 전술적 전투 사상자 처치(TCCC) 위원회는 가능한 경우 통기성 체스트 씰이 비통기성 체스트 씰보다 선호된다고 권고했다. 통기성 체스트 씰을 사용할 수 없는 경우 비통기성 체스트 씰을 대체 방법으로 사용할 수 있지만, 이후 긴장기흉이 발생하는지 환자를 주의 깊게 관찰해야 한다.

이 연구를 고려하여 병원 전 외상 소생술(PHTLS)은 개방 기흉 처치에 대해 다음과 같은 방법을 권장한다.

- 개방 가슴 상처 위에 통기성 체스트 씰을 부착한다.
- 통기성 체스트 씰을 사용할 수 없는 경우 상처 위에 랩이나 포일을 덮고 3면을 테이프로 붙인다.
- 이 중 어느 것도 사용할 수 없는 경우 비통기성 체스트 씰이나 바셀린 거즈와 같은 재료를 사용할 수 있지만, 이 방법은 긴장기흉이 발생할 수 있으므로 환자의 상태가 악화하는 징후가 있는지 주의 깊게 관찰해야 한다.
- 환자에게 빈맥, 빠른 호흡 또는 기타 호흡곤란의 징후가 나타나면 드레싱의 모서리를 몇 초간 제거하여 압력을 가하는 공기가 방출되도록 하고 필요에 따라 환기를 보조한다.
- 호흡곤란이 계속되면 긴장기흉이 발생했다고 가정하고 앞겨드랑선과 만나는 다섯 번째 갈비사이공간에 길이가 8cm의 대구경(10~16 게이지) 바늘을 사용하여 바늘감압을 시행한다.

이러한 처치로 적절하게 환자를 지지하지 못하면 기관내삽관 및 양압 환기가 필요할 수 있다. 양압을 사용하고 개방 상처를 밀봉하기 위해 드레싱을 시행한 경우 병원 전 처치 제공자는 긴장기흉이 발생하는지 환자를 주의 깊게 모니터링해야 한다. 호흡곤란이 심해지는 징후가 나타나면 상처를 덮고 있는 드레싱을 제거하여 축적된 압력을 감압해야 한다. 이러한 방법이 효과적이지 않으면 바늘감압을 고려한다.

양압 환기를 시행하는 경우 상처를 봉합하는 것은 기능적 환기 회복의 관점에서 훨씬 덜 중요하지만, 멸균드레싱은 추가적인 상처 부위 오염을 제한하는 관점에서 여전히 가치가 있다. 양압 환기는 폐를 직접 환기해 일반적으로 개방 기흉과 관련된 병태생리학을 효과적으로 처치한다.

긴장기흉

긴장기흉은 생명을 위협하는 응급 상황이다. 공기가 빠져나오지 않고 가슴막안으로 계속 유입되면 가슴속 압력이 높아진다. 가슴속 압

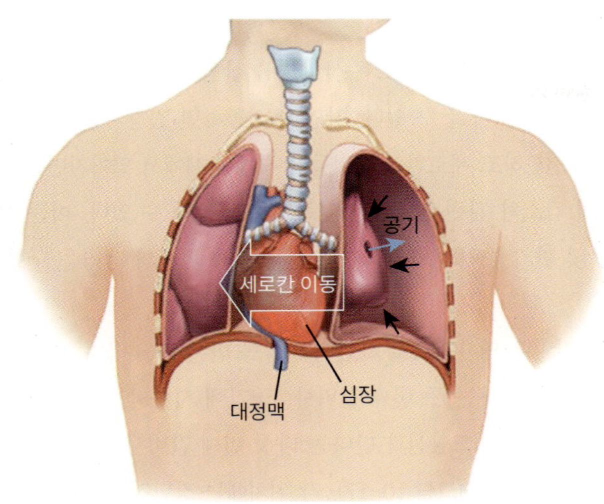

그림 10-16 긴장기흉. 가슴막안에서 빠져나가지 못한 공기의 양이 계속 증가하면 영향을 받은 쪽의 폐가 허탈 될 뿐만 아니라 세로칸이 반대쪽으로 이동한다. 그러면 반대쪽 폐가 압축되고 가슴속 압력이 증가하며 대정맥이 꼬여 심장으로의 혈액 복귀가 감소한다.
© National Association of Emergency Medical Technicians (NAEMT)

력이 상승하면 환기 기능 저하가 증가하고 심장으로 정맥혈복귀가 감소한다. 심박출량 감소와 함께 가스 교환이 악화하면 심각한 쇼크가 발생할 수 있다(**그림 10-16**). 가슴의 손상된 쪽의 압력이 증가하면 세로칸의 구조물이 손상된 반대쪽으로 밀릴 수 있다. 이러한 해부학적 왜곡은 가로막을 통과하는 아래대정맥의 꼬임으로 인해 심장으로 정맥혈복귀를 더욱 방해할 수 있다. 또한, 손상되지 않은 쪽의 폐 팽창이 점점 더 제한되어 호흡기 손상이 더 심해질 수 있다.

가슴 손상을 입은 모든 환자는 긴장기흉이 발생할 위험이 있다. 특히 기흉이 발생할 가능성이 있는 환자(예: 갈비뼈 골절 징후가 있는 환자), 기흉이 있는 것으로 알려진 환자(예: 가슴에 관통상을 입은 환자), 양압 환기를 받는 가슴 손상 환자 등이 고위험군에 해당한다. 이러한 환자는 순환 장애와 관련된 호흡 곤란이 증가하는 징후가 있는지 지속해서 모니터링하고 적절한 외상센터로 신속히 이송한다.

평가

환자평가 중에 발견되는 소견은 가슴막안에 축적된 압력의 양에 따라 달라진다(**Box 10-3**). 초기에 환자가 불안과 불편함을 보인다. 그들은 일반적으로 가슴 통증과 호흡곤란을 호소한다. 긴장기흉이 악화하면 불안, 빠른 호흡, 호흡곤란이 증가하고 심한 경우 청색증과 무호흡이 발생할 수 있다.

전형적인 소견은 손상된 쪽의 호흡음이 들리지 않는 것, 타진 시

Box 10-3 긴장기흉 징후

긴장기흉의 경우 다음과 같은 징후가 자주 논의되지만, 많은 징후가 나타나지 않거나 현장에서 파악하기 어려울 수 있다.

초음파

- 초음파에서 폐가 보이지 않음. 기흉은 긴장기흉으로 발달하기 전에 확인하고 처치할 수 있다. 그러나 호흡 상태에 대한 사전 평가와 상관없이 호흡 상태에 변화가 생기면 임상적 반복 및 초음파를 사용할 수 있는 경우 기흉에 대한 평가를 수행한다. **Box 10-2** 및 바늘감압 부분을 참조한다.

관찰

- 청색증은 현장에서 확인하기 어려울 수 있다. 어두운 조명, 피부색의 변화, 외상과 관련된 흙 및 혈액으로 인해 청색증이 잘 보이지 않는 경우가 많다.
- 목정맥 확장은 긴장기흉의 전형적인 징후로 설명된다. 그러나 긴장기흉 환자도 상당한 양의 혈액을 잃었을 수도 있으므로 목정맥의 확장이 눈에 띄지 않을 수 있다.

촉진

- 피부밑기종은 흔한 소견이다. 가슴안 내 압력이 증가하면 공기가 가슴벽의 조직을 통해 빠져나간다. 긴장기흉은 가슴 내 압력이 상당히 증가하기 때문에 피부밑기종은 종종 전체 가슴벽과 목 부위에서 촉지될 수 있으며 때로는 복벽과 얼굴에서도 나타날 수 있다.
- 기관 편위는 일반적으로 후기 징후이다. 이 징후가 존재하더라도 신체검사로 진단하기 어려울 수 있다. 목에서 기관은 근막과 기타 지지구조에 의해 목뼈에 부착되어 있으므로 기관편위는 가슴 내 현상에 더 가깝지만, 심할 경우 목정맥구멍파임에서 촉지될 수 있다. 기관편위는 병원 전 환경에서 흔히 관찰되지 않는다.

청진

- 손상된 쪽의 호흡음이 감소한다. 신체검사에서 가장 도움이 되는 부분은 손상된 쪽의 호흡음이 감소했는지 확인하는 것이다. 그러나 이 징후를 사용하려면 병원 전 처치 제공자는 정상 호흡음과 감소한 호흡음을 구별할 수 있어야 한다. 이러한 구별은 많은 연습이 필요하다. 환자를 접촉할 때마다 호흡음을 듣는 것이 도움이 될 것이다.

© National Association of Emergency Medical Technicians (NAEMT)

과공명음, 손상되지 않은 쪽으로 기관편위가 나타날 수 있으며 모두 혈류역학적 허탈이 진행되는 맥락에서 발생한다. 모든 환자의 청진을 지속해서 시행하면 병원 전 처치 제공자가 호흡음이 없거나 줄어든 것을 감지할 가능성이 높아진다. 현장에서 타진 시 과공명음을 확인하는 것은 종종 불가능하지만, 환자평가의 정확성을 위해 이 소견을 언급한다. 가능한 경우 일반적으로 환자가 누워있는 상태에서 두 번째와 세 번째 갈비사이 공간에서 초음파 검사를 시행하여 기흉의 징후를 확인하고 필요에 따라 반복 시행할 수 있다. 가슴 타진이나 초음파 검사를 위해 이송과 처치를 지연해서는 안 된다.

목정맥 팽대, 가슴벽 비빔소리, 청색증 등의 다른 신체적 소견이 나타날 수 있다. 가슴속 압력이 높아지고 맥압이 좁아지면서 빈맥과 빠른 호흡이 점점 더 두드러져 저혈압과 비보상성 쇼크가 나타난다.

처치

처치의 우선순위는 긴장기흉을 감압하는 것이다. 다음과 같은 세 가지 소견이 모두 있는 경우 감압을 시행한다.

1. 호흡곤란이 악화하거나 백마스크로 장비로 환기가 어려운 경우
2. 호흡음이 일방적으로 감소하거나 없어짐
3. 비보상성 쇼크(수축기 혈압 90mmHg 미만이고 맥압이 좁아짐)

임상적 상황과 병원 전 처치 제공자의 교육 수준에 따라 가슴막 감압을 시행하기 위한 몇 가지 방법이 있다. 감압을 시행할 수 없다면 (기본 소생술만 가능하고 제거할 폐쇄드레싱이 없는 경우) 고농도 산소(흡입산소농도≥94%)를 투여하면서 신속한 평가와 적절한 의료기관으로 신속하게 이송하는 것이 필수적이다. 양압 환기는 환자가 저산소 상태이고 산소 보충에 반응하지 않는 경우에만, 시행하며 이러한 상황은 긴장기흉을 급속히 악화시킬 수 있다. 환기를 조조하면 공기가 가슴막안으로 더 빠르게 축적할 수 있다. 전문 소생술은 환자를 의료기관으로 이송하는 것보다 빠르게 시행할 수 있는 경우에만 시행할 수 있다.

폐쇄드레싱으로 인해 의심되는 긴장기흉

개방 기흉 환자에게 폐쇄드레싱을 적용하면 잠시 개방하거나 제거해야 한다. 이렇게 하면 상처 부위를 통해 공기가 빠져나가 긴장기흉이 감압 될 수 있다. 긴장기흉의 증상이 재발하는 경우 이 절차를 이송 중에 주기적으로 반복해야 할 수 있다. 몇 초 동안 드레싱을 제거하는 것이 효과가 없거나 개방 상처가 없는 경우 전문소생술 제공자는 바늘감압을 시행해야 한다.

삽관된 환자에서 의심되는 긴장기흉

삽관된 환자의 경우 기관내관의 위치가 잘못되면 긴장기흉으로 오인 될 수 있다. 기관내관이 깊게 삽입되면 일반적으로 오른쪽 주기관지로 삽입이 되어 반대쪽 폐는 환기가 되지 않고 호흡음과 가슴벽 확장이 현저하게 감소할 수 있다. 이러면 가슴 감압술을 시행하기 전에 기관내삽관의 위치를 평가하고 확인한다.

바늘감압(바늘 가슴관삽입)

손상된 쪽의 가슴막안으로 주삿바늘을 삽입하면 압력을 받아 축적된 공기가 빠져나갈 수 있다. 감압이 성공하면 긴장기흉을 개방 기흉으로 전환하고 세로칸의 장기들이 허탈된 폐에서 멀어지면서 정맥 복귀혈 감소와 관련된 혈류역학 문제를 회복할 수 있다. 이는 산소 공급 및 환기 능력의 즉각적인 개선을 통해 환자의 생명을 구할 수 있다.

바늘감압은 역사적으로 가슴의 영향을 받은 쪽(젖꼭지 옆쪽)의 빗장중간선과 만나는 두 번째 갈비사이공간에 시행되었다. 그러나 최근의 증거는 앞겨드랑선과 만나는 다섯 번째 갈비사이공간(측면 접근) 것을 지지한다(**그림 10-17**). 각 위치에는 장단점이 있다. 빗장중간선에서의 감압은 병원 전 환경에서 접근하기 쉽다는 장점이 있지만, 이 위치의 가슴벽 두께로 인해 카테터가 가슴안에 도달하지 못하거나 환자를 이동하는 동안 카테터가 빠지거나 막힐 수 있다. 또한, 부주의하게 카테터를 빗장밑 혈관, 속가슴동맥, 심장 및 폐혈관으로 삽입하여 출혈을 유발할 위험이 적다. 이러한 이유로 현재 병원 전 긴장기흉 감압을 시행하기 위한 1차 위치로 측면 접근법이 권장되고 있다.

카테터를 앞겨드랑선 부위에 삽입하는 장점은 상대적인 안전성과 효과를 포함한다. 이 위치의 가슴벽은 남성과 여성 모두에서 체질량

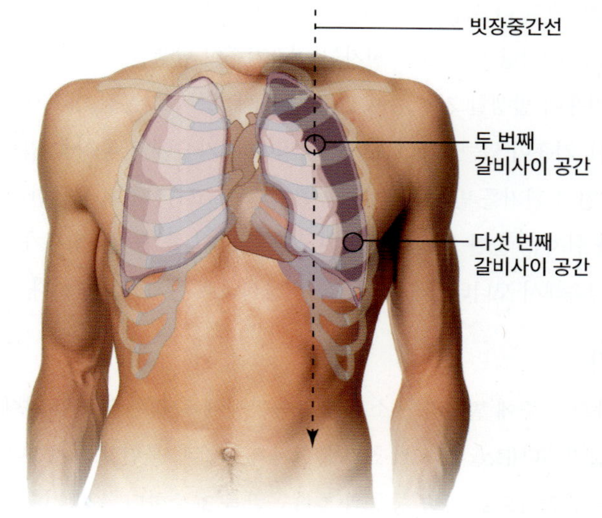

그림 10-17 긴장기흉이 의심되는 경우 처치를 위한 가슴안 바늘감압. 이 술기는 바늘 길이가 최소 8cm 이상인 대구경(10~16 게이지) 정맥 주삿바늘을 사용하여 수행한다. 주삿바늘은 앞겨드랑선과 만나는 다섯 번째 갈비사이공간에 위치해야 한다.

지수(BMI) 사분위에 걸쳐 더 얇다. 또한 이 위치에 더 높은 성공률이 보고되었으며 앞겨드랑선과 만나는 다섯 번째 갈비사이 공간에 삽입된 카테터는 꼬임이 문제가 될 수 있지만, 이송 중에 더 안정적이며 빠질 가능성이 적다는 증거가 있다.

선택한 위치와 관계없이 감압은 길이가 최소 8cm 이상인 대구경(10~16 게이지) IV 바늘을 사용하여 시행한다. 바늘과 카테터는 공기가 밀려 나올 때까지 삽입해야 하지만, 그 지점을 넘어서는 안 된다. 손상을 받은 쪽의 폐가 허탈되어 반대쪽으로 이동하므로 바늘감압을 시행하는 중에 손상을 입을 가능성은 거의 없다. 감압이 완료되면 바늘에서 속침을 제거하고 카테터가 빠지지 않도록 가슴에 테이프로 고정한다. 감압을 시행한 후 환자를 주의 깊게 모니터링한다. 한 연구에서는 혈관 카테터의 꼬임, 막히거나 빠짐으로 인한 기계적 실패율이 26%였으며 감압 시도의 43%는 궁극적으로 긴장기흉을 완화하는 데 실패한 것으로 나타났다.

이 절차를 성공적으로 수행하면 긴장기흉이 단순 개방 기흉으로 전환된다. 호흡 노력의 완화는 개방 기흉의 부정적인 영향보다 훨씬 더 크다. 감압 카테터의 지름이 환자의 기도보다 훨씬 작으므로 카테터를 통한 공기의 이동으로 인해 환기 노력이 크게 저하될 가능성은 거의 없다. 따라서 한 방향 판막을 만드는 것은 임상적 관점에서 볼 때 불필요할 수 있다. 상업용을 사용하는 것은 비용이 많이 들고 글러브를 이용하여 밸브를 만드는 것은 시간이 오래 걸린다. 필요에 따라 보조 환기와 보충 산소를 지속해서 공급하는 것이 적절하다. 바늘감압술이 실패하면 이 술기에 대한 교육을 받고 의료 지도를 받으면 손가락 가슴관삽입 또는 손가락 감압술이 방법이 될 수 있다.

일반적으로 양쪽 가슴에 긴장기흉이 발행하는 것은 삽관 및 양압 환기를 하지 않는 환자에게서 매우 드물게 발생한다. 환자를 재평가하는 첫 번째 단계는 기관내관의 위치를 확인하고 기관내관을 압박하는 꼬임이나 구부러짐이 없는지 확인하며 기관내관이 부주의로 주기관지로 삽입되지 않았는지 확인하는 것이다. 양압 환기를 시행하지 않는 환자에게 양쪽 가슴에 바늘감압을 시행하는 경우 극도의 주의를 기울여야 한다. 병원 전 처치 제공자의 평가가 잘못되면 양측 기흉이 생성되어 심각한 호흡곤란을 유발할 수 있다.

환자를 적절한 의료기관으로 신속하게 이송해야 한다. 이송 시간이 특히 짧은 경우가 아니라면 이송 중에 정맥 라인을 확보하고 환자의 상태가 악화하는지 자세히 관찰한다. 반복적인 감압과 기관내삽관이 필요할 수 있다.

튜브 가슴관삽입

일반적으로 가슴관삽입(튜브 가슴관삽입)은 시간, 절차적 합병증, 교육 문제 등의 이유로 병원 전 환경에서 수행하지 않는다. 바늘감압은 필요한 단계가 적고 사용하는 장비도 적기 때문에 튜브 가슴관삽입보다 더 빠르게 감압을 시행할 수 있다. 튜브 가슴관삽입의 발표된 합병증은 2.8~21%이며 여기에는 감염으로 인해 가슴막안에 고름이 고이거나 심장 또는 폐 손상, 가슴벽 피부밑조직이나 복막강 내 위치 이상 등이 발생한다. 이 술기를 시행하려면 상당한 교육이 필요하며 숙련도를 유지하기 위해서는 지속적인 연습이 필요하다.

가슴관을 삽입한 채 이송되는 환자는 특히 양압 보조 환기를 받는 경우 여전히 긴장기흉이 발생할 위험이 있다. 긴장기흉의 징후가 나타나기 시작하면 먼저 가슴관이나 연결 튜브에 꼬임이 없는지 확인한다. 다음으로 연결 튜브가 제대로 워터 씰 및 배액 장치에 올바르게 연결되어 있는지 확인한다. 확인된 문제가 없더라도 환자가 긴장기흉이 증가하는 징후가 있는 환자에게는 바늘감압이 필요할 수 있다. 이미 가슴관삽입이 되어 있다고 해서 지체하지 않는다(**Box 10-4**).

혈흉

혈흉은 혈액이 가슴막안으로 들어갈 때 발생한다. 이 공간에는 많은 양의 혈액(2,500~3,000mL)을 수용할 수 있으므로 혈흉은 대량 출혈의 원인이 될 수 있다. 실제로 가슴으로 대량 출혈이 발생하면 쇼크가 발생하며 충격을 받은 폐의 실제 허탈보다 더 큰 생리학적 결과를 초래할 수 있다(**그림 10-19**). "긴장혈흉"을 일으킬 만큼 충분한 혈액이 축적되는 경우는 드물다. 혈흉을 유발하는 기전은 다양한 유형의 기흉을 유발하는 기전과 같다. 출혈은 가슴벽 근육, 갈비사이 혈관, 폐 실질, 폐혈관 또는 가슴의 큰 혈관에서 발생할 수 있다.

평가

평가 결과 가슴으로 손실된 혈액의 양과 관련된 쪽의 폐 압박에 따라 환자가 어느 정도 고통스러워하는 것을 알 수 있다. 가슴 통증과 호흡곤란이 다시 특징으로 나타나며 일반적으로 심각한 쇼크의 징후가 나타난다. 병원 전 처치 제공자는 빈맥, 빠른 호흡, 혼란, 창백, 저혈압 등 쇼크 징후가 있는지 환자를 모니터링한다. 손상 부위의 호흡음이 감소하거나 없지만, 타진 시 둔탁음이 들린다(기흉의 과공명음과 비교). 기흉은 혈흉과 함께 나타날 수 있으며 심폐 기능 저하 가능성을 높인다. 순환 혈액량 감소로 인해 목정맥 확장이 나타나지 않

Box 10-4 튜브 가슴관삽입 문제 해결

가슴관 배액 시스템의 세 가지 기본 구성 요소

1. **밀봉**: 공기가 가슴막안에서 빠져나가는 것은 허용하지만, 되돌아오는 것은 허용하지 않는다. 밀봉은 일반적으로 공기가 가슴막안에서 빠져나가 흡기성 음압으로 상승할 때 거품이 발생하는 워터 실(water seal)이다.
2. **수집 장치**: 배액 물을 수집하고 측정한다. 배액되는 양의 변화를 관찰한다.
3. **흡인**: 배액 및 확장을 돕기 위해 음압을 제공한다. 흡인기가 올바르게 부착되어 있고 작동하는지 확인한다. 환자를 이송하기 전에 환자의 의료팀은 배액 시스템의 기본 작동을 재확인한다(**그림 10-18**).

가슴관 삽입 환자의 호흡 상태 변화

- 산소포화도측정을 포함한 활력 징후를 평가한다. 가슴관이 제대로 작동하지 않으면 환자는 빈맥, 빠른 호흡, 저산소증이 될 수 있다. 긴장기흉이 발생하면 피부밑기종, 호흡곤란 증가, 맥압 감소, 저혈압이 발생할 수 있다.
- 호흡음을 평가한다. 가슴관이 더 이상 기능하지 않고 대신 가슴 내부에 공기가 다시 축적되면 손상된 쪽에서 호흡음이 감소할 수 있다.
- 환기 노력을 평가한다. 가슴관이 올바르게 작동하지 않으면 환기 노력이 증가한다.
- 순환을 평가한다. 가슴관이 제대로 작동하지 않아 가슴 내부에 공기가 축적되면 환자는 빈맥이 발생할 수 있다. 긴장기흉이 발생하면 좁은 맥압이 좁아지고 저혈압이 발생할 수 있다.
- 의식 수준을 평가한다. 저산소증이나 쇼크 징후가 나타나면 환자는 불안해하고 동요할 수 있다. 이러한 합병증이 진행되면 환자의 의식 수준이 저하된다.

문제 해결 단계

- 이송하는 동안 가슴관이 빠지지 않았는지 드레싱과 튜브 삽관 부위를 확인한다.
- 가슴관이 단단히 연결되어 있고 꼬이거나 혈전 또는 고정장치가 없고 막히지 않았는지 확인한다.
- 체스트 씰(chest seal)이 손상되지 않고 작동하는지 확인한다. 환기할 때 거품이 발생하거나 변화가 있는지 확인한다.

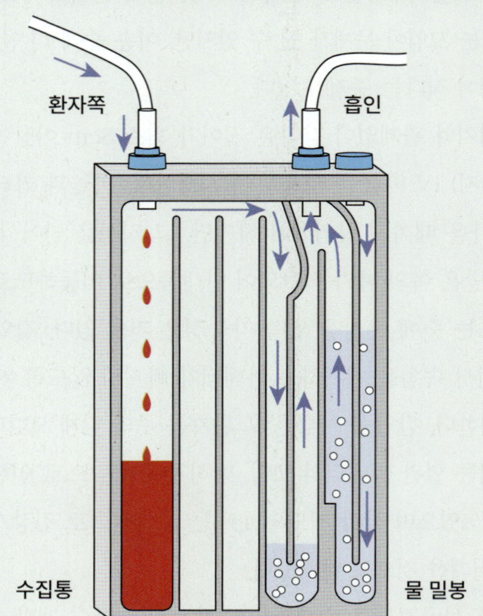

그림 10-18 가슴 배액 시스템은 음압을 제공하여 환자의 가슴 배액 및 팽창을 돕는다.
© National Association of Emergency Medical Technicians (NAEMT)

- 가슴관에 김이 서리거나 배액이 계속되고 있는지 평가한다.
- 흡인이 제대로 작동하는지 확인한다. 환기 주기 동안 계속 거품이 계속 발생하거나 음압 표시기가 나타나는지 확인한다.
- 환자의 환기 상태가 계속 악화하면 긴장기흉의 발생 징후가 있는지 면밀히 평가한다. 표시되면 배액 시스템에서 가슴관을 분리한다. 가슴관이 올바르게 배치되고 막히지 않으면 긴장기흉이 완화될 수 있다. 이 단계로 상태가 완화되지 않으면 바늘감압을 고려하고 의료 지도 의사의 의료 지도를 받는다.

© National Association of Emergency Medical Technicians (NAEMT)

는 경우가 많다.

처치

처치는 지속적인 관찰을 통해 생리학적 악화를 감지하고 적절한 지지를 제공하는 것이 포함된다. 고동도 산소를 투여하고 필요한 경우 기관내삽관을 시행하거나 백마스크로 보조 환기를 시행한다. 혈류역학 상태를 면밀히 모니터링한다. 무분별하게 많은 양의 결정질 용액을 투여하지 않고 적절한 관류를 유지하기 위해 정맥 라인을 확보하고 적절한 수액 처치를 시행한다. 가능한 경우 혈액제제 소생술이 적절할 수 있다. 즉각적인 수혈과 외과적 처치가 가능한 적절한 의료기관으로 신속하게 이송한다. 혈흉에 대한 가슴 바늘감압은 효과적이지 않으며 권장되지 않는다.

무딘 심장 손상

심장 손상은 주로 가슴 앞쪽에 충격이 가해지는 자동차 정면충돌과 같은 급감속 사고에서 가슴 앞쪽에 힘이 가해져 발생한다. 그러면 심장은 앞쪽의 복장뼈와 뒤쪽의 척추 사이에서 압박된다(**그림 10-20**). 이러한 심장 압박으로 인해 심실 내 압력이 정상보다 몇 배나 갑작스

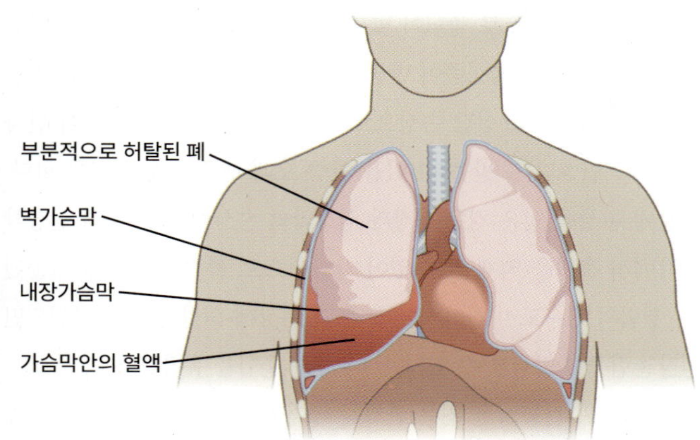

그림 10-19 혈흉. 가슴안으로 출혈과 관련된 혈액 손실(혈량저하증으로 이어짐)은 이 혈액으로 인해 폐가 압박되는 양보다 훨씬 더 심각한 문제이다.
© National Association of Emergency Medical Technicians (NAEMT)

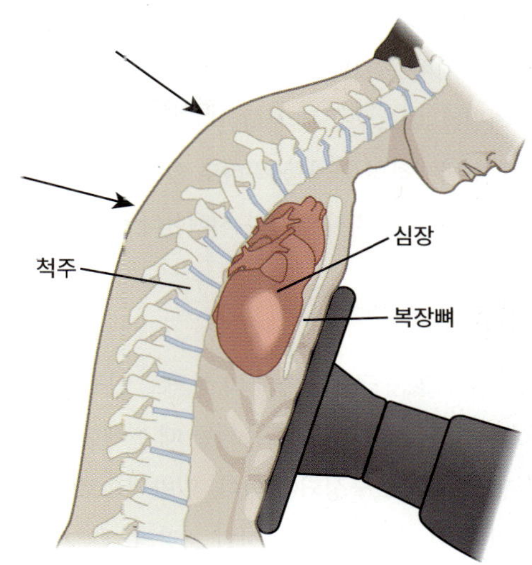

그림 10-20 심장은 복장뼈(복장뼈는 운전대나 대시보드에 부딪히면서)과 가슴벽 뒤쪽(가슴벽이 앞으로 계속 움직이면서) 사이에서 압박될 수 있다. 이 압박은 심근을 손상할 수 있다.
© National Association of Emergency Medical Technicians (NAEMT)

럽게 증가하여 다음과 같이 심장 타박상, 판막 손상 및 드물게 심장 파열이 발생할 수 있다.

- 심장 타박상: 심장 압박의 가장 흔한 결과가 심장 타박상이다. 심근 세포에 멍이 들고 심근 세포의 손상 정도도 다양하다. 이 손상은 종종 동빈맥과 같은 부정맥을 유발한다. 흔하지는 않지만, 심실빈맥 및 심실세동과 같은 심실조기수축 또는 비관류성 리듬이 발생할 수 있다. 심장의 중격 부위가 손상되면 심전도에 우각차단(RBBB)과 같은 심실 내 전도 이상이 나타날 수 있다. 많은 양의 심근이 손상되면 심장의 수축력이 손상되고 심박출량이 감소하여 심장성 쇼크가 발생할 수 있다. 일반적으로 외상 환경에서 발생하는 다른 형태의 쇼크와 달리 심장성 쇼크는 수액 투여로 개선되지 않으며 오히려 악화할 수 있다.
- 판막 파열: 심장 판막의 지지 구조물이나 판막 자체가 파열되면 일반적으로 판막이 기능을 상실하게 된다. 환자는 빠른 호흡, 거품소리(수포음) 및 새로 발생한 심잡음과 같은 울혈심부전(CHF)으로 증상 및 징후와 함께 다양한 정도의 쇼크 증상을 보일 수 있다.
- 심장 탈출은 동반한 무딘 심장막 파열: 드물게 발생하는 무딘 심장막 파열은 무딘 가슴 외상 환자의 0.4% 미만에서 발생한다. 이러한 환자는 혈류역학적 불안정성을 보일 수 있으며 특히 환자를 바로누운자세를 취해주면 심장이 심장막 파열 부위를 통해 탈출하여 심장 복귀가 손상될 수 있다.
- 무딘 심장 파열: 드물게 발생하는 무딘 심장 파열은 무딘 가슴 손상을 입은 환자의 1% 미만에서 발생한다. 이러한 환자의 대부분은 가슴안으로 대량출혈이나 치명적인 심장눌림증으로 인해 현장에서 사망한다. 생존한 환자는 일반적으로 심장눌림증이 나타난다.

평가

무딘 심장 손상의 가능성이 있는 환자를 평가한 결과 환자의 가슴 중앙에 정견으로 충격을 가한 기전이 나타난다. 복장뼈 위에 멍이 들거나 구부러진 운전대는 이러한 손상 기전을 의미한다. 다른 가슴 손상과 마찬가지로 환자는 가슴 통증과 호흡곤란을 호소할 가능성이 높다. 부정맥이 있는 경우 환자는 두근거림을 호소할 수 있다. 우려되는 신체 검진 소견으로는 복장뼈 위의 멍, 복장뼈 비빔소리, 복장뼈 불안정성 등이 있다. 부유 복장뼈(동요 복장뼈)가 있으면 복장뼈 양쪽의 갈비뼈가 골절되어 앞서 설명한 바와 같이 동요 가슴과 유사하게 호흡에 따라 모순 운동을 보일 수 있다. 판막 파열이 발생하면 저혈압, 목정맥 확장, 비정상적인 호흡음과 같은 급성 울혈심부전 징후와 함께 명치 부위에서 심한 잡음이 감지될 수 있다. 심전도 모니터링에서 부정맥(동빈맥, 심방세동, 조기심실수축 등)이 나타날 수 있다.

처치

핵심 처치 전략은 발생 가능성이 있는 무딘 심장 손상을 정확히 평가하고 임상 소견과 함께 평가 결과를 이송할 의료기관에 보고하는 것이다. 그동안 고농도 산소를 투여하고 적절하게 수액 처치를 시행하기 위해 정맥 라인을 확보한다. 환자에게 모니터를 부착하여 부정맥, ST 분절 상승을 모니터링한다. 부정맥이 있고 전문소생술(ALS)을 제공할 수 있다면 항부정맥 약물요법을 시행한다. 무딘 심장 손상에서 예방적 항부정맥 처치를 뒷받침하는 근거 자료는 없다. 항상 그렇듯이 환자에게 적절한 보조 환기를 시행한다. 바로 누운 상태에서 즉각적인 보상실패가 발생하면 환자를 똑바로 앉힌 상태로 유지한다. 항상 그렇듯이 보조 환기는 지시에 따라 시행한다.

심장눌림증

심장눌림증은 심장 또는 근위 대혈관의 상처로 인해 체액(보통 혈액)이 심장과 심장막 사이에 급성으로 축적될 때 발생한다. 심장막은 섬유질의 비탄성 조직으로 구성되어 있다. 일반적으로 심장막에는 앞서 서술한 바와 같이 가슴막안과 유사한 소량의 액체가 있다. 심장막은 비탄력적이기 때문에 심장막 내에 체액이 급격하게 축적되면 심장막 내 압력이 급격히 상승하기 시작한다. 이러한 심장막 내 압력 상승은 심장으로의 정맥복귀혈을 방해한다. 이는 결국 심박출량과 혈압 감소로 이어진다. 심장이 수축할 때마다 심장막으로 혈액이 추가로 유입되어 다음 수축을 준비하는 심장의 기능을 더욱 방해할 수 있다(**그림 10-21**). 이 상태는 무맥성 전기활동을 유발할 정도로 심해질 수 있으며 이는 생명을 위협하는 손상으로 모든 처치 단계에서 병원 전 단계에서 병원 전 처치 제공자가 최적의 결과를 달성하기 위해 협조적인 대응이 필요하다. 정상 성인의 심장막은 맥박 소실이 발생하기 전에 300mL의 체액을 수용할 수 있지만, 보통 50mL 정도만 있어도 심장 박동 복귀와 심박출량을 방해할 수 있다.

대부분의 경우 심장눌림증은 심장에 찔린 상처로 인해 발생한다. 이러한 손상 기전은 심실 중 한 곳을 관통하거나 심근의 열상을 초래할 수 있다. 우심실은 심장에서 가장 앞쪽에 있는 방이므로 관통성 외상에서 가장 흔하게 손상을 입는다. 손상의 해부학적 위치와 관계

없이 심장막 공간으로 출혈이 발생한다. 심장막 내 압력이 상승하면 생리학적으로 심장눌림증이 발생한다. 동시에 심장막 내의 압력이 증가하면 일시적으로 심장 손상으로 인한 추가 출혈을 방해하여 환자가 결정적인 처치를 받을 수 있을 만큼 오래 생존할 수 있도록 한다. 심장에 총상을 입은 경우 심장과 심장막의 손상이 너무 심해 심장막 공간에서 출혈을 억제할 수 없어 가슴안으로 출혈이 빠르게 배출된다. 찔림의 경우도 마찬가지이다. 무딘 손상에 의한 심실이 파열되면 심장눌림증이 발생할 수 있지만, 더 자주 출혈을 유발한다.

가슴 부위 관통상을 입은 환자를 평가할 때는 심장눌림증의 가능성을 염두에 두어야 한다. 빗장뼈를 따라 수평선과 유두에서 갈비뼈 가장자리까지 수직선을 그려서 형성된 직사각형 내에 관통상이 있는 경우 심장눌림증이 있거나 그렇지 않으면 다른 것으로 입증될 때까지 의심 지수를 높여야 한다(**그림 10-22**). 이러한 상처가 있는 환자를 처치하기 위해 적절한 의료기관으로 신속하게 이송을 시작하고 환자 상태를 보고해야 한다.

평가

평가에는 앞서 설명한 바와 같이 심장눌림증의 신체적 및 초음파 소견에 대한 인식과 함께 위험한 상처의 존재를 신속하게 인식하는 것이 포함된다(**Box 10-2**). Beck의 3 징후(Beck's triad)는 심장눌림증을 나타내는 소견으로 1) 멀어지거나 작아진 심장 소리(심장 주위의 체액으로 인해 판막이 닫히는 소리를 듣기 어려움), 2) 목정맥 확장

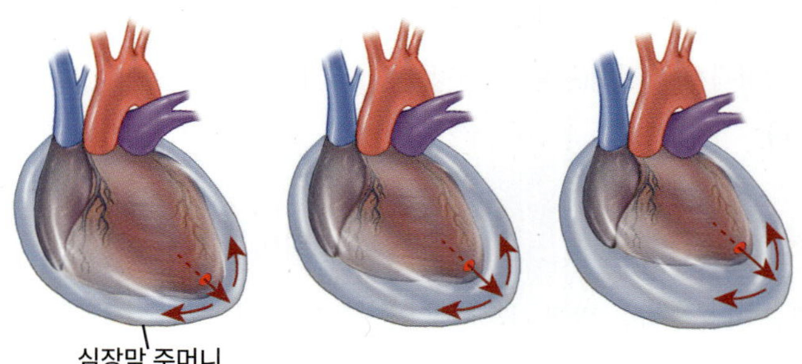

그림 10-21 심장눌림증. 심장 내 공간에서 심장막안으로 혈액이 유출되어 고이면서 심실 확장이 제한된다. 따라서 심실이 완전히 채워지지 않는다. 심장막안에 더 많은 혈액이 고이게 되면 혈액을 축적할 수 있는 심실 공간이 줄어들고 심박출량이 감소한다.

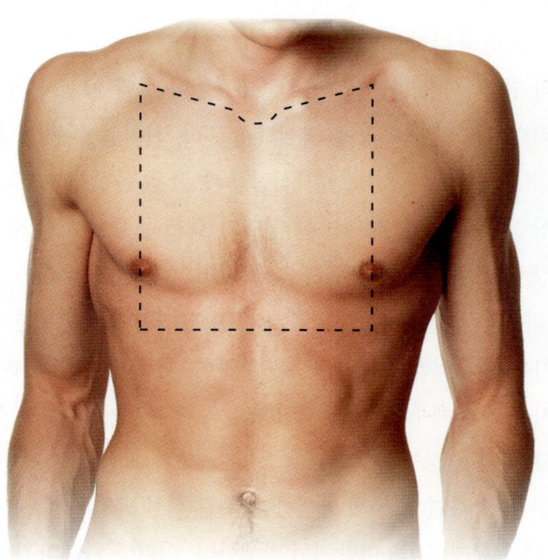

그림 10-22 관통상이 "심장 상자" 내에 발생하면 관통성 심장 손상을 의심하는 지수가 높아야 한다.

(심장막 안의 압력 증가로 인해 목정맥으로 혈액이 역류), 3) 저혈압
을 의미한다. 심장눌림증에서 설명되는 또 다른 신체적 소견은 모순
맥박이다(**Box 10-5**).

이러한 신체검사 징후 중 일부, 특히 감소한 심음이나 모순맥박을
현장에서 감지하기는 어렵다. 또한, 심장눌림증 환자 중 22~77%에서
만 Beck's triad가 나타난다. 따라서 병원 전 처치 제공자는 상처의
위치와 저혈압에 따라 높은 의심 지수를 유지하고 그에 따라 신속하
게 처치를 시행해야 한다.

처치

병원 전 처치 제공자는 환자를 즉시 외과수술이 가능한 의료기관으
로 신속히 이송하면서 모니터링을 시행한다. 병원 전 처치 제공자는
먼저 심장눌림증 존재할 가능성을 인식하고 이송할 의료기관에 응급
수술을 준비할 수 있도록 환자의 상태를 보고한다. 고농도의 산소를
투여하고 중심정맥압을 증가시켜 심장 충만을 개선할 수 있도록 정
맥 라인을 확보하여 적절하게 수액 소생술을 시작한다. 양압 환기는
정맥혈복귀를 감소시키고 혈류역학적 문제를 악화시킬 수 있으므로
가능하면 피해야 한다.

결정적인 처치를 위해서는 심장눌림증을 제거하고 심장 손상을 처
치해야 한다. 심장눌림증이 의심되는 환자는 가능한 한 즉시 외과수
술이 가능한 의료기관으로 즉시 이송한다. 심장막천자(심장막 공간
으로 바늘을 삽입)를 통해 심장막액의 일부를 배출하는 것이 효과적
인 일시적 처치 방법이다(**그림 10-23**). 심장막천자의 위험에는 심장
과 관상동맥의 손상으로 인한 심장눌림증 증가, 폐, 대혈관 및 간 손
상 등이 있다. 매우 드물게 현장 응급 상황에 대응하는 시스템에서
의사가 현장에 출동한 경우 소생술적 가슴절개(출혈을 조절하고 내
부 상처를 치료하기 위해 가슴을 여는 수술)를 현장에서 시행할 때도
있다.

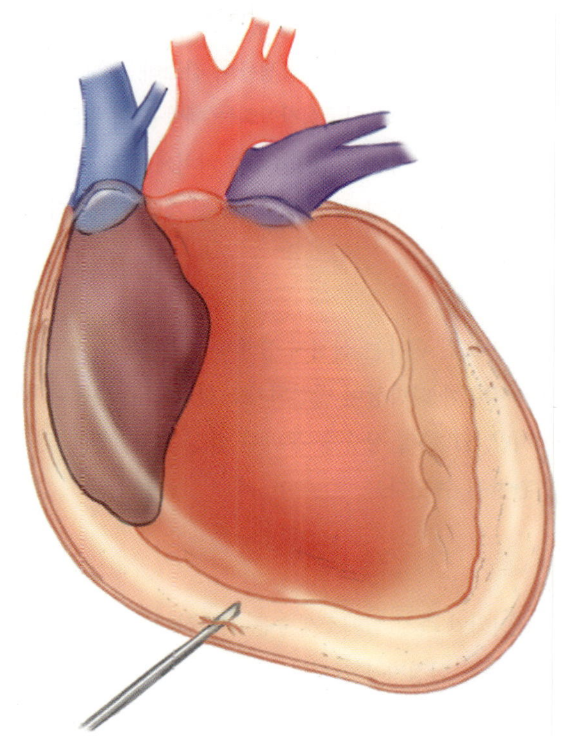

그림 10-23 심장막천자로 심장막액의 일부를 배출하는 것은 종종 심장눌림
증에 대한 효과적인 일시적 처치이다.
© National Association of Emergency Medical Technicians (NAEMT)

심장 진탕

심장 진탕이란 용어는 비관통성 가슴 손상으로 인한 갑작스러운 심
장사를 의미한다. 1990년대부터 미국에서 운영하는 국가 심장 소상
환자 등록의 220건 이상의 사례에 대한 데이터에 따르면 평균 발병
나이는 15세이고 사례의 95%는 남성이며 75%가 운동 중에 발생하는
것으로 나타났다. 대부분 전문가는 심장 주기의 전기적으로 취약한
부분에서 발생하는 상대적으로 경미한 비관통성 타격이 명치부위에
가해져 발생한다고 가정하지만, 다른 전문가들은 관상동맥 혈관 경련
이 발병에 영향을 미칠 수 있다고 생각한다. 손상 기전과 관계없이 그
결과 심실세동과 갑작스러운 심정지를 유발하는 심장 부정맥이다.

이 상태는 아마추어 스포츠 경기 중 야구공(가장 흔함), 아이스하
키 퍽, 라크로스 공 또는 소프트볼 같은 날아오는 물체에 환자가 가
슴 중앙을 맞아 경기 중에 가장 자주 발생한다. 그러나 신체 타격(격
투기), 저속 자동차 충돌, 야구공을 잡으려는 외야수 2명이 충돌한 후
에도 심장 진탕이 보고되었다. 충격 후 피해자는 한두 걸음 걷다가
갑자기 심정지로 바닥에 쓰러지는 것으로 알려져 있다. 일반적으로
부검 시 갈비뼈, 복장뼈 또는 심장에는 손상이 발견되지 않는다. 대

부분 피해자는 심장질환 병력이 없었다. 스포츠 경기 중 가슴벽 보호대를 사용한다고 해서 심장 진탕 발생률이 감소하는 것으로 입증되지 않았다. 미국심장협회와 미국심장학회는 예방을 위해 EMS에 신속한 신고를 포함하여 심장 진탕의 인식 및 처치에 대한 목격자 및 스포츠 경기 관계자의 교육 강화에 초점을 맞출 것을 권장한다.

평가

심장 진탕을 일으킨 환자는 심정지 상태에서 발견된다. 일부 피해자는 복장뼈에 경미한 타박상이 발견되기도 한다. 심실세동이 가장 흔한 리듬이지만, ST 분절 상승을 동반한 완전 심장차단과 좌각차단(LBBB)도 관찰될 수 있다.

처치

심정지가 확인되면 즉시 심폐소생술을 시작한다. 심장 진탕은 외상이나 출혈로 인한 심정지가 아니라 심근경색으로 인한 심정지와 유사한 방법으로 처치한다. 심장 리듬을 최대한 신속하게 파악하고 심실세동이 확인되면 신속한 제세동을 해야 한다. 예후는 좋지 않으며 생존 확률은 15% 이하이다. 이 상태의 거의 모든 생존자는 종종 목격자에 의한 신속한 심폐소생술과 즉각적인 제세동 처치를 받았다. 제세동기를 즉시 사용할 수 없는 경우 효과적이지는 않지만, 흉부타격법을 시도해 볼 수 있다. 흉부 타격을 시행하기 위해 심폐소생술과 제세동기 사용이 지연되어서는 안 된다. 즉각적인 제세동 시도가 실패하면 기도를 확보하고 정맥 라인을 확보한 후 에피네프린과 항부정맥 약물을 심정지 프로토콜에 설명된 대로 투여할 수 있다.

외상성 대동맥 파열

외상성 대동맥 파열은 상당한 힘의 감속 및 가속 기전으로 인해 발생한다. 고속 자동차 정면충돌과 높은 곳에서 추락하는 것이 그 예이다.

대동맥은 세로칸에 있는 심장의 윗부분에서 발생한다. 심장, 상행대동맥, 대동맥활은 가슴안에서 상대적으로 움직인다. 대동맥활이 하행대동맥으로 변화되면서 조직층으로 감싸고 척주에 부착된다. 따라서 하행대동맥은 상대적으로 움직이지 않는다. 고속 정면충돌과 같이 신체가 갑자기 감속하면 심장과 대동맥활은 고정된 하행대동맥에 비해 계속 앞으로 움직인다. 이러한 속도의 차이는 대동맥의 두 부분 사이의 접합부에서 대동맥벽에 전단력을 발생시킨다. 따라서 외상성 대동맥 손상의 일반적인 위치는 왼쪽 빗장밑동맥의 출발점 바로 원위부이다. 이 전단력은 대동맥벽에 다양한 정도로 파열시킬 수 있다(**그림 10-24**). 파열이 대동맥벽의 전체 두께를 통해 확장되면 환자는 가슴막안으로 빠르게 출혈이 발생한다. 그러나 파열이 대동맥벽의 바깥막은 손상되지 않고 부분적으로만 내측벽이 찢어졌다면 환자는 다양한 기간 생존할 수 있으며 생존하기 위해서는 신속한 평가와 처치가 필수적이다.

평가

대동맥 파열의 평가는 의심 지수에 달려 있다. 고에너지 감속 및 가속 기전과 관련된 상황에서는 높은 의심 지수를 유지해야 한다. 이러한 치명적인 손상의 경우 가슴 손상에 대한 외부 증거가 거의 없을 수 있다. 병원 전 처치 제공자는 기도와 호흡의 적절성을 평가해야 하며 가슴을 조심스럽게 청진하고 촉진해야 한다. 철저한 검사를 통해 양측 팔(왼쪽 팔보다 오른쪽 팔의 맥박이 더 강함) 또는 팔(위팔동맥)과 다리(넓적다리동맥)의 맥박이 다르다는 것을 확인할 수 있다. 혈압을 측정하면 대동맥 협착의 징후로 다리보다 팔에서 혈압이 더 높을 수 있다.

대동맥 파열의 확실한 진단을 내리기 위해서는 병원에서 방사선 촬영이 필요하다. 일반 가슴 방사선 촬영은 손상이 있음을 시사하는 다양한 징후를 보여줄 수 있다. 이 중 가장 신뢰할 수 있는 것은 세로칸의 확장이다(**그림 10-25**). 손상은 일반적으로 가슴 컴퓨터단층촬영(CT), 혈관조영술, 식도경유 심초음파검사를 통해 확인할 수 있다.

처치

현장에서 외상성 대동맥 파열을 처치하는 것은 도움이 된다. 적절한 손상 기전이 존재할 때 대동맥 파열을 의심할 수 있는 높은 의심 지수가 유지된다. 이송 시간이 매우 짧은 경우를 제외하고는 고농도 보충 산소를 투여하고 이송 중에 정맥 라인을 확보한다. 대동맥 파열의 손상 기전을 환자를 이송할 의료기관에 가능한 한 빨리 보고해야 한다. 이러한 손상을 성공적으로 처치하기 위해서는 엄격한 혈압 조절이 필수적이다(**Box 10-6**). 외상성 대동맥파열은 균형 잡힌 소생술이 임상적으로 중요한 또 다른 상황을 나타낸다. 수액 소생술로 혈압을 정상 또는 상승시키면 대동맥의 나머지 조직이 파열되어 빠른 대량 출혈을 초래할 수 있다. 이송 시간이 길어지면 혈압 관리는 일반적으로 오른쪽 팔에서 측정한 혈압 중 가장 높은 혈압을 기준으로 조절해야 한다. 베타차단제를 투여하면 혈압과 수축력을 모두 조절할 수 있다.

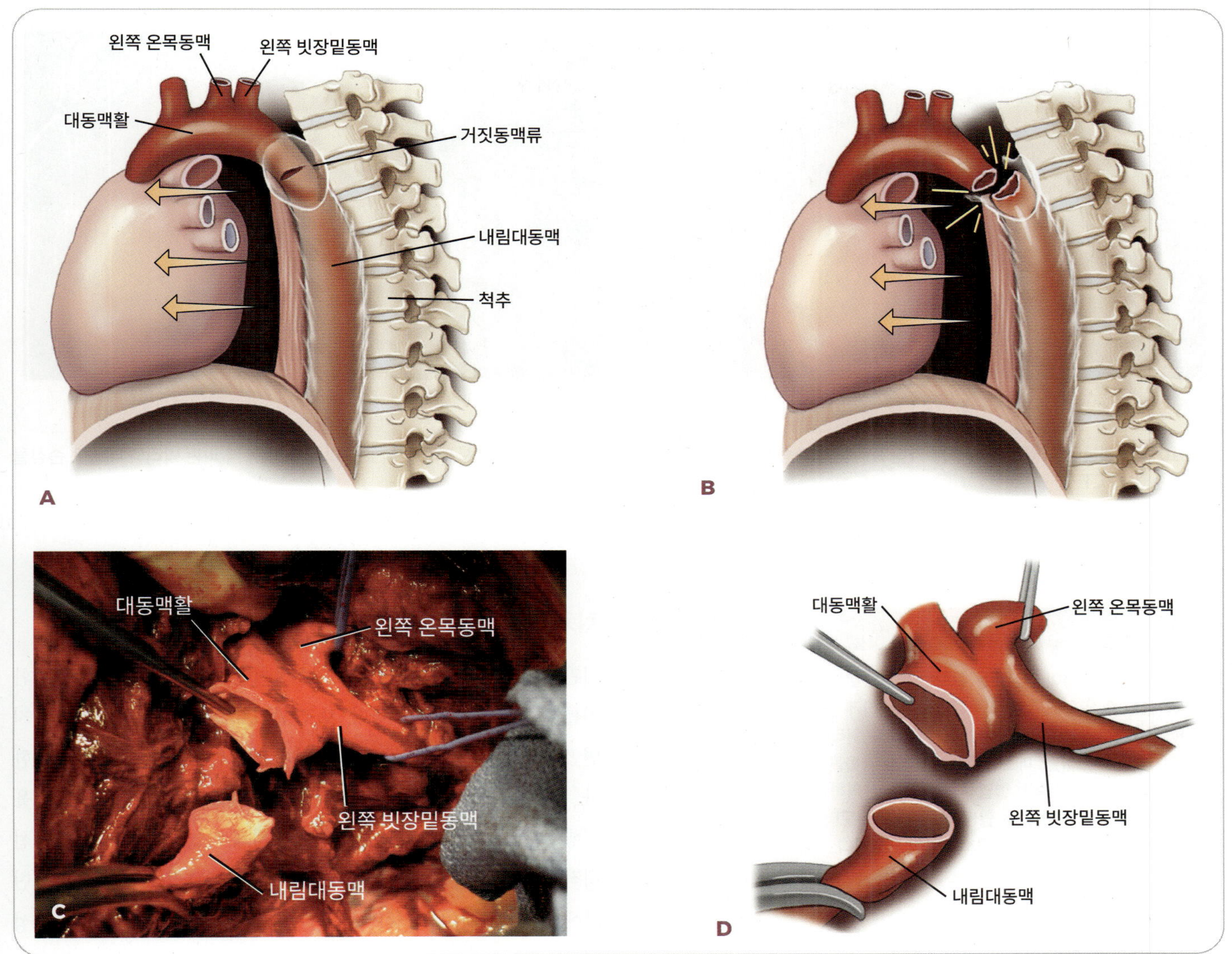

그림 10-24 **A.** 내림대동맥은 등뼈와 함께 움직이는 고정된 구조이다. 대동맥활, 대동맥 및 심장은 자유롭게 움직일 수 있다. 측면 충돌 시 몸통이 가속하거나 정면충돌 시 몸통이 급격히 감속하면 대동맥활-심장 복합체와 내림대동맥 사이의 운동 속도가 달라진다. 이러한 움직임으로 인해 가장 바깥층에 포함된 대동맥 내벽이 찢어져 거짓동맥류가 발생할 수 있다. **B.** 대동맥활과 내림대동맥의 교차점에서의 다열 또한 완전한 파열을 초래하여 가슴에 즉각적인 대량출혈을 일으킬 수 있다. **C**와 **D.** 외상성 대동맥 파열의 수술 사진 및 그림.

A, B, and D: © National Association of Emergency Medical Technicians (NAEMT); **C:** Courtesy of Norman McSwain, MD, FACS, NREMT-P.

기관기관지 파열

기관기관지 파열은 흔하지는 않지만, 잠재적으로 치명적인 상태이다. 폐의 모든 열상은 어느 정도 기도 파열을 동반하지만, 기관지 파열의 경우 기관 자체나 주기관지 또는 이차기관지 중 하나가 가슴속에서 파열된다. 이러한 파열로 인해 손상을 통해 세로칸이나 가슴막안으로 공기가 많이 유입된다(**그림 10-26**). 압력이 빠르게 축적되어 긴장기흉 또는 긴장 세로칸공기증이 발생하는데 이는 혈액이나 체액이 아닌 공기의 존재로 인해 발생한다는 점을 제외하면 심장눌림증과 유사하다. 긴장기흉의 일반적인 상황과 달리 바늘 가슴관삽입은 카테터를 통해 지속해서 공기의 흐름을 유발할 수 있어 긴장기흉을 완화하지 못할 수 있다. 이것은 이러한 기도를 통해 가슴막안으로 공기가 지속해 많이 흐르기 때문에 발생한다. 병변을 가로지르는 우선적인 공기 흐름과 압력으로 인해 호흡 기능이 크게 손상될 수 있다. 양압 환기의 느력은 긴장기흉을 악화시킬 수 있다. 관통성 외상보다 이 손상을 유발할 가능성이 더 높다. 그러나 고에너지 무딘 손상도 기관기관지 파옐을 유발할 수 있다.

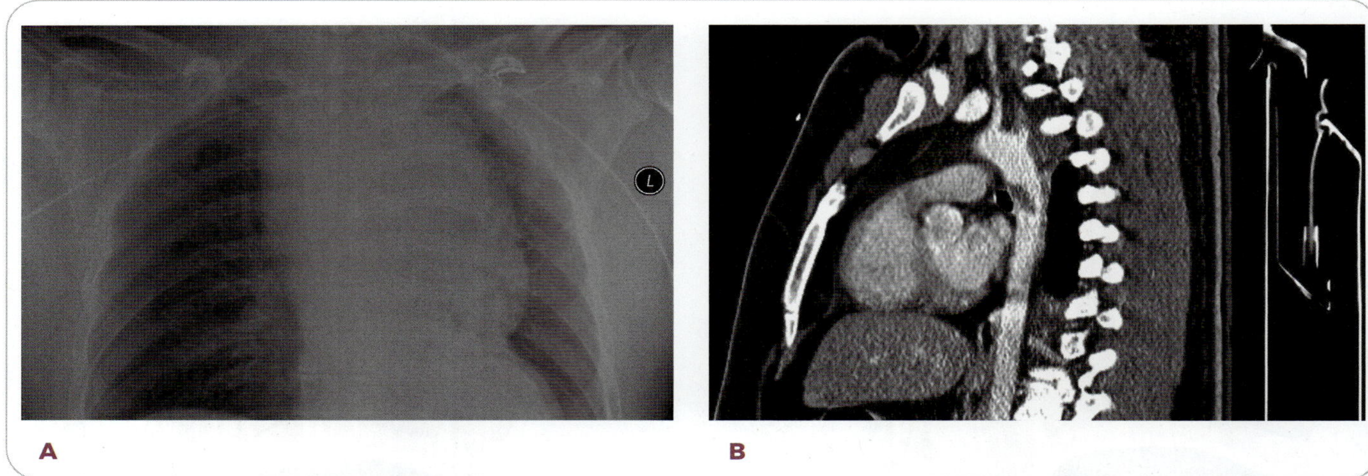

그림 10-25 대동맥 파열을 보여주는 가슴 X-ray 및 가슴 CT. **A.** 가슴 X-ray에서 대동맥 손상을 시사하는 세로칸 확장 **B.** 대동맥 피판 박리와 대동맥 손상을 보여주는 가슴 CT.

Courtesy of Dr. Mark Gestring, MD, FACS.

Box 10-6　혈압 유지

주의: 대동맥 파열이 의심되는 환자를 병원으로 이송할 때는 과도한 출혈이 발생할 수 있으므로 환자의 혈압을 급격하게 올리지 않는 것이 중요하다(3장 쇼크: 삶과 죽음의 병태생리학 참조). 이러한 환자 중 다수는 베타차단제(예: 에스몰롤, 메토프롤롤)와 같은 약물을 투여하여 혈압을 낮은 수준(일반적으로 수축기 혈압을 100mmHg 이하)으로 유지한다. 이러한 처치는 일반적으로 혈압을 훨씬 더 주의 깊게 모니터링할 수 있도록 동맥라인 삽입과 같은 침습적인 모니터링이 필요하다.

© National Association of Emergency Medical Technicians (NAEMT)

평가

기관기관지 파열 환자를 평가하면 환자가 명백한 고통을 겪고 있음을 알 수 있다. 환자는 창백하고 발한이 있을 수 있으며 호흡 보조근을 사용, 끙끙거림, 코 벌렁거림 같은 호흡 곤란의 증후를 보일 수 있다. 특히 가슴 위쪽과 목 주위에서 광범위한 피부밑기종을 확인할 수 있다(**그림 10-27**). 일반적으로 중요한 징후로 목정맥 확장이 중요한 소견으로 알려졌지만, 피부밑기종으로 인해 불분명해질 수 있으며 기관편위는 목정맥패임구멍에서 기관 촉진 시 확인할 수 있다. 환기 속도가 증가하고 산소포화도는 감소할 수 있다. 환자는 저혈압일 수도 있고 아닐 수도 있으며 피(객혈)를 토할 수 있다. 관통성 외상과 관련된 출혈은 무딘 손상의 경우에 나타나지 않을 수 있지만, 혈흉은 관통성 외상과 무딘 외상 모두에서 발생할 수 있다.

처치

기관기관지 파열을 성공적으로 처치하려면 보충 산소를 투여하고 환기를 신중하게 시행해야 한다. 보조 환기로 인해 환자가 더 불편해지면 산소만 투여하고 환자를 신속하게 적절한 의료기관으로 이송한다. 긴장기흉으로 진행되는 징후가 나타나는지 지속해서 모니터링을 시행하며 이러한 징후가 나타나면 신속하게 바늘감압을 시도한다. 선택적 주기관지 삽관과 같은 복잡한 전문 기도관리는 일반적으로 현장에서 불가능하며 이러한 시도는 주기관지 손상을 악화시킬 가능성이 있다.

외상성 질식

외상성 질식은 피해자가 신체적으로 목이 졸린 환자와 유사하기 때문에 그렇게 이름이 붙여졌다. 외상성 질식 환자는 목이 졸린 환자와 마찬가지로 얼굴과 목 부위(외상성 질식의 경우 가슴 위쪽)에 푸르스름하게 변색을 보인다. 그러나 목이 졸린 환자와 달리 외상성 질식 환자는 진정한 질식(공기 및 가스의 교환 중단)을 겪지 않는다. 외상성 질식 환자가 목 졸림 환자와 유사한 외모를 보이는 것은 두 환자 그룹 모두에서 나타나는 머리와 목의 정맥혈복귀 장애로 인해 발생한다.

외상성 질식의 발생 기전은 몸통이 짓눌려 가슴 내 압력이 급격히 증가하는 것이다. 이 압력으로 인해 혈액이 심장에서 역행 방향인 정

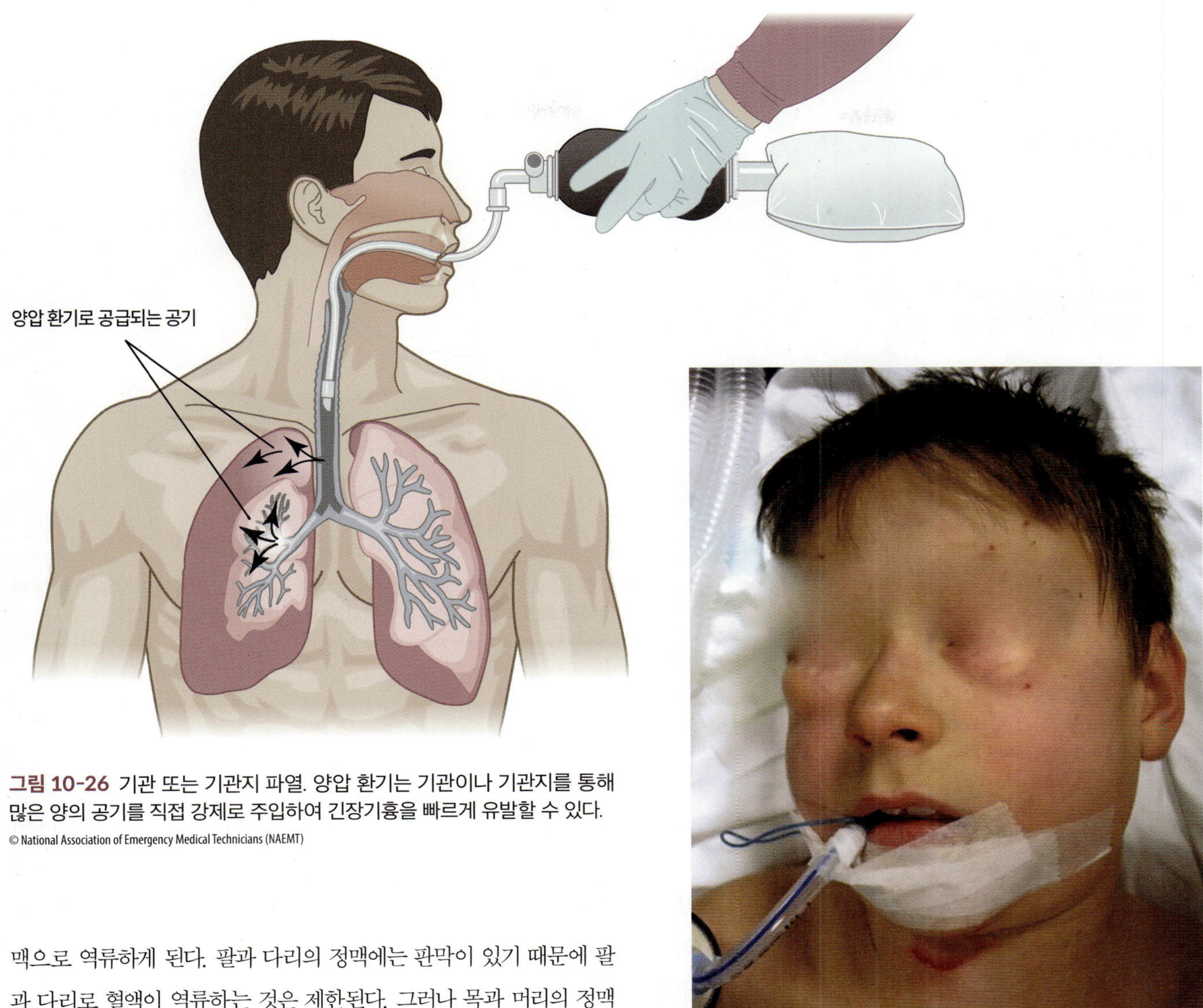

그림 10-26 기관 또는 기관지 파열. 양압 환기는 기관이나 기관지를 통해 많은 양의 공기를 직접 강제로 주입하여 긴장기흉을 빠르게 유발할 수 있다.
© National Association of Emergency Medical Technicians (NAEMT)

그림 10-27 목의 앞쪽에 외상을 입어 기관이 파열되어 얼굴(눈꺼풀)과 목에 피부밑기종이 발생한 환자.
Photograph provided courtesy of J.C. Pitteloud M.D., Switzerland

맥으로 역류하게 된다. 팔과 다리의 정맥에는 판막이 있기 때문에 팔과 다리로 혈액이 역류하는 것은 제한된다. 그러나 목과 머리의 정맥에는 이러한 판막이 없으므로 혈액이 먼저 목과 머리 쪽으로 유입된다. 피부밑 세정맥과 작은 모세혈관이 파열되고 혈액이 누출되어 피부가 자줏빛으로 변한다. 뇌와 망막의 작은 혈관이 파열되면 뇌와 눈의 기능 장애가 발생할 수 있다. 외상성 질식은 무딘 심장 파열의 지표로 보고된다.

평가

외상성 질식의 특징은 혈관의 부종과 팽만상태(즉 혈관이 부풀어 오르고 팽창하는 현상)로 피부가 붉게 착색되는 과도한 혈액이다. 이 증상은 으깸 수준 이상에서 가장 두드러지게 나타난다(**그림 10-28**). 손상을 입은 부위 이하의 피부는 정상이다. 이 손상을 유발하는 데 필요한 가슴에 가해지는 힘 때문에 이 장에서 이미 설명한 많은 손상과 척추 및 척수 손상이 나타날 수 있다.

처치

환자를 지지하고 고농도 산소를 투여하며 정맥 라인을 확보하고 필요한 경우 토조 환기를 시행한다. 적자색으로 변색은 일반적으로 생존자에서 1~2주 이내에 사라진다.

가로막 파열

흉복부 부위에 관통상을 입으면 가로막에 작은 열상이 발생할 수 있다. 가로막은 호흡에 따라 상승 및 하강하기 때문에 앞쪽의 유두 수준 또는 뒤쪽의 어깨뼈 끝 수준보다 낮은 부위에 발생하는 관통상은

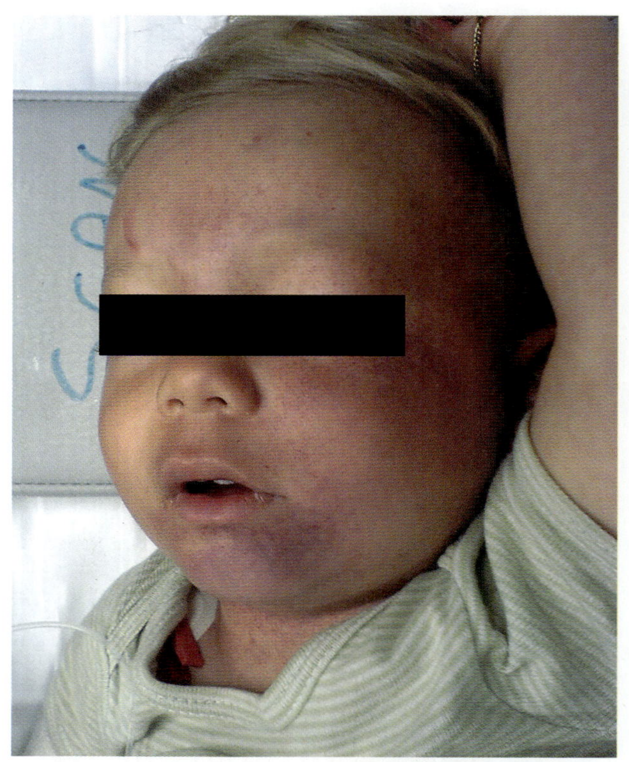

그림 10-28 외상성 질식이 발생한 어린이. 특히 턱에 자주색 변색이 있고 얼굴과 이마에 여러 개의 출혈점이 있는 것을 확인한다.

Photograph provided courtesy of J.C. Pitteloud M.D., Switzerland

가로막을 관통할 위험이 있다. 일반적으로 이러한 손상은 그 자체로는 심각한 문제를 일으키지 않지만, 향후 손상 부위를 통해 복부 장기의 탈장 및 조임이 발생할 위험이 있으므로 일반적으로 수술적 처치가 필요하다. 가슴 또는 복부 장기의 심각한 손상이 동반될 수 있으며 겉으로 보기에는 해가 없는 손상일 수 있다.

무딘 손상으로 발생한 가로막 파열은 복부에 충분한 힘을 가하여 복압을 급격하고 갑작스럽게 증가시켜 가로막을 파열시킬 만큼 충분히 증가시켰을 때 발생한다. 일반적으로 관통상에 동반되는 작은 열상과 달리 무딘 손상 기전에 의한 파열은 종종 크게 발생하며 복부 내장이 가슴안으로 급성 탈장될 수 있다(**그림 10-29**). 호흡곤란은 탈장된 장기가 폐에 가해지는 압력으로 인해 효과적인 환기를 방해하고 폐의 타박상으로 인해 발생한다. 이러한 환기 장애는 생명을 위협할 수 있다. 환기 기능 장애 외에도 갈비뼈 골절, 혈흉 및 기흉이 발생할 수 있다. 가로막의 파열을 통해 간, 비장, 위 또는 창자 등 복부 장기가 가슴안으로 밀려들어 가기 때문에 이런 장기 손상도 동반되어 나타날 수 있다. 이러한 환자는 심각한 통증을 겪고 있으며 신속한 처치가 필요하다.

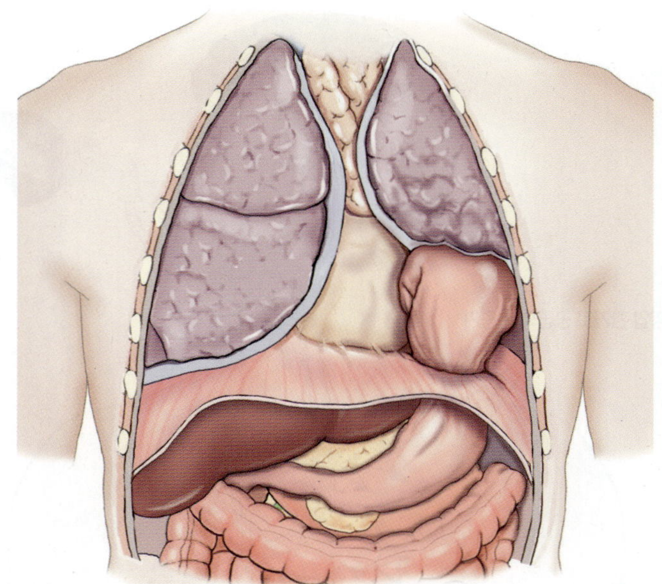

그림 10-29 가로막 파열로 인해 장이나 기타 구조물이 파열 부위를 통해 탈장하여 폐를 부분적으로 압박하고 호흡곤란을 유발할 수 있다.

© National Association of Emergency Medical Technicians (NAEMT)

평가

환자 평가 결과 불안하고 호흡이 빠르며 창백해 보이는 급성 호흡 곤란을 보인다. 환자는 가슴벽 타박상, 뼈 비빔소리 또는 피부밑기종이 있을 수 있다. 손상을 입은 쪽의 호흡음이 감소하거나 가슴 청진시 장음이 청진될 수 있다. 복부 장기가 가슴으로 탈장되면 복부가 홀쭉해 보일 수 있다.

처치

가로막 파열이 있을 수 있다는 사실을 즉시 인지해야 한다. 필요에 따라 고농도의 산소를 투여하고 보조 환기를 시행한다. 환자를 신속하게 평가하고 수술이 가능한 적절한 의료기관으로 신속하게 이송한다.

이송 지연

이송 지연 중 가슴 손상이 있거나 의심되는 환자를 처치하기 위한 우선순위는 기도 관리, 환기 및 산소공급, 출혈 조절, 적절한 수액 소생술을 제공하는 것이다. 이송 지연에 직면한 경우 병원 전 처치 제공자는 기관내삽관으로 기도를 확보하기 위한 역치가 낮아질 수 있다. 기관내삽관을 수행하기 위한 적응증에는 호흡곤란이 증가하거나 호흡부전(긴장기흉을 제거하거나 처치한 후)이 임박한 경우, 동요가슴,

개방기흉, 다발성 갈비뼈 골절이 포함된다. 산소포화도를 94% 이상으로 유지하기 위해 산소를 공급한다.

필요에 따라 보조 환기를 시행한다. 폐 타박상은 시간이 지남에 따라 악화하며 지속적양압환기기(CPAP), 이동식 인공호흡기를 사용한 호기말양압환기(PEEP), 호기말양압 밸브가 있는 백마스크를 사용하면 산소공급을 쉽게 시행할 수 한다. 심각한 가슴 손상이 있는 환자는 긴장기흉이 있거나 발생할 수 있으므로 지속적인 평가를 통해 특징적인 징후를 찾아야 한다. 호흡음이 감소하거나 없는 경우, 호흡 곤란이 악화하는 경우, 백마스크 장치를 짜는 데 어려움이 있는 경우, 인공호흡기를 사용하는 환자의 들숨 최대 압력이 증가하는 경우 및 저혈압이 있는 경우 가슴막감압을 시행한다. 환자에게 바늘감압이 필요하거나 개방 기흉이 있는 것으로 확인된 경우 일반적으로 항공의료전문가와 같이 적절한 자격을 갖춘 인원이 가슴관삽입술을 시행할 수 있다. 정맥 라인을 확보하고 수액을 신중하게 투여해야 한다.

가슴속, 태안 또는 복막뒤 출혈이 의심되는 환자는 심각한 머리 손상이 의심되지 않는 경우 수축기 혈압을 80~90mmHg 범위로 최대 2시간 동안 유지해야 한다. 과도한 수액 소생술을 시행하면 폐 타박상을 악화시킬 뿐만 아니라 내부출혈이 재발할 수 있다(3장 쇼크; 삶과 죽음의 병태생리학 참조).

다발성 갈비뼈 골절로 인한 심한 통증을 호소하는 환자는 정맥 내로 적절한 소량의 마약성 진통제를 투여하거나 케타민을 투여하면 도움이 될 수 있다. 다약성 진통제 투여로 인해 저혈압이나 호흡부전이 발생하면 수액 소생술과 보조 환기를 시행한다.

무딘 심장 손상과 관련된 부정맥이 있는 환자는 항부정맥 약물을 사용하면 도움이 될 수 있다. 시행한 모든 내용을 환자처치 보고서(PCR)에 상세하게 기록하고 환자의 상태와 처치 내용을 이송하는 의료기관에 보고한다.

요 약

- 가슴 손상 환자는 다기관 외상을 동반하는 경우가 많고 호흡기 및 순환계 손상 위험이 있으므로 신속하게 처치하고 결정적인 처치를 시행하기 위해 신속하게 이송해야 한다.

- 가슴 관통상에 대처할 때 병원 전 처치 제공자는 혈흉이나 기흉 또는 혈액기흉 모두를 처치할 준비를 해야 한다.

- 가슴에 무딘 손상이 발생한 경우 병원 전 처치 제공자가 주의해야 할 손상으로는 폐 타박상, 내장가슴막 파열, 갈비뼈 골절, 가슴의 주요 혈관의 전단 또는 파열, 가슴벽 파열 등이 있다. 관련 질환으로는 혈흉, 기흉 및 둔기에 의한 심장 또는 심장막 손상, 심장진탕, 치명적인 출혈 등이 있다. 맥박산소측정과 파형 호기말이산화탄소 분압측정은 환기 상태와 처치에 대한 반응을 평가하는 데 유용한 보조 장비이다.

- 병원 전 처치 제공자는 다음 세 가지 유형의 기흉을 인식하고 처치할 준비가 되어 있어야 한다.
  - 단순기흉은 가슴막안에 공기가 존재하는 것이다.
  - 개방기흉(흡인 가슴 상처)은 가슴벽의 손상으로 인해 환기 노력을 통해 외부에서 가슴막안으로 공기가 들어오고 나갈 수 없는 경우이다.
  - 긴장기흉은 공기가 계속 유입되어 가슴막안의 압력이 점진적으로 증가하여 가슴막안에 갇혀있을 때 발생한다. 긴장기흉의 징후는 현장에서 바늘감압으로 처치하면 치명적일 수 있는 문제를 해결할 수 있으므로 주의 깊게 확인한다.

- 무딘 가슴 손상 환자의 경우 다발성 외상 위험이 높으므로 이러한 환자를 이송할 때는 척추고정을 시행해야 한다.

- 심전도 모니터링을 통해 무딘 심장 손상을 예측할 수 있다.

- 가슴 외상이 의심되는 환자에게 고동도 산소를 추가로 투여하고 보조 환기의 필요성에 특히 주의를 기울여야 한다.

- 환자를 의료기관으로 이송 중에 정맥 라인을 확보하고 적절하게 수액 소생술을 시행한다.

- 많은 가슴 손상을 외과적 개입 없이 처치할 수 있지만, 가슴 손상 환자는 적절한 의료기관에서 평가 및 처치를 받아야 한다.

시나리오 재구성

당신과 동료는 건설 현장에서 쇠 파이프에 부딪혀 환자가 발생한 사고 현장으로 출동했다. 현장에 도착하자마자 현장 안전 관리자가 당신을 사고 발생 현장으로 안내한다. 현장 안전 관리자는 쇠 파이프를 이용해서 안전시설을 설치하던 중에 사고가 일어났다고 말했다. 환자의 동료가 말하기를 환자가 다른 쇠 파이프 기둥을 붙잡으려고 몸을 돌리다가 쇠 파이프 끝에 부딪혀 환자의 가슴에 관통했다고 하였다.

30대의 남성이 앞으로 몸을 숙이고 오른쪽 가슴을 부위에 수건을 대고 똑바로 앉아 있는 것을 발견했다. 당신은 환자에게 무슨 일이 일어났는지 물었고 환자는 당신에게 말을 하려고 하지만, 호흡하기 위해 5~6단어 후에 말을 멈춘다. 당신은 수건과 찢어진 옷을 제거한 후 약 5cm의 열상과 소량의 거품 섞인 혈액을 확인했다. 환자평가 결과 환자는 발한이 있고 노맥박은 빠르며 청진시 오른쪽의 호흡음이 감소했다. 다른 비정상적인 신체 소견은 없었다.

- 이 환자는 호흡곤란이 있는가?
- 환자에게 생명을 위협하는 손상이 있는가?
- 현장에서 어떤 처치를 수행해야 하는가?
- 이 환자를 이송하기 위해 어떤 방법을 사용해야 하는가?
- 예를 들어 농촌에서 장시간 환자를 이송하는 것은 처치 계획에 어떤 영향을 미치는가?
- 어떤 다른 손상이 의심되는가?

시나리오 해결책

현장 정보, 환자의 호소증상 및 신체검사를 통해 이 환자가 생명을 위협할 수 있는 심각한 손상을 입었을 수 있다고 의심하게 된다. 환자는 깨어있고 일관성 있게 말하고 있어 기도가 개방되어 있다는 것을 나타낸다. 환자는 완전한 문장을 말할 수 없어 심한 호흡 곤란을 겪고 있다. 발한과 빈맥으로 인해 혈류역학적 불안정성을 경험하고 있다. 상처의 위치, 거품이 나는 체액, 호흡음 감소는 개방 기흉이 있는 흡인성 가슴 상처를 나타낸다.

신속하게 개방 상처 부위에 3면 폐쇄드레싱을 적용하고 환자에게 보충 산소를 공급하고 필요에 따라 백마스크로 보조 환기를 고려한다. 이 시나리오에서 최 우선순위는 손상의 심각성을 인식하고 환자를 안정시킨 후 적절한 의료기관으로 신속하게 이송하는 것이다. 이 환자의 호흡 곤란과 소견을 고려할 때 합병증에 대한 위험이 상당히 높다. 가장 가까운 외상센터로 이송하는 것이 적절하고 이송 중에 정맥 라인을 확보한다.

호흡 곤란의 위험이 있으므로 환자의 환기 상태를 자세히 모니터링해야 한다 순환과 호흡 곤란의 징후가 나타나면 먼저 폐쇄드레싱을 제거하고 호전되지 않으면 손상된 가슴 부위에 바늘감압을 시행한다. 이송 시간이 길어지는 경우 항공 이송을 고려한다.

References

1. American College of Surgeons Committee on Trauma. Thoracic trauma. In: *Advanced Trauma Life Support, Student Course Manual*. 10th ed. American College of Surgeons; 2018.
2. Ghanta RK, Wall MJ, Mattox KL. Trauma thoracotomy: principles and techniques. In: Feliciano DV, Mattox KL, Moore EE, eds. *Trauma*. 9th ed. McGraw-Hill; 2020.
3. Livingston DH, Hauser CJ. Trauma to the chest wall and lung. In: Mattox KL, Feliciano DV, Moore EE, eds. *Trauma*. 5th ed. McGraw-Hill; 2004.
4. Howes DS, Bellazzini MA. Chronic obstructive pulmonary disease. In: Wolfson AB, Hendey GW, Ling LJ, et al., eds. *Harwood-Nuss' Clinical Practice of Emergency Medicine*. 5th ed. Wolters Kluwer/Lippincott Williams & Wilkins; 2010.
5. Wilson RF. Pulmonary physiology. In: Wilson RF. *Critical Care Manual: Applied Physiology and Principles of Therapy*. 2nd ed. Davis; 1992.
6. National Association of Emergency Medical Technicians. Advanced medical life support assessment for the medical patient. In: *Advanced Medical Life Support*, 3rd ed. Jones & Bartlett Learning; 2021:1-53.
7. Silverston P. Pulse oximetry at the roadside: a study of pulse oximetry in immediate care. *BMJ*. 1989;298:711.
8. Garrett PD, Boyd SY, Bauch TD, Rubal BJ, Bulgrin JR, Kinkler ES Jr. Feasibility of real-time echocardiographic evaluation during patient transport. *J Am Soc Echocardiogr*. 2003 Mar;16(3):197-201. doi: 10.1067/mje.2003.16
9. Roline CE, Heegaard WG, Moore JC, et al. Feasibility of bedside thoracic ultrasound in the helicopter emergency medical services setting. *Air Med J*. 2013;32(3):153-7. doi: 10.1016/j.amj.2012.10.013
10. Quick JA, Uhlich RM, Ahmad S, Barnes SL, Coughenour JP. In-flight ultrasound identification of pneumothorax. *Emerg Radiol*. 2016 Feb;23(1):3-7. doi: 10.1007/s10140-015-1348-z
11. Yates JG, Baylous D. Aeromedical ultrasound: the evaluation of point-of-care ultrasound during helicopter transport. *Air Med J*. 2017;36(3):110-115. doi: 10.1016/j.amj.2017.02.001
12. Pietersen PI, Mikkelsen S, Lassen AT, et al. Quality of focused thoracic ultrasound performed by emergency medical technicians and paramedics in a prehospital setting: a feasibility study. *Scand J Trauma Resusc Emerg Med*. 2021;29(1):40. doi: 10.1186/s13049-021-00856-8
13. Brun PM, Bessereau J, Levy D, Billeres X, Fournier N, Kerbaul F. Prehospital ultrasound thoracic examination to improve decision making, triage, and care in blunt trauma. *Am J Emerg Med*. 2014;32(7):817.e1-2. doi: 10.1016/j.ajem.2013.12.063
14. Kirkpatrick AW, Brown DR, Crickmer S, et al. Hand-held portable sonography for the on-mountain exclusion of a pneumothorax. *Wilderness Environ Med*. 2001;12(4):270-272. doi: 10.1580/1080-6032(2001)012[0270:hhpsft]2.0.co;2
15. Ziegler DW, Agarwal NN. The morbidity and mortality of rib fractures. *J Trauma Acute Care Surg*. 1994;37(6):975-979.
16. Pressley CM, Fry WR, Philip AS, et al. Predicting outcome of patients with chest wall injury. *Am J Surg*. 2012;204(6):900-904.
17. Flagel BT, Luchette FA, Reed RL, et al. Half-a-dozen ribs: the breakpoint for mortality. *Surgery*. 2005;138:717-725.
18. Jones KM, Reed RL, Luchette FA. The ribs or not the ribs: which influences mortality? *Am J Surg*. 2011;202(5);598-604.
19. Bulger EM, Arneson MA, Mock CN, Jurkovich GJ. Rib fractures in the elderly. *J Trauma*. 2000;48(6):1040-1046; discussion 1046-1047. doi: 10.1097/00005373-200006000-00007
20. Richardson JD, Adams L, Flint LM. Selective management of flail chest and pulmonary contusion. *Ann Surg*. 1982;196:481-487.
21. Di Bartolomeo S, Sanson G, Nardi G, et al. A population-based study on pneumothorax in severely traumatized patients. *J Trauma*. 2001;51(4):677-682.
22. Regel G, Stalp M, Lehmann U, et al. Prehospital care: importance of early intervention outcome. *Acta Anaesthesiol Scand Suppl*. 1997;110:71-76.
23. Barone JE, Pizzi WF, Nealon TF, et al. Indications for intubation in blunt chest trauma. *J Trauma*. 1986;26:334-337.
24. Mattox KL. Prehospital care of the patient with an injured chest. *Surg Clin North Am*. 1989;69(1):21-29.

25. Simon B, Ebert J, Bokhari F, et al. Management of pulmonary contusion and flail chest: an Eastern Association for the Surgery of Trauma practice management guideline. *J Trauma Acute Care Surg.* 2012 Nov;73(5 suppl 4):S351-S361.

26. Cooper C, Militello P. The multi-injured patient: the Maryland Shock Trauma Protocol approach. *Semin Thorac Cardiovasc Surg.* 1992;4(3):163-167.

27. Barton ED, Epperson M, Hoyt DB, et al. Prehospital needle aspiration and tube thoracostomy in trauma victims: a six-year experience with aeromedical crews. *J Emerg Med.* 1995;13:155-163.

28. Kheirabadi BS, Terrazas IB, Koller A, et al. Vented vs. unvented chest seals for treatment of pneumothorax (PTx) and prevention of tension PTx in a swine model. *J Trauma Acute Care Surg.* 2013;75:150-156.

29. Butler FK, Dubose JJ, Otten EJ, et al. Management of open pneumothorax in tactical combat casualty care: TCCC guidelines change 13-02. *J Special Ops Med.* 2013;13(3):81-86.

30. Kuhlwilm V. The use of chest seals in treating sucking chest wounds: a comparison of existing evidence and guideline recommendations. *J Spec Oper Med.* 2021;21(1):94-101.

31. Eckstein M, Suyehara DL. Needle thoracostomy in the pre-hospital setting. *Prehosp Emerg Care.* 1998;2:132.

32. Holcomb JB, McManus JG, Kerr ST, Pusateri AE. Needle versus tube thoracostomy in a swine model of traumatic tension hemopneumothorax. *Prehosp Emerg Care.* 2009;13(1):18-27.

33. American College of Surgeons Committee on Trauma. Thoracic trauma. In: *Advanced Trauma Life Support, Student Course Manual.* 10th ed. American College of Surgeons; 2018:66.

34. Netto FA, Shulman H, Rizoli SB, et al. Are needle decompressions for tension pneumothoraces being performed appropriately for appropriate indications? *Am J Em Med.* 2008;26;597-602.

35. Riwoe D, Poncia H. Subclavian artery laceration: a serious complication of needle decompression. *Em Med Aust.* 2011;23:651-653.

36. Inaba K, Branco BC Exkstein M, et al. Optimal positioning for emergent needle thoracostomy: a cadaver-based study. *J Trauma.* 2011;71:1099-1103.

37. Inaba K, Karamanos E, Skiada D, et al. Cadaveric comparison of the optimal site for needle decompression of tension pneumothorax by prehospital care providers. *J Trauma.* 2015;79(6):1044-1048.

38. Leatherman ML, Held JM, Fluke LM, et al. Relative device stability of anterior versus axillary needle decompression for tension pneumothorax during casualty movement: preliminary analysis of a human cadaver model. *J Trauma.* 2017;83(1):S136-S141.

39. Beckett A, Savage E, Pannell D, et al. Needle decompression for tension pneumothorax in tactical combat casualty care: do catheters placed in the midaxillary line kink more often than those in the midclavicular line? *J Trauma.* 2011;71:S408-S412.

40. Martin M, Satterly S, Inaba K, Blair K. Does needle thoracostomy provide adequate and effective decompression of tension pneumothorax? *J Trauma.* 2012;73(6):1410-1415.

41. Davis DP, Pettit K, Rum CD, et al. The safety and efficacy of prehospital needle and tube thoracostomy by aeromedical personnel. *Prehosp Emerg Care.* 2005;9:191-197.

42. Etoch SW, Bar-Natan MF, Miller FB, et al. Tube thoracostomy: factors related to complications. *Arch Surg.* 1995;130:521-525.

43. Newman PG, Feliciano DV. Blunt cardiac injury. *New Horizons.* 1999;7(1):26-34.

44. Sherren PB, Galloway R, Healy M. Blunt traumatic pericardial rupture and cardiac herniation with a penetrating twist: two case reports. *Scand J Trauma Resusc Emerg Med.* 2009;17:64.

45. Lindenmann J, Matzi V, Neuboeck N, Porubsky C, Ratzenhofer B, Maier A. Traumatic pericardial rupture with cardiac herniation. *Ann Thorac Surg.* 2010;89:2028-2030.

46. LeBlanc N, Tan L. Pericardial rupture with cardiac herniation following blunt thoracic trauma. *JTCVS Tech.* 2020 Dec;4:375–377. doi: 10.1016/j.xjtc.2020.08.011

47. Ivatury RR. The injured heart. In: Mattox KL, Feliciano DV, Moore EE, eds. *Trauma.* 5th ed. McGraw-Hill; 2004:555.

48. Symbas NP, Bongiorno PF, Symbas PN. Blunt cardiac rupture: the utility of emergency department ultrasound. *Ann Thorac Surg.* 1999;67(5):1274-1276.

49. Demetriades D. Cardiac wounds. *Ann Surg.* 1986;203(3):315-317.

50. Jacob S, Sebastian JC, Cherian PK, et al. Pericardial effusion impending tamponade: a look beyond Beck's triad. *Am J Em Med.* 2009;27:216-219.

51. Ivatury RR, Nallathambi MN, Roberge RJ, et al. Penetrating thoracic injuries: in-field stabilization versus prompt transport. *J Trauma.* 1987;27:1066.

52. Bleetman A, Kasem H, Crawford R. Review of emergency thoracotomy for chest injuries in patients attending a UK accident and emergency department. *Injury.* 1996;27(2):129-132.

53. Durham LA III, Richardson RJ, Wall MJ Jr, et al. Emergency center thoracotomy: impact of prehospital resuscitation. *J Trauma.* 1992;32(6):775-779.

54. Honigman B, Rohweder K, Moore EE, et al. Prehospital advanced trauma life support for penetrating cardiac wounds. *Ann Emerg Med.* 1990;19(2):145-150.

55. Lerer LB, Knottenbelt JD. Preventable mortality following sharp penetrating chest trauma. *J Trauma.* 1994;37(1):9-12.

56. Ho AM, Graham CA, Ng CS, et al. Timing of tracheal intubation in traumatic cardiac tamponade: a word of caution. *Resuscitation.* 2009;80(2):272-274. doi: 10.1016/j.resuscitation.2008.09.021

57. Möller CT, Schoonbee CG, Rosendorff C. Haemodynamics of cardiac tamponade during various modes of ventilation. *Br J Anaesth.* 1979;51(5):409-415. doi: 10.1093/bja/51.5.409

58. Wall MJ Jr, Pepe PE, Mattox KL. Successful roadside resuscitative thoracotomy: case report and literature review. *J Trauma.* 1994;36(1):131-135.

59. Coats TJ, Keogh S, Clark H, et al. Prehospital resuscitative thoracotomy for cardiac arrest after penetrating trauma: rationale and case series. *J Trauma.* 2001;50(4):670-673.

60. Zangwill SD, Strasburger JF. Commotio cordis. *Pediatr Clin North Am.* 2004;51(5):1347-1354.

61. Perron AD, Brady WJ, Erling BF. Commodio cordis: an underappreciated cause of sudden cardiac death in young patients: assessment and management in the ED. *Am J Emerg Med.* 2001;19(5):406-409.

62. Maron BJ, Estes NA 3rd. Commotio cordis. *N Engl J Med.* 2010;362(10):917-927.

63. Tainter CR, Hughes PG. Commotio cordis. In: StatPearls [Internet]. StatPearls Publishing. Updated September 28, 2021. Accessed February 10, 2022. https://www.ncbi.nlm.nih.gov/books/NBK526014/

64. 2010 American Heart Association Guidelines for Cardiopulmonary Resuscitation and Emergency Cardiovascular Care Science. *Circulation.* 2010;122:S745-S746.

65. Wall MJ, Ghanta RK, Mattox KL. Heart and thoracic vessels. In: Feliciano DV, Mattox KL, Moore EE, eds. *Trauma.* 9th ed. McGraw-Hill; 2020.

66. Fabian TC, Roger T. Sherman lecture: advances in the management of blunt thoracic aortic injury: Parmley to the present. *Am Surg.* 2009;75(4):273-278.

67. DuBose JJ, Scalea TM, O'Connor JV. Trachea, bronchi, and esophagus. In: Feliciano DV, Mattox KL, Moore EE, eds. *Trauma*. 9th ed. McGraw-Hill; 2020.

68. Rogers FB, Leavitt BJ. Upper torso cyanosis: a marker for blunt cardiac rupture. *Am J Emerg Med*. 1997;15(3):275-276.

Suggested Reading

Bowley DM, Boffard KD. Penetrating trauma of the trunk. *Unfallchirurg*. 2001;104(11):1032-1042.

Brathwaite CE, Rodriguez A, Turney SZ, et al. Blunt traumatic cardiac rupture: a 5-year experience. *Ann Surg*. 1990;212(6):701-704.

Helm M, Schuster R, Hauke J. Tight control of prehospital ventilation by capnography in major trauma victims. *Br J Anaesth*. 2003;90(3):327-332.

Lateef F. Commotio cordis: an underappreciated cause of sudden death in athletes. *Sports Med*. 2000;30:301-308.

Papadopoulos IN, Bukis D, Karalas E, et al. Preventable prehospital trauma deaths in a Hellenic urban health region: an audit of prehospital trauma care. *J Trauma*. 1996;41(5):864-869.

Rozycki GS, Feliciano DV, Oschner MG, et al. The role of ultrasound in patients with possible penetrating cardiac wounds: a prospective multicenter study. *J Trauma*. 1999;46:542-552.

Ruchholtz S, Waydhas C, Ose C, et al. Prehospital intubation in severe thoracic trauma without respiratory insufficiency: a matched-pair analysis based on the Trauma Registry of the German Trauma Society. *J Trauma*. 2002;52(5):879-886.

Streng M, Tikka S, Leppaniemi A. Assessing the severity of truncal gunshot wounds: a nation-wide analysis from Finland. *Ann Chir Gynaecol*. 2001;90(4):246-251.

가슴 외상 술기

바늘감압

원리: 환자의 호흡, 환기 및 순환에 영향을 미치는 긴장기흉으로 인한 가슴속 압력을 감소시킨다.

긴장기흉이 발생하여 가슴속 압력이 증가하는 환자의 경우 압력이 증가한 가슴안 쪽을 감압해야 한다. 이 압력이 완화되지 않으면 환자의 환기 능력이 점차 제한되고 정맥혈복귀가 저하되어 심박출량이 불충분해져 사망에 이를 수 있다.

폐쇄드레싱을 사용하여 개방기흉을 처치하고 긴장기흉이 발생하는 환자의 경우 일반적으로 개방 상처를 통해 감압하여 가슴에 기존 통풍구를 확보할 수 있다. 상처 부위의 폐쇄드레싱을 몇 초 동안 열면 가슴의 압력이 완화되면서 공기가 상처 밖으로 빠져나가기 시작한다.

이 압력이 해제되면 폐포 환기가 적절히 이루어지고 공기가 상처로 흡입되는 것을 막기 위해 폐쇄드레싱으로 상처를 다시 밀봉한다. 환자를 주의 깊게 모니터링하고 긴장기흉이 재발하는 징후가 나타나면 드레싱을 다시 제거하여 가슴안의 압력을 낮추어야 한다.

폐쇄 긴장기흉의 감압은 손상을 받은 가슴부위에 가슴관삽입을 통해 이루어진다. 가슴관삽입을 시행하는 방법에는 여러 가지가 있다. 바늘감압은 가장 신속한 방법이고 특별한 장비가 필요하지 않기 때문에 현장에서 가장 선호하는 방법이다.

바늘감압은 위험을 최소화하며 산소 공급과 순환을 개선하여 환자에게 큰 도움이 될 수 있다. 바늘감압은 다음 세 가지 기준을 충족하는 경우에만 실시해야 한다.

1. 호흡곤란이 악화하거나 백마스크 장비로 보조 환기가 곤란한 경우

2. 호흡음이 감소하거나 호흡음이 소실된 경우

3. 비보상 쇼크(수축기 혈압 90mmHg 미만)

바늘감압에 필요한 장비에는 주삿바늘, 주사기, 0.5인치 접착테이프 및 알코올 솜이 포함된다. 사용하는 주삿바늘은 길이가 최소 8cm 이상의 대구경 IV 카테터(10~14 게이지)를 사용할 수 있다. 더 큰 구경을 사용할 수 없는 경우 16 게이지 카테터를 사용할 수 있다.

병원 전 처치 제공자는 주삿바늘을 주사기에 연결하고 다른 병원 전 처치 제공자는 환자의 가슴을 청진하여 어느 쪽에 긴장기흉이 있는지 확인한다.

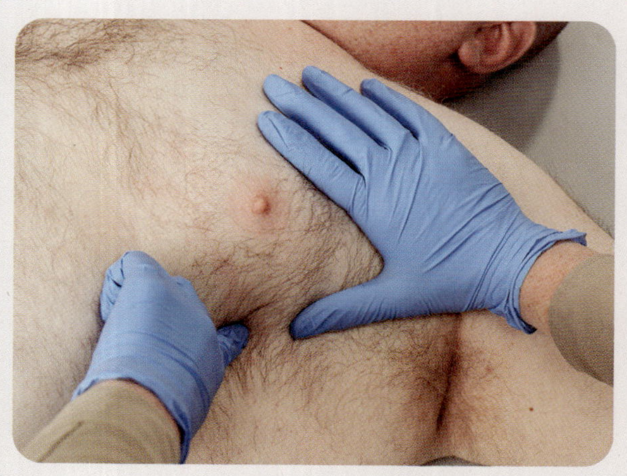

1 긴장기흉을 확인한 후 영향을 받은 쪽(빗장중간선과 두 번째 갈비사이공간 또는 앞겨드랑선과 다섯 번째 갈비사이공간이 만나는 지점)에 해부학적 랜드마크를 표시한다.

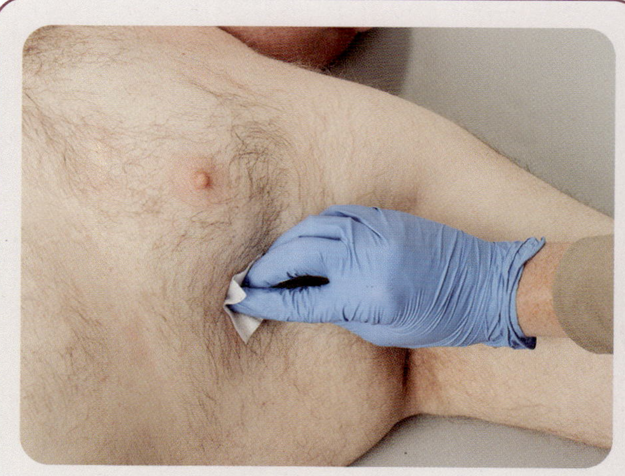

2 해당 부위를 알코올 솜으로 소독한다.

(다음 페이지에 계속)

가슴 외상 술기 (이어서)

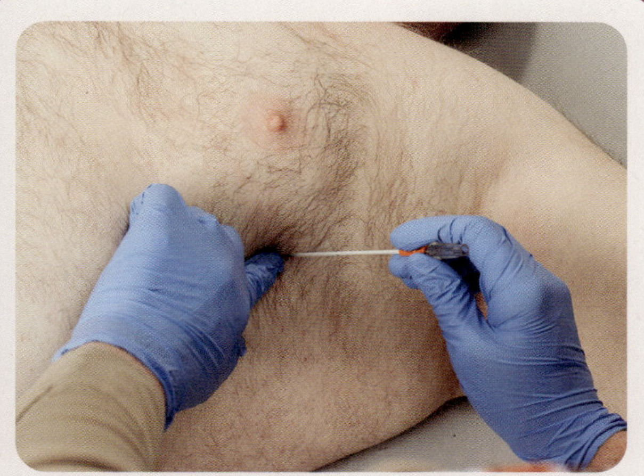

3 바늘을 삽입할 부위는 바늘을 잡지 않은 손의 손가락으로 확인하고 주삿바늘과 주사기는 갈비뼈의 윗부분에 위치한다.

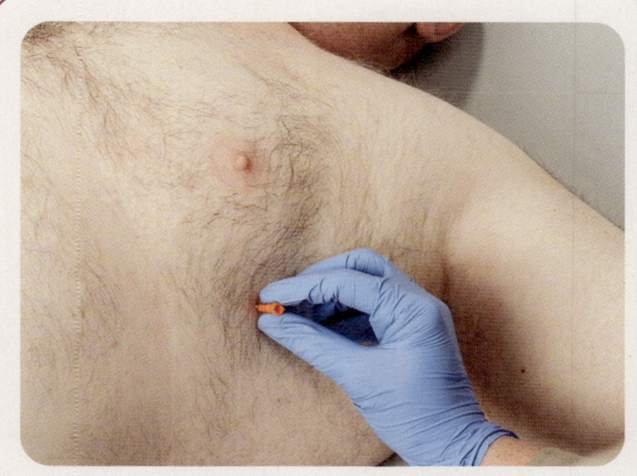

4 주삿바늘이 가슴안으로 들어가면 공기가 카테터를 통해 빠져나오면 바늘을 더 이상 삽입하지 않는다.

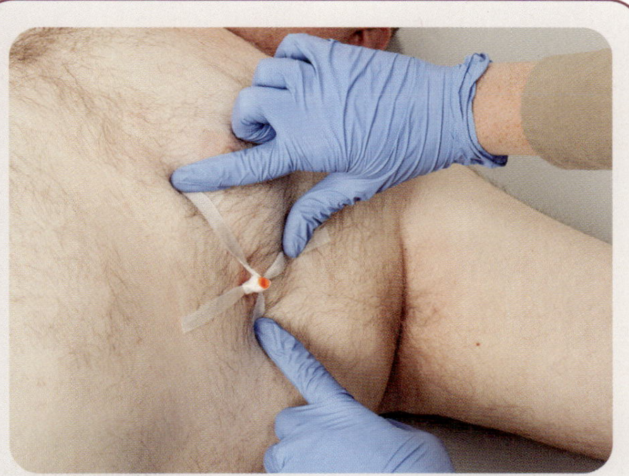

5 카테터가 빠지거나 꼬이지 않도록 주의해서 잡고 탐침을 제거한다. 탐침을 제거할 때 카테터 허브에서 공기가 빠져나오는 소리가 들려야 한다. 만약에 공기가 빠져나오지 않더라도 가슴 바늘감압을 시도했다는 것을 알 수 있도록 카테터를 제자리에 테이프로 고정한다.

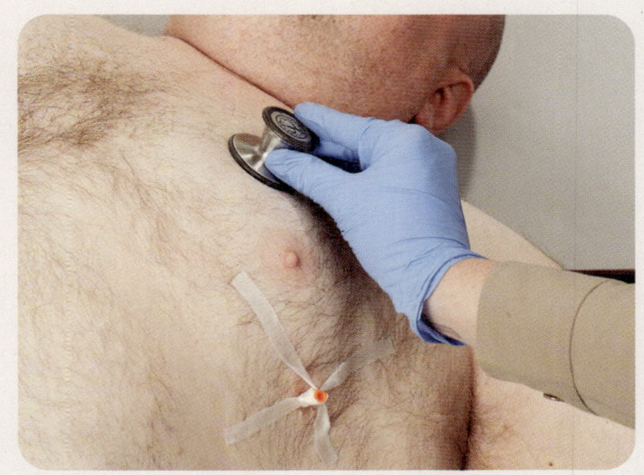

6 탐침을 제거한 후 카테터를 테이프로 제자리에 고정한다. 카테터를 고정한 후 가슴을 청진하여 호흡음이 증가했는지 확인한다. 환자를 모니터링하고 적절한 의료기관으로 이송한다. 병원 전 처치 제공자는 한 방향 밸브를 적용하는 데 시간을 낭비할 필요가 없다. 카테터가 혈전으로 막혀 긴장기흉이 재발하는 경우 바늘감압을 반복해서 시행할 수 있다.

복부 외상

Lead Editors
Thomas Scalea, MD
Emily Esposito, DO

학습 목표

이 장의 학습을 완료하면 다음과 같은 내용을 수행할 수 있다.

- 현장 평가 정보와 손상 기전을 분석하여 배 또는 골반 외상의 의심 수준을 결정할 수 있다.
- 복부 및 골반의 해부학적 구조를 이해하여 복부 손상 환자의 인지 및 분류에 도움을 줄 수 있다.
- 복부에 대한 무딘 손상 또는 관통상의 병태생리학적 영향을 예측할 수 있다.
- 복부 내 손상을 나타내는 신체검사 결과를 인식할 수 있다.
- 복부 손상의 외부 징후와 특정 복부 장기 손상 가능성을 연관시킬 수 있다.
- 복부 또는 골반 외상을 입은 상황에서 신속한 처치 및 이송에 대한 적응증을 파악할 수 있다.
- 찔린 쿨체, 내장 탈출, 외부 생식기 외상을 포함하여 복부 외상이 의심되는 환자에 대한 현장 처치 결정을 이해할 수 있다.
- 임신과 관련된 해부학적 및 생리학적 변화를 외상의 병태생리학적 처치와 연관시킬 수 있다.
- 임신부 외상이 태아에게 미치는 영향과 처치와 우선순위에 대해 논의할 수 있다.

시나리오

당신은 3시간 전에 넘어진 후 현재 복통이 점점 심해졌다는 20대 중반의 남성 환자가 있는 건설 현장으로 출동했다. 환자는 현장에서 나무 조각에 걸려 넘어지면서 쌓여 있던 각목에 왼쪽 가슴과 복부를 부딪쳤다고 말한다. 환자는 심호흡할 때 왼쪽 가슴우리 아래쪽에 중간 정도의 통증을 느끼며 가벼운 호흡곤란을 호소한다. 환자의 동료는 그가 나무어 걸려 넘어졌을 때 바로 도움을 요청하려고 하였지만, 그는 증상이 그리 심하지 않다고 말하여 기다리라고 말했다고 한다. 하지만 이후 그는 불편감이 점점 심해지고 있으며 지금은 어지럽고 힘이 빠지는 느낌이 든다고 말한다.

당신은 환자가 눈에 띄게 불편한 상태로 바닥에 앉아 있는 것을 발견한다. 환자는 왼쪽 가슴 아랫부분과 윗배를 움켜쥐고 있다. 환자는 기도가 개방되어 있고 호흡수는 28회/분, 맥박수는 124회/분, 혈압은 94/58mmHg이다. 환자의 피부는 창백하고 발한이 있다. 당신은 환자를 눕히고 신체검사를 한 결과 명백한 뼈 비빔소리 없이 왼쪽 아래 갈비뼈의 통증을 호소하였다. 복부는 팽창되지 않았고 촉진 시 부드럽지만, 왼쪽 윗배 부위에서 압통과 자발적인 근육 경직을 보였다. 외부출혈과 피부밑기종은 없다.

- 환자에게 발생할 수 있는 손상은 무엇인가?
- 이 환자를 처치할 때 우선순위는 무엇인가?
- 복막염의 징후가 있는가?

개요

복부는 외상에서 세 번째로 흔하게 손상되는 신체 부위이다. 무딘 복부 외상의 신체적 징후는 관통상보다 덜 분명하므로 복부 손상을 쉽게 놓칠 수 있다. 인지하지 못한 복부 손상은 외상 환자에서 예방할 수 있는 사망의 주요 원인 중 하나이다. 병원 전 평가의 한계로 인해 복부 손상이 의심되는 환자는 가장 가까운 적절한 의료기관으로 신속하게 이송하여 가장 좋은 처치 방법이다.

심한 복부 외상으로 인한 조기 사망은 일반적으로 관통상 또는 무딘 손상으로 인한 대량출혈로 발생한다. 몸통에 외상을 입은 후 설명할 수 없는 쇼크가 발생한 환자는 달리 입증될 때까지 복강 내 출혈이 있는 것으로 간주한다. 국소적인 증상과 징후가 없다고 해서 복부 외상의 가능성을 배제할 수는 없다. 증상이나 징후는 종종 발생하는 데 시간이 걸리며 특히 알코올, 약물, 외상성 뇌손상으로 인해 의식 수준이 변화된 환자에게서 파악하기가 특히 어렵다. 초기에 발견되지 않은 간, 비장, 결장, 소장, 위, 췌장 손상으로 합병증과 사망이 발생할 수 있다. 환자 평가 시 운동학을 고려하여 의심 지수를 높이고 병원 전 처치 제공자에게 복부 외상 및 복강 내 출혈 가능성을 알 수 있다. 복부 외상의 정확한 위치나 정도를 파악하는 것이 아니라 손상 가능성을 인식하고 임상 소견을 처치하고 적절한 의료기관으로 이송하는 것이 더 중요하다.

해부학

복부에는 소화기, 내분비, 비뇨생식기계의 주요 기관과 순환계의 주요 혈관이 있다. 복강은 가로막 아래에 위치하고 그 경계에는 앞복벽, 골반, 척추, 복부와 옆구리 근육이 포함된다. 복강은 복부의 많은 장기를 덮고 있는 복막과의 관계에 따라 두 영역으로 나뉜다. 복막강(실제 복강)에는 비장, 간, 쓸개, 위, 대장의 일부(횡행결장, 구불결장), 대부분 소장(주로 공장, 회장) 및 여성 생식기관(자궁 및 난소)으로 구성된다(**그림 11-1**). 복막뒤공간은 복막 뒤쪽에 있는 복강 내 구역으로 신장, 요관, 아래대정맥, 복부대동맥, 췌장, 십이지장의 대부분, 상행결장 및 하행결장, 직장을 포함한다(**그림 11-2**). 방광 및 남성생식기(음경, 고환, 전립샘)는 복막강보다 아래에 있다.

복부 일부는 가슴 아래에 있다. 이는 가로막의 돔 모양이 특히 숨을 내쉴 때 명치 부위의 장기가 가슴 아랫부분으로 올라갈 수 있게 한다. 흉복부라고도 하는 복부의 이 윗부분은 앞쪽과 옆구리는 갈비

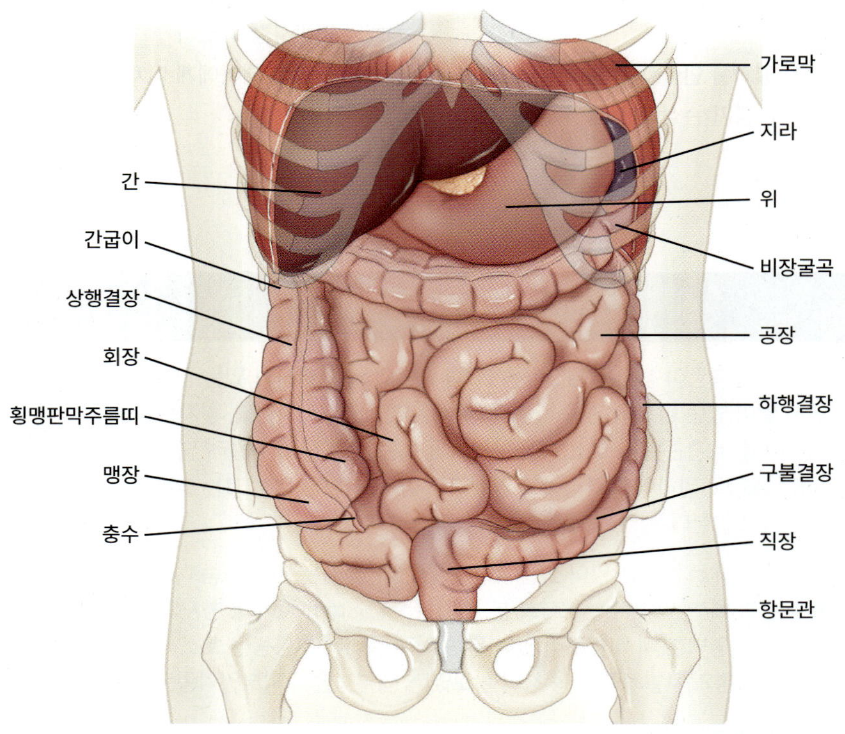

그림 11-1 복강 내 장기에는 고형장지(비장, 간), 위장관의 속이 빈 장기(위장, 소장, 결장), 생식기 등이 있다.

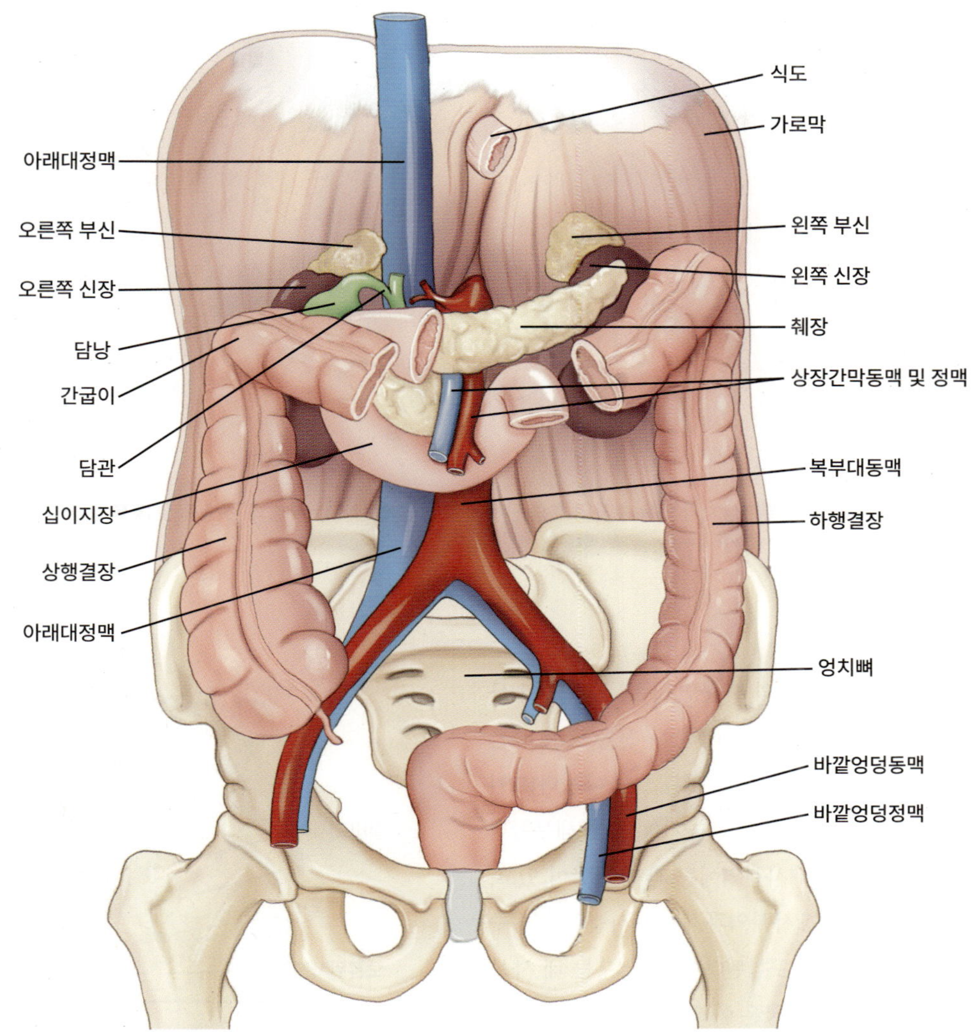

그림 11-2 복부는 복막강과 복막뒤공간으로 나뉜다. 복막뒤공간은 복막 뒤쪽의 복부 부분을 포함한다. 복막뒤 장기는 복강 내에 있지 않기 때문에 이러한 구조에 손상을 입어도 일반적으로 복막염이 발생하지 않지만, 큰 혈관 및 고형장기에 손상을 입으면 빠르게 대량출혈이 발생할 수 있다.

© National Association of Emergency Medical Technicians (NAEMT)

뼈, 뒤쪽은 척주에 의해 보호된다. 흉복부는 가로막으로 분리되는 앞쪽에는 간, 담낭, 비장, 위의 일부가 있고 뒤쪽에는 폐의 하엽이 있다. 또한 식도와 아래대정맥과 같은 큰 혈관은 가로막의 작은 구멍을 통해 가슴과 배 사이로 뻗어 있다. 이러한 위치 때문에 갈비뼈가 골절되는 것과 같은 힘이 복부 장기를 손상할 수 있다.

이러한 복부 장기와 가슴안 하부의 관계는 호흡 주기에 따라 변한다. 최대 날숨 시 가로막은 앞쪽으로 4번째 갈비 사이공간(남성의 경우 유두 수준), 측면으로는 6번째 갈비사이공간, 뒤쪽으로는 8번째 갈비사이공간까지 확장되어 가슴우리에서 복부 장기를 더 잘 보호한다. 반대로 최대 들숨 시 수축한 가로막의 돔은 6번째 갈비사이공간의 높이에 있으며 팽창된 폐는 가슴을 거의 채우고 이러한 복부 장기를 가슴아래에서 밀어낸다. 이러한 해부학적 위치 아래의 가슴에 관통상을 입은 환자는 복부 손상도 입었을 수 있다. 따라서 흉복부 관통상으로 손상된 장기는 손상 당시 환자가 들숨과 날숨 중 어떤 단계에 있었는지에 따라 다를 수 있다(**그림 11-3**).

복부의 가장 아래쪽 부분은 골반에 의해 사방이 보호된다. 이 부위에는 직장, 소장의 일부(특히 환자가 바로 서 있을 때), 방광 및 여성 생식기관이 있다. 골반 골절과 관련한 복막뒤 출혈은 복강 내 이 부위에서 가장 큰 문제이다.

가슴우리와 골반 사이의 복부는 앞쪽과 옆쪽의 복부 근육과 기타 연부조직에 의해서만 보호된다. 뒤쪽으로는 허리뼈와 척추의 길이를 따라 위치한 두껍고 강한 척추 주위 근육이 더 많은 보호 기능을 제

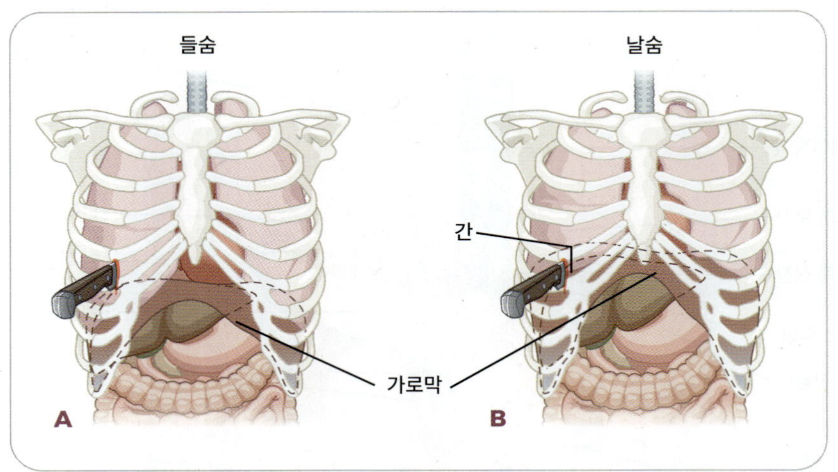

그림 11-3 찔린상처가 있는 환자의 호흡 단계에 따른 복부 장기와 가슴의 관계 **A.** 들숨 **B.** 날숨
© National Association of Emergency Medical Technicians (NAEMT)

공한다(**그림 11-4**).

　환자 평가를 위해 복부 표면을 네 개의 사분면으로 나눈다. 이 사분면은 칼돌기의 끝에서 두덩결합까지 가운데에 한 선을 긋고 다른 한 선은 배꼽 수준에서 이 정중선에 수직으로 선을 그어 나눈다(**그림 11-5**). 장기 위치와 통증 반응의 상관관계가 높기 때문에 해부학적 기준에 대한 지식이 중요하다. 오른위사분역에는 간과 담낭이 있고, 왼위사분역에는 비장과 위, 오른아래사부역과 왼아래사분역에는 주로 장, 원위 요관, 여성의 경우 난소가 포함된다. 장의 일부는 네 사분면 모두에 존재한다. 여성의 방광과 자궁은 아래 사분면 사이의 정중선에 있다.

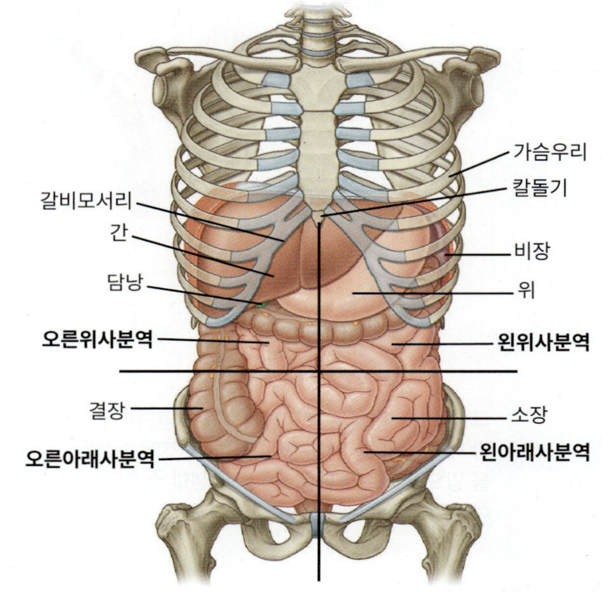

그림 11-5 신체의 다른 부위와 마찬가지로 통증, 압통 및 기타 징후가 명확하게 나타날수록 진단이 더 정확해진다. 가장 일반적인 확인 방법은 복부를 오른위, 왼위, 오른 아래, 왼 아래의 사분면으로 나눈다.
© National Association of Emergency Medical Technicians (NAEMT)

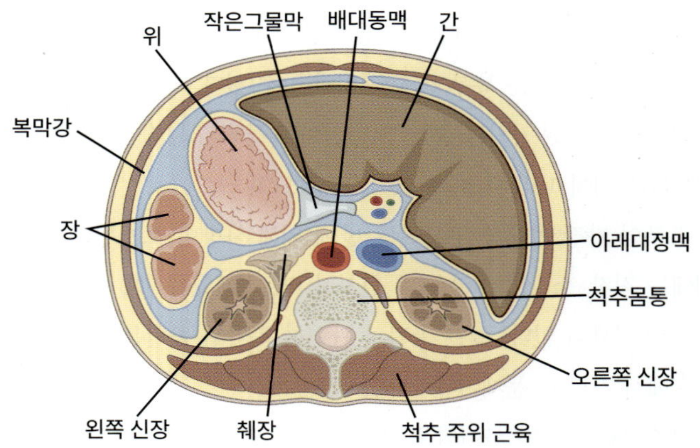

그림 11-4 복강의 이 횡단면은 장기의 앞뒤 방향 위치와 특히 앞쪽과 옆쪽의 상대적으로 제한된 보호 기능을 파악할 수 있게 해준다.
© National Association of Emergency Medical Technicians (NAEMT)

병태생리학

복부 장기를 속이 빈 장기, 고형장기, 혈관으로 나누며 이러한 구조에 대한 손상 징후를 설명하는 데 도움이 된다. 손상을 입으면 고형장기(간, 비장)와 혈관(대동맥, 대정맥)에서 출혈이 발생하지만, 속이 빈 장기(장, 담낭, 방광)는 주로 복막강이나 복막뒤공간으로 내용물이 유출된다(이 경우에도 출혈이 발생하지만, 고형장기만큼 심하지는 않은 경우가 많음). 복강 내로의 혈액 손실은 그 원인과 관계없이 출혈 쇼크의 발생에 기여하거나 주요 원인이 될 수 있다. 위장관으로부터 복막강으로 산, 소화 효소 및 세균이 방출되고 이를 인지하고 외과적 개입으로 즉시 처치하지 않으면 복막염(복막 또는 복강 내벽의 염증) 및 패혈증이 발생한다. 소변과 담즙은 일반적으로 무균 상태(세균이 포함되지 않음)이고 소화 효소가 포함되어 있지 않기 때문에 담낭이나 방광 천공은 장에서 유출된 물질만큼 빠르게 복막염을 일으키지는 않는다. 마찬가지로 복막강 내에는 산, 소화 효소 및 세균이 부족하므로 복강 내 혈액이 복막염을 유발하는 데 몇 시간이 걸릴 수 있다. 장 손상으로 인한 출혈은 장간막(복강의 후벽에 장을 부착하는 복막 조직의 주름)의 큰 혈관이 손상되지 않는 한 일반적으로 경미하다.

복부 손상은 관통상, 무딘 손상 또는 폭발 외상으로 인해 발생할 수 있다. 총상이나 찔린 상처와 같은 관통상 외상은 무딘 손상보다 쉽게 눈에 띈다. 관통상으로 인해 여러 장기가 손상될 수 있으며 발사체 유형의 손상과 관련된 높은 에너지와 환자를 찌르는 데 사용되는 대부분의 상대적으로 낮은 에너지를 고려할 때 총상보다 찔린 상처로 인해 더 일반적으로 손상될 수 있다. 총알이나 칼날과 같은 관통 물체의 잠재적 궤적을 머릿속으로 시각화하면 내부 장기의 손상 가능성을 식별하는 데 도움이 될 수 있다. 옆구리와 엉덩이에 관통상을 입으면 복강 내 장기도 함께 손상될 수 있다. 이러한 관통상은 주요 혈관이나 고형장기에서 출혈을 일으키고 관통상에서 가장 빈번하게 손상되는 장기인 장의 일부분에 천공을 일으킬 수 있다.

무딘 외상은 종종 관통성 외상으로 인한 손상보다 인식하기가 더 어렵다. 복부 장기에 대한 이러한 손상은 압박 또는 전단력으로 인해 발생한다. 압박 손상의 경우 복부 장기가 자동차 핸들과 척추 사이와 같은 단단한 물체 사이에 눌려 으깨어진다. 전단력은 지지하는 인대에 가해지는 찢어지는 힘으로 인해 고형장기가 파열되거나 혈관 파열을 일으킨다. 간과 비장은 쉽게 찢어지고 출혈이 발생할 수 있으며 출혈이 빠른 속도로 발생할 수 있다. 압박으로 인해 복강 내 압력이 증가하면 가로막이 파열되어 복부 장기가 가슴안으로 이동할 수 있다 **(그림 11-6)** (4장 외상의 물리학 및 10장 가슴 외상 참조). 복강 내 장기가 가슴안으로 밀려들어 가면 폐 팽창을 손상시키고 호흡 및 심장 기능에 영향을 미칠 수 있다. 가로막의 양쪽 절반의 파열은 똑같이 발생하는 것으로 알려졌지만, 오른쪽에 있는 간과 그 부착물이 복강 내 내용물이 오른쪽 가슴으로 탈장하는 것을 막아 오른쪽 가로막 손상의 진단을 더 어렵게 만들기 때문에 왼쪽 가로막의 절반의 파열이

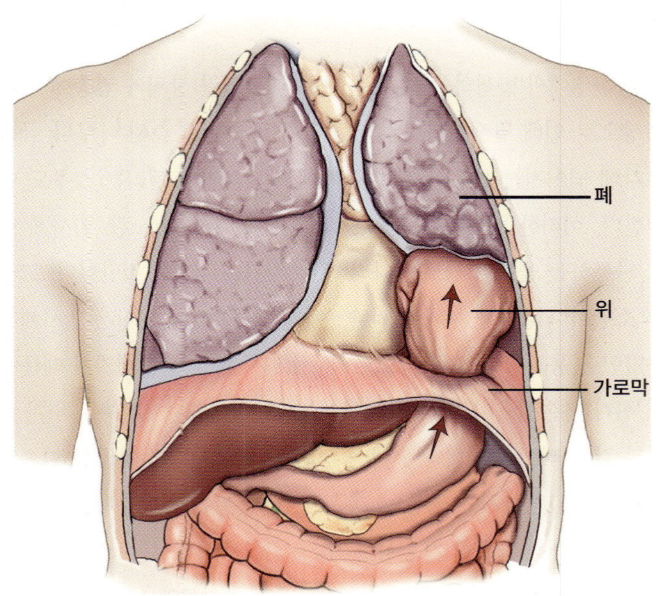

그림 11-6 복부 내부의 압력이 증가하면 가로막이 파열되어 위나 소장과 같은 복부 내 장기가 가슴으로 탈출할 수 있다.
© National Association of Emergency Medical Technicians (NAEMT)

더 자주 진단된다.

골반 골절은 골반에 인접한 많은 작은 혈관의 손상으로 인한 대량 출혈과 관련이 있을 수 있다. 골반 골절과 관련된 다른 손상으로는 방광 및 직장 손상, 남성의 요도 손상, 여성의 질 손상이 있다.

복부에 대한 일차 폭발 손상은 주로 장과 같은 속이 빈 장기에 영향을 미친다. 이는 장벽 괴사 또는 천공으로 지연된 방식으로 나타날 수 있다. 이차 폭발 손상은 관통 파편이나 파편이 복부에 부딪혀 발생할 수 있으며 삼차 폭발 손상은 무딘 외상과 유사하며 환자가 다른 물체에 부딪힐 때 발생한다.

평가

복부 손상의 평가는 특히 병원 전 환경에서 사용할 수 있는 진단 기능이 제한적이기 때문에 어려울 수 있다. 손상 기전, 신체검사 결과, 환자 또는 목격자의 이야기 등 다양한 정보를 바탕으로 복부 손상을 의심할 수 있는 지수를 형성해야 한다.

운동학

다른 유형의 외상과 마찬가지로 폭발, 무딘 손상, 관통상 여부와 관계없이 손상 기전에 대한 지식은 병원 전 처치 제공자가 복부 손상에 대한 의심 지수를 형성하는 데 중요한 역할을 한다.

관통성 외상

민간 환경에서 발생하는 대부분 관통상은 찔린 상처와 권총에 의한 총상으로 인해 발생한다. 예를 들어, 누군가가 돌출된 나무나 금속 조각에 넘어지는 경우와 같이 물체에 부딪치거나 찔리는 경우도 발생한다. 이러한 낮거나 중간 정도의 운동에너지 힘은 칼, 발사체 또는 관통하는 물체의 경로를 따라 복부 장기를 찢거나 절단한다. 고성능 소총이나 공격용 무기로 인한 손상과 같이 고속 손상은 발사체가 복막안을 통과할 때 일시적으로 더 큰 일시적 공동이 생기기 때문에 더 심각한 손상을 유발하는 경향이 있다. 발사체는 갈비뼈, 척추, 골반과 같은 뼈에 부딪혀 파편이 형성되어 내부 장기에 천공을 일으킬 수 있다. 찔린 상처는 권총, 소총 또는 산탄총에서 발사된 발사체에 비해 복막안을 관통할 가능성이 작다.

복막을 관통하는 찔린 상처로 간(40%), 소장(30%), 가로막(20%), 결장(15%)을 손상할 가능성이 가장 높지만, 총상은 소장(50%), 결장(40%), 간(30%), 복부 혈관(25%)을 손상시키는 경우가 가장 흔하다. 등의 근육이 두꺼우므로 등을 관통하는 외상은 전복벽의 손상보다 복막 내 구조물의 손상을 초래할 가능성이 작다. 전반적으로 복부에 찔린 상처를 입은 환자의 약 15%만이 외과적 개입이 필요하지만, 총상을 입은 환자의 약 85%는 복부 손상을 확실하게 처치하기 위해 수술이 필요하다. 접선 총상은 피부밑조직을 관통할 수 있지만, 복막안으로 들어가지 않는다. 폭발 장치로 인한 파편이 복막을 관통하여 내부 장기를 손상할 수도 있다.

무딘 손상

복부 장기를 손상할 수 있는 압축력과 전단력은 다양한 기전을 통해 발생한다. 환자는 자동차와 오토바이 충돌, 차량에 치이거나 부딪혔을 때 또는 높은 곳에서 추락한 후 상당한 감속 및 압축력을 받을 수 있다. 자동차 충돌 시에는 차량 탑승자와 관련하여 충격 위치를 고려해야 한다. 예를 들어 운전자의 측면 충돌은 정면충돌로 인한 감속 및 압축 손상과는 달리 비장 손상을 의심하게 된다. 복부 장기는 급격한 감속이나 심한 압박과 같은 심각한 운동 손상과 관련된 사고에서 가장 자주 손상되지만, 폭행, 계단에서 넘어지거나 스포츠 활동(예: 축구에서 태클을 당하는 경우)과 같이 해가 없는 것처럼 보이는 기전으로 인해 복부 손상이 발생할 수도 있다. 안전띠, 에어백, 스포츠 패딩 등 환자가 사용하는 모든 보호 장치나 장비에 주목한다.

고형장기를 압박하면 구조가 찢어질(예: 간 열상) 수 있지만, 장이

Box 11-1 고형장기 손상의 비수술적 처치

비장, 간 또는 신장 손상이 의심되는 경우 현대 외상센터에서는 더 이상의 외과적 치료가 필요하지 않다. 경험에 따르면 이러한 손상의 대부분은 쇼크가 발생하기 전에 출혈이 멈추고 외과적 치료 없이 치유되는 것으로 나타났다. 연구에 따르면 환자가 저혈량 쇼크나 복막염을 겪지 않는다면 심각한 고형장기 손상도 안전하게 관찰할 수 있는 것으로 나타났다. 환자는 병원에 입원하여 활력징후, 혈액검사, 복부검사 등을 자세히 모니터링하며 초기에는 중환자실에 입원하는 경우가 많다. 이와 같은 방법의 장점은 환자가 잠재적으로 불필요한 수술을 받지 않도록 방지한다는 것이다. 비장은 감염과 싸우는 데 중요한 역할을 하므로 비장을 제거하면 환자(특히 어린이)가 특정 세균 감염에 취약해진다.

이러한 비수술적 처치의 성공 사례는 소아의 비장 손상에 대해 처음 보고되었지만, 이 방법은 간이나 신장에 손상을 입은 환자뿐만 아니라 성인 환자에게도 종종 적용된다. 둔기에 의한 외상 후 비장 손상의 약 84%가 이러한 방식으로 치료될 수 있으며 외상센터에서는 90% 이상의 성공률을 보인다는 데이터도 있다. 마찬가지로 많은 간 손상이 비수술로 관리되며 성공률은 90% 이상이다. 비수술적 관리에는 단순한 관찰이 아닌 혈관 조형술을 통한 색전술이 포함될 수 있다.

이 술기의 실패 위험(재출혈, 외과적 처치가 필요한 쇼크 발생)은 손상 후 처음 며칠 동안 가장 높다. 병원 전 처치 제공자는 퇴원 후 재출혈이 발생한 환자에게 대응할 수 있으므로 이와 같은 방법을 숙지하고 있어야 한다.

© National Association of Emergency Medical Technicians (NAEMT)

나 방광과 같이 속이 빈 장기에 비슷한 힘이 가해지면 구조물이 파열되어 그 내용물이 복부로 유출될 수 있다. 전단력은 후복막에 고정된 상행결장과 이동성이 높은 소장이 복막이 결합하는 부위와 같이 다른 구조물에 연결된 부위에서 구조물이 찢어질 수 있다. 복부에 둔기에 의한 외상 후 가장 흔하게 손상되는 장기는 비장, 간 및 소장이다. 모든 고형장기 손상에 외과적 개입이 필요한 것은 아니다(**Box 11-1**). 이러한 유형의 고형장기 손상의 대부분은 저절로 출혈이 멈추는 경우가 많으므로 병원에서 주의 깊게 관찰할 수 있다.

폭발 손상

모든 원인(예: 군수품, 산업, 의료)에서 발생하는 폭발은 다양한 형태로 대량의 에너지를 생성한다. 수 밀리초 내에 폭발파라고 하는 강렬한 과압 충격이 환경(예: 공기, 물)을 통과한다. 이 충격은 반경 3제곱에 반비례하여 공기 중에서 빠르게 감소한다. 이 과압 충격에 근접해 있는 사람들은 1차 폭발 손상을 입는다. 그 직후에는 에너지가 충전된 파편이 뒤따르면 파편은 시간과 거리에 따라 그 수와 운동에너지가 빠르게 감소한다. 날아다니는 파편과 파편에 의한 이차적 손상을 2차 폭발 손상이라고 한다. 다음으로 폭발의 기체 생성물과 폭발풍

에 의해 생성된 물리적 움직임은 피해자를 주변 구조물로 밀어붙여 상당한 무딘 힘을 발생시켜 자동차 충돌이나 낙상으로 인한 손상과 유사한 손상을 유발할 수 있다. 이러한 무딘 손상 기전으로 인한 손상을 3차 폭발 손상이라고 한다. 마지막으로 폭발과 관련된 손상(예: 화약, 압착) 또는 질병(예: 먼지, 연기 또는 유독 가스로 인한 심리적 영향 또는 호흡 문제)을 포함하여 폭발과 관련된 다른 문제가 발생하며 신체의 모든 부위에 영향을 미칠 수 있다. 이와 관련된 손상을 4차 폭발 손상이라고 한다.

앞서 언급했듯이 폭발이 발생하는 환경은 물리적으로 중요하다. 공중에서 폭발이 일어나면 에너지를 방출하는 폭발파가 발생하여 이동하면서 공기를 압축한다. 1차 폭발의 에너지는 짧은 거리만 이동한 후 소멸한다. 반면에 밀폐된 공기 공간에서의 폭발은 폭발파가 구조물에 반사되어 2차 이상의 파동으로 피해자에게 재접촉하기 때문에 추가적인 손상을 유발할 수 있다. 수중 폭발로 인한 폭발파도 다르게 작용하여 더 큰 피해를 줄 수 있다. 물은 본질적으로 비압축성이기 때문에 수중 폭발로 인한 폭발파는 그 에너지가 천천히 소멸하고 공기 중보다 3배 더 멀리 이동한다.

복강에만 국한된 1차 폭발 손상은 장벽 손상으로 이어질 수 있으며 이는 지연된 방식으로 천공이 나타날 수 있다. 2차 폭발 손상은 복강을 관통할 수도 있고 그렇지 않을 수도 있지만, 추가적인 병원 검사가 필요한 관통상을 초래한다. 3차 폭발 손상은 비장, 신장, 간 열상 및 장 손상을 포함한 무딘 복부 손상을 초래한다.

병력

병력은 환자, 가족 또는 목격자로부터 얻을 수 있으며 환자 처치 기록지에 기록하고 의료기관에 전달해야 한다. 현장 사진을 확보하여 환자를 이송한 의료기관의 의료진과 공유하는 것은 손상 기전을 명확하게 전달하는 데 도움이 될 수 있다. SAMPLE 병력의 구성 요소(증상, 알레르기, 나이, 약물, 과거 병력, 마지막 식사, 손상 발생 전 사건) 외에도 손상의 기전과 사망률과 이환율을 잠재적으로 높일 수 있는 동반 질환의 존재 여부에 맞게 질문을 한다. 예를 들어, 자동차 충돌 사고의 경우 다음과 같은 사항을 확인하기 위한 질문을 할 수 있다.

- 충돌 유형, 차량 내 환자의 위치 또는 차량에서 이탈 여부
- 충돌 발생 시 예상 차량 속도
- 승객 공간 침범, 운전대 변형, 앞 유리 손상 및 구조 필요성 등 차량 손상 정도
- 안전띠, 에어백 전개, 어린이용 안전 시트 등 안전장치 사용 여부

관통상의 경우 다음과 같은 사항을 확인하기 위해 질문을 할 수 있다.

- 무기 종류(권총, 소총, 칼의 길이)
- 환자가 총에 맞거나 칼에 찔린 횟수
- 환자가 총에 맞은 거리
- 현장에서 출혈량(정확한 추정이 어려운 경우가 많음)
- 관통상 이전의 병력(총알 파편이 남아 있을 수 있음)

신체검사

일차평가

대부분의 심각한 복부 손상은 일차평가에서 확인된 이상 증상으로 나타나며 주로 호흡과 순환에서 나타난다. 관련된 손상이 없는 한 복부 외상 환자는 일반적으로 기도가 개방되어 있다. 호흡, 순환 및 장애 평가에서 발견되는 변화는 일반적으로 존재하는 쇼크의 정도와 일치한다. 초기 보상성 쇼크 환자는 호흡수가 약간 증가할 수 있지만, 중증 출혈성 쇼크 환자는 현저한 빠른 호흡을 보일 수 있다. 가로막 파열로 인해 복부의 내용물이 손상 부위 가슴안으로 탈장되면 호흡 기능이 손상되는 경우가 많으며 호흡음 청진시 가슴에서 장음이 들릴 수 있다. 마찬가지로 복강 내 출혈로 인한 쇼크는 다른 소견이 거의 없는 경미한 빈맥부터 심한 빈맥, 저혈압, 창백하고 차갑고 축축한 피부까지 다양하게 나타날 수 있다.

복강 내 출혈의 가장 신뢰할 수 있는 지표는 원인 불명의 저혈량 쇼크의 존재 여부이다. 장애를 평가할 때 병원 전 처치 제공자는 복부 외상으로 인한 보상성 쇼크 환자의 경우 경미한 불안이나 초조함과 같은 미묘한 징후만 발견할 수 있지만, 생명을 위협하는 출혈이 있는 거의 깨어나지 않거나 의식 상태에 심각한 저하가 있을 수 있다. 이러한 복강 평가에서 이상이 발견되면 즉시 이송을 준비하는 동안 복부를 노출하고 타박상이나 관통상과 같은 외상의 증거가 있는지 검사해야 한다.

이차평가

이차평가를 시행하는 동안 복부를 더 자세히 검사한다. 이 평가는 주로 복부의 시진 및 촉진을 포함하며 체계적으로 접근해야 한다.

시진

복부에 연부조직 손상과 팽창이 있는지 검사한다. 복부, 옆구리 또는 등에 연부조직 외상이 발견되면 복강 내 손상을 의심할 수 있다. 이

러한 소견에는 타박상, 찰과상, 찔린 상처, 총상, 명백한 출혈, 내장 적출, 찔린 물체 또는 타이어 자국과 같은 비정상적인 소견이 포함될 수 있다. "안전띠 징후"(어깨 및 허리벨트에 의한 복벽이 압박되어 복부에 반상출혈이나 찰과상이 나타나는 것)는 급격한 감속으로 인해 복부에 상당한 힘이 가해졌음을 나타내며(**그림 11-7**) 복강 내 손상 가능성을 8배 증가시킨다. 안전띠 징후가 있는 소아 환자의 복부 내 손상 발생률은 성인보다 더 높다. 안전띠와 관련된 손상은 일반적으로 장과 장간막이 안전띠와 복부 앞벽, 뒤쪽 척추 사이에 압박되고 으깨지기 때문에 장과 장간막에 발생하며 종종 지연되어 나타난다. 그레이-터너 징후(Grey-Turner's sign, 옆구리 반상출혈) 및 쿨렌징후(Cullen's sign, 배꼽 주위의 반상출혈)는 복막뒤 출혈을 나타내지만, 이러한 징후는 종종 지연되어 손상 후 처음 몇 시간 동안은 보이지 않을 수 있다.

복부의 윤곽을 관찰하여 복부가 평평하거나 팽창되었는지 평가해야 한다. 복부 팽창은 심각한 내부출혈을 나타낼 수 있지만, 성인의 복강은 뚜렷한 팽창 징후가 나타나기 전에 최대 1.5L의 체액을 보유할 수 있다. 복부 팽창은 백마스크 장비로 환기를 시행하는 동안 위에 공기가 가득 차서 발생할 수도 있다. 이러한 징후는 복강 내 손상을 나타낼 수 있지만, 심각한 내부 손상을 입은 일부 환자는 이러한 징후가 나타나지 않을 수 있다.

촉진

압통 부위를 확인하기 위해 복부 촉진을 시행한다. 이상적으로는 환자가 통증을 호소하지 않는 부위에서 촉진을 시작한다. 그런 다음 각 복부 사분면을 촉진한다. 압통 부위를 촉진하는 동안 병원 전 처치 제공자는 환자가 해당 부위의 복부 근육을 긴장시키는 것을 확인할 수 있다. 자발적 보호라고 하는 이 반응은 촉진으로 인한 통증으로부터 환자를 보호한다. 비자발적 보호는 복막염에 대한 반응으로 복벽 근육의 경축 또는 연축이 나타난다. **Box 11-2**에는 복막염의 존재와 일치하는 신체적 소견이 나열되어 있다. 자발적 보호와 달리 환자가 주의가 산만하거나(예: 대화 중) 복부를 몰래 촉진하는 경우(예: 장음을 청진하는 것처럼 하면서 청진기로 누르는 경우) 비자발적 보호가 남아있다. 반동 압통의 존재는 오랫동안 복막염을 나타내는 중요한 소견으로 여겨져 왔지만, 현재 많은 외과 의사는 복부를 깊숙이 누른 다음 빠르게 압력을 배는 이 동작이 과도한 통증을 유발한다고 생각한다. 반동 압통이 있는 경우 환자는 복압이 완화될 때 더 심한 통증을 느끼게 된다.

명백하게 손상을 입은 복부를 깊게 또는 강하게 촉진하면 통증이 발생할 뿐만 아니라 이론적으로 출혈이나 기타 손상을 악화시킬 수 있으므로 피해야 한다. 복부에 찔린 물체가 있는 경우 촉진 시 세심한 주의를 기울여야 한다. 실제로 이물질이 찔린 환자의 복부를 촉진하여 얻을 수 있는 유용한 추가 정보는 거의 없다.

압통은 복강 내 손상의 중요한 지표이지만, 여러 가지 요인으로 인해 압통을 평가하는 데 혼란을 줄 수 있다. 외상성 뇌손상 환자나 약물 또는 알코올의 영향을 받은 환자와 같이 의식 상태가 변화된 환자는 신뢰할 수 없는 검사를 할 수 있다. 즉, 심각한 내부 손상이 있는 경우에도 환자가 압통을 이야기하지 않거나 촉진에 반응하지 않을 수 있다. 소아와 노인 환자는 통증 반응 저하로 인해 복부 검사를 신뢰할 수 없을 가능성이 높다. 반대로 아래쪽 갈비뼈 골절이나 골반 골절 환자는 골절 또는 관련 내부 손상으로 인한 압통으로 검사 결과가 모호할 수 있다. 환자가 팔다리 또는 척추 골절과 같은 손상으로 인한 산만한 통증이 있는 경우 촉진 시 복부 통증이 유발되지 않을 수 있다.

병원 전 환경에서 골반 촉진은 환자 처치에 영향을 줄 수 있는 정보를 거의 제공하지 않는다. 이 평가를 수행하는 데 시간이 걸리면 불안정한 골절 부위에 형성된 혈전이 파괴되어 출혈을 악화시킬 수 있으므로 한 번만 시행한다. 이 평가를 하는 동안 골반을 부드럽게 촉진하여 불안정성과 압통을 평가한다. 이 평가에는 다음과 같은 두 단계가 포함된다.

1. 엉덩뼈 능선을 안쪽으로 누르기

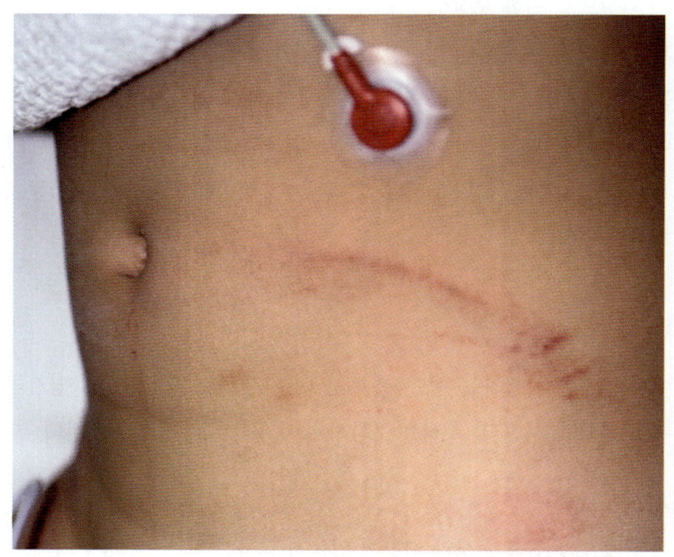

그림 11-7 환자가 안전띠에 부딪혀 감속할 때 발생하는 복부 "안전띠 징후"이다.
Courtesy of Peter T. Pons, MD, FACEP.

2. 두덩결합을 후방으로 누르기

검사 중 불안정성이나 통증이 발견되면 골반을 더 이상 촉진하지 말고 골반 고정대를 적용해야 한다.

청진

복막안 출혈이나 장 내용물의 유출은 장의 연동운동이 멈추는 장폐색을 유발할 수 있다. 이 경우 장음이 감소하거나 없어져 복부가 "조용한" 상태가 된다. 일반적으로 장음 청진은 병원 전 평가 도구로 유용하지 않다. 이 진단 징후는 환자의 병원 전 처치를 변경하지 않으므로 그 유무를 판단하는 데 시간을 낭비해서는 안 된다. 그러나 호흡음 청진시 가슴에서 장음이 들리면 가로막 파열을 고려할 수 있다.

타진

복부 타진 시 고음 또는 둔탁한 소리가 들릴 수 있지만, 이와 같은 정보는 외상 환자의 병원 전 처치에 변화를 주는 것이 아니므로 귀중한 시간만 소비하므로 병원 전 평가 도구로 권장하지 않는다. 환자가 기침할 때 복부 압통이 심하거나 타진 시 통증이 있는 경우 복막염의 주요 소견으로 볼 수 있다. 복막염의 징후는 **Box 11-2**에 요약되어 있다.

특별 검사 및 주요 지표

복부 손상을 입은 대부분 환자에게는 외과적 평가와 많은 경우 개입이 여전히 핵심적인 필요 사항이며 정확한 손상 내용을 파악하기 위해 시간을 낭비해서는 안 된다. 많은 환자에서 컴퓨터단층촬영(CT) 또는 외과적 검사를 통해 복부를 추가로 평가할 때까지 특정 장기 손상의 확인이 이루어지지 않는다.

응급실에서 초음파는 외상 환자의 복강 내 출혈을 평가하는 데 사용되는 주요 침상 검사 방식이 되었다. 외상 환자에서 시행하는 응급 초음파검사(FAST)는 복강 내 3곳(간과 신장 사이, 비장과 신장 사이, 방광 주변)의 부위와 4번째로 심장막 부위에서 심장 주위에 체액이 있는지 평가한다. 외상 환자에서 시행하는 확장된 응급 초음파검사

(eFAST)는 기흉이나 혈흉을 평가하기 위해 오른쪽 및 왼쪽 가슴 부위를 검사한다(**그림 11-8, Box 11-3**). 액체는 초음파를 장치로 다시 반사하지 않기 때문에 초음파상으로는 검은색으로 나타난다. 하나 이상의 부위에 체액이 있는 경우 걱정할 수 있지만, 초음파 검사는 혈액과 다른 유형의 체액(복수, 방광 파열로 인한 소변 등)을 구별할 수 없다.

복막강을 평가하는 데 사용되는 다른 방법과 비교할 때 FAST는 환자의 침상 옆에서 신속하게 수행할 수 있고 소생술을 방해하지 않으며 비침습적이고 방사선 노출이 없으며 CT보다 비용이 훨씬 저렴하다. FAST 검사의 가장 큰 단점은 손상 부위를 명확하게 진단하지 못하고 혈액일 수 있는 체액의 존재 여부만 알려준다는 것이다. FAST 검사의 또 다른 단점으로는 검사 및 판독이 시술자의 기술과 경험에 따라 달라질 수 있으며 비만, 피부밑공기가 있거나 이전에 수술받은 적이 있는 환자의 경우 유용성이 떨어질 수 있다는 점이다. 가장 중요한 것은 FAST 검사 결과가 음성이라고 해서 외과적 개입이 필요할 수 있는 손상을 포함한 손상의 존재를 배제할 수 없다는 것이다. FAST 검사에서 음성은 검사를 시행한 시점에 복부에 체액이 보이지 않았다는 의미일 뿐이다. 이 결과는 손상이 존재하지 않거나 복부에 혈액이 충분히 고이지 않았기 때문일 수 있다(외상 사고 현장에 대한 EMS의 신속한 대응을 고려할 때 실제로 발생할 가능성).

사용 편이성과 향상된 초음파 기술로 인해 일부 지상 또는 항공 응급의료서비스 시스템과 군대에서는 병원 전 단계에서 FAST를 시행하고 있다. FAST 검사는 현장에서 실행할 수 있는 것으로 입증되었지만, 병원 전 혈액제제 투여의 필요성을 결정하거나 대량 수혈 프로토콜 보다 신속하게 활성화하는 데 사용되고 있다. 그러나 복부 외상 환자의 개선된 결과를 입증한 병원 전 연구는 제한적이다. 응급실 환자를 대상으로 한 연구 결과에 따르면 몸통 외상이 의심되는 환자의 수술 치료 시간이 크게 단축되고 자원 사용이 개선되었으며 병원비용이 절감된 것으로 나타났다. FAST는 열악한 환경이나 다수 사상자 발생 상황에서도 유용할 수 있다. 그러나 이는 주로 병원으로의 이송을 지연시키거나 환자의 실제 상태에 대해 잘못된 확신을 줄 수 있으므로 PHTLS에서는 병원 전 일상적인 처치에는 FAST 사용을 권장하지 않는다.

이러한 다양한 구성 요소에도 불구하고 복부 손상을 평가하기는 어려울 수 있다. 다음은 복부 손상을 의심하게 하는 주요 지표이다.

- 외상의 명백한 징후(예: 연부조직 손상, 총상)
- 다른 명백한 원인이 없는 저혈량 쇼크의 존재

Box 11-2 복막염 진단을 뒷받침하는 신체검사 결과

- 촉진 또는 기침 시 현저한 복부 압통(국소적 또는 전신적)
- 비자발적 보호
- 타진 시 압통
- 장음이 감소하거나 없음

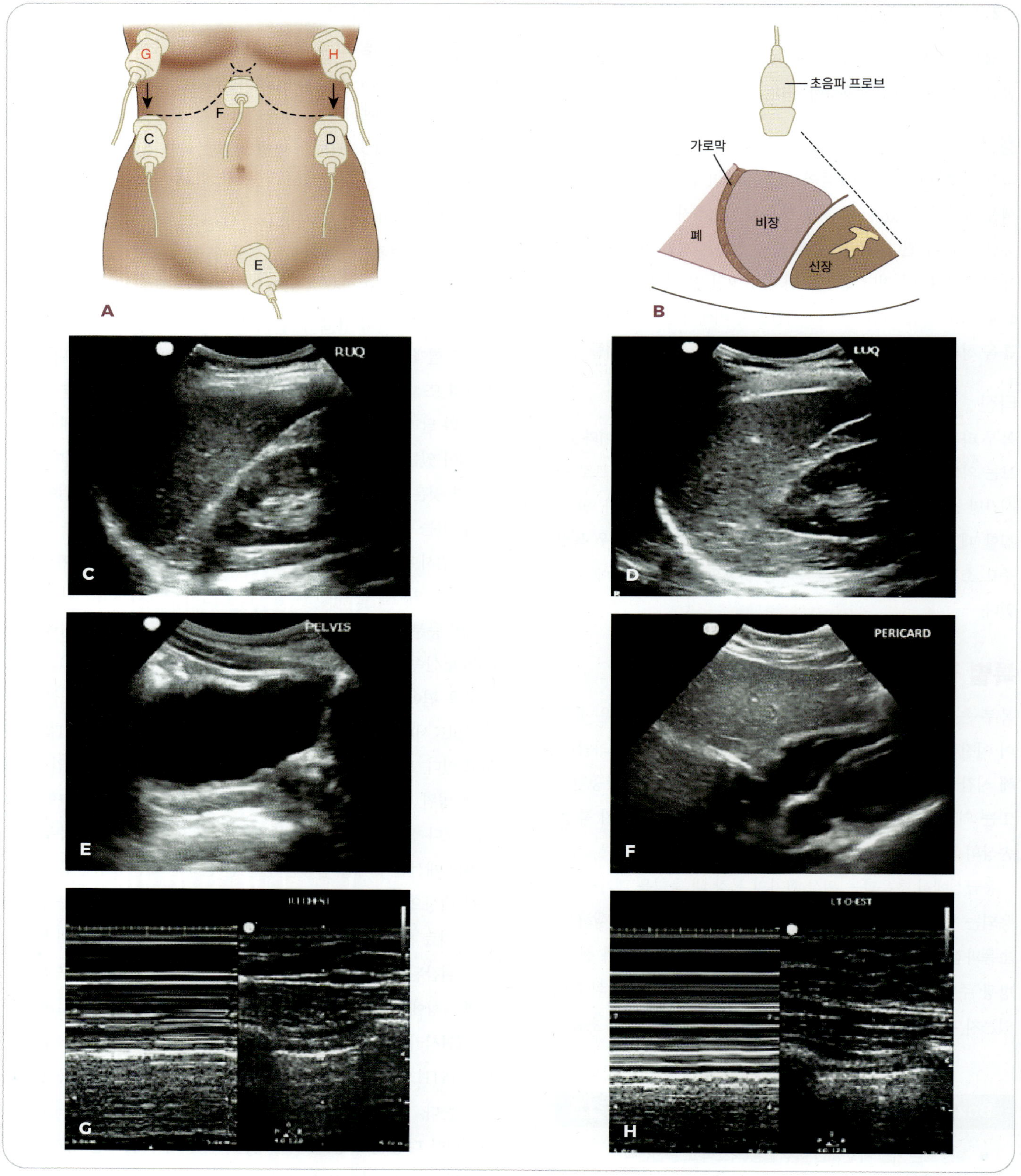

그림 11-8 외상 환자에서 시행하는 확장된 응급 초음파검사(eFAST). **A.** eFAST 검사를 시행하는 6 부위에 대한 프로브 위치. **B.** 비장 모양을 보기 위한 초음파 프로브 위치에 폐, 비장, 가로막 및 신장의 방향. **C.** 오른위사분역의 정상 모습. **D.** 왼위사분역의 정상 모습. **E.** 골반의 정상 모습. **F.** 심장막의 정상 모습. **G.** 오른쪽 가슴의 정상 모습. **H.** 왼쪽 가슴의 정상 모습

Box 11-3 eFAST 검사*

대부분의 심각한 복강 내 손상은 복강 내 출혈과 관련이 있으므로 외상 환자에게 eFAST 검사는 가치가 있다. 초음파로는 체액의 종류를 구별할 수 없지만, 외상 환자의 체액은 모두 혈액으로 추정된다.

방법
- 5구역의 초음파 영상을 이미지화하고 그중 3구역의 영상은 복강을 평가할 수 있다.
  1. 심장막
  2. 간 주위(모리슨 주머니)
  3. 비장 주위
  4. 골반
  5. 전흉부
- 누출된 체액은 초음파 영상에서 검은색으로 나타난다.
- 한 곳 이상의 영역에서 체액이 있으면 양성 영상을 나타낸다.

장점
- 신속한 수행 가능
- 침대 옆에서 검사 가능
- 소생술에 방해가 되지 않음
- 비침습적 검사
- 컴퓨터단층촬영(CT)보다 비용이 저렴

단점
- 비만 환자, 피부밑에 공기가 있거나 이전에 복부 수술을 받은 적이 있는 환자의 경우 검사가 어려울 수 있다.
- 검사 방법은 의료진에 따라 다르다.

*FAST and eFAST have been studied in several prehospital systems.[18-24]

© National Association of Emergency Medical Technicians (NAEMT)

- 다른 손상(예: 골절, 외부출혈)으로 설명할 수 없는 쇼크
- 복막염의 존재 유무

처치

복부 외상 환자에 대한 병원 전 처치의 중요한 점은 잠재적 손상의 존재를 인식하고 환자를 처치할 수 있는 가장 가까운 적절한 의료기관으로 신속하게 이송하는 것이다.

일차평가에서 확인된 생명 기능의 이상은 이송 중에 처치한다. 산소포화도를 94% 이상으로 유지하기 위해 보충 산소를 투여하고 필요한 경우 기도를 확보하며 필요하면 보조 환기를 시행한다. 외부출혈은 직접 압박이나 지혈대로 지혈한다.

복부 외상이 있는 환자는 종종 내부출혈을 조절하고 손상 부위를 치료하기 위해 수혈과 외과적 치료가 필요한 경우가 많으므로 가능

한 한 외상센터와 같이 즉각적인 수술이 가능한 의료기관으로 환자를 이송해야 한다. 특히 저혈압 또는 복막 징후와 관련된 복부 외상의 증거, 내장적출 또는 박힌 물체의 존재 등 신속한 외과적 개입이 필요하다는 것을 나타내는 소견이 있으면 즉시 즉각적인 외과적 처치를 해야 한다. 복강 내 손상을 입은 환자를 이용할 수 있는 수술실과 수술 팀이 없는 의료기관으로 이송하는 것은 신속한 이송의 목적에 어긋난다. 일반외과 전문의가 상주하는 병원이 없는 시골 지역의 경우 복부 외상을 입은 불안정한 환자의 생존을 위해서는 조기 외과적 개입이 중요하므로 구급차나 항공 이송을 통해 외상센터로 직접 이송하는 것을 고려해야 한다. 사례 보고에 따르면 병원 전 환경에서 고도로 훈련된 팀이 복부 외상 환자의 출혈을 조절하기 위해 병원에서 대동맥 내 풍선폐쇄술(REBOG)을 사용하여 결정적인 처치를 시행할 수 있는 의료기관으로 이송할 시간을 확보한 사례가 있다(**그림 11-9**). 전문 교육이 필요하고 결과에 대한 이점이 불분명하며 심각한 합병증이 발생할 가능성이 있으므로 대동맥 내 풍선폐쇄술은 병원 전 환경에서 시험 중이지만, 현재 PHTLS에서는 권장하지 않는다.

환자가 척추 또는 골반 손상을 일으킬 수 있는 무딘 외상을 입으면 안정화를 적절하게 수행한다. 척추 고정에 대한 적절한 지침은 9장 척추 외상을 참조한다. 골반 손상이 의심되는 혈류역학적으로 불안정한 무딘 외상 환자의 경우 병원 전 처치 제공자는 시트로 골반을 고정하거나 시판되는 골반고정대를 적용하여 골반을 안정화하는 것

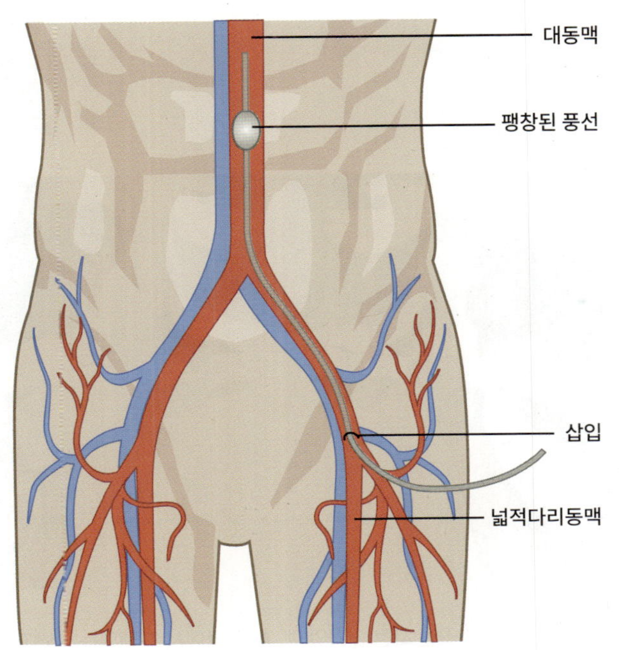

그림 11-9 몸통에 조절되지 않는 출혈에 대한 대동맥 내 풍선폐쇄술(REBOA).

© National Association of Emergency Medical Technicians (NAEMT)

이 좋다(**그림 11-10**). 이러한 방식으로 골반을 고정하면 골반 부피가 줄어들고 골절 조각이 안정화되어 최종 치료를 받을 수 있는 의료기관으로 이송하는 동안 심각한 출혈의 위험을 줄이는 데 도움이 된다. 골반고정대의 권장 적용에 대한 지침은 **Box 11-4**에 설명되어 있다.

이송 중에 정맥 라인을 확보한 후 결정질 수액을 투여할지 여부는 환자의 임상 증상에 따라 결정된다. 복부 외상 환자는 균형 잡힌 소생술이 필요한 주요 상황 중 하나이다. 정맥 내로 수액을 적극적으로 투여하면 환자의 혈압이 형성된 혈전을 파괴할 수 있는 수준까지 상승하여 혈액 응고와 저혈압으로 인해 멈췄던 출혈이 재발할 수 있다. 혈액 응고를 방해하고 저혈압으로 인해 멈추었던 출혈이 재발할 수 있다(정맥 내 수액 투여에 대한 자세한 내용은 3장 쇼크; 삶과 죽음의 병리학에서 확인할 수 있다). 결정질 수액 또는 혈액제제를 사용할 수 있는지에 관계없이 병원 전 처치 제공자는 복부나 골반의 출혈 부위에서 멈췄던 출혈이 다시 발생하지 않도록 정상 범위

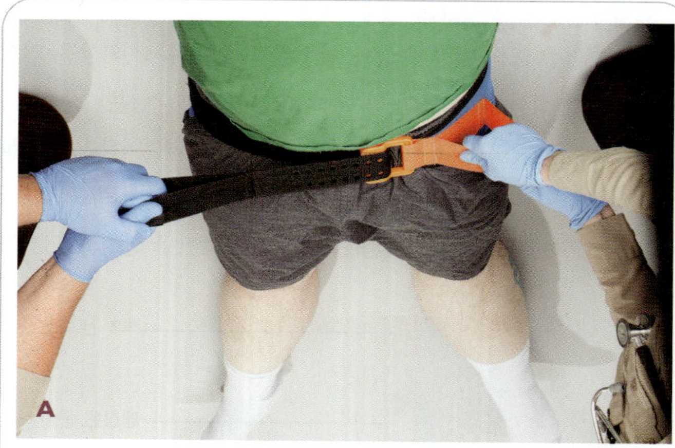

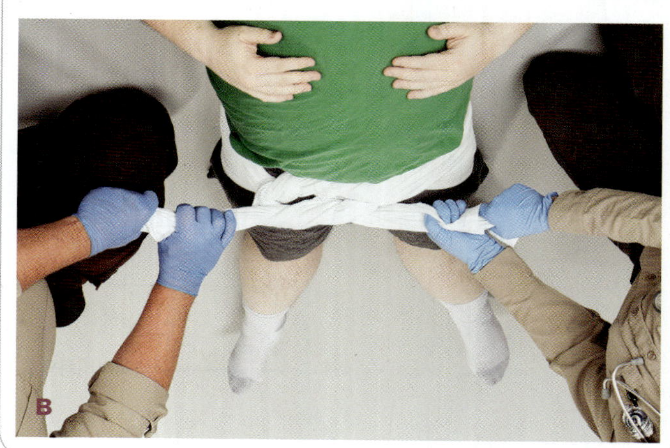

그림 11-10 병원 전 골반 고정 술기의 예. **A.** 시중에서 판매되는 골반고정대. **B.** 시트를 이용한 골반고정.

Box 11-4 골반고정대 적응증

다음과 같은 상황에서 골반 골절이 의심되는 경우 골반고정대를 적용해야 한다.

- 심각한 무딘 손상(예: 오토바이 충돌) 또는 다음 징후 중 하나 이상을 동반한 폭발 손상
  - 골반 통증
  - 골반 골절을 시사하는 신체검사 결과
  - 주요 하지 절단 또는 부분 절단
  - 쇼크
  - 무의식(통증 호소 또는 압통 소견이 없는 경우)

로 혈압을 유지하는 것이 아니라 중요한 장기에 관류를 제공할 수 있도록 혈압을 유지해야 한다. 외상성 뇌손상이 없는 경우 목표 수축기 혈압은 80~90mmHg(평균 동맥압 60~65mmHg)이다. 복강 내 출혈이 의심되고 외상성 뇌손상이 있는 환자의 경우 수축기 혈압을 최소 110mmHg으로 유지한다.

트라넥삼산(TXA)은 수년간 출혈을 조절하는 데 사용되어 온 혈전 안정화 약물로 병원 전 단계에서 사용하기 시작했다. 트라넥삼산은 플라스미노겐에 결합하여 플라스민으로 변하는 것을 방지하여 혈전 내 피브린 분해를 방지하는 작용을 한다. 현재 진행 중인 연구는 트라넥삼산의 적절한 병원 전 역할을 결정하는 데 도움이 될 것이다. 3장 쇼크: 삶과 죽음의 병태생리학 장에서 트라넥삼산에 대해 자세히 설명되어 있다.

특별한 고려 사항

박힌 물체

박힌 물체를 제거하면 추가적인 외상을 유발할 수 있고 박힌 물체가 출혈을 막고 있을 수 있으므로 병원 전 환경에서 복부에 박힌 물체를 제거하는 것은 금기이다(**그림 11-11**). 병원 전 처치 제공자는 환자의 복부에 박힌 물체를 움직이거나 제거해서는 안 된다. 병원에서 이러한 물체는 방사선 검사를 통해 물체의 모양과 위치가 확인되고 수혈 및 수술팀이 준비될 때까지 제거하지 않는다. 이러한 물체는 수술실에서 제거한다.

병원 전 처치 제공자는 현장에서나 이송 중에 더 이상 움직이지 않도록 박힌 물체를 손이나 기계적으로 고정할 수 있다. 때에 따라서

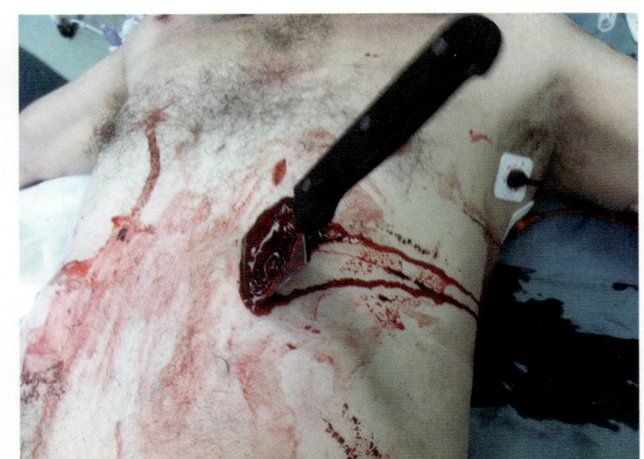

그림 11-11 병원 전 환경에서 복부에 찔린 물체를 제거하는 것은 금기이다.
Courtesy of Lance Stuke, MD, MPH.

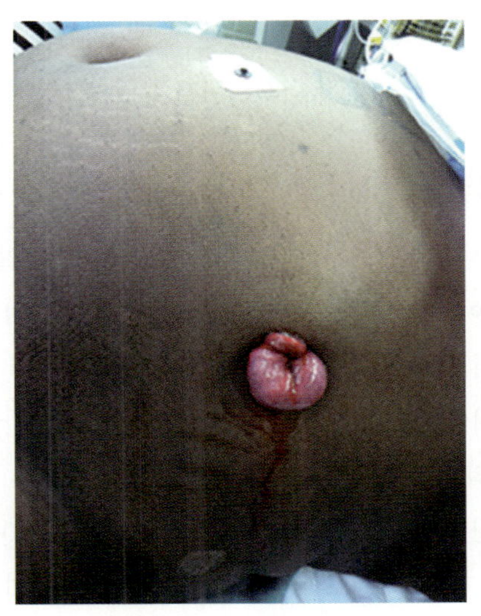

그림 11-12 복벽의 상처를 통해 장이 돌출된 경우
Courtesy of Lance Stuke, MD, MPH.

환자를 외상센터로 이송하기 위해 박힌 물체를 절단해야 할 수도 있다. 박힌 물체 주변에서 출혈이 발생하면 손으로 물체 주변과 상처 부위에 직접 압박을 한다. 특히 환자가 박힌 물체를 볼 수 있는 경우 환자의 심리적 지지가 중요하다.

이러한 환자에게 복부를 촉진하거나 타진하는 것은 물체의 원위 끝에서 추가적인 장기 손상을 일으킬 수 있으므로 시행하지 않는다. 박힌 물체가 있으면 외과 의사의 처치가 필요하므로 추가 검사는 필요하지 않다.

내장탈출

복부 내장탈출은 장, 조직 또는 기타 복부 장기의 일부가 개방 상처를 통해 복강 밖으로 돌출된 것을 말한다(**그림 11-12**). 가장 자주 육안으로 보이는 조직은 장을 덮고 있는 지방질의 그물막이다. 튀어나온 조직을 복강으로 다시 밀어 넣으려는 시도를 해서는 안 된다. 내장은 복부 표면에 돌출된 상태 그대로 두어야 한다.

처치는 돌출된 장이나 다른 장기가 더 손상되지 않도록 보호하는 데 중점을 두어야 한다. 대부분의 복부 내용물은 습한 환경이 필요하다. 장이나 다른 복부 장기가 건조해지면 세포사가 발생한다. 따라서 튀어나온 복부 내용물은 생리식염수(보통 정맥용 생리 식염수)를 적신 깨끗한 드레싱이나 멸균 드레싱으로 덮어야 한다. 이러한 드레싱은 건조하지 않도록 주기적으로 생리식염수로 다시 적셔주어야 한다. 젖은 드레싱은 환자를 따뜻하게 유지하기 위해 크고 건조한 폐쇄드레싱으로 덮을 수 있다.

복부 장기 탈출 환자에게는 심리적 지원이 매우 중요하므로 환자를 침착하게 유지하도록 주의를 기울여야 한다. 울며 소리를 지르거나 기침을 하는 등 복부 내 압력을 증가시키는 모든 행동은 장기를 바깥쪽으로 더 많이 밀어낼 수 있다. 이러한 환자는 신속하게 외상센터로 이송한다.

산과 환자의 외상

임신 중 이상은 서 있다가 넘어지는 것과 같은 경미한 것부터 자동차 충돌로 인한 관통상이나 고속 무딘 손상 등 심각한 것까지 다양하다. 임신 중 외상은 지난 수십 년 동안 증가하여 현재 미국에서 비산과적 산모 사망의 주요 원인이 되었다. 자동차는 임신 중 외상으로 인한 손상의 절반과 태아 사망과 관련된 외상의 82%를 차지한다. 이러한 사고 대부분은 부적절한 안전띠 사용이 주요 원인이다. 골반 골절은 태아 사망으로 이어지는 가장 흔한 모체 손상이다. 골반 골절이 있는 여성을 대상으로 한 연구에서 태아 사망률은 35%에 달했다. 사망 원인으로는 태아의 직접적인 손상(20%), 태반조기박리(32%), 모체 쇼크(36%) 등이 있었다. 모체의 생리학적 변화의 일부인 혈관 확장은 골반 골절 후 출혈의 위험을 증가시키며 이러한 모체의 사망률은 9%에 달한다. 직접적인 무딘 외상으로 인한 손상에는 태반조기박리와 자궁 파열이 포함될 수 있다. 태반조기박리는 경미한 손상의 1~6%, 중증 손상의 최대 절반에서 합병증을 유발하는 것으로 알려져 있다. 자궁 파열은 임신한 외상 환자의 1% 미만에서 발생한다. 관통상 후 모체의 사망률은 임신한 자궁이 모체의 내부 장기를 보호는 역할을 하므로 더 유리하다. 그러나 관통상 후 태아 사망률은 최대 73%에 이른다. 임신 중에 발생하는 해부학적 및 생리학적 변화에 대한 적절한 지식은 환자의 손상을 가장 효과적으로 인식하는 데 필수적이다.

해부학적 및 생리학적 변화

임신은 신체 시스템에 해부학적 및 생리학적 변화를 일으킨다. 이러한 변화는 보이는 손상 유형에 영향을 미칠 수 있으며 손상을 입은 임신한 환자의 평가를 특히 어렵게 만들 수 있다. 병원 전 처치 제공자는 두 명 이상의 환자를 처치하고 있으며 임신 기간 동안 여성의 해부학 및 생리학에 발생한 변화를 알고 있어야 한다.

　사람의 임신은 일반적으로 수정에서 출산까지 약 40주 동안 지속하며 이 임신 기간은 3기로 나눈다. 임신 1기는 12주까지이고 2기는 임신 28주까지이다.

　수정부터 착상, 태아가 자라면서 자궁은 임신 38주까지 계속 커진다. 약 12주까지 성장하는 자궁은 골반에 의해 보호된다. 임신 20주가 되면 자궁의 기저부가 배꼽에 위치하고 38주가 되면 칼돌기에 가까워진다. 이러한 해부학적 변화로 인해 자궁과 그 내용물은 무딘 손상 및 관통상에 더 취약해진다(**그림 11-13**). 자궁 손상에는 파열, 관통, 태반조기박리(태반 일부가 자궁벽에서 떨어져 나오는 경우), 조기 양막파열 등이 있다(**그림 11-14**). 태반과 임신한 상태의 자궁은 혈관이 매우 많으므로 이러한 구조에 손상을 입으면 심각한 출혈이 발생할 수 있다. 출혈은 자궁이나 복강 내부에 숨겨져 있을 수 있으므로 외부에서 보이지 않을 수 있다.

　임신 후기에는 복부의 뚜렷한 돌출이 분명하지만, 자궁을 제외한

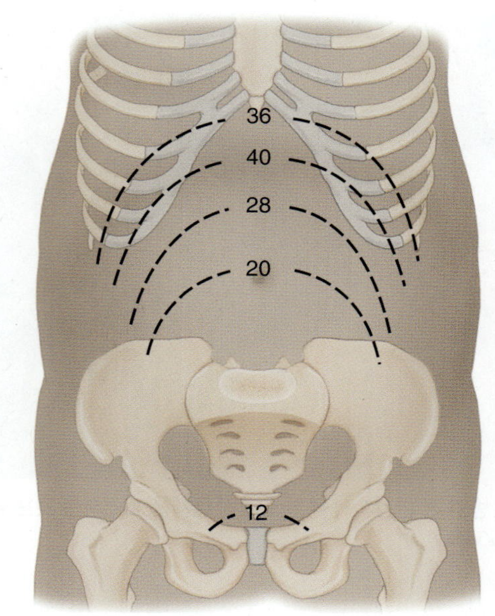

그림 11-13 자궁 바닥의 높이. 임신이 진행됨에 따라 자궁은 손상에 더 취약해진다.

© National Association of Emergency Medical Technicians (NAEMT)

나머지 복부 장기는 본질적으로 변하지 않는다. 자궁이 늘어나 결국 가장 큰 복강 내 장기가 된다. 이 얇은 벽 구조는 손상을 입기 쉽다. 임신 2기 후기와 3기 기간에는 자궁에 의해 장이 보호된다. 자궁의 크기와 무게가 증가하면 환자의 무게 중심이 바뀌고 낙상 위험이 증가하고 손상을 입을 수 있다. 임신하지 않은 무딘 외상 환자의 경우와 마찬가지로 비장이 가장 흔하게 손상되는 장기이다.

　이러한 해부학적 변화 외에도 임신 중에는 생리학적 변화가 발생

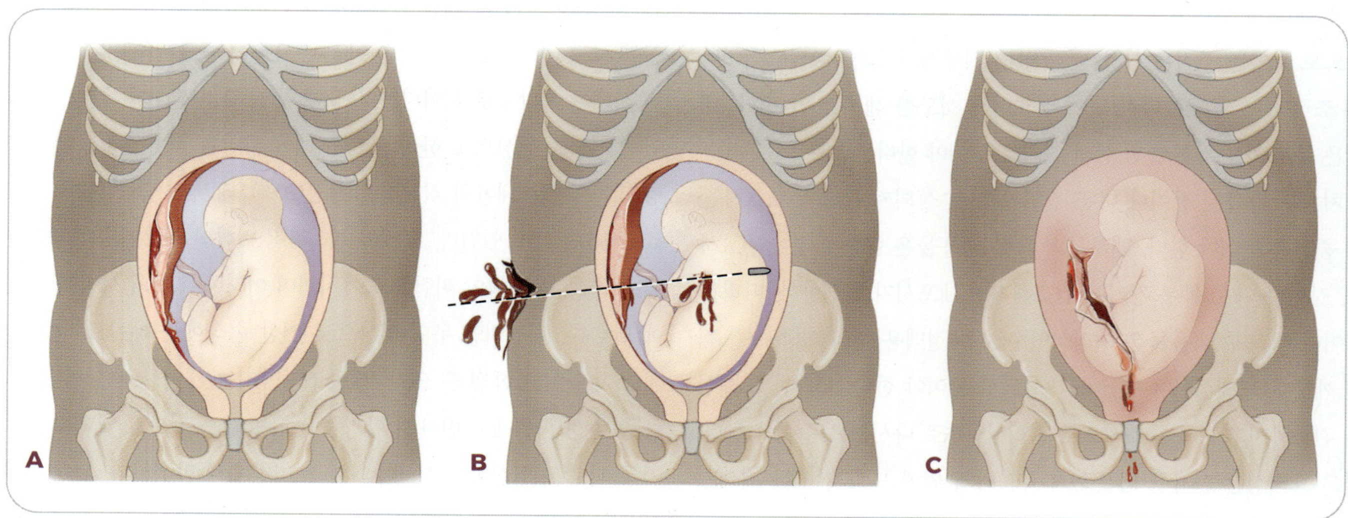

그림 11-14 자궁 외상의 그림. **A.** 태반조기박리. **B.** 자궁에 총상. **C.** 자궁 파열.

© National Association of Emergency Medical Technicians (NAEMT)

한다. 여성의 심박수는 일반적으로 임신 3기가 되면 정상보다 분당 15~20회 증가한다. 이로 인해 빈맥을 구분하기가 더 어려워진다. 수축기 혈압과 이완기 혈압은 일반적으로 임신 2기에는 5~15mmHg 떨어지지만, 만삭이 되면 정상으로 돌아오는 경우가 많다. 임신 10주가 되면 여성의 심박출량은 1~1.5L/분까지 증가한다. 임신 말기에는 여성의 혈액량이 약 50% 증가한다. 혈류량은 임신하지 않았을 때 60mL/분에서 만삭이 되면 600mL/분으로 증가한다. 이러한 심박출량과 혈액량의 증가로 인해 건강한 임신부는 혈량저하증의 징후와 증상이 나타나기 전에 1,200mL~1,500mL의 혈액을 잃을 수 있다. 저혈량 쇼크는 임신 3기 환자에게 조기산통을 유발할 수 있다. 순환 혈액량 손실에 반응하여 항이뇨호르몬과 함께 분비되는 옥시토신은 자궁 수축을 자극한다.

임신 중에는 혈장 부피가 적혈구 질량보다 훨씬 더 많이 증가하기 때문에 희석성 빈혈이 발생한다. 간은 과다대사 상태가 되어 응고 인자와 섬유소원 생성을 증가시킨다. 환자는 심부정맥혈전증(DVT)과 파종혈관내응고(DIC)가 발생할 가능성이 더 높다.

임신 3기에는 가로막이 2~4cm 상승하며 특히 환자가 바로누운자세일 때 경미한 호흡곤란이 나타날 수 있다. 바로누운자세에서 호흡곤란을 유발하는 경우 환자의 머리 부분을 30도 정도 올려주는 자세가 도움이 될 수 있다. 가슴관은 간이나 비장의 잠재적인 손상을 피하기 위해 2cm 더 높게 삽입해야 한다. 임신 중에는 장의 연동운동이 느려지므로 식사 후 몇 시간 동안 음식물이 위에 남아있을 수 있다. 따라서 임신한 환자는 특히 삽관 시 구토와 흡인에 대한 위험이 크다.

임신 중독증(자간증이라고도 함)은 임신 후기의 합병증이다. 자간전증은 부종과 고혈압이 특징인 반면, 자간증은 의식 상태 변화와 발작을 특징으로 하여 외상성 뇌손상과 유사하다. 임신과 관련된 잠재적 합병증과 당뇨병, 고혈압, 발작 병력 등 기타 의학적 상태에 대해 세심하게 신경학적 평가하고 질문을 하는 것이 중요하다.

평가

임신은 일반적으로 임신부의 기도를 변화시키지 않지만, 임신 3기의 환자를 긴척추고정판에 바로누운자세로 있으면 심각한 호흡곤란이 발생할 수 있다. 위장관의 연동운동이 감소하면 구토 및 흡인의 가능성이 높아진다. 호흡음 청진 및 맥박산소측정 모니터링을 포함하여 기도개방 여부 및 폐 기능을 평가한다.

다른 원인으로 인한 복액복막과 마찬가지로 자궁 손상과 관련된 복강 내 출혈은 몇 시간 동안 복막염을 일으키지 않을 수 있다. 손상으로 인한 출혈은 임신부의 심박출량과 혈액량 증가로 인해 가려질 수 있다. 따라서 미묘한 변화(예: 피부색, 의식 상태)에 대한 높은 의심 지수와 평가가 중요한 단서를 제공할 수 있다.

일반적으로 태아의 상태는 임신부의 상태에 따라 달라지지만, 임신부의 상태와 활력징후가 혈류역학적으로 정상으로 보이는데도 태아가 위험할 수 있다. 이는 신체가 자궁(태아)에서 중요한 장기로 혈액을 보내기 때문에 발생한다. 병원 전 환경에서는 정확한 원인을 파악할 수 없더라도 신경학적 변화를 평가하고 기록한다.

임신하지 않은 환자와 마찬가지로 장음 청진은 일반적으로 병원 전 환경에서 도움이 되지 않는다. 마찬가지로 현장에서 태아의 심음을 확인하기 위해 귀중한 시간을 소비하는 것이 유용하지 않으며 심음의 유무에 따라 병원 전 처치가 달라지지도 않는다. 외부 생식기에 질 출혈의 증거가 있는지 확인하고 환자에게 자궁 수축과 태아의 움직임에 대해 질문해야 한다. 자궁수축은 조기 진통이 시작되었음을 나타낼 수 있으며 태동 감소는 심각한 태아 곤란의 불길한 징후일 수 있다.

복부를 촉진하면 압통이 나타날 수 있다. 단단하고 딱딱하면서 부드러우면 태반조기박리를 시사하며 이는 약 70%의 사례에서 눈에 보이는 질 출혈과 관련이 있다.

처치

손상을 입은 임신한 환자의 경우 임신부의 상태에 집중해야 태아의 생존을 가장 잘 보장할 수 있다. 본질적으로 태아가 생존하려면 일반적으로 임신부가 생존해야 한다. 적절한 기도를 확보하고 호흡 기능을 보조하는 것이 우선시되어야 한다. 산소포화도를 95% 이상을 유지할 수 있도록 충분한 산소를 투여한다. 특히 임신 후기에는 환기가 필요할 수 있다. 구토를 예상하고 필요한 경우 흡인을 시행한다.

쇼크 처치의 목표는 기본적으로 모든 환자와 같으며 특히 보상되지 않은 쇼크의 증거가 있는 경우 신중하게 정맥 내로 수액을 투여한다. 임신 3기에 질 출혈이 있거나 판자같이 단단한 경우 태반조기박리 또는 자궁 파열을 나타낼 수 있다. 이러한 상태는 태아의 생명뿐만 아니라 임신부의 생명도 위협할 수 있는데 이는 과다출혈이 빠르게 발생할 수 있기 때문이다. 손상을 입은 임신한 환자에게 가장 적합한 목표 혈압을 정의하기 위한 좋은 데이터는 존재하지 않는다. 그러나 수축기 혈압과 평균 혈압을 정상적으로 회복시키면 임신부의 추가적인 내부출혈이 발생할 위험이 있더라도 태아의 관류가 개선될 가능성이 있다.

일부 여성은 바로누워자세로 있을 때 심각한 저혈압을 보일 수 있다. 임신 중 바로누운자세에서 저혈압은 일반적으로 임신 3기에 발생하며 커진 자궁이 아래대정맥을 압박하기 때문에 발생한다. 이로 인해 심장으로의 정맥혈복귀가 급격히 감소하고 혈액이 덜 채워지기 때문에 심박출량과 혈압이 떨어진다(**그림 11-15**).

바로누운자세에서 저혈압을 완화하기 위해 다음과 같은 방법을 사용할 수 있다(**그림 11-16**).

1. 임신부를 왼쪽으로 눕히거나(옆누운자세), 척추 움직임 제한이 필요한 경우 긴척추고정판 오른쪽 아래에 10~15cm 정도의 패딩을 대어준다.
2. 환자를 회전시킬 수 없다면 오른쪽 다리를 들어 올려 자궁을 왼쪽으로 이동시켜야 한다.
3. 손으로 자궁을 환자의 왼쪽으로 이동시켜 준다.

이 3가지 방법으로 대정맥의 압박을 줄여 심장으로의 정맥혈복귀를 증가시키고 심박출량을 개선한다.

임신한 외상 환자의 이송이 지연되어서는 안 된다. 모든 임신한 외상 환자는 경미한 손상만 입은 것으로 보이더라도 가장 가까운 적절한 의료기관으로 신속하게 이송한다. 이상적인 의료기관은 외과와 산부인과 처치가 즉시 가능한 외상센터이다. 임신부를 적절히 소생시키는 것이 임신부와 태아의 생존을 위한 열쇠이다.

비뇨생식기 손상

신장, 요관, 방광에 손상을 입으면 혈뇨가 나타나는 경우가 가장 흔하다. 이 징후는 일반적으로 환자에게 도뇨관을 삽입하지 않는 한 쉽게 확인할 수 없다. 신장은 심박출량의 상당 부분을 받기 때문에 이러한 장기에 무딘 손상이나 관통상을 입으면 환자의 생명을 위협하는 복막뒤출혈이 발생할 수 있다.

골반 골절은 방광과 질 또는 직장 벽의 열상과 관련될 수 있다. 깊은 서혜부나 회음부 열상을 동반한 개방 골반 골절은 심각한 외부출혈을 초래할 수 있으며 질이나 직장의 열상은 생명을 위협하는 합병증을 초래할 수 있다.

외부 생식기의 외상은 다양한 손상 기전으로 인해 발생할 수 있지만, 오토바이나 자동차 충돌시 튕겨 나오거나 산업 재해, 걸터앉은 유형의 손상 기전, 총상, 성폭력으로 인한 손상이 가장 흔하다. 이러한 장기에는 수많은 신경 말단이 있으므로 이러한 손상은 심각한 통증과 심리적 문제를 동반한다. 이 장기에는 수많은 혈관이 있으며 다량의 출혈이 발생할 수 있다. 일반적으로 이러한 유형의 출혈은 직접압박이나 압박 드레싱으로 조절할 수 있다. 특히 임신부의 출혈을 조절하기 위해 질 내부나 요도에 드레싱을 삽입해서는 안 된다. 출혈을 조절하기 위해 직접 압박이 필요하지 않으면 이러한 상처는 생리식염수를 적신 멸균 거즈로 덮어준다. 절단된 부위는 12장 근골격 외상에 설명된 대로 처치한다. 모든 생식기 손상에 대한 추가 평가는 병원에서 이루어져야 한다.

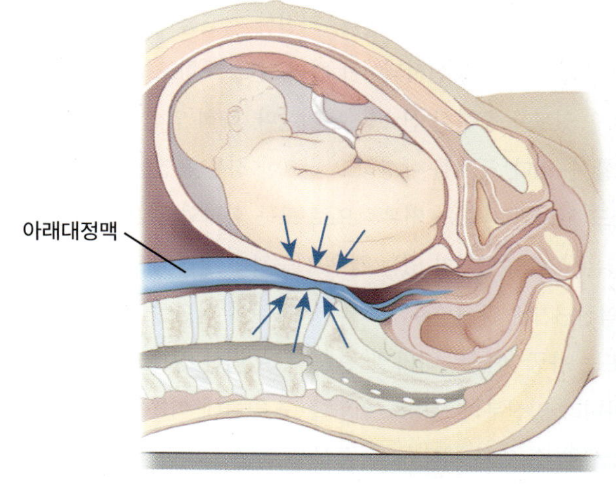

그림 11-15 만삭 자궁이 대정맥을 압박하는 경우

© National Association of Emergency Medical Technicians (NAEMT)

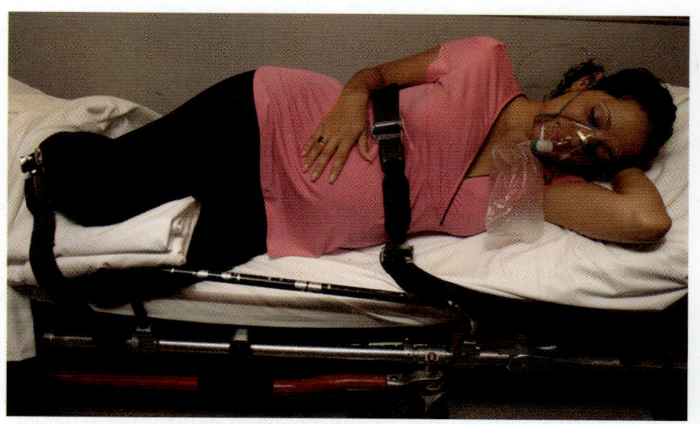

그림 11-16 임신부를 왼쪽으로 눕히면 자궁이 아래대정맥에서 떨어져 심장으로의 혈액 순환을 개선하여 혈압을 회복하는 데 도움이 된다.

© Jones & Bartlett Learning. Courtesy of MIEMSS.

요 약

- 복강 내 손상은 내부출혈과 복강 내로 위장관 내용물이 유출되어 생명을 위협하는 경우가 많다.
- 병원 전 현장에서 내부 장기 손상 정도를 확인할 수 없으므로 복부 또는 골반 외상의 징후와 함께 손상 기전을 파악하여 병원 전 처치 제공자의 의심 지수를 높여야 한다.
- 복부 외상 환자의 처치에는 산소 공급, 출혈 조절, 신속한 이송 준비 등이 포함된다. 몸통 손상을 입은 무딘 외상 환자에게는 척추 고정을 시행해야 한다. 혈류역학적으로 불안정한 경우 골반을 골반고정대로 고정해야 한다.
- 균형 잡힌 소생술은 중요한 장기에 관류를 제공하면서 잠재적으로 내부출혈을 악화시킬 위험을 최소화할 수 있다. 혈액 제제를 사용한 병원 전 소생술은 30일 사망률을 낮춘다는 연구 결과가 있지만, 이 프로그램은 자원 집약적이며 아직 널리 이용되지 않는다.
- 응급 외과적 개입이 생명을 구할 수 있으므로 복부 외상 환자는 즉시 수술이 가능한 외상센터로 이송한다.
- 임신의 해부학적 및 생리학적 변화는 외상의 징후 및 증상의 발현, 임신한 외상 환자의 처치에 영향을 미친다.
- 외상으로 인한 태아의 잠재적인 손상 관리는 임신부의 효과적인 소생술을 통해 이루어진다.

시나리오 재구성

당신은 3시간 전에 넘어진 후 현재 복통이 점점 심해졌다는 20대 중반의 남성 환자가 있는 건설 현장으로 출동했다. 환자는 현장에서 나무 조각에 걸려 넘어지면서 쌓여 있던 각목에 왼쪽 가슴과 복부를 부딪쳤다고 말한다. 환자는 심호흡할 때 왼쪽 가슴우리 아래쪽에 중간 정도의 통증을 느끼며 가벼운 호흡곤란을 호소한다. 환자의 동료는 그가 나무에 걸려 넘어졌을 때 바로 도움을 요청하려고 하였지만, 그는 증상이 그리 심하지 않다고 말하여 기다리라고 말했다고 한다. 하지만 이후 그는 불편감이 점점 심해지고 있으며 지금은 어지럽고 힘이 빠지는 느낌이 든다고 말한다.

당신은 환자가 눈에 띄게 불편한 상태로 바닥에 앉아 있는 것을 발견한다. 환자는 왼쪽 가슴 아랫부분과 윗배를 움켜쥐고 있다. 환자는 기도가 개방되어 있고 호흡수는 28회/분, 맥박수는 124회/분, 혈압은 94/58mmHg이다. 환자의 피부는 창백하고 발한이 있다. 당신은 환자를 눕히고 신체검사를 한 결과 명백한 뼈 비빔소리 없이 왼쪽 아래 갈비뼈의 통증을 호소하였다. 복부는 팽창되지 않았고 촉진 시 부드럽지만, 왼쪽 윗배 부위에서 압통과 자발적인 근육 경직을 보였다. 외부출혈과 피부밑기종은 없다.

- 환자에게 발생할 수 있는 손상은 무엇인가?
- 이 환자를 처치할 때 우선순위는 무엇인가?
- 복막염의 징후가 있는가?

시나리오 해결책

환자의 왼쪽 아래 갈비뼈와 왼쪽 위쪽 사분면에 압통이 있다. 이러한 소련은 가슴, 복강 내 장기 또는 두 장기의 손상을 나타낼 수 있다. 활력징후는 보상성 저혈량 쇼크와 일치하며 혈흉 또는 복강 내 출혈을 고려해야 한다. 아래쪽 갈비뼈의 압통은 비장 열상을 동반한 갈비뼈 골절로 복강 내 출혈이 발생했을 가능성이 높다.

산소를 투여하고 환자를 이송할 준비를 한다. 외상센터로 이송하는 중에 정먁 라인을 확보하고 수액을 투여하지만, 환자의 혈압을 고려할 때 적극적인 수액 투여는 혈압을 지나치게 높여 출혈을 증가시킬 수 있으므로 혈압이 80mmHg 미만으로 떨어지지 않는 한 수액 투여는 피해야 한다.

References

1. American College of Surgeons (ACS) Committee on Trauma. Abdominal trauma. In: *Advanced Trauma Life Support for Doctors, Student Course Manual*. 8th ed. ACS; 2008:111-126.

2. Banerjee A, Duane TM, Wilson SP, et al. Trauma center variation in splenic artery embolization and spleen salvage: a multicenter analysis. *J Trauma Acute Care Surg*. 2013;75(1):69-75.

3. Hemmila MR, Wahl WL. Management of the Injured Patient. In: Doherty GM, ed. *Current Surgical Diagnosis and Treatment*. McGraw-Hill Medical; 2008:227-228.

4. Aldemir M, Tacyildiz I, Girgin S. Predicting factors for mortality in the penetrating abdominal trauma. *Acta Chir Belg*. 2004;104:429-434.

5. American College of Surgeons (ACS) Committee on Trauma. Abdominal and pelvic trauma. In: *Advanced Trauma Life Support, Student Course Manual*. 10th ed. ACS; 2018:82-101.

6. Boese CK, Hackl M, Müller LP, et al. Nonoperative management of blunt hepatic trauma: a systematic review. *J Trauma Acute Care Surg*. 2015;79(4):654-660.

7. Centers for Disease Control and Prevention. Explosions and Blast Injuries: A Primer for Clinicians. Accessed February 28, 2022. https://www.cdc.gov/masstrauma/preparedness/primer.pdf

8. Ritenour AE, Blackbourne LH, Kelly JF, et al. Incidence of primary blast injury in US military overseas contingency operations: a retrospective study. *Ann Surg*. 2010;251(6):1140-1144.

9. U.S. Department of Defense, Blast Injury Research Coordinating Office. What Is Blast Injury. Last updated June 18, 2019. Accessed February 28, 2022. https://blastinjuryresearch.amedd.army.mil/index.cfm/blast_injury_101#:~:text=Tertiary%20blast%20injuries,Traumatic%20amputations

10. Champion HR, Holcomb JB, Young LA. Injuries from explosions: physics, biophysics, pathology, and required research focus. *J Trauma Acute Care Surg*. 2009 May 1;66(5):1468-1477.

11. Owers C, Morgan JL, Garner JP. Abdominal trauma in primary blast injury. *J British Surg*. 2011;98(2):168-179.

12. Velmahos GC, Tatevossian R, Demetriades D. The "seat belt mark" sign: a call for increased vigilance among physicians treating victims of motor vehicle accidents. *Am Surg*. 1999;65(2):181-185.

13. Rozycki GS, Ochsner MG, Schmidt JA, et al. A prospective study of surgeon-performed ultrasound as the primary adjuvant modality for injured patient assessment. *J Trauma Inj Infect Crit Care*. 1995;39(3):492-500.

14. Rozycki GS, Ochsner MG, Feliciano DV, et al. Early detection of hemoperitoneum by ultrasound examination of the right upper quadrant: a multicenter study. *J Trauma Inj Infect Crit Care*. 1998;45(5):878-883.

15. Rozycki GS, Ballard RB, Feliciano DV, et al. Surgeon-performed ultrasound for the assessment of truncal injuries: lessons learned from 1540 patients. *Ann Surg*. 1998;228(4):557-567.

16. Polk JD, Fallon WF Jr. The use of focused assessment with sonography for trauma (FAST) by a prehospital air medical team in the trauma arrest patient. *Prehosp Emerg Care*. 2000;4(1):82-84.

17. Bloom BA, Gibbons RC. Focused assessment with sonography for trauma. 2021 Jul 31. In: *StatPearls*. StatPearls Publishing; Published July 31, 2021. Accessed February 28, 2022. https://pubmed.ncbi.nlm.nih.gov/29261902/

18. Melanson SW, McCarthy J, Stromski CJ, et al. Aeromedical trauma sonography by flight crews with a miniature ultrasound unit. *Prehosp Emerg Care*. 2001;5(4):399-402.

19. Walcher F, Kortum S, Kirschning T, et al. Optimized management of polytraumatized patients by prehospital ultrasound. *Unfall-Chirurg*. 2002;105(11):986-994.

20. Strode CA, Rubal BJ, Gerhardt RT, et al. Wireless and satellite transmission of prehospital focused abdominal sonography for trauma. *Prehosp Emerg Care*. 2003;7(3):375-379.

21. Heegaard WG, Ho J, Hildebrandt DA. The prehospital ultrasound study: results of the first six months (abstract). *Prehosp Emerg Care*. 2009;13(1):139.

22. Partyka C, Coggins A, Bliss J, et al. A multicenter evaluation of the accuracy of prehospital eFAST by a physician-staffed helicopter emergency medical service. *Emerg Radiol*. 2021 Nov 24:1-8.

23. Partyka CL, Coggins A, Bliss J, et al. An evaluation of the accuracy of prehospital eFAST in the assessment of polytrauma by a physician-staffed helicopter emergency medical service. *medRxiv*. Jan 1, 2020. doi: 10.1101/2020.12.02.20242453

24. Press GM, Miller SK, Hassan IA, et al. Prospective evaluation of prehospital trauma ultrasound during aeromedical transport. *J Emerg Med*. 2014 Dec 1;47(6):638-645.

25. Yates JG, Baylous D. Aeromedical ultrasound: the evaluation of point-of-care ultrasound during helicopter transport. *Air Med J*. 2017 May 1;36(3):110-115.

26. Heegard WG, Hildebrandt D, Spear D, et al. Prehospital ultrasound by paramedics: results of field trial. *Acad Em Med*. 2010;17(6):624-630.

27. Jorgensen H, Jensen CH, Dirks J. Does prehospital ultrasound improve treatment of the trauma patient? A systematic review. *Eur J Emerg Med*. 2010;17(5):249-253.

28. Rooney KP, Lahham S, Lahham S, et al. Pre-hospital assessment with ultrasound in emergencies: implementation in the field. *World J Emerg Med*. 2016;7(2):117-123.

29. Sadek S, Lockey DJ, Lendrum RA, Perkins Z, Price J, Davies GE. Resuscitative endovascular balloon occlusion of the aorta (REBOA) in the pre-hospital setting: an additional resuscitation option for uncontrolled catastrophic haemorrhage. *Resuscitation*. 2016;107:135-138.

30. Shackelford S, Hammesfahr R, Morisette D. The use of pelvic binders in tactical combat casualty care. *J Spec Oper Med*. 2016 Nov 7:135-147.

31. Sondeen JL, Coppes VG, Holcomb JB. Blood pressure at which rebleeding occurs after resuscitation in swine with aortic injury. *J Trauma Acute Care Surg*. 2003;54(5):S110-S117.

32. Guyette FX, Sperry JL, Peitzman AB, et al. Prehospital blood product and crystalloid resuscitation in the severely injured patient: a secondary analysis of the Prehospital Air Medical Plasma Trial. *Ann Surg*. 2021;273(2):358-364. doi: 10.1097/SLA.0000000000003324

33. Pusateri AE, Moore EE, Moore HB, et al. Association of prehospital plasma transfusion with survival in trauma patients with hemorrhagic shock when transport times are longer than 20 minutes: a post hoc analysis of the PAMPer and COMBAT clinical trials. *JAMA Surg*. 2020;155(2):e195085. doi: 10.1001/jamasurg.2019.5085

34. Sperry JL, Guyette FX, Brown JB, et al; PAMPer Study Group. Prehospital plasma during air medical transport in trauma patients at risk for hemorrhagic shock. *N Engl J Med*. 2018 Jul 26;379(4):315-326. doi: 10.1056/NEJMoa1802345

35. Riesberg JC, Gurney JM, Morgan M, et al. The management of abdominal evisceration in tactical combat casualty care:

TCCC guideline change 20-02. *J Spec Oper Med*. 2021 Jan 1;21(4):138-142.

36. Krywko DM, Toy FK, Mahan ME, Kiel J. Pregnancy trauma. In: *StatPearls*. StatPearls Publishing. Updated Jul 2, 2021. Accessed 10/12/2021. https://www.ncbi.nlm.nih.gov/books/NBK430926/

37. Leggon RE, Wood GC, Indeck MC. Pelvic fractures in pregnancy: factors influencing maternal and fetal outcomes. *J Trauma*. 2002;53(4):796-804.

38. Mason SM, Schnitzer PG, Danilack VA, Elston B, Savitz DA. Risk factors for maltreatment-related infant hospitalizations in New York City, 1995–2004. *Ann Epidemiol*. 2018;28(9):590-596.

39. American College of Surgeons (ACS) Committee on Trauma. Chapter 12, Trauma in pregnancy and intimate partner violence. In: *Advanced Trauma Life Support, Student Course Manual*. 10th ed. ACS; 2018:229.

Suggested Reading

Beldowicz GC, Leshikar D, Cocanour CS. Trauma in pregnancy. In: Moore EE, Feliciano DV, Mattox KL, eds. *Trauma*. 9th ed. McGraw-Hill; 2020:709.

Berry MJ, McMurray RG, Katz VL. Pulmonary and ventilatory responses to pregnancy, immersion and exercise. *J Appl Physiol*. 1989:66(2):857.

Jones LA. Abdominal trauma. In: Stone C, Humphries RL, eds. *Current Diagnosis and Treatment Emergency Medicine*. 8th ed. McGraw-Hill; 2017.

Kim FJ, Donalisio da Silva R. Genitourinary tract. In: Moore EE, Feliciano DV, Mattox KL, eds. *Trauma*. 9th ed. McGraw-Hill; 2020:659.

Raja AS, Zabbo CP. Trauma in pregnancy. *Emerg Med Clin North Am*. 2012;30:937-948.

근골격 외상

Lead Editors
Gerard Slobogean, MD
Christopher Renninger, MD

학습 목표 이 장의 학습을 완료하면 다음과 같은 내용을 수행할 수 있다.

- 팔다리 손상 환자를 분류하고 데 사용되는 세 가지 범주를 나열하고 이 분류를 처치의 우선순위와 연관시켜 설명할 수 있다.
- 팔다리 외상과 관련한 일차평가 및 이차평가에 관해 설명할 수 있다.
- 긴뼈와 골반의 개방골절 및 폐쇄골절에서 출혈의 중요성에 관해 설명할 수 있다.
- 병원 전 환경에서 처치가 필요할 수 있는 팔다리 손상과 관련된 5가지 주요 병태생리학적 문제를 나열할 수 있다.
- 단일 외상 및 다기관 외상이 동반된 팔다리 외상 처치에 관해 설명할 수 있다.
- 팔다리 손상과 관련된 시나리오를 줬을 때 적절한 부목을 선택하여 고정할 수 있다.
- 넓적다리뼈 골절 처치와 관련된 특별히 고려할 사항을 설명할 수 있다.
- 절단 처치에 관해 설명할 수 있다.

시나리오

6월 어느 화창한 토요일 오후 당신은 오토바이 경기장에서 경기 중 사고가 발생했다는 신고를 받고 현장으로 출동하였다. 현장에 도착하자마자 당신은 경기장 안전 관리자의 안내를 받아 관중석 바로 앞 트랙의 한 구역으로 이동하여 경기 의료지원팀(2인 1조의 응급의료반응자)이 트랙에 바로누워 있는 한 명의 환자를 처치하고 있는 곳으로 이동한다.

응급의료반응자(EMR) 중 한 명이 환자는 350cc급 오토바이 14대가 경주를 하던 중 3대가 관중석 앞에서 충돌했다고 말한다. 다른 두 명의 운전자는 손상을 입지 않았지만, 이 환자는 오른쪽 다리와 골반에 심한 통증이 있어 일어서거나 움직일 수 없었다. 의식을 잃은 상태는 아니었고 다리 통증 외에 다른 호소증상은 없었다. 의료지원팀은 바로누운자서에서 환자의 오른쪽 다리를 도수로 고정하고 있었다.

환자를 평가한 결과 19세 남성으로 의식이 명료하고 과거 병력이나 외상 병력이 없는 것을 확인했다. 환자의 초기 활력징후는 혈압 104/68mmHg, 맥박 112회/분, 호흡 24회/분, 피부는 창백하고 발한 증상을 보였다.

환자는 코너를 돌아 앞으로 나오는 순간 다른 운전자와 충돌했으며 충돌로 인해 균형을 잃고 트랙을 가로질러 미끄러졌다고 말했다.

(다음 페이지에 계속)

시나리오 (이어서)

환자는 오른쪽 다리가 최소 한 대 이상의 오토바이에 치였다고 말했다. 환자의 오른쪽 다리를 시진한 결과 왼쪽과 비교하였을 때 짧아지고 개방 상처가 없으며 넓적다리 앞쪽 중간 부위에 압통과 타박상이 있었다.

- 이 사고로 인한 손상 기전을 통해 이 환자의 잠재적 손상에 대해 무엇을 알 수 있는가?
- 어떤 유형의 손상이 의심되며 처치의 우선순위는 무엇인가?

개요

근골격 손상은 외상 환자에게서 흔히 발생하지만, 즉각적으로 생명을 위협하는 경우는 드물다. 그러나 골격 외상은 팔다리나 골반 내 외부출혈 또는 내부출혈이 대량으로 발생하면 생명을 위협할 수 있다.

중증외상 환자를 처치할 때 병원 전 처치 제공자는 팔다리 손상과 관련하여 세 가지 주요 사항을 고려해야 한다.

1. 우선순위를 평가하고 유지한다. 심각해 보이지만 생명을 위협하지 않는 근골격 손상에 주의가 산만해지지 않도록 한다(**그림 12-1**).
2. 잠재적으로 생명을 위협할 수 있는 근골격 손상을 인식한다.
3. 손상의 기전과 근골격 손상을 유발한 힘 그리고 그 에너지 전달로 인한 다른 생명을 위협하는 손상의 가능성을 인식한다.

일차평가 중에 생명을 위협하거나 잠재적으로 생명을 위협할 수 있는 손상이 발견되면 이차평가를 시행해서는 안 된다. 일차평가 중에 발견된 모든 문제는 이차평가를 시작하기 전에 수정해야 한다(이후 논의 참조). 이것은 환자를 병원으로 이송할 때까지 이차평가를 연기하거나 때에 따라 응급실(ED)에 도착할 때까지 기다리는 것을 의미할 수 있다.

중증외상 환자는 환자의 이동을 쉽게 할 수 있도록 긴척추고정판이나 기타 동등한 장비에 고정하여 이송 중에 중증 손상 및 경증 손상 처치를 시행할 수 있다. 이러한 방비를 사용하면 적절한 경우 손상 부위별 부목을 적용하지 않고 전신을 고정하고 이송하면서 손상 부위를 처치할 수 있다. 척추 움직임 제한에 대한 자세한 내용은 9장 척추 외상에서 설명되어 있다. 병원 전 제공자는 이송 시간 지연의 위험과 명백한 변형이나 마찰음 없이 근골격계 통증이 있는 팔다리에 부목을 적용하는 것의 이점을 고려한다. 일반적으로 팔다리의 변형은 곧게 펴거나 일반적으로 재정렬한 다음 고정하고 이송해야 한다. 병원 전 처치 제공자는 외상 당시보다 더 많은 힘이나 손상을 입힐 가능성이 없으며 팔다리를 심하게 변형된 자세로 장시간 방치하는 것은 상당한 단점이 있다.

해부학과 생리학

인체의 전체적인 해부학과 생리학을 이해하는 것은 병원 전 처치 제공자의 지식 기반에서 중요한 부분이다. 이 교재에서는 해부학과 근골격계의 모든 해부학과 생리학을 다루지는 않지만, 기본적인 내용을 다루고 있다.

성인의 인체는 약 206개의 뼈로 이루어져 있다(**그림 12-2**). 골격은 몸통뼈대와 팔다리뼈대로 나뉜다. 몸통뼈대는 두개골, 척추, 복장뼈, 갈비뼈를 포함한 신체의 중앙 부분의 뼈로 구성된다. 팔다리뼈대는 팔과 다리의 뼈, 팔이음뼈, 골반(엉치뼈 제외)으로 구성된다.

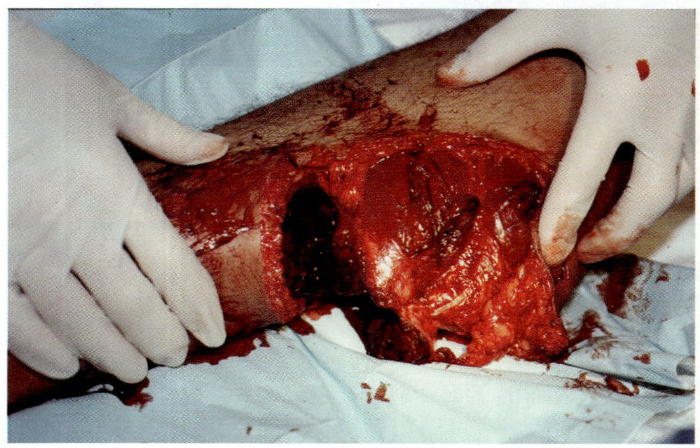

그림 12-1 일부 팔다리 손상을 겉으로 보기에는 심각해 보이지만, 즉시 생명을 위협하지는 않는다.

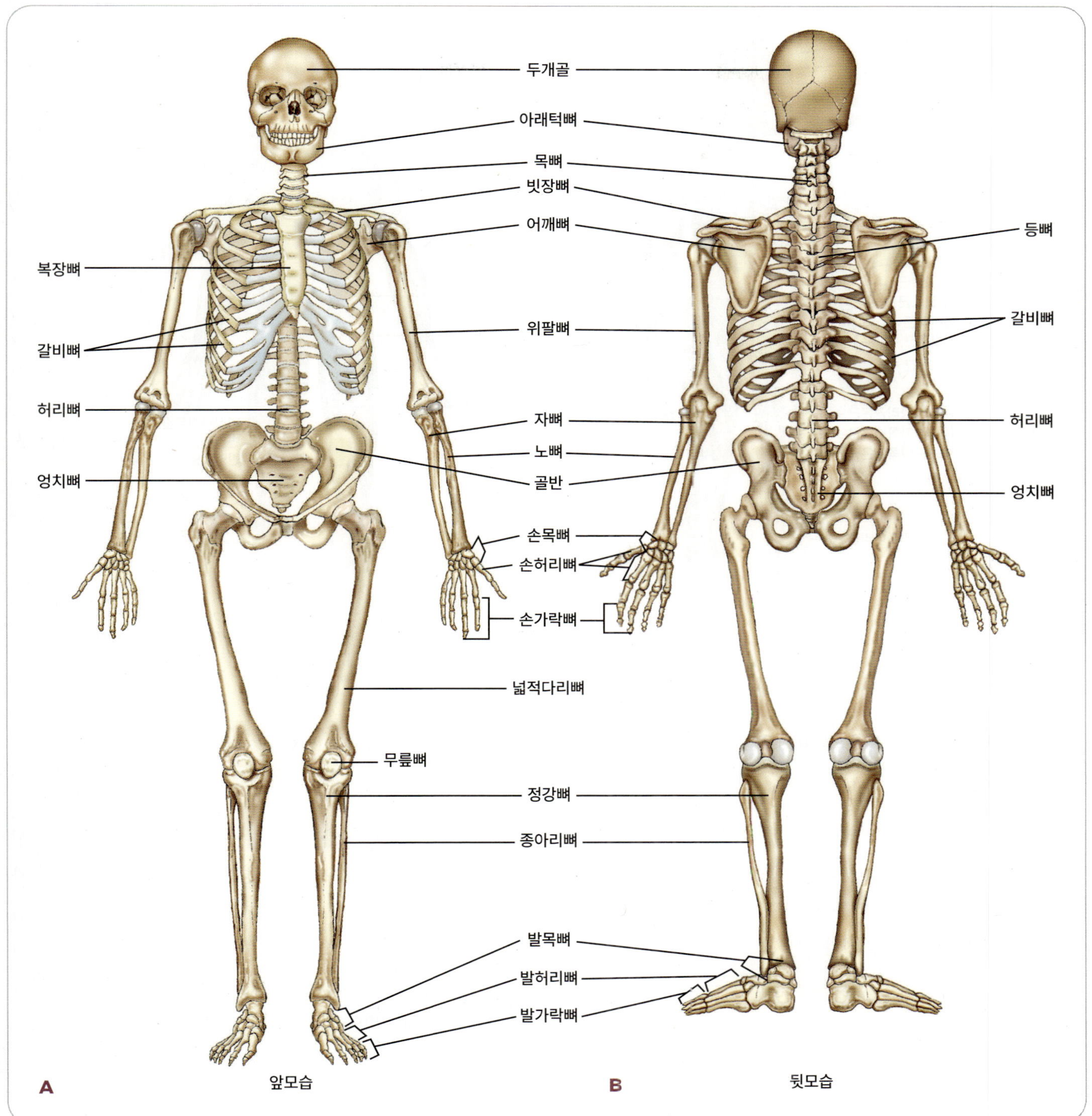

그림 12-2 인체 골격. **A.** 앞모습 **B.** 뒷모습.
© National Association of Emergency Medical Technicians (NAEMT)

인체에는 약 650개의 개별 근육이 있으며 이것은 근육의 기능에 따라 분류된다. 이 장에서 다루는 근육은 맘대로근육 또는 골격근이다. 이 근육은 골격계를 움직이기 때문에 골격근으로 분류된다.

이 범주에 속하는 근육은 신체의 구조를 자발적으로 움직인다(**그림 12-3**).

이 장에서 설명하는 다른 중요한 구조는 힘줄과 인대이다. 힘줄은

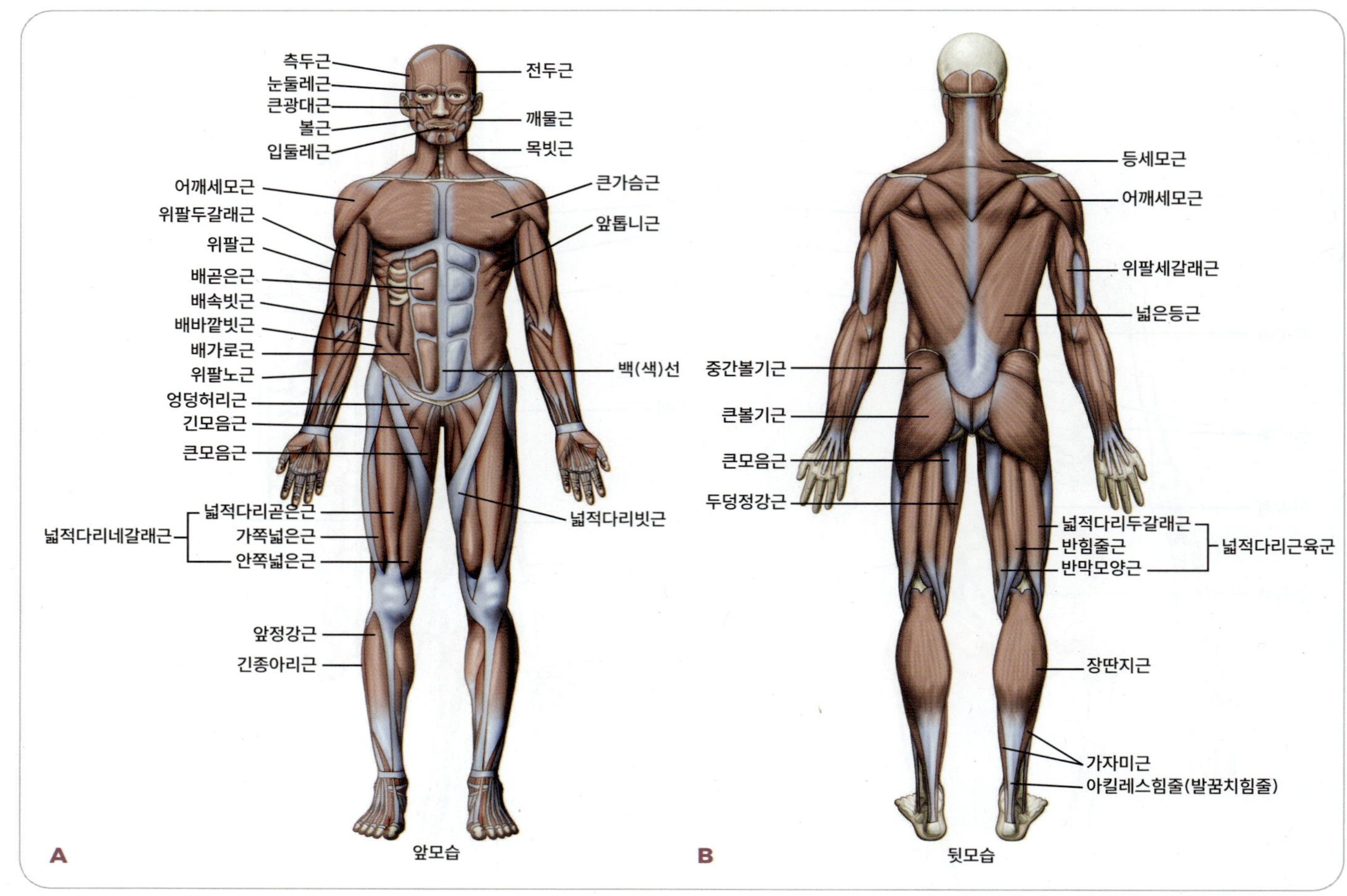

그림 12-3 인체의 주요 근육. **A.** 앞모습 **B.** 뒷모습.
© National Association of Emergency Medical Technicians (NAEMT)

뼈에 근육을 연결하는 질기고 비탄력적인 섬유질 조직으로 이루어진 띠이다. 힘줄은 근육 끝에 있는 흰색 부분으로 근육을 움직을 뼈에 직접 부착한다. 인대는 뼈와 뼈를 연결하는 질기고 섬유질 조직으로 관절을 서로 고정하는 역할을 한다.

평가

근골격 외상은 다음 세 가지 주요 유형으로 분류할 수 있다.

1. 골반 또는 팔다리의 외부출혈 또는 내부출혈과 같이 생명을 위협하는 근골격 손상

2. 다 계통의 생명을 위협하는 외상(생명을 위협하는 손상과 팔다리 골절)과 관련된 생명을 위협하지 않는 근골격 외상

3. 생명을 위협하지 않는 단일 근골격 외상(단일 팔다리 골절)

일차평가의 목적은 생명을 위협하는 손상을 파악하고 처치하는 것이다. 생명을 위협하지 않는 근골격 손상의 존재는 손상과 관련된 힘을 나타내는 지표가 될 수 있으며 병원 전 처치 제공자에게 다기관 외상의 가능성을 평가할 수 있도록 한다. 생명을 위협하지 않지만, 심각해 보이는 근골격 손상으로 인해 주의가 산만해지지 않도록 주의해야 한다. 이러한 손상으로 인해 병원 전 처치 제공자가 일차평가를 수행하는 데 방해를 받아서는 안 된다.

손상 기전

손상 기전을 이해하는 것은 외상 환자의 평가 및 처치에서 중요한 기능 중 하나이다. 손상 기전과 관련된 에너지(예: 서 있는 상태에서 넘어지는 것과 오토바이에서 고속으로 튕겨 나가는 것)를 신속하게 파악하면 병원 전 처치 제공자가 가장 심각한 손상이나 상태를 의심하고 인식하는 데 도움이 된다. 손상 기전을 결정하는 가장 좋은 방법은 환자에게서 직접 듣는 것이다. 환자가 반응이 없으면 목격자로부

터 손상에 대한 자세한 정보를 얻을 수 있다. 이러한 방법을 사용할 수 없는 경우 현장에서 관찰한 내용과 신체검사에서 발견된 손상 유형과 관련된 정보는 환자를 이송할 의료기관에 보고하고 환자처치보고서(PCR)에 기록해야 한다.

손상 기전에 따라 병원 전 처치 제공자는 환자가 입었을 수 있는 손상에 대해 높은 의심 지수를 가질 수 있다. 다양한 손상 유형에 대한 이러한 고려와 지식은 환자를 평가해야 하는 추가 손상을 떠올리게 할 수 있다. 다음과 같은 예를 고려한다.

- 환자가 창밖으로 다리부터 뛰어내리면 가장 먼저 의심되는 손상은 다리, 골반, 척추의 골절이다. 고려해야 할 이차 손상은 전단 손상 기전으로 인한 복부 손상이다.
- 오토바이를 타고 가다가 전봇대와 충돌하여 환자의 머리가 전봇대에 부딪히면 일차 손상에는 머리, 목뼈, 가슴 손상이 포함된다. 이차 손상에는 오토바이의 핸들에 넓적다리를 부딪쳐 넓적다리뼈 골절이 발생할 수 있다.
- 자동차 측면 충돌 시 탑승자의 경우 근골격 외상에는 팔 및 다리 골절과 골반 손상을 고려해야 한다. 고려해야 할 관련 손상 유형에는 머리 손상, 갈비뼈 또는 폐 손상과 복부 손상이 포함된다.

일차평가 및 이차평가

일차평가

환자 평가의 첫 번째 단계는 현장 안전을 확보하고 상황을 평가하는 것이다. 현장이 최대한 안전해지면 환자를 평가할 수 있다. 일차평가는 기도, 호흡, 순환 등 생명 유지에 필요한 요소를 기반으로 이루어진다.

변형된 골절이나 부분 절단은 시각적인 영향 때문에 병원 전 처치 제공자의 시선을 끌 수 있지만, 생명을 위협하는 상태를 먼저 고려해야 한다. 여전히 일차평가에서 가장 중요한 부분은 대량 출혈, 기도, 호흡, 순환, 장애 및 노출/환경(XABCDE)이다. 일차평가에서 생명을 위협하는 상태가 확인된 환자의 경우 이러한 문제가 해결될 때까지 근골격 외상 처치를 연기해야 한다. 대량 외부출혈은 근골격 원인으로 인한 경우가 많으므로 일차평가에서 일반적으로 직접 압박을 가한 후 즉시 근위부에 지혈대를 적용하는 방법으로 먼저 지혈해야 한다. 환자가 생명을 위협하는 손상을 입으면 병원 전 처치 제공자는 다음으로 기도, 호흡 및 순환을 평가하고 처치한다. 환자에게 생명을 위협하는 손상이 없는 경우 병원 전 처치 제공자는 이차평가를 진행할 수 있다.

이차평가

일차평가 중에 발생하는 팔다리의 대량 외부출혈을 평가하고 지혈하는 것을 제외하고 팔다리에 대한 평가는 이차평가 중에 시행한다. 신체검사를 쉽게 하려고 병원 전 처치 제공자는 주변 환경이 허용하는 한 일차평가에서 제거하지 않았던 옷을 제거하는 것을 고려한다. 손상 기전이 분명하지 않으면 골반과 손발을 포함한 팔과 다리를 모두 안전하게 노출하기 위해 모든 노력을 기울여야 한다. 또한, 환자나 목격자에게 손상이 어떻게 발생했는지 질문할 수 있다. 환자에게 팔다리에 통증이 있는지에 대해서도 질문해야 한다. 척수손상이 없는 한 심각한 근골격 손상을 입은 대부분 환자는 통증을 호소한다.

팔다리 평가에는 팔다리 통증, 쇠약 또는 비정상적인 감각을 평가하는 것이 포함된다. 특히 다음과 같은 사항에 주의를 기울인다.

- 뼈와 관절의 손상: 이 평가는 골절이나 탈구를 나타낼 수 있는 변형이 있는지 검사하고(**표 12-1**) 팔다리의 압통이나 비빔소리가 있는지 확인하기 위해 팔다리를 촉진한다. 이러한 신체적 소견이 없다고 해서 골절이나 기타 근골격 손상의 가능성을 배제할 수는 없다. 비빔소리는 골절된 뼈끝이 서로 마찰할 때 뼈가 갈리는 느낌을 말한다. 비빔소리는 손상 부위를 촉진하거나 팔다리를 움직여서 확인할 수 있다. 비빔소리는 '딱, 탁탁거리고 펑' 또는 포장에 사용

표 12-1 일반적인 관절 탈구와 변형		
관절	방향	변형
어깨곤절	앞	외전(벌림) 및 외회전
	뒤	내부 회전으로 고정
팔꿈치관절	뒤	뒤쪽으로 튀어나온 팔꿈치머리
엉덩관절	앞	신전, 외전, 외회전
	뒤	굴곡, 내전, 내회전
무릎관절	앞뒤	정상적인 윤곽 소실, 확장*
발목관절	외부에서는 가쪽이 가장 일반적임	외회전, 두드러진 내측 복사
목말밑관절	외부에서는 가쪽이 가장 일반적임	측면으로 전위된 발꿈치뼈

*평가 전에 자연적으로 감소할 수 있다.

Reproduced from American College of Surgeons Committee on Trauma. *Advanced Trauma Life Support*. 10th ed. Author; 2018:155.

하는 '뽁뽁이'가 터지는 소리와 비슷하다. 환자를 평가하는 동안 골절된 뼈가 서로 부딪히는 느낌은 추가 손상을 유발할 수 있으므로 일단 비빔소리가 발견되면 비빔소리를 유발할 수 있는 반복적인 조치를 시행해서는 안 된다. 비빔소리는 쉽게 잊히지 않는 뚜렷한 느낌이므로 일단 확인되면 즉시 고정한다.

- 연부조직 손상: 병원 전 처치 제공자는 부종, 열상, 찰과상, 혈종, 피부색 그리고 상처를 시진으로 검사한다. 겉으로 보이는 골절에 가까운 상처는 개방골절일 가능성을 고려한다. 일반적인 소견에서 나타나는 통증을 동반한 연부조직의 단단함과 긴장은 구획증후군의 존재를 나타낼 수 있다. 구획증후군은 팔다리를 위협하는 손상이므로 환자를 이송할 의료기관의 의료진에게 보고해야 한다(구획증후군의 처치는 이 장의 뒷부분에서 설명한다).

- 관류: 관류는 가장 원위부에서 만져지는 맥박(팔의 노동맥 또는 자동맥, 다리의 발등동맥 또는 뒤정강동맥)을 확인하고 손가락이나 발가락의 모세혈관 재충전 시간을 확인하여 평가한다. 팔다리에 원위부 맥박이 촉지되지 않으면 동맥 파열, 혈종이나 뼛조각에 의한 혈관 압박 또는 구획증후군을 나타낼 수 있다. 혈종이 크거나 커지면 큰 혈관에 손상이 있음을 나타낼 수 있다.

- 신경학적 기능: 병원 전 처치 제공자는 신경학적 평가에서는 팔다리의 운동 및 감각기능을 모두 평가해야 한다. 병원 전 환경의 대부분 상황에서는 전체 신경학적 기능을 평가하는 것으로 충분하다. **표 12-2**는 가장 흔한 손상 부위와 함께 가장 큰 신경운동 및 감각 분포를 보여준다. 신경 기능 장애가 있을 것으로 예상되는 부위에 손상이 없으면 병원 전 처치 제공자는 더 많은 질문을 하고 추가 검사의 필요성을 고려한다.

- 운동기능: 운동기능은 먼저 환자에게 조금이라도 쇠약감이 있는지를 물어봄으로써 평가할 수 있다. 팔의 운동기능은 환자가 주먹을 쥐었다 폈다 하는 것과 악력(환자가 병원 전 처치 제공자의 손가락을 꼭 쥐는 것)으로 평가하고 다리의 운동기능은 환자가 발가락을 움직이고 발로 검사자의 손을 밀고 당기게 하여 평가한다. 환자가 병원에 도착한 후 볼기 근육을 쥐어짜는 능력이 있다고 해서 전체 신경학적 검사 중 직장 검사의 필요성이 없어지는 것은 아니다.

- 감각기능: 감각기능은 감각의 결손이나 변화가 있는지 질문하여 평가할 수 있다. 감각기능은 각 팔다리의 가장 원위부에서 검사해야 한다. **표 12-2**와 **표 12-3**은 팔다리의 운동 및 감각 기능에 대한 보다 자세한 평가를 수행하는 데 필요한 정보를 제공한다.

부목 고정 후 팔다리의 관류 및 신경학적 기능에 대한 평가를 반복적으로 시행해야 한다.

관련 손상

이차평가를 수행하는 동안 손상 기전에 기반한 단서는 일반적으로 관련된 특정 손상 유형을 발견하는 데 도움이 될 수 있다. 이러한 손상 유형을 통해 병원 전 처치 제공자는 특정 골절과 관련된 잠재적인 손상을 평가할 수 있다. **표 12-4**는 관련 손상의 몇 가지 예이다.

특정 근골격 손상

팔다리 손상은 병원 전 환경에서 처치가 필요한 두 가지 주요 문제인 출혈과 맥박 소실을 초래한다.

출혈

출혈은 대량이거나 소량일 수 있다. 상처의 모양과 관계없이 손실된 혈액량과 손실 속도에 따라 환자가 혈액량 손실을 보상할 수 있는지

표 12-2 팔의 말초 신경 평가

신경	운동	감각	예상되는 손상 부위
자신경	집게손가락 벌림	새끼손가락	
정중 먼쪽 신경	엄지두덩 수축 및 대립	집게손가락 말단	손목 어긋남
정중 신경, 앞 뼈속신경	집게손가락 끝 굽힘	없음	위팔뼈 관절융기 골절(소아)
근육피부신경	팔꿈치 굽힘	노쪽 아래팔	어깨 앞쪽 탈구
노신경	엄지손가락, 손허리손가락 폄	첫 번째 갈퀴막공간	원위 위팔뼈, 앞쪽 어깨 탈구
겨드랑신경	삼각근	가쪽 어깨	어깨 앞쪽 탈구, 근위 위팔뼈 골절

Reproduced from American College of Surgeons Committee on Trauma. *Advanced Trauma Life Support*. 10th ed. Author; 2018:161.

표 12-3 다리의 말초 신경 평가

신경	운동	감각	손상
넓적다리신경	무릎 폄	앞무릎	두덩뼈 가지 골절
폐쇄신경	엉덩이 모음	넓적다리 안쪽	폐쇄 고리 골절
뒤정강신경	발가락 굽힘	발바닥	무릎 탈구
얕은 종아리신경	발목 뒤집힘(외번)	발등의 가쪽	종아리뼈 목 골절, 무릎 탈구
깊은 종아리신경	발목/발가락 등쪽굽힘	등쪽 첫 번째에서 두 번째 갈퀴막 공간	종아리뼈 목 골절, 구획증후군
궁둥신경	발목 등쪽굽힘 또는 바닥쪽굽힘	발	엉덩관절 후방 탈구
위볼기신경	엉덩관절 벌림	엉덩이 위	절구 골절
아래볼기신경	큰볼기근 엉덩관절 폄	엉덩이 아래	절구 골절

Reproduced from American College of Surgeons Committee on Trauma. *Advanced Trauma Life Support*. 10th ed. Author; 2018:161.

아니면 쇼크에 빠질지가 결정된다. 기억해야 할 좋은 규칙은 "경미한 출혈은 없으며 모든 적혈구가 중요하다."라는 것이다. 경미한 출혈이라도 충분히 오랫동안 방치하면 상당한 출혈로 이어질 수 있다.

외부출혈

외부 동맥 출혈은 생명을 위협할 수 있으므로 일차평가 중에 반드시 확인해야 한다. 일반적으로 이러한 유형의 출혈은 쉽게 알아볼 수 있지만, 환자 아래에 피가 숨겨져 있거나 두껍거나 어두운 옷을 입으면 평가가 어려울 수 있다. 명백한 출혈은 즉각적인 처치가 필요하며 환자의 기도와 호흡을 처치하는 동안 또는 그 전에 평가하고 지혈한다.

외부출혈량을 추정하기는 매우 어려울 수 있다. 경험이 부족한 사람은 외부출혈량을 과대평가하는 경향이 있지만, 외부출혈의 명백한 징후가 항상 명백한 것은 아니기 때문에 과소평가도 할 수 있다. 한 연구에 따르면 병원 전 현장에서 출혈량의 추정은 부정확하며 임상적으로 도움이 되지 않는다고 한다. 출혈량 추정이 부정확한 이유는 환자가 손상을 입은 현장에서 이동했거나, 손실된 혈액이 옷이나 흙에 흡수되었거나 물이나 비에 씻겨 내려갔을 수 있다는 점 등 여러 가지가 있다. 추정 출혈량의 정확성과 관계없이 외부출혈에 대한 병원 전 처치는 여전히 생명을 구하는 중요한 개입이다.

내부출혈

내부출혈은 근골격 외상에서 흔히 발생하며 종종 놓치는 경우가 많다. 내부출혈은 주요 혈관(대부분 신체의 긴뼈와 가까운 곳에 위치)

표 12-4 근골격 손상과 관련된 손상

근골격 손상	계류/관련 손상
빗장뼈 골절 어깨뼈 골절 어깨 골절/어깨 탈구	주요 가슴 손상, 특히 폐 타박상 및 갈비뼈 골절 어깨가슴 분리
팔꿈치 골절/탈구	위팔동맥 손상 정중신경, 자신경 및 노신경 손상
넓적다리뼈 골절	넓적다리 목 골절 무릎인대 손상 엉덩관절 후방 탈구
무릎후방 탈구	넓적다리 골절 엉덩관절 후방 탈구
무릎탈구 또는 정강뼈 정점 전위	오금동맥 및 신경 손상
발꿈치뼈 골절	척추 손상 또는 골절 목발뼈 및 발꿈치뼈 골절-탈구 정강뼈 정점 골절
개방골절	관련 비골격 손상의 높은 발생률

Reproduced from American College of Surgeons Committee on Trauma. *Advcnced Trauma Life Support*. 10th ed. Author; 2018:164.

손상, 근육 손상, 뼈 골절로 인해 발생할 수 있다. 팔다리가 지속해서 붓거나 차갑고 창백하며 맥박이 촉지되지 않는 팔다리는 주요 동맥이나 정맥의 내부출혈을 나타낼 수 있다. 심각한 내부출혈은 골절과 관련이 있을 수 있다. 개방골절은 상당한 양의 내부출혈과 외부출혈의 조합과 관련될 수 있지만, 특정 골절로 인한 출혈량에 대한 근거 데이터가 부족하다. 그런데도 넓적다리와 골반은 생명을 위협할 정도로 충분한 양의 출혈이 발생할 수 있다.

환자를 평가할 때는 팔다리 외상과 관련된 잠재적인 내부출혈과 외부출혈을 모두 고려해야 한다. 이를 통해 병원 전 처치 제공자는 쇼크 발생 가능성을 예측하고 전신 상태 악화 가능성에 대비하며 쇼크 발생을 최소화하기 위해 적절히 처치할 수 있다.

처치

외부출혈의 초기 처치는 상처 부위에 직접 압박을 가하는 것이다. 팔다리를 높인다고 해서 출혈이 느려지는 것은 아니며 근골격 외상에서는 이미 존재하는 손상을 악화시킬 수 있다(3장 쇼크: 삶과 죽음의 병태생리학에서 설명 참조). 직접 압박이나 압박 드레싱으로 외부출혈이 즉각적이고 완전히 조절되지 않으면 지혈대를 사용해야 한다(3장 쇼크: 삶과 죽음의 병태생리학에서 설명된 원칙을 따른다). 첫 번째 지혈대를 적용한 후에도 출혈이 조절되지 않으면 두 번째 지혈대를 첫 번째 지혈대 바로 위쪽에 적용한다. 서혜부나 겨드랑이와 같이 지혈대를 사용하기 어려운 출혈 부위에는 국소 지혈제 사용을 고려할 수 있다. 이러한 지혈제는 이송 시간이 오래 걸리는 상황에서도 사용을 고려할 수 있다.

지혈대 사용은 병원 전 출혈성 팔다리 손상 처치의 표준이다. 병원 전 지혈대 사용에 대한 자세한 내용은 3장, 쇼크: 삶과 죽음의 병태생리학을 참조한다.

팔다리 외상과 관련된 내부출혈은 대량일 수 있으며 일부 상황에서는 쇼크로 이어질 수 있다. 다른 모든 내부출혈과 마찬가지로 현장에서 팔다리 내부출혈을 지혈하기는 어렵고 효과도 미미할 수 있다. 골절을 고정하는 것이 도움이 될 수 있다. 불안정성이 있는 골반 골절의 경우 골반을 감싸는 골반고정대나 시트를 사용하면 골반 부피를 효과적으로 줄여 간접적으로 출혈을 줄일 수 있다.

생명을 위협하는 팔다리 출혈이 있는 환자의 출혈을 조절한 후 병원 전 처치 제공자는 일차평가를 재평가하고 기도, 호흡, 순환 및 소생술에 집중하여 환자의 상태를 가장 잘 치료할 수 있는 의료기관으로 신속하게 이송할 수 있다. 이송 중에 쇼크가 있는 환자에게 산소 투여 및 정맥 내 수액 소생술을 시작할 수 있다. 이대 내부출혈이 의심되는 경우 목표 수축기 혈압은 80~90mmHg (평균 혈압은 60~65mmHg)이고 외상성 뇌손상이 의심되는 환자의 경우 수축기 혈압을 110mmHg로 유지해야 한다는 점을 명심한다. 출혈이 경미하고 쇼크나 기타 생명을 위협하는 징후가 없는 환자의 경우 직접 압박으로 출혈을 조절할 수 있으며 이차평가를 시행한다.

맥박이 촉지되지 않는 팔다리

환자를 평가하는 동안 각 팔다리의 원위부 맥박을 확인하려고 할 때 고려할 한 가지 사항은 골절 부위 변형이 팔다리 관류 감소의 원인일 수 있다는 것이다. 일반적으로 일차평가(XABC)를 완료한 후 맥박이 없는 것으로 확인된 변형된 팔다리가 있는 경우 팔다리를 다치지 않은 팔다리의 일반적인 모양으로 재정렬을 시행한다. 그 후 맥박이 회복되었는지 재평가를 시행한다. 이 재정렬의 목적은 개방골절을 줄이거나 기능을 회복하거나 손상을 결정적으로 치료하는 것이 아니라는 점에 유의하는 것이 중요하다. 단순히 혈류를 위한 직접적인 경로를 제공하고 변형으로 인해 발생할 수 있는 혈관의 꼬임이나 압박을 제거하는 것이 목적이다.

맥박이 회복되거나 모세혈관 재충전이 적절한 경우 이 위치에서 팔다리를 부목으로 고정한다. 이와 관련 내용은 환자를 이송할 의료기관에 보고해야 한다.

구획증후군을 일으키는 것과 같은 손상 기전이 팔다리 근위부의 분리된 구획 내에서 출혈 및 관련 부기로 인한 원위부 폐쇄를 유발할 수도 있다. 맥박이 없는 팔다리를 평가할 때는 구획증후군에 대한 평가를 고려해야 한다. 구획증후군은 맥박이 없는 팔다리를 위협하는 손상이며 즉각적인 수술이 가능한 의료기관으로 이송하는 것이 중요하다.

골반 골절

심각한 골반 골절 또는 기타 골반 고리의 심각한 파열은 병원 전 처치 제공자에게 여러 가지 어려운 문제를 제시한다(**그림 12-4**). 첫 번째는 골반 골절로 인해 혈류역학적으로 불안정한 환자를 구별하는 것이다. 현장에서 손상 기전, 손상 중 신체에 가해진 에너지의 양 및 다리 변형 등을 고려하여 골반 손상을 평가하는 추가적인 방법이다. 잠재적으로 정확한 평가는 삶과 죽음의 차이를 의미할 수 있다. 정형외과에서 실제로 생명을 위협하는 손상은 거의 없지만, 골반 고리의 파열은 생명을 위협할 수 있다.

골반 골절에서 가장 심각한 즉각적인 문제는 처치가 매우 어려울

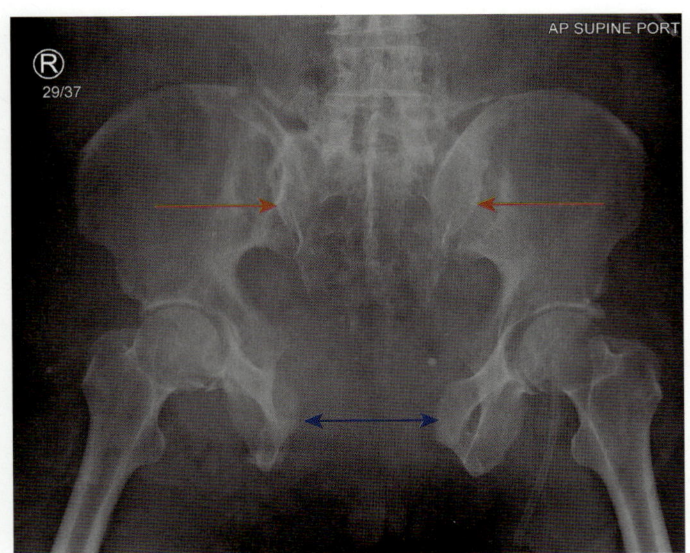

그림 12-4 심각한 골반 고리 파열. 파란색 화살표는 현저한 전방 결합 확대를 나타낸다. 빨간색 화살표는 후방에 양측 엉치엉덩뼈 손상을 보여준다.

Courtesy of Andrew Pollak, MD.

수 있는 내부출혈이다. 골반 골절은 경미하고 상대적으로 중요하지 않은 골절부터 대량의 내부출혈 및 외부출혈과 관련된 생명을 위협하는 손상까지 다양하다(**Box 12-1**). 골반 고리 골절은 9~20% 사이의 전체 사망률과 관련이 있다. 또한, 무딘 외상에 의한 골반 고리 골절이 있으면 사망의 독립적인 위험 요소이며 사망 확률이 두 배로 증가한다. 골반 골절이 있는 환자는 외상성 뇌손상, 긴뼈골절, 가슴 손상, 남성의 요도 파열, 비장 손상, 간 및 신장 손상을 동반하는 경우가 많다.

골반을 평가하기 위해 앞쪽에서 뒤쪽으로 그리고 옆에서 부드럽게 손으로 누르면 비빔소리와 불안정성을 확인할 수 있다. 두덩뼈 부위를 촉진하면 왼쪽과 오른쪽이 비대칭 골반을 확인할 수 있으며 이는 심각한 골반 고리 파열을 나타낸다. 신체검사로 골반 불안정성이 확인되면 출혈이나 응고를 악화시킬 수 있으므로 골반 안정성을 평가하기 위한 추가 검사는 금기이다.

골반의 개방골절은 직장이나 질에 열상을 입힐 수 있으며 외부출혈의 명백한 원인이 쉽게 드러나지 않을 수 있다. 골반 골절 유형을 구별하고 분류하거나 숨겨진 열상이 있어 개방골절인지 아닌지를 판단하는 것은 병원 전 처치 제공자의 역할이 아니다. 일차 목표는 생명을 위협하는 골반 골절을 구별하고 적절한 처치를 제공하는 것이다.

일부 골반 고리 골절은 골절 유형과 변위 정도에 따라 골반 부피

가 증가하여 생명을 위협할 수 있는 다량의 골반 내 출혈이 발생할 수 있습니다. 골반고정대를 적용하여 골반 내 부피를 제한하여 출혈을 감소시키기 위해서는 골반고정대가 제 역할을 할 수 있도록 적절하게 태치해야 한다. 골반고정대는 골반 내 부피를 제한하여 골반 골절과 관련된 출혈을 줄임으로써 혈류역학적으로 안정화를 위해 설계된 것이지 골반 골절을 안정화할 수 있도록 설계된 것은 아니다. 병원 전 환경에서 골반 고리 손상의 안전성과 불안정성을 확실하게 판별하기는 매우 어려운 것으로 입증되었다. 방사선 촬영 전에 골반고정대를 적용하면 병원과 중환자실 입원 기간이 줄어들고 초기 수혈 요구량이 감소할 수 있다는 증거는 제한적이다. 따라서 적절한 손상 기전이 있고 골반 고리 손상에 대한 임상적 우려(특히 혈류역학적 불안정성이 있는 경우)에서 합의된 권장 사항은 병원 전 환경에서 골반고정대를 적용하는 것이다.

골반고정대는 위골반문둘레가 아닌 넓적다리큰돌기에 위치해야 한다. 일반적으로 골반고정대가 너무 위쪽에 위치하면 복부를 압박할 수 있고 심한 경우 환기가 어려워질 수 있다. 적절한 위치를 확인

하면 체형과 관계없이 골반고정대에서 골반으로 압박을 전달할 수 있다. 적절한 배치를 통해 골반 부피가 감소하고 골반이 안정화되며 이상적으로는 지속적인 출혈을 감소시킬 수 있다.

넓적다리뼈 골절

넓적다리뼈 골절은 골반 손상과 마찬가지로 양쪽 넓적다리에 대량의 출혈이 동반되기 때문에 생명을 위협할 수 있다. 성인의 경우 넓적다리뼈 골절로 대량의 혈액을 잃으면 혈류역학적 불안정성과 쇼크가 발생할 수 있다. 생명을 위협하는 상태가 아니라면 넓적다리뼈 몸통 골절이 의심되는 경우 골절을 안정시키기 위해 견인부목을 적용해야 한다. 도수 또는 기계 장치를 사용하여 견인을 적용하면 내부출혈을 줄이고 환자의 통증을 줄이는 데 도움이 될 수 있다.

넓적다리뼈를 부목으로 고정하는 것은 넓적다리의 근육 구조로 인해 독특한 형태의 부목을 적용해야 하는 상황을 나타낸다. 넓적다리의 근육이 강하기 때문에 부목이나 견인으로 변형, 재정렬 및 고정이 어려운 경우가 많다.

견인부목 사용에 대한 금기 사항은 다음과 같다.
- 같은 쪽 발목 및 발의 박리 또는 절단
- 무릎 부위에 골절이 의심되는 경우(이 경우 견인부목을 단단한 부목으로 사용할 수 있지만, 견인을 적용해서는 안 된다.)

불안정성(골절 및 탈구)

관절을 지지하는 구조물의 파열, 골절, 주요 근육이나 힘줄 손상은 다친 팔다리의 불안정성을 유발한다.

골절

뼈가 부러지면 뼈를 고정하면 통증이 감소할 수 있다. 손상 당시 골절을 유발하기 위해 가해진 에너지는 병원 전 처치 제공자가 골절된 팔다리를 재정렬하고 부목이나 견인을 시행하고 고정하는 것보다 더 많은 손상을 유발한다.

일반적으로 골절은 폐쇄 또는 개방골절로 분류된다. 폐쇄골절은 골절된 뼈의 끝부분에 의해 피부가 손상되지 않지만, 개방골절은 피부의 연속성이 중단되어 뼈가 기능적 또는 잠재적으로 심하게 노출된다(**그림 12-5A**). 정형외과 의사는 골절 유형에 따라 골절을 분류할 수 있지만, 골절 유형에 대한 지식이 현장 처처에 영향을 미치지는 않지만, 관련 피부 무결성에 대한 지식은 영향을 줄 수 있다.

폐쇄골절

폐쇄골절은 뼈는 부러졌지만, 환자의 피부 손상이 없는 골절이다(예: 골절 부위의 피부가 손상되지 않은 경우, **그림 12-5B**). 폐쇄골절의 징후로는 통증, 압통, 변형, 혈종, 부종 및 비빔소리 등이 있다. 그러나 일부 환자에게서는 통증과 압통이 유일한 증상일 수 있다. 맥박, 피부색, 운동 및 감각기능은 골절이 의심되는 부위의 원위부에서 평가해야 한다. 환자가 자발적으로 팔다리를 움직일 수 있거나 다리의 경우 걸을 수 있다고 해서 항상 골절되지 않은 것은 아니며 외상성 사고로 인해 분비되는 아드레날린은 환자가 평상시에는 견딜 수 없는 통증을 견딜 수 있도록 동기를 부여할 수 있다. 또한 일부 환자는 통증에 대한 내성이 현저히 높다.

개방골절

개방골절은 일반적으로 날카로운 뼈끝이 안쪽에서 바깥쪽으로 피부를 관통하거나 드물게는 외상이나 물체가 골절 부위의 피부와 근육을 파열시킬 때 발생한다(바깥쪽에서 안쪽으로, **그림 12-5C**). 골절이 외부 환경에 노출되면 골절된 뼈의 끝이 피부 또는 환경으로부터 오염된 세균에 의해 오염된다. 이러한 오염은 골절의 치유를 방해할 수 있는 심각한 합병증인 골수염으로 이어질 수 있다. 개방골절과 관련된 피부 손상은 종종 심각한 출혈과 관련이 없지만, 지속적인 출혈은 골수 공간이나 조직 내부 깊숙이 있는 혈종의 감압으로부터 발생할 수 있다.

골절 가능성이 있는 부위 근처의 개방 상처는 개방골절로 간주하여 처치해야 한다. 일반적으로 튀어나온 뼈나 뼈끝을 의도적으로 원위치해서는 안 되지만, 부목을 적용하거나 고정하기 위해 골절된 팔다리를 다시 정렬하면 정상 위치로 돌아오는 때도 있다.

외상 환자에서 개방골절을 항상 쉽게 확인할 수 있는 것은 아니다. 상처에서 뼈가 튀어나온 것은 분명하지만, 골절이나 변형에 근접한 연부조직 손상은 골절된 뼈끝이 피부 표면을 뚫고 조직으로 다시 들어가서 발생했을 수 있다.

처치

골절 처치에서 가장 먼저 고려해야 할 사항은 출혈을 조절하고 쇼크를 처치하는 것이다. 직접 압박 및 압박 드레싱은 현장에서 발생하는 거의 모든 외부출혈을 조절할 수 있다. 개방 상처나 노출된 뼈끝 부분은 멸균 생리식염수나 물에 적신 멸균 드레싱으로 덮어야 한다. 통증 조절, 부목 적용, 골절 안정화, 변형된 팔다리의 재정렬을 통한 관

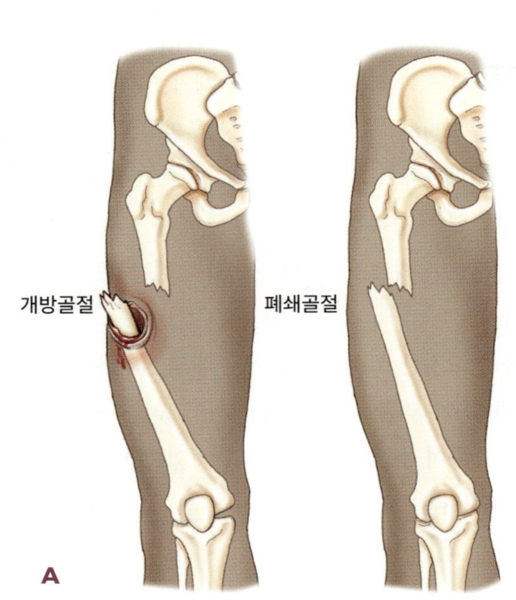

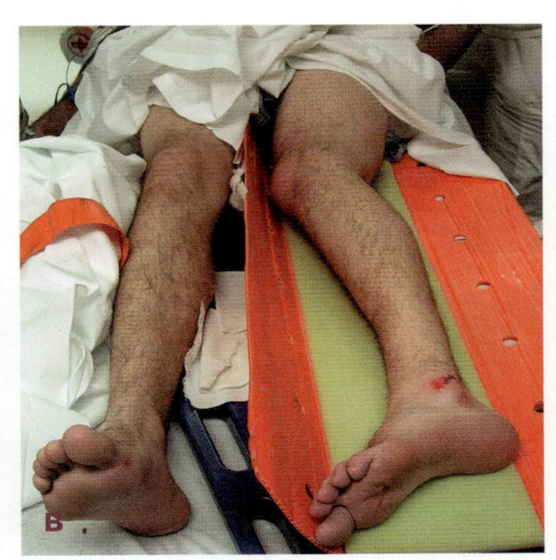

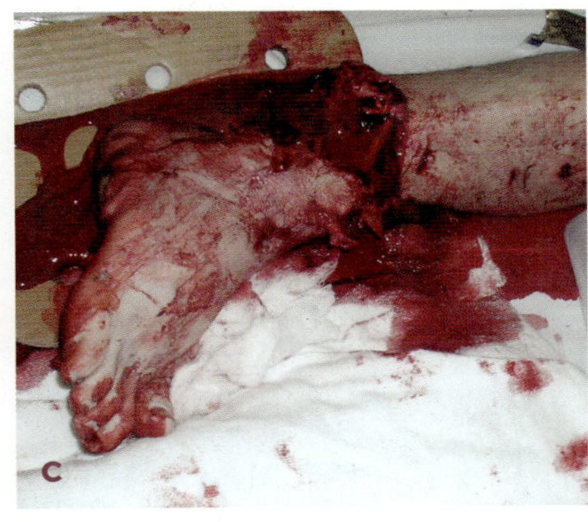

그림 12-5 **A.** 개방골절과 폐쇄골절 **B.** 넓적다리뼈의 폐쇄골절(참고: 왼쪽 다리의 안쪽돌림과 단축에 주목한다.) **C.** 정강뼈 개방골절.

A. © National Association of Emergency Medical Technicians (NAEMT); **B.** Courtesy of Norman McSwain, MD, FACS, NREMT-P; **C.** Courtesy of Peter T. Pons, MD, FACEP.

류 개선 등을 위해 부목 적용 시 변형된 팔다리를 재정렬하는 것을 고려한다. 개방골절의 뼈끝이 재정렬을 시행하거나 부목을 적용하는 동안 상처 안으로 들어가면 이 사실을 환자 처치보고서(PCR)에 기록하고 응급실 의료진에게 보고해야 한다. 최근 일부 문헌에서는 항생제 투여를 지지하며 일부 데이터에 따르면 항생제를 조기에 투여하면 감염률을 감소시킬 수 있다고 한다. 항생제 투여는 논란의 여지가 있다. 그러나 도시 또는 교외 환경에서 항생제를 현장에서 투여하면 감염률이 감소한다는 증거는 아직 없다.

부목을 적용하기 전에 일반적으로 손상을 입은 팔다리를 정상적인 해부학적 위치로 돌려놓아야 하며 필요한 경우 부드럽게 견인을 시행하여 팔다리를 가능한 한 정상 길이로 재정렬하는 등 합리적인 임상적 판단에 따라 최대한 노력해야 한다. 정상적인 해부학적 정렬로 돌아간 단축 골절은 부목을 대기가 더 쉽다. 둘째, 정렬을 회복하면 동맥이나 신경의 압박이 완화되고 관류 및 신경 기능이 개선될 수 있다. 또한 골절 부위를 해부학적 자세로 재정렬하면 출혈이 감소하고 통증 조절에도 도움이 된다.

개방골절이고 뼈가 노출된 경우 정상적인 해부학적 자세로 복원하기 전에 멸균증류수나 생리식염수로 뼈끝을 시간이 허락하는 한 부드럽게 헹구어 명백한 오염을 제거해야 한다. 개방골절은 수술실에서 세척과 이물질 제거가 필요하므로 이 조작 중에 뼈끝이 피부로 다시 들어가더라도 크게 걱정할 필요는 없다. 그러나 복원되기 전에 뼈가 노출되었었다는 사실은 환자를 이송하는 의료기관에 보고해야 하는 중요한 정보이다. 팔다리를 정상 위치로 복원하기 위해 두 번 이상 시도해서는 안 되며 복원을 실패한 경우 골절된 팔다리를 발견된 자세 그대로 부목으로 고정한다.

부목 고정의 주요 목적은 골절된 신체 부위의 움직임을 방지하는 것이다. 이렇게 하면 환자의 통증을 줄이고 골절된 부위를 안정시키는 데 도움이 된다. 팔다리의 긴뼈를 효과적으로 고정하려면 팔다리 전체를 고정해야 한다. 도수로 지지하면서 손상된 부위 위쪽의 관절과 뼈 아래쪽의 관절과 뼈를 모두 고정한다. 다양한 종류의 부목이 있으며 대부분의 부목은 개방 및 폐쇄골절 모두에 사용할 수 있다(**Box 12-2**). 부목을 적용한 후에는 팔다리의 추가 검사가 제한되므로 부목을 적용하기 전에 철저한 평가를 시행한다.

모든 유형의 부목을 적용할 때 다음과 같은 네 가지 추가 사항이 중요하다.

1. 필요한 경우 부목 안쪽에 패드를 대어 팔다리의 움직임을 방지하고 환자의 편안함을 제공하며 욕창을 예방할 수 있다.

Box 12-2 부목의 종류

다음과 같은 다양한 부목과 부목 재료를 사용할 수 있다(**그림 12-6**).

- 경성 부목(rigid splints)은 모양을 변화시킬 수 없다. 신체 부위를 부목의 모양에 맞게 적용해야 한다. 경성 부목의 예로는 판자 부목(나무, 플라스틱, 금속)과 긴척추고정판이 있다. 경성 부목은 긴뼈 손상에 가장 적합하다.
- 성형 부목(formable splints)은 손상된 팔다리의 모양에 맞게 다양한 모양으로 부목을 변형하여 사용할 수 있다. 성형 부목의 예로는 진공부목, 베개, 담요, 공기부목, 판지 부목, 철사형 사다리부목, 폼으로 덮인 성형 가능한 금속 부목이 있다. 성형 부목은 발목, 손목 및 긴뼈 손상에 가장 적합하다.
- 견인부목(traction splints)은 기계적 직렬식 견인력을 유지하여 골절을 재정렬하는 데 도움이 되도록 설계되어 있다. 견인부목은 넓적다리뼈 몸통 골절을 고정하기 위해 가장 많이 사용된다.

© National Association of Emergency Medical Technicians (NAEMT)

2. 장신구와 시계를 제거하여 추가 부종으로 인해 혈액 순환을 방해하지 않도록 한다. 비누, 로션 또는 수용성 젤과 같은 윤활제를 이용하면 꽉 끼는 반지를 쉽게 제거할 수 있다.

3. 부목을 고정하기 전과 후에 손상 부위의 원위부에서 신경혈관 기능을 평가하고 그 이후에도 주기적으로 평가한다. 맥박이 촉지되지 않는 팔다리는 혈관 손상 또는 구획증후군을 나타내므로 적절한 의료기관으로 신속하게 이송하는 것이 더욱 중요하다.

4. 부목을 고정한 후 가능하면 부종과 욱신거리는 것을 감소시키기 위해 팔다리를 들어 올리는 것을 고려한다. 얼음이나 냉찜질을 사용하여 통증과 부기를 줄일 수 있으며 골절이 의심되는 부위에 적용할 수도 있다.

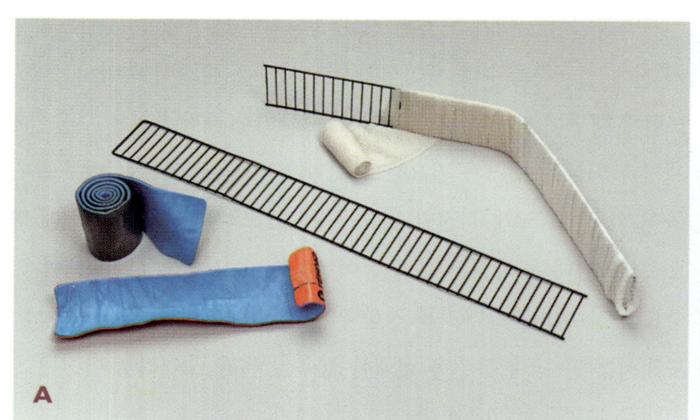

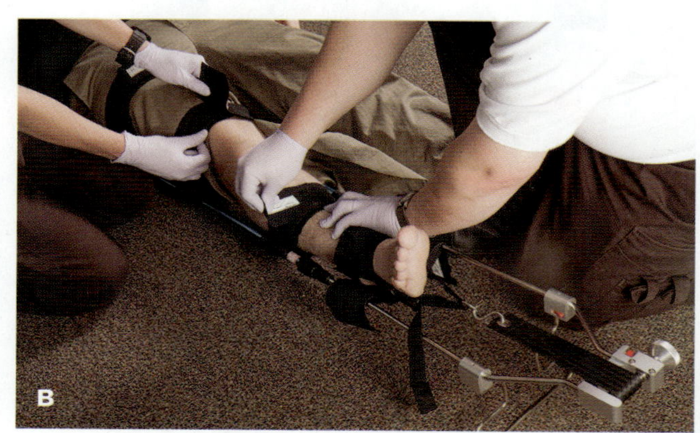

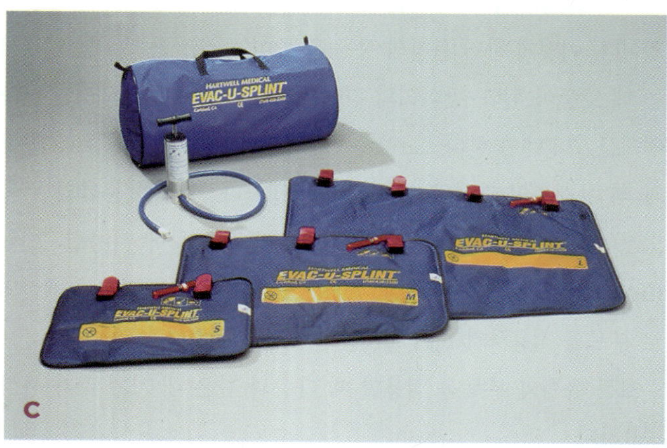

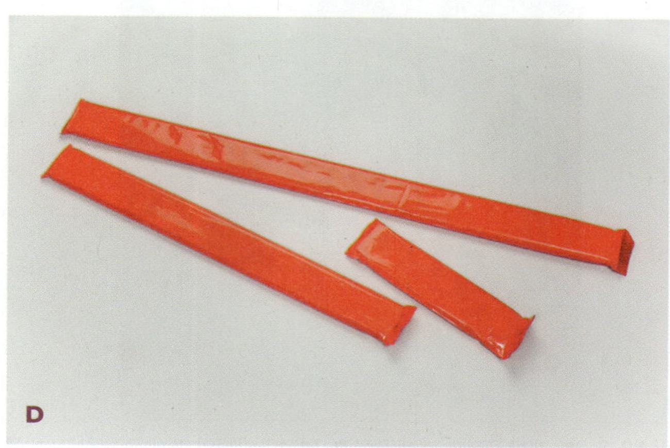

그림 12-6　**A.** 성형부목 **B.** 견인부목 **C.** 진공부목 **D.** 보드부목.

A & D. © National Association of Emergency Medical Technicians (NAEMT); B. © Jones & Bartlett Learning. Photographed by Darren Stahlman. C. Courtesy of Hartwell Medical.

탈구

관절은 인대에 의해 서로 연결되어 있다. 관절을 구성하는 뼈는 힘줄에 의해 근육에 부착되어 있다. 팔다리의 움직임은 근육의 수축(단축) 때문에 이루어진다. 근육 길이가 수축하면 뼈에 붙어있는 힘줄이 당겨져 관절에서 팔다리가 움직인다. 탈구는 일반적으로 관절에서 지지 구조와 안정성을 제공하는 인대의 심각한 손상으로 인해 관절에서 두 개의 뼈가 분리되는 것이다(**그림 12-7** 및 **그림 12-8**). 골절과 유사한 탈구는 병원 전 처치 제공자가 고정해야 하는 불안정한 부위를 만든다. 탈구는 심한 통증을 유발할 수 있다. 탈구는 X-ray 검사 없이는 임상적으로 골절과 구별하기 어려울 수 있으며 골절과도 관련이 있을 수 있다(골절-탈구). 관절의 변형은 탈구의 유형과 방향에 대한 단서를 제공한다.

병원 전 처치 제공자는 탈구를 적절하게 설명하기 위해서는 원위부를 기준으로 한다. 예를 들어, 무릎 탈구는 정강뼈가 넓적다리뼈와 관련하여 이동하는 방향을 기준으로 한다. 후방 무릎 탈구는 정강뼈가 넓적다리뼈보다 뒤쪽에 있다는 것을 의미한다.

이전에 탈구를 경험한 적이 있는 사람의 인대는 정상보다 느슨해져 있어 외과적 처치로 문제를 교정하지 않으면 더 자주 탈구가 발생할 수 있다. 탈구가 처음 발생한 환자와 달리 이러한 환자는 손상에 대해 잘 알고 있는 경우가 많으므로 평가와 안정화에 도움이 될 수 있다. 만성적이거나 잦은 탈구 환자라고 해서 반드시 현장에서 교정을 시도할 필요는 없다. 이러한 환자들은 자가 정복이 불가능할 때 탈구된 상태로 병원으로 이송하는 것이 처음 탈구된 환자보다 덜 위험하고 통증과 불편함의 관점에서 더 잘 견딜 수 있는 경우가 많다.

처치

일반적으로 탈구가 의심되는 부위는 발견된 자세 그대로 부목으로 고정해야 한다. 맥박이 없거나 약할 때 혈류를 회복시키기 위해 관절을 부드럽게 재정렬할 수 있다. 재정렬은 환자 팔다리의 혈관 상태를 개선할 수 있다. 그러나 의료기관으로 이송하는 시간이 짧은 경우에는 재정렬을 시도하기보다는 이송을 시작하는 것이 더 나은 결정이다. 이러한 조작은 환자에게 심한 통증을 유발할 수 있으므로 팔다리를 움직이기 전에 환자가 미리 준비를 해야 한다. 대부분의 탈구는 부목을 사용하여 고정해야 하며 어깨 손상에는 팔걸이를 사용한다. 손상을 입게 된 경위, 부목 고정 전후의 맥박, 운동, 감각, 피부색 등을 부목으로 고정하기 전과 후에 평가하고 기록한다. 이송 중에 얼음이나 냉찜질을 사용하여 통증과 부기를 줄일 수 있다. 통증을 줄이기 위해 필요한 경우 진통제를 투여할 수 있다.

탈구의 교정 시도는 프로토콜 또는 직접 의료 지도를 통해 허용되는 경우와 병원 전 처치 제공자가 적절한 방법에 대해 적절한 교육을 받은 경우에만 시행한다. 탈구에 대한 모든 교정 시도는 기록하고 환자를 이송하는 의료기관의 의사에게 보고해야 한다.

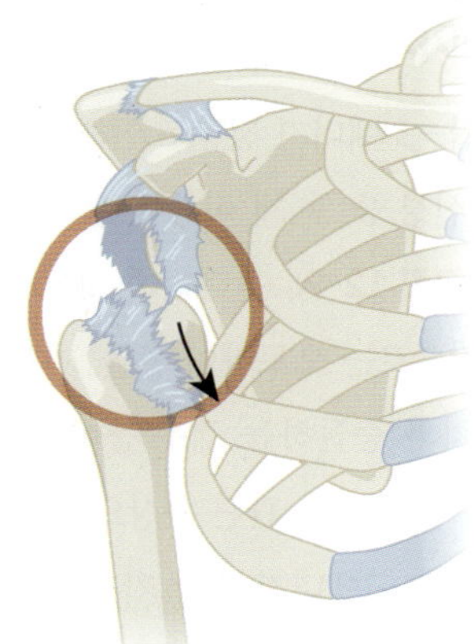

그림 12-7 탈구는 관절에서 뼈가 분리되는 것을 말하며 그림은 전형적인 전방 어깨탈구를 보여준다.

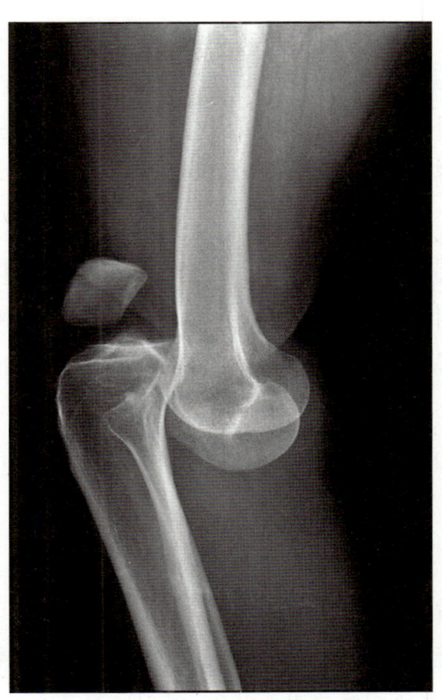

그림 12-8 넓적다리뼈보다 정강뼈가 앞쪽에 있는 오른쪽 전방 무릎탈구. 정강뼈(원위 부분)가 넓적다리뼈(근위 부분)의 전방으로 이동한 것을 확인할 수 있다.

특별한 고려 사항

심각한 다기관 외상 환자

팔다리의 손상을 포함한 다기관 외상 환자의 일차평가에서 우선순위를 준수한다고 해서 팔다리 손상을 무시하거나 팔다리 손상을 더 이상 위험으로부터 보호하지 말아야 한다는 의미는 아니다. 오히려 생명을 위협하지 않는 팔다리 손상을 입은 중증외상 환자에게는 팔다리보다 생명 유지가 우선이라는 의미이다. 소생술을 통해 생명 기능을 유지하는 데 중점을 두어야 하며 손상이 얼마나 극적으로 보이는지와 관계없이 팔다리 손상을 해결하기 위해 제한적인 처치만 취해야 한다. 환자를 긴척추고정판이나 진공부목과 같은 기타 전신을 고정할 수 있는 장비로 적절히 고정하면 모든 팔다리와 골격 전체가 해부학적인 자세로 고정되어 환자를 쉽게 이동시킬 수 있다. 일차평가에서 확인된 생명을 위협하는 문제에 대한 지속적인 처치가 필요하고 이송 시간이 짧은 경우 이차평가를 생략할 수 있다. 이차평가가 연기되면 병원 전 처치 제공자는 이차평가를 시행하지 못한 이유를 간단히 기록할 수 있다.

구획증후군

구획증후군은 팔다리 내의 압력 증가로 인해 팔다리로의 혈액 공급이 감소하여 팔다리를 위협하는 상태를 말한다. 팔다리의 근육은 근막이라고 하는 치밀한 결합조직으로 둘러싸여 있다. 이 근막은 근육이 포함된 팔다리에 수많은 구획을 형성한다. 근육의 근막은 신축성이 적기 때문에 구획 내부의 압력이 증가하면 구획증후군이 발생할 수 있다.

구획증후군의 가장 흔한 두 가지 원인은 골절이나 혈관 손상으로 인한 구획 내 출혈과 혈류가 감소하거나 차단된 후에 허혈성 근육 조직이 재관류 될 때 형성되는 제3공간의 부종이다. 그러나 부목이나 깁스를 너무 꽉 조이면 외부 압박으로 인해 구획증후군이 발생할 수 있다. 구획 내 압력이 모세혈관 압력 이상으로 증가하면 모세혈관을 통한 혈류가 손상된다. 이 혈관에 의해 혈액이 공급되는 조직에 허혈이 발생한다. 압력으로 인해 동맥 순환과 신경 기능까지 손상될 정도로 압력이 계속 높아질 수 있다.

구획증후군 발생의 두 가지 초기 징후는 1) 외상에 적합한 기준 통증보다 높고 통증 완화 조치에 반응하지 않는 통증과 2) 관련 팔다리의 감각 변화(비정상적인 감각 또는 감각 감소/부재)이다. 통증은 종종 손상에 비례하지 않은 것으로 설명된다. 이 통증은 해당 팔다리의 손가락이나 발가락을 수동적으로 움직일 때 극적으로 증가할 수 있다. 신경은 혈액 공급에 매우 민감하므로 혈류에 문제가 생기면 감각 이상으로 나타난다. 이러한 증상이 일반적으로 골절과 관련이 있다는 사실은 병원 전 처지 제공자가 변화를 구별할 수 있도록 기본 순환, 운동, 감각 평가에 이어 반복적인 재평가를 시행해야 한다는 점을 강조한다.

구획증후군의 다른 세 가지 전형적인 징후인 맥박소실, 창백함, 마비는 늦게 발견되는 소견이며 이는 명백한 구획증후군과 팔다리의 근육 괴사의 위험에 처해 있음을 나타낸다. 신체검사만으로 구획 압력을 판단하기는 어렵지만, 구획이 극도로 긴장되어 있고 촉진 시 단단하게 만져질 수 있다.

처치

병원에서는 구획증후군이 의심되는 팔다리의 구획 압력을 측정할 수 있다. 구획증후군은 피부와 근막을 통해 영향을 받은 구획을 절개하여 영향을 받은 근육 조직의 압력을 낮추는 응급 수술(근막절개술)을 통해 확실하게 처치해야 한다.

현장에서는 기본적인 처치만 시도할 수 있다. 단단히 고정한 부목이나 드레싱을 제거하고 원위부 관류 상태를 재평가한다. 팔다리에 부목을 고정하면 안정성을 제공한다. 팔다리를 높이는 것은 권장하지 않는다. 팔다리를 심장과 수평으로 유지하는 것이 이상적이다. 또한, 부목을 적용할 때 발목을 배 쪽으로 구부려 다리의 전방 구획 압력을 줄여야 한다. 장거리 이송 중에 구획증후군이 발생할 수 있으므로 이 문제를 조기에 파악하기 위해 지속적인 평가가 필수적이다.

심하게 훼손된(짓이겨진) 팔다리

심각하게 훼손된 팔다리는 고에너지 전달로 인해 1) 피부 및 근육, 2) 힘줄, 3) 뼈, 4) 혈관, 5) 신경 중 두 개 이상에 심각한 손상이 발생하는 복합 손상을 말한다(**그림 12-9**). 팔다리에 짓이겨진 손상이 발생하는 일반적인 손상 기전으로는 오토바이 충돌, 자동차에서 튕겨 나간 경우, 보행자가 자동차와 충돌하는 경우 등이 있다. 이러한 상황이 발생하면 환자는 외부출혈 또는 관련 손상으로 인한 출혈로 쇼크 상태에 빠질 수 있으며 이는 고에너지 손상 기전으로 인해 흔히 발생한다. 대부분의 팔다리 손상은 심각한 개방골절을 동반하며 절단이 필요한 경우가 많다. 일부 환자에서 팔다리를 살릴 수 있지만, 일반적으로 여러 번의 수술이 필요하며 장기간 신체장애가 흔하다.

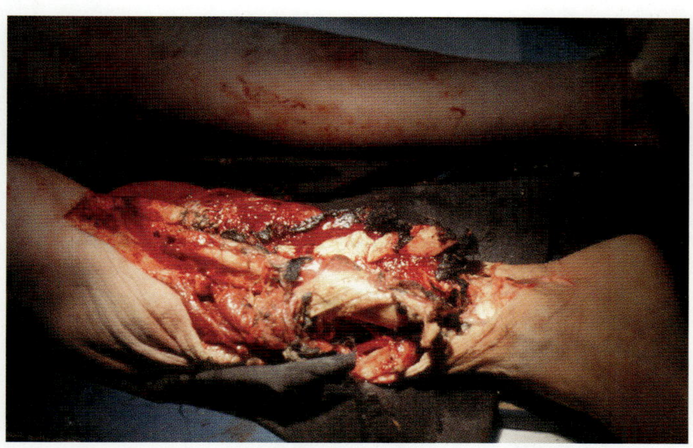

그림 12-9 두 차량 사이의 으깸손상으로 인해 짓이겨진 다리 손상 환자. 환자는 골절과 광범위한 연부조직 손상을 입었다.
Courtesy of Peter T. Pons, MD, FACEP.

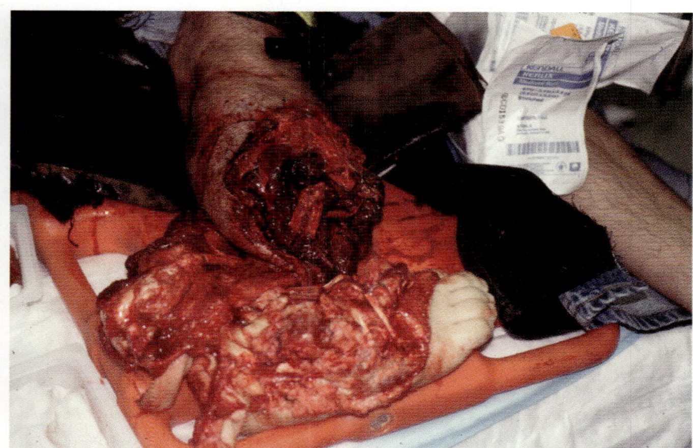

그림 12-10 오른쪽 다리가 기계에 끼여 완전히 절단되었다.
Courtesy of Peter T. Pons, MD. FACEP..

처치

팔다리가 짓이겨진 경우에도 생명을 위협하는 상태를 배제하거나 해결하기 위해 일차평가에 중점을 둔다. 지혈대 사용을 포함한 출혈 조절이 필요할 수 있다. 환자의 상태가 허락한다면 짓이겨진 팔다리를 부목으로 고정한다. 이러한 환자들은 Level I 외상센터로 이송해 치료하는 것이 가장 좋다.

절단

팔다리에서 조직이 완전히 분리되면 조직은 영양분과 산소 공급이 완전히 차단된 상태이다. 이러한 유형의 손상을 절단이라고 한다. 절단은 팔다리의 일부 또는 전부를 잃는 것이다. 모든 절단에는 다량의 출혈이 동반될 수 있지만, 부분 절단에서 출혈이 더 심하다. 혈관이 완전히 절단되면 혈관이 수축하고 근육 안으로 당겨지며 혈전이 형성되어 출혈이 감소하거나 멈출 수 있지만 혈관이 부분적으로만 절단되면 양쪽 끝이 수축하지 않고 손상된 혈관에서 혈액이 지속해서 분출될 수 있다.

절단은 종종 현장에서 명백하게 나타난다(**그림 12-10**). 이러한 유형의 손상은 목격자들의 큰 관심을 받으며 환자는 팔다리가 절단된 것을 알 수도 있고 모를 수도 있다. 병원 전 처치 제공자는 심리적으로 이 손상을 조심스럽게 다뤄야 한다(**Box 12-3**).

가능한 한 재접합 할 수 있도록 절단된 부위를 찾아야 한다. 특히 팔과 엄지손가락의 경우 더욱 그렇다. 다리 절단은 일반적으로 재접합 성공률이 낮으므로 보조기를 착용하고 외상성 절단 환자의 경우 재접합을 시행하지 않는 경우가 많다.

충분한 수의 병원 전 처치 제공자가 도움을 줄 수 없다면 절단된 팔다리를 찾기 전에 일차평가를 시행해야 한다. 절단된 팔다리의 모습은 끔찍할 수 있지만, 환자의 기도가 개방되지 않았거나 숨을 쉬지 않는다면 팔다리 절단은 생명을 위협하는 우선순위에 밀려 이차적인 문제이다.

절단은 매우 고통스러울 수 있으며 일차평가에서 생명을 위협하는 문제가 없다면 필요한 경우 통증 관리를 시행해야 한다(**그림 12-11**).

처치

절단된 부분을 관리하는 원칙은 다음과 같다.

1. 절단된 부위를 락테이트 링거액으로(LR) 부드럽게 헹구어 세척한다.
2. 락테이트 링거액으로 적신 멸균 거즈로 절단된 부위를 싸서 비닐봉지나 용기에 넣는다.
3. 비닐봉지나 용기에 라벨을 붙인 후 얼음을 채운 다른 용기에 넣는다.
4. 얼음 위에 직접 올려놓거나 드라이아이스와 같은 다른 냉각제

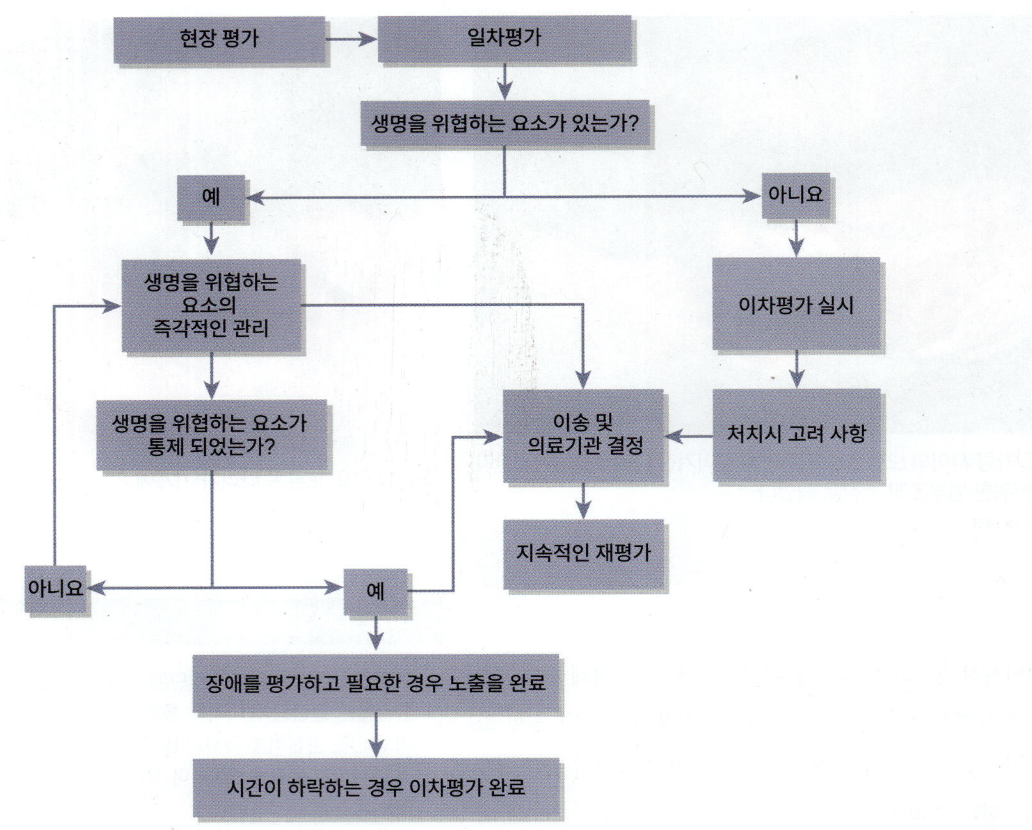

그림 12-11 일차평가 알고리즘
© National Association of Emergency Medical Technicians (NAEMT)

를 추가하여 절단된 부분을 얼리지 않는다.

5. 환자와 함께 가장 가까운 적절한 의료기관으로 절단된 부분을 이송한다.

절단된 부위에 산소가 공급되지 않는 시간이 길어질수록 성공적으로 접합될 가능성이 낮아진다. 절단된 신체 부위를 얼리지 않고 차갑게 하면 대사율이 감소하고 이 중요한 시간을 연장할 수 있다. 그러나 접합술이 성공적인 부착이나 궁극적인 기능 회복을 보장하는 것은 아니다. 특히 무릎 아래 절단의 경우 의족은 환자가 거의 정상에 가까운 생활을 재개할 수 있도록 해주기 때문에 다리 접합술을 거의 고려하지 않는다. 또한 일반적으로 건강하고 젊은 환자의 절단 부위가 깨끗하게 절단된 경우에만 보통 접합술을 고려한다. 흡연자는 담배의 니코틴이 강력한 혈관수축제로 작용하므로 접합된 부위의 혈류를 손상시킬 수 있으므로 접합이 성공할 가능성이 낮다. 손가락(특히 엄지손가락) 또는 손, 아래팔을 접합해야 하는 환자는 접합수술이 가능한 Level I 외상센터로 이송해야 한다. 궁극적으로 접합 수 있는지 아닌지는 수술팀의 결정에 달려있다.

분실된 절단 부위를 찾기 위해 환자 이송을 지연해서는 안 된다. 절단된 부분을 쉽게 찾을 수 없는 경우 경찰관이나 다른 구급대원이나 구조대원이 현장에 남아 절단된 부위를 찾아야 한다. 절단된 부위를 환자와 별도의 차량으로 이송하는 경우 병원 전 처치 제공자는 절단 부위를 이송하는 사람이 환자를 어느 의료기관으로 이송하는지와 절단된 부위를 찾은 후 어떻게 처리해야 하는지를 명확하게 이해하도록 설명을 해준다. 절단 부위를 찾는 즉시 환자를 이송하는 의료기관에 보고하고 가능한 한 빨리 절단 부위의 이송을 시작한다.

현장에서 절단

일반적으로 기계에 팔다리가 끼어서 구조하기 어려운 경우 팔다리는 추가적인 구조 전문 지식을 이용해 해결할 수 있다. 환자의 팔다리가 기계에 끼면 종종 간과되는 전문가는 기계를 수리하는 유지보수 담당자이다. 이 사람은 일반적으로 기계를 신속하게 분해해서 환자를 구출할 수 있는 전문 기술을 가지고 있다. 그러나 드물게는 환자의 팔다리가 끼어 있으면 현장 절단술이 끼어있는 팔다리를 구조할 수 있

Box 12-4 현장 절단 세트

절단 세트는 의료 지도 의의 차량에서 보관가능하며 현장 절단의 경우에 필수적이다. 다음 목록은 다양한 절단 세트의 예이다.

의료 기기

- Curved Mayo scissors ....1 each
- Curved hemostats..4 each
- Kelly clamps, regular ....2 each
- Needle holder, regular ....2 each
- Towel clamps ....4 each
- Forceps with teeth, regular..1 each
- Rake retractor, six prong, sharp....................................2 each
- Gigli saw handles..2 each
- Gigli saw wire...3 each
- Amputation knife...1 each
- Bone cutter ....1 each

일회용품

- Surgical gowns, sterile
- Surgical gloves, sterile
- Scalpel, #10 blade
- Sterile towels (4 pack)
- Lap pads (10 pack)
- Drapes

- Bone wax

봉합 물품

- 2-0 silk ties
- 0 silk ties
- 0 silk on atraumatic needle
- 2-0 silk on gastrointestinal (GI) needle, multipack
- 3-0 silk on GI needle, multipack

드레싱 물품

- Roller gauze
- Army Battle Dressing (ABD) pads, large
- Elastic bandages, 4 inch (10cm)
- Elastic bandages, 6 inch (15cm)

약물

- Neuromuscular blocking agents (succinylcholine, vecuronium, etc.)
- Ketamine
- Fentanyl

기도관리 (if not on EMS units)

- Intubation tray
- Endotracheal tubes

는 유일한 합리적인 선택일 수 있다. 지역 외상 체계는 적절한 장비를 갖춘 현장 절단 팀의 구성을 고려해야 한다(**Box 12-4**). 드물게 사용되기는 하지만, 이러한 팀이 생명을 구하는 것으로 나타났다. 미국에서 공식적인 현장 절단은 병원 전 처치 제공자의 업무 범위에 포함되지 않지만, 일부 끼인 팔다리는 작은 조직 한 가닥으로만, 연결되어 있을 수 있다. 이 조직을 절단할지 아니면 의사가 현장에 도착할 때까지 기다릴지는 의료 지도 의사의 의료지도를 받아 결정해야 한다. 상당한 절단이 필요한 경우 해부학적 지식과 전문적인 술기 능력이 필요하므로 숙련된 의사가 시행하는 것이 가장 이상적이다. 절단을 시행하기 위해 전신 마취 및 삽관 등 진정제를 투여해야 할 수도 있다.

으깸증후군

외상성 손상으로 팔다리가 짓눌리면 횡문근융해증이라는 반응이 나타날 수 있다. 이 상태는 영향을 받은 팔다리 근육이 죽고 미오글로빈이 방출되는 것과 관련이 있다. 임상적으로 횡문근융해증은 신부전, 말단 장기 손상 및 잠재적으로 사망을 초래할 수 있다. 이러한 미오글로빈 방출로 인한 충격의 시작은 팔다리에서 누르는 압력이 제거된 후이다.

근육에 외상을 입으면 미오글로빈과 칼륨을 모두 방출한다. 환자가 구출되면 손상된 팔다리에 갑자기 혈액이 재관류되고 동시에 미오글로빈과 칼륨 수치가 높아진 혈액이 손상된 부위에서 신체의 나머지 부분으로 순환한다. 혈액 내 칼륨 수치가 높아지면 생명을 위협하는 부정맥이 발생할 수 있으며 미오글로빈은 홍차 또는 콜라 색의 소변을 생산하여 결국 신부전을 초래할 수 있다. 이러한 현상이 복합적으로 나타나는 것을 일반적으로 으깸증후군이라고 한다.

으깸증후군은 제1차 세계대전에서 붕괴한 참호에서 구조된 독일 병사들에게서 처음 발견되었고 제2차 세계대전에서는 런던 공습 중 무너진 건물에서 구조된 환자들에게서 다시 나타났다. 2차 세계대전 당시 으깸증후군의 사망률은 90%가 넘었다. 한국전쟁 당시 사망률은 84%였으나 혈액투석의 등장 이후 사망률이 53%로 감소했다. 베트남전쟁에서 사망률은 50%로 거의 비슷했다.

그러나 으깸증후군의 중요성은 역사적 또는 군사적 관심에만 국한되어서는 안 된다. 지진 생존자의 약 3~20%가 으깸손상을 입었고 건물 붕괴로 인한 생존자의 약 40%가 으깸손상을 입는다. 1978년 중국 베이징에서 발생한 지진으로 35만 명 이상이 손상을 입었고 242,769명이 사망하였다. 이 중 48,000명 이상이 으깸증후군으로 사망했다. 일반적으로 으깸증후군의 기전에는 참호 붕괴, 건축물 붕괴 또는 차량 충돌로 인한 끼임이나 깔림이 포함된다.

으깸증후군 환자는 다음과 같이 구분된다.

- 장기간의 눌림(낌)
- 외상성 근육 손상
- 손상 부위의 혈액순환 장애

특히 외상성 횡문근융해증은 주로 노인인 환자가 넘어져 엉덩관절 골절되어 일어나지 못하거나 욕실에서 넘어져 욕조나 변기 옆에 끼인 환자에게서도 발생할 수 있다. 이러한 환자는 종종 딱딱한 표면에 같은 자세로 누워 몇 시간 또는 며칠 후에 발견될 수 있다. 장기간 근육에 환자의 체중이 가해지면 근육이 손상되고 외상성 횡문근융해증 소견이 나타난다.

처치

으깸증후군의 결과를 개선하기 위한 핵심은 조기에 적극적인 수액 소생술 시행하는 것이다. 병원 전 처치 제공자는 팔다리를 구출하는 과정에서 눌리거나 끼인 팔다리 내에 독소가 축적되고 있다는 사실을 기억하는 것이 중요하다. 눌리거나 끼였던 팔다리를 구출하면 축적되었던 독소는 독극물을 마신 것과 유사하게 중심 순환계로 흘러 들어간다. 따라서 팔다리를 구조하기 전에 축적된 미오글로빈과 칼륨의 독성 영향을 최소화하는 것이 성공 여부에 달려있다. 소생술은 구출하기 전에 시행해야 한다. 수액 소생술이 지연되면 환자의 50%에서 신부전이 발생하고 12시간 이상 지연되면 환자의 거의 100%에서 신부전이 발생한다. 일부 저자는 환자가 적절하게 소생할 때까지 구출을 지연해야 한다고 주장한다. 소생술이 제대로 이루어지지 않은 환자는 팔다리의 압박이 풀릴 때 대사에 의해 생성된 산과 칼륨이 혈류로 갑자기 방출되기 때문에 구출 중에 심정지가 발생할 수 있다.

수액 소생술은 시간당 최대 1,500mL의 속도로 생리식염수를 투여하여 시간당 150~200mL의 적절한 신장 배출량을 유지해야 한다. 정맥 내 수액 투여 시 링거스락테이트(LR) 용액은 칼륨이 포함되어 있으므로 소변량이 적절해질 때까지 투여하지 않는다. 구출하는 동안 투여하는 수액 1L당 중탄산나트륨 50mEq와 만니톨 10g을 추가하면 신부전 발생률을 낮추는 데 도움이 될 수 있다. 환자가 구출한 후에는 생리식염수 투여량을 시간당 500mL로 줄이고 수액 L당 1앰플의 중탄산나트륨을 희석해서 투여하거나 5% 포도당 수액(D5W)을 번갈아 가며 투여할 수 있다.

혈압이 안정되고 혈액량이 회복되면 고칼륨혈증 예방과 혈장 미오글로빈의 독성 영향에 주의를 기울여야 한다. 현장에서 고칼륨혈증은 심전도 모니터링에서 끝이 뾰족한 T 파가 발생하는 것으로 알 수 있다. 증가한 칼륨의 처치는 정맥 내로 중탄산나트륨 투여, 베타차단제(알부테롤) 흡입, 포도당 및 인슐린 투여(가능한 경우)하고 생명을 위협하는 심부정맥이 발생하면 정맥 내로 염화칼슘을 투여하는 고칼륨혈증에 대한 표준 프로토콜에 따라 시행한다. 소변을 알칼리화하면 신장을 어느 정도 보호할 수 있지만, 중요한 것은 증가한 소변 배출량(일반적으로 50~100mL/hr 범위)을 유지하는 것이다.

삠

삠은 인대가 늘어나거나 찢어지는 손상이다. 삠은 관절이 정상적인 운동 범위를 초과하여 갑자기 뒤틀려 발생한다. 삠은 심한 통증, 부종 및 혈종이 있는 것이 특징이다. 삠은 겉으로 보기에 골절이나 탈구와 비슷해 보일 수 있다. 삠과 골절의 확실한 구분은 X-ray 검사를 통해서만 가능하다. 병원 전 환경에서는 골절이나 탈구로 판명될 경우를 대비해 삠이 의심되는 경우 부목으로 고정하는 것이 좋다. 얼음이나 냉찜질이 통증을 완화하는 데 도움이 될 수 있다. 마약성 진통제의 사용은 일반적으로 필요하지 않거나 바람직하지 않으며 부목 적용, 거상, 냉찜질에 반응하지 않는 심각한 통증이 있는 경우에만 사용해야 한다.

처치

삠이 의심되는 경우의 일반적인 처치는 다음과 같다.

1. 일차평가에서 발견된 생명을 위협하는 모든 손상을 확인하고 처치한다.
2. 외부출혈을 지혈하고 환자의 쇼크를 처치한다.
3. 원위부의 신경혈관 기능을 평가한다.
4. 손상 부위를 지지한다.
5. 손상된 팔다리를 부목으로 고정한다.
6. 얼음이나 냉찜질로 통증과 부기를 조절한다.

7. 부목 고정 후 손상된 팔다리를 재평가하여 원위부 신경혈관 기능의 변화를 확인한다.

이송 지연

팔다리 외상을 입은 환자는 종종 동반된 손상이 있다. 복부 또는 가슴 손상으로 인해 내부출혈이 지속해서 발생할 수 있으며 이송 지연하는 동안 생명을 위협하는 모든 상태를 확인하고 새로운 변화가 나타나는지 확인하기 위해 일차평가를 자주 재평가를 한다. 활력징후를 주기적으로 측정해야 한다. 골반, 복부, 가슴에 심각한 내부출혈이 의심되지 않는 한 적절한 관류를 유지할 수 있는 속도로 정맥 내로 결정질 수액을 투여한다. 구획증후군이 의심되거나 맥박이 감소하거나 활동성 출혈이 발생한 상황에서는 자주 재평가를 시행한다.

장거리 이송 중에 병원 전 처치 제공자는 팔다리 관류에 더 많은 주의를 기울여야 한다. 혈액 공급이 손상된 팔다리를 병원 전 처치 제공자가 혈류 개선을 최적화하기 위해 해부학적 위치를 회복하려고 시도할 수 있다. 마찬가지로 이송 시간이 길어지는 경우 이송을 시작하기 전에 원위부 순환 장애를 동반한 탈구는 현장에서 교정을 고려할 수 있다. 맥박, 피부색, 체온, 운동 및 감각 기능을 포함한 원위부의 관류 상태를 주기적으로 평가한다. 잠재적으로 구획증후군이 발생할 가능성이 있는지 모니터링한다. 이러한 검사는 모든 변화를 포함하여 주의 깊게 시행하고 기록하며 환자를 이송할 의료기관의 의료진에게 보고해야 한다.

환자의 편안함을 보장하려는 조치를 해야 한다. 필요한 경우 환자가 편안하게 패드를 대고 부목을 적용한다. 특히 관류 장애를 동반한 팔다리는 압력에 의해서 궤양이 발생할 수 있으므로 팔다리에 압력이 가해질 수 있는 부위를 평가해야 한다. 필요하면 비경구 마약성 진통제를 투여하고 환기 속도, 혈압, 맥박산소포화도측정, 호기말이산화탄소분압을 주의 깊게 모니터링해야 한다.

오염된 상처는 생리식염수로 세척해서 입자가 큰 이물질(흙이나 풀)을 제거해야 한다. 이송 시간이 길어지거나 의료기관에서 치료받는 것이 지연되는 경우 개방골절 환자에게 항생제를 투여할 수 있다. 항생제 사용에 대한 지침이 있고 그람 양성(세팔로스포린이나 세파졸)이 일반적이며 많은 연구자는 더 심각하고 오염된 손상에 대해 그람음성(아미노글리코사이드)을 추가할 것을 권장한다. 페니실린은 농장에서 발생한 손상에 사용되었다. 신체 일부가 절단되면 차가운 상태로 유지해야 하지만, 물에 담가 얼거나 조직이 짓무르지 않도록 주기적으로 평가해야 한다.

요 약

- 다기관 외상 환자의 경우 먼저 일차평가와 팔다리의 외부출혈 또는 내부출혈을 포함하여 생명을 위협하는 모든 손상을 구별하고 처치하는 데 주의를 기울여야 한다.
- 병원 전 처치 제공자는 치명적이지 않은 눈에 보이는 상처나 환자의 요구사항으로 인해 생명을 위협하는 상황을 해결하는 데 주의가 분산되지 않도록 주의해야 한다.
- 환자를 완전히 평가하고 전신에 영향을 미치지 않는 단일 손상만 있는 것으로 확인되면 치명적이지 않은 손상을 처치해야 한다.
- 근골격 손상은 안정과 편안함 및 통증 완화를 위해 고정해야 한다.

- 손상 기전과 에너지 전달을 신속하게 파악하면 병원 전 처치 제공자가 가장 심각한 손상이나 상태를 의심하고 인식하는 데 도움이 된다.
- 골절 처치에서 가장 먼저 고려해야 할 사항은 출혈을 조절하고 쇼크를 처치하는 것이다.
- 일반적으로 탈구가 의심되는 부위는 발견된 자세 그대로 부목으로 고정한다.
- 으깸증후군은 장시간 눌러 허혈이 발생한 신체 부위에 재관류로 인해 발생한다. 손상된 근육 조직은 미오글로빈과 칼륨을 혈류로 방출하는데 이는 신장과 심장에서 독성을 일으킬 수 있다.

시나리오 재구성

6월 어느 화창한 토요일 오후 당신은 오토바이 경기장에서 경기 중 사고가 발생했다는 신고를 받고 현장으로 출동하였다. 현장에 도착하자마자 당신은 경기장 안전 관리자의 안내를 받아 관중석 바로 앞 트랙의 한 구역으로 이동하여 경기 의료지원팀(2인 1조의 응급의료반응자)이 트랙에 바로 누워 있는 한 명의 환자를 처치하고 있는 곳으로 이동한다.

응급의료반응자(EMR) 중 한 명이 환자는 350cc급 오토바이 14대가 경주를 하던 중 3대가 관중석 앞에서 충돌했다고 말한다. 다른 두 명의 운전자는 손상을 입지 않았지만, 이 환자는 오른쪽 다리와 골반에 심한 통증이 있어 일어서거나 움직일 수 없었다. 의식을 잃은 상태는 아니었고 다리 통증 외에 다른 호소증상은 없었다. 의료지원팀은 바로누운자세에서 환자의 오른쪽 다리를 도수로 고정하고 있었다.

환자를 평가한 결과 19세 남성으로 의식이 명료하고 과거 병력이나 외상 병력이 없는 것을 확인했다. 환자의 초기 활력징후는 혈압 104/68mmHg, 맥박 112회/분, 호흡 24회/분, 피부는 창백하고 발한 증상을 보였다.

환자는 코너를 돌아 앞으로 나오는 순간 다른 운전자와 충돌했으며 충돌로 인해 균형을 잃고 트랙을 가로질러 미끄러졌다고 말했다. 환자는 오른쪽 다리가 최소 한 대 이상의 오토바이에 치였다고 말했다. 환자의 오른쪽 다리를 시진한 결과 왼쪽과 비교하였을 때 짧아지고 개방 상처가 없으며 넓적다리 앞쪽 중간 부위에 압통과 타박상이 있었다.

- 이 사고로 인한 손상 기전을 통해 이 환자의 잠재적 손상에 대해 무엇을 알 수 있는가?
- 어떤 유형의 손상이 의심되며 처치의 우선순위는 무엇인가?

시나리오 해결책

일차평가를 완료하고 단일 근골격 손상임을 확인한 후 당신은 동료의 도움을 받아 오른쪽 넓적다리 몸통 골절에 견인부목을 적용할 수 있었다. 환자를 긴척추고정판에 고정한 후 구급차로 환자를 옮겨 병원으로 이송할 수 있었다. 구급차에 탑승한 후 비재호흡마스크를 이용해 산소를 투여하고 정맥 라인을 확보했다. 환자는 부목을 고정 후 통증이 많이 호전되었으며 지금은 진통제가 필요하지 않다고 말했다. 이송하는 동안 환자의 활력징후는 변하지 않았다.

References

1. Williams B, Boyle M. Estimation of external blood loss by paramedics: is there any point? *Prehosp Disaster Med.* 2007;22(6):502-506.
2. Shulman JE, O'Toole RV, Castillo RC, et al. Pelvic ring fractures are an independent risk factor for death after blunt trauma. *J Trauma.* 2010;68:930-934.
3. Pierrie SN, Seymour RB, Wally MK, Studnek J, Infinger A, Hsu JR; Evidence-based Musculoskeletal Injury and Trauma Collaborative (EMIT). Pilot randomized trial of pre-hospital advanced therapies for the control of hemorrhage (PATCH) using pelvic binders. *Am J Emerg Med.* 2021 Apr;42:43-48. doi: 10.1016/j.ajem.2020.12.082
4. Pap R, McKeown R, Lockwood C, Stephenson M, Simpson P. Pelvic circumferential compression devices for prehospital management of suspected pelvic fractures: a rapid review and evidence summary for quality indicator evaluation. *Scand J Trauma Resusc Emerg Med.* 2020;28(1):65.
5. van Leent EAP, van Wageningen BV, Sir Ö, Hermans E, Biert J. Clinical examination of the pelvic ring in the prehospital phase. *Air Med J.* 2019;38(4):294-297.
6. Zingg T, Piaget-Rosssel R, Steppacher J, et al. Prehospital use of pelvic circumferential compression devices in a physician-based emergency medical service: a 6-year retrospective cohort study. *Sci Rep.* 2020;10(1):1-8.
7. Yong E, Vasireddy A, Pavitt A, Davies GE, Lockey DJ. Pre-hospital pelvic girdle injury: improving diagnostic accuracy in a physician-led trauma service. *Injury.* 2016; 47(2):383-388.
8. Hsu S-D, Chen C-J, Chou Y-C, Wang S-H, Chan D-C. Effect of early pelvic binder use in the emergency management of suspected pelvic trauma: a retrospective cohort study. *Int J Environ Res Public Health.* 2017;14(10):1217. doi: 10.3390/ijerph14101217
9. Coccolini F, Stahel PF, Montori G, et al. Pelvic trauma: WSES classification and guidelines. *World J Emerg Surg.* 2017;12:5.
10. Scott I, Porter K, Laird C, Greaves I. Bloch M. The pre-hospital management of pelvic fractures: initial consensus statement. *Emerg Med J.* 2013;30(12):1070-1072.
11. McCreary D, Cheng C, Lin ZC, Nehme Z, Fitzgerald M, Mitra B. Haemodynamics as a determinant of need for pre-hospital application of a pelvic circumferential compression device in adult trauma patients. *Injury.* 2020;51(1):4-9.
12. Garner MR, Sethuraman SA, Schade MA, Boateng H. Antibiotic prophylaxis in open fractures: evidence, evolving issues, and recommendations. *J Am Acad Orthop Surg.* 2020 Apr 15;28(8):309-315. doi: 10.5435/JAAOS-D-18-00193
13. Seyfer AE, American College of Surgeons Committee on Trauma. *Guidelines for Management of Amputated Parts.* ACS; 1996.
14. Harbour PW, Malphrus E, Zimmerman RM, Giladi AM. Delayed digit replantation: what is the evidence? J Hand Surg Am. 2021 Oct;46(10):908-916. doi: 10.1016/j.jhsa.2021.07.007
15. Sharp CF, Mangram AJ, Lorenzo M, Dunn EL. A major metropolitan "field amputation" team: a call to arms . . . and legs. *J Trauma.* 2009;67(6):1158-1161.
16. Pepe E, Mosesso VN, Falk JL. Prehospital fluid resuscitation of the patient with major trauma. *Prehosp Emerg Care.* 2002 6:81.
17. Better OS. Management of shock and acute renal failure in casualties suffering from crush syndrome. *Ren Fail.* 1997:19:647.
18. Vanholder R, Borniche D, Claus S, et al. When the earth trembles in the Americas: the experience of Haiti and Chile 2010. *Nephron Clin Pract.* 2011;117(3):c184-c197. doi: 10.1159/000320200
19. Lameire N, Sever MS, Van Biesen W, Vanholder R. Role of the international and national renal organizations in natural disasters: strategies for renal rescue. *Semin Nephrol.* 2020 Jul;40(4):393-407. doi: 10.1016/j.semnephrol.2020.06.007
20. Michaelson M, Taitelman U, Bshouty Z, et al. Crush syndrome: experience from the Lebanon war, 1982. *Isr J Med Sci.* 1984;20:305-307.
21. Pretto EA, Angus D, Abrams J, et al. An analysis of prehospital mortality in an earthquake. *Prehosp Disaster Med.* 1994;9:107-117.
22. Collins AJ, Burzstein S. Renal failure in disasters. *Crit Care Clin.* 1991;7:421-435.
23. Sever MS, Vanholder R, Lameire N. Management of crush-related injuries after disasters. *N Engl J Med.* 2006; 354:1052-1063.

Suggested Reading

American College of Surgeons Committee on Trauma. Musculoskeletal trauma. In: ACS Committee on Trauma. *Advanced Trauma Life Support.* 10th ed. ACS; 2018:148-167.

Ashkenazi I, Isakovich B, Kluger Y, et al. Prehospital management of earthquake casualties buried under rubble. *Prehosp Disast Med.* 2005;20(2):122-133.

Coppola PT, Coppola M. Emergency department evaluation and treatment of pelvic fractures. *Emerg Med Clin North Am.* 2003;18(1):1-27.

특수 술기

넓적다리뼈 골절에 견인부목 적용

원칙: 넓적다리뼈 골절을 고정하여 넓적다리 내부출혈을 최소화한다.

이러한 유형의 고정은 넓적다리뼈 몸통 골절을 고정하기 위해 사용한다. 견인과 고정을 적용하면 근육 경련과 통증을 줄이는 동시에 골절된 뼈끝이 추가 손상을 일으키고 출혈을 증가시킬 가능성을 줄이는 데 도움이 된다. 견인부목은 환자의 상태가 안정적이고 시간이 허용하는 경우에만 적용해야 한다. 무릎이나 정강뼈에 골절이나 손상이 동반되면 견인부목을 사용할 수 없다. 아래 술기는 HARE 견인부목 사용법법을 설명한 것이다. SAGER 견인부목과 같은 다른 견인부목은 프로토콜이나 지침에 따라 사용할 수 있다.

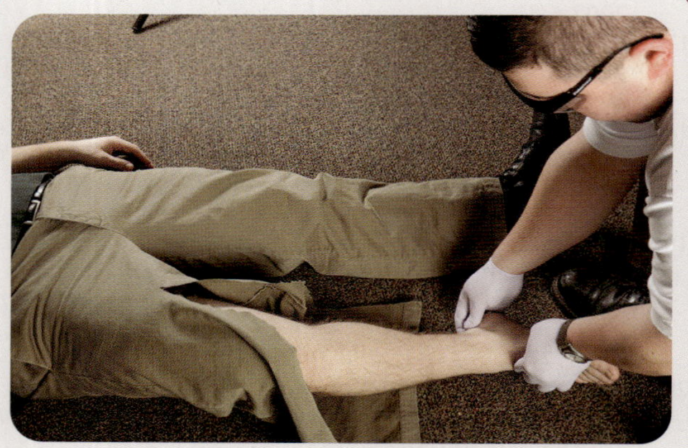

1　병원 전 처치 제공자는 환자에게 처치할 내용을 설명하고 골절된 다리를 노출하고 조작 전후에 환자의 신경혈관 상태를 평가한다.

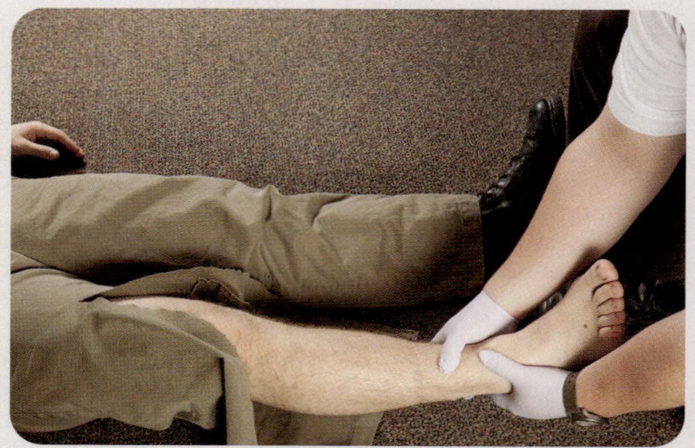

2　골절된 팔다리에 뚜렷한 변형이 있는 경우 두 번째 병원 전 처치 제공자가 발목과 발을 잡고 부드럽게 일직선이 되도록 견인하여 환자의 다리 길이를 원래대로 회복시킨다.

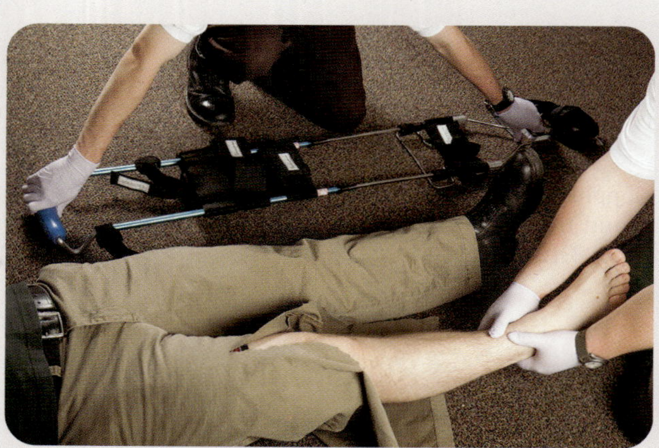

3　견인부목을 다치지 않은 다리에 대고 측정하여 적절한 길이(발뒤꿈치에서 약 20~25cm)로 조절한다.

(다음 페이지에 계속)

넓적다리뼈 골절에 견인부목 적용 (이어서)

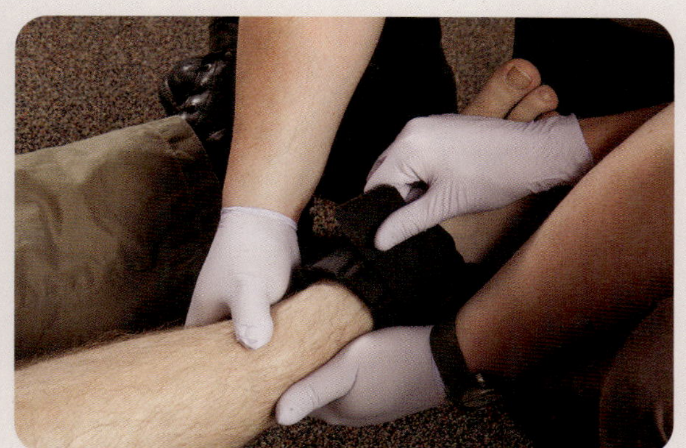

4 발목 고정끈을 골절된 발목에 적용하고 발목 고정끈은 필요에 따라 견인력을 유지하는 데 사용할 수 있다.

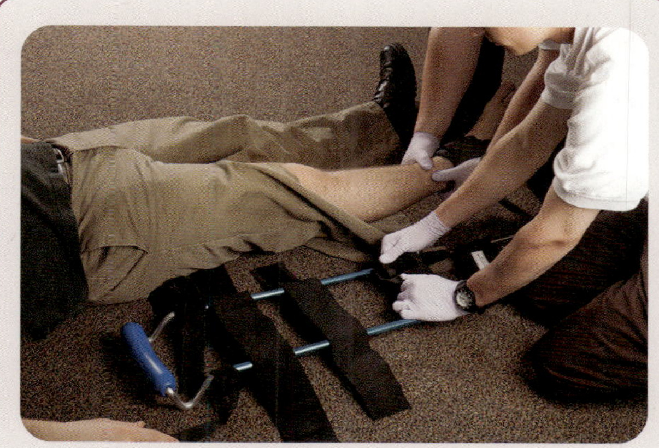

5 모든 고정끈의 벨크로를 열어놓는다.

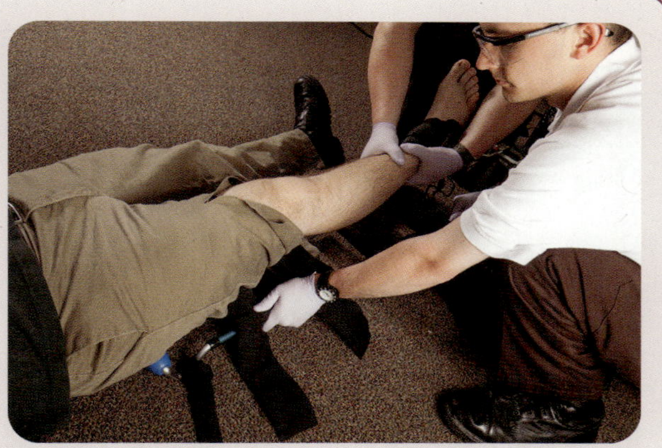

6 환자의 다리를 들어 올리고 견인부목의 근위 끝이 골반의 궁둥뼈결절에 위치시킨다.

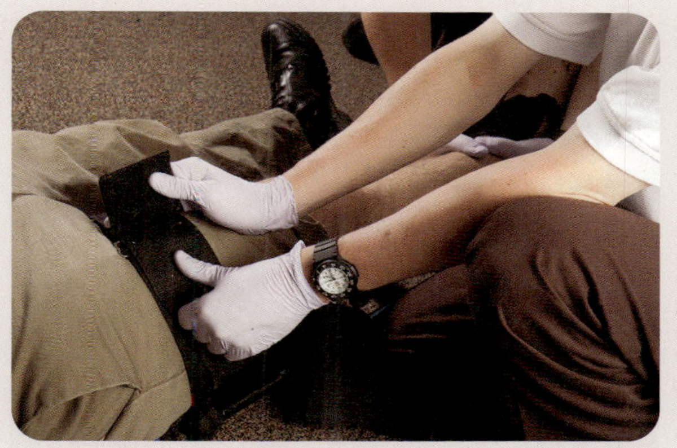

7 병원 전 처치 제공자는 근위부 고정끈을 넓적다리 근위부에 고정한다.

(다음 페이지에 계속)

넓적다리뼈 골절에 견인부목 적용 (이어서)

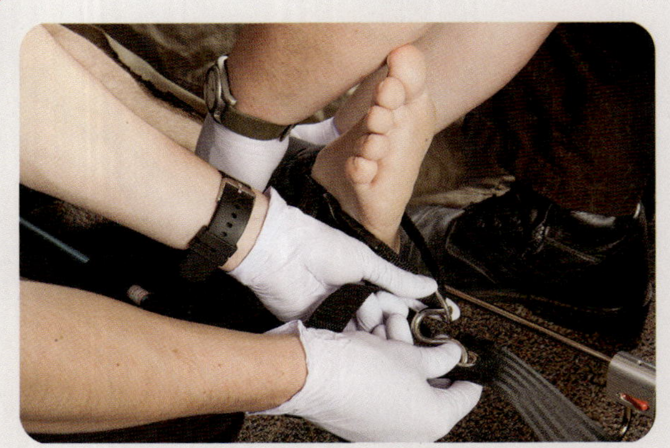

8　발목 고정끈과 견인부목의 원위부 끝에 있는 당김 고리에 연결한다.

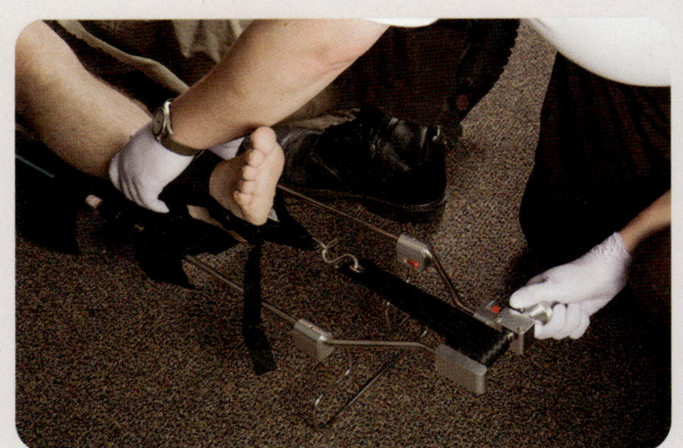

9　병원 전 처치 제공자는 도수 견인을 유지하면서 당김 고리를 천천히 돌려 견인을 시행한다. 환자의 골절된 다리를 다치지 않은 다리와 같은 길이로 견인이 되면 견인을 멈춘다.

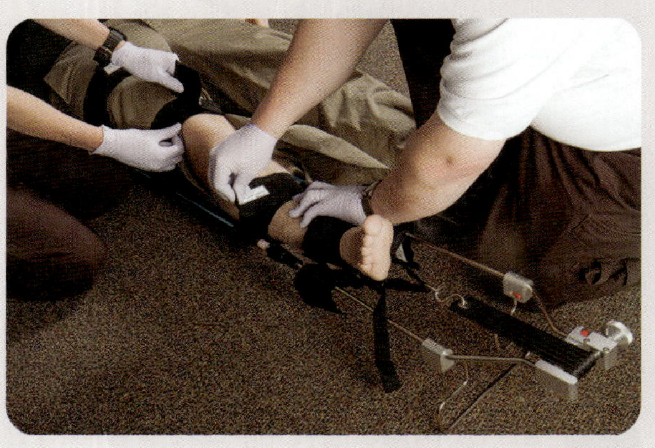

10　병원 전 처치 제공자는 남은 고정끈으로 다리를 견인부목에 고정한다.

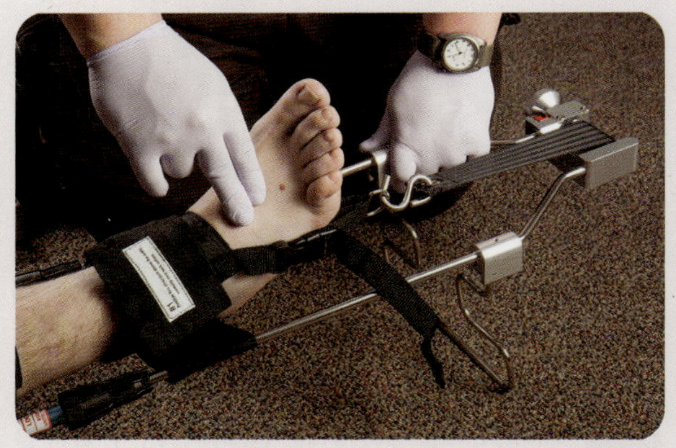

11　병원 전 처치 제공자는 환자의 신경혈관 상태를 재평가한다.

골반 고리 골절에 대한 골반고정대 적용

원칙: 골반 고리 골절을 고정하여 진행 중인 골반 내부출혈을 최소화한다.

이러한 유형의 고정은 골반 고리 골절에 사용한다. 골반고정대를 사용하면 골반을 고정하여 통증을 개선하고 골반 부피를 줄여 추가 손상과 출혈 증가를 예방하는 데 도움이 될 수 있다. 골반고정대는 불안정한 골반 고리 손상이 의심되는 모든 환자에게 안전하게 사용할 수 있다. 시중에서 판매되는 여러 가지 골반고정대 또는 클램프가 있는 시트 중 하나를 프로토콜 및 정책에 따라 사용할 수 있다.

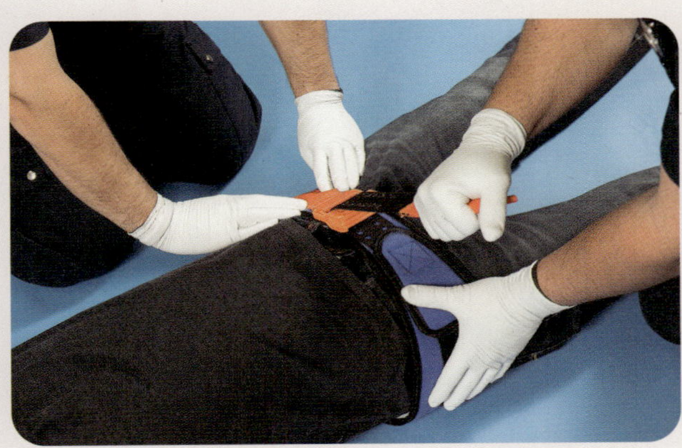

1 적용 전후에 환자의 신경혈관 상태를 평가한다. 골반고정대는 표준 통나무굴리기법을 사용하여 넓적다리큰돌기 수준에서 환자 아래에 배치한다. 그런 다음 사용하는 고정대 모델에 따라 벨크로 또는 래칫 조임 기전을 사용하여 고정대를 조여 고정한다. 장치를 고정한 후 혈압과 원위부 신경혈관 상태를 재평가한다. 흡인 시 환자의 가슴이 확장되는 기능을 쉽게 손상시킬 수 있으므로 고정대가 넓적다리큰돌기 높이보다 높게 위치하지 않도록 주의한다.

화상 손상

Lead Editors
Jennifer M. Gurney, MD, FACS
Spogmai Komak, MD
Brian H. Williams, MD, FACS

학습 목표   이 장의 학습을 완료하면 다음과 같은 내용을 수행할 수 있다.

- 화상 손상의 원인, 병태생리학, 전신 영향 및 임상적 결과를 설명할 수 있다.
- 화상 손상의 근본적인 체액 변화를 설명할 수 있다.
- 화상 깊이에 대한 최신 분류 체계를 정의할 수 있다.
- 얼음이 어떻게 화상 깊이를 더 깊게 만들 수 있는지 설명할 수 있다.
- 9의 법칙을 사용하여 화상 면적을 추정할 수 있다.
- 다양한 공식을 이용해 수액 소생술을 계산하고 이해할 수 있다.
- 미국 육군 외과 연구소(USAISR)의 10의 법칙을 사용하여 성인의 초기 수액 투여량을 계산할 수 있다.
- 화상을 입은 소아 환자에게 추가로 필요한 수액량을 설명할 수 있다.
- 소아 화상과 아동학대의 독특한 측면을 설명할 수 있다.
- 병원 전 처치를 위한 적절한 화상 드레싱에 관해 설명할 수 있다.
- 전기 손상의 고유한 우려 사항과 소생술에 미치는 영향에 관해 설명할 수 있다.
- 방사선 및 화학 화상 시 특별한 고려사항을 설명할 수 있다.
- 둘레 화상 환자의 우려 사항과 이러한 손상의 처치에 관해 설명할 수 있다.
- 연기 흡입의 세 가지 요소에 관해 설명할 수 있다.
- 중증 화상 손상 환자의 병원 전 처치 및 처치 우선순위에 관해 설명할 수 있다.
- 화상센터로 환자를 이송하는 기준에 관해 설명할 수 있다.

© Ralf Hiemisch/Getty Images

시나리오

당신은 주택 건물 화재 현장으로 도움 요청을 받고 출동했다. 당신과 동료가 도착했을 때 2층 주택이 완전히 불길에 휩싸여 지붕과 창문에서 짙은 검은 연기가 쏟아져 나오는 것을 목격했다. 당신은 응급의료반응자(EMR)가 처치하고 있는 환자가 있는 곳으로 이동했다. 환자는 반려견을 구하기 위해 불타는 건물에 다시 들어갔다가 소방관에 의해 의식이 없는 상태로 발견되어 구조되었다고 한다.

환자는 30대로 보이는 남성이고 옷 대부분이 불에 탔다. 환자는 얼굴에 화상을 입은 것이 분명하고 머리카락이 불에 그을렸다. 환자는 의식이 없고 자발적으로 호흡은 하고 있지만, 코골이 호흡을 하고 있다. 응급의료반응자는 환자에게 비재호흡마스크를 이용해 고유량의 산소를 공급하고 있었다. 신체검사 시 턱 밀어올리기 방법으로 기도를 유지하여 그는 쉽게 호흡하고 있다. 환자의 셔츠 소매는 불에 탔고 팔에는 둘레 화상이 있지만, 노동맥은 쉽게 확인할 수 있었다. 환자의 맥박수는 118회/분, 혈압은 148/94mmHg, 호흡수는 22회/

(다음 페이지에 계속)

분, 맥박산소측정기로 측정한 산소포화도는 92%이다. 신체검사 결과 환자는 머리 전체에 화상을 입었고 가슴 앞과 배에 물집이 생겼으며 오른쪽과 왼쪽 팔과 손 전체에 전층 화상을 입었다.

- 이 환자의 화상 정도는 어느 정도인가?
- 이 환자를 처치하기 위한 첫 번째 단계는 무엇인가?
- 병원 전 처치 제공자는 흡입 손상을 어떻게 인식할 수 있을까?

개요

급성 열 손상은 매년 전 세계적으로 약 18만 명이 목숨을 잃는 심각한 의학적 문제이다. 2020년에는 전 세계적으로 약 1,000만 명 이상의 사람들이 화상으로 치료받았다. 화재로 인한 치명적인 화상의 95% 이상이 저소득 및 중간 소득 국가에서 발생하며 어린이와 노인은 가장 취약한 계층으로 사망률이 가장 높다. 중증 화상은 심각한 외상성 손상으로 좋은 임상 결과를 얻기 위해서는 전 과정에 걸쳐 고도로 전문화된 처치가 필요하다. 화상 외상은 장기간의 중환자실 치료, 반복되는 패혈증, 다발성 장기 기능 장애 외에도 심각한 흉터와 기형을 동반하는 경우가 많다는 점에서 독특하다.

화상의 원인

화상의 대부분은 화염(55%)으로 인한 열 손상으로 발생하며 그다음이 화상(40%) 손상이다. 화재는 성인에게 가장 흔한 화상의 원인이지만, 뜨거운 액체로 인한 화상은 어린이와 노인에게 가장 흔한 화상이다. 주택 화재는 화상으로 인한 입원 환자의 약 4%를 차지하지만, 치사율은 12%(주택 화재로 입원한 환자의 경우)로 다른 원인으로 인한 화상 환자의 치사율 3%보다 훨씬 높으며 흡입 손상과 관련이 있을 것으로 추정된다. 저소득층에서 화재 및 화상 사망 위험이 증가하는 원인에는 현행 화재 안전 규정을 충족하도록 지어지지 않은 오래된 건물에 거주하거나 복잡한 주거 환경, 연기 감지기 부재 등 복합적인 요인이 있다.

노인과 어린이는 화상을 입기 가장 취약한 연령대이다. 열탕 화상은 1~5세 어린이에게 가장 흔하게 발생하는 화상이다. 아동학대는 침수 열탕 화상의 많은 부분을 차지한다. 고의적인 화상은 일반적으로 화상의 패턴과 부위에 따라 우발적인 화상과 구분할 수 있다. 비우발적인 화상은 어린이의 손이나 발이 끓는 물에 담겼을 때 장갑을 끼거나 스타킹을 신은 것처럼 가장자리가 선명하게 드러나는 경우가 많다. 어린이가 뜨거운 액체를 흘려서 생기는 화상은 머리, 몸통, 손과 발, 손바닥 표면에서 가장 많이 발생한다. 화상의 다른 원인으로는 저온, 전기, 화학물질 및 방사선 손상 등이 있다.

화상 손상의 병태생리학

피부는 열전도율이 상대적으로 낮으므로 열 손상에 대한 광범위한 방어막을 제공한다. 피부 내 열전달은 가열된 물질의 열 전도성, 열이 전달되는 면적, 물질의 온도에 의해 결정된다. 피부에 열이 급격하게 전달되면 피부 방어막 기능의 급속한 조절 장애로 인해 체온 조절, 감염 방지 및 체액 항상성 유지가 손상되어 화상으로 인한 손상이 발생한다. 화상 손상은 전신 순환의 변화로 인해 이차적인 형태의 분포성 쇼크를 유발한다. 화상으로 인해 발생한 쇼크는 복잡하고 다인성이지만, 혈관벽의 완전한 상실과 그에 따른 사이질로 단백질 손실은 저혈량 및 분포성 쇼크를 유발하는 병태생리학 일부이다. 모세혈관 투과성 증가로 인해 사이질 공간으로의 체액 이동이 증가하고 정수압과 삼투압의 불균형으로 인해 혈관 내 구획에서 체액이 빠르게 이동한다. 심한 화상 손상의 경우 체액, 전해질 및 단백질의 급격한 손실로 인해 유효 순환 혈장량 손실, 대량 부종 형성, 말단 장기 관류 감소 및 심혈관 기능 저하가 발생한다.

화상 손상의 체액 변화

화상으로 인한 손상은 피부계통의 파괴와 함께 인상적인 생리학적 변화를 특징으로 한다. 열 손상은 국소 및 전신 염증 반응으로 인한 항상성 파괴로 이어져 혈관 내 용적 고갈, 폐동맥의 압력 저하, 전신 혈관 저항 증가, 심근 수축력 저하를 특징으로 하는 분포성 및 저혈량 쇼크 생리학의 독특한 조합인 "화상 쇼크"로 절정에 이르게 된다.

직접적인 열 손상은 국소 충혈, 부종 및 그에 따른 모세혈관 누출로 나타나는 미세혈관 순환의 변화를 유발한다. 부종은 혈과 내피와 투과성에 미치는 영향으로 인해 발생하며 이는 다양한 매개체와 사이토카인(히스타민, 브래디키닌, 인터루킨)의 영향을 받아 화상 후 부종 형성의 초기 단계(12~24시간)를 주도하는 것으로 생각된다. 이러한 부종 형성은 심할 수 있으며 화상으로 인한 쇼크의 원인이 될 수 있다.

수액 투여는 혈관 내 용적과 관류를 회복하는 것을 목표로 하는 효과적인 소생술의 초석이다. 지난 세기 동안 화상 쇼크 소생술의 유형, 양, 지속시간 및 종료점에 대한 논의가 계속됐지만, 수액 소생술을 시행하지 않으면 큰 화상 상처는 균일하게 치명적인 결과를 초래한다. 1950년대 이전에는 저혈량 쇼크 또는 쇼크에 의한 신부전이 열 손상 후 사망의 주요 원인이었다. 목표 수액 소생술은 병원 전 환경에서 시작해야 한다. 과도한 소생술은 이환율과도 관련이 있으므로 병원 전 수액 소생술의 적시성과 비율을 이해하는 것은 화상 손상 후 첫 24시간 동안의 전반적인 소생술 처치에 중요한 요소이다. 화상으로 인한 손상에서 수액 소생술의 목표는 혈관 내 용적을 회복하고 화상 후 혈량저하증 환자를 지원하는 것이다.

여러 가지 소생술 공식을 사용할 수 있으며 수액 소생술에 사용하는 수액의 구성은 다양하다. 적절한 말단 장기 관류를 유지하는 데 필요한 최소한의 수액을 투여하고 화상을 입은 조직에서 손실된 세포 외 염분을 보충하는 것이 필수적이라는 데 의견이 일치한다.

화상 손상의 전신적 영향

화상으로 인한 손상 후 순환하는 카테콜아민의 여러 배 증가로 인해 극적인 대사 과다 반응을 일으킨다. 체표면적(TBSA)의 30%를 초과하는 화상은 사이토카인과 염증 매개 물질이 전신 순환계로 대량 방출되는 특징이 있다.

화상으로 인한 손상에 대한 초기 심혈관 반응은 말초혈관 저항의 상승과 함께 심박출량이 감소하는 것이다. 이러한 반응은 화상 손상 직후에 나타나며 이차적으로는 사이질 내로 체액이 이동하여 혈관 내 부피 감소로 나타난다. 수액 소생술을 시작하고 혈장량이 교체된 후에는 심박출량이 증가하여 약해진 대사 과다 반응으로 유발되는 과역동 상태로 인해 정상 심박출량을 초과한다.

카테콜아민, 바소프레신 및 앤지오텐신의 방출은 말초 및 내장의 혈관수축을 유발하여 말단 장기 기능에 영향을 줄 수 있다. 혈관 내 부피의 감소로 인해 사구체 여과율과 신장 혈류가 초기에 감소한다. 또한, 화상 손상 후에는 장간막 혈류 감소, 장 점막 완전성 감소 및 외피 모세혈관 누출이 발생한다. 이에 따라 위장관 기능 장애가 발생하고 세균이 문맥순환으로 전이된다.

다른 형태의 외상과 마찬가지로 화상 손상에서도 폐 기능이 변화한다. 소생술 후 호흡수와 일회호흡량이 증가하여 분당 환기량이 증가한다. 순환하는 사이토카인은 폐혈관 저항을 증가시켜 폐 모세혈관 정수압을 감소시키고 손상 초기 소생술 단계에서 폐 기능 장애를 일으킬 수 있다.

피부의 해부학

피부는 인체에서 가장 큰 기관이다. 피부는 외부 환경으로부터 보호, 체액 조절, 체온 조절, 감각 및 대사 적응을 포함한 여러 가지 복잡한 기능을 수행한다(**그림 13-1**). 피부는 평균 성인의 경우 약 1.5~2.0㎡를 덮고 있으며 표피와 진피의 두 층으로 구성되어 있다. 바깥쪽 표피는 눈꺼풀과 같은 부위에서 두께가 약 0.05mm이고 발바닥에서는 1mm 정도로 두꺼울 수 있다. 표피는 외배엽에서 유래하며 재생되어 치유할 수 있다. 표피는 진피 돌기(표피 능선)와 맞닿아 있는 표피 돌기(유두)를 포함하는 기저막 층을 통해 진피와 연결된다.

피부의 진피층은 중배엽에서 유래하며 유두 진피와 망상 진피로 나뉜다. 유두 진피는 생체 활성이 매우 높으므로 표면 부분층 화상이 일반적으로 깊은 부분층 화상보다 더 빨리 치유되는 이유이다(깊

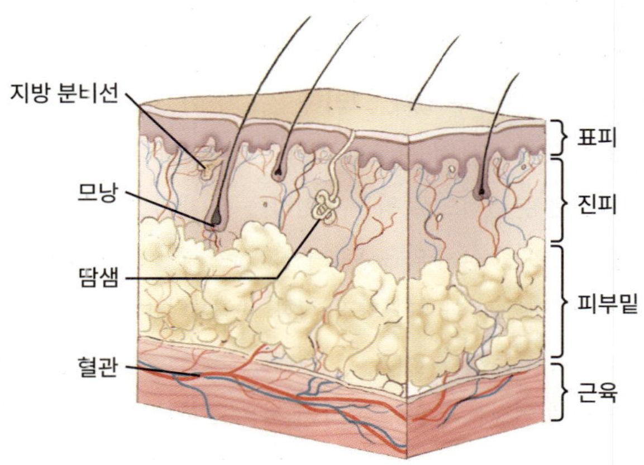

그림 13-1 정상 피부. 피부는 표피와 진피 두 층으로 구성된다. 피부밑층과 관련 근육은 피부 아래에 있다. 일부 층에는 땀샘, 모낭, 혈관 및 신경과 같은 구조가 포함되어 있다. 이러한 모든 구조는 체온 유지, 체온 손실, 체온 상승과 상호 관련이 있다.

© National Association of Emergency Medical Technicians (NAEMT)

은 화상에서는 유두 성분이 소실되기 때문).

더 깊은 진피는 표피보다 평균 10배 더 두껍다. 피부밑층 또는 피부밑조직은 지방과 결합 조직으로 구성되어 피부의 바깥층을 기저 구조물에 부착하는 데 도움을 준다. 피부밑층에는 또한 큰 혈관과 신경이 일부 포함되어 있다.

남성의 피부는 여성의 피부보다 두껍고 어린이와 노인의 피부는 평균 성인의 피부보다 얇다. 이러한 사실은 한 사람이 단일 화상 물질에 노출되어도 다양한 깊이의 화상을 입을 수 있는 이유, 왜 같은 화상에 노출된 성인은 표재성 손상만 입지만, 어린이는 심부 화상을 입을 수 있는 이유, 노인이 젊은 성인보다 더 심부 화상을 입는 이유를 설명해 준다. 입은 어린이가 성인보다 심부 손상이 발생하는지 또는 노인이 성인보다 심부 화상을 입을 수 있는지를 설명할 수 있다.

화상의 특성

화상 손상은 열이 가해져 피부, 피부밑조직, 지방, 근육 및 심지어 뼈까지 손상되어 발생한다. 급성 열 손상 후 세포 수준의 변화는 단백질의 변성과 형질막 무결성의 손실을 유발한다. 접촉 온도와 접촉시간은 화상 손상의 깊이를 결정하는 중요한 요인이다.

급성 열 손상은 손상 중심부에서 조직 괴사를 일으키고 주변에서는 점차 손상이 줄어든다. 열 손상의 깊이는 열 노출 정도와 열 침투 깊이에 따라 달라진다.

피부 손상은 즉각적인 손상과 지연성 손상의 두 단계로 발생할 수 있다. 즉각적인 손상은 급성 열 노출로 인해 형질막 무결성이 즉시 손실되고 단백질이 변성되는 것이다. 지연성 손상은 부적절한 소생술, 건조, 부종 및 상처 감염으로 인해 발생한다. 피부는 짧은 기간 동안 40℃의 온도를 견딜 수 있다. 그러나 온도가 이 지점을 초과하면 조직 파괴의 정도가 대수적(logarithmic)으로 증가한다.

전층 화상은 본질적으로 원을 형성하는 세 개의 조직 손상 영역이 있다(**그림 13-2**). 중심 구역을 응고구역(zone of coagulation)이라고 하며 이 구역은 조직 파괴가 가장 심한 구역이다. 이 구역의 조직은 괴사 상태이며 회복할 수 없다.

괴사 구역에 인접한 부위는 손상이 적은 구역이다. 정체구역(zone of stasis)이라고 하는 이 구역은 생존할 수 있는 세포와 생존 불가능한 세포가 모두 존재한다는 특징이 있다. 이 구역은 손상 직후 모세혈관 수축 및 허혈이 동반되어 혈류가 약한 경우가 많다. 이 부위의 괴사를 예방하기 위해서는 수액 소생술과 혈관수축 방지를 포함하

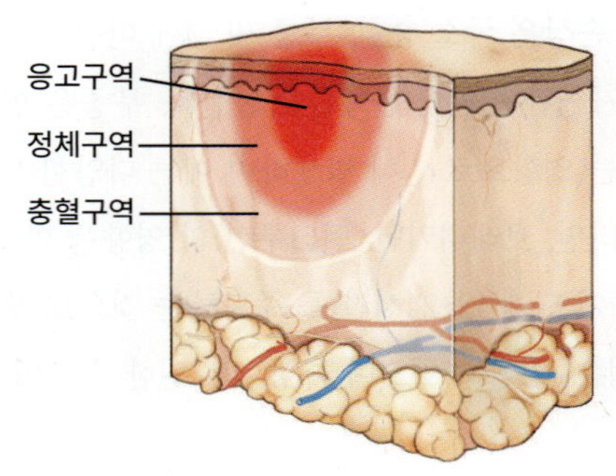

그림 13-2 화상 손상의 3개 구역
© National Association of Emergency Medical Technicians (NAEMT)

여 시기적절하고 적절한 화상 처치가 중요하다. 습윤 드레싱, 국소 항생제, 상처의 감염 여부를 자주 관찰하는 등 국소 상처 처치를 통해 손상된 세포가 조직 괴사로 진행되지 않도록 할 수 있다. 환자를 적절하게 소생시키지 못하면 손상된 조직의 세포가 죽고 조직 괴사가 발생한다.

정체구역에 손상을 입히는 흔한 실수는 목격자나 병원 전 처치 제공자가 손상 부위에 얼음을 대어 주는 것이다. 화상의 진행을 멈추는 것이 중요하지만, 피부에 얼음을 대면 혈관 수축이 일어나 손상된 조직에 꼭 필요한 재관류를 방해할 수 있다. 화상 부위에 얼음을 대어주면 통증이 감소할 수는 있지만, 조직이 추가로 손상될 수 있다. 작은 화상의 경우 이는 큰 문제가 되지 않지만, 큰 화상의 경우 국소 조직을 보호하고 저체온증을 예방하기 위해 얼음찜질을 자제해야 한다. 진통제는 경구 또는 비경구로 제공해야 한다.

가장 바깥쪽 손상 부위를 충혈구역(zone of hyperemia)이라고 한다. 이 구역은 세포 손상이 최소화되어 있으며 화상 손상에 의해 시작된 염증 반응으로 인해 이차적으로 혈류가 증가하는 것이 특징이다. 충혈구역은 생존할 수 있는 세포가 특징이며 저관류 또는 상처 감염으로 인한 추가 손상이 없는 한 일반적으로 회복된다. 화상 소생술의 목표 중 하나는 이 부위를 보존하여 환자에게 필요한 수술 및 피부 이식의 양을 줄이는 것이다.

화상 깊이

화상 깊이를 추정하는 것은 가장 경험이 많은 병원 전 처치 제공자라도 의외로 어려울 수 있다. 종종 부분층으로 보이는 화상이 전층 화상으로 발전할 수 있다. 또는 언뜻 보기에는 화상 표면이 부분층으로 보이지만, 후에 병원에서 죽은 조직 제거 후 표피가 분리되어 그 아래쪽에 흰색의 전층 화상으로 드러나는 경우도 있다. 병원 전 환경에서

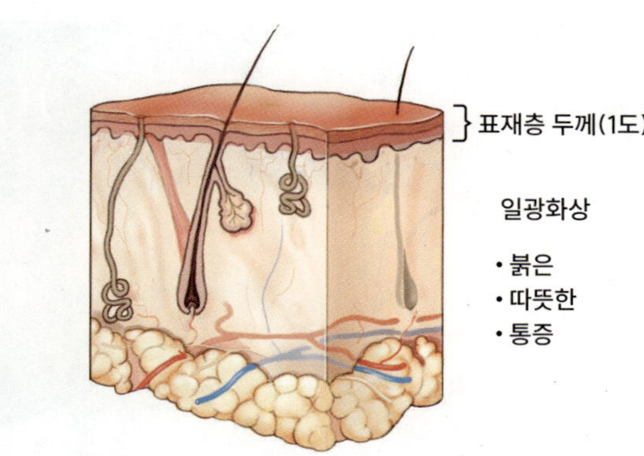

그림 13-3 표재 화상.
© National Association of Emergency Medical Technicians (NAEMT)

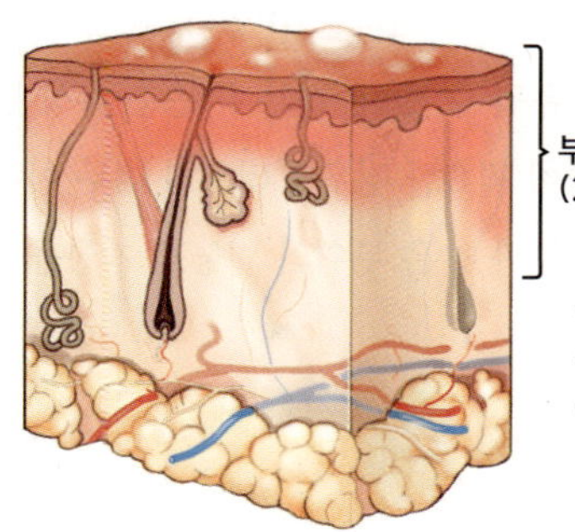

그림 13-4 부분층 화상.
© National Association of Emergency Medical Technicians (NAEMT)

는 환자의 소생술 요구에 따라 상처가 변할 수 있으므로 명확한 전층 화상 부위를 제외하고 화상 깊이를 추정하기가 훨씬 더 어렵다. 종종 환자에게 손상이 표면이거나 깊으며 최종 화상 깊이를 결정하기 위해 추가 평가가 필요하다고 간단히 설명하는 것이 가장 좋다. 또한, 병원 전 처치 제공자는 병원에서 상처를 초기에 평가하고 죽은 조직을 제거할 때까지 화상 깊이를 추정하려고 시도해서는 안 된다.

표재 화상

표재 화상은 단지 표피만 손상되며 붉고 통증이 있는 것이 특징이다 (**그림 13-3**). 이러한 화상은 유두 진피까지 확장되며 특징적으로 물집이 생기지 않는다. 이 상처는 압력을 가하면 희게 변하고 이 부위의 혈류가 인접한 정상 피부에 비해 증가한다. 표면 피부 상처는 일반적으로 흉터 형성 없이 2~3주 이내에 치유된다. 이러한 상처는 외과적 절제 및 이식이 필요하진 않다. 이 깊이의 화상은 수액 투여를 위해 사용되는 체표면적(TBSA)의 백분율을 계산할 때 포함되지 않는다.

부분층 화상

2도 화상이라고도 하는 부분층 화상은 표피와 기저 진피의 다양한 부분을 포함하는 화상을 말한다(**그림 13-4**). 부분층 화상은 다시 표재 또는 심부 화상으로 더 분류할 수 있다. 부분층 화상은 물집(**Box 13-1**)으로 나타나거나 반짝이거나 축축하게 보이는 피부가 벗겨진 화상 부위로 나타난다. 표재성 진피 화상은 유두 진피까지 확장된다. 이러한 상처는 압력을 받으면 화끈거리고 혈관 확장으로 인해 진피로 가는 혈류가 정상 피부보다 증가한다. 이러한 상처는 통증이 심하고 진피의 잔여물이 살아남기 때문에 이 화상은 종종 치유될 수 있지만

일반적으로 약 3주가 걸린다. 심부 부분층 화상을 입으면 대부분의 진피층이 파괴되고 생존 가능한 표피 세포는 거의 남지 않는다. 생존 불가능한 조직이 두껍고 생존 가능한 진피에 부착되어 있기 때문에 일반적으로 물집이 형성되지 않는다. 혈류가 저하되고 심부 부분층 화상과 전층 화상 상처를 구분하기가 어려운 경우가 많다. 그러나, 만지는 감각을 느낄 수 있다면 심부 부분층 화상 상처라는 것을 나타낸다. 3주 동안 치유되지 않는 심부 부분층 화상 상처는 절제와 이식을 받아야 한다.

부분층 화상의 경우 괴사 부위는 표피 전체와 얕은 진피의 다양한 깊이를 포함한다. 적절한 처치가 시행되지 않으면 정체구역은 괴사로 진행되어 화상이 더 커지고 잠재적으로 전층 화상으로 전환되어 절

제 및 이식이 필요한 더 넓은 부위로 이어질 수 있다. 표재 부분층 화상은 세심한 상처 처치로 치유될 수 있다. 심부 부분층 화상은 위치, 크기, 환자 요인에 따라 수술이 필요한 경우가 많으며 피부 이식을 통해 흉터를 최소화하고 특히 손과 같은 부위의 기능적 기형을 제한할 수 있다.

전층 화상

전층 화상은 조직 깊숙이 화상을 입어 표피와 진피가 완전히 파괴되어 상처를 다시 채울 표피 세포가 남지 않는다. 화염, 액체 또는 화학 원소와 장시간 접촉하여 발생할 수 있다. 전층 화상은 여러 가지 형태로 나타날 수 있다(**그림 13-5**). 이러한 처치는 환자의 인종이나 피부색과 관계없이 대부분 두껍고, 건조하며 흰색의 가죽 같은 화상으로 나타난다(**그림 13-6**). 이렇게 두껍고 가죽처럼 손상된 피부를 가피라고 한다. 심한 경우 피부가 검게 그을린 젓처럼 보이며 혈전(응고)이 보인다(**그림 13-7**). 전층 화상은 감각이 없고 건조하며 두껍고 가죽 같은 느낌이 든다.

　전층 화상 부위는 감각이 없더라도 일반적으로 부분층 화상 부위에 둘러싸여 있다. 또한 환자를 샤워시키고 상처를 세척하기 전에 심부 부분층 화상과 전층 화상을 구별하는 것은 어려울 수 있다. 전층 화상이 아닌 상처는 환자에게 심각한 통증을 유발한다. 또한 전층 화상은 조직의 유연성을 잃기 때문에 특히 가피(전층 화상 상처)가 둘레에 있는 경우 환자는 이러한 수축 효과를 느낄 수 있다. 가슴 주위에 둘레 전층 화상 상처가 생기면 가슴의 움직임과 환기를 방해하여 생명을 위협할 수 있다. 마찬가지로 팔다리 주위의 전층 화상 상처는 부종과 구획증후군을 유발할 수 있다. 이송 중에는 추가적인 부종을 방지하기 위해 전층 화상 상처가 있는 팔다리를 가능한 한 많이 올려야 한다. 전층 화상은 장애를 유발하고 생명을 위협할 수 있으므로 전층 화상을 입은 환자는 화상센터에서 관리해야 한다. 전문

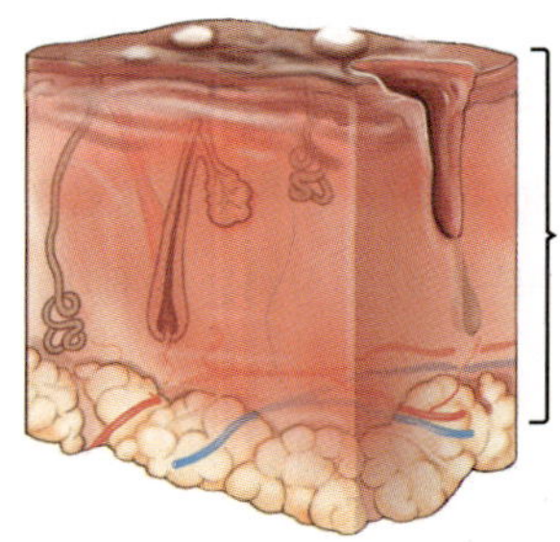

그림 13-5 전층 화상.
© National Association of Emergency Medical Technicians (NAEMT)

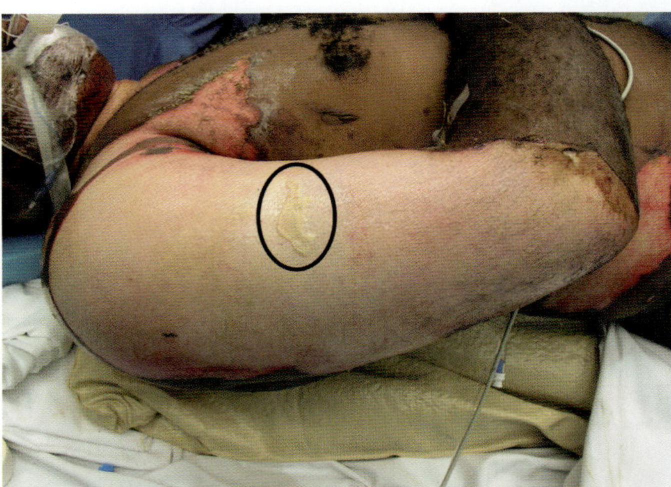

그림 13-6 이 환자는 부분층 화상 및 전층 화상을 입었으며 하얗고 가죽 같은 외관을 특징으로 한다.
Courtesy of Dr. Jeffrey Guy.

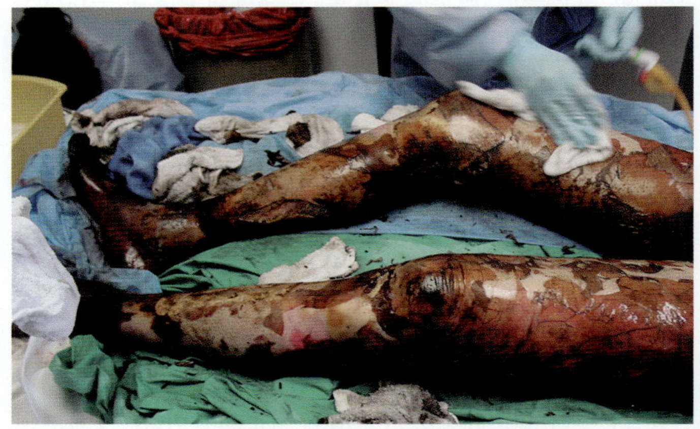

그림 13-7 피부가 그을리고 혈관에 혈전이 보이는 심부 전층 화상의 예이다.
Courtesy of Dr. Jeffrey Guy.

센터에서 신속한 외과적 절제와 집중 재활 치료가 필요하다.

피부밑 화상

피부밑 화상(이전에는 4도 화상이라 함)은 피부의 모든 층을 태울 뿐만 아니라 기저 지방, 근육, 뼈 또는 내부 장기까지 태우는 화상을 말한다(**그림 13-8** 및 **그림 13-9**). 이러한 화상은 실제로 심부 조직 손상을 초래하는 전층 화상이다. 이러한 화상은 피부와 기저 조직 및 구조의 손상으로 인해 극도로 쇠약해지고 손상될 수 있다. 죽은 조직과 상당한 괴사 조직 제거는 광범위한 연부조직 결함을 초래할 수 있다.

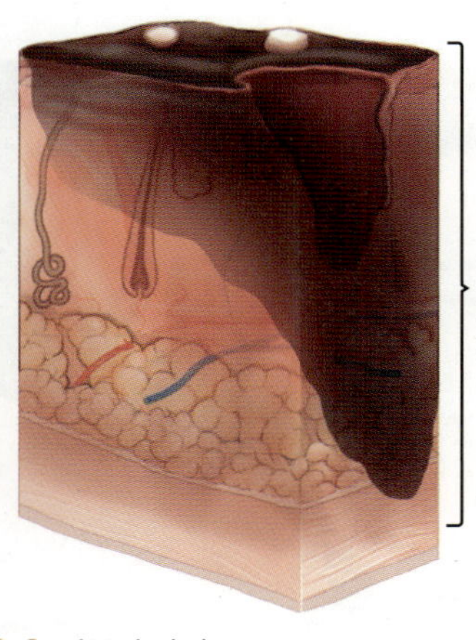

그림 13-8 피부밑 화상.
© National Association of Emergency Medical Technicians (NAEMT)

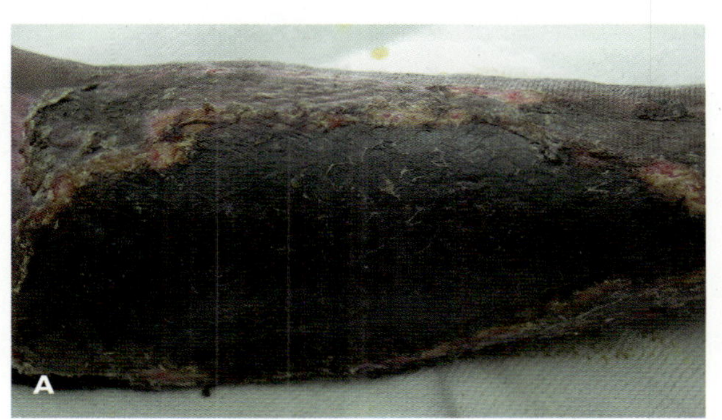
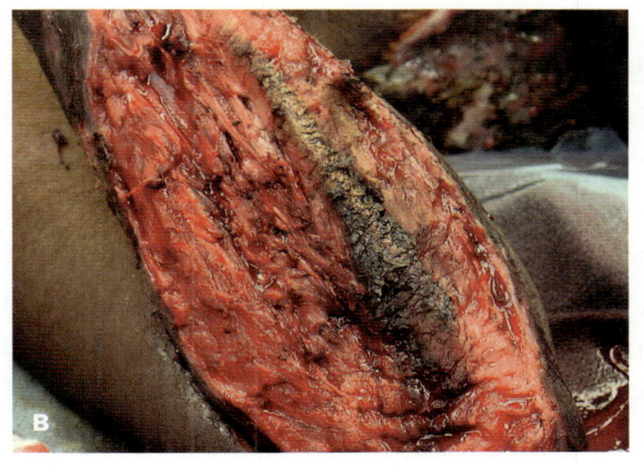

그림 13-9 피부밑 화상은 심부 조직 손상이 있는 전층 화상을 말한다. **A.** 피부. **B.** 피부밑지방, 근육 및 뼈.
Courtesy of Dr. Jeffrey G.y.

화상 평가

일차평가 및 소생술

일차평가의 목표는 생명을 위협하는 문제를 중요도에 따라 체계적으로 평가하고 처치하여 생명을 보존하는 것이다. 주요 화상 손상의 산만한 특성을 고려할 때 화상의 경우 일차평가 알고리즘을 정확하게 기억해야 한다. 화상 과정을 멈추고 현장이 안전한지 확인한 후 처치 알고리즘은 출혈 평가부터 시작한다. 화상 환자는 평가 및 소생술의 모든 단계에서 고유한 문제를 안고 있지만, 화상 환자 처치는 외상 처치 방법인 XABCDE(대량출혈, 기도, 호흡, 순환, 장애, 노출/환경)를 적용할 수 있다.

심한 화상은 매우 병적일 수 있으며 생존 가능성과 결과는 화상 부위의 체표면적에 따라 다르지만, 화상 자체가 즉시 생명을 위협하는 손상은 드물다. 화상의 전체적인 모양이 극적으로 보일 수 있으며 강한 냄새는 방해가 될 수 있다. 이런 것으로 인해 병원 전 처치 제공자는 주의를 분산시켜서는 안 된다. 숙련된 병원 전 처치 제공자는 환자가 화상 외에도 외상을 입었을 수 있으며 더 즉각적인 생명을 위협하는 덜 명백한 내부 손상이 있을 수 있다는 점을 고려해야 한다.

대량 외부출혈 지혈

화상 환자는 외상 환자이다. 주의를 산만하게 하는 화상으로 인한 손상의 특성을 고려할 때 이 기본적인 사실을 잊어서는 안 된다. 외상과 화상센터에서도 의료진은 화상 손상으로 인해 주의가 산만해져 외상 처치 알고리즘을 따르지 못할 수 있다(Box 13-2). 화상은 명백하고 때로는 위협적인 손상이지만, 생명을 위협할 수 있는 덜 명백

한 내부 손상을 평가하는 것이 중요하다. 예를 들어, 화상을 피하려고 건물 창문에서 뛰어내릴 수 있고 불타는 구조물이 무너져 환자에게 떨어지거나 자동차 충돌 사고로 불타는 차 안에 환자가 갇힐 수 있다. 이러한 모든 경우 환자는 화상과 골반 골절, 긴뼈 골절, 뇌손상, 흉복부 손상과 같은 외상성 손상을 모두 입었을 수 있다. 배제하거나 처치해야 하는 즉각적으로 생명을 위협하는 것은 관련 손상으로 인한 출혈이다.

기도

화상 손상은 급성 외상성 손상의 일부이며 모든 외상 환자와 마찬가지로 기도 처치 우선순위에 대한 주의가 가장 중요하다(Box 13-3). 화염에 대한 급성 노출로 인한 열 손상은 성대 수준 이상의 기도에 부종을 유발하여 기도를 폐쇄할 수 있다. 따라서 신중한 초기평가와 지속적인 평가가 필요하다. 이송 시간이 길어질 가능성이 높은 병원

Box 13-2 병원 전 화상 위험

- 화상 손상으로 인해 주의가 산만해져 출혈이나 기타 생명을 위협하는 손상을 인지하고 처치하지 못하는 경우
- 화상 및 출혈이 있는 환자에서 지나치게 적극적인 수액 소생술 시행
- 화상이 가장 생명을 위협하는 손상이 아닐 수 있음을 인지하지 못함
- 저혈압이 있는 화상 환자에서 출혈을 배제하지 못함
- 저체온증 예방 실패
- 화상 부위를 과대 또는 과소평가하고 환자를 과소 또는 과대 또는 과소 소생시키지 않음

전 처치 제공자는 기도 평가에 특히 주의를 기울여야 한다. 화상 환자의 기도 관리는 연기 손상의 우려가 있거나 밀폐된 공간에서 화재로 인한 초기 열 손상이 발생하면 더 어렵다. 미국 화상센터에 입원한 열 손상 환자의 30% 이상은 연기 흡입 손상을 동반한다. 상부 기도에 대한 직접적인 열 손상은 점막이 점진적으로 부어오르는 부종을 유발하여 흡입 시 공기 유입에 대한 저항이 증가할 수 있다. 처음에는 명백한 호흡곤란 징후가 없을 때 모든 환자에게 100% 가습된 산소를 공급해야 한다. 적절한 가슴 상승과 환기를 제한할 수 있는 몸통의 둘레 화상의 유무에 특히 주의하면서 환자를 자세하게 검사해야 한다.

기관내삽관은 급성 호흡곤란 환자, 호흡곤란이 증가하는 환자, 얼굴이나 목에 화상을 입어 부종과 기도 폐쇄를 일으킬 수 있는 환자에게 필요하다. 특히 폭발이나 감속 사고로 인해 화상을 입은 환자의 경우 목뼈 손상에 특히 주의를 기울여야 한다. 기도 폐쇄가 임박했다는 징후는 협착음, 심한 쉰 목소리, 침 흘림이다. 흡입 손상으로 인해 기도에 그을음이 생길 수도 있으므로 기침하거나 다량의 검은색/탄

Box 13-3 화상 환자의 기도 관리 위험성

- 기도의 열 손상 징후를 인지하지 못함. 쉰 목소리, 호흡곤란, 침 흘림, 조직 충혈/수포 등의 징후가 있을 수 있다.
- 기도를 조기에 확보하지 않음. 기도 부종이 악화하면 기관내삽관이 매우 어려워질 수 있다.
- 외과적 기도 유지에 대한 준비가 되어 있지 않은 경우
- 성대 아래에 커프가 있는 튜브가 아닌 후두마스크기도기 또는 임시 기도 장치를 배치한다. 화상 환자는 성대 부종과 관련된 문제를 우회하기 위해 확실하게 기도를 유지해야 한다.
- 기관내관 또는 반지갑상연골절개술을 고정하기 위해 테프를 사용한다. 테이프는 화상 환자의 피부에 달라붙지 않으므로 화상 환자에게 중요한 튜브를 고정할 때는 테이프를 사용하지 않는다.

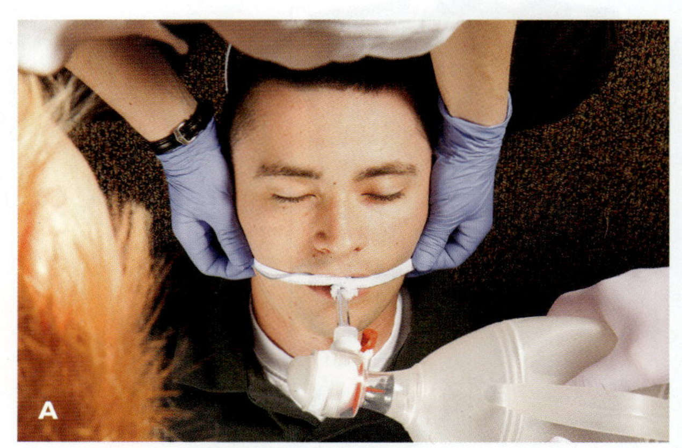

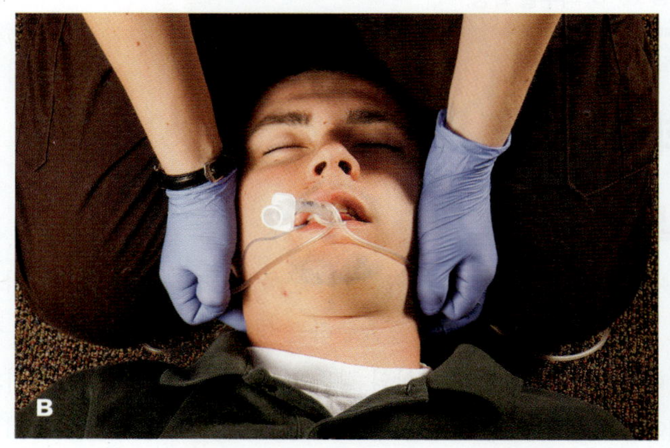

그림 13-10 병원 전 처치 제공자는 환자가 얼굴에 화상을 입은 경우 배꼽 테이프나 수액 세트를 사용하여 기관내관을 고정할 수 있다. **A.** 배꼽 테이프 **B.** 수액 세트.
© Jones & Bartlett Learning. Photographed by Darren Stahlman.

소질의 가래를 배출하는 환자는 기도 손상 여부를 자세히 모니터링해야 한다.

환자에게 기관내삽관을 시행하면 기관내관을 고정할 때 의도치 않은 이탈이나 발관을 방지하기 위해 특별한 예방 조치를 해야 한다. 얼굴에 화상을 입은 후에는 얼굴 피부가 벗겨지거나 진물이 나는 경우가 많으므로 테이프로 기관내관을 고정하는 것은 적합하지 않다. 기관내관을 두 개의 탯줄 테이프(**그림 13-10A**)를 사용하거나 수액 세트를 머리에 감아서 고정할 수 있다. 한쪽은 귀 위로 다른 한쪽은 귀 아래로 감아서 고정한다(**그림 13-10B**). 시중에서 판매되는 천이나 벨크로 제품을 이용할 수도 있다.

호흡

다른 외상 환자와 마찬가지로 갈비뼈 골절, 기흉, 폐쇄성 또는 개방성

가슴 손상과 같은 문제로 인해 호흡에 악영향을 미칠 수 있다. 가슴 우리 둘레 화상의 경우 가슴우리의 순응도가 점차 감소하여 환자의 공기 이동 및 환기 능력을 저해할 수 있다. 이 경우 즉시 신속한 가슴 벽의 가피절개를 시행하고 환자를 수술이 가능한 가장 가까운 의료 기관으로 이송해야 한다. 환자에게 기관절개가 필요하다는 징후는 백밸브로 환기가 어렵거나 환기의 압력 경보가 증가하는 경우이다. 기흉이 이미 배제되었고 환자의 몸통에 둘레 화상이나 전층 화상이 있는 경우 환기를 위해 가피절개가 필요할 수 있다. 가피절개는 딱딱하게 굳은 가피를 절개하여 환자의 호흡 운동에 따라 가슴벽이 확장되고 움직일 수 있도록 하는 수술 절차이다. 부분층 화상은 가슴벽에 이러한 수축 효과를 일으키지 않으므로 가피절개가 필요하지 않다.

순환

혈액 순환을 평가하고 처치하는 과정에는 혈압측정, 둘레 화상 평가 (이 장의 둘레 화상 부분 참조) 및 정맥 라인 확보가 포함된다. 팔다리에 화상을 입으면 혈압을 정확하게 측정하는 것이 어렵거나 불가능하며 혈압을 측정할 수 있더라도 전층 화상 및 팔다리의 부종으로 인해 전신 동맥혈압을 정확하게 반영하지 못할 수 있다. 환자의 동맥혈압이 적절하더라도 둘레 화상으로 인해 팔다리의 원위부 관류가 심각하게 감소할 수 있다. 화상을 입은 팔다리의 부종을 줄이기 위해서 이송 중에 팔다리를 올려준다.

체표면적 20% 이상의 화상을 입은 경우 대량 수액 소생술에 필요한 빠른 유속으로 수액을 투여할 수 있도록 두 개의 대구경 정맥 라인을 확보하는 것은 필수이다. 정맥 라인 확보는 화상을 입은 손상 부위나 화상 부위에 인접하지 않게 시행하는 것이 이상적이지만, 다른 부위에 시행할 수 없는 경우 화상 부위에서 정맥 라인을 확보할 수 있다. 카테터를 화상 부위나 화상 부위 근처에 삽입할 때는 카테터가 실수로 빠지지 않도록 특별한 조치를 해야 한다. 일반적으로 정맥 카테터를 고정하는 데 사용되는 접착테이프와 드레싱은 화상을 입은 조직 위나 인접한 곳에 부착하면 효과가 없다. 화상센터에서는 화상을 입은 환자에게 테이프가 잘 붙지 않기 때문에 정맥 카테터를 제자리에 봉합하는 경우가 많다. 카테터를 고정하는 다른 방법으로 켈릭스(Kerlix)나 코반롤(Coban rolls)로 부위를 감싸는 방법이 있다. 일부 환자의 경우 병원 전 처치 제공자가 정맥 라인을 확보하지 못할 수도 있다. 골내(IO) 주사는 수액이나 진통제를 투여하는 신뢰할 수 있는 대체 방법이다.

장애

화상 환자 특유의 생명을 위협하는 신경학적 장애의 원인은 일산화탄소 및 사이안화수소 가스 등 흡입된 독소의 영향이다. 이러한 독소는 질식을 유발할 수 있다(연기 흡입 손상 부분 참조).

다른 외상 환자와 마찬가지로 환자의 신경 및 운동 기능 장애를 평가한다. 팔다리에 화상을 입으면 드레싱을 시행한 후 긴뼈 골절을 확인하고 필요한 경우 부목을 적용한다. 척추 손상이 의심되는 경우 척추 움직임 제한을 시행한다.

노출/환경

다음 우선순위는 환자를 완전히 노출하는 것이다. 화상 부위가 점차 부어오르면 장신구가 압박 밴드 역할을 하여 말단 부위의 순환을 방해할 수 있으므로 즉시 제거해야 한다. 기계적 외상이 발생한 경우 옷에 가려져 있을 수 있는 손상을 확인하기 위해 환자의 모든 옷을 제거한다. 화상 환자의 옷을 제거하는 것이 잠재적으로 처치 효과가 있을 수 있다. 옷과 장신구에는 잔열이 남아있을 수 있으며 이는 환자에게 손상을 입힐 수 있다. 화학 화상을 입은 후 옷이 환자에게 화상을 입힌 물질이 스며들 수 있다. 화학 화상의 경우 잠재적으로 위험한 물질이 묻은 환자의 의복을 부적절하게 취급하면 환자와 병원 전 처치 제공자 모두에게 손상을 입힐 수 있다. 화학물질 냄새가 나는 옷은 주의해서 취급해야 하며 병원 전 처치 제공자는 보호안경을 포함한 보호 장비를 착용해야 한다.

넓은 면적의 화상을 입은 환자를 처치할 때 외부 온도를 조절하는 것이 중요하다. 넓은 면적의 화상을 입은 환자는 자신의 체온을 유지할 수 없으므로 저체온증에 매우 취약하다. 화상은 피부의 혈관 확장을 유발하여 열 손실을 증가시킨다. 또한 화상으로 인해 개방성 상처를 입으면 체액이 누출되어 증발로 인해 환자의 체온 손실이 더욱 악화한다. 환자의 체온을 유지하기 위해 모든 노력을 기울인다. 마른 시트 위에 담요를 여러 겹으로 환자를 덮는다. 이송하는 구급차 또는 항공기의 객실은 계절과 관계없이 따뜻하게 유지한다. 일반적으로 병원 전 처치 제공자가 적절하다고 느끼는 주변 온도는 너무 낮아서 환자가 저체온증에 걸릴 위험이 있다.

이차평가

일차평가를 완료한 후 다음 목표는 모든 외상 환자에 대한 이차평가를 완료하는 것이다. 화상 손상에 대한 이차평가는 다른 외상 환자에 대한 평가와 다르지 않다. 병원 전 처치 제공자는 머리부터 발끝까지 완전한 평가를 시행해야 한다. 앞서 언급했듯이 화상의 겉모습은 인상적일 수 있지만, 이러한 상처는 일반적으로 즉시 생명을 위협하지는 않는다. 다른 외상 환자와 마찬가지로 철저하고 체계적으로 이차평가를 시행해야 한다. 정맥 라인을 확보해야 하지만, 실패할 수도 있으므로 정맥 라인을 확보하기 위해 환자를 의료기관으로 이송하는 것이 지연되어서는 안 된다. 가장 가까운 의료기관으로 이송하는 시간이 60분 미만이면 정맥 라인을 확보하기 위해 이송을 지연해서는 안 된다. 정맥 라인을 확보화면 화상 면적에 따라 락테이트 링거 용액을 투여해야 한다. 이 초기 수액 투여 속도는 미 육군 외과 연구소(USAISR) 10의 법칙을 사용할 수 있다. 일반적으로 화상 면적에 10을 곱하여 초기 수액 투여 속도를 구할 수 있다. 평균 체중의 성인에서 30% 체표면적 화상을 입은 환자는 시간당 300mL, 40% 체표면적의 화상을 입은 환자는 시간당 400mL, 50% 체표면적의 화상을 입은 환자는 시간당 500mL의 수액을 투여해야 한다. 5세 이상의 어린이는 화상 면적과 어린이의 체격에 따라 시간당 100~250mL를 투여해야 한다.

화상 범위 추정(평가)

일차평가 및 이차평가를 완료하면 화상 상처에 대한 철저한 평가를 시행한다. 상처를 깨끗하게 하고 평가한다. 화상 면적을 추정하는 것은 환자를 적절하게 소생시키고 화상으로 인한 저혈량 쇼크와 관련된 합병증을 예방하는 데 필요하다. 화상 면적의 측정은 손상의 심각성과 중증도를 분류하기 위한 도구로도 사용된다. 가장 널리 적용되는 방법은 9의 법칙으로 성인의 주요 신체 부위를 전체 체표면적의 9%로 간주하는 원칙을 적용한다(**그림 13-11**). 회음부 또는 생식기 부위는 1%를 차지한다.

손바닥 법칙을 사용하여 화상 면적을 평가할 수도 있다(**그림 13-12**). 환자의 손바닥을 사용하는 것은 작은 화상 면적을 추정하기 위해 널리 받아들여지고 오랫동안 사용되었다. 그러나 손바닥을 정의하는 기준과 손바닥의 크기에 대한 통일된 기준은 없다. 손바닥의 평균 면적(펴진 손가락은 제외)은 남성의 경우 체표면적의 0.5%, 여성의 경우 체표면적의 0.4%이다. 손바닥과 함께 다섯 손가락을 다 폈을 때 손가락을 포함한 손바닥 면적을 모두 포함하면 남성의 경우 체

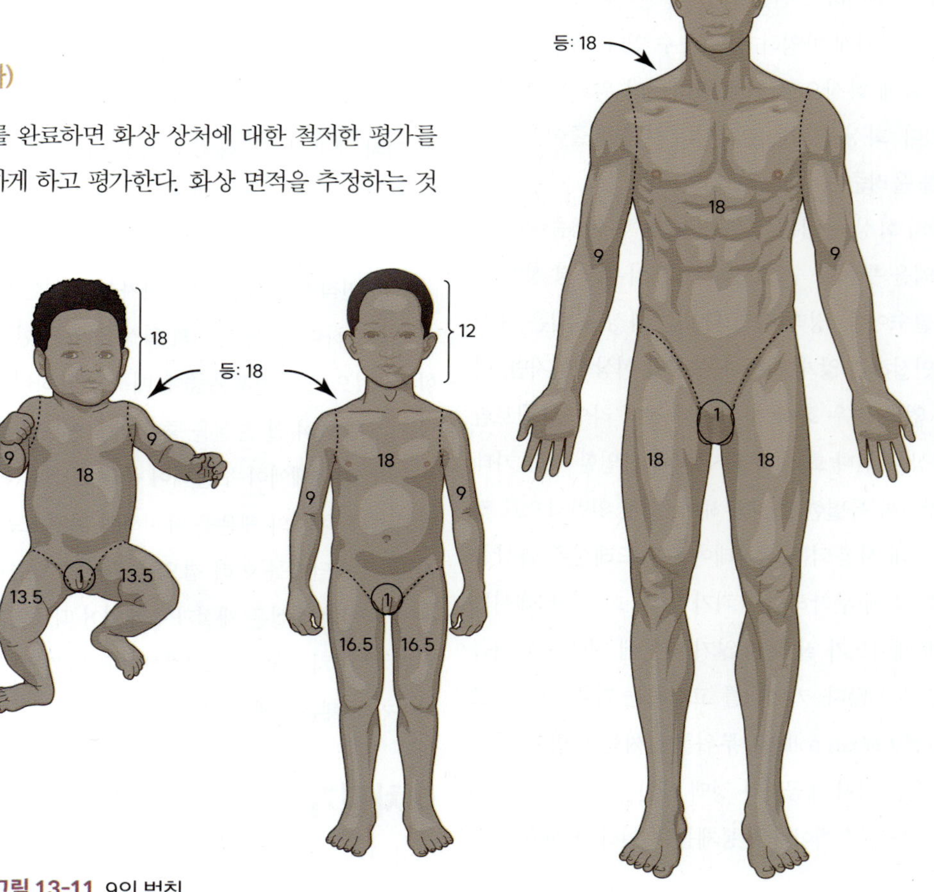

그림 13-11　9의 법칙.
© Jones & Bartlett Learning

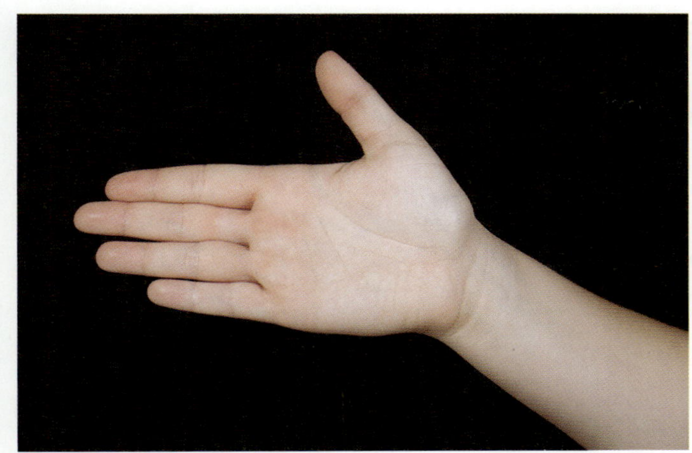

그림 13-12 손바닥 법칙은 환자의 손바닥과 손가락을 사용하여 작은 화상의 면적을 추정한다.
© Jones & Bartlett Learning. Photographed by Kimberly Potvin.

표면적의 0.8%, 여성의 경우 체표면적의 0.7%이다. 손바닥의 면적은 성별에 따라 다르고 환자의 체중에 따라 달라진다. 환자의 체질량지수(BMI)가 증가하면 신체의 체표면적이 증가하고 손바닥의 체표면적 비율은 감소한다. 대부분은 환자의 손바닥과 손가락을 합친 환자의 체표면적은 약 1%로 추정할 수 있다.

어린이의 화상 면적 추정치는 머리의 체표면적이 상대적으로 증가하기 때문에 성인의 화상 면적 추정치와 다르다. 또한, 어린이의 머리와 다리의 체표면적 비율은 나이에 따라 다르다. 룬드-브로더(Lund-Browder) 도표는 어린이의 나이 관련 변화를 고려한 도표이다. 이 도표를 사용하여 병원 전 처치 제공자는 화상 부위를 룬드-브로더 도표에 표시하여 화상 면적을 결정한다(**그림 13-13**). 이 방법을 사용하려면 화상 지도를 그린 다음 지도를 계산된 화상 면적으로 변환해야 한다. 이 방법은 복잡하므로 병원 전 상황에서 사용하기 어렵다.

드레싱

이송하기 전에 상처 부위에 드레싱을 시행해야 한다. 드레싱의 목적은 지속적인 오염을 방지하고 상처 부위의 공기 흐름을 줄여 통증을 조절하는 데 도움이 되도록 하는 것이다.

환자를 이송하기 전에 건조 멸균 시트나 수건 형태의 드레싱을 시행하면 충분하다. 그런 다음 멸균 화상 시트 위에 환자를 위치시키고 여러 겹의 담요로 덮어 환자의 체온을 유지할 수 있도록 한다. 화상 센터에서 환자를 평가할 때까지 국소항생제 연고와 크림을 바르지 않도록 한다.

이송

화상 외에 다발성 손상을 입은 환자는 먼저 외상센터로 이송하여 출혈 및 기타 생명을 위협하는 손상을 확인하고 필요한 경우 외과적 처치를 시행한다. 외상센터에서 안정되면 화상을 입은 환자는 화상센터로 이송하여 최종 화상 치료와 재활 치료를 받을 수 있다. 미국 화상협회와 미국 외과학회는 화상 환자를 화상 센터로 이송하기 위한 기준을 **그림 13-14**에 설명된 바와 같이 확인했다. 화상센터에 쉽게 접근할 수 없는 지역에서는 의료 지도 의사의 의료 지도에 따라 이송할 의료기관을 결정한다.

처치

초기 화상 처치

화상 환자 처치의 초기 단계는 화상의 진행 과정을 멈추는 것이다. 화상을 멈추는 가장 효과적이고 적절한 방법은 다량의 실온수로 세척하는 것이다. 화상 부위에 얼음을 적용하는 것은 화상을 멈추고 통증을 억제해 주지만, 국소 혈관 수축을 자극하여 울혈 구역의 조직 손상 정도를 증가시킬 위험이 있다(**Box 13-4**). 옷과 장신구는 잔열을 유지해 환자에게 지속해서 화상을 입힐 수 있으므로 모두 제거한다. 또한 장신구는 조직이 부어오르기 시작하면서 손가락이나 팔다리를 압착할 수 있다. 화상을 입어 피부에 달라붙은 옷은 제거하지 말고 실온의 물로 식혀야 한다.

최근 화상을 효과적으로 드레싱 하려면 멸균된 비접착성 드레싱을 적용한 후 깨끗하고 건조한 시트로 해당 부위를 덮어준다. 시트를 쉽게 구할 수 없는 경우 멸균 수술 가운, 수건 또는 Mylar 구조용 담요 등으로 대체할 수 있다. 드레싱은 지속적인 환경으로 인한 오염을 방지하는 동시에 노출된 신경 말단위로 공기가 흐르면서 환자가 통증을 느끼는 것을 방지하는 데 도움이 된다. 공기의 흐름이나 화상 피부의 접촉 또는 움직임은 환자에게 상당한 통증을 유발한다. 화상 과정을 멈추고 화상 상처의 공기 이동/오염을 방지하는 것과 균형을 이루어야 한다. 멸균 하이드로겔이 포함된 일부 상업용 드레싱은 두 가지 과정에 모두 사용할 수 있으며 병원 전 환경에서 유용할 수 있다.

병원 전 처치 제공자는 종종 화상 부위에 멸균 시트를 단순하게 적용하는 것에 만족하지 못하고 좌절하는 경우가 많았다. 그러나 국소 연고와 기존의 국소 항생제는 화상 부위를 직접 검사하는 데 방

화상 추정치 및 도표
연령 대 면적적

부위	출생~1세	1~4세	6~9세	10~14세	15세	성인	2도 화상	3도 화상	총	제공자 영역
머리	19	17	13	11	9	7	2			
목	2	2	2	2	2	2	2			
앞 몸통	13	13	13	13	13	13	7	5		
뒤 몸통	13	13	13	13	13	13	8			
오른 엉덩이	2½	2½	2½	2½	2½	2½				
왼 엉덩이	2½	2½	2½	2½	2½	2½	1.5			
생식기	1	1	1	1	1	1	1			
오른위팔	4	4	4	4	4	4				
왼위팔	4	4	4	4	4	4	1			
오른아래팔	3	3	3	3	3	3	1			
왼아래팔	3	3	3	3	3	3	2			
오른 손	2½	2½	2½	2½	2½	2½	2			
왼 손	2½	2½	2½	2½	2½	2½	2.5			
오른 넓적다리	5½	6½	8	8½	9	9½	4			
왼 넓적다리	5½	6½	8	8½	9	9½	4	2		
오른 종아리	5	5	5½	6	6½	7				
왼 종아리	5	5	5½	6	6½	7				
오른 발	3½	3½	3½	3½	3½	3½				
왼 발	3½	3½	3½	3½	3½	3½				
총							38	7	45%	

화상 도표

나이   39
성별   M
체중   Pce Burn Wt. 59.6 kg

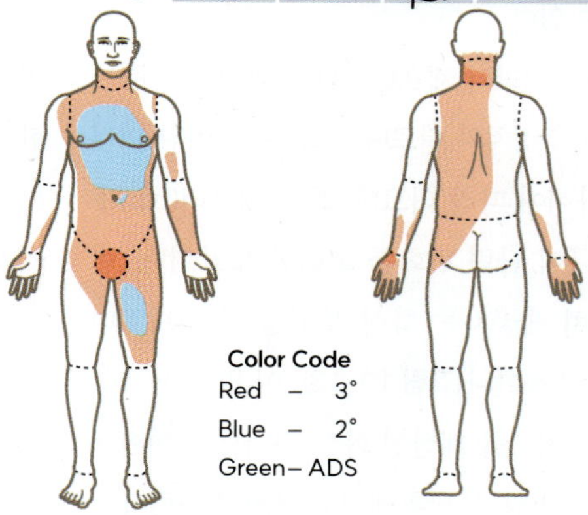

그림 13-13 작성된 룬드-브라우더(Lund-Browder) 차트의 예이다.

© National Association of Emergency Medical Technicians (NAEMT)

해가 되므로 사용해서는 안 된다. 이러한 국소 연고와 항생제를 바른 경우 화상센터에 입원할 때 화상 부위를 직접 눈으로 확인하고 화상 정도를 판단할 수 있도록 제거해야 한다. 또한, 일부 국소 약물은 상처 치유를 돕기 위해 사용되는 가공된 조직 제품의 사용을 복잡하게 만들 수 있다.

고농도 항균 코팅 드레싱은 화상센터에서 상처 치료의 주류를 이루고 있다(**그림 13-15**). 이 드레싱은 은, 유황 또는 꿀과 함께 사용된다. 일부 드레싱은 은으로 코팅되어 있는데, 이 은은 개방된 화상 상처에 바르면 며칠에 걸쳐 서서히 방출된다. 방출된 은은 상처를 오염시키고 감염시키는 일반적인 균에 대한 강력한 항균 효과가 있다. 최근에 이 드레싱은 화상센터에서 병원 전 처치에 이르기까지 적용되고 있다. 이 대형 항균 시트는 화상 부위에 빠르게 부착할 수 있으며 오염된 균을 박멸할 수 있다. 이 상처 처치 방법을 사용하면 병원 전 처치 제공자가 적용 후 30분 이내에 화상 상처 오염을 크게 줄이는 비약물성 장치를 적용할 수 있다. 야생 및 군에서 사용하는 드레싱의 장점은 크기가 작고 가볍다는 것이다. 서류 봉투 크기의 용기에 최소

화상센터 의뢰 기준

화상센터에서는 성인, 어린이 또는 모두를 치료할 수 있다.

화상센터에 의뢰해야 하는 화상 손상은 다음과 같다.

1. 전체 체표면적(TBSA)의 10%를 초과하는 부분층 화상
2. 얼굴, 손, 발, 생식기, 회음부 또는 주요 관절에 화상을 입은 경우
3. 모든 연령대의 3도 화상
4. 낙뢰 손상을 포함한 전기 화상
5. 화학 화상
6. 흡입 손상
7. 화상 처치를 복잡하게 하거나, 회복을 지연시키거나, 사망률에 영향을 미칠 수 있는 기저 질환이 있는 환자의 화상으로 인한 손상
8. 화상 및 동반되는 외상(예: 골절)이 있는 환자 중 화상 손상이 이환율 또는 사망률의 가장 큰 위험을 초래하는 경우. 이러한 경우 외상이 더 큰 즉각적인 위험을 초래하는 경우, 환자는 화상 병동으로 이송되기 전에 외상센터에서 먼저 안정될 수 있다. 이러한 상황에서는 의사의 판단이 필요하며 지역 의료 통제 계획 및 분류 프로토콜과 일치해야 한다.
9. 어린이를 돌볼 수 있는 자격을 갖춘 인력이나 장비가 없는 병원에서 화상을 입은 어린이
10. 특별한 사회적, 정서적 또는 재활 치료가 필요한 환자의 화상

중증도 결정

1도(표재)
표재성이고 붉으며 때때로 통증이 있다.

2도(부분층)
피부가 붉어지고 물집이 생기고 부어오를 수 있다. 매우 고통스럽다.

3도(전층)
희끄무레하거나 검게 그을리거나, 반투명하며 화상 부위에 핀으로 찌르는 듯한 감각이 없다.

전체 체표면적(TBSA) 비율

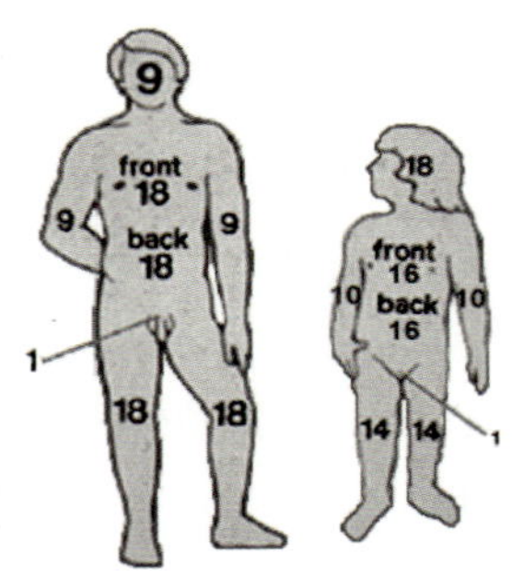

그림 13-14 화상 환자를 화상센터로 이송하거나 이송하기 위한 미국 화상 협회 기준
Courtesy of the American College of Surgeons.

Box 13-4 화상 냉각

잠재적으로 논란이 될 수 있는 주제는 화상 부위를 냉각하는 방법이다. 몇몇 연구자들이 다양한 냉각 방법이 화상을 입은 조직의 상처 치유에 미치는 영향뿐만 아니라 화상 조직의 미세한 외관에 미치는 영향을 평가했다. 한 연구에서 연구자들은 화상 냉각이 실험적으로 시행한 화상 상처에 유익한 효과가 있다는 결론을 내렸다. 냉각을 시행한 화상은 냉각하지 않은 화상보다 세포 손상이 적었다.

연구자들은 냉각이 화상을 입은 진피의 온도, 조직의 미세 구조, 상처 치유에 미치는 영향을 직접 측정할 수 있었다. 한 연구에서는 다양한 냉각 방법의 결과를 평가하였다. 연구자들은 15℃의 수돗물로 화상 부위를 식힌 경우와 시중에서 판매되는 젤을 바르는 경우를 비교했다. 각 방법은 화상 직후와 30분 지연 후에 적용했다. 즉각적인 수돗물 냉각은 화상 조직 내의 온도를 낮추는 데 거의 2배나 효과적이었다. 이 실험에서 냉각된 상처는 손상 후 3주 후에 미세한 더 나은 외관과 상처 치유를 보였다.

얼음으로 화상 부위를 과도하게 식히는 것은 해로우며 화상으로 인해 이미 손상된 조직의 손상을 증가시킬 수 있다. 이러한 사실은 동물 실험에서 입증되었는데, 얼음으로 즉시 화상 부위를 식히는 것이 수돗물을 사용하거나 아무런 처치를 하지 않는 것보다 더 해로운 것으로 나타났다. 1~8℃의 얼음물을 적용하면 냉각 처치를 전혀 하지 않은 화상보다 조직 파괴가 더 많이 발생했다. 반대로 12~18℃의 수돗물로 냉각하면 냉각되지 않은 상처에서 관찰된 것보다 조직 괴사가 적고 치유 속도가 빨랐다.

중요한 고려 사항은 냉각에 관한 연구가 실험동물을 대상으로 수행되었으며 화상을 입은 면적이 매우 제한적이었다. 평가된 화장 면적 중 가장 심한 화상의 체표면적은 10%이었다.

요약하면 화상 부위를 냉각하는 방법이 같은 것은 아니다. 병원 전 환경에서는 급성 화상 과정을 멈추기 위해 상온의 물로 냉각을 실시할 수 있지만, 너무 공격적인 냉각은 추가적인 조직 손상을 초래할 수 있으므로 그 이상은 실시하지 않아야 한다. 또한, 급성 화상 과정을 멈추는 것 이상의 지속적인 냉각은 심한 화상을 입은 환자에게 저체온증을 유발할 수 있다. 화상 냉각의 또 다른 잠재적 위험은 화상과 기계적 외상을 동시에 입은 환자의 경우 전신 저체온증이 응고를 형성하는 혈액의 능력에 예측 가능하고 해로운 영향을 미칠 수 있다는 것이다.

한의 무게로 보관할 수 있는 항균 드레싱은 성인 한 명 전체를 덮을 수 있다.

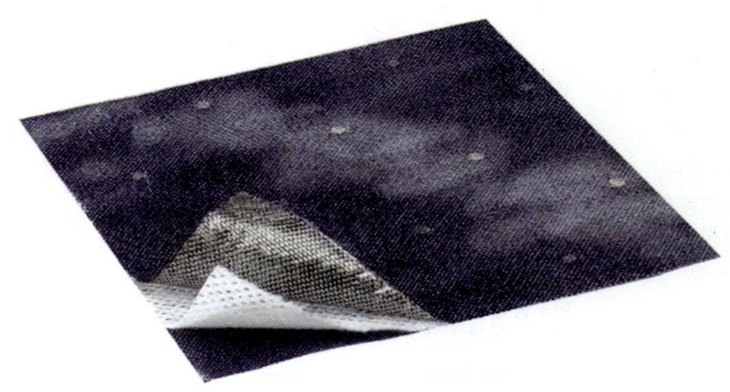

그림 13-15 액티코트 드레싱.
Courtesy of Smith & Nephew.

수액 소생술

화상 손상을 입으면 세포의 완전성이 직접적으로 파괴되고 매개체가 지속해 방출되어 혈관 투과성과 미세혈관 정수압이 증가한다. 이로 인해 혈관 내 공간에서 사이질로 체액이 대량으로 유출된다. 초기 수액 소생술의 근본적인 목표는 혈관 내 체액을 보충하고 처음 24~48시간 동안 혈량저하증이 발생하지 않도록 환자를 지원하는 것이다.

화상 손상의 수액 소생술은 혈관 내 용적 손실을 회복하는 것뿐만 아니라 예상되는 혈관 내 용적 손실을 실제 손실과 유사한 속도로 대체하는 것을 목표로 한다(**Box 13-5**). 외상 환자의 경우 병원 전 처치 제공자는 개방골절 또는 내부출혈로 인해 이미 손실된 용적을 대체한다. 이와는 대조적으로 화상을 입은 환자를 처치할 때는 환자가 이미 손실한 체액을 계산하여 보충하는 것이 목표일뿐만 아니라 화상 손상 후 첫 24시간 동안 환자가 잃을 것으로 예상되는 수분을 보충하는 것이다. 조기 수액 소생술은 화상 환자가 쇼크로 진행되는 것을 예방하는 데 목적이 있다. 화상 환자에게 소변 배출량을 유지하는 것은 필수적이며 적절한 소생술의 주요 지표이다. 체표면적의 20%를 초과해 화상을 입은 환자는 소변 배출량을 자세히 모니터링해야 하며 40%를 초과해 화상을 입은 모든 환자는 시간당 소변 배출량을 모니터링하기 위해 도뇨관을 삽입해야 한다. 화상 소생술은 소변 배출량에 따라 시행할 수 있으며 이 장에 제시된 공식은 시간당 평균 소변 배출량으로 모니터링할 수 있는 혈관 내 용적을 회복하는 것을 목표로 한다. 소변 배출량을 수액 소생술의 목표로 삼는 데 어려움이 있다면 중증 화상 환자에게 급성 신장 손상 및 무뇨증이 발생할 정도로 쇼크가 심할 경우 젖산 및 염기 결핍과 같은 소생술의 다른 평가 지표를 자세히 모니터링해야 한다.

화상 환자를 소생시키는 것은 새는 양동이에 물을 채우는 것에 비유할 수 있다. 양동이에서 일정한 속도로 물이 새고 있다. 양동이 안쪽 상단부근에 선이 그려져 있다. 목표는 물의 수위를 그려진 선에 맞추어 일정하게 유지하는 것이다. 처음에는 수심이 낮을 것이다. 양동이를 오래 방치할수록 수위가 낮아지고 보충해야 하는 물의 양이 많아진다. 용기에서 계속 누수가 발생하므로 양동이를 적절한 수준까지 채운 후에는 원하는 수준을 유지하기 위해 일정한 속도로 물을 계속 추가해야 한다.

화상 환자가 소생하지 못하거나 소생하지 않은 상태로 있는 시간이 길어질수록 환자는 더 심한 혈량저하 상태가 된다. 따라서 체액의 항상성을 유지하기 위해 더 많은 양의 수액이 필요하다. 환자가 소생한 후에도 혈관 공간은 양동이와 같은 방식으로 계속 누출된다. 이 항상성 지점과 평형을 유지하려면 지속해서 손실을 대체하기 위해 추가 수액을 공급해야 한다. 과소생술을 과소생술만큼이나 해로울 수 있으므로 투여되는 수액을 추적하는 것이 중요하다. 이송 시간이 1시간 이상인 환자의 경우 수액 소생술과 관련해 환자를 이송할 의료기관의 의사에게 의료 지도를 받는다. 일부 지역에서는 화상 소생술에 혈장을 사용하기 시작했으며 이 방법이 더 널리 사용됨에 따라 병원 전 환경으로 확대될 수 있다.

성인 환자

화상 환자의 수액 소생술 초기 처치에는 정맥 내 수액 투여, 특히 락테이트 링거액(lactated Ringer's solution)을 투여하는 것이 가장 좋다. 모든 소생술 공식은 소생술에 대한 생리학적 반응에 따라 조절되는 수액 소생술 양에 대한 초기 지침이다. 소변 배출량은 화상 소생술의 가장 좋은 모니터이며 목표 소변 배출량은 이상적인 체중의 0.5~1.0mL/kg/hr이다. 과도한 소생술은 부족한 소생술과 마찬가지로 많은 해로운 영향을 미칠 수 있으므로 피해야 한다. 수액 소생술을 위해 투여한 수액과 시간당 소변 배출량은 체표면적이 40%를 초과하는 화상을 입은 모든 환자를 모니터링해야 한다. 손상 후 처음 24시간 동안 투여하는 수액의 양은 일반적으로 2~4mL × 체중(kg) × 체표면적(부분 및 전층 화상)이다. 현재 권장 사항은 2mL/kg/%(체표면적)로 수액 소생술을 시작하는 것이다. 이는 시작 속도이며 이후 측정된 소변 배출량에 따라 투여 속도를 조절한다. 화상 환자에게 수액 소생술을 시행할 때 사용하는 몇 가지 공식이 있다. 가장 주목할 만한 것은 파크랜드 공식과 브룩 공식이다. 파크랜드 공식은 4mL × 체중(kg) × 화상 면적(%) 비율로 수액을 공급하는 공식이다. 이 수액의 절반은 화상 후 처음 8시간 이내에 투여해야 하고 나머지 절반은 8~24시간 사이에 투여해야 한다.

수액의 절반은 병원 전 처치 제공자가 환자를 처치하기 시작한 시점이 아니라 환자가 화상을 입은 시점부터 8시간 이내에 투여해야 한다는 점에 유의한다. 이 세부 사항은 초기 처치가 지연될 수 있는 야생이나 군대 환경에서 특히 중요하다. 예를 들어 환자가 화상을 입은 후 3시간 동안 수액 투여 없이 응급 처치를 받기 위해 내원하는 경우 계산된 전체 수액량의 절반을 향후 5시간 동안 투여해야 한다. 따라서 환자는 손상 후 8시간이 지나면 목표 수액량을 투여받게 된다.

화상 환자의 소생술에는 0.9% 생리식염수보다 락테이트 링거액을 사용하는 것이 좋다. 화상 환자는 일반적으로 다량의 수액을 정맥 내로 투여하는 것이 필요하다. 화상 소생술 과정에서 다량의 생리식염수를 투여받은 환자는 생리식염수 수액에 포함된 다량의 염화물로 인해 종종 고염소혈산증이 발생하는 경우가 있다. 화상 환자에게는 생리식염수를 투여하지 않는다.

수액 소생술 투여량 계산

화상 환자의 소생술을 위한 초기 수액 공급량은 브룩 공식[(2mL × 체중(kg) × 화상 면적(%)] 또는 파크랜드 공식[4mL × 체중(kg) × 화상 면적(%)]을 기준으로 한다.

예를 들어, 80kg인 남성이 체표면적 30%에 해당하는 전층 화상을 입었고 손상 직후 현장에서 처치하고 있다고 가정해 보겠다. 수액 소생술의 양은 파크랜드 공식을 사용하여 다음과 같이 계산할 수 있다.

$$\textbf{24시간 동안 투여할 수액량} = 4\text{mL} \times 체중(\text{kg}) \times 체표면적(\%)$$
$$= 4 \times 80 \times 30$$
$$= 9{,}600\text{mL}$$

24시간 동안 투여해야 할 수액량을 계산하고 이것을 2로 나누어 8시간 이 내에 투여할 수액량을 구한다.

$$\textbf{8시간 이내에 투여할 수액량} = 9{,}600\text{mL} \div 2 = 4{,}800\text{mL}$$

따라서 한 시간 동안 투여할 수액량은 8시간 이내에 투여할 수액량을 8로 나누면 된다.

$$\textbf{1시간 이내에 투여할 수액량} = 4{,}800\text{mL} \div 8\text{h} = 600\text{mL}$$

나머지 16시간 동안 투여할 수액량은 다음과 같다.

$$\textbf{16시간 동안 투여할 수액량} = 9{,}600\text{mL} \div 2 = 4{,}800\text{mL}$$

마지막 16시간 동안 시간당 투여할 수액량은 16으로 나누면 된다.

$$\textbf{1시간 이내에 투여할 수액량} = 4{,}800\text{mL} \div 16\text{h} = 300\text{mL}$$

화상 소생술을 위한 USAISR 10의 법칙

병원 전 환경에서 화상 환자의 수액 요구량을 계산하는 과정을 간소화하기 위해 미 육군 외과 연구소(USAIRS)의 연구원들은 초기 수액 소생술에 도움이 되는 10의 법칙을 개발했다. 화상 체표면적의 백분율(%)을 계산하여 10으로 반올림한다. 예를 들어, 체표면적의 37% 화상을 입은 환자의 체표면적을 반올림하여 40%로 한다. 그런 다음 백분율에 10을 곱하여 시간당 투여하는 수액량(mL)을 구한다. 따라서 앞의 예를 가지고 계산하면 $40 \times 10 = 400\text{mL/hr}$이다. 이 공식은 체중이 40~70kg인 성인에게 사용한다. 환자가 이 체중 범위를 초과하는 경우 체중이 70kg을 초과할 때마다 체중이 10kg씩 늘어날 때마다 시간당 100mL를 추가로 투여한다.

10의 법칙을 파크랜드 공식과 비교하면 계산된 수액량이 약간만 다르다는 것을 즉시 알 수 있다. 수액 요구량을 계산하는 데 어떤 방법을 사용하든 계산된 수액 요구량은 추정치이며 환자에게 제공되는 실제 수액량은 환자의 임상 반응에 따라 조정해야 한다. 임상 반응의 가장 좋은 지표는 소변 배출량, 정상 혈압, 뇌손상이 없는 경우 적절한 의식 상태이다.

소아 환자

화상을 입은 소아의 수액 소생술은 성인보다 더 적은 체표면적(10~20%)에 화상을 입은 후에 시작한다. 소아 환자는 비슷한 크기의 화상을 입은 성인보다 상대적으로 더 많은 양의 수액을 정맥 내로 투여해야 한다(때에 따라 5.8~6.2mL/kg/체표면적(%)인 것으로 보고됨). 어린이는 체중에 비해 체표면적이 크기 때문에 체액 손실이 비례적으로 더 크다. 또한 소아는 화상 소생 기간 적절한 혈당을 유지하기 위해 간에서 대사성 글리코겐 저장량이 적다. 이러한 이유로 어린이는 표준 유지 수액과 함께 5% 포도당이 함유된 수액(D5LR)을 정맥 내로 표준 속도로 투여해야 한다. 이송 시간이 1시간 이상인 소아 화상 환자는 저혈당 상태가 되지 않도록 혈당 검사를 시행한다. 또한 화상 범위가 넓은 소아 환자는 이송할 의료기관에 사전에 보고한다.

연기 흡입: 수액 소생술 및 기타 고려 사항

열 화상과 흡입 화상이 동반된 환자는 더 많은 양의 수액 소생술이 필요할 수 있다. 화상센터에서 기관지 내시경을 통해 진단이 이루어지기 때문에 병원 전 환경에서는 흡입 손상 유무를 판단하기 어려운 경우가 많다. 이러한 환자의 소생술은 흡입 손상이 없는 유사한 화상에 비해 훨씬 더 많은 수액이 필요한 것으로 보고되었다. 흡입 손상을 입은 환자는 협착음, 그을린 코털 등의 다른 징후가 있을 가능성이 높으며 병원 전 기도 및 호흡 관리가 필요할 수 있다.

연기 흡입 및 흡입 손상과 처치 고려사항에 대한 자세한 내용은 다음 부분에서 설명한다.

통증 조절

화상은 극도로 고통스러우므로 병원 전 환경에서부터 통증 완화를 위해 적절한 주의를 기울여야 한다. 통증을 조절하기 위해 적절한 용량의 펜타닐(1mcg/kg) 또는 모르핀(0.1mg/kg)과 같은 마약성 진통제를 투여해야 한다. 케타민 0.5mg/kg은 화상 환자에게 매시간 안전하게 사용하여 통증 조절을 강화하고 마약성 진통제 사용과 관련된 합병증 위험을 줄일 수 있다.

특별한 고려 사항

전기 손상

전기 손상은 겉으로 보이는 피부 손상만으로는 드러나지 않을 수 있는 기저 조직 파괴 및 괴사와 함께 치명적인 손상이 될 수 있다. 전기 손상의 중증도는 전압, 전류, 전류 흐름 경로, 접촉 시간 및 접촉 지점의 저항에 의해 결정된다.

전기 손상은 교류(AC) 또는 직류(DC)의 전류로 인해 발생한다. 전기 손상은 저전압(<1,000V) 또는 고전압(>1,000V)에서 발생할 수 있다. 전류는 일반적으로 저항이 가장 적은 경로(신경과 혈관을 통해)를 따라 흐르지만, 고전압 전류는 유입 지점과 접지 사이를 직접 통과할 수 있다. 전류는 유입 지점에 집중된 후 갈라졌다가 다시 모였다가 빠져나가기 때문에 접촉 부위와 빠져나가는 부위에서 가장 심각한 조직 손상이 발생한다(**그림 13-16**). 고전압 전기 손상은 종종 피부에 검은 금속 코팅을 남기는 검게 그을린 깊은 화상을 입는다. 조직 손상의 심각도는 접촉 부위 주변에서 가장 크며 전류의 경로와 관련하여 중요한 장기에 손상이 발생한다.

전기 화상을 치료할 때 병원 전 처치 제공자는 기저 조직의 손상을 과소평가하기 쉬우므로 일반적으로 수액 소생술 요구량은 체표면적을 측정하여 추정할 수 없다는 점을 명심해야 한다. 기저 조직 약화는 종종 광범위하며 근육 조직 손상을 수반한다. 종종 영향을 받은 근육을 둘러싼 근막이 팔다리에 부종을 제안하고 그 결과 영향을

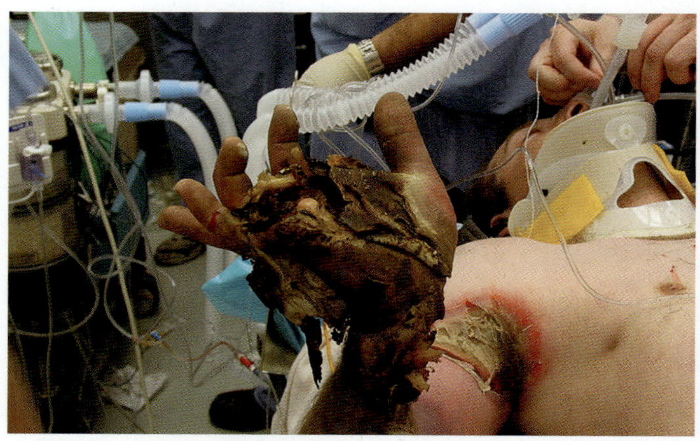

그림 13-16 고압 전선으로 인한 전기 손상 후 환자
Courtesy of Dr. Jeffrey Guy.

받는 구획의 압력이 상승한다. 이에 따라 영향을 받은 팔다리 내에 구획증후군이 발생할 수 있다.

초기 전기 손상으로 인한 이차적인 허혈이 지속되고 구획 압력이 지속해서 증가하면 6~8시간 후에 돌이킬 수 없는 근육 손상이 발생할 수 있다. 구획 내 근육 괴사는 사이토카인 매개체의 추가 방출을 초래하여 혈관 투과성을 증가시키고 손상 부위로 체액의 유출을 증가시킨다. 괴사한 근육에서 방출된 헤모글로빈은 신장을 통해 순환된다. 근육에서 발견되는 또 다른 분자인 미오글로빈이 방출되면 신장 집합관이 막혀 급성신부전으로 이어진다. 이 상태인 근색소뇨는 차 또는 콜라 색의 소변으로 나타난다(**그림 13-17**). 전신 손상을 입은 환자 이송 중 구획증후군에 대해 할 수 있는 처치는 한계가 있다. 환자를 이송하는 의료기관의 의료진에게 구획증후군에 대한 우려를 보고하는 것이 중요하다.

전기 손상과 으깸 손상은 많은 유사한 점이 있다. 두 손상 모두 많은 근육이 대량으로 파괴되고 그 결과 칼륨과 미오글로빈이 모두 방출된다(12장 근골격 외상 참조). 근육에서 칼륨의 방출되면 혈청 칼슘 수치가 많이 증가하여 심장 부정맥이 발생할 수 있다. 칼륨 수치가 높아지면 탈분극성 근육 이완제인 석시닐콜린의 투여가 매우 위험해질 수 있다. 급속연속기관삽관과 같이 환자에게 약물을 이용한 마비가 필요한 경우 베쿠로늄이나 로쿠로늄과 같은 비탈분극제를 사용할 수 있다. 석시닐콜린은 중증 고칼륨혈증의 위험이 있으므로 화상 또는 으깸 손상 환자에게 이차적으로 사용해서는 안 된다.

전기 손상을 입은 환자의 병원 간 이송을 위해 병원 전 처치 제공자가 출동할 수 있다. 전원을 해야 하는 전기 화상은 이송 전에 전해질을 검사해야 하며 도뇨관을 삽입한 상태로 이송한다. 근색소뇨

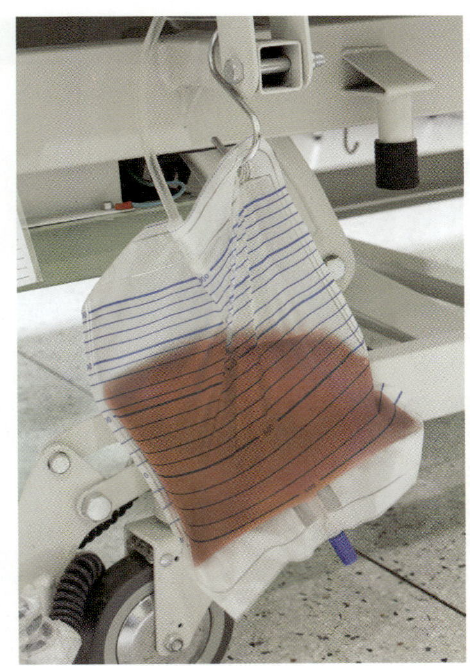

그림 13-17 고압 전선으로 인해 전기적 손상을 입은 환자의 소변. 환자는 광범위한 근육 파괴 후 근색소뇨가 있다.

© Suphatthra China/Shutterstock

가 있는 환자는 급성 신장 손상을 방지하기 위해 성인의 경우 시간당 100mL 이상, 어린이의 경우 1mL/kg 이상의 소변 배출량을 유지하기 위해 적극적인 수액 투여가 필요하다. 미오글로빈의 소변 내 용해도를 높이고 신장 손상 가능성을 줄이기 위해 중탄산나트륨을 투여하는 경우도 있지만, 급성 신장 손상 예방에 대한 실제 이점은 여전히 논쟁의 여지가 있으며 의도한 효과를 얻기 위해 소변을 적절한 pH로 알칼리화하기는 매우 어렵다. 병원 전 환경이나 병원 간 이송 중에는 소변 알칼리화를 시도해서는 안 된다.

전기 화상을 입은 환자는 기계적 손상도 동반할 수 있다. 전기 화상 환자의 약 15%는 외상성 손상을 동반한다. 이 비율은 다른 손상 기전으로 화상을 입은 환자보다 2배나 높다. 고막이 파열되어 청력 장애가 발생할 수 있다. 강렬하고 지속적인 근육 수축(근육 경련)은 어깨 탈구 및 척추와 긴뼈의 압박 골절을 초래할 수 있으므로 전기 손상 환자에게는 척추 움직임 제한을 고려해야 한다. 긴뼈 골절이 발견되거나 의심되는 경우 부목으로 고정해야 한다. 두개 내 출혈과 심장 부정맥도 발생할 수 있다.

전류가 가슴을 통과했다면 심장이 전류 일부를 받았을 수 있다. 현장에서의 심정지는 감전으로 인한 즉각적인 사망의 가장 흔한 원인이다. 환자가 심장 기능을 회복하더라도 심근 불안정성이 지속될 수

있다. 칼슘과 마그네슘 수치가 낮으면 이를 악화시킬 수 있다. 다른 병원에서 외상센터로 이송하는 환자는 이송 전에 심전도와 전해질 검사를 받아야 한다.

둘레 화상

몸통이나 팔다리의 둘레 화상은 두껍고 비탄성 가피가 형성되어 생명이나 팔다리를 위협하는 상태를 초래할 수 있다. 가슴둘레 화상은 가슴벽을 수축시켜 환자가 숨을 들이마시지 못해 질식할 수 있다. 팔다리 둘레 화상을 입으면 팔다리에 지혈대를 착용한 것과 같은 효과가 발생하여 팔다리에 맥박이 촉지되지 않을 수 있다. 따라서 모든 둘레 화상은 응급상황으로 처리하고 환자를 화상센터로 이송하거나 화상센터로 즉시 이송할 수 없는 경우 외상센터로 이송해야 한다. 앞서 설명한 바와 같이 가피절개는 더 깊은 조직을 확장하고 이전에 압박되어 종종 폐쇄된 혈관 구조를 감압할 수 있도록 화상 가피 절개를 통해 이루어지는 외과적 절개이다(**그림 13-18**).

연기 흡입 손상

화재로 인한 주요 사망 원인은 열 손상이 아니라 독성 연기 흡입이다. 밀폐된 공간에서 연기에 노출된 모든 환자는 흡입 손상의 위험이 있는 것으로 간주한다. 얼굴에 화상을 입거나 가래에 그을음이 있는 피해자는 연기 흡입 손상의 위험이 있지만, 이러한 징후가 없다고 해서 독성 흡입 손상을 배제할 수는 없다(**Box 13-6**). 노출 후 며칠 동안 징후와 증상이 나타나지 않을 수도 있으므로 높은 의심 지수를 유지하는 것이 매우 중요하다.

흡입 손상은 증기, 뜨거운 공기, 가스 또는 독성 연기로 인해 발생

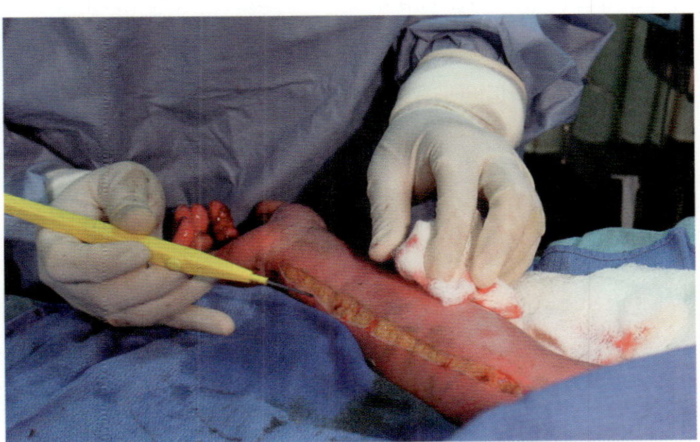

그림 13-13 둘레 화상의 수축 효과를 완화하기 위해 가피절개술을 시행한다.

Courtesy of Dr. Jeffrey Guy.

Box 13-6 연기 흡입/흡입 손상을 암시하는 단서

- 밀폐된 공간에서 발생한 화상
- 혼란 또는 동요
- 얼굴이나 가슴에 화상을 입은 경우
- 눈썹이나 코털의 탄 자국
- 심정지(저산소증 또는 일산화탄소)
- 가래의 그을음(탄소성 가래)
- 쉰 목소리, 목소리 소실 또는 협착음

Box 13-7 일산화탄소 중독의 증상

- 경증
  - 두통
  - 피로감
  - 구역
- 중등도
  - 심한 두통
  - 구토
  - 혼동
  - 기면/졸음
  - 심박수 및 호흡수 증가
- 중증
  - 경련
  - 혼수
  - 심정지

한다. 흡입 손상은 상부기도 손상, 하부기도 손상, 폐실질 손상 및 전신 독성을 초래할 수 있다. 화재 발생 환경에 따라 다양한 재료와 화학물질이 연소 과정의 일부가 될 수 있으며, 이러한 화합물이 함께 작용하여 손상과 이환율을 증가시킬 수 있다. 손상의 정도는 발화지점, 온도, 농도 및 생성된 가스의 용해도에 따라 영향을 받는다.

입인두, 기관지 부위 및 폐 실질에 부종이 형성되는 것은 연기 흡입 손상의 많은 영향을 설명한다. 지속적인 부종은 미세혈관 파열을 일으켜 가스 교환을 억제한다. 또한 부종이 입인두를 막아 환자의 호흡을 어렵고 하고 삽관을 어렵게 만들 수도 있다. 이것이 조기 삽관 및 기도 확보가 필수적인 이유 중 하나이다. 기도 또는 흡입 손상이 우려되는 경우 적극적인 수액 소생술과 그로 인한 부종 형성 전에 삽관을 시행해야 한다.

독성 가스 흡입 손상

임상적으로 중요한 두 가지 기체 생성물은 일산화탄소와 사이안화수소다. 두 분자는 모두 질식제로 분류되며 세포 저산소증에 의한 세포 사멸을 유발한다. 이러한 화합물 중 하나 또는 두 가지가 모두 포함된 연기로 인해 질식한 환자는 적절한 혈압이나 맥박산소측정기 측정값이 정상으로 측정되더라도 조직에 산소가 충분히 전달되지 않는다.

일산화탄소

일산화탄소는 나무, 종이, 면과 같은 일반적인 제품이 불완전 연소할 때 발생하는 무색, 무취의 기체이다. 자동차 배기가스에서도 생성될 수 있다. 일산화탄소는 산소보다 훨씬 큰 친화력으로 헤모글로빈에 결합한다. 헤모글로빈에 대한 이러한 경쟁적인 결합은 조직으로의 산소 전달을 감소시켜 특히 산소 소비량이 많은 조직(뇌와 심장)에서 심각한 저산소증을 유발한다. 일산화탄소 흡입 증상은 노출 기간 또는 심각도와 그에 따른 혈청 농도에 따라 달라진다. 증상은 경미한 두통

부터 혼란, 무의식, 심정지, 경련, 사망에 이르기까지 다양하다(**Box 13-7**). 일산화탄소 중독 환자는 전형적으로 붉은 체리 색 피부색이 나타난다고 가르친다. 안타깝게도 이는 종종 뒤늦게 나타나는 징후이므로 진단을 고려할 때 이에 의존해서는 안 된다. 진단은 동맥혈 또는 정맥혈에서 일산화탄소헤모글로빈의 직접 측정을 기반으로 해야 한다. 일산화헤모글로빈과 산소헤모글로빈을 구별할 수 없으므로 맥박산소측정기의 사용이 제한된다. 맥박산소측정기는 일산화탄소 중독으로 인한 심각한 세포 저산소증이 있는 환자에서 정상으로 판독될 수 있다. 맥박산소측정기는 일산화탄소 중독을 감지하는 데 사용해서는 안 되며 흡입 손상이 의심되는 환자에게 보충 산소 공급을 보류하는 것이 안전한지 판단하는 데 사용해서는 안 된다.

혈류 내 일산화탄소의 양을 비침습적으로 측정하는 휴대용 맥박 일산화탄소측정기는 병원 전 환경에서 사용할 수 있다(**그림 13-19**). 이 측정 장비는 맥박산소측정기와 모양과 작동 방식이 비슷하다. 환자는 일반적으로 10~20%의 일산화탄소헤모글로빈 농도에서 경미한 증상을 호소한다. 혈중 일산화탄소 농도가 증가하면 증상이 점차 악화한다. 혈중 이산화탄소 농도가 50~60%를 초과하면 경련, 혼수 및 사망에 이를 수 있다.

일산화탄소 중독의 처치는 일산화탄소 발생원으로부터 환자를 이동시켜 산소를 투여하는 것이다. 실내 공기(산소 21%)를 호흡할 때 인체는 일산화탄소를 절반 농도로 줄이는 데 250분이 걸린다. 환자에게 100% 산소를 공급하면 일산화탄소헤모글로빈의 반감기는 40~60분으로 줄어든다. 일산화탄소 중독이 의심되는 모든 환자는

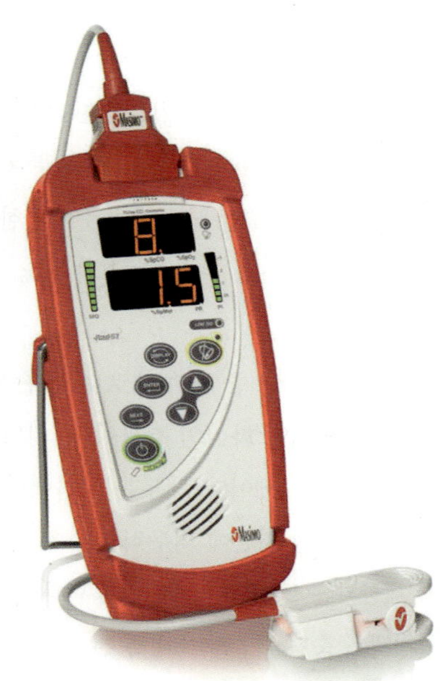

그림 13-19 병원 전 일산화탄소 측정기(Rad-57).
Courtesy of Masimo Corporation.

맥박산소측정기 측정값과 관계없이 100% 산소를 공급해야 한다.

고압 산소 요법에 대해서는 논란의 여지가 있지만, 정상 산소 요법(100% 산소)으로 일산화탄소 제거가 예상대로 이루어지지 않는 경우 고려해야 한다. 고압산소 치료는 2~3기압에서 여러 부분으로 구성된 일반적인 요법으로 고압 챔버에서 제공한다. 제한된 연구에 따르면 고압산소 치료를 통해 일산화탄소 중독으로 인한 신경학적 합병증이 개선된 것으로 나타났다. 고압산소 요법을 시행하기로 결정하였으면 지체해서는 안 된다. 이러한 환자에서 정상 산소 상태로 빠르게 복귀하는 것이 예후 개선과 관련이 있으며 환자가 높은 일산화탄소 수치를 오래 있을수록 뇌와 심장에 더 많은 손상이 발생한다. 7건의 무작위 임상시험을 검토한 결과 고압산소 치료와 100% 산소 치료를 비교했다. 그 결과 신경학적 후유증 개선과 관련하여 엇갈린 결과가 나왔다. 현재 흡입 손상 환자에서 고압산소 치료의 역할은 논란의 여지가 있으며 정상 압력의 산소 처치로 충분한 산소 공급이 이루어지지 않고 일산화탄소 노출로 인해 심각한 기저 신경학적 손상이 있는 경우에만 환자별로 고려해야 한다.

사이안화물

사이안화물 가스는 플라스틱이나 폴리우레탄이 연소할 때 생성된다. 사이안화물 중독은 세포의 에너지 생산 과정을 방해하여 세포가 산소를 사용하는 것을 못 하게 한다. 사이안화수소는 사이토크롬 C산화 효소의 가역적 억제로 인해 발생하는 조직 무산소증과 함께 세포

산소화를 억제한다. 환자는 혈액에 충분한 양의 산소가 있음에도 불구하고 질식으로 사망할 수 있다. 사이안화물 중독의 증상으로는 의식 수준 변화, 어지럼, 두통, 빈맥 또는 빠른 호흡 등이 있다. 화재 현장에서 일산화탄소에 중독된 환자도 사이안화물 중독의 위험에 노출된 것으로 간주한다.

사이안화물 중독의 치료는 해독제를 신속하게 투여하는 것이다. 사이안화물 해독제는 사이안화물 분자에 직접 결합하여 해가 없는 물질로 변화시키는 약물이다. 히드록소코발라민(시아노키트)은 사이안화물에 직접 결합하여 독성이 없는 사이아노코발라민(비타민 B12)을 형성하여 사이안화물을 해독한다. 히드록소코발라민은 미국과 유럽에서 병원 전에 사용할 수 있다. 사이안화물 중독이 의심되는 경우 자유롭게 사용해야 한다. 유럽에서 사이안화물 중독에 사용되는 두 번째 해독제는 디이코발트에데테이트이지만, 사이안화물 중독이 발생하지 않은 상태에서 이 약물을 투여하면 코발트 중독이 발생할 위험이 있다.

역사적으로 "Lilly 키트" 또는 "Pasadena 키트"는 미국에서 사용되는 전통적인 사이안화물 해독제 키트였으며 일부 환경에서는 여전히 활용될 수 있다. 대부분의 병원 전 시스템에는 시아노키트가 갖춰져 있어야 하지만, 병원 전 처치 제공자는 릴리 키트에 대해 알고 있어야 한다. 이 사이안화물 중독 치료 방법은 1930년대에 개발되었으며 치사량의 21배에 달하는 사이안화물에 중독된 동물을 해독하는 데 효과적인 것으로 밝혀졌다. 이 해독제 치료의 목표는 환자의 혈액에서 두 번째 독성(메트헤모글로빈)이 형성되도록 유도하는 것이다. 이렇게 유도된 독성 물질은 사이안화물과 결합하여 신체가 사이안화물을 천천히 해독하고 배설할 수 있도록 한다.

Lilly 키트에는 지정된 순서대로 투여하는 세 가지 약물이 포함되어 있다. 첫 번째 약물은 질산염이나 아밀질산염 또는 질산나트륨이다(둘 다 키트에 제공됨). 아밀질산염은 앰풀을 개봉하면 기체가 방출되어 환자가 흡입하게 되며 질산나트륨은 정맥 내로 투여하는 것이 더 효과적이고 병원 전 처치 제공자가 아밀질산염 가스 누출을 피할 수 있으므로 선호되는 투여 방법이다. 질산염 약물은 환자의 헤모글로빈 일부를 메트헤모글로빈이라는 형태로 변화시켜 세포의 미트콘드리아에서 사이안화물을 독성 작용 부위에서 멀리 끌어내린다. 사이안화물이 메트헤모글로빈과 결합하면 미토콘드리아는 다시 한 번 세포에 필요한 에너지를 생산하기 시작할 수 있다. 안타깝게도 메트헤모글로빈은 헤모글로빈처럼 세포에 산소를 운반하지 못하기 때문에 독성이 있다. 이러한 산소 전달 감소는 환자가 연기 흡입으로

인해 일산화탄소 농도 증가와 관련된 조직의 저산소증을 악화시킬 수 있다.

　키트의 세 번째 약물은 티오황산나트륨으로 질산염이 메트헤모글로빈과 결합할 수 있도록 정맥 내로 투여한다. 메트헤모글로빈의 티오황산나트륨과 사이안화물은 티오시안산염으로 대사되어 환자의 소변으로 안전하게 배설된다. 메트헤모글로빈의 독성과 Lilly 키트 전체를 투여하는 데 필요한 시간 때문에 하이드록소코발라민이 사이안화물 중독 치료에 선호되는 해독제이다.

독성에 의해 유발된 폐 손상

간단히 말해서 연기는 불완전 연소로 인해 생성되는 화학적 먼지이다. 연기 속의 화학 물질은 기도 및 폐의 내벽과 반응하여 기도와 폐의 내벽 세포를 손상한다. 암모니아, 염화수소, 이산화황과 같은 화합물은 흡입 시 부식성 산과 알칼리를 형성하고 물과 반응한다. 이러한 독성 물질은 기관과 세기관지를 둘러싸고 있는 세포의 괴사를 유발한다. 일반적으로 이러한 세포는 섬모라고 하는 작은 털 같은 구조가 있다. 이 섬모에는 점액이 덮여 있으며 정상적으로 흡입한 이물질을 포집하여 인두로 운반하고 인두에서 위장관으로 삼켜진다. 흡입 손상 후 며칠이 지나면 이 세포는 죽는다. 이렇게 괴사한 세포에서 나온 조직파편과 세포가 일반적으로 포집하는 조직파편은 제거되지 않고 축적된다. 그 결과 분비물이 증가하고 점액과 세포 조직파편으로 기도가 막히고 생명을 위협하는 폐렴의 발병률이 증가한다.

병원 전 처치

연기에 노출된 환자를 처치하는 데 있어 가장 중요한 요소는 기관내삽관의 필요성을 결정하는 것이다. 기도 폐쇄의 징후를 인식하기 위해서는 기도유지 상태를 지속해서 재평가한다. 목소리의 변화, 분비물 제거의 어려움, 침 흘림은 기도 폐쇄가 임박했다는 징후이다. 환자의 기도 개방이 의심스러운 경우 병원 전 처치 제공자는 기관내삽관을 시행하여 기도를 확보할 수 있다. 때에 따라서는 기도를 유지하기 위해 급속연속기관삽관이 필요할 수 있다. 환자의 이송 시간이 긴 경우 확실하게 기도 유지를 제공할 수 있는 기관내삽관이 필요할 수 있다. 연기를 흡입한 환자는 피부에 화상이 없더라도 화상센터로 이송한다. 이송 시간이 길어지는 경우 이송할 의료기관의 의료진에게 보고는 물론 확실한 기도 관리를 제공할 수 있는 의료기관으로 이송하는 것도 고려해야 한다. 이러한 환자는 숙련된 병원 전 처치 제공자라도 삽관이 어려울 수 있으므로 외과적 기도 확보가 가능한 의료진이

준비되어 있어야 한다.

　연기를 흡입한 환자는 피부 화상이 없더라도 화상센터로 이송해야 한다. 화상센터는 더 많은 양의 연기 흡입 환자를 치료하며 고유한 방식의 기계적 환기와 때로는 고압 산소 요법을 제공한다.

아동 학대

화상 손상은 어린이 사망 원인 중 세 번째로 흔한 손상이다. 전체 아동학대의 약 20%는 의도적인 화상의 결과이다. 의도적으로 화상을 입은 어린이의 대부분은 1~2세이다. 대부분 국가에서 의료인은 아동학대가 의심되는 경우 관련 기관에 의무적으로 신고해야 한다. 따라서 병원 전 처치 제공자는 병원의 의료진에게 학대 우려를 알리고 의무 보고에 대한 정책을 숙지해야 하며 병원 전 처치 제공자가 직접 신고해야 할 수도 있다.

　아동 학대에서 볼 수 있는 가장 흔한 형태의 화상은 강제 침수로 인한 이차적인 화상이다. 이러한 손상은 일반적으로 성인이 배변 훈련과 관련된 벌로 어린이를 뜨거운 물에 담글 때 발생한다. 침수 화상은 피부가 장시간 노출로 인해 심부 화상을 입는 경우가 많다(물의 온도가 다른 형태의 화상보다 많을 수 있음). 손상의 심각성을 결정하는 요인으로는 환자의 나이, 물의 온도, 노출 시간 등이 있다. 어린이는 손이나 발에 장갑 모양, 양말 모양으로 심부 부분층 또는 전층 화상을 입을 수 있다. 화상이 대칭적이고 스플래시 패턴이 없는 경우 병원 전 처치 제공자는 특히 의심된다(**그림 13-20** 및 **그림 13-21**). 의도적인 화상을 입으면 어린이는 두려움이나 고통으로 인해 팔과 다리를 강하게 구부려 방어 자세를 취하게 된다. 이로 인해 화상 패턴은 오금(무릎), 전주와(팔꿈치), 서혜부에 굴곡 자국을 남긴다. 화상을 입은 조직과 화상을 입지 않은 조직 사이에 뚜렷한 경계선이 나타나면 이는 고의로 담근 것을 나타낸다(**그림 13-22**).

　우발적인 화상의 경우 화상의 깊이가 다양하고 가장자리가 불규칙하며 심한 화상 부위에서 멀리 떨어진 작은 화상을 입어 튀긴 자국을 나타낸다. 우발적인 화상의 일반적인 기전은 전자레인지에 데운 국물에 의한 것이다.

접촉 화상

접촉 화상은 우발적이든 의도적이든 어린이 화상 중 두 번째로 흔한 기전이다. 모든 신체 표면에는 어느 정도의 굴곡이 있다. 우발적인 접촉 화상이 발생하면 화상을 일으키는 기구가 굴곡진 인체의 표면과 접촉하게 된다. 화상을 일으키는 기구가 굴곡진 표면에서 벗어나거나

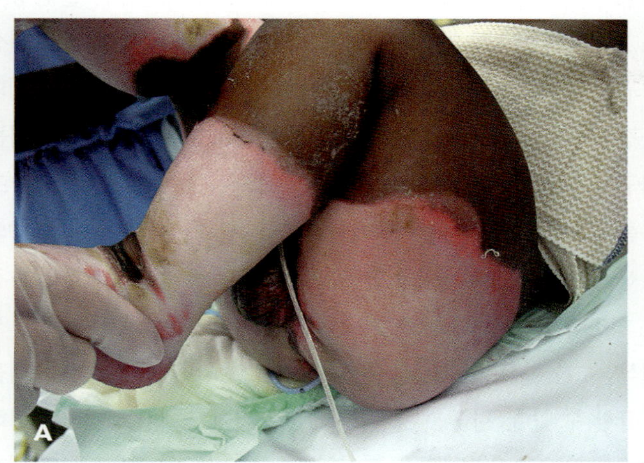

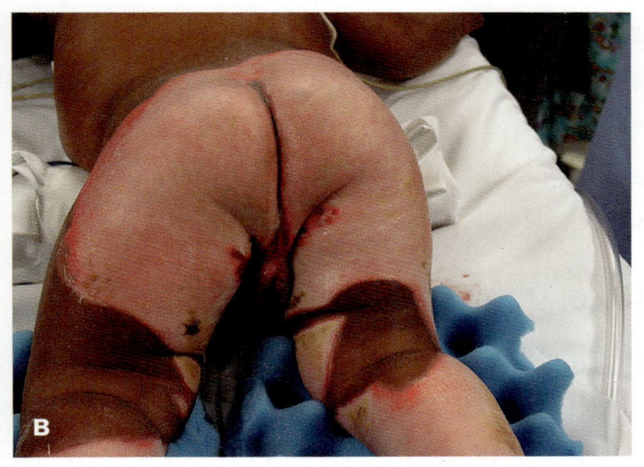

그림 13-20 화상 패턴의 직선과 튄 자국이 없는 것은 이 화상이 학대의 결과임을 나타낸다. **A.** 옆면 **B.** 뒷면.
Courtesy of Dr. Jeffrey Guy.

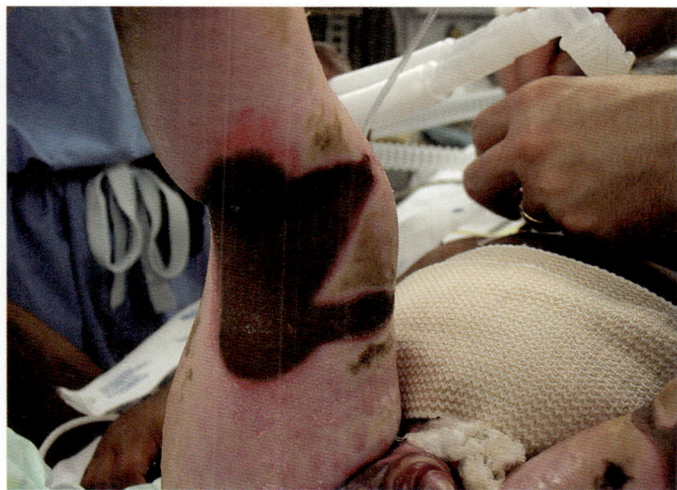

그림 13-21 굴곡 부위가 남아 있고 화상을 입은 피부와 화상을 입지 않은 피부 사이의 경계선이 뚜렷한 것은 어린이가 손상 전에 몸을 구부리고 방어적인 자세를 취하고 있었음을 나타낸다. 이러한 자세는 화상이 우발적으로 발생하지 않았다는 것을 나타낸다.
Courtesy of Dr. Jeffrey Guy.

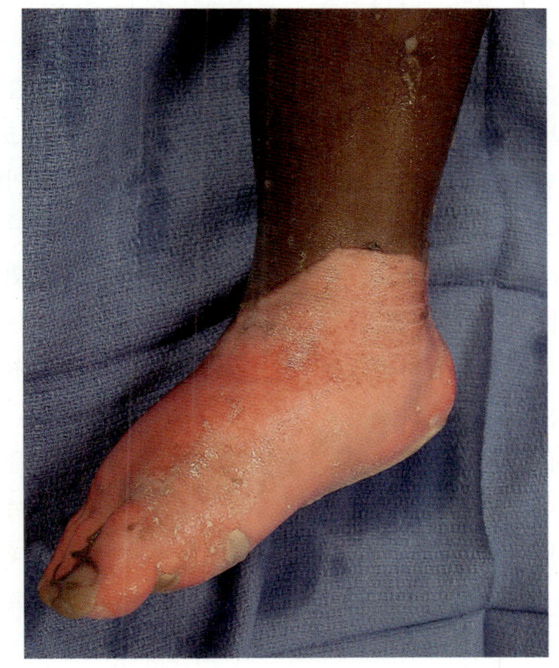

그림 13-22 어린이의 발에 양발 형태의 화상을 입은 것은 아동 학대와 일치하는 고의적인 침수 화상 손상을 나타낸다.
Courtesy of Dr. Jeffrey Guy.

피해자가 뜨거운 물체에서 물러난다. 그 결과 화상의 가장자리와 깊이가 불규칙하다. 어린이가 의도적인 접촉 화상을 입으면 화상을 입힌 도구가 어린이의 피부를 누르게 되어 화상을 입은 조직과 화상을 입지 않은 조직 사이에 균일한 깊이의 뚜렷한 경계선이 생긴다. 접촉 화상과 관련된 일반적인 물체로는 고데기, 스팀다리미, 라디에이터, 냄비와 프라이팬 등이 있다.

방사선 화상

방사선 화상은 환자가 방사선 노출 사실을 항상 인지하지 못하기 때문에 진단하기 어려울 수 있다. 다양한 형태의 방사선으로 인한 화상의 심각성은 대상 조직이 흡수하는 에너지의 양에 따라 달라진다. 다양한 형태의 방사선은 전자기, X-선, γ선 및 미립자가 포함된다. 이러한 다양한 형태의 방사선은 조직에 다양한 정도의 에너지를 전달한다. 전자기 방사선은 조직을 통과할 수 있고 심각한 손상을 일으키지 않지만, 중성자 노출과 같은 다른 형태의 방사선은 조직에 흡수되어 심각한 손상을 일으킨다. 흡수 조직에 손상을 입히는 것은 방사선의 흡수이다. 방사선의 흡수 용량은 실제 방사선량보다 더 심한 손상을 입힌다. 서로 다른 형태의 방사선 등가선량에 노출하더라도 개인에 미치는 영향은 크게 달라진다.

현재 방사선 피폭의 가장 흔한 원인은 산업재해 또는 직업적 사고 이다. 그러나 전 세계적으로 테러의 위협이 증가함에 따라 방사선 분산 장치(방사성 물질이 추가된 재래식 폭발물) 또는 소형 즉석 핵 장치의 폭발이 발생할 가능성이 있으므로 모든 병원 전 처치 제공자는 이러한 유형의 손상에 대해 어느 정도 인지하고 있어야 한다(자세한 내용은 18장 폭발 및 대량살상무기 참조).

대도시 지역에서 핵무기가 폭발하면 많은 사람이 다치고 죽는 재앙적인 사고가 발생할 수 있다. 핵폭발로 인한 손상 기전은 폭발에 대한 접근성에 따라 달라지며 초기 화염 폭풍으로 인한 열 화상, 초음속 파괴 폭발로 인한 무딘 손상 및 관통성 외상, 방사능 생성으로 인한 장기 손상 등이 있다. 열 화상과 방사선 화상의 조합으로 인한 사망률은 같은 규모의 열 화상 또는 방사선 화상 단독으로 인한 사망률보다 더 높다. 핵무기 폭발 후 열 화상과 방사선 화상의 조합은 사망률에 시너지 효과를 발휘한다.

방사성 물질은 위험하며 초기 우선순위는 위험 물질에 노출된 환자와 같다. 적절한 개인보호장비를 착용하고 환자를 오염원으로부터 이동시킨 후 오염된 의복을 벗기고 물로 충분히 세척한다. 제거한 의복은 오염된 것으로 간주하고 주의해서 취급해야 한다. 오염된 부위에서 방사능 잔해나 입자를 제거할 때 오염되지 않은 신체 표면에 손상이 발생하지 않도록 조심스럽게 세척을 시행한다. 가이거 계수기를 사용한 전신 조사에 따라 오염이 정상 상태로 최소화될 때까지 세척을 계속한다.

이 접근방식의 예외는 방사선 손상과 더불어 심각한 외상을 입은 환자이다. 이러면 즉시 옷을 제거하고 명백한 오염을 세척하며 동시에 외상성 손상을 안정시켜야 한다. 병원 전 처치 제공자는 환자의 손상이 아무리 심각하더라도 방사선 손상에 노출되지 않도록 지속해서 예방 조치를 취하는 것이 중요하다. 구토 및 설사와 관련된 급성 방사성 손상은 다량의 방사선 중독을 나타내며 치사율이 높다. 이러한 환자는 병원 전 환경에서 수액 소생술로 지지적 처치를 시행하고 방사선 독성 처치에 전문성을 갖춘 병원으로 신속하게 이송해야 한다.

핵사고가 발생한 후에는 정맥 주사용품, 주입 펌프 및 환자를 이송할 의료기관이 부족할 수 있다. 병원 전 처치 제공자는 환자에게 정맥 라인을 확보하고 수액 소생술을 시행할 수 없는 경우 경구 수액

공급으로 환자를 소생시킬 수 있다. 실제로 경구 소생술은 열 손상에도 고려되고 있으며 일부 병원에서는 대량의 정맥 내 수액 투여 대신 경구 소생술을 사용한 결과를 평가하고 있지만, 아직 병원 전 단계의 환경에는 도입되지 않았다. 그러나 자원이 제한된 비상 상황에서는 경구 수분 보충 및 소생술을 반드시 고려해야 하며 현재 및 향후 조사를 통해 이 요법이 결과를 개선하는지 여부를 알 수 있다. 대량의 화상 또는 방사선 사상자가 발생한 재난 발생 후와 같이 제한적인 경우 협조적인 환자에게는 소변 배출량을 유지하기 위해 균형 잡힌 생리식염수를 마시도록 권장하거나 코위관 또는 비장관을 통해 수액을 공급할 수 있다. 경구용 평형염액에는 모이어 염액[(물 1리터에 염화소듐 4g(염분 0.5티스푼)], 중탄산나트륨 1.5g(중조 0.5티스푼)과 세계보건기구의 경구 수액제(WHOORS)가 있다. 동물 연구에 따르면 체표면적 40%의 화상을 입은 환자에서 이러한 소생술 전략으로 고무적인 결과를 얻었다. 위장관으로 평형염액을 20mL/kg의 비율로 투여하면 표준 정맥 수액 소생술과 동등한 소생술 효과를 얻을 수 있었다.

화학 화상

모든 병원 전 처치 제공자는 화학물질 손상 처치의 기본 사항을 숙지하고 있어야 한다. 도시 환경의 병원 전 처치 제공자는 산업 현장에서 화학물질 사고에 출동하는 반면, 시골 지역에서 근무하는 병원 전 처치 제공자는 농업에 사용되는 물질과 관련된 사고에 출동할 수 있다. 매일 수많은 위험 물질이 고속도로와 철도를 통해 도시와 농촌으로 운송된다. 군의 병원 전 처치 제공자는 무기나 소이탄, 장비 연료나 유지 보수에 사용되는 화학물질, 민간 시설물 파손 후 화학물질 유출로 인한 화학 화상 환자를 처치할 수 있다.

화학 물질로 인한 손상은 일반적으로 매우 짧은 시간 동안 노출되는 열 손상과 달리 가해 물질에 장시간 노출되어 발생하는 경우가 많다. 화학물질 손상의 심각성은 화학 물질의 특성, 화학 물질의 농도, 접촉 시간, 화학 물질의 작용기전이라는 네 가지 요인에 의해 결정된다.

화학 작용제는 산성, 염기성, 유기물 또는 무기물로 분류된다. 산은 pH7(중성)과 0(강산) 사이의 화학물질이고 염기는 pH7~14 (강염기)인 화학 물질이다(**그림 13-23**). 산은 응고 괴사라는 과정을 통해 조직을 손상하고 손상된 조직은 응고되어 산이 더 깊은 침투를 막는 장벽으로 변한다. 이와 대조적으로 알칼리 화상은 액화 괴사라는 과정을 통해 조직을 파괴한다. 염기는 조직을 액화시켜 화학물질이 더

깊숙이 침투하여 점점 더 깊은 조직 손상을 일으킨다. 알칼리 작용제는 조직의 단백질을 녹여 알칼리성 단백질을 형성하는 데 이 알칼리성 단백질은 용해되어 영향을 받은 조직 깊숙한 곳까지 추가 반응을 일으킬 수 있다. 유기 용액은 세포벽의 액체막을 녹여 세포 구조를 파괴하고 주로 이 기전을 통해 손상을 일으킨다. 반면 무기 용액은 세포 외부에 남아 있다. 화학 화상은 표면에 나타나는 것보다 훨씬 더 깊을 수 있다. 충분한 때로는 지속적인 세척이 필요할 수 있다. 알칼리 손상의 경우 표면 pH를 확인하여 8 미만이어야 한다. 이송 시간이 긴 환자의 경우 알칼리 손상을 입으면 지속해서 세척이 필요할 수 있다.

병원 전 처치

화학물질에 노출된 환자를 처치할 때 가장 우선시되는 것은 개인 및 현장의 안전이다. 다른 응급 상황과 마찬가지로 병원 전 처치 제공자는 항상 자신을 먼저 보호해야 한다. 화학물질 위험에 노출될 가능성이 있는 경우 현장 안전을 확보하고 특수 보호복이나 호흡 장비가 필요한지 또는 특수 훈련을 받은 인력이나 장비가 필요한지 결정한다. 장비와 구급차가 오염되지 않도록 한다. 오염된 구급차는 다른 환자에게 노출 위험을 초래한다. 가능한 한 빨리 화학물질이 무엇인지 파악하도록 한다.

액체 또는 분말 형태의 화학물질로 오염되었을 수 있으므로 환자의 모든 의복을 제거하고 오염된 의복은 주의해서 폐기한다. 피부에 미립자 물질이 묻어 있으면 솔을 이용해서 털어낸 후 다량의 물로 환자를 세척한다. 세척은 유해 물질의 농도를 희석하고 남아있는 물질을 씻어낸다. 세척의 핵심은 다량의 물을 사용하는 것이다. 흔히 범하는 실수는 1~2L의 물로 환자를 씻었고 바닥에 물이 고이기 시작하면 세척 과정을 중단하는 것이다. 소량의 물로만 세척할 경우 오염 물질이 환자의 체표면 전체에 퍼져 씻겨 내려가지 않는다.

세척액이 적절히 흘러내리고 배출되지 않으면 오염된 세척액이 환자 아래에 고여 이전에 노출되지 않았거나 손상되지 않은 신체 부위에 손상을 입힐 수 있다. 병원 전 환경에서 세척액 배출을 촉진하는 간단한 방법의 하나는 환자를 긴척추고정판에 눕힌 다음 기울이거나 머리 부분을 들어 올리는 것이다. 긴척추고정판의 낮은 부위에 큰 플라스틱 통이나 비닐봉지를 놓아 오염된 세척액을 모을 수 있도록 한다.

화학 화상에서 중화제는 병원 전 처치 제공자가 사용해서는 안 된다. 이러한 중화제는 중화 과정에서 발열 반응으로 열을 발산하는 경우가 많다. 따라서 병원 전 처치 제공자는 의도치 않게 화상 외에 열 화상을 일으킬 수 있다. 시중에 판매되는 대부분의 오염 제거 용액은 사람이 아닌 장비의 오염을 제거할 목적으로 만들어진 것이다.

눈의 화학 화상

알칼리 굴질 노출로 인한 눈 손상이 발생할 수 있다. 눈은 조금만 노출되어도 시력과 안구 기능을 위협할 수 있다. 즉시 다량의 세척액으

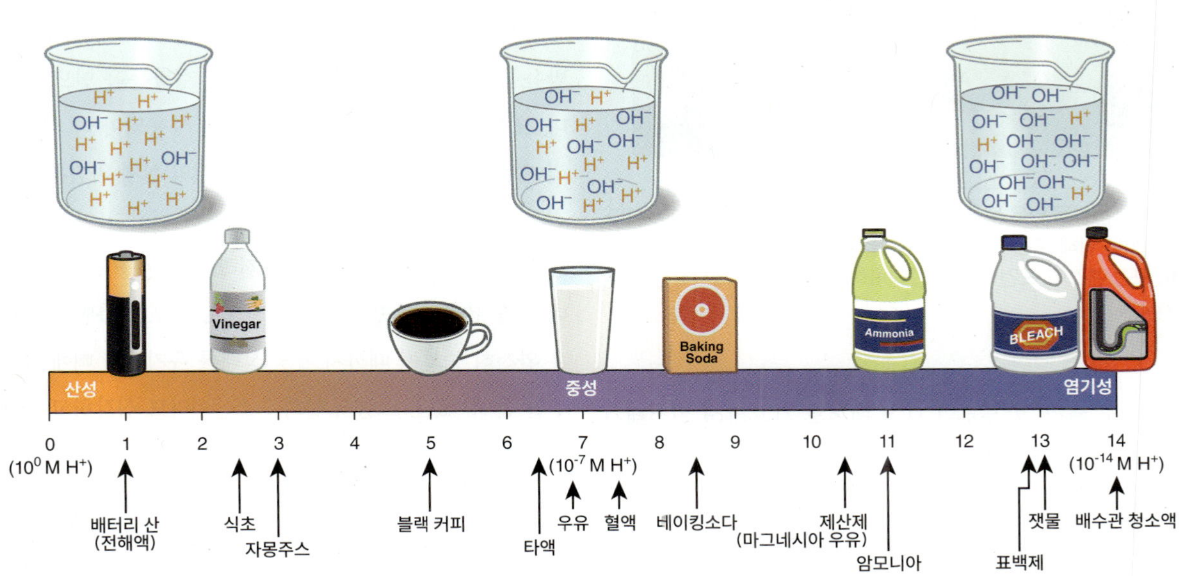

그림 13-23 화학물질은 수조 또는 수산화 이온의 양에 따라 산성, 중성 또는 염기로 분류된다. 많은 가정용품이 산성 또는 염기성이며 취급 시 주의가 필요하다.

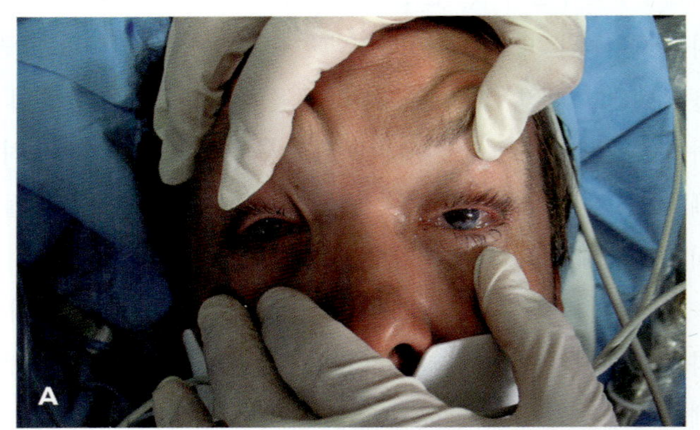

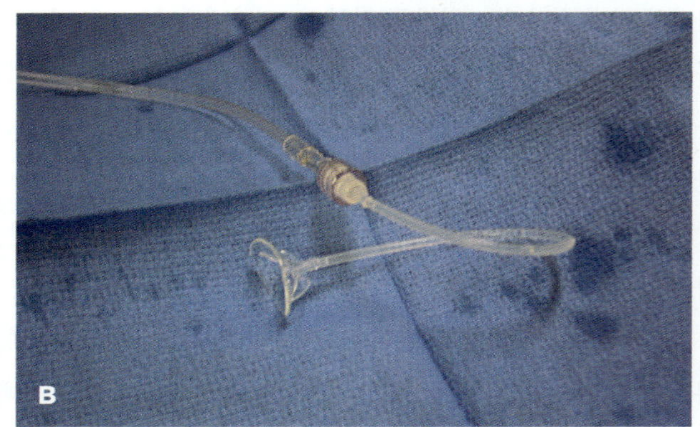

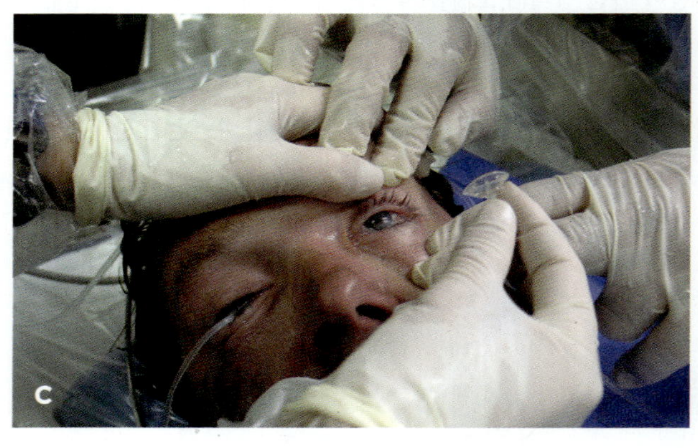

그림 13-24 화학 손상을 입은 눈은 다량의 생리식염수로 즉시 세척해야 한다. 적절한 안구 세척을 위해 모건 렌즈를 눈에 넣을 수 있다. **A.** 눈에 화학 화상을 입은 경우. **B.** 모건 렌즈 **C.** 모건 렌즈를 삽입하여 환자의 눈을 세척하는 경우.

Courtesy of Dr. Jeffrey Guy.

입관을 수액 세트에 연결하여 세척할 수 있다. 프로파라카인과 같은 안과용 국소 마취제를 바르면 병원 전 처치 제공자가 환자를 쉽게 처치할 수 있다. 이러한 환자는 안과 전문의가 있는 의료기관으로 이송한다.

특정 화학물질에 대한 노출

시멘트는 알칼리성 물질로 작업자의 옷에 묻거나 신발에 떨어질 수 있다. 분말 시멘트는 환자의 땀과 반응하여 열을 발산하고 피부를 과도하게 건조하거나 건조하게 하는 반응을 일으킨다. 이러한 노출은 일반적으로 시멘트에 접촉한 후 몇 시간 또는 다음 날에 화상을 입게 된다. 초기 처치는 시멘트 가루를 솔로 떨어낸 후 다량의 물로 세척하는 것이다.

휘발유 및 등유와 같은 연료는 장시간 노출되면 접촉 화상을 유발할 수 있다. 이러한 유기 탄화수소는 세포막을 용해해 피부와 기저 조직을 괴사시킬 수 있다. 연료를 덮어쓴 환자의 오염 제거는 다량의 물로 세척하는 것이다. 휘발유 접촉 노출은 전층 조직 손상을 초래할 수 있다. 장시간 노출되거나 중증도의 노출은 전신 독성을 초래할 수 있다. 국소 손상을 통해 독성 물질이 흡수되면 중증 심혈관, 신장, 폐, 신경 및 간의 합병증이 발생할 수 있으며 이러한 환자는 중환자실에 입원하여 지속적인 모니터링과 실험실 평가를 시행한다. 전신 독성이 의심되는 경우 상처를 통해 독성 물질이 지속해서 흡수될 우려가 있는 경우 신속한 외과적 죽은 조직 제거가 필요할 수 있다.

불화수소산은 가정, 산업 및 군사 환경에서 널리 사용되는 위험한 물질이다. 주로 냉매 제조에 사용되지만, 제초제, 의약품, 하이옥탄휘발유, 알루미늄, 플라스틱, 전기 부품, 형광등을 만드는 데도 사용된다. 또한, 유리와 금속을 에칭하는 데 사용되며 녹 제거제와 자동차 휠 세척제로도 사용된다. 이 화학 물질의 실제 위험은 불소 이온으로 전해질, 특히 칼슘과 마그네슘에 심각한 변화를 일으킨다. 불소 이온은 칼슘 및 마그네슘과 같은 양전하는 이온을 킬레이트화하여 세포 내 칼슘 유출을 유발하고 결과적으로 세포를 사멸시킨다. 불소 이온은 완전히 중화될 때까지 활성 상태를 유지하며 뼈에 효과적으로 침투할 할 수 있다. 소량의 불화수소산이라도 심각하고 잠재적으로 치명적인 저칼슘혈증을 유발할 수 있다. 저칼슘혈증은 심장 부정맥을 빠르게 유발한다. 처치하지 않고 방치하면 불화수소산은 조직을 액화시키고 환자의 뼈에서 칼슘을 침출하여 치명적인 심장 부정맥을 일으킬 수 있다. 불산 노출에 대한 초기 처치는 물로 세척한 후 응급

로 눈을 세척해야 한다. 가능하면 모건 렌즈를 사용하여 지속해서 세척하여 안구 오염을 제거한다(**그림 13-24**). 눈의 화학 화상을 처치하려면 5L 이상의 세척액으로 지속적인 세척이 필요할 수 있다. 모건 렌즈를 사용할 수 없는 경우 수액 세트를 사용하여 수동으로 지속해서 세척을 하거나 양쪽 눈에 문제가 있는 경우 생리식염수 백에 코삽

실에서 글루콘산칼슘 젤을 바르는 것이다. 불화수소산 화상을 입은 환자는 즉시 추가 처치를 받을 수 있도록 화상센터로 이송한다.

인으로 의한 손상은 군사 환경에서 종종 발생한다. 백린(WP)은 군수품 생산에 사용되는 강력한 방화제이다. 공기에 노출되면 격렬하게 연소하여 화려한 화염과 짙은 연기를 발생시킨다. 모든 약제가 연소하거나 산소가 부족해질 때까지 계속 연소한다. 피부에 닿으면 백린은 심부 화학 화상 및 열 화상을 일으킨다. 이러한 화상은 외과적 절제 또는 구리 용액으로 신속한 처치가 필요하지만, 특히 병원 전 환경에서는 거의 사용할 수 없다.

초기 처치는 백린에 노출 시 환자에게 산소 공급을 중단하는 것이다. 의복에 발화할 수 있는 인 입자가 남아 있을 수 있으므로 모든 의복을 신속하게 제거한다. 손상을 입은 부위는 물이나 생리식염수로 적신 드레싱을 시행하고 이송하는 동안 드레싱이 건조하지 않도록 축축하게 유지한다. 드레싱이 건조되면 남아있는 백린이 재점화되어 드레싱에 불이 붙고 환자에게 화상을 입힐 수 있다.

하이포아염소산염 용액은 가정용 표백제 및 산업용 세척제를 생산하는 데 사용된다. 이 용액은 강알칼리성 용액이지만, 일반적으로 사용되는 용액은 4~6%이며 신체의 넓은 부위가 화학물질에 노출되지 않는 한 일반적으로 치명적이지는 않다. 유황 겨자와 질소 겨자는 발포제 또는 수포 작용제로 분류되는 화합물이다. 이러한 물질은 화학

무기로 사용됐으며 화학 테러의 위협으로 인식되고 있다. 이러한 화학 물질은 노출 시 피부에 화상을 입히고 물집을 일으킨다. 이 물질은 피부에 자극을 주고 폐와 눈에 자극을 유발한다. 노출 후 환자는 목과 눈에 작열감을 호소한다. 피부 침범은 노출되고 몇 시간 후에 붉어지며 오염된 부위에 물집이 생긴다. 심하게 노출되면 환자는 피부 전층 괴사 및 호흡부전이 발생한다. 현장에서의 주요 처치는 의도하지 않은 교차 오염을 방지하기 위해 오염을 제거하는 것이다.

수포제에 노출된 환자를 처치할 때 병원 전 처치 제공자는 적절한 글러브, 보호복 및 호흡 장비를 착용해야 한다. 환자는 오염을 제거하고 물과 생리식염수로 세척해야 한다. 특수 훈련을 받은 구조대원이 오염을 제거하기 위해 사용하는 다른 약제에는 희석된 하이포아염소산염 용액과 시중에서 구할 수 있으며 흡수제 역할을 하는 백토 분말을 사용할 수 있다. 환자가 화상센터에 도착하면 추가적인 전문 처치가 필요하다.

최루가스 및 이와 유사한 화학 물질은 폭동 진압 작용제로 알려져 있다. 폭동 진압 작용제는 피부, 점막, 폐, 눈에 자극을 일으켜 노출된 사람을 빠르고 짧게 무력화시킨다. 손상 정도는 약제에 노출된 정도에 따라 결정된다. 자극의 지속 시간은 일반적으로 30~60분 동안 지속된다. 처치는 폭동 진압 작용제에 노출된 사람을 노출원에서 구출하여 오염된 의복을 제거하고 환자의 피부와 눈을 세척하는 것이다.

요 약

- 화상의 크기와 관계없이 모든 화상은 심각하다.
- 생명을 위협할 수 있는 화상에는 큰 열 화상, 전기 화상 및 화학 화상이 포함된다.
- 기계적 외상(예: 관통상, 무딘 손상)과 달리 신체는 화상을 입은 손상을 견딜 수 있는 적응 기전이 거의 없으므로 입원이 필요한 화상은 화상센터에서 처치해야 한다.
- 화상은 피부에만 국한된 것이 아니라 전신에 걸쳐 발생하는 매우 심각한 손상이다. 심각한 화상을 입은 환자는 심혈관계, 폐, 위장, 신장 및 면역체계의 기능 장애를 겪게 된다.
- 적절한 수액 소생술을 제공하지 않으면 불응성 쇼크, 다기관 기능 장애, 심부 화상으로 이어질 수 있다. 따라서 화상 손상 후 생존을 최적화하는 데 병원 전 처치 제공자의 역할이 매우 중요하다.
- 화상은 복잡하고 위험하지만, 빠르게 치명적인 경우는 드물다. 심한 연기 흡입과 큰 열 화상을 입은 환자는 사망하는 데 몇 시간 또는 며칠이 걸릴 수 있다. 화상 환자는 다른 기계적 외상도 동반할 가능성이 높다. 화상 환자에 대한 외상 우선순위는 같으며 의료진은 화상 처치로 인해 주의가 분산되어서는 안 된다.

- 인상적인 화상은 생명을 위협할 수 있는 다른 손상으로부터 병원 전 처치 제공자의 주의를 분산시킬 수 있다. 일차 및 이차평가를 수행하면 이러한 손상(예; 기흉, 심장눌림증, 비장 파열)을 놓칠 가능성을 줄일 수 있다.
- 최우선 순위는 개인 및 현장 안전이다. 종종 손상 원인은 병원 전 처치 제공자에게 손상을 입힐 위험이 여전히 존재한다.
- 고기능 부위(손, 얼굴, 관절, 회음부)의 작은 화상이라도 흉터 형성으로 인한 장기적인 장애를 초래할 수 있다.
- 화상센터 이송 기준을 숙지하면 모든 환자가 화상 후 최대한의 기능 회복을 달성하는 데 도움이 된다.
- 화상 환자의 주요 사망 원인은 연기 흡입으로 인한 합병증(질식, 열 손상, 지연된 독성 유발 폐 손상 등)이다. 환자는 48시간 이상 호흡부전 증상이 나타나지 않는 경우가 많다. 피부에 화상을 입지 않았더라도 연기 흡입 환자는 화상센터로 이송해야 한다.
- 화학 물질이나 방사성 물질과 같은 위험 물질로 인한 화상 환자는 병원 전 처치 제공자와 의료진에게 해당 물질이 의도치 않게 오염되지 않도록 오염 제거를 시행해야 한다.

시나리오 재구성

당신은 주택 건물 화재 현장으로 도움 요청을 받고 출동했다. 당신과 동료가 도착했을 때 2층 주택이 완전히 불길에 휩싸여 지붕과 창문에서 짙은 검은 연기가 쏟아져 나오는 것을 목격했다. 당신은 응급의료반응자(EMR)가 처치하고 있는 환자가 있는 곳으로 이동했다. 환자는 반려견을 구하기 위해 불타는 건물에 다시 들어갔다가 소방관에 의해 의식이 없는 상태로 발견되어 구조되었다고 한다.

환자는 30대로 보이는 남성이고 옷 대부분이 불에 탔다. 환자는 얼굴에 화상을 입은 것이 분명하고 머리카락이 불에 그을렸다. 환자는 의식이 없고 자발적으로 호흡은 하고 있지만, 코골이 호흡을 하고 있다. 응급의료반응자는 환자에게 비재호흡마스크를 이용해 고유량의 산소를 공급하고 있었다. 신체검사 시 턱 밀어올리기 방법으로 기도를 유지하여 그는 쉽게 호흡을 하고 있다. 환자의 셔츠 소매는 불에 탔고 팔에는 둘레 화상이 있지만, 노동맥은 쉽게 확인할 수 있었다. 환자의 맥박수는 118회/분, 혈압은 148/94mmHg, 호흡수는 22회/분, 맥박산소측정기로 측정한 산소포화도는 92%이다. 신체검사 결과 환자는 머리 전체에 화상을 입었고 가슴 앞과 배에 물집이 생겼으며 오른쪽과 왼쪽 팔과 손 전체에 전층 화상을 입었다.

- 이 환자의 화상 정도는 어느 정도인가?
- 이 환자를 처치하기 위한 첫 번째 단계는 무엇인가?
- 병원 전 처치 제공자는 흡입 손상을 어떻게 인식할 수 있을까?

시나리오 해결책

환자는 심각한 손상을 입었다. 환자가 불에 탄 건물에서 얼굴에 화상을 입고 호흡이 곤란한 상태로 쓰러진 채 발견되었다는 점을 고려할 때 환자가 다량의 연기를 흡입했을 가능성이 높다고 생각해야 한다.

기도 부종과 흡입 손상이 있는지 평가하고 재평가한다. 기도 개방을 염두에 두어야 하지만, 현재 환자는 스스로 기도를 관리하고 있다. 기도 관리를 가장 잘할 수 있는 사람은 환자라는 점을 염두에 두고 환자를 이송하는 데 필요한 시간과 기도 부종이 있는 환자의 기도 관리 어려움 사이에 균형을 맞춰야 한다. 이송이 길어지거나 지연될 때 기관내삽관으로 기도를 확보하고 기관내관을 고정한다. 환자는 연기에 노출되어 질식 우려가 있으므로 100% 산소 공급이 필요하다. 환자에게 휴대용 일산화탄소 모니터에서 일산화탄소헤모글로빈 수치가 16%이며 환자가 100% 산소를 공급받고 있으므로 이미 치료 중이다. 시안화합물 중독 가능성이 있는 연기 흡입 처치에 관한 프로토콜을 참조한다.

양쪽 팔에 심부 전층 화상을 입어 정맥 라인을 확보할 수 없다. 양쪽 다리 모두 화상을 입지 않았으며 골절의 흔적도 없다. 왼쪽 정강뼈에 골내(IO) 주사를 시도하여 젖산 링거액을 투여한다.

환자는 머리 전체, 양쪽 팔, 가슴에 화상을 입었다. 각 팔다리는 체표면적의 약 9%이고 가슴은 18%, 머리는 약 9%의 화상을 입었다. 따라서 추정되는 체표면적은 약 45%이다. 이 환자의 체중은 80kg이다. USAISR 10의 법칙을 사용하여 환자의 초기 수액 필요량을 계산한다.

$$45\%(\text{체표면적}) \times 10\text{mL/hr} = 450\text{mL/hr}(\text{초기 수액 투여 속도})$$

환자가 1시간 이상 이송해야 하는 경우 혈류역학 및 소변 배출량에 따라 수액 투여 속도를 조절해야 한다. 장거리 이송 시 환자를 이송할 화상센터의 의료진에게 보고하고 필요한 경우 수액 소생술에 관해 의료 지도를 받는다.

References

1. World Health Organization. Burns: Key facts. Published March 6, 2018. Accessed November 21, 2021. https://www.who.int/news-room/fact-sheets/detail/burns/
2. Vyrosek SB, Annest JL, Ryan GW. Surveillance for fatal and non-fatal injuries—United States, 2001. *MMWR Surveill Summ*. 2004;53(7):1-57.
3. Herndon DN. *Total Burn Care*. 5th ed. Elsevier; 2018:15-26.
4. Goodwin CW, Dorethy J, Lam V, Pruitt BA Jr. Randomized trial of efficacy of crystalloid and colloid resuscitation on hemodynamic response and lung water following thermal injury. *Ann Surg*. 1983 May;197(5):520-531.
5. Evans EI, Purnell OJ, Robinett PW, Batchelor A, Martin M. Fluid and electrolyte requirements in severe burns. *Ann Surg*. 1952;135:804-817.
6. Shires GT. Proceedings of the Second NIH Workshop on Burn Management. *J Trauma*. 1979;19(11 suppl):862-863.
7. Schwartz SL. Consensus summary on fluid resuscitation. *J Trauma*. 1979;19(11 suppl):876-877.
8. Moyer CA, Margrave HW, Monafo, WW. Burn shock and extravascular sodium deficiency: treatment with Ringer's solution with lactate. *Arch Surg*. 1965;90:799-811.
9. Mortiz AR, Henrique FC Jr. Studies of thermal injury: the relative importance of time and surface temperature in the causation of cutaneous burn injury. *Am J Pathol*. 1947;23:695-720.
10. Robinson MC, Del Becarro EJ. Increasing dermal perfusion after burning by decreasing thromboxane production. *J Trauma*. 1980;20:722-725.
11. Heggers JP, Ko F, Robson MC, et al. Evaluation of burn blister fluid. *Plast Reconstr Surg*. 1980;65:798-804.
12. Pruitt BA Jr, Goodwin CW, Mason AD Jr. Epidemiological, demographic and outcome characteristics of burn injury. In: Herndon DN, ed. *Total Burn Care*. 2nd ed. WB Saunders; 2002:16-32.
13. Rossiter ND, Chapman P, Haywood IA. How big is a hand? *Eurns*. 1996;22(3):230-231.
14. Berry MG, Evison D, Roberts AH. The influence of body mass index on burn surface area estimated from the area of the hand. *Burns*. 2001;27(6):591-594.
15. de Camara DL, Robinson MC. Ultrastructure aspects of cooled thermal injury. *J Trauma*. 1981;21:911-919.
16. Jandera V, Hudson DA, de Wet PM, Innes PM, Rode H. Cooling the burn wound: evaluation of different modalities. *Burns*. 2000;26:265-270.
17. Sawada Y, Urushidate S, Yotsuyanagi T, Ishita K. Is prolonged and excessive cooling of a scalded wound effective? *Burns*. 1977;23(1):55-58.
18. Venter TH, Karpelowsky JS, Rode H. Cooling of the burn wound: the ideal temperature of the coolant. *Burns*. 2007;33:917-922.
19. Dunn K, Edwards-Jones VT. The role of Acticoat with nanocrystal-line silver in the management of burns. *Burns*. 2004;30(suppl):S1.
20. Wright JB, Lam K, Burrell RE. Wound management in an era of increasing bacterial antibiotic resistance: a role for topical silver treatments. *Am J Infect Control*. 1998;26:572-577.

21. Yin HQ, Langford R, Burrell RE. Comparative evaluation of the antimicrobial activity of Acticoat antimicrobial dressing. *J Burn Care Rehabil*. 1999;20:195-200.

22. Chung KK, Salinas J, Renz EM, et al. Simple derivation of the initial fluid rate for the resuscitation of severely burned adult combat casualties: in silico validation of the rule of 10. *J Trauma*. 2010;69:S49-S54.

23. Merrell SW, Saffle JR, Sullivan JJ, Navar PD, Kravitz M, Warden GD. Fluid resuscitation in thermally injured children. *Am J Surg*. 1986;152:664-669.

24. Graves TA, Cioffi WG, McManus WF, Mason AD Jr, Pruitt BA Jr. Fluid resuscitation of infants and children with massive thermal injury. *J Trauma*. 1988;28:1656-1659.

25. Carvajal HF. Fluid therapy for the acutely burned child. *Compr Ther*. 1977;3:17-24.

26. Herndon DN. *Total Burn Care*. 2nd ed. WB Saunders; 2002.

27. Navar PD, Saffle JR, Warden GD. Effect of inhalation injury on fluid resuscitation requirements after thermal injury. *Am J Surg*. 1985;150:716-720.

28. Lalonde C, Picard L, Youn YK, Demling RH. Increased early postburn fluid requirement and oxygen demands are predictive of the degree of airway injury by smoke inhalation. *J Trauma*. 1995;38(2):175-184.

29. RxList. Anectine: warnings. Reviewed January 31, 2011. Accessed September 1, 2013. http://www.rxlist.com/anectine-drug/warnings-precautions.htm

30. Dash S, Arumugam PK, Muthukumar V, Kumath M, Sharma S. Study of clinical pattern of limb loss in electrical burn injuries. *Injury*. 2021 Jul;52(7):1925-1933. doi: 10.1016/j.injury.2021.04.028

31. Herndon DN. *Total Burn Care*. 5th ed. Elsevier; 2018:398-400.

32. Forbes WH, Sargent F, Roughton FJW. The rate of carbon monoxide uptake by normal men. *Am J Physiol*. 1945;143:594-608.

33. Mellins RB, Park S. Respiratory complications of smoke inhalation in victims of fires. *J Pediatr*. 1975;87(1):1-7. doi: 10.1016/s0022-3476(75)80059-x

34. Weaver LK, Hopkins RO, Chan KJ, et al. Hyperbaric oxygen for acute carbon monoxide poisoning. *N Engl J Med*. 2002;347(14):1057-1067.

35. Juurlink DN, Buckley NA, Stanbrook MB, Isbister GK, Bennett M, McGuigan MA. Hyperbaric oxygen for carbon monoxide poisoning. *Cochrane Database Syst Rev*. 2005;(1):CD002041.

36. Han S, Cho YS. Hyperbaric oxygen therapy in carbon monoxide poisoning: still controversial. *J Emerg Med*. 2021 Nov;61(5):619-620.

37. Chen KK, Rose CL, Clowes GH. Comparative values of several antidotes in cyanide poisoning. *Am J Med Sci*. 1934;188:767-781.

38. Feldstein M, Klendshoj NJ. The determination of cyanide in biological fluids by microdiffusion analysis. *J Lab Clin Med*. 1954;44:166-170.

39. Vogel SN, Sultan TR. Cyanide poisoning. *Clin Toxicol*. 1981;18:367-383.

40. Herndon DN, Traber DL, Niehaus GD, et al. The pathophysiology of smoke inhalation in a sheep model. *J Trauma*. 1984;24:1044-1051.

41. Till GO, Johnson KJ, Kunkel R, et al. Intravascular activation of complement and acute lung injury. *J Clin Invest*. 1982;69:1126-1135.

42. Thommasen HV, Martin BA, Wiggs BR, Quiroga M, Baile EM, Hogg JC. Effect of pulmonary blood flow on leukocyte uptake and release by dog lung. *J Appl Physiol Respir Environ Exerc Physiol*. 1984;56:966-974. doi: 10.1152/jappl.1984.56.4.966

43. Trunkey DD. Inhalation injury. *Surg Clin North Am*. 1978;58:1133-1140.

44. Haponik E, Summer W. Respiratory complications in the burned patient: diagnosis and management of inhalation injury. *J Crit Care*. 1987;2:121-143.

45. Cahalane M, Demling R. Early respiratory abnormalities from smoke inhalation. *JAMA*. 1984;251:771-773.

46. Herndon DN. *Total Burn Care*. 5th ed. Elsevier; 2018:16-19.

47. Hight DW, Bakalar HR, Lloyd JR. Inflicted burns in children: recognition and treatment. *JAMA*. 1979;242:517-520.

48. U.S. Department of Justice, Office of Justice Programs, Office of Juvenile Justice and Delinquency Prevention. Burn injuries in child abuse. Published May 1997. Reprinted June 2001. Accessed December 17, 2013. https://www.ojp.gov/pdffiles/91190-6.pdf

49. Başaran A, Narsat MA. Clinical outcome of pediatric hand burns and evaluation of neglect as a leading cause: a retrospective study. *Ulus Travma Acil Cerrahi Derg*. 2022 Jan;28(1):84-89.

50. Chadwick DL. The diagnosis of inflicted injury in infants and young children. *Pediatr Ann*. 1992;21:477-483.

51. Adronicus M, Oates RK, Peat J, et al. Nonaccidental burns in children. *Burns*. 1998;24:552-558.

52. Purdue GF, Hunt JL, Prescott PR. Child abuse by burning: an index of suspicion. *J Trauma*. 1988;28:221-224.

53. Lenoski EF, Hunter KA. Specific patterns of inflicted burn injuries. *J Trauma*. 1977;17:842-846.

54. Brooks JW, Evans EI, Ham WT, Reid JD. The influence of external body radiation on mortality from thermal burns. *Ann Surg*. 1953;136:533-545.

55. American Burn Association. Radiation injury. In: *Advanced Burn Life Support Course*. ABA; 1999:66.

56. Michell MW, Oliveira HM, Vaid SU, et al. Enteral resuscitation of burn shock using intestinal infusion of World Health Organization oral rehydration solution (WHO ORS): a potential treatment for mass casualty care. *J Burn Care Rehabil*. 2004;25:S48.

57. Bromberg BF, Song IC, Walden RH. Hydrotherapy of chemical burns. *Plast Reconstr Surg*. 1965;35:85-95.

58. Leonard LG, Scheulen JJ, Munster AM. Chemical burns: effect of prompt first aid. *J Trauma*. 1982;22(5):420-423.

59. Alam M, Moynagh M, Orr DS, Lawlor C. Cement burns—the Dublin national burns experience. *J Burns Wounds*. 2007;7:33-38.

60. Mozingo DW, Smith AD, McManus WF, Mason AD. Chemical burns. *J Trauma*. 1988;28(5):642-647.

61. Mistry D, Wainwright D. Hydrofluoric acid burns. *Am Fam Physician*. 1992;45:1748-1754.

62. Willems JL. Clinical management of mustard gas casualties. *Ann Med Milit Belg*. 1989;3S:1-61.

63. Papirmeister B, Feister AJ, Robinson SI, et al. The sulfur mustard injury: description of lesions and resulting incapacitation. In: Papirmeister B, Feister A, Robinson S, Ford R, eds. *Medical Defense Against Mustard Gas*. CRC Press; 1990:13.

64. Sidell FR, Takafuji ET, Franz DR. *Medical Aspects of Chemical and Biological Warfare*. Washington, DC: Office of the Surgeon General; 1997.

소아 외상

Lead Editors
Jessica Naiditch, MD, FACS, FAAP
Katherine Remick, MD, FAAP, FACEP, FAEMS
David Tuggle, MD, FACS, FAAP

학습 목표   이 장의 학습을 완료하면 다음과 같은 내용을 수행할 수 있다.

- 특별한 어린이 손상 유형을 설명하는 소아의 해부학적 및 생리학적 차이를 설명할 수 있다.
- 소아 환자의 기도 관리와 적절한 조직으로 산소 공급 회복의 특별한 중요성에 관해 설명할 수 있다.
- 소아 혼자의 나이별 활력징후를 구분할 수 있다.
- 소아 환자에게서 발견되는 다양한 손상을 처치하는 방법에 관해 설명할 수 있다.
- 사고가 아닌 외상을 암시하는 소아 외상의 징후를 설명할 수 있다.

시나리오

당신은 교통량이 많은 고속도로에서 발생한 자동차 충돌 사고 현장으로 출동했다. 두 대의 차량이 정면충돌하였다. 차량 탑승자 중 한 명은 어린이용 보조 의자에 부적절하게 고정된 어린이이다. 사고 당시 날씨와 관련된 요인은 없었다.

현장에 도착했을 때 경찰이 사고 주변 지역의 교통을 통제하고 있었다. 당신의 동료와 다른 도착한 구급대원이 환자를 평가하는 동안 당신은 어린이에게 다가간다. 약 2세의 정도의 남자아이가 비스듬히 기울어진 어린이용 보조 의자에 앉아 있었다. 어린이가 앉아 있는 앞좌석 머리 받침대 뒤쪽에 피가 묻어있는 것을 확인한다. 머리, 얼굴, 목 부위에 찰과상과 경미한 출혈이 있음에도 불구하고 어린이는 매우 침착해 보인다.

당신은 "엄마, 엄마"라고 약하게 반복해서 말하는 2세 남아의 일차 및 이차평가를 시행한다. 맥박수는 180회/분이고 노동맥이 위팔동맥보다 약하며 촉진으로 측정한 혈압은 50mmHg이다. 호흡수는 분당 18회이며 약간 불규칙하지만, 비정상적인 소리는 들리지 않는다. 계속 환자를 평가하면서 "엄마"라는 말을 하지 않고 멍하니 허공을 응시하는 것을 확인한다. 또한 동공이 약간 확장되어 있고 피부가 창백하고 땀이 나는 것을 알 수 있다. 자신을 소아의 유모라고 밝힌 한 여성이 당신에게 아이의 엄마가 오는 중이니 기다려 달라고 말한다.

- 이 환아의 처치 우선순위는 무엇인가?
- 이 어린이에게 가장 가능성이 높은 손상은 무엇인가?
- 이 환아에게 가장 적절한 의료기관은 어디인가?

© Ralf Hiemisch/Getty Images

개요

미국 질병통제예방센터(CDC)에서 매년 발표하는 데이터에 따르면 손상이 미국 어린이 사망의 가장 흔한 원인이다.

미국 질병통제예방센터에 따르면 2019년 한 해 동안 19세 미만의 어린이 7,000명 이상이 의도하지 않은 손상으로 사망했다. 이러한 사망 원인의 주요 원인은 차량 충돌, 질식, 익사, 중독, 화재, 낙상 등이었다. 이러한 사망과 관련하여 이용할 수 있는 데이터를 면밀히 평가한 결과 안타깝게도 아동기 손상은 종종 예방할 수 있는 경우가 많다. 더욱 충격적인 사실은 어린이 그룹 간에 의도하지 않은 손상으로 인한 사망률에 인종적, 민족적 격차가 크다는 사실이다. 예를 들어 2010~2019년까지 차량 충돌로 인한 손상으로 인한 사망률은 흑인 어린이는 9% 증가했지만, 백인 어린이는 24% 감소했다. 중독으로 인한 사망률은 같은 기간 동안 히스패닉 어린이의 경우 50%, 흑인 어린이의 경우 24% 증가했지만, 백인 어린이의 경우 9% 감소했다(그림 14-1). 이러한 데이터가 가장 취약한 집단에 대한 위험을 가장 효과적으로 줄일 수 있는 방식으로 예방 전략과 개입을 목표로 하는 데 사용될 수 있기를 바란다.

소아 처치의 모든 측면과 마찬가지로 손상을 입은 어린이를 적절히 평가하고 처치하려면 소아 성장 및 발달의 고유한 특성(미성숙한 해부학 및 발달하는 생리학을 포함)뿐만 아니라 손상의 고유한 기전에 대한 철저한 이해가 필요하다.

"어린이는 작은 성인이 아니다"라는 속담은 사실이다. 어린이는 손상 당시의 신체적, 심리·사회적 발달에 따라 뚜렷하고 재현할 수 있는 손상 유형, 다양한 생리적 반응 및 특별한 처치가 필요한 경우가 있다.

이 장에서는 소아 외상 환자의 특수한 특성을 설명하는 것으로 시작하여 최적의 외상 처치와 그 근거를 검토한다. 소아 외상의 고유한 특성은 병원 전 처치 제공자가 이해하는 것이 중요하지만, 일차평가 및 이차평가를 이용한 기본적인 기본 생명 유지 및 전문 생명 유지를 위한 처치 방법은 나이나 크기와 관계없이 모든 환자에게 동일하다.

소아 외상 환자

소아 외상의 인구 통계

소아 환자의 고유한 요구와 급성 손상을 입은 어린이 환자를 평가할 때 특별한 주의가 필요하다. 소아 인구에서는 무딘 손상(vs. 관통상)의 상대적 발생률이 가장 높으며 관통상은 손상의 7.8%에 불과하다. 관통상은 종종 신체의 단일 기관에 손상을 입히지만, 무딘 외상은 여러 기관에 손상을 입히는 경향이 더 크다.

낙상, 자동차에 치인 보행자, 차량 충돌로 인한 탑승자 손상은 미

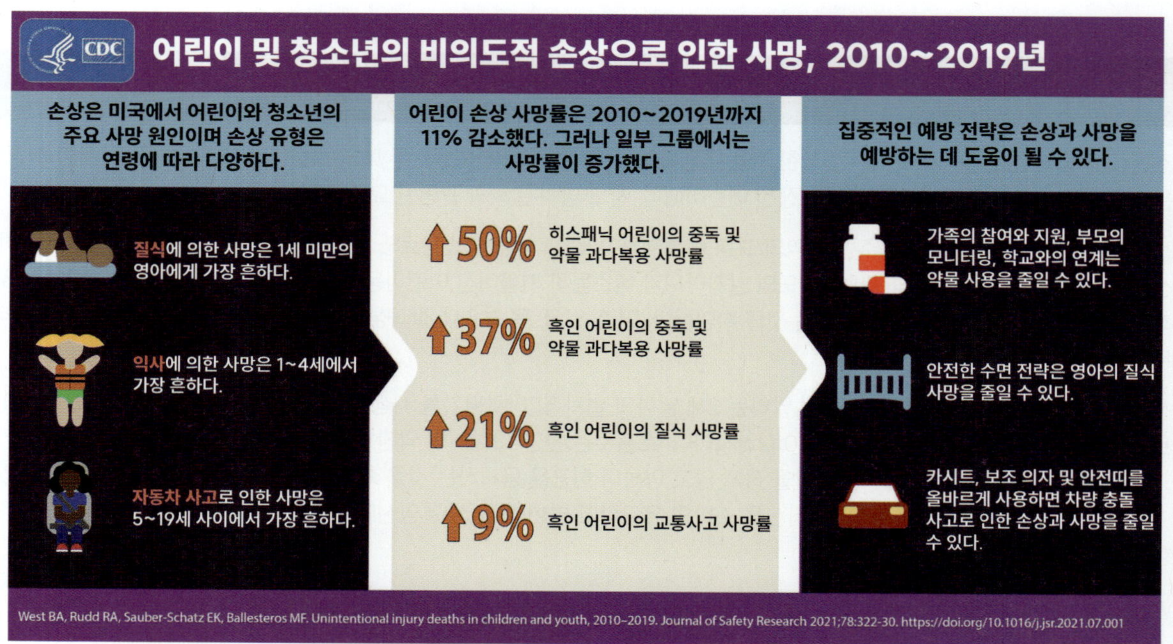

그림 14-1 어린이 및 청소년의 비의도적 손상으로 인한 사망, 2010~2019년

국에서 소아 손상의 가장 흔한 원인이며 15세 미만 어린이의 경우 낙상으로만 연간 240만 건 이상의 손상을 입는다. 세계보건기구(WHO)는 전 세계적으로 매년 약 83만 명의 어린이가 외상으로 사망하고 수천만 명의 어린이가 치명적이지 않은 손상으로 입원하는 것으로 추정한다. 미국에서와 교통 관련 사고가 소아 사망의 가장 흔한 원인이며 화상, 살인, 낙상이 그다음으로 흔한 원인이다.

이 장 전체에서 설명할 여러 가지 이유로 인해 주요 소아 외상에서는 다기관 손상이 예외가 아니라는 규칙이다. 외상에 대한 최소한의 외부 증거가 있더라도 생명을 위협할 수 있는 내부 손상이 여전히 존재할 수 있으므로 적절한 장비를 갖춘 외상센터에서 평가해야 한다.

외상 및 소아 외상의 물리학

어린이의 체구가 작기 때문에 자동차 펜더, 범퍼 및 낙상으로 인한 힘이 가해지는 표면적이 더 작다. 체지방으로 인한 완충 작용이 적고, 결합 조직의 탄력성 증가하며 내장이 신체 표면에 근접해 있기 때문에 어린이는 성인과 같은 방식으로 이러한 힘을 분산시키는 능력이 제한되므로 에너지가 장기에 더 쉽게 전달된다. 또한 어린이의 골격은 불안전하게 석회화되어 있고 여러 개의 활성화된 성장점을 포함하고 있으며 성인보다 더 탄력적이다. 따라서 외부 손상의 명백한 증거 없이도 심각한 내부 손상이 있을 수 있다.

일반적인 손상 유형

어린이의 고유한 해부학적 및 생리학적 특징과 연령에 따른 일반적인 손상 기전이 결합하여 뚜렷하지만, 예측 가능한 손상 유형이 나타난다(표 14-1). 부적절한 안전띠 사용 또는 앞좌석에 탑승한 어린이는 에어백의 충격으로 인해 심각한 손상을 초래할 수 있다(Box 14-1). 외상을 입은 환자는 시간이 매우 중요한 경우가 많으며 이러한 유형을 잘 알고 있으면 병원 전 처치 제공자가 손상을 입은 어린이에 대한 처치 신속하게 결정하는 데 도움이 될 수 있다. 예를 들어 폐쇄 머리 손상을 동반한 무딘 소아 외상은 혈량저하증 및 저혈압보다 무호흡, 저환기 및 저산소증을 훨씬 더 흔하게 유발한다. 따라서 소아 외상 환자를 위한 임상 처치 지침에는 기도와 호흡에 대한 집중적인 처치가 더욱 강조되어야 한다.

열 항상성

어린이의 체표면적과 체질량 사이의 비율은 출생 시 가장 높고 영유아기와 아동기에 걸쳐 감소한다. 따라서 체온이 바르게 손실될 수 있는 표면적이 많아지면 어린이에게 추가적인 스트레스를 줄 뿐만 아니

표 14-1 소아 외상과 관련된 일반적인 손상 유형	
외상 유형	**손상 유형**
자동차 충돌 (어린이는 동승자)	억제되지 않은: 다기관 외상(가슴 및 복부 포함), 머리 및 목 손상, 두피 및 얼굴 열상
	억제된: 가슴 및 복부 손상, 하부 척추 골절
자동차 충돌 (어린이는 보행자)	저속: 다리 골절
	고속: 다기관 외상(가슴 및 복부 포함), 머리 및 목 손상, 다리 골절
높은 곳에서 추락	낮음: 팔 골절
	중간: 머리 및 목 손상, 팔다리 골절
	높음: 다기관 외상(가슴 및 복부 포함), 머리 및 목 손상, 팔다리 골절
자전거에서 넘어짐	헬멧 미착용: 머리 및 목 열상, 두피 및 얼굴 열상, 팔 골절
	헬멧 착용: 팔 골절
	핸들에 충돌: 복부 내부 손상

Modified from American College of Surgeons Committee on Trauma. Pediatric trauma. In: *ATLS® Advanced Trauma Life Support® Student Course Manual*. 10th ed. ACS; 2018:186-213.

> ### Box 14-1 안전띠 및 에어백과 관련된 소아 손상
>
> 50개 주 모두에서 어린이용 카시트 또는 어린이 보호 장치 사용을 의무화하는 법률이 시행되고 있지만, 어린이 보호 장치가 종종 부적절하게 설치된다는 증거가 있다. 또한 조수석 에어백이 장착된 앞좌석에 어린이가 탑승한 경우 어린이는 적절하게 안전띠를 착용했는지와 관계없이 심각한 손상을 입을 가능성이 높다. 조수석 에어백에 노출된 어린이는 에어백이 없는 앞좌석 탑승자보다 심각한 손상을 입을 가능성이 두 배 더 높다.
>
> 2점식 허리 안전띠를 착용했거나 안전띠를 부적절하게 착용한 어린이는 자동차 충돌 시 장기 손상의 위험이 증가한다. 이러한 유형의 안전띠 손상은 췌장, 대동맥 및 허리 손상을 유발할 수 있으며 이러한 어린이는 심각한 다기관 외상의 위험에 처할 수 있다. 자동차 충돌 후 허리 안전띠에 고정되어 자동차 충돌 후 복벽에 멍이 든 채로 발견된 어린이는 달리 확인될 때까지 복강 내 손상을 입었다고 가정하는 것이 합리적이다.
>
> 어린이와 관련된 모든 자동차 충돌 사고의 약 1%에서 어린이가 전개된 조수석 에어백에 노출된다. 1세대 에어백이 전개된 차량 충돌 사고에 연루된 어린이 중 최대 14%가 심각한 손상을 입었다. 에어백 기술이 개선됨에 따라 에어백 전개 중 손상 위험은 여전히 크지만, 10%로 감소했다. 이러한 손상에는 경증의 상체 및 얼굴 화상, 열상 또는 가슴, 목, 얼굴 및 팔의 손상이 포함될 수 있다.

라 대사 장애와 쇼크에 대한 어린이의 생리학적 반응이 달라질 수 있다. 심각한 저체온증은 중증의 응고병증과 잠재적으로 돌이킬 수 없는 심혈관 허탈을 초래할 수 있다. 또한 저체온증의 임상 징후 중 상당수는 보상되지 않은 쇼크가 임박한 경우와 유사하므로 병원 전 처치 제공자의 임상적 평가를 혼란스럽게 할 수 있다.

심리 사회적 문제

손상을 입은 어린이에게 심리적인 영향은 큰 도전이 될 수 있다. 특히 아주 어린 아이의 경우 스트레스, 통증 또는 기타 위협으로 인해 어린이가 무서운 사건을 처리하는 능력이 손상되면 퇴행적인 심리적 행동이 나타날 수 있다. 낯선 환경에서 낯선 사람을 만나면 어린이는 병력 청취, 신체검사 및 처치에 완전히 협조하는 데 한계가 있을 수 있다. 이러한 특성을 이해하고 손상을 입은 어린이를 위로하고 달래려는 의지는 좋은 관계를 형성하고 어린이의 생리적 상태를 종합적으로 평가하는 데 가장 효과적인 수단인 경우가 많다.

어린이의 부모 또는 보호자(유모)도 특별한 주의가 필요한 경우가 많으며 "부모도 환자"로 간주할 수 있다. 모든 환자의 처치는 효과적인 의사소통에서 시작하지만 이러한 '부모 환자'를 대할 때 의사소통이 더욱 중요하다. 단순히 위로의 말이나 오랜 인내로 이루어질 수도 있지만, 부모나 보호자의 요구 사항을 잘 알지 못한다면 어린이 환자를 위한 효과적인 병원 전 처치 제공자가 될 수 없다.

부모 또는 주 보호자는 자녀의 손상 및 처치 계획에 대한 정보를 요구하거나 자녀의 상태에 대한 정보를 요구할 수 있다. 이를 무시하면 부모는 화를 내거나 공격적으로 변하여 효과적인 처치에 심각한 장애를 초래할 수 있다. 그러나 부모를 처치 과정에 참여시키면 부모는 자녀를 처치하는 팀의 실질적 구성원으로 역할을 할 수 있다.

가족 중심 치료의 개념은 의료 전문가와 가족 간의 협력 관계를 구축하고 이러한 관계를 활용하여 양질의 응급의료서비스를 제공하는 데 도움을 주는 역동적인 접근 방식이다. 가족 중심 치료는 가족 구성원의 상태에 대한 가족의 지식이 치료의 질과 의사소통을 향상하고 가족을 팀의 일원으로 포용하는 데 중요한 도구라는 점을 인식한다. 또한 부모 또는 보호자의 참여는 어린이에게 부모가 안전한 사람으로 보증된다는 신호를 보내어 아동의 협력 가능성을 높인다. 의료진은 어린이가 아프거나 다칠 때마다 보호자도 영향을 받으며 보호자 역시 환자로 간주해야 한다는 점을 기억해야 한다.

회복 및 재활

소아 외상 환자의 경우 경미한 손상도 이후의 성장과 발달에 영향을 미칠 수 있는 특징이 있다. 해부학적으로 성숙한 성인과 달리 소아는 손상에서 회복해야 할 뿐만 아니라 정상적인 성장을 지속해야 한다. 특히 영구적인 장애, 성장 기형 또는 이후의 비정상적인 발달 측면에서 손상이 이 과정에 미치는 영향을 과대평가할 수 있다. 경미한 외상성 뇌손상을 입은 어린이는 뇌 기능, 심리적 적응 또는 기타 조절 기관에 장기간 장애를 겪을 수 있다. 이러한 장애는 형제자매와 부모에게 상당한 영향을 미쳐 이혼을 포함한 가족 기능 장애의 발생률이 높아질 수 있다.

급성 손상 단계에서 부적절하거나 최적의 치료가 이루어지지 않으면 어린이의 즉각적인 생존뿐만 아니라 장기적인 삶의 질에 이르기까지 광범위한 결과를 초래할 수 있다. 따라서 급성 손상을 입은 어린이를 처치하고 이송 결정을 내릴 때 손상에 대한 높은 의심 지수를 유지하고 임상적 상식을 사용하는 것이 매우 중요하다.

병태생리학

손상을 입은 어린이의 최종 결과는 손상 후 처음 순간에 제공되는 처치의 질에 따라 결정될 수 있다. 이 중요한 시기에 조직적이고 체계적인 일차평가는 불필요한 이환율을 피하고 치명적일 수 있는 손상을 간과하는 것을 방지하기 위한 최선의 방법이다. 성인 환자와 마찬가지로 어린이에서 즉시 사망에 이르는 가장 흔한 세 가지 원인은 저산소증, 대량출혈, 심각한 중추신경계 외상이다. 이 부문에서는 이 세 가지 즉시 사망 원인에 대해 자세히 설명한다. 신속한 분류, 응급처치와 안정화와 가장 적절한 치료 센터로의 이송은 의미 있는 회복 가능성을 최적화할 수 있다.

저산소증

어린이의 기도가 개방되어 있고 정상적으로 작동하는지 확인했다고 해서 특히 중추신경계 손상, 저환기 또는 관류저하가 있는 경우 산소 보충 및 보조 환기가 필요하지 않은 것은 아니다. 상태가 양호해 보이는 어린이도 경미한 빠른 호흡에서 탈진 및 무호흡 상태로 빠르게 악화할 수 있다. 기도를 확보한 후에는 환기 속도와 깊이를 주의 깊게 평가하여 적절한 환기가 이루어지고 있는지 확인해야 한다. 환기가 불충분한 경우 고농도 산소를 공급하는 것만으로는 저산소증이 지속되거나 악화하는 것을 예방할 수 없다.

외상으로 손상된 뇌에 일시적인 저산소중이 미치는 영향은 특별한 주의가 필요하다. 어린이는 의식 수준(LOC)에 심각한 변화가 있을 수 있지만, 뇌 저산소중을 피하면 완전한 기능 회복 가능성이 매우 높다.

적극적인 기도 관리가 필요한 소아 환자는 전문 기도유지 장비로 기도유지를 시행하기 전 예방산소투여를 실시해야 한다. 이 산소화되는 탈질소화는 폐포 질소를 산소로 대체하여 폐포 내 산소 보유량을 확보함으로써 산소혈색소 포화도를 최소화하면서 무호흡을 가능한 한 지속할 수 있도록 시도한다. 이렇게 하면 기도 확보와 관련된 술기를 시행할 때 안전하게 시행할 수 있는 시간이 향상된다. 여러 번 또는 장기간 기도 확보를 시도하는 동안 저산소 상태가 지속하면 단순히 백마스크 장비로 환기를 시행하고 신속하게 이송하는 것보다 어린이에게 더 해로울 수 있다. 백마스크 장비를 이용한 환기와 같은 기본적인 생명유지술로 환기와 산소 공급이 적절하게 이루어지고 있다면 전문 기도유지를 시도하는 것은 불필요하며 잠재적으로 해로울 수 있다.

출혈

대부분의 소아 손상은 즉각적인 대량출혈을 일으키지 않는다. 그러나 대량출혈을 초래하는 손상을 입은 소아는 손상 직후 또는 병원에 도착한 직후 사망하는 경우가 많다. 이러한 사망은 다발성 내부 장기 손상으로 인해 발생하는 경우가 많으며 적어도 한 가지 이상의 심각한 손상으로 인해 급성 출혈이 발생한다. 이러한 출혈은 단순 열상이나 타박상처럼 경미한 것일 수도 있고 비장 파열, 간 열상 또는 신장 파열과 같이 생명을 위협하는 출혈일 수도 있다.

손상을 입은 어린이는 전신 혈관 저항을 증가시켜 출혈을 보상하지만, 말초 관류의 감소로 이어진다. 소아는 기존의 말초 혈관 질환에 의해 혈관수축이 제한되지 않기 때문에 생리학적으로 이러한 반응에 더 능숙하다. 혈압 측정으로는 쇼크의 초기 징후를 파악하는 것은 부적절한 방법이다. 빈맥은 두려움이나 통증의 결과로 나타날 수 있지만, 달리 입증될 때까지 출혈이나 혈량저하증에 의한 이차적인 것으로 간주해야 한다. 맥압이 좁아지고 빈맥이 증가하면 쇼크가 임박했다는 첫 번째 미세한 징후일 수 있다.

또한, 병원 전 처치 제공자는 호흡 노력의 변화, 의식 수준 감소, 피부 관류 감소(체온 저하, 피부색 저하, 모세혈관 재충전 시간 지연)에서 알 수 있는 장기 관류의 비효율적인 징후에 세심한 주의를 기울여야 한다. 성인과 달리 어린이에서 이러한 출혈의 초기 징후는 미묘하고 파악하기 어려울 수 있으므로 쇼크를 늦게 인지할 수 있다. 병원 전 처치 제공자가 이러한 초기 징후를 놓치면 어린이는 보상 기전이 실패할 정도로 충분한 순환 혈액량을 잃을 수 있다. 이런 일이 발생하면 심박출량이 급감하고 장기 관류가 감소하며 어린이는 빠르게 보상 능력이 저하되어 종종 돌이킬 수 없는 치명적인 저혈압과 쇼크로 이어질 수 있다. 따라서 무딘 외상을 입은 모든 어린이는 활력징후가 비정상적으로 나타나기 훨씬 전에 출혈이 진행 중임을 알릴 수 있는 미묘한 징후를 발견할 수 있도록 주의 깊게 모니터링해야 한다.

비보상 쇼크로 빠르게 전환되는 주된 이유는 적혈구의 손실과 그에 상응하는 산소 운반 능력의 손실이다. 결정질 수액 투여로 손실된 혈관 내 부피를 회복하면 일시적으로 혈압이 상승할 수 있지만, 체액이 모세혈관막을 통과하면서 순환량이 빠르게 소실된다. 혈액이 손실되고 혈액 내 부피를 결정질 수액으로 대체하면 혈류에 남아있는 적혈구가 희석되어 조직에 산소를 운반하는 혈액의 능력이 감소한다. 따라서 20mL/kg 이상의 결정질 수액을 볼루스로 1회 이상 투여해야 하는 어린이는 상태가 급속히 악화할 수 있으며 혈관 내 체적 소생술과 병행하여 산소 전달 능력을 회복하기 위해 적혈구 수혈이 필요할 수 있다. 지속해서 출혈 징후가 있는 어린이 환자에게는 혈액 제제의 조기 투여를 고려해야 한다. 이는 두 번의 수액을 볼루스로 투여하기 전에 시작할 수 있다.

그러나 일단 정맥 라인이 확보되면 심각한 쇼크 상태가 아닌 손상을 입은 어린이에게 실수로 과도한 수액 소생술을 시행하는 경향이 있다. 생리식염수는 산성을 띠기 때문에 상온에서 투여하면 냉각 및 경미한 산증을 유발할 수 있으며 이는 응고를 저해하여 진행 중인 출혈을 악화시킬 수 있다. 중등도의 출혈이 있고 말단 장기의 관류저하의 증거가 없으며 활력징후가 정상인 어린이의 경우 수액 소생술은 20mL/kg의 생리식염수를 1~2회 이하로 투여하는 것으로 제한해야 한다. 1회의 볼루스로 투여하는 혈관 내 구성 성분은 대략 어린이 혈액량의 25%에 해당한다. 따라서 두 번 이상의 볼루스로 투여가 필요한 경우 병원 전 처치 제공자는 이전에 발견하지 못한 지속적인 출혈의 원인이 있는지 어린이를 재평가해야 한다.

외상성 뇌손상을 입은 어린이의 경우 이차 뇌손상의 원인으로 알려져 있고 예방할 수 있는 저혈압을 예방하기 위해 수액 소생술을 실시해야 한다. 뇌관류압은 두개내압과 평균 동맥압(혈액을 두개골로 유도하는 압력)의 차이이다. 외상성 뇌손상은 두개내압을 증가시킬 수 있다. 따라서 혈액에 산소가 충분히 공급되더라도 전신 혈압이 낮으면 산소가 공급된 혈액이 뇌로 관류되지 않아 저산소성 뇌손상이 발생할 수 있다. 의인성 뇌부종을 예방하기 위해 과도한 수액 소생술은 피해야 하지만, 저혈압이 한 번만 발생해도 사망률이 150%까지 증가시킬 수 있으므로 수액 소생술로 저혈압을 예방하거나 신속하게 처치해야 한다. 어린이의 활력징후를 주의 깊게 평가하고 처치 후 지속해서 재평가하여 처치를 결정해야 한다.

저장성 결정질 수액(예: 포도당 용액)은 뇌부종을 증가시키는 것으로 알려져 있으므로 등장성 결정질 용액은 외상성 뇌손상이 있는 어린이의 소생술을 위해 선택해야 하는 수액이다. 또한, 고장성 결정질 수액(예: 고삼투식염수)은 광범위한 모니터링이 이루어지는 소아 중환자실에서 뇌부종 치료에 유용할 수 있지만, 현재까지 현장에서 투여했을 때 소아 외상 환자의 결과가 개선된 것으로 입증된 증거는 없다. 탈출증이 임박한 상황에서 동공이 수축하거나 글래스고혼수척도 점수가 현저하게 감소한 증거(2점 이상 하락)가 있는 경우 병원 전 환경에서 이송 지연이 필요한 경우 고장식염수 투여를 고려할 수 있다.

중추신경계 손상

심각한 중추신경계 외상 후 병태생리학적 변화하는 몇 분 안에 시작된다. 조기에 적절한 소생술을 실시하는 것이 중추신경계 외상을 입은 어린이의 잠재적 생존율을 극대화하는 열쇠이다. 일부 중추신경계 손상은 압도적으로 치명적이지만, 치명적인 신경학적 손상을 입은 많은 어린이는 이차 손상을 예방하기 위한 신중하고 체계적인 노력 후에 완전하게 기능적인 회복을 이룰 수 있다. 이러한 회복은 관류저하, 저환기, 과다환기 및 허혈이 발생하는 것을 예방함으로써 가능하다. 적절한 환기와 산소 공급(과다환기를 피하면서)은 저혈압을 피하는 것만큼이나 외상성 뇌손상의 처치에 중요하다.

중추신경계 손상 정도에 따라 어린이는 성인보다 사망률이 낮고 생존 가능성이 높다. 그러나 뇌 이외의 손상이 추가로 발생하면 어린이가 좋은 결과를 얻을 가능성이 줄어드는데, 이는 관련 손상으로 인한 쇼크가 잠재적으로 부정적인 영향을 미칠 수 있음을 보여준다.

외상성 뇌손상이 있는 어린이는 종종 의식 변화를 보이며 초기 평가 시 목격하지 못한 의식 소실 기간이 지속될 수 있다. 의식 소실 병력은 잠재적인 중추신경계 손상의 가장 중요한 예후 인자 중 하나이므로 모든 사례에 대해 기록해야 한다. 손상을 목격하지 못한 경우 사고에 대한 기억 상실이 의식 상실을 대신하는 것으로 사용된다. 또한, 다음을 포함하여 기본적인 신경학적 상태에 대한 완전한 기록이 중요하다.

1. 글래스고혼수척도 점수(소아용으로 수정됨)
2. 동공 반응
3. 감각 자극에 대한 반응
4. 운동 기능

이는 신경 손상에 대한 초기 소아 외상 평가에서 필수적인 단계이다. 적절한 기준선 평가가 없으면 지속적인 후속 조치와 평가가 매우 어려워진다.

목뼈 손상 가능성이 있는 소아 환자의 경우 병력 청취에 세심한 주의를 기울이는 것이 특히 중요하다. 어린이의 골격은 여러 개의 성장점이 불완전하게 석회화되어 척수가 늘어나거나 타박상 또는 무딘 손상을 방사선촬영으로 진단하지 못하는 경우가 많다. 이러한 상태는 방사선학적 이상이 없는 척수 손상(SCIWORA)이라고 한다. 의료기관에 이송되기 전에 해결되는 일시적인 신경학적 결손은 심각한 척수 손상을 나타내는 유일한 지표일 수 있다. 빠른 증상 해결에도 불구하고 방사선학적 이상이 없는 척수 손상을 입은 어린이는 최초 손상 후 최대 4일까지 척수 부종이 발생할 수 있으며 처치하지 않고 방치하면 치명적인 신경학적 장애를 초래할 수 있다.

평가

일차평가

소아 환자의 작고 다양한 신체 크기(표 14-2), 혈관의 지름 감소 및 순환량 감소, 기도의 독특한 해부학적 특성으로 인해 기본 생명 유지에 사용되는 표준 절차는 종종 매우 까다롭고 기술적으로 어렵게 만든다. 효과적인 소아 외상 소생술을 위해서는 적절한 크기의 기도기, 후두경 날, 기관내관, 성문위기도기, 코위관, 혈압계 커프, 산소마스크, 백마스크 장비 및 관련 장비를 사용할 수 있어야 한다. 지나치게 큰 정맥 카테터나 부적절한 크기의 기도기를 사용하는 것은 소아 환자에게 신체적 손상을 입힐 수 있을 뿐만 아니라 적절한 의료기관으로 이송하는 것이 지연될 수 있으므로 득보다 실이 더 클 수 있다. 색상으로 구분된 길이별 소생술 가이드(이 장의 뒷부분에서 설명)는 실용적인 약물 및 장비에 대한 참조를 제공한다.

모든 연령대의 어린이에 대한 신속한 평가는 첫인상에서 시작된다. 어린이의 경우 병원 전 처치 제공자는 발달 단계와 시각 및 청각, 외모에 대한 이해를 바탕으로 중증도(즉, 아프거나 아프지 않은)를 신속하게 판단하기 위해 신속한 접근 방식을 사용해야 한다. 환자와 처

표 14-2 소아 환자의 키와 몸무게 범위

그룹	나이	평균 기준 범위	
		평균키(cm)	평균 몸무게(kg)
신생아	0~1개월	51~63	4~5
영아	1개월~1세	56~80	4~11
유아	1~2세	77~91	11~14
취학 전 아동	3~5세	91~122	14~25
학령기 아동	6~12세	122~165	25~63
청소년	12~15세	165~182	62~80

© National Association of Emergency Medical Technicians (NAEMT)

음 접촉할 때 소아 평가 삼각구도(PAT)를 사용하면 중증도 수준을 설정하고 처치의 긴급성을 결정하며 생리학적 문제의 일반적인 범주를 파악하는 데 도움이 된다(**그림 14-2**).

　소아 평가 삼각구도의 구성 요소는 외모, 호흡 상태 및 피부 순환이다. 일반적으로 이 검사는 환자가 얼마나 심각한지에 대한 초기 인상을 만들기 위해 멀리서 실시한다. 첫 번째 단계는 TICLS(근육 강도, 상호작용, 친밀감, 보는 상태, 언어 상태/우는 상태) 도구를 사용하여 어린이의 전반적인 외모를 평가하는 것이다.

- 근육 강도. 자발적으로 움직이고 앉거나 서 있다(적절한 나이)
- 상호 작용. 의식이 명료하고 주변 환경에 있는 사람들과 활동에 주의를 기울이며 장난감/물건(예: 펜라이트)에 손을 뻗는다.
- 안정감. 보호자에 대한 반응이 다름
- 보기/시선. 병원 전 처치 제공자와 눈을 맞추고 시각적으로 추적
- 말/울음. 울음소리가 강하거나 나이에 맞는 언어를 사용함

두 번째 단계는 호흡을 평가하는 것이다. 이 단계에는 비정상적인 기도 소리와 비정상적인 체위, 가슴 뒤 당김과 코 벌렁거림이 있는지 평가한다.

　셋째 병원 전 처치 제공자는 창백함, 반점 형성, 청색증을 찾아 피부로의 혈액 순환을 평가해야 한다. 이 세 가지 소아 평가 삼각구도 구성 요소를 결합하면 일반적인 기본 인상을 형성할 수 있다. 일반적인 주요 인상은 아프거나 아프지 않은 급성 발작 또는 손상을 보상할 수 있는 어린이의 능력에 대한 임상 의사의 전반적인 평가이다.

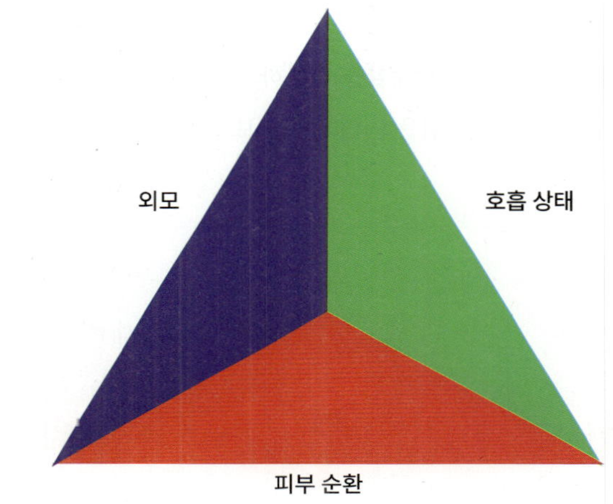

그림 14-2 소아 평가 삼각구도(PAT)

Used with permission cf the American Academy of Pediatrics. Pediatric Education for Prehospital Professionals. American Academy of Pediatrics; 2000.

러한 유형의 손상 발생률도 낮다. 초기 우선순위는 대량 외부출혈을 확인하고 직접 압박으로 조절하거나 지혈대를 적용하여 출혈을 조절하는 것이다. 외부출혈이 해결되었거나 출혈이 없는 경우 병원 전 처치 제공자는 어린이의 기도를 관리해야 한다.

기도

손상을 입은 성인과 마찬가지로 급성 손상을 입은 어린이의 경우 현장 안전을 확보하고 대량 출혈을 해결하거나 배제한 다음 우선순위는 기도 처치이다. 그러나 손상을 입은 어린이의 처치를 복잡하게 만드는 몇 가지 해부학적 차이점이 있다. 소아는 후두부와 혀가 상대적으로 크고 기도가 앞쪽에 있다. 또한 어린이가 작을수록 머리뼈와

안정화 우선순위

소아의 경우 즉각적인 대량출혈로 인한 생존율이 낮다. 다행히도 이

얼굴 중간 사이의 크기 차이가 더 크다. 따라서 상대적으로 큰 후두부는 목뼈를 수동적으로 굴곡시킨다(**그림 14-3**). 이러한 요인으로 인해 어린이는 성인보다 해부학적 기도 폐쇄의 위험이 더 높다. 외상이 없는 경우 소아 환자의 기도는 냄새 맡는 자세(sniffing position)라고 하는 얼굴 중간의 약간 전방 위쪽에 위치하는 것이 가장 잘 보호된다(**그림 14-4**). 그러나 외상이 있는 경우 중립 자세로 목뼈를 고정하여 냄새 맡는 자세에서 발생하는 목뼈 5번과 6번(C5, C6)의 굴곡과 C1~C2의 신전을 방지하여 고정하는 것이 목뼈를 가장 잘 보호한다. 이 자세에서 필요한 경우 턱들어올리기법으로 쉽게 기도 개방을 시행할 수 있다.

기도 유지 중에 목뼈를 도수로 고정하고 시중에서 구입하거나 수건 롤과 같은 단단한 목뼈 고정 장치를 사용하여 어린이가 고정될 때까지 유지한다. 또한, 영아의 몸통 아래에 2~3cm 두께의 패드나 담요를 대어주면 목의 급격한 굽힘을 완화하고 기도를 유지하는 데 도움이 될 수 있다. 손상을 입은 어린이에게 보조 환기가 필요한 경우 고

유량(최소 15L/분)의 100% 산소를 백마스크에 연결하여 환기를 시행하는 것이 최선의 선택일 수 있다. 적절하게 맞는 산소마스크와 "압착-배출-배출" 타이밍 기술을 사용한다. 가슴의 상승과 하강을 관찰하고 호기말이산화탄소분압 모니터링이 가능한 경우 35~40mmHg 수준으로 유지한다. 작은 어린이의 경우에도 가중하면 1인 환기보다 2인 백마스크 환기를 시행한다. 저산소증이 교정되지 않은 상태에서 삽관을 시행하면 손상을 입은 어린이에게 더 나쁜 결과를 초래할 수 있다. 따라서 삽관을 시도하기 전에 저산소증을 교정하고 기도 유지를 최적화하기 위해 모든 노력을 기울여야 한다. 어린이가 의식이 없는 경우 입인두기도기 삽입을 고려할 수 있지만, 구토의 위험이 있으므로 정상 구역반사를 보이는 어린이에게는 사용하지 않는다. 성문위기도기인 후두마스크와 후두튜브기도기도 마찬가지이며 자원과 인력이 제한적이거나 이송 시간이 길어 2인 백마스크 환기의 유용성이 제한될 것으로 예상되는 소아 외상 환자의 기도를 유지하기 위해 성문위기도기의 크기가 적절하다면 삽관을 고려할 수 있다. 특히 체중이 20kg 미만인 아주 어린 소아의 경우 이러한 장치는 상대적으로 큰 소아의 후두개를 기도 안으로 밀어 넣어서 의인성 상기도 폐쇄를 일으킬 수 있다. 기관내삽관과 비교하여 성문위기도기는 신속하게 삽입할 수 있다는 이점이 있다.

어린이의 후두는 성인에 비해 크기가 작고 약간 더 앞쪽과 머리 쪽에 위치하여 삽관 시도 시 성대를 시각적으로 확인하기가 더 어렵다(**그림 14-5**). 기관내삽관은 기도 손상이 있는 어린이에게 가장 신뢰할 수 있는 환기 수단이지만, 기도 관리를 엄격하게 통제해야 하는 경우(예: 심한 머리 손상), 기도 폐쇄가 임박한 경우, 백마스크 환기를

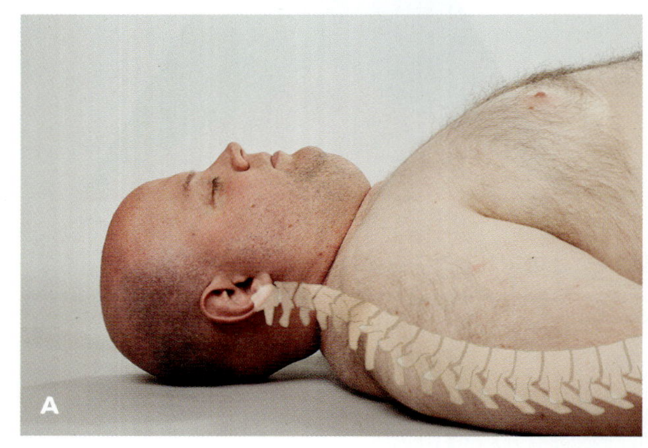
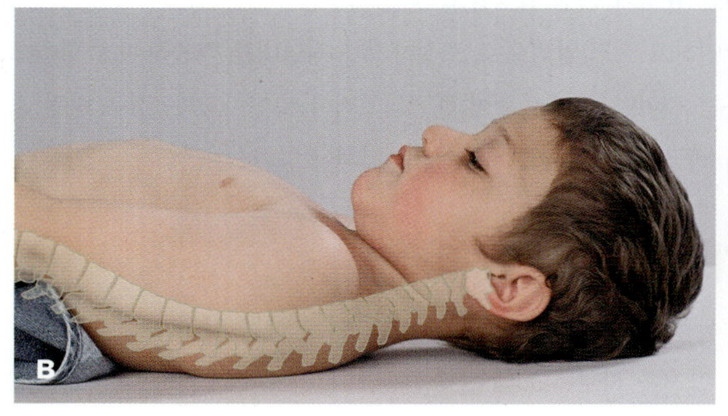

그림 14-3 **A.** 어린이는 성인보다 후두부가 크고 어깨 근육량이 적다. **B.** 평평한 표면에 어린이를 위치시키면 이러한 요인으로 인해 목이 굴곡된다.

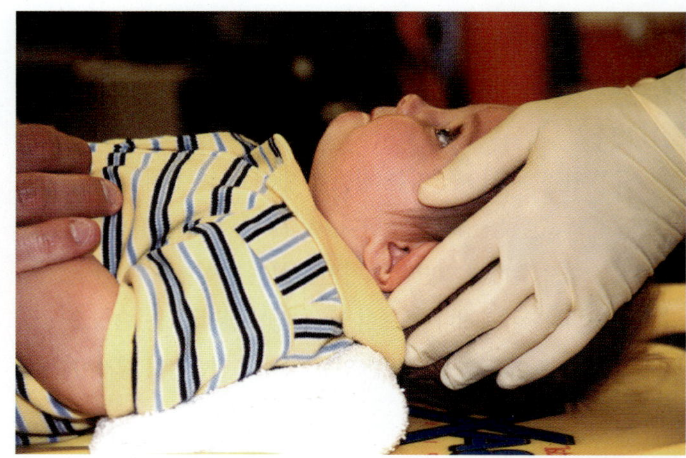

그림 14-4 냄새 맡는 자세

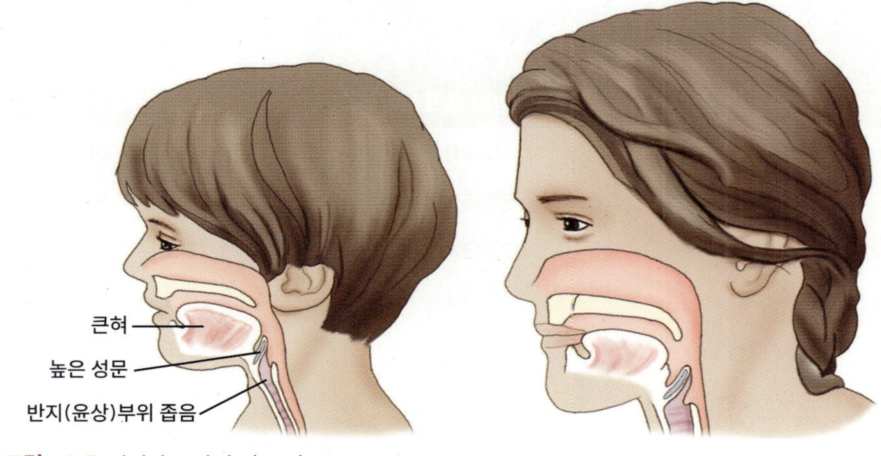

그림 14-5 성인과 소아의 기도 비교
© National Association of Emergency Medical Technicians (NAEMT)

효과적으로 유지할 수 있는 자원이 부족한 경우에만 사용해야 한다. 어린이에게는 코기관삽관을 권장하지 않는다. 이 술기는 환자가 자발적으로 호흡을 해야 하고 비교적 신속하게 후방의 코인두 각을 맹목적으로 통과해야 하며 어린이에게 더 심한 출혈을 일으킬 수 있다. 또한, 두개골 바닥 골절이 있는 환자의 경우 실수로 머리덮개뼈를 관통할 수 있다.

외과적 반지갑상연골절개는 일반적으로 어린이 외상 환자 처치에서 시행하지 않지만, 큰 소아(보통 12세)에게는 고려할 수 있다. 이 방법은 술기에 대해 특별히 교육을 받고 이를 수행할 수 있는 의료인만 시행할 수 있다.

호흡

모든 외상 환자와 마찬가지로 심각한 외상을 입은 어린이는 일반적으로 85~100%의 산소 농도(FiO$_2$ 0.85~1.0)로 산소 보충이 필요하다. 이 농도는 보충 산소와 적절한 크기의 투명한 플라스틱 소아용 마스크를 사용하면 유지된다. 어린이에게 저산소증이 생기면 신체는 환기 속도를 증가시키고 가슴 움직임 노력과 목과 복부의 보조 근육 사용 증가를 포함하여 환기 노력을 격렬하게 증가시켜 보상한다. 대사 요구량이 증가하면 환자의 심박출량을 증가하는 비율이 호흡 노력을 유지하는 데 사용되므로 심한 피로를 유발하고 환기부전을 초래할 수 있다. 호흡곤란은 보상성 호흡 노력에서 호흡부전, 호흡 정지, 궁극적으로는 저산소성 심정지로 빠르게 진행될 수 있다. 중추 청색증은 말초성 청색증보다 상당히 늦게 발생하며 종종 호흡부전의 일관성이 없는 징후이다. 병원 전 처치 제공자는 호흡부전이 임박했음을 확인하기 우해 이 소견에만 의존해서는 안 된다.

호흡곤란 징후를 조기에 인지하여 어린이의 환기 상태를 평가하고 보조 환기를 제공하는 것은 소아 외상 환자 처치의 핵심 요소이다. 4세 미만 영우아의 정상적인 환기율은 일반적으로 성인 2~3배이다(**표 14-3**).

호흡곤란과 쇼크의 첫 징후는 호흡의 노력이나 어려움을 동반하는 빠른 호흡일 수 있다. 호흡곤란이 심해지면 얕은 호흡이나 최소한의 가슴 움직임 등 추가적인 징후와 증상이 나타난다. 호흡음은 감소하거나 거의 들리지 않고 코나 입에서 공기 교환이 감소하거나 최소화될 수 있다. 환기 노력이 더 힘들어지면 다음과 같은 증상이 나타날 수 있다.

- 숨을 쉴 때마다 머리가 움직임
- 헐떡거르 거나 끙끙거리는 소리
- 콧구멍 확장
- 협착음 또는 코골이 호흡
- 복장위, 빗장위, 갈비밑 또는 갈비사이 수축
- 목과 복벽 근육과 같은 호흡 보조 근육 사용
- 가슴이 내려갈 때 복부 팽창(가슴과 복부 사이의 시소 효과)

어린이의 환기 효과는 다음과 같은 지표를 사용하여 평가해야 한다.

- 호흡 속도와 깊이(분당 용량) 및 노력은 환기의 적절성을 나타낸다.
- 분홍색 피부는 환기가 적절하게 이루어지고 있음을 나타낸다.
- 피부가 거무스름하거나 회색, 청색증 또는 얼룩덜룩하면 산소 공급과 관류가 충분하지 않음을 나타낸다.

표 14-3 소아 환자의 환기 속도

그룹	나이	환기 속도(회/분)	백마스크 장비로 보조 환기가 필요할 수 있음을 나타내는 환기 속도(회/분)
신생아	0~1개월	30~60	< 30 또는 > 60
영아	1개월~1세	30~53	< 30 또는 > 53
유아	1~2세	22~37	< 22 또는 > 37
취학 전 아동	3~5세	20~28	< 20 또는 > 28
학령기 아동	6~12세	18~25	< 18 또는 > 25
청소년	12~15세	12~20	< 12 또는 > 20

Data from American Heart Association (AHA). Vital signs in children. *Pediatric Advanced Life Support*. AHA; 2020.

- 불안, 안절부절못함, 전투적 행동은 저산소증의 초기 징후일 수 있다.
- 기면, 의식 수준 저하, 무의식은 저산소증의 진행된 징후일 수 있다.
- 호흡음은 공기 교환의 깊이를 나타낸다.
- 쌕쌕거림(천명음), 거품소리(수포음) 또는 삑삑호흡음은 비효율적인 산소공급을 나타낸다.
- 맥박산소측정 및 호기말이산화탄소분압측정 수치의 감소는 호흡부전을 나타낸다.

환기에 대한 신속한 평가에는 환자의 환기 속도(특히 빠른 호흡), 환기 노력(노력의 정도, 콧구멍 확장, 호흡 보조 근육 사용, 수축과 시소 효과), 청진(공기 교환, 양측의 대칭, 병적 소리), 피부색, 의식 상태 평가가 포함된다.

초기에 빠른 호흡과 호흡 노력 증가를 보이는 어린이의 경우 환기 속도가 정상화되고 호흡 노력이 눈에 띄게 줄어드는 것을 탈진 또는 임박한 호흡부전을 나타낼 수 있으므로 즉시 호전되는 징후로 판단해서는 안 된다. 환자의 임상적 상태 변화와 마찬가지로 이것이 생리학적 상태의 호전 또는 악화인지 확인하기 위해 주기적으로 재평가해야 한다.

병원 전 처치 제공자는 어린이의 일반적 인상, 소아 평가 삼각구도(PAT) 사용 및 어린이의 호흡 노력 평가를 종합하여 보조 환기가 필요한 어린이를 신속하게 구별할 수 있다. 소아 평가 삼각구도에 따라 외모가 양호해도 호흡 노력이 증가하고 있는 어린이는 호흡곤란 상태이므로 기도 위치(척추 안정화), 보충 산소공급 및 재평가에 주의를 기울여야 한다. 외모가 좋지 않고 호흡 노력이 증가한 어린이는 호흡부전 상태이므로 보조 환기가 필요한 대상자로 간주해야 한다. 주된 문제는 산소 농도보다는 흡기량 때문에 고농도 산소(FiO_2 0.85~1.0)를 공급할 수 있는 저장주머니를 연결한 백마스크 장비를 사용하여 보조 환기를 시행하는 것이 가장 좋다. 어린이의 기도는 매우 작기 때문에 분비물, 혈액, 체액 및 이물질의 증가로 인해 폐쇄되기 쉬우므로 조기에 주기적으로 흡인해야 한다. 또한, 코로 호흡하는 영아의 경우 콧구멍을 흡인한다.

영아에게 마스크 밀착을 시행할 때 턱 아래의 연부조직을 압박하면 혀가 연구개 쪽으로 밀려 기도가 폐쇄될 위험이 커지므로 주의해야 한다. 단단하지 않은 부드러운 기관에 압력을 가하는 것도 피해야 한다. 어린이의 크기와 나이에 따라 한 손 또는 두 손을 사용하여 마스크를 밀착시킬 수 있다. 일반적으로 모든 연령대에 걸쳐 두 손을 사용하는 것이 좋다. 올바른 크기의 백마스크 장비를 사용하여 적절하게 마스크를 밀착시키고 적절한 일회 호흡량을 제공하며 과다팽창과 압력 손상의 위험을 최소화해야 한다. 가슴 상승이 보일 때까지만 백마스크를 사용하여 적절하게 환기를 시행한다. 환기의 적절성은 호기말이산화탄소를 35~40mmHg 사이로 유지하는 것을 목표로 모니터링하여 평가할 수도 있다. 어린이에게 환기를 너무 세게 하거나 너무 많은 양의 일회 호흡량으로 환기를 시행하면 위 팽창이 발생할 수 있다. 결과적으로 위 팽창은 역류, 흡인 또는 가로막 운동을 제한하여 적절한 환기를 방해할 수 있다. 어린이의 세로칸이 더 잘 움직이기 때문에 공격적인 환기는 긴장기흉으로 이어져 심각한 호흡곤란과 갑작스러운 심혈관 허탈을 초래할 수 있다. 이러한 움직임은 외상성 대동맥 손상으로부터 어린이를 보호하지만, 긴장기흉에 대한 취약성을 증가시킨다. 더 세로칸의 움직임이 많을수록 쉽게 압박되어 성인보다 호흡 손상과 심혈관 허탈이 더 일찍 발생할 수 있다.

어린이의 호흡 상태 변화는 미묘할 수 있지만, 환기가 불충분하여 저산소증이 발생할 때까지 호흡이 빠르게 악화할 수 있다. 환자의 호흡은 일차평가의 한 부분으로 평가해야 하며 지속해서 적절한지 확인하기 위해 주기적으로 주의 깊게 재평가해야 한다. 맥박산소측정을 관찰하고 산소포화도를 94% 이상으로 유지하기 위해 노력한다.

어린이에게 수동으로 환기를 시행할 때마다 환기 속도를 신중하게 조절하는 것이 중요하다. 실수로 환자에게 환기를 과도하게 시행하면 혈중 이산화탄소 농도를 감소시키고 뇌혈관 수축을 유발한다. 이는 외상성 뇌손상 환자의 예후를 악화시킬 수 있다. 또한 과다환기 압력으로 인해 위 흡입을 유발할 수 있다. 팽창된 위는 더 유연한 소아 가슴을 밀어 올려 일회 호흡량을 제한할 수 있다. 환기 부족과 저산소증을 방지하기 위해 일회 호흡량을 전달할 때 가슴이 상승하는지 확인한다.

순환

출혈을 지혈한 후 기도개방을 적절하게 시행하고 호흡을 확인한 다음 순환평가를 진행한다. 어린이의 심박수를 평가하여 빈맥, 정상 또는 서맥으로 구분한다. 소아가 서맥인 경우 기도를 재평가한다. 심박수가 정상이거나 빠른 경우 저관류 징후(창백함, 반점 형성, 모세혈관 재충전 시간 지연)가 있는지 확인한다.

출혈성 손상을 입은 어린이는 말초 혈관 저항을 증가시켜 평균 동맥압을 유지함으로써 적절한 순환량을 유지할 수 있다. 이러한 보상기전의 임상적 증거로는 모세혈관 재충전 지연, 말초 부위 창백, 반점 형성, 차가운 말초 부위 피부, 말초 맥박의 강도 감소 등이 있다. 어린이에서 순환량의 약 30%가 손실되면서 심각한 저혈압 징후가 나타난다. 저혈압은 혈량저하증의 후기 징후이다. 출혈성 손상을 입은 어린이는 생리적 예비력이 증가하기 때문에 약간의 비정상적인 활력징후만 보인다. 초기 빈맥은 심리적 스트레스, 통증 또는 두려움으로 인한 것일 수 있지만, 외상을 입은 어린이에게서는 항상 혈량저하증에 의한 이차적인 것으로 간주해야 한다. 어린이가 빈맥이 있지만, 혈압이 정상이라면 보상성 쇼크일 수 있다. 저관류의 징후가 있는지 살펴보고 자주 재평가를 시행한다. 말초혈관 저항이 증가해도 순환량 손실을 보상하기에 충분하지 않으면 혈압이 떨어진다. 진행성 쇼크의 개념은 손상을 입은 어린이의 초기 처치에서 가장 중요한 관심사

이며 신속한 평가로 처치를 위해 적절한 외상센터로 이송해야 하는 주요 징후이다.

저혈압을 동반한 빈맥이 있는 어린이는 생명을 위협하는 심각한 응급상황(비 보상성 쇼크)을 경험하고 있다. 모든 외부출혈을 지혈하고 팔다리 손상으로 인해 심각한 출혈이 발생한 경우 지혈대를 적용함으로 생명을 구할 수 있다. 가능한 한 빨리 수액 소생술을 시작해야 하지만, 외상센터로 이송이 지연되어서는 안 된다. 이송 중에 정맥라인 확보와 수액 투여를 시작할 수 있다.

기도 평가에서와 마찬가지로 심박수나 혈압을 한 번만 측정하는 것은 생리학적 안정성과 같지 않다. 활력징후와 관류 상태의 연속적인 측정과 변화 추세는 급성 손상 단계에서 어린이의 혈류역학적 상태를 측정하는 데 매우 중요하다. 활력징후를 자세히 모니터링하는 것은 임박한 쇼크 징후를 인식하고 임상적 악화를 방지하기 위해 적절한 처치를 수행하는 데 절대적으로 필요하다. **표 14-4** 및 **표 14-5** 는 소아의 연령대별 맥박과 혈압의 정상 범위를 제공한다. **Box 14-2** 는 소아 활력징후 및 정상 범위에 대한 추가 논의를 제공한다.

장애

출혈, 기도, 호흡, 순환을 평가한 후 일차평가에는 신경학적 상태 평가가 포함되어야 한다. AVPU 척도(명료, 언어 자극에 대해 반응, 통증 자극에 대한 반응, 무반응)는 어린이의 신경학적 상태를 간단하고 빠르게 평가할 수 있는 도구이지만, 글래스고혼수척도(GCS)보다 정보가 적다. 동공의 크기가 같고, 둥글며 빛에 반응하는지를 확인하기 위해 동공에 대한 면밀한 검사와 글래스고혼수척도 평가를 병행해야 한다. 성인과 마찬가지로 글래스고혼수척도 점수는 신경학적 상태에 대한 보다 철저한 평가를 제공하며 각 소아 외상 환자에 대해 계산해야 한다. 소아 외상 환자의 경우 다양한 발달 단계를 고려할 수 있도록 글래스고혼수척도를 수정할 수 있다(**표 14-6**).

글래스고혼수척도의 운동 구성 요소 점수는 총 글래스고혼수척도를 평가하는 것만큼이나 유용할 수 있다. 운동 반응 구성 요소의 중요성에 대한 자세한 내용은 6장 환자 평가 및 관리를 참조한다.

글래스고혼수척도 점수를 자주 반복 측정하며 손상 후 기간 신경학적 상태의 진행과 개선을 기록하는 데 사용해야 한다. 시간이 허락한다면 이차평가에서 운동 및 감각 기능에 대한 보다 철저한 평가를 수행해야 한다.

표 14-4 소아 환자의 맥박수

그룹	나이	활동시 맥박수 (회/분)	안정시 맥박수 (회/분)	심각한 문제 가능성을 나타내는 맥박수*(회/분)
신생아	0~1개월	120~205	100~160	< 100 또는 > 160
영아	1개월~1세	110~180	90~160	< 80 또는 > 150
유아	1~2세	98~140	80~120	< 60 또는 > 140
취학 전 아동	3~5세	80~120	65~100	< 60 또는 > 130
학령기 아동	6~12세	75~118	60~90	< 50 또는 > 120
청소년	12~15세	60~100	50~90	< 45 또는 > 100

*서맥 또는 빈맥

Data from American Heart Association (AHA). Vital signs in children. *Pediatric Advanced Life Support*. AHA; 2020.

표 14-5 소아 환자의 혈압

그룹	나이	예상 혈압 범위(mmHg)	수축기 혈압의 하한선(mmHg)
신생아	0~1개월	수축기: 67~84 이완기: 35~53 평균 동맥압: 45~60	> 60
영아	1개월~1세	수축기: 72~104 이완기: 37~56 평균 동맥압: 50~62	> 70
유아	1~2세	수축기: 86~106 이완기: 42~63 평균 동맥압: 49~62	> 70
취학 전 아동	3~5세	수축기: 89~112 이완기: 46~72 평균 동맥압: 58~69	> 75
학령기 아동	6~12세	수축기: 97~120 이완기: 57~80 평균 동맥압: 66~79	> 80
청소년	12~15세	수축기: 110~131 이완기: 64~83 평균 동맥압: 73~84	> 90

Data from American Heart Association (AHA). Vital signs in children. *Pediatric Advanced Life Support*. AHA; 2020.

Box 14-2 소아 활력징후 및 정량적 기준

소아 또는 어린이라는 용어는 신체 발달, 정서적 성숙과 신체 크기 등 다양함 범위가 포함된다. 환자에 대한 접근 방식과 여러 손상의 영향은 영아와 청소년기 사이에서 크게 다르다.

대부분의 해부학적 및 치료 용량 고려 사항에서 어린이의 체중은 실제 나이보다 더 정확한 지표로 사용된다. **표 14-2**에는 다양한 나이의 건강한 어린이의 평균 키와 몸무게가 나와 있다.

허용할 수 있는 활력징후 범위는 소아 집단 내에서 나이에 따라 다르다. 어린이에게는 성인 기준을 지침으로 사용할 수 없다. 성인의 호흡 속도가 분당 30회인 경우 빠른 호흡이고 맥박이 분당 120~140회이면 빈맥이다. 이 두 가지 모두 성인에서 놀라울 정도로 높은 것으로 간주하며 중요한 병리학적 소견이다. 그러나 영아의 경우 같은 결과가 정상 범위 내에 있을 수 있다.

연령대별 활력징후의 정상 범위는 모든 소아청소년과 진료에서 일관되지 않을 수 없다. 이전에 정상 활력징후 병력이 없는 손상을 입은 소아의 경우 경계선 활력징후는 특정 소아에게 생리학적으로 허용되는 징후일지라도 병리학적인 것으로 간주할 수 있다. **표 14-4** 및 **표 14-5**의 지침은 소아 환자의 활력징후를 평가하는 데 도움이 될 수 있다. 이 표는 해당 연령대의 어린이 대부분이 해당하는 통계학적으로 일반적인 범위를 나타낸다.

시중에 판매되는 몇 가지 물품은 소아 활력징후 및 장비 크기에 대한 참조 가이드 역할을 한다. 여기에는 소아의 키에 근거한 소생술 테이프와 여러 슬라이드 규칙형 플라스틱 저울, 모바일 애플리케이션이 포함된다. 다음 가이드라인 공식을 사용하여 1~10세까지 예상되는 결과를 추정할 수도 있다.

허용 가능한 최저 수축기 혈압(mmHg) = 70 + [2 × 소아의 나이(세)]
총 혈관 혈액량(mL) = 80mL × 소아의 체중(kg)

소아의 정량적 활력징후는 중요하지만, 평가에 사용되는 정보 중 하나일 뿐이다. 활력징후가 정상적인 어린이도 중증의 호흡곤란이나 보상되지 않는 쇼크로 빠르게 악화할 수 있다. 활력징후는 손상의 기전 및 다른 임상 소견에 따라 고려해야 한다.

노출/환경

어린이는 잠재적으로 생명을 위협할 수 있는 다른 손상이 있는지 평가해야 한다. 그러나 손상을 확인하기 위해서는 노출이 중요하고 필요하지만, 어린이는 옷을 벗기려고 하면 겁을 먹을 수 있다. 유아 또는 미취학 어린이가 심각한 손상을 입지 않았으면 머리부터 발끝까지 신체검사하는 것이 덜 겁을 줄 수 있다. 각 부위를 노출하면서 설명하고 가능하면 부모가 참석하도록 한다. 또한, 어린이는 체표면적이 넓기 때문에 저체온증에 걸리기 쉽다. 다른 손상을 확인하기 위한 검사가 완료되면 체온을 유지하고 추가 열 손실을 방지하기 위해 어린이를 덮어야 한다.

이차평가

소아 환자에 대한 이차평가는 생명을 위협하는 상태가 확인되고 처치 시행한 후에만 일차평가에 이어 실시해야 한다. 머리와 목에 명백한 변형, 타박상, 찰과상, 천자, 화상, 압통, 열상 또는 부종이 있는지 검사를 시행해야 한다. 가슴 부위를 재평가한다. 호흡곤란이나 비정상적인 호흡음으로 나타나는 잠재적인 폐 타박상은 대량 수액 소생술을 시행한 후에 분명해질 수 있다. 외상 환자는 손상 당시 금식(NPO)인 경우가 드물다. 두개골 바닥 골절 가능성이 있는 심각한 얼굴 및 머리 외상이 있는 경우 코위관이나 입위관 삽입이 필요할 수 있으며 프로토콜이 허용하는 경우 코위관 삽입은 금기라는 점을 염두에 두어야 한다. 위 감압은 기도가 막혔거나 외상 후 발작이 있는 어린이에게 특히 중요하다.

복부 검사는 팽창, 압통, 변색, 반상출혈 및 종괴의 유무에 중점을 두어야 한다. 엉덩뼈능선을 주의 깊게 촉진하면 불안정한 골반 골절이나 복막과 비뇨생식기 손상을 의심할 수 있을 뿐만 아니라 숨겨진 출혈의 위험이 증가할 수 있다. 불안정한 골반에 주목해야 하지만, 골반을 반복적으로 검사하면 추가 손상과 출혈이 증가할 수 있으므로 시행해서는 안 된다. 환자를 이동하거나 이송하는 동안 적절한 척추 움직임 제한을 시행해야 한다.

각 팔다리를 검사하고 촉진하여 압통, 변형, 혈액 공급 감소, 신경학적 결손을 배제한다. 여러 개의 성장판이 있는 어린이의 불안정하게 석회화된 골격은 성장판 손상이 발생할 가능성이 높다. 따라서 부종, 통증, 압통 또는 운동 범위 감소가 있는 부위는 방사선 검사로 평가를 시행할 때까지 골절된 것으로 간주하고 처치한다. 성인과 마찬가지로 어린이의 경우 팔다리의 정형외과적 손상은 사망률에는 거의 영향을 미치지 않지만, 장기적인 변형 및 장애를 초래할 수 있다.

처치

외상성 손상을 입은 소아 환자의 생존을 위해서는 신속한 심폐 평가와 나이에 따른 적극적인 처치, 소아 외상을 처치할 수 있는 의료기관으로 신속한 이송이 핵심이다. 색상으로 구분된 길이 기반 소생 테이프(Broselow 소생술 테이프)는 환자의 키를 신속하게 파악하여 체중, 사용할 장비의 크기, 소생술에 사용하는 약물의 적절한 투여량을 상관관계로 추정할 수 있는 가이드 역할을 하기 위해 고안되었다. 또한 대부분의 병원 전 단계 시스템에는 소아 외상 환자를 위한 적절한

표 14-6 소아 글래스고혼수척도			
	점수	> 1 세	< 1 세
눈 뜨기 반응	4	자발적으로	자발적으로
	3	언어 명령에 따라	소리지르다
	2	통증에 따라	통증에 따라
	1	눈뜨지 않음	눈뜨지 않음
운동 반응	6	지시를 따름	자연스러운 움직임
	5	통증 부위를 인식	통증 국소화
	4	자극시 움츠림	자극시 움츠림
	3	비정상적인 굴곡	비정상적인 굴곡
	2	비정상적인 신전	비정상적인 신전
	1	전혀 움직이지 않음	전혀 움직이지 않음
		> 5세	2~5세	0~23개월
언어 반응	5	적절하게 답변	나이 수준에 적절한 대답	적절하게 웃고 떠들기
	4	지남력 상실 및 대화	부적절한 단어	울음
	3	부적절한 단어	울음 또는 비명	부적절한 울임 또는 비명
	2	이해할 수 없는 소리	끙끙대다	끙끙대다
	1	반응 없음	반응 없음	반응 없음

Modified from Low A, Hulme J. *ABC of Transfer and Retrieval Medicine*. John Wiley & Sons; 2014.

의료기관을 선택하기 위한 지침이 있다. 모든 외상센터가 손상을 입은 어린이를 적절하게 처치할 수 있는 역량(즉, 소아 준비성)을 갖춘 것은 아니다. 소아 전문외상센터는 손상을 입은 어린이의 사망률을 두 배나 낮추는 것과 관련이 있다. 외상은 여전히 어린이 사망의 주요 원인이므로 2023년부터 모든 ACS 인증 외상센터는 오아 준비 상태의 결함을 평가하고 해결하기 위한 계획을 개발해야 한다. 현장에 도착하기 전에 프로토콜을 검토하여 위급한 어린이에 대한 신속한 결정을 내려야 한다.

심각한 외부출혈 지혈

외상 환자의 일차평가에서 외부출혈을 확인하고 지혈해야 한다. 다량의 외부출혈이 있는 경우 기도를 확보하기 전에 이 출혈을 지혈해야 한다. 출혈 조절은 직접 압박으로 지혈할 수 있다. 출혈 부위에 4 × 4인치 거즈 패드를 대고 압력을 유지하면 된다. 이송 중에 압력을 지속해서 유지해야 한다. 직접 압박으로 출혈을 적절하게 지혈하지 못하면(또는 팔다리의 경우) 지혈대를 적용할 수 있다. 일부 지혈대는 너무 크거나 어린이나 영아에게는 효과가 없을 수 있다. 래칫 또는 윈들러스 스타일의 지혈대가 필요할 수 있다. 대량 출혈을 조절하는 것은 필수적이다. 환자에게 출혈이 계속되면 관류가 개선되지 않고 출혈 쇼크로 진행된다.

기도

환기, 산소 공급 및 관류는 성인과 같이 어린이 손상 환자에게도 필수적이다. 따라서 손상을 입은 어린이의 초기 소생술의 주요 목표는 가능한 한 신속하고 적절하게 조직으로 산소 공급을 회복하는 것이다. 현장 안전을 확보하고 대량 외부출혈을 해결한 후 평가 및 소생술의 최우선 순위는 기도를 개방하고 유지하는 것이다.

흡인, 도수 기도 개방, 보조기도기를 사용하여 기도를 개방하고 유

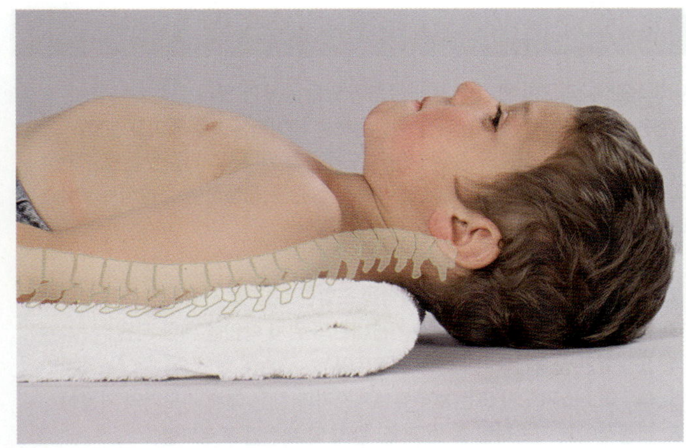

그림 14-6 어린이의 몸통 아래에 적절한 패딩을 대어주거나 어린이의 후두부가 움푹 팬 척추고정판을 사용한다.
© National Association of Emergency Medical Technicians (NAEMT)

Box 14-3 소아 기관내삽관

소아 환자의 기관내삽관 시 목뼈 고정에 세심한 주의를 기울여야 한다. 병원 전 처치 제공자는 동료가 기관내삽관을 시행하는 동안 어린이의 척추를 중립 자세로 유지해야 한다.

소아 기도의 가장 좁은 부위는 반지고리이며 생리적 커프를 형성한다. 이러한 차-이로 인해 이전에는 소아에게 커프가 없는 기관내관을 사용했지만, 최근 권고안에서는 모든 연령대에 커프가 있는 튜브를 사용할 것을 권장하고 있다. 커프가 있는 튜브를 사용하면 병원 전 처치 제공자가 밀봉 강도와 어린이의 산소 공급 및 환기 상태에 따라 커프를 완전히 팽창시키거나 부분적으로 또는 전혀 팽창시키지 않을 수 있다. 의인성 기관 손상을 예방하려면 커프 압력이 25cmH₂O를 넘지 않아야 한다. 커프가 있는 기관내관의 적절한 크기는 소아의 새끼손가락 또는 외부 콧구멍의 지름을 사용하거나 다음 공식을 사용하여 추정할 수 있다.

$$(나이 \div 4) + 3.5$$

일반적인 반지연골 압박은 더 이상 권장되지 않지만, 소아의 후두 앞쪽 구조물이 더 잘 보이게 하려고 약간의 반지연골 압박을 시도해 볼 수 있다. 그러나 소아의 기관연골고리는 비교적 부드럽고 유연하므로 과도한 반지연골 압박은 기도를 완전히 폐쇄할 수 있다.

응급 상황에서 소아 환자에게 삽관을 시행하는 동안 발생하는 실수는 기관내관을 너무 깊게 삽입해서 오른쪽 주기관지에 위치시키는 것이다. 기관내관은 절대로 기관내관 크기의 3배를 초과하여 삽입해서는 안 된다. 예를 들면, 3.0cm의 기관내관은 9cm 이하의 깊이에서 입술에 위치해야 한다.

기관내관을 삽입한 후에는 항상 가슴과 명치부위를 청진하고 가능한 경우 호기말이산화탄소분압측정기를 사용하여 모니터링해야 한다. 특히 환자가 움직인 후에는 기관내관 위치를 자주 재평가해야 한다. 청진을 통해 기관내관 삽입을 확인하는 것 외에도 다른 폐 손상이 있는 소아에게 성공적으로 삽관을 시행한 경우 양압 환기로 인해 긴장기흉이 발생할 위험이 더 커질 수 있다.

지해야 한다. 성인과 마찬가지로 소아 환자의 초기 처치에는 목뼈를 중립 자세로 고정하는 것이 포함한다. 머리 부위에 오목한 부분이 있는 특수 소아용 척추고정판을 사용하지 않는 한 불균형적으로 큰 후두부 때문에 목뼈가 약간 굴곡되지 않고 일직선으로 유지되도록 소아의 몸통 아래에 적절한 패딩(2~3cm)을 배치해야 한다(**그림 14-6**). 기도 위치를 조절하고 유지할 때 목과 기관의 연부조직을 압박하지 않도록 해야 한다.

기도 유지를 도수로 시행하고 구역 반사가 없으면 입인두기도기를 삽입할 수 있다. 이 장비는 성인처럼 입인두 뒤쪽에서 90° 또는 180° 돌리지 말고 설압자를 이용하여 혀의 방향과 평행하게 조심스럽고 부드럽게 삽입한다. 혀를 누르기 위해 설압자를 사용하면 소아 환자에게 도움이 될 수 있다.

기관을 직접 눈으로 보면서 기관내삽관을 시행하는 것은 이송 지연 시 필요할 수 있다(**Box 14-3**). 그러나 이 절차는 백마스크 장비로 충분한 산소 공급을 유지할 수 없는 경우에만, 숙련된 제공자가 시행해야 한다. 중요한 것은 백마스크장비로 보조 환기를 받은 소아 환자보다 현장에서 초기에 삽관을 시행한 소아 환자의 생존율이나 신경학적 결과가 개선되었다는 데이터가 없다는 것이다. 오히려 결과가 같거나 더 나쁘다는 몇 가지 증거도 있다. 병원 전 삽관을 여러 번 시도하는 것은 심각한 합병증과 관련이 있다(**Box 14-4**).

여러 가지 성문위기도기가 성인 외상 환자에게 효과적인 기도유지 장치로 입증되었지만, 크기가 크고 작은 크기가 없기 때문에 어린 소아(122cm 미만)를 위한 기도유지 장비로 적합하지 않다. 후두마스크기도기, i-gel, 후두튜브기도기는 기도가 성인과 더 유사한 8세 이상의 어린이에게 대체 기도유지 장비로 사용할 수 있다. 그러나 초기 연구에 따르면 기관내삽관 대신 성문위기도기를 사용한 어린이에서 결과가 개선되지 않는 것으로 나타났다. 또한 백마스크 환기는 소아들에서 성문위기도기와 비교해 개선된 결과와 관련이 있다.

소아 환자의 경우 기관내삽관의 이점보다 위험이 클 수 있으므로 특히 백마스크 환기로 적절한 환기와 산소 공급이 가능한 어린이의 경우 삽관을 시도하기 전에 신중하게 고려해야 한다. 기관내삽관과 관련된 위험에 대한 고려는 비시각화 전문 기도유지 장비를 추가로 사용할 수 있게 되었고 병원 전 처치에 추가됨에 따라 점점 더 중요해지고 있다.

호흡

어린이의 분당 환기량과 호흡 노력을 주의 깊게 평가해야 한다. 경미

Box 14-4　병원 전 소아 삽관: 중요한 논쟁

외상성 뇌손상을 입은 소아를 처치할 때 가능한 한 빨리 기관내관을 삽입하는 것이 도움이 되리라는 것은 직관적으로 보일 수 있다. 후향적 연구에 따르면 병원에 도착하기 전에 기관 삽관을 받은 성인 외상성 뇌손상 환자의 생존율이 개선된 것으로 나타났다. 후속 연구에서는 급속연속기관삽관(RSI)을 평가하여 성인과 소아 삽관의 효율성과 성공률이 개선되었음을 입증했다. 그러나 많은 후향적 및 전향적 사례 관리 연구에서 병원 전 단계 백마스크 장비를 이용한 환기와 비교하여 병원 도착 전 삽관이 생존율이나 신경학적 결과를 개선하지 못했으며 오히려 해로울 수 있다는 사실이 밝혀졌다. 병원 전 환경에서의 소아 기도 관리에 대한 체계적인 검토에 따르면 백마스크 장비를 이용한 환기는 모든 형태의 전문 기도관리와 비교하여 생존율 향상 및 합병증 감소와 관련이 있는 것으로 나타났다.

장시간의 저산소증은 삽관 과정과 관련이 있으며 외상센터로 이송되는 환자의 삽관 후 과도한 환기 기간과 관련이 있는 경우가 많다.

병원 전 단계에서 소아 삽관을 뒷받침하는 데이터는 제한적이고 모호하다. 자발 호흡을 하는 소아의 경우 약물의 도움을 받거나 받지 않는 삽관은 권장되지 않는다. 병원 전 단계에서 소아에게 삽관을 시행하는 응급의료서비스 프로그램은 최소한 다음이 포함되어야 한다.

1. 긴밀한 의료 지도와 감독
2. 실제로 실습해 보는 수술실 경험을 포함한 실습 및 지속적인 교육
3. 환자 모니터링, 약물 보관 및 기관내관의 위치 확인을 위한 자원
4. 표준화된 급속연속기관삽관 프로토콜
5. 후두마스크기도기 또는 후두튜브기도기와 같은 대체 기도기의 가용성
6. 집중적이고 지속적인 질 보장, 질 관리 및 재점검 프로그램

한 저산소증에서 호흡 정지로 빠르게 악화할 가능성이 있으므로 호흡곤란과 환기 노력 증가가 관찰되면 보조 환기를 시행한다. 고농도의 산소(FiO_2 0.85~1.0)를 공급할 수 있는 저장주머니가 연결된 소아용 백마스크 장비를 사용한다. 지속적인 맥박산소측정은 기도, 호흡을 지속해서 평가하기 위한 보조 장비이다. 85~100%의 산소 농도를 제공할 수 있도록 산소 저장주머니가 연결된 백마스크 장비를 사용해야 한다. 맥박산소측정기를 이용해 기도와 호흡을 지속해서 평가하고 산소포화도를 94% 이상으로 유지한다.

삽관을 시행하는 소아 환자의 경우 성대를 통과하는 기관내관을 직접 눈으로 확인하고 양쪽 호흡음이 들리며 환기 시 명치부위에서 소리가 들리는지 청진 등을 포함하여 다양한 방법을 사용하여 기관내관의 위치를 확인해야 한다. 지속해서 호기말이산화탄소분압($ETCO_2$) 모니터링을 시행하여 기관내관 위치를 확인하고 저산조증만큼이나 외상성 노손상 회복에 해로울 수 있는 극단적인 고탄산혈증 및 저탄산혈증을 피하고자 호기말이산화탄소분압을 35~40mmHg를 목표로 유지한다.

긴장기흉

어린이는 성인보다 긴장기흉으로 인한 급성 심혈관계 허탈에 더 취약하다. 긴장기흉이 있는 대부분의 어린이는 산소 공급 및 환기에서 감지할 수 있는 변화가 발생하기 전에 정맥혈복귀 감소로 인한 이차적인 급성 심장 보상실패가 나타난다. 특히 백마스크 장비나 전문 기도 유지를 시행하고 양압 환기를 시작한 후 급격하게 보상 실패가 나타나는 어린이는 긴장기흉에 대해 신속하게 평가를 시행한다.

목정맥 확장은 목뼈보호대를 착용했거나 출혈로 인한 혈량저하증으로 판단하기 어려울 수 있다. 기관 편위는 긴장기흉의 후기 징후이며 목정맥구멍패임에서 기관을 촉진해야만 확인할 수 있다. 이러한 소아 환자에서 심혈관 손상과 관련하여 호흡음이 들리지 않는 것은 응급 바늘감압 또는 손가락 가슴관삽입이 필요한 징후를 나타낸다. 삽관된 소아 환자의 경우 왼쪽에서 호흡음이 감소하면 오른쪽 주기관지 삽관을 의미할 수 있지만, 급성 심장 보상실패와 관련된 경우 이러한 호흡음은 긴장기흉을 나타낼 수 있다. 이러한 미묘한 차이를 구별하기 위해서는 환자의 기도 및 호흡 상태를 주의 깊게 재평가해야 한다.

성인을 대상으로 한 연구는 긴장기흉이 의심되면 가슴관삽입을 지지하지만, 체계적 검토에 따르면 바늘감압과 손가락 가슴관삽입 중 어느 것이 더 나은 결과를 가져온다고 확실히 밝혀진 것은 없다. 소아 환자의 긴장기흉에 대해 이 두 가지 중재법을 비교한 연구는 아직 없다. 숙련된 의사를 대상으로 한 설문조사에 따르면 어린 소아 환자에게는 바늘감압을 시행하고 소아 환자에게는 가슴관삽입을 선호하는 것으로 나타났다. 소아 환자의 긴장기흉에 대한 바늘감압은 빗장중간선과 만나는 두 번째 갈비뼈사이 공간에 시행해야 한다. 이 접근법은 중간겨드랑선과 만나는 다섯 번째 갈비사이 공간에 바늘감압을 시행하는 것에 대한 성인의 권장 사항이 변경된 것과는 대조적이다. 바늘감압 및 가슴관삽입에 대한 자세한 내용은 10장 가슴 외상을 참조한다. 세로칸이 빠르게 정상 위치로 돌아오고 정맥복귀혈이 빠르게 회복되기 때문에 가슴감압은 소아에게 더 즉각적으로 효과적인 경우가 많다. 병원 전 처치 제공자는 혈관 카테터를 삽입한 후 이탈되지 않도록 주의 깊게 관찰한다.

순환

소아 환자의 외부출혈이 지혈되면 관류를 평가한다. 외부출혈을 지혈하는 방법으로는 직접 손으로 압력을 가하고 압박 드레싱 사용, 팔다리에 대량출혈이 발생한 경우 지혈대를 사용한다. 외부출혈을 조절하는 것은 단순히 흡수성 드레싱으로 여러 겹 덮는 것으로 해결할 수 있는 문제가 아니다. 초기에 적용한 드레싱이 혈액으로 젖으면 드레싱을 교체하는 것보다 기존에 적용한 드레싱 위에 드레싱을 추가하는 것이 좋다. 동시에 상처 부위를 압박하거나 상처 패킹 또는 지혈대 적용 등 지속해서 출혈을 지혈하기 위한 추가 처치를 고려한다.

소아의 혈관계는 일반적으로 심각한 손상이 일어날 때까지 정상 혈압을 유지할 수 있으며 이 시점에서 소생술에 반응하지 않는 경우가 많다. 수액 소생술은 보상성 저혈량 쇼크의 징후가 있을 때마다 시작해야 하며 비보상성 쇼크가 나타나는 소아 환자에게는 즉시 시작해야 한다. 생리식염수를 20mL/kg 볼루스(bolus)로 먼저 투여한다. 출혈 쇼크가 의심되는 소아에게는 혈액 및 트라넥삼산(TXA)를 조기에 투여하는 것을 프로토콜에 따라 고려한다.

출혈 쇼크 또는 혈량저하증의 징후를 보이는 소아 외상 환자의 경우 생존을 위한 핵심 요소는 적절한 양의 수액 소생술과 적절한 의료 기관으로 신속하게 이송을 시작하는 것이다. 정맥 라인을 확보하거나 정맥 내로 수액을 투여하기 위해 이송을 지연해서는 안 된다.

혈관 확보

중증 저혈압이나 쇼크 징후가 나타나는 소아 환자의 수액을 보충할 때는 심장 전부하가 더 이상 감소하지 않도록 우심방에 충분한 양의 수액을 공급해야 한다. 정맥 라인을 확보하기 위한 가장 적절한 초기 부위는 팔오금(팔꿈치 아래팔 앞쪽)과 발목의 두렁정맥이다. 바깥 목정맥은 정맥 라인을 확보할 수 있지만, 좁은 공간에서는 기도 유지가 우선시되어야 하고 목뼈보호대로 인해 접근하기 어려울 수 있다.

불안정하거나 불안정할 가능성이 있는 소아 환자의 경우 말초 정맥 라인 확보를 90초에 2회 시도하는 것으로 제한한다. 말초혈관 확보에 실패하면 골내(IO) 주사를 시행한다(**Box 14-5**).

소아 환자에게 빗장밑정맥 또는 속목정맥에 카테터를 삽입하는 것은 병원 내에서 가장 잘 통제된 상황에서만 시행하며 병원 전 환경에서 시도해서는 안 된다.

어떤 소아 환자에게 정맥 라인 확보가 필요한지 결정하는 것은 손상의 중증도, 병원 전 처치 제공자의 경험, 이송 시간 등 여러 요인에 따라 달라진다. 소아 환자에게 혈관확보가 필요하거나 이송 중에 수액 소생술이 필요한지 불확실한 경우 의료 지도 의사의 의료 지도를 받아야 한다.

수액 요법

등장성 결정질 용액은 혈량저하 소아 환자에게 초기 투여하는 수액이다. 수액을 선택할 때는 다량의 조직 손상이 있는 경우 응고병증과

Box 14-5 소아 골내 주입

골내 주입(IO)은 모든 연령대의 손상을 입은 어린이에게 수액 소생술을 시행할 수 있는 대체 부위를 제공할 수 있다. 이는 약물 주입, 혈액 또는 다량의 수액 투여를 위한 효과적인 경로이다.

골내 주입을 위해 가장 접근하기 쉬운 부위는 정강뼈 거친면 바로 아래 내측 정강뼈이다. 피부를 소독하고, 다리를 적절히 고정한 후 정강뼈 거친면에서 1~2cm 아래, 정강뼈 앞쪽 안쪽 부위를 선택한다. 이 술기에는 특수 제작된 골내 주삿바늘이 가장 적합하지만, 척추 천자 주삿바늘이나 골수 주삿바늘도 사용할 수 있다. 18~20게이지의 척추 천자 주삿바늘은 뼈의 피질을 통하여 골수로 들어갈 때 주삿바늘이 막히는 것을 방지하는 투관 침이 있기 때문에 잘 작동한다. 응급상황에서는 14~20게이지 모든 주삿바늘을 사용할 수 있다.

다양한 기계 장치를 사용하여 골내 주삿바늘을 삽입의 어려움을 덜어주는 시중에서 판매되는 다양한 장치가 있다. 예를 들어 한 장비는 고속 드릴을 사용하여 특수 설계된 골내 주삿바늘을 삽입할 수 있고 다른 장비는 스프링이 장착된 기전을 사용한다. 주삿바늘은 뼈에 90°의 각도로 위치시키고 피질을 통해 골수까지 강하게 삽입한다.

주삿바늘이 골수 나에 적절히 삽입되었다는 증거는 다음과 같다.

1. 주삿바늘이 피질을 통과한 후 부드러운 "팡" 소리가 들리고 저항이 느껴지지 않는다.
2. 골수가 주삿바늘로 흡인된다.
3. 수액이 피부밑 침윤의 증거가 없이 골수 내로 주입된다.
4. 주삿바늘이 안전하게 고정되어 있고 느슨해지거나 흔들리지 않는다.

경피경유정맥관삽입(정맥 라인 확보)에 실패하면 초기 소생술 중에 골내 주입을 고려래야 한다. 골수 공간은 유속이 제한되어 있으므로 수액 및 약물 투여는 압력을 가한 상태에서 이루어져야 하며 초기 소생술 후 골내 경로만으로는 충분하지 않은 경우가 거의 없다.

삽입 부위의 적절한 위치는 중요하며 소아 환자에게는 더욱 중요하다. 랜드마크를 제대로 구별하지 못하면 골내 주입 위치가 잘못되어 소생술이 비효율적이거나 수액이 전신 순환으로 유입되지 않고 팔다리의 연부조직에 대량으로 주입되면 구획증후군이 발생할 수 있다.

전해질 농도(예; 칼륨)를 악화시킬 수 있는 산도를 고려해야 한다. 결정질 수액이 혈관 내 공간에 머무는 시간이 상대적으로 짧음으로 전혈을 이용한 소생술이 훨씬 더 효과적인 이유 중 하나이다. 이에 대해서는 3장 쇼크: 삶과 죽음의 병태생리학에서 자세히 설명한다.

과거에는 혈액제제를 투여하기 전에 생리학적으로 필요한 경우 20mL/kg의 수액 투여로 수액 소생술을 시작하고 결정질 수액을 볼루스로 반복하는 것이 일반적이었다. 그러나 현재 권장 사항은 출혈 쇼크가 의심되는 경우 혈액제제를 더 일찍 시작할 것을 권장한다. 이는 적혈구 또는 전혈 투여로 이루어질 수 있으며 이러한 중증 손상 환자에게 처음으로 투여되는 수액일 수도 있다. 결정질 수액을 볼루스 투여하는 것은 일시적으로 순환계를 채웠다가 순환계에서 누출되기 때문에 일시적으로 심혈관 안정성을 회복시킬 수 있다. 그러나 순환하는 적혈구가 교체되고 산소 운반이 회복될 때까지 저산소로 인한 손상이 계속될 수 있다.

통증 조절

성인과 마찬가지로 병원 전 환경에서 소아 환자의 통증 관리를 고려해야 한다. 적절한 소량의 마약성 진통제는 신경학적 또는 복부 검사에 영향을 미치지 않는다. 모르핀과 펜타닐 모두 투여할 수 있는 약물이지만, 이것은 병원 전 처치 지침이나 의료 지도 의사의 지시에 따라서만 투여해야 한다. 저혈압 및 저환기의 부작용으로 인해 정맥 내로 마약성 진통제를 투여받는 모든 소아 환자는 맥박산소측정과 지속적인 활력징후를 모니터링해야 한다. 일반적으로 벤조다이아제핀은 호흡 억제에 대한 상승효과로 인해 호흡정지를 일으킬 수 있으므로 마약성진통제와 같이 투여해서는 안 된다. 케타민 사용에 대한 프로토콜을 사용할 수 있는 경우 병원 전 단계에서도 유용한 대안이 될 수 있다.

이송

가장 적절한 의료기관으로 적시에 도착하는 것이 어린이 생존에 핵심 요소일 수 있으므로 소아 환자 처치에서 분류는 중요한 고려 사항이다.

예방할 수 있는 소아 외상 사망의 비극은 지난 30년간 보고된 여러 연구를 통해 밝혀졌다. 소아 외상 사망의 대부분은 예방할 수 있거나 잠재적으로 예방 가능한 것으로 분류할 수 있는 것으로 추정된다. 이러한 통계는 지속적이고 조율된 고품질의 처치를 제공할 수 있는 지역의 소아 외상센터를 설치하는 주요 동기 중 하나이었다. 최근

연구에 따르면 성인 외상센터가 반드시 소아를 위한 준비가 되어 있지 않다. 소아를 처치할 준비가 되어 있지 않은 외상센터에서 처치를 받은 손상을 입은 어린이는 사망률이 2배나 증가한다. 미국 외과학회 외상위원회는 검증된 모든 외상센터에서 소아청소년과 처치를 시행할 수 있도록 통합할 것을 지지한다. 가능하면 EMS 시스템은 중증 손상을 입은 어린이를 처치할 수 있는 외상센터로 먼저 이송해야 한다. 심박수, 호흡수, 혈압 등 생리적 이상을 조기에 발견하면 다기관 손상을 의심하고 소아 외상센터의 필요성이 높아질 것이다.

많은 도시 지역에는 소아 외상센터와 성인 외상센터가 모두 있다. 다발성 외상을 입은 소아 외상 환자는 외상을 입은 소아를 전문적으로 처치할 수 있는 소아 외상센터에서 초기 소생술과 결정적인 처치를 받을 수 있는 것이 가장 이상적이다. 성인 외상센터를 우회하여 소아 외상센터로 이송하는 것이 적절할 수 있다. 그러나 많은 지역사회에서 가장 가까운 소아 전문 외상센터는 몇 시간 떨어진 거리에 있거나 없을 수 있다. 이러면 소아 외상센터로 이송하기 전에 조기 소생술과 평가를 통해 소아의 생존 가능성을 높을 수 있으므로 심각한 외상을 입은 소아는 가장 가까운 성인 외상센터로 이송한다.

근처에 소아 전문 외상센터가 없는 지역에서는 성인 외상센터에서 근무하는 의료진이 성인과 소아 외상 환자의 소생술과 처치의 경험이 있어야 한다. 두 시설 모두 가까운 곳에 없는 지역에서는 병원 전 분류 지침에 따라 중증 손상을 입은 어린이 외상 환자를 치료할 수 있는 가장 가까운 적절한 의료기관으로 이송한다.

시골 지역에서 신속한 이송을 위해 항공 이송을 고려할 수 있다. 소아 외상센터로의 지상 이송이 빠른 도시 직역에서는 항공 이송의 이점을 제공한다는 증거가 거의 없다. 항공 이송을 이용하는 것은 환자와 승무원 모두 상당한 위험에 노출된다는 것이 점점 더 분명해지고 있다. 이러한 자원을 활용할지를 결정할 때는 이러한 우려를 신중하게 고려해야 한다.

많은 응급의료와 외상 시스템에서는 지침에 따라 소아 환자 분류 기준을 사용한다. 모든 병원 전 처치 제공자는 사용하고 있는 분류 프로토콜을 숙지하고 있어야 한다.

특별한 손상

외상성 뇌손상(TBI)

미국에서 0~4세 사이의 어린이와 청소년 중 매년 약 3,000명이 외상성 뇌손상으로 사망하고 29,000명이 입원한다. 가장 심각한 뇌손상

의 대부분은 예방으로만 칠할 수 있지만, 초기 초기를 통해 이차 뇌손상을 최소화하고 결과적으로 어린이의 손상 중중도를 줄일 수 있다. 이차적 손상을 예방하기 위해서는 적절한 환기, 산소 공급 및 적절한 관류가 필요하다. 중증 외상성 뇌손상을 입은 소아 환자의 회복은 일반적으로 성인보다 나은 것으로 간주하지만, 기능적, 인지, 행동 이상을 포함한 다양한 장애가 지속해서 나타난다.

초기 신경학적 평가 결과는 예후에 유용하다. 그러나 초기 신경학적 평가가 정상이더라도 심각한 뇌손상을 입은 어린이는 뇌부종, 관류저하 및 이차적 손상에 취약할 수 있다(**Box 14-6**). 또한, 비사고적 외상의 피해자는 외상의 외부 증거가 거의 없지만, 상당한 두개내손상을 입었을 수도 있다. 이송 중에 기준 글래스고혼수척도 점수를 자주 재평가하고 기록한다. 보충 산소를 공급하고 가능하면 맥박산소측정기로 모니터링해야 한다.

저산소증과 마찬가지로 저혈압을 동반한 혈량저하증은 기존의 외상성 뇌손상의 결과를 급격히 악화시킬 수 있다. 이러한 손상과 관련된 외부출혈은 지혈하고 내부출혈을 제한하기 위해 어린이의 골절된 팔다리 부목으로 고정해야 한다. 이러한 소아 환자는 정맥 내 수액소생술을 통해 정상 혈액량을 유지하도록 노력해야 한다. 드물게 6개월 미만의 영아는 머리뼈 봉합과 숫구멍이 열려 있으므로 두개내출혈로 인해 혈량저하 상태가 될 수 있다. 숫구멍이 열려 있는 영아는 두개내혈종이 확대되는 것을 더 잘 견딜 수 있으므로 급속한 확대가 일어나기 전까지는 증상이 나타나지 않을 수 있다. 숫구멍이 튀어나온 영아는 더 중증 외상성 뇌손상을 입은 것으로 간주한다.

글래스고혼수척도가 8점 이하인 소아 환자의 경우 기관내삽관을 시행하는 것이 아니라 적절한 산소 공급과 환기를 목표로 한다. 기관내삽관을 장시간 시도하는 것은 저산소증의 기간이 길어지고 적절한 의료기관으로 이송을 지연시킬 수 있다. 소아 환자에게 가장 좋은 기도 유지는 가장 안전하고 효과적이다. 구토가 발생할 경우 흡인을 준비하면서 백마스크 장비로 환기를 시행하는 것이 외상성 뇌손상을 입은 소아 환자에게 가장 좋은 기도유지 방법인 경우가 많다.

동공이 느리게 반응하거나 반응하지 않는 경우 전신성 고혈압, 서맥과 비정상 호흡 패턴과 같이 두개내압 증가의 증상과 징후가 있는 소아 환자는 일시적으로 경미한 과다환기를 시행하면 두개내압을 낮추는 데 도움이 될 수 있다. 그러나 과다환기의 효과는 일시적이며 중추신경계로의 산소 공급을 감소시켜 실제로 추가적인 이차 뇌손상을 유발할 수 있다. 소아 환자에게 진행 중인 뇌탈출 징후(뇌 부위 손상으로 인한 한쪽이 쇠약과 같은 원위부 신경학적 이상)가 나타나지

소아 환자, 특히 스포츠 활동을 하는 소아 환자의 뇌진탕 또는 경미한 외상성 뇌손상 문제는 매우 중요한 주제가 되었다. 2006년~2013년까지 응급실 표본 데이터베이스에 따르면 미국 응급실에서 외상성 뇌손상 진단을 받은 소아 환자 수는 610만 명(2.83%)에 달하며 연구 기간 소아 외상성 뇌손상 환자 수는 34.1% 증가했다. 과거에는 소아 운동선수가 뇌진탕을 당하면 잠시 경기에 출전하지 못하게 한 후 가능한 한 빨리 경기에 복귀하도록 했다. 하지만 머리와 뇌에 반복적으로 충격을 받으면 인지, 행동, 기능에 장기적인 장애가 생길 수 있다. 뇌진탕을 입은 소아 선수는 경기에서 제외되어야 하며 경기가 진행되는 동안 그리고 자격을 갖춘 의사의 경기 참가 허가를 받을 때까지 경기에 참여해서는 안 된다.

뇌진탕에 대한 인식은 매우 중요하다. 한때 뇌진탕은 잠시 의식을 잃었다가 정상 기능으로 돌아오는 것으로 생각되었지만, 이제는 의식 소실이 진단을 내리는데 필요하지 않다는 것을 이해하게 되었다. 뇌진탕은 두통, 구역, 균형 문제, 멍하거나 어리벙벙한 느낌, 혼돈, 느리거나 반복적으로 질문하는 등 다양한 증상과 불만을 수반할 수 있다. 스포츠 경기 현장에 있는 의료진은 신경학적 검사뿐만 아니라 표준 작업 평가 도구를 사용하여 소아 운동선수의 뇌진탕을 평가할 수 있는 공식적인 방법을 갖출 것을 권장한다.

뇌진탕에서 완전히 회복하는 데는 1주일 이상이 걸릴 수 있으며 때에 따라 몇 개월이 걸릴 수도 있다. 소아 운동선수가 뇌진탕에서 완전히 회복되어 무증상이 될 때까지 경기 복귀를 허용해서는 안 된다. 증상이 사라진 후에는 증상의 재발을 평가하기 위해 반복적인 평가와 함께 등급이 매겨진 구조화된 형식으로 활동과 놀이를 재개할 수 있다. 증상이 재발하는 것은 불완전한 회복을 의미하며 소아 운동선수는 증상이 호전될 때까지 스포츠 참여를 자제해야 한다. 경기 복귀 방향은 자격을 갖춘 의사가 결정해야 하며 뇌진탕을 당한 어린이는 철저한 평가 없이 경기에 복귀해서는 안 된다.

않는 한 과다환기는 시행하지 않는 것이 좋다. 삽관이 시행된 소아 환자는 호기말이산화탄소분압 모니터링을 통해 약 35mmHg로 유지하도록 한다. 호기말이산화탄소분압이 25mmHg 미만인 경우 과다환기는 신경학적 결과 악화와 관련이 있다. 호기말이산화탄소분압을 사용할 수 없으면 호흡수를 소아의 경우 25회/분, 영아의 경우 30회/분으로 유지한다.

이송 지연하는 동안 프로토콜이 허용하는 경우 두개내압 상승의 증거가 있는 소아에게 소량의 만니톨(0.5~1.0g/kg) 또는 고장식염수를 투여하면 도움이 될 수 있다. 그러나 불충분한 수액 소생술 시행 중에 만니톨을 투여하면 혈량저하와 쇼크가 악화할 수 있다. 의료 지도 의사의 의료 지도를 받지 않았거나 프로토콜에서 허용하지 않는 한 현장에서 만니톨을 투여해서는 안 되며, 이 경우 위험과 이점을 신중하게 비교해야 한다. 그런데도 병원 전 환경에서 고장식염수 또는 만니톨을 사용하는 것은 뇌탈출증이 임박한 경우에만 사용해야 한다. 짧은 발작은 외상성 뇌손상 후 발생할 수 있으며 환자의 안전,

산소공급 및 보조 환기를 시행하는 것 외에는 병원 전 처치 제공자의 특별한 처치가 필요하지 않은 경우가 많다. 그러나 재발성 발작이 우려되는 경우 미다졸람(0.1mg/kg)과 같은 벤조다이아제핀을 정맥 내로 투여해야 할 수 있다. 모든 벤조다이아제핀은 환기 저하 및 저혈압의 잠재적 부작용과 신경 학적 검사를 애매하게 할 수 있으므로 이러한 환자에게는 매우 주의해서 사용한다.

척수 외상

소아 환자의 척추 움직임 제한을 시행해야 하는 적응증은 손상 기전과 신체검사 소견을 근거로 한다. 머리, 목 또는 몸통의 격렬하거나 갑작스러운 움직임을 암시하는 다른 손상의 존재 또는 변형, 통증, 신경학적 결손과 같은 척추 손상의 특정 징후가 있는지에 따라 결정된다. 성인 환자와 마찬가지로 척추 손상이 의심되는 소아 환자의 경우 적절한 병원 전 처치는 머리를 중립 자세로 유지하고 도수 고정 후 적절한 크기의 목뼈보호대를 착용시킨 후 머리, 목, 몸통, 골반, 다리가 중립 자세를 유지할 수 있도록 적절한 장비에 고정하는 것이다. 신경학적 결손이 빠르게 회복되는 소아 환자는 SCIWORA가 있을 수 있으며 지연된 이차 후유증에 취약할 수 있다. 이러한 환자들은 병원에 도착 전에 증상이 해결되더라도 척추 움직임 제한을 유지해야 한다. 이는 어린이의 환기 또는 입을 벌리는 능력을 손상하거나 다른 소생술에 지장을 주지 않으면서 이루어져야 한다.

어린이는 의사소통할 수 없거나 스스로 평가에 참여할 수 없으므로 척추 움직임 제한을 시행할 수 있는 기준이 더 낮다. 현장에서 어린이의 척추 움직임 제한을 임상적으로 제거하는 것의 안정성을 검증한 연구는 아직 없다. 앞서 설명한 것과 같은 미성숙함은 고정에 대한 어린이의 두려움과 협력 부족에 기여한다. 척추 움직임 제한을 시행하려는 시도에 강하게 거부하는 어린이는 발생한 척추 손상을 악화시킬 위험이 높아질 수 있다. 소아를 억제하지 않고 조용히 누워있도록 설득할 수 있다면 억제하지 않는 것이 타당할 수 있다. 그러나 환자의 안전을 위해 척추 움직임 제한을 중단하는 결정은 신중하고 철저하게 문서화된 근거와 이송 중 또는 이송 직후 지속적인 신경학적 상태에 대한 평가에 의해 뒷받침되어야 한다. 이러한 결정은 의료 지도 의사의 의료 지도를 받은 후 결정하는 것이 가장 이상적이다.

대부분의 작은 소아를 딱딱한 평면에 위치시키면 뒤통수가 상대적으로 크기 때문에 목이 수동적으로 굴곡 된다. 소아 환자의 몸통 아래에 충분한 패딩(2~3cm)을 넣어 몸통을 들어 올려 머리가 중립 자세기 되도록 해야 한다. 패딩은 어깨에서 골반까지 연속적이고 평평해야 하며 등뼈, 허리뼈, 엉치뼈, 꼬리뼈가 앞뒤로 움직일 가능성 없이 평평하고 안정적인 고정판 위에 있도록 몸통의 측면 가장자리까지 확장되어야 한다. 또한 구토 시 흡인을 피하기 위해 척추 고정판을 움직이거나 환자와 척추고정판을 옆으로 돌려야 할 때 측면 움직임이 발생하지 않도록 소아의 측면과 척추고정판 가장자리 사이에 패딩을 배치해야 한다.

다양한 새로운 소아 고정 장비를 사용할 수 있다. 병원 전 처치 제공자는 정기적으로 연습하고 병원 전 단계에서 사용되는 모든 특수 장비뿐만 아니라 성인용 장비를 사용하여 소아 환자를 고정하는 방법을 숙지하고 있어야 한다. 소아 환자에게 조끼 형태의 장비를 사용하는 경우 호흡 억제를 예방할 수 있도록 적절하게 고정해야 한다. 과거에는 영아나 소아 환자가 발생한 경우 카시트에 고정하는 것이 권장되었다. 현재 미국 고속도로 교통안전국(NHTSA)에서는 소아 환자를 카시트 대신 적절한 크기의 소아용 고정 장비에 고정하여 이송할 것을 권장하고 있다. 손상을 입은 소아를 카시트에 똑바로 세운 자세로 유지하면 환자의 머리가 척추에 가하는 축 방향 하중이 증가하므로 카시트보다 표준 척추고정 장비를 사용하는 방법이 선호된다. 고정하지 않은 어린이는 보호자의 무릎에 앉혀서 이송해서는 안 되며 카시트에서 적절하게 고정하여 이송한다.

가슴 손상

어린이의 가슴우리는 매우 탄력적이기 때문에 가슴의 골격 구조에 대한 손상은 적지만, 폐 타박상, 기흉 또는 혈흉과 같은 근본적인 폐 손상의 위험은 여전히 존재한다. 소아기에 갈비뼈 골절은 드물지만, 갈비뼈 골절이 있는 경우 가슴속 손상 위험이 높다. 비빔소리는 평가를 통해 확인할 수 있으며 기흉의 징후일 수 있다. 사망 위험은 갈비뼈가 골절된 개수에 따라 증가한다. 높은 의심 지수는 이러한 손상을 확인하는 열쇠이다. 가슴과 몸통에 외상을 입은 모든 소아 환자는 호흡곤란과 쇼크 징후가 있는지 주의 깊게 모니터링 한다. 무딘 외상 후 소아 환자의 몸통에 생긴 찰과상이나 타박상은 병원 전 처치 제공자에게 소아 환자가 가슴 외상을 입었다는 유일한 단서가 될 수 있다.

또한, 충격이 심한 무딘 가슴 외상을 입은 소아 환자를 의료기관으로 이송하는 동안 소아 환자의 심장 리듬을 모니터링 한다. 모든 경우에서 가슴 외상 환자를 처치하는 데 중요 사항은 환기, 산소 공급 및 적절한 의료기관으로 적시에 주의해서 이송하는 것이다.

복부 손상

복부에 무딘 손상, 불안정한 골반, 외상 후 복부팽창, 복부경직 또는 압통, 기타 설명할 수 없는 쇼크가 있는 경우 복강 내 출혈과 관련이 있을 수 있다. 소아 환자의 복부에 "안전띠 징후" 또는 핸들 자국이 있는 경우 심각한 내부 손상을 나타내는 경우가 많다(**그림 14-7**).

복부 손상 처치의 병원 전 핵심 요소에는 목표 수액 소생술, 보충적 고농도 산소 공급과 적절한 의료기관으로 신속한 이송과 이송 중 지속해서 주의 깊은 모니터링이 포함된다. 복강 내 손상을 입은 소아 환자에게 병원 전 처치 제공자가 제공할 수 있는 결정적인 처치는 아직 없으므로 소아 환자를 가장 가까운 적절한 의료기관으로 신속하게 이송하기 위해 모든 노력을 기울여야 한다.

팔다리 외상

성인의 골격에 비해 어린이의 골격은 활발하게 성장하고 있으며 연골 조직과 대사적으로 활발한 성장판으로 구성되어 있다. 골격을 함께 유지하는 인대 구조는 종종 인대가 부착된 뼈보다 더 강하고 기계적 파괴를 더 잘 견딜 수 있다. 따라서 골격 외상을 입은 어린이는 긴뼈 골절, 탈구 또는 변형이 발생하기 전에 심한 외상을 입는 경우가 많다. 불완전(생나무)골절이 흔하며 영향을 받은 팔다리를 움직일 때 뼈의 압통과 통증으로만 나타날 수 있다.

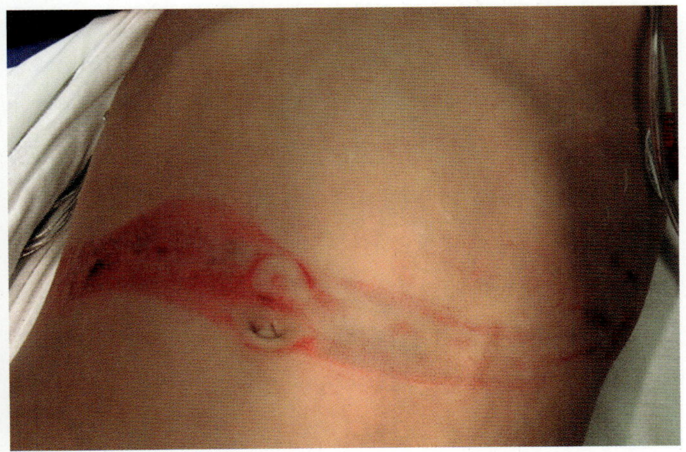

그림 14-7 비장이 파열된 6세 환자의 "안전띠 징후". 안전띠 징후는 종종 심각한 복부 내 손상과 관련이 있다.

Courtesy of Dr. Jeffrey Guy.

관통상 이외의 손상으로 인한 일차 관절 손상은 골간 또는 골단 부위의 손상에 비해 흔하지 않다. 성장판과 관련된 골절은 급성 손상 단계에서 주의 깊게 구별하고 처치해야 적절한 치유를 보장할 뿐만 아니라 계속 성장함에 따라 후속 변위 또는 변형을 예방할 수 있다는 점에서 독특하다. 어린이의 신경 혈관 손상과 정형외과적 손상과의 연관성을 항상 고려해야 하며 말초혈관 및 신경학적 평가를 주의 깊게 시행한다. 종종 잠재적으로 쇠약해질 수 있는 손상의 존재 여부는 방사선 또는 말초 관류의 감소가 조금이라도 의심되는 경우 동맥조영술을 통해서만 확인할 수 있다.

때때로 팔다리 손상과 관련된 겉으로 보이는 심한 변형 때문에 생명을 위협할 수 있는 손상에 관한 관심이 분산되어서는 안 된다. 조절되지 않은 출혈은 팔다리 외상으로 인해 가장 생명을 위협하는 결과이다. 성인 및 소아 다발성 외상 환자 모두 일차평가, 소생술, 신속하게 처리를 완료한 후 즉시 적절한 의료기관으로 이송을 시작하는 것이 사망률을 줄이는 데 가장 중요하다. 소아 환자의 소생술을 방해하지 않고 이송 중에 부목을 적용할 수 있다면 긴뼈 골절로 인해 발생한 출혈과 통증을 최소화하는 데 도움이 되지만, 생명을 위협하는 손상에 대한 주의는 항상 최우선으로 유지한다.

화상 손상

화상은 자동차 충돌과 익사에 이어 소아 외상 사망 원인 중 세 번째로 높은 비율을 차지한다. 손상을 입은 어린이를 처치하는 일은 항상 병원 전 처치 제공자에게 상당한 신체적, 감정적 어려움을 초래하며 이러한 어려움은 화상을 입은 소아 환자를 처치할 때 더욱 증가한다. 화상을 입은 소아 환자는 기도에 부종이 발생할 수 있고 팔다리의 화상으로 인해 정맥 라인 확보가 어려울 수 있으며 통증으로 인해 히스테리 증상을 보일 수 있다.

다른 소아 외상과 마찬가지로 일차평가를 따라야 하지만, 일차평가의 모든 단계는 열 손상이 없는 소아보다 더 복잡할 수 있다. 건물화재와 관련된 대부분의 사망은 연부조직 화상과 직접적인 관련이 없으며 연기 흡인으로 인해 이차적으로 발생한다. 어린이가 불이 난 건물에 갇히면 침대 밑이나 벽장 속에 숨는 경우가 많다. 이러한 어린이는 사망하는 경우가 많으며 시신을 수습해도 화상을 입지 않은 경우가 많고 일산화탄소나 사이안화수소 중독 및 저산소증으로 사망하는 경우가 많다.

열로 인한 기도의 부종은 화상 환자에게 항상 우려되는 문제이지만, 특히 소아에게 더욱 그렇다. 소아는 기도의 지름이 작으므로 1mm의 부종이 발생하면 지름이 더 큰 성인보다 소아는 훨씬 더 심한 기도 폐쇄를 일으킬 수 있다. 기도에 부종이 발생한 소아 환자는 앉아서 몸을 앞으로 기울여 침을 흘리거나 쉰 목소리 또는 목소리 변화를 호소할 수 있다. 이러한 증상이 나타나면 신속하게 의료기관으로 이송을 준비하고 시작해야 한다. 이송 중에 보충 산소를 투여하고 증상이 진행되거나 어린이가 호흡 정지 또는 심정지가 발생할 경우 기도를 유지하기 위한 처치를 준비한다.

기관내관을 삽입한 경우 기관내관이 의도치 않게 이탈되거나 빠지지 않도록 보호한다. 소아 화상 환자가 실수로 기관내관을 제거한 경우 부종이 진행되어 병원 전 처치 제공자는 다시 삽관하지 못할 수 있으며 그 결과는 치명적일 수 있다. 얼굴에 화상을 입은 소아 환자에게는 일반적인 테이프로 기관내관을 얼굴에 고정해서는 안 된다. 기관내관은 두 조각의 배꼽 테이프로 고정해야 하며 한 조각은 귀 위에 다른 조각은 귀 아래에 부착한다. 배꼽 테이프를 대신할 수 있는 효과적인 대안은 수액 세트이다. 이러한 물품을 사용할 수 없지만, 보조자가 있다면 책임을 지고 기관내관을 고정할 처치 제공자를 지정한다.

수액 소생술

소아 화상 환자의 쇼크 발생을 예방하기 위해서는 정맥 라인을 신속하게 확보하는 것이 중요하다. 소아 환자에게 수액 소생술이 지연되면 특히 화상을 입은 영아의 경우 임상 결과가 심하게 악화하고 사망률이 증가하는 것과 관련이 있다.

기도를 확보하고 적절한 환기와 산소를 공급한 후에는 정맥 라인을 신속하게 확보하는 것이 중요하다. 소아는 혈관 내 용적이 상대적으로 작으므로 수액 소생술이 지연되면 저혈량 쇼크가 빠르게 진행될 수 있다. 중증 화상의 경우 필요한 수액을 대량으로 투여하기 위해 일반적으로 두 개의 말초정맥 라인 확보가 필요하다. 하나의 큰 구경 정맥 카테터를 삽입하기도 어려운 경우가 많으므로 두 개의 정맥 카테터를 삽입하기는 더 어렵다. 팔다리에 화상을 입으면 적절한 수액 소생술을 위해 필요한 정맥 라인을 확보하는 것이 어렵거나 불가능할 수 있다.

화상을 입은 성인 환자와 마찬가지로 화상을 입은 어린이의 경우 손상 시점부터 수액 필요량을 계산하므로 수액 소생술 시작이 30분이라도 지연되면 저혈량 쇼크가 발생할 수 있다. 과도한 수액 투여는 호흡기 합병증과 과도한 부종을 유발하여 화상 처치를 복잡하게 만들 수 있다.

수액 소생술을 시작할 때 화상 환자에게 일반적으로 투여하는 수액의 양은 화상을 입은 전체 체표면적(TBSA)을 기준으로 계산되며 이후 소생술은 관류 및 소변 배출량에 따라 결정된다. 체표면적은 성인 전장 화상 부상자를 기준으로 수액 소생술에 필요한 수액량을 신속하고 정확하게 추정하는 "9의 법칙"과 함께 사용된다. 이 화상 범위를 추정하는 방법의 전제는 성인 신체 주요 부위(예: 머리, 팔, 몸통 앞부분)가 각각 체표면적의 9%를 차지한다는 것이다. 어린이의 해부학적 부위는 성인과 비례적으로 다르며 어린이는 머리가 크고 팔다리가 작다. 어린이 화상의 체표면적을 과대평가하는 경향이 있다. 표재성 화상(온전한 홍반성 피부)은 체표면적을 계산하는 데 포함되지 않는다는 점을 기억한다. 소아 화상 면적을 추정할 때는 9의 법칙이 아닌 룬드-브로더(Lund-Browder chart) 차트와 같은 나이별 도표를 사용해야 한다. 이 도표를 사용하면 각 다리는 13.5%, 팔은 9%, 가슴과 등은 각각 18%, 머리는 18%로 추정할 수 있다. 만약 룬드-브로더 차트와 도표를 사용할 수 없는 경우 "손바닥 법칙"을 사용할 수 있다. 이 방법을 사용하면 소아 환자의 손바닥과 손가락의 크기는 체표면적의 약 1%를 차지한다. 이 방법은 신체 부위 전체가 아닌 국소적인 부위에 대한 화상 면적을 추정할 때 유용하다(이러한 화상 면적 추정 방법에 대한 자세한 내용은 13장 화상 손상을 참조한다).

수액 소생술에 필요한 정맥 내 수액 투여량은 화상을 입은 체표면적의 비율에 따라 결정된다(13장 화상 손상 참조). 소아에게는 두 가지 중요한 고려 사항이었다. 첫째 작은 소아는 글리코겐 저장량이 제한되어 있다. 글리코겐은 본질적으로 포도당 분자가 서로 연결된 상태이며 탄수화물 저장에 사용된다. 저장된 글리코겐은 스트레스를 받을 때 동원된다. 이러한 제한된 글리코겐 저장량이 고갈되면 소아는 빠르게 저혈당이 발생할 수 있다. 둘째, 소아는 부피 대 표면적 비율이 크고 성인의 일반적인 체형은 원통형이지만, 어린이는 원 모양과 비슷하다(**그림 14-8**). 임상적 의미는 어린이가 화상을 입었을 때 더 많은 정맥 내 수액이 필요하다는 것이다. 병원 도착 전 초기 소생술의 경우 의식 상태에 변화가 있는 소아는 혈당을 확인해야 한다. 소아에게 빈맥이 있고 관류가 불량한 경우 20mL/kg 수액을 볼루스로 투여해야 한다. 투여한 총 수액량은 병원 도착 즉시 의료진에게 보고한다.

말초 정맥 라인이 확보되면 정맥 라인이 부주의로 빠지지 않도록 조치를 해야 한다. 정맥 라인을 고정하기 위해 일반적으로 사용하는 반창고나 드레싱이 화상 부위 조직에 부착되지 않을 수 있기 때

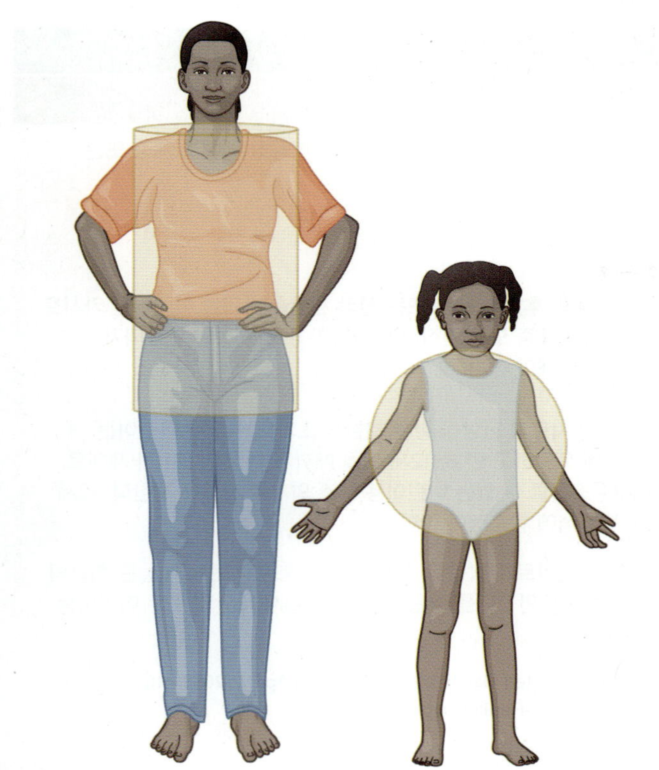

그림 14-8 성인의 일반적인 모양은 원통형이지만, 어린이는 용적 대 표면적 비율이 크고 원 모양과 비슷하다.
© National Association of Emergency Medical Technicians (NAEMT)

문에 화상 부위 또는 화상 부위 인접한 부위에 정맥 라인을 확보하고 고정하는 데 종종 부착되지 않는 경우가 많다. 가능하면 정맥 라인은 Kerlix 드레싱으로 고정하지만, 부종이 발생하면 드레싱이 압박 밴드가 되는 것을 방지하기 위해 화상 부위 드레싱을 자주 모니터링한다.

말초 정맥 라인을 확보할 수 없는 경우 불안정하거나 의식이 없는 소아 환자들에게 골내(IO)로 수액 투여를 한다. 이전에는 3세 미만의 소아 환자에게만 권장되었지만, 이제는 성인뿐만이 아니라 나이가 많은 소아에게도 골내로 수액을 투여한다.

학대

소아 화상의 약 10%는 비사고성 화상이다. 이 중 최대 50%의 어린이는 반복적인 학대를 경험할 수 있으며 이 중 30%는 결국 학대로 인해 사망한다. 병원 전 처치 제공자 사이에서 이 문제에 대한 인식이 높아지면서 이러한 소아 외상의 원인을 더 잘 발견할 수 있다. 손상을 둘러싼 상황과 손상 유형 자체를 세심하게 기록하면 관련 기관이 가해자를 기소하는 데 도움이 될 수 있다.

어린이가 화상을 입는 가장 흔한 두 가지 기전은 열탕 화상과 접촉 화상이다. 열탕 화상은 비우발적 화상의 가장 흔한 원인이다. 열탕 화상은 일반적으로 대소변을 가릴 수 있는 나이의 어린이에게 발생한다. 일반적인 시나리오는 아이가 변기가 아닌 다른 곳에서 소변이나 대변을 본 후 끓는 물이 담긴 욕조에 몸을 담그는 경우이다. 이러한 열탕 화상은 화상을 입은 조직과 화상을 입지 않은 조직이 뚜렷하게 구분되고 아이가 끓는 물을 피하려고 다리를 자주 올리기 때문에 굴곡 주름이 생기는 유형이 특징이다(13장 화상 손상 참조).

접촉 화상은 학대로 인해 발생한 화상의 두 번째로 흔한 기전이다. 접촉 화상을 입히는 데 흔히 사용되는 물품으로는 고데기, 다리미, 라이터, 담배 등이 있다. 담배 화상은 지름이 1cm가 약간 넘는 원형의 균일한 상처로 나타난다. 이러한 손상을 감추기 위해 가해자는 일반적으로 옷으로 가려지는 부분, 두피의 헤어라인 상부 또는 겨드랑이에 화상을 입힐 수 있다.

신체의 모든 표면은 어느 정도 굴곡이 있어서 실수로 뜨거운 물건이 신체 표면에 떨어지면 초기 접촉 지점이 생기고 접촉 지점에서 멀어지게 된다. 그 결과 화상의 경계가 불규칙하고 깊이가 고르지 않게 된다. 반대로 뜨거운 물건을 고의로 사용하여 화상을 입히는 경우 해당 물건이 신체 부위를 눌러 화상을 입게 된다. 화상은 뚜렷하고 규칙적인 경계선과 균일한 깊이의 화상 유형을 보인다(13장 화상 손상 참조).

학대를 의심하는 높은 지수가 중요하며 학대가 의심되는 모든 환자는 보고해야 한다. 다양한 가구의 위치, 고데기의 존재 유무, 욕조물의 깊이 등 주변 환경을 세심하게 관찰한다. 현장에 있었던 사람들의 이름을 기록한다. 화상으로 인한 학대가 의심되는 소아 환자는 화상의 크기와 관계없이 소아 화상 치료 경험이 풍부한 의료기관에서 치료받아야 한다.

아동학대 및 방임은 이 장의 뒷부분에서 더 자세히 설명한다.

자동차 손상 예방

미국 소아과학회(AAP)는 어린이를 위한 최적의 차량 내 안전띠 착용을 정의했다(**표 14-7**). 미국 소아과학회는 만 2세까지 어린이는 항상 유아용 카시트에 고정되어 좌석 뒤쪽을 향하도록 하는 것을 권장한다. 컨버터블 시트의 후면 무게 또는 신장 제한을 초과한 어린이는 카시트 제조업체에서 허용하는 최대 체중과 신장을 기준으로 가능한 오랫동안 안전띠가 있는 전방을 향한 시트를 사용해야 한다. 그런

표 14-7 카시트의 종류

연령	시트 종류	일반적인 사용법
영아 및 유아	■ 뒤쪽을 보도록 장착하는 전용 ■ 뒤쪽을 보도록 장착하지만 전환 가능	모든 영유아는 만 2세 이상이거나 카시트 제조업체에서 허용하는 최고 체중 또는 신장에 도달할 때까지 뒷좌석에 탑승해야 한다.
유아 및 취학 전 아동	■ 전환 가능 ■ 안전띠가 있는 전방을 보도록 장착	방향을 전환할 수 있는 시트의 후향식 체중 또는 신장 제한을 초과한 어린이는 카시트 제조업체에서 허용하는 최고 체중 또는 신장까지 가능한 한 오랫동안 안전띠가 장착된 전향식 카시트를 사용해야 한다.
학령기 아동	■ 어린이용 보조의자	체중이나 키가 차량용 안전 시트의 전방을 향한 제한을 초과하는 모든 어린이는 일반적으로 키가 145cm에 도달하고 만 8~12세가 될 때까지 차량 안전띠가 제대로 맞을 때까지 벨트 위치를 조절할 수 있는 어린이용 보조 의자를 사용해야 한다. 13세 미만의 모든 어린이는 뒷좌석에 탑승해야 한다.
큰아이들	■ 안전띠	어린이가 차량용 안전띠를 올바르게 착용할 수 있을 만큼 충분히 큰 아이들은 최상의 보호를 위해 항상 허리 및 어깨 안전띠를 사용해야 한다. 13세 미만의 모든 어린이는 뒷좌석에 탑승해야 한다.

Reproduced from American Academy of Pediatrics (AAP). Car seats: information for families. Updated March 6, 2018. Accessed April 2, 2018. https://www.healthychildren.org/English/safety-prevention/on-the-go/Pages/Car-Safety-Seats-Information-for-Families.aspx

다음 8~12세까지 안전띠를 착용할 수 있는 어린이용 카시트를 사용한다. 이때부터 표준 3점식 성인용 안전띠를 사용할 수 있다. 절대로 허리를 고정하는 2점식 벨트만 사용해서는 안 된다. 모든 어린이는 13세가 될 때까지 뒷좌석에 앉아야 한다.

차선책은 8세 미만의 어린이는 어린이용 카시트나 보조 의자를 사용하지 않고 8세 이상의 어린이가 3점식 안전장치를 사용하지 않는 것으로 정의된다(Box 14-1). 한 검토 연구에 따르면 이러한 지침을 준수했을 때 적절하게 안전띠를 착용한 어린이의 복부 손상 위험성은 안전띠를 착용하지 않은 소아보다 3.5배 낮았다. 뒷좌석에 소아를 앉히는 보호 효과는 앞좌석의 3점식 안전띠로 고정하는 것 보다 뒷좌석에 앉아 허리를 고정하는 2점식 안전띠만 매더라도 사망 위험이 최소 30% 감소하는 것으로 나타났다. 손상 예방에 대한 자세한 내용은 16장 손상 예방을 참조한다.

아동 학대 및 방임

아동 학대(학대 또는 우발적 외상)는 소아기 손상의 중요한 원인이다. 2018년 미국에서 입증된 아동 학대 사례는 약 678,000건, 학대로 인한 사망자는 1,738명이었다. 병원 전 처치 제공자는 상황에 따라 아동 학대 가능성을 항상 고려한다.

병원 전 처치 제공자는 다음과 같은 상황 중 하나라도 발견되면 학대 또는 방치를 의심한다.

- 병력과 신체적 손상 정도가 일치하지 않거나 보고된 병력이 자주 변경되는 경우
- 가족의 부적절한 반응
- 손상 발생 시간과 의학적 처치를 요청하는 사이의 간격이 길어진 경우
- 어린이의 발달 수준과 일치하지 않는 손상 병력. 예를 들어 신생아가 침대에서 굴러떨어졌다는 병력은 신생아가 발달적으로 몸을 뒤집을 수 없으므로 의심할 수 있다.

다음과 같은 특정 유형의 손상은 학대를 암시한다(그림 14-9).

- 다양한 단계의 다발성 골절 또는 타박상(손바닥, 아래팔, 정강뼈 부위 및 보행 중인 어린이의 이마는 일반적인 낙상으로 자주 다치는 부위에서 제외). 우발적으로 발생한 타박상은 골격의 융기 부위에 발생하며 고의적인 상해로 인한 타박상은 엉덩이, 복부 또는 등에 나타날 수 있다.
- 물린 자국, 담배 화상, 밧줄 자국, 손자국 또는 특이한 형태의 손상과 같은 비정상적인 손상
- 특이한 부위에 뚜렷하게 구분된 화상이나 열탕 화상(13장 화상 손상 참조)

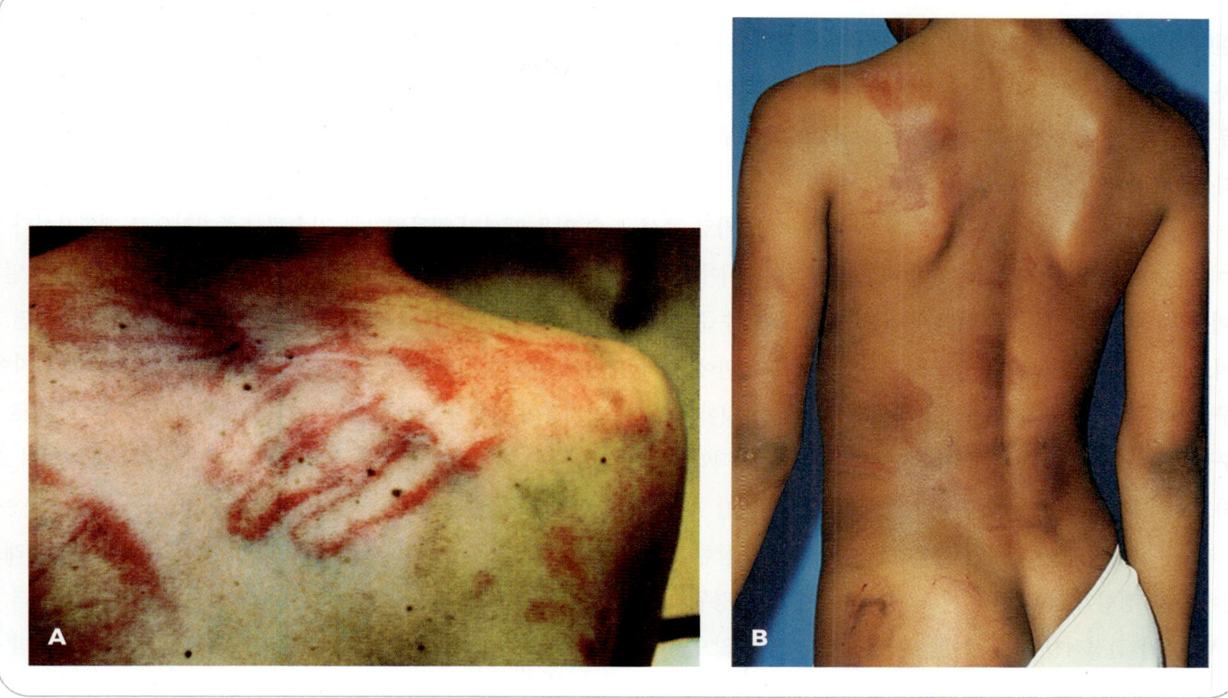

그림 14-9 비사고성 외상 가능성 지표. **A.** 손자국과 비슷한 타박상 **B.** 여러 단계의 치유 단계에 있는 타박상.

A: Courtesy of Moose Jaw Police Service; **B:** Courtesy of Ronald Dieckmann, MD.

TEN-4-FACESp 타박상 임상 결정 규칙은 방임과 관련된 타박상을 구별하는 데 매우 민감하고 구체적인 도구이다(**그림 14-10**).

- TNE: 몸통(가슴, 복부, 등, 볼기, GU 부위, 엉덩이), 귀 또는 목의 멍
- FACES: 코뼈, 턱의 각도, 뺨(지방 부분), 눈꺼풀, 결막밑 부위의 멍
- 4: "TEN-4-FACES" 4세 미만 어린이의 타박상 또는 4개월 이하 영아의 모든 타박상
- p: 무늬가 있는

많은 국가에서 병원 전 처치 제공자는 잠재적인 아동학대를 발견할 경우 법적으로 신고 의무가 있다. 일반적으로 선의로 소아의 최선의 이익을 위해 행동하는 의료진은 법적 조치로부터 보호받는다. 신고 절차는 다양하므로 병원 전 처치 제공자는 자신이 근무하는 지역에서 아동학대를 담당하는 기관을 알고 있어야 한다.

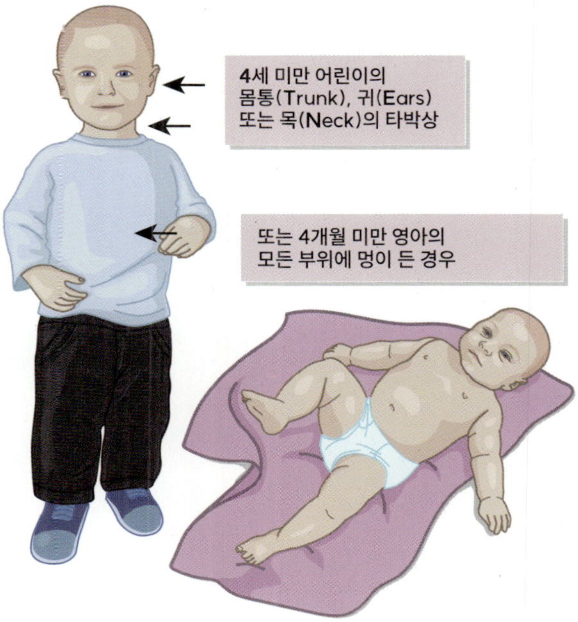

이송 지연

때에 따라 환자 위치, 분류 결정 또는 환경적 고려 사항으로 인해 이송이 길어지거나 지연되어 병원 전 처치 제공자가 소아 환자의 지속적인 소생술을 시행해야 하는 상황이 발생할 수 있다. 현장 자원(예: 혈액)이 부족하고 진단 및 처치 개입을 수행할 수 없으므로 이것이

그림 14-10 TEN-4-FACESp 타박상 임상 결정 규칙은 학대와 관련된 멍을 식별하는 데 매우 민감하고 구체적인 도구이다.

© National Association of Emergency Medical Technicians (NAEMT)

차선책일 수 있지만, 이 장에서 논의한 원칙을 체계적으로 적용하여 많은 어린이를 외상센터에 도착할 때까지 안전하게 처치할 수 있다. 소아 환자를 이송하는 의료기관과 무선 또는 휴대전화로 연락이 가능한 경우 병원 전 처치 제공자와 의료기관의 외상팀원 모두에게 지속적인 의사소통과 피드백이 중요하다.

처치는 일차평가의 구성 요소에 대한 지속적인 연속 평가로 구성된다. 소아 환자의 척추 움직임 제한이 전체적으로 유지되어야 한다. 상당히 이송 지연하는 경우 심각한 불편을 피하고 의식 수준 변화 및 잠재적으로 욕창이 있는 환자의 경우 단단한 척추고정판에서 이동시켜 구급차 주들것에서 척추 움직임 제한을 유지하는 것이 좋다. 이러면 구급차 주들 것을 이용해서 이송하는 동안 척추 움직임 제한을 유지하고 이차 척수 손상을 제한하기 위해 세심한 주의를 기울여야 한다. 기도유지가 시행되지 않는 경우 기관내삽관을 포함한 소아 기도유지에 대해 경험이 많은 병원 전 처치 제공자가 있는 경우 어린이의 상태에 따라 결정적인 기도 유지를 시행한다. 그렇지 않으면 백 마스크 장비를 이용해 적절한 산소 공급과 환기를 제공할 수 있다면 허용할 수 있는 처치 방법이다.

특히 머리 손상을 입은 어린이의 경우 맥박산소측정과 호기말이산화탄소분압을 모니터링 한다. 쇼크 징후가 있는 경우 소아가 호전되거나 결정적인 처치를 제공할 수 있는 의료기관으로 이송될 때까지 20mL/kg의 락테이티드 용액(LR) 또는 생리식염수를 볼루스로 투여한다.

글래스고혼수척도 점수를 조기에 계산하고 연속적으로 재평가한다. 다른 손상에 대한 평가를 지속하고 어린이의 체온을 정상으로 유지하기 위한 모든 표준 처치를 시행한다. 골절 부위는 신경혈관 평가를 시행한 후 부목으로 고정하여 안정화한다. 소아 환자를 안전하게 이송되거나 결정적인 처치를 제공할 수 있는 의료기관으로 이송할 수 있을 때까지 일차평가를 지속해서 주기적으로 재평가한다.

소아 환자의 상태에 변화가 있거나 보상되지 않으면 즉시 일차평가를 재평가해야 한다. 예를 들어 산소포화도를 모니터링하면 기관내관이 여전히 기도에 잘 고정되어 있는지, 그렇다면 소아 환자에게 긴장기흉이 발생한 것은 아닌지, 기관내관이 오른쪽 주기관지로 삽입된 것은 아닌지? 소아가 충분한 수액을 투여받았는데도 여전히 쇼크 상태인 경우 심장눌림증, 중증의 심장 타박상 또는 복강 내 손상이나 두피 열상과 같은 잠재적 출혈의 원인이 있을 수 있는가? 글래스고혼수척도 점수가 변경되었는가? 진행성 뇌손상을 암시하고 더 적극적인 처치가 필요한 편측마비와 같은 징후가 있는가? 팔다리의 순환과 신경학적 기능이 여전히 정상인가? 소아 환자의 체온이 정상인가? 무선 통신이 가능한 경우 소생술과 이송 과정에서 지속해서 의료 지도를 받는다.

기본에 주의를 기울이고 지속해서 재평가함으로써 어린이가 결정적인 처치를 받을 수 있는 의료기관으로 이송될 때까지 적절한 소생술을 시행할 수 있다.

요 약

- 병원 전 환경에서 소아 환자에 대한 일차평가와 처치에는 소아 환자의 고유한 특성을 설명하기 위해 수정된 표준 외상 생명 유지 원칙의 적용이 필요하다.

- 외상성 뇌손상은 외상으로 인한 사망의 가장 주요 원인이며 소아 환자에게 기도 유지가 필요한 가장 흔한 손상이다.

- 어린이는 "작은 성인"으로 생각해서는 안 된다. 소아는 고유한 해부학적 및 발달 단계에 따른 고려 사항이 있으며 환자와 보호자 모두 심리적 지원이 필요할 수 있다.

- 소아 평가 삼각구도(PAT)는 병원 전 처치 제공자가 아프거나 아프지 않은 일반적인 인상을 형성하는 데 도움이 된다. 소아 평가 삼각구도의 세 가지 구성 요소는 외모, 호흡 상태 및 피부 순환이다.

- 소아는 성인보다 용적 손실을 보상하는 능력이 더 오래 지속되지만, 보상 능력이 떨어지면 갑자기 심각하게 악화한다.

- 외상 징후가 거의 또는 전혀 없이도 심각한 내부 장기 및 혈관 손상이 발생할 수 있다.

- 다음과 같은 징후가 있는 소아 환자는 불안정한 상태이므로 지체 없이 적절한 의료기관, 이상적으로는 소아 외상센터로 이송해야 한다.
  - 호흡기 손상
  - 쇼크 또는 불안정한 순환 징후
  - 의식상태 변화
  - 머리, 가슴 또는 복부에 심각한 무딘 외상이 있는 경우
  - 다발성 골절 또는 심각한 골절(갈비뼈 또는 골반)의 증거가 있는 경우
  - 비사고성 외상에 대한 우려

- 손상 병력이 소아 환자의 증상과 일치하지 않을 때는 항상 학대나 비사고성 외상의 가능성을 고려해야 한다.

시나리오 재구성

당신은 교통량이 많은 고속도로에서 발생한 자동차 충돌 사고 현장으로 출동했다. 두 대의 차량이 정면충돌하였다. 차량 탑승자 중 한 명은 어린이용 보조 의자에 부적절하게 고정된 어린이이다. 사고 당시 날씨와 관련된 요인은 없었다.

현장에 도착했을 때 경찰이 사고 주변 지역의 교통을 통제하고 있었다. 당신의 동료와 다른 도착한 구급대원이 환자를 평가하는 동안 당신은 어린이에게 다가간다. 약 2세의 정도의 남자아이가 비스듬히 기울어진 어린이용 보조 의자에 앉아 있었다. 어린이가 앉아 있는 앞좌석 머리 받침대 뒤쪽에 피가 묻어있는 것을 확인한다. 머리, 얼굴, 목 부위에 찰과상과 경미한 출혈이 있음에도 불구하고 어린이는 매우 침착해 보인다.

당신은 "엄마, 엄마"라고 약하게 반복해서 말하는 2세 남아의 일차 및 이차평가를 시행한다. 맥박수는 180회/분이고 노동맥이 위팔동맥보다 약하며 촉진으로 측정한 혈압은 50mmHg이다. 호흡수는 분당 18회이며 약간 불규칙하지만, 비정상적인 소리는 들리지 않는다. 계속 환자를 평가하면서 "엄마"라는 말을 하지 않고 멍하니 허공을 응시하는 것을 확인한다. 또한 동공이 약간 확장되어 있고 피부가 창백하고 땀이 나는 것을 알 수 있다. 자신을 소아의 유모라고 밝힌 한 여성이 당신에게 아이의 엄마가 오는 중이니 기다려 달라고 말한다.

- 이 환아의 처치 우선순위는 무엇인가?
- 이 어린이에게 가장 가능성이 높은 손상은 무엇인가?
- 이 환아에게 가장 적절한 의료기관은 어디인가?

References

1. National Center for Injury Prevention and Control, Centers for Disease Control and Prevention. 10 leading causes of death reports, 2005–2018. Updated September 22, 2021. Accessed March 4, 2022. https://www.cdc.gov/injury/wisqars/LeadingCauses.html

2. Centers for Disease Control and Prevention. Injuries among children and teens. Last reviewed September 22, 2021. Accessed February 23, 2022. https://www.cdc.gov/injury/features/child-injury/index.html

3. American College of Surgeons. National Trauma Data Bank 2013: Pediatric Report. American College of Surgeons; 2016. Accessed March 12, 2018. https://www.facs.org/~/media/files/quality%20programs/trauma/ntdb/ntdb%20pediatric%20annual%20report%202016.ashx

4. National Center for Injury Prevention and Control, Centers for Disease Control and Prevention. Updated November 20, 2020. Accessed March 4, 2022. https://wisqars.cdc.gov/nonfatal-leading

5. Peden M, Oyegbite K, Ozanne-Smith J, et al., eds. *World Report on Child Injury Prevention*. World Health Organization; 2008.

6. Bachman SL, Salzman GA, Burke RV, Arbogast H, Ruiz P, Upperman JS. Observed child restraint misuse in a large, urban community: results from three years of inspection events. *J Safety Res*. 2016 Feb;56:17-22.

7. Grisoni ER, Pillai SB, Volsko TA, et al. Pediatric airbag injuries: the Ohio experience. *J Pediatr Surg*. 2000;35(2):160-162.

8. Durbin DR, Kallan M, Elliott M, et al. Risk of injury to restrained children from passenger air bags. *Traffic Injury Prev*. 2003;4(1):58-63.

9. Durbin DR, Kallan M, Elliott M, et al. Risk of injury to restrained children from passenger air bags. *Annu Proc Assoc Adv Auto Med*. 2002;46:15-25.

10. Ferguson SA, Schneider LW. An overview of frontal air bag performance with changes in frontal crash-test requirements: findings of the Blue Ribbon Panel for the evaluation of advanced technology air bags. *Traffic Inj Prev*. 2008;9(5):421-431.

11. Arbogast KB, Kallan MJ. The exposure of children to deploying side air bags: an initial field assessment. *Ann Proc Assoc Adv Automot Med*. 2007;51:245-259.

12. EMSC-Partnership for Children, National Association of Emergency Medical Technicians. Guidelines for Providing Family-Centered Care. Published July 2000. Accessed March 22, 2022. https://www.nh.gov/safety/divisions/fstems/ems/documents/emscguidelines.pdf

13. Gausche M, Lewis RJ, Stratton SJ, et al. Effect of out-of-hospital pediatric endotracheal intubation on survival and neurological outcome: a controlled clinical trial. *JAMA*. 2000;283(6):783-790.

14. Davis DP, Hoyt DB, Ochs M, et al. The effect of paramedic rapid sequence intubation on outcome in patients with severe traumatic brain injury. *J Trauma Injury Infec Crit Care*. 2003;54(3):444-453.

15. Davis DP, Dunford JV, Poste JC, et al. The impact of hypoxia and hyperventilation on outcome after paramedic rapid sequence intubation of severely head-injured patients. *J Trauma Injury Infect Crit Care*. 2004;57(1):1-8.

16. York J, Arrillaga A, Graham R, Miller R. Fluid resuscitation of patients with multiple injuries and severe closed-head injury: experience with an aggressive fluid resuscitation strategy. *J Trauma Injury Infect Crit Care*. 2000;48(3):376-380.

17. Manley G, Knudson MM, Morabito D, et al. Hypotension, hypoxia, and head injury: frequency, duration, and consequences. *Arch Surg*. 2001;136(10):1118-1123.

18. Chesnut RM, Marshall LF, Klauber MR, et al. The role of secondary brain injury in determining outcome from severe head injury. *J Trauma*. 1993;34(2):216-222.

19. Luten R. Error and time delay in pediatric trauma resuscitation: addressing the problem with color-coded resuscitation aids. *Surg Clin North Am*. 2002;82(2):303-314.

20. Fernández A, Ares MI, Garcia S, Martinez-Indart L, Mintegi S, Benito J. The validity of the pediatric assessment triangle as the first step in the triage process in a pediatric emergency department. *Pediatr Emerg Care*. 2017 Apr;33(4):234-238.

21. Gausche-Hill M, Eckstein M, Horeczko T, et al. Paramedics accurately apply the pediatric assessment triangle to drive management. *Prehosp Emerg Care*. 2014;18(4):520-530.

22. American College of Surgeons Committee on Trauma. Pediatric trauma. In: ACS Committee on Trauma. *Advanced Trauma Life Support for Doctors, Student Course Manual*. 8th ed. ACS; 2008:225-245.

23. Sokol KK, Black GE, Azarow KS, Long W, Martin MJ, Eckert MJ. Prehospital interventions in severely injured pediatric patients: rethinking the ABCs. *J Trauma Acute Care Surg*. 2015;79(6):983-989.

24. Kragh JF Jr, Cooper A, Aden JK, et al. Survey of trauma registry data on tourniquet use in pediatric war casualties. *Pediatr Emerg Care*. 2012 Dec;28(12):1361-1365.

25. Chou R, Totten AM, Pappas M, et al., eds. *Glasgow Coma Scale for Field Triage of Trauma: A Systematic Review* [Report No.: 16(17)-EHC041-EF]. Agency for Healthcare Research and Quality; 2017.

26. Van de Voorde P, Sabbe M, Rizopoulos D, et al.; PENTA study group. Assessing the level of consciousness in children: a plea for the Glasgow Coma Motor subscore. *Resuscitation*. 2008;76(2):175-179.

27. Newgard C, Lin A, Olson L, et al. Evaluation of emergency department pediatric readiness and outcomes among US trauma centers. *JAMA Pediatr*. 2021;175(9):947-956. doi: 10.1001/jamapediatrics.2021.1319

28. National Vital Statistics System, Centers for Disease Control and Prevention. Deaths: final data for 1997. *Morb Mortal Wkly Rep*. 1999;47(19):1.

29. Ehrlich PF, Seidman PS, Atallah D, et al. Endotracheal intubation in rural pediatric trauma patients. *J Pediatr Surg*. 2004;39:1376-1380.

30. Winchell RJ, Hoyt DB. Endotracheal intubation in the field improves survival in patients with severe head injury. *Arch Surg*. 1997;132(6):592-597.

31. Davis DP, Ochs M, Hoyt DB, et al. Paramedic-administered neuromuscular blockade improves prehospital intubation success in severely head-injured patients. *J Trauma Injury Infect Crit Care*. 2003;55(4):713-719.

32. Pearson S. Comparison of intubation attempts and completion times before and after the initiation of a rapid sequence intubation protocol in an air medical transport program. *Air Med J*. 2003;22(6):28-33.

33. Hansen ML, Lin A, Eriksson C, et al. A comparison of pediatric airway management techniques during out-of-hospital cardiac arrest using the CARES database. *Resuscitation*. 2017;120:51-56.

34. Gerritse BM, Draaisma JM, Schalkwijk A, van Grunsven PM, Scheffer GJ. Should EMS-paramedics perform paediatric tracheal intubation in the field? *Resuscitation*. 2008;79(2):225-229.

35. Weihing VK, Crowe EH, Wang HE, Ugalde IT. Prehospital airway management in the pediatric patient: a systematic review. *Acad Emerg Med*. 2021. doi: 10.1111/acem.14410

36. Davis BD, Fowler R, Kupas DF, Roppolo LP. Role of rapid sequence induction for intubation in the prehospital setting: helpful or harmful? *Curr Opin Crit Care*. 2002;8(6):571-577.

37. Heins M. The "battered child" revisited. *JAMA*. 1984;251(24):3295-3300. doi: 10.1001/jama.251.24.3295

38. Davis DP, Valentine C, Ochs M, et al. The Combitube as a salvage airway device for paramedic rapid sequence intubation. *Ann Emerg Med*. 2003;42(5):697-704.

39. Fukuda T, Sekiguchi H, Taira T, et al. Type of advanced airway and survival after pediatric out-of-hospital cardiac arrest. *Resuscitation*. 2020;150:145-153.

40. Hernandez MC, Antiel RM, Balakrishnan K, Zielinski MD, Klinkner DB. Definitive airway management after prehospital supraglottic rescue airway in pediatric trauma. *J Pediatr Surg*. 2018;53(2):352-356.

41. Inaba K, Karamanos E, Skiada D, et al. Cadaveric comparison of the optimal site for needle decompression of tension pneumothorax by prehospital care providers. *J Trauma*. 2015;79(6):1044-1048.

42. Leatherman ML, Held JM, Fluke LM, et al. Relative device stability of anterior versus axillary needle decompression for tension pneumothorax during casualty movement: preliminary analysis of a human cadaver model. *J Trauma*. 2017;83(1):S136-S141.

43. McCarthy A, Curtis K, Holland AJ. Paediatric trauma systems and their impact on the health outcomes of severely injured children: an integrative review. *Injury*. 2016;47(3):574-585.

44. Lerner EB, Drendel AL, Cushman JT, et al. Ability of the physiologic criteria of the field triage guidelines to identify children who need the resources of a trauma center. *Prehosp Emerg Care*. 2017;21(2):180-184.

45. Larson JT, Dietrich AM, Abdessalam SF, Werman HA. Effective use of the air ambulance for pediatric trauma. *J Trauma Injury Infect Crit Care*. 2004;56(1):89-93.

46. Eckstein M, Jantos T, Kelly N, Cardillo A. Helicopter transport of pediatric trauma patients in an urban emergency medical services system: a critical analysis. *J Trauma Injury Infect Crit Care*. 2002;53(2):340-344.

47. Englum BR, Rialon KL, Kim J, et al. Current use and outcomes of helicopter transport in pediatric trauma: a review of 18,291 transports. *J Pediatr Surg*. 2017;52(1):140-144.

48. Polites SF, Zielinski MD, Fahy AS, et al. Mortality following helicopter versus ground transport of injured children. *Injury*. 2017;48(5):1000-1005.

49. Brown JB, Leeper CM, Sperry JL, et al. Helicopters and injured kids: improved survival with scene air medical transport in the pediatric trauma population. *J Trauma Acute Care Surg*. 2016;80(5):702-710.

50. National Center for Injury Prevention and Control, Centers for Disease Control and Prevention. Injuries among Children and Teens. https://www.cdc.gov/traumaticbraininjury/data/index.html#:~:text=Children%20(birth%20to%2017%20years,related%20deaths1%20in%202019

51. Goh MS, Looi D, Goh J, et al. The impact of traumatic brain injury on neurocognitive outcomes in children: a systematic review and meta-analysis. *J Neurol Neurosurg Psychiatry*. 2021. doi: 10.1136/jnnp-2020-325066

52. Halstead ME, Walter KD, Council on Sports Medicine and Fitness. Clinical report—sport-related concussion in children and adolescents. *Pediatrics*. 2010;126:597-615.

53. McCrory P, Meeuwisse W, Aubry M, et al. Consensus statement on concussion in sport: the 4th International Conference on Concussion in Sport held in Zurich, November 2012. *J Sci Med Sport*. 2013;16(3):178-189.

54. Centers for Disease Control and Prevention (CDC). Sports-related recurrent brain injuries—United States. *Morb Mortal Wkly Rep*. 1997;46(10):224-227.

55. Halstead ME, Walter KD, Moffatt K; Council on Sports Medicine and Fitness. Sport-related concussion in children and adolescents. *Pediatrics*. 2018;142(6):e20183074. doi: 10.1542/peds.2018-3074

56. Carmona Suazo JA, Maas AI, van den Brink WA, et al. CO_2 reactivity and brain oxygen pressure monitoring in severe head injury. *Crit Care Med*. 2000;28(9):3268-3274.

57. Adelson PD, Bratton SL, Carney NA, et al. Guidelines for the acute medical management of severe traumatic brain injury in infants, children, and adolescents. Chapter 4. Resuscitation of blood pressure and oxygenation and prehospital brain-specific therapies for the severe pediatric traumatic brain injury patient. *Pediatr Crit Care Med*. 2003;4(suppl 3):S12-S18.

58. De Lorenzo RA. A review of spinal immobilization techniques. *J Emerg Med*. 1996;14(5):603-613.

59. Valadie LL. Child safety seats and the emergency responder. *Emerg Med Serv*. 2004;33(7):68-69.

60. U.S. Department of Transportation, National Highway Traffic Safety Administration. Working group best-practice recommendations for the safe transportation of children

in emergency ground ambulances. DOT HS 811 677. September 2012. Accessed March 22, 2022. https://www.nhtsa.gov/staticfiles/nti/pdf/811677.pdf

61. Williams FN, Herndon DN, Hawkins HK, et al. The leading causes of death after burn injury in a single pediatric burn center. *Crit Care*. 2009;13(6):183.

62. Hollén L, Coy K, Day A, Young A. Resuscitation using less fluid has no negative impact on hydration status in children with moderate sized scalds: a prospective single-centre UK study. *Burns*. 2017;43(7):1499-1505.

63. Müller Dittrich MH, Brunow de Carvalho W, Lopes Lavado E. Evaluation of the "early" use of albumin in children with extensive burns: a randomized controlled trial. *Pediatr Crit Care Med*. 2016;17(6):e280-e286.

64. Loos MHJ, Almekinders CAM, Heymans MW, de Vries A, Bakx R. Incidence and characteristics of non-accidental burns in children: a systematic review. *Burns*. 2020;46(6):1243-1253. doi: 10.1016/j.burns.2020.01.008

65. Peck MD, Priolo-Kapel D. Child abuse by burning: a review of the literature and an algorithm for medical investigations. *J Trauma*. 2002;53(5):1013-1022.

66. Hettiaratchy S, Dziewulski P. ABC of burns: pathophysiology and types of burns. *BMJ*. 2004;328(7453):1427-1429.

67. Hight DW, Bakalar HR, Lloyd JR. Inflicted burns in children: recognition and treatment. *JAMA*. 1979;242:517.

68. American Academy of Pediatrics Committee on Injury and Poison Prevention. Selecting and using the most appropriate car safety seats for growing children: guidelines for counseling parents. *Pediatrics*. 2002;109(3):550.

69. Nance ML, Lutz N, Arbogast KB, et al. Optimal restraint reduces the risk of abdominal injury in children involved in motor vehicle crashes. *Ann Surg*. 2004;239(1):127-131.

70. Bauer M, Hines L, Pawlowski E, et al. Using Crash Outcome Data Evaluation System (CODES) to examine injury in front vs. rear-seated infants and children involved in a motor vehicle crash in New York State. *Inj Epidemiol*. 2021;8(1):32. doi: 10.1186/s40621-021-00328-8

71. Pierce MC, Kaczor K, Aldridge S, et al. Bruising characteristics discriminating physical child abuse from accidental trauma. *Pediatrics*. 2010;125:67-74.

Suggested Reading

EMSC Partnership for Children, National Association of EMS Physicians. Model pediatric protocols: 2003 revision [no authors listed]. *Prehosp Emerg Care*. 2004;8(4):343.

© Ralf Hiemisch/Getty Images

노인 외상

Lead Editors
Danielle Hashmi, DO
Angel Ramon Lopez, MD
Robert D. Barraco, MD, MPH, FACS, FCCP

학습 목표   이 장의 학습을 완료하면 다음과 같은 내용을 수행할 수 있다.

- 노인 인구의 외상 역학에 관해 설명할 수 있다.
- 노화의 해부학적 및 생리학적 영향을 노인 외상 원인과 병태생리학적인 요인으로 설명할 수 있다.
- 노인 환자의 기존 의학적 문제와 외상성 손상의 상호 작용과 이러한 상호 작용이 외상의 병태생리학 및 징후에 어떻게 차이를 일으키는지 설명할 수 있다.
- 노인 외상의 병태생리학 및 증상에 대한 특정 약물의 생리학적 효과에 관해 설명할 수 있다.
- 노인 인구에서 사용하는 평가 방법과 고려 사상을 젊은 인구에서 사용되는 것과 비교하여 설명할 수 있다.
- 가능한 한 가장 편안하게 노인 환자를 안전하고 효과적으로 척추 고정을 시행하기 위한 척추 고정 방법을 수정하여 시연할 수 있다.
- 노인 외상 환자의 처치와 젊은 외상 환자의 처치를 비교하여 설명할 수 있다.
- 현장과 노인 환자 평가 시 학대와 방임의 증상과 징후가 있는지 평가할 수 있다.

시나리오

당신은 78세 여성이 계단에서 넘어졌다는 신고를 받고 현장으로 출동했다. 그녀의 딸은 불과 15분 전에 전화 통화를 했으며 어머니를 모시고 쇼핑하러 어머니의 집에 가고 있었다고 말한다. 집에 도착했을 때 쓰러져 있는 어머니를 발견하고 즉시 119에 도움을 요청했다.

당신이 현장에 도착했을 때 계단 아래에 누워 있는 환자를 발견했다. 환자를 처음 보았을 때 환자가 노령의 여성임을 알 수 있었다. 척추를 중립 자세로 고정하는 동안 환자가 당신의 명령에 반응하지 않는다는 것을 확인했다. 이마의 눈에 띄는 열상이 있고 왼쪽 손목에 명백한 변형이 있으며 외부출혈은 없다. 환자는 당뇨병이 있음을 나타내는 의료정보용 팔찌를 착용하고 있다.

- 낙상으로 인해 의식상태가 변화되었는가? 아니면 선행 사건이 있었는가?
- 환자의 나이, 병력, 복용 중인 약물이 손상과 어떻게 상호작용하여 병태생리와 증상이 젊은 환자와 다르게 나타나는가?
- 노인 외상 환자를 외상센터로 이송하기 위한 추가 기준이 있는가?

개요

노인 인구는 미국에서 가장 빠르게 증가하는 연령층이다. 2019년 현재 미국 인구의 16%인 5,400만 명 이상이 65세 이상이며 2060년에는 이 숫자가 9,470만 명에 달할 것으로 예상되며 80세 이상 인구는 같은 기간 3배 증가할 것으로 예상된다. 마찬가지로 전 세계 60세 이상 인구는 2015년 9억 명(세계 인구의 12%)이 조금 넘었고 2050년까지 20억 명(세계 인구의 22%) 이상으로 증가할 것으로 예상된다.

노인의 손상은 병원 전 또는 병원 내 처치에서 고유한 문제를 일으킨다. 환자의 나이가 처치 결과에 미치는 영향을 조사한 초기 데이터 중 일부는 1990년에 발표된 후향적 연구인 미국 외상 외과학회(ACSCT)의 중증 외상 처치 결과에 관한 연구에서 나온 것이다. 65세 이상 환자의 결과 데이터를 젊은 환자의 결과 데이터와 비교했다. 사망률은 45~55세 사이에 증가했으며 75세에는 두 배로 증가했다. 이러한 나이의 사망 위험은 손상의 중증도와 관계없이 발생했다. 노인 외상 환자는 젊은 환자에 비해 사망률이 높다는 연구 결과가 계속 발표되고 있다. 사망률과 이환율이 증가하지만, 역사적으로 노인 환자는 유사한 손상을 입은 젊은 환자에 비해 외상센터에서 처치를 받을 가능성이 낮다.

노인 인구가 계속 증가함에 따라 외상성 손상을 입는 노인 환자 수가 증가하고 있다. 외상은 55~64세 사망의 세 번째 주요 원인이며 65세 이상에서는 일곱 번째 주요 사망 원인이다. 이 연령대의 외상 관련 사망은 전체 외상 사망의 35%를 차지한다. 2050년에는 전체 외상 환자의 약 40%가 노인 환자가 될 것으로 예상된다. 특정 기전과 손상 유형은 노인 인구에게 고유하다. 자동차 사고가 외상 사망의 전체 주요 원인이지만, 75세 이상의 환자에게서는 낙상이 주요 사망 기전이다.

이 장에서는 노인 외상 환자의 고유한 요구 사항과 증가한 위험 수준을 강조하는 것을 목표로 한다. 특히 노화 과정과 공존하는 의학적 문제가 외상과 외상 처치 대한 노인 환자의 반응에 미치는 영향을 이해해야 한다. 이 장에서 설명하는 특별한 고려사항은 65세 이상이거나 신체적으로 나이가 더 들어 보이거나, 일반적으로 노인 인구와 관련된 의학적 문제를 가진 중년 외상 환자의 평가와 처치에 포함되어야 한다. 외상성 손상을 조기에 인지하고 신속하게 처치하는 것이 노인 외상 환자 처치에서 가장 중요하다.

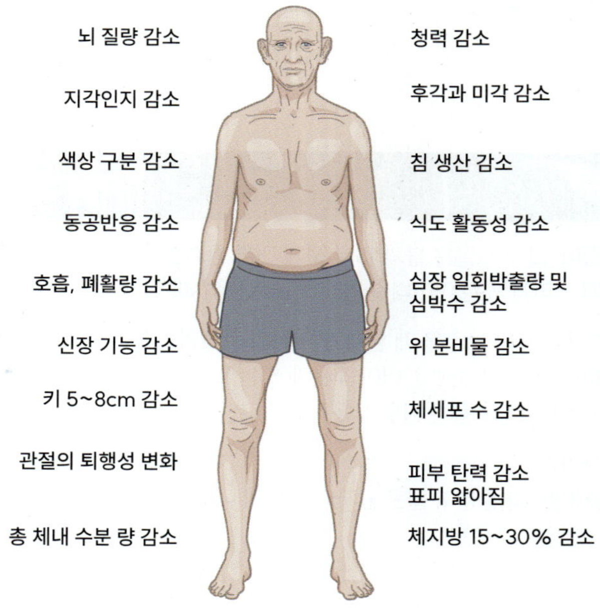

노화의 해부학 및 생리학

노화 과정은 신체 구조, 신체 구성 및 장기 기능의 변화를 일으켜 병원 전 처치 중에 고유한 문제를 일으킬 수 있다. 노화 과정은 사망률과 이환율에 영향을 미친다.

노화 또는 노쇠는 초기 성인기에 시작되는 자연스러운 생물학적 과정이다. 이 시기에는 장기 시스템이 성숙해지면서 생리학적 성장의 전환점에 도달한다. 신체는 항상성(인체 내부 환경이 상대적으로 일정하게 유지되는 상태)을 유지하는 능력을 점차 상실하고 사망에 이를 때까지 수년에 걸쳐 생존력이 감소한다.

노화 과정은 세포 수준에서 발생하며 해부학적 구조와 생리학적 기능 모두에 반영된다. 노년기는 일반적으로 허약함, 느린 인지 과정, 심리적 기능 장애, 정력 감소, 만성 및 퇴행성 질환의 출현, 감각의 예민함 감소 등의 특징이 있다. 기능적 능력이 저하되고 피부 주름, 모발 색상 및 양의 변화, 골관절염, 반응 시간 및 반사 신경 둔화 등 노년기의 잘 알려진 외부 증상과 징후가 나타난다(**그림 15-1**). 그러나 노화가 진행된다고 해서 삶의 질이 반드시 저하되는 것은 아니라는 점에 유의하는 것이 중요하다.

만성 질환의 영향

심각한 의학적 문제 없이 고령에 도달하는 사람도 있지만, 노인은 일하고 정상적인 생활을 하는 데 제약이 되는 건강 상태를 가질 가능성이 훨씬 더 높다(**표 15-1**). 역사적으로 노인들은 미국의 다른 연령

그림 15-1 노화로 인한 변화
© National Association of Emergency Medical Technicians (NAEMT)

표 15-1 만성 질환을 앓고 있는 환자 비율

만성 질환의 수	55~64세	65세 이상
만성 질환 1가지 이상	69.5%	85.6%
만성 질환 2가지 이상	37.1%	56.0%
만성 질환 3가지 이상	14.4%	23.1%

참고: 만성 질환에는 관절염, 현재 천식, 암, 심혈관 질환, 만성폐쇄폐질환 및 당뇨병이 포함된다.

Data from Centers for Disease Control and Prevention. Percent of U.S. adults 55 and over with chronic conditions. Accessed May 23, 2022. https://www.cdc.gov/nchs/health _policy/adult_chronic_conditions.htm

대보다 응급실(ED)을 포함한 의료 지원을 더 높은 비율로 소비한다. 노인 환자는 젊은 환자보다 더 높은 빈도로 응급의료서비스를 이용한다.

나이가 들어감에 따라 추가적인 의학적 문제가 발생할 수 있으며 종종 누적된 부정적인 결과를 초래할 수 있다. 신체에 미치는 총 영향은 일반적으로 각 개별 영향을 합한 것보다 크다. 각 질환이 진행되어 신체의 중요한 기능의 질이 감소함에 따라 경미한 해부학적 또는 생리학적 손상을 견딜 수 있는 능력이 크게 감소한다(**Box 15-1**).

환자가 소아, 중년 또는 노인인지 아닌지와 관계없이 일반적으로 심각한 외상으로 인한 우선순위는 처치의 필요성 및 생명을 위협하는 상태는 같다. 그러나 이러한 기존의 신체적 조건으로 인해 노인 환

Box 15-1 예방 관리

예방적 관리는 특히 노년층의 건강을 최적으로 유지하는 핵심 요소이다. 안타깝게도 일부 노인은 재정적 여유가 부족하여 예방 치료를 받지 못하는 경우가 있다.

© National Association of Emergency Medical Technicians (NAEMT)

자는 종종 덜 심각한 손상으로 사망하고 젊은 환자보다 더 빨리 사망한다. 데이터에 따르면 기존의 질환은 노인 외상 환자의 사망률에 영향을 미치며 외상 환자에게 더 많은 질환이 있을수록 사망률이 높아진다(**표 15-2**). 몇몇 질환은 외상에 반응하는 생리학적 능력을 방해하기 때문에 사망률을 증가시킨다(**표 15-3**).

표 15-2 기존 질병(PED)의 수 및 외상 후 환자 결과

기존 질병의 수	생존	사망	사망률(%)
0	6,341	211	3.2
1	868	56	6.1
2	197	36	15.5
3개 이상	67	22	24.7

Data from Milzman DP, Boulanger BR, Rodriguez A, Soderstrom CA, Mitchell KA, Magnant CM. Pre-existing disease in trauma patients: a predictor of fate independent of age and injury severity score. *J Trauma.* 1992;32:236–244.

표 15-3 기존 질병(PED)의 유병률 및 외상 후 관련 사망률

기존 질병	환자 수	기존 질병(%)	합계(%)	사망률(%)
고혈압	597	47.9	7.7	10.2
폐 질환	286	23	3.7	8.4
심장 질환	223	17.9	2.9	18.4
당뇨병	198	15.9	2.5	12.1
비만	167	13.4	2.1	4.8
암	80	6.4	1	20
신경계 장애	45	3.6	0.6	13.3
신장병	40	3.2	0.5	37.5
간 질환	41	3.3	0.5	12.2

Data from Milzman DP, Boulanger BR, Rodriguez A, Soderstrom CA, Mitchell KA, Magnant CM. *Pre-existing disease in trauma patients: a predictor of fate independent of age and injury severity score. J Trauma.* 1992;32:236–244.

귀, 코, 목구멍(ENT)

충치, 잇몸 질환 및 치아 손상으로 인해 다양한 보철물이 필요하다. 보철, 틀니, 고정식 또는 탈부착이 가능한 의치 등도 특별한 문제를 일으킬 수 있다. 이러한 이물질은 쉽게 부서지고 흡인되어 기도를 막을 수 있다.

노인들은 구강 건조증을 경험할 가능성이 더 높다. 침샘의 꽈리세포 수가 약간 감소하여 최대 침 생산량이 최대 50%까지 감소할 수 있다. 이는 씹고 삼키는 데 다양한 영향을 미칠 수 있으며 혈량저하증의 증가나 부재를 정확하게 입증하지 못한다. 또한 특정 약물은 구강 건조와 관련이 있는 것으로 입증되었다.

얼굴 윤곽의 변화는 부분적으로 치아가 없으므로(무치악) 아래턱뼈의 흡수로 인해 발생한다. 이러한 흡수는 입안 내부를 수축시키는 특징적인 모양을 유발하며 백마스크 장비로 밀착시키거나 기관내삽관 중에 기도를 충분히 시각화하는 능력에 악영향을 미칠 수 있다.

코 인두 조직은 나이가 들면서 점점 더 약해진다. 이러한 변화가 외상 초기에 발생할 수 있는 위험 외에도 코인두기도기 삽입과 같은 처치를 주의 깊게 시행하지 않으면 다량의 출혈을 유발할 수 있다.

호흡계

노인의 환기 기능은 부분적으로 가슴벽의 탄력성 감소와 기도의 경직으로 인해 감소한다. 가슴벽과 폐의 순응도는 나이가 들수록 감소하며 이로 인해 호흡 노력이 증가할 수 있다. 이는 가슴 외상으로 인한 호흡부전의 위험 증가와 관련이 있다. 저산소증에 대한 심장 반응이 둔화하면 호흡부전을 구별하기가 더 어려워질 수 있다. 호흡계의 효율성이 떨어지면 노인은 호흡에 더 큰 노력을 기울이고 일상 활동을 수행하기 위해 더 큰 노력이 필요하다.

폐의 폐포 면적은 나이가 들면서 감소한다. 예를 들어 70세 노인은 폐포 면적이 16% 감소한다. 이미 감소한 폐포 면적은 산소 흡수량을 더욱 감소시킨다. 또한, 신체가 노화됨에 따라 헤모글로빈을 산소로 포화시키는 능력이 감소하여 기준 산소포화도가 낮아지고 사용할 수 있는 산소 보유량이 감소한다. 기계적 환기 장애와 가스 교환을 위한 표면 감소로 인해 노인 외상 환자는 외상과 관련된 생리학적 손실을 보상하려는 능력이 떨어진다.

노인의 기도와 폐의 변화는 항상 노화와 관련이 있는 것은 아니다. 평생 환경 독소에 만성적으로 누적 노출되면 직업적 위험이나 담배 연기로 인해 발생할 수 있다. 이는 만성폐쇄폐질환(COPD)으로 이어질 수 있다. 기침 및 구역반사가 손상되고, 기침 강도가 약해지거나 식도괄약근 긴장이 약해지면 흡인성 폐렴의 위험이 커진다. 섬모(기관지에서 이물질과 점액을 밀어내는 호흡기 세포의 털 같은 돌기)의 수가 감소하면 노인은 흡인된 미세먼지로 인한 문제에 더 취약해진다.

호흡기에 영향을 미치는 또 다른 요인은 척주 만곡의 물리적 변화이다. 주로 척주후만증이 증가하고 전후방 또는 동반되는 만곡 변화는 종종 인체 역학 장애와 추가적인 환기 기능 저하로 이어진다(**그림 15-2**).

가로막에 영향을 미치는 변화도 환기 문제를 일으킬 수 있다. 가슴벽이 경직되면 가로막의 움직임에 더 많이 의존하여 음압의 흡입 압력을 얻을 수 있다. 가로막에 대한 의존도가 높아지면 노인은 복부 내 압력 변화에 특히 민감해진다. 따라서 누운자세나 과식으로 인한 배부름은 환기 부족을 유발할 수 있다.

가슴벽 손상은 노인 환자의 이러한 근본적인 호흡기 변화를 더욱 악화시킬 수 있다. 실제로 갈비뼈 골절이 있는 노인 외상 환자는 젊은 환자보다 사망률과 폐렴과 같은 합병증 위험이 현저히 높다. 기저 폐 질환과 노화로 인한 생리학적 변화의 조합으로 인해 노인 환자는 외상 후 호흡기 손상에 취약할 수 있다.

심혈관계

2019년 미국에서 65세 이상 인구의 주요 사망 원인은 심장병이었다. 실제로 심장병은 다른 연령대에서는 주요 사망 원인이 아니었음에도

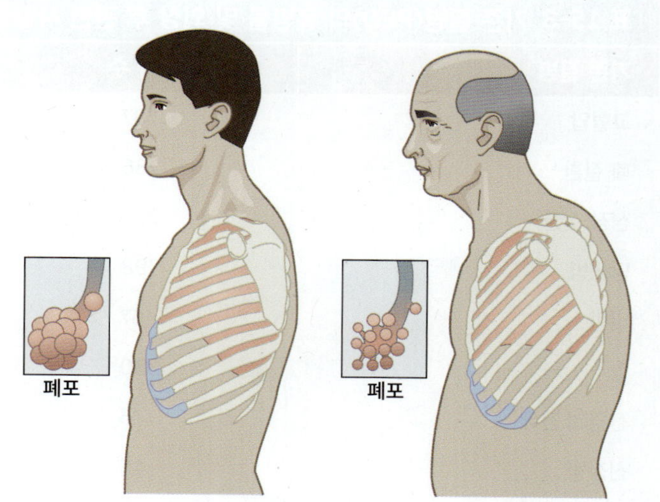

그림 15-2 척추 굽이는 앞뒤로 척추가 굽어져 호흡 곤란을 일으킬 수 있다. 폐포 표면적이 감소하면 폐에서 교환되는 산소의 양을 감소시킬 수 있다.

모든 연령대의 사망 원인을 합친 것보다 더 많은 사망을 차지할 정도로 이 연령대에서 많은 사망을 차지했다.

나이와 관련된 동맥 탄력의 감소는 말초 혈관 저항의 증가로 이어진다. 심근과 혈관은 적절하게 기능하기 위해 탄성, 수축성 및 확장(신축성) 특성에 의존한다. 심장벽의 순응도가 감소하여 심박출지수가 매년 약 1%씩 감소한다. 동시에 혈관 저항은 매년 1%씩 증가한다. 나이가 들어감에 따라 심혈관계는 체액을 체내로 이동시키는 효율성이 떨어진다.

죽상경화증은 혈관이 좁아지는 질환으로 동맥 내에 지방 침전물이 쌓이면서 동맥벽의 내층이 두꺼워지는 상태이다. 플라크라고 하는 이러한 침전물은 혈관의 구경을 감소시켜 저항을 증가시키고 혈액이 앞으로 이동하는 것을 더 어렵게 만든다. 관상동맥에서도 이와 같은 내강 협착이 발생한다. 미국 인구의 거의 50%가 65세까지 관상동맥 협착증을 앓고 있다.

이러한 협착의 결과 중 하나는 미국 성인에게 흔히 발생하는 고혈압이다. 동맥벽이 석회화되면 내분비 및 중추 신경계 자극에 대한 순응도와 반응 능력이 저하된다. 혈액 순환 감소하면 모든 중요한 장기에 악영향을 미칠 수 있으며 심장질환의 흔한 원인이다. 이는 노인 외상 환자의 기준 혈압이 젊은 환자보다 높을 수 있으므로 중요하다. 노인 외상 환자의 평가 및 처치에서 흔히 발생하는 함정은 "정상"으로 보이는 혈압을 쇼크의 징후로 인식하지 못하는 것이다.

나이가 들어감에 따라 심장 자체의 섬유 조직과 크기가 증가(심근 비대)한다. 심장의 전도계 세포의 위축은 심장 부정맥의 발생률을 증가시킨다. 저혈압에 반응하는 심장의 정상적인 반사는 나이가 들수록 감소하여 노인 환자가 저혈압을 보상하기 위해 심박수와 일회박출량을 증가시키는 능력을 감소시킨다. 박동조율기를 사용하는 환자와 베타차단제를 복용하는 환자는 외상에 의한 스트레스에 따른 산소 소비량 증가를 충족하기 위해 심박수와 심박출량을 조절하는 능력이 감소한다.

노인 외상 환자의 경우 혈액 순환이 감소하면 세포 저산소증이 발생한다. 세포 저산소증은 부정맥, 급성 심부전이 발생할 뿐만 아니라 심지어 급사를 초래할 수도 있다. 노인의 경우 카테콜아민에 반응하는 심장 수축 반응이 감소하기 때문에 출혈이나 다른 쇼크의 원인을 보상하는 신체의 능력이 현저히 저하된다. 또한 총 순환 혈액량이 감소하여 외상으로 인한 혈액 손실에 대한 생리학적 예비량이 줄어든다. 심장의 확장기 기능 장애로 인해 환자가 혈량저하 상태에서 감소하는 심박출량을 증가시키기 위해 심방 충만에 더 의존하게 된다.

심부전 증가와 함께 혈액 순환 및 순환 방어 반응이 감소하면 노인 외상 환자의 쇼크를 처치하는 데 심각한 문제가 발생한다. 심혈관계의 순응도가 떨어지기 때문에 수액 소생술시 주의 깊게 모니터링해야 한다. 저혈압과 쇼크를 처치할 때는 과도한 수액 소생술로 혈액량 과부하가 발생하지 않도록 주의를 한다.

신경계

나이가 들어감에 따라 뇌의 무게와 신경세포의 수는 감소한다. 뇌의 무게는 약 20세에 최고치(1.4kg)에 도달한다. 80세가 되면 뇌는 무게의 약 10%가 감소하며 뇌 위축이 진행된다. 또한 경막 연결정맥이 더 늘어나서 찢어지기 쉽다. 그 결과 경막외출혈의 빈도가 낮아지고 경막밑출혈의 빈도는 높아진다. 신체는 감소한 뇌의 크기를 뇌척수액을 증가시켜 보상한다. 뇌 주위의 추가 공간은 뇌를 타박상으로부터 보호할 수 있지만, 가속 또는 감속 손상에 대한 반응으로 더 많은 뇌의 움직임을 허용한다. 또한 머리 저장 공간이 증가하면 증상이 거의 없거나 전혀 없는 노인 환자의 경우 뇌 주위에 상당한 양의 혈액이 축적될 수 있다.

특정 신경을 따라 신경 자극이 전달되는 속도도 감소한다. 이러한 감소는 행동과 생각에 약간의 영향을 미친다. 반사 신경은 느리지만 상당한 정도는 아니다. 특히 파킨슨병과 같은 질병을 앓고 있는 환자의 경우 보상기능이 손상되어 낙상 발생률이 높아질 수 있다. 말초 신경계도 신경 자극의 둔화로 인해 영향을 받아 떨림과 불안정한 걸음걸이를 유발한다.

일반적인 정보 및 어휘 능력은 향상하거나 유지되지만, 정신 및 근육 활동(정신운동 능력)이 필요한 기술은 감소할 수 있다. 언어 이해력, 산술 능력, 생각의 유창성, 경험적 평가 및 일반적인 지식과 관련된 지적 기능은 학습 활동을 계속하는 사람의 경우 60세 이후에도 증가하는 경향이 있다. 치매 및 알츠하이머병과 같은 관련 질환이 있는 사람은 예외이다.

치매는 일상생활에 지장을 초래하는 인지 능력의 저하를 총칭하는 용어이다. 알츠하이머병은 가장 흔한 형태의 치매이다. 가장 일반적으로 기억력, 주의력, 의사소통 능력 및 판단력이 손상될 수 있지만, 증상은 다양할 수 있다. 치매는 미국에서 65세 이상 인구 10명 중 1명이 앓고 있다. 치매는 노인 사망의 다섯 번째 주요 원인이며 장애를 일으키는 주요 원인이다. 치매로 인한 인지 장애는 일반적으로 점진적으로 나타난다.

섬망은 치매와는 다르다. 섬망은 부주의, 인지 기능 장애 및 의학적 원인과 관련된 변동하는 경과를 특징으로 하는 갑작스럽고 급격한 정신 상태의 변화이다. 섬망은 일반적으로 근본적인 급성 과정이 교정되면 되돌릴 수 있다. 그러나 섬망은 사망률과 이환율 증가와 관련이 있다. 예일대학교의 한 연구에 따르면 중환자실 입원 시 섬망과 관련된 사망률이 1년간 증가한 것으로 나타났다. 최근 메타 분석에 따르면 섬망은 특히 중환자실 환자의 사망률 증가와 관련이 있을 수 있다는 지속적인 연구 결과가 발표되었다.

노인 환자는 정신 건강에도 상당한 부담을 안고 있다. 우울증은 노인에게 흔하다. 우울증, 치매, 기질성 뇌 질환을 고려할 수 있지만, 노인 외상 환자를 평가할 때는 외상성 뇌손상, 저산소증, 쇼크를 먼저 고려하는 것이 중요한다(8장 머리와 목 외상 참조).

감각 변화

시각 및 청각

전반적으로 남성이 청각 장애를 겪을 확률이 더 높지만, 시각 관련 장애는 남녀 모두 비슷한 발생률을 보인다(**Box 15-2**).

시력 저하는 모든 연령대에서 문제가 되지만, 특히 노인에게는 훨씬 더 문제가 될 수 있다. 시력이 나빠지면 처방전을 제대로 읽지 못하거나 운전 능력에 악영향을 미칠 수 있다. 또한, 노인은 시력, 색상 구별 능력 및 야간 시력도 점진적으로 감소한다. 눈의 수정체 세포는 원래의 분자 구조로 회복할 수 없다. 결국 수정체는 두께와 굴곡을 증가시키는 능력을 상실하게 된다. 그 결과 40세 이상에서는 거의 보편적으로 원시(노안)가 발생하여 독서를 위해 안경이 필요하다.

눈의 다양한 구조가 변화하기 때문에 노인은 어두운 환경에서 보는 데 더 어려움을 겪는다. 나이가 들면 눈의 수정체는 혼탁해져 빛을 투과할 수 없게 된다. 이러한 점진적인 과정을 통해 백내장이 발생하거나 수정체가 혼탁해져 눈에 들어오는 빛을 차단하고 왜곡시켜 시야를 흐리게 만든다. 80세 이상 인구의 절반 이상이 백내장의 영향을 받는다. 이러한 시력 저하는 특히 야간 운전 시 자동차 충돌 위험을 높인다.

점진적인 청력 저하(노년 난청)도 노화의 특징이다. 노년 난청은 일반적으로 내이로의 소리 전도 손실로 인해 발생하며 보청기를 사용하면 이러한 손실을 어느 정도 보완할 수 있다. 이러한 청력 손실은 많은 사람이 한꺼번에 말을 하거나 사이렌 소리와 같은 시끄러운 주변 소음이 있을 때와 같이 복잡한 소리를 구별하려고 할 때 가장 두드러지게 나타난다.

통증 인식

노화 과정과 당뇨병과 같은 질병의 존재로 인해 노인은 통증을 정상적으로 인지하지 못할 수 있으며 이로 인해 과도한 더위와 추위에 노출되어 손상 위험이 커질 수 있다. 많은 노인은 관절염과 같은 만성 통증을 유발하는 질환을 앓고 있다. 매일 통증을 느끼며 생활하면 통증에 대한 내성이 증가하여 환자가 손상 부위를 식별하지 못할 수 있다. 특히 평소 통증이 있는 환자를 평가할 때 병원 전 처치 제공자는 통증이 증가했거나 통증 부위가 확대된 부위를 찾아야 한다. 또한 외상 발생 이후 통증의 특징이나 악화 요인을 기록하는 것도 중요하다.

신장계통

노화에 따른 일반적인 변화로는 신장의 여과 수준 감소와 배설 능력 감소가 있다. 50세 이후에는 신장의 질량이 급격히 감소하고 60세 이후에는 신장단위의 손실로 인해 사구체여과율(GFR)이 감소한다. 일반적으로 신장에서 제거되는 약물을 투여할 때는 이러한 변화를 고려한다. 크레아틴 제거는 근육량이 감소함에 따라 감소하기 때문에 혈청 크레아티닌보다 신장 기능에 대한 더 신뢰할 수 있는 예측 인자가 된다. 또한, 나이와 관련된 죽상경화성 혈관 변화는 신장 혈류의 비율을 감소시켜 사구체여과율에 더 많은 영향을 미칠 수 있다. 만성 신부전은 일반적으로 노인에게 영향을 미치며 환자의 전반적인 건강 상태와 외상을 견딜 수 있는 능력을 저하한다. 예를 들어 신장 기능 장애는 만성 빈혈의 원인 중 하나이며 이는 환자의 생리적인 예비력을 떨어뜨릴 수 있다.

Box 15-2 노화에 따른 감각 변화의 영향

시각 및 청각 변화는 매우 미묘할 수 있으며 오랜 기간에 걸쳐 발생하여 환자가 변화가 발생했다는 사실을 인식하지 못할 수도 있다. 주치의의 예방 검진에는 미묘한 감각 변화를 평가하기 위한 선별 검사가 포함되어야 한다.

근골격

뼈는 나이가 들면서 무기질을 잃고 뼈의 소실(골다공증)은 성별에 따라 다르다. 젊은 성인기에는 여성이 남성보다 뼈 질량이 더 많다. 그러나 뼈 소실은 여성에서 더 빠르고 폐경 후 가속화된다. 골다공증 발병률이 높으므로 노인 여성은 특히 넓적다리뼈(엉덩관절) 목 골절이 발생할 확률이 더 높다. 골다공증의 원인으로는 에스트로젠 감소, 활동량 저하, 칼슘의 부적절한 섭취 및 비효율적인 사용 등이 있다.

골다공증은 엉덩관절 골절이나 척추뼈의 자연 압박 골절의 주된 원인이다. 발병률은 남성의 경우 연간 1%, 85세 이상 여성의 경우 2%에 달한다.

노인은 추간판의 높이가 감소하기 때문에 젊은 성인기보다 키가 작아지는 경우가 있다. 추간판이 평평해지면서 20~70세 사이에 키가 약 5cm 감소한다. 가슴 부위의 척주후만증(척주굽이)도 키 감소의 원인이 될 수 있으며 종종 골다공증으로 인해 발생한다(**그림 15-3**). 뼈에 구멍이 많아지고 약해지면 앞쪽에 침식이 발생하고 척추의 압박 골절이 발생할 수 있다. 등뼈의 굴곡이 심해지면서 머리와 어깨가 앞으로 밀린 것처럼 보인다. 특히 폐기종과 같은 만성폐쇄폐질환이 있는 경우 호흡 보조 근육의 발달이 증가하기 때문에 척주후만증이 더 두드러질 수 있다.

관절염은 노인에게도 흔한 질환이다. 골관절염(OA)은 관절에 영향을 미치는 퇴행성 질환으로 관절 운동에 매끄러운 표면을 제공하는 연골이 손상되는 질환이다. 류마티스관절염(RA)은 자가 면역 반응

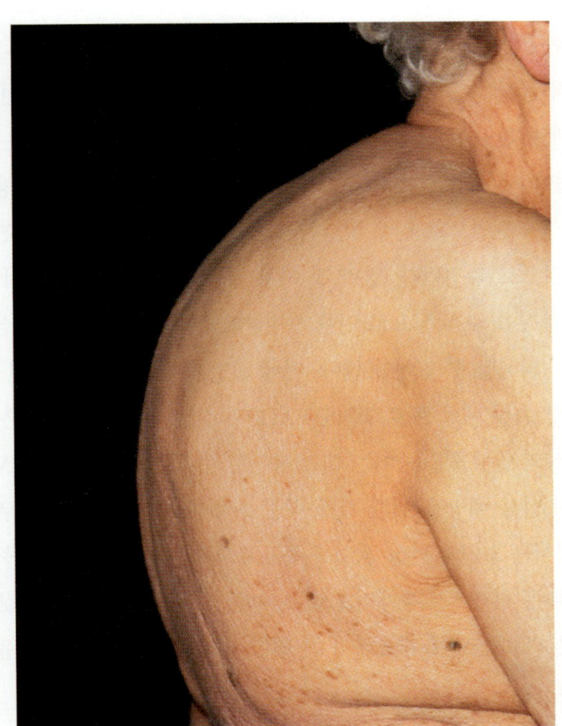

그림 15-3 일반적인 골다공증으로 인한 척주후만증
© Dr. P. Marazzi/Science Source

으로 인한 염증성 질환으로 관절의 부종과 변형이 생길 수 있다. 이러한 만성 질환은 신체의 움직임 감소와 만성 통증을 유발할 수 있다. 노인 환자를 평가하고 이송할 때는 이러한 제한 사항을 고려해야 한다.

성장 호르몬의 절대 수치는 노화와 함께 단백 동화 호르몬에 대한 반응성 감소와 함께 감소한다. 이러한 현상이 복합적으로 작용하여 노인의 근육량이 감소한다. 근육 소실은 근육 세포의 절대적인 수와 세포 크기의 감소로 현미경으로 확인할 수 있다.

근골격계와 관련된 결손(예: 지형 변화에 따라 엉덩관절이나 무릎을 적절하게 구부리지 못하는 경우)은 노인이 낙상하기 쉬운 원인이 된다. 근육 피로는 움직임, 특히 낙상에 영향을 미치는 많은 문제를 일으킬 수 있다. 신체의 정상적인 자세 변화는 흔하며 척추의 노화에 따른 변화는 신체의 굴곡이 더 심해진다. 어느 정도의 골다공증은 노화와 함께 보편적으로 발생한다. 이러한 점진적인 뼈 흡수로 인해 뼈는 덜 유연해지고 부서지기 쉬우며 쉽게 부러진다. 운동량 감소로 인한 근력 감소와 함께 뼈의 강도가 감소하면 경미하거나 중간 정도의 힘으로도 다발성 골절이 발생할 수 있다. 노인에게 가장 흔한 골절 부위는 넓적다리뼈 몸쪽 부위(엉덩관절), 위팔뼈 및 손목이다. 손상의 기전으로 낙상 발생률이 증가하면 등쪽굽힘 자세로 손을 앞쪽으로 뻗으면서 넘어지게 되어 노뼈 먼쪽 부위의 콜레스골절(Colles' fracture)이 자주 발생한다.

척추 전체는 나이가 들면서 주로 골다공증, 골증식증 및 지지 인대의 석회화 등의 영향으로 인해 변화한다. 이러한 석회화로 인해 척추 운동 범위가 감소하고 척추관이 좁아진다. 척추관이 좁아지고 골증식 질환으로 인해 이러한 환자는 척추뼈가 실제로 부러지지 않더라도 경미한 외상으로 척수나 신경이 압박될 가능성이 커진다. 골다공증과 자세 변화의 복합적인 힘으로 인해 낙상이 증가한다. 노인 환자는 가벼운 낙상에도 골절이 발생할 수 있다.

피부

피부와 결합 조직의 현저한 변화는 노화와 관련이 있으며 외상에 대한 반응과 직접적인 상처 치유에 어려움을 초래한다. 세포 수가 감소하고 조직 강도가 떨어지며 피부의 기능 상태가 손상된다. 피부가 노화되면서 땀샘과 기름샘이 소실된다. 땀샘의 소실은 신체의 체온 조절 능력을 감소시킨다. 기름을 생성하는 기름샘의 소실은 피부를 건조해지고 쉽게 벗겨지게 만든다. 피부와 모발에 색을 내는 멜라닌의 생산이 감소하여 노화로 인해 창백해진다. 피부가 기저 결합조직의

변화로 인해 얇아지고 반투명하게 보이고 비교적 경미한 외상으로 인한 손상을 입기 쉽다. 피부가 얇아지고 건조해지면 경미한 손상과 미생물에 대한 저항력이 감소하여 상처로 인한 감염률이 증가한다. 탄력을 잃으면 피부가 늘어나 주름이 생기고, 특히 얼굴 근육과 같이 많이 사용하는 부위에 주름이 생기기 쉽다. 또한, 피부가 얇아지면 상대적으로 낮은 에너지 전달에 반응하여 심각한 조직 손실과 손상이 발생할 가능성이 커진다.

지방 조직의 손실은 노인이 저체온증에 걸리기 쉬운 원인이 될 수 있다. 나이가 들면서 피부 두께가 감소하는 것도 체온조절 기능 장애의 원인이 된다. 그러나 저체온증은 노년층에서 잠재적인 패혈증, 갑상샘저하증 또는 페노티아진 과다 복용의 가능성도 시사한다. 또한 지방조직의 손실로 인해 머리, 어깨, 척추, 엉덩이, 엉덩관절, 발꿈치와 같은 뼈 돌출부에 대한 패딩이 줄어들게 된다. 추가 패딩 없이 장시간 고정하면 해당 부위에 조직 괴사와 궤양이 발생할 수 있으며 처치 및 이송 중 통증과 불편함이 증가할 수 있다. 따라서 노인 환자를 고정하고 이송하는 동안 피부 손상으로 인한 합병증을 고려해야 한다.

영양과 면역체계

노화로 인해 체질량의 감소하고 신진 대사율이 감소하면 칼로리 요구량이 감소한다. 그러나 비효율적인 이용으로 인해 단백질 요구량은 오히려 증가할 수 있다. 이러한 상반된 변화는 종종 노인 외상 환자의 영양실조를 초래할 수 있다. 은퇴한 개인의 재정 상태도 양질의 영양 섭취에 영향을 미칠 수 있다.

면역체계의 기능 능력은 노화에 따라 감소한다. 전반적으로 면역 반응과 관련된 장기(가슴샘, 간, 비장)의 크기가 모두 줄어든다. 감염에 대한 세포 매개 및 체액 반응도 감소한다. 노인 인구에서 흔히 나타나는 기존의 영양 문제와 함께 감염에 대한 취약성이 증가한다. 패혈증은 노인 환자에서 심각한 외상이나 경미한 외상 후 사망에 이르는 흔한 원인이다.

평가

2019년 65세 이상 인구의 26%가 전년도에 응급실을 방문했다. 기본적인 병원 전 평가는 모든 환자에게 동일하지만, 노인 환자를 평가할 때 염두에 두어야 할 특정 고려 사상이 있다. 이 부분에서는 이러한 고려 사항과 함께 이 환자 집단에서 가장 흔한 손상 기전 및 유형에 관해 설명한다.

외상의 물리학

낙상

낙상은 노인의 외상성 사망 및 장애의 주요 원인이다. 매년 65세 이상 인구 4명 중 1명이 낙상으로 인해 3백만 명이 응급실을 방문하고 약 3만 명의 사망자가 발생했다. 남성과 여성의 낙상 빈도는 비슷하지만, 여성은 골다공증이 더 심하므로 심각한 손상을 입을 가능성이 두 배 이상 높다. 낙상은 서 있는 자세에서 발생하더라도 심각한 손상과 생명을 위협하는 외상을 초래할 수 있으며 낙상 환자의 최대 20~30%는 중등도에서 중증의 손상을 입는다.

낙상의 원인은 여러 가지가 있다. 낙상은 자세와 걸음걸이의 변화로 인해 발생한다. 백내장, 녹내장 및 야간 시력 상실로 인한 시력 저하는 안전한 보행에 필요한 시각적 신호의 상실에 이바지한다. 중추 및 말초 신경계 질환과 심혈관 질환으로 인한 혈관 불안정성은 낙상을 더욱 가속한다. 노인이 넘어지기 쉬운 기존 질환과 함께 사용되는 벤조다이아제핀, 베타 차단제, 항우울제와 같은 약물은 낙상을 더욱 악화시킨다. 후자는 코로나19 팬데믹 이후 특히 중요할 수 있다. 특히 사회적 고립으로 인해 노인 인구에서 불안과 우울증 발병률이 증가한 것으로 나타났다. 마지막으로 환경적 요인도 낙상의 중요한 원인이다. 미끄러운 바닥, 깔개, 계단, 잘 맞지 않는 신발, 어두운 조명과 같은 환경의 물리적 장벽은 추가적인 위험을 초래한다.

긴뼈 골절이 손상의 대부분을 차지하며 엉덩관절 골절로 인한 사망률과 이환율이 가장 높다. 엉덩관절 골절로 인한 사망률은 손상 후 1년이 지나면 20%이며 2년이 지나면 33%로 증가한다. 사망률은 여러 가지 원인으로 인해 발생하지만, 이동성 감소의 영향과 관련이 있는 것으로 추정된다. 병원 전 처치 제공자는 노인 환자의 낙상 발생률, 부상률 및 낙상으로 인한 합병증의 심각성을 고려할 때 심각한 손상을 의심할 수 있어야 한다. 미국 질병통제예방센터의 노인 사고, 사망 및 손상 예방 프로그램(STEADI)과 같은 예방 프로그램은 이러한 손상의 발생률을 줄이는 데 효과적일 수 있다. 또한, 많은 EMS 기관에서 낙상 예방을 위해 가정 방문을 한다. 그러나 다기관 무작위 시험에서는 노인의 낙상 감소를 목표로 하는 다인자 예방 전략의 시행에 따른 결과에서 통계적으로 유의미한 차이를 발견하지 못했으며 낙상은 의료 산업에 계속해서 큰 영향을 미치고 있다는 점에 유의해야 한다.

차량으로 인한 외상

2000년부터 2018년까지 노인 운전자의 수는 60% 이상 증가했다. 2010년부터 2019년까지 이 연령대의 차량 사고 사망자는 31% 증가했지만, 보행자 사고 사망자는 55% 이상 증가했다. 안타깝게도 나이가 증가함에 따라 차량 충돌로 인한 손상 위험도 증가한다. 주행 거리당 사망자 수를 비교하면 70~74세 운전자부터 사망률이 증가하며 85세 이상 운전자에서 가장 높은 사망률을 보인다(**Box 15-3**).

이러한 높은 사망률은 특정 생리학적 변화에 기인한다. 특히, 시각 및 청각 장애와 함께 기억력과 판단력의 미묘한 변화로 인해 반응 시간이 지연될 수 있다. 음주로 인한 사고는 다른 환자 집단에 비해 덜 자주 보고되지만, 모든 환자가 음주 관련 검사를 받는 것은 아니므로 이러한 통계는 추론에 불과하다.

노인 보행자는 전체 보행자 손상의 10%, 전체 보행자 사망자의 20%를 차지한다. 보행 속도가 느리기 때문에 교통 신호가 허용하는 시간이 너무 짧아 노인이 횡단보도를 안전하게 건너기 어려울 수 있다.

노인 학대

전 세계 데이터에 따르면 60세 이상 인구의 15%가 학대를 경험한 것으로 나타났다. 여기에는 방임, 신체적, 성적, 정서적 학대, 재정적 착취가 포함된다. 노인 인구의 취약성에도 불구하고 학대 사례는 제대로 보고되지 않고 있다. 자세한 내용은 노인 학대 부문을 참조한다.

화상

60세 이상의 환자는 모든 화상 중증도 범주에서 사망률이 더 높다. 또한 노인 환자는 화상 및 입원과 관련된 합병증에 직면할 가능성이 더 높다. 가장 흔한 합병증으로는 폐렴, 요로감염, 호흡 부전 등이 있다. 젊은 환자 집단과 달리 60세 이상 환자는 화상 크기가 훨씬 작으면서도 사망률이 더 높다. 60~69세 환자의 경우 체표면적이 40%인 경우 사망률이 50%를 초과하고 70~79세 환자의 경우 체표면적이 30%인 경우 사망률이 50%를 초과하며 80세 이상 환자의 경우 체표면적이 20%인 경우 사망률이 50%를 초과한다. 손상 기전은 화염에 의한 손상, 화상 또는 뜨거운 물체와의 접촉이 가장 흔하다.

외상성 뇌손상

노인 환자의 외상성 뇌손상(TBI) 발생률이 높아 미국에서 매년 12,000명이 사망하는 것으로 추정된다. 노인 환자의 경우 젊은 환자에 비해 외상성 뇌손상으로 인한 사망률이 높으며 손상 후 장기 요양 시설과 재활 치료의 필요성도 증가한다.

뇌 위축으로 인해 최소한의 임상 소견으로도 상당히 큰 경막밑출혈이 존재할 수 있다. 머리 외상과 저혈량 쇼크가 함께 발생하면 사망률이 더 높아진다. 노인 환자의 경우 기존 질환이나 그 치료가 정신 상태 변화의 원인이 될 수 있다. 혼동이 급성인지 만성인지 확실하지 않으면 손상을 입은 환자가 외상성 뇌손상을 입었다고 가정하는 것이 가장 안전하며 가능하면 먼저 외상센터로 이송하여 검사받아야 한다. 항응고제를 사용하면 경미해 보이는 손상이 심각한 외상성 뇌손상을 초래할 수 있으므로 항응고제 사용은 고려해야 할 또 다른 중요한 요소이다. 환자가 항응고제나 혈액 희석제를 복용하고 있는지를 확인하는 것은 초기 평가에서 필수적인 요소이다.

일차평가

대량 출혈

외상 환자에서 생명을 위협하는 출혈의 교정 가능한 원인을 찾는다. 심한 출혈이 있는 외부 부위는 조기에 인지해야 한다.

기도

현장 안전을 확보하고 대량 출혈을 조절한 후 노인 환자의 기도평가를 진행한다. 부분 기도 폐쇄 또는 완전 기도 폐쇄로 인한 저산소증으로 인해 이차적으로 의식 변화가 나타날 수 있다. 입안에 틀니, 부러지거나 빠진 치아와 같은 이물질이 있는지 확인한다.

호흡

다른 성인과 마찬가지로 분당 10회 미만 또는 30회 이상의 속도로 호흡하는 노인 환자는 분당 호흡량이 적절하지 않으며 적절한 기도 유지가 필요하다. 대부분의 성인에서 분당 12~20회의 호흡수는 정상이

Box 15-3 노인 운전자

미국 의사협회(AMA)는 미국고속도로교통안전국(NHTSA)의 지원을 받아 노인 운전자 평가 및 상담을 위한 의사의 가이드라는 프로그램을 제작했다. 이 프로그램은 NHTSA 웹사이트에서 온라인으로 이용할 수 있다.(https://one.nhtsa.gov/people/injury/olddrive/olderdriversbook/pages/contents.html.

며 적절한 분당 호흡량이 있음을 의미한다. 그러나 노인 환자의 경우 일회 호흡량이 감소하면 분당 12~20회의 호흡 속도에서도 분당 호흡량이 부적절할 수 있다. 이러한 변화로 인해 환기 속도가 정상이더라도 호흡음을 즉시 평가해야 한다. 일회 호흡량 감소로 인해 호흡음이 더 잘 들리지 않을 수 있다는 점에 유의한다.

노인 환자의 폐활량은 종종 50%까지 감소한다. 척추의 전후방 변화로 인해 안정 시 환기-관류 불일치가 발생한다. 저산소증은 젊은 환자보다 쇼크의 결과로 발생할 가능성이 훨씬 더 높다. 또한 노인 환자는 가슴우리의 운동이 감소한다. 모세혈관에서 산소 및 이산화탄소 교환의 감소가 현저하고 저산소혈증은 점진적으로 진행되는 경향이 있다.

순환

일부 결과는 개별 환자의 사건 발생 전 또는 기저 상태를 알아야만 적절하게 해석할 수 있다. 일반적으로 정상으로 간주하는 활력징후 및 기타 소견의 예상 범위는 모든 개인에게 "정상"이 아니며 편차는 노인 환자에게서 훨씬 더 흔하다. 일반적인 범위는 대부분 성인 개인차를 포함할 만큼 아주 넓지만, 모든 연령대의 개인은 이러한 기준을 벗어날 수 있으므로 노인 환자에서 이러한 편차를 예상해야 한다.

약물 복용이 이러한 변화에 영향을 미칠 수 있다. 예를 들어, 일반 성인의 경우 수축기 혈압 120mmHg는 정상으로 간주하며 일반적으로 큰 문제가 되지 않는다. 그러나 일반적으로 수축기 혈압 150mmHg 이상인 만성 고혈압 환자의 경우 수축기 혈압이 120mmHg이면 보상 저하가 발생할 정도의 잠복성 출혈(또는 저혈압을 유발하는 다른 손상 기전)을 시사하는 것을 우려할 수 있다. 마찬가지로, 베타 차단제와 같은 약물의 효과와 순환하는 카테콜아민(에피네프린)에 대한 심장의 약화한 반응으로 인해 노인 환자의 경우 심박수는 외상을 나타내는 지표로 적절하지 않다. 정량적 정보나 객관적 징후를 다른 결과와 분리하여 사용해서는 안 된다. 이러한 변화가 발생했거나 심각한 병리학적 소견이라는 사실을 인지하지 못하면 환자에게 좋지 않은 결과를 초래할 수 있다.

모세혈관 재충전 시간 지연은 말초 동맥 질환으로 인한 순환 효율 저하로 인해 노인 환자에게서 흔하며 급성 순환계 변화를 나타내는 신뢰할 수 있는 지표가 아닐 수 있다. 팔다리의 운동, 감각 및 순환 기능이 약간 감소하면 노인 환자에서 정상적인 결과를 나타낼 수 있다.

장애

노인 환자의 신경학적 손상에 대한 의심 수준을 높이기 위해 모든 소견을 종합적으로 검토해야 한다. 노인 환자의 경우 시간과 장소에 대한 지남력은 신중하고 완전한 질문을 통해 평가해야 한다. 노인은 사고력, 기억력, 지남력(과거와 현재에 대한)에 큰 차이가 있을 수 있다. 현장에 있던 사람이 노인 환자(모든 환자)의 기본 정신 상태를 설명할 수 없다면 현재 나타나는 모든 결함은 급성 신경학적 손상, 저산소증, 저혈압 또는 이 세 가지가 복합적으로 작용한 것으로 간주해야 한다. 노인 환자의 기본 정신 상태를 파악하는 것은 매우 중요하며 환자나 가족 또는 간병인으로부터 정보를 얻는 것이 포함될 수 있다.

노출/환경

노인은 주변 환경 변화에 더 취약하다. 노인은 열 생산과 열 발산 모두에 장애가 있어 환경 온도 변화에 대응하는 능력이 떨어진다. 체온 조절은 전해질 불균형, 기초대사율 저하, 떨림 능력 감소, 동맥경화증, 약물이나 알코올의 영향과 관련이 있을 수 있다. 고체온은 뇌혈관 질환(뇌졸중) 또는 이뇨제, 항히스타민제, 항파킨슨제 등의 약물로 인해 발생할 수 있다. 저체온은 대사량 감소, 체지방 감소, 말초혈관 수축 감소, 영양의 부족과 관련이 있다.

이차평가

노인 외상 환자의 이차평가는 젊은 환자와 같은 방법으로 생명을 위협하는 치명적인 문제를 해결한 후에만 실시한다. 그러나 여러 가지 요인으로 인해 노인 환자의 평가가 복잡해질 수 있으므로 병원 전 처치 제공자는 노인 환자를 평가할 때 노화의 변화가 증상에 어떤 영향을 미칠 수 있는지 고려해야 한다.

의사소통 문제

노화 과정의 정상적인 생물학적 영양부터 병원 전 처치 제공자와 환자 관계에 대한 세대 간 기대에 이르기까지 노인 환자와 의사소통할 때 많은 요인이 작용한다. 노인과 가장 잘 소통하는 방법을 이해하면 병원 전 처치 제공자가 신속하고 효과적인 처치를 제공하는 데 도움이 된다.

- 노인 환자의 청각 또는 시각 장애로 인해 추가적인 인내가 필요할 수 있으며 공감과 연민은 필수이다. 의사소통이 어렵거나 불가능하다고 해서 환자의 지능을 과소평가해서는 안 된다.

- 중요한 다른 사람이나 간병인이 참여해야 할 수도 있다. 환자가 자세한 병력을 확실하게 제공할 수 없는 경우 중요한 정보를 수집하기 위해 환자의 허락을 받아 간병인이나 배우자 또는 동료에게 정보를 얻을 수도 있다. 모든 논의에 환자를 적절히 참여시키는 것을 잊지 않는다. 일부 노인 환자는 친척이나 지원자의 도움 없이는 정보 제공을 꺼릴 수 있다. 어떤 환자는 다른 사람이 동석하는 것을 원하지 않는 예도 있으므로 이를 인정하고 존중해야 한다.
- 노인 환자의 감소한 청각, 시각, 이해력 및 거동 장애가 병력 청취 및 신체검사에 영향을 미칠 수 있다는 것을 기억한다. 소음, 산만함, 장애가 환자와의 상호 작용에 영향을 미칠 수 있다. 예를 들어, 환자가 평가 및 검사 중에 구두 지시를 듣지 못하거나 이해하지 못하여 급성 결손을 제대로 평가하기 어려울 수 있다.
- 환자를 존중하고 경멸하는 것으로 해석될 수 있는 언어는 피한다. 환자가 부를 때 낮추거나 무시하는 것으로 간주할 수 있는 단어는 피해야 한다. 특히 응급상황에서는 환자가 질문을 처리하는 데 몇 초가 더 걸릴 수 있다. 환자에게 한 번에 한 가지씩 질문하고 환자가 응답할 때까지 기다렸다가 다른 질문을 한다.

생리적 변화

병원 전 처치 제공자는 노인 연령대에서 자주 발생하는 생리적 차이에 대비해야 한다.

- 생리적 변화는 젊은 환자에 비해 병태생리학적 변화로 이어진다. 발열, 통증, 압통과 같은 심각한 질병의 전형적인 소견은 노인 환자에게서 나타나는 데 더 오래 걸릴 수 있으며 나타나는 징후와 증상을 혼동할 수 있다. 또한 많은 약물이 질병과 손상에 대한 생리적 반응에 부정적인 영향을 미칠 수 있다. 병원 전 처치 제공자는 종종 환자의 병력에만 의존해야 한다.
- 이해력 저하 또는 신경학적 장애는 많은 노인 환자에게 심각한 문제이다. 이러한 장애는 섬망에서 알츠하이머병과 같은 치매에 이르기까지 다양하다. 이러한 환자들은 자신을 표현하는 데 어려움을 겪을 뿐만 아니라 정보를 받거나 평가에 도움을 주는 데도 어려움을 겪을 수 있다. 노인 환자는 안절부절못하고 때로는 전투적일 수도 있다.
- 노인 환자는 영양이나 수분이 부족할 수 있다. 환자의 악력이나 피부 탄력, 체온을 느낄 수 있도록 환자와 악수하고 영양 상태를 확인한다. 환자가 건강해 보이는지, 말라 보이는지 아니면 쇠약해 보이는가? 노인 환자는 갈증 반응이 감소하고 체지방량(15~30%)과 총체액량이 감소한다.

- 노인 환자는 골격근 무게가 감소하고 뼈가 납작해지고 약해지며 관절의 퇴행성 변화와 골다공증 등이 있다. 노인은 비교적 경미한 손상에도 골절이 발생할 확률이 높으며 척추, 엉덩관절, 갈비뼈에 골절이 발생할 위험이 크다. 환자가 쉽게 일어나거나 앉는 것은 근력에 대한 단서를 제공하므로 관찰해야 한다.
- 노인 환자는 심근 세포가 퇴화하고 박동조율 세포 수가 적다. 노인은 심장과 주요 동맥의 탄력이 떨어지기 때문에 부정맥이 발생하기 쉽다. 베타 차단제, 칼슘 채널 차단제, 이뇨제를 광범위하게 사용하면 이 문제가 더 복잡해진다. 노인 환자는 손상 후 종종 폐 손상이 없음에도 불구하고 저산소증과 함께 낮은 심박출량을 나타낸다. 심박수, 일회박출량 및 심장 예비력이 모두 감소하여 외상 후 이환율과 사망률이 증가한다. 조기 보상 기전 실패로 나타내는 징후를 평가할 때 기준 활력징후를 고려한다. 건강한 사람에게는 "정상"인 혈압이 동반 질환이 있는 노인 환자에게는 심각한 저혈압을 나타낼 수 있다.

환경적 요인

환자가 발견되는 환경은 환자의 건강에 대해 많은 것을 알려줄 수 있다. 만성 기저 질환은 환경적 요인과 열악한 생활 조건으로 인해 악화할 수 있다. 노인 환자의 경우 날씨 관련 질환도 고려한다. 더위 및 추위 관련 사망률은 나이가 들수록 증가하며 특히 75세 이상의 경우 더욱 증가한다.

- 상황에 맞지 않는 환자의 행동 문제나 징후가 있는지 확인하고 외모와 몸단장을 살펴본다. 환자의 옷차림과 몸단장이 환자가 발견된 장소와 상황에 적절한가? 환자가 일상생활을 정상적으로 수행할 수 있어 보이는가? 생활공간이 깨끗하고 잘 관리되고 있는가? 노인 학대 뜨는 방임의 가능성은 없는가? 생활환경의 적절한 온도 조절과 의복이 기후와 일치하는가?

상세한 병력

약물

환자의 약물에 대한 지식은 병원 전 처치를 결정하는 데 중요한 정보를 제공할 수 있다. 노인 외상 환자의 기존 질환은 중요한 발견이다. 다음 약물은 노인들이 자주 사용하고 노인 외상 환자의 신체검사 및 처치에 영향을 미칠 가능성이 있으므로 특히 관심을 가져야 한다.

- 베타 차단제(예: 프로프라놀롤, 메토프롤롤)는 환자의 절대적 또는 상대적 서맥을 유발할 수 있다. 이러한 상황에서는 쇼크 발생의 증후로 빈맥이 나타나지 않을 수 있다. 약물이 신체의 정상적인 교감

신경 보상 기전을 억제하면 환자의 순환계 악화의 실제 수준을 가릴 수 있다. 이러한 환자는 겉으로 보기에는 경고 없이 신속하게 보상을 상실할 수 있다.

- 칼슘 채널 차단제(예: 딜티아젬)는 말초혈관 수축을 방지하고 저혈량 쇼크를 가속할 수 있다.
- 비스테로이드소염제(예: 이부프로펜)는 혈소판 기능 장애를 유발하고 출혈을 증가시킬 수 있다.
- 항응고제 및 항혈소판제(예: 클로피도그렐, 아스피린, 와파린, 다비가트란, 아픽사반, 리바록사반)는 출혈을 증가시킬 수 있다. 외상으로 인한 출혈은 환자가 항응고제를 복용 중일 때 더 활발하게 일어나고 조절하기 어렵다. 더 중요한 것은 내부출혈이 빠르게 진행되어 쇼크와 사망으로 이어질 수 있다는 것이다.
- 혈당강하제(예: 인슐린, 메트포르민, 로지글리타존)는 손상을 초래한 사건과 인과 관계가 있을 수 있으며 사용 사실을 인지하지 못할 때 의식 상태에 영향을 미치며 혈당 안정화를 어렵게 만들 수 있다.
- 약초 및 보충제를 포함한 일반 의약품이 자주 사용된다. 처방전 없이 구매할 수 있는 약물을 "의약품"으로 간주하지 않는 환자들은 이러한 약품이 의약품 목록에 포함되지 않는 경우가 많다. 따라서 환자에게 사용 여부에 대해 구체적으로 질문해야 한다. 이러한 약물은 규제가 없으며 예측할 수 없는 효과와 약물 상호작용이 있을 수 있다. 이러한 약물의 합병증으로는 출혈(마늘) 및 심근경색(에페드린/마황)이 있다.

노인 외상 환자의 약물 목록을 평가하는 것은 환자가 인지 능력이 저하되어 있거나 약물 이름이 어려운 광범위한 약물 목록을 가지고 있는 경우 어려울 수 있다. 일부 지역 사회에서 EMS 기관에서 생명 파일 프로젝트(www.folife.org)와 같은 프로그램을 홍보하고 있다. 이 프로그램은 환자의 병력에 관한 세부 사항을 냉장고 문과 같이 직관적인 위치에 부착하는 것을 권장한다. 환자는 병력 기록 양식을 작성하여 냉장고에 부착해 놓으면 병원 전 처치 제공자가 쉽게 알 수 있다(**그림 15-4**). 또한 병원과 의사가 사용하는 전자 의무기록 시스템에는 환자에게 처방한 최근 약물 목록이 포함되어 있어 이러한 정보를 확인할 수 있다.

노인 환자는 또한 5가지 이상의 약물을 복용하는 것을 설명하는 데 사용하는 용어인 다중 약물 요법을 시행하는 비율이 더 높다. 실제로 노인 환자의 거의 절반 이상이 다중 약물 요법의 정의에 해당한다. 이는 이러한 환자에서 이환율의 중요한 원인이 될 수 있다. 노인 6

명 중 1명은 약물로 인한 부작용을 경험한다. 미국 노인병학회는 다중 약물 요법과 그 합병증을 해결하기 위해 노력의 하나로 노인 환자의 잠재적으로 부적절한 약물 사용을 식별하기 위한 비어스 기준(Beers criteria)을 마련했다. 병원 전 처치 제공자는 특히 외상성 손상을 입은 노인 환자의 경우 가정 내 약물 복용이 미치는 영향을 인식해야 한다.

노인 환자는 여러 가지 약물을 복용하는 경우가 많으므로 환자의 외상, 의식 상태 변화 또는 활력징후 변화의 가능한 원인으로 약물 상호작용 또는 의도하지 않은 과다 복용 가능성을 고려한다.

외상성 손상을 유발할 수 있는 건강 상태

여러 가지 의학적 상태가 외상성 사건, 특히 의식 수준이나 신경학적 결손을 초래할 수 있는 사건에 취약하게 만들 수 있다. 일반적인 예로는 뇌전증, 부적절한 약물 투여로 인한 저혈당증, 항고혈압제로 인한 실신, 급성 관상동맥증후군으로 인한 부정맥 그리고 뇌졸중 등이 있다. 만성 질환의 발병률은 나이가 들수록 증가하기 때문에 노인 환자는 젊은 환자에 비해 의학적 문제로 인한 외상을 입을 가능성이 더 높다. 병원 전 처치 제공자는 다음과 같이 외상성 손상을 촉발한 의학적 문제를 가리킬 수 있는 일차 및 이차평가에서 다음과 같은 단서에 주목한다.

- 목격자는 피해자가 충돌 전에 의식을 잃은 것처럼 보였다고 함
- 당뇨병과 같은 기저 질환을 나타내는 환자 인식 팔찌 착용
- 심전도 모니터링 중에 나타나는 불규칙한 심박동 또는 부정맥이 발견되는 경우

병원 전 처치 제공자는 이 정보를 제공하는 유일한 출처일 수 있으며 이 모든 정보는 환자를 이송할 수 있는 적절한 의료기관을 선택하는 데 도움이 된다.

처치

대량 출혈

심한 외부출혈은 대량 출혈로 이어질 수 있다. 생명을 위협하는 이 출혈을 인지하고 신속하게 지혈해야 한다. 출혈 부위에 직접 압박을 가하거나 팔다리에 심한 출혈이 있는 경우 직접 압박으로 지혈되지 않으면 출혈을 조절하기 위해 지혈대를 사용한다.

FILE OF LIFE

KEEP INFORMATION UP TO DATE !!
Review At Least Every Six Months !
MEDICAL DATA REVIEWED AS OF___MO.____YR.
Name:　　　　　　　　　　　　　　　　Sex:
　　　　　　　　　　　　　　　　　　　M F
Address:
Doctor:　　　　　　　　　Phone #:
Doctor:　　　　　　　　　Phone #:
EMERGENCY CONTACTS
Name:　　　　　　　　　　Phone #:
Address:
Name:　　　　　　　　　　Phone #:
Address:

KEEP INFORMATION UP TO DATE !!
Review At Least Every Six Months !
MEDICAL DATA REVIEWED AS OF　　MO.　　YR.
Name:　　　　　　　　　　　　　　　Sex:
　　　　　　　　　　　　　　　　　　M F
Address:
Doctor:　　　　　　　Phone #:
Preferred Hospital:

EMERGENCY CONTACTS
Name:　　　　　　　　Phone #:
Address:
Name:　　　　　　　　Phone #:
Address:

MEDICAL DATA
Use pencil for ease in making changes.

Special Conditions/Remarks:

Medication	Dosage	Frequency

Pharmacy:　　　　　　Phone:
Date of Birth:
Blood Type:　　　　Religion:
Health Care Proxy on file at:
Living Will on file at:
® FILE OF LIFE　　SEE BACK OF CARD FOR ADDITIONAL INFORMATION

Use Pencil for ease in making changes
Recent Surgery:　　　　　　　　**Date:**

Do you have an EMS-NO CPR Directive or a DNR form ?
YES ☐　　NO ☐　　**Where is it located ?**

MEDICAL CONDITIONS
Check all that exist

☐ No known medical conditions　　☐ Hemodialysis
☐ Abnormal EKG　　☐ Hemolytic Anemia
☐ Adrenal Insufficiency　　☐ Hepatitis-Type [　　]
☐ Angina　　☐ Hypertension
☐ Asthma　　☐ Hypoglycemia
☐ Bleeding Disorder　　☐ Laryngectomy
☐ Cancer　　☐ Leukemia
☐ Cardiac Dysrhythmia　　☐ Lymphomas
☐ Cataracts　　☐ Memory Impaired
☐ Clotting Disorder　　☐ Myasthenia Gravis
☐ Coronary Bypass Graft　　☐ Pacemaker
☐ Dementia ☐ Alzheimer's ☐　　☐ Renal Failure
☐ Diabetes/Insulin Dependent　　☐ Seizure Disorder
☐ Eye Surgery　　☐ Sickle Cell Anemia
☐ Glaucoma　　☐ Stroke
☐ Hearing Impaired　　☐ Tuberculosis
☐ Heart Valve Prosthesis　　☐ Vision Impaired
☐ Other:

ALLERGIES

☐ Aspirin　　☐ Insect Stings　　☐ Penicillin
☐ Barbiturate　　☐ Latex　　☐ Sulfa
☐ Codeine　　☐ Lidocaine　　☐ Tetracycline
☐ Demerol　　☐ Morphine　　☐ X-Rays Dyes
☐ Horse Serum　　☐ Novocaine　　☐ No Known Allergies
☐ Environmental:
☐ Other:

MEDICAL INSURANCE
Med Ins Co:
Policy #:
Other Med Ins Co:
Policy #:
Medicaid #:　　　　　Medicare #:

그림 15-4 생명의 파일
Courtesy of the File of Life Foundation.

기도

노인에게 흔히 볼 수 있는 틀니는 기도 유지에 영향을 미칠 수 있다. 일반적으로 틀니는 마스크로 입 주위를 더 잘 밀착할 수 있도록 그대로 두어야 한다. 그러나 부분 틀니는 응급상황에서 쉽게 빠지기 때문에 기도를 완전 또는 부분 폐쇄를 유발할 수 있으므로 제거한다.

코 인두 점막 조직이 약하고 항응고제를 사용할 가능성이 있는 노인 외상 환자는 코인두기도기 삽입으로 인한 출혈 위험이 크다. 이러한 출혈은 환자의 기도를 더욱 손상해 흡인을 유발할 수 있다.

관절염은 턱관절과 목뼈에 영향을 미칠 수 있다. 이러한 부위의 유연성이 감소하면 기관내삽관과 같은 기도 유지 술기가 더 어려워질 수 있다.

기도 관리의 목적은 조직으로 적절한 산소 공급을 위해 기도를 개방하고 유지하는 것이다. 노인 외상 환자는 생리적 예비력이 크게 제한되어 있으므로 백마스크 장비 또는 전문 기도 유지술을 통한 조기 기계적 환기를 고려한다.

호흡

모든 외상 환자에게는 가능한 한 빨리 보충 산소를 공급하고 산소포화도는 일반적으로 94% 이상으로 유지한다. 노인 인구는 만성폐쇄폐질환(COPD) 유병률이 높다. 환자가 중증 만성폐쇄폐질환을 앓고 있더라도 일상적인 도시 또는 교외에서 이송 중에 고농도 산소를 투여해도 환자의 호흡 충동에 해로울 가능성은 낮다. 그러나 병원 전 처치 제공자는 환자가 기면(졸린 상태) 또는 호흡수가 감소하는 것을 확인하면 전문 기도 유지를 고려하여 백마스크 장치를 사용하여 보조 환기를 시행할 수 있다.

노인은 가슴벽의 경직이 증가한다. 또한 가슴벽 근력이 감소하고 연골의 유연성이 감소하여 가슴우리의 유연성이 떨어진다. 이러한 변화와 기타 변화가 폐 용적 감소의 원인이 된다. 노인 환자는 젊은 외상 환자보다 더 일찍 백마스크 장치를 이용한 보조 환기가 필요할 수 있다. 증가한 가슴벽 저항을 극복하기 위해 백마스크에 가해지는 기계적 힘을 약간 증가시켜야 할 수도 있다. 그러나 기준치의 낮은 폐 용적에서 알 수 있듯이 백마스크 보조 환기를 제공할 때 위 팽창이나 기흉과 같은 의도하지 않은 결과를 초래할 수 있으므로 많은 일회 호흡량은 필요하지 않은 경우가 있다.

호기말이산화탄소분압을 측정하는 호기말이산화탄소분압측정기는 호흡 상태를 평가하는 데 사용되는 또 다른 도구일 수 있다. 중증 외상을 입은 노인 외상 환자의 호기말이산화탄소분압 측정값은 이용할 수 있는 다른 임상 정보와 연관되어야 한다.

순환

노인은 심혈관계 예비력이 부족할 수 있다. 순환 혈액량 감소, 만성 빈혈 가능성 그리고 기존에 앓고 있던 심근 및 관상동맥 질환으로 인해 환자는 소량의 출혈에도 거의 견디지 못한다.

노인 환자는 피부가 이완되거나 항응고제 및 항혈소판제 복용으로 인해 더 큰 혈종이 발생하기 쉽고 잠재적으로 더 심각한 내부출혈이 발생할 수 있다. 개방 상처를 직접 압박하여 출혈을 조기에 조절하고 골절을 안정화하거나 고정하고 외상센터로 신속하게 이송하는 것이 필수적이다. 수액 소생술은 손상 기전과 전반적인 쇼크 양상에 따라 심각한 출혈이 의심되는 지수에 따라 실시한다. 동시에 노인 환자는 과도한 체액 부하를 견디는 능력이 떨어지므로 정맥 내 수액 과다 투여는 피해야 한다. 소변 배출량은 특히 병원 전 환경에서 노인 환자의 관류량을 측정하는 데 좋지 않은 척도이다.

척추 움직임 제한

다발성 무딘 손상을 입은 외상 환자의 경우 목뼈, 등뼈 및 허리뼈를 보호하는 것이 표준 처치이다. 의식상태가 정상이고 주의를 산만하게 하는 손상이 없는 환자의 경우 척추 손상의 구체적인 증거가 없는 한 척추 움직임 제한은 필요하지 않다. 노인 환자의 경우 이러한 기준은 외상 상황뿐만 아니라 기도 개방을 유지하려는 시도가 우선시되는 급성 내과적 문제에도 적용되어야 한다. 목뼈의 퇴행관절염이 있는 노인 환자는 척추에 손상을 입지 않았더라도 기도 유지를 위해 목의 위치를 조작하는 과정에서 척추 손상을 입을 수 있다. EMS 제공자는 척추 움직임 제한의 잠재적 중요성을 이해하는 것 외에도 프로토콜을 숙지하고 있어야 한다.

병원 전 처치 제공자는 중증의 척주후만증이 있는 노인 환자에게 목뼈보호대를 착용시킬 때 실수로 기도나 목동맥을 압박하지 않도록 주의해야 한다. 표준 목뼈보호대가 환자에게 적합하지 않으면 수건을 말아서 머리 고정대처럼 사용하는 것이 더 바람직할 수 있다.

척주후만증이 있는 노인 환자를 고정할 때 환자의 머리 아래와 어깨 사이에 패딩을 대어 주어야 할 수 있다(**그림 15-5**). 진공 매트리스(전신형 진공부목)는 환자의 해부학적 구조에 맞게 형성하여 압력 지점을 줄이고 적절한 지지와 더 편안함을 제공할 수 있다. 허약한 노인 환자는 피부가 얇고 지방 조직이 부족하므로 누워 있을 때 압력

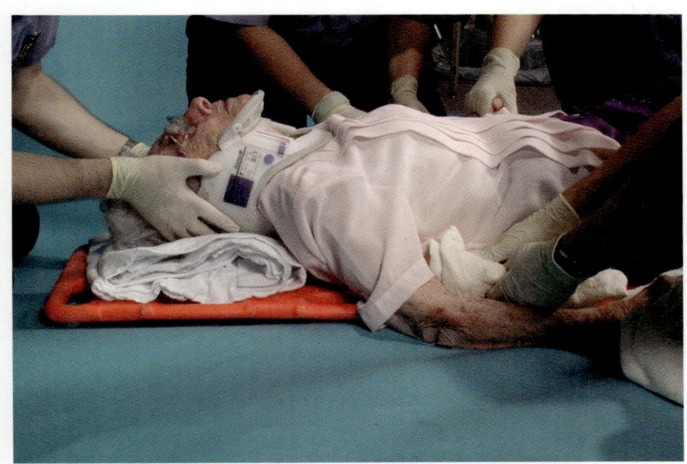

그림 15-5 긴척추고정판을 사용할 때 척추후만증 환자의 척추 움직임 제한을 달성하기 위한 올바른 방법이다. 가슴 척주후만 변형으로 인해 형성된 공간을 채우기 위해 머리 뒤에 패딩을 넣는다.
© Jones & Bartlett Learning

궤양(욕창)이 발생할 가능성이 더 높다. 환자가 긴척추고정판에 고정되어 있는 경우 추가 패딩이 필요할 수 있다. 환자가 긴척추고정판에 누워 있을 때 항상 압박 지점이 있는지 확인하고 적절하게 패딩을 적용하는 것이 좋다. 다리 고정 끈을 적용할 때 노인 환자는 엉덩관절과 무릎의 운동 범위가 감소하여 다리를 완전히 펴지 못할 수 있다. 이 경우 이송 중에 편안함과 안전을 위해 다리 아래에 패딩을 대어주어야 할 수 있다.

체온 조절

노인 환자는 처치 및 이송 중에 저체온증과 고체온증이 있는지 자세히 모니터링해야 한다. 철저한 평가를 위해 환자를 노출하는 것이 적절하지만, 노인은 특히 열 손실이 발생하기 쉽다. 신체검사가 완료되면 체온을 보호하기 위해 담요 또는 기타 사용할 수 있는 물품으로 환자를 덮어준다.

파킨슨병, 우울증, 정신병 및 메스꺼움을 치료하는 데 사용되는 약물 등 다양한 약물의 영향으로 환자가 고열에 더 취약해질 수 있다. 환자를 통제된 환경으로 신속하게 옮길 수 없는 경우 냉각요법을 고려한다(자세한 내용은 19장 환경 외상 I : 더위와 추위 참조).

극심한 더위와 추위 속에서 장시간 구출하면 노인 환자가 위험에 처할 수 있으므로 신속하게 대처한다. 노인 외상 환자를 외부에서 가온 또는 냉각하는 방법을 고려하며, 환자의 약해진 피부 구조와 적용 부위에 직접적인 열 손상 가능성에 따라 위험의 균형을 맞춰야 한다.

따라서 열원 또는 냉각 원과 환자의 피부 사이에 시트나 환자의 옷 일부를 놓아야 한다.

법적 고려 사항

노인 외상 환자를 처치할 때 몇 가지 법적인 고려 사항이 문제가 될 수 있다. 대부분의 미국에서 배우자, 형제자매, 자녀, 자녀의 배우자와 부모는 성인을 위한 의료 결정을 내릴 때 자동으로 법적 지위를 갖지 않는다. 위임장이나 법원이 지정한 후견인은 개인의 재정 문제에 대한 권한을 가질 수 있지만, 반드시 개인의 의료 결정에 대한 통제권을 갖는 것은 아니다. 법원이 임명한 후견인은 현지 법률 및 임명에 대한 구체적인 책임에 따라 의료 결정을 내릴 권한이 없을 수도 있다. 이러한 권한은 성년후견인 또는 의료에 대한 영구 위임장이 명시되어 있고 그러한 제삼자의 권한에 대한 명확한 문서가 있는 경우에만, 존재하는 것으로 간주한다.

외상 현장에서 처치를 제공하는 동안에는 이러한 미세한 법적 구분을 하기 어려울 수 있다. 구급차가 출동하고 도움 요청이 이루어졌기 때문에 의식이 없거나 의식상태가 저하된 환자의 경우 처치에 대한 묵시적 동의 개념이 적용된다. 환자의 친척이 병원 전 처치 제공자의 처치를 반대하거나 환자 진료를 방해하려고 시도하는 경우 경찰에 도움을 요청한다. 또한, 병원 전 처치 제공자는 의료 지도를 통해 의료 지도 의사가 직접 대화하도록 할 수 있다. 현장에서 병원 전 처치 제공자가 내린 결정을 명확하게 기록한다.

노인 학대 신고

2019년부터 미국의 모든 주에서 병원 전 처치 제공자를 포함한 의료 종사자는 노인 학대가 의심되는 경우 신고해야 할 법적 의무가 있다. 추가 설명이 필요하거나 누군가가 병원 전 처치를 방해하는 사람이 있는 경우 경찰에 신고하고 도움을 요청한다. 법은 일반적으로 경찰관이 현장에서 적시에 결정을 내릴 수 있도록 프로토콜을 제공하며 시간이 허락하는 경우 나중에 병원에서 설명할 수 있도록 한다. 이러한 사건은 구급활동일지에 빠짐없이 완벽하게 기록한다.

노인 학대

노인 학대에 대한 보편적인 정의는 없다. 그러나 미국 국립 노인학대센터와 질병통제예방센터에서는 노인에게 해를 끼치는 행위 또는 행위의 부재를 포함하는 용어로 사용한다. 여기에는 신체적, 정서적, 성적 학대뿐만 아니라 재정적 착취와 방임도 포함된다.

노인 학대는 드문 일이 아니지만, 보고되지 않는 경우가 많다. 미국 질병통제예방센터에 따르면 60세 이상 인구 10명 중 1명은 매년 어떤 형태로든 학대를 경험한다. 남성은 여성보다 치명적이지 않은 폭행과 살인의 비율이 더 높으며 안타깝게도 노인 환자 인구의 살인 비율은 증가하고 있다. 학대 피해자가 학대자에 대한 의존 또는 기타 이유로 신고를 꺼리는 학대에 대한 명확하고 보편적인 정의의 부재, 의무 신고자에 대한 주마다 다른 규정 등 여러 가지 요인으로 인해 신고율이 저조한 것으로 나타났다.

미국 예방 서비스 태스크 포스는 노인 학대 선별 검사를 권고할 충분한 증거를 찾지 못했다. 그러나 이러한 징후를 인식하고 학대 의심 사례를 신고하는 능력이 학대의 악순환을 끊는 데 중요한 역할을 할 수 있으므로 병원 전 처치 제공자가 알아두어야 할 학대 징후가 있다. 여기에는 불안 및 우울증과 같은 정서적 징후와 다음과 같은 신체적 징후가 포함된다.

- 골절된 뼈
- 타박상
- 열악한 생활환경
- 치료되지 않은 욕창궤양
- 상처
- 찢어지거나 얼룩진 옷

학대 유형

학대는 다음과 같이 여러 가지 유형으로 분류할 수 있다.

- 신체적 학대에는 신체적 손상을 초래하는 폭행, 물리적인 힘 또는 신체적 강압뿐만 아니라 강제적으로 먹이기 및 화학적 구속 수단도 포함된다. 신체적 학대의 징후는 물체(예: 벽난로 부지깽이)가 남긴 자국과 같이 명백할 수도 있고 미묘할 수도 있다. 노인 학대의 징후는 아동학대 징후와 유사하다(**그림 15-6**). (14장 소아 외상 참조)
- 정서적 학대는 언어적 학대, 어린애 취급, 협박, 위협 또는 감각 자극 박탈의 형태로 나타날 수 있다.
- 금전적 착취에는 귀금속 절도 또는 횡령뿐만 아니라 후견인 또는 위임장의 부적절한 사용도 포함될 수 있다.
- 성폭행 또는 성적 학대에는 동의할 능력이 없는 노인을 대상으로 한 동의하지 않은 성적 접촉 및 모든 성적 상호 작용이 포함된다.
- 방임은 영양, 생활환경 유지, 개인 간병과 같은 노인을 돌보는 의무

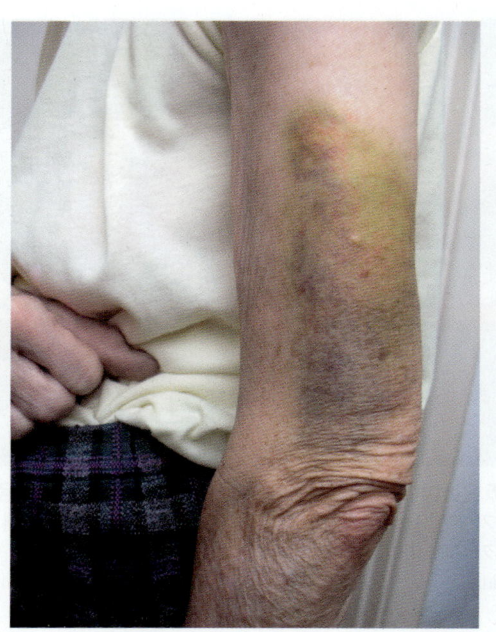

그림 15-6 다양한 치유 단계에 있는 타박상은 신체적 학대를 암시한다. 예를 들어 70세 남성이 간병인의 집에서 여기에 묘사된 것과 같은 타박상을 입고 응급실로 이송되면 병원 전 처치 제공자는 학대 가능성을 고려해야 한다.

를 이행하지 않는 것을 말한다.

COVID-19가 노인 학대에 미치는 영향

노인들은 COVID-19로 인해 심각한 질병에 더 취약할 뿐만 아니라 바이러스 확산을 줄이기 위해 시행된 조치로 인해 부정적인 결과를 초래할 수 있다. 사회적 거리 두기로 인해 노인 인구가 학대 위험에 더 많이 노출되는 여러 가지 부작용이 발생하고 있다. 필수적이지 않은 것으로 간주되는 사업체의 폐쇄로 인해 의료, 재정 및 개인적 필요에 대한 접근성 문제가 발생한다. 이는 치매와 같은 기저 질환을 악화시킬 수 있을 뿐만 아니라 팬데믹 기간 노인 가족, 친구 또는 이웃을 돌볼 준비가 되어 있거나 준비되어 있지 않을 수 있는 간병인에게 추가적인 부담을 줄 수 있다. 주식 시장 하락은 은퇴 자금 손실로 이어져 재정적 어려움으로 이어지고 노년층은 재정적 착취의 위험에 처할 수 있다. 이러한 요인으로 인해 노인 학대에 직면할 위험이 증가하고 학대가 신고될 가능성이 낮은 상황에 처할 수도 있다.

중요 사항

많은 학대를 받은 환자는 보복에 대한 두려움이나 개인을 보호하고 싶어서 거짓 진술을 하도록 공포에 떨게 된다. 가족 구성원에 의한 노

Box 15-4 노인 학대 및 방치 신고

대부분의 지역에서 EMS 제공자는 노인 학대, 방치 및 착취가 의심되는 경우 법적으로 의무적으로 신고해야 한다. 의무 신고자는 병원 직원과 같은 중개자에게 의존하지 않고 학대 조사를 담당하는 기관에 직접 신고해야 한다. 개인이 즉각적인 위험에 처해 있거나 성폭행을 당한 경우 경찰에 신고해야 한다. 학대 또는 방임의 결과로 보이는 사망이 발생한 경우 의무 신고자는 경찰에 반드시 신고해야 한다.

의무 신고자는 의심되는 학대, 방치 및 착취를 신고하지 않을 경우 이에 대한 책임을 진다. 신고자는 신고와 관련된 민형사상의 책임으로부터 보호받으며 신원을 기밀로 유지할 수 있다. 신고자는 HIPAA에 따라 보호되는 정보라도 해당 사건과 관련된 의료 정보를 고유할 수 있다. 노인 학대 신고 의무화에 관한 법률은 정부 차원에서 제정되어 있다. 모든 병원 전 처치 제공자는 관련 법률을 숙지하고 있어야 한다.

© National Association of Emergency Medical Technicians (NAEMT)

인 학대의 경우 가정환경에서 쫓겨나는 것에 대한 두려움으로 인해 노인 환자가 학대의 원인에 대해 거짓말을 할 수 있다. 다른 노인 학대의 경우 감각 기능 저하 또는 치매로 인해 학대에 대한 적절한 설명이 어려울 수 있다. 병원 전 처치 제공자는 학대를 구별하고 환자가 이야기한 내용을 확인해야 한다. 학대 이력이나 학대와 일치하는 소견은 환자처치보고서에 기록한다.

학대 상황을 파악하고 신고하면 환자에 대한 추가적인 외상을 줄일 수 있다. 학대 의심 지수가 높으면 사회복지 서비스 및 공공 안전 기관에 보호 서비스를 의뢰할 수 있다(**Box 15-4**).

조치

손상을 입은 환자의 병원 전 처치에서 가장 큰 어려움 중 하나는 외상센터에서 제공되는 전문외상처치 및 기타 전문적인 처치의 혜택을 가장 많이 받을 수 있는 환자를 정의하는 것이다. 앞서 언급한 여러 가지 이유로 인해 기존 분류 기준의 신뢰성이 떨어질 수 있다. 미국 질병통제예방센터의 손상 환자 현장 분류 지침에 따르면 55세 이상의 외상 환자는 외상센터로 이송하는 것을 고려할 것을 권장한다.

손상을 입은 노인 환자와 젊은 환자 간의 차이와 결과의 차이로 인해 외상센터로 이송해야 하는 노인을 구별하는 데 고유한 기준이 필요한지 여부를 결정하기 위해 많은 연구가 진행되고 있다. 일부 연구에서는 노인 전용 분류 기준을 사용하면 외상센터 이송 기준을 충족하는 노인의 수가 증가한다는 결과가 나왔지만, 다른 연구에서는 그 증가를 입증하지 못했다.

이송 지연

노인 외상 환자에 대한 대부분의 처치는 손상을 입은 환자의 병원 전 처치에 대한 일반적인 지침을 따른다. 그러나 이송 지연하는 경우 몇 가지 특수한 상황이 존재한다. 예를 들어 해부학적 손상이 덜 심각한 노인 환자는 외상센터로 직접 이송한다.

병원 전 환경에서 장기간에 걸쳐 쇼크를 치료하려면 이송 중 활력징후를 주의 깊게 재평가해야 한다. 국소 압박으로 출혈을 조절한 후 수액 소성술은 심장 기능이 손상된 환자의 잠재적인 과부하를 피하면서 혈관 내 용적 상태의 소생술을 최적화하기 위해 생리학적 반응에 맞게 조절해야 한다.

노인 환자는 긴척추고정판에 고정되어 이송 지연 시 압력으로 인한 피부 손상 위험이 커진다. 약해진 피부 구조와 혈류 공급 장애로 인해 노인 환자는 젊은 외상 환자보다 조기에 합병증을 유발할 수 있다. 이송 지연하기 전에 환자의 피부를 보호하기 위해 적절히 패딩 처리된 긴척추고정판, 진공부목 또는 구급차 주들것에 환자를 눕히는 것을 고려한다. 외곽 지역에 있는 구급대는 피부 손상 가능성을 제한하면서 환자를 고정할 수 있는 특수 설계된 저압 긴척추고정판이나 진공부목을 구매해서 사용하는 것을 고려한다.

이송 지연해야 하는 노인 환자에게는 환경 제어가 필수적이다. 신체 노출을 제한하고 차량 온도를 조절하는 것은 저체온증을 제한하고 합병증을 예방하는데 중요한다.

마지막으로 외곽 지역에서 노인 외상 환자를 이송하는 것은 항공 이송을 적절하게 활용할 수 있다. 헬기를 이용한 환자 이송은 환경에 노출되는 시간을 줄일 수 있으며 쇼크 지속 시간을 줄이고 조기 수술 및 수혈을 시행할 수 있는 외상센터로 신속한 이송을 보장할 수 있다.

예방

모바일 통합 의료 및 지역사회 프로그램을 통해 병원 전 처치 제공자는 노인의 외상을 예방하는 노력에 더 많은 역할을 할 수 있다. 현재 많은 지역 사회의 의료 프로그램은 만성 질환을 앓고 있는 환자에게 초점을 맞추고 있으며 이들 중 다수는 노인 환자이다. 이러한 프로그램은 노인 환자의 낙상 위험과 같은 안전 위험을 파악하고 손상을 예방하기 위한 교육 및 개입을 할 특별한 기회가 될 수 있다. EMS 시스템과 병원 전 처치 제공자는 지역사회의 건강을 개전하기 위해 이러한 유형의 프로그램을 고려한다.

요 약

- 노인 인구가 빠르게 증가하고 있다.
- 손상을 입은 환자 처치에 대한 일반적인 지침은 같지만, 손상을 입은 노인 환자 처치에는 몇 가지 특별한 접근 방식이 있다.
- 노화, 만성 질환 및 약물 복용과 관련된 해부학적 및 생리학적 변화는 특정 유형의 외상 가능성을 높이고 외상을 복잡하게 만들며 쇼크에 대한 보상 능력을 저하할 수 있다. 노인 환자는 생리적 예비력이 떨어지고 신체적 감소해서 신체적 손상을 잘 견디지 못한다.
- 노인 외상 환자의 병력과 복용 중인 약물에 대한 지식은 우수한 처치를 제공하는 데 필수적이다.

- 노인 외상 환자의 경우 여러 가지 요인으로 인해 조기 악화 징후를 가릴 수 있으며 이로 인해 명백한 경고 없이 갑작스럽고 급격한 기능 저하가 발생할 가능성이 커진다.
- 노인 외상 환자의 경우 초기 증상에 나타나는 것보다 더 심각한 손상이 발생했을 수 있다.
- 병원 전 처치 제공자는 노인 학대의 징후를 인식하고 의심되는 경우 적절한 기관에 신고한다.
- 노인 외상 환자를 외상센터로 직접 이송하기 위한 분류 기준을 낮게 적용하는 것이 중요하다.

시나리오 재구성

당신은 78세 여성이 계단에서 넘어졌다는 신고를 받고 현장으로 출동했다. 그녀의 딸은 불과 15분 전에 전화 통화를 했으며 어머니를 모시고 쇼핑하러 어머니의 집에 가고 있었다고 말한다. 집에 도착했을 때 쓰러져 있는 어머니를 발견하고 즉시 119에 도움을 요청했다.

당신이 현장에 도착했을 때 계단 아래에 누워 있는 환자를 발견했다. 환자를 처음 보았을 때 환자가 노령의 여성임을 알 수 있었다. 척추를 중립 자세로 고정하는 동안 환자가 당신의 명령에 반응하지 않는다는 것을 확인했다. 이마의 눈에 띄는 열상이 있고 왼쪽 손목에 명백한 변형이 있으며 외부출혈은 없다. 환자는 당뇨병이 있음을 나타내는 의료정보용 팔찌를 착용하고 있다.

- 낙상으로 인해 의식상태가 변화되었는가? 아니면 선행 사건이 있었는가?
- 환자의 나이, 병력, 복용 중인 약물이 손상과 어떻게 상호작용하여 병태생리와 증상이 젊은 환자와 다르게 나타나는가?
- 노인 외상 환자를 외상센터로 이송하기 위한 추가 기준이 있는가?

시나리오 해결책

노인 환자의 외상을 평가할 때 외상이 일차적으로 발생했는지 아니면 뇌졸중, 심근경색 또는 실신과 같은 의학적 문제로 인해 이차적으로 발생했는지 즉시 판단할 수 있는 것은 아니다. 병원 전 처치 제공자는 외상성 손상을 유발했을 수 있는 이전 의학적 문제의 징후를 찾아야 한다.

일차평가 결과 이 환자는 기도가 개방되어 유지하고 있으며 분당 16회의 환기 속도로 호흡하고 있다. 대량 외부출혈은 없으며 이마 열상으로 인한 출혈은 직접 압박으로 쉽게 지혈할 수 있다. 환자의 심박수는 84회/분이고 혈압은 154/82mmHg이다. 당신은 환자의 머리와 척추를 도수 고정하고 긴척추고정판에 패딩을 적용하여 고정한다. 환자가 당뇨병을 앓고 있으므로 혈당 수치를 확인하여 의식 상태에 대한 교정 가능한 원인이 있는지 확인한다. 환자의 나이와 명백한 외상성 뇌손상, 추락의 정도를 고려하여 가장 가까운 외상센터로 신속하게 이송한다.

References

1. U.S. Census Bureau. State and county quick facts. Updated July 1, 2021. Accessed January 25, 2022. https:// www.census.gov/quickfacts/fact/table/US#viewtop

2. Mather M, Jacobsen L, Pollard K, Population Reference Bureau. Aging in the United States. *Popul Bull.* 2015;70(2):2-17. Accessed January 25, 2022. https:// www.prb.org/resources/population-bulletin-vol-70-no-2 -aging-in-the-united-states/

3. United Nations, Department of Economic and Social Affairs, Population Division. *World Population Prospects: The 2015 Revision; Key Findings and Advance Tables.* United Nations; 2015.

4. Champion H, Copes WS, Sacco WJ, et al. The Major Trauma Outcome Study: establishing national norms for trauma care. *J Trauma.* 1990;30(11):1356-1365.

5. Hashmi A, Ibrahim-Zada I, Rhee P, et al. Predictors of mortality in geriatric trauma patients: a systematic review and meta-analysis. *J Trauma Acute Care Surg.* 2014;76(3):894-901.

6. Lane P, Sorondo B, Kelly JJ. Geriatric trauma patients: are they receiving trauma center care? *Ann Emerg Med.* 2003;10(3):244-250.

7. Centers for Disease Control and Prevention, National Center for Injury Prevention and Control, Web-Based Injury Statistics Query and Reporting System (WISQARS). Ten leading causes of death by age group, United States—2018. Accessed January 25, 2022. https://www.cdc.gov/injury /images/lc-charts/leading_causes_of_death_by_age_group _2018_1100w850h.jpg

8. American College of Surgeons Committee on Trauma. *Advanced Trauma Life Support, Student Course Manual.* 9th ed. American College of Surgeons; 2012:272-284.

9. Caterino J, Brown N, Hamilton M, et al. Effect of geriatric-specific trauma triage criteria on outcomes in injured older adults: a statewide retrospective cohort study. *J Am Geriatr Soc.* 2016;64(10):1944-1951.

10. Jacobs D. Special considerations in geriatric injury. *Curr Opin Crit Care.* 2003;9(6):535-539.

11. U.S. Department of Health and Human Services, Centers for Disease Control and Prevention, National Center for Health Services. Hospitalizations for patients aged 85 and over in the United States, 2000–2010. Published 2015. Accessed January 25, 2022. https://www.cdc.gov/nchs /data/databriefs/db182.pdf

12. Roberts D, McKay M, Shaffer A. Increasing rates of emergency department visits for elderly patients in the United States, 1993 to 2003. *Ann Emerg Med.* 2008;51(6):769-774.

13. Jones C, Wasserman E, Li T, et al. The effect of older age on EMS use for transportation to an emergency department. *Prehosp Disaster Med.* 2017;13:1-8.

14. Smith CH, Boland B, Daureeawoo Y, Donaldson E, Small K, Tuomainen J. Effect of aging on stimulated salivary flow in adults. *J Am Geriatr Soc.* 2013;61(5):805-808. doi: 10.1111/ jgs.12219

15. American College of Surgeons Committee on Trauma. *Advanced Trauma Life Support, Student Course Manual.* 10th ed. American College of Surgeons; 2018:214-224.

16. Smith T. Respiratory system: aging, adversity, and anesthesia. In: McCleskey CH, ed. *Geriatric Anesthesiology.* Williams & Wilkins; 1997.

17. Bergeon E, Lavoie A, Clas D, et al. Elderly trauma patients with rib fractures are at greater risk of death and pneumonia. *J Trauma.* 2003;54(3):478-485.

18. Jacobs D, Plaisier BR, Barie PS, et al. Practice management guidelines for geriatric trauma: the EAST Practice Management Guidelines Work Group. *J Trauma.* 2003;54(2):391-416. doi: 10.1097/01.TA.0000042015.54022.BE

19. Deiner S, Silverstein JH, Abrams K. Management of trauma in the geriatric patient. *Curr Opin Anaesthesiol.* 2004;17(2):165-170.

20. Carey J. *Brain Facts: A Primer on the Brain and Nervous System.* Society for Neuroscience; 2002.

21. Alzheimer's Association. 2017 Alzheimer's disease facts and figures. *Alzheimer's Dement.* 2017;13:325-373.

22. Pisani M, Kong S, Kasl S, et al. Days of delirium are associated with 1 year mortality in an older intensive care unit population. *Am J Crit Care Med.* 2009;180:1092-1097.

23. Aung Thein M, Pereira J, Nitchingham A, Caplan G. A call to action for delirium research: meta-analysis and regression of delirium associated mortality. *BMC Geriatrics.* 2020;20(325):1-12.

24. U.S. Department of Health and Human Services, National Institutes of Health, National Eye Institute. Facts about cataracts. Updated August 3, 2019. Accessed January 25, 2022. https://www.nei.nih.gov/learn-about-eye-health/eye -conditions-and-diseases/cataracts

25. EPOS Group. Incidence of vertebral fracture in Europe: results from the European Prospective Osteoporosis Study (EPOS). *J Bone Miner Res.* 2002;17:716-724.

26. Blackmore C. Cervical spine injury in patients 65 years old and older: epidemiologic analysis regarding the effects of age and injury mechanism on distribution, type, and stability of injuries. *Am J Roentgenol.* 2002;178:573-577.

27. Administration for Community Living. 2020 profile of older Americans. Published May 2021. Accessed January 25, 2022. https://acl.gov/sites/default/files/Aging%20and %20Disability%20in%20America/2020ProfileOlder Americans.Final_.pdf

28. Bhasin S, Gill TM, Reuben DB, et al. A randomized trial of a multifactorial strategy to prevent serious fall injuries. *N Engl J Med.* 2020;393(2):129-140.

29. Centers for Disease Control and Prevention. Facts about falls. Last reviewed August 6, 2021. Accessed January 25, 2022. https://www.cdc.gov/falls/facts.html

30. Centers for Disease Control and Prevention. STEADI: Stopping Elderly Accidents, Deaths & Injuries. Accessed January 25, 2022. https://www.cdc.gov/steadi/materials.html

31. Centers for Disease Control and Prevention, National Center for Injury Prevention and Control, Division of Unintentional Injury Prevention. Older adult drivers. Updated December 7, 2020. Accessed August 29, 2021. https:// www.cdc.gov/transportationsafety/older_adult_drivers /index.html

32. National Highway Traffic Safety Administration. Traffic safety facts: 2019 data: pedestrians. Published May 2021. Accessed August 30, 2021. https://crashstats.nhtsa.dot.gov/ Api/Public/ViewPublication/813121

33. Joseph CB. Physician's guide to assessing and counseling older drivers: second edition. *J Med Libr Assoc.* 2013;101(3):230-231. doi: 10.3163/1536-5050.101.3.017

34. Yon Y, Mikton CR, Gassoumis ZD, Wilber KH. Elder abuse prevalence in community settings: a systematic review and meta-analysis. *Lancet Glob Health.* 2017 Feb;5(2):e147-e156.

35. National Center for Elder Abuse. Welcome to the National Center on Elder Abuse. Accessed August 30, 2021. https:// ncea.acl.gov/

36. American Burn Association. 2016 National Burn Repository. Accessed January 25, 2022. https://ameriburn.org/wp-content/uploads/2017/05/2016abanbr_final_42816.pdf

37. Richmond R, Aldaghlas TA, Burke C, et al. Age: is it all in the head? Factors influencing mortality in elderly patients with head injuries. *J Trauma*. 2011;71(1):E8-E11.

38. Berko J, Ingram D, Saha S, et al. Deaths attributed to heat, cold, and other weather events in the United States, 2006–2010. *Natl Health Stat Rep*. 2014;76.

39. Maher R, Hanlon J, Hajjar E. Clinical consequences of polypharmacy in elderly. *Expert Opin Drug Saf*. 2014;13(1):57-65.

40. American Geriatrics Society. 2019 updated AGS Beers criteria for potentially inappropriate medication use in older adults. *J Am Geriatr Soc*. 2019;67:674-694. doi: 10.1111/jgs.15767

41. National Association of Emergency Medical Technicians, American Geriatrics Society, Snyder, DR. *Geriatric Education for Emergency Medical Services*. 2nd ed. Jones & Bartlett Learning; 2015.

42. American Bar Association. Adult Protective Services reporting chart. Published December 2019. Accessed January 25, 2022. https://www.americanbar.org/content/dam/aba/administrative/law_aging/2020-elder-abuse-reporting-chart.pdf

43. Centers for Disease Control and Prevention. Preventing Elder Abuse. Updated June 2, 2021. Accessed September 1, 2021. https://www.cdc.gov/violenceprevention/elderabuse/fastfact.html

44. U.S. Preventive Services Task Force. Intimate Partner Violence, Elder Abuse, and Abuse of Vulnerable Adults: Screening. Published October 23, 2018. Accessed September 1, 2021. https://www.uspreventiveservicestaskforce.org/uspstf/recommendation/intimate-partner-violence-and-abuse-of-elderly-and-vulnerable-adults-screening

45. Makaroun LK, Bachrach RL, Rosland AM. Elder abuse in the time of COVID-19: increased risks for older adults and their caregivers. *Am J Geriatr Psychiatry*. 2020;28(8):876-880. doi: 10.1016/j.jagp.2020.05.017

46. Sasser SM, Hunt RC, Faul M. Guidelines for field triage of injured patients: recommendations of the National Expert Panel on Field Triage 2011. *Morb Mortal Wkly Rep*. 2012;61(1):1-20.

47. Ichwan N, Darbha S, Shah M, et al. Geriatric-specific triage criteria are more sensitive than standard adult criteria in identifying need for trauma center care in injured older adults. *Ann Emerg Med*. 2015;65(1):92-100.

48. Phillips S, Rond P, Kelly S, et al. The failure of triage criteria to identify geriatric patients with trauma: results from the Florida Trauma Triage Study. *J Trauma*. 1996;40(2):278-283.

Suggested Reading

American College of Surgeons Committee on Trauma. Geriatric trauma. In: *Advanced Trauma Life Support, Student Course Manual*. 10th ed. American College of Surgeons; 2018:214-225.

American Geriatrics Society, Snyder DR. *Geriatric Education for Emergency Medical Services*. 2nd ed. Jones & Bartlett Learning; 2015.

Reske-Nielsen C, Medzon R. Geriatric trauma. *Emer Med Clin North Am*. 2016;34(3):483-500.

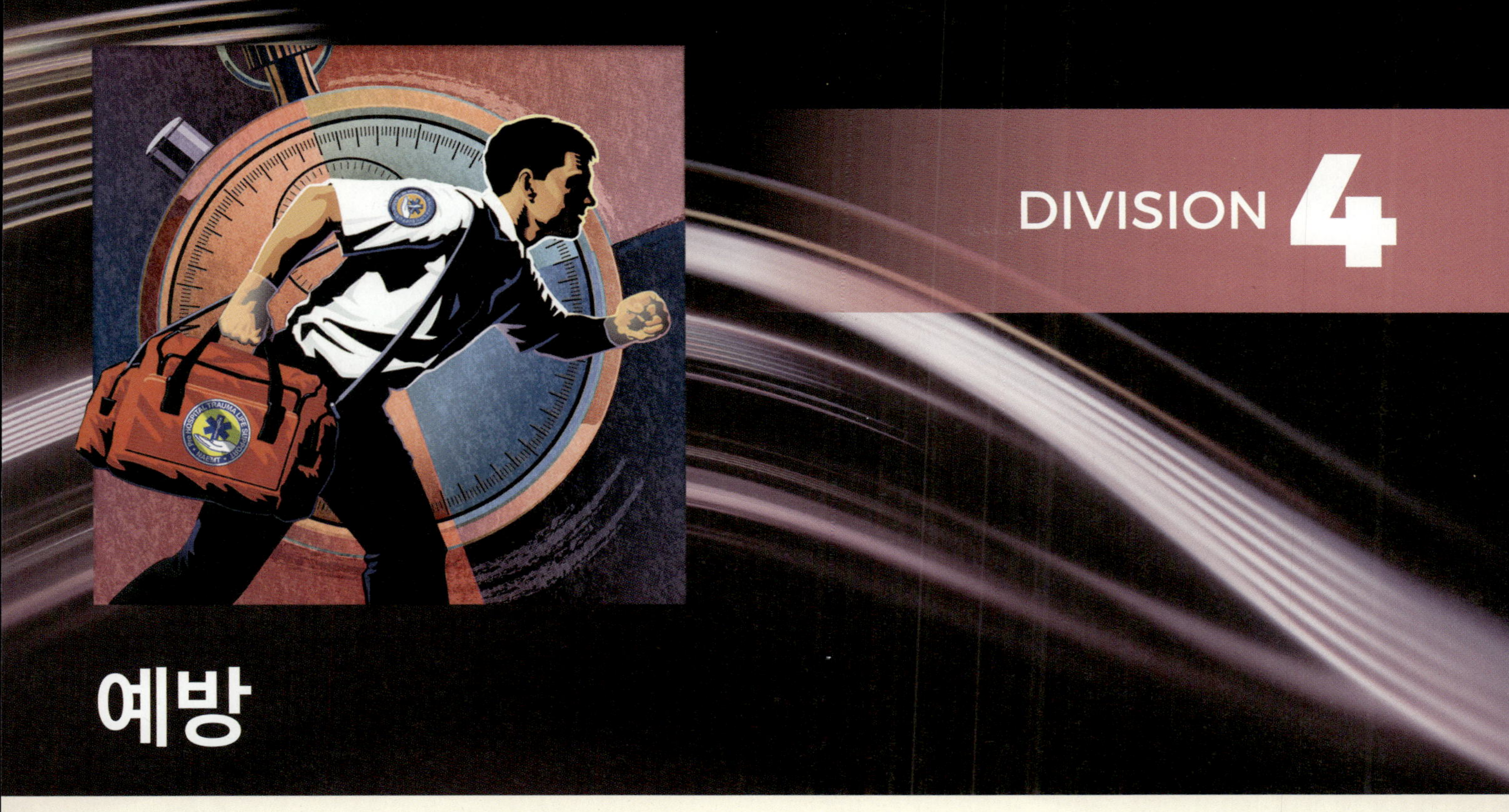

예방

제 16 장   손상 예방

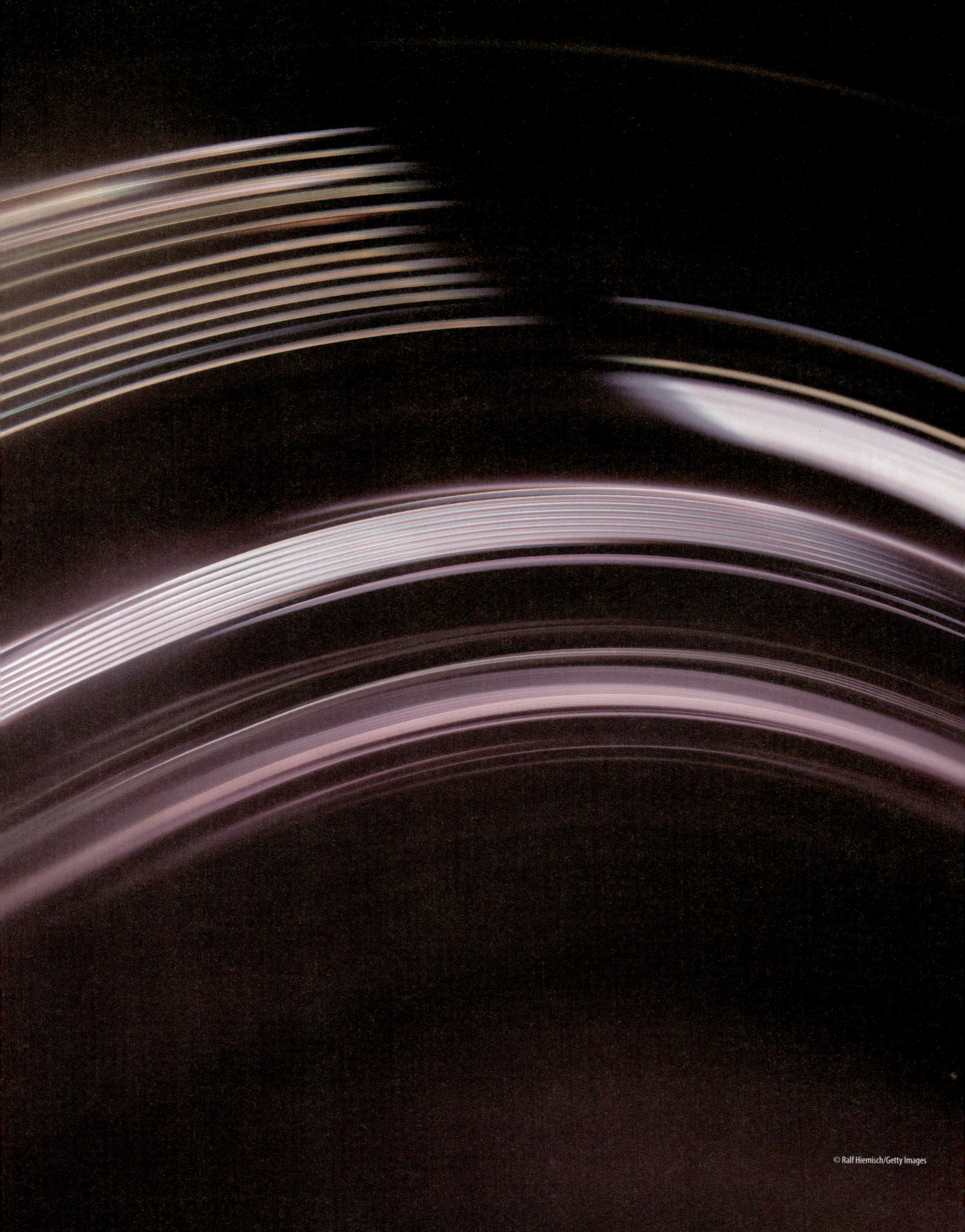

손상 예방

Lead Editors
Heidi Abraham, MD, EMT-B, EMT-T, FAEMS
Thomas Colvin, NREMT-P
Nancy Hoffmann, MSW

학습 목표   이 장의 학습을 완료하면 다음과 같은 내용을 수행할 수 있다.

- 손상의 원인으로서 에너지의 개념을 설명할 수 있다.
- 관심이 있는 손상 유형에 대한 해든 매트릭스(Haddon Matrix)를 작성할 수 있다.
- 병원 전 처치 제공자가 정확하고 세심한 현장 평가와 수집한 데이터 문서화의 중요성을 손상 예방 조치의 성공과 연관시킬 수 있다.
- 지역사회 또는 EMS 기관에서 손상 예방 프로그램의 개발, 실행 및 평가를 지원할 수 있다.
- 친한 동료의 폭력의 확산과 EMS가 주의해야 할 단서에 관해 설명할 수 있다.
- 다음을 포함하여 손상 예방에 있어 EMS의 역할을 설명하고 옹호한다.
  - 개인
  - 가족
  - 지역사회
  - 전문가
  - 조직
  - 단체 연합
- 병원 전 처치 제공자가 손상의 위험을 줄이기 위해 시행할 수 있는 전략을 파악할 수 있다.

시나리오

당신과 동료는 자동차 충돌 현장에서 도착해서 비만 환자를 차량 운전석에서 신속하게 구출하기 위해 노력하고 있다. 환자는 충돌 당시 안전띠를 매지 않은 상태였다. 당신과 동료는 모두 도로에 있기 때문에 승인된 안전 조끼를 착용하고 장비를 확인하고 있다. 경찰관이 현장에 도착해서 교통 통제를 하고 있으며 구급차가 주차되어 있어 다가오는 차량으로부터 최대한 보호받을 수 있다. 환자의 무게로 인해 사용 중인 전동 주들것에 환자를 적절히 고정하였다. 전동 주들것을 사용하면 당신과 동료의 몸에 과도한 부담을 주지 않고 환자를 구급차로 안전하게 들어 올릴 수 있다.

구급차에 탑승한 후에는 환자실의 의자에 앉아 몸을 고정하고 환자를 계속 처치하는 동안 동료는 차량을 안전하게 운전하여 병원으로 이동한다. 구급차가 병원에 무사히 도착하면 응급실 의료진에게 환자를 인계한다. 환자 인계 후 서류를 작성하는 동안 병원 전 처치 제공에 대한 전반적인 국가 손상 및 사망 통계를 고려한다. 당신과 동료가 손상 예방의 모든 측면에 세심한 주의를 기울인 덕분에 관련된 모든 사람이 안전하게 출동을 마무리할 수 있었다.

- 자동차 충돌 및 기타 외상성 손상의 원인으로 인한 손상과 사망을 방지하기 위한 사고 예방이 현실적인 접근 방식인가?
- 안전띠 및 안전 시트 사용과 관련된 법규 준수가 손상과 사망을 예방하는 데 영향을 미친다는 증거가 있는가?
- 병원 전 처치 제공자로서 우리는 자동차 충돌로 인한 사망과 손상을 예방하기 위해 무엇을 할 수 있는가?

개요

현대 EMS 시스템 개발의 주요 원동력은 1966년 미국 국립과학원(NAS)/국립 연구위원회(NRC)에서 발간한 백서 사고 사망 및 장애, 현대 사회의 방치된 질병이었다. 이 백서는 미국 내 손상 관리의 미비점을 조명하고 "사고"로 인해 손상을 입은 환자를 위한 현장 처치와 신속한 이송을 위한 공식적인 시스템을 시작하는 데 도움이 되었다. 이 새로운 교육계획은 아프거나 다친 환자에게 병원 전 처치를 제공하는 더욱 효율적인 시스템을 구축하는 데 중요한 역할을 했다.

백서 발간 이후 미국에서 손상으로 인한 사망 및 장애 발생률은 감소했다. 그러나 이러한 진전에도 불구하고 손상은 주요 공중보건 문제로 남아 있다. 2020년 미국에서 손상으로 인한 사망자는 278,345명에 달하며 수백만 명이 어느 정도 손상의 영향을 받았다. 손상은 모든 연령대의 주요 사망 원인이다. 특히 어린이, 청소년, 45세 미만의 성인 등 일부 연령층에서는 손상이 주요 사망 원인이다.

손상은 전 세계적인 문제이기도 하다. 세계보건기구(WHO)는 매년 손상 관련 사망자가 440만 명에 달하며 2019년에는 전 세계적으로 약 310만 명이 예방할 수 있는 손상으로 사망한 것으로 추정한다(살인이나 자살은 제외).

손상을 입은 환자를 돌보고자 하는 열방으로 인해 많은 사람이 EMS 분야로 몰리고 있다. PHTLS 과정은 병원 전 처치 제공자에게 환자 평가 및 손상 처치에 효율적이고 효과적으로 대처할 수 있도록 교육한다. 손상을 입은 환자를 돌보기 위해 잘 훈련된 병원 전 처치 제공자가 항상 필요하다. 그러나 손상에 대처하는 가장 효율적인 방법은 손상을 처음부터 예방하는 것이다. 모든 수준의 의료 종사자는 손상 예방에 적극적인 임무를 수행하여 지역사회뿐만 아니라 자신을 위해서도 최고의 결과를 얻을 수 있다.

1966년 미국 국립과학원/국립 연구위원회 백서의 저자들은 이 백서를 집필할 당시 손상 예방의 중요성을 인식했다.

> 손상 문제에 대한 장기적인 해결책은 예방이다. --- 사고 예방을 위해서는 가정, 학교 및 직장에서의 교육과 더불어 뉴스 매체를 통한 잦은 안전 촉구, 응급처치 교육 및 공청회, 규제 기관의 검사와 감시가 필요하다.

광견병이나 홍역과 같은 일부 질병의 예방은 매우 효과적이어서 한 건의 사례가 발생해도 머리기사가 된다. 공중보건당국은 예방이 질병을 개선하는 데 가장 큰 효과를 가져온다는 사실을 잘 알고 있다. 병원 전 처치 제공자를 위한 교육 과정에는 병원 전 처치 제공자가 자신의 손상을 예방하는 방법으로 현장 안전 및 개인보호장비에 대한 공식적인 교육이 오랫동안 포함됐다. EMS 시스템이 지역사회 예방 전략에서 더욱 적극적인 임무를 수행하도록 박차를 가하기 위해 EMS 공동체에 의해 그리고 EMS 공동체를 위해 개발된 미래를 위한 EMS 과제에서는 "지역사회 건강을 개선하고 신속하게 의료 자원을 더욱 적절하게 사용하기" 위해 추가로 발전시켜야 할 14가지 중 하나로 예방을 꼽았다. 후속 문서인 EMS 과제 2050 응급의료 서비스의 미래를 위한 사람 중심 비전은 비전 선언문에서 EMS가 다음을 지원하는 역할을 간략하게 설명한다. "예방, 대응 및 임상 치료에 대한 데이터 기반의 증거 기반 및 안전한 접근 방식을 통해 지역사회 주민과 방문객의 건강"을 지원하는 역할을 설명한다.

EMS 시스템은 사후 대응에만 국한된 분야에서 지역사회 응급의료와 같은 추가적인 측면을 포함하고 예방에 더욱 중점을 두는 광범위한 의료 분야로 변모하고 있다. 현장의 실무자들은 EMS의 핵심 임무의 일환으로 일차적 손상 예방(PiP)을 지원하지만, 설문조사에 참여한 응답자 중 50% 미만이 임상 진료 중에 일차적 손상 예방을 시행하고 있다. 이 장에서는 병원 전 처치 제공자에게 손상 예방의 핵심 개념을 소개한다.

손상의 개념

손상의 정의

손상 예방에 대한 논의는 손상이라는 용어의 정의로 시작한다. 손상은 이제 일반적으로 특정 형태의 물리적 에너지가 방출되거나 정상적인 에너지 흐름에 장애가 발생하여 발생하는 해로운 사건으로 정의된다. 손상의 원인은 매우 다양하므로 처음에는 연구와 예방에 있어 큰 장애물이었다. 예를 들어 노인의 낙상으로 인한 엉덩관절 골절과 젊은 성인의 머리에 자해로 인한 총상을 입는 것의 공통점은 무엇인가? 또한 노인 여성의 낙상으로 인한 넓적다리뼈 골절과 오토바이 충돌로 인한 젊은 남성의 넓적다리뼈 골절을 어떻게 비교할 수 있는가? 차량 충돌, 칼에 찔림, 자살, 익사 등 모든 가능한 손상 원인에는 피해자에게 에너지가 전달된다는 한 가지 공통점이 있다.

질병으로서의 손상

질병 과정은 수년간 연구되었다. 이제 질병이 발생하려면 1) 질병을 유발하는 병인, 2) 병인이 서식할 수 있는 숙주, 3) 병인과 숙주가 함

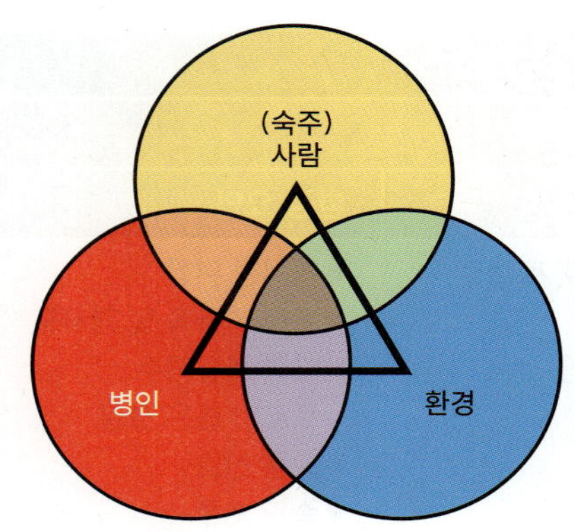

그림 16-1 역학의 삼각구조
© National Association of Emergency Medical Technicians (NAEMT)

께 모일 수 있는 적절한 환경이라는 세 가지 요소가 동시에 존재하고 상호 작용해야 질병이 발생한다는 것이 이해되었다. 공중보건 전문가들은 이 "역학적 3요소"를 인식한 후 질병을 퇴치할 방법을 발견했다 (**그림 16-1**). 숙주에게 백신을 접종하거나 항생제로 병원체를 파괴하거나, 위생 개선을 통해 환경 전파를 줄이거나, 이 세 가지를 모두 조합하여 특정 전염병을 박멸할 수 있었다.

1940년대 후반에 이르러서야 손상 과정에 관한 중요한 연구가 이루어졌다. 손상 연구의 선구자들은 명백히 다른 결과에도 불구하고 질병과 손상이 놀라울 정도로 유사하다는 것을 보여주었다. 둘 다 모두 역학 3요소의 세 가지 요소가 필요하므로 둘 다 질병으로 취급된다.

1. 손상이 발생하려면 숙주(즉, 사람)가 존재해야 한다. 질병과 마찬가지로 숙주의 감수성은 개인마다 일정하게 유지되는 것이 아니라 내부 및 외부 요인에 따라 달라진다. 내부 요인으로는 지능, 성별, 반응 시간 등이 있다. 외부 요인에는 중독이나 사회적 신념이 포함되고 같은 사람 내에서도 시간이 지남에 따라 감수성이 달라진다.

2. 앞서 설명한 것처럼 손상의 원인은 에너지이다. 에너지를 방출하는 물체에 노출되는 속도, 모양, 재료와 시간 등이 모두 숙주의 내성 수준을 초과하는지에 영향을 미친다.

3. 숙주와 병인은 둘이 상호 작용할 수 있는 환경에서 함께 있어야 한다. 일반적으로 환경은 물리적 요소와 사회적 요소로 나뉜다. 물리적 환경 요소는 직접 보고 만질 수 있으며 사회적 환경 요소에는 태도, 신념 및 판단이 포함된다. 예를 들어 청소년은 다른 연령대에 비해 사회적 요소가 더 크기 때문에 위험을 감수하는 행동(물리적 요소)에 참여할 가능성이 더 높다.

숙주, 병인 및 환경의 특성은 시간과 상황에 따라 변화한다. 공중보건 전문가인 톰 크리스토펠과 수잔 스카보 갤러거는 이러한 역학 관계를 다음과 같이 설명하였다.

> 예를 들어 역학 삼각구도의 구성 요소를 끊임없이 돌아가는 바퀴라고 생각하면 이해하기가 쉬울 것이다. 각 바퀴 안에는 파이 모양의 부분이 있으며 각 부분에는 좋은 상황과 나쁜 상황의 변수가 하나씩 있다. 세 바퀴는 서로 다른 속도로 회전하므로 서로 다른 특성이 서로 다른 시간과 다른 조합으로 상호 작용한다. 어떤 조합은 손상이 발생하지 않으리라 예측하고 어떤 조합은 재난을 예측한다.

손상의 경우 숙주는 호기심 많고 잘 움직이는 2세 어린이, 병인은 물이 가득 찬 수영장에 비치볼이 가장자리 너머에 떠 있는 경우, 환경은 베이비시터가 전화를 받기 위해 수영장 문을 열어둔 채로 뛰어가는 경우일 수 있다. 숙주, 병인, 환경이 모두 한꺼번에 모이면 의도하지 않은 손상(이 경우 익사)이 발생할 수 있다.

해든 매트릭스(HADDON MATRIX)

윌리엄 J. 해든 주니어 박사는 손상 예방 과학의 아버지로 여겨진다. 1960년대 중반 그는 역학 3요소 개념을 통해 손상을 다음과 같은 세 가지 시간적 단계로 구분할 수 있다는 사실을 알아냈다.

1. 사고 전: 손상 전
2. 사고: 해로한 에너지가 방출되는 시점
3. 사고 후: 손상의 여파(또한 1장, PHTLS: 과거, 현재, 미래 참조).

각 시간적 단계에서 역학 3요소의 세 가지 요인을 조사하여 해든은 9개의 셀의 "단계 요인" 매트릭스를 만들었다(**표 16-1**). 이 격자는 해든 매트릭스로 알려지게 되었다. 이 매트릭스는 손상 발생 확률을 높이거나 낮추는 사건이나 행동을 그래픽으로 묘사하는 수단을 제공한다. 또한 예방 전략을 식별하는 데에도 사용할 수 있다. 해든 대트릭스는 여러 요인이 손상으로 이어질 수 있으므로 손상의 심각성을 예방하거나 줄일 여러 기회가 존재한다는 것을 보여준다. 이 매트릭스는 손상이 단일 원인, 불운 또는 운명의 결과라는 통념을 없애는 데 중요한 역할을 했다.

표 16-1은 구급차 충돌 사고에 대한 해든 매트릭스를 나타낸다. 대트릭스의 각 셀에 포함된 구성 요소는 검사 중인 손상에 따라 다르다. 사고 전 단계에는 충돌 가능성에 이바지할 수 있는 요인이 포함되지만, 에너지는 여전히 통제되고 있다. 이 단계는 몇 초에서 몇 년까지 지속될 수 있다. 사고 단계는 손상의 심각성에 영향을 미치는 요

표 16-1 구급차 충돌 사고에 대한 해든 매트릭스

	역학의 삼각구도		
시간 단계	숙주 요인	병인 요인	환경 요인
사고 전 단계	■ 운전자의 시력 ■ 경험과 판단 ■ 교대 근무당 구급차에 있는 시간 ■ 피로 수준 ■ 적절한 영양 섭취 ■ 스트레스 지수 ■ 회사 및 지역사회 운전 법규 준수 ■ 운전자 교육 과정의 질	■ 브레이크, 타이어 등의 유지 보수 ■ 장비 결함 ■ 구급차의 높은 무게 중심 ■ 속도 ■ 제어의 용이성	■ 가시성 위험 ■ 도로의 굴곡 및 경사도 ■ 표면 마찰계수 ■ 도로의 좁은 갓길 ■ 교통 신호 ■ 속도 제한
사고 단계	■ 안전띠 사용 ■ 신체 상태 ■ 손상 임계값 ■ 탈출	■ 속도 기능 ■ 구급차 크기 ■ 자동 구속 장치 ■ 접촉면의 경도와 날카로움 ■ 느슨한 물건(클립보드, 손전등)의 경도 및 날카로움 ■ 안전한 운전 습관 실천(속도, 라이트, 사이렌 사용, 추월, 교차로, 후진) ■ 운전 중 동료의 습관 훈련(전방 주시, 교차로 통과) ■ 안전한 주차	■ 가드레일 부족 ■ 중앙 분리대 ■ 도로와 움직이지 않는 물체 사이의 거리 ■ 속도 제한 ■ 기타 교통 상황 ■ 안전띠 사용에 대한 태도 ■ 탈출 경로 유지 ■ 환경이 안전하다고 가정을 하지 않음 ■ 날씨
사고 후 단계	■ 나이 ■ 신체 상태 ■ 손상의 유형 또는 정도	■ 연료 시스템 무결성 ■ 함정	■ 비상 통신 기능 ■ EMS 출동 시간과 품질 ■ EMS 직원 교육 ■ 구출 장비의 가용성 ■ 지역사회의 외상 처치 시스템 ■ 지역사회의 재활 프로그램

Data from Blau G, Chapman S, Boyer E, Flanagan R, Lam T, Monos C. Correlates of safety outcomes during patient ambulance transport: a partial test of the Haddon Matrix. *J Allied Health*. 2012;41(3):e69-72. PMID: 22968779.

인을 나타낸다. 이 기간에 제어되지 않은 에너지가 방출되고 에너지 전달이 신체의 허용 범위를 초과하면 손상이 발생한다. 사고 단계는 일반적으로 매우 짧으며 몇 초 동안만 지속될 수 있고 몇 분 이상 지속되는 경우는 드물다. 사고 후 단계의 요인은 손상이 발생한 후 결과에 영향을 미친다. 사고 유형에 따라 몇 초에서 숙주의 남은 수명까지 지속될 수 있다(1장 PHTLS: 과거, 현재, 미래 참조).

앞서 언급했듯이 해든 매트릭스의 주요 목적은 손상 위험을 인식하여 손상을 예방하는 것이다. 공중보건 프로그램에서는 1차, 2차, 3차 예방이라는 용어를 사용하고 있다.

- 1차 예방은 손상이 발생하기 전에 이를 예방하는 것을 목표로 한다. 이러한 유형의 예방 활동에는 위험을 감수하는 행동을 최소화하고 교육 프로그램과 헬멧, 어린이용 안전 시트, 차량 고정 시스템과 같은 보호 장비 사용이 포함된다.
- 2차 예방은 외상성 뇌손상 후 저산소증이나 저혈압이 발생하지 않도록 하거나 이미 발생하면 가능한 한 빨리 교정하는 등 급성 손상의 진행을 막기 위해 취하는 조치를 말한다.
- 3차 예방은 손상(또는 질병) 후 사망 및 장기적인 장애를 최소화하는 데 초점을 둔다. 적극적이고 공격적인 재활 프로그램이 이 범주에 속한다.

스위스 치즈 모형

영국의 심리학자 제임스 리즌은 사고가 어떻게 발생하는지에 대한 또 다른 사고방식을 제안했다. 그는 이 과정을 스위스 치즈에 비유했다. 모든 상황에서 손상을 입히거나 오류를 일으킬 수 있는 잠재적인 위험이 존재한다. 이를 방지하기 위해 일반적으로 일련의 안전장치 또는 장벽이 있다. 그는 이러한 각 보호 장벽이나 안전장치를 스위스 치즈 조각에 비유했다. 치즈의 구멍은 위험이나 오류로 인해 손상을 입을 가능성을 높이는 결함이나 실패이다. 이러한 결함은 조직이나 관리의 결함으로 인해 발생하거나(잠재적 결함) 시스템의 감독을 소홀히 한 결과 발생하거나(잠재적 결함) 누락 또는 위임 행위의 결과로 발생할 수 있다(적극적 결함). 모든 위험에는 궤적이 있으며 후속 피해가 발생하기 위해서는 일반적으로 일련의 실패가 발생해야 하고 그 궤적이 모든 안전장치가 실패하고 손상이 발생할 수 있도록 정렬된 구멍이나 실패와 교차해야 한다고 주장한다(**그림 16-2**).

손상의 분류

손상을 세분화하는 일반적인 방법은 의도에 따라 분류하는 것이다. 손상은 의도적 또는 비의도적 원인으로 인해 발생할 수 있다. 이는 손상을 보는 논리적인 방법이지만, 손상 예방 노력의 어려움을 강조한다.

의도적 손상은 일반적으로 대인 관계 또는 자기 주도적 폭력 행위와 관련이 있다. 살인, 자살, 폭력, 성폭력, 가정 폭력, 아동 학대, 전쟁 등의 문제가 이 범주에 속한다.

과거에는 의도하지 않은 손상을 사고라고 했다. 미국 국립과학원(NAS)/국립 연구위원회(NRC) 백서의 저자들은 당시의 어휘인 우발적 사망 및 장애를 적절하게 언급했다. 이제 손상이 발생하려면 특정 요인이 복합적으로 작용해야 한다고 믿기 때문에 의료진은 이제 사고라는 용어 차량 충돌, 익사, 추락, 감전 등의 사고로 인해 의도하지 않은 손상과 관련된 예방 가능성의 정도를 정확하게 설명하지 못할 수도 있다는 사실을 깨닫고 있다. EMS 시스템은 자동차 사고(MVA) 대신 자동차 충돌 또는 충돌(MVC)이라는 용어를 사용함으로써 이 개념을 수용했다. 그러나 대중적인 용어 사용은 훨씬 더 느리게 변화했다. 뉴스 기자들은 여전히 자동차 사고나 우발적인 총격 사건으로 손상을 입은 사람을 묘사한다. 사고라는 용어는 손상이 우발적으로 발생했으므로 피할 수 없었다는 의미를 내포하고 있다. 대체 용어의 사용은 사람들이 손상과 관련된 사고를 평가할 때 예방 가능성을 고려하도록 유도하기 위한 것이다.

또한 이 두 가지 일반적인 손상 분류가 중복될 수 있다는 점도 유의해야 한다. 예를 들어, 자동차 충돌 사고가 자살을 시도하는 운전자로 인해 발생했을 수 있다. 자동차 사고로 분류하는 것만으로는 운전자에게 해를 끼치려는 의도가 없다는 것을 의미하지만, 운전자가 자살을 생각했다는 사실을 알았다면 충돌 또는 충돌을 유발하려는 의도가 분명하게 드러난다.

문제의 범위

손상은 전 세계적으로 주요한 보건 문제로 매년 440만 명이 사망하며(**Box 16-1**), 교통사고 약 135만 명, 자살로 약 70만 명, 대인 폭력으로 약 52만 명이 사망한다. 손상 관련 사망의 원인은 발생 기전과 영향을 받는 연령대 측면에서 국가마다 다르다. 경제적, 사회적, 발달적 문제로 인해 손상 관련 사망의 원인은 국가마다, 심지어 같은 국가 내에서도 지역마다 다르다.

예를 들어, 서태평양의 저소득 및 중간 소득 국가에서는 손상 관련된 주요 사망 원인으로 차량 충돌 손상, 익사, 자살이지만, 아프리카에서는 차량 충돌 손상, 전쟁, 대인 폭력이 주요 원인이다. 아프리카 대륙의 고소득 국가에서는 5~29세 사이의 주요 사망 원인이 차량 충돌 손상이었다. 미주 저소득 및 중간 소득 국가의 같은 연령대에서는 대인 폭력이 주요 원인이다. **그림 16-3**은 손상이 전 세계 질병 부담

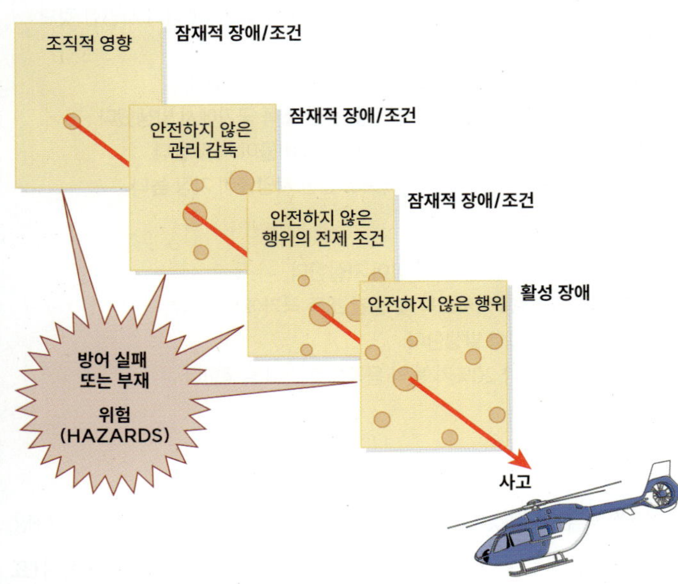

그림 16-2 스위스 치즈 모델은 방어, 장벽 및 안전장치가 사고 궤적에 의해 어떻게 뚫릴 수 있는지에 대한 모델이다.

Box 16-1 전 세계 손상 관련 통계

전반적인 손상

- 손상과 관련된 상위 사망 원인은 다음과 같다.
  1. 교통사고 손상
  2. 폭력 행위
  3. 낙상
  4. 익사
  5. 화상
  6. 중독
  7. 자살
- 손상은 전 세계 사망의 9%, 전체 장애의 16%를 차지한다.
- 5~29세 주요 사망 원인 상위 10개 중 3개가 손상과 관련이 있다.
- 교통사고 손상은 2030년까지 7번째 주요 사망 원인이 될 것으로 예상된다.
- 남성은 여성보다 두 배나 많은 손상으로 사망하며 치명적인 화상으로 인한 손상은 예외이다
- 아프리카 남성의 손상 관련 사망률이 가장 높다.
- 손상 관련 사망의 약 90%가 저소득 및 중간 소득 국가에서 발생한다.
- 손상은 조기 사망 또는 장애로 인한 잠재적 수명 손실의 12%를 차지한다.

교통사고 손상

- 매년 약 135만 명이 교통사고로 인한 손상으로 사망하고 2천만~5천만 명 이상이 손상 또는 장애를 입었다.
- 교통사고 손상은 5~29세 어린이와 청소년의 주요 사망 원인이다.
- 25세 미만 남성의 교통사고 사망률은 여성보다 거의 3배 가까이 높다.
- 저소득 국가는 고소득 국가보다 교통사고로 인한 사망자 수가 3배 이상 많다.
- 아프리카와 동남아시아가 교통사고 손상으로 인한 사망자 중 가장 높은 비율을 차지한다.
- 충돌 가능성과 그 결과의 심각성은 속도 증가와 직접적으로 연관되어 있다.

화상

- 매년 약 18만 명의 사망자가 화상으로 사망하고 대부분 저소득 및 중간 소득 국가에서 발생한다.
- 동남아시아 여성의 화재 관련 화상 사망률이 가장 높다.
- 5세 미만 어린이와 노인은 화재 관련 사망률이 가장 높다.
- 치명적이지 않은 화상으로 인한 손상은 전 세계적으로 질병의 주요 원인이다.

익사 손상

- 201년에는 약 236,000명이 익사로 사망한 것으로 추산된다.

- 익사 사망자의 90% 이상이 저소득 및 중간 소득 국가에서 발생한다.
- 다양한 연령대 중 5세 미만 어린이의 익사 사망률이 가장 높으며 익사 사망의 50% 이상을 차지한다.
- 미국에서 익사는 1~14세 어린이의 비의도적 손상으로 인한 사망의 두 번째 주요 원인이다.
- 공식적인 전 세계 데이터 분류에는 홍수나 수상 운송 사고로 인한 익사 사망이 고려되지 않아 전 세계 익사 사망자 수가 과소평가 되어 있다.

낙상

- 매년 684,000명이 낙상으로 사망하는 것으로 추정된다.
- 낙상 관련 사망자의 80% 이상이 저소득 및 중간 소득 국가에서 발생한다.
- 전 세계 모든 지역에서 65세 이상의 성인, 특히 여성의 낙상 사망률이 가장 높다.
- 낙상은 현재 비의도적인 손상으로 인한 사망의 두 번째 주요 원인이다.
- 전 세계적으로 낙상은 교통사고로 인한 손상, 익사, 화상, 중독을 모두 합친 것보다 더 많은 손상 후유증을 남긴다.

중독

- WHO 데이터에 따르면 2016년 전 세계에서 106,683명이 의도하지 않은 중독으로 사망한 것으로 추산된다.
- 치명적인 중독 사고의 80% 이상이 저소득 및 중간 소득 국가에서 발생했다.
- 유럽 지역이 전 세계 중독 사망자의 3분의 1 이상을 차지한다.
- 뱀에게 물리는 것은 대부분 잘 알려지지 않은 공중보건 문제이다. 신뢰할 수 있는 데이터를 확보하기는 어렵지만, 매년 5백만 건 이상의 뱀물림 사고가 발생하며 이로 인해 최대 270만 건의 독에 중독되고 8만~10만 명이 사망하는 것으로 추정된다.

폭력

- 2019년 전 세계적으로 대인 폭력으로 인해 약 415,000명이 사망한 것으로 추정된다.
- 사망자의 대부분은 15세~49 남성과 여성에서 발생했다.
- 전체 살인 사건 중 95%가 저소득 및 중간 소득 국가에서 발생했다.
- 미주 지역에서 15~29세 남성의 대인 폭력 비율이 가장 높다.
- 여성 중 아프리카에서 대인 폭력으로 인한 사망률이 가장 높다.

자살

- 매년 전 세계적으로 약 70만 명이 자살한다.
- 전체 자살 중 77%가 저소득 및 중간 소득 국가에서 발생한다.
- 자살은 전생에 걸쳐 발생한다.
- 전 세계 자살의 약 20%가 농약 음독으로 인해 발생한다.

에서 주도적인 역할을 한다는 것을 보여준다.

2019년 미국에서 36,000명 이상의 사람이 차량 충돌로 사망했다. 이 중 승용차 탑승자의 47%가 안전띠를 착용하지 않았다. 음주 관련 충돌 사고로 인한 사망자는 10,142명으로 하루에 28명, 즉 52분마다 한 명씩 목숨을 잃었다. 미국에서는 의도하지 않은 손상이 전체 사망 원인 중 4번째로 큰 비중을 차지하며 매년 약 20만 명이 사망한다(**표 16-2**). 손상은 미국뿐만 아니라 전 세계 대부분의 선진국 청소년에게 특히 심각한 문제이다. 미국에서 손상은 모든 질병을 합친 것보다

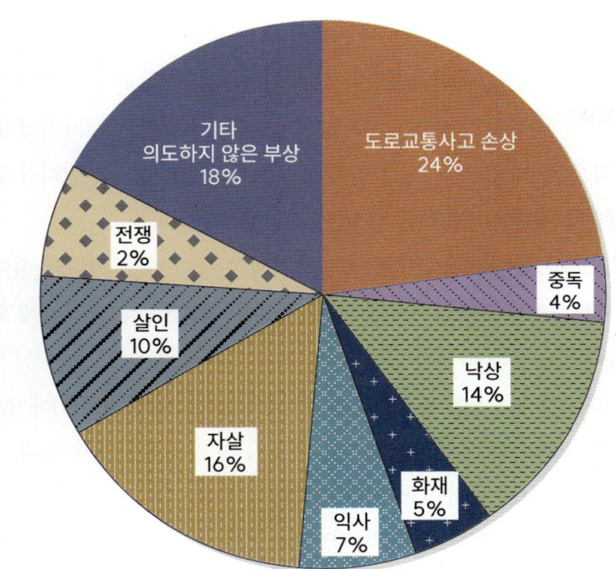

그림 16-3 전 세계 손상 사망률의 원인별 분포

Data from World Health Organization. Injuries and violence: the facts 2014. n.d. https://apps.who.int/iris/bitstream/handle/10665
/149798/9789241508018_eng.pdf

더 많은 어린이와 청소년을 사망에 이르게 하며 1~44세 사이의 주요 사망 원인으로 남아 있다. 이 연령대의 고의적 상해에는 두 번째 주요 사망 원인인 자살과 살인이 포함된다. 자살 건수는 계속 증가하고 있다. 같은 그룹의 비의도적인 상해 사망에도 비의도적 중독(예: 아편유사제 과다 복용), 차량 충돌 및 비의도적 낙상이 포함된다. 아편유사제 과다 복용으로 인한 사망자만 2019년에 49,860명에 달했다.

안타깝게도 손상으로 인한 사망은 빙산의 일각에 불과하다. 손상은 또한 모든 연령, 인종, 사회경제적 계측에 걸쳐 장애를 일으키는 주요 원인이다. 손상으로 인해 매년 2,900만 건의 응급실 방문이 필요하며 가족, 친구, 동료, 지역사회에 더 많은 영향을 미친다.

손상으로 인한 잠재 수명 손실 기간(YPLL)을 조사하면 그 영향을 더욱 실감할 수 있다. 잠재 수명 손실 기간은 조사 대상 그룹의 고정 연령(일반적으로 65세 또는 70세 그룹의 기대 수명)에서 사망 시 연령을 빼서 계산한다. 경제협력기구(OECD)와 대부분의 미국 연방 및 주 정부 기관에서는 75세를 기준으로 삼는다. 예를 들어 70세에 사망하는 사람의 기대 수명은 5이지만, 10세에 사망하는 어린이의 기대 수명은 65세이다. 따라서 손상은 모든 연령대의 사람들이 사망하거나 장애가 발생하더라도 어린이, 청소년 및 청년층에게 불균형적으로 영향을 미친다. 즉, 손상은 1~44세 사이의 미국인 사망의 주요 원인이기 때문에 다른 어떤 사망 원인보다 더 많은 잠재 수명 손실 기간을 유발한다. 2020년에는 손상으로 인해 약 490만 년의 세월을 빼앗겼다(**그림 16-4**). 의도하지 않은 중독(주로 아편유사제 과다 복용)이 그중 140만 년을 차지했다.

손상의 심각성에 대한 세 번째 척도는 재정적으로 입증할 수 있다. 손상으로 인한 경제적 손실은 환자와 직계 가족을 훨씬 넘어서는 영향을 미친다. 손상으로 인한 비용은 넓은 범위에 걸쳐 있다. 손상 비용은 국가 및 기타 기관, 다른 가입자에게 비용을 전가하는 민간 보험 프로그램, 환자뿐만 아니라 고용주가 부담하기 때문에 모든 사회 구성원이 그 영향을 받는다. 결과적으로 개인이 심각한 손상을 입으면 모두가 비용을 지불한다. 2019년 미국 질병통제예방센터는 직접 의료비용(3,270억 달러)과 업무 손실 잠재 수명 손실 기간 가치, 삶의 질 손실 비용을 포함하여 손상 비용으로 4조 2,000억 달러가 발생한 것으로 추정했다. 세계보건기구의 데이터에 따르면 예방 활동이 좋은 투자임을 알 수 있다.

- 오토바이 헬멧에 1달러를 투자할 때마다 32달러의 의료비를 절약

표 16-2 연령대별 손상 관련 사망 원인 순위(2020년)

	\+ 1	1-4	5-9	10-14	15-24	25-34	35-44	45-54	55-64	65 +	모든 연령
					연령대						
의도하지 않은 손상	4위	1위	1위	1위	1위	1위	1위	3위	4위	8위	4위(200,955)
의도적 손상											
자살	*	*	10위	2위	3위	2위	4위	7위	9위	*	*
살인	*	3위	4위	4위	3위	2위	7위	10위	*	*	*

*해당 데이터 없음/상위 10대 사망 원인에 포함되지 않거나 사용할 수 있는 데이터

Data from Centers for Disease Control and Prevention, National Center for Injury Prevention and Control. 10 leading causes of death, United States, 2020, all races, both sexes. Web-based Injury Statistics Query and Reporting System (WISQARS) website. Accessed March 2, 2022. https://www.cdc.gov/injury/wisqars/

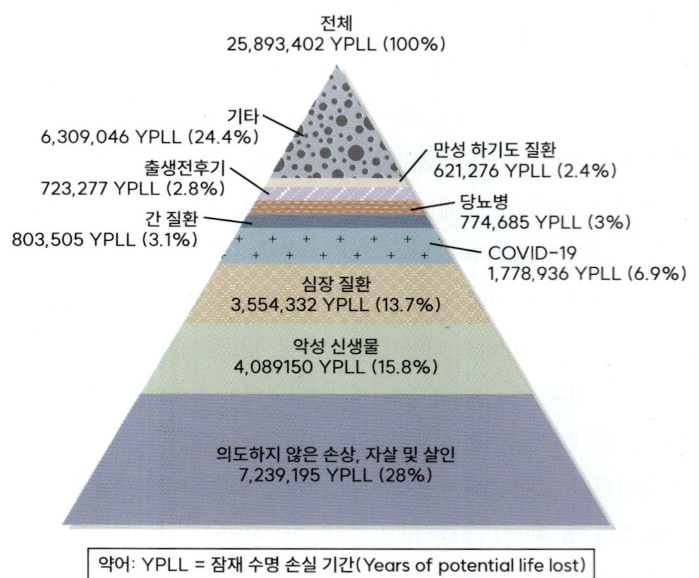

그림 16-4 75세 이전에 잃어버린 잠재 수명 손실 기간

Data from Centers for Disease Control and Prevention, National Center for Injury Prevention and Control. Years of potential life lost (YPLL) before age 75, 2020 United States, all races, both sexes, all deaths. Web-based Injury Statistics Query and Reporting System (WISQARS) website. Accessed March 2, 2022. https://www.cdc.gov/injury/wisqars/

할 수 있다.

- 안전띠는 튕겨 나갈 위험과 중상 또는 치명적인 손상을 입을 위험을 40%~65% 감소시키며 1975년~2008년까지 약 255,000명의 생명을 구했다.

이환율, 사망률 및 경제적 스트레스 측면에서 손상으로 인한 피해는 너무 과도하다. 크리스토펠과 갤러거는 다음과 같이 말했다.

손상은 항상 공공의 안녕에 위협이 되어 왔지만, 20세기 중반까지만 해도 전염병은 사람의 이환율과 사망률에 미치는 끔찍한 영향을 무색하게 했다. 다른 분야에서 공중보건이 개선되면서 손상을 "방치된 전염병"이라고 부린 정도로 공중 보건의 주요 위협으로 남았다.

사회는 의료계의 모든 분야에서 예방 활동을 강화할 것을 촉구하고 있다. 미국의 구급차협회에 따르면 미국에서만 840,600명에 달하는 병원 전 처치 제공자가 있는 만큼 EMS 시스템은 지역 사회에서 손상 예방 노력에 크게 기여할 수 있다.

친한 동료의 폭력

친한 동료의 폭력(IPV)은 현재 또는 이전의 친한 동료에 의한 신체적 폭력, 성폭력, 심리적 공격 또는 스토킹으로 정의된다. CDC의 친한 동료 및 성폭력 설문조사에서는 성폭력 및 친한 동료 폭력에 대한 자료를 수집한다. 미국에서는 여성의 1/3 이상(36.4%)이 친한 동료

에 의한 성폭력(18.3%), 신체적 폭력(30.6%), 스토킹(10.4%)을 경험한 것으로 나타났다. 마찬가지로 남성의 약 1/3이 평생 교제 중 성폭력(8.2%), 신체적 폭력(31%), 스토킹(2.2%)을 경험한 것으로 나타났다. 마지막으로 여성의 36.4%가 친한 동료로부터 한 번 이상 심리적 공격 행위를 경험했다고 답해 남성(34.2%)보다 높았다.

직업군의 특성상 응급구조사는 환자와 현장의 다른 사람들 사이의 역학 관계를 관찰할 수 있는 독특한 위치에 있다. 친한 동료에 의한 폭력의 징후는 다음과 같다.

- 지나치게 보호적인 동료. 가해자는 피해자가 학대에 관해 이야기할지도 모른다는 생각에 피해자를 혼자 두는 것을 주저할 수 있다.
- 학대자가 질투하거나 통제하는 행동
- 지나치게 소심한 환자. 눈을 마주치는 것을 피하거나 질문을 할 때 동료에게 미루는 환자를 만날 수 있다.
- 설명할 수 없는 손상이나 반복적인 손상. 환자는 눈이나 목에 멍이 든 것에 관해 설명하지 않으려 하거나 치유 단계에 따라 신체에 멍이 들거나 골절 병력이 있을 수 있다.

친한 동료의 폭력이 의심되는 경우 경찰에 신고를 한다. 구급대원도 이러한 출동에서 2차 피해자가 될 수 있는 특수한 위치에 있다. 이러한 출동에서는 항상 자신의 안전에 특히 주의를 기울이고 높은 수준의 상황 인식을 유지한다. 가해자와 대면하는 것은 EMS 요원의 의무가 아니라는 점을 기억한다. 이는 위험한 행동이다.

EMS 제공자의 손상

EMS 제공자는 손상을 초래할 수 있는 다양한 상황에 노출되어 있다. 이러한 현장에서는 정서적, 신체적 위기에 처한 사람들이 포함되기 때문에 EMS 제공자와 경찰관의 노력에도 불구하고 안전이 보장되지 않는 경우가 많다. EMS 제공자가 업무 중 폭행을 당하거나 총에 맞거나 다른 방식으로 공격을 당했다는 보고가 정기적으로 접수되고 있다. 응급 업무의 특성상 손상을 입을 수 있는 상황이 많다. 현장으로 출동하는 것만으로도 위험할 수 있다. 환자 들기, 위험한 환경 및 전염병에 대한 노출, 수면 부족 및 업무로 인한 스트레스도 손상을 초래할 기회를 제공한다. 직면한 비극적인 상황은 종종 우울증, 불안, 외상 후 스트레스 장애(PTSD)를 유발하며 이는 병원 전 처치 제공자에게 심각한 신체적 영향을 미칠 뿐만 아니라 추가적인 심리적 스트레스를 유발할 수 있다.

수면 부족은 병원 전 처처 제공자의 건강과 업무 수행에 분명한 영향을 미치는 중요한 요소이다. 깨어 있는 시간이 길어질수록 피로와

졸음이 심해지고 반응시간, 의학적 의사 결정 및 판단력 장애가 커지며 실수, 본인 또는 타인의 손상, 심지어 사망의 가능성도 커진다. 수면 부족은 알코올 중독과 비교되어 18시간 동안 잠을 자지 않으면 혈중알코올농도(BAC) 0.05%와 비슷하고 24시간 동안 잠을 자지 않으면 혈중알코올농도 0.1%와 가까워진다.

또한, 수면 부족은 병원 전 처치 제공자의 건강에 심각한 영향을 미칠 수 있으며 중요한 개인 및 가족 관계에 지장을 줄 수 있다. 수면 부족은 과민성, 불안, 우울증으로 이어질 수 있다.

2011년에 발표한 연구에서는 2003~2007년까지 응급구조사와 구급대원의 치명적인 손상과 치명적이지 않은 손상을 검토했다. 연구자는 미국 노동통계청의 치명적인 산업재해 인구조사 데이터와 국가전자 손상 감시 시스템의 직업적 부분을 검토했다. 그 결과 해당 기간 99,400명의 치명적이지 않은 손상과 65명의 사망자를 발견했다. 대부분의 사망자는 자동차 충돌(45%)이나 항공기 추락(31%)과 같은 교통 관련 사고였다. 정규직에 해당하는 EMS 종사자의 사망률은 10만 명당 7명이었다. 일반적으로 급여를 받는 EMS 제공자의 사망률은 인구 10만 명당 6.3명이다. 이에 비해 같은 기간 소방관의 사망률은 10만 명당 6.1명, 전체 근로자의 사망률은 10만 명당 4명이었다. 이번 보고서에서 유일하게 다행인 점은 10년 전 보고서보다 사망자 수가 낮아졌다는 점이다.

이 수치는 충격적인 진실을 드러낸다. 개리슨에 따르면

> EMS 종사자에게 가장 위험한 시간은 이동 중인 구급차 안에 있거나 차량 충돌 현장에서 작업할 때 다른 차량이 접근하는 것이다.

EMS 제공자가 손상 및 손상 예방의 개념을 알고 이해하여 구급차에 내재한 위험을 파악하고 수정할 수 있도록 하는 것이 중요하다. 교육 첫날부터 교육생들은 현장에서 병원 전 처치 제공자보다 더 중요한 사람은 없으므로 자신의 안전을 최우선으로 해야 한다고 것을 배운다. 구급차 안에서 안전띠를 착용하는 것은 안전을 위한 첫걸음이다.

국가 EMS 안전 문화 프로젝트는 2009년 미국 EMS 자문위원회(NEMSAC)가 미국 교통부 산하 고속도로 안전관리국(NHTSA)에 EMS 안전 향상을 위한 전략을 수립하라는 권고에 따라 시작되었다. 미국 응급의학회(ACEP)와 어린이 EMS(EMSC) 프로그램은 소방 및 EMS 그룹의 다른 주요 참여자와 함께 이 프로젝트에 참여하여 6가지 핵심 요소를 포함하는 전략에 합의했다.

- 실수나 아차사고에 대한 보고를 장려하여 향후 오류를 방지할 수 있도록 하는 정의로운 문화
- 전국 기관 간의 지원 및 자원 조정
- 병원 전 처치 제공자와 환자 안전 데이터 시스템을 통해 이러한 문제의 범위를 더 잘 이해할 수 있음
- 이러한 주제에 대한 더 나은 교육을 포함하도록 EMS 교육의 변화
- 충분한 증거를 바탕으로 한 안전기준 공포
- 사고 보고 및 조사

해결책으로로서의 예방

가장 이상적인 것은 처음부터 손상이 발생하지 않도록 예방하여 손상 발생 후 처치할 필요가 없도록 하는 것이다. 손상을 예방하면 환자와 가족이 고통과 경제적 어려움에서 벗어날 수 있다. 미국 질병통제예방센터(CDC) 산하 국립 손상 예방통제센터(NCIPC)는 상위 5대 주요 원인으로 인한 사망의 최대 40%가 예방할 수 있는 것으로 추정하고 있다.

숙주, 병인 및 환경은 언제든지 변할 수 있으므로 의료진이 항상 모든 개별 손상을 예측하거나 예방할 수는 없다. 그러나 고위험군(병원 전 처치 제공자 포함), 고위험 제품, 고위험 환경을 식별하는 것은 가능하다. 고위험군 또는 환경에 초점을 맞춘 예방 노력은 가능한 한 광범위한 사회에 영향을 미친다. 의료 제공자는 다양한 방법으로 예방을 추구할 수 있다. 일부 전략은 미국과 전 세계에서 성공적인 것으로 입증되었다. 그러나 다른 전략은 한 지역에서는 효과가 있지만 다른 지역에서는 효과가 없는 예도 있다. 손상 예방 전략을 실행하기 전에 해당 전략의 효과 여부를 판단하는 데 중점을 두어야 한다. 재창조할 필요는 없지만, 의료 제공자는 성공의 가능성을 높이기 위해 예방 전략을 수정해야 할 수도 있다. 이를 위한 방법은 다음 부문에서 검토한다.

손상 예방의 개념

목표

손상 예방 프로그램의 목표는 이전에 파악된 사회 구성원의 지식, 태도 및 행동에 변화를 가져오는 것이다. 잠재적인 피해자에게 단순히 정보를 제공하는 것만으로는 손상을 예방할 수 없다. 프로그램은 사회의 태도에 영향을 미치고 가장 중요한 행동의 변화를 가져올 수 있는 방식으로 실행되어야 한다. 행동의 변화는 장기적으로 지속되기를 바란다. 이 작업은 기념비적이지만, 극복할 수 없는 것은 아니다.

개입할 기회

예방 전략은 손상 사건에 미치는 영향에 따라 마련할 수 있다. 이러한 전략은 해든 매트릭스의 시간적 단계와 일치한다. 일차 개입으로 알려진 사고 발생 전 개입은 손상 발행을 예방하기 위해 노력한다. 음주 운전자가 운전하지 못하게 하기 위한 조치, 운전 중 문자 메시지를 금지하는 법, 신호등 설치 조치 등은 충돌 사고를 예방하기 위해 고안된 것이다. 사고 단계 개입은 발생한 손상의 타격을 완화하여 손상의 심각성을 줄이기 위한 것이다. 안전띠 작용 의무화, 차량에 쿠션이 있는 대시보드와 에어백 설치, 어린이 안전 시트에 관한 법률 시행 등은 충돌 사고로 인한 손상의 심각성을 줄이기 위한 수단이다. 사고 후 개입은 손상을 입은 환자의 생존 가능성을 높일 수 있는 수단을 제공한다. 체력 단련을 장려하고 충돌 시 폭발하지 않는 차량용 연료 시스템을 설계하며 고품질의 EMS 시스템을 구현하는 것은 손상을 입은 환자의 회복 시간을 단축하기 위한 것이다.

병원 전 시스템은 전통적으로 지역사회의 개입을 사고 발생 후 단계로 제한해 왔다. 그 결과 수많은 생명을 구했지만, 손상이 발생할 때까지 기다리는 데 내재한 한계로 인해 최상의 결과를 얻지 못했다. EMS 시스템은 손상 주기에 더 일찍 진입하는 방법을 모색해야 한다. 해든 매트릭스를 사용하면 EMS 시스템은 다른 공중보건 및 공공 안전 기관과 협력하여 손상이 발생을 예방하거나 충격을 환화할 수 있는 기회를 파악할 수 있다.

잠재적 전략

손상 예방을 위한 최선의 전략은 없다. 가장 효과적인 선택은 손상의 유형에 따라 다르다. 그러나 해든은 여러 지점에서 손상을 유발하는 사건의 사슬을 끊기 위해 고안된 10가지 일반 전략 목록을 개발했다 (**표 16-3**). 이러한 전략은 통제되지 않은 에너지의 방출을 방지하거나 최소한 신체가 더 잘 견딜 수 있는 양으로 줄이는 방법을 나타낸다. **표 16-3**은 사고 전 단계, 사고 단계 및 사고 후 단계에서 취할 수 있는 대응책과 숙주, 병인 또는 환경을 대상으로 하는 대응책도 제시한다. 이 목록은 완전한 것이 아니며 현재 직면하고 있는 특정 문제에 대한 가장 효과적인 선택을 결정하는 데 도움이 되는 출발점 역할을 할 뿐이다.

대부분의 손상 예방 전략은 능동적이거나 수동적이다. 수동적 전략은 개인의 조치가 거의 또는 전혀 필요하지 않다. 스프링클러 시스템과 차량 에어백이 그 예이다. 능동적 전략은 보호 대상자의 협력이 필요하다. 예를 들어, 수동 안전띠 착용, 오토바이 또는 자전거 헬멧 착용 등이 그 예이다. 수동적 조치는 일반적으로 사람들이 보호를 받기 위해 의식적으로 무언가를 할 필요가 없으므로 더 효과적이다. 하지만, 수동적 전략은 비용이 많이 들거나 입법 또는 규제 조치가 필요할 수 있으므로 일반적으로 실행하기가 더 어렵다. 때로는 능동적 전력과 수동적 전략의 조합이 최선의 선택이 될 수도 있다.

전략 실행

손상 예방 전략을 실행하기 위한 네 가지 일반적인 접근 방법은 손상 예방의 4E(교육, 집행, 기술, 형평성)로 알려져 있다. 이러한 각 요소는 아래에 설명되어 있다.

교육

교육 전략은 정보를 전달하기 위한 것이다. 교육 대상은 고위험 활동에 참여하는 개인, 추가 예방 법안이나 규제를 제정할 권한이 있는 정책 입안자, 손상 예방에 적극적으로 참여하는 방법을 배우는 병원 전 처치 제공자 등이 될 수 있다.

한때 사회는 대부분의 손상이 단순히 사람의 실수로 인한 것이라고 믿었기 때문에 교육이 예방 프로그램을 실행하는 주요 수단이었다. 이러한 가정은 어느 정도 사실이지만, 많은 사람이 에너지와 환경이 손상을 유발하는 데 어떤 역할을 하는지 인식하지 못했다. 그러나 교육은 여전히 자주 사용되며 네 가지 전략 중 가장 쉽게 실행하는 방법일 것이다.

경험에 따르면 교육 전략은 여러 가지 이유로 인해 압도적인 성공을 거두지 못했다. 우선 대상들이 메시지를 듣지 못할 수도 있다. 메시지를 듣더라도 일부는 노골적으로 거부하거나 행동을 바꿀 만큼 충분히 수용하지 않을 수 있다. 메시지를 받아들인다고 해도 산발적으로 받아들이거나 시간이 지남에 따라 열의가 줄어들 수 있다. 그러나 교육은 다음 네 가지 영역에서 손상을 줄이는 데 특히 유용할 수 있다.

1. 어린아이들에게 나중에 평생 간직할 수 있는 기본적인 안전 행동과 기술을 가르친다. 예를 들면 연기 감지기가 경보음을 울릴 때 적절하게 대응하거나 응급상황에서 119에 도움을 요청하는 방법, 안전띠 매기 등이 있다.
2. 특정 연령대의 특정 유형과 원인에 대해 교육한다. 교육은 이러한 그룹에 사용할 수 있는 유일한 전략일 수 있다.

표 16-3 손상 대책을 위한 기본 전략

전략	가능한 대책	전략	가능한 대책
위험의 초기 생성을 방지한다.	■ 폭죽, 삼륜 전지형 차량 또는 각종 독극물을 제조하지 않는다. ■ 고등학교 미식축구장에서 스피어링을 제거한다.	물질적 장벽으로 보호해야 할 위험과 위험 요소를 분리한다.	■ 수영장의 모든 면에 울타리를 설치한다. ■ **스포츠 및 직업적 위험에 대비해 보호안경 착용을 권장한다.** ■ 고속도로 중앙분리대를 설치한다. ■ 위험한 기계 주변에 보호막을 설치한다. ■ 인도와 도로 사이에 가드레일을 설치한다. ■ 차량 문에 강화 패널을 설치한다. ■ **의료 종사자가 사용한 주삿바늘을 폐기물 통에 직접 버리도록 요구한다.** ■ **오토바이, 자전거, 고위험 스포츠 활동 시 헬멧 착용을 의무화한다.**
위험 요소에 포함된 에너지의 양을 줄인다.	■ 자동차 엔진의 마력을 제한한다. ■ 독성 약품을 더 작고 안전한 양으로 포장한다. ■ **속도 제한을 준수한다.** ■ 도로에 개인 소유 차량의 수를 줄이기 위해 대중교통 개선을 의무화한다. ■ **가정용 온수기의 온도를 낮추도록 권장한다.** ■ 총기의 총구 속도를 제한한다. ■ 폭죽의 화약량을 제한한다.		
		위험의 기본 특성을 수정한다.	■ 차량에 에어백을 제공한다. ■ 접을 수 있는 스티어링 칼럼을 제공한다. ■ 분리형 기둥을 제공한다. ■ 아기 침대 칸막이를 너무 좁게 만들어 아기의 목을 조이지 않도록 한다. ■ 분리형 야구 베이스를 도입한다. ■ **노약자 가정에 깔개를 제거한다.**
이미 존재하는 위험 요소의 방출을 방지한다.	■ **총기는 총기함에 보관하거나 총기 자물쇠를 사용한다.** ■ 안전요원이 근무하지 않을 때는 수영장과 해변을 폐쇄한다. ■ **욕조와 샤워실에는 미끄럼 방지 표면을 사용하도록 권장한다.** ■ 모든 유해 가정용 약품 및 화학물질은 어린이 보호용 용기를 사용하도록 한다. ■ **차량 내에서 휴대전화 사용 제한하거나 핸즈프리 모델을 사용한다.** ■ 회전식 농기계에 안전 보호막 설치를 의무화한다. ■ 차량 핸들링을 개선한다.	보호해야 할 대상을 위험에 더 잘 견디도록 만든다.	■ **골다공증을 줄이기 위해 칼슘 섭취를 권장한다.** ■ **직접 압박, 가슴압박 심폐소생술, 기타 교육과 같은 캠페인을 홍보하여 대중에게 응급상황을 대처하는 방법을 가르친다.** ■ 운동선수의 근골격계 조절을 장려한다. ■ 뇌전증과 같은 질환을 치료하여 화상, 익사, 낙상으로 이어질 수 있는 사고를 예방한다. ■ 지진에 취약한 지역의 내진 건축 규정을 확인한다.
위험의 비율 또는 공간 분포를 수정한다.	■ **안전띠와 어린이용 안전 시트를 사용해야 한다.** ■ 잠김 방지 브레이크를 제공한다. ■ 축구화에 짧은 클리트 사용을 권장하여 무릎에 갑작스러운 힘이 전달되지 않고 발이 회전할 수 있도록 한다. ■ 차량용 에어백 설치를 의무화한다. ■ 차량에 유압식 범퍼를 제공한다. ■ 작업자의 추락을 방지하기 위해 안전띠를 제공한다. ■ **난연성 잠옷 사용을 권장한다.**	위험으로 인해 이미 발생한 피해에 대응하기 시작한다.	■ **응급의료서비스를 제공한다.** ■ **공항, 체육관, 학교 등 공공장소에 AED를 비치한다.** ■ 환자를 적절한 교육을 받은 병원 전 처치 제공자에게 안내하는 시스템을 도입한다. ■ **응급상황에 대응할 수 있도록 학교 프로토콜을 개발한다.** ■ **주민들에게 응급처치 교육을 제공한다.** ■ 자동 스프링클러 시스템을 설치한다.
위험 요소와 보호해야 할 요소를 시간 또는 공간적으로 분리한다.	■ 통행량이 많은 교차로에 보행자용 육교를 설치한다. ■ 도로변에 전봇대나 나무가 없도록 한다. ■ 보호자가 없는 수역 근처에 놀이 공간을 만들지 않는다. ■ 자전거 도로를 설치한다. ■ 살충제를 사람이 없는 시간에 살포한다. ■ 인도를 설치한다. ■ 위험 물질을 운반하는 트럭은 교통량이 적은 도로를 따라 운행한다. ■ **가정에서 연기 감지기 설치를 권장한다.**	피해 대상을 안정화, 수리 및 복구한다.	■ 손상 처치 초기 단계에서 재활 계획을 수립한다. ■ 하반신 마비 환자를 위한 직업 재활을 활용한다.

*나열된 예는 설명을 위한 것일 뿐이며 PHTLS, NAEMT 및 미국 외과학회 외상위원회의 공식 권장 사항은 아니다.

굵게 표시된 것은 EMS 제공자의 교육 및 리더십을 제공할 수 있는 기회를 나타낸다.

3. 위험과 허용할 수 있는 위험에 대한 대중의 인식을 변화시켜 사회적 규범과 태도를 변화시킨다. 이러한 접근 방식은 음주 운전과 관련하여 사용되었으며 현재는 자전거, 스쿠터, 스케이트보드를 타거나 롤러블레이드를 탈 때 헬멧을 착용하는 것과 관련하여 이루어지고 있다.

4. 정책 변화를 촉진하고 소비자들이 더 안전한 제품을 요구하도록 교육한다.

손상 예방을 위한 단일 접근 방식인 교육 프로그램은 실망스러운 결과를 가져왔다. 많은 약물과 마찬가지로 교육도 일정 기간이 지난 후 다시 교육해야 지속적인 효과를 얻을 수 있다. 그러나 다른 형태의 실행 전략과 결합하면 교육은 유용한 도구가 될 수 있다. 교육은 종종 시행 및 기술 전략을 위한 길을 닦는 출발점 역할을 한다.

시행

시행은 법의 설득력을 활용하여 간단하지만, 효과적인 예방 전략의 준수를 강제하고자 한다. 법적 명령은 요구하거나 금지할 수 있으며 다음과 같이 개인의 행동, 제품 또는 환경 조건을 대상으로 할 수 있다.

- 사람들에게 적용되는 법적 요건으로는 안전띠 착용 의무화, 소아용 안전 시트 착용 의무화, 헬멧 착용 의무화 등이 있다.
- 사람들에게 적용되는 금지 사항으로는 음주 운전 법규, 제한 속도 및 폭행 법규 등이 있다.
- 제품에 적용되는 법적 요건에는 연방 자동차 안전 표준과 같은 설계 및 성능 표준이 포함된다.
- 제품에 적용되는 금지 사항에는 위험한 동물이나 인화성 섬유에 대한 제한이 포함된다.
- 장소에 적용되는 법적 요건에는 고속도로를 따라 이정표와 가드레일 설치, 수영장 주변에 펜스 설치 등이 있다.
- 장소에 적용되는 금지 사항에는 학교와 공항 터미널에서의 총기 조지 금지가 포함된다.
- 특정 대상 그룹 및 장소에 적용되는 법적 요건에는 교통량이 많은 사고 현장에서 공공 안전 및 구조대원이 눈에 잘 띄는 옷을 착용해야 한다는 정부의 요구사항이 포함된다.

사람들이 법의 혜택을 받으려면 법을 준수해야 하므로 법의 실행은 적극적인 대응책이다. 지침이 개인의 자유를 침해한다고 생각하거나 적발될 가능성이 거의 없거나 법 위반으로 인한 불이익을 받지 않으면 대상자는 지침을 준수할 가능성이 낮을 수 있다.

사회 전체가 법을 준수하거나 최소한 법의 테두리 안에서만, 지키려는 경향이 있으므로 교육보다 법 집행이 더 효과적인 경우가 많다. 교육과 함께 법을 집행하는 것이 단독으로 시행하는 것보다 더 나은 결과를 가져오는 것으로 보인다. 오토바이 헬멧 착용에 관한 법률은 손상 예방에 있어 법 집행의 역할에 대한 흥미로운 사례 연구를 제공한다. 오토바이 운전자에 대한 헬멧 착용과 관련된 법이 폐지된 주에서는 심각한 손상과 사망자 비율이 증가했다.

기술

가장 효과적인 손상 예방 방법은 파괴적인 에너지 방출을 숙주로부터 영구적으로 분리되는 것이다. 수동적 대응책은 개인의 노력을 거의 또는 전혀 들이지 않고도 이러한 목표를 달성할 수 있다. 기술 전략은 제품이나 환경에 손상 방지 기능을 구축하여 숙자기 호보를 받기 위해 다른 행동을 할 필요가 없도록 하는 것이다. 기술 전략은 실제로 필요한 사람들에게 도움이 되며 매번 그렇게 한다. 건물의 자동 스프링클러 시스템, 보트의 부양 선체, 구급차의 예비 경보와 같은 조치는 모두 숙주가 거의 또는 전혀 노력하지 않고도 생명을 구할 수 있도록 고안된 것이다.

기술은 손상 예방에 대한 완벽한 해답인 것 같다. 이는 수동적이고 효과적이며 일반적으로 네 가지 4Es 중 가장 방해가 적다. 안타깝게도 실행하는 데 가장 많은 비용이 드는 경우가 많다. 제품에 안전성을 설계하면 일반적으로 비용이 더 많이 들고 입법 또는 규제를 시작해야 할 수도 있다. 제조업체가 감당할 수 있는 비용이나 고객이 기꺼이 지급할 수 있는 비용보다 더 많은 비용이 들 수도 있다. 사회는 제품에 얼마나 많은 안전 기능을 탑재하기를 원하는지 그리고 이러한 노력을 재정적으로 얼마나 지원할 의향이 있는지를 결정한다.

교육의 새로운 계획 시행 및 기술 전략보다 선행되어야 한다. 궁극적으로 가장 효과적인 대응책은 네 가지 실행 전략을 모두 통합한 대응책일 수 있다.

형평성

형평성은 흔히 손상 예방의 네 번째 E로 설명된다. 형평성은 인구 내 손상 위험의 격차를 줄이기 위해 노력할 때 다른 세 가지 요소에 모두 적용된다는 점에서 다른 세 가지 요소와 구별된다.

교육 측면에서는 고위험군을 대상으로 한 교육이 이루어질 수 있도록 노력해야 한다. 메시지가 대상 고객에게 효과적으로 전달되려면 청중이 접근하기 쉬운 형식과 문화적으로 적합한 방식으로 전달되어야 한다.

예를 들어, 사람들이 가정 내 실내 난방기의 위험성을 이해하도록 돕는 것은 대체 난방 수단을 확보하기 위한 노력이 함께 이루어지지 않는다면 효과적이지 않다. 위험에 대중의 인식을 바꾸려면 커뮤니티에서 위험의 정도와 완화에 대한 대화가 필요하다. 헬멧을 쓰지 않고 스케이트보드를 타지 말라고 말하는 것은 머리 손상과 스케이트보드 사고의 결과에 대한 정확한 정보를 제공하고 헬멧을 구하는 방법을 알려주는 것과 병행할 때보다 효과가 떨어진다.

특히, 위험에 처한 집단이 직면한 다양한 문제를 고려하지 않아 불평등이 발생하는 경우가 많으므로 외상으로 인한 손상 위험을 완화하기 위한 모든 개입의 형평성 렌즈를 적용한다.

공중 보건 접근법

손상과 손상 예방에 관해 많은 것이 밝혀졌다. 안타깝게도 손상에 대해 알려진 사실과 실제로 시행되고 있는 조치 사이에는 큰 차이가 존재한다. 손상은 전 세계 모든 사회에서 복잡한 문제이다. 안타깝게도 한 사람이나 한 기관의 노력만으로는 별다른 영향을 미치지 못하는 경우가 많다. 공중 보건 접근 방법을 취함으로써 질병에 대처하는 데 성공을 거두었으며 이와 같은 접근 방법은 손상 예방에도 진전을 보인다. 다른 공공 및 민간 기관과 힘을 합친 EMS 기관은 스스로 할 수 있는 것만큼, 혹은 그 이상의 성과를 거둘 수 있었다. 파트너십은 복잡하고 난해한 문제를 해결하기 위해 커뮤니티의 전문성을 한데 모으는 역할을 한다.

공중 보건 접근 방법은 다음과 같이 4단계 과정을 통해 지역사회 기반 질병을 퇴치하기 위한 지역사회 기반 연합을 구성한다.

1. 감시
2. 위험 요소 파악
3. 개입 평가
4. 실행

이 연합은 역학, 의료계, 공중보건학교, 공공보건기관, 지역사회 지지 프로그램, 경제학, 사회학 그리고 사법제도와 같은 다양한 분야의 전문가로 구성되어 있다. EMS 시스템은 손상 예방에 대한 공중보건 접근 방식에서 중요한 위치를 차지한다. 놀이터의 안전을 개선하기 위한 연합에 참여한다고 해서 끔찍한 차량 충돌 사고 현장에서 즉각적인 처치 효과가 나타나지 않을 수도 있지만, 그 결과는 훨씬 더 광범위하게 나타날 것이다.

감시

감시는 지역사회 내에서 자료를 수집하는 과정이다. 인구 기반 자료를 수집하면 손상의 실제 규모와 지역사회에 미치는 영향을 파악하는 데 도움이 된다. 지역사회는 시, 군, 구 또는 구급차 서비스 자체일 수 있다. 프로그램에 대한 지원, 적절한 자원 분배 그리고 여러 전문 분야의 틈에 포함할 사람을 정하는 것도 문제의 범위를 이해하는데 달려있다.

지역사회 내에서 이용할 수 있는 정보 출처는 다음과 같다.

- 사망률 데이터
- 입원 및 퇴원 통계
- 의료 기록
- 외상 등록
- 경찰 보고서
- EMS 출동 기록지
- 보험 보고서
- 현재 진행 중인 연구 목적으로 수집된 고유한 감시 데이터

위험 요인 확인

문제를 파악하고 조사한 후에는 올바른 집단에 예방 전략을 지시하기 위해 누가 위험에 처해 있는지 알아야 한다. 손상 예방에 대한 "샷건" 접근 방식은 표적화된 접근 방식보다 성공률이 낮다. 원인과 위험 요인을 파악하면 누가, 언제, 어디서 어떤 유형의 손상을 입었는지 알 수 있다. 치명적인 차량 충돌 시 음주 운전과 같은 위험 요인이 명백한 예도 있다. 다른 경우에는 손상 사고와 관련된 실제 위험 요인을 발견하기 위한 연구가 필요하다. EMS 시스템은 손상이 발생한 현장에서 공중 보건의 "눈과 귀" 임무를 수행하여 다른 사람이 발견할 수 없는 위험 요인을 식별할 수 있다. 그런 다음 위험 요인이 적절하게 확인되면 해든 매트릭스로 도표로 표시할 수 있다.

개입 평가

위험 요인이 명확해지면 개입 전략이 등장하기 시작한다. 해든의 10가지 손상 예방 전략 목록이 출발점이 될 수 있다(**표 16-3** 참조). 지역사회마다 특성이 다르지만, 약간의 수정을 거치면 한 지역사회의 손상 예방의 새로운 계획이 다른 지역에서도 효과가 있을 수 있다. 잠재적인 가입이 선택되면 네 가지 중 하나 이상을 사용하는 시범 프로그램을 통해 본격적인 실행의 성공 여부를 알 수 있다.

실행

공중보건 접근 방법의 마지막 단계는 개입의 실행과 평가이다. 유사한 프로그램 실행에 관심이 있는 다른 사람들이 따를 수 있도록 세부 실행 절차가 준비되어 있다. 평가 자료 수집은 프로그램의 효율성을 측정한다. 다음 세 가지 질문에 답하면 프로그램의 성공 여부를 판단하는 데 도움이 될 수 있다.

1. 태도, 기술 또는 판단력이 바뀌었는가?
2. 행동에 변화가 생겼는가?
3. 행동 변화가 긍정적인 결과로 이어졌는가?

공중보건 접근 방식은 손상과 같은 질병을 퇴치할 수 있는 입증된 수단을 제공한다. 여러 전문 분야의 공동체에 기반을 둔 노력을 통해 "누가, 무엇을, 어디서, 언제, 왜"를 파악하고 손상 문제를 해결하기 위해 행동 계획을 개발할 수 있다. EMS 시스템은 손상에 대해 알려진 사실과 이에 대한 조치 사이의 격차를 좁히는 데 훨씬 더 실질적인 임무를 수행해야 한다. 이러한 접근 방법은 연속적인 고리로 생각할 수 있다. 손상 관리 전략을 실행한 후에도 지속적인 감시가 이루어진다. 이러한 데이터는 전략을 수정하거나 변경하는 데 사용된다. 손상 예방의 성공은 위험에 처한 더 많은 인구로 확대될 수 있다.

손상 예방에서 EMS의 역할 변환

전통적으로 의료 분야에서 병원 전 처치 제공자의 역할은 거의 전적으로 사건 발생 개인에 대한 일대일 처치에 집중되었다. 손상의 원인이나 손상을 예방하기 위해 병원 전 처치 제공자가 할 수 있는 일을 이해하는 데는 거의 중점을 두지 않았다. 그 결과 환자는 같은 환경으로 돌아갔다가 다시 손상을 입을 수 있다. 또한 다른 사람이 손상을 입지 않도록 하기 위한 지역사회 차원의 예방 프로그램 개발에 도움이 될 수 있는 정보가 문서로 만들어지지 않아 공중보건 부문에서 사용할 수 없는 상태로 남아 있을 수 있다.

손상에 대한 공중보건 접근 방식은 보다 사전 예방적이다. 손상을 예방하기 위해 숙주, 인자 및 환경을 변경하는 방법을 결정하기 위해 노력한다. 공중 보건은 감시를 수행하고 개입을 실행하는 연합을 통해 지역 사회 전체의 예방 프로그램을 개발하기 위해 노력한다. 미래를 위한 EMS 의제는 EMS 시스템과 공중보건 사이의 긴밀한 연계를 통해 건강관리의 두 의료 부문을 더욱 효과적으로 만들 수 있는 방안을 만들 것이다. 지역사회 응급의료 실천은 EMS가 손상 및 질병 예방의 이러한 측면에 더 많이 관여하게 된 한 가지 방법이다.

병원 전 처치 제공자는 지역사회 전반의 손상 예방 프로그램 개발에 더욱 적극적인 임무를 수행할 수 있다. EMS 시스템은 지역사회에서 독보적인 위치를 차지하고 있다. 미국에서만 100만 명이 넘는 응급구조사가 있으며 기본 및 전문 응급구조사가 지역사회 수준에 널리 분포되어 있다. 병원 전 처치 제공자는 지역사회에서 신뢰할 수 있는 평판을 얻고 있어 주목받는 본보기가 되고 있다. 또한, 이들은 가정과 사업체에서도 쉽게 환영받는다. 손상 예방에 대한 공중보건 접근 방식의 모든 단계에 EMS가 있으면 도움이 된다.

일대일 개입

EMS 시스템은 귀중한 손상 예방 개입을 수행하기 위해 환자 처처에 대한 일대일로 접근 방식을 포기할 필요가 없다. 일대일 접근 방식을 통해 EMS 시스템을 손상 예방 새로운 계획을 수행할 수 있게 한다. 병원 전 처치 제공자는 고위험군 환자에게 직접 손상 예방 메시지를 전달할 수 있다. 성공적인 교육 프로그램의 한 가지 지표는 행동을 변화시키기에, 충분한 열정을 가지고 정보를 받아들이는 것이다. 병원 전 처치 제공자는 자신의 역할 모델 지위를 활용하여 중요한 예방 메시지를 전달할 수 있다. 사람들은 암묵적으로 롤 모델을 존경하고 그들의 말에 귀를 기울이며 그들이 하는 행동을 모방한다.

현장 예방 상담은 "가르칠 수 있는 순간"을 활용한다. 가르칠 수 있는 순간이란 중요한 의학적 개입이 필요하지 않은 환자나 환자의 가족이 롤 모델의 말을 더 잘 받아들일 수 있는 상태에 있을 때를 말한다. 병원 전 처치 제공자는 의학적 개입이 거의 또는 전혀 필요하지 않다는 것이 명백해지면 현장에 있는 시간이 낭비되었다고 생각할 수 있다. 그러나 이 시기가 일차 예방을 시행하기에 가장 좋은 시기일 수 있다.

모든 도움 요청에서 손상 예방 상담을 받을 수 있는 것은 아니다. 심각하고 생명을 위협하는 신고는 급성 치료에 집중해야 한다. 하지만 구급차 출동 중 95%는 생명을 위협하지 않는다. 구급차 출동 중 상당수는 경미한 처치가 필요한 경우이다. 이러한 위급하지 않은 출동에는 일대일 예방 상담이 적절할 수 있다.

환자와 상호작용은 일반적으로 처치가 거의 또는 필요하지 않은 짧은 만남이다. 하지만 환자와 가족에게 향후 손상을 예방하는 방법을 논의하고 시연할 수 있는 충분한 시간을 제공한다. 병원 전 처치 제공자는 환자의 환경에 들어가는 유일한 의료 종사자이기 때문에 손상을 입을 수 있는 상황을 볼 수 있다는 점에서 독특한 위치에 있다. 불이 들어오지 않는 전구를 교체하는 할아버지의 추락을 방지할 수 있도록 어두운 복도 바닥에 깔아 놓은 미끄러운 카펫을 제거하는 것의 중요성에 관해 이야기하는 롤 모델을 통해서 할아버지의 추락을 방지할 수 있을 것이다. 병원 전 처치 제공자는 병원으로 이동하는 동안 세심한 주의를 기울여야 한다. 예방하는 방법을 이야기하는 것은 날씨나 스포츠에 관해 이야기하는 것보다 더 가치 있는 주제이다. 교육 시간은 1~2분 소요되며 처치나 이송에 방해가 되지 않는다.

병원 전 처치 제공자가 현장에서 손상 예방 상담을 할 수 있도록 훈련하는 교육 프로그램이 개발되었다. 이러한 유형의 프로그램을 더욱 개발하고 평가하여 어떤 프로그램이 가장 가치 있고 따라서 병원 전 처치 제공자의 기본 교육에 포함할 가치가 있는지 파악한다.

지역사회 개입

손상 예방에 대한 공중보건 접근 방식은 지역사회를 기반으로 하며 여러 전문 분야의 팀을 포함한다. 병원 전 처치 제공자는 이러한 팀의 중요한 구성원이 될 수 있는 전문성을 갖추고 있다. 지역사회 전반의 예방 전략은 손상 문제에 따라 "누가, 언제, 무엇을, 어디서, 왜"를 적절히 해결하기 위한 데이터에 의존한다. 앞서 설명한 것처럼 여러 정보 출처에서 필요한 데이터를 제공한다. 병원 전 처치 제공자는 다른 어떤 팀원보다 손상 당시 환자와 환경과의 상호작용을 조사할 기회가 많다. 이를 통해 환자가 응급실에 도착할 때까지 나타나지 않았던 고위험 개인, 고위험 태도 또는 고위험 행동을 식별할 수 있다.

병원 전 처치 제공자는 다음 두 가지 방법으로 의료시설로 이송가는 도중에 획득한 문서를 사용할 수 있다.

1. 환자를 이송하는 구급대원이 데이터를 즉시 사용할 수 있다. 응급의학 전문의와 간호사도 손상 예방에 대한 역할을 개선하고 강화해야 한다. 이미 논의되거나 시연된 내용을 알고 있는 경우 이들의 "가르칠 수 있는 순간"은 병원 전 처치 제공자의 현장 상담을 강화하고 보완할 수 있다.

2. 공중보건의 다른 사람들은 병원 전 처치 제공자의 손상 데이터를 소극적으로 사용하여 포괄적인 지역사회 전반의 손상 예방 프로그램을 개발하는 데 도움을 줄 수 있다.

병원 전 처치 제공자는 일반적으로 지역사회 전체 예방 프로그램을 지원하기 위해 문서화 작업을 하지 않는다. 지역사회 전반의 예방 프로그램 개발에 도움이 되는 정보를 언제, 어떻게 문서화해야 하는지 알기 위해서는 공중보건 팀의 다른 구성원들과 대화를 시작한다.

EMS 시스템의 리더는 공중보건 분야의 다른 사람들과 협력하여 손상에 대한 완전한 문서화를 촉진하는 문서화 정책을 개발해야 한다.

EMS는 지역사회에 큰 영향을 미치는 실행 가능하고 효과적인 손상 예방 프로그램의 선봉장이 될 수 있다. 이 프로그램은 소아 사망을 예방하고자 하는 소수의 EMS 전문가의 열망으로 만들어졌다. 노스캐롤라이나, 플로리다, 사우스캐롤라이나, 오리건, 버지니아의 서비스 및 개인은 EMS의 손상 예방 모범 사례로 니콜라스 로즈클랜즈 상을 통해 손상 예방 프로그램을 설계, 조정 및 실행한 공로로 인정받았다.

병원 전 처치 제공자가 환자를 교육할 기회가 존재하지만, 데이비드 재슬로우 박사와 동료들의 연구에 따르면 소수의 병원 전 처치 제공자만이 교육 가능한 순간을 활용하고 있는 것으로 나타났다. 연구 결과에 따르면 33%만이 손상 위험 행동을 수정하는 방법을 정기적으로 환자에게 교육하고 19%만이 적절한 보호 장치 사용에 대한 교육을 정기적으로 제공하는 것으로 나타났다.

EMS 제공자를 위한 손상 예방

"사고 현장에서 가장 중요한 사람은 누구인가?" EMS 교육생들은 항상 교육 초반에 이 질문을 받으면서 자신의 안전에 대해 생각하게 된다. 항상 한두 명의 학생이 "환자"라고 대답한다. 이러한 잘못된 답변은 강사가 손상 예방이 병원 전 처치 제공자가 제공할 수 있는 가장 가치 있는 서비스라는 점을 강조하기 위해 교육 과정 전반에 걸친 지침을 시작하도록 가르칠 수 있는 순간을 제공한다.

테러 활동이나 위험 물질 유출로 인한 적대적인 환경은 안타깝게도 뉴스에 자주 등장한다. 많은 테러 공격에는 현장에 도착한 구급대원과 구조대원을 죽이거나 다치게 하려고 고안된 2차 폭발물이 포함된다. 그러나 병원 전 처치 제공자의 일상적인 활동에서도 경력이나 삶이 끝날 수 있는 손상을 입을 수 있는 충분한 기회를 제공한다. 미국 노동통계국은 EMS에서 "일반적인" 위험에 대해 정확하게 묘사하고 있다.

EMT와 구급대원은 날씨와 관계없이 실내와 실외에서 근무한다. 이들은 무릎을 꿇고 몸을 구부리거나 무거운 물건을 들어야 한다. 이 EMT와 구급대원은 사이렌 소리로 인한 소음성 난청과 환자를 들어올리다 허리 손상을 입을 위험이 있다. 또한 EMT와 구급대원은 B형 간염, AIDS와 같은 질병에 노출될 수 있으며 약물 과다 복용자나 정신적으로 불안정한 환자의 폭력에도 노출될 수 있다. 생사를 넘나드는 상황과 고통받는 환자를 상대하는 업무는 육체적으로 힘들 뿐만 아니라 스트레스도 많이 받는다.

병원 전 처치 제공자는 도움을 요청하는 응급 환자를 처치하고 이송하는 동안 손상이나 사망에 대한 상당한 위험에 노출된다. 현장과 이동 중인 구급차에서 손상과 관련된 위험은 안전띠를 착용하거나 야광 의류와 같은 적절한 예방 조치를 활용하여 최소화할 수 있다.

병원 전 처치 제공자는 일상적인 업무의 위험에 안주할 수 있다. 안일함이란 잠재적인 위험에 직면해 있음에도 불구하고 인식하지 못하는 안전감 또는 안정감을 말한다. 일부 EMS 종사자에게 나타나는 젊은이 특유의 이상주의와 무적함도 상황을 더욱 악화시킨다. 예방 정책을 수립하고 절차를 준수하며 긍정적인 성과에 보상을 제공함으로써 손상 예방 문화 또는 더 나아가 안전 문화를 조성하기 위해서는 관리가 필요하다. 병원 전 처치 제공자도 손상 예방 원칙을 동등하게 준수해야 한다. 관리자나 병원 전 처치 제공자가 새로운 계획에 실패하면 잠재적으로 치명적인 결과를 초래할 수 있다.

고려해야 할 다른 요소로는 개인의 경험 수준과 피로도가 있다. 운전자는 차량을 안전하게 운전할 수 있도록 충분한 준비와 교육을 받아야 하며 EMS 종사자는 안전한 운행을 유지하기 위해 충분히 잘 수 있도록 모니터링 한다. 구급차 충돌 사고에 연루된 EMS 종사자의 공통 요소를 조사한 한 연구에 따르면 구급차 충돌 사고에 연루된 운전자가 젊은 EMS 종사자일 확률이 더 높았으며 수면 문제를 보고한 EMS 종사자일 사고 발생 확률이 높았다.

영국 수면학회의 닐 스탠리 박사는 "기상 후 15분에서 30분 동안은 그 누구도 정말 중요한 일을 해서는 안 된다"라고 말한다. 이는 EMS 종사자가 밤에 깨어 있든 잠을 자고 있든 관계없이 즉시 대응해야 하며 "정상적으로" 기능해야 한다는 점을 고려할 때 EMS에 심각한 영향을 미친다. 미국 도로교통안전국은 EMS의 피로와 관련된 증거를 검토하고 피로 위험 관리를 위한 권장 사항을 개발하기 위해 패널을 만든 EMS 피로 프로젝트를 지원했다. 패널의 권장 사항 중 5가지 사항은 다음과 같다.

- 피로/졸음 조사 도구를 사용하여 EMS 종사자의 피로를 측정하고 모니터링한다.
- EMS 종사자의 교대 근무 시간을 24시간보다 짧게 유지한다.
- EMS 종사자가 피로 대책으로 카페인을 섭취할 수 있도록 허용한다.
- EMS 종사자에게 근무 중 낮잠을 잘 기회를 제공하여 피로를 완화한다.
- EMS 종사자에게 피로 및 피로 관련 위험을 완화하기 위한 교육 및 훈련을 제공한다.

패널은 EMS 시스템에서 피로 완화 프로그램을 구현하려면 진정한 효과를 달성하기 위해 여러 가지 전략이 필요하다고 언급했다. 그러나 피로의 유병률과 피로 완화가 의료진과 환자 안전 모두에 미치는 중요성이 실행에 걸림돌이 되는 장애물보다 더 크다는 점을 고려해야 한다.

병원 전 처치 제공자는 가장 소중한 자산일 뿐만 아니라 가장 비싼 자산이기도 하다. 직원이 손상을 입지 않아야 서비스, 지역사회 그리고 가장 중요한 병원 전 처치 제공자에게 이익이 된다. 사내 손상 예방 프로그램은 그 자체로 가치가 있다. 많은 EMS 및 법 집행 기관은 손상의 즉각적인 처치와 재활을 위해 운동 트레이너를 직원으로 두는 것의 이점을 깨닫고 있다. 이러한 기관 중 96%는 운동 트레이너가 1년 이내에 근로자의 보상비용에 영향을 미쳐 전체 의료비용을 최대 50%까지 절감했다고 보고했다. 업무 복귀가 훨씬 빨라진다는 것은 병원 전 처치 제공자에게 심리적으로도 큰 도움이 된다.

자넷 키네 박사와 동료들은 교육, 실행, 기술 구현 전략을 활용하는 사내 예방 프로그램을 언급한다. 프로그램의 다양성은 EMS 시스템과 관련된 위험과 예방 관련 새로운 계획의 필요성을 보여준다. 또한, EMS 지역사회 간의 다양성을 보여준다. 모든 EMS 시스템이 유사하더라도 개별 서비스는 위험 요소와 예방 우선순위가 다르다.

네 가지 Es는 EMS 종사자에게 같게 적용된다. 교육 프로그램은 건강을 증진하고 허리 손상을 예방하며 폭력적인 환자의 잠재력에 대한 인식을 높인다. 시행 프로그램은 필수 체력 프로그램을 도입하고 폭력적인 환자를 안전하고 효과적으로 다루기 위한 프로토콜을 수립한다. 기술의 새로운 계획은 장비의 위치와 좌석의 위치를 평가하여 구급차 뒷좌석의 안전띠 사용률을 높이는 데 중점을 둔다. 채용 전 신체검사 및 체력 강화는 허리 손상을 줄이는 데 도움이 된다.

소규모의 사내 손상 예방 프로그램은 직원의 건강 개선이라는 가장 중요한 결과 이상의 보상을 얻을 수 있다. 작은 성공은 더 크고 복잡한 노력에 참여할 수 있는 토대를 마련한다. 이것은 모든 직원에게 손상 예방에 관한 귀중한 현장 학습 도구를 제공한다. 또한, 사내 예방 프로그램은 사내 프로그램 실행 및 평가를 지원하는 지역사회의 다른 공중 보건 기관에 EMS 시스템을 소개한다.

요 약

- 손상을 예방하는 가장 효율적이고 효과적인 방법은 처음부터 손상을 입지 않도록 예방하는 것이다.
- 질병과 손상은 비슷하다. 두 가지 모두 역학 삼각구도의 3요소인 숙주, 매개 요인, 환경이 존재해야 한다.
- 해든 매트릭스는 사고 전, 사고 단계, 사고 후 단계에서 역학 3요소를 조사하여 손상 위험을 예측하는 데 도움이 된다.
- 스위스 치즈 모델에 따르면 모든 위험에는 궤적이 있으며 일반적으로 일련의 실패가 발생해야 후속 피해가 발생할 수 있다.
- 손상은 의도적이거나 의도하지 않은 것으로 분류된다.
- 경제적, 사회적 및 발달적 문제로 인해 손상 관련 사망의 원인은 국가마다, 심지어 같은 국가 내에서도 지역마다 다르다.
- 손상은 1~44세 미국인 사망의 주요 원인이다. 손상은 다른 어떤 사망 원인보다 더 많은 잠재적 생명 손실의 원인이 된다.
- 친한 동료의 폭력은 현재 또는 과거 친한 동료에 의한 신체적 폭력, 성폭력, 심리적 공격 또는 스토킹으로 정의된다. 병원 전 처치 제공자는 친한 동료의 폭력이 의심되는 경우 해당 경찰서에 신고한다.
- 손상 예방 프로그램은 이전에 확인된 사회 부분의 지식, 태도 및 행동에 변화를 가져오는 것을 목표로 한다.
- 대부분의 손상 예방 전략은 능동적(보호 대상자의 협조가 필요함)이거나 수동적(의식적인 노력이 필요하지 않음)이다.
- 손상 여방의 4E는 교육, 집행, 기술 및 형평성이다.
- 공중보건 접근 방식은 1) 감시, 2) 위험 요소 식별, 3) 개입 평가, 4) 실행의 4단계 과정을 통해 지역사회 기반 질병에 대처하기 위한 지역사회 기반 연합을 구축한다.
- 병원 전 처치 제공자는 지역사회 전반의 손상 예방 프로그램 개발에 더욱 적극적인 임무를 수행할 수 있다. 역할 모델을 활용하여 중요한 예방 메시지를 전달할 수 있으며 가르칠 수 있는 순간을 활용한다.
- 자해 여방은 병원 전 처치 제공자가 할 수 있는 가장 가치 있는 서비스이다.

시나리오 재구성

당신과 동료는 자동차 충돌 현장에서 도착해서 비만 환자를 차량 운전석에서 신속하게 구출하기 위해 노력하고 있다. 환자는 충돌 당시 안전띠를 매지 않은 상태였다. 당신과 동료는 모두 도로에 있기 때문에 승인된 안전 조끼를 착용하고 장비를 확인하고 있다. 경찰관이 현장에 도착해서 교통 통제를 하고 있으며 구급차가 주차되어 있어 다가오는 차량으로부터 최대한 보호받을 수 있다. 환자의 무게로 인해 사용 중인 전동 주들것에 환자를 적절히 고정하였다. 전동 주들것을 사용하면 당신과 동료의 몸에 과도한 부담을 주지 않고 환자를 구급차로 안전하게 들어 올릴 수 있다.

구급차에 탑승한 후에는 환자실의 의자에 앉아 몸을 고정하고 환자를 계속 처치하는 동안 동료는 차량을 안전하게 운전하여 병원으로 이동한다. 구급차가 병원에 무사히 도착하면 응급실 의료진에게 환자를 인계한다. 환자 인계 후 서류를 작성하는 동안 병원 전 처치 제공에 대한 전반적인 국가 손상 및 사망 통계를 고려한다. 당신과 동료가 손상 예방의 모든 측면에 세심한 주의를 기울인 덕분에 관련된 모든 사람이 안전하게 출동을 마무리할 수 있었다.

- 자동차 충돌 및 기타 외상성 손상의 원인으로 인한 손상과 사망을 방지하기 위한 사고 예방이 현실적인 접근 방식인가?
- 안전띠 및 안전 시트 사용과 관련된 법규 준수가 손상과 사망을 예방하는 데 영향을 미친다는 증거가 있는가?
- 병원 전 처치 제공자로서 우리는 자동차 충돌로 인한 사망과 손상을 예방하기 위해 무엇을 할 수 있는가?

시나리오 해결책

당신과 동료가 자동차 충돌 현장에서 안전을 유지할 수 있었던 것은 소속 부서의 안전 프로토콜을 기억하고 따랐기 때문이다. 당신은 비상등이나 경광등을 켜는 것이 항상 운전자의 주의를 끄는데 충분하지 않다는 것을 알고 있었기 때문에 현장에서 작업하는 동안 다른 운전자에게 더 잘 보이도록 승인된 야광 조끼를 착용했다. 또한, 당신은 환자를 적절히 들어 올리는 기술과 절차를 기억하고 준수했으며 구급차의 환자칸에서 안전띠를 착용하여 안전을 확보했다.

또한, 당신 팀은 최근 구급차 후면의 반사판 디자인을 변경하여 멀리서도 구급차를 확인할 수 있도록 했다. 야간에 볼 수 있는 시야를 확보하기 위해 구급차 외부에 빨간색과 흰색 조명을 파란색 조명으로 교체했다. 이러한 조치는 모두 현장에서 시야와 관련된 문제를 줄이고 탑승자 안전을 확보하는 데 매우 도움이 되는 것으로 입증되었다.

References

1. National Academy of Sciences/National Research Council. *Accidental Death and Disability: The Neglected Disease of Modern Society*. National Academy of Sciences/National Research Council; 1966.
2. National Center for Health Statistics. *Health, United States, 2000—With Adolescent Health Chartbook*. National Center for Health Statistics; 2000.
3. National Center for Health Statistics, Centers for Disease Control and Prevention. All injuries. Updated January 22, 2022. Accessed March 2, 2022. https://www.cdc.gov/nchs/fastats/injury.htm
4. National Center for Health Statistics, Centers for Disease Control and Prevention. Accidents or unintentional injuries. Reviewed January 24, 2022. Accessed March 2, 2022. https://www.cdc.gov/nchs/fastats/accidental-injury.htm
5. National Safety Council. International overview. Accessed March 2, 2022. https://injuryfacts.nsc.org/international/international-overview/
6. Peden M, McGee K, Sharma G. *The Injury Chart Book: A Graphical Overview of the Global Burden of Injuries*. World Health Organization; 2002.
7. Centers for Disease Control and Prevention, National Center for Injury Prevention and Control. Ten leading causes of death by age group, United States—2018. Accessed March 2, 2022. https://www.cdc.gov/injury/images/lc-charts/leading_causes_of_death_by_age_group_2018_1100w850h.jpg
8. National Safety Council. Injury Facts: International overview. Published 2020. Accessed April 7, 2022. https://injuryfacts.nsc.org/international/international-overview/#:~:text=According%20to%20the%20World%20Health,3%2C159%2C000%20died%20from%20preventable%20injuries%20
9. National Highway Traffic Safety Administration, U.S. Department of Health and Human Services, Health Resources and Services Administration, Maternal and Child Health Bureau. *Emergency Medical Services Agenda for the Future*. National Highway Traffic Safety Administration; 1999.
10. EMS Agenda 2050 Technical Expert Panel.. *EMS Agenda 2050: A People-Centered Vision for the Future of Emergency Medical Services* (Report No. DOT HS 812 664). National Highway Traffic Safety Administration; 2019.
11. Jaslow D, Ufberg J, Marsh R. Primary injury prevention in an urban EMS system. *J Emerg Med*. 2003;25(2):167-170. doi: 10.1016/s0736-4679(03)00165-3. PMID: 12902003
12. Martinez R. Injury control: a primer for physicians. *Ann Emerg Med*. 1990;19:72-77.
13. Christoffel T, Gallagher SS. *Injury Prevention and Public Health: Practical Knowledge, Skills, and Strategies*. Aspen; 1999.
14. Reason J. Human error: models and management. *BMJ*. 2000;320:768-770.
15. Cohen L, Miller T, Sheppard MA, Gordon E, Gantz T, Atnafou R. Bridging the gap: bringing together intentional and unintentional injury prevention efforts to improve health and well being. *J Safety Res*. 2003;34:473-483.
16. Centers for Disease Control and Prevention. Road traffic injuries and deaths: a global problem. Last reviewed December 14, 2020. Accessed March 2, 2022. https://www.cdc.gov/injury/features/global-road-safety/index.html
17. World Health Organization. Injuries and violence. Published March 19, 2021. Accessed March 2, 2022. https://www.who.int/news-room/fact-sheets/detail/injuries-and-violence
18. World Health Organization. Global status report on road safety 2018: summary. World Health Organization; 2018. https://www.who.int/publications/i/item/9789241565684
19. World Health Organization. Burns. https://www.who.int/news-room/fact-sheets/detail/burns#:~:text=Burns%20are%20a%20global%20public,and%20South%2DEast%20Asia%20regions. Published March 5, 2018. Accessed March 28, 2022.
20. World Health Organization. Drowning. Published April 27, 2021. Accessed March 2, 2022. https://www.who.int/news-room/fact-sheets/detail/drowning
21. World Health Organization. Falls. Published April 26, 2021. Accessed March 2, 2022. https://www.who.int/news-room/fact-sheets/detail/falls
22. World Health Organization. Guidelines for establishing a poison centre. Published January 14, 2021. Accessed March 2, 2022. https://www.who.int/publications/i/item/9789240009523
23. World Health Organization. Snakebite envenoming. Published May 17, 2021. Accessed March 2, 2022. https://www.who.int/news-room/fact-sheets/detail/snakebite-envenoming

24. Institute for Health Metrics and Evaluation. Interpersonal violence: level 3 cause. Accessed March 2, 2022. https://www.healthdata.org/results/gbd_summaries/2019/interpersonal-violence-level-3-cause

25. World Health Organization. Suicide. Published June 17, 2021. Accessed March 2, 2022. https://www.who.int/news-room/fact-sheets/detail/suicide

26. Federal Highway Administration. *Highway statistics, 2019.* U.S. Department of Transportation; 2020.

27. Department of Transportation, National Highway Traffic Safety Administration. Seat belts. Accessed March 2, 2022. https://www.nhtsa.gov/risky-driving/seat-belts

28. Department of Transportation, National Highway Traffic Safety Administration. Drunk driving. Accessed March 2, 2022. https://www.nhtsa.gov/risky-driving/drunk-driving

29. Centers for Disease Control and Prevention, National Center for Injury Prevention and Control. Fatal injury data. Web-based Injury Statistics Query and Reporting System (WISQARS). Reviewed February 10, 2022. Accessed March 2, 2022. https://www.cdc.gov/injury/wisqars/fatal.html

30. Centers for Disease Control and Prevention, National Center for Injury Prevention and Control. Injuries and violence are leading causes of death. Reviewed February 28, 2022. Accessed March 2, 2022. https://www.cdc.gov/injury/wisqars/animated-leading-causes.html

31. Centers for Disease Control and Prevention. Drug overdose deaths. Reviewed March 3, 2021. Accessed March 2, 2022. https://www.cdc.gov/drugoverdose/deaths/index.html

32. U.S. Department of Health and Human Services. Injury and violence. Accessed March 2, 2022. https://www.healthypeople.gov/2020/leading-health-indicators/2020-lhi-topics/Injury-and-Violence

33. Organisation for Economic Co-operation and Development. Potential years of life lost. Accessed March 2, 2022. https://data.oecd.org/healthstat/potential-years-of-life-lost.htm

34. Peterson C, Miller GF, Barnett SB, Florence C. Economic Cost of Injury—United States, 2019. *Morb Mortal Wkly Rep.* 2021;70:1655-1659.

35. Houry D. Saving lives and protecting people from injuries and violence. *Ann Emerg Med.* 2016 Aug;68(2):230-232.

36. National Center for Injury Prevention and Control, Division of Violence Prevention. Intimate partner violence: definitions. Reviewed October 9, 2021. Accessed March 2, 2022. https://www.cdc.gov/violenceprevention/intimatepartnerviolence/index.html

37. Smith SG, Zhang X, Basile KC, Merrick MT, Wang J, Kresnow M, Chen J. National Intimate Partner and Sexual Violence survey: 2015 data brief – updated release. Published November 2018. Accessed March 2, 2022. https://www.cdc.gov/violenceprevention/pdf/2015data-brief508.pdf

38. VanDale K. Sleep deprivation in EMS. Fire Engineering website. Published February 1, 2013. Accessed March 2, 2022. https://www.fireengineering.com/firefighting/sleep-deprivation-in-ems/

39. Patterson PD, Weaver MD, Frank RC, et al. Association between poor sleep, fatigue, and safety outcomes in emergency medical services providers. *Prehosp Emerg Care.* 2012;16:86-97.

40. Reichard A, Marsh S, Moore P. Fatal and nonfatal injuries among emergency medical technicians and paramedics. *Prehosp Emerg Care.* 2011;15(4):511-517.

41. Page D. Studies show dangers of working in EMS. *Journal of Emergency Medical Services.* Published October 31, 2011. Accessed March 2, 2022. https://www.jems.com/operations/studies-show-dangers-working-ems/

42. Garrison HG. Keeping rescuers safe. *Ann Emerg Med.* 2002;40:633-635.

43. Erich J. Creating a culture of safety. *EMS World.* 2014;42(1):15-16.

44. Centers for Disease Control and Prevention. Up to 40 percent of annual deaths from each of five leading US causes are preventable. Published May 1, 2014. Accessed March 2, 2022. https://www.cdc.gov/media/releases/2014/p0501-preventable-deaths.html

45. National EMS Advisory Council. Strategy for a national EMS culture of safety DRAFT 3.1. Published May 16, 2012. Accessed March 2, 2022. https://www.ems.gov/pdf/nemsac/may2012/ems_culture_of_safety-draft_3-1_05162012.pdf

46. Mertz KJ, Weiss HB. Changes in motorcycle-related head injury deaths, hospitalizations, and hospital charges following repeal of Pennsylvania's mandatory motorcycle helmet law. *Am J Public Health.* 2008;98(8):1464-1467.

47. Bledsoe GH, Li G. Trends in Arkansas motorcycle trauma after helmet law repeal. *South Med J.* 2005;98(4):436-440.

48. Chenier TC, Evans L. Motorcyclist fatalities and the repeal of mandatory helmet wearing laws. *Accid Anal Prev.* 1987;19(2):133-139.

49. Centers for Disease Control and Prevention. Ambulance crash-related injuries among emergency medical services workers—United States, 1991–2002. *Morb Mortal Wkly Rep.* 2003;52(8):154-156.

50. Todd KH. *Accidents Aren't: Proposal for Evaluation of an Injury Prevention Curriculum for EMS Providers—A Grant Proposal to the National Association of State EMS Directors.* Department of Emergency Medicine, Emory University School of Medicine; 1998.

51. National Association of State EMS Officials. 2020 National Emergency Medical Services Assessment. Published May 27, 2020. Accessed March 2, 2022. https://nasemso.org/wp-content/uploads/2020-National-EMS-Assessment_Reduced-File-Size.pdf

52. Kinnane JM, Garrison HG, Coben JH, et al. Injury prevention: is there a role for out-of-hospital emergency medical services? *Acad Emerg Med.* 1997;4(4):306-312.

53. California Paramedic Foundation. EPIC Medics. Accessed March 2, 2022. https://caparamedic.org/epic-medics/

54. Hawkins ER, Brice JH, Overby BA. Welcome to the world: findings from an emergency medical services pediatric injury prevention program. *Pediatr Emerg Care.* 2007:23(11):790-795.

55. Griffiths K. Best practices in injury prevention. *J Emerg Med Serv.* 2002;27(8):60-74.

56. Krimston J, Griffiths K. Best practices in injury prevention. *J Emerg Med Serv.* 2003;28(9):66-83.

57. Jaslow D, Ufberg J, Marsh R. Primary injury prevention in an urban EMS system. *J Emerg Med.* 2003;25(2):167-170.

58. U.S. Department of Labor. Emergency medical technicians and paramedics. In: U.S. Department of Labor, Bureau of Labor Statistics, eds. *Occupational Outlook Handbook, 2004–2005 Edition.* U.S. Department of Labor; 2004.

59. Federal Emergency Management Agency, U.S. Fire Administration. *EMS Safety: Techniques and Applications.* International Association of Fire Fighters, FEMA contract EMW-91-C-3592. Federal Emergency Management Agency; 1994.

60. Studnek JR, Fernandez AR. Characteristics of emergency medical technicians involved in ambulance crashes. *Prehosp Disaster Med.* 2008;23(5):432-437.

61. Patterson PD, Higgins JS, Van Dongen HPA, et al. Evidence-based guidelines for fatigue risk management

in emergency medical services. *Prehosp Emerg Care*. 2018;22(Suppl 1):89-101.

62. Kilpatrick D. Athletic trainers: a new hope for firefighter recovery. Fire Engineering website. Published December 1, 2016. Accessed March 2, 2022. https://www.fireengineering.com/firefighting/athletic-trainers-a-new-hope-for-firefighter-recovery/

63. Kilpatrick D. The cost efficiency of athletic trainers. Firehouse website. Published December 1, 2016. Accessed March 2, 2022. https://www.firehouse.com/safety-health/health-fitness/article/12268580/the-cost-efficiency-of-athletic-trainers

Suggested Reading

American College of Surgeons Committee on Trauma. *Advanced Trauma Life Support, Student Course Manual*. 10th ed. American College of Surgeons; 2018.

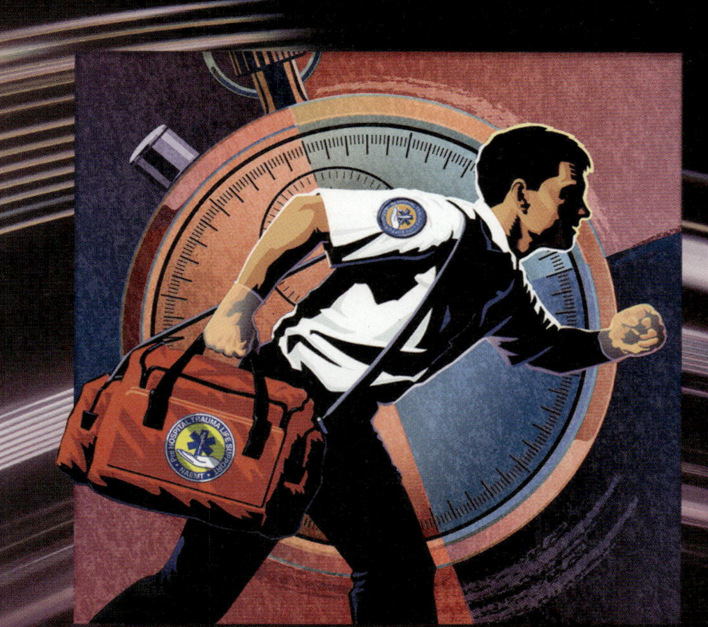

다수 사상자와 테러

제 17 장　재난 관리

제 18 장　폭발과 대량살상무기

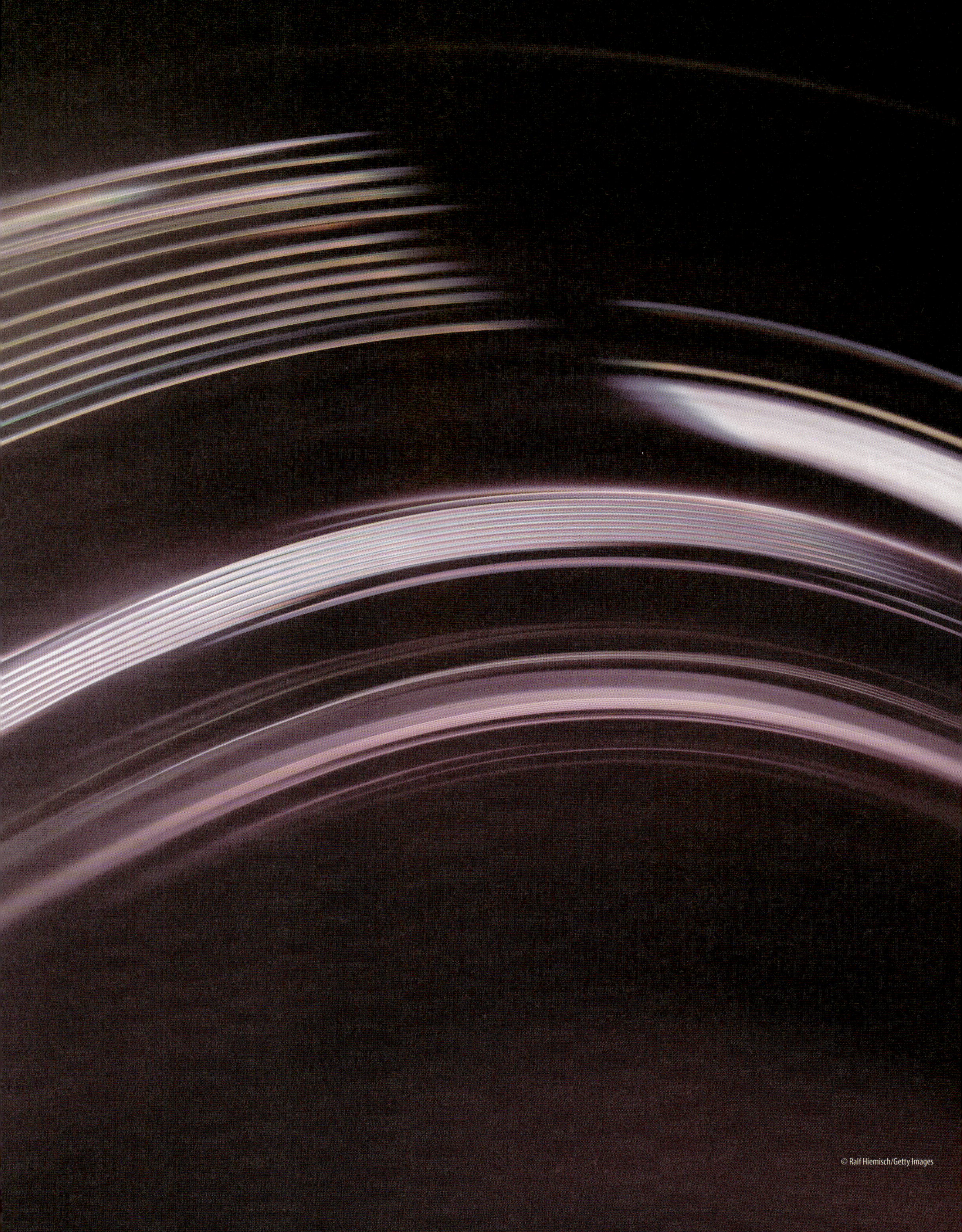
© Ralf Hiemisch/Getty Images

재난 관리

Lead Editor
Faizan H. Arshad, MD

학습 목표 이 장의 학습을 완료하면 다음과 같은 내용을 수행할 수 있다.

- 재난 주기의 5단계를 파악할 수 있다.
- 종합적인 비상 관리 과정을 설명할 수 있다.
- 재난 대응 과정에서 흔히 발생하는 일반적인 함정을 주제로 논의할 수 있다.
- 재난에 대한 의료 대응을 구성하는 요소를 이해하고 설명할 수 있다.
- 재난 대응이 병원 전 처치 제공자의 심리적 안녕에 영향을 어떤 영향을 미칠 수 있는지 인식할 수 있다.

시나리오

당신은 대규모 기상 이변으로 인해 지역 사회 전체가 침수되어 대피소로 사용 중인 지역 고등학교로 출동하였다. 도로 폐쇄와 정전에 대한 주민의 우려를 해결하기 위해 시장과 고위 관계자들이 고등학교에서 진행되는 회의에 참석했다.

현장으로 출동하던 중 체육관의 관람석이 붕괴하여 다수의 사상자가 발생했다는 신고가 여러 건 접수되었다는 상황실의 연락을 받았다. 경찰과 소방 인력도 현장으로 출동 중이지만 현재 집중 호우와 관련된 사고로 인해 가용 자원이 제한적이다.

- 어떤 안전 및 보안 문제가 발생할 것으로 예상하는가?
- 어떤 중증도 분류 시스템을 이용해야 하는가?
- 이 사건에 대한 대응을 어떻게 구성해야 하는가?

개요

재난은 기존의 비상 대응과 비교할 때 시간이 오래 걸리고 여러 기관이 관여할 수 있으며 의료 및 심리·사회적 문제를 포함할 수 있다. 또한, 초기 대응이 끝난 후에도 인프라 재건 등 재난 대응 단계가 장

기화할 수 있으며 이는 초기 대응이 종료된 후에도 계속될 수 있다.

유엔 재난위험경감사무국은 재난을 다음과 같이 정의하였다.

지역 사회 또는 사회의 기능에 심각한 장애가 발생하여 광범위한 인적, 물적, 경제적 또는 환경적 손실을 초래하며 이는 영향을 받는 지

역 사회 또는 사회가 전체 자원을 사용하여 대처할 수 있는 능력을 초과한다.

이 광범위한 정의는 의료 문제 또는 응급의료 대응에 대한 구체적인 언급을 제공하지는 않지만, 상당한 규모의 재난에 대한 전반적인 지역 사회 및 사회 정치적 대응을 포함한다.

의학적 관점에서 재난의 정의는 더욱 세분화할 수 있다. 재난은 의료지원을 요청하는 환자 수가 응급의료 시스템의 일반적인 자원으로 감당할 수 있는 수준을 초과하거나 때로는 외부의 도움이 필요한 상황으로 정의된다. 이 개념은 병원과 병원 전 환경을 포함한 모든 의료 환경에 적용된다. 이러한 상황을 일반적으로 다수 사상자 사고(MCI)라고 한다. 다수 사상자 사고는 한 명 이상의 사상자가 발생했지만, 표준 지역 자원으로 처리할 수 있는 사건인 "다수 사상자 사고"를 지칭하는 데에도 사용한다. 이 교재에서 다수 사상자 사고는 지역 사회의 가용 자원을 압도하는 다수 사상자 사고를 지칭하는 데 사용된다.

이러한 정의는 1) 재난은 특정 희생자 수에 의존하지 않으며, 2) 재난의 영향이 의료 대응의 가용 자원을 초과하고 일반적으로 인프라의 혼란이 발생한다는 두 가지 핵심 개념을 설명한다는 점을 이해하는 것이 중요하다. 간단히 말해 모든 다수 사상자 사고는 재난의 구성 요소이지만, 모든 재난이 다수 사상자 사고는 아니다.

다음 재난의 시간, 장소 또는 복잡성을 예측하기는 어렵다. 그런데도 모든 재난은 원인과 관계없이 유사한 의료 및 공중 보건 결과를 초래한다. 재난마다 이러한 결과가 발생하는 정도와 재난 발생 지역의 의료 및 공공 보건 인프라를 붕괴시키는 정도는 다르다. 재난 대응의 기본 원칙은 가용 자원을 가지고 최대한 많은 사람에게 최대의 이익을 제공하는 것이다. 이 목표는 개별 환자에게 최대의 이익을 주는 것이 목표인 일반적인 의료 서비스와 다르다.

자연 재난과 테러 행위를 포함한 인위적 재난은 가능한 모든 재난 위협을 포괄한다. 대량살상무기(WMDs)는 다수의 사상자를 발생시키는 동시에 환경을 오염시킬 수 있는 특히 불길한 위협이다(18장 폭발 및 대량살상무기 참조).

일관되고 원칙적이며 이상적으로 예행연습을 거친 재난 관리에 대한 접근 방식이 전 세계적으로 받아들여지고 있다. 이 전략은 다수 사상자 사고 대응을 위한 틀을 형성한다. 다수 사상자 사고 대응의 주요 목표는 재난으로 인한 이환율(부상과 질병)과 사망률을 줄이는 것이다. 모든 병원 전 처치 제공자는 환자 처치, 현장 관리, 지속적인 작전 위협으로 인한 잠재적 복잡성을 고려하여 다수 사상자 사고 대

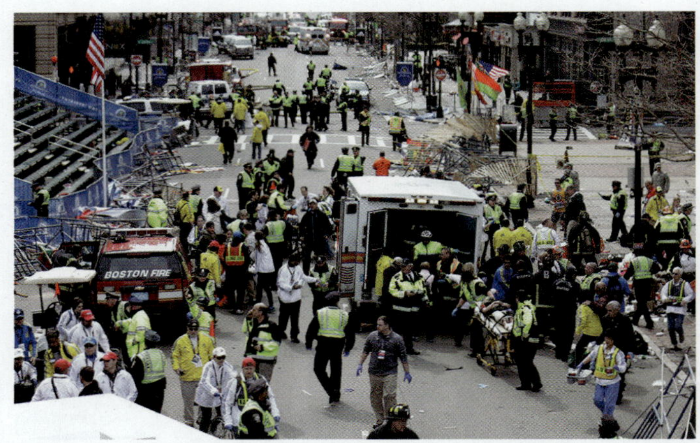

그림 17-1 보스턴 마라톤 대회 폭탄 테러 현장에서 다수 사상자 관리.
© Charles Krupa/File/AP Photo

응의 핵심 원칙을 훈련에 통합해야 한다(**그림 17-1**).

재난 주기

재난에 대한 이론적 근거가 제안되었다. 이 근거를 사용하여 재난의 사건 순서를 분석할 수 있다. 이 개념적 설명은 재난의 전체적인 과정에 대한 개요를 제공할 뿐만 아니라 대응 과정을 개발하기 위한 기초를 제공한다. 재난 대응의 5단계는 다음과 같이 설명된다.

1. 정지 기간 또는 재난 간 기간은 위험 평가 및 완화 활동을 수행하고 잠재적인 사건에 대한 대응 계획을 개발, 테스트 및 실행해야 하는 재난 또는 다수 사상자 사고 사이의 시간을 나타낸다. 정보 수집도 재난 간 기간의 구성 요소이다.

2. 두 번째 단계는 전조(재난 전) 단계 또는 경고 단계이다. 이 단계에서는 특정 사고가 임박했거나 발생할 가능성이 높은 것으로 확인되었다. 여기에는 허리케인과 같은 자연적인 기상 조건 또는 총기 난사 사건이나 적대적인 가해자 사건과 같이 폭력적이고 잠재적으로 폭력적인 상황이 활발하게 전개되고 있음을 반영할 수 있다. 이 기간에 후속 사건의 영향을 완화하기 위해 특정 조치를 할 수 있다. 이러한 방어 조치에는 물리적 구조물 강화, 대피 계획 시작, 사건 발생 후 대응을 위한 공중 보건 자원 동원 등의 조치가 포함될 수 있다. 그러나 모든 사건에 경고 단계가 있는 것은 아니라는 점에 유의해야 한다. 예를 들어 지진은 예고 없이 발생할 수 있다.

3. 세 번째 단계는 충격 단계 또는 실제 사건이 발생하는 시기이다. 이 기간에는 발생하는 사건의 영향이나 결과를 변경하기 위해

할 수 있는 일이 거의 없는 경우가 많다.

4. 네 번째 단계는 응급, 구조 또는 구호 단계로 충격이 발생한 직후의 기간이다. 이 단계에서 대응이 이루어지며 적절한 관리와 개입을 통해 예방 가능한 사망을 줄일 수 있다. 응급의료대응자, 병원 전 처치 제공자, 구조대, 의료지원 서비스의 기술을 총동원하여 사건의 생존자 수를 최대로 늘릴 수 있다.

5. 다섯 번째 단계는 복구 또는 재건 단계로 의료, 공중보건, 지역 사회 인프라(물리적, 정치적)의 조율된 노력을 통해 재난의 영향을 극복하고 재건하기 위해 지역 사회 자원이 요청되는 시기이다. 이 기간은 지역 사회가 완전히 회복되기까지 가장 길고 때로는 수개월에서 수년까지 지속될 수도 있다.

재난 주기(**그림 17-2**)를 이해하면 병원 전 처치 제공자는 지역 사회에서 발생할 수 있는 위험과 사건에 대비하여 어떤 준비를 했는지 평가할 수 있다. 사건이 발생한 후에는 사후 조치 보고서를 비판적으로 평가하고 실무자의 개별 대응과 다른 사람들의 대응을 평가하여 대응 과정의 효율성을 결정하고 향후 개선 영역을 식별할 기회가 이어진다. 이러한 개념은 규모와 관계없이 모든 재난에 적용된다.

재난 주기의 단계별 기간은 해당 지역 사회에서 사건이 발생하는 빈도, 사건의 성격, 지역 사회의 준비 정도에 따라 달라진다. 예를 들어 일부 지역에서 정지 기간이 매우 길 수 있지만(수년 단위로 측정) 다른 지역에서는 몇 달 또는 며칠 단위로 측정될 수 있다(예: 허리케인). 미국 남동부 주에서는 매년 허리케인에 대비하여 약 6~8개월의 정지 기간을 두고 허리케인 발생에 대비한다. 이와는 대조적으로 뉴잉글랜드주에서는 허리케인이 강타한 적이 있지만, 정지 기간이 더 긴 드문 사건이다. 마찬가지로 구조 및 복구 단계는 특정 사건에 따라 크게 달라질 수 있다. 비행기 추락과 같은 사고의 구조 및 복구는 몇 시간에서 며칠 만에 완료되지만, 대규모 홍수의 구조 및 복구까지는 몇 주에서 몇 개월 또는 그 이상이 걸릴 수 있다.

종합적인 응급 상황 관리

재난 주기에 대한 지식은 종합적인 응급 상황 관리와 관련된 단계를 구현하는 데 사용될 수 있다. 종합적인 응급 상황 관리를 관리하는 데 필요한 구체적인 단계를 정의하며 완화, 준비, 대응, 복구 및 예방의 다섯 가지 구성 요소로 이루어져 있다.

- 완화(Mitigation): 응급 상황 관리의 이 구성 요소는 일반적으로 재난 주기 중 정지 기간 단계에서 발생한다. 지역 사회에서 다수 사상

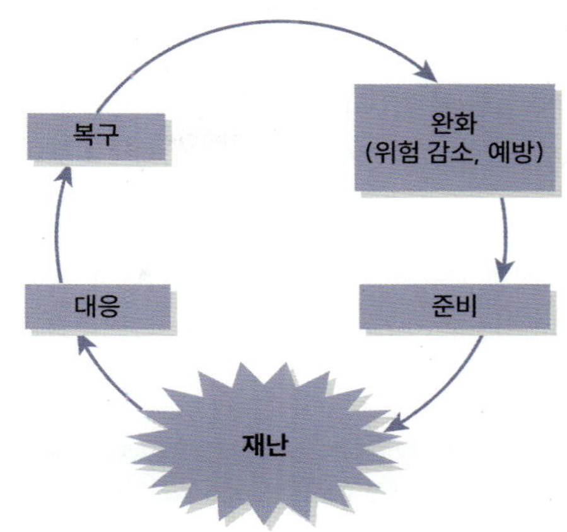

그림 17-2 재난 주기. 정지 단계는 완화 및 대비 화살표로 표시된다. 경고 단계는 사고가 발생하기 직전에 나타난다. 그다음에는 구조 및 복구 단계가 이어진다.
© National Association of Emergency Medical Technicians (NAEMT)

자 사고의 잠재적인 위험 또는 다수 사상자 사고의 발생 가능성이 있는 원인을 파악하고 평가한다. 그런 다음 이러한 위험으로 인해 사고가 발생하지 않도록 예방하거나 예기치 못한 일이 발생할 때 그 영향을 최소화하는 조치를 한다.

- 준비(Preparedness): 이 단계에서는 사고의 사전 파악과 필요한 물품(요구 사항, 특별한 도움이 필요한 사람을 위한 내구성이 있는 의료 장비, 대응 장비, 사고 관리에 필요한 인력, 특정 시나리오가 전개될 때 채택할 구체적인 사고 조치 계획 등)이 포함된다.

- **대응(Response)**: 이 단계에서는 준비 단계에서 확인된 다양한 자원을 활성화하고 배치하여 실제 사고를 관리한다. 일반적으로 이 기간에는 기존의 병원 전 처치 제공자가 활동한다.

- **복구(Recovery)**: 이 구성 요소는 지역 사회를 사고 발생 이전의 기능 상태로 되돌리는 데 필요한 조치를 다룬다.

이 과정은 일반적으로 재난 관리에 적용되지만, 각 응급 대응자의 개별 응급 준비에도 같은 단계를 사용할 수 있다.

개인 준비

각 지역 사회와 정부 기관이 잠재적 재난에 대비하기 위해 종합적인 계획 과정을 수립하는 것이 중요하듯이 각 병원 전 처치 제공자는 재난으로 인해 발생할 수 있는 많은 문제에 개인적, 직업적 자원에서 대처할 준비가 되어 있어야 한다.

병원 전 처치 제공자는 실제 사고 발생 전에 재난 대응에 수반될 수 있는 여러 잠재적 위험에 대해 완전히 이해하고 이러한 위험으로

부터 자신을 보호하는 데 필요한 조처를 할 준비가 되어 있어야 한다. 건물 붕괴, 위험 물질 사고, 총기 난사/적대 행위, 대량살상무기 및 환자 처치에 미치는 잠재적 영향, 적절한 개인보호장비, 전반적인 사고 관리 등의 문제에 대한 지식의 격차를 사전에 파악하여 해결해야 한다. 정기적인 교육과 기관 간 훈련은 기술과 역량을 유지하고 다양한 분야의 최초반응자와 함께 공동 대응을 연습할 수 있는 사전 예방적인 방법이다.

재난은 일반적인 운영 기간을 초과할 수 있으며 병원 전 처치 제공자는 자신의 역할, 책임, 잠재적으로 장기화할 수 있는 부재에 대해 가족과 논의해야 한다. 이러한 논의에는 재난 발생 시 가족들이 해야 할 일과 안전을 보장하기 위해 어디로 가야 하는지에 대해 준비도 포함된다. 재난이 발생하기 전에 지역 EMS 시스템에서 물품과 장

Box 17-1 비상용품 목록

모든 가정에는 응급상황에 대비한 기본적인 물품(최소 3일분)이 준비되어 있어야 한다. 다음은 비상용품 키트에 포함되어야 하는 몇 가지 기본 품목 목록이다. 개인이 이 목록을 검토하고 거주 지역과 가족의 고유한 필요 사항을 고려하여 각자의 특정 요구 사항을 충족하는 비상용품 키트를 만드는 것이 중요하다. 또한 개인이 최소 두 개의 비상용품 키트를 준비해야 하는데, 하나는 집에는 풀 키트로, 다른 하나는 직장, 차량 또는 기타 시간을 보내는 장소에 작은 휴대용 키트로 준비해야 한다. 처방한 약도 비상용품 키트를 계획할 때 고려해야 할 중요한 요소이다.

- 물: 사람과 애완동물 당 하루 약 3.7L(대피용 3일분, 가정에서는 2주분)
  - 더운 기후, 임산부 및 아픈 사람을 위해 이보다 더 많은 물을 저장하는 것을 고려
  - 효과적인 정수 필터를 추가하는 것이 좋음
- 식품: 애완동물용 식품을 포함한 부패하지 않고 준비하기 쉬운 식품(대피용 3일분, 가정용 2주분)(Box 17-2 참조)
  - 비상 상황시 식량이 부족해지는 것보다 나눠 먹을 수 있는 여분의 식량을 준비하는 것이 낫다는 것을 기억한다.
- 충전기가 있는 휴대전화
- 미국 해양대기청(NOAA) 채널에 주파수를 맞출 수 있는 라디오와 여분의 건전지
- 손전등 및 여분의 건전지
- 구급상자(Box 17-3 참조)
- 도움을 요청할 수 있는 호루라기
- 오염된 공기를 정화할 수 있는 방진 마스크, 플라스틱 시트와 고정할 수 있는 테이프
- 개인위생을 위한 물티슈, 쓰레기봉투, 끈
- 렌치나 펜치(멀티툴 장치)
- 식품용 캔 따개(키트에 통조림 식품이 포함된 경우)
- 지역 지도

비상용품 키트에 추가할 수 있는 추가 품목

- 분유, 이유식, 기저귀, 젖병, 젖꼭지, 냉장 보관이 필요하지 않은 약품 등 유아를 위한 물품
- 특수 식품, 의치 용품, 여분의 안경, 보청기 건전지, 정기적으로 사용하는 처방한 약 및 비처방약, 흡입기 및 기타 필수 장비를 포함하여 노인, 특별한 도움이 필요한 사람 또는 심각한 알레르기가 있는 사람을 위한 품목
  - 처방한 약 및 안경
  - 보험증서 사본, 통장, 신분증과 같은 중요한 서류는 방수되는 휴대용 용기에 보관

- 현금 및 거스름돈
- 응급처치 책 또는 www.ready.gov에서 제공하는 정보 등 비상시 참고 자료
- 1인당 침낭이나 담요(기후에 따른 추가 침구류 고려)
- 긴팔 셔츠, 긴 바지, 튼튼한 신발 등 갈아입을 옷을 준비(필요한 경우 여벌의 옷을 준비)
- 가정용 염소계 표백제 및 약품 점적기(물과 표백제를 9 : 1로 희석하면 표백제를 소독제로 사용할 수 있다. 응급상황시에는 물 3.7L에 가정용 액체 표백제 16방울을 섞어 사용할 수 있다. 향이 나거나 색소가 첨가된 표백제는 사용하지 않는다.)
- 소화기(A-B-C형)
- 방수 용기에 담긴 성냥
- 종이와 연필
- 어린이를 위한 게임기나 책, 좋아하는 장난감, 인형 등
- 주방용품: 수동식 캔 따개, 휴대용 식기 세트, 일회용 컵, 접시, 다용도 칼, 설탕과 소금, 알루미늄 포일과 랩, 재밀봉할 수 있는 비닐봉지, 종이 타월
- 위생 및 위생용품: 샴푸, 탈취제, 치약, 칫솔, 빗, 솔, 립밤, 자외선 차단제, 콘택트렌즈 및 소모품, 정기적으로 복용하는 모든 의약품, 화장지, 물티슈, 비누, 손 소독제, 액체 세제, 여성용품, 비닐 쓰레기봉투, 소독제, 가정용 염소계 표백제, 뚜껑이 단단한 중형 플라스틱 물통
- 바늘과 실
- 갈 수 있는 장소와 전화번호가 표시된 지역 지도
- 열쇠와 신분증(자동차나 집 열쇠, 운전 면허증, 여권, 신분증 사본) 등
- 신용카드 사본
- 처방전 사본
- 소형 텐트, 나침반 및 삽

휴대하거나 이동하기 쉬운 용기에 물건을 포장하고 용기에 명확하게 라벨을 붙인 후 찾기 쉬운 장소에 보관한다. 예를 들어, 더플 백, 배낭, 뚜껑이 달린 쓰레기통은 좋은 용기이다. 재난 상황에서 가족들이 집에서 대피하거나 피난을 갈 수도 있기 때문에 재난 용품 키트를 빨리 찾을 수 있어야 한다. 자동차의 연료는 가족들이 안전한 장소로 신속하게 대피할 수 있도록 가득 채워 놓는다. 재난이 발생한 후 적절한 물품을 준비하면 가족이 자택에 갇히거나 대피하는 시간을 견디는 데 도움이 될 수 있다.

영아, 노인, 반려동물 등 키트를 사용할 모든 사람의 요구 사항을 충족시킬 수 있는지 확인한다. 어린이를 포함하여 키트를 사용할 수 있는 모든 사람과 같이 키트를 구성하는 것이 좋다. 키트는 어린이의 성장과 발달뿐만 아니라 처방 변경, 유효 기간 검토 등을 고려하려 매년 재구성한다.

비를 조달하는 것처럼 병원 전 처치 제공자는 가족의 요구를 충족시킬 수 있는 충분한 물품을 확보해야 한다(Box 17-1, Box 17-2, Box 17-3). 병원 전 처치 제공자는 연장 근무 기간 누가 어린이와 애완동물을 돌볼 것인지 계획해야 한다. 이러한 조치는 의료진과 가족 모두를 안심시키는 데 도움이 되며, 특히 재난이 장기화하는 동안 필요한 경우 의료진이 계속 근무할 수 있도록 한다.

가족 통신 계획을 세우는 방법을 비롯하여 재난 발생 시 개인 및 가족 준비에 관한 정보가 포함된 추가 자원은 미국 연방재난관리청(FAMM)이 후원하는 준비된 캠페인이 있으며 온라인(www.ready.gov.)에서 확인할 수 있다.

다수 사상자 사고(MCI) 관리

재난 대응의 중요한 전제는 모든 재난이 지역적이라는 점을 기억하는 것이다. 가용 자원의 가변성은 도시, 교외, 시골 지역에 따라 엄청나게 다를 것이다. 일반적으로 총 피해자의 수 외에도 손상의 심각성과 다양성은 다수 사상자 사고에 영향을 받은 지역 사회 외부의 자원과 지원이 필요한지를 결정하는 데 중요한 요소가 된다.

오늘날의 복잡한 재난, 특히 테러 및 대량살상무기(WMD: 화학, 생물학, 방사능, 핵)와 관련된 재난은 엄격하고 위험한 환경을 초래할 수 있다. 엄격한 환경이란 자원, 공급품, 장비, 인력, 이송 및 정치적, 물리적, 사회적, 경제적 여건의 기타 측면이 제한되는 환경을 말한다. 이러한 제한으로 인해 지역과 자원 인프라에 따라 즉각적인 처치의 가용성과 적절성에 대한 제약이 달라질 수 있다. 병원 전 처치 제공자는 재난에 대항할 때 아프거나 손상을 입은 환자 개개인에게 같은 수준의 처치를 제공할 수 없다는 점을 예상해야 한다. 특정 기준을 충족하는 환자에게 신속하게 의미 있는 처치를 제공하면 소생할 수 있는 환자의 결과를 최적화할 가능성이 가장 높다.

다수 사상자 사고와 관련된 응급의료 문제에는 다음 다섯 가지 요소가 포함된다.

Box 17-2 식품 키트

- 최소 3일분의 부패하지 않은 식품
- 냉장, 조리 또는 조리가 필요 없고 물이 거의 또는 전혀 필요하지 않은 식품을 선택
- 캔을 딸 수 있는 도구와 식기
- 갈증을 유발할 수 있는 짠 음식은 피함
- 가족이 먹을 음식을 선택
- 권장 식품은 다음과 같다.
  - 바로 먹을 수 있는 통조림 고기, 과일 및 채소
  - 단백질, 과일 바
  - 건조 시리얼 또는 그래놀라
  - 땅콩버터
  - 말린 과일
  - 견과류
  - 크래커
  - 통조림 주스
  - 부패하지 않도록 저온살균 우유
  - 고열량 식품
  - 비타민
  - 유아용 식품
  - 스트레스를 해소할 수 있는 식품
- 조리를 할 수 있는 프로판 스토브 또는 그릴(여분의 프로판 탱크 포함)

Data from Federal Emergency Management Agency. Ready America. n.d. www.ready.gov; and Centers for Disease Control and Prevention. Emergency preparedness and response. n.d. https://emergency.cdc.gov/

Box 17-3 구급 상자

응급상홍에서는 가족이 베이거나 화상을 입거나 기타 손상을 입을 수 있다. 구급상자에는 다음과 같은 물품이 포함되어야 한다.
- 라텍스 글러브 또는 멸균 글러브 두 세트
- 출혈을 막기 위한 멸균 드레싱
- 소독용 세정제/비누 및 항생 물티슈
- 감염 예방을 위한 항생제 연고
- 감염 예방을 위한 화상 연고
- 다양한 크기의 붕대
- 눈을 씻어내거나 일반 오염 제거제로 사용할 수 있는 안구 세척액
- 체온계
- 인슐린, 심장약, 천식에 필요한 흡입기와 매일 복용하는 처방 약(유효 기간을 고려하여 주기적으로 약을 교체)
- 혈당, 혈압측정기, 소모품 및 처방된 의료용품
- 지팡이, 보행기, 정전 시 사용할 수 있는 의료 장비

기타 유용한 물품
- 충전할 수 있는 휴대전화
- 가위
- 핀셋
- 바셀린 또는 기타 윤활제 튜브
- 비처방약
  - 아스피린 또는 비아스피린 진통제(아세트아미노펜)
  - 지사제
  - 제산제(배탈용)
  - 완화제

Data from Federal Emergency Management Agency. Ready America. n.d. www.ready.gov; and Centers for Disease Control and Prevention. Emergency preparedness and response. n.d. https://emergency.cdc.gov/

- 수색 및 구조: 이 활동에는 사건의 영향을 받은 사람들을 체계적으로 찾고 위험한 상황에서 구조하는 과정이 포함된다. 상황에 따라 구출 문제가 수반되는 경우 특수 훈련을 받은 팀을 투입해야 하는 경우가 많다.
- 환자 분류 및 초기 안정화: 손상이나 질병의 심각성에 따라 각 피해자를 체계적으로 평가 및 분류하고 생명 또는 팔다리를 위협하는 즉각적인 문제를 해결하기 위해 초기 의료 서비스를 제공하는 과정이다.
- 환자 추적: 이것은 환자를 고유하게 식별하고 최초 접촉부터 수색 및 구조, 대피, 분류 및 이송, 궁극적으로 최종 치료에 이르기까지 추적하는 시스템이다.
- 결정적인 처치: 이 구성 요소는 환자의 손상을 처치하는 데 필요한 특정 의료 서비스를 제공하는 것이 포함된다. 이 처치는 일반적으로 병원에서 제공되지만, 병원이 사상자들로 인해 과부하가 걸리거나 병원이 사고로 직접적인 영향을 받거나 피해를 본 경우 주요 사건에서 대체 의료 시설을 사용할 수 있다.
- 대피: 이것은 재난 피해자와 손상을 입은 환자를 재난 현장에서 안전한 장소 또는 결정적인 처치를 받을 수 있는 의료기관으로 이송하는 과정이다.

다수 사상자 사고와 관련된 공중 보건 문제에는 다음이 포함된다.
- 물(안전한 식수 공급 보장)
- 음식(쉽게 부패하지 않고 냉장 보관이나 조리가 필요 없는 음식이 이상적임)
- 대피소(대피할 수 있는 안전한 장소)
- 위생(사람과 동물의 배설물, 고형 폐기물, 폐수와의 접촉으로부터 보호)
- 보안 및 안전
- 교통
- 의사소통(전염성 질병에 대한 정보를 포함하여 영향을 받는 인구에 대한 정보)
- 풍토병 및 유행병(풍토병은 특정 지역이나 사람에게 항상 존재하지, 일반적으로 낮은 빈도로 발생하는 질병이지만, 유행병은 위험에 처한 인구에게 빠르게 발병하고 확산하는 질병)

의료 및 공중 보건 재난 대응 활동은 하나의 조직 구조인 사고지휘 시스템을 통해 조정된다.

국가 사고관리체계(NIMS)

국가 사고관리체계는 사고의 원인, 규모, 위치, 복잡성과 관계없이 사고 관리에 대한 포괄적이고 체계적인 접근 방식을 위한 템플릿을 제공하기 위해 개발되었다. 국가 사고관리체계는 모든 위험과 사건에 대한 일련의 대비 개념과 원칙을 제공한다. 이는 통신 및 정보관리시스템의 공통 운영 구조와 상호 운영을 위한 필수 원칙을 설명한다. 또한 표준화된 자원 관리 절차를 제공한다. 국가 사고관리체계는 사고 현장 지휘체계를 사용하여 사고에 직접 대응하고 감독한다.

재난지휘체계(ICS)

재난 대응에는 다양한 조직이 참여할 수 있다. 재난지휘체계는 다양한 유형의 기관(경찰, 소방, EMS 등) 및 유사한 기관의 여러 관할 구역이 공통 언어와 조직 구조를 사용하여 재난 또는 기타 주요 사고에 대한 대응을 관리하면서 효과적으로 협력할 수 있게 하려고 만들어졌다(그림 17-3). 자세한 내용은 5장 현장 관리에서 확인할 수 있다. 다양한 대응 기관의 대표자들은 일반적으로 현장 지휘 본부에 모여 기관 간 의사소통과 의사결정을 촉진하고 지휘 과정을 통합하기 위해 협력한다.

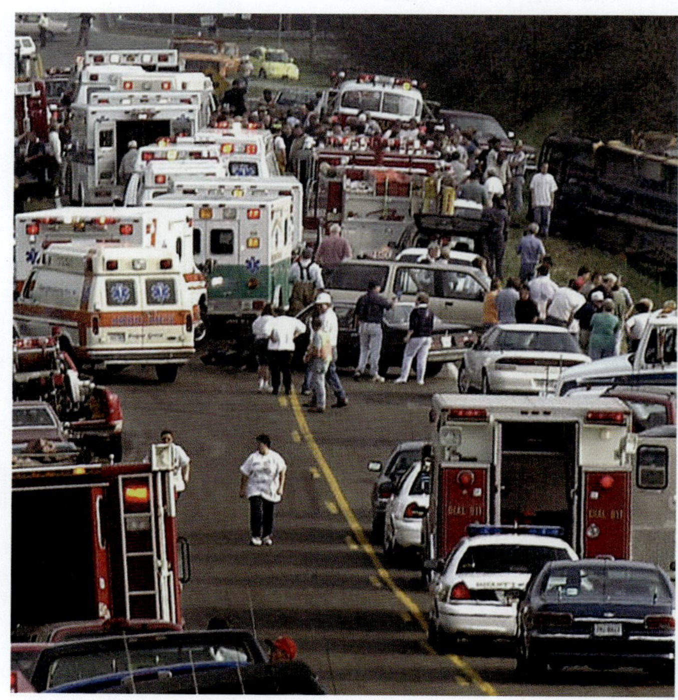

그림 17-3 재난지휘체계(ICS)를 사용하면 재난 현장에서 소방, 경찰 및 EMS 자산을 통합할 수 있다.

재난지휘체계는 사건의 특정 성격이나 주요 대응 기관(경찰, 소방 또는 의료기관)과 관계없이 항상 수행해야 하는 여러 가지 기능이 있다는 것을 인식하고 있다. 사고지휘체계는 이러한 필수 기능을 중심으로 구성되어 있으며 구성 요소는 다음과 같다.

- 지휘
- 안전 책임자
- 정보 책임자
- 연락 책임자
  - 계획
  - 물류
  - 운영
  - 재정

이러한 기능은 모든 사고에 다양한 수준으로 적용되며 현재 병원 전 단계부터 병원 내까지 모든 유형의 의료 환경에서 재난에 대한 대응을 조직하는 데 사용되고 있다.

의학적 관점에서 몇 가지 중요한 재난지휘체계의 원칙이 다수 사상자 사고 대응에 도움이 될 것이다.

1. 재난지휘체계는 가급적 첫 번째 응급 구조대원이 현장에 도착하는 즉시 조기에 구축해야 한다. 지휘권을 확립하는 것은 모든 구조대원에게 중요한 첫 단계이며 현장에 도착하면 지휘권이 감독관에게 이양될 수 있다는 것을 기억한다.
2. 독립적으로 일하는 경우가 많은 의료 및 공중 보건 대응자는 다수 사상자 사고 동안 다른 기관과 대응을 더 잘 통합하기 위해 재난지휘체계 관리 원칙을 구현해야 한다.
3. 재난지휘체계를 구현하면 사고에 대한 전반적인 대응 내에서 의료 대응을 효과적으로 통합할 수 있다.

재난지휘체계에 대한 자세한 정보 및 교육은 FEMA 웹사이트에서 확인할 수 있다.

재난지휘체계의 특징

재난지휘체계는 긴급한 사고를 관리하기 위한 표준적이고 전문적이며 체계적인 접근 방식을 제공한다. 재난지휘체계를 사용하면 비상 대응 기관이 더욱 안전하고 효율적으로 운영할 수 있다. 표준화된 접근 방식은 여러 기관의 자원 사용을 촉진하고 조정하여 공통의 목표를 향해 노력한다. 또한 각 상황에 맞는 고유한 접근 방식을 개발할 필요가 없으므로 재난지휘체계 또는 재난 발생 시 귀중한 시간을 절약할 수 있다. 재난지휘체계는 대규모 사건과 관련하여 흔히 생각하지만, 지역 사회에서 더 자주 발생하고 여러 최초 대응 기관의 통합이 필요한 일상적인 다수 사상자 사고에도 사용할 수 있다. 예를 들어 2~3대의 차량이 관련된 교통사고는 일상적인 다수 사상자 사고의 한 예이다.

사고를 효과적으로 관리하려면 권한과 책임의 계층 구조를 제공하고 공식적인 의사소통 채널을 구축하는 조직 구조가 필요하다. 명령 체계를 사용하면 조직 내 모든 사람의 구체적인 책임과 권한이 명확하게 규정되고 사전 정의되어 이질적인 그룹이 더 쉽게 함께 운영할 수 있다.

담당 기관

관할권 권한은 일반적으로 단일 초점이 있는 사건에서는 문제가 되지 않는다. 여러 관할 구역이 관련되거나 단일 관할 구역 내의 여러 기관이 사건의 다양한 측면에 대한 권한을 가지고 있는 경우 문제가 더 복잡해질 수 있다. 책임이 중복되는 경우 재난지휘체계는 단일 지휘체계를 사용할 수 있다. 이 접근 방식은 서로 다른 기관의 대표자들이 하나의 계획을 위해 함께 일하고 모든 조치가 완전히 조율되도록 한다. 지휘는 재난지휘체계에서 선택한 용어이지만, 오해의 소지가 있을 수 있다. 사고는 관리된다는 것이고 참여 인원은 지휘가 이루어지는 것임을 기억하는 것이 중요하다. 사고 지휘는 개인이 수행하든 통합 지휘를 통해 수행하든 관리 및 리더십 위치이다. 지휘 구조는 전략적 목표를 설정하고 사고의 영향에 대한 포괄적인 이해를 유지하며 현장을 효과적으로 관리하는 데 필요한 전략을 파악하는 역할을 담당한다. 지휘 기능은 단일 또는 통합의 두 가지 방식 중 하나로 구성된다.

단일 명령은 가장 전통적인 명령 기능이며 사고 지휘관이라는 용어로 이어진다. 단일 관할 구역 내에서 사고가 발생하고 관할 또는 기능 기관의 중복되지 않는 경우 해당 관할 기관에서 단일 사고 지휘관을 파악하고 지정하여 전반적인 사고 관리 책임을 부여한다. 그렇다고 해서 다른 기관이 대응하지 않거나 사고 관리를 지원하는 역할이 없다는 의미는 아니다.

단일 명령은 단일 관할 구역의 단일 부서가 사고 관리와 관련된 전략적 목표를 책임질 때 가장 적합하다. 단일 지휘는 초기에 통합 지휘를 통해 관리되었던 사고의 후기 단계에서도 적절하다. 시간이 지남에 따라 많은 사고가 안정화되면서 전략적 목표는 단일 관할 구역 또는 분야 내에서 점점 더 집중된다. 이러한 상황에서는 통합 지휘체계를 단일 지휘체계로 전환하는 것이 적절하다.

모든 기관과 관할 구역이 동의하는 경우 다기관 및 다중 관할 구역 사고에서 단일 사고 지휘관을 지정하는 것도 허용된다. 그러나 이 경우 지휘관은 신중하게 선택해야 한다. 현장 지휘관은 사고 행동 계획(IAPs)의 기반이 되는 전략적 사고 목표를 개발할 책임이 있다. 사고 행동 계획은 사고 관리를 위한 전반적인 전략을 반영하는 일반적인 목표를 포함하는 구두 또는 서면 계획이다. 사고 지휘관은 사고 행동 계획과 사건 해결에 필요한 자원과 관련된 모든 요청에 대한 책임이 있다.

관할권이 겹치거나 법적 책임이 있는 여러 기관이 같은 사건에 연루되면 통합 지휘는 여러 가지 이점을 제공한다. 이 접근 방식에는 각 기관의 대표자가 협력하여 지휘 권한을 공유한다. 이들은 함께 일하며 의사 결정 과정에 직접 참여한다. 통합 지휘는 협력을 보장하고 혼란을 방지하며 목표와 목적에 대한 합의를 보장하는 데 도움이 된다. 통합 지휘의 예로는 위험 물질 방출과 관련된 상황을 들 수 있다. 소방서는 화재 통제, 위험 물질 확산 방지 및 구조를 담당하고 경찰서는 대피 및 지역 보안을 담당하며 공공사업소는 현장 청소를 담당한다.

모든 위험 및 모든 위험 시스템

재난지휘체계는 화재, 홍수, 토네이도, 비행기 추락, 위험 물질 사고, 총기 난사 또는 적대적인 공격자 사건, 공중 보건 비상사태, 폭발 또는 기타 모든 유형의 응급 상황에서 자원을 관리하는 데 적용할 수 있는 모든 위험 및 모든 위험 시스템으로 발전했다. 이러한 종류의 시스템은 명령, 통제 및 통신에 대한 요구 사항이 유사한 대규모 공공 행사 또는 대규모 집회 행사와 같은 많은 비응급 상황을 관리하는 데에도 사용되었다. 재난지휘체계의 유연성 덕분에 필요한 구성 요소를 사용하여 필요에 따라 관리 구조를 확장할 수 있다. 여러 기관과 조직의 운영이 사고 관리에 원활하게 통합될 수 있다.

일상적인 적용성

재난지휘체계는 주요 사고뿐만 아니라 일상적인 작업에도 사용할 수 있고 사용해야 한다. 모든 사고에서 지휘체계를 확립해야 한다. 일상적인 시스템을 정기적으로 사용하면 표준 절차 및 용어에 익숙해질 수 있다. 일상적인 상황에서 재난지휘체계를 자주 사용하면 대형 사고에 더 쉽게 적용할 수 있다.

명령의 통일성

단일 지휘체계는 각 직속 상사가 한 명만 있는 관리 개념이다. 모든 명령과 과제는 해당 상사로부터 직접 전달되며 모든 보고는 같은 상사에게 이루어진다. 이 접근 방식은 한 사람이 여러 상사로부터 명령받을 때 발생할 수 있는 혼란을 제거한다. 지휘체계가 일원화되면 문제 해결뿐만 아니라 인명 및 재산 손실 가능성도 줄인다. 각 사람에게 한 명의 상사만 두도록 함으로써 지휘의 통일성은 전반적인 책임감을 높이고 프리랜서를 방지하며 의사소통의 흐름을 개선하며 운영 문제를 조정하는 데 도움을 주고 실무자의 안전을 강화할 수 있다. 재난지휘체계가 반드시 직급 위주의 시스템이 아니다. 직급이 낮은 사람이 일시적으로 더 높은 직급에 배치되더라도 각 상황에 맞는 적절한 직급에 최고의 자격을 갖춘 사람을 배치해야 한다. 이 개념은 시스템의 효과적인 적용을 위해 매우 중요하며 모든 참여자가 반드시 수용해야 한다. 또한 국가 사고관리체계의 핵심 구성 요소인 운영, 계획, 물류 및 재정/행정 부분의 지휘관 및 재난지휘체계 직책에 대한 일련의 국가 자격 인증 표준이다.

통제 범위

통제 범위는 조직 내 모든 수준에서 한 명의 감독관에게 보고하는 부하 직원의 수를 의미한다. 통제 범위는 전략 수준부터 운영/전술 수준 및 업무 수준까지 모든 수준의 재난지휘체계와 관련이 있다.

대부분의 상황에서 한 사람이 효과적으로 감독할 수 있는 인원은 3~7명에 불과하다. 응급상황 발생 시 역동적인 특성으로 인해 재난지휘체계에서 명령 또는 감독할 책임이 있는 개인은 일반적으로 5명 이상을 직접 감독해서는 안 된다. 실제 통제 범위는 사고의 복잡성과 수행되는 작업의 성격에 따라 달라져야 한다. 예를 들어, 위험 물질과 관련된 복잡한 사고의 경우 통제 범위는 세 가지에 불과할 수 있지만, 덜 강도 높은 작업의 경우 통제 범위가 일곱 가지까지 늘어날 수 있다.

모듈식 조직

재난지휘체계는 유동적이고 모듈식으로 설계되었다. 재난지휘체계 조직 구조는 지휘, 운영, 계획, 물류, 재정 및 행정을 미리 정의되어 있으며 필요에 따라 인력을 배치하고 운영할 준비가 되어 있다. 실제로 재난지휘체계는 특정 사고에 필요한 도구만 사용하는 조직의 도구 상자로 특징지어지는 경우가 많다. 재난지휘체계에서 이러한 도구는 직책, 직무 설명, 직책 간의 관계를 정의하는 조직 구조로 구성된다.

일부 직책과 기능은 자주 사용되는 반면, 다른 직책과 기능은 복잡하거나 특수한 상황에서만 필요하다. 어떤 직책에는 원하는 역할에 누군가를 배정하기만 하면 활성화할 수 있다.

공통 용어

재난지휘체계는 조직 내에서 응급 상황과 관련된 모든 기관에서 공통 용어를 사용하도록 권장한다. 공통 용어는 각 단어에 하나의 정의가 있으며 응급 상황을 관리하는 데 사용되는 두 단어의 정의가 같지 않음을 의미한다. 모두가 같은 용어를 사용하여 같은 생각을 전달하므로 모든가 그 의미를 이해할 수 있다. 각 업무에는 하나의 책임이 있으며 각 업무에 대한 책임자가 누구인지 모두가 알고 있다.

통합된 의사소통

통합된 의사소통은 응급 상황에 부닥친 모든 사람이 감독관과 팀원과 소통할 수 있도록 보장한다. 재난지휘체계는 모든 수준에서 지휘체계에서 위아래로 의사소통을 지원해야 한다. 메시지는 지휘체계를 통해 효율적으로 위아래로 전달되어야 한다.

통합 사고 대응 계획

재난지휘체계는 사고에 관련된 모든 사람이 하나의 전체적인 계획을 따르도록 한다. 조직의 여러 구성 요소는 서로 다른 기능을 수행할 수 있지만, 모든 노력은 같은 중요한 목표와 목적을 달성하는 데 이바지한다. 발생하는 모든 것은 전체 대응 내에서 조정된다. 소규모 사고의 경우 지휘부는 행동 계획을 수립하고 사고 우선순위, 목표, 전략 및 전술을 모든 참여 부서에 전달한다. 모든 참여 기관의 대표자가 정기적으로 만나 계획을 개발하고 업데이트한다. 크고 작은 사고에서 사고와 관련된 사람들은 자신의 구체적인 역할이 무엇이며 전체 계획에 어떻게 부합하는지 이해한다.

지정된 사고 시설

지정된 사고 시설에는 특정 기능이 항상 수행되는 장소가 지정된다. 예를 들어 지휘는 항상 현장 지휘 본부를 기반으로 한다. 준비 지역, 재활 지역, 사상자 집결 장소, 처치 지역, 헬기 착륙장은 모두 특정 기능이 수행되는 지정된 구역이다. 특정 사고에 필요한 시설은 특정 사고 행동 계획 또는 사전에 정의된 재난지휘체계의 계획에 따라 설정된다.

자원 관리

자원 관리에는 사고와 관련된 자원을 할당하고 추적하는 표준 시스템을 사용ᄒ-는 것이 수반된다. 재난지휘체계의 자원 관리 시스템은 다양한 자원 할당을 추적한다. 대규모 사고의 경우 단위(unit)는 종종 사고 장소로 직접 이동하지 않고 대기 장소로 파견된다. 대기 장소는 사고 현장과 가까운 곳에 여러 대원을 예비로 배치하여 필요시 바로 투입할 수 있도록 준비할 수 있는 장소이다.

재난지휘체계의 구성

재난지휘체계 구조는 응급사고에서 수행되는 모든 범위의 의무, 책임 및 기능을 확인한다. 일부 구성 요소는 거의 모든 사건에 사용되지만, 다른 구성 요소는 가장 규모가 크고 복잡한 상황에만 적용된다. 재난지휘체계 조직의 다섯 가지 구성 요소는 지휘, 운영, 계획, 물류 및 재정/행정이다.

재난지후 체계 조직도는 기본적일 수도 있고 더 많은 구성 요소가 필요할 때 복잡성을 추가할 수도 있다. 재해지휘체계 조직도의 각 블록은 기능 영역과 작업 설명을 나타낸다. 직책은 주어진 상황에 필요한 추가 구성 요소를 결정하는 사고 지휘부에 의해 필요에 따라 배치한다.

지휘

재난지휘치계 조직도에서 첫 번째 구성 요소는 지휘이다(**그림 17-4**). 지휘는 재난지휘체계에서 모든 사고에 대해 항상 채워져야 하는 유일한 직책으로 명확하게 정의된 리더가 있으면 사고 관리에 여러 가지 이점이 있기 때문이다. 지휘는 첫 번째 팀이 현장에 도착할 때 설정되고 마지막 팀이 현장을 떠날 때까지 유지된다.

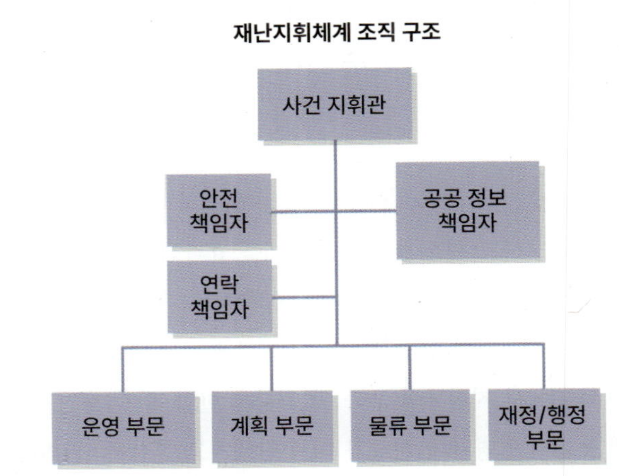

그림 17-4 재난지휘체계의 조직도.
© National Association of Emergency Medical Technicians (NAEMT)

재난지휘체계 구조에서 지휘(단일 또는 통합)는 사고 관리에 대한 최종적인 책임을 지며 사고 현장에서 모든 활동을 지휘하는 데 필요한 권한을 갖는다. 지휘는 다음 작업을 직접 담당한다.

- 전략 결정
- 사고 전술 선택
- 실행 계획 수립
- 재난지휘체계 조직 개발
- 자원 관리 및 추가 자원 요청
- 자원 활동 조정
- 현장 안전 제공
- 사고에 대한 정보 공개
- 외부 기관과의 협력

현장 지휘소

현장 지휘소는 사고에서 본부 역할을 한다. 지휘체계의 기능은 현장 지휘소에 집중되어 있으므로 지휘부와 모든 직접 지원 인력은 항상 현장 지휘소에 배치되어야 한다. 지휘소가 설치되는 즉시 모든 팀에 위치를 전파한다.

사건 현장과 관련하여 지휘소는 근처의 안전한 장소에 있어야 한다. 대형 사고의 경우 특수 차량이나 건물에 설치하는 경우가 많다. 이 위치는 지휘체계 관계자들이 불필요한 방해를 받지 않고 활동할 수 있도록 해준다. 지리적으로 분산된 대형 사고의 경우 지휘소는 사고 현장으로부터 어느 정도 떨어져 있을 수 있다.

지휘 본부 관계자

지휘체계 관계는 현장 본부에 직접 보고하는 기능을 수행하며 조직의 다른 주요 부서에 위임할 수 없다. 안전 책임자, 연락 책임자 및 언론(공보) 책임자는 항상 지휘 본부 참모의 일부 인력이다. 또한, 보좌관, 비서와 고문은 지휘 참모 구성원을 위해 직접 일하도록 배정될 수 있다.

안전 책임자

안전 책임자는 사고 현장에서 안전 문제를 효과적으로 관리할 책임이 있다. 안전 책임자는 위험한 상황을 식별하고 평가하여 안전하지 않은 관행을 주의하며 안전 절차가 적절하게 준수되는지 확인하는 등 안전 측면에서 지휘부의 눈과 귀 역할을 한다. 안전 책임자는 사고 발생 초기에 임명된다. 사고가 더 복잡해지고 현장에 투입되는 자원의 수가 증가하면 자격을 갖춘 인력을 보조 안전 책임자로 추가로 지정할 수 있다.

연락 책임자

연락 책임자는 외부 기관의 대표자와 연락 창구 기능을 하는 지휘부의 대표이다. 연락 담당관은 해당 기관의 대표와 정보를 교환하는 역할을 담당한다. 사고가 진행 중일 때는 지휘부가 현장 지휘소를 방문하는 모든 사람을 직접 만날 시간이 없을 수도 있다. 연락 담당관은 이러한 상황에서 지휘부를 대표하여 정보를 입수하여 제공하거나 사람들을 적절한 위치나 기관으로 안내하는 역할을 한다. 연락 지역은 지휘소와 인접해야 하지만, 지휘소 내부에 있어서는 안 된다.

공공 정보 책임자

공공 정보 책임자(PIO)는 사고 정보를 수집하여 언론 및 기타 적절한 기관에 공개할 책임이 있다. 주요 사고 발생 시 대중 및 언론과의 소통은 정보 전달에 있어 매우 중요하다. 지휘부는 사고 관리를 최우선 과제로 삼아야 하므로 공공 정보 책임자는 언론사 요청에 대한 연락 담당자 임무를 수행하여 지휘부가 사고에 집중할 수 있도록 한다. 언론사 본부는 현장 지휘 본부 내부가 아니라 근처에 설치한다. 공공 정보 책임자를 지정하면 특히 여러 기관이 관련된 복잡한 사고 발생 시 일관되고 조율된 메시지를 전달하는 데 도움이 된다.

일반 직원의 역할

현장 지휘관은 전체 현장 지휘부 조직에 대한 전반적인 책임을 지지만, 현장 지휘관의 책임 중 일부 요소는 지휘 참모진이 처리할 수 있다. 사고가 너무 크거나 너무 복잡하여 한 사람이 효과적으로 관리하기 어려운 경우 현장 지휘관은 운영의 일부를 감독할 사람을 지정할 수 있다. 긴급 사고에서 발생하는 모든 것은 재난지휘체계 내의 주요 기능 구성 요소로 나눌 수 있다.

- 운영
- 계획
- 물류
- 재정/행정

이 네 부서의 책임자를 통칭하여 재난지휘체계의 참모진이라고 한다. 지휘부는 이 네 가지 직책 중 어떤 직책을 활성화해야 하는지, 언제 활성화할지, 각 직책에 누가 배치되어야 하는지 결정한다. 재난지휘 체계의 조직에는 기능 영역 또는 직무 설명을 나타내며 항상 인력이 배치되어야 하는 직책을 의미하지 않는다는 점을 기억한다.

재난지휘체계 총괄 참모진에 속한 네 명의 담당자가 배치되면 현장 지휘소에서 작전을 수행할 수 있지만, 이러한 구조가 꼭 필요한 것은 아니다. 대규모 사고가 발생한 네 개의 기능별 부문은 서로 다른 위치에서 운영될 수 있지만, 항상 지휘부와 직접 연락을 취하게 된다.

운영

운영 부서는 사고 완화와 직접적으로 관련된 모든 조치를 관리할 책임이 있다. 운영반은 갇힌 사람을 구출하고 손상을 입은 환자를 처치하며 응급 상황을 완화하는 데 필요한 모든 조치를 한다.

소규모 사고의 경우 지휘부는 운영 부서의 기능을 직접 감독할 수 있다. 복잡한 사건의 경우 지휘부는 전략에 집중하고 임무 완수에 필요한 전술에 집중할 수 있도록 별도의 운영 책임자가 책임을 맡게 된다.

작전은 전략적 목표와 긴급 운영 작전 수행 방법을 개괄적으로 수행하는 사고 행동 계획에 따라 수행된다. 대부분의 사고에서 사고 행동 계획은 비교적 간단하며 몇 개의 단어나 문구로 표현할 수 있다. 대규모 사고에 대한 사고 행동 계획은 정기적으로 업데이트되고 현장 지휘관이 일일 브리핑에 사용되는 긴 문서가 될 수 있다.

계획

계획 부서는 사고와 관련된 정보의 수집, 평가, 배포 및 사용을 담당한다. 계획 부서는 사전 계획, 건물 설계도면, 지도, 항공사진, 도표, 참고 자료, 상황판을 사용한다. 또한, 사고 행동 계획을 개발하고 업데이트하는 일도 담당한다. 계획 부서는 누가 무엇을 해야 하는지 개발하고 필요한 자원을 확인한다.

현장 지휘부는 정보를 획득하고 관리 및 분석이 필요한 경우 계획 부서를 활성화한다. 계획 책임자는 현장 지휘부에 직접 보고한다. 계획 부서에 배정된 개인은 현장 상황을 조사하고 이용할 수 있는 정보를 검토하여 예상되는 사건의 경과를 예측하고 전략 및 전술에 대한 권장 사항을 준비한다. 또한, 계획 부서는 대규모 사고 발생 시 자원을 파악하고 지휘부에 정기적인 상황 및 자원 상황 보고서를 제공한다.

물류

물류 부서는 사고 발생 시 물품, 서비스, 시설과 물품 제공을 담당한다. 물류 책임자는 지휘부에 직접 보고하며 사고에 대한 보급 책임자 역할을 한다. 이 부서의 책임 중에는 차량에 연료를 공급하고 구조대원에게 음식과 음료를 제공하며 특수 장비를 배치하는 것도 포함된다.

재정/행정

재정/행정 부서는 명령에 따라 직접 관리되는 네 번째 주요 재난지휘체계 구성 요소이다. 이 부문은 사고 발생 시 회계 및 재정적 측면과 사고 후 발성할 수 있는 모든 법적 문제를 담당한다. 재정 및 회계 문제는 일반적으로 사고 이후에 해결되기 때문에 대부분의 사고에는 이 부서에 인력이 배치되지 않는다. 하지만 즉각적인 재정 관리가 필요한 대규모의 장기간 지속하는 사고에서 특히 외부 자원을 신속하게 조달해야 할 때는 재정/행정 부서가 필요할 수 있다. 자연 재난이나 위험 물질 사고가 발생했을 때 화주, 운송업체, 화학물질 제조업체 또는 보험회사로부터 보상을 받을 수 있는 경우 재정/행정 부서를 설립할 수 있다. 이에 대한 훌륭한 예는 대부분의 의료기관이 코로나 19 팬데믹을 해결하기 위해 시작한 대응이다. 각 개인 병원, 요양원, EMS 기관 또는 NIMS 구조를 사용한 기타 기관은 정부에서 환급을 위한 비용을 추적해야 하는 등 대응과 관련된 수많은 재정적 문제를 해결하기 의해 재정/행정 부서를 설립했을 것이며 이 중 일부는 재정/행정 부서가 처음 시작될 당시에는 정의되지도 않은 상태였을 것이다.

재난 발생 시 의료 대응

재난 대응에는 여러 가지 동시 목표가 있을 수 있지만, 의료 대응의 특정 구성 요소를 결합하면 재난 피해자의 사망률과 이환율을 최소화하는 데 도움이 된다. 이 장에서는 이러한 조치를 차례대로 설명하지만, 실제 재난 발생 시에는 많은 조치가 동시에 수행된다는 점을 기억하는 것이 중요하다(**Box 17-4**). 또한 전반적인 대응은 사고 발생 위치와 프로토콜 및 가용 자원에 따라 달라질 수 있다는 점을 언급하는 것이 중요하다. 대응을 위한 지휘체계나 구조는 국제적 배치에 따라 상당히 다를 수 있다.

초기대응

첫 번째 단계는 EMS 대응 시스템의 신고 및 활성화이다. 이 단계는 일반적으로 사건 목격자에 의해 신고가 이루어지고 나서 경찰, 소방, 응급의료기관의 대응을 요청하는 방식으로 수행된다(**그림 17-5**).

사고 현장에 가장 먼저 도착한 병원 전 처치 제공자는 전체 응급의료 대응의 발판을 가련하는 여러 가지 중요한 기능을 수행한다. 구조대원으로서의 일반적인 업무와 달리 이러한 업무에는 환자 처치 시작이 포함되지 않는다. 현장에 가장 먼저 도착한 병원 전 처치 제공

Box 17-4 재난에 대한 의료 대응의 기본 단계

재난에 대한 의료 대응에는 다음과 같은 기본 단계가 포함된다.

1. 신고 및 EMS 활성화
2. 초기 대응
3. 현장에서 EMS 대응
4. 상황 평가
   a. 원인
   b. 사상자 수
   c. 추가 자원
      Ⅰ. 의료
      Ⅱ. 기타
5. 상황과 요구 사항 전달
6. 의료체계 활성화
   a. 의료기관에 알림
7. 수색 및 구조
8. 분류(기도 및 생명을 위협하는 출혈 지혈)
9. 사상자 확인
10. 치료
11. 이송
12. 재분류

© National Association of Emergency Medical Technicians (NAEMT)

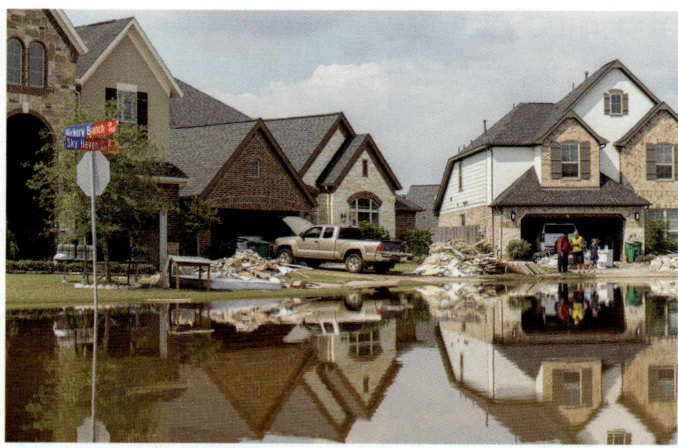

그림 17-5 허리케인이나 홍수와 같은 자연 재난이 발생하면 소방본부 상황실로 전화가 쇄도한다. 2017년 텍사스에서 발생한 허리케인 하비로 인한 폭풍 피해 모습.

© Michelmond/Shutterstock

수색 및 구조

이 시점에서 환자 처치를 현장에서 시작할 수 있다. 일반적으로 이 과정은 피해를 본 현장에서 사상자를 찾아 안전한 장소로 대피시키는 수색 및 구조 활동으로 시작된다. 재난 현장 근처의 지역 주민과 생존자 스스로가 가능한 경우 즉각적인 수색 및 구조 자원이 되는 경우가 많으며 이들은 공공 안전 요원이 도착하기 전에 이미 희생자 수색을 시작했을 수도 있다. 경험에 따르면 지역 사회가 재난 현장에 대응하여 피해자를 돕는 과정을 시작할 수 있다.

많은 국가와 지역 사회에서 국가와 지역 재난 대응 계획의 필수적인 부분으로 공식적이고 전문적인 수색 및 구조팀을 만들었다. 이 팀의 구성원은 제한된 공간 환경 대한 전문 교육을 받고 특정 사고에 따라 활성화된다. 이 수색 및 구조팀에는 일반적으로 다음이 포함된다.

- 의료전문가로 구성된 간부
- 위험 물질, 구조 공학, 중장비 운전, 수색 및 구조 방법에 대한 지식을 갖춘 전문가
- 훈련된 구조견과 조련사

중요한 것은 전문 팀을 활성화하는 데 시간이 걸릴 수 있으며 열악한 환경에서는 즉흥적인 대응이 필요한 경우가 많다. 예를 들어, 건설 현장에서 발생한 다수 사상자 사고에서는 현지 건설 회사가 재난 현장에서 무거운 잔해를 옮기는 데 사용할 수 있는 장비, 도구와 자재를 포함한 귀중한 수색 및 구조 자산을 제공할 수 있다.

자는 전반적인 현장 평가를 수행해야 한다. 이 평가의 목표는 잠재적인 위험을 평가하고 전체 사상자 수를 추정하여 현장 필요한 추가 의료 자원을 결정하고 수색 및 구조팀과 같은 특수 인력과 장비가 필요한지를 평가하는 것이다. 시간에 따라 실무자는 구급대원과 구조대원에게 의도적으로 해를 가하기 위해 고안된 이차 폭발물의 징후도 주의 깊게 확인한다.

기본 평가가 완료되면 평가 결과를 상황실에 보고하고 필요한 자원을 요청한다. 이후 병원 전 처치 제공자는 부상자를 분류하고 분류 결과에 따라 한곳으로 모으고 현장에 도착하는 구급차, 지원 인력 및 공급 물품을 배치할 적절한 위치를 선정한다.

또한 대응하는 EMS 기관은 사고 인근 지역에서 환자를 수용할 수 있는 병원에 사고에 대해 알리고 예상 사상자 수와 각 사상자의 중증도를 전달하여 의료기관이 적절하게 준비하고 재난 계획을 활성화할 수 있도록 하는 것이 중요하다. 재난 대응의 현장 구성 요소는 재난 피해자를 위한 전체 생존 사슬의 첫 번째 연결 고리이며 EMS 기관은 상황실에 즉시 통보할 책임이 있다.

분류

환자를 파악하고 대피시키려면 환자 분류 장소로 이동시켜 평가하고 중증도를 분류할 수 있다. 분류라는 용어는 "분류한다"라는 뜻의 프랑스어이다. 의학적 관점에서 볼 때 분류란 손상 중증도에 따라 사상자를 분류하는 것을 의미한다. 이 과정은 1800년대 초 나폴레옹의 외과 군의관이자 나폴레옹 전쟁 중 기본 구급차를 개발한 것으로 유명한 도미니크 라레 남작(Baron Dominique Larrey)에 의해 처음 설명되었다. 래리는 다음과 같이 말했다.

> 심각한 손상을 입은 사람들은 계급과 관계없이 가장 먼저 처치를 받아야 한다. 경미한 손상을 입은 사람은 중증 손상을 입은 사람이 수술받거나 드레싱을 받을 때까지 기다릴 수 있지만, 그렇지 않으면 중증 손상을 입은 사람은 몇 시간 동안 생존하지 못하거나 드물게는 다음 날까지 생존하지 못할 수도 있다.

래리 이후 더 연구되고 확장된 이 개념은 즉각적인 처치와 생명을 구하는 처치가 필요한 환자에게 우선순위를 부여하는 역할을 한다.

환자 분류는 모든 재난 의료 대응의 중요한 임무 중 하나이다. 앞서 언급한 바와 같이 재난이 아닌 상황에서 일반적인 환자 분류의 목적은 개별 환자에게 가장 큰 이익을 주는 것이다. 이 의무는 일반적으로 가장 아픈 환자를 찾아 처치하는 것을 의미한다. 다수 사상자 발생 시 환자 분류의 목표는 가장 많은 사람에게 최선의 처치를 제공하는 것이다. 현장에서 다수 사상자 분류는 훈련받은 중증도 분류 담당자가 시행해야 한다. 중증도 분류 담당자는 어떤 사람이 치명적인 손상을 입었는지 또는 어떤 사람이 생존 가능성이 희박한지에 대한 어려운 결정을 내릴 수도 있으므로 현장에서 환자를 평가하고 처치에 대한 다양한 임상 경험이 있어야 한다. 일반적으로 현장 경험이 많은 구급대원이 이 요건을 충족하며 현장 경험이 있는 의사도 이 역할을 할 수 있다. 그런데도 모든 병원 전 처치 제공자는 환자 분류를 기본적으로 수행할 수 있어야 하며 다양한 중증도 분류 알고리즘을 수행할 수 있도록 충분한 연습을 해야 한다. 어린이와 특별한 도움이 필요한 환자 등 취약 계층을 다루는 전문 교육은 매우 유용할 수 있다.

환자를 평가하고 분류할 수 있는 다양한 방법이 있다. 한 가지 방법은 신속한 생리적 및 정신 상태를 평가하는 것이다. 이 분류 과정을 START 분류 알고리즘(단순 분류와 신속한 처치)이라고 한다. 이 분류 방법은 환자의 호흡 상태, 관류 상태 및 정신 상태를 평가하여 결정적인 처치를 시행할 수 있는 의료기관으로 초기에 이송 우선순위를 결정한다(5장 현장 관리 **Box 5-6** 참조). 다른 분류 방법으로 MASS(이동, 평가, 분류, 이송), Smart, JumpStart(소아 분류 방법), Sacco 분류 방법이 있다.

국제 지침을 제공하고 분류 과정에 일관성을 부여하기 위해 미국 질병통제예방센터는 다양한 분야의 전문가 그룹을 소집하여 현재 SALT로 알려진 합의 기반 분류 방법을 개발했다(5장 현장 관리 **Box 5-7** 참조). 이 분류 방법은 환자의 이동 능력에 따라 환자를 분류하고 환자의 소생술 처치 필요성 평가, 해당 처치 시행, 궁극적으로 처치와 이송이 포함된다.

정확한 환자 분류 방법과 관계없이 모든 분류 과정은 궁극적으로 환자를 4가지 손상 중증도 중 하나로 분류한다. 우선순위가 가장 높은 환자는 손상이 심각하지만, 생존 가능성이 있는 것으로 확인된 환자이며 일반적으로 즉시 처치가 필요하고 빨간색으로 분류한다. 중등도의 손상을 입고(보행할 수 없을 수 있음) 처치가 잠시 지연되더라도 견딜 수 있는 환자는 지연 환자로 분류되며 노란색으로 구분한다. "보행이 가능한 환자"라고도 하는 비교적 경미한 손상을 입은 환자는 최소 피해자로 분류되며 녹색으로 구분한다. 현장에서 사망했거나 손상이 너무 심해 사망이 불가피한 환자는 사망 또는 예상 환자로 분류하고 검은색으로 표시한다. 주목할 점은 일부 분류 방법, 특히 SALT에서는 치명적인 손상을 입은 환자와 사망한 환자를 구분하여 사망할 것으로 예상되는 환자는 회색으로 분류한다는 것이다. 특정 도시 대응 기관에서는 인구 밀도와 대응 지역으로 인해 사고 발생 시 의료 환자(주황색 태그)를 식별하는 것이 중요하다는 점에 주목했다. 예를 들어 흡입된 파편으로 인해 구조물이 붕괴한 후 만성 폐쇄성 폐질환이 악화한 환자는 외상성 손상은 없지만, 긴급한 이송이 필요할 수 있다. 외상 환자는 외상 처치가 가능한 시설에 과부하가 걸릴 수 있으므로 비외상 상태를 파악하면 해당 환자를 대체 시설로 안내할 수 있다.

이 모든 색상 분류는 재난 현장에서 "재난 분류표"를 사용하는 것을 의미하며 환자 분류가 완료되면 환자에게 부착한다. 색상 분류는 환자 분류에 대한 즉각적인 시각적 참조를 제공한다. 일부 환자 분류 방법에서는 긴급, 응급, 경증, 사망 또는 예상 환자를 각각 ClassⅠ, ClassⅡ, ClassⅢ, ClassⅣ로 분류하는 분류 방법을 사용하기도 한다.

중증도 분류 담당자는 중증 손상 환자를 처치하기 위해 분류를 일시적으로 중지하려는 유혹을 피하는 것이 중요하다. 이 초기 분류 단계에서 처치는 쉽고 빠르게 진행할 수 있고 노동 집약적이지 않은 초치로 제한된다. 일반적으로 도수 기도 개방, 바늘감압, 화학적 해독제 투여, 상처 패킹 및 지혈대 사용을 포함한 외부출혈 지혈과 같은 처치만 시행해야 한다는 것을 의미한다. 백마스크 장치 환기, 폐쇄식 가슴 압박, 정맥로 확보, 기관내삽관과 같은 처치는 분류 과정에서 시행하지 않는 경우가 많다. 이 원칙에 대한 한 가지 제한적인 예외는 전술적 사건에 대응하는 동안 성문위기도기를 사용하는 경우가 있다는 것이다.

환자 분류가 완료되면 환자들은 분류 우선순위에 따라 부상자 집결 장소로 모이게 된다. 구체적으로 모든 긴급 환자(빨간색), 응급(노란색), 비응급 환자(녹색)별로 모이게 된다. 부상자 집결 장소는 피해자를 쉽게 이동하고 신속하게 처치를 제공할 수 있을 만큼 재난 현장과 가까운 곳이어야 하지만, 지속적인 위험으로부터 안전할 수 있도록 사고 현장으로부터 충분히 멀리 떨어져 있어야 한다. 중요한 고려사항은 다음과 같다.

- 재난 현장과의 접근성
- 위험 요소 및 오염된 환경으로부터 안전한 곳
- 기후 조건으로부터 보호(가능한 경우)
- 재난 피해자와 담당자가 쉽게 볼 수 있는 곳
- 지상, 공중, 수상 대피를 위해 출입로가 편리한 곳
- 대기 중인 구급차의 배기가스로부터 안전한 거리

추가 의료진과 자원이 현장에 도착해서 사용할 수 있으면 환자 분류 우선순위에 따라 부상자 집결 장소에서 의료지원 및 처치가 제공된다. 이러한 장소는 현장에 출동한 의사가 손상을 입은 환자를 추가로 평가하고 처치할 수 있도록 배정될 수 있는 적절한 장소이다.

마지막으로 이송 자원이 확보되면 환자는 다시 한 번 분류 우선순위에 따라 결정적인 처치를 받을 수 있도록 의료기관으로 이송한다(**그림 17-6**). 이송이 가능한 경우 추가 처치를 제공하기 위해 긴급 환자는 현장에 대기하지 않는다(**그림 17-7**). 필요한 처치는 의료기관으로 이송하는 동안에 시행해야 한다.

눈에 보이는 심각한 손상으로 인해 구급대원은 종종 즉각적인 처치와 이송을 위해 개별 환자를 앞으로 이동시키고 분류 과정을 생략하는 경향이 있다. 모든 피해자를 분류하여 구조 가능한 피해자를 먼저 처치할 수 있도록 이러한 경향을 피해야 한다. 그런데도 다음과 같은 특정 시나리오에서는 분규 과정을 우회하는 것을 고려할 수 있다.

1. 악천후로 인해 구조대원과 사상자에게 과도한 위험을 초래하는 경우
2. 보조 조명을 사용할 수 없는 어둠 또는 일몰이 임박한 경우
3. 자연적이거나 부자연스러운 사건으로 인한 지속적인 손상 위험
4. 즉시 이용할 수 있는 분류 시설 또는 분류 담당자가 없는 경우
5. 법 집행 시나리오에서 피해자를 사고 현장에서 이송을 위해 환자 집결 지점까지 신속하게 이동해야 하는 전술적 상황

마지막으로 분류는 역동적이고 지속적인 과정으로 생각해야 한다. 환자를 평가하고 분류한 후에는 나머지 처치에 대한 해당 분류를 수행하지 않을 수 있다. 예를 들어 주요 팔다리 상처와 출혈이 동반된 환자는 처음에는 긴급 환자로 분류할 수 있지만, 상처에 압박을 가하

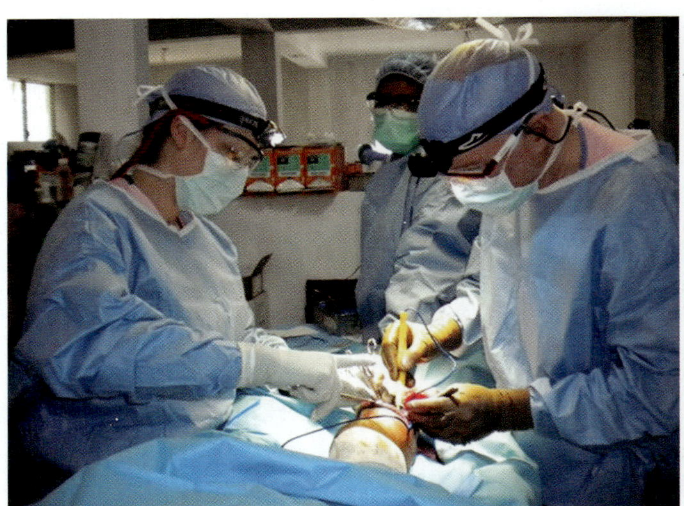

그림 17-6 2010년 아이티 대지진 이후 아이티의 한 병원에서 의료 서비스를 받고 있다.

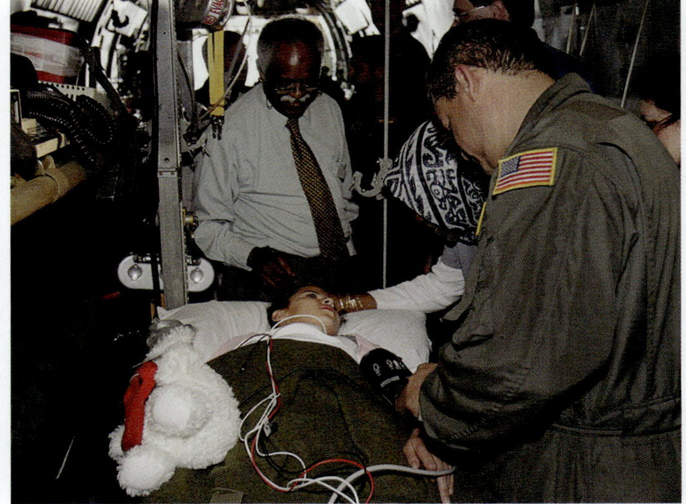

그림 17-7 환자 수송을 위해 개조된 군용 수송기 내부.

고 출혈이 조절된 후에는 비응급 환자로 재분류할 수 있다. 또는 처음에는 긴급 환자로 분류했던 환자가 급격히 악화하여 이후 지연 환자로 재분류할 수도 있다.

환자가 이송을 기다리는 동안 현장에서 재분류를 시행해야 한다. 또한 환자는 이송 목적지에 도착한 후 응급 수술의 우선순위에 따라 재분류를 시행할 수 있다.

처치

초기에는 환자 수가 가용 자원을 초과하기 때문에 현장에서의 처치는 일반적으로 도수로 기도를 개방하고 긴장기흉 완화, 외부출혈 지혈, 화학물질에 대해 해독제를 투여하는 것으로 제한된다. 적절한 자원이 현장에 도착하거나 병원으로 이송하는 동안에만 정맥 라인 확보나 골절 부위 부목 고정과 같은 추가 처치를 제공한다.

이송

다수 사상자 사고 현장에서 의료기관으로 환자를 이송하고 추적하는 데는 다양한 이송 방법을 이용하기 때문에 부서 간의 협조가 필요하다. 긴급 및 응급 환자는 헬기나 구급차를 이용해 의료기관으로 이송한다. 다수 사상자가 발생한 사고에서 경미한 환자는 버스 및 승합차 등의 차량을 이용해서 더 쉽고 신속하게 관리할 수 있으며 때에 따라 환자를 평가 및 처치를 위해 병원이 아닌 다른 장소로 이송할 수 있다. 그러나 이러한 대체 이송 수단을 사용하는 경우 충분한 물품과 장비를 갖춘 병원 전 처치 제공자가 같이 탈 수 있도록 배정해야 한다. 각 환자의 이동 경로와 이송된 의료기관을 정확하게 환자 추적일지 또는 추적 시스템을 통해 정확하게 기록한다.

중증외상 환자 발생에 효과적으로 대응하는 데 있어서 또 다른 중요한 문제는 이송이 시작된 후 환자의 목적지에 대한 의사결정 과정과 관련이 있다. 최근의 사례에 따르면 쉽게 움직일 수 있거나 이동할 수 있는 환자들은 가능한 모든 교통수단을 이용하여 재난 현장을 떠나 주변 병원으로 직접 이동하는 경우가 많다. 이로 인해 재난 현장에서 가장 가까운 병원에 많은 수의 보행이 가능한 환자가 도착하는 경우가 종종 있다. 예를 들어 2017년 라스베이거스 하베스트 음악 페스티벌 총격 사건에서는 우버 및 리프트 등 애플리케이션 기반 택시 서비스를 이용한 것으로 유명하다.

병원 전 처치 제공자는 재난 현장에서 가장 가까운 병원은 첫 번째로 환자를 이송하는 구급차가 도착하기 전에도 환자들로 붐빌 수 있다는 사실을 병원 전 의료진이 이해해야 한다. 환자를 가장 가까운

병원으로 이송하기 전에 응급실 상황과 구급차로 이송된 환자를 수용하고 처치할 수 있는 능력을 확인하기 위 통신 채널을 구축해야 한다. 가장 가까운 병원이 혼잡할 경우 EMS 시스템은 필요할 때 환자를 더 먼 의료기관으로 이송할 수 있다. 환자를 여러 기관으로 분산하면 궁극적으로 모든 수용 병원이 제공할 수 있는 환자 처치를 최적화할 수 있는 능력을 더 잘 보존할 수 있다. 환자의 상태에 따라 외상, 화상, 이식 센터 등 전문 처치 시설에 대한 배려도 고려해야 한다.

그러나 병원 수가 제한된 지역 사회에서는 EMS가 환자를 가장 가까운 병원으로 이송하는 것 외에 다른 선택의 여지가 없을 수 있다. 일부 지자체에서는 재난 의료 통제 센터가 병원과 직접 연락하여 급성 손상 환자를 처리할 수 있는 역량을 파악한다.

의료 지원팀

재난의 규모가 커서 추가 현장 자원이 필요한 경우, 일부 병원에서는 재난 대응팀을 구성하면 EMS 현장 대응을 강화하고 현장 처치를 제공함으로써 병원 전 처치 제공자가 사상자 집결지에서 의료 서비스를 제공하는 업무에서 벗어나 환자 이송을 수행할 수 있도록 한다. 기관은 주변 지역 사회와 기존 협약을 맺고 상호 지원을 활용하여 병원 전 치료 역량을 추가로 제공할 수 있다(**그림 17-8**). 또한 주 또는 연방 정부의 외부 자원이 필요한 경우 많은 지자체에서 다른 응급의료 대응팀을 이용할 수 있다.

미국에서는 도시 의료 대응 시스템(MMRS)의 결과로 많은 도시에 도시 의료 대응 시스템 태스크포스 또는 대응팀이 만들어졌다. 도시 의료 대응 시스템은 테러 또는 공중보건 비상사태에 대응하기 위해

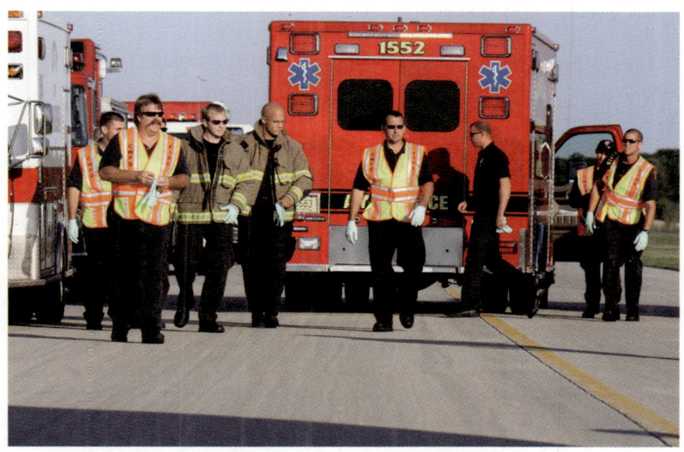

그림 17-8 대규모 비상 상황이 발생하면 주변 지역사회의 기관이 상호 지원을 제공할 수 있다.

미국 보건복지부(DHHS)에서 개발하고 자금을 지원했다. 목표는 다양한 지역 대응 기관과 서비스를 통합하여 이러한 사건에 대한 대응을 강화하는 것이다. 이러한 대응 자산은 응급의학과, 외상외과, 외과 세부 전문 분야 및 간호 분야의 의료 인력으로 구성된다. 도시 의료 대응 시스템 태스크 포스는 주 및 연방 기금을 통해 구매한 자원으로 대응할 수 있다. 이러한 대응팀은 의료 시설을 보강 및 보충하거나 환자에게 급증하는 환자 수용 능력과 의료 서비스를 제공하기 위해 설치된 이동식 의료 시설에 인력을 배치하는 데 사용할 수 있다.

미국 정부는 더 큰 규모로 국가 재난 의료시스템을 통해 재난 의료지원팀(DMATs)을 동원할 수 있는 역량을 갖추고 있다. 재난 의료지원팀은 현장 처치를 제공할 뿐만 아니라 이동식 의료시설을 만들 수 있으며 이 중 일부는 재난 지역의 자원이 과부하 되었을 때 외과적 처치를 수행하고 환자의 중요한 처치 요구를 충족할 수 있는 능력을 갖추고 있다. 재난 의료지원팀 요청은 일반적으로 지역 비상 관리자가 주 비상 관리 당국에 주지사 사무실이 연방 정부를 거쳐 국가 재난 의료 시스템의 대응 프로그램을 담당하는 DHHS에 요청하는 등 적절한 채널을 통해 이루어져야 한다. 일부 주에서는 주 전체 비상사태에 대응할 수 있는 유사하게 조직되고 구조화된 팀이 있다.

테러 및 대량살상무기의 위협

테러는 구급 및 구조대원에게 가장 어려운 다수 사상자 사고를 일으킬 수 있다. 자살 폭탄 테러범부터 재래식 무기, 군사 무기, 대량살상무기(화학, 생물학, 방사능, 핵무기)에 이르기까지 테러 위협은 다양하다. 테러 사건은 인간이 만든 모든 재난 중에서 가장 많은 사상자와 사망자를 발생시킬 가능성이 높다(특수 무기에 관한 자세한 내용은 18장 폭발 및 대량살상무기를 참조).

테러리스트들은 안타깝게도 민간인 사상자를 발생시키는데 놀라운 기지를 보여주었다. 2001년 9월 11일 테러 공격 당시 테러리스트들은 연료가 가득한 여객기를 이용해 막대한 인명 및 재산 피해를 발생시켰다.

특히 대량살상무기와 관련된 테러리스트 위협의 독특한 특징 중 하나는 심리적 인명 피해가 주로 발생한다는 점이다. 테러리스트는 목표를 달성하기 위해 많은 사람을 죽일 필요 없이 의료 인프라를 압도할 수 있는 공황과 공포 분위기를 조성하기만 하면 된다. 1995년 3월 도쿄에서 발생한 사린 테러 당시 총 5,000명의 환자가 병원에 내원했다. 이 중 사린가스로 인해 신체적 영향을 받은 환자는 1,000명 미만이었고 나머지는 심리적 스트레스와 의사에 진료를 받고 싶어 했다. 2001년 미국에서 발생한 탄저균 사건에서도 실제 탄저균 노출이 아닌 비특이적 호흡기 증상으로 응급실에 내원한 환자 수가 급격히 증가했다.

폭발과 폭탄 테러는 전 세계적으로 테러리스트에 의한 재난에서 가장 빈번하게 발생하는 대량 인명 피해의 원인으로 일차 사건과 응급구조대원에게 피해를 주기 위한 이차 폭발 장치 모두에서 계속되고 있다. 이러한 폭탄 테러의 대부분은 사망률이 낮은 비교적 작은 폭발물로 구성된다. 그러나 건물, 수도관, 가스 배관 또는 이동 중인 차량에 전략적으로 설치할 때 그 영향은 훨씬 더 커질 수 있다(**그림 17-9**). 높은 이환율과 사망률은 폭발의 강도뿐만 아니라 표적이 된 건물의 붕괴로 이어지는 후속 구조적 손상과도 관련이 있다. 더 큰 위협은 재래식 소이탄과 방사성 물질을 결합한 "더러운 폭탄"과 같이 재래식 폭발물에 화학, 생물학 또는 방사능 물질을 결합한 폭발물일 수 있다.

환경을 오염시키는 대량살상무기의 경우 가장 큰 물류 관련 난제가 될 수 있다. 구급대원과 구조대원은 오염 위험으로 인해 환자 이송에 제한받을 수 있다. 병원 전 처치 제공자는 손상의 정도를 판단할 뿐만 아니라 오염 가능성과 오염 제거 및 초기 안정화 필요성을 평가하기 위해 환자 분류를 수행할 수 있는 준비와 장비를 갖추어야 한다. 동시에 병원 전 처치 제공자는 적절한 개인보호장비를 사용하여 잠재적 오염으로부터 자신을 보호하기 위한 적절한 조치를 해야 한다.

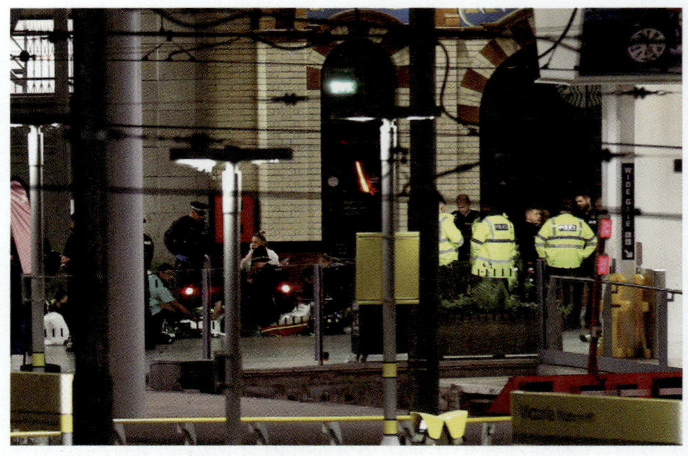

그림 17-9 2017년 맨체스터 폭탄 테러

오염 제거

오염 제거는 위험 물질 및 대량살상무기와 관련된 모든 재난에 대한 중요한 고려 사항이다(**그림 17-10**). 많은 희생자가 발생하고 알려지지 않은 물질이 사용되며 다수의 우려되는 환자가 발생하는 테러 사건은 오염되었거나 오염되었을 가능성이 있는 사상자가 발생할 가능성을 크게 높인다(자세한 내용은 18장 폭발 및 대량살상무기 참조). 일반적으로 환자가 오염되었다고 판단되는 경우 결정적인 처치를 받을 수 있는 의료기관으로 이송하기 전에 오염 제거를 시행해야 한다. 오염 제거 과정에서 현장 보안과 인력은 오염 물질을 포함하고 안전하게 폐기하는 것과 마찬가지로 중요한 고려 사항이다.

처치 구역

위험 물질 및 대량살상무기와 관련된 재난에 대응할 때는 분류 및 사상자 처치 지역은 오염 지역으로부터 최소 270m 정도 떨어진 곳을 기준으로 바람이 불어오는 방향과 높은 곳에 배치하는 것이 중요하다.

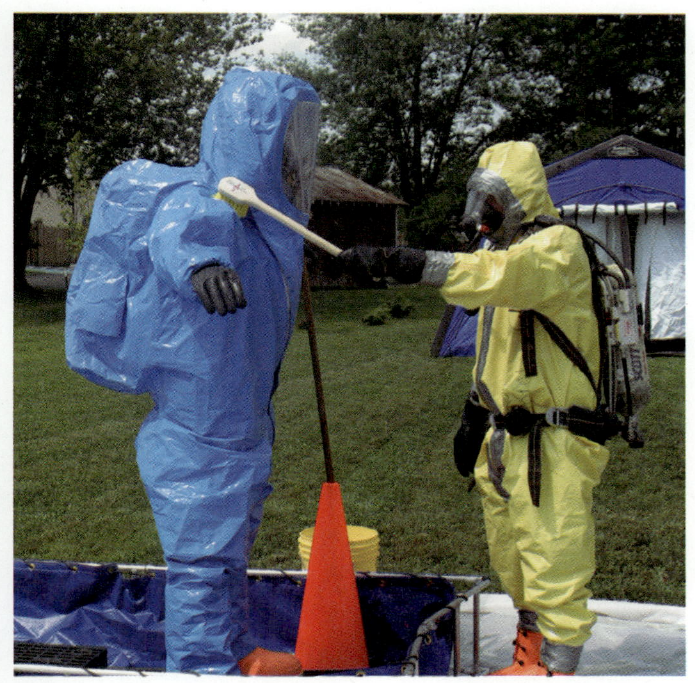

그림 17-10 레벨 B 개인보호장비를 착용한 대원이 전방통제지역(warm zone)에서 레벨 A 개인보호복을 착용한 대원의 오염 제거를 한다.

© Jones & Bartlett Learning

재난에 대한 심리적 반응

심리적 트라우마 및 기타 심리적 후유증은 자연 재난이나 인간에 의해 의도하지 않은 재난과 같은 사고의 빈번한 부작용이다. 반대로 테러의 목적 중 하나는 심리적 고통, 트라우마, 불안을 유발하는 것이다. 모든 구급대원이나 구조대원에게 좋은 심리적 건강 상태를 유지하는 것은 신체 건강을 유지하는 것만큼이나 중요하다.

정신 건강에 영향을 미치는 재난의 특징

모든 재난이 같은 수준의 심리적 영향을 미치는 것은 아니다. 정신 건강에 가장 큰 영향을 미치는 것으로 보이는 재난 특징은 다음과 같다.

- 사전 경고가 거의 없거나 전혀 없음
- 개인 안전에 대한 심각한 위협
- 알려지지 않은 잠재적인 건강에 영향
- 불확실한 사고의 지속 시간
- 사람의 실수나 악의적 의도
- 테러 대상과 관련된 상징성

심리적 반응에 영향을 미치는 요인

재난을 경험한 모두 사람은 피해자든 구급대원과 구조대원이든 어느 정도 영향을 받는다. 다행히도 그렇다고 해서 대부분의 개인이 정신 건강 장애가 발생한다는 의미는 아니다. 하지만 피해자와 구급대원과 구조대원은 모두 영향을 받은 모든 개인은 피해자와 구급대원과 구조대원 모두 사건에 대해 어떤 유형의 심리적 또는 정서적 반응을 보일 수 있다.

마찬가지로 회복력을 증진하고 이러한 비상사태로부터 지역 사회의 회복을 도울 수 있는 개인적 대응과 집단적 대응이 모두 존재한다. 재난에 대한 개인의 대응에 영향을 미치는 요인은 다음과 같다.

- 사고에 대한 신체적, 심리적 접근성
- 끔찍하거나 기괴한 상황에 대한 노출
- 재난으로 인해 이전보다 건강 상태 저하
- 손실 규모
- 이전 트라우마 병력

트라우마에 대한 집단적 대응에 영향을 미치는 요인은 다음과 같다.

- 지역 사회의 혼란 정도

- 재난 전 가족과 지역사회의 안정성
- 지역 사회 리더십
- 복구 노력의 문화적 민감성

재난으로 인한 심리적 후유증

재난 후 심리적 반응은 가벼운 스트레스 반응부터 외상 후 스트레스 장애(PTSD), 주요 우울증, 급성 스트레스 장애 또는 자살에 이르기까지 매우 다양하다. 외상 후 스트레스 장애는 끔찍하거나 끔찍한 사고에 노출된 후 발생하는 정신 건강 상태로 사건에 대한 회상, 악몽, 불안, 놀람 반응의 증가, 소음이나 촉감에 대한 민감성, 사고에 대한 통제할 수 없는 생각 등의 증상이 나타날 수 있다.

중재

비교적 간단한 몇 가지 조치를 통해 개인이 사건의 심리적 영향을 최소화하고 재난 이전 수준의 기능으로 복귀하는 데 도움을 줄 수 있다.

- 개인은 가능한 한 빨리 일상적인 활동으로 복귀해야 한다.
- 정신 건강 장애 진단을 받지 않은 사람의 경우 재난에 대한 심리적 반응과 이러한 반응이 개인과 유가족에게 어떤 영향을 미칠 수 있는지 설명하는 교육 자료를 제공하는 것이 도움이 될 수 있다.
- 위기 상담을 제공하고 치료가 필요한 경우 치료를 의뢰한다.
- 정신 건강 문제가 진단되면 인지 행동치료, 트라우마 정보에 기반한 치료, 안구 운동 둔감과 및 재처리 요법, 약물치료 등 치료적 중재가 도움이 될 수 있다.

EMS 제공자 스트레스

EMS 제공자는 스트레스의 이차 피해자가 될 수 있으며 다른 심리적 후유증을 경험할 수 있다. 이러한 후유증은 사고 발생 중이나 사고 발생 후에도 업무 수행에 부정적인 영향을 미칠 수 있다. 개인 건강은 물론 가족 및 직장 관계에도 부정적인 영향을 미칠 수 있다. 직장 상사와 동료는 사고 대응에 참여한 개인의 스트레스 및 심리적 고통의 발생이나 징후에 주의를 기울여야 한다.

사고 후 스트레스를 예방하고 관리하기 위한 여러 가지 중재 전략이 자주 사용된다. 여기에는 보고, 스트레스 해소, 슬픔을 관리하기 위한 부문이 포함된다. 이러한 과정을 통칭하여 위기 상황 스트레스 관리(CISM)라고 한다. 위기 상황 스트레스 관리의 가치는 주로 EMS 제공자에게 의무적으로 개입해야 할 때 의문이 제기되어 왔다. 위기

상황 스트레스 관리는 참여 의사가 있는 EMS 제공자에게 선택적으로 제공할 수 있지만, 일부 상황에서는 실제로 해를 끼칠 수 있으므로 모든 EMS 제공자에게 의무적으로 시행해서는 안 된다. 심리적 응급처치, 목사, 동료 지원, 직원 지원 프로그램, 건강 검진 등의 대체 프로그램은 위기 상황 스트레스 관리의 일부 한계를 해결하고 EMS 제공자가 심리적으로 불만이 있거나 고통의 징후를 보이고 도움을 받을 수 있는 상황에서 즉각적으로 개입할 수 있는 효과적인 도구를 팀에게 제공한다.

작업자의 스트레스 징후

EMS 제공자에게 나타나는 일반적인 스트레스 징후에는 생리적, 정서적, 인지, 행동적 요소가 있다.

생리적 징후

- 휴식 후에도 지속되는 피로
- 구역
- 미세한 떨림
- 틱
- **감각 이상**
- 어지럼
- 위장 장애
- 심장 두근거림
- 질식 또는 질식할 것 같은 느낌

정서적 징후

- 불안
- 과민성
- 압도당하는 느낌
- 자신 또는 타인에 대한 비현실적인 피해 예상
- 무관심
- 죄책감

인지 징후

- 기억상실
- 의사 결정의 어려움
- 명칭 실어증(일반적인 사물이나 친숙한 사람의 이름을 기억하지 못함)
- 집중력 문제 또는 산만함
- 집중 시간 감소
- 계산 능력 저하

행동 징후

- 불면증
- 과잉 경계
- 쉽게 울음
- 부적절한 유머
- 의식적인 행동
- 회피/사회적 고립

현장에서 스트레스 관리

다음과 같은 현장 개입은 스트레스를 줄이는 데 도움이 될 수 있다.

- 외상성 자극에 대한 노출 제한
- 합리적인 운영 시간
- 적절한 휴식 시간(**그림 17-11**)
- 합리적인 식단
- 규칙적인 운동 프로그램
- 개인 시간
- 공감하는 동료와의 대화
- 스트레스 징후 모니터링

재난 교육 및 훈련

공식적인 교육 및 훈련 프로그램의 개발과 실행은 다수 사상자 사고 발생 시 효과적으로 대응할 수 있는 병원 전 처치 제공자의 능력을 향상할 것이다. 병원 전 처치 제공자는 재난 및 다수 사상자 관리에서 완화 및 대비, 수색 및 구조, 분류, 응급처치, 이송, 재난 후 복구

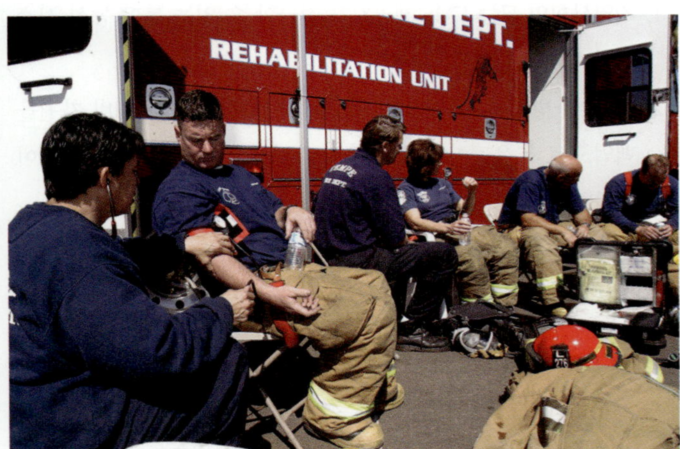

그림 17-11 현장에서 적절한 휴식 시간을 가지면 스트레스 해소에 도움이 된다.
© Jones & Bartlett Learning. Courtesy of MIEMSS.

등 다양한 임무를 수행할 수 있다. 교육 및 훈련에 관한 준비는 다양한 구조화된 학습 환경뿐만 아니라 비구조화 학습 환경에서도 이루어질 수 있다. 교육 효과와 비교 대응으로 측정할 때 각각의 장단점이 있다.

독립적인 훈련은 재난 대비의 기초이다. 문헌뿐만이 아니라 인터넷을 통해서도 다양한 자료를 이용할 수 있다. 미국 질병통제예방센터, 공공보건 기관, 연방재난관리청(FEMA) 및 군대는 모든 개인에게 인터넷 기반 학습 기회와 자료를 제공한다. 교육 과정은 시간적 여유가 있는 일정에 따라 독립적으로 이수할 수 있다. 그러나 이 방법은 직접인 실습 경험을 제공하지 않는다.

그룹 교육은 재난 대응과 관련하여 특정 팀을 대상으로 진행된다. 교육 프로그램을 광범위하게 이용할 수 있으며 사고 지휘체계 및 대량살상무기 대비에 대한 이해를 포함한다. 수많은 전문가와 전문 기관은 공중보건, 응급의학, 중환자 처치, 외과와 내과 전문 분야를 포함하여 모든 수준의 병원 전 처치 제공자를 포함하여 각자의 전문 진료 범위에 맞는 교육 프로그램과 모듈을 개발했다. 병원 전 처치 제공자를 위한 이러한 유형의 프로그램 중 한 가지 예로 NAEMT의 모든 위험 재난 대응 과정이 있다(**Box 17-5**).

시뮬레이션은 효과적인 재난 대응에 필수적으로 다양한 배경을 가진 많은 사람을 한자리에 모을 수 있는 훈련 기회를 제공한다. 두 가지 예로는 탁상 훈련과 실제 현장 훈련이 있다. 탁상 훈련은 재난 대응을 테스트하고 평가하는 데 비용 효율적이고 매우 유용한 방법이다. 이름에서 알 수 있듯이 이 훈련은 테이블을 중심으로 진행되며 다양한 참가자가 예상되는 대응 조치를 말로 지시한다. 탁상 연습을 통해 여러 분야의 기관이 실시간으로 소통하고 상호 작용할 수 있다. 이러한 활동에는 숙련된 진행자가 목표를 통해 참가자를 안내하고 연습이 끝날 때 그룹에 건설적인 피드백을 제공하는 형태의 지도가 필요하다.

현장 훈련은 지역사회 재난 대응 계획을 실제 실행 및 수행을 포함

하는 가장 현실적인 훈련이다. 현장 훈련을 통해 서면으로 정의된 목표를 달성할 수 있는 신체적 역량을 실시간으로 평가를 할 수 있다. 이상적인 훈련은 피해자를 충격 및 손상이 발생한 지점에서 EMS 대응 시스템을 통해 의료시설에서 결정적인 처치를 받을 수 있도록 이송하는 것이다. 그러나 이러한 훈련은 노동 집약적이고 시간이 오래 걸리며 잠재적으로 많은 비용이 든다.

실제 대응 시 예상되는 모든 적절한 기관과 참여자가 포함된 다분야 훈련이 정기적으로 실시되어야 한다. 이러한 방식으로 각 기관은 재난 발생 시 각자의 역할, 책임 및 역량을 배우고 이해할 기회를 갖게 된다.

재난 대응의 일반적인 함정

다수 사상자 사고 발생 후 사후 조사를 통해 이러한 사고에 대한 의료 대응과 관련된 일관된 문제를 확인했다. 이러한 문제는 이러한 사건에 대한 대응에 대한 후속 평가와 재난 대응 인프라를 강화하기 위한 기금을 받기 위해 미국 정부가 의무화한 위험, 취약성 및 요구 사항 평가를 수행한 지역 사회에서 확인되었다.

대비

지역 사회의 EMS 제공자로서 병원 전 처치 제공자는 다수 사상자 발생 시 발생할 수 있는 참혹한 상황에 대비하고 다양한 방법으로 이러한 사고에 대비한다. 탁상 훈련은 유용한 준비 방법이 될 수 있지만, 실무자가 필요한 임무를 수행할 수 있는 능력이나 EMS 기관이 적시에 효율적인 방식으로 자원과 자산을 현장에 가져올 수 있는 능력을 실제로 테스트하지는 못한다. 실제와 같은 기능적 재난 훈련에서 피해자를 평가한 후 분류하고 처치를 시행한 후 의료기관으로 이송하고 응급의료 지원 시스템을 통해 추적하는 훈련은 실제와 같은 방식으로 필요한 응급의료 대응을 테스트하는 데 더 효과적이다. 급증하는 환자를 수용하고 피해자에게 필요한 수의 인력, 구급차 및 기타 장비를 공급할 수 있는 능력은 지역 사회 전체가 적절히 대처해야 한다.

안타깝게도 실시간으로 급증하는 사고에 대응하는 능력을 테스트하는 기관은 거의 없으며 대신 탁상형 훈련에 의존하여 대응 능력을 측정한다. 여러 기관이 참여하는 지역사회 차원의 훈련은 조직의 다수 사상자 사고에 대응하는 대비 수준을 더욱 확실하게 예측할 수 있다. 또한 다수 사상자 사고는 매우 다양할 수 있으며 대형 화재 경보에 대한 대응은 총기 난사 사건에 대한 대응과는 크게 다를 수 있다. 모든 위험에 대응하기 위한 기본 접근 방법에는 위험 취약성 분석을 수행하여 특정 지역에 영향을 미칠 가능성이 가장 높은 잠재적 다사 사상자 사고 또는 재난 시나리오를 식별하고 우선순위를 정하는 것이 포함된다. 위험 취약성 분석은 주변 지역사회에 영향을 미칠 가능성이 높은 위험이나 위험을 쉽게 확인할 수 있는 체계적인 위험 평가 도구이다. 또한 이 분석은 발생 가능성이 가장 높은 사고 또는 지역사회에 가장 큰 혼란을 초래하는 사고에 가장 효과적으로 대처할 수 있도록 대응 새로운 계획 및 자원을 조정한다.

통신

통합 통신 시스템의 부재는 다수 사상자 사고에 대한 조정된 대응 능력을 크게 저해한다. 개별 통신 시스템은 효과적이지만, 단일 통신 방식에 의존하는 것은 실패를 위한 준비이다. 예를 들어 2001년 9월 11일 세계무역센터에 있는 중앙 통신 센터가 파괴된 후 휴대전화 사용은 효과적이지 못했다. 또한, 서로 다른 무선 기술이나 주파수로 인해 경찰, 소방 및 EMS 기관이 서로 통신할 수 없는 것도 다수 사상자 사고에 효과적으로 대응할 수 있는 능력을 떨어뜨리는 한계이다.

기본 통신을 위해 선택한 자원과 관계없이 시스템의 이중화는 가장 중요하다. 유선전화 시스템, 휴대전화 시스템, 위성 전화 시스템, VHF 무전기 및 800~900MHz의 주파수 시스템은 모두 어느 정도의 취약성을 가지고 있으며 특정 사고로 인해 손상될 수 있다. 따라서 지속적이고 효과적인 통신을 보장하기 위해서는 다양한 통신 방법을 확보하는 것이 중요하다.

통신 기능을 유지하려면 다음 두 가지 원칙이 필수적이다.

1. 지역사회의 모든 EMS 제공자가 접근할 수 있는 통합 통신 시스템이 있어야 한다.
2. 한 통신 방식이 실패하거나 비활성화될 경우 다른 예비 자원을 백업으로 효율적이고 효과적으로 사용할 수 있도록 시스템이 이중화가 되어 있어야 한다.

또 다른 일반적인 문제는 통신 내용을 기록하는 방법으로 코드를 사용하는 것이다. 안타깝게도 모든 기관이 사용할 수 있는 합의된 단일 비상 코드 세트가 없으므로 대응 기관이 다른 기관과 함께 현장에서 서로 다른 의미가 있는 코드를 사용하게 될 수도 있다. 이러한 이유로 사고 현장 지휘체계와 국가 사고관리체계(NIMS)는 사고 발생 시 의미의 혼동을 피하고자 일반 용어를 사용할 것을 권장한다.

현장 안전

현장 안전은 다수 사상자 사고에서 계속 증가하는 문제가 되고 있다. 현장 안전 및 보안은 다음과 같은 이유로 중요하다.

1. 추가 사상자를 초래하는 2차 사고로부터 긴급 대응팀을 보호하기 위해(예: 최초 대응자를 대상으로 하는 2차 폭발물)
2. 구경꾼의 방해를 받지 않고 긴급 대응팀 및 피해자가 안전하게 출입할 수 있게 하려고
3. 현장 및 잠재적인 물리적 증거를 보호하고 확보하기 위해

재난 발생 시에는 사고 대응으로 인해 자원이 부족할 수 있으므로 현장 보안이 중요한 과제가 될 수 있다. 병원 전 단계 및 의료계는 필요한 경우 보안 및 병력 보호를 받을 수 있도록 현지 경찰과 협력이 필요하다.

직접 파견 지원

일부 다수 사상자 사고에서는 영향을 받은 관할 구역의 공식적인 지원 요청 없이 인접 지역이나 심지어 멀리 떨어진 지역사회의 공공 안전 및 EMS 기관(모든 유형의 의료 인력)이 현장에 출동하는 경우가 있다. 이러한 자체 파견 구급대원은 좋은 의도를 가지고 있지만, 진행 중인 사고에 복잡성을 더할 수 있다. 자체 파견 지원의 경우 사고 지휘체계와 효과적으로 통합할 수 없으므로 조율된 구조 활동에 부담을 줄 수 있다. 또한 자체 파견된 긴급 구조대원이 가져온 호환되지 않는 무선 시스템으로 인해 통신 문제가 더욱 어려워질 수 있다.

이상적으로 공공 안전 및 EMS 기관은 책임 관할 구역과 현장 지휘관이 특별히 요청하는 경우에만 재난 현장으로 출동한다. 또한 현장에 대한 접근을 통제하고 가능한 한 빨리 모든 대응팀과 자원봉사자가 자격을 갖추고 사고 대응에 더 잘 통합될 수 있도록 안내할 수 있는 대기 구역을 마련하는 것이 도움이 된다.

공급 및 장비 자원

대부분의 EMS 기관은 일상적인 소모품 사용 계획을 세우고 일일 예상 수요에 따라 소모품을 구매한다. 대규모 재난이 발생하면 이러한 자원이 빠르게 고갈되고 기존 공급망에 차질이 생길 수 있다. 재난 발생 시 소모품 보충을 위해 예비 자원을 확보하는 것은 고품질 환자 처치라는 지속적인 임무를 수행하는 데 필수적이다. 공급품은 적시에 사용할 수 있어야 하며 적절하게 분배 방법이 마련되어 있어야 한다. 분배 계획은 다른 임무를 맡고 있을 수 있으므로 배치된 병원 전

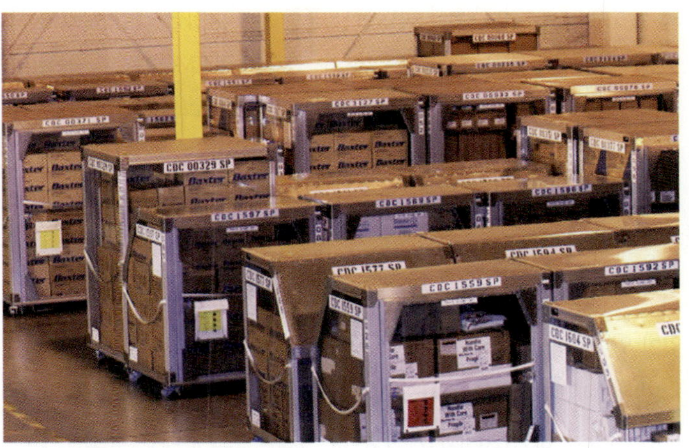

그림 17-12 도시 의료 대응 시스템 기금을 지원받도록 지정된 지역사회에서는 이러한 사태에 대비하여 지역사회 비축 의약품을 구매했거나 구매 중이다.

Courtesy of Strategic National Stockpile Communications Team/Centers for Disease Control and Prevention

처치 제공자에게 의존해서는 안 된다.

EMS 기관은 또한 의약품 보충 계획을 위한 계획을 수립해야 한다. 도시 의료 대응 시스템(MMRS)은 기금을 받을 수 있도록 지정된 지역사회에서는 이러한 사태에 대비하여 비축했거나 구매하고 있다(**그림 17-12**).

병원에 알리지 않음

다수 사상자 사고에 대응하는 혼란스러운 상황 속에서 병원 전 의료 대응을 시작하기 위해 수행해야 하는 수많은 작업을 수행하는 것 외에도 환자 유입에 대비하기 위해 병원에 직접 연락하는 것을 간과하는 경우가 많다. 병원 알림 및 활성화는 EMS 기관의 다수 사상자 사고 계획에서 필수적인 부분이어야 하며 그렇지 않으면 병원에 통보되지 않거나 너무 늦게 사고 상황이 전달되어 환자 유입을 최적화할 수 없다. 현장 처치에서 병원 처치로 조정되고 원활하게 전환이 이루어질 수 있도록 EMS 기관은 병원 통보를 다수 사상자 사고 계획의 일부로 포함하는 것이 필수적이다. 구조대가 재난지휘체계를 구현하는 것처럼 병원에도 병원 사고 지휘 시스템이라는 고유한 재난지휘체계가 있으며 이를 활성화하고 의료 시설에 추가 자원을 활용하는 임무를 수행할 수 있다. 또한 현장에서 병원으로 병원에서 현장으로 지속적인 통신을 통해 사고의 현재 상황과 특정 병원으로 환자가 몰리는 것을 모니터링하는 데 중요하다.

미디어

미디어는 종종 재난 대응의 물리적 및 운영 과정에 해를 끼치는 것으

로 간주한다. 그러나 소셜 미디어를 포함한 미디어는 책임감 있게 사용할 경우 재난 대응 시 자산이 될 수 있으므로 EMS 기관은 소셜 미디어를 포함한 미디어와 협력하는 것이 좋다. 미디어는 일반 대중에게 정확한 정보를 전파하여 사고 발생 전, 사고 중 또는 사고 후에 적절한 행동 지침을 제공하는 데 도움이 될 수 있다. 미디어의 목적은 대중에게 정보를 전달하는 것이며 병원 전 기관은 미디어와 협력하여 제공된 정보가 적시에 정확하고 대응 과정에 도움이 되도록 할 책임이 있다.

미디어 대응에 대한 교육을 받고 사고에 대해 말할 수 있는 권한을 가진 지정된 공보관(PIO)을 지정하는 것은 사고에 대한 정보를 원하는 다양한 미디어 담당자와 소통하는 방법이다. 특히 중요한 것은 각 대응 기관에 공보관이 존재할 가능성이 높다는 사실을 인식하는 것이다. 통합명령체계에 따라 단일 공보관이 하나의 일관된 메시지를 전달하는 것이 이상적이지만, 여러 기관의 공보관이 전달하는 모든 메시지는 서로 일관성이 있어야 한다. 항상 그렇듯이 개별 대응자는 소셜 미디어에 잠재적인 현장 사진을 공유할 때 주의를 기울여야 한다. 소셜 미디어 정책을 준수하는 것은 작전 대응 시 항상 고려해야 할 사항이며 미디어의 정보 요청은 기관 내 지정된 공보관에게 전달해야 한다.

요 약

- 재난은 자연적인 기후 또는 지질학적 사건으로 인해 발생하지만, 인간의 의도적이거나 비의도적인 행위로 인해 발생할 수도 있다.

- 재난은 예측할 수 없지만, 적절한 대비를 통해 상상할 수 없는 상황을 관리할 수 있는 상황으로 바꿀 수 있다.

- 재난지휘체계(ICS)를 사용하면 다양한 유형의 기관(예: 소방, 경찰, EMS)과 유사한 기관의 여러 관할 구역이 공통 언어와 조직 구조를 사용하여 재난 또는 기타 주요 사고에 대한 대응을 관리하면서 효과적으로 협력할 수 있다.

- 병원 전 처치 제공자는 환자 분류의 개념을 이해하며 가용한 자원으로 가장 많은 사람에게 처치를 제공할 수 있도록 해야 한다.

- 이송은 인근 병원이 환자를 수용할 수 있는지와 특정 환자의 경우 더 나은 처치를 제공할 수 있는 외상센터로 이송하는 것이 도움이 될 지와 같은 요소를 고려한다.

- 재난이 다양한 규모로 발생하고 다양한 원인으로 인해 발생하지만, 다음과 같이 재난 관리를 방해하는 일반적인 함정이 확인되었다.

  - 부적합한 준비

- 통신 장애
- 부적절한 현장의 안전 조치
- 자체 파견 지원
- 공급 및 장비 부족
- 미디어 홍보 부족

- 재난 대응은 피해자와 구급대원과 구조대원 등 관련자들에게 심리적 충격을 줄 수 있다. 기관은 신체 건강을 유지하는 것만큼이나 중요한· 정신 건강을 유지할 수 있도록 영향을 받은 직원과 자발적인 디브리핑을 고려한다. 정신 건강의 중요성이 더욱 주목받음에 따라 기관에서는 직원 지원 프로그램, 동료 상담, 위기 핫라인, 정신 건강 및 회복력 교육 및 인식 강화, 지속적인 감시 및 건강 검진 등 더 많은 자원을 제공하고 있다.

- 재난 주기를 이해하는 것은 대비 및 예방 노력에 중요하다. 일반적으로 재난 대응에는 휴지기, 전조(경고) 단계, 충격 단계, 구조, 응급 또는 구호 단계, 복구 또는 재건 단계의 5가지 단계가 있다.

- 다수 사상자 사고에 대응할 때 가장 좋은 결과는 문제 영역을 확인하고 개선하기 위해 연습, 테스트 및 평가를 거친 잘 구축된 재난 계획을 수립하는 데서 비롯된다.

시나리오 재구성

당신은 대규모 기상 이변으로 인해 지역 사회 전체가 침수되어 대피소로 사용 중인 지역 고등학교로 출동하였다. 도로 폐쇄와 정전에 대한 주민의 우려를 해결하기 위해 시장과 고위 관계자들이 고등학교에서 진행되는 회의에 참석했다.

현장으로 출동하던 중 체육관의 관람석이 붕괴하여 다수의 사상자가 발생했다는 신고가 여러 건 접수되었다는 상황실의 연락을 받았다. 경찰과 소방 인력도 현장으로 출동 중이지만 현재 집중 호우와 관련된 사고로 인해 가용 자원이 제한적이다.

- 어떤 안전 및 보안 문제가 발생할 것으로 예상하는가?
- 어떤 중증도 분류 시스템을 이용해야 하는가?
- 이 사건에 대한 대응을 어떻게 구성해야 하는가?

시나리오 해결책

고등학교에서 도움 요청을 받고 출동하는 동안 미리 계획된 상호 지원 자원이 동시에 파견되어 지원한다. 지역 병원에도 다수 사상자 사고 관련 내용이 통보되었다. 가장 먼저 도착한 구급대원으로서 통합지휘체계가 구축되고 있는 현장 지휘 본부에 보고한다. 훈련한 대로 현장과 의학적 필요성에 대한 전반적인 평가를 수행하고 해당 정보를 다시 출동팀에 전달한다.

분류 팀 리더가 사상자 분류를 시작한다. 치료 구역은 붕괴 현장으로부터 안전한 거리에 설치한다. 사상자들이 치료 구역에 도착하면 부상 정도에 따라 분류한다. 병원 전 처치 제공자는 손상에 대한 적절한 처치와 2차 분류를 시작한다. 상호 원조 자원이 준비 구역에 도착하면 임무를 부여받고 배치된다. 이송 차량이 도착하면 부상자를 병원으로 이송한다. 모든 환자는 이 과정의 각 단계를 통해 추적 및 파악된다. 수용 인원과 환자 수와 관련하여 병원과 지속해 소통한다.

모든 사상자가 사고 현장에서 이송하면 소방, 경찰, 관련 기관이 붕괴 원인을 조사하기 시작한다.

References

1. United Nations Office for Disaster Risk Reduction. Disaster. Accessed January 18, 2022. https://www.undrr.org/terminology/disaster

2. Starr GA, Allen TW, Stewart CE. Chapter 4. Disaster Medicine. In: Stone C, Humphries RL, eds. *CURRENT Diagnosis & Treatment Emergency Medicine*. 7th ed. McGraw Hill; 2011. Accessed January 31, 2022. https://accessemergencymedicine.mhmedical.com/content.aspx?bookid=385§ionid=40357217

3. Cuny FC. Introduction to disaster management: lesson 5–technologies of disaster management. *Prehosp Disaster Med*. 1993;6:372-374.

4. Phillips SJ, Knebel A, eds. *Mass Medical Care with Scarce Resources: A Community Planning Guide*. Prepared by Health Systems Research, Inc., an Altarum company, under contract No. 290-04-0010. AHRQ Publication No. 07-0001. Agency for Healthcare Research and Quality; 2007.

5. Federal Emergency Management Agency. ICS resource center. Accessed January 18, 2022. http://training.fema.gov/EMIWeb/IS/ICSResource/index.htm

6. U.S. Department of Agriculture. ICS 300 – Lesson 4: Unified Command. Accessed January 18, 2022. https://www.usda.gov/sites/default/files/documents/ICS300Lesson04.pdf

7. Auf der Heide E. The importance of evidence-based disaster planning. *Ann Emerg Med*. 2006;47:34-49.

8. Larrey DJ. *Memoires de Chirurgie Militaire, et Campagnes*. Vols. 1-4. J. Smith, Publisher; 1812-1817.

9. Burkle FM, ed. *Disaster Medicine: Application for the Immediate Management and Triage of Civilian and Military Disaster Victims*. Medication Examination Publishing; 1984.

10. Burkle FM, Hogan DE, Burstein JL. *Disaster Medicine*. Lippincott, Williams & Wilkins; 2002.

11. Lerner EB, Schwartz RB, Coule PL, et al. Mass casualty triage: an evaluation of the data and development of a proposed national guideline. *Disaster Med Public Health Preparedness*. 2008;2(Suppl 1):S25-S34.

12. Super G. *START: A Triage Training Module*. Hoag Memorial Hospital Presbyterian; 1984.

13. Arshad FH, Williams A, Asaeda G, et al. A modified Simple Triage and Rapid Treatment algorithm from the New York City (USA) Fire Department. *Prehosp Disaster Med*. 2015;30(2):1-6.

14. Burkle FM, Newland C, Orebaugh S, et al. Emergency medicine in the Persian Gulf: part II–triage methodology lessons learned. *Ann Emerg Med*. 1994;23:748-754.

15. Bloch YH, Schwartz D, Pinkert M, et al. Distribution of casualties in a mass-casualty incident with three local hospitals in the periphery of a densely populated area: lessons learned from the medical management of a terrorist attack. *Prehosp Disast Med*. 2007;22:186-192.

16. Hick JL, Ho JD, Heegaard WG, et al. Emergency medical services response to a major freeway bridge collapse. *Disaster Med Public Health Preparedness*. 2008;2(Suppl 1):S17-S24.

17. Bledsoe BE. Critical incident stress management (CISM): benefit or risk for emergency services? *Prehosp Emerg Care*. 2003;7(2):272-279. doi: 10.1080/10903120390936941

18. Assistant Secretary for Preparedness and Response. Tracie Healthcare Emergency Preparedness Information Gateway. Lessons Learned From the Pulse Nightclub Shooting: An Interview with Staff from Orlando Regional Medical Center. Accessed April 8, 2022. https://files.asprtracie.hhs.gov/documents/aspr-tracie-lessons-learned-from-the-pulse-nightclub-shooting-508.pdf

19. Assistant Secretary for Preparedness and Response. Tracie Healthcare Emergency Preparedness Information Gateway. Healthcare Response to a No-Notice Incident: Las Vegas. Published March 28, 2018. Accessed April 8, 2022. https://files.asprtracie.hhs.gov/documents/aspr-tracie-no-notice-incident-las-vegas-webinar-ppt-508.pdf

20. Assistant Secretary for Preparedness and Response. Tracie Healthcare Emergency Preparedness Information Gateway. ASPR TRACIE Technical Assistance (TA) Request. August 9, 2019. Accessed April 8, 2022. https://files.asprtracie.hhs.gov/documents/aspr-tracie-ta---after-action-reports--real-life-events---8-9-19-final.pdf

21. American College of Emergency Physicians. Unsolicited medical personnel volunteering at disaster scenes. Published June 2002. Reaffirmed October 2008. Revised October 2017. Accessed January 18, 2022. https://www.acep.org/patient-care/policy-statements/unsolicited-medical-personnel-volunteering-at-disaster-scenes/

Suggested Reading

Briggs SM. *Advanced Disaster Medical Response: Manual for Providers*. 2nd ed. Cine-Med Inc; 2014.

De Boer J, Dubouloz M. *Handbook of Disaster Medicine: Emergency Medicine in Mass Casualty Situations*. Van der Wees; 2000.

Eachempati SR, Flomenbaum N, Barie PS. Biological warfare: current concerns for the health care provider. *J Trauma*. 2002;52:179-186.

Emergency Medicine Clinics of North America. 1996;14(2) (entire issue).

Feliciano DV, Anderson GV Jr., Rozycki GS, et al. Management of casualties from the bombing at the Centennial Olympics. *Am J Surg*. 1998;176(6):538-543.

Hirshberg A, Holcomb JB, Mattox KL. Hospital trauma care in multiple-casualty incidents: a critical view. *Ann Emerg Med*. 2001;37(6):647-652.

Hogan DE, Burstein JL, eds. *Disaster Medicine*. 2nd ed. Lippincott, Williams & Wilkins; 2016.

Slater MS, Trunkey DD. Terrorism in America: an evolving threat. *Arch Surg*. 1997;132(10):1059-1066.

Stein M, Hirshberg A. Medical consequences of terrorism: the conventional weapon threat. *Surg Clin North Am*. 1999;79(6):1537-1552.

U.S. Department of Homeland Security, Federal Emergency Management Agency. Accessed January 18, 2022. www.fema.gov

제18장

폭발과 대량살상무기

Lead Editors
Daniel P. Nogee, MD
Faizan H. Arshad, MD

학습 목표   이 장의 학습을 완료하면 다음과 같은 내용을 수행할 수 있다.

- 대량살상무기(WMD) 사건의 완화와 관련하여 필수적으로 고려해야 할 사항을 논의할 수 있다.
  - 현장 평가
  - 사고 지휘
  - 개인보호장비
  - 환자 분류
  - 오염제거 원칙
- 특정 대량살상무기와 관련된 손상 기전, 평가 및 처치, 이송 시 고려 사항에 관해 설명할 수 있다.
  - 폭발 및 소이 작용제
  - 화학 작용제
  - 생물학적 작용제
  - 방사성 작용제
- 추가 연구를 위해 자원에 접근하고 활용하는 방법을 이해할 수 있다.

시나리오

더운 여름 저녁 당신은 유명한 카페 밖에서 폭발이 발생했다는 신고를 받고 현장으로 출동하였다. 이 카페는 평소에도 손님으로 붐비고 일반적으로 야외 테이블에도 많은 손님이 앉는다는 것을 알고 있다. 응급의료상황관리자는 이 사고와 관련하여 여러 건의 신고 전화를 받았지만, 피해자 수는 아직 파악되지 않았다고 알려준다. 다른 공공 안전 기관도 현장으로 출동했다.

현장에 도착해서 당신은 현장에 도착한 첫 번째 병원 전 처치 제공자라는 것을 알았다. 사고 현장에 아직 사고 지휘 본부가 설치되지 않았다. 수십 명의 사람들이 카페에서 대피하고 있다. 많은 사람이 명백한 출혈이 있는 피해자를 도와 달라고 간청하고 있다. 다른 희생자들은 의식 상태가 불안정한 채 바닥에 누워있다.

- 가장 먼저 무엇을 해야 하는가?
- 행동 절차를 결정할 때 우선순위는 무엇인가?
- 많은 사람을 어떻게 돌볼 것인가?

개요

대량살상무기(WMD)와 관련된 사고에 대비하는 것은 EMS 시스템의 어려운 과제이다. 다양한 유형의 대량 살상무기를 기억하기 위해 다양한 암기법이 사용되지만, 아마도 가장 기억하기 쉬운 방법은 화학(**C**hemical), 생물학(**B**iologic), 방사성(**R**adiologic), 핵(**N**uclear) 및 폭발(**E**xplosive)을 나타내는 약자인 CBRNE일 것이다.

이러한 사건은 어디에서나 예고 없이 발생할 수 있다는 것을 역사가 증명하고 있다.

- 1995년 오클라호마시의 머러 연방정부 청사 폭탄 테러로 168명이 사망하고 700명의 부상자가 발생했다. 사망자의 80%는 폭발물의 직접적인 영향보다는 건물 붕괴로 인해 발생했다. 오클라호마시의 한 병원으로 이송된 환자의 1/3은 EMS로 이송되었다. 이송된 환자 중 64%는 입원이 필요했지만, 스스로 응급실에 내원한 환자 중 입원이 필요한 환자는 6%에 불과했다.
- 2001년 9월 11일 테러리스트들이 여객기를 폭탄으로 사용한 세계무역센터 테러로 1,100명 이상의 부상자가 발생했으며 이 중 1/3이 병원 전 처치 제공자에 의해 병원으로 이송되었다. EMS 제공자가 부상자의 29%를 차지했다.
- 2004년 스페인 마드리드에서 발생한 다중 열차 폭탄 테러로 190명이 사망하고 2,051명이 손상을 입었다.
- 2005년 런던에서 지하철 3대와 이층 버스 1대에서 폭탄이 폭발하여 52명이 사망하고 779명 이상이 부상을 입었다.
- 2013년 보스턴 마라톤 대회 폭탄 테러로 3명이 사망하고 약 264명이 손상을 입었다.
- 2015년 프랑스 파리에서 발생한 총기 난사 사건과 자살 폭탄 테러범에 의해 130명이 사망하고 수백 명이 손상을 입었다.
- 2016년 6월 플로리다주 올랜도의 펄스 나이트클럽에서 한 총격범이 군중을 향해 총기를 난사하여 성인 49명이 사망하고 53명이 손상을 입었다.
- 2016년 프랑스 니스에서 한 테러리스트가 바스티유의 날을 기념하기 위해 모인 군중 사이로 대형 화물트럭을 고의로 몰고 돌진하여 86명이 사망하고 458명이 손상을 입었다.
- 2017년 맨체스터 아레나 폭탄 테러로 22명이 사망하고 약 250명이 손상을 입었다. 이 사건의 희생자 중 다수는 어린이였다.
- 2017년 뉴욕에서 테러리스트가 고의로 빌린 화물 트럭을 몰고 의도적으로 자전거 도로를 주행해서 8명이 사망하고 12명이 손상을 입었다.
- 2017년 10월 루트 91 하베스트 컨트리 페스티벌 총격 사건으로 58

명이 사망하고 500명 이상이 손상을 입어 미국 역사상 최악의 총기 난사 사건으로 기록되었다.

재래식 폭발물이 대량살상무기 사고의 가장 일반적이고 가능성이 높은 형태이지만, 전 세계 EMS 시스템은 화학 및 생물학적 위험 사건으로 인해 어려움을 겪고 있다. 1995년 도쿄 지하철에서 발생한 사린 가스 공격으로 12명이 사망하고 5,000명 이상이 병원에서 치료를 받았으며 이들 중 다수는 무증상이었지만, 가스 누출 가능성을 우려했다. 도쿄 소방서는 1,364명의 소방관을 피해 지하철 16곳에 출동시켰으며 135명(10%)의 EMS 제공자가 신경작용제에 직간접적으로 노출되어 피해를 보았다. 유엔은 시리아 내전 기간 강력한 화학무기 사린(2015), 염소(2014), 유황 겨자(2015)의 사용을 포함하여 여러 건의 화학 공격 혐의를 조사했으며 이에 따라 민간인과 최초반응자 중 사상자가 발생했다.

미국에서 생명을 위협하는 생물테러 공격으로 많은 사상자가 발생한 적은 없지만, 그렇다고 해서 EMS 시스템이 생물테러 위협에 대비하지 않는다는 의미는 아니다. 1998년과 1999년 동안 미국 전역에서 200건 이상의 사고에서 약 6,000명이 탄저균 관련 사건으로 피해를 입었다. 2001년 가을에 배달된 탄저균이 포함된 편지로 인해 탄저병이 발생한 사례는 22건에 불과했지만, 의심스러운 소포와 분말에 대한 공공 안전 기관에 도움을 요청하는 내용이 수없이 많이 접수되었다.

생물테러 사건은 아니지만, COVID-19 팬데믹은 지역, 지방 및 국가 차원에서 EMS와 재난 대응 자원에 상당한 부담을 주었다. 팬데믹 초기에는 많은 요양원과 요양 시설에서 대규모 확진자가 발생하여 주방위군과 연방재난의료지원팀(DMAT)을 비롯한 EMS 기관과 재난 대응 조직이 다수 사상자 분류, 물류 지원, 환자 처치를 제공해야 했다. 효과적인 개인보호장비의 제한된 가용성으로 인해 팬데믹 초기에 EMS 및 응급실 직원을 포함한 많은 구급대원이 COVID-19에 걸려 한정된 의료 자원에 더 큰 부담을 주었다. 2003년 토론토에서 발생한 중증급성호흡기증후군(SARA)과 2013~2016년 아프리카에서 발생한 에볼라 바이러스병(EVD)과 같이 의료 자원에 국지적인 부담을 주었지만, COVID-19 팬데믹의 엄청난 규모는 감염병 발생이 EMS 및 기타 의료 자원에 미칠 수 있는 부담을 부각했다. COVID-19 팬데믹으로 인한 전 세계적인 혼란은 바이러스 기능 향상 연구에 중점을 둔 실험실에서 의도적으로 감염성 바이러스를 방출했을 때의 잠재적 영향에 대해 조명했다.

테러리스트가 방사능 오염에 대한 공포와 손상을 일으킬 수 있는 방사능 확산 장치(더티 폭탄)를 터뜨릴 수 있다는 추측이 가능해지면서 언젠가 EMS가 방사능 대량살상무기 사건에 대응해야 할지도 모른다는 위협이 커지고 있다.

대량살상무기는 전통적으로 앞서 언급한 CBRNE 무기로 여겨졌지만, 다양한 형태와 모양으로 만들 수 있다. 예를 들어, 테러리스트가 의도적으로 바퀴 달린 차량을 몰고 군중을 향해 돌진하는 "의도적인 차량 공격"은 안타깝게도 지난 몇 년 동안 더 흔해졌는데 이는 기존의 CBRNE 공격보다 무기(차량)와 표적(군중)을 쉽게 구할 수 있기 때문으로 보인다.

또한 한 명 이상의 사람들이 소형 무기(예: 권총, 소총, 기타 사용 가능한 비군용 또는 군용 총기)로 민간인을 공격하는 총기 난사 또는 공공 집단 총격 사건은 미국 및 해외에서 점점 더 흔하며 심각해지고 있다. 총기 난사 사건 자체는 대량살상무기로 간주하지 않지만, 총기 난사 사건은 EMS 제공자에게 매우 유사한 문제를 일으키므로 대량살상무기 사건의 맥락에서 고려된다.

소규모 총격 사건에 비해 총기 난사 사건은 피해자의 손상과 의료진의 치료 사이의 시간이 길어지고 많은 피해자로 인해 지역 의료 자원이 과부하되어 대량 출혈로 인해 더 많은 사상자가 발생할 수 있다. 총기 난사 사건에 대응하는 병원 전 처치 제공자는 가해자의 직접적인 표적이 될 수 있어 현장 안전에 대한 우려가 제기된다.

2013년 하트포드 컨센서스 컨퍼런스를 통해 대규모 총격 사건에 대비하고 이를 완화하기 위한 THREAT 체제가 만들어졌다. 이는 위협 억제, 출혈 조절, 신속한 구조, 의료진에 의한 평가, 최종 처치를 위한 이송으로 구성된다. 민간인에게 외상 중심 의료 교육을 제공하는 지혈 캠페인, 표적이 될 가능성이 높은 지역에 대규모 외상 치료 자원(지혈대, 붕대 등) 사전 배치, 병원 전 처치 제공자를 위한 TCCC/TECC 등 적극적인 총격범 관련 의료 교육, 경찰/공공 안전 기관과 연계한 대응 훈련 등 다각적인 접근 방식이 대규모 총격 사건에서 사상자를 줄이는 데 도움이 될 수 있다.

일반적인 고려 사항

현장 평가

현장을 적절하게 평가할 수 있는 병원 전 처치 제공자의 능력은 개인의 안전과 동료의 안전을 보장하는 데 매우 중요하다. 대량살상무기 사건은 응급 서비스 대응에 심각한 위협이 된다. 고폭발물 폭발의 경우 화재, 위험 물질 유출, 전선 위험, 파편 또는 침하(분화구 생성)의 위험이 발생할 수 있다. 오클라호마시티 폭탄 테러로 인해 응급구조대원 1명이 건물 파편에 맞아 사망했다. 2001년 세계무역센터 테러 당시 건물이 붕괴하면서 소방관 343명, 응급구조사 15명, 경찰관 3명 등 많은 EMS 제공자가 사망했다.

화학 물질 공격은 1차 원인인 무기뿐만 아니라 피해자의 피부, 의복과 개인 소지품의 오염에 의한 2차 노출로 인해 잠재적으로 병원 전 처치 제공자가 오염물질에 노출될 수 있다. 생물학적 작용제는 전달 형태에 따라 원인 물질(예: 에어로졸화된 탄저균 포자)로 인한 질병 또는 전염성 질병(예: 페스트 또는 천연두)의 전염 위험을 초래할 수 있다. 병원 전 처치 제공자와 환자 모두에게 또 다른 위험은 추가 장치의 가능성이다. 예를 들어, EMS 제공자가 사고 현장에 도착한 후 폭발하도록 설정된 두 번째 폭탄을 설치하여 손상뿐만 아니라 혼란과 공황 상태를 가중할 수 있다.

병원 전 처치 제공자가 폭발물 또는 대량살상무기와 관련된 사건 현장에 출동하여 현장을 평가할 때는 이러한 모든 요소를 고려해야 한다. 이러한 현장에 진입하기 전에 모든 관련 기관의 대응팀은 바람이 부는 오르막 방향에서 접근하고 사고 현장으로부터 안전한 거리를 두고 대기해야 한다. 많은 대량살상무기, 특히 화학 및 생물학적 작용제는 흡입 위험이 있고 바람이 부는 방향에서는 의도하지 않게 노출될 가능성이 높으므로 바람을 등지고 접근하는 것이 중요하다. 액체 화학물질이 유출되는 사고 시 유출수에 노출되는 것을 피하고자 오르막 쪽에 위치를 선택한다.

그런 다음 병원 전 처치 제공자는 사고 현장으로부터 안전한 거리에서 현장을 평가하여 잠재적인 위험을 경고하는 단서를 찾아야 한다. 눈에 코이는 증기, 유출된 액체 또는 지속해서 확산 가능성에 주목해야 하며 이러한 관찰은 적극적인 위험을 나타낸다. 환자 평가의 일부로 환자가 어떻게 나타나는지 살펴보는 것이 반드시 포함되어야 하며 특히 다수의 사상자가 발작을 일으켜 화학 또는 생물학적 작용제가 방출되었을 가능성을 시사하는 등 환자의 징후와 증상에 주의를 기울여야 한다. 병원 전 처치 제공자는 적절하고 안전한 대응을 위한 적절한 조치를 하고 현장에서 대응하는 인력의 보호 조치를 강화하며 환자에게 효과적인 처치를 제공할 수 있도록 재난지휘체계를 통해 평가한 내용을 전달해야 한다.

잠재적으로 오염 가능성이 있는 현장에 대한 접근과 출입을 통제해야 한다. 목격자와 자원봉사자가 현장에 들어가 오염 물질에 노출

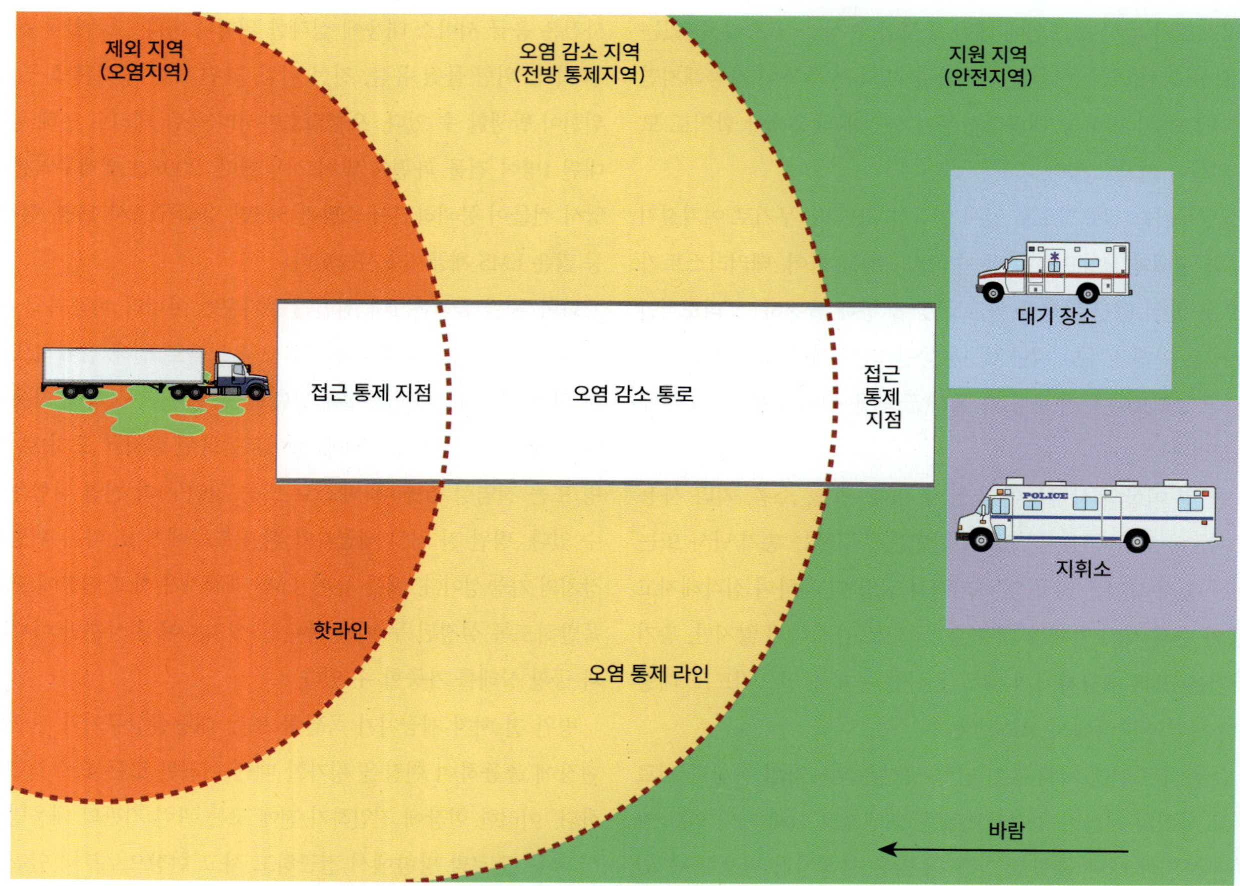

그림 18-1 대량살상무기 또는 위험 물질 사고 현장은 일반적으로 오염지역, 전방 통제지역, 안전지역으로 나뉜다. 지휘소와 대기 장소는 둘 다 안전지역 내에 위치해야 한다.
© National Association of Emergency Medical Technicians (NAEMT)

될 경우 사상자 수가 증가할 수 있으므로 현장에 들어가도록 허용해서는 안 된다. 또한 사고 피해자가 스스로 이동하여 응급실로 내원하는 환자는 위험한 화학물질이나 물질을 더 확산시킬 수 있으므로 현장에서 대피하려는 피해자를 통제해야 한다. 위험 물질 사고와 유사하게 오염 물질의 확산과 노출을 방지하고 환자 평가 및 처치를 위한 안전한 구역을 제공하기 위해 통제된 출입구와 이동 통로를 확보한 현장 통제구역(오염지역, 전방 통제지역, 안전지역)을 설정해야 한다 (**그림 18-1**, 개인보호장비 부분 참조).

재난지휘체계(ICS)

재난지휘체계는 효과적인 대응을 보장하기 위해 사용할 수 있는 모든 자원을 조정하는 관리 구조를 제공한다. 재난지휘체계는 5장, 현장 관리 및 17장, 재난 관리에서 자세히 설명한다. 규모나 복잡성과 관계없이 모든 사고에는 지정된 사고 지휘관이 있으며 이 지휘관은

다른 관할 기관의 지원을 받을 때까지 병원 전 처치 제공자 중 가장 먼저 대응할 수 있다. 병원 전 처치 제공자는 기관 간 환경에서 재난 지휘체계를 숙지하고 실행을 연습할 수 있는 기회를 갖는 것이 중요하다.

개인보호장비

대량살상무기 사건에 대응할 때는 적절한 개인보호장비(PPE)를 착용해야 한다. 개인보호장비에 대한 요구 사항은 관련된 특정 작용제 및 병원 전 처치 제공자의 특정 역할과 훈련 수준에 따라 표준 근무복부터 공기호흡기(SCBA)가 장착된 완전 밀폐형 복장에 이르기까지 다양하다. 이 장비는 호흡기, 피부 및 점막에 관해 규정된 수준으로 보호하여 구급대원과 구조대원이 위험 물질에 노출되지 않고 보호하도록 설계되었다. 모든 유형의 위험 물질을 다룰 때 개인보호장비는 일반적으로 다음과 같은 수준으로 설명된다(**그림 18-2**).

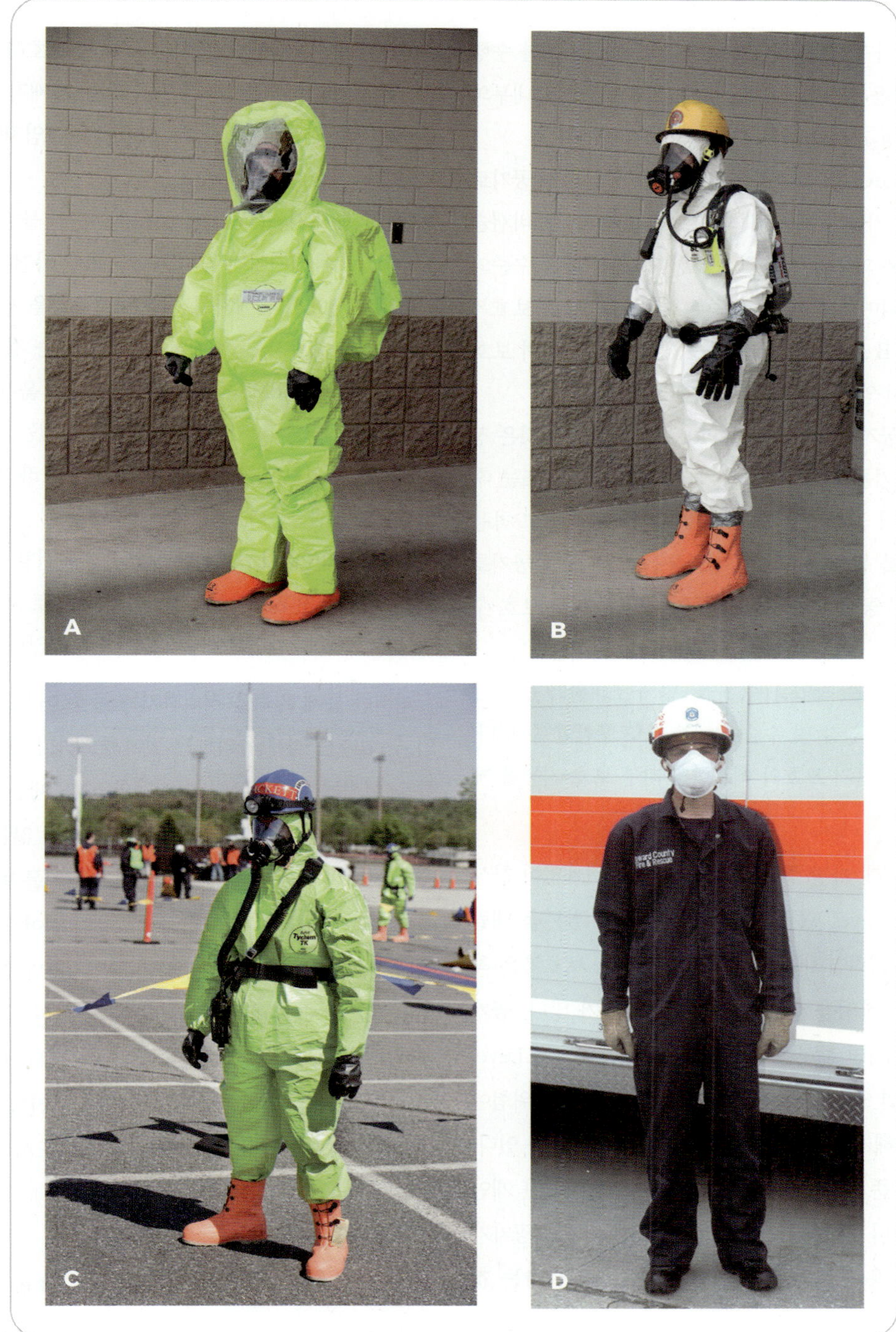

그림 18-2 개인보호장비. **A.** Level A, **B.** Level B, **C.** Level C, **D.** Level D.
A-C. Courtesy of Rick Brady; **D.** © Jones & Bartlett Learning. Courtesy of MIEMSS.

- **Level A**: 이 레벨은 가장 높은 수준의 호흡기와 피부 보호 기능을 제공한다. 호흡기는 양압으로 EMS 제공자에게 공기를 공급하는 공기호흡기(SCBA) 또는 공기 공급식 호흡기(SAR)로 보호된다. 착용자를 완전히 감싸는 내화학성 방호복은 피부와 점막을 보호한다. 이 보호복을 착용하는 데는 상당한 시간이 걸리므로 병원 전 처치 제공자가 환자에게 접근하여 도움을 줄 수 있는 능력이 지연된다. 이러한 유형의 혼란스러운 상황에 대응하는 병원 전 처치 제공자는 인내심을 가지는 것이 필요하다. 또한 이러한 수준의 보호복을

착용하고 벗을 수 있도록 지원하기 위해 추가 인력을 투입해야 한다. 숙련된 EMS 제공자가 Level A 보호복을 착용하고 임무를 수행할 수 있는 시간은 사용 가능한 공기 공급과 밀폐된 보호복 내부의 열과 습도 그리고 특정 기관의 프로토콜에 의해 제한된다.

- **Level B**: 호흡기는 Level A 보호복과 양압으로 공급되는 공기로 보호된다. 비말 보호 기능만 제공하는 슈트, 장갑, 장화 등 비캡슐형 내화학성 보호복은 피부와 점막을 보호한다. 가장 높은 수준의 호흡기 보호가 제공되며 피부 보호 수준은 낮다. Level A 보호복과 마찬가지로 Level B 보호복도 입고 벗는 데 시간이 걸리며 보호복을 착용한 상태에서 임무를 수행하는 시간이 제한된다.
- **Level C**: 호흡기는 공기 정화 호흡기(APR)로 보호된다. 이것은 정화통을 통해 주변 공기를 양압으로 빨아들여 얼굴마스크 또는 후드에 전달하는 전동식 공기 정화 호흡기(PAPR)일 수도 있고 착용자가 착용한 마스크를 통해 호흡하여 정화통을 통해 주변 공기를 빨아들이는 무동력식 공기 정화 호흡기일 수도 있다. 피부 보호 수준은 Level B와 같다.
- **Level D**: 이 수준은 표준 작업복(즉, 구급 및 구조대원의 표준 근무복)을 의미하며 가운, 장갑 및 수술용 마스크도 포함할 수 있다. Level D는 최소한의 호흡기 보호와 최소한의 피부 보호 기능을 제공한다.

병원 전 처치 제공자에게 가장 좋은 보호는 위협과 관계없이 항상 가장 높은 보호 수준의 Level A를 착용하는 것이라고 결론을 내릴 수 있다. 그러나 이는 합리적인 대응이 아니다. Level A 보호복은 착용하기가 번거롭고 수동 작업을 수행하기 어려운 경우가 많다. 공기 호흡기(SCBA)를 사용하려면 충분한 훈련과 경험이 필요하다. Level A 보호복은 착용하면 열 스트레스와 신체적 피로에 노출될 위험이 있다. EMS 제공자와 피해자 간의 의사소통을 어렵게 만들 수 있다. 추정되는 위협, 훈련 수준, 실무자의 운영 책임에 따라 적절한 개인보호장비를 선택해야 한다. 가장 중요한 것은 병원 전 처치 제공자가 선택한 개인보호장비 사용에 대한 교육을 받고 연습해야 한다는 것이다.

통제지역

개인보호장비는 의심되거나 알려진 환경의 위험과 위협의 근접성을 기준으로 선택된다. 위협에 대한 근접성은 종종 다음과 같은 통제구역으로 설명된다.

- **오염지역(Hot zone)**은 건강과 생명에 즉각적인 위협이 있는 지역이다. 여기에는 유해 가스, 증기, 에어로졸, 액체 또는 분말로 오염된 환경이 포함된다. EMS 제공자를 보호하는 데 적합한 개인보호장비는 해당 물질에 노출될 수 있는 잠재적 경로와 해당 물질을 기준으로 결정된다. Level A 보호복은 오염지역에서 가장 자주 사용된다.
- **전방 통제지역(Warm zone)**은 원인 물질의 농도가 제한되는 지역으로 특징지어진다. 대량살상무기 사건 현장의 경우 이 지역은 오염지역에서 피해자를 이동시켜 오염을 제거하는 지역이다. 병원 전 처치 제공자는 이 지역에서 작업하는 경우 오염물질이 오염지역에서 피해자, EMS 제공자, 장비에 묻어 옮겨지기 때문에 이 지역에서 작업하는 경우 여전히 노출될 수 있는 위험이 있다. 물질에 노출될 수 있는 잠재적인 노출 경로에 따라 개인보호장비를 착용하는 것을 권장한다.
- **안전지역(Cold zone)**은 오염지역과 전방 통제지역의 외곽 지역으로 오염되지 않아 노출 위험이 없으므로 표준 예방조치 이외의 특별한 수준의 개인보호장비가 필요하지 않다.

이러한 통제 지역을 정의하기는 종종 어렵고 정적이기보다는 동적일 수 있다는 점에 유의하는 것이 중요하다. 통제 지역의 역동성에 영향을 미치는 요인으로는 피해자와 EMS 제공자의 활동과 주변 상황 등이 있다. 예를 들어, 완전히 무력화되지 않는 한, 오염된 피해자는 공황 상태에 빠지거나 인근 병원에서 처치를 받으려는 의도로도 안전지역에 있는 병원 전 처치 제공자를 향해 걸어가거나 현장을 완전히 떠날 수 있다. 각 구역 지정에 따라 오염지역과 전방 통제지역, 안전지역으로 지정되지만, 바람 방향이 바뀌면 병원 전 처치 제공자는 적절한 개인보호장비를 착용하지 못하거나 신속하게 대피할 수 없는 경우 노출 위험에 처할 수 있다. 대량살상무기 사건에 대한 대응 계획을 계획하거나 대응할 때 이러한 비상 상황을 반드시 예상해야 한다.

환자 분류

병원 전 처치 제공자는 대량살상무기 사건 발생 후 평가와 처치가 필요한 수많은 피해자를 마주하게 될 가능성이 높다. 모든 EMS 시스템은 피해자를 신속하게 분류하는 방법을 파악하고 연습해야 한다. 대량살상무기 사건에서 환자 분류의 목적은 가장 많은 희생자에게 최선의 처치를 시행하는 것이다.

현장 분류는 일반적으로 쉽게 측정할 수 있는 생리학적 기준에 따라 환자의 중증도를 분류하여 신속한 처치 및 의료기관으로 이송해야 하는 피해자를 파악한다. 여러 가지 분류 방법과 기준을 사용할 수 있다. 환자 분류 방법에는 START(단순 분류 및 신속한 처치) 분류법, MASS(이동, 평가, 분류, 이송) 분류법, SALT(이동 능력에 따른 분류, 인명 구조의 필요성 평가, 분류 및 이송의 필요성 평가) 분류법이 있다.

어떤 환자 분류 방법을 사용하든 병원이나 외상센터를 포함한 모든 수준의 처치와 병원 전 처치 제공자 사이에서 인정받고 익숙하게 사용하기 위해서는 일상적인 EMS 운영에 사용해야 한다.

오염 제거의 원칙

환자와 병원 전 처치 제공자 모두 건강에 위험을 초래할 수 있는 물질에 노출된 후에는 오염제거가 필요할 수 있다. 이러한 사람들은 지정된 오염 제거 구역에서 현장 오염 제거 절차를 수행해야 한다. 오염 제거 구역은 일반적으로 조건이 허용하는 경우 맞바람이 부는 오르막 지역에 위치해야 한다. 증기나 가스에만 노출된 것으로 알려지면 이차 오염을 방지하기 위한 오염 제거가 필요하지 않지만, 피해자의 의복은 제거해야 한다.

오염 제거는 2단계 절차로 진행되며 먼저 모든 의류, 장신구와 신발을 제거하고 나중에 식별할 수 있도록 봉투에 담아 태그를 붙여 보관한다. 이러한 품목은 사고 조사에서 증거 자료로 사용될 수 있으며 오염 제거가 성공적으로 완료되면 소유자에게 돌려줄 수 있다. 의복을 제거하는 간단한 행위만으로도 대부분의 오염 물질을 제거할 수 있다. 남아 있는 고체 오염 물질은 조심스럽게 털어내고 액체 오염물질은 닦아서 제거한다. 두 번째 단계는 물과 중성 세제로 피부 표면을 씻어 피부에 묻은 오염 물질을 제거하는 것이다. 피부에 강한 세제나 표백제를 사용하지 말고 부드럽게 문지른다. 피부를 화학적 또는 물리적으로 자극하면 문제의 오염 물질의 흡수가 증가할 수 있다. 방사능 사고 중 오염 제거는 세척으로 인한 오염된 유출수가 발생할 수 있으므로 건식 오염 제거가 이차 오염 제거에 대부분 효과적이기 때문에 오염 제거는 거의 항상 건식으로 이루어진다. 쉽게 모일 수 있는 피부 주름, 겨드랑이, 샅굴 부위, 엉덩이, 발 부분은 특히 주의해야 한다. 방사능 오염 제거는 거의 항상 건조하며 세척 시 오염 물질 유출로 이어질 수 있지만, 이차 오염 제거에 대부분 효과적이다.

반응성 피부 오염 로션(RSDL), 플러스 어스 및 기타 다양한 제품을 포함한 특수 오염 제거제에는 유해 화학 물질이 피부를 통해 완전히 흡수되기 전에 중화시킬 수 있는 활성 성분이 함유되어 있다. 정확한 작용 기전과 사용 절차는 제품마다 다르지만, 일반적으로 이러한 성분은 피부 오염 제거 과정의 일부로 포함되며 기존에 사용하던 비누와 물 또는 희석된 치아염소산나트륨(표백제) 용액 대신 추가로 사용된다. 실험실 및 동물 모델에서 이러한 특수 오염 제거제를 사용하면 전신 독성을 줄이고 생존율을 개선할 수 있다고 한다. 개별 EMS 기관은 이러한 제품 중 하나 이상을 오염 제거에 추가하여 사용하는 것을 고려하고 미국 보건복지부(DHHS)는 유용한 의료 대책 데이터베이스와 연구를 지원하는 링크가 포함된 "화학 위험 응급의료 관리" 웹사이트를 운영하고 있다.

오염된 부피 부위가 누락되지 않도록 체계적으로 오염 제거를 수행해야 한다. 특히 증상이 있는 환자의 경우 눈에서 콘택트렌즈를 제거하고 다량의 물이나 생리식염수로 점막을 세척해야 한다. 걸을 수 있는 환자는 병원 전 처치 제공자의 지시에 따라 스스로 오염 제거를 수행할 수 있어야 한다. 보행이 불가능한 환자는 적절한 개인보호장비를 착용한 EMS 제공자의 도움을 받아 들것에 누워있는 환자의 오염을 제거해야 한다. 시기적절하고 효과적인 오염 제거는 환자 처치 결과를 개선하는 데 매우 중요하지만, 현장 보안(오염된 환자가 오염되지 않은 지역으로 돌아다니지 않도록 하기 위해), 오염지역 의료진(가능한 경우 오염 제거 전에 환자를 안정시키기 위해), 지속 가능한 작업-휴식 주기를 유지할 수 있는 충분한 오염 제거 팀 등 많은 자원과 훈련된 인력이 필요하다(특히 주변 온도가 따뜻한 경우 완전한 개인보호장비를 착용하고 오염 제거를 수행하는 것은 육체적으로 지칠 수 있음).

생명을 위협하는 다양한 위험 물질에 노출되는 시간을 줄이기 위해 신속한 오염 제거가 필요할 수 있다. 모든 병원 전 처치 제공자는 환자와 구조대원 모두의 노출 시간을 최소화하기 위해 공식 위험 물질/오염제거 팀이 도착하기 전이라도 시행할 수 있는 신속한 오염 제거 절차를 숙지하고 있어야 한다.

오염 제거 구역을 계획하고 설정할 때 고려해야 할 사항은 다음과 같다.

- 옷을 벗어야 하는 모든 환자 또는 제공자에게 프라이버시 제공
- 세척 및 샤워를 위해 가능한 경우 따뜻한 물을 사용할 수 있도록 준비
- 오염 제거 완료 시 의복을 대신할 수 있는 적절한 대체품 제공
- 피해자에게 개인 소지품을 돌려주거나 필요한 폐기에 관한 최종 결정이 나려질 때까지 개인 소지품이 안전하게 보관한다는 것을 보장
- 가능한 경우 폐수를 적절하게 처리

피해자의 오염 제거가 완료된 후에는 환자가 오염 제거를 받았다는 사실을 기록하는 방법을 마련해야 한다. 이 시점에서 피해자를 돌려보내지 않고 일정 기간 관찰하여 독성 징후가 발생하거나 재발하는지 여부를 확인하여 불안전한 오염 물질 제거와 반복적인 체적 및 처치가 필요한지 결정한다.

폭발, 폭발물 및 소이제

폭발물로 인한 손상을 이해하는 것은 민간과 군사 환경의 모든 병원 전 처치 제공자에게 필수적이다. 병원 전 처치 제공자는 의도하지 않은 폭발물과 산업용 폭발물 그리고 우편물 폭탄, 로켓 추진 수류탄, 대인 지뢰, 공중 투하 집속탄, 강화 폭발 무기, 사제폭발물(IEDs) 등 다양한 대인 폭발물로 인한 손상의 병태생리학을 이해할 수 있어야 한다. 1983년부터 2002년까지 미국에서 주류, 담배 및 화기 단속국(ATF)이 보고한 36,110건의 폭탄 테러 사건에 관한 연구에 따르면 "미국의 경험에 따르면 폭탄 테러에 사용되는 물질은 쉽게 구할 수 있으며 의료진은 이에 대비해야 한다."라고 결론을 내렸다.

폭발은 주로 가스 누출이나 화재로 인해 가정에서 발생하며 광업, 철거 현장, 화학물질 제조, 연료 또는 곡물과 같이 분진 발생 물질을 취급하는 많은 산업 현장에서 발생하는 직업적 위험 요소이다. 산업 폭발은 화학물질 유출, 화재, 장비 유지보수 결함 또는 전기, 기계 오작동으로 발생하며 화재, 유독가스, 건물 붕괴, 이차 폭발, 파편으로 다수 사상자를 발생시킬 수 있다. 폭발의 또 다른 일반적인 원인은 보일러와 같은 가압 밀폐 용기의 파열로 내부 압력이 높은 압력을 견딜 수 있는 용기의 능력을 초과할 때 발생한다. 화재와 폭발을 초래하는 메스암페타민의 불법 제조는 지난 20년 동안 증가했으며 EMS 제공자에게 폭발 및 화학적 위험을 초래할 수 있다. 1995년~2010년까지 작업 현장 관련 사망사고를 분석한 결과 의도치 않은 화재 및 폭발 사고가 2,373건 발생했고 최소 1명이 사망했으며 이 중 다수 사상자가 발생한 사고는 12% 미만이었다.

전 세계적으로 테러리스트들이 민간인을 대상으로 폭탄, 특히 사제폭발물을 점점 더 많이 사용하고 있다. 이러한 장치는 저렴하고 쉽게 구할 수 있는 재료로 만들어지며 전 세계의 이목을 집중시키는 파괴적인 혼란을 초래한다. EMS 제공자는 화학, 생물학 또는 핵 공격보다 재래식 폭발물에 의한 손상을 입을 가능성이 훨씬 더 높다. 1970년~2014년까지 전 세계적으로 폭발물을 사용한 테러 공격은 58,000건 이상 발생했으며 2000년대 초반부터 매년 테러로 폭발 건수가 많

이 증가하고 있다. 이 중 약 5%가 자살 폭탄 테러였으며 공격할 때마다 사망자와 부상자의 수가 많이 증가했다.

민간인에 대한 폭탄 공격이 발생하면 민간과 군의 EMS 제공자가 모두 출동할 수 있으므로 모든 병원 전 처치 제공자는 이러한 빈번한 상황에서 자신의 역할을 숙지하고 있어야 한다.

현재 미국은 일반적으로 다른 국가에 비해 폭탄 공격에 많이 노출되지는 않았지만, 2019년에는 총 715건의 폭발 사고(의도적 폭탄, 우발적 폭발, 의도가 확인되지 않았거나 아직 조사 중인 사건 포함)가 발생했으며 이 사고로 인해 16명이 사망했고 86명이 손상을 입었다.

폭발물의 종류

병원 전 처치 제공자는 폭발 테러 사고의 사상자를 평가할 때 폭발 장치의 유형과 위치를 고려해야 한다. 폭발물은 폭발 속도에 따라 고성능 폭약과 저성능 폭약 중 하나로 분류된다.

고성능 폭약

고성능 폭약은 거의 즉각적으로 반응한다. 고성능 폭약은 매우 빠르게 폭발하고 에너지를 방출하도록 설계되었기 때문에 충격파 또는 과압 현상을 일으킬 수 있으며 이로 인해 일차 폭발로 손상을 초래할 수 있다. 초기 폭발은 순간적인 압력 상승을 일으켜 초음속으로 바깥쪽으로 이동하는 충격파를 생성하지만, 매우 빠르게 감소한다. 고성능 폭발로 인한 과압은 주변 압력이 14.7psi인 것에 비해 제곱 인치당 400만psi를 초과할 수 있다. 충격파는 엄청난 양의 에너지가 빠르게 방출될 때 생성되는 폭발파의 선행 전선이자 필수 구성요소로 파편 추진, 환경 파편 생성, 강렬한 열복사를 동반한다(**Box 18-1**). 충격파 또는 압력파는 발생지점에서 전파되며 폭발 지점으로부터 거리가 멀어질수록 빠르게 소멸한다. 이 파동을 폭발로 인해 발생하는 바람과 혼동해서는 안 된다.

고성능 폭약의 일반적인 예로 2, 4, 6-TNT, 니트로글리세린, 다이너마이트, 질산암모늄 연료유, 젤리그나이트와 플라스틱 폭발물 셈텍스 등 TNT보다 1.5배 위력을 가진 최신 폴리머 결합 폭약이 있다. 고성능 폭약은 뼈와 연부조직을 분쇄하고 폭발로 인한 압력 손상을 일으키며 탄도 속도로 파편(파편화)을 날려 보낼 수 있는 날카롭고 부서지는 효과(파괴력)가 있다. 특히 폭발물이 노후화(셈텍스)되거나 때에 따라 습기가 있는 경우(다이너마이트)에는 높은 폭발력이 낮은 폭발을 일으킬 수 있다는 점에 유의해야 한다. 그러나 그 반대는 사실이 아니며 저성능 화약이 고성능 폭발을 일으킬 수는 없다.

BOX 18-1 폭발 관련 용어

- **폭풍파**: 폭풍파는 고체(또는 액체)에서 기체로 갑자기 전환될 때 발생한다. 이 사고는 폭발 주변 지역의 대기압을 거의 순간적으로 상승시켜 고도로 압축된 공기 분자가 음속보다 빠르게 이동하는 결과를 초래한다. 이 파동은 시간과 거리에 따라 빠르게 소멸한다.
- **충격파**: 폭풍파의 앞쪽 가장자리는 충격파이다. 이 고속 파동은 초음속으로 이동한다. 충격파는 에너지를 전달하여 경로에 있는 물체에 부딪히고 통과하여 손상을 일으킨다.
- **응력파**: 응력파는 고주파, 초음속, 세로 방향의 압력파로 조직이 작고 빠른 왜곡과 함께 높은 국소적 힘을 생성한다. 미세혈관 손상을 일으키고 조직 경계면에서 강화/반사되어 특히 폐, 귀, 장과 같은 가스로 가득 찬 장기에서 손상 가능성을 높인다.
- **전단파**: 전단파는 응력파보다 속도가 느리고 지속 시간이 긴 저주파 횡파를 말한다. 횡파는 변위된 입자가 파동이 진행하는 방향에 수직으로 움직이는 파동이다. 횡파는 조직의 비동기적 움직임을 유발한다. 손상 정도는 비동기적 움직임이 조직 고유의 탄성을 극복하는 정도에 따라 달라지며 그 결과 조직이 찢어지고 장기가 파열될 수도 있다.
- **폭발풍**: 고성능 폭발물이 폭발하면 폭발의 힘으로 인해 폭발 지점 바로 주변의 모든 공기를 밖으로 밀려나면서 갑작스러운 진공 상태가 만들어진다. 폭발의 힘이 소진되면 밀려났던 모든 공기가 진공에 반응하여 다시 밀려 들어온다. 그 결과 강력한 바람이 발생하여 물체와 파편이 폭발지점 쪽으로 다시 빨려 들어갈 수 있다.

저성능 화약

저성능 폭약(예: 화약)이 활성화되면 고체 상태에서 기체 상태로 비교적 느리게 변화하며(폭발보다는 연소에 더 특징적인 작용) 일반적으로 초속 2,000m/s 미만으로 움직이는 폭발파를 생성한다. 저성능 폭약의 예로는 파이프 폭탄, 화약, 화염병과 같은 순수 석유 기반 폭탄이 있다. 용기 파열 및 휘발성 화합물의 점화로 인한 폭발도 저성능 폭약의 유형에 속한다. 저성능 폭약은 에너지를 훨씬 더 천천히 방출하므로 과압을 발생시킬 수 없다.

폭발물의 종류와 양에 따라 장치 폭발과 관련된 폭발의 크기가 결정된다. 따라서 현장에 대한 접근 방식과 EMS 제공자 및 장비를 배치할 위치를 결정하는 것은 매우 중요하다. 의심스러운 장치 또는 잠재적인 이차 폭발이 발생할 때 현장에서 안전한 거리를 유지해야 한다(폭발 가능 크기에 따른 안전거리에 관한 지침은 5장, 현장 관리의 **표 5-1** 참조).

손상 기전

폭발 후 외상성 손상은 일반적으로 1차, 2차, 3차 폭발 손상의 세 가지 범주로 나뉜다. 폭발로 인해 직접적으로 발생하는 손상 외에도 폭발물 또는 오염 물질과 관련된 합병증 또는 독성 효과로 인해 발생하는 4차 및 5차 손상으로 분류되는 추가 점주의 손상이 설명되어 있다. 이러한 손상은 개별적으로 설명되어 있지만, 폭발 피해자에게는 복합적으로 발생할 수 있다(4장 외상의 물리학 **표 4-1**에는 폭발이 인체에 미치는 영향이 요약되어 있다).

1차 폭발 손상

1차 폭발 손상은 고성능 폭약의 폭발과 폭발 과압파가 신체 또는 조직과 상호작용하여 응력 및 전단파를 생성하여 발생한다. 응력파는 1) 작고 빠른 왜곡으로 높은 국소적 힘을 생성하고, 2) 미세 혈관 손상을 일으키며, 3) 조직 접합 면에서 강화되고 반사되어 특히 폐, 귀, 위장 등 공기로 채워진 장기에서 손상 가능성을 높이는 초음속 비틀림파(횡파)이다. 응력파에 의한 손상은 1) 폐포와 같은 섬세한 구조물의 압력 차, 2) 기체로 채워진 구조물의 빠른 압축과 그에 따른 재팽창, 3) 조작가스 접합 면에서의 파동 반사로 인해 발행한다.

비틀림파는 조직의 비동기적 움직임을 유발하는 더 낮은 속도와 더 긴 지속 시간을 가진 횡파이다. 손상의 정도는 동시에 일어나지 않는 운동이 조직 그유의 탄성을 극복하는 정도에 따라 달라지며 그 결과 조직의 찢어지고 부착 부위의 파열을 일으킬 수 있다. 그러나 근육, 뼈 및 고형 장기 손상은 충격파 단독으로 인한 것보다 폭발의 2차, 3차 및 4차 영향으로 인해 발생할 가능성이 훨씬 더 높다.

피해자가 폭발에 얼마나 근접했는지 그리고 밀폐된 공간에서 폭발이 발생하는 경우 충격파에 대한 차폐 또는 증강 여부에 따라 피해자는 1차 폭발 손상을 입을 수 있다.

1차 폭발 손상은 폐, 장, 중이 등 가스로 채워진 장기에서 발생한다. 조직 손상은 기체-액체 경계면에서 발생하며 아마도 장기 내 기체가 빠르게 압축되어 해당 장기가 급속한 압축이 발생한 후 빠르게 팽창하여 조직 손상이 발생한다. 폐 손상은 폐 타박상 또는 혈기흉으로 나타나며 환자가 손상으로 즉시 의식을 잃지 않으면 저산소혈증을 초래한다(**Box 18-2**). 폐포-모세혈관 경계면이 파괴되어 동맥기체 색전증이 발생하여 뇌 또는 심장 색전 합병증을 유발할 수 있다. 장 손상은 장벽의 혈종이나 장 천공을 포함할 수 있다. 고막 파열 또는 중이 소골의 파열도 발생할 수 있으며 이는 1차 폭발 손상의 가장 흔한 형태이다(4장 외상의 물리학 참조). 폭발 후 청력 손실은 흔하며 일시적이거나 영구적일 수 있다.

폐에 대한 1차 폭발 손상의 증거는 폭발 후 몇 분 후에 관련 손상으로 사망한 환자에서 생존한 환자보다 더 자주 발견되지만, 밀폐된

BOX 18-2 폭발성 폐 손상: 병원 전 처치 제공자가 알아야 할 사항

미국에서 폭발 관련 손상을 입은 환자를 처치한 경험이 있는 민간 병원 전 처치 제공자는 거의 없다. 폭발성 폐 손상(BLI)은 고유한 분류, 진단 및 처치 문제를 일으키며 고성능 폭약의 폭발로 인한 폭발파가 신체에 미치는 직접적인 결과이다. 밀폐된 공간에서 폭발이 일어났거나 폭발과 가까운 곳에 있는 사람은 더 높은 위험에 노출된다. 폭발성 폐 손상은 호흡 곤란과 저산소증을 특징으로 하는 임상 진단이다. 폭발성 폐 손상은 드물지만, 가슴에 명백한 외부 손상 없이 발생할 수 있다. 폭발성 폐 손상은 즉각적으로 나타나지 않는 경우가 많지만, 전반적인 소생 과정에서 몇 시간에 걸쳐 발생한다.

임상적 양상

- 증상으로는 호흡곤란, 객혈, 기침, 가슴 통증 등이 나타날 수 있다.
- 징후로는 빠른 호흡, 저산소증, 청색증, 무호흡, 쌕쌕거림, 호흡음 감소, 혈류역학적 불안정성 등이 나타날 수 있다.
- 체표면적 10% 이상의 화상, 두개골 골절, 몸통 관통상 또는 머리 손상을 입은 피해자는 폭발성 폐 손상에 걸릴 가능성이 더 높을 수 있다.
- 혈흉이나 기흉이 발생할 수 있다.
- 폐 및 혈관의 파열로 인해 공기가 동맥 순환으로 유입되어(공기 색전) 중추신경계, 망막 동맥 또는 관상 동맥에 색전증이 발생하여 뇌졸중과 유사한 증상을 유발할 수 있다.
- 폭발 폐 손상의 임상적 증거는 초기 평가 시점에 나타나는 경우가 많지만, 소생술 과정에서 초기 손상 후 몇 시간 후에 나타나는 경우가 더 많아 폭발 후 24~48시간 후에 발생하는 것으로 보고되었다.
- 다른 손상이 동반될 수 있다.

병원 전 처치 고려 사항

현장 안전은 병원 전 처치 제공자에게 장상 중요한 고려 사항이지만, 이와 같은 사고는 완전히 안전하다고 선언하기 전에 모든 유형의 EMS 제공자가 현장에 진입해야 한다. 병원 전 처치 제공자는 주변 환경을 계속 주시하고 추가 장치에 대한 가능성에 대해 관찰하며 1차 폭발의 결과로 발생할 수 있는 다른

위험을 고려해야 한다. 환자 평가 및 처치 단계는 직간접적인 위협 가능성이 완화되고 병원 전 처치 제공자가 TCCC 및 TECC의 지침에 따라 안전한 운영 환경을 갖췄다고 가정할 때 다음과 같다.

- 초기 분류, 외상 소생술 및 환자 이송은 다수 사상자에 대한 표준 프로토콜을 따라야 하며 여기에는 XABCDE를 이용한 일차평가 또는 MARCH 알고리즘(대량 출혈, 기도, 호흡, 순환, 머리 및 저체온증 관리)에 다른 평가 및 처치가 포함된다.
- 환자의 위치와 주변 환경에 유의한다. 밀폐된 공간에서 폭발이 발생하면 폐 손상을 포함한 1차 폭발 손상의 발생률이 높아진다.
- 폭발성 폐 손상이 의심되거나 확인된 모든 환자는 저산소소혈증을 예방할 수 있는 충분한 고유량 산소를 공급받아야 한다.
- 임박한 기도 손상은 즉각적인 처치가 필요하다.
- 환기 부전이 임박하거나 발생하면 환자에게 기관내삽관을 시행해야 하지만, 병원 전 처치 제공자는 기계적 환기와 양압이 폭발성 폐 손상 환자의 폐포 파열, 기흉, 공기색전증의 위험을 증가시킬 수 있다는 것을 인지해야 한다.
- 공기색전증이 의심되는 경우 고유량 산소를 투여하고 환자를 반좌측 또는 왼쪽 옆누운자세를 취해준다.
- 혈흉 또는 기흉의 임상적 증거가 있거나 의심되는 경우 면밀한 관찰이 필요하다. 임상적으로 긴장기흉이 있는 환자의 경우 가슴감압을 시행해야 한다. 항공으로 이송하는 폭발성 폐 손상이 의심되는 환자는 면밀한 관찰이 필요하다.
- 폭발성 폐 손상 환자에게 수액을 과도하게 투여하면 체액 과부하가 발생하고 폐 상태가 악화할 수 있으므로 수액 투여는 신중하게 이루어져야 한다.
- 다수 사상자 발생에 대한 대응 계획에 따라 폭발성 폐 손상 환자는 가장 가까운 적절한 의료기관으로 신속하게 이송한다.

Data from Centers for Disease Control and Prevention, National Center for Injury Prevention and Control, Division of Injury Response. Blast injuries: fact sheets for professionals. Published March 1, 2012. Accessed January 26, 2022. https://stacks.cdc.gov/view/cdc/21571

공간에서 폭발 후 생존한 부상자 사이에서 폐 1차 폭발 손상이 더 자주 발생하는 것으로 나타났다. 1차 폭발 손상은 다른 심각한 손상과도 관련이 있으며 사고 초기 생존자에서 사망 위험이 증가한다는 것을 나타낸다. 베이루트에서 발생한 야외 폭발 후 생존자의 0.6% 만이 1차 폭발 손상의 증거를 보였으며 이 중 11%는 사망했다. 예루살렘에서 발생한 밀폐된 공간 폭발 사고 생존자의 38%가 1차 폭발 손상의 증거를 보였으며 사망률은 약 9%였다. 마찬가지로 런던 지하철에서 발생한 3개의 폭탄 중 2개는 넓은 터널에서 폭발하여 각각 6명과 7명의 사망자가 발생했다. 지하철에서 폭발한 세 번째 폭탄은 좁은 터널에서 폭발하여 26명의 사망자를 발생시켰다. 이와 같은 개방된 공간과 밀폐된 공간에서 발생한 폭발 사고에서 사망률 차이는 폭발파가 주변 지역으로 분산되지 않고 희생자에게 반사되어 발생했다.

2차 폭발 손상

2차 폭발 손상은 날아다니는 파편과 폭발 파편으로 인해 발생한다. 2차 폭발 손상은 테러리스트 폭탄 테러 및 저성능 폭발 사고에서 가장 흔하게 발생하는 손상 유형이다. 이러한 파편은 파편화되도록 설계된 군용 무기와 같이 폭탄 자체의 구성요소일 수도 있고 못, 나사, 볼트로 보강된 사제폭탄 일부일 수도 있다. 폭발풍에 의해 날아다니는 파편에 의해서도 2차 폭발 손상이 발행할 수 있다(**Box 18-1**). 노출된 고막의 50%를 파열시킬 정도로 충분한 과압(약 5psi)을 생성하는 데 필요한 힘은 시속 233km의 폭발풍을 일시적으로 발생시킬 수 있다. 심각한 1차 폭발 손상을 초래하는 과압과 관련된 폭발풍은 시속 1,337km를 초과할 수 있다. 이러한 폭발풍은 지속 기간은 짧지만, 강력한 힘으로 파편을 먼 거리까지 날려 관통상과 무딘 손상을 유발할 수 있다.

3차 폭발 손상

3차 폭발 손상은 폭발풍에 의해 피해자가 넘어지거나 고정된 물체와 충돌하여 발행한다. 이에 따라 무딘 손상 및 관통성 외상과 같은 모든 범위의 손상이 발생할 수 있다.

4차 및 5차 효과

폭발 이후에는 4차 영향이 나타날 수 있다. 이러한 손상으로 연료, 금속으로 인한 화상 및 독성, 구조물 붕괴로 인한 외상, 토양이나 환경오염으로 인해 상처가 오염되어 패혈성 증후군이 발생할 수 있다.

　방사선, 화학 물질 또는 생물학적으로 강화된 폭발물(예: 더러운 폭탄)의 위협이 증가함에 따라 방사선, 화학 물질 또는 생물학적 작용제와 자살 폭탄 테러범의 뼛조각과 같은 발사체에 의한 손상을 포함하는 5차 폭발 손상이 발생했다.

손상 유형

병원 전 처치 제공자는 익숙한 관통상, 무딘 손상, 열상 그리고 1차 폭발 손상을 입은 생존자와 직면할 수 있다. 손상 환자의 수와 유형은 폭발의 크기, 구성, 환경, 위험에 처한 잠재적 피해자의 위치와 수 등 여러 요인에 따라 달라진다.

　폭탄 테러의 유형에 따라 다양한 사망률이 나타났다. 폭탄 테러를 조사한 연구에 따르면 폭탄 테러로 구조물 붕괴로 인해 피해자 4명 중 1명, 밀폐 공간에서 폭탄 테러로 12명 중 1명, 개방 공간 폭탄 테러로 25명 중 1명이 테러 직후 사망했다. 추가 연구에 따르면 밀폐된 공간에서 폭발이 발생하면 사망률이 더 높은 것으로 나타났다. 연부조직 손상, 정형외과 외상, 외상성 뇌손상이 생존자 사이에서 주로 발생한다(**Box 18-3**).

　18명의 생존자는 목동맥 및 목정맥 열상, 얼굴 및 무릎 동맥 열상, 신경, 건, 인대 절단 등 심각한 연부조직 손상을 입었다. 17명의 생존자는 장부분 절단, 신장, 비장, 간 열상, 기흉, 폐 타박상 등 심각한 내부 장기 손상을 입었다. 골절 환자 중 37%는 다발성 골절이 있었고 머리 손상 진단을 받은 환자 중 44%는 병원에 입원해야 했다.

평가 및 처치

외상 환자에 대한 일반적인 평가와 처치는 대량살상무기로 인한 사상자에게도 적용할 수 있으며 다른 장에서 다루고 있다. 그러나 이 환자 집단에서 고유한 것은 1차 폭발 손상의 가능성이다. 1차 폭발

Box 18-3 폭탄 테러: 손상 유형

- 근골격 손상이 생존자 수술의 대부분을 차지한다.
- 사망자 중 폭발로 인한 폐 손상이 가장 많다(17%~47%).
- 폭발로 인한 뇌 및 안구 외상은 해당 장기의 표면적이 작음에도 불구하고 흔하다.
- 4곳 이상의 신체 부위에 대한 외부 손상 또는 광범위한 화상(체표면적의 10% 초과)은 심각한 내부 손상을 나타내는 지표이다.
- 귀 손상(고막 천공)은 흔히 발생하며 대부분 양측에 발생한다.
- 밀폐된 공간에서 발생한 폭발이 개방된 공간에서 발생한 폭발보다 사망률이 훨씬 높다(15.8% vs 2.8%).

Data from Frykberg ER, Tepas JJ III. Terrorist bombings: lessons learned from Belfast to Beirut. *Ann Surg.* 1988;208:569-576; Turégano-Fuentes F, Caba-Do ussoux P, Jover-Navalón JM, et al. Injury patterns from major urban terrorist bombings in trains: the Madrid experience. *World J Surg.* 2008;32(6):1168-1175.

손상은 병원 전 처치 제공자가 객혈과 폐 타박상, 긴장기흉 또는 동맥 가스색전증 환자를 만날 가능성을 증가시킬 수 있다. 1차 폭발 손상 생존자 중 임상 증상이 즉시 나타나거나 24~48시간 지연되어 나타날 수 있다. 폐내 출혈과 국소 폐포 부종으로 인해 혈액이 섞인 분비물이 발생하고 환기-관류 불일치, 폐내 션트 증가, 순응도 저하가 발생한다. 저산호혈증이 발행하여 호흡량이 증가한다. 이는 비관통성 가슴 외상의 다른 기전에 의해 유발되는 폐 타박상과 병태생리학적으로 유사하다. 갈비뼈 골절이 있으면 가슴에 3차 또는 4차 손상을 의심해야 한다.

　1차 폭발 손상은 즉각적으로 드러나지 않는 경우가 많으므로 현장에서 1) 거품 같은 분비물 및 호흡 곤란 모니터링, 2) 지속해서 산소포화도 측정, 3) 산소 공급 등의 처치가 이루어져야 한다. 산소포화도 감소는 증상이 시작되기 전에도 1차 폭발성 폐 손상의 위험 신호이다. 과다 수액 투여가 발생하지 않도록 주의하면서 수액 투여를 신중하게 관리해야 한다.

　폭발 피해자의 경우 다발성 외상의 가능성이 높아진다. 이러한 환자의 처치 원칙은 다른 기전으로 인한 외상에 대한 원칙과 유사하다. 손상 환경의 뉘앙스가 1차 손상과 2차 및 상위 손상의 상대적 우위에 큰 영향을 미칠 수 있으므로 환자는 외형에 비례하지 않은 내부 손상을 나타낼 수 있다. 예를 들어, 폭발에 가까웠지만 콘크리트 벽으로 보호된 환자는 1차 폭발 영향으로 인해 심각한 내부 손상을 입었을 수 있지만, 폭발에서 멀리 떨어져 있어 날아온 파편으로 인한 2차 폭발 손상을 입은 환자보다 덜 심각한 손상을 입은 것으로 보일 수 있다. 병원 전 처치 제공자는 모든 손상을 입은 환자를 자세히 관찰하고 활력징후를 자주 재평가하며 필요에 따라 더 높은 범주로 재분류해야 한다.

이송 고려 사항

이송이 필요한 환자는 추가 평가 및 처치를 위해 적절한 의료기관으로 이송해야 한다. 이러한 환자는 종종 지정된 외상센터로 이송하는 것이 필요하다. 병원 전 처치 제공자는 폭발 사고 후 환자 이송의 역학에 대해 알고 있어야 한다. 병원에 도착하는 환자는 일반적으로 보행이 가능한 환자가 먼저 도착하고 중증 환자는 구급차를 이용해 나중에 도착한다.

이와 같은 두 가지 방식의 환자 이송은 오클라호마시티 폭탄 테러에서 입증되었다. 폭탄 테러 발생 후 5~30분 후에 환자들이 응급실에 도착하기 시작했으며 중증 손상을 입은 환자는 도착하는 데 더 오랜 시간이 걸렸다. 또한 다른 재난과 마찬가지로 오클라호마시티에서 지리적으로 가장 가까운 병원에서 대부분의 희생자를 수용했다. 첫 번째 환자 유입에 압도된 인근 병원은 2차 유입 시 도착한 중증 환자를 관리하는 데 어려움을 겪을 수 있다. 오클라호마시티에서 응급실에 도착한 전체 환자 수는 60~90분 동안 시간당 220명이었으며 환자의 64%가 사고 발생 반경 2.4km 이내에 있는 응급실을 내원했다. 병원 전 처치 제공자는 폭탄 테러 현장에서 구급차로 이송할 환자를 어느 의료기관으로 이송할지 결정할 때 후자의 사실을 고려해야 한다. 폭탄 테러 현장에 가장 가까운 많은 병원이 자체적으로 상당한 피해를 입은 경우 환자 분포 패턴이 훨씬 더 복잡하고 예측하기 어렵다. 예를 들어, 2020년 베이루트 항구에서 발생한 질산암모늄 폭발 사고 당시 항구에서 가장 가까운 세 곳의 병원은 폭발로 인한 피해자를 수용할 수 없을 정도로 구조적 손상을 입어 실제로 환자와 손상을 입은 직원을 다른 의료기관으로 이송해야 했다. 다른 병원(반경 5km 이내 병원)은 폭발 후 54시간 동안 환자가 너무 많이 몰려 일부 병원은 수술실이나 중환자실에 입원한 환자만 기록했다. 상처 봉합과 같은 일차 진료를 받은 환자들은 등록되지 않은 환자였으며 폭발의 영향을 입은 환자 수가 상당히 적게 집계되었다.

소이제

소이제는 일반적으로 군대에서 장비, 차량 및 구조물을 태우는 데 사용된다. 테러리스트는 사제폭발물의 치사율을 높이기 위해 이를 사용할 수 있다. 가장 흔히 알려진 세 가지 소이제는 테르밋, 마그네슘, 백린이다. 이 세 가지 물질은 모두 매우 높은 온도에서 연소하는 인화성 화합물이다.

테르밋

테르밋은 알루미늄과 산화철 분말로 1,982℃에서 격렬하게 연소하며 용해된 철 분말이다. 주요 손상 기전은 부분 화상 또는 전층 화상이다. 일차 및 이차평가는 화상을 처치하기 위한 개입으로 수행된다. 테르밋 상처는 다량의 물로 세척한 후 잔여 입자나 물질은 나중에 제거할 수 있다.

마그네슘

마그네슘은 분말 또는 고체 형태의 금속으로 매우 뜨겁게 타는 성질이 있다. 마그네슘은 부분 화상 또는 전층 화상을 유발할 수 있을 뿐만 아니라 조직액과 반응하여 알칼리 화상을 유발할 수 있다. 같은 화학 반응으로 수소 가스가 생성되어 상처 부위에 거품이 생기거나 피부밑기종이 발생할 수 있다. 마그네슘 분진을 흡입하면 기침, 빠른 호흡, 저산소증, 쌕쌕거림, 폐렴, 기도 화상 등의 호흡기 증상이 나타날 수 있다. 상처에 남아있는 마그네슘 입자는 물과 반응하므로 상처에서 죽은 조직제거 또는 미립자를 제거할 수 있을 때까지는 세척을 시행하지 않는 것이 좋다. 다른 의심되는 물질의 오염 제거와 같은 다른 이유로 세척이 필요한 경우 상처에서 마그네슘 입자를 씻어내거나 제거할 수 있도록 주의해야 한다.

백린

백린(WP)은 공기에 노출되면 자연 발화하여 노란색 불꽃과 흰 연기를 발생시키는 고체이다. 백린이 피부와 닿으면 부분 화상 또는 전층 화상을 유발할 수 있다. 백린 탄약의 폭발로 인해 백린이 피부에 박힐 수 있다. 이 물질은 공기에 노출되면 피부에서 계속 연소한다. 병원 전 처지 제공자는 환부를 물에 담그거나 생리식염수로 적신 드레싱을 해당 부위에 적용해서 피부 화상 가능성을 줄일 수 있다. 백린은 지용성이므로 이 환자에게 기름기가 많은 드레싱을 피해야 하며 이러한 드레싱을 시행하면 전신 흡수 및 독성의 가능성이 증가할 수 있다. 전신 흡수 치명적인 심장, 간, 신장 손상을 초래할 수 있다. 백린이 다시 점화되면 불이 붙을 수 있으므로 오염된 의복을 제거해야 한다. 백린은 자외선을 비추면 형광을 내기 때문에 철저한 오염 제거에 사용할 수 있다. 황산구리는 백린과 반응하면 피부에서 쉽게 확인할 수 있는 검은색 화합물을 생성하기 때문에 역사적으로 백린을 중화하고 제거를 쉽게 하는 데 사용됐다. 그러나 황산구리 사용으로 인한 합병증, 특히 혈관 내 용혈(혈관 내 적혈구 파괴)로 인해 황산구리는 선호도가 떨어졌으며 질산은의 국소 적용은 피부와 상처에 묻은 백린을 더 안전하고 효과적으로 오염을 제거할 수 있다.

화학 물질

산업 단지 사고, 유조차 또는 철도 차량 유출 사고, 화학물질 운반 트럭, 군용 무기, 테러 공격 등 다양한 시나리오에서 병원 전 처치 제공자가 화학 물질에 노출될 수 있다(**Box 18-4**). 1984년 인도 보팔에서 발생한 유니온 카바이드 산업 사고와 1995년 도쿄에서 발생한 사린 가스 공격이 이러한 사고의 예이다.

화학 작용제의 물리적 특성

물질의 물리적 성질은 화학적 구조, 환경 온도 및 대기 압력에 의해 영향을 받는다. 이러한 요소는 물질이 고체, 액체 또는 기체 상태로 존재하는지를 결정한다. 화학 작용제의 물리적 상태를 이해하는 것은 가능한 노출 경로와 전파 및 오염 가능성에 대한 단서를 제공하기 때문에 병원 전 처치 제공자에게 중요하다.

고체는 부피와 모양이 고정된 물질 상태이며 분말은 고체의 한 예이다. 녹는점까지 가열하면 고체는 액체가 되고 끓는점까지 가열되면 액체는 기체가 된다. 고체 입자와 액체 입자는 먼지 입자나 액체 미스트와 유사하게 공기 중에 부유할 수 있다. 이를 에어로졸이라고 한다. 증기는 단순히 기체 상태의 고체 또는 액체이지만, 기술적으로

0℃ 및 정상 대기압(1기압, 14.7psi)으로 정의되는 표준 온도 및 압력에서 고체 또는 액체로 발견될 것으로 예상된다. 따라서 일부 고체 및 액체는 실온에서 증기를 방출할 수 있다. 고체가 액체 상태를 건너뛰고 증기를 방출하는 과정을 승화라고 한다. 고체나 액체가 상온에서 기체 형태로 증발할 가능성은 물질의 휘발성이라 정의한다. 휘발성이 높은 물질은 실온에서 쉽게 기체로 전환된다.

이러한 물리적 특성은 1차 및 2차 오염과 가능한 노출 경로에 영향을 미친다. 1차 오염은 화학물질이 방출되는 지점에서 화학물질에 노출되는 것으로 정의된다. 예를 들어, 1차 오염은 정의에 따라 오염 지역에서 발생한다. 가스, 증기, 액체, 고체 및 에어로졸은 모두 1차 오염의 원인이 될 수 있다.

2차 오염은 피해자, 구급대원과 구조대원 또는 오염된 장비나 잔해에 의해 화학물질이 발생지로부터 이동한 후 노출되는 것으로 정의된다. 2차 오염은 일반적으로 전방통제 지역에서 발생하지만, 노출된 피해자가 스스로 대피할 수 있는 경우 더 먼 곳에서도 발생할 수 있다. 고체와 액체(때로는 에어로졸)는 일반적으로는 2차 오염에 기여한다. 기체와 증기는 일반적으로 물질 흡입으로 인해 손상을 유발하고 피부에 침착되지 않기 때문에 2차 오염을 영향을 미치지 않는다. 그러나 증기는 옷에 묻은 가스를 배출하여 다른 사람을 위험에 노출할 수 있다.

휘발성은 2차 오염의 위험에 중요한 역할을 한다. 휘발성이 높은 물질일수록 지속성이 낮다고 간주하며 이는 기화가 되기 때문에 물리적 오염이 오래 지속될 가능성이 낮다는 것을 의미한다. 이러한 화학 물질은 쉽게 분산되어 바람에 의해 날아갈 수 있다. 휘발성이 낮은 물질은 더 지속적인 것으로 간주한다. 이러한 물질은 기화하지 않거나 매우 느린 속도로 기화하기 때문에 노출된 표면에 오랫동안 남아 2차 오염의 위험을 높인다. 예를 들어, 신경 작용제인 사린은 비지속성 작용제지만, 신경작용제 VX는 지속성 작용제이다.

개인보호장비

개인보호장비는 화학물질에 대한 노출될 위험에 따라 선택된다. Level A는 사용 중인 특정 위험물질과 그 농도를 알기 전까지는 오염 지역에 진입하는 EMS 제공자에게 적합하다. 위험물질이 확인되면 사고지휘관은 특히 오염 제거를 수행하거나 전방 통제지역에서 작업하는 대응자의 경우 더 낮은 수준의 개인보호장비(Level B, Level C)로 전환하기로 할 수 있다. 특히 기관별 프로토콜에 따라 대응 요원이 안전하게 활동할 수 있는 구역을 항상 결정해야 한다.

Box 18-4 화학 작용제의 분류

- 시안화물(혈액제 또는 질식제)
  - 시안화수소(Hydrogen cyanide), 염화시아노겐(cyanogen chloride)
- 신경작용제
  - 타분(GA), 사린(GB), 소만(GD), 사이클로사린(GF), VX, 일부 농약
- 폐 독성 물질(질식 또는 폐 작용제)
  - 염소, 포스겐, 디포스겐, 암모니아
- 수포제
  - 유황 머스터드, 루이사이트
- 무능화작용제
  - BZ(3-퀴누클리딘일 벤질레이트)
- 누액제(폭동 진압제)
  - CN 및 CS(최루 가스제), 올레오레신 캡사이신(OC 또는 후추 스프레이)
- 구토제
  - 아담사이트(Adamsite)

평가 및 관리

현장의 안전을 확인한 후 병원 전 처치 제공자는 먼저 피해자가 오염 제거를 받고 있는지 확인한다. 액체 상태의 화학물질에 피부가 노출되었을 가능성이 있는 환자는 물로 오염을 제거해야 한다. 가능한 경우 비누를 사용할 수도 있지만, 일반적으로 다량의 물로 세척하는 것으로 충분하다. 가스에 노출되었다고 해서 샤워로 오염을 제거해야 하는 것은 아니지만, 지속적인 노출을 피하고 잔류 증기가 갇혀 있을 수 있는 의복을 벗어야 하며 이는 나중에 가스를 방출하여 현장이나 병원에서 의료진에게 위험을 초래할 수 있다.

피해자의 오염이 적절하게 제거되면 병원 전 처치 제공자는 아직 구체적으로 확인되지 않은 위험 물질에 노출된 징후와 증상을 보이는 환자를 만날 가능성이 높다. 화학물질에 노출된 피해자는 다음과 같은 부위에 영향을 미치는 노출 징후와 증상을 나타낼 수 있다.

- 호흡계, 산소화 및 환기에 영향을 미침
- 눈과 상기도 손상을 유발하는 점막
- 신경계, 발작이나 혼수상태 및 의식 수준 변화를 초래
- 위장관, 구토 또는 설사 유발
- 피부, 화끈거림과 물집을 유발하는 경우

현재 나타나는 증상과 징후를 평가하고 개선 또는 진행 여부를 평가하는 것이 중요하다. 임상 소견이 악화하는 환자는 오염물질을 불완전하게 제거했을 가능성이 높으므로 오염 물질이 완전히 제거되었는지 확인하기 위해 오염 제거를 반복적으로 실시해야 한다.

환자에게 즉시 필요한 인명 구조 개입을 결정하기 위해 일차평가가 필요하다. 그런 다음 이차평가를 통해 화학물질의 특성을 나타내는 증상군을 식별하는 데 확인하고 특정 해독제를 제안할 수 있다. 특정 종류의 화학물질이나 독소에 노출되었음을 시사하는 이러한 임상 징후와 증상을 중독 증후군이라고 한다.

자극성 가스 중독 증후군에는 점막 화상 및 염증, 기침, 호흡 곤란 등이 포함된다. 염소, 포스젠, 암모니아 등이 원인 물질로 작용할 수 있다.

질식 중독 증후군은 세포의 산소 결핍으로 인해 발생한다. 이는 산소가 부족한 대기에서와 같이 산소가 부족하거나 일산화탄소 중독에서와 같이 세포에 산소가 제대로 전달되지 않거나 사이안화물 중독에서와 같이 세포 수준에서 산소를 활용하지 못해서 발생할 수 있다. 징후와 증상으로는 호흡곤란, 가슴 통증, 부정맥, 실신, 발작, 혼수, 사망 등이 있다.

콜린성 중독 증상은 콧물, 호흡기 분비물, 호흡 곤란, 메스꺼움, 구토, 설사, 심한 발한, 동공수축, 의식 상태 변화, 발작, 혼수상태 등이 특징적으로 나타난다. 살충제와 신경 작용제는 이러한 콜린성 증상과 징후를 유발할 수 있다.

대부분의 경우 병원 전 처치 제공자는 손상의 구체적인 화학적 원인을 알지 못한 상황에서 지지 요법을 시작한다. 문제를 일으킨 물질이 적절하게 확인되거나 중독 증상 또는 임상 증상을 통해 그 물질의 정체를 알 수 있는 경우 해당 물질에 대한 특화된 처치를 제공할 수 있다. 사이안화물 및 신경 작용제 피해자는 작용제별 해독 요법의 혜택을 받을 수 있는 환자의 예이다.

이송 고려 사항

오염된 환자는 오염이 제거될 때까지 이송해서는 안 된다. 오염된 환자를 이송하면 이송 차량과 처치 제공자가 교차 오염되므로 오염이 제거될 때까지 이송을 중단해야 한다. 이로 인해 구급차를 이용한 환자 이송 능력이 저하되고 현장 출동 시간이 길어져 질병 또는 손상을 입은 환자 이송이 지연될 수 있다. 오염된 환자의 오염이 제거될 때까지 이송을 중단하는 것과 같이 항공 이송에도 같게 적용한다.

환자는 추가 평가와 처치를 시행하기 위해 적절한 의료기관으로 이송해야 한다. 일부 화학물질 중독 영향은 8~24시간 동안 나타나지 않을 수 있으므로 최적의 의료기관으로 이송하는 것이 특히 중요하다. 지역 사회는 화학물질에 의해 손상을 입은 환자 처치하기 위해 선호하는 의료기관을 지정할 수 있다. 이러한 의료기관은 전문 교육을 받거나 중환자 치료가 가능하고 특정 해독제를 구비하고 있어 이러한 환자를 더 잘 관리할 수 있다. 이송 역학과 관련하여 폭발 사고에 대해 앞서 언급한 것과 유사한 고려사항이 이러한 환자에게도 적용된다.

사고 현장에서 가까운 응급실은 보행이 가능 환자와 스스로 응급실을 방문한 환자에 의해 과부하가 걸릴 수 있다. 사린가스 사고 후 도쿄의 한 병원에 내원한 640명의 환자 중 541명이 구급차 지원 없이 응급실에 도착했다. 사건 발생지에서 가장 가까운 병원에 가장 많은 외래 환자가 몰렸을 가능성이 높다. 구급차를 통해 이송되는 환자의 목적지를 결정할 때 이러한 요소를 고려해야 한다.

특정 화학 물질 선택

사이안화물

병원 전 처치 제공자는 특정 플라스틱이나 섬유가 타는 화재에 대응하거나 사이안화물이 대량으로 발견될 수 있는 특정 산업 단지에 출동할 때 사이안화물을 가장 흔히 접하게 된다. 사이안화물은 화학 합성, 전기도금, 광물 추출, 염색, 인쇄, 사진, 농업, 제지업, 섬유와 플라스틱 제도에 사용된다. 그러나 사이안화물은 군용 비축물자에도 포함되어 있으며 일부 테러리스트 웹사이트에서는 사이안화물 분산시키는 장치를 만드는 방법을 제공하고 있다.

사이안화수소는 휘발성이 매우 높은 액체이므로 대부분 증기나 기체로 접하게 된다. 따라서 실외보다 환기가 잘 안되는 밀폐된 공간에서 다수 사상자가 발생할 가능성이 더 크다. 쓴 아몬드 냄새가 이 작용제와 연관되어 있지만, 이것은 사이안화수소 노출의 신뢰할 수 있는 지표가 아니며 모든 사람이 이 냄새를 감지할 수 있는 것은 아니다.

사이안화물의 작용 기전은 세포 수준에서 대사 또는 호흡을 정지시켜 빠르게 세포 사멸을 초래한다. 사이안화물은 세포의 미토콘드리아에 결합하여 세포 대사에서 산소 사용을 방지한다. 사이안화물 중독 환자는 실제로 산소를 흡입하고 혈액으로 흡수할 수 있지만, 세포 수준에서 산소를 사용할 수는 없다. 따라서 환기 중인 환자는 비청색성 저산소증의 증거를 보이게 된다.

가장 영향을 받는 기관은 중추신경계와 심장이다. 경증의 사이안화물 중독 증상으로는 두통, 어지럼, 졸림, 메스꺼움, 구토, 점막 자극 등이 있다. 중증의 사이안화물 중독 증상으로는 의식 변화, 부정맥, 저혈압, 발작 및 사망이 포함된다. 높은 수준의 사이안화물 가스를 흡인한 후 몇 분 이내에 사망할 수 있다.

처치

고농도 산소 공급, 수액 또는 혈관수축제로 저혈압을 교정하고 발작 관리 등 지지요법이 중요하다. 사이안화물 중독이 확인되었거나 의심되는 환자에게는 사이안화물 해독제 키트를 사용할 수 있다거나 중독 증상이 나타나는 환자에게 사용한다.

하이드록소코발라민(프로비타민 B_{12})은 사용하기 쉽고 한 번만 약물을 투여하면 되고 그 자체로 독이 되는 중간 화학 물질을 생성하지 않기 때문에 사이안화물 중독에 대한 현장에서 해독제로 선호되는 약물이다. 최신 사이안화물 해독제 키트에는 사이안화물과 결합하여 무독성인 시아노코발라민(비타민 B_{12})을 형성하는 정맥 주사용 하이드록시코발라민이 포함되어 있다.

이전에 사용하던 사이안화물 해독제 키트에는 아질산염과 티오황산염이라는 두 가지 약물이 포함되어 있다. 아질산아밀을 흡입하거나 정맥 라인으로 아질산나트륨을 투여하면 메트헤모글로빈(그 자체로도 충분히 높은 농도에서는 사망에 이를 수 있는 독성 물질)이 생성되어 혈류에서 사이안화물과 결합하여 환자의 세포 호흡에 독이 될 가능성이 없게 만든다. 아질산염을 투여한 후 티오황산나트륨을 정맥 라인으로 투여하면 사이안화물이 신장에서 배설되는 무해한 티오시안산염으로 전환되는 것을 돕는다.

신경작용제

신경작용제는 원래 살충제로 개발되었지만, 인체에 미치는 영향이 알려지면서 1900년대 초중반에 다양한 종류가 개발되었다. 이 치명적인 화학 물질은 많은 국가의 군수 비축물자에서 찾을 수 있다. 신경작용제는 테러 조직에 의해 제조되어 사용되기도 했는데 1994년 일본 마쓰모토와 1995년 일본 도쿄 지하철에서 발생한 신경작용제 유출 사건은 가장 악명 높은 사건이다. 최근에는 유엔 사찰단이 2013년 시리아 내전에서 민간인을 대상으로 신경작용제 사린이 사용된 것을 확인했으며 이로 인해 최초반응자를 포함한 다수의 사상자가 발생했다. 일반적으로 사용되는 살충제(예: 말라티온, 카바릴)와 일반적인 치료제(예: 피조스티그민, 피리도스티그민)는 신경작용제와 특성을 공유하여 유사한 임상 효과를 유발한다.

신경작용제는 일반적으로 실온에서 액체 상태이고 사린은 가장 휘발성이 강한 신경작용제이다. VX는 휘발성이 가장 낮으며 유성 액체로 발견된다. 중독의 주요 경로는 증기 흡입(일반적으로 휘발성 또는 비지속성 작용제)과 피부를 통해 흡수(일반적으로 VX)이다. 신경작용제는 매우 적은 용량으로도 손상을 입히거나 사망에 이르게 할 수 있다. 현재까지 개발된 신경작용제 중 가장 강력한 신경작용제인 VX는 소량의 작은 방울을 피부에 떨어뜨리는 것만으로도 피해자는 사망할 수 있다. 신경작용제는 액체이기 때문에 오염된 옷, 피부 및 기타 물체와의 접촉으로 인한 2차 오염의 위험이 있다.

신경작용제의 작용 기전은 아세틸콜린을 분해하는 데 필요한 효소인 아세틸콜린에스테라아제를 억제하는 것이다. 아세틸콜린은 콜린성 수용체를 자극하는 신경전달물질이다. 아세틸콜린 수용체는 평활근, 골격근, 중추신경계 및 대부분 외분비샘에서 발견된다. 이러한 콜린성 수용체 중 일부는 무스카린 부위(실험적으로 무스카린에 의해 자극되기 때문)라고 불리며 대부분 평활근과 땀샘에서 발견된다. 다른 부위는 니코틴 부위(실험적으로 니코틴에 의해 자극되기 때문)라고 하며 대부분 골격근에서 발견된다. 기억을 돕는 방법으로 DUMBELS(설사, 배뇨, 동공수축, 서맥, 기관지염, 기관지 연축, 구토, 눈물 흘림, 타액 분비, 발한)은 신경작용제 독성의 무스카린 효과와 관련된 증상을 나타낸다. 기억을 돕는 방법으로 MTWHF[동공 확대(드물게 나타남), 빈맥, 쇠약, 고혈압, 고혈당, 떨림]는 니코틴 수용체의 자극과 관련된 증상을 나타낸다(**Box 18-5**). 무스카린 수용체와 니코틴 수용체에 모두의 결과인 중추신경 효과에는 혼동, 경련, 혼수상태가 포함된다.

임상 효과는 신경작용제 노출 용량과 경로(흡입 또는 피부)에 따라 다르며 무스카린 효과 또는 니코틴 효과 중 어느 것이 우세한지에 따라 달라진다. 소량의 증기 노출은 주로 눈, 코, 기도에 자극을 유발한다. 다량의 증기에 노출되면 빠르게 의식 소실, 발작, 무호흡, 근육 이완으로 이어질 수 있다. 동공수축은 증기 노출을 나타내는 가장 민감한 지표이다. 피부 노출의 증상도 노출량과 발병 시간에 따라 다르다. 소량으로도 최대 18시간 동안 증상을 나타내지 않을 수 있다. 피부 노출 부위에 기저 근육의 경련과 국소적 발한이 발생할 수 있으며 위장관 증상으로 메스꺼움, 구토, 설사가 나타날 수 있다. 다량의 피부 노출은 수 분 내에 증상이 나타나며 증기 노출과 유사한 효과를 나타낸다.

신경작용제의 임상 증상으로는 콧물, 가슴 압박감, 동공수축, 호흡곤란, 과도한 침 분비 및 발한, 메스꺼움, 구토, 복부 경련, 불수의적 배뇨 및 배변, 근육 경련, 혼동, 발작, 이완성 마비, 혼수, 호흡부전 및 사망이다.

처치

신경작용제 중독의 처치에는 오염 제거(**그림 18-3**), 일차평가, 해독제 투여 및 지지요법이 있다. 기관지 수축과 다량의 분비물로 인해 환기 및 산소 공급이 어려울 수 있다. 환자는 자주 흡인이 필요할 수 있으

며 이러한 증상은 해독제 투여 후 개선된다. 신경작용제 중독 처치를 위한 세 가지 치료 약물은 아트로핀, 염화프랄리독심, 벤조다이아제핀이다.

아트로핀은 니코틴 부위에는 거의 영향을 미치지 않지만, 수용체 부위에서 경쟁적 길항 작용을 통해 신경작용제의 무스카린 효과를 대부분 역전시키는 항콜린성 약물이다. 아트로핀은 폐 증상이 있는 노출된 환자에게 사용한다. 동공수축만으로는 아트로핀 투여의 적응증이 아니며 또한 아트로핀은 안구 이상을 교정하지 않는다. 아트로핀은 지역 프로토콜에 따라 투여한다. 환자의 호흡 또는 환기 능력이 개선되거나 호흡기 분비물이 마를 때까지 사용한다. 중증도에서 중증 노출의 경우 초기 투여량을 4~6mg으로 시작하여 몇 시간 내에 걸쳐 10~20mg의 아트로핀을 투여하는 것은 드문 일이 아니다.

염화프랄리독심(2-PAM 염화물)은 옥심이다. 프랄리독심은 신경작용제와 아세틸콜린에스테라아제 사이의 결합을 분리하여 효소를 재활성화하여 주로 니코틴성 수용체에 대한 신경작용제의 영향을 줄이는 데 도움을 준다. 옥심 치료는 방출되는 신경작용제에 따라 노출 후 몇 분에서 몇 시간 내로 시작해야 효과가 있으며 그렇지 않으면 아세틸콜린에스테라아제와 신경작용제 간의 결합이 영구화(노화)되어 환자의 회복이 지연될 수 있다.

벤조다이아제핀 치료는 발작을 관리하고 간질 상태와 관련된 뇌손상 및 기타 생명을 위협하는 영향을 줄이기 위해 시작한다. 발작이 시작되었는지와 관계없이 심각한 신경작용제 중독 징후가 있는 모든 환자에게 권장된다. 미다졸람은 근육 내 또는 정맥 라인으로 투여 후 생체 이용률이 빠르고 높으므로 선호되는 벤조다이아제핀 약물이다. 동물실험에서 얻은 증거에 따르며 초기 중독 후 투여가 지연되면 발

Box 18-5　신경 작용제 암기법

암기법 **DUMBELS**(설사, 배뇨, 동공수축, 서맥, 기관지루, 기관지 연축, 구토, 눈물 흘림, 타액 분비, 발한)는 신경 작용제 독성의 무스카린 효과와 관련된 증상을 나타낸다.

압기법 **MTWHF**[동공확대(드물게 보임), 빈맥, 쇠약, 고혈압, 고혈당, 떨림]는 니코틴 수용체의 자극과 관련된 증상을 나타낸다.

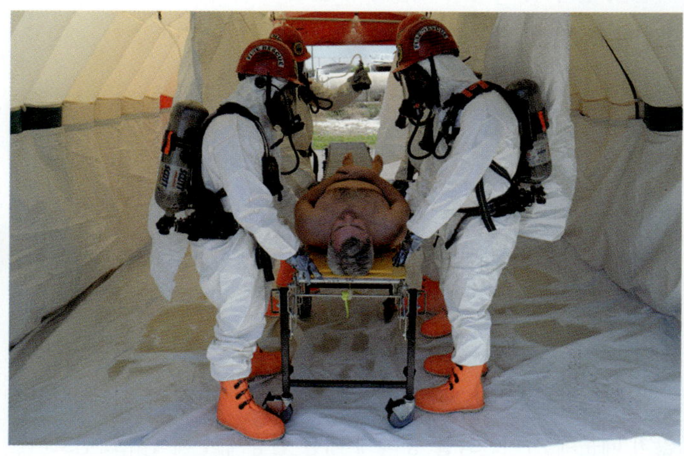

그림 18-3　신경 작용제로 인한 오염 제거

작 종료 및 신경보호 효과가 감소하는 것으로 나타났다. 미다졸람을 사용할 수 없는 경우 디아제팜(바륨) 또는 로라제팜(아티반)을 대체 약물로 사용할 수 있지만, 미다졸람보다 효과가 떨어질 수 있다.

아트로핀과 프랄리독심은 듀오도트(DuoDote)라는 단일 자가 주사기에 함께 포장되어 있다. 아트로핀의 용량은 2.1mg이고 프랄리독심의 용량은 600mg이다. 이 자가 주사기는 신경작용제에 노출되었을 때 신속하게 근육 주사를 시행하기 위한 것이다. 총투여용량은 이러한 약물의 사용 지침 및 적정 효과에 따라 결정된다. 과거에는 아트로핀과 프랄리독심은 Mark-1 키트로 판매되는 개별 자가 주사기로 공급되었다. 이러한 키트는 대부분 두 가지 해독제가 포함된 단일 자가 주사기로 대체되었다. 피아제팜은 신경작용제용 경련 해독제(CANA, **그림 18-4**)로 판매되는 10mg 자가 주사기로도 제공된다.

5~10분 간격으로 1~3개의 자가 주사기를 사용해 최대 6mg의 아트로핀을 투여하면 대부분의 경증에서 중등도 신경작용제로 발생한 환자의 호흡기 분비물을 건조할 수 있는 임상적 종점까지 치료하는 데 충분할 수 있다. 그러나 중독 정도가 더 심각한 경우에는 대부분의 병원 전 처치 제공자가 휴대하는 것보다 훨씬 많은 양의 아트로핀, 프랄리독심, 벤조디아제핀이 필요할 수 있다. 환자가 여러 개의 자가 주사기를 사용한 후 몇 분 이내에 임상적 안정에 도달하지 못한 경우

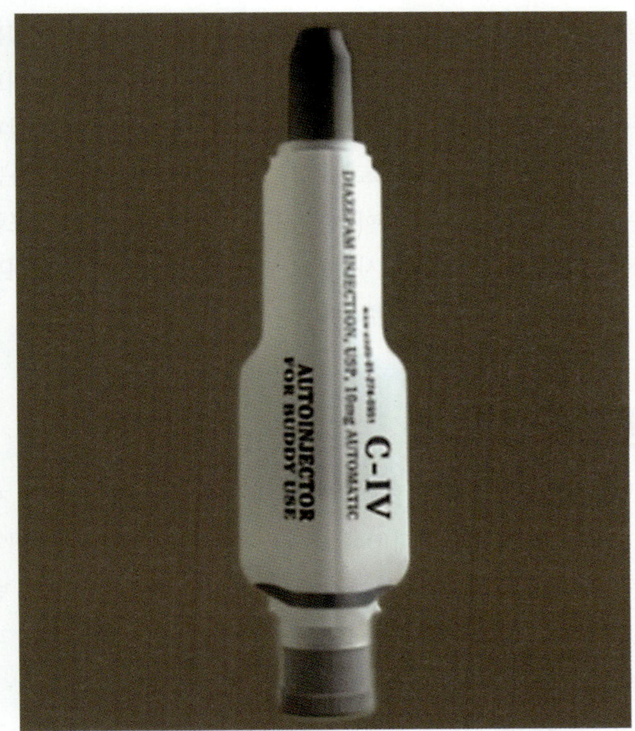

그림 18-4 신경 작용제 경련 해독제(CANA)
Courtesy of the USDHHS Radiation Emergency Medical Management.

병원에서 최종 처치를 받을 수 있을 때까지 아프로핀과 벤조디아제핀을 추가로 정맥 내 투여하는 것을 고려한다. 국가 전략 물품(SNS)에서 관리하는 CHEMPACK 시스템은 신경작용제로 인한 다수 사상자 사고의 신속하고 효과적인 처치를 위해 자가 주사기와 아프로핀, 프랄리독심, 벤조디아제핀 다회용 바이알을 포함한 신경작용제 의료 대책을 대량으로 배포했다. 병원 전 처치 제공자는 중증 또는 다수의 신경작용제에 감염된 환자를 이송할 곳을 고려하기 위해 가장 가까운 CHEMPACK 자원의 위치를 숙지해야 한다.

폐 독성 물질

염소, 포스겐, 암모니아, 이산화황 및 이산화질소를 포함한 폐 독성 물질은 수많은 산업 제조 현장에서 사용되고 있다. 포스겐은 군사용으로 비축됐으며 제1차 세계대전에서 가장 치명적인 화학 작용제로 사용되었다. 시리아 내전 중 화학 공격을 조사하는 유엔 조사관들은 염소가 여러 사건에서 무기로 사용되었다고 의심했지만, 확실하게 확인할 수는 없었다.

폐 독성 물질은 기체, 증기, 에어로졸화된 액체 또는 고체일 수 있다. 작용제의 특성은 손상을 유발하는 능력에 영향을 미친다. 예를 들어, 2㎛ 이하의 에어로졸화된 입자는 폐포에 쉽게 접근하여 손상을 유발하지만, 그보다 큰 입자는 폐포에 도달하기 전에 걸러진다. 작용제의 수용성도 손상 유형에 영향을 미친다. 수용성이 높은 암모니아와 이산화황은 눈, 점막 및 상기도에 자극과 손상을 유발한다. 수용성이 낮은 포스겐과 산화질소는 눈, 점막 및 상기도에 즉각적인 자극과 손상을 덜 유발하는 경향이 있어 피해자에게 경각심을 거의 주지 않고 이러한 물질에 장기간 노출될 수 있다. 장기간 노출되면 폐포가 손상될 가능성이 커져 상기도 손상뿐만 아니라 폐포 허탈 및 비심인성 폐부종이 발생할 수 있다. 염소와 같은 적당히 수용성인 작용제는 상기도와 폐포에 자극을 줄 수 있다.

폐 독성 물질에 따라 손상 기전은 다양하다. 예를 들어, 암모니아는 점막의 수분과 결합하여 강염기인 수산화암모늄을 형성한다. 염소와 포스겐은 물과 결합하여 염산을 생성하여 조직에 손상을 일으킨다. 폐 독성 물질은 전신적으로 흡수되지 않지만, 상기도에서 폐포에 이르기까지 폐 시스템의 구성 요소를 파괴해 피해자를 손상한다.

수용성이 높은 작용제는 눈, 코, 입에 화끈거림을 유발한다. 눈물, 콧물, 기침, 호흡곤란, 성문 자극 또는 후두경련으로 인한 이차적인 호흡곤란이 발생할 수 있다. 기관지연축은 기침, 쌕쌕거림 및 호흡곤란을 유발할 수 있다. 수용성이 낮아 폐포 손상을 유발하는 작용제

는 다량 노출 시 폐포 상피를 즉시 손상시켜 급성 호흡부전으로 사망에 이를 수 있으며 노출량이 적더라도 용량에 따라 경미한 비심인성 폐부종에서 전격성 급성 호흡곤란 증후군으로 진행되며 이차적으로 호흡곤란이 지연(24~48시간)되어 나타날 수 있다.

처치

폐 독성 물질의 관리에는 환자를 해당 물질로부터 제거, 다량의 물로 세척하여 오염 제거(특히 암모니아의 경우 기체, 액체, 고체에 노출되는 경우), 일차평가, 지지요법이 포함되며 환기와 산소 공급을 극대화하기 위한 중재가 필요할 수 있다. 눈 자극은 다량의 생리식염수로 세척하여 처치할 수 있다. 콘택트렌즈를 착용하고 있는 경우 렌즈를 제거한 후 세척한다. 다량의 기도 분비물이 있는 경우 흡인이 필요할 수 있다. 기관지수축은 흡인한 β 아드레날린 작용제에 반응할 수 있다. 저산소증은 고유량 산소를 제공하여 교정하고 기관내삽관을 시행한 후 양압환기가 필요할 수 있다. 병원 전 처치 제공자는 다량의 분비물, 성문 주위의 염증, 후두연축으로 인해 이차적으로 기도 관리가 어려워질 수 있으므로 이에 대비해야 한다. 포스젠에 노출된 모든 피해자는 증상이 지연되어 나타날 수 있으므로 정확한 평가와 진단을 위해 의료기관으로 이송한다.

수포 작용제

수포 작용제에는 유황 겨자, 질소 겨자, 루이사이트 등이 있다. 이러한 작용제는 많은 국가에서 군사 작전을 위해 비축해 왔다. 유황 겨자는 제1차 세계대전에서 처음으로 도입되었으며 이라크가 쿠르드족을 상대로 사용했고 1980년 이란과의 분쟁에서도 사용된 것으로 알려졌다. 최근에는 시리아 전쟁에서 사용된 것으로 의심되고 있다. 수포 작용제는 비교적 제조가 쉽고 저렴하다.

유황 겨자는 기름기가 있는 투명한 황갈색 폭탄이나 분무기로 에어로졸화할 수 있다. 휘발성이 낮으므로 표면에 1주일 이상 존재할 수 있다. 이러한 지속성으로 인해 이차 오염이 쉽게 일어날 수 있다. 이 작용제는 피부와 점막을 통해 흡수되어 노출 후 3~5분 이내에 직접적인 세포 손상을 일으키지만, 임상 증상과 징후가 나타나려면 노출 후 1~12시간(보통 4~6시간)이 걸릴 수 있다. 증상 발현이 지연되면 피해자가 노출 사실을 인지하기 어려워 이차 오염 가능성이 높아지는 경우가 많다. 따뜻하고 촉촉한 피부는 피부 흡수 가능성을 높여 서혜부와 겨드랑이 부위가 특히 취약하다. 눈, 피부, 상기도에는 홍반과 부종부터 수포 형성, 전층 괴사에 이르기까지 다양한 소견이

나타날 수 있다. 상기도 침범은 기침과 기관지연축을 유발할 수 있다. 고용량 노출 시 구역, 구토, 골수 억제 등이 나타날 수 있다.

유황 겨자에 노출되면 처치는 비누와 물을 사용한 오염 제거, 일차평가 및 지지요법이 포함되며 겨자 작용제의 효과에 대한 해독제는 존재하지 않는다. 실제로 유황 겨자로 인한 세포 손상은 노출 후 몇 분 이내에 발생하므로 오염을 제거한다고 해서 노출된 환자의 임상 경과가 바뀌지 않는다는 점에 유의해야 한다. 이는 주로 의도치 않은 교차 오염을 방지하기 위해 시행하는 것이다. 눈과 피부는 노출이 인지되는 즉시 다량의 물로 오염을 제거하여 작용제의 추가 흡수를 최소화하고 이차 오염을 방지해야 한다. 소포와 물집의 액체는 이차 오염원이 아니다. 폐 기관지수축은 분무형 β 작용제로 호전될 수 있다. 피부 상처는 국소 상처 처치와 관련하여 화상으로 간주하고 처치해야 한다.

루이사이크는 비슷한 증상을 보이지만 유황 겨자보다 작용 시작이 훨씬 빠르게 작용하여 눈, 피부 및 호흡기에 즉각적인 자극과 통증을 유발한다. 유황 겨자와 달리 루이사이크는 골수 억제를 일으키지 않는다. 또한 이 작용제는 모세혈관 누출로 인한 이차적인 혈관 내 체액 고갈의 결과인 루이사이크 쇼크라는 독특한 증상이 있다.

유황 겨자와 마찬가지로 이러한 노출 환자의 병원 전 처치는 오염 제거, 일차평가 및 지지요법이 포함된다. 영국산 항루이사이트(BAL)는 루이사이트에 노출된 환자를 병원에서 처치할 때 사용할 수 있는 해독제이다. 저혈량 쇼크 또는 폐 증상이 있는 환자에게 정맥 내로 투여한다. 영국산 항루이사이트 연고를 국소적으로 바르면 점막과 피부 손상을 예방하는 것으로 보고되었다. 병원 전 처치 제공자는 독성 비소 화합물과 활성 루이사이트 또는 위험한 분해 산물이 포함되어 있을 수 있으므로 루이사이트로 인한 피부에 발생한 물집 내부의 액체와 접촉하지 않도록 주의한다.

생물학적 제제

전염성 질병에 노출되는 형태의 생물학적 작용제는 병원 전 처치 제공자에게 애일 위협이 된다(**Box 18-6**). 결핵, 인플루엔자, 사람면역결핍바이러스(HIV), 메티실린 내성 황색포도상구균(MRSA), SARS 변종, 수막알균, 기타 수많은 균의 감염 또는 전파를 방지하기 위해 적절한 감염 관리 절차가 마련되어 있어야 한다.

여기에 언급된 질병은 현재 알려진 전염 능력에 따른 것이다. 그러나 바이러스 기능은 실험실에서 잠재적으로 조작될 수 있다. 이러

Box 18-6 생물학적 대량살상무기 작용제의 분류

- 세균 작용제
  - 탄저병
  - 브루셀라증
  - 마비저
  - 페스트
  - Q 열
  - 야토병
- 바이러스성 작용제
  - 천연두
  - 베네수엘라 말 뇌염
  - 니파 바이러스
  - 바이러스성 출혈열(에볼라바이러스병, 황열, 한타 바이러스)
  - 바이러스 기능 향상 연구와 관련된 새로운 위협
- 생물학적 독소
  - 보툴리눔
  - 리신
  - 포도상구균 장독소 B
  - T-2 진균독소

한 조작으로 인해 감염성과 독성이 많이 증가한 변종 바이러스가 생성될 수 있다. 이러한 병원체를 의도적 또는 우발적으로 환경에 방출하면 최근의 COVID-19 팬데믹보다 더 큰 팬데믹을 유발할 수 있다. COVID-19 팬데믹의 원인이 된 SARS CoV-2 바이러스가 실험실에서 방출된 것인지 동물 저장고에서 인간에게 전염된 것인지에 대한 확실한 결론을 내릴 수 있는 증거는 없지만, 이번 사건은 팬데믹을 유발하기 위한 의도적인 바이러스 배포 또는 바이러스를 조작하거나 연구하는 과정에서 발생한 실험실 사고로 인해 향후 그러한 사건이 발생할 가능성을 상기시켜 준다.

생물학적 테러 사건에 대비하면 EMS 시스템 준비의 복잡성이 증가한다. 의도적인 테러 행위에는 에어로졸화된 포자, 에어로졸화된 살아있는 균 또는 에어로졸화된 생물학적 독소와 같이 질병이나 질환을 유발할 가능성이 있는 생물학적 작용제의 전달이 포함될 수 있다. 페스트, 탄저병, 천연두 등 병원 전 처치 제공자가 일반적으로 볼 수 없는 병원균을 가진 환자를 만날 수 있으므로 적절한 개인보호장비와 예방 조치가 필요하다. 익숙한 감염관리 절차는 이러한 잠재적 전염성 환자를 안전하게 처치하는 데 효과적이다. 병원 전 처치 제공자가 명백한 누출 사건에 대응하는 경우 다른 위험 물질 사고와 마찬가지로 피해자의 오염 제거 및 개인보호장비에 대한 적절한 예방조치가 필요하다. 그러나 이 전체 과정은 발표가 지연되는 상황에서 훨씬 더 복잡해진다. 잠복기의 다양성으로 인해 오염원을 파악하고 확산을 통제하기가 더 어려워진다.

농축된 생물학적 작용제와 감염된 환자

병원 전 처치 제공자는 두 가지 방법으로 생물테러를 경험할 수 있다. 첫 번째 시나리오는 생물학적 작용제로 확인되었거나 추정되는 물질이 명백하게 유출되는 경우이다. 1998년과 1999년에 있었던 탄저균 사칭 사건과 2001년 탄저균 편지가 좋은 예이다. 병원 전 처치 제공자는 백색 가루를 뒤집어쓰거나 탄저병이 의심되는 사람을 수없이 만났다. 이러한 상황에서 병원 전 처치 제공자는 의심스러운 물질에 오염된 환경이나 환자를 마주하게 된다. 알 수 없는 에어로졸 물질을 배달하는 장치와 같은 의심스러운 활동으로 인해 EMS 시스템이 호출될 수 있다. 이러한 사고에서 위험의 성격은 일반적으로 알려지지 않았으므로 개인 안전을 위한 예방 조치가 항상 가장 중요해야 한다. 이러한 사건은 달리 입증될 때까지 대량살상무기 사건으로 간주하고 처리해야 한다. 의심스러운 물질이 실제로 감염성 균 도는 독소의 농축 에어로졸인 경우 생물학적 작용제에 적합한 개인보호장비를 착용하고 오염을 제거한다.

이 상황에서 병원 전 처치 제공자는 피부나 의복에 생물학적 작용제로 의심되는 물질에 오염된 피해자를 돌보게 된다. 의심되는 생물학적 작용제와 직접 접촉하는 사람, 환자 또는 병원 전 처치 제공자는 노출된 모든 의복을 벗고 노출된 피부를 비누와 물로 철저히 씻어야 한다. 피해자의 피부나 의복에서 임상적으로 유의미한 물질이 다시 에어로졸화될 가능성은 거의 없으며 병원 전 처치 제공자에게 미치는 위험은 무시할 수 있다. 그러나 일반적인 관행에 따라 오염 가능성이 있는 의복은 일반적으로 얼굴과 머리 위로 당겨서 벗지 말고 대신 잘라내어 오염 물질을 흡입할 위험을 최소화 한다. 그런 다음 물 또는 비누와 물을 사용하여 오염 제거를 진행할 수 있다. 적절한 공중보건 관련 기관의 담당자와 상의하여 항생제 예방조치의 필요성을 결정한다.

두 번째 시나리오는 원거리에서 은밀하게 발생한 생물테러 사건의 피해자인 환자에 대한 대응이다. 환자가 직장에서 은밀한 공격을 받은 후 탄저균 포자를 흡입했고 며칠이 지난 지금 폐 탄저균 증상이 나타나고 있을 수 있다. 테러리스트가 자신에게 천연두 접종했을 수 있으며 의심스러운 발진이 있는 환자의 도움을 받고 출동할 수도 있다. 이러면 적절한 감염 관리 절차에 대한 지식과 생물학적 위험에 적

Box 18-7　개인보호장비 착용 순서

필요한 예방 조치(예: 표준 예방 조치 및 접촉, 비말 또는 공기 감염 격리)에 따라 사용되는 개인보호장비(PPE)의 유형에 따라 다르다.

1. 가운
- 목에서 무릎, 팔에서 손목 끝까지 몸통을 완전히 덮고 등을 감싸준다.
- 목뒤와 허리에 고정한다.

2. 마스크 또는 호흡보호구
- 머리와 목의 중앙에 타이 또는 신축성 밴드를 고정한다.
- 얼굴과 턱 아래에 꼭 맞게 착용한다.
- 마스크가 잘 맞는지 확인한다.

3. 보호안경 또는 얼굴 가리개
- 얼굴과 눈 위에 씌우고 맞게 조절한다.

4. 글러브
- 격리 가운의 손목을 덮을 정도로 길게 늘인다.

안전한 작업 수칙을 준수하여 자신을 보호하고 오염 확산을 제한한다.

- 얼굴에 손을 대지 않는다.
- 접촉하는 표면을 제한한다.
- 장갑이 찢어지거나 심하게 오염되면 장갑을 교체한다.
- 손 위생을 시행한다.

Reproduced from Centers for Disease Control and Prevention. PPE sequence. October 16, 2014. https://www.cdc.gov/hai/pdfs/ppe/ppe-sequence.pdf

합한 개인보호장비의 적절한 착용 및 탈의를 통해 개인 및 공공의 안전을 보장할 수 있다(**Box 18-7, Box 18-8**). 이 시나리오에서 환자의 오염 제거는 노출이 과거에 며칠 전에 발생했기 때문에 필요하지 않다.

　모든 병원 전 처치 제공자는 감염 관리 목적을 위해 개인보호장비에 대해 잘 알고 있어야 한다. 전염 가능성과 전염 경로에 따라 다양한 종류의 개인보호장비가 권장된다. 모든 환자를 처치하는 데 사용되는 표준 예방 조치에 추가하여 전염 기반 개인보호장비를 사용한다. 여기에는 접촉, 비말, 에어로졸 예방 조치가 포함된다.

접촉 시 주의 사항

이 보호 수준은 직접 또는 간접 접촉에 의한 미생물 전파 가능성을 줄이기 위해 권장된다. 접촉 예방 조치에는 글러브와 가운 착용이 포함된다.

　일반적으로 접촉 예방 조치가 필요한 균에는 바이러스성 결막염, 메티실린 내성 황색포도상구균(MRSA), 옴, 단순포진 또는 대상포진 바이러스 등이 있다. 생물 테러로 인해 발생할 수 있는 엄격한 접촉

Box 18-8　개인보호장비 제거 순서

호흡보호구를 제외하고는 출입구 또는 관련 지역의 대기실에서 개인보호장비를 벗는다. 오염된 지역에서 나와 문을 닫은 후 호흡보호구를 벗는다.

1. 글러브
- 글러브의 바깥쪽이 오염된 경우
  - 장갑을 낀 반대쪽 손으로 바깥쪽을 잡고 벗긴다.
  - 벗은 장갑을 장갑 낀 손으로 잡는다.
  - 장갑을 벗지 않은 손의 손가락을 손목의 남은 장갑 아래로 밀어넣는다.
  - 첫 번째 장갑 위로 장갑을 벗깁니다.
  - 장갑을 쓰레기통에 버린다.

2. 보호안경
- 보호안경 또는 얼굴 가리개의 외부가 오염된 경우
  - 제거하려면 헤드밴드나 이어피스를 잡고 제거한다.
  - 지정된 용기에 넣거나 폐기물 용기에 넣는다.

3. 가운
- 가운의 앞면과 소매가 오염된 경우
  - 가운을 묶은 끈을 푼다.
  - 가운 안쪽만 만지도록 목과 어깨에서 당겨서 벗긴다.
  - 가운을 뒤집는다.
  - 접거나 말아 폐기물 용기에 버린다.

4. 마스크 또는 호흡보호구
- 마스크나 호흡보호구의 앞면이 오염된 경우-만지지 않는다.
  - 아래쪽, 위쪽 끈 또는 고무줄을 잡고 제거한다.
  - 폐기물 용기에 버린다.

개인보호장비를 벗은 후에는 손을 씻는다. 개인보호구를 벗는 과정에서 손이 오염되면 즉시 손을 씻거나 알코올 성분 소독제를 사용한다.

Data from Centers for Disease Control and Prevention, Atlanta. Sequence for putting on personal protective equipment (PPE). https://www.cdc.gov/hai/pdfs/ppe/ppe-sequence.pdf

예방 조치가 필요한 균에는 환자가 폐 증상이나 심한 구토 및 설사를 하지 않는 한 가래톳페스트, 마르부르크바이러스병, 에볼라와 같은 바이러스성 출혈열이 포함되며 이 경우 공기 전염 예방 조치도 같이 시행해야 한다.

비말 주의 사항

이 보호 수준은 감염된 사람이 대화, 재채기, 기침할 때 또는 흡인과 같은 일상적인 처치 중에 배출되는 큰 비말 핵($5\mu m$ 이상)에 의해 전염되는 것으로 알려진 미생물의 전염 가능성을 줄이기 위해 권장된다. 이러한 비말은 노출된 눈, 코, 입의 점막에 붙어 감염된다. 비말은 크기가 크기 때문에 공기 중에 떠다니지 않으므로 접촉은 보통 0.9m 이하로 정의되는 가까운 거리에서 있어야 한다. 비말 감염 예방 조치

에는 글러브, 가운, 보호안경, 외과용 마스크 착용이 포함된다. 비말은 공기 중에 떠다니지 않으므로 추가적인 호흡기 보호구나 공기 여과 장치가 필요하지 않다.

이 범주에서 일반적으로 발생하는 균에는 인플루엔자, 폐렴미코플라스마, 침습성 인플루엔자균 또는 나이세리아수막염균이 포함된 패혈증이나 수막염을 유발한다. 폐렴 흑사병은 생물 테러 사고의 결과로 발생할 수 있는 균의 한 예이다.

에어로졸 주의 사항

이 수준의 보호는 공기를 통한 미생물 전파 가능성을 줄이기 위해 권장된다. 일부 균은 작은 비말 핵(5㎛ 미만)에 부착되어 공기 중에 부유하거나 먼저 입자에 부착될 수 있다. 이 경우 미생물은 환경 조건에 따라 발생원 주변 또는 발생원으로부터 더 먼 곳까지 기류에 의해 광범위하게 분산될 수 있다. 이러한 확산을 방지하기 위해 이러한 환자는 날숨 환기를 여과할 수 있는 병원 내 음압 격리실에 격리된다.

에어로졸 예방 조치에는 글러브, 가운, 보호안경, N-95 마스크(**Box 18-9**)와 같이 접합성 테스트를 거친 밀착형 고성능 미립자 공기 필터(HEPA) 마스크가 포함된다. 에어로졸 예방 조치가 필요한 질병의 예로는 결핵, 홍역, 수두 및 중증 급성 호흡기 증후군(SARS), SARS-CoV-2를 포함한 변종 사스 등이 있다. 폐 증상을 동반하는 천연두와 바이러스 출혈열은 생물 테러 사건과 관련이 있을 수 있는 예이다.

선택된 제제

미국 질병통제예방센터는 대중에게 미치는 영향에 따라 생물테러 작용제를 우선순위에 따라 분류한다(**표 18-1**).

> ### Box 18-9 생물학적 제제 주의 사항
>
> 생물학적 사건과 관련된 많은 질병은 농축된 물질에 노출될 위험이 없다면 표준 예방 조치 외에 추가적인 보호 조치가 필요하지 않다. 예를 들면 탄저균이나 보툴리눔과 같은 생물학적 독소를 흡입한 환자이다. 그러나 대부분 특정 생물학적 작용제는 며칠 동안 확인되지 않을 가능성이 높다. 탄저균과 같은 일부 작용제는 사람 간에 전염되지 않지만, 병원 전 처치 제공자는 다음과 같은 최악의 상황을 가정하고 에어로졸 예방 조치를 포함하여 사용할 수 있는 모든 예방 조치를 취해야 한다.

탄저

탄저는 탄저균에 의해 발생하는 질병이다. 탄저균은 포자를 형성하는 박테리아이므로 식물성 세포 또는 포자 형태로 존재할 수 있다. 식물성 세포는 숙주 균에서 잘 살지만, 수십 년 동안 환경에서 생존할 수 있는 포자와 달리 체외에서 오래 생존할 수 있다.

탄저는 자연적으로 발생하며 감염된 동물 또는 탄저균에 오염된 동물성 제품과 접촉한 사람이 감염되어 피부병 형태로 나타나는 경우가 가장 많다. 탄저 류포자는 무기화되어 여러 국가의 군사 비축품에 보관된 것으로 알려져 있다. 1979년 스베르들롭스크의 소련 군사 시설에서 에어로졸화된 탄저병 포자가 실수로 유출되는 사건으로 인해 약 79건의 폐 탄저 감염 사례가 발생했으며 68명이 사망한 것으로 보고되었다. 2001년 탄저균 포자에 오염된 편지가 미국 우체국을 통해 저명한 국회의원과 언론사에 발송되었다. 비록 22건(폐 11건, 피부 11건)과 5명의 사망자가 발생했지만, 수천 명의 사람들이 항생제를 이용한 예방적 치료가 필요했다. 예를 들어, 워싱턴 DC 상공에 탄저균 포자 100kg을 살포한다면 13만 명에서 300만 명의 사망자가 발생할 수 있는 것으로 추산된다.

탄저균에 노출되는 경로는 호흡기, 위장관, 피부의 상처 등이 있다. 호흡기를 통해 탄저균에 노출되면 흡입 또는 폐탄저병이 발생한다. 위장관을 통한 노출은 위장관 탄저병을 유발하고 피부 감염은 피부 탄저병을 유발한다.

위장관 탄저병은 드물게 발생하며 포자에 오염된 음식물 섭취로 인해 탈생한다. 환자는 구역, 구토, 불쾌감, 출혈성 설사, 급성 복통 등의 비특이적 증상을 보이며 사망률은 약 50%이다. 피부 탄저병은 포자나 균이 피부의 손상 부위에 침착한 후 발생한다. 이로 인해 구진이 발생하고 이후 궤양이 생겨 국소 부종을 동반한 건조하고 검은 가피가 생긴다. 항생제 치료하지 않으면 사망률이 20%에 이르지만, 항생제를 사용하면 사망하는 경우는 드물다.

테러 공격의 효과를 극대화하기 위해 탄저균을 포자 형태로 확산시킬 가능성이 높다. 탄저균 포자의 크기는 약 1~5㎛로 포자가 에어로졸 형태로 공기 중에 부유할 수 있다. 에어로졸화된 포자는 폐로 흡입되어 폐포에 침착될 수 있다. 그런 다음 대식세포에 의해 섭취되어 세로칸 림프샘으로 운반되어 포자가 발아하여 독소를 생산하며 급성 출혈성 세로칸염(가슴안 중앙의 림프샘으로 출혈)을 유발하고 종종 사망에 이르게 한다. 포자 흡입 후 증상의 시작은 다양하며 대부분 피해자는 1~7일 이내에 증상이 나타나지만, 최대 60일의 잠복기

표 18-1 생물테러 작용제에 대한 CDC 위험 분류

분류	위험	작용제
A	분류 A작용제는 다음과 같은 이유로 국가 안보에 위험을 초래하는 작용제이다. ■ 사람 간 전파 또는 전염의 용이성 ■ 높은 사망률의 위험 ■ 공중 보건에 중대한 영향을 미칠 가능성 ■ 광범위한 대중의 공황 및 사회적 혼란 발생 위험 ■ 공중 보건 대비를 위한 특별 조치의 필요성	탄저 보툴리누스중독 흑사병(페스트) 두창 야토병 바이러스성 출혈열 ■ 필로바이러스 ■ 아레나바이러스
B	분류 B작용제는 다음으로 인해 위험을 초래하는 작용제이다. ■ 전파의 용이성 ■ 중간 정도의 이환율과 낮은 사망률 초래 ■ CDC의 진단 역량 및 질병 감시를 구체적으로 강화할 필요가 있는 경우	브루셀라증 클로스트리디움 퍼프린젠스 식품 안전 위협(예: 살모넬라 종, 대장균) 마비저 멜리오이드증 앵무새병 Q열 리신 독소 포도알균장독소 B 발진티푸스 바이러스성 뇌염 물 안전 위협(예: 장염비브리오 콜레라, 크립토스포리디움 파붐)
C	분류 C작용제는 신종 병원체로 확인되었으며 다음과 같은 이유로 위험을 초래하는 병원체이다. ■ 대량 확산을 위해 조작될 수 있는 가능성 ■ 가용성 ■ 생산 용이성 ■ 높은 이환율 및 사망률 발생 가능성 ■ 건강에 중대한 영향을 미칠 가능성	신종 감염병 ■ 한타 바이러스 ■ 니파 바이러스

Data from Centers for Disease Control and Prevention. Bioterrorism agents/diseases. Accessed December 3, 2021. https://emergency.cdc.gov/agent/agent-list-category.asp

가 있을 수 있다. 초기에는 발열, 오한, 호흡곤란 기침, 가슴 통증, 두통, 구토 등 비특이적 증상이 나타난다. 며칠이 지나면 증상이 호전되다가 발열, 호흡곤란, 발한, 쇼크, 사망으로 급속히 악화한다. 2001년 탄저균 공격 이전에는 탄저균 흡입으로 인한 사망률이 90%에 달하는 것으로 알려졌지만, 당시 사건의 결과에 따르면 조기 항생제 치료와 중환자 치료를 받으면 사망률이 현저히 낮아질 수 있다고 한다.

흡입 탄저는 전염성이 없으며 병원 전 처치 제공자에게 위험을 초래하지 않는다. 에어로졸화된 포자에 노출될 때만 감염될 위험이 있다. 흡입 탄저균에 감염된 것으로 알려진 환자를 처치하는 경우 표준 예방조치만 시행하면 되지만, 특정 작용제를 알 수 없는 경우 에어로졸 예방 조치가 필요하다. 병원 전 처치 제공자는 지지 요법을 제공하고 중환자 치료가 가능한 의료기관으로 환자를 이송한다.

처치

탄저균 포자는 파괴하기가 매우 어렵고 피해자의 피부나 옷에 쉽게 묻을 수 있어 병원 전 처치 제공자에게 감염 위험을 초래할 수 있다. 탄저균 유출이 확인되었거나 의심되는 피해자(예: 의심스러운 흰색 가루가 들어 있는 편지)는 Level A 개인보호장비를 착용한 대응자가 현장에서 오염을 제공하여 이송 장비가 오염되거나 피해자의 피부나 옷에 묻은 탄저균 포자에 의해 의료진이 감염되는 것을 방지해야 한다.

항생제 예방 처치는 포자에 노출된 개인에게만 필요하다. 지역 공중보건 담당자가 적절한 항생제 및 예방 치료 기간을 결정한다. 최신 권장 사항에 따르면 경구용 시프로플록사신 또는 독시사이클린으로 60일간 치료하고 노출 후 백신을 접종할 것을 권장한다.

탄저균 백신은 존재하며 1998년에 미군을 위한 예방접종 프로그램이 시행되었다. 현재 예방접종은 6번의 초기 접종과 매년 추가 접종이 필요하다. 현재 이 백신은 포자에 노출될 위험이 높은 군인과 실험실 및 산업 근로자에게만 권장된다. 미국 질병통제예방센터는 탄저균에 노출될 위험이 있는 탄저균 사고 발생 시 EMS 제공자가 사용할 수 있도록 국가 전략 비축용으로 수만 명분의 탄저균 백신을 구매했다.

흑사병

흑사병은 페스트균에 의해 발생하는 질병이다. 자연적으로 발생하며 벼룩과 설치류에서 발견된다. 감염된 벼룩이 사람을 물면 가래톳 흑사병에 걸릴 수 있다. 이 국소 감염을 치료하지 않으면 환자는 전신 질환이 발생하여 패혈증과 사망에 이를 수 있다. 많은 환자가 폐 증상(폐렴흑사병)으로 진행될 수 있다. 흑사병은 1346년 당시 유럽 인구의 약 3분의 1에 해당하는 2,000만~3,000만 명의 목숨을 앗아간 흑사병의 원인이 되었다. 흑사병균은 동물 매개체를 거치지 않고 직접 에어졸화할 수 있는 기술이 개발되어 군사적 목적으로 무기화되었다. 세계보건기구는 최악의 시나리오에서 인구 5백만 명이 거주하는 도시에 50kg의 흑사병균이 에어로졸로 방출되면 15만 명에서 폐렴흑사병이 발병하고 3만 6천 명의 사망자가 발생할 수 있다고 보고한다.

감염된 벼룩에게 물려 자연적으로 발생하는 흑사병은 발열, 오한, 쇠약감, 목, 서혜부 또는 겨드랑이의 림프절이 급격히 부어오르는 증상이 2~8일 이내에 발생한다. 치료를 받지 않은 환자는 전신 질환으로 악화하여 사망에 이를 수 있다. 12%는 가슴 통증, 호흡곤란, 기침, 객혈을 호소하는 폐렴흑사병으로 발전하는 것으로 알려져 있으며 이러한 환자는 전신 질환으로 사망할 수도 있다.

테러리스트가 무기로 사용하여 발생하는 전염병은 에어로졸화된 균에 의해 발생할 가능성이 높으므로 임상적으로 폐렴 형태의 질병으로 나타날 수 있다. 에어로졸화된 흑사병 균을 흡입하면 1~6일 이내에 증상이 나타난다. 환자는 발열, 기침, 호흡곤란과 함께 피가 섞인 가래 또는 묽은 가래를 보인다. 오심, 구토, 설사, 복통도 나타날 수 있다. 감염된 림프선은 일반적으로 나타나지 않는다. 항생제를 사용하지 않으면 호흡기 증상 발생 후 2~6일 이내에 사망한다.

현재 폐렴흑사병을 예방할 수 있는 백신은 없다. 이 질병의 치료에는 항생제 및 지지요법이 포함되며 종종 중환자 치료가 필요하다. 알려진 폐렴흑사병 환자에게 무방비 상태로 밀접 노출된 개인에게는 항생제 요법이 권장된다.

흑사병 환자는 전염병 위험이 있다. 피부 증상과 징후만 있는 환자의 경우(가래톳흑사병) 병원 전 처치 제공자를 보호하기 위해 접촉 예방 조치를 시행하는 것이 적절하다. 환자가 테러 공격 후 더 가능성이 높은 시나리오인 흑사병(폐렴흑사병)의 폐 징후를 보이는 경우 병원 전 처치 제공자는 호흡기 비말 보호에 적합한 개인보호장비를 착용해야 한다. 비말 예방 조치에는 외과용 마스크, 보호안경, 글러브와 가운이 포함된다. 흑사병균이 명백하게 전달되는 현장에 출동하는 구급대원과 구조대원은 오염지역이나 전방 통제지역에 들어갈 때 위험한 환경에 적합한 Level A 개인보호복을 착용해야 한다.

처치

흑사병 피해자는 현장에서 지지요법으로 처치를 시행한다. 폐렴흑사병 환자를 응급실에서 적절히 격리하고 의료진이 적절한 개인보호장비를 준비할 수 있도록 도착 전에 환자를 이송할 의료기관에 보고하는 것이 중요하다. 환자에게 외과용 마스크를 착용시키는 것이 이차 전파 가능성을 줄일 수 있다.

차량과 장비의 오염 제거는 전염성 질병 환자를 이송한 후 필요한 것과 유사하다. 접촉 표면은 미국 환경보호청(EPA)에서 승인한 소독제나 1:1,000으로 희석한 표백제 용액으로 닦아야 한다. 흑사병균이 1차 에어로졸이 용해된 후에도 장기적으로 환경에 위협이 된다는 증거는 없다. 이 균은 열과 햇빛에 민감하며 살아있는 숙주 밖에서 오래 살지 못한다. 흑사병균은 포자를 형성하지 않는다.

두창

두창은 질병의 중증도에 따라 대두창과 소두창라고도 한다. 자연적으로 발생하는 이 바이러스성 질병은 1977년에 박멸되었지만, 러시아 바이러스 준비 연구소와 미국 질병통제예방센터 등 최소 두 곳의 실험에 여전히 존재한다. 소련 정부는 1980년에 폭탄과 미사일에 사용할 두창 바이러스를 대량으로 생산하고 군사적 목적으로 더 치명적인 바이러스 변종을 개발하는 프로그램을 시작했다고 주장했다. 소련이 해체된 후 두창 바이러스의 주인이 바뀌었을 수 있다는 우려가 있다.

두창 바이러스는 입인두 또는 호흡기 점막에 침입하여 피해자 감염시킨다. 12~14일의 잠복기를 거친 후 환자는 발열, 무력감, 두통, 요통 등의 증상을 보인다. 그런 다음 환자는 입안 점막에서 시작하여 특징으로 둥글고 팽팽한 수포와 농포가 있는 전신 피부 발진으로 빠르게 진행되는 반구진 발진이 발생한다. 발진은 몸통보다 머리와 팔다리에 더 조밀하게 발생하는 경향이 있으며(원심성) 병변의 단계에 따라 균일하게 나타난다(**그림 18-5**). 이 사진을 보면 두창은 수두와 구별할 수 있으며(**Box 18-10**) 수두는 몸통에서 시작하여 몸통(구심성)에서 더 조밀하게 발생하고 다양한 발달 단계의 병변(새로운 병변은 오래된 병변과 같이 나타남)을 보인다(**그림 18-6**). 자연 발생한 두

창으로 인한 사망률은 약 30%이다. 사람면역결핍바이러스(HIV)와 같이 면역력이 저하된 환자에서 자연적으로 발생하는 두창의 경과에 대해서는 알려진 바가 거의 없다.

두창은 주로 감염된 환자의 입인두에서 튀어나온 비말핵과 직접 접촉으로 전파되는 전염성 질환이다. 오염된 의복과 침구류도 바이러스를 퍼트릴 수 있다. 환자는 발진이 나타나기 약간 전부터 전염성이 있지만, 입인두의 발진이 미미한 경우에는 전염성이 항상 분명하지 않을 수 있다. 두창 환자를 처치할 때 병원 전 처치 제공자는 접촉 및 에어로졸 예방 조치에 적합한 개인보호장비를 착용해야 한다. 여기에는 N95 마스크, 보호안경, 가운이 포함된다. 두창 환자를 처치하는 사람은 예방 접종을 받는 것이 가장 이상적이다.

미국의 두창 예방접종 프로그램은 1972년에 중단되었다. 이 예방접종 프로그램이 제공하는 잔류 면역은 알려지지 않았으며 40년 전에 마지막으로 예방접종을 받은 사람은 현재 두창에 걸릴 가능성이 높다고 한다. 두창 바이러스 예방접종은 미국 국방성과 국무부 일부 직원에게 제공된다. 또한, 미국 보건복지부 산하의 공중 보건 두창 대응팀의 프로그램에 따라 백신이 제공되고 있다. 현재 이 백신은 임상 시험에 참가하는 일반 대중에게만 제공된다. 공중보건 비상사태가 발생하면 미국은 일반인을 대상으로 대량 예방 접종을 할 수 있는 백신을 비축하고 있다. 노출 후 4일 이내에 백신을 접종하면 질병에 걸리는

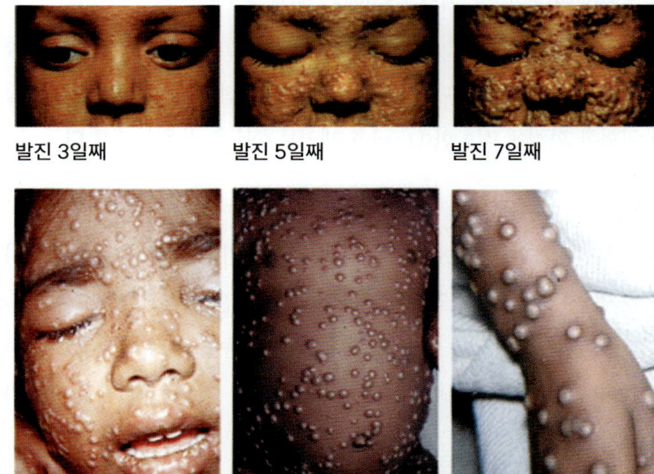

발진 3일째 · 발진 5일째 · 발진 7일째

신체 일부의 모든 병변이 같이 발전한다.

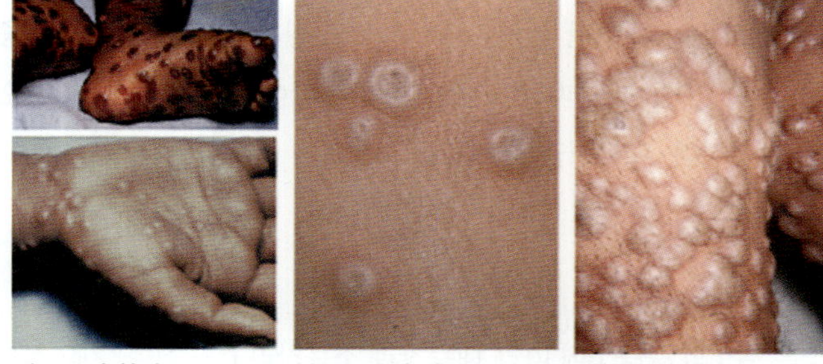

대부분의 환자는 손바닥이나 발바닥에 병변이 있다. · 배꼽모양의 병변 · 융합성 병변

그림 18-5 두창.
Courtesy of the Centers for Disease Control and Prevention.

Box 18-10 수두와 두창 구별하기

수두는 두창과 혼동될 가능성이 가장 높은 질환이다. 수두의 특징은 다음과 같다.

- 전구 증상이나 경미한 전구 증상이 없다.
- 병변은 표재성 소포로 "장미 꽃잎에 맺힌 이슬" 같다.
- 병변에는 소낭이 나타나며 신체의 어느 한 부분에 여러 단계(구진, 수포, 딱지)의 병변이 있다.
- 구심성 분포로 몸통에 병변이 가장 많이 집중되고 말단 팔다리에 병변이 가장 적다. 병변은 얼굴과 두피에도 나타날 수 있으며 간혹 전신에 똑같이 영향을 받는다.
- 첫 번째 병변은 얼굴이나 몸통에 나타난다.
- 환자가 독성을 보이거나 혼수상태에 빠지는 경우는 드물다.
- 병변은 황반에서 구진, 수포, 딱지로 빠르게 진행된다(24시간 이내).
- 손바닥과 발바닥에는 거의 나타나지 않는다.
- 환자는 신뢰할 수 있는 수두 예방 접종 기록이 없다.
- 이러한 환자 중 50~80%는 발진이 나타나기 10~21일 전에 수두 또는 대상포진에 노출된 것을 기억한다.

Modified from Centers for Disease Control and Prevention, National Center for Emerging and Zoonotic Infectious Diseases (NCEZID), Division of High-Consequence Pathogens and Pathology (DHCPP). Evaluating patients for smallpox: acute, generalized vesicular or pustular rash illness protocol. 2016. https://www.cdc.gov/smallpox/clinicians/algorithm-protocol.html

것을 어느 정도 예방하고 치명적인 결과를 예방할 수 있는 것으로 나타났다.

처치

두창 환자를 처치하기 위해 병원 전 처치 제공자는 지지요법을 제공한다. 권장되는 개인보호장비를 항상 착용해야 하며 감염 관리 절차를 위반하지 않는 것이 중요하다. 적절한 격리 시설과 적절한 훈련을 받은 직원이 있는 의료기관을 파악해야 한다. 환자를 이송할 의료기관에 연락하여 두창에 걸린 환자 또는 감염이 의심되는 환자가 있음을 알리고 바이러스 전파 방지를 위해 적절한 예방 조치를 취할 수 있도록 해야 한다. 두창 환자가 확인되면 매우 중요한 공중보건 비상상태로 간주한다.

감염 관리 절차를 위반하지 않고 개인보호장비를 적절하게 탈의

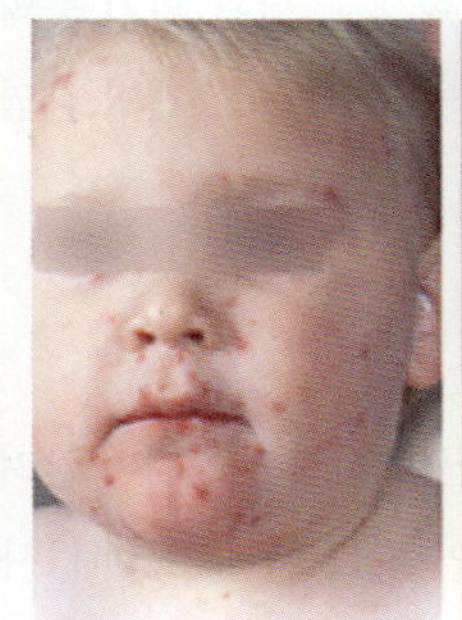
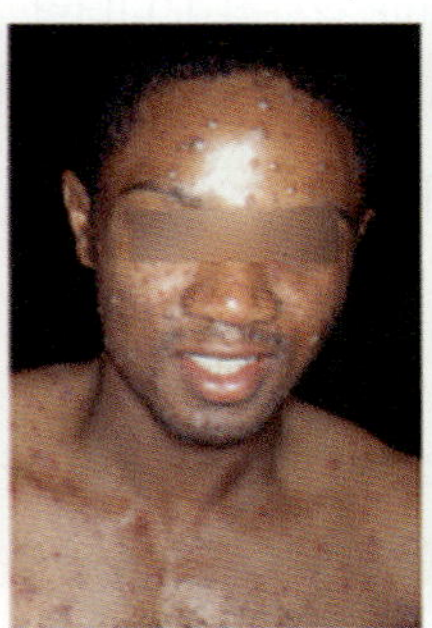
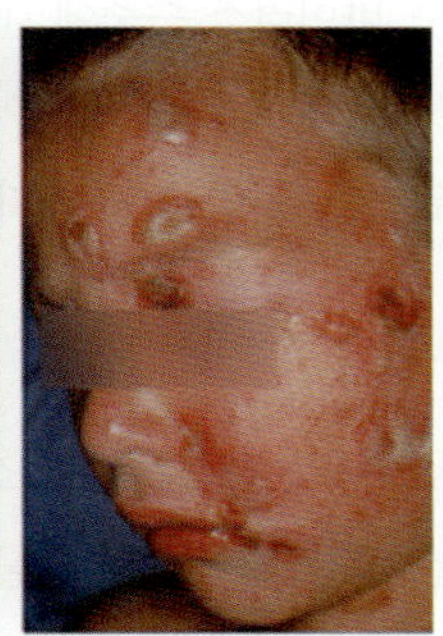

수두에 걸린 건강한 어린이　　수두에 걸린 건강한 성인　　병변의 세균성 초감염

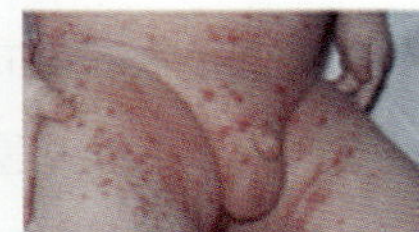
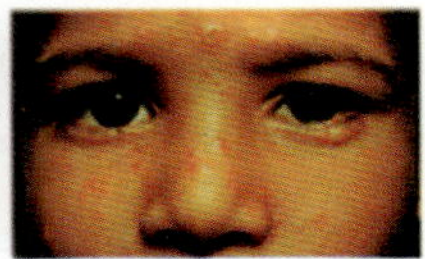
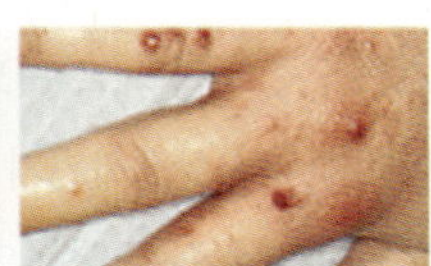

발진 부위　　발진 3일째　　단계에 따른 병변의 발전

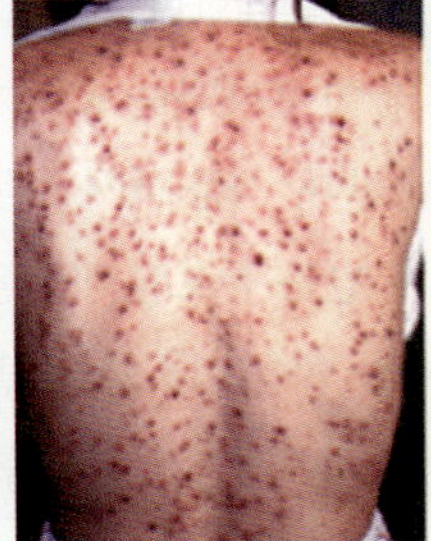
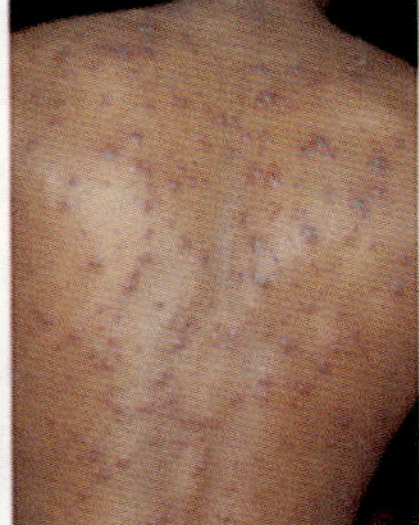
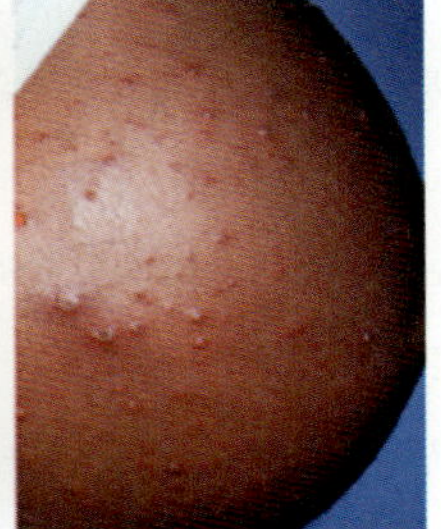

수두에 걸린 건강한 성인　　수두에 걸린 건강한 성인　　수두에 걸린 임산부

그림 18-6 수두
Courtesy of the Centers for Disease Control and Prevention.

하는 것은 병원 전 처치 제공자의 안전을 위해 중요하다. 오염된 모든 일회용 의료 폐기물은 다른 규제 의료 폐기물과 마찬가지로 적절하게 폐기물 통에 담아 라벨을 부착하고 폐기해야 한다. 재사용할 수 있는 의료 장비는 사용 후 표준 프로토콜에 따라 고압증기멸균 소독이나 높은 수준의 소독을 시행하고 세척한다. 주변 환경은 미국 환경보호청(EPA)에 등록된 세제와 소독제로 세척한다. 구급차의 공기 오염 제거 또는 훈증 소독은 필요하지 않다.

에볼라 바이러스 및 기타 바이러스성 출혈열

바이러스성 출혈열(VHF)은 여러 가지 바이러스에 의해 발생하는 임상 증후군으로 발열, 권태감, 출혈성 증상(가장 심한 경우 응고 병증, 정맥천자 부위 및 점막 출혈, 점상 출혈, 반상출혈 등)이 임상적으로 나타나는 것이 특징이다. 감염으로 인해 사망하는 감염자의 비율로 정의되는 치사율은 바이러스성 출혈열 바이러스에 따라 크게 다르며 같은 바이러스가 발생하더라도 90%를 초과할 수 있다. 바이러스성 출혈열을 유발하는 바이러스의 예로는 에볼라 바이러스, 마르부르크 바이러스, 황열 바이러스 및 라사 바이러스 등이 있다. 구소련이 무기화된 바이러스성 출혈열 바이러스에 관한 연구를 수행했으며 현재 테러리스트 조직이 바이러스성 출혈열을 악용하기 위한 자체 프로그램을 개발하고 있을 수 있다.

에볼라 바이러스는 필로바이러스(바이러스 입자의 필라멘트 모양에서 유래)의 일종으로 1976년 현재 남수단과 콩고민주공화국의 국경 근처에서 발생한 두 번의 바이러스성 출혈열 발생 환자에서 처음 분리 및 확인되었다. 에볼라라는 이름은 후자의 발생지 근처의 작은 강 이름에서 유래했다. 이후 과학적 연구를 통해 1989년 버지니아주 러스턴의 검역 시설에 수용된 연구용 원숭이들 사이에서 발생한 레스턴 에볼라 바이러스를 포함하여 여러 발병을 일으킨 에볼라 바이러스의 여러 변종이 확인되었다. 두창과 달리 에볼라 바이러스는 동물, 특히 박쥐에서 자연적으로 전염된 것으로 알려져 언제든 새로운 발병이 발생할 수 있다. 에볼라 바이러스는 2014년 서아프리카 전역으로 확산하여 2013~2016년까지 미국 및 서방 국가에서 보고된 28,000건 이상의 사례 중 11,000명 이상이 사망하면서 전 세계적으로 주목을 받기 시작했다.

임상적으로 에볼라 바이러스에 감염되면 2~21일의 잠복기를 거쳐 발열, 오한, 전신 권태감 및 근육통 등의 증상이 나타나고 복통, 구토, 설사 등의 위장관 증상과 두통, 혼동 등의 신경학적 증상 그리고

기침, 가슴 통증, 호흡곤란 등의 호흡기 증상이 나타나는 에볼라바이러스병(EVD)에 걸린다. 질병이 최고조에 달하면 심한 경우 출혈성 증상과 전신 응고병증이 나타날 수 있다. 사망은 주로 위장관 부피 손실로 인한 다발성 장기부전, 패혈증, 전해질 이상, 저혈량 쇼크로 인해 발생한다. 치사율은 변종과 발병 사례에 따라 크게 다르지만, 2013~2016년 서아프리카 발병의 최종 치사율은 40% 미만이었으나 발병 초기에는 약 75%, 일부 이전 발병에서는 90% 이상이었다. 이러한 치사율의 개선은 주로 위장관 부피와 전해질 손실을 적극적으로 보충하는 등 에볼라바이러스병 환자에 대한 처치가 개선되었기 때문으로 추정된다.

처치

전염성이 매우 강한 바이러스의 특성으로 인해 에볼라바이러스병이 의심되는 환자를 이송하는 것은 EMS 종사자에게 상당한 위험을 초래한다. 증상이 있는 환자의 체액에는 매우 많은 양의 활성 바이러스가 포함되어 있으며 소량의 노출만으로도 감염될 수 있다. 서아프리카에서 발병한 발병 사례를 검토한 결과 의료 종사자 중 3.9%가 에볼라바이러스병 환자를 돌보다 감염된 것으로 나타났다. 미국 질병통제예방센터는 현재 이용할 수 있는 최상의 증거를 바탕으로 에볼라바이러스병 환자 이송 시 개인보호장비 사용에 대한 구체적인 지침을 발표했다. 간단히 말해 미국 질병통제예방센터는 산업안전보건청(OSHA)은 Level C 보호복과 유사한 여러 겹(일회용 수술복, 불 침투성 가운, 앞치마, 여러 겹의 장갑과 신발 덮개)으로 피부 보호와 전동식 호흡 보호장비 및 N95 마스크 등 호흡기와 점막 보호를 권장한다. 이러한 권장 사항은 또 다른 발병이 발생할 때 업데이트될 수 있다. 에볼라바이러스병 개인보호장비에 대한 광범위한 교육과 경험이 있는 숙련된 관찰자가 착용과 탈의 절차를 직접 감독할 것을 강력히 권장한다.

조지아주 애틀랜타의 그레디 병원과 네브래스카주 오마하의 네브래스카 메디컬센터에 소속된 EMS 기관은 2013~2016년 에볼라바이러스병이 발생하기 전에 전염성이 높은 중증 환자를 이송하기 위한 장비와 계획을 개발했으며 이후 실제 및 의심되는 에볼라바이러스병 환자를 처치하고 이송한 경험에 대한 보고서를 발표했다. 이 보고서에는 다음과 같이 에볼라바이러스병 환자 이소에 대한 구체적이고 유용한 권고 사항이 다수 포함되어 있다.

- 적절한 개인보호장비 사용[(착용/탈의 절차에 엄격한 주의를 기울이고 장거리 이송 시 의료진 보호와 편안함을 위해 음압 마스크보다 전동식 호흡 보호 장비 착용(PAPR)을 권장]
- 환자칸과 구급차 운전실을 즉석 양압 시스템으로 분리
- 구급차 환자칸 내의 모든 장비와 표면을 두꺼운 플라스틱 시트로 덮어 오염을 제한
- 오염 제한 보호복 또는 캡슐 내에서 환자 추가 격리
- 소독용 물티슈를 사용하여 구급차와 장비의 오염을 주의해서 제거 (바이러스 입자를 에어로졸화할 수 있는 가압된 물로 표면을 분사하는 것과 반대)

2013~2016년 발병에서 얻은 경험을 바탕으로 현재 에볼라바이러스병 환자의 의학적 처치는 주로 증상 조절과 경구 위장관 수액 및 전해질 손실 보충에 중점을 두고 있다. 항바이러스제, 면역조절제, 백신 등 생존율을 개선할 수 있는 여러 가지 새로운 치료법이 있지만, 그 효과는 아직 연구 중이다. 정맥 라인으로 수액 투여, 전해질, 세포 수, 바이러스 수준에 대한 검사실 모니터링, 항생제, 삽관/환기 등의 사전 지지요법도 도움이 될 수 있지만, 이러한 조치는 의료진의 감염 위험을 많이 증가시킨다.

보툴리눔 독소

보툴리눔 독소는 클로스트리듐 보툴리눔 세균에 의해 생성되며 알려진 가장 독성이 강한 물질이다. 신경 작용제인 VX보다 15,000배, 사린보다 10만 배 더 독성이 강하다. 보툴리눔 독소는 미국, 구소련, 이라크, 이란, 시리아, 북한 등에서 군사용으로 무기화되었다. 도쿄 지하철 사린 테러를 일으킨 옴진리교는 1995년에 보툴리눔 독소 에어로졸을 살포하려고 시도했지만, 성공하지 못했다. 독소를 농축하고 안정화하여 살포하기가 어렵다는 보고가 있지만, 테러리스트가 보툴리눔 에어로졸을 점적으로 살포하면 0.5km 이내에 있는 사람의 10%를 무력화하거나 사망에 이르게 할 수 있는 것으로 추정된다. 또한 이 독소는 많은 사람을 중독시키려는 시도로 식품에 넣을 수도 있다.

자연적으로 세 가지 형태의 보툴리누스중독이 존재한다. 상처를 통한 보툴리누스중독은 클로스트리듐 보툴리눔이 존재하는 조직이 파괴된 더러운 상처에서 독소가 흡수될 때 발생한다. 식품 매개 보툴리누스중독은 부적절하게 조리되거나 가정에서 만든 통조림 식품을 통해 세균이 증식하고 독소를 생성하고 피해자가 이를 섭취할 때 발생한다. 장내 보툴리누스중독은 독소가 위장관 내에서 생산되고 흡수될 때 발생한다. 이 세 가지 자연 발생 형태 외에도 에어로졸화된 보툴리눔 독소로 인해 흡입 보툴리누스중독이라고 하는 인공적인 형태의 보툴리누스중독이 발생할 수 있다.

오염 경로와 관계없이 보툴리눔 독소는 신경근 접합부로 운반되어 비가역적으로 결합하여 신경전달물질인 아세틸콜린의 정상적인 방출을 방해하고 하행 이완마비를 유발한다. 증상이 시작되는데 걸리는 시간은 몇 시간에서 며칠이다. 모든 환자는 복시와 다발성 뇌신경 결손이 나타나 시력, 언어, 삼킴에 어려움을 겪게 된다. 하행 마비의 정도와 속도는 독소의 용량에 따라 달라진다. 환자는 피로해지고 머리와 목 근육을 조절하는 능력을 상실하고 구역반사 소실, 호흡근 마비로 진행되어 호흡부전이 발생하여 기관내삽관 및 수개월의 기계적 환기가 필요할 수 있다. 치료를 받지 않은 환자는 일반적으로 상기도 폐쇄 또는 부적절한 환기로 사망한다. 보툴리눔 독성의 전형적인 세 가지 특징은 1) 뇌신경 결손을 동반한 하행 대칭성 이완마비, 2) 발열 소실, 3) 감각이 분명해지는 것이다. 몇 주에서 수개월이 지나면 새로운 축삭돌기가 발달하여 신경이 차단된 근육에 신경을 공급하면서 회복될 수 있다.

처치

보툴리누스중독 환자에 대한 처치는 병원에서 항독소를 투여하는 것이다. 항독소를 조기에 투여하면 악화를 최소화할 수는 있지만, 이미 발생한 마비를 되돌릴 수는 없다. 이 항독소는 미국 질병통제예방센터에서 구할 수 있다.

보툴리누스중독 환자를 처치하는 병원 전 처치 제공자는 기도 관리 및 부적절 환기에 주의해야 한다. 환자 스스로 분비물을 관리하지 못하거나 기도 유지를 못할 수 있다. 가로막 마비로 인해 환자가 적절한 일회 호흡량을 생성하지 못할 수 있다. 환자가 바로누운자세를 취하면 이러한 증상이 악화할 수 있다. 호흡곤란을 겪는 환자는 기관내삽관을 시행하고 적절하게 환기를 시행한다.

보툴리눔 독성은 전염성 질환이 아니기 때문에 보툴리눔 독성 증상을 보이는 환자 관리에는 표준 예방조치가 적절하다. 보툴리눔 에어로졸은 환경에서 쉽게 분해되며 테러 목적으로 전달된 후 2일이 지나면 상당 부분 비활성화될 것으로 예상된다. 명백한 에어로졸 확산 사고에 대해 대응자는 오염지역 및 전방 통제지역에서 작업하는 경우 위험한 환경에 적합한 Level A 개인보호복을 착용한다.

에어로졸은 평균 기상 조건에서 약 2일 동안 지속될 수 있으므로 보툴리눔 에어로졸에 노출된 피해자는 옷을 제거한 후 비누와 물로 씻어 오염을 제거한다. 장비는 0.1% 차아염소산 표백제 용액을 사용하여 오염을 제거할 수 있다. 환자는 병원 도착 후 격리할 필요는 없지만, 기계적 환기가 필요한 환자에게는 중환자 처치가 필요할 수 있다.

방사선 재난

2011년 9월 11일 테러 공격 이후 방사선 응급 상황을 관리해야 하는 EMS 시스템의 가능성에 대한 새로운 고려가 이루어졌다. 역사적으로 계획은 군용 핵무기의 전략적 교환이나 드물게 발생하는 원자력 발전소 사고에 대한 민방위 대비에 중점을 두었다. 그러나 현재 테러리스트가 재래식 폭발물을 사용하여 방사성 물질을 환경으로 확산시키는 급조된 핵폭발 장치 또는 방사능 분산 장치(RDD)를 배치할 가능성에 대한 인식이 높아지고 있다. 냉전 시대에 우려했던 대규모 핵 거래는 오늘날에는 가능성이 낮아졌지만, 지난 수십 년 동안 소규모 국가들 사이에서 핵무기가 확산하면서 불량 국가나 테러리스트 단체가 핵무기를 획득하여 민간인을 공격하는 데 사용할 수 있다는 우려가 제기되고 있다.

방사선 사고는 드물지만, 1944년 이후 미국에서는 243건의 방사선 사고가 발생했으며 1,342명의 사상자가 심각한 피폭 기준을 충족했다. 전 세계적으로는 403건의 방사선 사고가 발생하여 133,617명의 피해자 중 심각한 피폭자는 2,965명이었으며 120명의 사망자가 발생했다. 1986년 체르노빌 사고로 인해 2005년 기준 116,500~125,000명의 피폭 사상자와 50명에 가까운 사망자가 발생했으며 추가 암 발생으로 사망한 사람까지 포함하면 4,000명에 달하는 것으로 추정된다. 1987년 브라질 고이아니아에서 발생한 사고는 의료 방사선 치료에 사용되는 고방사성 동위원소인 세슘-137을 보관하던 용기가 깨지면서 내부에 있던 방사성 물질이 퍼진 사건이다. 오염된 129명 중 20명이 입원했고 4명이 사망했으며 약 125,000명이 방사능 오염 검사를 받았다. 방사성 동위원소의 방출은 피해자들이 방사능 중독으로 지역 병원에 내원한 지 16일이 지나서야 발견되었으며 이러한 인식 지연으로 인해 오염된 피해자 수가 증가했을 가능성이 높다. 일본 후쿠시마 원자력 발전소는 2011년 인근 지진과 쓰나미로 인해 심각한 피해를 입어 여러 개의 원자로가 파괴되고 방사능이 환경으로 방출되었다. 이 사고로 인해 주변 지역 주민과 환경에 미치는 건강상의 영향을 완전히 평가하기까지는 몇 년에서 수십 년이 걸릴 것이다.

방사선 재난은 피해자와 EMS 제공자 모두에게 공포와 혼란을 일으킬 수 있다. 위험 요소 및 관리 원칙을 숙지하면 적절하게 대응할 수 있고 공황과 혼돈을 줄이는 데 도움이 된다(**Box 18-11**).

전리방사선 및 방사성 오염에 노출될 수 있는 다음과 같은 몇 가지 시나리오에서 발생할 수 있다. 예를 들면 1) 핵무기 폭발, 2) 핵폭발이 아닌 재래식 폭발물을 터뜨려 방사성 물질을 분산시키는 더러운 폭

Box 18-11 방사선 재난 관리 원칙

1. 현장의 안전을 평가한다.
2. 모든 환자는 방사선 손상을 고려하기 전에 외상으로 인한 손상을 의학적으로 안정시켜야 한다. 그런 다음 환자는 외부 방사선 노출 및 오염 여부를 평가한다.
3. 외부 방사선원이 충분히 크면 조직 손상을 일으킬 수 있지만, 환자가 방사능에 노출되지는 않는다. 외부 방사선에 치명적으로 노출된 환자라도 병원 전 처치 제공자에게 위협이 되지 않는다.
4. 환자는 피부나 옷에 묻은 방사성 물질에 오염될 수 있다. 표면 오염의 90% 이상은 옷을 제거하면 오염 물질을 제거할 수 있다. 나머지는 비누와 물로 씻어낼 수 있다.
5. 병원 전 처치 제공자는 보호복, 장갑, 마스크 등 최소한의 표준 예방 조치를 준수하여 방사능 오염으로부터 자신을 보호해야 한다.
6. 노출 후 4시간 이내에 구역, 구토 또는 피부 홍반이 생기는 환자는 외부 방사선에 많이 노출되었을 가능성이 높다.
7. 상처 부위의 방사능 오염은 흙으로 처리하고 가능한 한 빨리 물로 세척한다. 금속성 이물질은 만지지 않는다.
8. 요오드화칼륨(KI)은 방사성 요오드가 방출된 경우에만 사용할 수 있다. 요오드화칼륨은 일반적인 방사선 해독제가 아니다.
9. 시간, 거리, 차폐의 개념은 방사선 노출로 인한 부작용을 예방하는 데 핵심적인 요소이다. 방사선 노출은 영향을 받은 부위에서 노출을 줄이고 방사선원으로부터 거리를 늘리며 금속 또는 콘크리트 차폐물을 사용하여 최소화할 수 있다.

Modified from Department of Homeland Security Working Group on Radiological Dispersion Device (RRD) Preparedness. Medical preparedness and response subgroup. May 1, 2003. https://www.hsdl.org/?abstract&did=437718

탄(dirty bomb) 또는 방사선 분산 장치 폭발, 3) 원자로 파괴 또는 사고 유발, 4) 핵폐기물을 잘 못 처리하는 것이다.

방사선 재난의 의학적 영향

방사선 재난과 관련된 손상과 위험은 복잡한 요인에 의해 발생한다. 핵폭발의 경우 1차, 2차, 3차 폭발로 인해 폭발 손상, 열 손상, 건물 붕괴로 인해 사상자가 발생한다. 피해자는 방사선이 인체를 통과하여 손상을 일으키지만, 오염은 일으키지 않는(X-ray 촬영과 유사) 방사선 검사로 인해 방사선 손상을 입을 수 있다. 낙진으로 인해 피부와 옷에 침착될 수 있는 외부 방사능 오염, 피해자가 흡입, 섭취하거나 상처에 침착될 수 있는 방사성 미립자 오염을 통한 내부 방사능으로 인해 추가로 방사선 손상을 입을 수 있다.

원자로 사고는 특히 원자로가 임계점에 도달한 상황에서 핵폭발 없이도 다량의 전리방사선을 발생시킬 수 있다. 폭발, 화재 및 가스 방출로 인해 방사성 가스 또는 미립자 물질이 발생할 수도 있으며 이로 인해 구급대원과 구조대원이 방사성 입자에 의한 오염 위험에 노출될 수 있다.

방사능 분산 장치(RDD)가 폭발해도 일반적으로는 즉각적인 손상을 유발할 만큼 충분한 방사선이 방출되지 않는다. 그러나 방사성 분산 장치는 피해자와 EMS 제공자를 오염시킬 수 있는 방사성 미립자를 분산시키고 기존 폭발물로 인한 손상을 처치하기 어렵게 만들어 병원 전 처치 제공자의 처치를 복잡하게 만들 수 있다. 방사성 분산 장치는 방사능을 우려하는 시민과 EMS 제공자에게 혼란과 공포를 일으켜 피해자를 돕기 위한 노력을 방해할 수 있다.

전리방사선은 원자와 상호작용하고 에너지를 축적하여 세포에 손상을 입힌다. 이러한 상호작용은 이온화를 초래하여 세포핵을 직접적으로 손상시켜 세포 사멸 또는 기능 상실을 일으키거나 간접적으로 체내 수분과 상호작용하여 독성 분자를 생성하고 세포 구성 요소를 손상할 수 있다. 단시간에 다량의 투과성 전리방사선(γ 선 및 중성자)에 빠르게 노출되면 급성 방사선 질환을 일으킬 수 있다. 전리방사선의 종류에는 α입자, β 입자, γ 선, 중성자가 있다.

α 입자는 상대적으로 커서 피부를 통과할 수 없다. 온전한 피부나 옷은 α 입자를 방출하는 외부 오염으로부터 피부를 적절하게 보호한다. α입자 입자로 인한 전리방사선은 α 입자 방사체를 흡입하거나 섭취하여 내부로 유입되는 경우에만, 문제가 된다. α입자 방사선은 내부로 유입되면 인접 세포에 심각한 국소 세포 손상을 일으킬 수 있다.

β 입자는 작은 입자로 α 입자보다 더 깊숙이 침투할 수 있으며 피부 기저부를 손상시켜 β 화상을 유발할 수 있으며 피부의 더 깊은 층에 영향을 미칠 수 있다. β 입자 방사선은 핵 낙진에서 가장 빈번하게 발견되며 β 입자는 또한 국소 방사선 손상을 초래한다.

γ 선은 X선과 유사하며 조직을 쉽게 투과할 수 있다. γ 선은 핵폭발과 함께 낙진으로 방출된다. γ 선은 방사선 분산 장치에 존재할 수 있는 일부 방사성 핵종에서 방출될 수도 있다. γ 방사선은 전신 노출이라는 결과를 초래할 수 있다. 전신 피폭은 급성 또는 만성 방사선 질환을 유발할 수 있다(**Box 18-12**, **표 18-2** 및 **표 18-3**).

중성자는 γ 선의 20배에 달하는 파괴 에너지로 조직에 쉽게 투과하여 세포의 원자 구조를 파괴할 수 있다. 중성자는 핵폭발 시 방출되지만, 낙진 위험은 없다. 중성자는 또한 전신 방사선 노출을 유발하며 급성 방사선 질환을 일으킬 수 있다. 중성자는 안정적인 금속을 방사성 동위원소로 전환할 수 있다. 이 능력은 피폭 당시에 금속성 물체가 달린 장신구나 금속성 물체를 소지하고 있는 환자에게 중요하다.

전신 피폭량은 그레이(Gy)로 측정하고 라드(rad; 방사선 흡수선량)은 그레이로 대체된 친숙한 선량 단위로 사용하기도 하며 1Gy는

100rad에 해당한다. 램(rem; 방사선 등가 선량)은 선량에 다양한 유형의 방사선을 고유한 특수 증착 패턴을 고려한 양호도(quality factor)를 곱한 값으로 표시된다. 램은 시버트(Sv)로 표기할 수 있고 1Sv는 100rem이다.

방사선은 빠르게 분열하는 세포에 가장 쉽게 영향을 미치므로 세포 주기 속도가 빠른 골수 및 위장관에 손상을 입힐 수 있다. 고선량은 중추신경계에 직접적인 영향을 미칠 수 있다. 전신 피폭 선량에 따라 피폭으로 인한 의학적 결과가 결정된다. 최대 1Gy의 전신 피폭을 받은 환자는 일반적으로 손상 징후가 나타나지 않는다. 1~2Gy의 경우 환자의 절반 미만이 오심과 구토를 일으키고 많은 사람이 백혈구 감소증에 걸리며 사망은 최소화된다. 2Gy 이상의 피폭을 받은 대부분 피해자는 병에 걸려 입원이 필요하며 6Gy 이상에서 피폭되면 사망률이 높아진다. 30Gy 이상의 선량에서는 신경학적 증후가 나타나고 사망할 가능성이 가장 높다.

백혈구감소는 일반적으로 불쾌감, 오심, 구토를 특징으로 하는 전구 단계에서 처음 나타나는 임상 증상을 보이며 진행된다. 이후에는 환자가 본질적으로 증상이 없는 잠복기가 이어진다. 잠복기의 기간은 전체 흡수된 방사선량에 따라 다르다. 방사선량이 많을수록 잠복기는 짧아진다. 잠복기 이후에는 손상된 장기에 의해 나타나는 후속 질병 단계가 이어진다. 골수 손상은 총 선량이 0.7~4.0Gy일 때 발생하며 며칠에서 몇 주에 걸쳐 백혈구 수치가 감소하고 감염에 대한 면역력이 감소한다. 혈소판이 감소하면 쉽게 멍이 들고 출혈이 생길 수 있으며 적혈구 감소로 빈혈이 발생할 수 있다. 6~8Gy에서는 위장관에 영향을 미쳐 설사, 체액 감소, 혈변이 발생한다. 30Gy 이상에서는 신경혈관 증후군의 증상이 나타나며 오심과 구토의 전구 증상을 경험하고 몇 시간만 지속되는 짧은 잠복기, 의식 상태의 급격한 악화, 혼수상태, 사망할 수 있으며 때로는 혈류역학적 불안정을 동반하기도 한다. 이 정도의 피폭량은 핵폭발 후에 발생할 수 있지만, 피해자는 폭발과 관련된 손상으로 인해 사망했을 가능성이 높다. 피해자는 폭발이 발생하지 않았지만, 원자로 노심이 임계점에 도달한 원자력 발전 시설에서도 이러한 고선량에 피폭될 수 있다.

모든 방사선 사고나 테러 사건이 고선량 방사선 피폭으로 이어지는 것은 아니다. 저선량 방사선 노출은 방사선 확산 장치 폭발 후 발생 가능성이 높으며 방사선으로 인한 이차적인 급성 손상을 일으키지는 않을 가능성이 높다. 선량에 따라 환자는 향후 암 발병 위험이 증가할 수 있다. 방사선 확산 장치 폭발의 급성 영향은 재래식 폭발에 의한 영향 외에도 스트레스 반응, 공포, 급성 우울증, 심리적인 영향이 있을 수 있으며 이는 EMS 기관과 의료 인프라에 상당한 부담을 줄 수 있다.

환자는 α, β, γ선을 방출하는 물질에 오염될 수 있지만, 가장 흔한 오염 물질은 α 및 β 방사선을 방출한다. 앞서 설명한 바와 같이 γ 방사선만 전신에 피폭을 유발할 수 있다. α 및 β 방사선은 투과력이 제한적이지만, 국소 조직 손상을 유발할 수 있다. 환자의 옷을 제거하고 비누와 물로 씻으면 쉽게 오염을 제거할 수 있다. 환자를 처치하는 병원 전 처치 제공자에게 방사선학적 위험을 초래할 정도로 환자가 오염이 되는 것은 불가능하므로 생명을 위협하는 외상성 손상을 처치하는 것이 즉각적인 우선순위이며 오염 제거를 위해 지연해서는 안 된다.

설명한 바와 같이 방사선 입자는 피부나 오염된 상처를 통해 흡입, 섭취 또는 흡수될 수 있다. 이러한 유형의 방사선 노출은 방사선 노출의 급성 영향을 초래하지는 않지만, 지연된 영향을 초래할 수 있다. 호흡기 보호장비 없이 공기 중 방사성 입자 위험 지역에서 활동하는 피해자나 EMS 제공자는 내부 오염을 확인하기 위해 후속 평가가 필

표 18-2 급성 방서선 증후군

특징	라드(Rad)는 선량 범위에 따른 전신 조사 또는 내부 흡수의 영향(1 rad = 1 centigray; 100 rad = 1 gray)					
	0~100 (0~1 Gy)	100~200 (1~2 Gy)	200~600 (2~6 Gy)	600~800 (6~8 Gy)	800~3,000 (8~30 Gy)	> 3,000 (> 30 Gy)
증후군 전구기						
구역, 구토	없음	5~50%	50~100%	75~100%	90~100%	100%
발병 시간	—	3~6시간	2~4시간	1~2시간	< 1시간	N/A
지속 시간	—	< 24시간	< 24시간	< 48시간	48시간	N/A
림프구 수	영향을 받지 않음	최소한으로 감소	< 1,000 at 24 hr	< 500 at 24 hr	몇 시간 내에 감소	몇 시간 내에 감소
중추신경계기능	손상 없음	손상 없음	일상적인 작업 수행 6~20시간 동안 인지 기능 장애	단순하고 일상적인 작업 수행 >24시간 인지기능 장애	빠른 무력화: 몇 시간의 명확한 간격을 가질 수 있음	
증후군의 잠복기						
증상 없음	> 2주	7~15일	0~7일	0~2일	없음	없음
질병 발현						
징후/증상	없음	중증도의 백혈구 감소증	중증 백혈구 감소증, 자반, 출혈, 폐렴, 300 rad 노출 후 탈모	설사, 발열, 전해질 불균형	경련, 실조, 떨림, 졸음증	
발병 시간	—	> 2주	2일~4주	2일~4주	1~3일	1~3일
위험 기간	—	없음	4~6주: 최대한 효과적으로 의료 개입	2~14일	1~46시간	
기관계	없음	—	조혈: 호흡기계(점막)	위장관 점막 계통	중추신경계	
입원 기간	0%	< 5% 45-60일	90% 60~90일	100% 100일 이상	100% 주, 개월	100% 며칠, 몇 주
사망률	없음	최소한	적극적인 치료 시 낮음	높음	매우 높음: 중요한 신경학적 증상은 치사량을 나타낸다.	

Abbreviations: CNS, central nervous system; d, day(s); GI, gastrointestinal; hr, hour(s); N/A, not available; wk, week(s)

Modified from Armed Forces Radiobiology Research Institute. *Medical Management of Radiological Casualties*. Author; 2003.

표 18-3 방사선 조사 후 지연 효과로 나타나는 증상

일반적	위장관	피부과	혈액학
두통	식용부진	부분 및 전층 피부 손상	림프구 감소
피로	구역	탈모	호중구 감소
쇠약	구토	궤양	혈소판 감소
	설사		자반
			기회감염

Modified from Armed Forces Radiobiology Research Institute. *Medical Management of Radiological Casualties*. Author; 2003.

요하며 흡입한 방사성 핵종의 영향을 희석하거나 차단하기 위해 의학적 개입이 필요할 수 있다.

개인보호장비

병원 전 처치 제공자는 방사선 재난이 발생한 후 전리방사선에 노출될 위험이 있는 환경에서 임무를 수행할 수 있다. 방사선 위험은 방사선 사건의 유형에 따라 크게 달라진다.

병원 전 처치 제공자가 화학 및 생물학적 위험 상황에서 사용할 수 있는 개인보호장비는 방사성 미립자 오염으로부터 어느 정도 보호할 수 있다. 그러나 원자로 손상이나 원전 폭발과 같은 고에너지 방사선원으로부터는 보호할 수 없다.

방사능은 기체, 에어로졸, 고체 또는 액체 형태로 존재할 수 있다. 방사성 가스가 존재하는 경우 공기호흡기(SCBA)가 가장 높은 수준의 보호 기능을 제공한다. 에어로졸이 존재하는 경우 오염된 입자의 흡입으로 인한 내부 오염을 방지하기 위해 공기 정화기(APR)가 적절할 수 있다. N95 마스크는 흡입된 미립자로부터 약간의 보호 기능을 제공할 수 있다. 표준 방수복은 α 방사선을 방출하는 입자로부터 보호하고 β 방사선에 대해서는 어느 정도 보호할 수 있지만, γ이나 중성자에 대해서는 보호하지 못한다. 이러한 유형의 방호복은 개인으로부터 미립자 물질을 제거하는 데 도움이 되지만, 고에너지 외부 방사선에 노출되었을 때 급성 방사선 질병의 위험으로부터 보호하지는 못한다.

병원 전 처치 제공자가 착용하는 일반적인 개인보호장비 중 어떤 것도 고에너지 방사선원으로부터 보호하지 못한다. 이러한 유형의 방사선은 핵폭발의 첫 1분 동안 발생하거나 중요한 원자로 노심 또는 세슘-137과 같은 고에너지 방사선원(방사선 분산 장치로 분산될 수 있는 방사선원)에서 발생한다. 이러한 방사선원으로부터 자신을 보호하는 가장 좋은 방법은 노출 시간을 줄이고 방사선원으로부터 일정한 거리를 유지하고 차폐하는 것이다. 구급대원과 구조대원을 보호하기 위해 새로운 재질의 저준위 γ선으로부터 보호할 수 있는 개인보호장비가 개발되고 있다.

화학 작용제로부터 보호하기 위해 착용하는 불충분한 개인보호장비와는 달리 방사선 방출 가스 또는 미립자의 흡입, 섭취 및 피부 흡수는 병원 전 처치 제공자나 피해자가 즉시 무능화되지는 않는다. 방사성 물질로 오염될 가능성이 있는 환경에서 업무를 수행하는 모든 의료진은 내부 오염 여부를 확인하기 위해 방사선 조사를 받아야 하며 필요한 경우 적극적인 처치를 받는다.

가능한 경우 선량률 측정기 또는 경보기를 착용해야 한다. 정상 및 응급 상황이 발생한 작업 환경에서 허용 가능한 전리방사선에 대한 선량 기준이 있다. 전리방사선의 선량률을 측정하여 EMS 제공자가 급성 방사선 질환이나 허용할 수 없을 정도로 높은 암 발병률의 위험에 처하는 것을 방지할 수 있다. 방사선 노출 수치와 한도에 대한 지침은 사고 지휘관에게 문의한다.

평가 및 처치

방사선 재난으로 손상을 입은 환자는 손상 기전에 따라 일차 및 이차평가를 시행해야 한다. 병원 전 처치 제공자는 핵폭발 사고나 방사선 분산장치 폭발로 인해 폭발 손상과 열 손상을 입은 환자를 평가할 수 있다(**Box 18-13**). 외상성 손상 처치에 우선순위를 두고 방사선학적 측면은 이차적으로 고려해야 한다. 방사성 미립자 오염을 제거하기 위해 피해자의 오염 제거가 권장되지만, 외상성 손상으로 즉각적인 처치가 필요한 경우 처치가 지연되어서는 안 된다. 환자가 즉각적인 처치가 필요한 심각한 손상 징후를 보이지 않는 경우 환자의 오염을 먼저 제거할 수 있다.

원자로 사용 후 핵연료봉 관련사고나 핵 장치 폭발로 인해 방사성 요오드가 환경에 존재하는 경우 EMS 제공자와 피해자에게 요오드화칼륨을 투여하면 갑상샘에 방사성 요오도가 암 발생 가능성을 높이는 것을 예방하는 데 도움이 될 수 있다. 재난에 대한 자세한 정보가 있을 때 병원 또는 관련 기관에서 권장하는 차단 요법 및 탈조합 처치를 권장할 수 있다. 차단 요법은 방사성 물질의 영향을 방해하기 의해 고안되었지만, 탈조합 처치는 물질과 결합하여 제거할 수 있는 약물을 사용하여 체내에서 방사성 물질을 제거하는 것을 목표로 한다.

이송 시 고려사항

환자는 외상 및 방사선 손상을 처치할 수 있는 가장 가까운 적절한 응급의료센터로 이송해야 한다. 모든 병원은 방사선 비상 관리 계획을 수립해야 하지만, 지역사회에서 오염 제거 시설을 갖추고 외상을 처치할 수 있으며 외부 및 내부 방사성 오염 가능성과 전신 피폭으로 인한 합병증에 효과적으로 대처할 수 있는 교육을 받은 직원이 있는 기관을 파악한다.

Box 18-13 방사선 노출에 대한 처치 및 오염 제거 고려 사항

처치 고려 사항

- 외상이 있는 경우 처치한다.
- 외부 방사성 오염 물질이 있는 경우 오염을 제거한다(생명을 위협하는 문제를 처치한 후).
- 방사성 요오드(예: 원자로 사고)에 있는 경우 최초 24시간 이내에만, 예방적 목적으로 요오드화칼륨(루골 용액) 투여를 고려한다(이후에는 효과가 없음).
- http://www.orau.gov/reacts/guidance.htm 참조

오염 제거 고려 사항

- 오염이 없는 노출은 오염 제거가 필요하지 않다.
- 오염에 노출되면 표준 예방 조치, 환자 의복을 제거하고 물로 오염 제거가 필요하다.
- 내부 오염 여부는 병원에서 결정한다.
- 오염 제거 전에 환자를 처치하면 의료기관이 오염될 수 있으므로 이송하기 전에 오염 제거를 시행한다.
- 생명을 위협하는 손상이 있는 경우 처치 후 오염을 제거한다.
- 생명을 위협하는 문제가 없는 경우 오염을 제거한 후 처치한다.

Modified from Armed Forces Radiobiology Research Institute, Medical Management of Radiological Casualties. Author; 2003.

요 약

- 테러리스트 정권이 제조한 대량살상무기는 문명사회에 심각한 위협이 된다.

- 병원 전 처치 제공자는 산업 사고로 인한 폭발 및 화학물질과 방사성 물질에 접촉할 수 있다.

- 병원 전 처치 제공자의 안전이 가장 중요하다. 이들은 개인보호장비의 수준과 오염 제거의 기본 사항에 대한 실무 지식을 갖추고 있어야 한다.

- 최근 테러 공격에서는 폭발물과 총기가 주로 사용되었다. 고성능 폭약이 폭발 현장에 근접한 생존자에게 1차 폭발 손상을 입히고 파편으로 인한 2차 손상을 입힌다.

- 화학 작용제는 피부와 폐를 손상할 수 있을 뿐만 아니라 작용제에 대한 단서를 제공하는 특정 독성 증상으로 나타나는 전신 질환을 유발할 수도 있다. 이러한 작용제 중 일부는 해독제를 사용한다.

- 생물학적 작용제는 독성이 강한 균 또는 생물체가 생성하는 독소일 수 있다. 병원 전 처치 제공자가 사용하는 보호 예방 조치의 유형은 특정 작용제에 따라 다르다.

- 여러 종류의 방사선이 존재한다. 이러한 물질에 노출되면 급성 방사선 질환이 발생할 수 있으며 이는 일반적으로 방사선 유형과 노출 기간에 따라 달라진다.

시나리오 재구성

더운 여름 저녁 당신은 유명한 카페 밖에서 폭발이 발생했다는 신고를 받고 현장으로 출동하였다. 이 카페는 평소에도 손님으로 붐비고 일반적으로 야외 테이블에도 많은 손님이 앉는다는 것을 알고 있다. 응급의료상황관리자는 이 사고와 관련하여 여러 건의 신고 전화를 받았지만, 피해자 수는 아직 파악되지 않았다고 알려준다. 다른 공공 안전 기관도 현장으로 출동했다.

현장에 도착해서 당신은 현장에 도착한 첫 번째 병원 전 처치 제공자라는 것을 알았다. 사고 현장에 아직 사고 지휘 본부가 설치되지 않았다. 수십 명의 사람들이 카페에서 대피하고 있다. 많은 사람이 명백한 출혈이 있는 피해자를 도와 달라고 간청하고 있다. 다른 희생자들은 의식 상태가 불안정한 채 바닥에 누워있다.

- 가장 먼저 무엇을 해야 하는가?
- 행동 절차를 결정할 때 우선순위는 무엇인가?
- 많은 사람을 어떻게 돌볼 것인가?

시나리오 해결책

언제나 그렇듯이 최우선 순위는 안전이다. 현장을 평가하고 구급대원과 구조대원에게 위협이 될 수 있는 2차 폭발 장치가 있는지 확인한다. 다른 위험 요소가 존재하는지, 파편, 노출된 전선, 위험 물질이 우출된 곳이 있는지 확인한다.

지휘체계와 소통하고 사고지휘체계를 사용한다. 현장에 가장 먼저 드착한 구급대원이므로 상황실에서는 정보를 얻기 위해 당신에게 의존하게 된다. 현장의 관련 세부 사항, 위험 요소 확인, 피해자 수, 현장과 피해자를 관리하는 데 필요한 자원의 수를 설명한다. 구경꾼을 주의 깊게 관찰하여 독극물의 증거가 있는지 확인한다. 호흡 곤란 환자가 비정상적으로 많은가? 피해자가 구토와 경련을 일으키는가? 폭발물 폭발과 더불어 독극물이 확산하였다는 증거가 있는가? 당신이 관찰한 내용을 바탕으로 상황실과 근무 중인 상급자가 다른 팀과 기관에 상황을 알리고 필요한 자원을 파견할 수 있다. 사전에 계획된 재난 대응 계획이 활성화될 수 있다.

모든 구급대원과 구조대원의 개인 안전이 보장되고 정보가 전달되견 다른 권한 있는 기관의 지시가 있을 때까지 사고 지휘관 임무를 수행할 준비를 한다.

가능한 한 빨리 사고에 적절한 개인보호장비를 착용한 다음 START 알고리즘을 사용하여 처치 및 이송을 위해 분류할 의도로 피해자에게 접근한다. 초기에 피해자의 의학적 처치 없이 피해자를 즉시(immediate), 긴급(urgent), 지연(delayed), 기대(expectant)로 분류한다. 폭발 피해자는 구급대원과 구조대원의 지시나 질문을 듣지 못할 스 있다는 점을 기억한다. 다른 지원이 도착하면 지휘 및 통제 기능을 맡을 상급자가 도착할 때까지 사고 현장 지휘체계의 임무를 수행해도록 직원에게 지시한다.

References

1. Chason R, Wiggins O, Tan R. Dozens of cases, and 10 deaths. Inside Maryland's worst coronavirus outbreak. W*ashington Post*. April 5, 2020. Accessed October 31, 2021. https://www.washingtonpost.com/local/maryland -news/pleasant-view-coronavirus-outbreak-carroll -county/2020/04/04/4a4bb2c2-7520-11ea-87da-77a8 136c1a6d_story.html

2. Torrey J, Orr J, Florance J. Rapid deployment of national guard alternative healthcare facility with isolation unit capabilities in response to covid-19. *Mil Med*. 2021;186(1-2):258-264.

3. Weiden MD, Zeig-Owens R, Singh A, et al. Pre-COVID-19 lung function and other risk factors for severe COVID-19 in first responders. *ERJ Open Res*. 2021;7(1):00610-2020. doi: 10.1183/23120541.00610-2020

4. Turner CD, Lockey DJ, Rehn M. Pre-hospital management of mass casualty civilian shootings: a systematic literature review [published correction appears in *Crit Care*. 2017 Apr 13;21(1):94]. *Crit Care*. 2016;20(1):362. doi:10.1186/ s13054-016-1543-7

5. Jacobs LM, Wade DS, McSwain NE, et al. The Hartford Consensus: THREAT, a medical disaster preparedness concept. *J Am Coll Surg*. 2013;217(5):947-953. doi: 10.1016/j .jamcollsurg.2013.07.002

6. Hogan DE, Waeckerle JF, Dire DJ, et al. Emergency department impact of the Oklahoma City terrorist bombing. *Ann Emerg Med*. 1999;34:160-167.

7. Kennedy K, Aghababian R, Gans L, et al. Triage: techniques and applications in decision making. *Ann Emerg Med*. 1996;28(2):136-144.

8. Garner A, Lee A, Harrison K. Comparative analysis of multiple-casualty incident triage algorithms. *Ann Emerg Med*. 2001;38:541-548.

9. Lerner EB, Schwartz RB, Coule PL, et al. Mass casualty triage: an evaluation of the data and development of a proposed national guideline. *Disaster Med Public Health Preparedness*. 2008;2(suppl 1):S25-S34.

10. Thors L, Koch M, Wigenstam E, Koch B, Hägglund L, Bucht A. Comparison of skin decontamination efficacy of commercial decontamination products following exposure to VX on human skin. *Chem Biol Interact*. 2017;273: 82-89.

11. Taysse L, Daulon S, Delamanche S, Bellier B, Breton P. Skin decontamination of mustards and organophosphates: comparative efficiency of RSDL and fuller's earth in domestic swine. *Hum Exp Toxicol*. 2007;26(2):135-141.

12. U.S. Department of Health and Human Services. Medical Countermeasures Database. Chemical Hazards Emergency Medical Management website. Updated August 16, 2021. Accessed January 31, 2022. https://chemm.hhs.gov /medical_countermeasures.htm

13. Hurst G, ed. *Field Management of Chemical and Biological Casualties Handbook*. 5th ed. Borden Institute, Walter Reed Army Medical Center; 2016.

14. Kapur GB, Hutson HR, Davis MA, Rice PL. The United States twenty-year experience with bombing incidents: implications for terrorism preparedness and medical response. *J Trauma*. 2005;59:1436-1444.

15. Melnikova N, Orr MF, Wu J, Christensen B. Injuries from methamphetamine-related chemical incidents—five states, 2001–2012. *Morb Mortal Wkly Rep*. 2015;64(33):909-912.

16. Pierce B. How rare are large, multiple-fatality work-related incidents? *Accid Anal Prev*. 2016;96:88-100.

17. Edwards DS, Mcmenemy L, Stapley SA, Patel HD, Clasper JC. 40 years of terrorist bombings: a meta-analysis of the casualty and injury profile. *Injury*. 2016;47(3):646-652.

18. U.S. Bomb Data Center. *Explosives Incident Report (EIR)— 2019*. Redstone Arsenal, AL: U.S. Bomb Data Center; 2019. https://www.atf.gov/file/143481/download

19. Arnold J, Halpern P, Tsai M. Mass casualty terrorist bombings: a comparison of outcomes by bombing type. *Ann Emerg Med*. 2004;43:263-273.

20. DePalma RG, Burris DG, Champion HR, et al. Blast injuries. *N Engl J Med*. 2005;352(13):1335-1342.

21. Centers for Disease Control and Prevention. Explosions and blast injuries: a primer for clinicians. Updated May 9, 2003. Accessed January 31, 2022. https://www.cdc.gov /masstrauma/preparedness/primer.pdf

22. Wightman JM, Gladish JL. Explosions and blast injuries. *Ann Emerg Med*. 2001;37:664-678.

23. Armed Forces Radiobiology Research Institute (AFRRI). *Medical Management of Radiological Casualties*. AFRRI; 2003.

24. Plurad DS. Blast injury. *Mil Med*. 2011 Mar;176(3):276-282. doi: 10.7205/milmed-d-10-00147

25. Almogy G, Mintz Y, Zamir G, et al. Suicide bombing attacks: can external signs predict internal injuries? *Ann Surg*. 2006;243(4):541-546.

26. Garner MJ, Brett SJ. Mechanisms of injury by explosive devices. *Anesthesiol Clin*. 2007;25(1):147-160.

27. Avidan V, Hersch M, Armon Y, et al. Blast lung injury: clinical manifestations, treatment, and outcome. *Am J Surg*. 2005;190(6):927-931.

28. Frykberg ER, Tepas JJ, Alexander RH. The 1983 Beirut Airport terrorist bombing: injury patterns and implications for disaster management. *Am Surg*. 1989;55:134-141.

29. Katz E, Ofek B, Adler J, et al. Primary blast injury after a bomb explosion in a civilian bus. *Ann Surg*. 1989;209: 484-488.

30. Kluger Y, Nimrod A, Biderman P, et al. Case report: the quinary pattern of blast injury. *J Emerg Mgmt*. 2006;4(1): 51-55.

31. Sorkine P, Nimrod A, Biderman P, et al. The quinary (Vth) injury pattern of blast (Abstract). *J Trauma*. 2007;56(1):232.

32. Nelson TJ, Wall DB, Stedje-Larsen ET, et al. Predictors of mortality in close proximity blast injuries during Operation Iraqi Freedom. *J Am Coll Surg*. 2006;202(3):418-422.

33. Mallonee S, Shariat S, Stennies G, et al. Physical injuries and fatalities resulting from the Oklahoma City bombing. *JAMA*. 1996;276:382-387.

34. Arnold JL, Tsai MC, Halpern P, et al. Mass-casualty, terrorist bombings: epidemiological outcomes, resource utilization, and time course of emergency needs (Part I). *Prehosp Disaster Med*. 2003;18(3):220-234.

35. Halpern P, Tsai MC, Arnold JL, et al. Mass-casualty, terrorist bombings: implications for emergency department and hospital emergency response (Part II). *Prehosp Disaster Med*. 2003;18(3):235-241.

36. U.S. Bomb Data Center. *Explosive incidents 2007: 2007 USBDC explosives statistics*. U.S. Bomb Data Center; 2007.

37. Caseby NG, Porter MF. Blast injury to the lungs: clinical presentation, management and course. *Injury*. 1976;8:1-12. doi: 10.1016/0020-1383(76)90002-4

38. Leibovici D, Gofrit ON, Shapira SC. Eardrum perforation in explosion survivors: is it a marker of pulmonary blast injury? *Ann Emerg Med*. 1999;34:168-172.

39. Coppel DL. Blast injuries of the lungs. *Br J Surg*. 1976;63: 735-737.

40. Cohn SM. Pulmonary contusion: review of the clinical entity. *J Trauma*. 1997;42:973-979.

41. Peleg K, Limor A, Stein M, et al. Gunshot and explosion injuries: characteristics, outcomes, and implications for care of terror-related injuries in Israel. *Ann Surg*. 2004;239(3):311-318. doi: 10.1097/01.sla.0000114012 .84732.be

42. Mansour HA, Bitar E, Fares Y, Makdessi AA, et al. The Beirut Port explosion: injury trends from a mass survey of emergency admissions. *Lancet*. 2021;398:21-22.

43. Tappan J. Magnesium and thermite poisoning. Medscape. Updated August 22, 2019. Accessed January 31, 2022. http://emedicine.medscape.com/article/833495-overview

44. Irizarry L. White phosphorus exposure. Medscape. Updated January 6, 2022. Accessed January 31, 2022. http://emedicine.medscape.com/article/833585-overview

45. Sidell FR, Takafuji ET, Franz DR, eds. *Medical Aspects of Chemical and Biological Warfare, TMM Series. Part 1: Warfare, Weaponry and the Casualty*. Office of the Surgeon General, TMM Publications; 1997.

46. Walter FG, ed. *Advanced HAZMAT Life Support*. 2nd ed. Arizona Board of Regents; 2000.

47. U.S. Army, Medical Research Institute of Chemical Defense. *Medical Management of Chemical Casualties Handbook*. U.S. Army Research Institute; 2000.

48. Greenfield RA, Brown BR, Hutchins JB, et al. Microbiological, biological and chemical weapons of warfare and terrorism. *Am J Med Sci*. 2002;323(6):326-340.

49. Okumura T, Takasu N, Ishimatsu S, et al. Report on 640 victims of the Tokyo subway sarin attack. *Ann Emerg Med*. 1996;28(2):129-135.

50. Centers for Disease Control and Prevention. Emergency Preparedness and Response—Specific Hazards: Facts about Cyanide. Last reviewed April 4, 2018. Accessed March 23, 2022. https://emergency.cdc.gov/agent/cyanide/basics/facts .asp#:~:text=Cyanide%20sometimes%20is%20 described%20as,CK%20(for%20cyanogen%20chloride)

51. Sellstrom A, Cairns S, Barbeschi M. Report of United Nations Mission to Investigate Allegations of the Use of Chemical Weapons in the Syrian Arab Republic on the Alleged Use of Chemical Weapons in the Ghouta Area of Damascus on 21 August 2013. United Nations. Published September 16, 2013. Accessed January 31, 2022. https://digitallibrary. un.org/record/756814?ln=en

52. Reddy SD, Reddy DS. Midazolam as an anticonvulsant antidote for organophosphate intoxication—a pharmacotherapeutic appraisal. *Epilepsia*. 2015;56(6):813-821.

53. Rotenberg JS, Newmark J. Nerve-agent attacks on children: diagnosis and management. *Pediatrics*. 2003;112: 648-658.

54. McDonough JH, Capacio BR, Shih TM. Treatment of nerve-agent-induced status epilepticus in the nonhuman primate. In: *U.S. Army Medical Defense—Bioscience Review, June 2–7*. U.S. Army Medical Research Institute; 2002.

55. U.S. Department of Health and Human Services. CHEMPACK: Chemical Hazards Emergency Medical Management. Updated August 16, 2021. Accessed October 31, 2021. https://chemm.hhs.gov/chempack.htm

56. United Nations, Security Council. Organization for the Prohibition of Chemical Weapons-United Nations Joint Investigative Mechanism. Fourth report of the Organization for the Prohibition of Chemical Weapons-United Nations Joint Investigative Mechanism. Published October 21, 2016. Accessed January 31, 2022. http://undocs .org/S/2016/888

57. Tuorinsky SD. *Textbooks of Military Medicine: Medical Aspects of Chemical Warfare*. Borden Institute, Walter Reed Army Medical Center; 2008.

58. Lipsitch M. Why Do Exceptionally Dangerous Gain-of-Function Experiments in Influenza? *Methods Mol Biol*. 2018;1836:589-608. doi: 10.1007/978-1-4939-8678-1_29

59. Ingelsby TV, Henderson DA, Bartlett JG, et al. Anthrax as a biological weapon: medical and public health management. *JAMA*. 1999;281(18):1735-1745.

60. Keim M, Kaufmann AF. Principles for emergency response to bioterrorism. *Ann Emerg Med*. 1999;34(2):177-182.

61. U.S. Congress, Office of Technology Assessment. Proliferation of weapons of mass destruction, Pub. No. OTA-ISC-559. U.S. Government Printing Office; 1993.

62. Inglesby TV, O'Toole T, Henderson DA, et al. Anthrax as a biological weapon, 2002: updated recommendations for management. *JAMA*. 2002;287:2236-2252.

63. Kman NE, Nelson RN. Infectious agents of bioterrorism: a review for emergency physicians. *Emerg Med Clin North Am*. 2008;26:517-547.

64. Stern EJ, Uhde KB, Shadomy SV, Messonnier N. Conference report on public health and clinical guidelines for anthrax. *Emerging Infect Dis*. 2008;14(4). https://wwwnc -origin.cdc.gov/eid/article/14/4/07-0969-f1

65. World Health Organization. Health Aspects of Chemical and Biological Weapons. World Health Organization; 1970.

66. Inglesby TV, Dennis DT, Henderson DA. Plague as a biological weapon: medical and public health management. *JAMA*. 2000;283(17):2281-2290.

67. Henderson DA, Inglesby TV, Bartlett JG. Smallpox as a biological weapon: medical and public health management. *JAMA*. 1999;281(22):2127-2137.

68. Centers for Disease Control and Prevention. *Smallpox Response Plan and Guidelines*. Version 3.0, Guide C, Part 1. Centers for Disease Control and Prevention; 2008:1-13.

69. Centers for Disease Control and Prevention. *Smallpox Response Plan and Guidelines*. Version 3.0, Guide F. Centers for Disease Control and Prevention; 2003:1-10.

70. Basler CF. Molecular pathogenesis of viral hemorrhagic fever. *Semin Immunopathol*. 2017;39(5):551-561.

71. Cenciarelli O, Gabbarini V, Pietropaoli S, et al. Viral bioterrorism: learning the lesson of Ebola virus in West Africa 2013–2015. *Virus Res*. 2015;210:318-326.

72. Feldmann H, Geisbert TW. Ebola haemorrhagic fever. *Lancet*. 2011;377:849-862.

73. Coltart CE, Lindsey B, Ghinai I, Johnson AM, Heymann DL. The Ebola outbreak, 2013–2016: old lessons for new epidemics. *Philos Trans R Soc Lond B Biol Sci*. 2017;372(1721):20160297. doi: 10.1098/rstb.2016.0297

74. Duraffour S, Malvy D, Sissoko D. How to treat Ebola virus infections? A lesson from the field. *Curr Opin Virol*. 2017;24:9-15.

75. Centers for Disease Control and Prevention, National Center for Emerging and Zoonotic Infectious Diseases, Division of Healthcare Quality Promotion. Guidance on personal protective equipment (PPE) to be used by healthcare workers during management of patients with confirmed Ebola or persons under investigation (PUIs) for Ebola who are clinically unstable or have bleeding, vomiting, or diarrhea in U.S. hospitals, including procedures for donning and doffing PPE. Reviewed August 30, 2018. Accessed January 31, 2022. https://www.cdc.gov/vhf /ebola/healthcare-us/ppe/guidance.html

76. Lowe JJ, Jelden KC, Schenarts PJ, et al. Considerations for safe EMS transport of patients infected with Ebola virus. *Prehosp Emerg Care*. 2015;19(2):179-183.

77. Isakov A, Miles W, Gibbs S, Lowe J, Jamison A, Swansiger R. Transport and management of patients with confirmed or suspected Ebola virus disease. *Ann Emerg Med*. 2015;66(3):297-305.

78. Franz DR, Jahrling PB, Friedlander AM, et al. Clinical recognition and management of patients exposed to biological warfare agents. *JAMA*. 1997;278(5):399-411.

79. Arnon SS, Schechter R, Inglesby TV, et al. Botulinum toxin as a biological weapon: medical and public health management. *JAMA*. 2001;285:1059-1070.

80. Hogan DE, Kellison T. Nuclear terrorism. *Am J Med Sci*. 2002;323(6):341-349.

81. World Health Organization, International Atomic Energy Agency, United Nations Development Programme. Chernobyl: the true scale of the accident. Published September 5, 2005. Accessed January 31, 2022. https://www.who .int/news/item/05-09-2005-chernobyl-the-true-scale-of -the-accident

82. Flynn DF, Goans RE. Nuclear terrorism: triage and medical management of radiation and combined-injury casualties. *Surg Clin North Am*. 2006;86(3):601-636.

Suggested Reading

Centers for Disease Control. Blast injuries: fact sheet for professionals. http://www.emergency.cdc.gov/blastinjuries

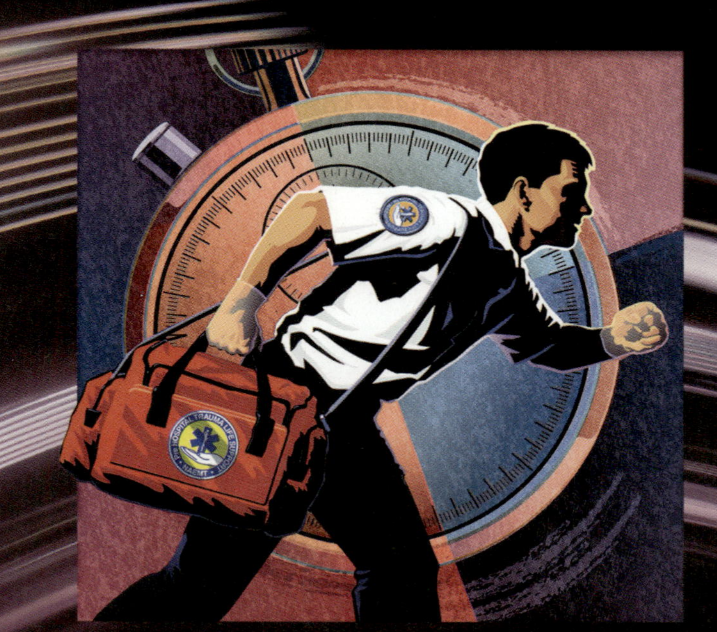

특별한 고려 사항

CHAPTER 19 환경 외상 I: 더위와 추위

CHAPTER 20 환경 외상 II: 낙뢰 , 익사 , 잠수 및 고도

CHAPTER 21 야생 외상 처치

CHAPTER 22 민간 전술적 응급의료지원 (TEMS)

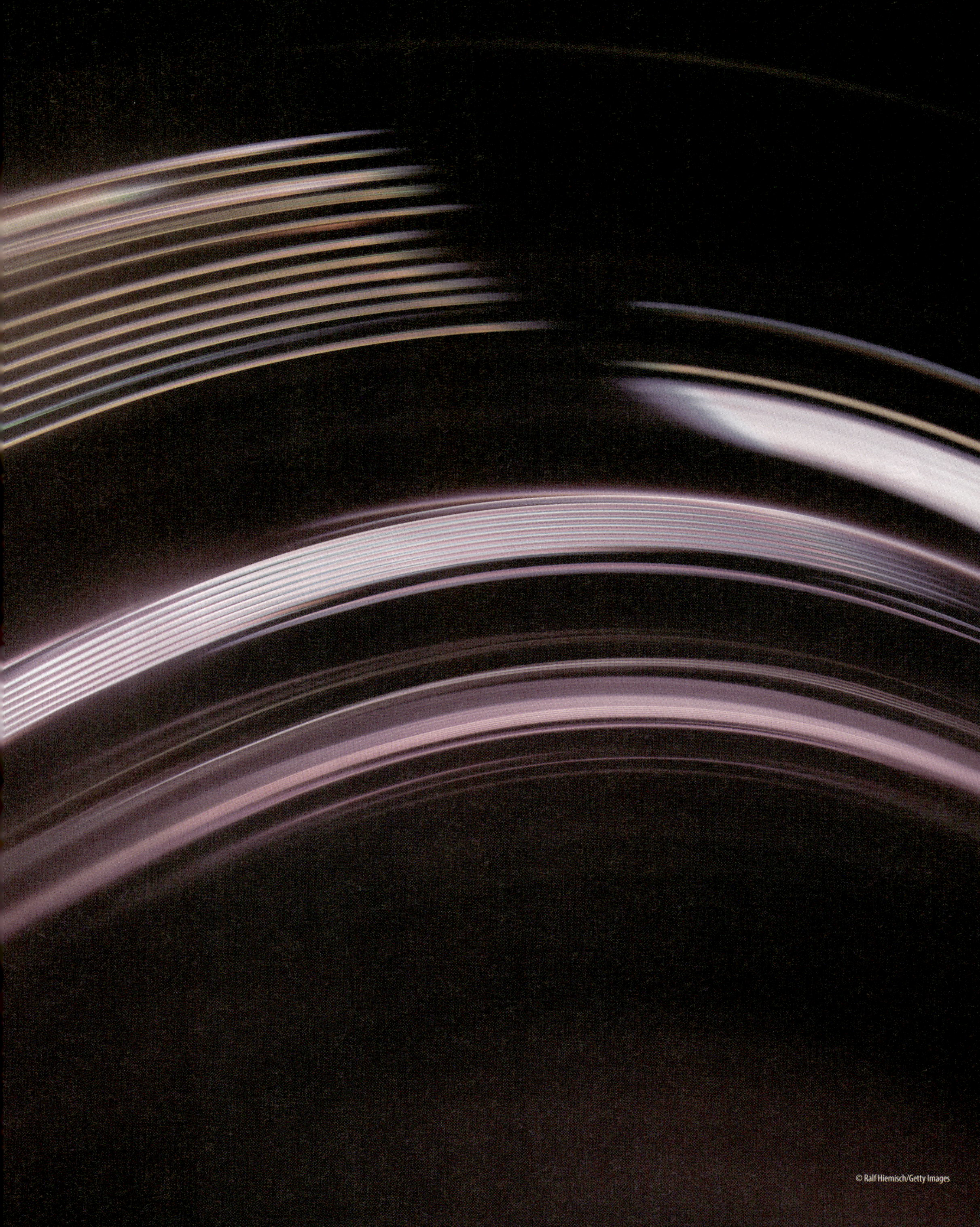

© Ralf Hiemisch/Getty Images

환경 외상 I: 더위와 추위

Lead Editors
Seth Hawkins, MD
R. Bryan Simon, RN

학습 목표   이 장의 학습을 완료하면 다음과 같은 내용을 수행할 수 있다.

- 열사병이 생명을 위협하는 응급 상황으로 간주하는 이유를 설명할 수 있다.
- 열사병과 운동 관련 저나트륨혈증의 유사점과 차이점을 구분할 수 있다.
- 열사병에 대한 가장 효과적이고 신속한 냉각 방법 두 가지를 설명할 수 있다.
- 병원 전 처치 제공자가 열사병에 걸릴 위험에 처하게 하는 다섯 가지 요인을 나열할 수 있다.
- 따뜻하거나 추운 환경에서 탈수를 예방하기 위한 수분 공급 지침에 관해 설명할 수 있다.
- 경증 저체온과 중증 저체온 처치의 차이점을 설명할 수 있다.
- 경증, 중등도, 중증 동상의 징후를 나열하고 동상 진행을 예방하는 방법에 관해 설명할 수 있다.
- 심정지 상태의 저체온증 환자를 적극적으로 따뜻하게 해야 하는 이유를 설명할 수 있다.

시나리오

기온이 38.9℃에 이르는 무더운 여름 오후이다. 지난 30일 동안 매일 기온이 37.8℃를 넘는 매우 습한 날씨였다. 주변 환경의 높은 온도로 인해 EMS 제공자들이 수많은 환자를 응급실로 이송해야 하는 열 관련 질환이 많이 발생했다.

17시에 당신과 동료는 차 안에서 의식을 잃은 남성 환자가 있다는 신고를 받고 출동한다. 당신이 현장에 도착했을 때 백화점 야외 주차장에 주차된 차량에서 의식이 없고 손상이 없는 76세 남성을 발견했다. 환자의 기도, 호흡, 순환(ABC) 및 의식 수준을 신속하게 평가한 결과 환자가 말을 할 수 있지만, 비논리적이고 비이성적인 말을 하고 있다는 것을 알 수 있었다.

- 이 환자의 의식 저하의 잠재적 원인은 무엇인가?
- 열 관련 진단을 뒷받침하는 특징적인 징후는 무엇인가?
- 현장에서 응급실로 이송하는 동안 이 환자를 어떻게 처치를 시행해야 하는가?

개요

이 장에서는 고온 및 저온 노출을 인식하고 처치하는 데 중점을 둔다. 미국에서 모든 환경 손상으로 인한 이환율과 사망률이 가장 높은 것은 열 손상으로 인해 발생한다.

극심한 더위와 추위는 여름과 겨울 동안 많은 사람에게 영향을 미칠 수 있는 손상과 잠재적으로 사망이라는 공통된 결과를 초래한다. 외상을 입은 환자가 저체온증(중심체온이 35℃ 미만) 또는 열 관련 질환(고체온증)으로 병원에 내원하여 중심체온이(38.5℃) 이상인 경우 사망률이 많이 증가한다는 사실을 아는 것이 매우 중요하다. 특히 고온과 저온 모두에 취약한 사람은 아주 어린 어린이, 노인, 도시 지역에 거주하는 빈곤층, 특정 약물을 복용하는 사람, 야외에서 일하는 직업군(예: 농업 종사자), 만성질환자, 알코올 중독 또는 기타 중독이 있는 사람이다. 열 관련 또는 추위 관련 응급상황이 발생할 상대적 위험은 야생 환경에서 더 높을 수 있지만, 미국에서 열 및 추위와 관련된 손상의 대부분의 EMS 출동은 도시 환경에서 발생한다. 따라서 모든 EMS 제공자는 이러한 내용을 잘 알고 있어야 한다(**Box 19-1**). 또한 환경이 극한으로 치닫는 기간 야생 오지에서 취미활동 및 고위험 모험 활동에 관한 관심이 확대됨에 따라 야생 지역에서 더 많은 사람이 열 관련 및 추위 관련 손상과 사망의 위험에 노출된다.

역학

열 관련 질환

미국에서 매년 약 618명이 불볕더위와 관련된 질환으로 사망한다. 2020년은 2016년과 같이 1880년 이후 기록된 역사상 가장 더운 해였고, 그 이전 7년은 역대 가장 더운 7년이었으며 측정할 수 있고 결과적으로 지구 온난화를 초래한 기후 변화 추세를 이어가고 있다. 허리케인, 번개, 토네이도, 홍수, 지진을 모두 합친 것보다 더 많은 사망

Box 19-1　병원 전과 병원 밖

이 문서는 병원 전 처치에 초점을 맞추고 있지만, 병원 전이라는 용어가 모든 상황에서 정확한 것은 아니다. 연구에 따르면 야생 지대 및 기타 외딴 야외 환경에서 처치를 받는 대부분의 사람은 일반적으로 병원에 즉시 접근할 수 없으므로 병원으로 이송되지 않는 것으로 나타났다. 따라서 일부 조직에서는 이러한 환경에서 제공되는 의료서비스를 병원 밖 의료서비스라고 한다.

자가 열 스트레스로 인해 발생하고 있다. 또한 주기적인 계절적 불볕더위(기온이 32.2℃ 이상인 날씨가 3일 이상 연속되는 경우)가 발생하면 이환율과 사망률이 매우 높아질 수 있다. 미국 질병통제예방센터(CDC)는 폭염 노출로 인해 총 10,527명의 사망자(2004~2018년)가 발생했다고 보고했다(연평균 702명).

저온 관련 질환

온화하거나 추운 날씨 조건으로 인해 미국에서 매년 평균 774명이 사망한다. 이 사망자 중 거의 절반이 65세 이상에서 발생했다. 나이를 고려하면 저체온증으로 인한 사망은 여성보다 남성에서 약 2.5배 더 자주 발생했다. 저체온증으로 인한 사망은 나이가 들면서 점차 증가하며 15세 이후에는 남성이 여성보다 3배 더 높다. 우발적 저체온증의 주요 요인으로는 도시 빈곤, 사회경제적 조건, 알코올 섭취, 영양실조, 나이(영아, 노인) 등이 있다.

저체온증은 일반적으로 서늘하거나 추운 날씨와 관련이 있지만, 일반적으로 춥다고 생각하지 않지만, 체온이 35.6℃ 이하로 떨어지는 조건에서도 발생할 수 있다. 예를 들어, 노인과 영아의 경우 여름철 집에서 에어컨 온도를 적응 기전에 비해 너무 낮게 켜놓으면 저체온증에 걸릴 수 있다. 수영이나 서핑을 즐기는 사람들은 여름철에 체온보다 낮은 물에 노출되면 저체온증에 걸릴 수 있으며 영하로 떨어지지는 않지만, 낮은 기온과 바람이 강하게 불고 비가 내리는 경우 저체온증을 발생시킬 수 있는 조건을 초래할 수 있다. 따라서 저체온증은 단순히 추운 날씨와 관련된 질병이 아니라는 점을 인식하는 것이 중요하다.

해부학

피부

신체의 가장 큰 기관인 피부는 외부 환경과 접하고 보호막 역할을 한다. 피부는 미생물의 침입을 방지하고 체액 균형을 유지하며 체온을 조절하는 역할을 한다. 피부는 표피, 진피, 피부밑조직의 세 가지 조직층으로 구성되어 있다(**그림 19-1**). 가장 바깥층인 표피는 혈관이 없는 상피 세포로만 구성되어 있다. 표피 아래에는 더 두꺼운 진피가 있다. 진피는 표피보다 20~30배 더 두껍고 혈관, 신경, 피지선 및 땀샘을 포함하는 결합조직으로 이루어져 있다. 가장 안쪽 층인 피부밑조직은 지방 조직뿐만 아니라 탄성 및 섬유 조직의 조합이다. 이 층

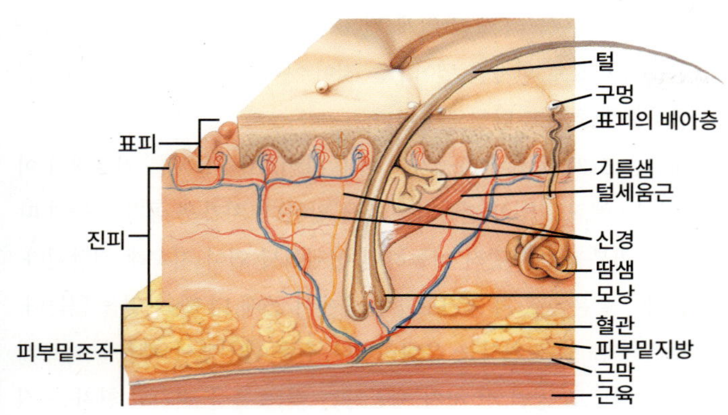

그림 19-1 피부는 표피, 진피, 피부밑조직의 세 가지 조직층과 관련 근육으로 구성되어 있다. 일부 층에는 땀샘, 모낭, 혈관 및 신경과 같은 구조가 포함되어 있다. 이러한 모든 구조는 체온 유지, 체온 손실 및 상승과 연관되어 있다.
© Jones & Bartlett Learning

아래에는 골격근이 있다. 피부, 신경, 혈관 및 기타 기본 해부학적 구조는 체온을 조절하는 데 중요한 역할을 한다.

생리학

체온 조절 및 체온 균형

인간은 항온 동물 또는 온혈 동물로 간주한다. 항온 동물의 주요 특징은 다양한 환경 온도와 관계없이 자신의 내부 체온을 환경 온도보다 높은 수준으로 일정하게 조절할 수 있다는 것이다.

인체는 본질적으로 따뜻한 내부 핵심과 외피로 나뉜다. 뇌와 가슴 및 복부 장기는 내부 핵심에 포함되며 피부와 피하층은 외피를 구성한다. 외피는 인체의 중심체온을 조절하는 데 중요한 역할을 한다. 중심체온은 열 생산과 열 발산 기전의 균형을 통해 조절된다. 피부 표면 온도와 외피의 두께는 환경 온도에 따라 달라진다. 외피는 혈액이 피부에서 또는 피부로 이동하기 때문에 온도가 낮을수록 두꺼워지고 온도가 높을수록 얇아진다. 혈관 수축으로 유도되는 이 외피 또는 조직 단열은 가벼운 비즈니스 정장을 입는 것과 거의 같은 수준의 보호 기능을 제공하는 것으로 추정된다.

신진대사에 의한 열 생산은 활동 수준에 따라 달라진다. 외부 온도 변화와 관계없이 신체는 일반적으로 37°C±0.6°C의 온도에서 약 0.6°C의 좁은 온도 범위 내에서 유지된다. 정상 체온은 뇌의 시상하부에서 조절되는 항상성 기전에 의해 좁은 범위에서 유지된다. 정상적인 체온은 뇌의 시상하부에서 조절되는 항상성 기전에 의해 좁은 범위에서 유지된다. 시상하부는 체온조절 중추로 알려져 있으며 체온의 신경학적 및 호르몬 조절을 제어하는 신체의 체온 조절기 역할을 한다. 뇌에 외상을 입으면 시상하부가 손상되어 체온 조절에 불균형이 생길 수 있다.

인간은 체온을 조절하는 행동 조절과 생리적 체온 조절이라는 두 가지 시스템을 가지고 있다. 행동 조절은 개인의 열 감각과 편안함에 의해 좌우되며 열로 인한 불편함을 줄이기 위한 의도적인 노력(예: 옷을 더 입거나 벗고 추운 환경에서 피난처를 찾는 것)이 특징이다. 행동 조절에서 열 정보가 뇌로 전달되는 감각 피드백의 처리는 잘 알려지지 않지만 열 감각과 편안함의 피드백은 환경 온도 변화에 대한 생리적 반응보다 더 빠르게 반응한다.

열 생산 및 열 균형

기초대사율은 주로 신진대사의 부산물로 생성되는 열로 주로 중요한 큰 기관과 골격근 수축에서 발생한다. 생성된 열은 순환계의 혈액을 통해 전신으로 전달된다. 이 장의 뒷부분에서 설명하는 것처럼 열전달 및 심폐 시스템에 의한 체내 열 발산은 열 질환의 평가 및 처치에 중요하다.

떨림은 근육의 긴장을 증가시켜 근육 수축과 이완을 반복함으로써 신진대사율을 증가시키며 이는 신체의 열 생성 기전 중 가장 강력한 것이다. 중심체온이 37°C일 때 피부 냉각으로 인해 떨림이 발생할 수 있지만, 일반적으로 떨림은 중심체온이 34.4~36.1°C로 떨어질 때 시작되어 중심체온이 30°C가 될 때까지 계속된다. 최대로 떨면 열 생산량이 휴식 상태의 5~6배로 증가한다.

열 생산과 열 손실 반응을 제어하는 생리학적 체온 조절 시스템은 잘 설명되어 있다. 체온 조절의 두 가지 원칙은 신체가 중심체온을 조절하는 방식을 이해하는 데 중요한 역할을 한다. 열 경사도는 두 물체 사이의 온도 차이(고온 대 저온)이다. 열평형은 접촉하고 있는 두 물체가 같은 온도 상태가 되는 것이다. 물체가 같은 온도 차이를 말한다. 열평형은 서로 접촉하는 두 물체가 같은 온도에 있는 상태로 따뜻한 물체에서 차가운 물체로 열이 전달되어 물체가 같은 온도가 될 때까지 이루어진다.

체온이 상승하면 정상적인 생리학적 반응은 피부 혈류를 증가시키고 땀을 흘리기 시작하는 것이다. 대부분의 체온은 전도, 대류, 복사 및 증발로 피부 표면에서 환경으로 전달된다. 열은 높은 온도에서 낮은 온도로 전달되기 때문에 신체는 더운 날씨에는 복사와 전도를 통해 인체가 열을 얻을 수 있다.

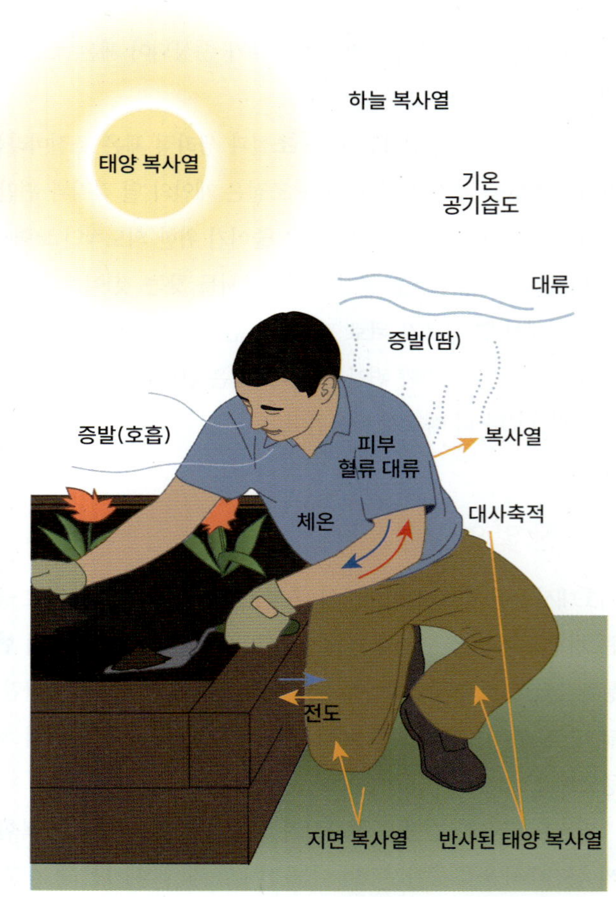

그림 19-2 인간이 환경과 열에너지를 교환하는 방법
© National Association of Emergency Medical Technicians (NAEMT)

체온을 유지하고 발산하는 방법은 병원 전 처치 제공자에게 중요한 개념이다. 고체온증 또는 저체온증 환자를 효과적으로 처치하려면 열과 냉기가 어떻게 신체로 전달되고 신체에서 어떻게 방출되는지 이해해야 한다(**그림 19-2**). 열과 냉기가 신체에서 전달되는 방법은 다음과 같다.

- 복사는 전자기 에너지의 형태로 열을 잃거나 얻는 것으로 따뜻한 물체에서 차가운 물체로 에너지가 전달되는 것을 말한다. 열 질환 환자는 태양으로부터 직접 추가적인 체온을 얻을 수 있다. 복사열 원은 환자를 평가하고 처치할 때 환자를 차갑게 하거나 따뜻하게 하기 위한 처치에 영향을 미치므로 병원 전 처치 제공자는 복사열 원을 이해하고 관리해야 한다.

- 전도는 넘어진 후 차가운 잔디밭에 누워 있는 환자와 같이 서로 직접 접촉하는 두 물체 사이에 열이 전달되는 것을 말한다. 환자는 일반적으로 차가운 공기에 노출되었을 때보다 차가운 바닥에 누워

있을 때 체온을 더 빨리 잃게 된다. 따라서 병원 전 처치 제공자는 단순히 담요로 환자를 덮어주는 것이 아니라 차가운 지면으로부터 환자를 보호하고 단열해야 한다.

- 대류는 고체 물체에서 공기나 물과 같이 고체 물체를 가로질러 이동하는 매질로 열이 전달되는 것을 말한다. 차가운 공기가 물이 따뜻한 피부를 가로질러 이동하면 신체에서 열이 지속해 전달된다. 신체는 같은 온도의 공기보다 물속에서 25배 더 빨리 열을 잃는다. 젖은 옷을 입은 환자는 온화하거나 추운 환경에서 체온을 빠르게 잃게 되므로 병원 전 처치 제공자는 젖은 옷을 벗기고 환자를 건조하게 유지하여 체온을 유지해야 한다. 병원 전 처치 제공자는 열 관련 질환 환자를 효과적으로 처치하기 위해 환자의 피부를 적시고 부채질하여 체온을 빠르게 발산하는 대류 열 손실 원리를 이용한다.

- 땀이 액체에서 증기로 증발하는 것은 상대 습도나 공기 중의 수분에 따라 신체에서 열 손실을 일으키는 매우 효과적인 방법이다. 수분과 함께 내쉬는 호흡, 피부, 점막에서 발생하는 열 손실을 모두 불감 상실이라고 하며 증발로 인해 발생한다. 이 불감 상실은 일반적으로 기초 열 생산량의 약 10%이지만, 체온이 상승하면 이 과정이 더 활발해져(감각적 손실) 땀이 생성된다. 증발로 인한 열 손실은 사막과 같이 서늘하고 건조하며 바람이 많이 부는 환경에서 증가한다. 대류와 증발은 중심체온을 조절하기 위해 신체에 의해 조절되기 때문에 다른 열전달 방법보다 더 중요하다.

체온이 정상 체온 범위(37℃±0.6℃)를 벗어나 상승(고체온증)하거나 하락(저체온증)하는 것은 다양한 내부 및 외부 원인으로 인해 발생할 수 있으며 합병증 없이 정상 체온으로 회복될 수 있다. 고체온증은 주로 다음과 같은 세 가지 방법의 하나로 발생한다.

- 지속적인 운동에 대한 정상적인 반응으로 생성된 열이 중심체온을 상승시키고 열 발산 반응(예: 발한, 피부로의 혈류 증가)을 위한 자극할 때

- 열 생산량과 환경으로부터 얻은 열의 합이 신체의 열 발산 능력보다 큰 경우

- 발열로 인한 경우

앞의 두 가지 방법과 달리 발열은 일반적으로 뇌의 온도 조절 설정점(체온 설정)의 변화로 인해 염증에 반응하여 발생하며 신체는 체온을 더 높게(37.8℃~41.1℃) 상승시킴으로써 이에 대응한다. 새로운 체온 조절 설정점 온도에 도달하기 위해 일시적으로 열 생산이 증가하여 침입하는 감염균에 덜 우호적인 환경을 만들려고 시도한다.

항상성

이러한 해부학적 구조와 생리학적 시스템은 온도 변화에 노출되었을 때 신체가 적절하게 기능할 수 있도록 상호 작용하도록 설계되었다. 신체는 말초 및 내부 영역에서 체온 조절 중추 및 뇌의 다른 영역으로 신경학적 피드백이 지속해 전달되고 그에 따른 반응이 나타난다. 이러한 모든 시스템은 상호 작용하여 신체에서 항상성이라고 하는 일정하고 안정적인 내부 상태를 유지한다. 그러나 때때로 항상성이 유지되지 않을 수도 있다. 예를 들어, 과도한 체온을 낮추기 위해 심혈관계 및 체온 조절 중추에서 불균형이 발생할 수 있으며 그 결과 땀을 통해 체액이 과도하게 손실되어 급성 탈수를 유발하고 열 질환의 증상과 징후를 유발할 수 있다.

열 질환의 위험 요인

인간을 대상으로 한 수많은 연구에서 더운 환경에 대한 내성에는 개인차가 큰 것으로 나타났다. 이러한 차이는 신체적 특성과 열 관련 질환 위험 증가와 관련된 의학적 상태로 부분적으로 설명할 수 있다 (**Box 19-2**). 열 생산이 신체의 열 발산 능력을 초과하는 모든 상황에서는 열 손상으로 이어질 수 있다는 점을 인식하는 것이 중요하다.

열 관련 질환의 주요 위험 요인으로는 알코올 섭취, 약물 복용, 탈수, 높은 체질량 지수, 비만, 부적절한 식이, 부적절한 복장, 낮은 체력, 수면 부족, 고령, 심혈관 질환, 피부 손상, 이전 열 관련 질환의 병력, 겸상적혈구 형질, 낭포성 섬유증, 바이러스 질환, 가장 더운 시간대의 운동이 있다. 일시적인 조건에는 서늘한 기후에 출발하여 도착 시 더운 기후에 적응하지 못한 채 여행하는 사람들에게 영향을 미치는 질환이 포함된다. 열 관련 질환의 위험에 노출되는 다른 일시적 요인으로는 열, 구토, 설사를 유발하는 감기 및 기타 질환과 식이 및 수분 섭취 부족을 포함한 일반적인 질병이 있다. 군인이나 소방관의 경우 누적 노출도 위험 요인으로 알려져 있으며 완화되지 않는 한 추가 노출 일수가 늘어날수록 위험이 증가한다.

만성 질환으로 간주하는 요인으로는 체력 수준, 신체 크기, 나이, 건강 상태, 약물 사용 등이 있으며 이러한 요인은 열 질환에 걸릴 위험이 더 크다.

비만, 체력 및 체질량 지수

유전적 요인으로 인한 비만과 낮은 체력 수준 또는 일상적인 신체 활동이 불충분한 좌식 생활 방식은 열 노출에 대한 내성을 감소시킨다. 체력은 체온 조절을 유지하는 데 필요한 심박출량을 유지할 수 있는 심혈관 예비력을 제공하며 신체 활동에 대한 지속적인 내성과 고열에 대한 땀 분비 증가를 통해 더 빨리 적응할 수 있게 해준다. 과체중인 사람은 열에 노출되면 피부 혈관이 확장되고 발한이 증가하는 정상적인 반응을 보인다. 하지만 체력 저하, 열 적응력 부족, 단열성 증가, 땀샘 분포 변화 등이 복합적으로 작용하면 움직임에 필요한 에너지 비용이 증가하고 열 질환에 걸릴 위험이 커진다.

나이

체온 조절 능력과 더위에 대한 내성은 나이가 들수록 감소하며, 특히 65세 이상의 경우 더욱 그렇다. 이러한 사람들은 저체중을 유지하고

Box 19-2 열 질환 위험 요인

내부 열 생산 증가시키는 요소

- 신체 활동
- 감염에 대한 반응(발열)
- 갑상샘항진증
- 불안 및 떨림 상태(파킨슨, 정신병, 조증, 약물 금단-아편 및 알코올)
- 약물 과다 복용(코카인, 카페인, LSD, 염산펜시클리딘, 메스암페타민, 엑스터시)

열 방출을 방해하는 요소

- 높은 주변 온도
- 높은 습도
- 비만(단열 효과, 발산 효율 저하)
- 혈관 확장 장애
- 당뇨병
- 알코올 중독
- 약물 복용: 이뇨제, 진정제, 베타 차단제, 항히스타민제, 페노티아진, 항우울제
- 땀 배출 능력 장애(낭성섬유증, 피부 질환, 화상 치유)
- 무겁거나 꽉 끼는 옷

열 스트레스 탈수에 대한 신체 반응을 저해하는 요소

- 열사병 이전 사건
- 최근 위장관 또는 호흡기 감염
- 저칼륨혈증
- 심혈관 질환

Abbreviations: GI, gastrointestinal; LSD, lysergic acid diethylamide.

Data from Hawkins SC, Simon RB, Beissinger JP, Simon D. Vertical Aid: Essential Wilderness Medicine for Climbers, Trekkers, and Mountaineers. The Countryman Press; 2017; Hall B, Hall J. Sauer's Manual of Skin Diseases. 10th ed. Lippincott Williams & Wilkins; 2010; Krakowski A, Goldenberg A. Exposure to radiation from the sun. In: Auerbach PS, ed. Auerbach's Wilderness Medicine. 7th ed. Mosby Elsevier; 2017; and Lipman GS, Gaudio FFG, Eifling KP, Ellis MA, Otten EM, Grissom CK. Wilderness Medical Society practice guidelines for the prevention and treatment of heat-related illness: 2019 update. Wilderness Environ Med. 2019;30(4):S33-S46.

체력 수준을 향상함으로써 더위에 대한 내성을 향상할 수 있다.

영유아는 성인보다 체표면적이 전체 체중보다 차지하는 비율이 훨씬 커서 열 관련 질환에 걸릴 위험이 훨씬 더 크므로 특별한 주의가 필요하다. 또한 영유아는 체온 조절 능력이 미숙하여 고온에 노출되었을 때 체온을 적절하게 유지할 수 없다.

건강 상태

당뇨병, 갑상샘 질환, 신장 질환과 같은 기저 질환이 있는 경우 열 과민증 및 열 질환의 위험이 높아질 수 있다. 피부 혈류와 순환 요구를 증가시키는 심혈관 질환 및 순환계 문제는 열 노출로 악화한다. 이러한 극한의 환경 조건에서 심장 질환과 폐 질환은 높은 주변 온도로 인해 악화하는 증상과 징후를 나타낼 수 있다. 개인에게 나타나는 경미한 형태의 열 질환으로는 땀구멍이 막히거나 염증이 생겨 열에 대한 내성이 감소하는 것으로 알려진 적색땀띠가 있다.

약물

특정 처방한 약 또는 일반의약품을 복용하면 열 질환에 걸릴 위험이 커질 수 있다(**Box 19-2**). 특정 약물은 대사성 열 생산을 증가시키고 체온 저하와 갈증을 억제하며 심장 예비력을 감소시키고 신장 전해질 및 체액 균형을 변화시킬 수 있다. 진정제 및 마약류 약물은 정신 상태에 영향을 미치고 논리적 추론과 판단에 영향을 미쳐 열에 노출되었을 때 의사 결정 능력을 억제할 수 있다.

탈수

총체액량(TBW)은 인체에서 가장 큰 구성 요소로 체중의 50~75%를 차지한다. 예를 들어 75kg의 남성은 체중의 60%에 해당하는 약 45L의 수분을 함유하고 있다. 수분 과다 섭취(수분 과잉) 또는 수분 부족으로 인한 정상적인 체내 수분 균형(수분 공급)의 과도한 변화는 항상성을 변화시켜 특정 징상과 징후를 유발한다. 탈수는 저장성 체액 손실로 인한 저장성 혈량저하증으로 정의되며 더위와 추위에 노출될 때 심각한 결과를 초래할 수 있으며 설사, 구토, 발열 등의 위험한 부작용으로 나타나기도 한다.

탈수는 노인 환자에서 볼 수 있듯이 여러 날에 걸쳐 발생하는 열 질환의 경우나 운동선수, 군인, 소방관처럼 땀을 많이 흘리는 신체 활동 중에 흔히 발견되는 증상이다. 노인의 경우 탈수 현상은 수분 섭취량이 적어서 발생하는 경우가 많지만, 운동선수, 군인, 소방관은 일상 활동 중에 수분 섭취량이 충분하지 않아 고갈된 총체액량을 보충하지 못한다. 어린이(15세 이하)와 65세 이상의 노인은 특히 탈수에 취약하다.

체수분은 땀, 눈물, 소변, 대변을 통해 매일 손실된다. 일반적으로 수분 섭취와 수분이 함유된 음식 섭취는 이러한 손실을 대체한다. 열, 설사 또는 구토를 동반하여 아프거나 열에 노출되면 탈수가 발생한다. 때때로 이뇨제와 같이 체액과 전해질을 고갈시키는 약물을 복용하면 탈수가 발생할 수 있다.

열에 노출되면 체내 수분이 주로 인체에서 열을 제거하는 주요 수단인 땀으로 손실된다. 개인은 시간당 0.8~1.4L의 땀을 흘릴 수 있으며 열에 순응한 일부 운동선수는 더운 환경에서 경기하는 동안 시간당 3.7L까지 땀을 흘릴 수 있다. 열 질환의 발병을 피하기 위한 핵심은 체액 균형을 유지하고 일상 활동 중 특히 중등도에서 열에 노출되는 신체 활동 중 탈수를 최소화하는 것이다. 탈수의 증상과 징후는 비특이적이며 때로는 식별하기 어렵다.

경중에서 중등도의 급성 탈수(체중의 2~6%)를 동반하면 갈증, 쇠약, 피로, 두통, 어지러움, 불안감, 열에 대한 내성 감소, 진하고 냄새가 나는 소변, 소변 배출량 감소, 인지 기능저하, 근력과 유산소 신체 능력 감소를 경험한다. 탈수가 심한 환자는 빈맥, 창백하고 땀이 나는 피부, 쇠약, 오심 등 저혈량 쇼크와 유사한 증상 및 징후가 나타난다.

열에 노출되는 동안 수분을 자주 섭취하도록 권장하는 경우 입으로 수분을 보충할 수 있는 속도는 위 배출 속도와 소장에서의 수분 흡수 속도에 따라 제한된다. 위장에서 소장으로 수분이 비워져 혈류로 흡수되는 속도는 시간당 최대 약 1~1.2L이다. 또한 땀으로 인한 체중 감소로 인해 총 체중의 5%가 탈수되면 위 배출량은 약 20~25% 감소한다. 다양한 수분 보충 전략과 고려 사항에 대해서는 이 장의 뒷부분에서 자세히 설명한다.

탈수의 증상과 징후

다음은 영유아, 어림이, 성인에게 나타나는 가장 흔한 탈수 증상 및 징후이지만, 사람마다 다른 증상이 나타날 수 있다.

- 배뇨 횟수 감소 및 짙은 색 소변
- 갈증
- 피부 건조
- 피로
- 가벼운 현기증

- 두통
- 어지럼
- 혼동
- 입안 및 점막 건조
- 심박수 및 호흡수 증가

영아 및 어린이의 경우 다음과 같은 추가 증상이 나타날 수 있다.

- 입안 및 혀 건조
- 울 때 눈물이 나지 않음
- 3시간 이상 기저귀가 젖지 않음
- 움푹 들어간 복부, 눈 또는 뺨
- 숫구멍 함몰(영아의 경우)
- 고열
- 무기력
- 과민성
- 꼬집었다가 풀었을 때 편평해지지 않는 피부(피부 텐팅)

열로 인한 손상

열 관련 장애는 열 질환이 있는 환자에게서 경증부터 중증까지 다양하게 나타날 수 있다. 병원 전 진료 제공자는 경미한 증후군(예: 열 발진, 운동 관련 근육 경련)에서 시작하여 주요 열 관련 질환(예: 열사병)으로 진행될 수 있다. 대부분의 열 노출에서 환자는 중심체온을 적절히 발산하고 중심체온을 정상 범위 내로 유지할 수 있다. 그러나 열 관련 질환으로 인해 EMS에 도움을 요청하는 경우 병원 전 처치 제공자가 환자를 평가하는 동안 경미한 열 관련 질환이 주요 열 질환의 증상 및 징후와 함께 나타날 수 있다(**표 19-1**).

경미한 열 관련 질환

경미한 열 관련 질환에는 적색땀띠, 열 부종, 운동 유발 근육(열) 경련, 열 실신 등이 있다. 이러한 질환은 생명을 위협하는 문제는 아니지만, 평가와 처치가 필요하다.

적색땀띠

"땀띠" 및 "열 발진"이라고도 하는 적색땀띠는 일반적으로 제한적인 옷을 입고 땀을 많이 흘리는 부위의 피부에 나타나는 붉고 소양감이 있는 구진성 발진이다(**그림 19-3**). 이 상태는 땀샘의 염증으로 인해 땀 관이 막혀 발생한다. 결과적으로 감염된 부위는 땀을 흘릴 수 없어 피부 표면의 양에 따라 열 질환에 걸릴 위험이 높아진다.

처치

처치는 해당 부위를 식히고 건조하며 해당 부위에 땀을 유발하는 추가 질환을 예방하는 것으로 시작된다. 예를 들어, 환자를 더위와 습기를 피해 서늘하고 건조한 환경으로 옮긴다. 시원한 물로 샤워하고 해당 부위를 건조하면 발진을 완화하는 데 도움이 된다. 가려움증을 완화하기 위해 항히스타민제를 투여할 수 있다.

열 부종

열 부종은 체온 조절 혈류의 필요성 증가를 보상하기 위해 혈장 부피가 팽창하는 열 적응 초기 단계에서 손, 발, 발목에 나타나는 경미한 의존성 부종이다. 이러한 형태의 부종은 과도한 수분 섭취나 심장, 신장 또는 간 질환을 나타내지 않는다. 다른 질병이 없는 경우 이 상태는 임상적으로 중요하지 않으며 자체적으로 제한된다. 열 부종은 여성에게서 더 자주 관찰된다.

처치

처치는 몸을 조이는 옷을 느슨하게 하고 꽉 조이거나 몸을 조이는 장신구를 제거하고, 다리를 들어 올리는 것으로 이루어진다. 이뇨제는 필요하지 않으며 열 질환의 위험을 증가시킬 수 있다.

운동 관련 근육(열) 경련

운동 관련 근육 경련은 모든 온도에서 발생할 수 있으며 특별히 체온 상승과 관련이 없다. 운동 관련 근육 경련은 종아리 근육뿐만 아니라 복부와 팔다리의 수의근에서도 흔히 볼 수 있는 단기적이고 고통스러운 근육 수축으로 나타나며 주로 따뜻하거나 더운 온도에서 장시간 신체 활동을 한 후 관찰되는 경우가 많다. 이러한 경련은 땀을 많이 흘리는 운동 중 또는 운동 회복 기간에 개인에게 발생한다. 민무늬근, 심장, 가로막, 숨뇌 근육(입 모양, 씹기, 삼키는 것과 관련된 근육)은 관여하지 않는다. 근육 경련은 단독으로 일어나거나 열 탈진과 함께 발생할 수 있다.

근육 경련의 원인은 알려지지 않지만, 체내 수분 손실, 나트륨 및 기타 전해질 손실과 함께 신경 근육의 피로가 복합적으로 작용하는 것으로 알려져 있다. 덥고 습한 환경에서 적절한 열 적응 없이 운동하거나 체력 수준을 넘어서는 운동을 하거나 땀을 많이 흘릴 때 더 흔히 나타난다.

표 19-1 일반적인 열 관련 질환

질환	원인/문제	증상 및 징후	처치
운동 관련 근육(열) 경련	땀으로 손실된 수분과 전해질을 보충하지 못하면 전해질과 근육에 문제가 생길 수 있다.	종아리, 허벅지, 복부 등 주로 운동 시 많이 사용되는 근육에 나타나는 통증과 연축성 근육 경련	서늘한 곳으로 이동하여 휴식을 취하고 스포츠음료나 나트륨이 함유된 음료(예: 토마토 주스)를 마시도록 권장한다. 탈수, 열 탈진, 열사병 또는 운동 관련 저나트륨혈증에 대한 증상이나 징후가 있는 사람은 이송한다.
탈수	땀 손실을 수분으로 대체하지 못함	갈증, 메스꺼움, 과도한 피로, 두통, 혈량저하증, 체온 조절 감소, 신체적 및 정신적 능력 감소	땀으로 손실된 수분을 이온 음료로 대체하고 체중과 수분 손실이 회복될 때까지 서늘한 곳에서 휴식을 취한다. 일부 환자의 경우 정맥 내로 수액 투여가 필요하다.
열탈진	불충분한 수분 섭취로 인한 과도한 열 부담, 정맥 저류로 인한 심혈관계 문제, 심장 충만 시간 감소, 심박출량 감소 등을 처치하지 않으면 열사병으로 진행될 수 있음	소변 배출량 삼소, 빈맥, 빠른 호흡, 쇠약, 불쾌감, 불안정한 걸음걸이, 극심한 피로, 창백/차가움/축축한 피부, 두통, 현기증(실신 가능), 오심, 구토, 정상 체온 또는 경미한 상승, 발한	활동을 중단하고, 열 스트레스를 제거하고, 환자를 서늘한 곳에 바로누운자세를 취해주고, 제한적인 의복을 적시고, 몸에 물을 뿌리고 부채질하고, 이온 음료와 같은 약간 염분이 있는 수분을 섭취하도록 권장하고 0.9% 생리식염수나 젖산 링거액을 정맥 내로 투여한다.
열사병	중심체온이 40.5°C를 초과하는 높은 체온, 세포 파괴, 다발성 장기 기능 장애, 체온 조절 중추 기능 장애를 동반한 신경학적 장애	혼란, 비이성적 행동 또는 섬망을 포함한 정신 상태 변화, 떨림, 처음에는 빈맥, 나중에는 서맥, 저혈압, 빠르고 얕은 호흡, 건조하거나 축축하고 뜨거운 피부, 의식 상실, 발작 및 혼수상태 등	응급상황: 환자를 물에 담그거나 적셔 신속하고 즉각적으로 냉각시키거나 환자를 차갑고 젖은 시트로 감싸고 부채질한다. 전신에 냉찜질하거나 뺨, 손바닥, 발바닥에 화학적 냉찜질 팩을 적용한다. 체온이 39°C가 될 때까지 계속 시행한다. 중심체온이 낮아지면 필요한 경우 쇼크 처치를 시행하고 기도를 유지하며 즉시 응급실로 이송한다.
운동 관련 저나트륨혈증	낮은 혈장 나트륨 농도(<135mmol/L), 일반적으로 더운 환경에서 장시간 활동하는 경우, 식수(> 1.5L/h) 또는 땀 배출량을 초과하는 경우, 부적절한 아르기닌 바소프레신 분비, 땀으로 손실된 나트륨을 대체하지 못하는 경우 등에 나타남	두통, 오심, 구토, 불쾌감, 현기증, 운동 실조, 정신 상태 변화, 다뇨증, 폐부종, 두개내압 징후, 발작, 혼수, 중심체온(39°C 미만), 열탈진 및 탈수 증상을 모방한다.	저장상 및 등장성 수액 섭취를 제한하고 짠 음식이나 식염수를 제공한다. 반응이 없는 환자는 비재호흡마스크로 분당 15L 산소를 공급한다. 혈청 나트륨 수치를 측정할 수 있고 130mmol/L 미만인 경우 3% 고장성 식염수 100mL를 10분 간격으로 3회 투여하거나 신경학적 증상이 종료될 때까지 정맥 내로 고장성 생리식염수를 투여한다. 명료한 환자는 앉은 자세, 반응이 없는 자세는 왼쪽 누운 자세로 신속하게 이송한다.

Modified from Schimelpfenig T, Richards G, Tartar S. Management of heat illnesses. In: Hawkins SC, ed. *Wilderness EMS*. Wolters Kluwer; 2018; Bennett BL, Hew-Butler T, Rosner MH, Myers T, Lipman GS. Wilderness Medical Society Practice guidelines for treatment of exercise-associated hyponatremia: 2019 update. *Wilderness Environ Med*. 2020;31(1):50-62.

처치

처치는 서늘한 환경에서 휴식을 취하고 경련이 발생한 부위의 근육을 스트레칭하거나 염화나트륨이 함유된 액체 및 음식을 섭취한다(예: 300~500mL의 물 또는 스포츠음료에 소금 1/8~1/4 티스푼을 희석, 300~500mL의 물과 소금 1~2정 또는 짠 스낵). 정맥 내 수액 투여는 거의 필요하지 않지만, 지속적인 중증의 광범위한 근육 경련은 정맥 내로 생리식염수를 투여하면 더 빠르게 완화될 수 있다. 소금 정제는 위장 장애를 유발할 수 있으므로 단독으로 사용하지 않는다.

열 실신

열 실신은 더운 환경에서 장시간 서 있을 때 나타나며 저혈압으로 인해 어지럼, 쇠약 또는 일시적인 의식 상실을 초래한다. 열에 노출되면

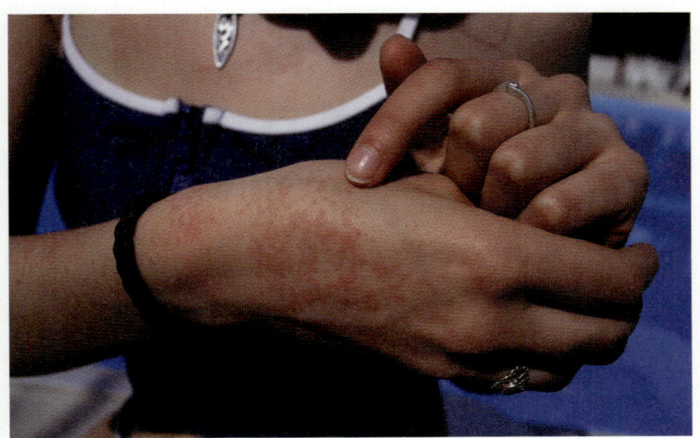

그림 19-3 열 발진.
© Ian west/Alamy Stock Photo

다리의 말초혈관이 확장되고 기립성 정맥혈 저류로 인해 저혈압을 유발한다. 열 실신은 종종 행군 중인 군인에게 자주 발생하며 장시간 운동을 마친 후 선수에게 나타날 수 있다. 열 실신의 또 다른 일반적인 이름은 열 관련 체위성 저혈압이다.

처치

열 스트레스에서 벗어나 시원한 환경으로 옮기고 환자를 누운 자세로 쉬게 한다. 조이는 옷을 느슨하게 하거나 제거하고 탈수가 의심되는 경우 입이나 정맥 내로 수분을 보충한다. 낙상이 발생하면 환자의 손상 여부를 철저하게 평가해야 한다. 심장 또는 신경학적 장애의 병력이 있는 환자는 실신의 원인에 대한 추가 평가가 필요하다. 이송 중 활력징후와 심전도 모니터링하는 것이 필수적이다.

주요 열 관련 질환

주요 열 관련 질환으로는 운동 관련 허탈, 열 탈진, 열사병(전형적인 형태와 운동성 형태)이 있으며 계속 방치할 때 생명에 위협이 될 수 있다.

운동 관련 허탈

이 장애는 격렬한 운동 후 허탈 될 때 발생한다. 운동 중에는 다리 근육의 수축은 정맥혈이 심장으로 돌아가는 것을 돕는다. 조깅이 끝났을 때와 같이 운동을 멈추면 심장으로 혈액이 돌아가는 데 도움이 되는 근육 수축이 현저히 느려진다. 이로 인해 심장으로 돌아가는 정맥혈이 감소하여 뇌로 가는 심박출량이 감소하게 된다. 이 장애는 마라톤, 울트라 마라톤, 철인 3종 경기를 완주하는 경우 종종 나타난다.

평가

징후와 증상으로는 서 있거나 걷기 어려움, 구역, 가벼운 현기증, 어지럼, 실신 등이 있다. 환자는 누우면 상태가 호전되지만, 서거나 앉으려고 하면 어지러워질 수 있다(기립저혈압). 땀을 많이 흘리는 것은 드문 일이 아니다. 호흡과 맥박이 빨라질 수 있으며 환자의 중심 체온은 정상이거나 약간 높을 수 있다. 탈수를 배제하기는 어렵지만, 이러한 유형의 운동 후 허탈은 혈량저하증으로 인한 것이 아니다. 이와는 대조적으로 운동 중에 발생하는 허탈은 다른 원인(예: 심혈관 질환)에 대한 즉각적인 평가가 필요하다.

처치

환자를 서늘한 환경으로 옮겨 누운 자세에서 다리를 올리고 휴식을 취하게 한다. 중등도에서 중증의 탈수 시 필요한 경우 정맥 내로 수액을 투여하고 의식이 있고 삼킬 수 있는 경우 입으로 시원한 액체를 공급한다. 이러한 환자 중 상당수는 탈수가 아닌 운동 종료 시 정맥 환류 감소로 인해 허탈이 나타날 수 있으므로 추가 평가가 완료되거나 수동적 냉각이 완료될 때까지 정맥 내로 수액을 투여하는 것을 보류하는 것이 좋다. 모든 형태의 허탈과 마찬가지로 다른 질환(예: 열사병, 운동 관련 저나트륨혈증, 심장 또는 신경학적 원인)을 배제하기 위한 추가 평가가 필요하다. 이송 중 활력징후와 심전도 모니터링은 부정맥을 감지하는 데 필요하다.

열탈진

열탈진은 병원 전 처치 제공자가 볼 수 있는 가장 흔한 열 관련 질환이다. 이 상태는 며칠에 걸쳐 노출되거나(노인에게 자주 나타남) 급성으로(운등선수에게 자주 나타남) 발생할 수 있다. 열탈진은 체온 조절을 위한 열 발산, 피부 혈류량 증가, 혈장량 감소, 혈관 확장으로 인한 심장으로 정맥혈 체온 조절(열 방출) 피부 혈류 증가, 혈장 부피 감소, 혈관 확장으로 인한 정맥혈복귀 감소, 땀으로 인한 염분과 수분 고갈로 인한 순환계 부하 증가를 지원하기에 불충분한 심박출량으로 인해 발생한다. 열탈진은 고온, 이뇨제 등 약물 사용, 불충분한 수분 섭취, 기존 심장부전 등의 복합적인 요인으로 인해 열탈진이 발생하는 경우가 많다.

심한 열탈진과 열사병을 구분하기 어려울 수 있지만, 의식 상태를 빠르게 평가하면 신경학적 관련 정도를 파악할 수 있다. 열탈진은 효과적으르 처치하지 않으면 생명을 위협하는 형태의 열 관련 질병인 열사병으로 이어질 수 있다. 열탈진은 열사병의 증거가 없을 때 제외하는 진단이다. 이러한 환자는 응급실에서 추가적인 신체 검진 및 검사실 평가가 필요하다.

평가

열탈진의 증상과 징후는 구체적이거나 민감하지 않다. 이러한 증상과 징후로는 피로, 어지럼, 두통, 불쾌감, 저혈압, 빠른 맥박 등이 대표적이다. 중심체온은 38.5~40℃로 측정될 수 있지만, 정상 또는 약한 상승할 수 있다. 열탈진의 급성기에는 혈압이 낮고 맥박과 환기 속도가 빨라지고 노동맥 맥박이 약하게 느껴질 수 있다. 환자는 일반적으로 땀이 나고 창백하며 잿빛으로 보인다.

　이러한 환자는 다른 체액 및 나트륨 손실 상태(예: 저나트륨혈증, 이후 설명 참조)의 증상과 징후를 보일 수 있으므로 과거 열 질환 병력과 현재 열 노출 사고에 대해 잘 파악하는 것이 중요하다. 열탈진이 열사병으로 진행될 수 있으므로 재평가하는 것이 중요하다. 의식 상태 및 성격 변화(예: 혼동, 지남력 장애, 비이성적 또는 비정상적 행동)가 있는지 지속해서 확인한다. 이러한 변화는 즉시 생명을 위협하는 열사병을 나타내는 고체온의 진행성 징후로 간주해야 한다.

처치

환자를 더운 환경(예: 햇볕, 뜨거운 노면, 뜨거운 차량)에서 즉시 그늘이나 에어컨이 있는 시원한 장소(예: 구급차)로 옮긴 후 누운 자세를 취해주고 열 발산을 방해하는 모든 것을 제거한다. 환자의 심박수, 혈압, 호흡수, 가능한 경우 직장 체온을 평가하고 특히 생명을 위협하는 열사병의 초기 지표인 중추신경계 상태 변화에 주의를 기울여야 한다.

　입으로 수분을 섭취할 수 있고 흡인의 위험이 없는 모든 환자는 입으로 수분 보충을 고려해야 한다. 이온 음료가 가장 이상적이지만, 음료는 희석하지 않은 상태에서 당 함량이 높으므로 물과 1:1로 희석해야 한다. 다량의 입안 수액 보충은 오심, 구토, 복부 팽만감을 증가시킬 수 있다. 일반적으로 혈압, 맥박, 직장체온이 정상적이면 정맥 내 수액 투여는 필요하지 않다. 그러나 입으로 수분을 섭취할 수 없는 환자의 경우 정맥 내로 수액을 투여하면 열탈진에서 빠르게 회복할 수 있다. 정맥 내 수액 투여가 필요한 경우 젖산 링거액(LR)이나 생리식염수(NS)를 사용해야 한다. 정맥 내 수액 투여는 탈수로 인한 위 배출과 소장에서의 흡수 지연으로 인해 입으로 수액을 섭취하는 것보다 더 빠르게 수액을 보충할 수 있다.

　운동성 열탈진에서 환자는 대부분 누워서 휴식을 취하고 입으로 수분을 보충하면 회복된다. 이러한 환자에게 정맥 내 수액 투여를 결정하기 전에 병원 전 처치 제공자는 탈수의 증상과 징후, 기립성(체위) 맥박, 혈압 변화, 입으로 수분을 섭취할 수 있는 능력에 대해 철저하게 평가해야 한다. 지속적인 의식 상태 변화는 열사병, 저나트륨혈증, 저혈당 및 기타 의학적 문제에 대한 추가 평가가 필요하다. 운동성 열탈진 환자에게 권장되는 정맥 내 수액 투여는 경미한 저혈당 환자의 경우 생리식염수 또는 5% 포도당(5/DW)을 투여한다. 그러나 장시간 운동(4시간 이상)을 한 환자, 특히 탈수의 명백한 임상 징후가 없는 환자나 다량의 물을 섭취한 운동선수에게서 열탈진이 의심되는 경우 정맥 내로 다량의 수액을 투여하지 않도록 병원 전 처치 제공자는 주의해야 한다. 이러한 유형의 환자는 운동 관련 저나트륨혈증(낮은 혈청 나트륨 수치)이 있을 수 있으며 입으로 수분을 공급하거나 정맥 내로 수액을 투여하면 희석으로 인해 저나트륨혈증이 더 심해져서 생명을 위협하는 상태를 초래할 수 있다. 열 관련 질병 또는 운동 관련 저나트륨혈증에 대해 환자를 정확하게 평가하는 최선의 방법에 대한 정보는 운동 관련 저나트륨혈증에 대한 논의를 참조한다.

　열탈진은 열사병과 구별하기 어려울 수 있고 열사병 환자는 중심체온을 빠르게 낮춰야 하므로 모든 열탈진 환자에게 적극적인 냉각 조치를 취하는 것이 최선의 처치이다. 능동 냉각은 물이나 젖은 천으로 머리와 상반신을 적신 다음 부채질하거나 바람을 불어줌으로써 대류에 의한 체열 발산을 증가시켜 간단하고 신속하게 수행할 수 있다. 체온을 낮추는 것을 통해 의식 상태도 개선될 수 있다. 의식이 없거나 빠르게 회복되지 않는 모든 환자는 즉시 생명의 위협하는 열사병 상태의 징후이므로 신속하게 이송한다. 이송 중에 적절한 환경 온도 조절과 활력징후, 의식 상태를 모니터링하는 것이 필수이다.

열사병

열사병은 가장 응급하고 생명을 위협하는 형태의 열 질환으로 간주하며 병원 전 처치 제공자가 직면하는 가장 시간에 민감한 생명을 위협하는 질환 중 하나이다. 열사병은 고열의 한 형태로 체온 조절 시스템의 장애로 인해 열을 발산하고 체온을 낮추는 신체의 생리적 시스템에 장애가 발생하는 질환이다. 열사병은 중심체온이 40℃ 이상으로 상승하고 중추신경계 기능 장애로 인한 섬망, 경련 또는 혼수상태를 초래하는 것이 특징이다.

　열사병과 열탈진을 비교했을 때 가장 큰 차이점은 신경학적 장애로 의식 상태 변화가 나타나는 것을 병원 전 처치 제공자가 확인할 수 있다. 병태생리적 변화는 종종 다발성 장기부전을 초래한다. 이러한 병태생리학적 변화는 장기 조직 온도가 임계 수준 이상으로 상승할 때 발생한다. 세포막이 손상되어 세포 부피, 신진대사, 산-염기 균형 및 막 투과성에 장애가 발생하여 궁극적으로 세포사와 함께 세포 및 전체 장기 기능 장애를 유발한다. 열사병 환자의 합병증 정도는 중심체온의 상승 정도와 전적으로 관련이 없다.

이러한 전신 병태생리학적 기능 장애는 병원 전 처치 제공자가 열사병을 조기에 인지해야 하는 근본적인 이유이다. 열사병을 조기에 인지하면 적극적인 전신 냉각을 통해 중심체온을 빠르게 낮추고 관련 열사병 이환율 및 사망률을 낮출 수 있다.

이환율과 사망률은 중심체온이 상승한 기간과 직접적인 관련이 있으며 긍정적인 환자 예후는 중심체온을 38.9℃ 이하로 얼마나 빨리 낮출 수 있는지와 직접적인 관련이 있다. 열사병은 병원 전 적극적인 처치와 병원 내 처치에도 불구하고 치명적인 경우가 많으며 생존한 환자 중 상당수는 영구적인 신경학적 장애를 입을 수 있다.

열사병은 전형적인(비운동성) 열사병과 운동성 열사병이라는 두 가지 임상 양상으로 나타난다(**표 19-2**).

전형적인 열사병은 영아, 열이 나는 어린이, 노숙자 또는 적절하게 에어컨을 사용할 수 없는 사람, 노인, 알코올 중독자, 만성질환이 있는 환자에게 가장 흔히 나타나는 질환이다. **Box 19-2**에 나열된 위험 요소(예: 약물 복용)에 의해 악화할 수 있다. 전형적인 증상은 며칠 동안 에어컨 없이 고온 다습한 실내 온도에 노출되어 탈수 및 높은 중심체온을 유발하는 환자에게서 나타난다. 종종 이 환자는 땀이 나지 않는 무한증을 보이기도 한다. 이는 특히 여름철 폭염이 지속되는 대도시에서 효과적인 가정 내 환기가 불가능하거나 사용하지 않을 때 흔히 발생한다. 현장 평가는 전형적인 열사병을 식별하는 데 도움이 되는 정보를 제공한다.

운동성 열사병(EHS)은 체력이 부족하거나 더위에 적응하지 못한 사람(예: 산업 근로자, 운동선수, 군인, 소방관, 기타 공공 안전 요원)이 덥고 습한 환경에서 단기간 격렬한 신체 활동을 할 때 흔히 나타나는 예방 가능한 질환이다. 이러한 환경에서는 체내 열 생산이 급격히 증가하고 신체가 열을 발산하는 능력이 제한될 수 있다. 거의 모든 운동성 열사병 환자는 전형적인 열사병 환자의 피부가 건조하고 뜨거우며 붉어지는 것과 달리 실신할 때 땀에 흠뻑 젖고 창백한 피부를 보인다. 격렬한 활동 중에 수분을 섭취하면 탈수 속도를 늦추고 중심체온이 상승하는 속도를 감소시킬 수 있지만, 탈수가 심하지 않은 경우에도 고열과 운동성 열사병이 발생할 수 있다.

적극적으로 실신한 후 10분 이내에 신속하게 처치를 시작하면 운동성 열사병으로 인한 사망은 발생하지 않는다. 운동성 열사병으로

표 19-2 전형적인 열사병과 운동성 열사병

	전형적	운동성
환자 특징	노인	남성(15~45세)
건강 상터	만성 질환	건강
동시에 진행 중인 활동	앉아 있는	격결한 운동
약물 복용	이뇨제, 항우울제, 항고혈압제, 항콜린제, 항정신병약	보통 없음
발한	나지 않을 수 있음	일반적으로 남
젖산 산증	대개는 없으며 있는 경우 예후가 좋지 않음	흔함
고칼륨혈증	일반적으로 없음	자주 있음
저칼륨혈증	흔하지 않음	자주
저혈당	흔하지 않음	일반적으로
크레아틴	약간 상승	크게 상승
횡문근융해	경증	자주 중증

Modified from Knochel JP, Reed G. Disorders of heat regulation. In: Kleeman CR, Maxwell MH, Narin RG, eds. *Clinical Disorders of Fluid and Electrolyte Metabolism*. McGraw-Hill; 1987.

사망이 발생할 수 있는 몇 가지 일반적인 이유는 **Box 19-3**에 나와 있다. "먼저 냉각을 시행하고 그다음 이송" 한다는 방침은 중심체온을 낮추기 시작하는 데 지연이 발생하지 않도록 하기 위한 것이다.

평가

증상과 징후의 양상은 고열의 정도와 지속 시간에 따라 다르다. 열사병 환자는 일반적으로 피부가 뜨겁고 붉어진다. 환자가 발견된 장소와 전형적인 열사병인지 운동성 열사병인지에 따라 땀을 흘릴 수도 있고 흘리지 않을 수도 있다. 혈압이 높아지거나 낮아질 수 있으며 노동맥은 일반적으로 빠르고 약하며 가늘고 이러한 환자의 25%는 저혈압이 발생한다. 환자의 의식 수준은 혼란스러운 상태부터 무의식에 이르기까지 다양하며 특히 체온을 낮추는 동안 발작이 나타날 수 있다. 병원에서 확인된 바와 같이 직장 체온은 40~46.7℃일 수 있지만, 체온이 40℃ 미만인 환자도 열사병에 걸릴 수 있다.

열사병과 다른 열 관련 질환을 구별하는 핵심은 의식 상태의 변화이다. 얄반적으로 체온이 상승하고 종종 상당히 높다. 만졌을 때 열

**Box 19-3 운동성 열사병(EHS)으로 인한 일반적인
사망 원인**

1. 부정확한 체온 측정 또는 오진. 이는 종종 다른 유사한 의학적 상태를
배제할 수 없기 때문이다. 입안, 겨드랑이, 고막 체온 측정은 체온 상
승 정도를 과소평가할 수 있으므로 병원 전 처치 제공자는 직장 체온
에만 의존하여 고열 정도를 판단하고 고위험군 환자의 경우 높은 의
심 지수를 유지해야 한다.
2. 처치를 받지 않거나 처치가 지연되는 경우. 운동성 열사병의 가능성
을 인지하지 못하고 효과적인 처치를 제공하기 위한 대응을 지연하
면 재앙적인 결과를 초래할 수 있다.
3. 비효율적인 전신 냉각 방법. 30분 이내에 중심 체온을 40℃ 미만
으로 빠르게 낮추는 것이 중요하다. 이 목표는 열사병 처치의 "황금
30분"으로 알려져 있으며 신속한 전신 냉각을 시행할 수 있는 표준
이다.
4. 즉시 이송. 운동성 열사병의 경우 현장에서 중심체온을 낮추기 위해
전신 냉각을 시작하고 이 처치가 시작될 때까지 이송하지 않는 것이
중요하다. 직장 체온 측정과 함께 이송 중에도 냉각을 계속하여 중심
체온이 40℃ 미만으로 떨어지도록 해야 한다.

이 나면서 의식 상태 변화(혼동, 방향 감각 상실, 무의식 또는 공격적)
에 변화가 있는 환자는 열사병으로 추정하고 체온을 낮추기 위해 즉
시 적극적으로 처치를 한다.

처치

열사병은 시간에 매우 민감한 응급 상황이며 환자를 열원으로부터
즉시 이동시켜야 한다. 동료가 환자의 기도, 호흡, 순환을 평가하고
안정시키는 동안 당신은 현장에서 즉시 환자 냉각을 시작해야 한다.
옷을 제거하기 전이라도 가능한 모든 수단(예를 들면, 정원 호스, 생
수, IV 생리식염수 백)을 써서 즉시 환자 냉각을 시작해야 한다. 얼음
적용과 찬물에 담그는 것은 가장 빠른 냉각 방법이지만, 병원 전 환
경에서는 이러한 방법이 제한될 수 있다.

1950년대 후반부터 찬물이나 얼음물에 담그면 혈관 수축이 일어
나 신체에서 열 손실을 줄이고 떨림이 시작되어 내부 열이 발생하여
열 교환이 제한될 것으로 생각되어 왔다. 현재의 경험적 증거는 이러
한 환자의 냉각 속도가 둔화할 것이라는 우려를 반박한다. 따라서 가
능하다면 이러한 형태의 냉각을 열사병 환자에게 보류해서는 안 된
다. 많은 프로토콜과 교육과정에서 반동 떨림(체온 상승)이나 "급격
한 증가" 또는 "증가 후 하강"을 방지하여 환자가 저체온에 빠지는 것
을 방지하기 위해 체온을 39℃ 미만으로 적극적으로 낮추지 말 것을
권장한다. 근거를 기반으로 한 야생의학회 고열 관리 지침에서는 이
러한 이론적 우려를 뒷받침하는 증거는 없지만, 열사병에서 능동적

냉각을 중단하는 임계값(39℃)으로 제시하고 있다.

찬물과 얼음을 즉시 사용할 수 없는 경우 환자의 과도한 옷을 벗
기고 머리부터 발끝까지 환자를 적신 다음 피부에 지속해서 부채질
한다. 이 과정은 현장에서 구급차로 환자를 이송할 준비를 하기 전에
지체하지 말고 즉시 시작해야 한다. 환자를 적시거나 부채질하는 것
은 증발 및 대류에 의한 열 손실을 유발하는 가장 효과적인 냉각 방
법이다. 전신 냉각 중에 빠르게 의식을 회복하는 환자는 일반적으로
예후가 좋다. 병원 전 처치 제공자가 열사병 환자에게 제공할 수 있
는 가장 중요한 처치는 기도, 호흡, 순환 유지와 함께 즉각적이고 신
속한 전신 냉각을 통해 중심체온을 낮추는 것이다.

환자는 에어컨이 작동되는 구급차를 이용해 이송해야 한다. 의료
기관까지 이송하는 시간이 짧더라도 열사병 환자를 구급차 내부가
따뜻한 상태로 환자를 이송하는 것은 잘못된 행동이다. 환자의 옷을
제거하고 차가운 물로 적신 시트로 환자를 덮은 후 실내에서 부채질
해주는 것이 좋다. 이용할 수 있고 시간이 허락한다면 냉찜질을 혈관
이 피부 표면에 가장 가깝게 노출된 서혜부, 겨드랑이, 목 주위에 시
행하는 것이 좋다. 냉찜질을 사용에 대해 광범위하게 권장되는 것은
훨씬 덜 효과적인 중심체온 냉각 방법이다. 얼음찜질만으로는 전신을
덮지 않는 한 중심체온을 빠르게 낮추기에는 충분하지 않으며 추가
냉각 방법으로만 고려해야 하며 환자 처치의 우선순위가 되어서는
안 된다.

가능하면 이송 중에는 5~10분마다 환자의 직장 체온을 측정하여
효과적인 냉각이 이루어지는지 확인한다. 환자의 체온을 측정하는
다른 부위(입안, 피부, 겨드랑이)는 환자의 중심체온을 적절하게 반영
하지 못하므로 처치를 결정하는 데 사용해서는 안 된다. 고유량의 산
소를 공급하고 필요하면 백마스크로 보조 환기를 시행하고 환자의
심전도를 모니터링한다.

열사병 환자는 일반적으로 광범위한 수액 소생술이 필요로 하지
않으며 일반적으로 초기에는 정맥 내로 1.0~1.5L의 생리식염수를 투
여한다. 500mL의 수액을 투여하고 활력징후를 평가한다. 수액 투여
량은 처음 1시간 동안 1~2L를 초과하지 않아야 하며 프로토콜을 따
르거나 의료 지도 의사의 의료 지도를 받는다. 이러한 환자는 저혈당
이 자주 발생하고 50% 포도당액을 정맥 내로 투여할 수 있으므로 혈
당을 모니터링한다. 프로토콜에 따라 발작을 일으키는 경우 5~10mg
의 다이아제팜 또는 벤조다이아제핀을 투여할 수 있다. 기도 개방을
유지하고 흡인을 예방하기 위해 환자를 회복 자세로 이송한다.

운동 관련 저나트륨혈증

운동 관련 저나트륨혈증(EAH)은 수분 중독으로도 알려져 있으며 등산객, 전문 등반가, 마라톤 선수, 울트라 마라톤 선수, 철인 3종 경기 선수, 오지 탐험가, 군 보병 등에서 장시간의 신체 활동 후 점점 생명을 위협하는 질환으로 점점 더 많이 보고되고 있다. 이러한 야외 활동의 인기가 높아짐에 따라 1980년대 중반에 처음 보고된 이후 경증에서 중증 운동 관련 저나트륨혈증 발생률이 꾸준히 증가했다. 현재 지구력 활동으로 인해 심각한 합병증 중 하나로 알려져 있으며 사고 관련 사망의 중요한 원인으로 지목되고 있다.

운동 관련 저나트륨혈증은 일반적으로 장시간 활동 시 과도한 수분 섭취(시간당 1.4L 이상)와 관련이 있다. 두 가지의 주요 발생 기전은 1) 과도한 수분 섭취와 2) 항이뇨호르몬(ADH)이라고도 하는 아르기닌 바소프레신(AVP)의 지속적인 분비로 인한 소변 배설 장애이다. 운동 관련 저나트륨혈증은 증상 발현에 따라 경증 또는 중증의 두 가지 형태로 나타날 수 있다.

심각한 경우 혈장 나트륨 농도가 낮아지면 혈액-뇌장벽 가로지르는 삼투압 균형이 깨져 뇌로 수분이 빠르게 유입되어 뇌부종이 발생한다. 머리 외상(8장 머리와 목 외상 참조)에서 두개내압 증가의 증상 및 징후와 유사한 방식으로 저나트륨혈증으로 인한 두통, 구토, 불쾌감, 혼동, 발작 등 신경학적 증상이 진행되어 혼수상태, 영구적 뇌손상, 뇌줄기 탈장 및 사망에 이르게 된다. 이러한 환자는 운동 관련 저나트륨혈증 뇌병증(EAHE)에 걸린 것으로 알려져 있다.

증상이 있는 운동 관련 저나트륨혈증 뇌병증 환자는 일반적으로 혈청 나트륨 농도가 126mEq/L(정상 범위 135~145mEq/L) 미만이며 장시간의 지속적인 활동에서 자주 나타나는 것처럼 저나트륨혈증이 빠르게(48시간 미만) 진행된다. 또는 경미한 형태의 운동 관련 저나트륨혈증은 일반적으로 쉽게 확인할 수 있는 증상(예: 쇠약, 오심, 구토, 두통 또는 무증상) 없이 혈청 나트륨 농도가 135~128mEq/L로 나타내며 휴식, 음식 및 전해질 수액으로 자기 제한적이다. 초기에는 경미한 증상과 징후가 나타나더라도 환자는 운동 관련 저나트륨혈증 뇌병증으로 진행될 수 있다. 지속적인 운동이 끝나면 위장관 내에 남아 있는 수분의 흡수로 인해 혈청 나트륨 농도가 급격히 떨어지는 것으로 알려져 있다. 이는 지속적인 활동을 마친 후 일시적으로 의식이 명료해진 후 활동 중단 후 약 30분 이내에 운동 관련 저나트륨혈증 뇌병증의 임상 징후가 급격히 나타나는 이유를 설명할 수 있다.

연구에 따르면 울트라마라톤 선수의 18~23%와 하와이 철인 3종 경기 완주자의 29%가 운동 관련 저나트륨혈증에 걸렸다고 한다. 2003년에는 그랜드 캐니언 국립공원(GCNP)의 등산객에서 32건의 운동 관련 저나트륨혈증이 보고되었으며 2004년~2009년까지 그랜드 캐니언 국립공원에서 발생한 모든 치명적이지 않은 열 관련 사고의 19%가 저나트륨혈증으로 인한 것이었다.

운동 관련 저나트륨혈증은 다음과 같은 상황에서 발생할 수 있다.

1. 지속적인 운동으로 인해 나트륨과 수분이 과도하게 손실되어 탈수 및 나트륨 고갈이 발생할 수 있다.
2. 혈장 나트륨을 유지하면서 물로만 과다수분 공급하여 나트륨 농도가 희석된다.
3. 땀으로 의한 과도한 나트륨과 체액 손실과 물만으로 과다 수분을 공급하는 경우이다.

증거에 따르면 운동 관련 저나트륨혈증은 장에서 흡수되지 않고 남아 있는 체액이 아니라 세포 외 공간에 체액이 저류되어 발생하는 것으로 나타났다. 일반적으로 이러한 환자는 스포츠 이온 음료를 섭취하지 않았거나 염분이 함유되지 않은 에너지 보충제를 먹었거나 땀으로 인한 나트륨 손실 또는 과도한 수분 섭취로 인한 희석의 균형을 맞추기에 부족한 양의 염분을 섭취한 경우이다.

다음은 운동 관련 저나트륨혈증의 발병과 관련된 몇 가지 주요 위험 요소이다.

1. 활동 또는 운동 시간(4시간 이상) 또는 느린 속도의 달리기/느린 속도의 운동
2. 여성(하체 체중으로 설명 가능)
3. 체질량지수(BMI)가 낮거나 높은 경우
4. 활동이나 운동 중 과도한 수분 섭취(시간당 1.5L 이상)
5. 신장 여과 기능을 감소시키는 비스테로이드성 항염증성(NSAIDS) 사용

운동 관련 저나트륨혈증은 증상이 비특이적이고 경미한 열 관련 질환에서 나타나는 증상과 유사하므로 "기타 열 관련 질환"으로 분류되었다. 많은 지속적인 운동과 수일간의 모험 활동이 따뜻하거나 더운 환경에서 진행되기 때문에 운동 관련 저나트륨혈증의 증상과 징후는 일종의 열 관련 질환으로 간주하며 환자는 저혈량증과 과도한 체온에 대처하는 표준 프로토콜에 따라 처치한다. 열 관련 질병의 증상과 징후는 일종의 고체온 질환으로 간주하며 환자는 추정되는 저혈량증 및 과도한 체온을 다루는 표준 프로토콜로 관리한다. 고열, 땀으로 인한 탈수, 정신 상태 변화를 교정하기 위해 체온을 낮추고 정맥 내로 수액을 투여하는 표준 프로토콜은 희석성 저나트륨혈증

을 악화시키고 환자를 발작과 혼수상태에 빠뜨릴 위험이 있다. 열탈진 환자와 달리 운동 관련 저나트륨혈증 환자에게 수액을 투여하고 휴식을 취하면 환자 상태가 악화할 수 있다.

이 "기타 열 관련 질환"은 의료진과 대중을 대상으로 예방, 조기 인식 및 처치에 대한 교육을 강화한 덕분에 오늘날 EMS 및 응급실에서 빨리 인식하고 올바르게 치료하고 있다(Box 19-4). 도시 또는 야생 환경에서 신체적 인내를 해야 하는 사건에서 직접 지원하거나 출동에 대응하는 병원 전 처치 제공자는 오늘날 운동 관련 저나트륨혈증이 더 자주 발생한다는 사실을 알아야 한다. 일반적으로 탈수는 장시간의 격렬한 활동에서 더 흔하게 발생하며 운동 또는 업무 관련 작업 수행 능력 저하와 심각한 열 관련 질환으로 이어질 수 있다는 점을 기억하는 것이 중요하다. 그러나 수분 과다복용으로 인한 증상으로 나타나는 저나트륨혈증은 더 위험하고 잠재적으로 생명을 위협할 수 있는 질병이다. 이러한 차이는 수분 보충 전략의 긴장감을 보여준다. 갈증을 수분 공급의 지표로 삼아 기다리면 경미한 탈수에 걸릴 수 있지만, 갈증 위험과 관계없이 수분을 보충하면 과다수분공급을 하여 운동 관련 저나트륨혈증에 걸릴 수 있다. 이 문제에 대한 자세한 내용은 이 장의 뒷부분에 있는 수분 보충 부문을 참조한다.

평가

저나트륨혈증은 지구력 운동선수 집단에서 다양한 증상과 징후가 나타날 수 있다(표 19-1 참조). 중심체온은 일반적으로 정상이지만 주변 온도, 체열 발산 및 최근 운동 강도에 따라 낮거나 약간 높아질 수 있다. 심박수와 혈압은 중심체온, 운동 강도, 저혈량증 또는 쇼크에 따라 낮거나 정상 이거나 높을 수 있다. 환기 속도는 정상 범위 내에서 약간 상승할 수 있다. 운동 관련 저나트륨혈증에서 관찰되는 과다환기는 시력 장애, 어지럼, 손 저림, 팔다리 감각 이상 등의 증상을 유발할 수 있다. 특징적인 평가 및 소견으로는 정신 상태 변화, 피로, 권태감, 두통, 매스꺼움 등이 있다. 다른 형태의 신경학적 변화로는 언어

둔화, 운동 실조, 비특이적 행동, 투쟁, 공포감, 두려움 등의 인지적 변화가 있다. 이러한 환자들은 종종 "임박한 멸망"을 느낀다고 한다.

처치

처치의 첫 번째 단계는 질환을 인식하고 중증도를 결정하는 것이다. 처치 방법은 운동 관련 저나트륨혈증의 중증도와 혈청 나트륨 농도를 측정에 사용할 수 있는 휴대용 진단 도구에 따라 결정된다. 그림 19-4는 운동 관련 저나트륨혈증 또는 열 관련 질환 여부를 판단하기 위해 환자를 평가하는 알고리즘을 제공한다. 경미한 증상은 보이는 환자를 관찰하여 운동 관련 저나트륨혈증 뇌병증으로 더 이상 진행되지 않도록 하고 과도한 체액이 정상적으로 이뇨 될 때까지 기다리는 등 보존적인 처치를 한다.

증상이 있는 환자는 기도를 유지하고 두개내압에 대한 체위 영향을 최소화하기 위해 바로 선 자세를 유지한다. 이러한 환자는 병원으로 이송하는 중에 분출성 구토를 하는 것으로 알려져 있다. 의식이 없는 환자는 회복 자세를 취해 구토에 대비하고 적극적인 기도 관리를 고려해야 한다. 고유량의 산소를 공급하고 정맥 라인을 확보하여 정맥 라인이 유지될 정도로 수액을 투여하고 발작 여부를 모니터링한다.

필요한 경우 항경련제(예: 의료 지침에 따라 벤조다이아제핀을 정맥 내로 투여)를 투여한다. 환자의 중증도와 의료기관 이송 시간에 따라 투여할 생리식염수의 양은 의료 지도를 받아 결정한다. 이러한 환자는 이미 체액 과부하 상태이므로 저나트륨혈증과 체액 과부하 정도를 악화시킬 수 있으므로 정맥 내로 저장성 수액을 투여하는 것은 금기이다.

운동 관련 저나트륨혈증 뇌병증(예: 뇌부종 및 폐부종)의 증상 및 징후가 있는 환자는 혈장 나트륨 농도를 증가시켜야 한다. 현재 병원 전 환경에서 처치에 대한 합의된 방법은 뇌부종을 급격히 감소시키기 위해 3% 고장성 생리 식염수를 10분에 걸쳐 100mL를 일시에 투여하는 것이다. 이 용액을 사용할 수 있는 경우 각 용량을 투여할 때마다 나트륨이 2~3mEq/L씩 증가한다. 임상적으로 개선이 나타나지 않으면 의료 지도를 받아 최대 2회까지 3% 고장성 생리식염수 100mL를 추가로 투여할 수 있다. 이러한 중증 운동 관련 저나트륨혈증 뇌병증 환자는 고장성 생리식염수를 투여받지 않으면 예후가 좋지 않다. 의료기관으로 이송하는 동안 환자를 진정시키고 정신 상태의 변화나 발작이 있는지 계속 모니터링한다.

Box 19-4 운동 관련 저나트륨혈증(EAH) 및 운동 관련성 저나트륨혈증 뇌병증(EAHE) 처치 지침

야생의학회는 격렬한 활동에 참여하는 환자를 병원 전 환경에서 병원 전 처치 제공자가 어떻게 처치해야 하는지에 중점을 두고 운동 관련 저나트륨혈증 및 운동 관련 저나트륨혈증 뇌병증 처치를 위한 실무 지침을 발표했다.

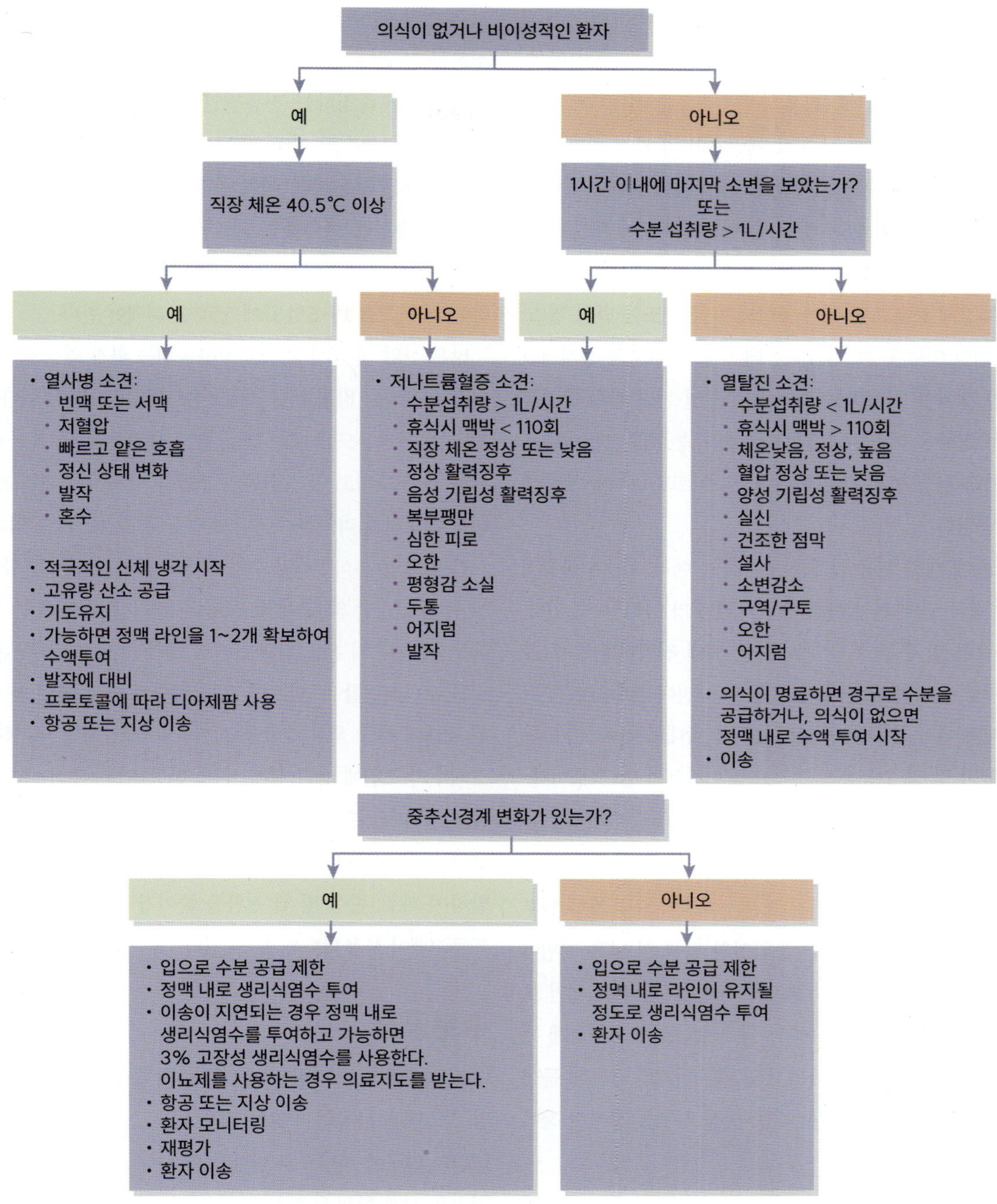

그림 19-4 열탈진, 열사병, 저나트륨혈증에 대한 처치 알고리즘
© National Association of Emergency Medical Technicians (NAEMT)

열 관련 질환 예방

열 스트레스는 미국에서 중요한 공중보건 요소이기 때문에 열 관련 질환을 예방하는 방법은 모든 지역 사회, 특히 열이 많은 직업 환경에서 일해야 하는 사람들에게 매우 중요하다. 예를 들어, 2006~2015년까지 미국에서는 총 1,000명의 소방관(자원봉사자, 경력자, 야생 소방관 포함)이 업무 중 사망했으며 이는 연평균 100명의 소방관이 사망했다. 2015년에는 90명의 소방관이 업무 중 사망했으며 60명 (66.7%)이 스트레스나 과로로 인해 현장에서 사망했고 열 질환도 이 범주도 이 범주에 포함되었다.

병원 전 처치 제공자와 해당 EMS 기관은 워크숍, 교육 자료, 기관 웹사이트 또는 뉴스레터, 지역 신문 등 다양한 형식의 열 스트레스 예방 전략에 대한 지역 사회 교육 파트너로서 좋은 자원이 될 수 있다.

일반 대중과 마찬가지로 병원 전 진료 제공자의 열 관련 질병은 직업적 위험에 해당하므로 EMS 및 기타 공공 안전 요원은 예방 전략을 사용하여 적절하고 관련성이 있는 경우 높은 주변 온도에 노출될 것에 대비해야 한다. 이러한 전략에는 행정 정책, 절차, 공학적 제어, 장비 사용 및 의료 감시 프로그램 등이 포함되며 급성 또는 만성 열 노출로 인한 전반적인 영향을 최소화하는 데 도움이 되도록 설계되었다. 간단한 예방 절차를 실행하는 것만으로도 열 관련 질환 발생률을 낮추는 데 큰 영향을 미칠 수 있다. **Box 19-5**는 병원 전 처치 제공자, 소방관, 기타 공공 안전 요원을 위한 열 스트레스 예방 전략에 대한 개요를 제공한다.

개인의 열 노출에 대한 허용 한계를 초과하는 여러 요인이 복합적으로 작용하여 결국 열 관련 질환의 증상과 징후가 나타날 수 있다. 체력, 열 순응, 생활 및 근무 환경, 개인위생, 체내 전해질과 수분 유지 및 보충을 위한 음식과 음료의 사용 등을 사전에 준비하면 중간 정도에서 더운 환경에서 근무할 수 있는 능력을 극대화할 수 있다. 환경, 수분 보충, 체력 및 열 순응은 필수적으로 이해해야 할 요소이다.

환경

병원 전 처치 제공자와 기타 공공 안전 요원은 직업적 요구 사항 일부로 고온 환경에 노출된다. 훈련 또는 응급상황 발생 시 많은 직원이 방호복, 위험 물질 보호복 또는 화학/생화학적 보호복과 같은 개인 보호복을 입고 작업하는 동안 높은 수준의 열 스트레스에 직면하게 된다. 이러한 열 스트레스는 환기가 잘되지 않거나 밀폐된 공간에 들어가거나 덥고 습한 날 햇볕이 내리쬐는 다중 충돌 사고 현장에서 작업을 해야 하는 경우 더욱 심해진다.

개인 보호복은 체온을 발산하는 신체의 능력을 저하하고 과중한 작업 중에 땀이 증발하는 것을 방지한다. 육체적으로 힘든 작업을 하는 동안 내부 열 생성과 외부 열 노출로 인해 땀을 많이 흘리는 사람은 탈수 및 열 질환에 걸릴 위험이 높다. 따라서 개인 보호복을 사용하면 열 순응과 체력을 통해 얻을 수 있는 생리학적 이점이 감소한다.

이러한 위험은 환경적 열 조건을 측정하고 해당하면 고온 환경에서 작업할 때 권장되는 휴식 및 수분 보충 지침을 준수함으로써 최소화할 수 있다.

열부하를 측정하는 전통적인 도구 중 하나는 열 스트레스 지수(Heat stress index) 이다(**그림 19-5**). 이 지수는 주변 온도와 상대 습도의 조합을 사용한다. 이는 주변 온도만 사용하는 것보다 잠재적인 전신 열 손상을 예측하는 데 더 좋은 방법이다. 직사광선이 비치는 곳, 열을 많이 방출하는 표면 근처 또는 두꺼운 보호복을 입고 작업하는 경우 **그림 19-5**의 표에 5.5℃를 더해야 한다.

많은 산업 및 군사 환경에서 사용되는 환경 열을 측정하기 위해 더 널리 사용되는 방법은 습구흑구온도지수(WBGT) 이다(**표 19-3**). 이 지수는 주변 온도에 대한 건구, 습도 측정은 습구, 복사열을 측정하기 위한 흑구 그리고 공기 이동의 조합을 사용하여 환경 조건의 영향을 더욱 정확하게 파악한다. 5단계 습구흑구온도 지수 범위의 온도에는 시간별 작업/휴식(분) 및 수분 섭취에 대한 지침이 통합되어 있다. 색상 플래그(깃발 없음, 녹색, 노란색, 빨간색, 검은색)는 5가지의 습구흑구온도지수의 온도 범위를 각각 나타낸다. 습구흑구온도지수는 매시간 모니터링할 수 있으며 모든 직원이 하루 종일 볼 수 있도록 야외 깃대에 해당 색상 깃발을 게시한다. 해당하면 이러한 습구흑구온도지수의 조건에 따라 복장, 신체 활동, 업무/휴식 주기, 수분 섭취량을 적절히 조정할 수 있다. 이와 같은 통합적 습구흑구온도지수 시스템과 관련 정책을 다양한 공공 안전 장소 및 훈련 현장에서 쉽게 개발하여 피로, 손상 및 열 질환을 줄이기 위한 효과적인 열 질환 예방 프로그램이 사용되도록 할 수 있다.

수분공급

수분 섭취에 대한 지침을 제공하는 데 습구흑구온도지수(WBGT) 깃발 시스템을 사용하지 않는 경우 미국 스포츠의학회(ASCM)에서 수년간의 연구를 바탕으로 발행한 또 다른 훌륭한 자료를 제시했다. 이 지침은 신체 활동을 하는 모든 사람에게 쉽게 적용할 수 있다. 특히 따뜻한 환경에서 활동하거나 갈증을 느낄 때 물과 스포츠 이온 음료를 쉽게 마실 수 있도록 하여 과도한 탈수(체중 2% 이상 감소)를 예방하기 위한 수분 보충 지침을 기관 내에 수립해야 한다(**Box 19-6**). 이상적으로 수분 보충 프로그램은 신체 활동 전후에 측정한 체중 감소 그리고 땀 손실, 체질량, 운동 강도를 기반으로 최적화되어야 한다.

Box 19-5 병원 전 처치 제공자의 열 관련 질환 예방

체력 수준을 향상하고 더위에 적응하면 열 질환으로 인한 심각한 결과를 예방할 수 있다.

유산소 운동을 통해 높은 수준의 체력을 유지하는 것은 열 스트레스로부터 자신을 보호하는 가장 좋은 방법 중 하나이다. 건강한 병원 전 처치 제공자는 순환계가 잘 발달하여 있고 혈액량이 증가한다. 이 두 가지 모두 체온을 조절하는 데 중요하다. 건강한 병원 전 처치 제공자는 땀을 더 빨리 흘리기 시작하므로 더 낮은 심박수와 체온으로 작업할 수 있다. 그들은 고온에 적응하지 못한 병원 전 처치 제공자보다 더위에 두 배 더 빨리 적응한다. 적응력을 잃는 속도도 더 느리고 빠르게 회복된다.

열 순응에 필요한 시간은 노출 시기와 빈도에 따라 다르며 열에 노출된 후 10~14일 이내에 신체가 다음과 같은 방식으로 변화하면서 적응하는 것으로 나타났다.

- 땀 생성 증가
- 심박수 감소
- 혈액 순환 개선
- 체온 감소

병원 전 처치 제공자로서 당신은 고온 환경에서 근무 시간을 점차 늘리고 수분을 보충하고 필요에 따라 휴식을 취함으로써 적응할 수 있다. 고온 환경에서 주기적으로 작업하거나 운동을 하면 열 순응이 유지된다.

작업 현장

열 스트레스 지수(그림 19-5 참조)는 온도와 습도가 결합하여 중간 정도의 열 스트레스 또는 높은 열 스트레스 조건을 만드는지 방법을 보여준다. 태양이나 주변 화염으로 인한 복사열이 높거나 바람이 불지 않을 때 또는 열심히 일하여 대사열이 많이 발생할 때는 열 스트레스에 대해 주의해야 한다. 열 스트레스 지수는 장시간의 고된 작업, 탈수 또는 개인 보호복과 장비의 영향은 고려하지 않는다.

열에 대한 스트레스가 있는 상황에서는 일하거나 운동하는 방법을 변경해야 한다. 자신의 페이스를 조절한다. 체력, 적응력, 내열성에는 개인차가 있다. 너무 무리하게 운동하면 열 관련 질환에 걸릴 수 있다.

가능하면 다음을 수행해야 한다.

- 열원 근처에서 작업하지 않는다.
- 서늘한 아침이나 저녁 시간에 더 열심히 작업한다.
- 피로를 최소화하기 위해 도구나 작업을 변경한다.
- 자주 휴식을 취한다.
- 가장 중요한 것은 손실된 수분을 보충하여 수분을 유지하는 것이다.

수분공급

체액을 유지하는 것은 신체 활동 중에 발생하는 땀과 체내 열을 제거하는 데 필수적이다. 탈수와 열 질환의 위험을 최소화하려면 운동이나 육체 활동 전이나 중간 또는 후에 수분을 보충해야 한다. 야생의학회는 과도한 수분 섭취와 운동 관련 열사병의 발병을 예방하는 동시에 적절한 수분 섭취를 보장하기 위해 적절한 수분 섭취(갈증 시)를 권장하고 있다. 병원 전 처치 제공자는 하루 종일 자신의 갈증 정도를 모니터링하고 체중이 2% 이상 감소하지 않도록 필요한 양만큼 수분을 섭취해야 한다. 개인의 특징(예: 체중, 유전적 요인, 열 순응 상태, 신진대사 상태)은 특정 활동의 땀 배출량에 영향을 미친다. 이러한 요인으로 인해 개인별 땀 배출 속도와 배출량이 크게 달라진다. 예를 들어, 장거리 달리기의 경우 여름철에 시간당 평균 1.4~1.9L의 땀을 흘리지만, 축구 선수는 시간당 1.9L에서 하루에 최대 8.5L의 땀을 흘리는 것으로 알려져 있다. 신체 활동을 하는 동안 탈수가 체중의 2%(활동 전에 옷을 벗은 상태의 체중)를 초과하지 않도록 자주 수분을 보충하는 것이 필요하다.

작업 전에 더위에 대비해 수분을 충분히 섭취해야 한다. 작업 전에 물, 주스 또는 이온 음료 200~500mL를 마신다. 신체 활동 전에 다량의 수분을 과도하게 섭취하는 것은 생리학적으로 이점이 없다. 미국 스포츠의학회는 이제 신체 활동 몇 시간 전에 천천히 수분을 섭취하고 체중 1kg당 약 5~7mL를 섭취할 것을 권장한다. 목표는 짚 색깔(담황색)에 가까운 맑은 소변을 배출하고 탈수 상태에서 활동을 시작하는 것을 방지하는 것이다.

작업 중에는 갈증을 느끼면 시간마다 여러 차례 수분을 섭취한다. 땀을 흘리는 속도와 시간당 필요한 물의 양은 개인마다 다를 수 있다. 다음과 같은 사항에 주의해야 한다. 시간당 개인별 땀 손실량을 확인하지 않은 상태에서 1.4L 이상을 초과하는 과도한 수분을 장시간 섭취하지 않도록 주의한다. 현재 미국 스포츠의학학회에서는 시간당 0.4~0.8L의 수분 섭취를 권장하며 서늘하거나 따뜻한 온도 조건에서의 활동과 체중이 가볍거나 무거운 사람에 따라 개인의 꽘 배량에 따라 수분 섭취량을 조정할 것을 권장하고 있다.

더위 속에서 일하는 동안 신체에 가장 필요한 것은 물이다. 연구 결과에 따르면 근로자는 향이 옅은 음료가 있을 때 더 많이 마시는 것으로 나타났다. 탄수화물과 이온 음료로 수분 보충의 일부를 제공하면 체액을 유지하고 에너

온도(℃) 대 상대적 습도 (%)

℃	90%	80%	70%	60%	50%	40%
26.6	85	84	82	81	80	79
29.4	101	96	92	90	86	84
32.2	121	113	105	99	94	90
35		133	122	113	105	98
37.7			142	129	118	109
40.5				148	133	121
43.3						135

온도	가능한 열 질환
26.7~32℃	장시간 노출과 신체활동에 따른 피로 발생 가능성이 있음
32~40.5℃	일사병, 열경련, 열탈진 발생 가능성이 있음
40.5~54.5℃	일사병, 열경련, 열탈진, 열사병 발생 가능성이 있음
54.5℃ 이상	지속된 노출에 의해 열사병이 발생 가능성이 높음

열지수(heat index)의 계산 특성에 따라, 위의 표는 ± 0.7℃의 오차가 있을 수 있다.

그림 19-5 열 스트레스 지수
Courtesy of the National Weather Service, Pueblo, Colorado. https://www.weather.gov/pub/

(다음 페이지에 계속)

Box 19-5 병원 전 처치 제공자의 열 관련 질환 예방 (이어서)

지와 전해질 수준을 유지하는 데 도움이 된다. 안타깝게도 많은 이온 음료에는 다량의 설탕이 함유되어 있어 실제로 섭취한 수분의 흡수를 늦출 수 있다. 작업 후에는 손실된 수분을 보충하기 위해 계속 물을 마셔야 한다. 땀을 많이 흘리는 활동(예: 화재 진압)으로 인해 손실된 수분을 신속하고 완벽하게 회복하려면 체중 1kg이 감소할 때마다 약 1.5L의 수분을 마셔야 한다. 수액이 나트륨과 칼륨이 포함되어 있거나 이러한 전해질이 포함된 음식을 섭취하면 수분 공급 효과가 향상된다.

감자, 자두 주스, 당근 주스, 바나나와 감귤류 등 칼륨이 풍부한 식품을 규칙적으로 섭취하고 레모네이드, 오렌지 주스, 토마토 주스 등 수분 섭취량을 다양하게 늘린다. 카페인은 소변으로 수분 손실을 증가시키기 때문에 커피나 콜라와 같은 카페인 음료의 양을 제한한다. 알코올 성분의 음료는 탈수를 유발하므로 마시지 않는다. 일반적인 바이러스 질환을 예방하려면 응급상황을 제외하고는 물병을 같이 사용하지 않는다.

소변의 양, 색깔 및 농도를 관찰하여 수분 보충 상태를 재평가할 수 있다. 진하고 농축된 소변의 양이 적고 배뇨 시 통증이 있다면 심각한 수분 보충이 필요하다는 신호이다. 탈수의 다른 징후로는 빠른 심박수, 쇠약, 과도한 피로, 어지럼 등이 있다. 체중이 몇 kg 급격히 감소하는 것은 탈수의 확실한 징후이다. 업무에 복귀하기 전에 수분을 보충한다. 탈수 상태에서 계속 작업을 하면 열사병, 근육 융해 및 신부전과 같은 심각한 결과를 초래할 수 있다.

의류

개인 보호복은 보호와 편안함 사이의 균형을 유지해야 한다. 호주 연구진은 개인보호장비를 착용하고 작업을 하는 것은 열을 차단하는 것이 아니라 열을 내보내는 것이라는 결론을 내렸다. 열부하의 약 70%는 힘든 작업 중에 발생하는 신진대사 열로 인해 내부에서 발생하고 30%만이 환경으로부터 발생한다. 공기의 흐름을 원활하게 하려고 헐렁한 옷을 입는다. 더운 환경에서 땀이 증발할 수 있도록 면 티셔츠와 속옷을 입는다. 단열을 방해하고 공기 흐름을 제한하며 열 스트레스를 유발할 수 있는 옷을 여러 겹 겹쳐 입지 않는다.

개인 차이

더위에 대한 반응은 사람마다 다르다. 소방관과 같은 일부 구급 및 구조대원은 근무 환경과 장비 요구 사항으로 인해 열 관련 질환에 걸릴 위험이 더 높다. 다른 이유로는 내열성과 땀 배출량의 유전적 차이, 신진대사 열 생산을 증가시키는 과체중, 질병, 불법 약물 및 약물 복용 등이 있으며 더운 환경에서 근무할 때 신체 반응에 영향을 미칠 수 있다. 처방 약이나 일반의약품을 복용 중이거나 질병이 있는 경우 의사나 약사에게 문의한다. 문제 발생 시 도움을 줄 수 있는 동료와 함께 항상 훈련하고 협력해야 한다. 서로에게 수분 섭취를 상기시키고 서로를 지켜본다. 동료에게 열 관련 질환이 나타나면 즉시 처치를 시작한다.

요약

예방

■ 유산소 운동을 통해 체력을 향상하거나 유지한다.

■ 열에 적응한다.

작업 중

■ 주변 환경(예: 온도, 습도, 바람)에 유의한다.

■ 자주 휴식을 취하고 갈증을 해소하기 위해 주기적으로 수분을 섭취한다.

■ 옷을 여러 겹 겹쳐 입지 않는다.

■ 일정한 속도를 유지한다.

수분 보충

■ 수분 보충 목표는 체중의 2% 이상 탈수(땀 손실)를 예방하는 것이다.

■ 작업 전에는 물, 주스 또는 이온 음료를 여러 컵 마신다.

■ 작업 중에는 수시로 수분을 섭취한다.

■ 작업 후에는 수분을 보충하기 위해 계속 물을 마신다.

■ 당신만이 탈수를 예방할 수 있다는 사실을 기억한다.

동료

■ 항상 동료와 같이 작업하거나 훈련한다.

음료

■ 탄수화물(5~10%)과 전해질(예: 나트륨 20~50mEq/L, 칼륨 2~5mEq/L)이 함유된 이온 음료는 수분 섭취를 촉진하고 에너지를 공급하며 소변으로 배출되는 수분 손실을 줄여준다. 탄수화물은 또한 장시간 힘든 작업을 하는 동안 면역 기능과 정신 상태를 유지하는 데 도움이 된다. 카페인과 알코올이 함유된 음료는 소변 생성을 증가시켜 수분 보충을 방해한다.

Modified from U.S. Department of Agriculture, U.S. Forest Service: Heat Stress Brochure, American College of Sports Medicine. Position stand: exercise and fluid replacement. *Med Sci Sports Exerc.* 2007;39(2):377.

운동

고온 환경에서 효과적으로 내열성을 높이려면 병원 전 처치 제공자는 개별화된 프로그램(예: 걷기, 조깅, 자전거 타기, 수영, 계단 오르내리기, 타원형 운동기구 사용)을 통해 유산소 능력을 증가시켜야 한다. 이러한 프로그램은 고온 환경에서 신체 활동과 열 발산 기전(체온조절)의 요구를 충족시키는 데 필요한 심박출량을 유지할 수 있는 심장 예비력을 제공한다. 미국 스포츠의학회, 미국 심장협회, 보건복지부가 협력하여 건강과 웰빙을 유지하기 위한 전국적인 신체 활동 권장 사항을 업데이트했다.

열 순응

공공 안전 조직 내에 열 순응을 위한 정책과 지침을 마련해야 한다. 열 순응은 약 8~14일 동안 하루에 60~120분 동안 열에 노출되는 운동으로 달성할 수 있다. 열 순응의 이점은 업무 수행 능력 향상, 내열성 향상, 생리적 긴장 감소이다. 이러한 적응에는 혈액량 증가, 박출량 증가, 특정 활동 수준에서 심박수 감소, 땀의 나트륨 농도 감소, 체내의 나트륨 보존, 발한 시작 시간 단축, 땀 배출량 증가 등이 포함된다(**Box 19-7**). 지구력 운동선수, 군 보병 등 열에 잘 견디는 사람들은 열 순응이 향상되어 바람직한 것으로 간주하지만, 시간당 1~2L의

표 19-3 더운 날씨 훈련 시 수분 보충 지침								
		쉬운 작업		적당한 작업		힘든 작업		
열 범주	WBGT 지수 (℃)	일/휴식(분)	수분 섭취 (mL/hr)	일/휴식 (분)	수분 섭취 (mL/hr)	일/휴식 (분)	수분 섭취 (mL/hr)	
1	25.5~27.7	NL	500mL	NL	750mL	20/20	750mL	
2	27.8~29.3	NL	500mL	50/10	750mL	30/30	1,000mL	
3	29.4~31.0	NL	750mL	40/20	750mL	30/30	1,000mL	
4	31.1~32.1	NL	750mL	30/30	750mL	20/40	1,000mL	
5	>32.2	50/10	1,000mL	20/40	1,000mL	10/50	1,000mL	

		쉬운 작업	보통 작업	힘든 일
		딱딱한 표면에서 4km/h로 14kg 미만의 무게를 들고 걷는 경우	딱딱한 도면에서 5.6km/h로 19kg 미만의 무게를 들고 걷는 경우 부드러운 모래 위를 4km/h로 걷기, 맨손 체조	딱딱한 표면에서 6km/h로 18kg 미만의 무게를 들고 걷는 경우 짐을 들고 부드러운 모래 위를 4km/h로 걷기

Abbreviations: kph, kilometers per hour; lb, pound; mph, miles per hour; NL, no limit to work time; WBGT, wet-bulb globe temperature.

참고: 작업/휴식 시간 및 수분 보충량은 지정된 열 범주에서 최소 4시간 동안 작업할 때 성능과 수분 공급을 유지한다. 개인마다 필요한 수분량은 다를 수 있다. 휴식은 최소한의 신체 활동(앉거나 서 있는)을 의미하며 가능하면 그늘에서 이루어진다.

주의: 시간당 수분 섭취량은 1.4L를 초과하지 않아야 한다. 일일 수분 섭취량은 11.4L를 초과하지 않아야 한다. 보호복 착용 시: 습한 기후에서는 WBGT 지수에 2.75℃를 추가한다. 의복 위에 개인보호장비를 착용하는 경우 쉬운 작업의 경우 WBGT 지수에 5.5℃를 추가하고 중간 정도 및 힘든 작업의 경우 WBGT 지수에 11℃를 추가한다.

Current version of WBGT, hydration, and work/rest guidelines as updated by U.S. Army Research Institute for Environmental Medicine (USARIEM) and published by Montain SJ, Latzka WA, Sawka MN. *Mil Med*. 1999;64:502.

땀을 더 많이 흘리면 체액 손실이 커져 탈수가 발생할 수 있다. 따라서 더 위에 잘 적응하는 사람의 땀 손실량이 많을수록 더위에 노출되는 동안, 특히 경구 수분 공급 일정을 엄격하게 지키지 않는 경우 수분 공급 요구량이 증가한다. **Box 19-8**은 열 순응 지침에 대한 개요를 제공한다.

응급 사고 재활

극도로 더운 환경에서 작업하는 동안 적절한 예방 조치(예: 수분 보충, 열 순응)를 취하더라도 EMS 종사자는 때때로 신체적 한계에 부딪히게 된다. 특히 소방관은 작업 환경에 따라 다양한 개인보호장비를 착용할 수 있다. 이러한 개인보호장비는 무겁고 제한적인 경우가 많아 현장에서 겪는 열 스트레스를 많이 증가시킬 수 있다. 재활은 과로 후가 아니라 과로 시점 이전에 이루어져야 한다. 재활에는 다음과 같은 원칙이 적용된다.

- 극한의 기후 조건에서 벗어나기
- 휴식 및 회복
- 필요한 경우 냉각 또는 재가온
- 수분 보충(체액 보충)
- 열량 및 전해질 보충
- 의료 모니터링
- 팀원 추적(책임)

한랭으로 의한 손상

탈수

탈수는 특히 신체 활동이 증가한 추운 날씨에 매우 쉽게 발생한다. 탈수는 다음과 같은 세 가지 주요 원인으로 발생한다.

- 땀의 증발
- 차가운 공기의 건조로 인한 호흡기 열 및 체액 손실 증가

Box 19-6 탈수를 최소화하기 위한 수분공급 지침

일반 원칙

특히 운동이나 신체 활동이 많은 활동을 할 때는 수분 섭취를 유지하는 것이 중요하다. 땀을 얼마나 많이 흘리느냐에 따라 필요한 수분 섭취량은 달라진다. 기억해야 할 일반적인 원칙은 다음과 같다.

1. 운동 전과 운동 중 그리고 목이 마를 때 물을 마신다.
2. 손실된 수분을 보충하기 위해 물과 이온 음료를 마신다.
3. 운동 전후의 체중을 측정하여 수분 섭취량이 충분한지, 부족한지, 과한지 확인한다.

운동하지 않을 때도 충분히 마신다. 평상시에는 수분 섭취를 잘하지 않다가 운동을 하면 더 빨리 탈수될 수 있다.

체중

체중은 수분 보충(또는 탈수)을 결정하는 데 사용되는 요소이다. 신체 활동 중에 손실된 수분을 보충하는 것이 중요하다. 이 수분을 보충하지 않으면 운동 후 체중이 감소한다. 반대로 신체 활동 중에 과도한 양의 물을 마시면 수분 섭취로 인해 체중이 증가할 수 있다. 이상적으로는 운동 전후의 체중이 거의 같아야 하며 이는 적절한 수분 수준을 유지했음을 나타낸다.

운동 중 수분을 충분히 섭취하지 않으면 운동 후에 수분을 보충해야 한다. 탈수를 체중 감량 방법으로 사용하지 않는다.

음료의 종류

충분한 양의 수분을 마시는 것을 기억하는 것 외에도 어떤 종류의 수분을 마셔야 하는지 아는 것이 중요하다. 격렬한 운동 중에 물만 마시면 전해질 불균형을 초래할 수 있다. 이온 음료는 땀으로 손실된 전해질을 보충하기 위해 고안된 제품이다. 그러나 대부분 스포츠음료에는 탄수화물이 과도하게 함유되어 있으므로 경구용 수분 보충제는 탄수화물 함량이 6%를 넘지 않아야 한

다. 많은 시판 스포츠음료는 물로 희석하여 이 탄수화물 농도에 도달할 수 있다. 운동 중에는 저나트륨혈증을 나타낼 수 있는 손과 발의 부종, 두통, 복부 팽만감에 주의한다.

또한, 운동선수이거나 격렬한 신체 활동이 필요한 직업에 종사하는 경우 식단에 적당량의 소금을 포함하여 신체의 염화나트륨 필요량 증가를 충족하는 데 도움이 되도록 한다.

수분 섭취 권장 사항

수분 보충(물 및 이온 음료)을 위한 권장 사항은 다음과 같다(**표 19-4**).

표 19-4 수분 섭취 권장 사항	
시간	**수량**
운동 4시간 전	0.5~0.6L
운동 10~15분 전	0.2~0.4L
60분 미만의 운동 중	15~20분마다 0.1~0.2L
60분 이상의 운동 중	15~20분마다 이온 음료 0.1~0.2L
운동 후(2시간 이내)	체중 0.5kg 감소마다 0.6~0.7L

Data from American College of Sports Medicine. Selecting and effectively using hydration for fitness. Accessed October 25, 2021. https://www.yumpu.com/en/document/read/46203304/selecting-and-effectively-using-hydration-for-fitness-american

---

Box 19-7 열 순응의 이점

1. 열 쾌적성: 개선됨
2. 중심체온: 감소
3. 피부 혈류: 더 빨라짐
4. 심박수: 감소
5. 염분 소실(땀 및 소변): 감소
6. 운동 능력: 향상
7. 발한: 더 일찍 그리고 더 많이
8. 체열 생성: 감소
9. 갈증: 개선
10. 장기 보호: 개선됨

Reproduced from the Heat Acclimatization Guide, Ranger and Airborne School Students. Accessed October 25, 2021. https://www.usariem.army.mil/assets/docs/partnering/HeatAcclimatizationGuide.pdf

- 한랭 유발 이뇨

한랭 유발 이뇨는 장시간 추위에 노출되었을 때 피부 혈관 수축으로 인해 발생하는 정상적인 생리적 반응이다. 이는 혈액을 차가운 신체 말단에서 체내의 깊은 정맥으로 혈액을 순환시켜 체온 손실을 줄이기 위한 신체의 반응이다. 이러한 반응으로 인해 중심 혈액량을 증가시켜 평균 동맥압, 일회박출량, 심박출량이 증가한다. 증가한 혈액

량은 잦은 배뇨로 나타나는 이뇨 작용을 일으킬 수 있다. 한랭 유발 이뇨는 혈장량을 7~15% 감소시켜 혈중 농축과 급성 탈수를 유발할 수 있으며 이는 정상보다 거의 두 배에 달하는 체액 손실로 이어진다.

더위에 노출될 때와 마찬가지로 추운 환경에서 작업하는 동안 목이 마르면 수분 보충 지침을 준수하고 수분을 섭취해야 관련 피로 및 신체적, 인지적 변화와 함께 탈수를 최소화할 수 있다. 추운 환경에서는 갈증이 억제되기 때문에 탈수는 심각한 위험이다.

경미한 한랭 관련 질환

접촉 동결 손상

차가운 물질이 보호되지 않은 피부에 닿으면 즉시 국소 동상을 일으킬 수 있다. 금속 표면, 알코올, 휘발유, 부동액, 얼음 또는 눈을 손으로 만지지 않는다. 평가와 처치에 대해서는 동상 부분을 참조한다(**Box 19-9**).

Box 19-8 열 순응 지침

다음은 더운 환경에서 신체 활동에 대비하여 건강하고 체력이 좋은 보병 장병들을 위해 고안된 더위 적은 지침의 수정 버전이다.

더운 날씨에 대해 걱정해야 하는가?

시원하거나 온화한 기후에서 일하는 데 익숙하다면 더운 날씨에 노출되면 작업을 완료하기가 훨씬 더 어려워질 수 있다. 더운 날씨는 피로를 느끼게 하고 회복을 더 어렵게 만들며 열 관련 질환의 위험을 높인다. 같은 능력을 갖춘 사람이라도 더운 날씨에서 일하는 데 익숙한 사람은 더위에 노출되었을 때 더 큰 내성과 신체 능력을 발휘한다.

열 순응이란 무엇인가?

열 순응은 생리적 부담(예: 심박수, 체온)을 줄이고 신체 작업 능력을 개선하며 편안함을 개선하고 중요한 장기(뇌, 간, 신장, 근육)를 열 손상으로부터 보호하는 생리학적 적응을 말한다. 열 순응에서 가장 중요한 생리학적 적응은 더 일찍 더 많이 땀을 흘리는 반응이며 이 반응을 개선하기 위해서는 발한이 필요하다.

열 순응은 기후와 신체 활동 수준에 따라 다르다. 가볍거나 짧은 육체적 작업만 수행하는 개인은 해당 작업을 수행하는 데 필요한 수준의 열 적응을 달성할 수 있다. 더 힘들거나 장기간의 작업을 시도하는 경우 더위 속에서 해당 작업을 성공적으로 수행하려면 추가적인 순응과 체력 향상이 필요하다.

어떻게 열에 순응할 수 있는가?

열 순응은 반복적인 더위 노출이 체온을 상승시키고 땀을 많이 흘리게 할 만큼 충분한 스트레스를 유발할 때 발생한다. 생존에 필요한 수준으로 신체 활동을 제한한 채 더위 속에서 휴식을 취하면 부분적인 적응만 이루어진다. 주어진 더운 환경에서 운동 강도에 맞는 최적의 열 적응을 달성하려면 더위 속에서의 신체 활동이 필요하다.

일반적으로 열 순응을 유도하려면 매일 약 8~14일의 열 노출이 필요하다. 열 적응하려면 근력 운동보다 심폐지구력이 필요한 운동(예: 조깅)과 함께 매일 최소 1시간~2시간(1시간씩 2회로 나누어 노출 가능)의 열 노출이 필요하다. 매일 운동 강도나 지속 시간을 서서히 늘린다. 필요한 신체 활동에 맞는 적절한 훈련 일정에 따라 운동한다.

열 순응의 이점은 약 1주일간 유지되다가 더위 노출이 끝나면 약 3주가 지나면 약 75%가 사라지면서 감소한다. 하루나 이틀 동안 시원한 날씨가 이어진다고 해서 더운 날씨에 적응하는 데 방해가 되지는 않는다.

얼마나 빨리 열에 순응할 수 있을까?

평균적으로 개인의 경우 더위에 적응하려면 약 8~14일 동안 더위에 노출되고 육체적 노동이 점진적으로 증가해야 한다. 순응 둘째 날에는 생리학적 스트레스의 현저한 감소가 관찰된다. 1주와 2주가 끝날 무렵에는 각각 60% 이상, 80% 이상의 생리학적 적응이 완료된다. 체력이 약한 사람이나 열 노출에 비정상적으로 취약한 사람은 완전히 적응하는 데 며칠 또는 몇 주가 더 필요할 수 있다.

신체적으로 건강한 사람은 약 1주일이면 더위에 적응할 수 있다. 그러나 고온에서 견딜 수 있는 내성을 극대화하려면 몇 주 동안 더위 속에서 생활하고 일해야 할 수도 있다.

가장 좋은 열 적응 전략은 무엇인가?

1. 더운 날씨에 노출되기 전에 체력을 극대화하고 더위에 적응한다. 서늘한 아침이나 저녁 시간에 체력단련 등 환경에 맞는 유지 관리 프로그램을 통해 체력을 유지한다.
2. 훈련과 더위 적응을 통합한다. 하루 중 가장 시원한 시간대에 훈련하고 한낮에는 더위에 적응한다. 온화한 기후에서 달성할 수 있는 것보다 평소 훈련 강도와 시간을 줄여서 천천히 시작한다. 고온에서 견딜 수 있는 정도에 따라 훈련 강도와 열 노출을 점차 늘린다. 인터벌 트레이닝을 사용하여 활동 수준을 조절한다.
3. 새로운 기후가 익숙한 기후보다 훨씬 더운 경우 처음 2일 동안은 달리기, 걷기 등의 레크리에이션 활동이 적절하다. 3일째가 되면 조금 더 높은 강도에서 달리기를 20~40분을 통합해서 할 수 있다.
4. 땀으로 손실된 수분을 보충하기 위해 충분한 물을 섭취한다. 시간당 0.9L 이 상의 땀을 흘리는 것이 일반적이다. 결과적으로 더위에 적응한 사람은 수분을 섭취하지 않으면 탈수 증상이 더 빨리 나타난다. 탈수는 열 적응과 체력 향상으로 인한 체온 조절 능력의 많은 이점을 무력화시킨다.

Data from Sawka MN, Kolka MA, Montain SJ. *Ranger and Airborne School Students' Heat Acclimatization Guide*. U.S. Army Research Institute of Environmental Medicine; 2003.

동상

동상은 종종 전조 증상으로 국소 조직에서 피부가 창백해지고 무감각해지는 가역적인 징후를 나타낸다. 동상은 일반적으로 뺨, 코, 귓불에 나타난다. 경미한 동상은 추위에 계속 노출되지 않는 한 제한적이고 동결 조직 손상으로 병원 전 처치 제공자의 처치와 의료기관으로 이송이 필요하지 않다.

저온 두드러기

저온 두드러기는 추위에 노출된 후 피부의 가려움증, 발적, 부종이 빠르게(수분 이내) 시작되는 것이 특징인 질환이다. 작열감이 두드러지게 나타날 수 있다. 히스타민의 국소적 방출로 인해 발생하는 이 증상은 염좌 및 타박상을 처치하기 위한 냉찜질을 시행하는 동안 피부에 얼음을 직접 적용할 때 관찰된다. 저온두드러기 병력이 있는 사람은 전신 아나필락시스로 인해 사망할 수 있으므로 찬물에 몸을 담그는 것을 피하는 것이 좋다. 처치에는 추위를 피하고 항히스타민제를 복용하는 것이 포함된다.

Box 19-9 동상 예방

외딴 곳이나 혹독한 환경에서 여행하거나 대응하는 사람들을 위해 야생의학회는 동상 예방 및 처치에 대한 자세한 진료 지침을 제공한다.

동창

동창은 만성적인 추위 노출로 인해 손가락의 신근 피부 표면 또는 모든 피부 표면(주로 발, 손, 다리, 허벅지)에 발생하는 가렵고 압통이 있는 푸르스름한 붉은 융기로 나타나는 동결되지 않은 저온 손상이다(그림 19-6). 동창은 온대 습한 기후에서 추위에 노출된 후 몇 시간 후에 발생한다. 때때로 햇빛 노출로 인해 악화하기도 한다. 추위는 피부의 소동맥과 정맥을 수축시키고 다시 따뜻해지면 혈액이 조직으로 누출되어 피부가 부어오른다.

동창은 말초 순환이 좋지 않은 사람들에게서 발생할 가능성이 더 높다. 가족력, 당뇨병, 흡연, 고지혈증, 영양부족(예: 신경성 식욕부진), 결합조직 질환, 골수 장애로 인한 말초 혈관 질환 등이 원인이 될 수 있다. 수포는 몇 시간에 걸쳐 가렵고 푸르스름한 부종으로 나타나며 7~14일 이내에 가라앉는다. 심한 경우 물집, 고름집, 딱지, 궤양이 발생할 수 있다. 때때로 병변이 고리 모양으로 나타날 수 있으며 두꺼워지고 수개월 동안 지속될 수 있다.

추위에서 벗어나면 증상이 가라앉는다. 적절한 장갑과 의복으로 환자를 추위로부터 보호하는 것이 처치의 핵심이다.

자외선(태양광) 각막염(설맹)

눈에 반사되는 밝은 빛에 노출되지 않도록 보호하지 않으면 피부와 눈에 자외선으로 인한 화상을 입을 위험이 높아진다. 이러한 위험은 고도가 높을수록 크게 증가한다. 태양 각막염은 노출 단계에서 교묘하게 발생하며 각막 및 결막 상피 화상은 2시간 이내에 발생하지만, 노출 후 6~12시간이 지나야 뚜렷하게 나타난다.

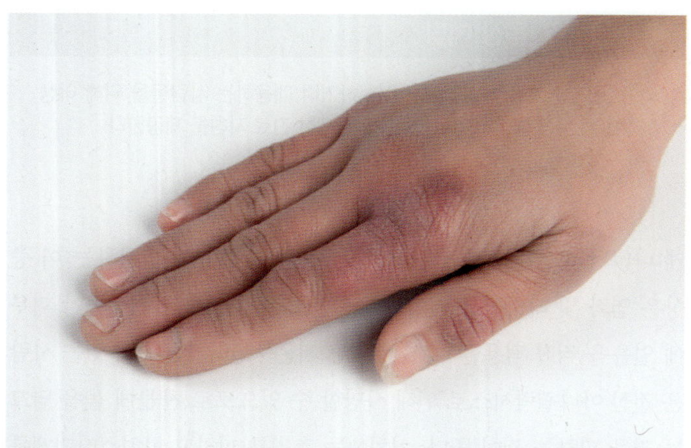

그림 19-6 동창은 발, 손, 다리, 넓적다리에 가장 흔하게 발생한다.
© kungfu01/Shutterstock

설맹은 과도한 눈물, 심한 통증, 충혈, 눈꺼풀 부종, 빛을 볼 때의 통증, 두통, 눈의 이물감, 시력 저하(흐릿함) 등의 증상에 따라 처치한다. 병원 전 처치 제공자는 추가 자외선 노출을 방지할 수 있는 다른 방법(예: 선글라스)이 없는 경우 영향을 받은 눈에 드레싱을 적용한 후 환자를 이송하는 것을 고려한다. 가능한 경우 국소 안과 마취제를 사용하여 증상을 완화할 수 있다. 손상의 중증도를 파악하고 항생제 및 진통제를 투여할지 결정하기 위해 의료기관에서의 평가와 처치가 필요하다.

주요 한랭 관련 질환

국소적인 피부 한랭 손상

저온 손상은 신체의 말초 부위에서 발생하며 동결(예: 동상) 또는 동결되지 않은(예: 동창, 침족병) 손상으로 분류된다. 국소적인 저온손상은 한랭 노출에 대한 적절한 준비, 저온 손상의 조기 인지 및 효과적인 처치를 통해 예방할 수 있다. 그러나 팔다리 손실의 위험이 있는 가장 심한 형태의 저온 손상인 동상은 이 부분에서 가장 우려되는 주요 손상이다.

저온 손상을 유발하는 요인에 대한 이해를 통해 예방하는 것이 중요하다. 니코틴, 알코올 중독, 노숙자, 주요 정신 질환은 여전히 중요한 발병 요인이다. 꽉 끼거나 조이는 옷, 너무 많은 양말, 꽉 끼는 신발은 동상 발병을 예측할 수 있는 요인이다. 겨울철에 실시하는 모험적인 스포츠 및 기타 여가 활동이 증가함에 따라 국소 저온 손상이 더 자주 발생한다.

병원 전 처치 제공자는 추운 환경에 장시간 노출된 환자의 체온 손실을 방지하고 노출된 피부를 동상으로부터 보호를 한다. 예를 들어, 차량에서 구출이 필요한 환자, 환자를 움직일 수 없는 상황, 연부조직 부종이 있는 환자의 경우 추운 환경에서 혈액 순환 장애로 인해 국소적 저온 손상의 발생률이 증가할 수 있다. 동상이나 다른 저온 손상을 입은 모든 환자를 처치하는 데 있어 우선순위는 환자가 추위에 더 이상 노출되지 않도록 보호하고 저체온증 예방 및 처치에 집중하는 것이다.

동결되지 않은 저온손상

동결되지 않은 저온손상(NFCI)은 얼지는 않지만, 추운 온도에서 조직에 손상을 입히는 증후군이다. 대부분 침수발 및 참호발과 관련된 이 증후군은 팔다리에 영향을 미칠 수 있다. 동결되지 않은 저온 손상은 장시간(수 시간에서 수일) 습하고 추운 환경에 노출되어 말초 조직이 손상되어 발생하며 조직의 동결은 수반되지 않지만, 동상과 같은 동결 손상과 공존할 수 있다. 이 증후군은 주로 발에 발생하며 두 가지 유형의 동결되지 않은 저온 손상으로 나타난다. 다음과 같은 손상은 임상적으로 같지만, 서로 다른 환경 조건으로 인해 발생한다. 참호발은 주로 보병 작전 중 군인에게서 발생하며 장기간의 추위 노출과 발의 혈액 순환 제한이 복합적으로 작용하여 발생하고 물에 잠기는 것과는 관련이 없다. 참호발은 물에 잠기는 것을 포함하지 않는다. 침수발은 차갑거나 차가운 물에 팔다리를 장기간 담가서 발생한다. 노숙자, 알코올 중독자, 노인, 등산객, 사냥꾼, 수일간 모험 스포츠를 즐기는 선수, 해양 생존자에게서 침수발이 나타날 수 있다. 부츠나 신발을 벗고 발을 검사하지 않거나 동결되지 않은 저온 손상에 대한 공식적인 의료 교육이 부족하므로 춥거나 습한 환경에 노출된 사람을 평가하는 동안, 이 증후군이 인식되지 않는 경우가 많다. 침수발은 침수 깊이에 따라 무릎 위까지 확장될 수 있다.

이 증후군은 0~15℃ 범위의 온도에서 수 시간 동안 다리가 차가워진 결과로 발생한다. 발 피부에 연부조직 손상이 발생하는데 이를 짓무름이라 한다. 피부가 손상되면 감염에 취약해진다. 이차 허혈 손상으로 인한 말초 신경과 혈관에 가장 큰 손상이 나타난다. 경중의 동결되지 않은 저온 비동결 저온 손상은 처음에는 자체적으로 제한되지만, 장기간 추위에 계속 노출되면 돌이킬 수 없게 된다. 발이 젖고 차가우면 위험이 높아지고 젖은 양말은 단열 효과가 떨어지고 물은 같은 온도의 공기보다 더 효과적으로 냉각되기 때문에 손상의 진행이 가속화된다. 꽉 끼는 옷, 부츠, 장시간 움직이지 않는 자세, 저체온증, 웅크린 자세 등 팔다리의 혈액 순환을 감소시키는 모든 요인이 손상의 원인이 될 수 있다. 동결되지 않은 저온 손상은 다음과 같이 4단계로 분류된다.

- **최소**: 발로 가는 혈류의 증가와 약간의 감각 변화로 인한 충혈은 손상 후 2~3일 후에도 남아있을 수 있다. 이 상태는 자체적으로 제한되며 7일 후에도 손상 징후가 남지 않는다. 종종 추위에 대한 민감성이 남아있을 수 있다.
- **경중**: 부종, 충혈, 경미한 감각 변화는 손상 후 2~3일 동안 지속된다. 손상 7일이 지나면 발바닥 표면과 발가락 끝에 무감각증이 나타나며 4~9주 동안 지속된다. 물집과 피부 손상은 관찰되지 않으며 걸을 때 통증을 유발하지 않으면 보행이 가능하다.
- **중등도**: 부종, 충혈, 물집, 반점이 손상 2~3일 후에 나타난다. 7일이 지나면 발등 및 발바닥 표면과 발가락 모두에서 무감각증이 나타난다. 부종은 2~3주 동안 지속되며 통증과 충혈은 최대 14주까지

지속된다. 일부 물집이 벗겨지지만, 심부 조직의 손상은 없다. 일부 환자는 영구적인 손상을 입을 수 있다.
- **중증**: 심한 부종, 주변 조직으로 혈액 유출(혈관 외 유출), 괴저가 손상 후 2~3일 후에 나타난다. 발 전체에 대한 완전한 무감각증이 7일이 지나도 남아 있으며 팔다리의 마비와 근육 소모가 나타난다. 손상은 다리 아래쪽까지 이어진다. 이 심각한 손상은 조직 손실을 초래하여 자동 절단(죽은 조직을 비수술적으로 절단하는 것)을 초래한다. 괴저는 조직 손실이 완료될 때까지 지속적인 위험이다. 환자는 장기간의 회복 기간과 영구적인 장애를 겪을 것으로 예상된다.

평가

환자가 경중이거나 중등도의 추위에 노출되었으므로 저체온증을 배제하고 탈수 여부를 평가하는 것은 필수이다. 이 두 가지 국소적 한랭 손상의 공통점은 손상이 발생하는 동안 무감각 또는 무감각이 발생할 정도로 팔다리가 차가워진다는 점이며 동상이 아니더라도 동결되지 않은 저온 손상은 교묘하고 잠재적으로 장애를 유발할 수 있는 손상이다.

동결되지 않은 저온 손상 처치의 핵심은 평가 중 이를 감지하고 인식하는 것이다. 일차평가 시 손상된 조직은 창백함, 부종, 짓무름이 나타나고 무감각하며 맥박이 없고 움직이지 않지만, 얼지 않은 상태로 보인다. 환자는 걸으려고 할 때 서툴고 비틀거린다고 호소한다. 추위에서 벗어난 후 재가온 중 또는 재가온 후에 허혈 조직의 재관류가 시작되면서 말초 혈류가 증가한다. 팔다리의 색이 흰색에서 얼룩덜룩한 옅은 파란색으로 변하면서 차갑고 무감각한 상태가 유지된다. 일반적으로 수동적으로 발을 따뜻하게 한 후에도 이러한 증상이 변하지 않으면 참호발 또는 침수발로 진단한다. 재가온 후 24~36시간이 지나면 심한 타는 듯한 통증과 함께 충혈이 발생하고 원위부가 아닌 근위부의 감각이 다시 나타난다. 이것은 정맥혈관 확장으로 인해 발생한다. 관류가 증가함에 따라 손상 부위에 부종과 물집이 생긴다. 충혈이 나타난 후에도 피부는 관류가 잘 이루어지지 않으면 손상이 진행됨에 따라 피부가 벗겨질 수 있다. 손상을 입은 팔다리에서 48시간이 지나도 맥박이 없다면 심하고 깊은 손상을 입은 것으로 조직 소실이 심하고 괴저가 발생할 가능성이 높다는 것을 의미한다.

처치

동결되지 않은 저온 손상이 감지되면 우선순위는 환자 또는 팔다리의 추가 냉각을 차단하고 손상 부위의 추가 손상을 방지하며 환자를

이송하는 것이다. 환자가 다친 다리로 걷지 못하게 하고 신발과 양말을 조심스럽게 벗긴다. 손상된 부위 또는 팔다리를 느슨하고 건조한 멸균 드레싱을 시행하고 추위로부터 보호하며 이송 중에 손상된 조직을 수동적으로 재가온하기 시작한다. 담요의 무게로 인해 손상 부위가 더 악화할 수 있다. 적극적인 재가온은 필요하지 않다. 환부를 마사지하면 조직이 더 손상될 수 있으므로 마사지를 하지 않는다. 필요하면 정맥 내로 수액을 투여하여 탈수 환자를 처치하고 재평가한다. 이송 시간에 따라 조직이 재관류하기 시작하면서 수동적 재가온 중에 심한 통증이 발생할 수 있다.

동결 저온 손상

동상(조직 손실 없음)으로 시작된 말초 조직의 저온 노출의 연속선상에서 동상은 경미한 조직 파괴부터 중증의 혈관 수축으로 인한 조직 손실까지 다양하다. 동상에 가장 취약한 신체 부위는 귀, 코와 같이 표면적 대비 질량 비율이 큰 조직이거나 손, 손가락, 발, 발가락 및 남성 생식기와 같이 신체 중심에서 가장 멀리 떨어진 부위이다. 발과 발가락은 가장 흔하게 영향을 받는 부위이다. 발과 발가락은 혈관 수축 시 혈액이 쉽게 우회시키는 동정맥 모세혈관 연결부위를 포함하기 때문에 저온 손상에 가장 취약한 구조이다. 바람직하지 않은 온도에 대한 신체의 정상적인 반응은 피부 표면으로의 혈류를 감소시켜 환경과의 열 교환을 줄이는 것이다. 우리 몸은 말초 혈관을 수축시켜 따뜻한 혈액을 몸의 중심부로 보내 정상적인 체온을 유지하는 방식으로 이를 수행한다. 이 혈류가 감소하면 말단 부위로 전달되는 열의 양이 크게 줄어든다.

추위에 노출되는 기간이 길어질수록 말초 부위로의 혈류가 더 많이 감소한다. 신체는 팔다리 및 피부 체온을 손실하면서 중심체온을 보존한다. 조직에서 발생하는 열 손실이 해당 부위에 공급되는 열보다 커진다.

팔다리가 15℃로 냉각되면 최대 혈관 수축과 최소 혈류량이 발생한다. 10℃까지 냉각이 계속되면 저온 유발 혈관 확장(CIVD)과 혈류량 증가로 인한 조직 온도 상승으로 인해 혈관 수축이 중단된다. 저온 유발 혈관 확장은 5~15분 주기로 재발하여 추위로부터 신체를 어느 정도 보호를 제공한다. 같은 추운 환경에 노출되었을 때 동상에 대한 감수성은 개인마다 차이가 있으며 이는 저온 유발 혈관 확장의 양으로 설명할 수 있다.

세포에는 피부 온도가 약 -2.2℃에 도달할 때까지 조직이 동결되지 않도록 막아주는 전해질과 기타 용질이 포함되어 있으므로 조직은 0℃에서도 얼지 않는다. 영하의 기온에서 팔다리를 보호하지 않고 방치하면 세포내액과 세포외액이 얼 수 있다. 그 결과 얼음 결정이 형성된다. 얼음 결정이 형성되면 팽창하여 국소 조직에 손상을 입힐 수 있다. 혈전이 형성되어 손상 부위로의 혈액 순환을 더욱 방해할 수 있다.

추위에 노출된 유형과 지속 시간은 동결 손상 정도를 결정하는 가장 중요한 두 가지 요소이다. 동상은 손상의 깊이와 임상 증상에 따라 분류된다. 대부분은 아주 경미하거나 심한 노출을 제외하고는 해동 후 최소 24~72시간이 지나야 손상 정도를 알 수 있다. 피부가 짧지만, 강렬한 추위에 노출되면 표재성 손상이 발생하지만, 장시간 노출되면 팔다리 전체에 심한 동상이 발생할 수 있다. 직접적인 저온 손상은 일반적으로 회복할 수 있지만, 재가온 과정에서 영구적인 조직 손상이 발생한다. 더 심하면 조직을 적절하게 재가온하더라도 미세혈관 혈전증이 발생하여 괴저 및 괴사의 초기 징후로 이어질 수 있다. 손상된 부위가 얼었다 녹았다가 다시 동결되면 두 번째 동결은 더 많은 양의 심각한 혈전증과 혈관 손상 및 조직 손실을 유발한다. 따라서 병원 전 처치 제공자는 초기 현장 처치 중 해동된 조직이 다시 얼지 않도록 해야 한다.

전통적인 동상 분류 방법은 다음과 같이 동결 후 초기 신체 소견과 재가온 후 병원에서 촬영한 영상을 바탕으로 화상과 유사한 4가지 손상 정도로 분류한다(**그림 19-7** 및 **그림 19-8**).

- 1도 동상(First-degree frostbite): 이 표피 손상은 차가운 공기나 금속에 잠깐 접촉한 피부로 손상이 제한된다. 피부가 하얗거나 손상 부위에 노르스름한 반점이 나타난다. 물집이나 조직 손실은 없다

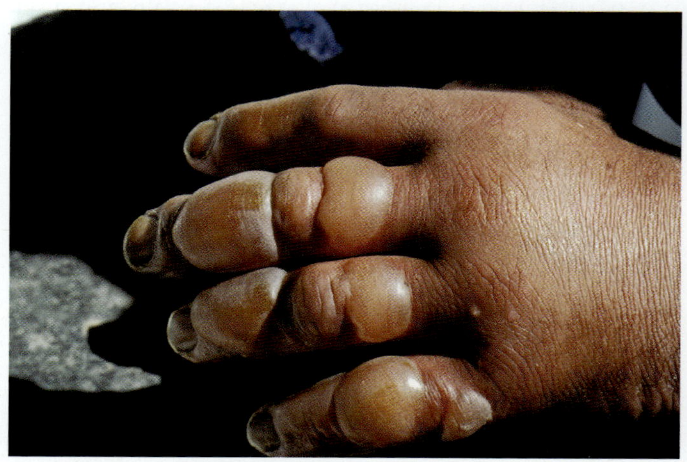

그림 19-7 동상 손상 24시간 후 부종과 물집 형성
© ANT Photo Library/Science Source

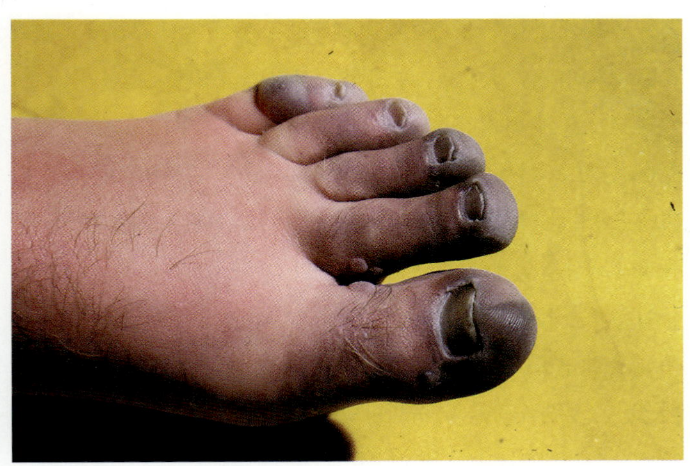

그림 19-8 해동 하루 후 출혈성 수포를 동반한 심부 2도 및 3도 동상.
© ANT Photo Library/Science Source

없으며 피부 빠르게 해동되고 감각이 무뎌지며 주변 부종과 함께 붉게 나타나고 7~10일 이내에 치유된다.

- 2도 동상(Second-degree frostbite): 이 정도의 동상은 표피와 진피 표면이 모든 손상된다. 처음에는 1도 손상과 비슷해 보이지만, 더 깊은 조직까지 동결이 발생한다. 조직은 만졌을 때 뻣뻣한 느낌이 들지만, 그 아래 조직은 압력을 받게 된다. 해동은 빠르게 진행되며 해동 후에는 홍반과 부종으로 둘러싸인 투명한 액체 또는 유백색 액체와 함께 표재성 피부 물집 또는 수포가 발생한다. 영구적인 조직 손실은 없으며 3~4주 안에 치유된다.
- 3도 동상(Third-degree frostbite): 이 손상 정도는 표피와 진피층이 포함된다. 동결된 피부는 뻣뻣하고 움직임이 제한된다. 조직이 해동된 후 피부는 혈액으로 가득 찬 물집(출혈성 수포)과 함께 부풀어 오르는데 이는 심부 조직에 혈관 손상이 있음을 나타내며 부기로 인해 움직임이 제한된다. 피부 손실이 서서히 진행되어 미라화 및 피부가 벗겨지고 치유가 느리다.
- 4도 동상(Fourth-degree frostbite): 이 단계에서는 조직이 진피까지 완전히 동결되어 근육과 뼈까지 포함된다. 동결 시에는 움직일 수 없고 해동 시에는 수동적으로 움직이며 고유한 근육 기능이 없다. 피부 관류가 불량하고 물집과 부종이 발생하지 않는다. 조직 괴사의 초기 징후가 분명하다. 조직의 박리와 생존 불가능한 조직의 자가 절단과 함께 느린 미라화 과정이 진행된다.

동상의 전통적 분류는 손상의 정도에 따라 4가지로 분류되지만, 병원 전 처치 제공자에게는 표면 또는 심부 동상으로 분류하기가 가장 쉽다. 표재성 동상(1도와 2도)은 피부와 피부밑조직에 영향을 미치며 재가온 하면 투명한 물집이 생긴다. 심부 동상(3도와 4도)은 피부, 근육 및 뼈에 영향을 미치며 피부를 다시 재가온 하면 출혈성 물집이 생긴다. 중증도 수준과 예상되는 조직 손실은 팔다리마다 다를 수 있다. 절단 위험을 확인하기 위해 재가온 후 동결된 조직을 검사하는 추가 분류 방법이 도입되었다.

특정 상황에서는 동상이 빠르게 발생할 수 있으며 병원 전 처치 제공자는 다음과 같이 대응할 수 있다.

- 탄화수소 액체(예: 휘발유, 부탄, 프로판)를 피부에 쏟은 경우 영하의 온도에서 급속한 증발과 전도를 일으킬 수 있음
- 따뜻한 피부로 극도로 차가운 금속을 만지는 경우
- 의료용 헬기의 회전날개 바람으로 인한 노출된 피부의 심한 체감온도

평가

도착 시 현장 안전을 평가한 다음 환자의 기도, 호흡, 순환을 평가한다. 환자를 추운 곳에서 습기, 추위, 바람으로부터 보호되는 장소로 옮겨 체온이 더 떨어지지 않도록 한다. 동상 환자는 탈수, 저혈량증, 저체온증, 저혈당증, 외상성 손상과 같은 추가적인 의학적 질환이 있을 수 있다. 체온 손실을 최소화하기 위해 젖은 옷을 벗겨야 한다. 의심스러운 경우 저체온증을 먼저 처치한다. 표재성 동상은 일반적으로 환경 조건, 환자의 주요 통증 또는 무감각 호소 부위, 같은 부위의 피부 변색 등을 종합하여 평가한다. 노출 시 환경 조건은 영하로 유지되어야 한다.

동상으로 인한 손상은 피부가 얼어 장갑이나 신발로 덮여 있을 때 손상 부위에 통증이 없을 수 있으므로 발견하기 어렵다. 동상 부위를 발견하려면 이전에 서술한 바와 같이 동상이 의심되는 신체 부위를 직접 육안으로 검사해야 한다. 해당 부위를 부드럽게 촉진하면 기저 조직이 유연하거나 딱딱한지 확인할 수 있다. 환자나 병원 전 처치 제공자는 얼어 있는 부위를 문지르거나 마사지하면 얼은 조직에 추가 세포 손상을 일으킬 수 있으므로 주의를 한다. 표재성 동상 환자는 일반적으로 동상 부위를 조작하는 동안 불편함을 호소한다. 심부 동상 환자의 경우 얼어붙은 조직을 단단하고 일반적으로 만질 때 통증이 없다. 손상 부위를 평가한 후 재가온 방법에 관한 결정은 일반적으로 응급실까지의 이송 시간을 고려하여 재가온 방법을 결정한다.

병원 전 단계에서 동상 환자의 재가온에 관해 알래스카주 EMS 프로토콜은 다음과 같이 명시되어 있다.

1. 이송 시간이 짧은 경우(최대 1~2시간) 병원 전 단계에서 부적절한 재가온 또는 재냉각으로 인한 위험은 심부 동상 처치 지연으

로 인한 위험보다 더 크다.

2. 이송 시간이 길어질 때(1~2시간 이상) 동상 부위가 자연적으로 녹는 경우가 많다. 동상 부위를 따뜻한 물로 빠르게 녹이는 것보다 저체온증을 예방하는 것이 더 중요하다. 그렇다고 해서 동상에 걸린 팔다리의 재가온을 방지하기 위해 차갑게 유지한다는 것을 의미하는 것은 아니다. 환자를 따뜻하게 유지하면 동상 부위가 다시 따뜻해질 것을 예상하고 어떤 대가를 치르더라도 동상 부위가 다시 얼지 않도록 보호를 한다.

처치

표재성 동상 또는 동창이 있는 환자는 따뜻한 손으로 환자의 귀를 덮거나 손가락을 겨드랑이 또는 서혜부에 손가락을 넣는 것처럼 환부를 따뜻한 신체 표면에 대도록 한다. 표재성 동상은 정상 체온으로만 따뜻하게 하면 된다.

병원 전 환경에서 심부 동상을 처치하려면 먼저 저체온증이 있는지 평가하고 처치를 한다. 열 손실을 최소화하기 환자의 환부에 지지요법과 적절한 대피소를 제공한다. 환자가 손상된 발로 걷지 않도록 한다. 환자가 움직이는 동안 손상되기 쉬운 조직을 추가 손상으로부터 보호하고 동상 부위를 평가한다. 동상 부위에서 옷과 장신구를 제거하고 감각이 상실되었는지 확인한다.

골절 원위부에 동상이 있는 경우 저항이 없는 한 팔다리를 해부학적 자세로 정렬을 시도한다. 원위부 순환을 방해하지 않는 방법으로 골절 부위를 부목으로 고정한다.

환부를 자연 건조하고 조직을 문지르지 않는다. 손상된 부위가 압박되지 않도록 건조한 멸균 드레싱을 느슨하게 시행한다. 손가락과 발가락은 멸균 거즈로 개별적으로 분리하여 보호하고 물집은 터트리지 않는다. 부종을 줄이기 위해 손과 발을 부목으로 고정하고 올려준다.

통증을 조절하기 위해 진통제가 필요할 수 있으며 조직이 해동되기 전에 투여를 시작해야 한다. 탈수를 처치하고 혈액의 점도와 모세혈관 응집형성을 줄이기 위해 정맥 내로 생리식염수 250mL를 투여한다. 적절한 의료기관으로 신속하게 이송한다.

현장에서 심부 동상 환자를 재가온하려는 시도는 환자의 최종 회복에 위험할 수 있으며 이송 지연(2시간 이상)하지 않는 한 권장하지 않는다. 이송 지연해야 하는 경우 환부를 37~39℃ 이하의 따뜻한 물에서 부드럽고 유연해질 때까지(~30분) 해동한다. 재동결이 우려되는 경우 해동하지 않는다. 동상에 걸린 조직은 감각이 감소하거나 없어

추가 손상이 발생할 수 있으므로 해동하는 동안 손상 부위가 수조의 측면이나 바닥에 닿지 않도록 하여 손상된 팔다리를 보호한다.

프로토콜에 따라 허용되는 경우 이부프로펜(12mg/kg 최대 800mg) 또는 아스피린(71~81mg)을 투여한다. 이부프로펜 같은 비스테로이드성 약물은 염증과 통증을 줄이고 혈관수축을 유발하는 물질의 생성을 억제하는 데 도움이 된다.

이송하는 동안 환자의 의식 수준과 기타 손상에 따라 가능한 경우 따뜻한 음료(무알코올성)를 제공하여 환자에게 수분을 공급한다. 니코틴은 혈관 수축을 더 유발함으로 흡연은 권장하지 않는다.

사고성 저체온증

저체온증은 직장 체온계로 직장에 적어도 15cm 이상 삽입하여 측정한 결과 중심체온이 35℃ 이하인 상태로 정의된다. 저체온증은 환자가 항상성을 유지하거나 정상적인 신체 기능으로 돌아갈 수 있을 만큼 충분한 열을 생산하지 못하는 중심체온의 감소로 볼 수 있다.

저체온증은 차가운 주변 공기, 찬물에 담그거나 찬물에 잠기는 등 다양한 상황에서 발생할 수 있으며 수술 중에 의도적으로 유발하거나 외상성 뇌손상과 같은 일부 질환의 처치 방법으로 사용할 수 있다. 저체온증은 특히 외상 환자의 경우에 적절한 환경에서도 발생할 수 있다. 침수(머리만 물 밖으로 나온 경우) 저체온증은 일반적으로 준비나 계획 없이 실수로 추운 환경에 노출되었을 때 발생한다. 예를 들어, 얼음물에 빠진 사람은 즉시 한랭 쇼크 헐떡임 반사, 운동 능력 소실, 저체온증, 익사 등의 침수로 인한 손상의 위험에 처하게 된다. 이러한 익수 사고의 독특한 측면은 저산소증과 저체온증으로 이어질 수 있다(이후 논의 및 20장, 환경 외상 II: 낙뢰, 익사, 다이빙 및 고도를 참조).

차가운 공기나 차가운 물에서 신진대사 열 생산이 열 손실과 일치할 수 있다면 저체온증으로 진행을 지연시킬 수 있다. 바다나 기타 극한 상황에서도 생존한 사례가 많이 보고되고 있으며 극심한 추위에 노출되어도 생존할 수 있다. 나이, 성별, 체성분(예: 체표면적 대 체질량지수), 떨림의 시작과 강도, 체력 수준, 영양 상태, 음주 등 많은 요인이 추위에 노출된 후 생존에 영향을 미치는 것으로 알려져 있다.

저혈당증은 저체온증의 진행 단계에서 발생할 수 있으며 침수로 인해 발생한 저체온증에서 더 흔할 수 있다. 저혈당증은 떨림 과정에서 수축하는 근육에 의해 연료 공급원인 혈당과 근육 내 글리코겐이 빠르게 고갈되기 때문에 발생한다. 떨림으로 인해 혈당 저장량이 고갈

되면 신체의 체온조절중추 역할을 하는 뇌의 시상하부에 주요 연료가 부족해진다. 따라서 음주한 사람은 알코올이 체내 포도당 생성을 차단하고 열 생성을 위한 최대 떨림을 억제하기 때문에 저체온증에 걸릴 위험이 더 커진다. 따라서 저체온증 환자의 저혈당을 신속하게 평가하고 효과적으로 처치해야 재가온 중 신진대사와 떨림을 효과적으로 증가시킬 수 있다.

동상과 달리 사망으로 이어질 수 있는 저체온증은 기온이 영하를 훨씬 넘는 환경에서 발생할 수 있다. 일차 저체온증은 일반적으로 건강한 사람이 악천후에 처해 있고 과도한 급성 또는 만성적인 추위에 노출될 분비가 되어 있지 않으며 무의식적으로 중심체온이 35℃ 이하로 떨어졌을 때 발생한다. 일차성 저체온증으로 인한 사망은 추위 노출의 직접적인 결과이며 검시관은 사고, 타살 또는 자살로 기록한다.

이차성 저체온증은 갑상샘저하증, 부신저하증, 외상, 암, 패혈증 등 환자의 전신 질환으로 인해 발생하는 정상적인 결과로 간주한다. 이차성 저체온증과 관련된 다양한 의학적 질환은 **Box 19-10**을 참조한

Box 19-10 이차성 저체온증과 관련된 질환

체온 조절 장애
- 중추 부전
- 신경성 식욕부진
- 뇌졸중
- 중추신경계 손상
- 시상하부 기능이상
- 대사 부전
- 신생물
- 파킨슨병
- 약리학적 효과
- 거미막밑출혈
- 독소
- 말초 부전
- 급성 척수 가로절단
- 열 생산 감소
- 신경병증
- 내분비 부전
- 알코올성 또는 당뇨병케톤산증
- 부신저하증
- 뇌하수체저하증
- 젖산산증
- 에너지 부족

- 극심한 신체활동
- 저혈당
- 영양실조
- 신경근 손상
- 최근 출산 및 고령으로 활동량이 적은 경우
- 떨림 장애

열 손실 증가
- 피부 질환
- 화상
- 약물 및 독소
- 의인성 원인
- 응급 분만
- 차가운 수액 투여
- 열사병 치료
- 기타 관련 임상 상태
- 암종증
- 심폐 질환
- 주요 감염(박테리아, 바이러스, 기생충)
- 다발성 외상
- 쇼크

Data from ECC Committee, Subcommittees and Task Forces of the American Heart Association. 2005 American Heart Association Guidelines for cardiopulmonary resuscitation and emergency cardiovascular care. *Circulation.* 2005;112(24): ivi-203; and American Heart Association. 2010 guidelines for cardiopulmonary resuscitation and emergency cardiovascular care. *Circulation.* 2010;122:S640-S656.

다. 이러한 유형의 저체온증을 인식하지 못하거나 부적절하게 처치할 경우 2시간 이내에 치명적일 수 있다. 이차성 저체온증 환자의 사망은 종종 기저 질환으로 인해 발생하며 저체온증에 의해 악화한다. 다른 손상의 합병증으로 인한 이차성 저체온증과 중심체온이 32℃ 미만인 중증 처제온증의 경우 사망률이 50%를 넘는다.

외상 후 경미한 저체온증은 모든 기상 조건에서 매우 흔하게 발생하므로 병원 전 처치 제공자는 외상 환자의 추가 체온 손실을 방지하기 위해 신속하게 조치를 취해야 한다.

저체온증과 외상 환자

외상센터에서 저체온증 환자를 받는 것은 매우 흔한 일이며 이러한 환자는 일차평가 중에 추가적인 체온 손실이 발생하는 것을 경험하게 된다. 병원 전 환경에서 시작되는 저체온증의 발생은 외상이 체온 조절에 미치는 영향과 열 생산의 주요 기전인 떨림 억제와 관련이 있다. 많은 환자에서 추운 응급실이나 외상센터에서 노출된 환자, 차가운 수액 투여, 복강 또는 흉강 개복, 열 생성 떨림을 방지하는 마취제 및 신경근차단제 사용, 수술실 환경에서의 추위 노출 등 다양한 원인으로 인해 병원 도착 후에도 열 손실이 계속된다.

병원 전 환경에서 외상 환자는 가능한 한 빨리 차가운 바닥에서 벗어나 따뜻한 구급차로 옮겨야 한다. 구급차 내 온도는 환자의 열 손실을 최소화하고 너무 더운 주변 작업 환경으로 인해 업무에 지장을 받을 수 있는 병원 전 처치 제공자의 업무 수행 능력을 극대화할 수 있도록 조절한다. 야생의학외는 이 두 가지 고려 사항의 이상적인 균형으로 구급차 내부 온도를 24℃로 권장한다. 정맥 내 따뜻한 수액(37.8~42.2℃) 투여는 환자의 체온을 유지하는 데 도움이 된다.

저체온 외상 환자의 사망률이 높은 원인 중 하나는 저체온증, 산증, 응고병증(혈액이 정상적으로 응고되지 않음)의 조합과 관련이 있다. 이것은 외상 환자의 치명적인 삼중고라고 한다. 응고병증은 환자를 다시 따뜻하게 하면 가역적이기 때문에 외상과 저체온증 모두에 대해 환자를 평가하고 처치하는 것이 필수적이다. 한 연구에 따르면 Level Ⅰ 외상센터에 입원한 외상 환자의 57%가 연속적인 치료 중 어느 시점에서 저체온증이 발생했다. 외상 환자의 중심체온이 32.2℃ 이하로 떨어지면 사망률이 40~100%에 이르는 것으로 보고되었다. 이 비율은 중등도 중심체온이 28~32.2℃에서 일차성 저체온증(비외상성) 환자의 사망률이 20%인 것과 대조된다. 따라서 외상 환자의 저체온증과 관련된 사망률은 매우 중요하여 일부 연구자들은 경증, 중등도, 중증 저체온증의 표준 정의를 넘어 특별한 외상 저체온증 분류

표 19-5 저체온증의 분류	
분류	**중심체온(℃)**
경증 저체온증	35-32℃
중등도 저체온증	32-28℃
중증 저체온증	28-24℃
심각한 저체온증	< 24℃

Data from Zafren K, Giesbrecht GG, Danzl DF, et al. Wilderness Medical Society practice guidelines for the out-of-hospital evaluation and treatment of accidental hypothermia. *Wilderness Environ Med.* 2014;25:426.

를 만들었다(**표 19-5**).

　외상, 저체온증 및 사망률 증가의 이러한 관계는 최근 전투 사상자를 포함하여 수십 년 동안 보고됐다. 그러나 최근의 임상 연구에 따르면 저체온증은 외상 환자의 사망에 대한 독립적인 위험 요인이 아니라 손상 중증도 또는 다발성 장기 기능장애 증후군과 더 밀접한 관련이 있는 것으로 보고되었다. 한 연구에서는 외상 환자의 저체온증 중증도에 영향을 미칠 수 있는 병원 전 특정 관행이 있다고 보고했다. 이러한 관행에는 저체온증을 예상하고 환자의 젖은 옷을 벗기지 않으며 체온을 자주 측정 측정하고 따뜻하게 실내 온도 유지, 따뜻한 수액만 정맥 내로 투여하는 것 등이 포함된다. 의도적으로 유도한 저체온증의 잠재적 처치 효과는 현재 연구 중이다(**Box 19-11**).

침수 저체온증

물에 잠기는 동안 신체에서 열이 증가하거나 열이 손실되지 않으면 수온은 열 중성 수온으로 간주한다. 열 중성 수온은 33~35℃로 이 온도는 알몸으로 목 높이의 물속에 수동적으로 서 있는 사람이 최소 1시간 동안 거의 일정한 중심체온을 유지할 수 있는 온도이다. 열 중성 수온에 있는 사람은 갑작스러운 찬물에 노출되었을 때 발생하는 초기 침수 쇼크 및 저체온증의 위험이 거의 없다.

　열 중성 하한보다 낮은 수온에 잠기면 즉각적인 생리학적 변화로 피부 온도가 급격히 떨어지고 말초혈관 수축으로 인한 떨림이 발생하며 신진대사 증가, 호흡 증가, 심박수 증가, 심박출량 증가, 평균 동맥압이 증가한다. 체내 열 손실을 상쇄하려면 신체 활동을 증가시키거나 몸을 떨거나 둘 다를 통해 열을 생산해야 한다. 그렇지 않으면 중심체온이 계속 감소하고 떨림이 멈추며 이러한 생리학적 반응은 중심체온이 감소함에 따라 비례하여 감소한다.

　침수 저체온증의 가장 큰 위험은 보통 수온이 25℃ 미만일 때 시작된다. 물의 열 발산 능력이 공기보다 25배나 더 크기 때문에 물속에서는 더 빠르게 저체온증에 걸릴 위험이 있다. 그러나 차가운 물에서 체온유지를 위해 수영과 같은 신체 활동을 계속하면 결국 신체를 둘러싼 차가운 물로 대류 열 손실이 증가하여 저체온증이 더 빨리 시작될 수 있으므로 해가 된다. 이러한 이해를 바탕으로 여러 명의 익수자가 함께 있는 경우 열 손실 방지 자세(HELP) 또는 몸을 움츠리는 자세를 사용하여 찬물에 잠기는 동안 열 손실을 최소화하도록 개인에게 권장하고 있다(**그림 19-9**).

　사고성 저체온증에서 정상적으로 신경학적 회복을 보인 영아의 기록된 최저 중심체온은 15℃이다. 성인의 경우 사고성 저체온증 생존자의 기록된 최저 중심체온은 13.7℃이다. 이 사례는 29세 여성에서 발생했는데, 이 여성은 심각한 저체온증 증상이 근육 수축에 영향을 미치기 전까지 40분 이상 자가 구조에 어려움을 겪었다. 구조대가 도착하기 전까지 80분 이상 물에 잠겨 있었고 병원으로 이송하는 동안 심폐소생술이 시행되었다. 3시간 동안 지속해 재가온을 시행한 후 중심체온이 정상으로 회복되었고 정상적인 생리학적 기능을 회복하여 생존했다.

활력증후가 거의 감지할 수 없는 수준으로 감소했을 수 있으므로 저체온증 환자의 초기 인상은 환자가 사망한 것처럼 보일 수 있다. 저체온증 환자를 처치하는 병원 전 처치 제공자는 환자의 체온이 35℃ 이상으로 회복되고 심폐 및 신경 기능의 증거가 없거나 생존 불가능 징후(기도 내 얼음, 가슴벽 동결, 참수 등)가 나타날 때까지 처치를 중단하고 환자의 사망을 선언해서는 안 된다. 29세의 저체온증 생존자는 현장에서 장시간의 심폐소생술을 시행한 후 완전한 신경 기능을 회복하고 퇴원한 환자의 예에 불과하다. 이 사례와 유사한 결과를 초래한 다른 사례에서 얻을 수 있는 교훈은 저체온증 환자의 초기 인상은 환자가 사망한 것처럼 보일 수 있지만, 이러한 초기 인상은 돌이킬 수 없는 소생 불능의 징후가 없는 한 기본 또는 전문 소생술을 보류할 충분한 근거가 되지 못한다는 것이다. 환자는 체온이 올라갈 때까지 죽은 것이 아니라는 것을 처치 제공자는 명심해야 한다.

의도적이든 비의도적이든 미국에서는 레크리에이션 및 상업 활동과 사고로 인해 일 년 내내 냉수 침수가 발생한다. 초기 익수 사고에서 치명적인 익사 없이 생존하더라도 수온에 따라 저체온증의 위험에 처할 수 있다. 일반인들은 일반적으로 매우 차가운 물에서 저체온증이 발생하는 데 걸리는 시간을 과소평가하며 저체온증이 사망까지 짧은 시간 내에 빠르게 발생한다고 믿는다. 그러나 침수로 인해 급사하는 경우는 저체온증이 아니라 공황 또는 저온 쇼크 반응으로 인해 물을 흡인하거나 일시적인 근육 마비/기능장애가 발생하여 치명적인 익사로 이어지는 경우가 많다. 이해해야 할 핵심 사항은 1) 저온 쇼크가 초기에 가장 큰 위협이며 2) 환자는 이러한 초기 생리학적 반응에서 생존하기 위해 헐떡임 반사와 호흡을 조절하는 데 더 집중해야 한다는 것이다(**Box 19-12**). 냉수 침수에 대한 신체의 반응은 사망에

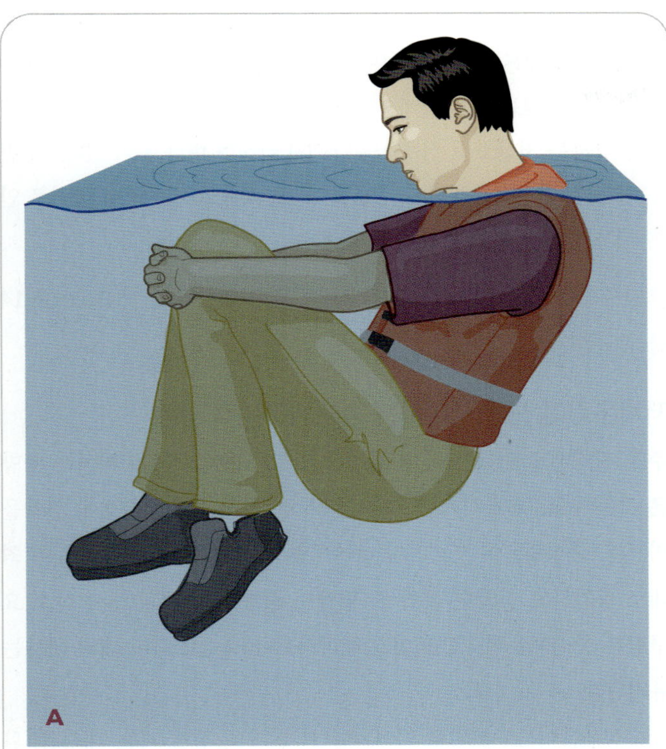

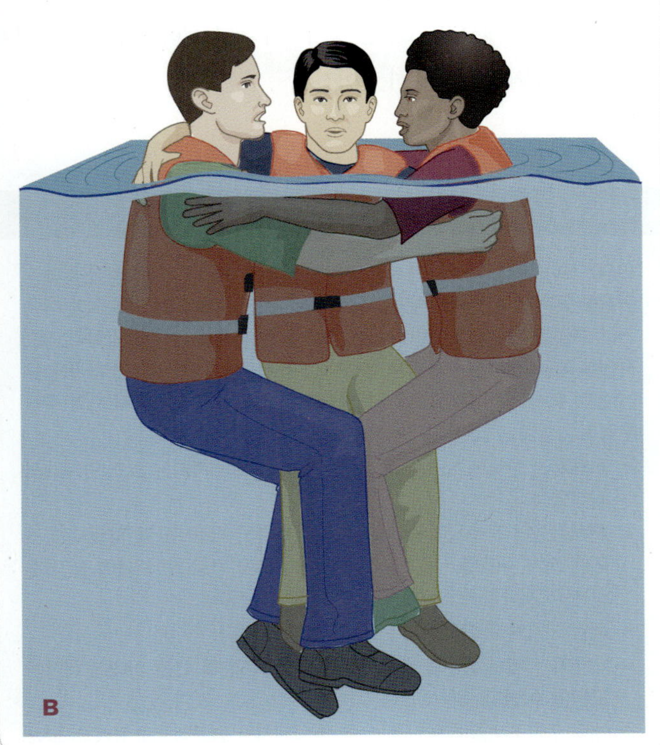

그림 19-9 차가운 물에서 생존자의 냉각 속도를 낮추는 기술. **A.** 열 방출을 줄이는 자세(HELP) **B.** 몸을 움츠리는 방법

Box 19-12 1-10-1 원칙

사람이 얼음처럼 차가운 물에 잠기면 저체온 쇼크나 저체온증의 발병 여부는 신체의 크기, 수온, 물에 잠긴 사람의 신체 부위 등 여러 요인에 따라 달라진다. 하지만 일반적으로 냉수 침수에 대한 환자의 생리학적 반응은 1-10-1 원칙으로 설명할 수 있다.

- **1분:** 저체온 쇼크의 위험은 약 1분 후에 사라진다. 환자는 당황하지 말고 호흡을 조절하며 기도를 깨끗이 유지하는 데 집중해야 한다.
- **10분:** 약 10분이 지나면 팔, 다리 및 기타 신체 부위를 움직일 수 없게 된다. 이 시간 동안 가능하면 스스로 구조하거나 구조대가 도착할 때까지 생존 가능한 자세를 취해야 한다.
- **1시간:** 저체온증으로 의식을 잃기까지 최대 1시간이 걸린다. 당황하거나 불필요하게 몸부림치면 이 시간이 단축된다. 구명조끼를 착용하면 심장이 멈추기까지 1시간 정도 더 버틸 수 있다.

이르는 4단계로 나눌 수 있다. 다음 4단계 모두에서 사망자가 발생한 것으로 보고되었다는 점에 유의한다.

- 첫 번째 단계-저온 쇼크 반응: 이 단계는 물에 잠긴 후 빠르게(1~2분 이내) 발생하는 심혈관 반사로 시작된다(20℃보다 차가운 물에서 발생할 수 있음). 빠른 피부냉각, 말초혈관 수축, 헐떡임 반사, 숨을 참지 못하는 증상, 과다호흡, 빈맥으로 시작된다. 헐떡임 반사는 개인의 머리 위치가 물 위 또는 물 아래인지에 따라 흡인 및 익사로 이어질 수 있다. 이러한 반응은 실신 또는 경련으로 인한 익사, 미주신경마비, 심실세동 등 여러 가지 상태로 인해 물에 잠긴 후 몇 분 이내에 즉각적인 급사 또는 사망으로 이어질 수 있다.

- 두 번째 단계-저온 무력화: 피해자가 저온 쇼크 단계에서 살아남으면 이후 5~15분 동안 말초 조직, 특히 팔다리에 상당한 냉각이 일어난다. 이러한 냉각은 팔다리의 미세한 운동 능력에 해로운 영향을 미치며 손가락 경직, 협응력 저하, 근력 상실을 유발하여 수영, 구조를 위해 줄 잡기 또는 기타 생존 운동 능력을 거의 불가능하게 만든다.

- 세 번째 단계-저체온증의 시작: 첫 번째 단계와 두 번째 단계에서 익사하지 않고 생존하면 30분 이상 물에 잠기면 지속적인 열 손실과 중심체온 저하로 저체온증에 걸릴 위험이 있다. 피해자가 피로와 저체온증으로 인해 수면 위에 머무를 수 없는 흡인 및 표류가 발생한다. 개인이 차가운 물에서 얼마나 오래 생존할 수 있는지는 여러 요인에 따라 달라진다. 수온 0℃에서 익수자는 1시간 이상 생존할 수 없으며 수온 15℃에서는 6시간 후 생존하는 경우는 흔하지 않다.

- 네 번째 단계-구조 붕괴: 이 단계에서는 겉으로 보기에 안정적이고 의식이 있는 상태임에도 불구하고 생존자 구조의 모든 기간(구조 전, 구조 중, 구조 후) 동안 사망자가 관찰되었다. 증상은 실신에서 심정지에 이르기까지 다양하며 재가온 쇼크 또는 구조 후 최대 24시간까지 모든 단계에서 사망이 발생할 수 있다. 구조 붕괴의 세 가지 원인으로는 1) 중심체온 저하, 2) 동맥혈압 저하, 3) 심실세동을 유발하는 저산소증, 산증 또는 pH의 급격한 변화 등이 있다. 네 번째 단계에서 생존해서 회복된 환자 중 최대 20%가 구조 붕괴로 인해 사망하는 것으로 알려져 있다.

냉수 침수 생존에 대한 자세한 내용은 **Box 19-13** 및 **Box 19-14**를 참고한다.

저체온증이 신체에 미치는 병태생리학적 영향

추운 환경에 노출되든 물에 잠기든 저체온증이 신체에 미치는 영향은 모든 주요 장기 시스템, 특히 심장, 신장 및 중추신경계에 영향을 미친다. 중심체온이 35℃까지 낮아지면 혈관수축, 떨림, 대사율이 최대로 증가하고 심박수, 호흡수, 혈압이 증가한다. 대뇌 대사 산소 요구량은 중심체온이 1℃ 떨어질 때마다 6~10% 감소하며 대뇌 대사는 유지된다.

중심체온이 30~35℃로 떨어지면 인지 기능, 심장 기능, 대사율, 환기 속도, 떨림 속도가 모두 현저하게 감소하거나 완전히 억제된다. 이 시점에서는 신체에서 열 소실을 방지하기 위한 생리학적 방어 기전이 압도되어 중심체온이 급격히 떨어진다.

Box 19-13 냉수에서 생존 지침

미국 해안경비대와 기타 수색 구조(SAR) 기관에서는 개인이 차가운 물에서 얼마나 오래 생존할 수 있는지 추정하는 데 도움이 되는 지침을 사용한다. 이 지침은 다음과 같은 변수의 영향을 바탕으로 중심체온 냉각 속도를 추정하는 수학적 모델이다.

- 수온 및 바다 상태
- 옷의 단열 효과
- 체성분(지방, 근육, 뼈의 양)
- 물에 잠긴 신체 부위 정도
- 물속에서 신체의 활동(예: 과도한 운동) 및 자세(예: HELP, 몸을 움츠림)
- 떨림에 의한 열 생성

Box 19-14 자가 구조

1960~1970년대의 초기 연구에 따르면 실수로 차가운 물에 빠졌을 때는 안전한 곳까지 원거리를 헤엄쳐서 스스로 구조하기보다는 제자리에 머물거나 구명조끼를 입고 가만히 떠 있거나 체온 유지를 유해 헤엄치지 않고 잔해에 매달리는 것이 더 나은 선택이었다. 최근 연구에 따르면 차가운 물(수온이 10~13.9℃)에 실수로 잠겼을 때 다음과 같은 조건에서 자가 구조 수영이 가능한 방법이라고 한다.

- 피해자가 찬물에 노출된 후 처음 몇 분 이내에 저제온 쇼크 단계에서 살아있다.
- 저체온증이 진행됨에 따라 의사결정 능력이 저하되므로 피해자가 조기에 자가 구조를 시도하거나 구조를 기다리기로 한다. 물에 잠긴 후 30분이 지나면 구조 성공률이 현저히 낮아진다.
- 해당 지역의 구조대원이 구조할 가능성은 낮다.
- 피해자는 체력 수준과 수영 능력에 따라 수영 후 45분 이내에 해안에 도달할 수 있다.
- 개인 구명조끼를 착용한 냉수 침수 피해자는 평균적으로 10℃의 물에서 약 800m를 수영할 수 있어야 일반적인 저체온증보다는 근육 냉각과 팔의 피로로 인한 무력화가 발생하기 전에 구조될 수 있다.
- 찬물에서 수영할 수 있는 거리는 따뜻한 물에서 수영할 수 있는 거리의 약 1/3이다.

중심체온이 29.4℃가 되면 심박출량과 대사율이 약 50% 감소한다. 환기와 관류가 부적절하고 신진대사 요구를 따라가지 못해 세포의 저산소증과 젖산을 증가시켜 대사성 및 호흡성 산증을 유발한다. 중심부와 뇌에 산소 공급과 혈류가 유지된다.

서맥은 심장박동조율기 세포의 탈분극에 대한 추위의 직접적인 영향과 전도 시스템을 통한 전파 속도 저하로 인해 많은 환자에서 발생한다. 심근이 차가울 때는 아트로핀과 다른 심장 약물을 사용해도 심박수를 증가시키는 데 효과가 없는 경우가 많다. 중심체온이 30℃ 이하로 떨어지면 심근은 과민 반응을 일으킨다. PR, QRS 및 QTC 간격이 연장되고 ST분절 및 T파 변화, J(또는 오스본)파가 나타날 수 있으며 급성 심근경색 같은 다른 심전도 이상을 모방할 수 있다. J파는 저체온증 환자에서 눈에 띄는 심전도 특징이며 중등도에서 중증의 저체온증 환자(32.2℃ 미만)의 약 1/3에서 나타난다. J파는 QRS 복합체와 ST 분절의 초기 부분 사이의 "혹과 같은" 편향으로 설명된다. J파는 aVL, aVF 및 좌측 전흉부 리드에서 가장 잘 보인다(**그림 19-10**).

심방세동과 극단적 서맥이 발생하고 28.3~32.2℃에서 지속될 수 있다. 중심체온이 26.7~27.8℃에 도달하면 심장의 물리적 자극으로 인해 심실세동(VF)이 발생할 수 있다. 심폐소생술 또는 환자를 평가하거나 이동시 거칠게 다루는 것만으로도 심실세동을 유발할 수 있다. 중심체온이 매우 낮은 상태에서는 맥박과 혈압을 감지할 수 없고 관절이 뻣뻣해지며 동공이 고정되고 확장된다. 재가온이 완료되고 생명 징후(심전도, 맥박, 호흡 및 중추신경계 기능)가 나타나지 않을 때까지 환자가 사망한 것으로 간주해서는 안 된다.

급성으로 추위에 노출되면 혈관 수축 시 혈액의 단락으로 인해 신장 혈류가 증가한다. 이로 인해 환자가 더 많은 소변을 생성하고 결과적으로 탈수 상태가 될 수 있는 한랭이뇨 현상이 발생할 수 있다. 27~30℃에서는 신장 혈류가 50% 감소한다. 이 중등도에서 중증의 저체온 수준에서는 심박출량 감소로 인해 신장 혈류량과 사구체 여과율이 감소하고 결국 급성신부전이 발생한다.

평가

현장 도착 즉시 현장 안전을 평가하는 것이 필수적이다. 모든 구급대원과 구조대원은 이러한 환경에서 작업하는 동안 추위에 노출되지 않도록 최대한의 안전과 보호를 받아야 한다. 환경 조건(예: 바람, 습기, 온도)이 저체온증을 의심할 만한 조건이 아니어도 저체온증을 의심해야 한다.

환자를 대피소로 조심스럽게 이동시키거나 현장에서 바람을 차단하는 단열재를 사용하여 더 이상 체온이 떨어지지 않도록 보호한다. 이렇게 하면 추가적인 열 손실을 방지할 수 있다. 그리고 환자의 기도, 호흡, 순환을 평가한다. 중등도에서 중증의 저체온증 환자의 경우 맥박이 매우 약하거나 없을 수 있으므로 최대 60초 동안 환자의

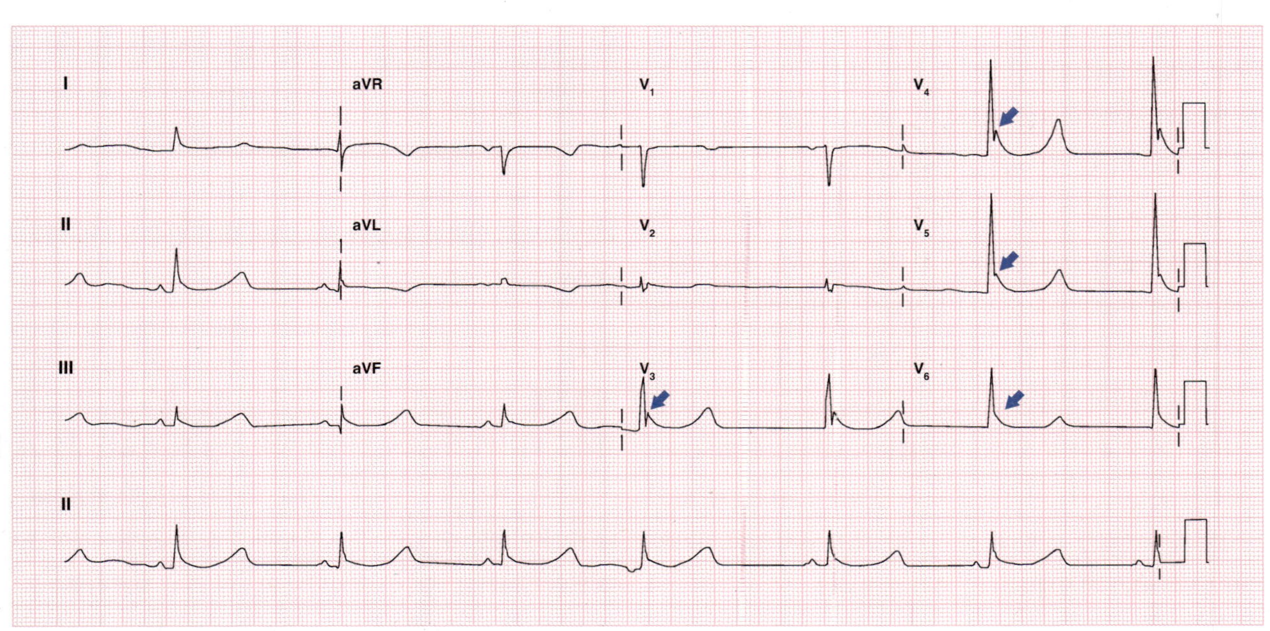

그림 19-10 저체온증 환자의 오스본 또는 J파

Data from *12-Lead ECG: The Art of Interpretation*, courtesy of Tomas B. Garcia, MD.

맥박을 주의 깊게 평가한다. 의식이 있는 일부 환자는 피로, 무기력, 메스꺼움, 어지럼 등을 호소할 수 있다. 신경학적 기능을 자주 평가하고 모니터링해야 한다. 중증 저체온증 환자는 일반적으로 느린 호흡, 혼미, 혼수상태를 보일 수 있다.

저체온을 정확하게 측정하려면 낮은 온도까지 측정할 수 있는 직장 체온계가 필요한 경우가 많다. 그러나 직장 체온은 일반적으로 현장에서 평가하거나 대부분 병원 전 단계에서 활력징후로 널리 사용하지는 않는다. 체온계를 사용할 수 있는 구급차에는 일반적으로 최저 35.6℃까지 측정할 수 있는 구강 또는 직장(영아용) 체온계가 비치되어 있다. 전자 체온계는 저체온증 상황에서는 정확한 체온을 측정하는 데 유용하지 않다. 고막 적외선 체온 측정은 일반적으로 측정값에 영향을 줄 수 있는 바깥귀길이 아닌 고막에서 측정하기 때문에 일반적으로 정확하다. 또한 귀에는 귀지와 혈액이 없어야 한다. 따라서 병원 전 처치 제공자는 현장 상황, 환자의 정신 상태, 활력징후 및 기도, 호흡, 순환에 의존해야 한다. **표 19-6**은 중심체온이 감소할 때 예상되는 생리학적 반응이다.

저체온증 의심 환자를 평가할 때는 떨림과 징과 정신 상태 변화의 징후가 중요하다. 경증 저체온증(중심체온이 32.2℃ 이상인 경우) 환자는 떨림이 있고 보통 의식 수준 변화(예: 혼동, 어눌한 말투, 걸음걸이 변화, 서투름)의 징후를 보인다. 행동이 느리고 일반적으로 거동하지 않고 앉거나 누워 있는 상태로 발견된다. 경찰이나 병원 전 처치 제공자는 이 상태를 약물이나 알코올 중독으로 오해하거나 노인 환자의 경우 뇌졸중으로 오해할 수 있다. 그러나 환자의 의식 수준은 저체온증의 정도를 나타내는 신뢰할 수 있는 지표는 아니며 일부 환자는 중심체온이 26.7℃ 미만인 상태에서도 의식을 유지하기도 한다.

환자의 중심체온이 32.2℃ 이하로 떨어지면 중등도의 저체온증이 나타나고 환자는 추위를 호소하지 않을 수이다. 떨림이 없을 수 있으며 환자의 의식 수준이 크게 저하되어 의식을 잃을 수도 있다. 환자의 동공이 느리게 반응하거나 동공이 확장되어 고정될 수 있다. 환자의 맥박이 약해지거나 없을 수 있으며 경증에서 중등도의 저혈압이 나타날 수 있다. 환자의 호흡은 분당 2회 정도로 느려질 수 있고 심전도 검사에서 가장 흔한 부정맥인 심방세동이 나타날 수 있다. PR 간격, QR 간격 및 QTC 간격이 연장된 다른 부정맥이 나타날 수 있으며 J(오스본) 파가 존재할 수 있다. 심근은 약 27.8℃에서 점차 차가워지고 과민해짐에 따라 심실세동이 더 자주 관찰된다.

대뇌 대사의 변화로 인해 환자가 의식을 잃기 전에 역설적으로 옷을 벗는 것이 관찰될 수 있다. 이는 환자가 추운 환경에서 옷을 벗으

표 19-6 저체온증의 특징		
분류	**중심체온**	**생리학적 반응**
경증 저체온증	35~32℃	• 떨림, 제자리걸음 • 혈관수축 • 호흡수 증가 • 무감각증 • 구음장애 • 운동실조 • 저온 이뇨
중등도 저체온증	32~28℃	• 떨림임 멈추고 점차 약해지고 뻣뻣해짐 • 조정력이 상실된 근육 • 호흡수 감소 • 느린 맥박 • 심각한 저환기 • 기도 보호 반사 감소 • 산소 소비량이 절반으로 감소 • 혼란 • 졸음증
중증 저체온증	28~24℃	• 분당 환기량 감소 • 기관지 분비물 증가 • 기관지 경련이 발생할 수 있음 • 약한 맥박 • 부정맥 • 느린 호흡 • 혼수
심각한 저체온증	< 24℃	• 사망 • 심정지

© National Association of Emergency Medical Technicians (NAEMT)

려는 시도로 임박한 온도 조절 실패에 대한 반응을 나타내는 것으로 생각된다.

처치

저체온증 환자의 병원 전 처치는 추가 체온 손실 방지하고 부드럽게 환자를 다루며 병원으로 신속한 이송 시작 및 필요한 경우 재가온을 시행한다. 여기에는 환자를 차가운 곳에서 따뜻한 구급차로 옮기거나 즉시 이송할 수 없는 경우 따뜻한 장소로 옮기는 것이 포함된다. 맥박을 평가하고 맥박이 촉지되지 않으면 즉시 심폐소생술을 시작해야 한다. 환자의 불필요한 움직임과 동작을 피하고자 젖은 옷은 가위로 절단하여 제거한다. 환자를 이동시키거나 처치 시 심실부정맥

이 발생하는 것에 대한 우려 때문에 중요한 처치가 지연되어서는 안된다. 이러한 우려는 중증 저체온증 환자(중심체온이 30℃ 미만)에서 더욱 현실적으로 나타난다. 환자를 차가운 바닥으로부터 단열되고 따뜻한 담요나 침낭으로 완전히 덮은 다음 전도, 대류, 증발에 의한 열 손실을 방지하기 위해 바람을 막아준다.

의식이 있고 명료한 환자는 알코올이나 카페인이 함유된 음료는 피해야 한다. 저혈당을 예상하고 환자의 혈당 수치를 평가한다. 혈당 수치가 정상인 경증 저체온증 환자에게는 따뜻한 고열량 또는 포도당이 함유된 수액을 공급한다. 혈당 수치가 낮은 중등도 저체온증 환자의 경우 프로토콜에 따라 정맥 내로 포도당을 투여하고 5분마다 혈당 측정을 반복해서 시행하고 추가로 포도당 투여가 필요한지 확인한다.

저체온증 환자는 조직으로의 산소 전달이 감소하기 때문에 산소를 보충하는 것이 도움이 될 수 있다. 산소 헤모글로빈 해리 곡선은 중심체온 감소에 따라 왼쪽으로 이동한다. 이는 적절한 수준의 헤모글로빈포화도를 나타내는 맥박산소측정 수치가 세포 수준에서 적절한 산소 공급을 반영하지 못할 수 있음을 의미한다. 산소를 따뜻하게 공급하고 가습할 수 있다면(42.2~46.1℃) 환자에게 더 많은 도움이 될 수 있다.

반응이 없는 저체온증 환자의 경우 수동적 재가온만으로는 중심체온을 높이는데 충분하지 않다. 이러한 환자는 기도를 보호하기 위해 보조기도기가 필요하며 이는 턱의 강직에 따라 시행한다. 병원 전 처치 제공자는 전문 기도유지를 시행하는 동안 치명적인 부정맥을 유발할 위험이 낮으므로 주저하지 말고 기도를 확실하게 유지해야 한다. 거칠게 다루지 않고 기관내삽관을 성공적으로 시행할 수 없는 경우 백마스크로 환기를 지속해서 시행하고 다른 전문 기도유지 장비(예: 후두튜브기도기, 후두마스크기도기, 코기관내삽관) 사용을 고려한다. 최소한 입인두기도기 또는 코인두기도기를 삽입한 후 백마스크 환기를 시행해야 한다.

정맥 내로 5% 포도당이 포함된 생리식염수를 42.8℃로 따뜻하게 데워 환자를 자극하지 않고 투여한다. 저체온증 환자에게 차가운(실온) 수액을 투여하면 환자를 더 차갑게 만들거나 재가온이 지연될 수 있으므로 투여해서는 안 된다. 생리식염수 및 포도당 용액을 사용할 수 없는 경우 따뜻한 결정질 용액을 사용한다. 500~1,000mL의 따뜻한 수액을 투여하고 수액 백을 환자 아래에 놓아 압력을 가하여 수액을 투여함으로써 수액이 얼거나 차가워지는 것을 방지한다. 따뜻한 수액의 재가온 효과는 기껏해야 미미하며 병원 전 처치 제공자

는 현명한 판단을 통해 수액 투여(입안 또는 정맥 내)가 환자에게 흡인, 기침, 고통스러운 자극의 위험을 감수할 가치가 있는지를 결정해야 한다. 환자의 팔다리에 핫팩을 대거나 마사지하는 것은 권장하지 않는다.

일반적으로 능동적 외부 재가온은 가슴 부위만 일어나며 팔다리에는 능동적인 재가온은 일어나지 않는다. 이러한 접근 방식은 말초순환이 증가하여 중심체온이 재가온하기 전에 팔다리에서 가슴으로 차가운 혈액이 더 많이 되돌아오는 것을 방지한다. 말초혈액의 복귀가 증가하면 산증과 고칼륨혈증이 증가하고 중심체온이 감소(잔류저체온)할 수 있다. 이는 소생술을 복잡하게 만들고 심실세동을 촉진할 수 있다.

2020 AHA 심폐소생술 및 응급 심혈관 치료를 위한 지침

특수 상황에서의 심정지-우발적 저체온증

저체온증 환자의 소생술에 대한 지침은 수십 년에 걸쳐 발전해 왔다. 미국심장협회의 응급 심혈관 치료 지침의 가장 최근 개정판은 2020년 순환기 학회지에 발표되었다. 이 지침은 우발적 저체온증으로 인한 이차적 심정지와 관련하여 2015년에 발표한 지침을 변경하지 않았다.

저체온증 환자는 병원 전 처치 제공자에게 많은 어려움을 줄 수 있으며 특히 의식이 없는 중등도 또는 중증 저체온증 환자는 더욱 그렇다. 중증 저체온증은 중심체온이 30℃ 미만으로 정의되기 때문에 심박출량 감소와 동맥압 감소로 인해 맥박이나 호흡을 감지할 수 없어 임상적으로 사망한 것처럼 보일 수 있다. 지금까지는 환자의 생존 가능성에 따라 이러한 환자에게 BLS 또는 ALS 처치를 시작할지를 결정하는 것이었다. 또한 이러한 환자가 일차적으로 저체온증에 노출되었는지 또는 이전에 내과 질환이나 외상성 손상을 입었는지를 결정하기 어려울 수 있다. 병원 전 처치 제공자의 다른 우려 사항은 잠재적인 과민성 심근이 있는 저체온증 환자를 거친 취급으로부터 보호하고 맥박이 감지되지 않는 환자에게 가슴압박을 시작하는 것이며 이 두 가지 처치로 인해 심실세동이 일어날 수 있다.

일차 또는 이차 저체온증을 유발한 상황과 관계없이 일반적으로 이송 거리가 짧은 도시 환경이든 이송이 상당히 지연될 가능성이 있는 오지의 환경이든 임상 증상에 근거하여 인명 구조 절차를 보류해

서는 안 되며 이 경우 환자 처치가 연장되어야 할 수도 있다(이후 논의 참조).

경증에서 중증 저체온증 처치를 위한 BLS 지침

저체온증이 있는 환자는 가능하면 수평 자세를 유지해야 하며, 특히 초기 처치 시에는 저혈압과 후유증이 악화하지 않도록 주의해야 한다. 저체온증 환자는 한랭이뇨 작용으로 체액이 고갈된 경우가 많다. 저체온증 환자의 경우 호흡과 맥박을 촉지하거나 감지하기 어려울 수 있다. 따라서 처음에는 호흡을 평가한 다음 최대 60초 동안 맥박을 확인해서 다음 중 하나를 확인하는 것이 좋다.

- 호흡 정지
- 맥박이 없는 심정지(무수축, 심실빈맥, 심실세동)
- 서맥(CPR 필요)

숨을 쉬지 않는 경우 환자가 명백히 사망한 경우(예: 참수, 사후경축)가 아니라면 즉시 구조 호흡을 시작한다. 맥박이 없고 순환 징후가 감지되지 않은 저체온증 환자에게는 즉시 가슴 압박을 시작한다. 맥박이 감지되는지 의심스러운 경우 가슴 압박을 시작한다. 환자가 다시 체온이 회복할 때까지 BLS 처치를 보류하지 않는다. 환자가 심정지 상태로 판단되면 최신 BLS 지침을 따른다.

무맥성 심실빈맥 또는 심실세동이 있는 경우 자동심장충격기(AED)를 사용해야 한다. 현재 응급 심혈관 처치 지침(**그림 19-11**)에서는 이러한 환자에게 최대 5주기(2분)의 심폐소생술(1주기는 가슴 압박 30회와 2회 인공호흡)을 시행한 후 AED가 도착하면 심전도 리듬을 분석하고 필요한 경우 제세동을 시행하는 것을 권장한다. 제세동 가능한 리듬이 확인되면 1회 제세동을 시행한 후 5주기의 심폐소생술을 계속 시행한다. 저체온즌 환자가 1회 제세동에도 맥박이 감지되는 반응을 보이지 않으면 추가 제세동 시도를 연기하고 추가 제세동을 시도하기 전에 환자를 30℃ 이상으로 재가온하는 데 중점을 두고 효과적인 심폐소생술에 집중한다.

저체온증 환자에게 가슴 압박을 시행하는 경우 추운 환경에서는 가슴벽의 탄력이 감소하기 때문에 더 큰 힘이 필요하다. 중심체온이 30℃ 미만인 경우 정상적인 동방결절 리듬으로의 전환은 일반적으로 이 중심체온이 재가온이 이루어질 때까지 회복되지 않는다.

환자가 다시 체온을 회복하고 반응이 없을 때까지 환자를 사망으로 선언하지 않는 것의 중요하다는 것은 아무리 강조해도 지나치지 않다. 저체온증 피해자를 대상으로 한 연구에 따르면 추위는 중요한 장기를 보호하는 효과가 있다고 한다.

저체온증 처치를 위한 ACLS 지침

현장에서 중중 저체온증을 처치하는 데는 여전히 논란의 여지가 있다. 그러나 ACLS 시행에 대한 지침은 정상체온 환자와는 다르다. 저체온증으로 의식이 없는 환자는 기도 보호가 필요하며 기관내삽관을 시행해야 한다. 심실세동이 발생하는 것을 우려하여 기도확보를 지연시키지 않는다. 앞서 언급한 바와 같이 제세동이 필요한 리듬이 감지되면 이상형 제세동기의 경우 120~200J 또는 단상형 제세동기의 경우 360J로 1회 제세동을 시행한 후 즉시 심폐소생술을 다시 시행한 다음 중심체온이 30℃ 이상이 될 때까지 심장 약물 및 후속 제세동 시행을 연기해야 한다. 가능하면 따뜻하고 가습된 산소 공급과 따뜻한 수액을 정맥 내로 투여하여 적극적인 재가온을 시작하고 추가 열 손실을 방지할 방법으로 환자를 이송한다. 경중 저체온증 환자에게는 수동적 재가온이 적절하다는 점에 유의한다. 그러나 중등도에서 중증의 저체온증 환자에게는 일반적으로 응급실, 수술실 또는 중환자실에서 시행하는 절차로 능동적 재가온을 적극적으로 시행해야 한다. 이러한 환자에 대한 수동적 재가온만으로는 병원 전 환경에서 중심체온을 높이는데 완전히 부적절하며 EMS 제공하는 추가 열 손실 방지하는 효과적인 처치에 집중한다.

저체온증 환자에게 ACLS 처치를 시행하는 경우 어려운 점은 심장이 ACLS 약물, 페이싱 및 제세동에 반응하지 않을 수 있다는 것이다. 또한 ACLS에 사용되는 약물(예: 에피네프린, 아미오다론, 리도카인, 프로카인아마이드)은 중증 저체온증 환자에게 반복적으로 투여하면 순환계에 독성 수준으로 축적될 수 있으며 특히 환자가 재가온 되었을 때 더욱 그렇다. 따라서 중심체온이 30℃ 미만인 환자의 경우 정맥 내 약물 투여를 보류하는 것이 좋다. 저체온증 환자가 처음에 중심체온이 30℃ 이상이거나 심한 저체온증 환자가 이 온도 이상으로 재가온된 경우 정맥 내로 약물을 투여할 수 있다. 그러나 ACLS에서 표준 약물 투여 간격보다 더 긴 약물 투여 간격이 권장된다. 중심체온이 30℃ 이상으로 상승하면 현재 ACLS 지침에 따라 반복적인 제세동을 시행해야 한다.

마지막으로 환자의 손상이 생명과 양립할 수 없는 경우 가슴 압박이 불가능할 정도로 몸이 얼어붙으면 입과 코가 얼음으로 막힌 경우에만 현장에서 실시하는 BLS와 ACLS 처치를 보류해야 한다. **그림 19-11**은 맥박이 있는 환자와 맥박이 없는 환자 모두에 대한 경증, 중등도 및 중증 저체온증 환자에 대한 지침이다.

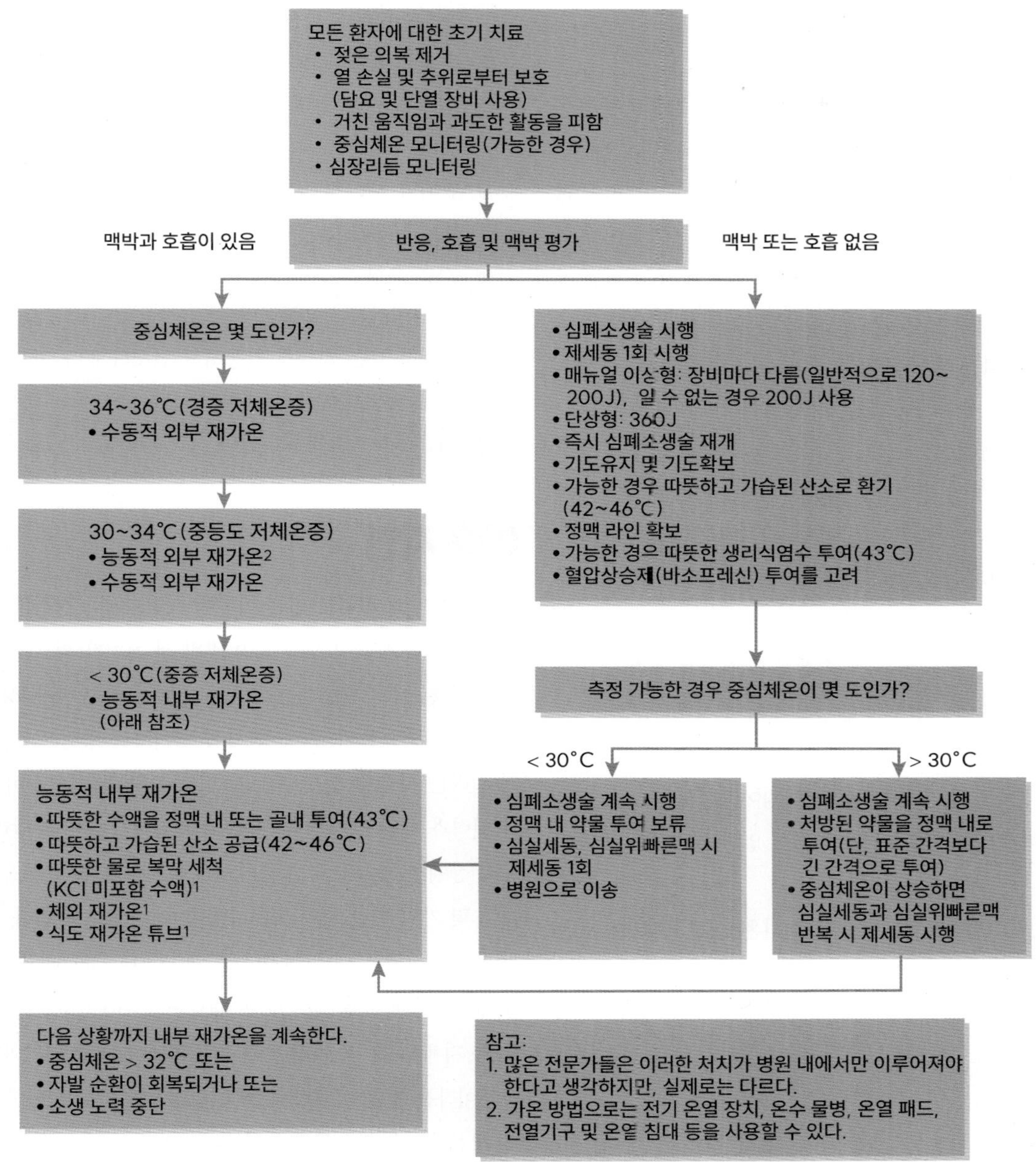

그림 19-11 2010년 심폐소생술 및 응급심혈관 치료 지침의 미국심장협회(AHA) 저체온증 알고리즘에서 수정되었다. 참고: 복막 세척, 체외 재가온 및 식도 재가온 튜브는 일반적으로 병원에서만 시행할 수 있는 시술이다.

Data from American Heart Association. Environmental trauma I: heat and cold. In Handbook of Emergency Cardiovascular Care for Healthcare Providers. AHA; 2006.

추위와 관련된 손상 예방법

현장에 있을 때는 환자, 본인 및 병원 전 처치 제공자의 추위와 관련된 손상을 예방하는 것이 중요하다. 저온 관련 손상을 예방하기 위한 권장 사항은 다음과 같다.

1. 일반적으로 저온 손상과 관련된 위험 요소에 유의한다.
 • 피로
 • 탈수
 • 영양 결핍
 • 추운 날씨에 대한 경험 부족
 • 흡연
 • 차가운 바람

2. 춥고 습하며 바람이 많이 부는 환경에서 건조한 상태를 유지할 수 없는 경우 가능한 한 빨리 대피할 곳을 찾는다.

3. 저온 손상 관련 병력이 있는 사람은 이후 저온 손상에 걸릴 위험이 더 높다.

4. 탈수를 피한다.

5. 추운 환경에서는 음주를 피한다.

6. 실수로 차가운 물에 빠졌을 경우 다른 사람들과 함께 모여 몸을 움츠리는 방법을 사용한다. 20℃ 미만의 차가운 물에서 가만히 있고 해안 근처(45분 거리 미만)가 아니라면 수영을 시도하지 않으면 생존할 가능성이 더 높다.

7. 다음과 같은 방법으로 추운 환경에서 생존 가능성을 높인다.
   - 생존에 대한 의지 유지
   - 적응력과 즉흥적인 대처 능력
   - 긍정적인 태도를 유지하고 일시적인 상황이라고 믿음
   - 침착한 상태를 유지

8. 겨드랑이나 서혜부에 손가락을 넣어 체온을 이용해 따뜻하게 한다. 발가락이나 발은 다른 사람의 배 위에 올려놓을 수 있다.

9. 추운 날씨에 예기치 않은 차량 내 비상 상황에 대비하여 방한복(예: 신발, 양말, 장갑, 겨울 모자, 단열 바지와 재킷, 바람막이)을 차 안에 보관한다. 젖은 옷은 열 손실을 악화시킬 수 있으므로 습기를 흡수하는 옷은 피한다(예: 양모나 양털 사용).

10. 항상 장갑을 착용한다. 추운 날씨에 맨손으로 금속 물체를 만지면 동상이 빠르게 발생할 수 있다. 벙어리장갑은 모든 손가락 주위에 따뜻한 공기를 가둘 수 있어 일반 장갑보다 효과적이다.

11. 풍속냉각지수(**그림 19-12**)는 풍속과 기온으로 구성되어 있음을 이해하고 극한의 추위에 대비하여 단열 의류와 방풍 의류를 착용한다.

12. 발에서 신발로 흡기를 전달하는 양말로 발을 건조하게 유지한다.

13. 굽이 낮은 신발을 신고 눈 위를 걷지 않는다. 적절한 신발과 방한복이 없는 경우 안전한 곳에서 머물도록 한다.

14. 눈 위에 직접 눕거나 쉬지 않는다. 나뭇가지, 침낭, 판초 또는 사용 가능한 모든 재료로 단열한다. 야외에서는 침낭을 사용한다.

15. 옷에 땀이 남아 있으면 열 손실을 증가시키고 떨림을 유발할 수 있으므로 땀을 흡수하고 유지하는 옷을 입지 않는다.

16. 로션을 사용할 때는 오일 기반 제품(예: 챕스틱, 바셀린)을 사용한다. 얼굴, 손, 귀에 수성 로션을 바르면 동창과 동상에 걸릴 위험을 증가시킨다.

17. 추운 날씨로부터 다리를 보호할 때는 생식기 부위를 보호해야 한다. 운동복 바지, 긴 속옷, 라이크라 타이츠, 고어텍스 바지 또는 이러한 의류를 조합하여 사용한다.

18. 동상을 예방하려면 다음과 같이 한다.
   - 혈액 순환을 방해하는 꽉 끼는 옷, 장갑, 부츠를 착용하지 않는다.
   - 손가락, 발가락, 얼굴을 주기적으로 움직여 체온을 유지하고 마비된 부위가 있는지 확인한다.
   - 저온 손상 및 저체온증의 경고 징후를 관찰할 수 있는 동료와 함께 일하거나 운동한다.
   - 적절한 보온 의류를 착용하고 건조하게 유지하며 항상 여분의 속옷, 양말, 신발을 휴대한다.
   - 저림과 무감각에 주의한다.

이송 지연

때때로 환자의 위치로 인해 이송이 지연되거나 적절한 의료기관으로 이송하는 데 시간이 오래 걸려 병원 전 처치가 필요할 수 있다. 따라서 병원 전 처치 제공자는 신속한 이송을 하는 것 이상으로 처치 방법을 고려해야 할 수 있다. 환자를 처치하는 방법은 결정적인 치료까지 걸리는 시간, 승인된 프로토콜, 보유하고 있는 장비와 소모품, 추가 인력과 자원, 환자의 위치, 손상의 심각성에 따라 달라질 수 있다.

이 장에서 논의된 각 환경의 중등도에서 중증 손상을 입은 환자에 대한 몇 가지 연장 처치 고려사항이 여기에 나와 있다. 모든 환자 처치와 같이 최우선 순위는 현장 안전, XABCDEs(대량 출혈, 기도, 호흡, 순환, 장애, 노출/환경)이며 때로는 MARH(대량 출혈, 기도, 호흡, 순환, 저체온증) 및 이러한 환경에 적절한 표준 평가와 처치 절차의 사용이라는 것을 이해해야 한다. 환경적인 스트레스(더위 또는 추위)를 제거하는 데 특별한 주의를 기울인다. 의료 지도가 가능한 경우 항상 초기에 의료 지도를 요청하고 처치를 시행하는 동안에 의료 지도 의사의 의료 지도를 받는다. 나열된 절차 중 업무 범위를 벗어나는 처치는 자격을 갖춘 다른 의료진에 의해서만 시행한다.

모든 기관에서 심폐소생술 중단에 대한 지침을 마련하고 있다는 사실을 아는 것이 중요하다. 미국심장협회는 BLS 또는 ALS 소생술의 보류 또는 중단으로 인해 발생하는 윤리적 문제에 대해 의견을 발표했다. 야생의학회는 일단 심폐소생술을 시작하면 의식이 있는 환자에게 소생에 성공할 때까지, 구조자가 지칠 때까지, 구조자가 위험에 처할 때까지, 환자가 더욱 확실한 처치를 위해 인계할 때까지 또는 환자가 장시간(30분)의 소생술에도 불구하고 반응이 없을 때까지 계속할 것을 권장한다. 또한 미국 응급의학협회는 병원 밖 환경에서의 심폐

풍속 냉각 도표(Wind Chill Chart)

온도 (°F)

풍속 (MPH) \ Calm	40	35	30	25	20	15	10	5	0	−5	−10	−15	−20	−25	−30	−35	−40	−45
5	36	31	25	19	13	7	1	−5	−11	−16	−22	−28	−34	−40	−46	−52	−57	−63
10	34	27	21	15	9	3	−4	−10	−16	−22	28	−35	−41	−47	−53	−59	−66	−72
15	32	25	19	13	6	0	−7	−13	−19	−26	−32	−39	−45	−51	−58	−64	−71	−77
20	30	24	17	11	4	−2	−9	−15	−22	−29	−35	−42	−48	−55	−61	−68	−74	−81
25	29	23	16	9	3	−4	−11	−17	−24	−31	−37	−44	−51	−58	−64	−71	−78	−84
30	28	22	15	8	1	−5	−12	−19	−26	−33	−39	−46	−53	−60	−67	−73	−80	−87
35	28	21	14	7	0	−7	−14	−21	−27	−34	−41	−48	−55	−62	−69	−76	−82	−89
40	27	20	13	6	−1	−8	−15	−22	−29	−36	−43	−50	−57	−64	−71	−78	−84	−91
45	26	19	12	5	−2	−9	−16	−23	−30	−37	−44	−51	−58	−65	−72	−79	−86	−93
50	26	19	12	4	−3	−10	−17	−24	−31	−38	−45	−52	−60	−67	−74	−81	−88	−95
55	25	18	11	4	−3	−11	−18	−25	−32	−39	−46	−54	−61	−68	−75	−82	−89	−97
60	25	17	10	3	−4	−11	−19	−26	−33	−40	−48	−55	−62	−69	−76	−84	−91	−98

동상 발생 시간 : ☐ 30분 ☐ 10분 ☐ 5분

$$풍속 냉각 (°F) = 35.74\ 0.6215T − 35.75(V^{0.16}) + 0.4275T(V^{0.16})$$
Where, T = 기온 (°F) V = 풍속(mph)

그림 19-12 풍속 냉각 지수
Courtesy of the National Weather Service.

소생술 중단에 대한 지침을 제공한다(6장, 현장 평가 및 처치 참조). 의료 지도가 가능한 경우 가능한 한 일찍 환자와 관련된 의료 지도를 시작하여 환자의 특수한 상황에 따라 총 20분이 지난 후에 심폐소생술 중단을 고려한다[심폐소생술을 20~30분 이상 연장할 수 있는 추가 상황(예: 찬물 침수, 낙뢰)에 대해서는 20장, 환경 외상 II: 낙뢰, 익사, 잠수 및 고도를 참조].

열 관련 질환

열사병

가능한 한 빨리 전신 냉각을 시행한다. 물을 사용할 수 있는 모든 방법을 활용한다. 시원한 물에 목까지 몸을 담그거나(신체 조절 유지 및 기도 보호) 전신에 물(예: 수액, 식염수, 생수 등)을 뿌리고 지속해서 바람(자연 바람, 부채질, 선풍기)을 제공한다. 가능하면 환자 상태를 의료 지도 의사에게 보고하고 추가 의료 지도를 받는다. 직장 체온이 38.9℃에 도달하면 신체의 냉각을 중단하고 환자가 떨거나 저체온증이 생기지 않도록 보호한다. 병원 전 처치 제공자가 도착하기 전에 목격자나 최초반응자가 이미 얼음찜질을 시작하면 환자의 직장 체온이 38.9℃에 도달할 때까지 얼음찜질을 계속 시행하는 것을 고려하고 의료 지도 의사에게 보고한다.

환자를 냉각시키면서 반응이 없는 환자의 기도를 유지하고 고유량의 산소를 백마스크에 연결하여 보조 환기를 시작한다. 정맥 라인을 확보하고 생리식염수 500mL를 투여한 후 활력징후를 평가한다. 환자에게 생리식염수 500mL를 투여할 때마다 활력징후를 평가해야 한다. 처음 1시간 동안 총 수액 투여량은 1~2L를 초과하지 않아야 한다. 병원 전 단계 처치가 길어지는 경우 그다음 1시간 동안 1L의 수액을 추가로 투여하는 것을 고려할 수 있다.

다음 우선순위는 프로토콜에 따라 다이아제팜과 포도당을 투여하여 발작과 저혈당을 처치하는 것이다. 환자를 회복 자세로 눕히고 의식 수준, 활력징후, 직장체온, 혈당 측정 등의 평가를 계속한다. 남은 이송 시간 동안 지지 요법과 기본적인 신체의 요구사항을 제공한다.

운동 관련 저나트륨혈증

혈중 나트륨 농도가 낮은 것으로 추정되는 경우 이를 교정한다. 환자가 입으로 음식을 섭취할 수 있는 경우 감자칩, 프레첼 또는 기타 짠 음식이나 스포츠음료, 기타 나트륨이 함유된 음료를 제공한다. 입으로 공급하는 나트륨 용액은 적절한 고장성 생리식염수 치료제로 입증되었다. 현장에서 물 반 컵(125mL, 9% 생리식염수)에 고체형 부용 큐브 3~4개를 용해하여 이 용액은 준비할 수 있다. 소금 정제만 투여하는 것은 권장하지 않으며 소금 정제와 함께 수분을 추가로 섭취해야 하며 나트륨 수치가 지나치게 높아질 위험이 있다.

그런 다음 정맥 라인을 확보하고 생리식염수를 정맥 라인이 유지될 정도의 속도로 투여한다. 환자를 의료기관으로 이송하는 데 예상되는 지연 시간 또는 심한 탈수 또는 횡문근융해증의 존재 여부에 따라 의료 지도 의사의 의료 지도를 받아 250mL/h 이상으로 수액을 투여한다. 저장성 수액은 뇌부종을 악화시키고 상태를 악화시켜 발작, 혼수, 사망으로 이어질 수 있으므로 사용하지 않는다. 중증 증상이나 징후(발작 또는 혼수)가 있는 환자에게는 푸포세마이드(가능한 경우 이뇨제)를 투여하여 세포 외 체수분 함량을 줄이는 동시에 정맥 내로 생리식염수를 250~500mL/h로 투여하여 나트륨을 공급하는 것을 고려한다.

뇌부종과 두개내압 증가를 평가한다. 기준 글래스고혼수척도 점수를 설정하고 진행성 뇌부종 및 두개내압 상승에 대해 10분마다 재평가한다(뇌부종에 대한 권장 사항에 따라 처치한다. 자세한 내용은 8장, 머리와 목 외상 장 참조).

메스꺼움과 분출성 구토를 처치할 준비를 한다. 대형 쓰레기봉투의 한쪽 면을 잡고 봉투의 가장자리에서 약 30cm 아래에 환자의 머리가 들어갈 구멍을 만든다. 구멍을 통해 환자의 머리를 넣어 환자가 봉투 중앙을 내려다볼 수 있도록 한다. 또한 이뇨가 시작되면 소변을 관리할 수 있도록 준비한다. 큰 쓰레기봉투를 기저귀로 사용하거나 양동이 또는 기타 용기를 사용한다.

환자가 폐 질환의 징후를 보이거나, 무기력하거나 숨이 차면 산소를 보충 공급한다(코삽입관으로 2~4L/분). 반응이 없는 환자의 기도를 개방하고 백마스크에 산소를 연결하여 분당 10회(과다환기 시행하지 않음)로 보조 환기를 시작한다(자세한 내용은 8장, 머리와 목 외상 참조).

환자의 혈당 수치를 평가하고 저혈당 환자에게 프로토콜에 따라 정맥 내로 포도당을 투여한다. 발작을 모니터링하고 항경련제(예: 프로토콜에 따라 초기에 정맥 내 또는 근육 내로 다이아제팜 2~5mg)를 투여한다. 의식이 없는 환자는 회복 자세를 취해주고 지속해서 평가를 시행한다.

한랭과 관련된 질환

동상

저체온증이 있는 경우 환자를 보호하고 처치한다. 재가온 절차를 시작하기 전에 정맥 내로 수액 소생술을 시작하거나 최소한 정맥 라인을 확보한다. 정맥 라인을 확보할 수 없는 경우 골강 내로 수액을 투여할 수 있다. 이송이 지연되는 상황에서는 능동적 재가온을 고려한다. 신속하고 적극적인 재가온은 조직에 내 얼음 결정의 직접적인 손상을 되돌릴 수 있지만, 손상의 중증도를 변화시키지는 못할 수 있다. 수동적 해동에 비해 결과를 크게 악화할 수 있으므로 해동된 조직이 재동결되지 않도록 하는 것이 중요하다. 능동적 재가온을 시행해야 하는 경우 언제 어디에서 시작해야 하는지가 주요 고려 사항이다.

표준 재가온 절차는 동상에 걸린 조직이 용기의 측면이나 바닥에 닿지 않도록 충분히 큰 용기에 37~39℃의 온수에 동상 조직을 담그는 것이다. 영향을 받은 팔다리를 담근다. 물은 보통 손에 닿았을 때 뜨겁지 않고 따뜻하게 느껴져야지 한다(여기에 제시된 온도 범위는 이전에 권장했던 온도 범위보다 낮다). 가능하면 구강 또는 직장 체온계를 사용하여 수온을 측정한다. 권장 온도보다 낮은 온도는 조직이 해동은 되지만, 빠른 해동과 조직 생존에는 도움이 되지 않는다. 온도가 높을수록 통증이 심해지고 화상을 입을 수 있다. 강한 건조한 열원(예: 모닥불 근처에 놓는 등)으로 재가온하지 않는다. 조직이 부드럽고 유연해질 때까지 계속 담그며 최대 30~60분이 소요될 수 있다. 담그는 동안 손상된 부위를 직접 문지르거나 마사지하지 말고 팔다리를 적극적으로 움직이면 도움이 된다. 따뜻하게 온수에 담그는 것이 불가능한 경우 추가 조직 손상을 방지하기 위해 손가락이나 발가락 사이에 멸균 거즈를 끼워 느슨하게 멸균 드레싱을 시행하고 물집은 터뜨리지 않는다.

급속 해동 시 극심한 통증이 발생한다. 필요한 경우 프로토콜에 따라 정맥 내로 진통제를 투여한다(아스피린은 라이증후군의 위험이 있으므로 소아 환자에게는 금기이다).

손상된 부위의 피부색, 환부의 온기, 감각이 정상으로 회복되는 것은 모두 좋은 징후이다. 손상된 모든 부위를 따뜻한 바람으로 건조하고(손상 부위를 수건으로 닦지 않는다) 피부에 알로에베라를 바르고 발가락이나 손가락 사이에 멸균 거즈를 대고 드레싱을 시행한 후 팔다리를 부목으로 고정한 후 들어 올려준다. 특히 야외에서 환자를 이송 장소로 옮길 때는 팔다리를 단열재로 덮고 방풍 및 방수 소재(예: 쓰레기봉투)로 감싸 체온을 유지한다.

저체온증

능동적 재가온 처치를 시작한다. 핵심은 환자를 주변 환경으로부터 단열시키고 젖은 옷을 제거한 후 마른 옷으로 갈아입혀 추가적인 열 손실을 방지하는 것이다. 정맥 라인을 확보하고 가온한 수액(40~42°C)을 투여한다.

떨림은 외부 재가온 방법에 비해 이송 시간이 짧은 일반적인 병원 전 환경에서 경증 저체온증이 있는 비외상 환자를 재가온시키는 가장 좋은 방법이다. 최대로 몸을 떨 수 있는 저체온증 환자는 시간당 최대 3~4℃까지 중심체온을 올릴 수 있다. 외부 열원을 종종 사용지만 최소한의 이점만 제공할 수 있다. 중등도에서 중증 저체온증 환자의 경우 이러한 열원은 저체온증 단열 랩(나중에 설명)과 함께 사용할 때 이송 지연하는 상황에서 여전히 중요한 고려 사항이다. 외부 열원과 관련된 몇 가지 고려 사항은 다음과 같다.

- 마스크로 따뜻하게(최대 42.2℃) 가습된 산소를 공급하면 환기 중 열 손실을 방지하고 호흡기를 통해 가슴으로 열을 어느 정도 전달할 수 있다.

- 신체 간 접촉은 열전달에 도움이 될 수 있지만, 많은 연구에서 경증의 저체온증 환자를 제외하고는 아무런 이점을 보여주지 못했다.

- 전기 및 휴대용 온열 패드는 추가적인 이점을 제공하지 않는다.

- 강제로 공기를 따뜻하게 덥히는 것은 냉각 후 중심체온이 다시 떨어지는 것(잔류 저체온)을 최소화하는 데 어느 정도 이점이 있으며 경증 저체온증 환자에게는 떨림과 유사한 효과적인 가온을 제공한다.

열 손실을 최소화하기 위해 야외 환경에서 모든 저체온증 환자를 보온한다. 환자의 체온을 보호할 수 있는 여러 겹의 체온저하 랩을 준비한다. 바닥에 방수 기능이 있는 대형 비닐 시트를 깔아준다. 방수포 위에 침낭, 담요 등의 단열층을 추가한다. 단열층 위에 외부 열원과 함께 환자를 눕힌다. 환자 위에 두 번째 단열층을 덮는다. 저체온증 랩의 왼쪽을 먼저 환자 위로 접은 다음 오른쪽을 접는다. 열 손실을 방지하기 위해 환자의 머리를 덮고 환자를 평가할 수 있도록 얼굴 부위만 열어둔다.

환자의 저혈당 여부를 평가한다. 환자에게 포도당을 투여하면 떠는 동안 근육의 대사에 충분한 연료(당)를 공급할 수 있어 저혈당을 예방할 수 있다. 의식이 명료한 환자는 따뜻하고 당분이 많은 수분을 입으로 섭취할 수 있게 한다.

요 약

- 병원 전 처치 제공자는 이 장에 설명하는 것과 같은 환경적 응급 상황에 필연적으로 직면하게 된다.

- 병원 전 환경에서 신속한 평가 및 처치를 제공하기 위해 병원 전 처치 제공자는 일반적인 환경 응급상황에 대한 기본 지식을 갖추고 있어야 한다. 또한 피부의 역할과 뇌의 체온 조절 기전을 포함하여 신체가 체온을 조절하는 방법을 이해한다.

- 체온을 유지하고 발산하는 방법은 병원 전 처치 제공자에게 중요한 개념이다. 병원 전 처치 제공자는 고체온증 또는 저체온증 환자를 효과적으로 처치할 수 있도록 열과 냉기가 신체에서 어떻게 전달되는지(예: 전도, 복사, 대류, 증발)를 이해한다.

- 열 관련 질환의 경우 병원 전 처치 제공자는 열사병 환자를 효과적이고 신속한 전신 냉각으로 처치하여 중심체온을 빠르게 낮춰야 한다.

- 저온 관련 질환의 경우 병원 전 처치 제공자는 중등도에서 중증의 저체온증이 있는 모든 환자를 부드럽게 관리해야 하며 시간을 들여 추운 환경에서 환자를 벗어나게 하고 체온을 모니터링하면서 수동적 재가온을 시작해야 한다. 핵심은 추가적인 체온 소실을 방지하는 것이다.

- 병원 전 처치 제공자는 일반적으로 중심체온이 30℃ 미만일 때 약물과 제세동이 효과가 없다는 점을 기억한다.

- 소생술이 소용없다는 명백한 징후(예: 가슴 동결, 기도 내 얼음)가 나타나지 않는 한 환자는 체온이 올라갈 때까지 사망한 것이 아니다.

- 병원 전 처치 제공자는 더위 및 추위와 관련된 손상으로부터 자신을 보호하는 방법과 다른 사람의 안전을 옹호하는 방법을 알고 있어야 한다. 중요한 예방 개념에는 수분 보충, 체력, 열 순응, 추운 날씨에 대한 적절한 복장, 위험 요인 피하기 등이 포함된다.

- 효과적인 구조자가 되려면 자신의 안전을 유지해야 한다는 점을 기억한다. 구조 시도 중 구조대원이 목숨을 잃는 경우가 너무 많다.

시나리오 재구성

기온이 38.9℃에 이르는 무더운 여름 오후이다. 지난 30일 동안 매일 기온이 37.8℃를 넘는 매우 습한 날씨였다. 주변 환경의 높은 온도로 인해 EMS 제공자들이 수많은 환자를 응급실로 이송해야 하는 열 관련 질환이 많이 발생했다.

17시에 당신과 동료는 차 안에서 의식을 잃은 남성 환자가 있다는 신고를 받고 출동한다. 당신이 현장에 도착했을 때 백화점 야외 주차장에 주차된 차량에서 의식이 없고 손상이 없는 76세 남성을 발견했다. 환자의 기도, 호흡, 순환(ABC) 및 의식 수준을 신속하게 평가한 결과 환자가 말을 할 수 있지만, 비논리적이고 비이성적인 말을 하고 있다는 것을 알 수 있었다.

- 이 환자의 의식 저하의 잠재적 원인은 무엇인가?
- 열 관련 진단을 뒷받침하는 특징적인 징후는 무엇인가?
- 현장에서 응급실로 이송하는 동안 이 환자를 어떻게 처치를 시행해야 하는가?

시나리오 해결책

76세의 이 남성은 쇼핑센터에서 아내가 돌아오기를 차 안에서 기다리고 있었다. 이 남성은 체액 손실(땀 남)을 상쇄할 수 있는 효과적인 수분 공급 없이 고열에 노출되어 탈수 상태이다. 체질량 지수가 30 이상인 이 환자는 비만으로 인해 열 관련 질환의 위험이 더 높다.

아내는 남편이 고혈압으로 이뇨제, 관상동맥 질환으로 베타 차단제, 파킨슨병 치료제로 항콜린제를 먹고 있다는 추가 병력을 알려주었다. 세 가지 약물 모두 열 관련 질환의 위험 요소로 알려져 있다. 이 환자는 에어컨이 작동되지 않는 차 안에서 발견되었기 때문에 AVPU척도를 사용하여 ABC와 의식 수준을 신속하게 평가해야 한다. 비이성적이고 비논리적인 진술, 나이, 장소 등을 고려할 때 열사병이 의심되는 상황이다.

무딘 손상이나 관통상이 있는지 신속하게 평가한다. 다음으로 노인 환자는 심장질환이나 신경학적 장애(예: 뇌졸중)와 같은 기저 질환의 악화 여부를 평가해야 한다. 이 환자의 세 가지 질환은 모두 고열로 인해 악화하여 사망 위험이 증가하는 것으로 알려져 있다. 이 환자는 즉시 전신 냉각을 받는 것이 중요하다.

(다음 페이지에 계속)

시나리오 해결책 (이어서)

환자를 앞좌석의 직사광선이 비치치 않는 곳으로 옮기고 여분의 옷을 벗긴다. 당신은 외상 처치 가방에 들어 있는 생리식염수를 사용하여 환자의 머리부터 발끝까지 적시기 시작한다. 동료에게 에어컨을 작동시켜 대류 열전달을 증가시키기 위해 환자의 몸 전체에 공기 흐름을 증가시킨다. 들것을 이용해 환자를 구급차로 이동할 준비를 한다. 이 고열 환자를 위해 구급차의 환자 칸에 얼음물과 차가운 물 수건을 준비한다.

환자를 차량에서 구급차로 신속하게 옮긴다. 이송을 시작하면 차가운 물수건으로 환자의 전신을 적시고 머리 위쪽에서 부채질한다. 환자에게 고유량 산소를 공급하고 정맥 라인을 확보하며 정맥 라인이 유지될 정도로 수액을 투여하며 심전도를 모니터링한다. 고체온 (40℃ 이상)을 확인하기 위해 직장 체온을 측정할 준비를 한다. 고체온이 확인되면 500mL의 생리식염수를 정맥 내로 볼루스로 투여한다. 열사병을 앓고 있는 76세 남자 환자의 활력징후를 측정하고 이송할 의료기관으로 환자 상태를 보고한다.

References

1. Centers for Disease Control and Prevention/National Center for Health Statistics. Compressed mortality file. Updated November 19, 2018. Accessed October 25, 2021. https://www.cdc.gov/nchs/data_access/cmf.htm
2. Centers for Disease Control and Prevention. Heat-related deaths—Chicago, Illinois, 1996–2001, and United States, 1979–1999. *Morb Mortal Wkly Rep.* 2003;52(26):610.
3. National Center for Environmental Health (NCEH)/Agency for Toxic Substances and Disease Registry (ATSDR), Coordinating Center for Environmental Health and Injury Prevention (CCEHIP). Natural disasters and severe weather: extreme heat. Updated June 30, 2021. Accessed October 25, 2021. https://www.cdc.gov/disasters/extreme heat/index.html
4. Meiman J, Anderson H, Tomasallo C. Hypothermia-related deaths—Wisconsin, 2014, and United States, 2003–2013. *Morb Mortal Wkly Rep.* 2015;64(6):141-143.
5. Centers for Disease Control and Prevention. Hypothermia-related deaths—United States, 2003. *Morb Mortal Wkly Rep.* 2004;53(8);172.
6. O'Brien KK, Leon LR, Kenefick RW. Clinical management of heat-related illnesses. In: Auerbach PS, ed. *Auerbach's Wilderness Medicine.* 7th ed. Mosby Elsevier; 2017.
7. Dow J, Giesbrecht GG, Danzl DF, et al. Wilderness Medical Society practice guidelines for the out-of-hospital evaluation and treatment of accidental hypothermia: 2019 Update. *Wilderness Environ Med.* 2019;30(Suppl 4):S47-S69.
8. Lugo-Amador NM, Rothenhaus T, Moyer P. Heat-related illness. *Emerg Med Clin North Am.* 2004;22:315-327.
9. Ulrich AS, Rathlev NK. Hypothermia and localized injuries. *Emerg Med Clin North Am.* 2004;22:281-298.
10. Centers for Disease Control and Prevention. Hypothermia-related deaths—United States, 2003. *Morb Mortal Wkly Rep.* 2004;53(8):172.
11. Brown DJA, Brugger H, Boyd J, et al. Accidental hypothermia. *N Engl J Med.* 2012;367(20);1930-1938.
12. Hawkins SC. Wilderness EMS systems. In: Hawkins SC, ed. *Wilderness EMS.* Wolters Kluwer; 2018.
13. Leon LR, Kenefick RW. Pathophysiology of heat-related illnesses. In: Auerbach PS, ed. *Auerbach's Wilderness Medicine.* 7th ed. Mosby Elsevier; 2017.
14. Freer L, Handford C, Imray CHE. Frostbite. In: Auerbach PS, ed. *Auerbach's Wilderness Medicine.* 7th ed. Mosby Elsevier; 2017.
15. Danzl DF, Huecker MR. Accidental hypothermia. In: Auerbach PS, ed. *Auerbach's Wilderness Medicine.* 7th ed. Mosby Elsevier; 2017.
16. National Aeronautics and Space Administration. 2020 Tied for Warmest Year on Record, NASA Analysis Shows. Published January 14, 2021. Accessed October 25, 2021. https://www.nasa.gov/press-release/2020-tied-for-warmest-year-on-record-nasa-analysis-shows
17. Vaidyanathan A, Malilay J, Schramm P, Saha S. Heat-related deaths—United States, 2004–2018. *Morb Mortal Wkly Rep.* 2020;69:729-734. doi: 10.15585/mmwr.mm6924a1
18. Centers for Disease Control and Prevention. Hypothermia-related deaths—United States, 1999–2002 and 2005. *Morb Mortal Wkly Rep.* 2006;55(10):282-284.
19. Hawkins SC, Simon RB, Beissinger JP, Simon D. *Vertical Aid: Essential Wilderness Medicine for Climbers, Trekkers, and Mountaineers.* The Countryman Press; 2017.
20. Hardy JD. Thermal comfort: skin temperature and physiological thermoregulation. In: Hardy JD, Gagge AP, Stolwijk JAJ, eds. *Physiological and Behavioral Temperature Regulation.* Charles C. Thomas; 1970.
21. Pozos RS, Danzl DF. Human physiological responses to cold stress and hypothermia. In: Pandolf KB, Burr RE, eds. *Medical Aspects of Harsh Environments.* Vol 1. Office of the Surgeon General, Borden Institute/TMM Publications; 2001:351-382.
22. Stocks JM, Taylor NAS, Tipton MJ, Greenleaf JE. Human physiological responses to cold exposure. *Aviat Space Environ Med.* 2004;75:444-457.
23. Wenger CB. The regulation of body temperature. In: Rhoades RA, Tanner GA, eds. *Medical Physiology.* Little, Brown; 1995.
24. Nunnelely SA, Reardon MJ. Prevention of heat illness. In: Pandolf KB, Burr RE, eds. *Medical Aspects of Harsh Environments.* Vol 1. Office of the Surgeon General, Borden Institute/TMM Publications; 2001:209-230.
25. Hall B, Hall J. *Sauer's Manual of Skin Diseases.* 10th ed. Lippincott Williams & Wilkins; 2010.

26. Krakowski A, Goldenberg A. Exposure to radiation from the sun. In: Auerbach PS, ed. *Auerbach's Wilderness Medicine*. 7th ed. Mosby Elsevier; 2017.

27. Lipman GS, Gaudio FFG, Eifling KP, Ellis MA, Otten EM, Grissom CK. Wilderness Medical Society practice guidelines for the prevention and treatment of heat-related illness: 2019 update. *Wilderness Environ Med*. 2019;30(4):S33-S46.

28. Yeo T. Heat stroke: a comprehensive review. *AACN Clin Issues*. 2004;15:280-293.

29. Wenger CB. Section I: human adaption to hot environments. In: Pandolf KB, Burr RE, eds. *Medical Aspects of Harsh Environments*. Vol 1. Office of the Surgeon General, Borden Institute/TMM Publications; 2001:51-86.

30. Sonna LA. Practical medical aspects of military operations in the heat. In: Pandolf KB, Burr RE, eds. *Medical Aspects of Harsh Environments*. Vol 1. Office of the Surgeon General, Borden Institute/TMM Publications; 2001:293-309.

31. Tek D, Olshaker JS. Heat illness. *Emerg Med Clin North Am*. 1992;10(2):299-310.

32. Wallace RF, Kriebel D, Punnett L, et al. The effects of continuous hot weather training on risk of exertional heat illness. *Med Sci Sports Exerc*. 2005;37(1):84-90.

33. Schimelpfenig T, Richards G, Tartar S. Management of heat illnesses. In: Hawkins SC, ed. *Wilderness EMS*. Wolters Kluwer; 2018.

34. Bedno SA, Li Y, Han W, et al. Exertional heat illness among overweight U.S. Army recruits in basic training. *Aviat Space Environ Med*. 2010;81(2):107-111.

35. Kenefick RW, Cheuvront SN, Leon LR, O'Brien KK. Dehydration and rehydration. In: Auerbach PS, ed. *Auerbach's Wilderness Medicine*. 7th ed. Mosby Elsevier; 2017.

36. Armstrong LE, Hubbard RW, Jones BH, Daniels JT. Preparing Alberto Salazar for the heat of the 1984 Olympic marathon. *Phys Sportsmed*. 1986;14:73-81.

37. Johnson RF, Kobrick JL. Psychological aspects of military performance in hot environments. In: Pandolf KB, Burr RE, eds. *Medical Aspects of Harsh Environments*. Vol 1. Office of the Surgeon General, Borden Institute/TMM Publications; 2001.

38. Sawka MN, Pandolf KB. Physical exercise in hot climates: physiology, performance, and biomedical issues. In: Pandolf KB, Burr RE, eds. *Medical Aspects of Harsh Environments*. Vol 1. Office of the Surgeon General, Borden Institute/TMM Publications; 2001.

39. Dutchman SM, Ryan AJ, Schedl HP, et al. Upper limits of intestinal absorption of dilute glucose solution in men at rest. *Med Sci Sport Exerc*. 1997;29:482-488.

40. Neufer PD, Young AJ, Sawka MN. Gastric emptying during exercise: effects of heat stress and hypohydration. *Eur J Appl Physiol*. 1989;58:433-439.

41. Bouchama A, Knochel JP. Medical progress: heatstroke. *N Engl J Med*. 2002;346(25):1978-1988.

42. Adams T, Stacey E, Stacey S, Martin D. Exertional heat stroke. *Br J Hosp Med (London)*. 2012;73(2):72-78.

43. Case DJ, Armstrong LE, Kenny GP, O'Connor FG, Huggins RA. Exertional heat stroke: new concepts regarding cause and care. *Curr Sports Med Rep*. 2012;11(3):115-123.

44. Casa DJ, McDermott BP, Lee E, Yeargin SW, Armstrong LE, Maresh CM. Cold-water immersion: the gold standard for exertional heat stroke treatment. *Exerc Sport Rev*. 2007;35(3):141-149.

45. Holtzhausen LM, Noakes TD. Collapsed ultra-endurance athlete: proposed mechanisms and an approach to management. *Clin J Sport Med*. 1997;7(4):292-301.

46. Gardner JW, Kark JA. Clinical diagnosis, management and surveillance of exertional heat illness. In: Pandolf KB, Burr RE, eds. *Medical Aspects of Harsh Environments*. Vol 1. Office of the Surgeon General, Borden Institute/TMM Publications; 2001:231-279.

47. Asplune CA, O'Connor FG, Noakes TD. Exercise-associated collapse: an evidence-based review and primer for clinicians. *Br J Sports Med*. 2011;45:1157-1162.

48. Nichols AW. Heat-related illness in sports and exercise. *Curr Rev Musculoskelet Med*. 2014;7:355-365.

49. Bennett BL, Hew-Butler T, Rosner MH, Myers T, Lipman GS. Wilderness Medical Society practice guidelines for treatment of exercise-associated hyponatremia: 2019 update. *Wilderness Environ Med*. 2020;31(1):50-62.

50. Rosner MH. Exercise-associated hyponatremia. *Semin Nephrol*. 2009;29(3):271-281.

51. Rosner M, Bennett B, Hoffman M, Hew-Butler T. Exercise induced hyponatremia. In: Simon E, ed. *Hyponatremia: Evaluation and Treatment*. Springer; 2013.

52. Leon LR, Helwig BG. Heat stroke: role of the systemic inflammatory response. *J Appl Physiol*. 2010;109(6):1980-1988.

53. Gaffin SL, Hubbard RW. Pathophysiology of heatstroke. In: Pandolf KB, Burr RE, eds. *Medical Aspects of Harsh Environments*. Vol 1. Office of the Surgeon General, Borden Institute/TMM Publications; 2001:161-208.

54. Semenza JC, Rubin CH, Flater KH, et al. Heat-related deaths during the July 1995 heat wave in Chicago. *N Engl J Med*. 1996;335(2):84-90.

55. Miller KC, Casa DJ, Adams WM, et al. Roundtable on preseason heat safety in secondary school athletics: prehospital care of patients with exertional heat stroke. *J Athl Train*. 2021;56(4):372-382.

56. Belval LN, Casa DJ, Adams WM, et al. Consensus statement: prehospital care of exertional heat stroke. *Prehosp Emerg Care*. 2018;22(3):392-397. doi: 10.1080/10903127.2017.1392666

57. Knochel JP, Reed G. Disorders of heat regulation. In: Narins RE, ed. *Maxwell and Kleenman's Clinical Disorders of Fluid and Electrolyte Metabolism*. 5th ed. McGraw-Hill; 1994.

58. Hawkins SC. Environmental emergencies. In: Pollak AN, ed. *Caroline's Emergency Care in the Streets*. 8th ed. Jones & Bartlett Learning; 2018.

59. Armstrong LE, Crago AE, Adams R, et al. Whole-body cooling of hyperthermic runners: comparison of two field therapies. *Am J Emerg Med*. 1996;14:335-358.

60. Costrini A. Emergency treatment of exertional heatstroke and comparison of whole-body cooling techniques. *Med Sci Sports Exerc*. 1984;22:15-18.

61. Gaffin SL, Gardner J, Flinn S. Current cooling method for exertional heatstroke. *Ann Intern Med*. 2000;132:678. doi: 10.7326/0003-4819-132-8-200004180-00023

62. Miller KC, Casa DJ, Adams WM, et al. Roundtable on preseason heat safety in secondary school athletics: prehospital care of patients with exertional heat stroke. *J Athl Train*. 2021;56(4):372-382.

63. Speedy DB, Noakes TD. Exercise-associated hyponatremia: a review. *Emerg Med*. 2001;13(1):17-27.

64. Backer HD, Shopes E, Collins SL, Barkan H. Exertional heat illness and hyponatremia in hikers. *Am J Emerg Med*. 1999;17(6):532-539.

65. Gardner JW. Death by water intoxication. *Mil Med*. 2002;164(3):432-434.

66. Noakes TD, Goodwin N, Rayner BL, et al. Water intoxication: a possible complication during endurance exercise. *Med Sci Sports Exerc*. 1985;17:370-375.

67. Rosner MH, Kirven J. Exercise-associated hyponatremia. *Clin J Am Soc Nephrol*. 2007;2:151-161.

68. Adrogue HJ, Madias NE. Hyponatremia. *N Engl J Med.* 2000;342(21):1581-1589.

69. Hiller WDB. Dehydration and hyponatremia during triathlons. *Med Sci Sports Exerc.* 1989;21(Suppl 5):S219-S221.

70. Speedy DB, Noakes TD, Rodgers IR. Hyponatremia in ultra-distance triathletes. *Med Sci Sports Exerc.* 1999;31:809-815.

71. Laird RH. Medical care at ultra-endurance triathlons. *Med Sci Sports Exerc.* 1989;21(Suppl 5):S222-S225.

72. Collins S, Reynolds B. The other heat-related emergency. *JEMS.* 2004;29(7):74-88.

73. Backer HD, Shopes E, Collins SL, Barkan H. Exertional heat illness and hyponatremia in hikers. *Am J Emerg Med.* 1999;17:532-539.

74. Noe RS, Choudhary E, Cheng-Dobson J, Wolkin AF, Newman SB. Exertional heat-related illnesses at the Grand Canyon National Park, 2004–2009. *Wilderness Environ Med.* 2013;24:422-428.

75. American College of Sports Medicine. Position stand: exercise and fluid replacement. *Med Sci Sports Exerc.* 2007;39(2):377-390.

76. Hew-Bulter T, Ayus JC, Kipps C, et al. Statement of Second International Exercise-Associated Hyponatremia Consensus Development Conference, New Zealand, 2007. *Clin J Sport Med.* 2008;18(2):111-121.

77. Ayus JC, Arieff A, Moritz ML. Hyponatremia in marathon runners. *N Engl J Med.* 2005;353:427.

78. U.S. Fire Administration. Firefighter fatalities in the United States in 2015. Federal Emergency Management Agency. Published October 2016. Accessed October 25, 2021. https://www.usfa.fema.gov/downloads/pdf/publications/ff_fat15.pdf

79. U.S. Department of Agriculture, U.S. Forest Service. Heat stress brochure. Accessed October 25, 2021. http://www.fs.fed.us/fire/safety/fitness /heat_stress/hs_pg1.html

80. Brazaitis M, Skurvydas A. Heat acclimation does not reduce the impact of hyperthermia on central fatigue. *Eur J Appl Physiol.* 2010;109:771-778.

81. Cheung SS, McLellan TM. Heat acclimation, aerobic fitness, and hydration effects on tolerance during uncompensable heat stress. *J Appl Physiol.* 1998;84:1731-1739.

82. Garrett AT, Goosens NG, Rehrer NJ, Patterson MJ, Cotter JD. Induction and decay of short-term heat acclimation. *Eur J Appl Physiol.* 2009;107:659-670.

83. Montain SJ, Latzka WA, Sawka MN. Fluid replacement recommendations for training in hot weather. *Mil Med.* 1999;164(7):502-508.

84. Parson KC. International standards for the assessment of the risk of thermal strain on clothed workers in hot environments. *Ann Occup Hyg.* 1999;43(5):297-308.

85. American College of Sports Medicine. Position stand on the recommended quantity and quality of exercise for developing and maintaining cardiorespiratory and muscular fitness, and flexibility in adults. *Med Sci Sports Exerc.* 1998;30(6):975-981.

86. Haskell WL, Lee IM, Pate RR, et al. Physical activity and public health: updated recommendation for adults from the American College of Sports Medicine and the American Heart Association. *Med Sci Sports Exerc.* 2007;39(8):1423-1424.

87. Sawka MN, Kolka MA, Montain SJ. *Ranger and Airborne School Students' Heat Acclimatization Guide.* U.S. Army Research Institute of Environmental Medicine; 2003.

88. Eichna LW, Park CR, Nelson N, et al. Thermal regulation during acclimatization in a hot, dry (desert type) environment. *J Appl Physiol.* 1950;163:585-597.

89. Federal Emergency Management System, U.S. Fire Administration. Emergency Incident Rehabilitation. Published February 2008. Accessed October 25, 2021. http://www.usfa.fema.gov/downloads/pdf/publications /fa_314.pdf

90. Hostler D. First responder rehab: good, better, best. *JEMS.* 2007;32(12):98-112; quiz 114.

91. Paterson R, Drake B, Tabin G, Butler FK Jr, Cushing T. Wilderness Medical Society practice guidelines for treatment of eye injuries and illnesses in the wilderness: 2014 update. *Wilderness Environ Med.* 2014;25:S19-S29.

92. Ulrich AS, Rathlev NK. Hypothermia and localized injuries. *Emerg Med Clin North Am.* 2004;22(2):281-298.

93. Thomas JR, Oakley EHN. Nonfreezing cold injury. In: Pandolf KB, Burr RE, eds. *Medical Aspects of Harsh Environments.* Vol 1. Office of the Surgeon General, Borden Institute/TMM Publications; 2001:467-490.

94. Montgomery H. Experimental immersion foot: review of the physiopathology. *Physiol Rev.* 1954;34(1):127-137.

95. Francis TJR. Nonfreezing cold injury: a historical review. *J R Nav Med Serv.* 1984;70:134-139.

96. Imray CHE, Handford C, Thomas OD, Castellani JW. Nonfreezing cold-induced injuries. In: Auerbach PS, ed. *Auerbach's Wilderness Medicine.* 7th ed. Mosby Elsevier; 2017.

97. Wrenn K. Immersion foot: a problem of the homeless in the 1990s. *Arch Intern Med.* 1991;151:785-788.

98. Ramstead KD, Hughes RB, Webb AJ. Recent cases of trench foot. *Postgrad Med J.* 1980;56:879-883.

99. Laskowski-Jones L, Jones L. Management of cold injuries. In: Hawkins SC, ed. *Wilderness EMS.* Wolters Kluwer, 2018.

100. Biem J, Koehncke N, Classen D, Dosman J. Out of cold: management of hypothermia and frostbite. *Can Med Assoc J.* 2003;168(3):305-311.

101. Vogel JE, Dellon AL. Frostbite injuries of the hand. *Clin Plast Surg.* 1989;16:565-576.

102. Mills WJ. Clinical aspects of freezing injury. In: Pandolf KB, Burr RE, eds. *Medical Aspects of Harsh Environments.* Vol 1. Office of the Surgeon General, Borden Institute/TMM Publications; 2001.

103. McIntosh SE, Hamonko M, Freer L, et al. Wilderness Medical Society Practice guidelines for the prevention and treatment of frostbite. *Wilderness Environ Med.* 2011;22;156-166.

104. Cauchy E, Davis CB, Pasquier M, Meyer EF, Hackett PH. A new proposal for management of severe frostbite in the austere environment. *Wilderness Environ Med.* 2016;27:92-99.

105. Zafren K, Giesbrecht G. State of Alaska Cold Injuries Guidelines. Department of Health and Social Services, Juneau, Alaska. Revised July 2014. Accessed October 25, 2021. http://mra.org/wp-content/uploads/2016/05/Alaska -DHSS-EMS-Cold-Injuries-Guidelines-June-2014.pdf

106. McIntosh SE, Freer L, Grissom CK, Pandey P, Dow DD, Hackett PH. Wilderness Medical Society practice guidelines for the prevention and treatment of frostbite: 2019 update. *Wilderness Environ Med.* 2019;30(4):S19-S32.

107. Sessler DI. Mild preoperative hypothermia. *N Engl J Med.* 1997;336:1730-1737.

108. Giesbrecht GG. Cold stress, near drowning and accidental hypothermia: a review. *Aviat Space Environ Med.* 2000;71:733-752.

109. Stocks JM, Taylor NAS, Tipton MJ, Greenleaf JE. Human physiological responses to cold exposure. *Aviat Space Environ Med.* 2004;75:444-457.

110. Gilbert M, Busund R, Skagseth A, et al. Resuscitation from accidental hypothermia of 13.7°C with circulatory arrest. *Lancet.* 2000;355:375-376.

111. Danzl DF, Pozos RS, Auerbach PS. Multicenter hypothermia survey. *Ann Emerg Med.* 1987;16(9):1042-1055.

112. Tsuei BJ, Kearney PA. Hypothermia in the trauma patient. *Injury Int J Care Injured.* 2004;35:7-15.

113. Stoner HB. Effects of injury on the responses to thermal stimulation of the hypothalamus. *J Appl Physiol.* 1972;33(5):665-671.

114. Ferrara A, MacArthur J, Wright H. Hypothermia and acidosis worsen coagulopathy in the patient requiring massive transfusion. *Am J Surg.* 1990;160:515-518.

115. Epstein M. Renal effects of head-out immersion in man: implications for understanding volume homeostasis. *Physiol Rev.* 1978;58:529-581.

116. Jurkovich G. Hypothermia in the trauma patient. *Adv Trauma.* 1989;4:111-140.

117. Jurkovich GJ. Environmental cold-induced injury. *Surg Clin N Am.* 2007;87(1):247-267.

118. Bennett BL, Giesbrect G, Zafren K, et al. Management of hypothermia in tactical combat casualty care: TCCC guideline proposed change 20-01 (June 2020). *J Spec Oper Med.* 2020;20(3):21-35.

119. Beilman GJ, Blondett JJ, Nelson AB. Early hypothermia in severely injured trauma patients is a significant risk factor of multiple organ dysfunction syndrome but not mortality. *Ann Surg.* 2009;249:845-850.

120. Mommsen P, Andruszkow H, Fromke C, et al. Effects of accidental hypothermia on posttraumatic complications and outcome in multiple trauma patients. *Injury.* 2013;44(1):86-90.

121. Lapostolle F, Sebbah JL, Couvreur J. Risk factors for the onset of hypothermia in trauma victims: the Hypotrauma study. *Crit Care.* 2012;16(4):R142. doi: 10.1186/cc1144

122. Trentzsch H, Huber-Wagner S, Hildebrand F, et al. Hypothermia for prediction of death in severely injured blunt trauma patients. *Shock.* 2012;37(2):131-139.

123. Nolan JP, Morley PT, Vanden Hoek TL, et al. Therapeutic hypothermia after cardiac arrest: an advisory statement by the Advance Life Support Task Force of the International Liaison Committee on Resuscitation. *Circulation.* 2003;108:118-121.

124. Alzaga AG, Cerdan M, Varon J. Therapeutic hypothermia. *Resuscitation.* 2006;70:369-380.

125. Nolan JP, Neumar RW, Adrie C, et al. Post-cardiac arrest syndrome: epidemiology, pathophysiology, treatment, and prognostication: a scientific statement from the International Liaison Committee on Resuscitation; the American Heart Association Emergency Cardiovascular Care Committee; the Council on Cardiovascular Surgery and Anesthesia; the Council on Cardiopulmonary, Perioperative, and Critical Care; the Council on Clinical Cardiology; the Council on Stroke. *Resuscitation.* 2008;79:350-379.

126. Nolan JP, Hazinski MF, Billi JE, et al. Part 1: executive summary: 2010 International Consensus on Cardiopulmonary Resuscitation and emergency cardiovascular care science with treatment recommendations. *Resuscitation.* 2010;81S:e1-e25.

127. Crompton EM, Lubomirova I, Cotlarciuc I, Han T, Sharma SD, Sharma P. Meta-analysis of therapeutic hypothermia for traumatic brain injury in adult and pediatric patients. *Crit Care Med.* 2017;45(4):575-583.

128. Andres PJD, Sinclair HL, Rodriguez A, et al. Hypothermia for intracranial hypertension after traumatic brain injury. *N Engl J Med.* 2015;373:2403-2412.

129. Finkelstein RA, Alam HB. Induced hypothermia for trauma: current research and practice. *J Intensive Care Med.* 2010;25(4):205-206.

130. Carlson LD. Immersion in cold water and body tissue insulation. *Aerospace Med.* 1958;29:145-152.

131. Giesbrecht GG, Steinman AM. Immersion into cold water. In: Auerbach PS, ed. *Auerbach's Wilderness Medicine.* 7th ed. Mosby Elsevier; 2017.

132. Wittmers LE, Savage M. Cold water immersion. In: Pandolf KB, Burr RE, eds. *Medical Aspects of Harsh Environments.* Vol 1. Office of the Surgeon General, Borden Institute/TMM Publications; 2001:531-552.

133. Tipton MJ. The initial responses to cold-water immersion in man. *Clin Sci.* 1989;77:581-588.

134. Keatinge WR, McIlroy MB, Goldfien A. Cardiovascular responses to ice-cold showers. *J Appl Physiol.* 1964;19:1145-1150.

135. Mekjavic IB, La Prairie A, Burke W, Lindborg B. Respiratory drive during sudden cold water immersion. *Respir Physiol.* 1987;70(1):121-130.

136. Sempsrott J, Schmidt AC, Hawkins SC, Cushing TA. Drowning and submersion injuries. In: Auerbach PS. *Auerbach's Wilderness Medicine.* 7th ed. Mosby Elsevier; 2017.

137. Wissler EH. Probability of surviving during accidental immersion in cold water. *Aviat Space Environ Med.* 2003;74:47-55.

138. Tikuisis P. Predicting survival time at sea based on observed body cooling rates. *Aviat Space Environ Med.* 1997;68:441-448.

139. Hayward JS, Errickson JD, Collis ML. Thermal balance and survival time prediction of man in cold water. *Can J Physiol Pharmacol.* 1975;53(1):21-32.

140. Ducharme MB, Lounsbury DS. Self-rescue swimming in cold water: the latest advice. *Appl Physiol Nutr Metab.* 2007;32:799-807.

141. Van Mieghem C, Sabbe M, Knockaert D. The clinical value of the ECG in noncardiac conditions. *Chest.* 2004;125(4):1561-1576.

142. Vanden Hoek TL, Morrison LJ, Shuster M, et al. Part 12.9: cardiac arrest in special situations: accidental hypothermia: 2010 American Heart Association guidelines for cardiopulmonary resuscitation and emergency cardiovascular care. *Circulation.* 2010;122:S829-S861.

143. Panchal AR, Bartos JA, Cabañas JG, et al. Part 3: adult basic and advanced life support: special circumstances of resuscitation: accidental hypothermia. 2020 American Heart Association guidelines for cardiopulmonary resuscitation and emergency cardiovascular care. *Circulation.* 2020;142(16):S366-S468.

144. Morrison LJ, Kierzek G, Diekema DS, et al. Part 3: Ethics. 2010 American Heart Association Guidelines for cardiopulmonary resuscitation and emergency cardiovascular care. *Circulation.* 2010;122:S665-S675.

145. Danzl DF, Lloyd EL. Treatment of accidental hypothermia. In: Pandolf KB, Burr RE, eds. *Medical Aspects of Harsh Environments.* Vol 1. Office of the Surgeon General, Borden Institute/TMM Publications; 2001:491-529.

146. Southwick FS, Dalglish PH. Recovery after prolonged asystolic cardiac arrest in profound hypothermia: a case report and literature review. *JAMA.* 1980;243:1250-1253.

147. Bernard MB, Gray TW, Buist MD, et al. Treatment of comatose survivors of out-of-hospital cardiac arrest with induced hypothermia. *N Engl J Med.* 2002;346(8):557-563.

148. Reuler JB. Hypothermia: pathophysiology, clinical setting, and management. *Ann Intern Med.* 1978;89:519-527.

149. Armstrong LE. Cold, windchill, and water immersion. In: Armstrong LE. *Performing in Extreme Environments.* Human Kinetics; 2000.

150. Wilderness Medical Society. Myocardial infarction, acute coronary syndromes, and CPR. In: Forgey WW, ed. *Practice*

Guidelines for Wilderness Emergency Care. 5th ed. Globe Pequot Press; 2006.

151. National Association of EMS Physicians. Position paper of the National Association of EMS Physicians: termination of resuscitation in nontraumatic cardiac arrest. *Prehosp Emerg Care*. 2011;15(4):542. doi: 10.3109/10903127 .2011.598621

152. Siegel AJ, d'Hemecourt P, Adner MM, Shirey T, Brown JL, Lewandrowski KB. Exertional dysnatremia in collapsed marathon runners: a critical role for point-of-care testing to guide appropriate therapy. *Am J Clin Pathol*. 2009;132(3):336-340.

153. Auerbach PS, Constance BB, Freer L. *Field Guide to Wilderness Medicine*. 4th ed. Mosby Elsevier; 2013.

Suggested Reading

Auerbach PS, ed. *Auerbach's Wilderness Medicine*. 7th ed. Mosby Elsevier; 2017.

Hawkins SC, Simon RB, Beissinger JP, Simon D. *Vertical Aid: Essential Wilderness Medicine for Climbers, Trekkers, and Mountaineers*. The Countryman Press; 2017.

Hawkins SC. *Wilderness EMS*. Wolters Kluwer; 2017.

환경 외상 II: 낙뢰, 익사, 잠수 및 고도

Lead Editors
Seth C. Hawkins, MD
Justin Sempsrott, MD

학습 목표   이 장의 학습을 완료하면 다음과 같은 내용을 수행할 수 있다.

- 야외에서 발생하는 낙뢰와 관련된 안전상의 위험을 설명할 수 있다.
- 다수의 낙뢰 사상자 발생 시 "역" 분류법을 설명할 수 있다.
- 고소병의 주요 위험 요소를 파악할 수 있다.
- 익사 사고의 적절한 초기 ABC(기도, 호흡, 순환) 처치에 관해 설명할 수 있다.
- 치명적이니 않은 익사 사고의 처치에 관해 설명할 수 있다.
- 익사 사고를 예방하는 다섯 가지 방법을 확인할 수 있다.
- 제I형 감압병과 제II형 감압병의 증상과 징후를 비교할 수 있다.
- 제II형 감압병과 동맥기체색전증에 대한 주요 처치 방법에 관해 설명할 수 있다.
- 급성 고산병과 고소뇌부종(HACE)의 유사점과 차이점에 관해 설명할 수 있다.

시나리오

어느 해안 마을에서 4인 가족이 쌀쌀한 겨울날 반려견과 함께 해변을 산책하고 있었다. 아들이 물가를 고무공을 던지자, 개가 쫓아갔다. 순식간에 해안을 거친 파도에 강아지가 휩쓸려 갔다. 17세의 아들은 개를 구하기 위해 가장 먼저 물로 뛰어들었지만, 물에 휩쓸려 버리고 말고 이 장면을 부모와 누나가 목격했다.

소년의 아버지와 어머니는 바닷가에 비치된 부력 장치를 잡고 소년을 따라 파도 속으로 들어가 도와주었다. 19세의 딸은 해변에 남아 휴대전화로 도움을 요청했다. 개는 결국 해안으로 돌아왔다. 부모는 아들이 차가운 물속에 잠긴 채 반응이 없는 것을 발견한 후 아들을 꺼냈다. 딸의 신고 후 7분 이내에 구급대가 현장에 도착했다.

구급차에서 내릴 때 의식을 잃은 10대 소년이 파도가 밀려오는 모래사장에 얼굴을 옆으로 돌린 채 반쯤 엎드린 채 누워 있는 것을 목격했다. 소년은 아직 파도가 밀려오는 지역에 있으며 파도에 휩쓸릴 수 있다. 당신은 현장에 도착한 119구조대와 함께 피해자에게 접근한다.

- 이 상황에서 환자에게 어떻게 접근해야 하는가?
- 환자의 맥박이나 호흡이 없는 경우 즉시 시행해야 할 처치는 무엇인가?
- 현장에서 해결해야 할 환자에 대한 다른 우려 사항은 무엇인가?

개요

매년 전 세계적으로 낙뢰, 익사, 스쿠버 다이빙, 고지대 등반 등 다양한 환경 조건으로 인해 심각한 이환율과 사망률이 발생할 수 있다(19장, 환경 외상 I: 더위 및 추위 참조). 병원 전 처치 제공자는 각 유형의 환경과 관련된 장애를 알아야 하고 이와 관련된 해부학, 생리학 및 병태생리학을 이해하며 환자 평가 및 처치를 신속하게 수행하는 방법을 알고 있어야 한다. 동시에 자신과 다른 공공 안전 요원의 손상을 예방하는 방법을 알고 있어야 한다.

낙뢰 관련 손상

낙뢰는 뇌우 시즌에 인명과 재산에 대한 가장 널리 퍼져 있는 위협이며 1959년 이후 미국에서 홍수에 이어 두 번째로 많은 폭풍 관련 사망자가 발생한 원인이다. 전 세계에서 매일 5만 건 이상의 뇌우가 발생하며 초당 100회 이상 낙뢰가 지구를 강타한다. 낙뢰는 매년 약 75,000건의 산불을 일으키고 전체 화재의 40%를 발화하는 것으로 보고되고 있다. 가장 파괴적인 형태는 번개는 구름에서 지상으로 떨어지는 낙뢰이다(**그림 20-1**). 미국의 실시간 낙뢰 감지 시스템에 따르면 구름에서 지상으로 낙뢰가 발생하는 횟수는 연간 약 2,000만 회에 달하며 여름 오후에는 시간당 최대 50,000번의 번개가 치는 것으로 추정된다. 미국에서 낙뢰는 6월부터 8월까지 가장 빈번하게 발생하지만, 플로리다와 멕시코만 남동부 해안에서는 일 년 내내 발생하며 플로리다와 텍사스는 낙뢰로 인한 사망의 25%를 차지한다. 전 세계적으로 낙뢰에 안전한 구조물과 예방 교육이 부족하므로 농촌 지역에 거주하는 사람이 가장 큰 위험에 처해 있다. 그 결과 매년 24,000명의 사망자가 발생하는 것으로 추정되며 낙뢰는 전 세계적으로 사망자보다 약 10배 더 많은 손상을 유발한다.

1950년대 이후로 미국에서 낙뢰로 인한 사망자 수는 감소했는데 이는 농촌 지의 야외 작업 인구 감소, 다가오는 폭풍에 대한 경보시스템 개선, 낙뢰 안전에 대한 공공 교육 증가, 의료서비스 개선 등의 이유로 보인다. 20세기 초반에 낙뢰로 인한 연간 사망자 수가 400명에 달했지만, 1968년부터 2010년까지 연간 평균 사망자 수는 79명이었으며 최근 보고서에 따르면 현재 낙뢰로 인한 사망자는 매년 약 30명에 불과하고 약 400명이 손상을 입는 것으로 나타났다. 2006~2019년 데이터에 대한 연구에 따르며 골퍼가 낙뢰로 인한 사망자의 대부분을 차지한다는 일반적인 믿음으로 밝혀졌으며 이 기간에 개인이 낚시 중 사망자는 골퍼보다 4배, 해변 활동/캠핑 사망자는 골퍼보다 2배 더 많은 것으로 나타났다. 6월부터 8월까지 낙뢰 활동과 낙뢰로 인한 사망자가 가장 많았으며 주말(금요일~일요일)이 가장 흔했다.

낙뢰로 인한 가장 큰 위협은 신경 및 심폐 손상이다. 병원 전 및 병원 내 처치를 위한 낙뢰 손상 예방 및 처치에 대한 야생의학회(WMS)의 임상 지침을 이용할 수 있다. 이러한 의학적 처치에 대한 권장 사항은 근거의 질에 따라 등급이 매겨진다(2장, 황금 원칙, 선호 및 비판적 사고 참조).

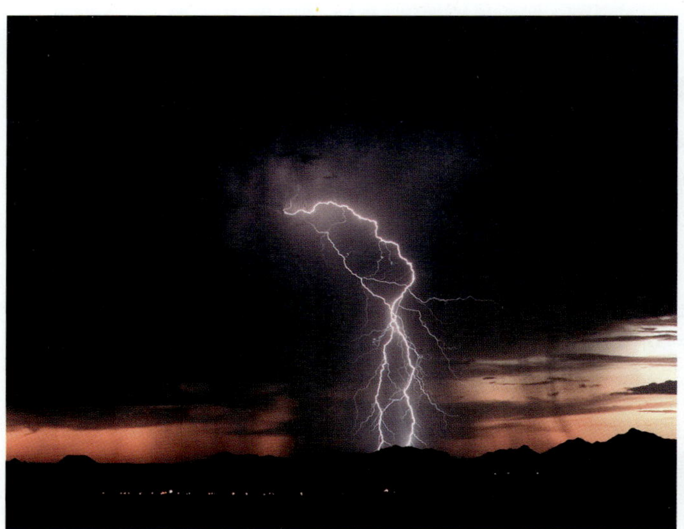

그림 20-1 줄무늬 번개 패턴이 있는 구름에서 땅으로 떨어지는 낙뢰

© Jhaz Photography/Shutterstock

역학

미국 국립해양대기청(NOAA) 자료에 따르면 2006년부터 2019년까지 낙뢰로 인한 사망자는 418명이었다. 이 사망자 중 79%가 남성이었다.

머리나 다리에 화상을 입은 경우 사망 위험이 더 높으며 일부 분석에 따르면 낙뢰 생존자의 약 74%가 영구적인 장애를 겪는 것으로 나타났다. 그러나 다른 연구에서는 영구적인 손상이 훨씬 적다고 보고하는 등 이 발견은 논란의 여지가 있다. 낙뢰로 사망한 사람 중 52%는 야외 있었다(이 중 25%는 야외 작업 중). 플로리다 낙뢰 사고에 대한 한 연구에서는 낙뢰 피해자의 63%가 1시간 이내에 사망했다.

손상 기전

낙뢰로 인한 손상은 다음과 같은 6가지 기전으로 인해 발생할 수 있다.

- 직접적인 낙뢰는 사람이 피난처를 찾을 수 없는 야외 환경에 있을 때 발생하고 이는 사람과 관련된 낙뢰의 3~5%에 불과하다.

- 측면 섬광 또는 비말 접촉은 낙뢰가 물체(예: 땅, 건물, 나무)에 부딪혀 피해자 또는 여러 명의 피해자에게 튈 때 발생한다. 전류는 1차 낙뢰 물체에서 튀어 사람에게 튈 수 있다. 사람에서 사람으로, 나무에서 사람으로, 심지어 실내에서 전화선을 통해 전화 통화 중인 사람에게도 튀는 경우가 있다(전화기와 전선이 얼굴에 가까이 있는냐에 따라 튀는 접촉이 아닌 직접 접촉이 될 수도 있다).

- 접촉은 낙뢰에 직접 맞거나 물체가 튀어서 사람이 직접 접촉한 때 발생한다. 이는 전체 낙뢰 손상의 3분의 1을 차지한다. 카라비너와 같은 금속 장비를 몸에 지니고 있거나 뇌우를 동반할 수 있는 등반 구조 중 빌레이와 같은 구조 시스템에 묶여 있는 구조대원의 경우 야생의학회(WMS)와 등반 의학 전문가들은 개별적으로 묶는 것을 권장한다. 또한 카라비너, 얼음 도구, 등산/스키 스틱과 같은 금속 물체는 격리하고 직접적인 접촉을 피해야 한다.

- 보폭전압(Step voltage)은 낙뢰가 지면이나 근처 물체에 부딪혀 전류가 방사형으로 바깥쪽으로 퍼지면서 그 과정에서 사람의 몸을 통과할 때 발생한다. 인체의 조직은 지면보다 저항이 적기 때문에 전류는 저항이 가장 적은 경로를 따라 한쪽 다리로 들어와 다른 쪽 다리로 이동한다. 접지 전류는 낙뢰 손상의 대부분을 차지한다. 보폭전압은 전압 또는 접지전류라고도 한다.

- 상향 방전(upward streamer)은 전류가 지상에서 피해자를 통과할 때 발생하지만, 하향 낙뢰와 연결되지 않을 때 발생한다. 이 흐르는 에너지는 전체 낙뢰에 비해 적으며 낙뢰 손상의 약 1~15%를 차지한다. 상향 방전은 최근에 확인된 낙뢰 접촉 형태이다.

- 낙뢰로 의해 생성된 충격파로 인해 폭발 손상 또는 기타 무딘 손상이 발생할 수 있으며 이는 사람을 9m까지 밀어낼 수 있다. 또한 산불, 건물 화재 및 폭발을 일으키는 낙뢰로 인해 부상을 입을 수 있다.

다음은 전기 및 낙뢰 전류로 인한 손상 중증도를 결정하는 6가지 알려진 요소에 의해 결정된다.

- 회로 유형
- 노출 시간
- 전압
- 전류량
- 조직의 저항
- 전류 방향

낙뢰나 다른 고전압 전원이 인체에 접촉하면 인체 내에서 발생하는 열은 전류량, 조직 저항 및 접촉 시간에 정비례한다. 다양한 조직의 저항(예: 신경 < 혈액 < 근육 < 피부 < 지방 < 뼈)이 증가함에 따라 전류가 통과할 때 발생하는 열도 증가한다.

낙뢰 손상은 고전압 전기 손상과 비슷하다고 생각하기 쉽다. 그러나 두 가지 손상 기전에는 상당한 차이가 있다. 낙뢰는 직류(DC)로 산업 및 가정용 전기 손상의 원인이 되는 교류(AC)와는 달리 직류(DC)이다. 번개는 3,000~50,000Å 범위의 전류로 수백만 볼트의 전하를 생성하며 신체에 노출되는 시간은 순간적(10~100m/s)이다. 낙뢰의 온도는 지름에 따라 다르지만, 평균 온도는 약 8,000℃이다. 이에 비해 고전압 전기 노출은 낙뢰보다 전압이 훨씬 낮은 경향이 있다. 그러나 낙뢰 손상과 고전압 전기 손상을 구별하는 핵심 요소는 신체 내에서 전류에 노출 기간이다. 그 결과 더 오랜 시간 동안 전기적 손상에 노출되어 결과적으로 더 깊은 화상을 입게 되고 심부 근육 및 신장 손상의 위험이 더 커진다. 이로 인한 심장 부정맥은 심실세동이 더 흔하게 발생한다.

때때로 번개는 최대 0.5초 동안 지속되는 장시간 낙뢰를 일으키는 드문 낙뢰 패턴으로 인해 고전압 전기에서 볼 수 있는 손상 패턴을 보일 수 있다. 고온 낙뢰라고 하는 이러한 유형의 낙뢰는 인체 조직에 깊은 화상을 입히고 나무를 부러트리며 화재를 일으킬 수 있다. 낙뢰는 신체에 상처를 입히기도 하지만, 피해자를 강타한 후 낙뢰가 지나가는 더 일반적인 경로는 신체 위를 지나가는 것이다. 이를 섬락(flashover) 전류라고 한다. 섬락 전류는 눈, 귀, 코, 입에도 들어갈 수 있다. 섬락 전류 흐름이 많은 피해자가 낙뢰에서 살아남는 이유라는 이론이 있다. 또한 섬락 전류는 피부의 수분을 증발시키거나 피해자의 옷이나 신발 일부를 폭발시킬 수 있는 것으로 알려져 있다. 엄청난 섬락 전류는 큰 자기장을 생성하여 신체 내에 이차 전류를 유도하고 심정지 및 기타 내부 손상을 유발할 수 있는 것으로 생각된다.

낙뢰로 인한 손상

낙뢰 손상은 경미한 표재성 손상부터 중증의 다발성 외상 및 사망에 이르기까지 다양하다. **표 20-1**에는 낙뢰 손상의 일반적인 증상과 징후가 나열되어 있다. 낙뢰로 인한 회복 가능성이나 예후를 판단하는 도구로서 피해자를 경증, 중등도, 중증의 세 가지 손상 범주 중 하나로 분류할 수 있다.

<table>
<tr><td colspan="3" style="background:#1a1a2e;color:#fff">표 20-1 낙뢰 손상: 일반적인 증상과 징후 및 처치법</td></tr>
<tr><td>손상</td><td>증상 및 징후</td><td>처치</td></tr>
<tr><td>경증</td><td>팔다리에 이상한 감각, 혼란, 기억상실, 일시적 의식 상실, 청각 장애 또는 실명, 고막 파열</td><td>현장 안전, XABCD 평가, 병력 및 이차평가, 심전도 모니터링, 산소 공급 및 경미한 부상을 입은 모든 환자 이송</td></tr>
<tr><td>중등도</td><td>지남력장애, 전투적임, 마비, 골절, 무딘 손상, 다리 맥박소실, 척수 쇼크, 발작, 일시적인 심폐정지, 혼수</td><td>현장 안전, XABCDEs 평가, 병력 및 이차평가, 심전도 모니터링, 필요시 조기 심폐소생술 시행(CAB), 산소공급 및 모든 환자 이송</td></tr>
<tr><td>중증</td><td>경증 및 중등도 증상 및 징후, 이관으로 체액 누출, 심장 세동 또는 심장무수축</td><td>심폐소생술(CAB) 및 ALS 시행, 다수의 환자 발생 시 '역분류법 사용</td></tr>
</table>

Abbreviations: CAB, circulation, airway, breathing; CPR, cardiopulmonary resuscitation; ECG, electrocardiogram; XABCDE, exsanguinating hemorrhage, airway, breathing, circulation, disability, expose/environment.

Data from O'Keefe Gatewood M, Zane RD. Lightning injuries. *Emerg Med Clin North Am*. 2004;22:369-403; and Cooper MA, Andrews CJ, Holle RL, Blumenthal R, Aldana NN. Lightning-related injuries and safety. In: Auerbach PS, ed. *Auerbach's Wilderness Medicine*. 7th ed. Mosby Elsevier; 2017:71-118.

경증 손상

경증 손상을 입은 환자는 의식이 명료하고 영향을 받은 팔이나 다리에 불쾌하고 감각 이상을 느낀다고 호소한다. 더 심각한 낙뢰의 경우 피해자는 머리를 맞았다고 이야기하거나 원인을 알 수 없는 폭발이 자신을 강타했다고 진술한다.

환자는 다음과 같은 증상을 보이며 현장에 나타날 수 있다.

- 혼란(단기 또는 몇 시간에서 며칠)
- 기억상실(단기 또는 수 시간에서 며칠)
- 일시적인 난청
- 실명
- 일시적 의식상실
- 일시적 감각 이상
- 근육통
- 피부 화상(드물게 발생)
- 일시적 마비

피해자는 활력징후가 정상이거나 경미한 일시적 고혈압을 보이며 회복은 대개 점진적이고 완전하다.

중등도 손상

중등도의 손상을 입은 환자는 진행성 단일 또는 다기관 손상을 입었으며 그중 일부는 생명을 위협할 수 있다. 이 범주의 일부 환자는 영구적인 장애가 있을 수 있다. 환자는 다음과 같은 증상을 가지고 현장에 나타날 수 있다.

- 즉각적인 영향
  - 발작
  - 난청
  - 심정지 및 심장 손상
  - 폐 손상
  - 혼란, 기억상실
  - 시각상실
  - 어지럼
  - 충격파로 인한 타박상
  - 무딘 손상(예: 골절)
  - 가슴 통증, 근육통
  - 고막 파열
  - 두통, 구역, 뇌진탕 후 증후군
- 지연 효과
  - 신경학적 증상 및 징후
  - 기억력 결핍
  - 주의력 결핍
  - 신경심리학적 변화
  - 코딩 및 검색 문제
  - 주의산만
  - 성격 변화
  - 과민성
  - 만성 통증
  - 발작

낙뢰의 충격 부위에 따라 뇌의 호흡 중추에 영향을 미치는 낙뢰는 저산소혈증으로 인한 이차 심정지로 이어질 수 있는 장기간의 호흡 정지를 초래할 수 있다. 이 분류에 속하는 피해자는 즉각적인 심폐정지를 경험할 수 있지만, 심장의 고유한 자동성으로 인해 자발적으로 정상 심장 리듬으로 돌아올 수 있다. 즉각적인 심폐정지가 가장 큰 위협이므로 병원 전 처치 제공자는 모든 낙뢰 피해자에게 즉시 CAB(순환, 기도, 호흡) 순서로 즉각적인 생명을 위협하는 상황에 대비해야 하며 사고 발생한 후 최대 3일까지 발생할 수 있는 이차 심장 문제가 있을 수 있으므로 심전도를 지속해서 모니터링해야 한다.

중증 손상

낙뢰로 인한 급사의 기전은 심장 및 호흡 정지가 동시에 일어나는 것이다. 직접적인 낙뢰로 인해 심각한 손상(심혈관 또는 신경계 손상)을 입었거나 심폐소생술이 지연된 피해자는 예후가 좋지 않다. 현장에 도착한 병원 전 처치 제공자는 무수축 또는 심실세동을 동반한 심정지 환자를 발견할 수 있다. 낙뢰는 대규모 직류 전기충격을 일으켜 심근 전체를 동시에 탈분극시킨다. 미국 심장협회는 초기 평가에서 사망한 것으로 보이는 환자에게 적극적인 심폐소생을 할 것을 권장한다. 이는 낙뢰로 인한 심정지 후 회복이 잘 되었다는 많은 보고와 이 범주에 속하는 피해자가 일반적으로 젊고 심장질환이 없다는 사실에 근거한 것이다. 1980년에 발표된 자료에 따르면 심폐소생술을 받은 낙뢰 환자의 23%만이 생존한 것으로 나타났는데 이 통계는 현대 의학 문헌에서 여전히 공유되고 있지만, 최근의 심폐소생술 기반 소생술의 혁신을 설명하지 못할 수도 있다. 심정지의 모든 원인 중에서 번개는 초기 손상이 일시적이고 가역적일 수 있으므로 회복에 대한 좋은 예후 중 하나일 수 있다.

낙뢰 후 전기 활동이 자발적으로 회복되면서 초기 심정지가 관찰되는 경우는 드물지 않지만, 숨뇌의 호흡중추가 마비되어 호흡 정지가 지속되면 이차적 저산소성 심정지가 발생할 수 있다. 장기간의 심장 및 신경학적 허혈이 발생하면 이러한 환자를 소생시키기가 매우 어려울 수 있다. 다른 일반적인 소견으로는 뇌척수액과 혈액이 이관에 보이는 고막 파열, 안구 손상, 연부조직 타박상, 두개골 골절, 갈비뼈 골절, 팔다리 골절 및 척추 골절을 포함한 낙상 등으로 인한 다양한 형태의 무딘 손상이 있다. 이 범주에 속하는 많은 환자는 화상의 증거가 없다. 낙뢰로 인한 피부 화상을 입은 환자의 경우 일반적으로 전체 체표면적 20% 미만인 것으로 보고된다.

낙뢰 피해자에게는 중추신경계 손상이 흔히 발생하며 이는 네 가지 그룹으로 분류된다.

- 제1그룹 중추신경계 효과(즉시 및 일시적): 의식 상실(75%), 감각 이상(80%), 허약감(80%), 혼란, 기억상실 및 두통
- 제2그룹 중추신경계 효과(즉시 및 장기적): 저산소성 허혈 신경병증, 두개내출혈, 심정지 후 뇌경색
- 제3그룹 중추신경계 효과(지연성 신경 증후군 가능성): 운동 신경 질환 및 운동 장애
- 제4그룹 중추신경계 효과(낙상 및 폭발로 인한 외상): 경막밑혈종, 경막외혈종, 거미막밑출혈

평가

현장에 도착하면 다른 출동과 마찬가지로 병원 전 처치 제공자 및 기타 공공 안전 요원의 안전을 최우선으로 고려해야 한다. 구조대원은 해당 지역에 낙뢰가 발생할 가능성이 여전히 있는지 확인한다. 폭풍이 다가오거나 지나간 후에도 낙뢰는 주 폭풍에서 16km 떨어진 곳까지 실제 위협으로 남아 있으므로 "청천벽력"이라고 불을 정도로 항상 눈에 보이지 않는 위험 요소가 존재한다. 실제로 이러한 현실은 예기치 않은 사건에 대해 "느닷없이" 또는 "맑고 푸른 하늘에서"라는 속담의 근원이기도 하다.

맑은 날에는 낙뢰가 칠 수 있으므로 목격자가 없으면 손상 기전이 불분명할 수 있다. 손상 기전이 확실하지 않으면 응급상황에 대비하여 즉시 XABCDE's(대량출혈, 기도, 호흡, 순환, 장애, 노출/환경) 및 생명을 위협하는 상태가 있는지 평가한다. 낙뢰에 맞은 환자(다른 손상 기전으로 인해 감전된 환자와는 대조적으로)는 전하를 가지고 있지 않으므로 환자를 만지는 것은 환자 처치에 위험이 없다. 환자의 심장 리듬을 심전도로 모니터링한다. QT 간격 연장 및 일시적인 T파 역전과 같은 비특이적인 ST분절 및 T 파의 변화를 보이는 것이 일반적이지만, Q파 또는 ST분절 상승을 동반한 심근경색의 보가 구체적인 증거는 거의 보이지 않는다.

환자가 안정되면 이러한 유형의 외상으로 발생할 수 있는 광범위한 손상을 과악하기 위해 머리부터 발끝까지 상세한 평가가 필요하다. 팔과 다리에 일시적인 마비(벼락 마비)가 발생할 수 있으므로 환자의 상황 인식 능력과 모든 팔다리의 신경 기능을 평가해야 한다. 낙뢰 피해자는 자율신경 기능 장애로 인해 동공이 확장되어 머리 외상과 유사한 것으로 알려져 있다. 피해자의 절반 이상이 어떤 형태로든 안구 손상을 입었으므로 눈을 평가한다. 이관에서 혈액과 뇌척수액이 있는지 확인한다. 피해자의 절반은 고막이 한쪽 또는 양쪽이 파열되어 있다. 낙뢰 손상의 모든 피해자는 단단한 물체에 부딪히거나 낙하

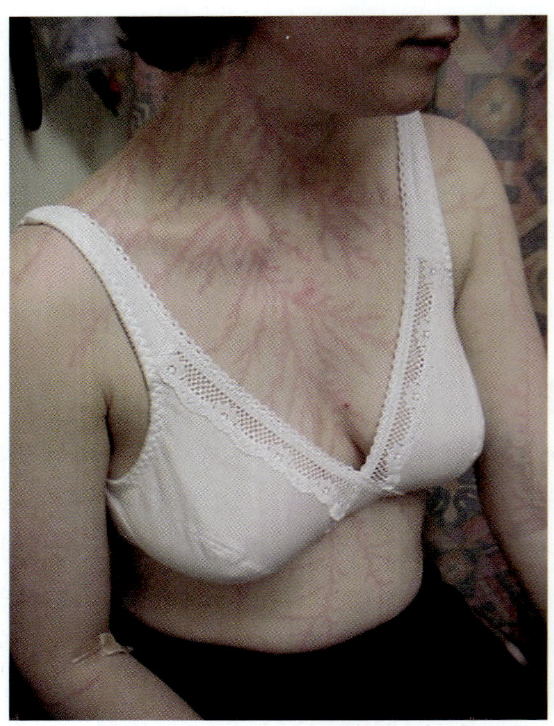

그림 20-2 리히텐베르크 모양.

물에 맞아 무딘 손상 또는 근육 경련으로 인한 탈구와 같은 기타 근골격계 손상을 입을 가능성이 높다. 평가 시 척추 손상의 가능성을 고려하고 프로토콜에 따라 처치를 시행한다.

　피부 표면부터 전층 화상에 이르기까지 화상의 징후가 있는지 피부를 평가한다. 낙뢰 화상은 처음 몇 시간 내에 발생하기 때문에 현장에서 겉으로 드러나지 않을 수도 있다. 화상은 낙뢰 생존자의 절반 미만에서 발생하며 대부분은 표재성 화상이다. 피부에 리히텐베르크 도형(Lichtenberg's figures)으로 알려진 깃털 모양이 나타나는 것이 일반적이지만, 이러한 패턴은 화상이 아니며 24시간 이내에 사라진다(**그림 20-2**). 옷에 불이 붙거나 장신구 또는 기타 물체의 가열로 인해 화상을 입은 경우가 더 흔하다.

　사고로 인해 다수의 환자가 발생하면 즉시 환자 분류 원칙에 따라 중증도 분류를 시행한다. 일반적인 환자 분류 원칙에는 제한된 인력과 자원을 중등도 및 중증 환자에게 집중하고 호흡과 혈액 순환이 없는 환자는 신속하게 우회하는 것이다. 그러나 낙뢰 환자가 다수 발생한 경우 이러한 환자는 호흡 정지 또는 심정지 상태이며 신속하게 처치하면 회복될 가능성이 높으므로 "역" 분류를 시행하고 사망자 소생술을 가장 먼저 시행한다. 반면에 낙뢰를 맞고 살아남은 다른 환자들은 관련 외상이나 내부출혈이 없는 한 상태가 악화할 가능성이 거의 없다.

처치

낙뢰 손상 환자 처치할 때 우선순위는 현장에서 자신과 동료의 안전을 확보하고 피해자의 XABCDE 여부를 평가하는 것이다. 자발 호흡이나 순환이 없으면 현재 지침에 따라 최대 효과적인 심폐소생술을 5주기(2분)까지 시행하고 자동심장충격기(AED)나 심전도 모니터로 심장 리듬을 평가한다. 자동심장충격기는 일부 기록된 사례에서 도움이 되는 것으로 입증되었다. 낙뢰로 인한 심폐정지 시에는 다른 장에서 설명한 대로 미국심장협회의 최신 ACLS 및 PALS 지침에 따라 ALS 조치를 한다. 쇼크와 저체온증을 평가하고 처치한다. 중등도 및 중증 손상을 입은 모든 환자에게 고유량 산소를 공급한다. 낙뢰에 의한 손상을 입은 환자는 기존의 고전압 전기 손상 환자와 달리 조직 파괴가 심하지 않고 화상을 입어 많은 양의 수액이 필요로 하지 않으므로 정맥 내 수액 공급은 정맥 라인을 유지(KVO)할 속도로 시작해야 한다. 활력징후가 불안정하거나 관련 외상을 입은 환자는 적절하게 수액 소생술을 시행할 수 있다.

　골절 부위를 고정하고 필요한 경우 척추 움직임 제한을 시행한 후 이송을 준비한다. 경미하거나 중증 손상을 입은 낙뢰 피해자는 추가 평가 및 관찰을 위해 응급실로 이송해야 한다. 병원까지의 거리, 이송 시간 및 병원 전 처치 제공자의 전반적인 위험과 환자의 이득을 고려하여 지상 또는 항공으로 환자를 이송한다.

　앞서 언급한 바와 같이 낙뢰 피해자는 조기에 효과적인 소생술을 받으면 긍정적인 결과를 얻을 확률이 높다. 그러나 이러한 환자가 20~30분 이상 지속되는 BLS 또는 ALS 절차를 통해 맥박을 회복할 수 있다는 증거는 거의 없다. 소생술을 중단하기 전에 기도를 확보하고 호흡을 보조하며 저혈량증, 저체온증 및 산혈증을 교정하여 환자를 안정시키기 위해 모든 노력을 기울인다.

예방

일 년 내내 뇌우가 자주 발생하기 때문에 낙뢰가 자주 발생한다. 병원 전 처치 제공자와 일반인 모두 예방과 낙뢰에 대한 여러 가지 오해와 상식에 대해 교육을 받아야 한다(**Box 20-1**). 국립기상청(NWS), 국립해양대기청(NOAA), 국립 낙뢰 안전연구소(NLSI), 미국적십자사(ARC), 연방재난관리청(FEMA) 등의 기관에서 수많은 낙뢰 예방 관련 자료를 제공한다.

　낙뢰 손상 예방 및 처치를 위한 공식 지침은 야생의학회(WMS), 미국심장협회(AHA), 국제 산악응급의료위원회(ICMEM), 국제등산연맹

Box 20-1 낙뢰에 대한 오해와 진실

일반적인 오해

낙뢰에 대한 다음과 같은 일반적인 상식은 모두 잘못된 것이다.

- 낙뢰는 항상 치명적이다.
- 주요 사망 원인은 화상이다.
- 낙뢰를 맞은 피해자는 화염에 휩싸이거나 재로 변한다.
- 피해자는 낙뢰를 맞은 후에도 전류가 흐르거나 충전된 상태를 유지한다.
- 폭풍이 치는 동안 건물 안에 있으면 낙뢰로부터 100% 보호된다.
- 폭풍우가 치는 동안 건물 안에 있으면 낙뢰로부터 100% 보호된다.
- 낙뢰는 같은 장소를 두 번 떨어지지 않는다.
- 고무 밑창이 신발과 비옷을 착용하면 사람을 보호할 수 있다.
- 차량의 고무 타이어는 사람을 손상으로부터 보호한다.
- 금속 장신구를 착용하면 벼락을 맞을 위험이 커진다.
- 낙뢰는 항상 가장 높은 물체에 떨어진다.
- 비가 내리지 않는 한 번개는 위험하지 않다.
- 낙뢰는 천둥 없이도 발생할 수 있다.

환자 처치에 관한 오해

병원 전 처치 제공자가 알고 있는 몇 가지 잘못된 상식과 오해는 환자의 처치와 결과에 부정적인 영향을 미칠 수 있다.

- 낙뢰로 즉시 사망하지 않은 피해자는 괜찮을 것이다.
- 피해자에게 겉으로 드러나는 손상 징후가 없다면 피해가 그다지 심각하지 않을 수 있다.
- 낙뢰 손상은 다른 고전압 전기 손상과 유사하게 처치해야 한다.
- 낙뢰 피해자는 몇 시간 동안 소생술을 받으면 성공적으로 회복될 수 있다.

Box 20-2 산악 지역의 병원 전 처치 제공자를 위한 예방 지침

산악 지역에서 응급처치를 제공하는 병원 전 처치 제공자는 특히 고도가 높고 외딴 지역에서 공원 관리자, 수색 및 구조대, 기타 공공 안전 요원으로 근무하는 종사자는 낙뢰 위험에 더 많이 노출된다. 이러한 병원 전 처치 제공자를 위한 몇 가지 일반적인 예방 지침은 다음과 같다.

- 산악 지형에서 천둥과 번개는 주로 여름철 늦은 오후와 밤에 발생하므로 일기 예보를 참고한다. 따라서 정오까지 등산하고 오후 2시에는 내려간다는 말이 있다. 낙뢰의 위험을 줄이기 위해 오후 중반까지 낮은 고도로 내려오라는 의미로 사용한다.
- 산에서 낙뢰를 피할 수 있는 가장 좋은 장소는 산장이나 산악 대피소이다. 열린 문과 창문에서 멀리 떨어진다.
- 텐트는 낙뢰로부터 보호하지 못하며 텐트 기둥이 피뢰침 역할을 할 수 있다.
- 큰 동굴이나 계곡은 안전하지만, 작은 동굴은 입구나 측벽에 가까이 있으면 보호가 거의 되지 않는다.
- 젖은 하천 바닥은 개방된 공간보다 더 위험하다.
- 산등성이와 정상, 송전탑, 스키 리프트에 접근하지 않는다.
- 야외에서 낙뢰가 치는 경우 큰 나무 아래는 위험하므로 접근하지 않는다. 숲에서는 작은 나무들 사이로 들어가는 것이 가장 좋다.
- 야외에서 낙뢰가 치는 상황에 노출되면 앉거나 눕지 않는다. 발이나 무릎을 모으고 웅크린 자세로 지면에 접촉하는 면적을 최대한 작게 유지하여 접지 전류로 인한 손상을 최소화하는 것이 가장 좋다. 병원 전 처치 제공자는 무릎을 꿇거나 앉을 수 있는 마른 팩과 같은 단열재를 사용하여 자신과 지면 사이에 접촉을 피해야 한다.
- 여러 사람이 함께 있는 경우 서로 보이지 않을 정도의 거리를 유지하여 접지 전류나 사람 사이의 섬광으로 인한 손상자 수를 줄인다.
- 폭풍이 오기 전에 사전 경고를 받고 예방 조치를 취할 수 있도록 소형 휴대용 낙뢰 탐지기를 사용하는 것을 고려한다.

의료위원회(CIMCF) 등 국내 및 국제 의료위원회와 단체에서 발표하고 있다(**Box 20-2**).

병원 전 처치 제공자 및 기타 공공 안전 요원은 폭풍 경보를 제공하고 하루 종일 업데이트되는 악천후 경보에 대한 절차를 수립하여 예방의 한 가지 방법으로 활용한다. 야외에서 100% 안전한 곳은 없다. 구급차는 큰 건물이 없을 때 병원 전 처치 제공자에게 가장 안전한 대피소이다.

공교육에서 사용되는 모토 중 하나는 "보이면 피하고 들리면 도망가라"이다. 또 다른 유용한 규칙은 "30-30 규칙"이다. 번개를 본 후 천둥소리가 들리기까지 시간이 30초 이하면 위험에 처한 것이므로 적절한 대피소를 찾아야 한다. 이 규칙에 따르면 뇌우는 여전히 위협적이며 폭풍이 지나간 후에도 최대 16~20km까지 낙뢰가 칠 수 있으므로 마지막 번개나 천둥 후 30분이 지난 후에야 야외 활동을 재개하는 것이 안전하다고 간주한다. 번개 근접 거리의 또 다른 측정은 번개 후 천둥소리가 날 때까지 5초마다 번개가 1.6km 떨어져 있다는 "섬광 소리"의 법칙이다. 30-30 법칙에 대한 일부 잘못된 가르침에 따르면 마지막 천둥소리 후 30분이 지나면 폭풍의 위치가 48km 이상 떨어져 있다고 한다.

"섬광 소리(flash-to-bang)" 규칙에서 설명하는 것처럼 섬광과 천둥소리 사이의 시간이 30초 이하면 폭풍은 9.7km 밖에 떨어져 있지 않으며 이는 폭풍에서 번개가 치는 16.1~24.1km 거리 내에 있는 것이다.

낙뢰 예방에 대한 자세한 내용은 **Box 20-3**을 참조한다. 낙뢰 피해자를 위한 지원에 대한 정보는 **Box 20-4**를 참조한다.

Box 20-3 낙뢰 안전 지침

다음은 폭풍우 발생 시 번개 안전에 대한 지침이다.

- 낙뢰에 안전한 차량이나 구조물을 찾는다.
  - 완전히 밀폐된 금속 차량인 자동차는 낙뢰에 안전한 대피소이다. 비행기, 버스, 승합차, 운전석이 대부분 금속으로 된 밀폐형 건설 장비 등 기타 모든 금속 이동 운송 관련 차량도 안전하다. 그러나 주의할 점은 차량의 외부 금속 차폐가 손상되어서는 안 된다는 점이다. 이는 곧
    - 차량의 창문은 올려야 한다.
    - 라디오 다이얼, 금속 문손잡이, 양방향 라디오 마이크 등 외부 물체와 연결되는 내부 물체와 접촉해서는 안 된다.
  - 내부에서 외부로 관통하는 다른 모든 물체와 접촉하지 않는다.
  - 유리섬유 및 기타 플라스틱으로 만들어진 차량과 오토바이, 트랙터, 골프 카트, 전지형 차량과 같이 밀폐된 덮개가 없는 소형 탑승 기계 또는 차량은 안전하지 않다.
  - 금속 재질의 건물은 번개에 안전한 장소이다. 벽돌과 목재로 만든 크고 영구적인 구조물도 마찬가지이다. 다시 한번 주의할 점은 번개가 지나가는 경로의 일부가 되지 않도록 주의해야 한다는 것이다. 즉, 모든 전기 회로, 스위치, 동력 장비, 금속 문과 창문, 난간 등을 피해야 한다. 버스 정류장, 정자, 야구장 더그아웃과 같이 기둥으로 받쳐진 작은 구조물은 안전하지 않다.

다음은 실내에서 번개 안전을 위한 지침이다.

- 창문, 열린 문, 벽난로, 욕조와 샤워기, 싱크대, 가전제품 같은 금속 물체에서 멀리 떨어진다.
- 라디오와 컴퓨터의 전원을 끄고 유선전화는 비상시에만 사용한다.
- 폭풍우가 오기 전에 모든 수도꼭지를 잠그고 전기 제품과 장비의 전원을 끈다.

다음은 야외에서 낙뢰 안전을 위한 지침이다.

- 휴대용 라디오, 휴대전화 또는 기타 전자 신호/통신 장치를 사용하지 않는다.
- 자전거, 트랙터, 울타리 등 금속 물체를 피한다.
- 나무와 같이 높은 물체를 피하고 최대한 몸을 웅크린다.
- 송전선, 수송관 및 스키 리프트 근처를 피한다.
- 개방된 장소를 피한다.
- 개방된 대피소(예: 간이 차고, 버스 차고)는 측면 섬광이나 지면 타격이 발생할 수 있으므로 전체 규모에 따라 피한다.
- 유인할 수 있는 골프채와 스키 폴을 버린다.
- 대규모 야외 행사에서는 근처에 있는 버스나 미니 밴 등으로 대피한다.
- 가능하면 지면에 닿는 면적을 최소화한다. 지면과 접촉을 최소화하기 위해 두 발로 웅크리고 귀를 막고 앉아 있는 번개 자세를 취하거나 당신과 지면 사이에 배낭 및 비전도 물체를 깔고 앉는다. 무릎을 꿇거나 다리를 꼬고 앉는 것도 편안한 자세이다.
- 키가 큰 나무 근처에 서 있거나 껴안거나 쪼그려 앉지 않는다. 작은 나무가 있는 지역을 찾는다.
- 물이 없는 배수로를 찾아 대피한다.
- 물에 있는 경우 즉시 물 밖으로 나와 물에서 멀리 떨어진 내륙으로 이동한다. 수영이나 보트 타기 또는 물 위에 있는 가장 높은 물체 근처에 가지 않는다.

Box 20-4 낙뢰 손상을 입은 생존자

낙뢰 피해 생존자를 위한 지원은 국제 낙뢰 및 감전 생존자 협회(LS&ESSI, Inc.)에서 제공한다. 이 비영리 지원 단체는 생존자, 가족 및 기타 이해관계자들로 구성되어 있다. 미국 전역과 13개 이상의 국가에 회원들이 있다(www.lightning-strike.org).

익사

익사는 미국에서 흔한 사고로 매년 4,000명 이상이 익사로 사망한다. 익사는 모든 연령대에서 예방 가능한 사망의 주요 원인으로 꼽히지만, 특히 어린이들 사이에서 유행병처럼 흔하다. 세계보건기구(WHO)는 2019년 익사로 인한 사망자가 약 23만 6,000명에 달하며 이는 전 세계 모든 손상 관련 사망의 7%를 차지하여 의도하지 않은 손상 사망의 세 번째 주요 원인으로 추정하고 있다. 이 통계에는 치명적이지 않은 익사나 홍수, 자살 또는 살인으로 인한 사망은 포함되지 않았으며 많은 중간 및 저소득 국가에서는 익사 후 병원에 도착하지 못해 사망하는 때도 있으므로 실제 익사로 인한 전 세계의 부담은 과소평가 되어 있을 가능성이 높다.

이전에는 익사를 공기로 호흡하는 포유류가 액체에 잠겨 사망하는 결과로 정의했다. 이제 익사는 결과가 아닌 과정으로 이해한다. 과거에는 건식 익사, 습식 익사, 이차 익사, 지연 익사 및 익사 직전 등 여러 가지 수식어가 사용되었다. 이러한 용어 중 특히 문화적, 국제적 맥락에서 보편적으로 통용되거나 의학적으로 인정되는 정의는 없다. 2002년 세계 익사 학술대회에서 채택된 업데이트된 정의에 따르면 익사는 일반적으로 물과 같은 액체 매체에 잠기거나 잠긴 결과 때문에 호흡 장애가 발생하는 과정이다.

물에 잠기거나 물에 잠겼으나 처음에는 생존했지만, 나중에 사망한 환자를 정의하고 분류하고자 하는 욕구가 항상 있었다. 부검 시 염분이나 폐에 물이 있는지에 따라 분류 체계는 익사의 주요 병태생리와 최종적인 공통 경로인 뇌 무산소증에서 벗어나게 된다. 이환율과 관계없이 뇌졸중에서 살아남은 사람을 뇌졸중 직전이라고 하지

않는 것처럼 건성 익사, 이차 익사, 익사 직전과 같은 용어는 의미가 없으며 이는 세계보건기구, 국제소생술연락위원회, 야생의학회, 미국 질병통제예방센터, 미국심장협회, 미국적십자사, 미국 응급의학회에서도 채택하고 있다.

익사 과정은 환자의 기도가 수면 아래로 내려가거나(침수) 얼굴 위로 물이 튀면서(침수, 흡인을 통한 손상) 호흡 장애로 시작된다. 익사 과정에는 치명적인 익사(환자가 사망), 이환율이 있는 비치명적 익사(환자는 생존하지만, 손상 또는 질병이 남음), 이환율이 없는 비치명적 익사(사망 또는 명백한 심각한 손상 또는 질병이 없음)의 세 가지 결과 또는 수식어만 있다. 익사 분류와 관련된 추가 고려 사항은 다음과 같다.

- 호흡 장애 없이 물에 잠기거나 물에 잠겼지만, 물에서 구조가 필요한 환자와 관련된 사고는 익사가 아닌 수난 구조로 간주한다.
- 번개와 마찬가지로 야생의학회(WMS)는 야생 의학 분야 내에서 가장 최근의 권장 사항과 그 근거를 평가하는 데 도움이 되는 익사에 대해 합의 기반 처치 지침을 개발했다.

역학

익사는 미국 내 모든 연령대에서 의도치 않은 손상으로 인한 사망의 다섯 번째 주요 원인이지만, 특히 어린 연령대에서 압도적으로 많이 발생한다. 익사는 1~4세의 의도하지 않은 손상으로 인한 사망의 주요 원인이고, 5~14세의 경우 손상 사망의 두 번째 주요 원인이며 15~24세의 손상 사망의 세 번째 주요 원인이다. 욕조, 세면대, 변기 등에서 익사할 위험에 노출된 영아(1세 미만)의 손상 사망의 세 번째 주요 원인이다. 미국 질병관리본부에 따르면 2010년부터 2019년까지 미국에서 매년 평균 3,957건의 의도하지 않은 치명적인 익사 사고가 발생했으며 매년 약 8,080건이 비치명적인 익사로 응급실에서 치료를 받는 것으로 추정된다. 매년 347명은 보트 관련 사고로 익사하여 사망했다.

치명적인 익사 사고는 자연 수역(호수, 강, 바다)에서 가장 많이 발생하며 수영장과 욕조가 그 뒤를 따른다. 이에 비해 미국 응급실에서 치료받은 의도하지 않은 비치명적인 익사 사고는 수영장에서 가장 많이 발생했고 그다음으로 자연환경과 욕조가 그 뒤를 이었다. 치명적이지 않은 손상률은 4세 이하 어린이와 모든 연령대의 남성에서 가장 높았다. 익사로 사망한 환자의 80%는 남성이었다.

익사 사고를 당한 어린이 4명 중 1명이 치명적이지 않은 익사 사고로 응급처치를 받았고 그 결과 뇌손상이 없는 경우부터 돌이킬 수

없는 다양한 정도의 뇌손상을 입었다.

치명적인 신경학적 손상은 모든 연령대의 익사 생존자들이 가장 두려워하는 결과이며 익사는 폐를 통한 신경학적 질환이라는 자명한 이치를 보여준다. 익사 후 생존과 장기 기능의 주요 결정 요인은 중추 신경계 손상의 정도이다.

익사의 위험 요소

특정 요인으로 인해 익사 위험이 커질 수 있다. 이러한 요인을 인식하면 경계심이 높아지고 이러한 발생을 사고를 최소화하기 위한 예방 전략과 정책을 수립하는 데 도움이 된다. 영유아의 주요 위험 요인은 부적절한 감독이며 청소년과 성인의 경우 위험한 행동과 약물 또는 알코올 사용이다.

익사 위험 요소는 다음과 같다.

- 저산소성 의식 상실을 유발하는 호흡 행동. 수중 수영 거리를 늘리기 위해 일부 수영 선수는 수중으로 들어가기 직전에 의도적으로 과다호흡을 하여 동맥혈이산화탄소분압($PaCO_2$)을 낮춘다. 만성폐쇄폐질환이 없는 환자의 경우 체내 이산화탄소 수치가 호흡을 자극하기 때문에 동맥혈이산화탄소분압이 감소하면 숨을 참는 동안 숨을 쉬기 위해 시상하부의 호흡 중추로 전달되는 피드백을 감소시킨다. 그러나 이러한 수영 선수는 과다호흡을 해도 동맥혈산소분압(PaO_2)이 크게 변하지 않기 때문에 익사할 위험이 있다. 수중에서 계속 수영하면 이 개인이 수중에서 수영을 계속하면 동맥혈산소분압이 크게 감소하여 의식을 잃고 뇌 저산소증이 발생할 수 있다. 이 상태를 얕은 수심에서 의식 상실, 다이빙 상황에서 상승 저산소증, 수면 의식 상실 및 의식 상실성 무호흡이라고 부르기도 하지만, "저산소 의식 상실"이라는 용어가 이 상태를 설명하는 데 일반적으로 사용된다.
- 우발적인 냉수 침수로 인한 저온 쇼크가 발생한다. 익사 위험이 더 큰 또 다른 상황은 찬물에 잠기는 경우(머리를 내밀기)이다. 찬물에 침수되면 발생하는 생리학적 변화는 여러 상황에 따라 신체에 치명적인 결과를 초래하거나 보호 효과를 가져올 수 있다. 냉수 침수 후 몇 분 이내에 심혈관계 허탈과 급사로 인한 부작용이 더 흔하며 이를 "저온 쇼크"라고 한다(자세한 내용은 19장, 환경 외상 I: 더위와 추위를 참조).
- 나이. 익사는 호기심이 많은 성격과 부모의 감독 소홀로 인해 영유아에서 가장 많이 발생하는 등 젊은 층에서 유행하는 것으로 알려져 있다. 4세 미만 어린이의 익사율이 가장 높다.
- 성별. 남성이 익사 사고의 80%를 차지하며 나이에 따라 두 번의 최

고 발생 시기가 있다. 남성의 경우 2세에 첫 번째 최고 발생률을 보이고 10세까지 감소하다가 18세에 다시 급격히 증가하여 최고조에 이른다. 나이가 많은 남성은 수중 활동에 더 많이 노출되고 물가에서 술을 더 많이 마시며 위험을 감수하는 행동을 더 많이 하므로 익사할 위험이 더 높을 수 있다.

- 인종. 미국의 인종차별 역사로 인해 많은 나이 든 아프리카계 미국인들은 수영장 출입이나 수영 강습을 받지 못했다. 조부모나 부모가 수영하지 않는다면 자녀를 위한 수영 강습은 가족에게 우선순위가 낮아질 수 있다. 오늘날 아프리카계 미국인 어린이는 백인 어린이보다 더 자주 익사한다. 아프리카계 미국인 어린이는 연못, 호수 및 기타 자연 수원에서 익사하는 경향이 있다. 백인 어린이들 보다 익사가 더 자주 발생한다. 그러나 수영장에서 익사 사고가 발생하면 5~19세 사이의 아프리카계 미국인 어린이는 백인 어린이보다 5.5배 더 자주 익사하며, 특히 11세~12세 사이에서는 아프리카계 미국인 어린이가 백인 어린이보다 10배 더 자주 익사하는 등 그 격차가 가장 크다. 전반적으로 아프리카계 미국인 남자 어린이의 익사율은 백인 남자의 3배에 달하며 군대에서는 아프리카계 미국인 병사가 백인 병사보다 62% 더 자주 익사하는 것으로 추정된다. 잘 알려지지 않은 여러 가지 이유로 이민자, 히스패닉 및 기타 소수 민족의 익사 비율도 더 높다.
- 위치. 익사는 일반적으로 뒷마당에 있는 수영장이나 호수, 연못, 바다와 같은 자연 지역에서 발생하지만, 양동이와 욕조에서도 발생한다. 우물이 있는 시골 지역의 주택은 어린아이가 익사할 위험이 7배나 높다. 다른 위험한 장소로는 물통, 분수대, 지하 저수조 등이 있다.
- 알코올과 약물. 음주는 판단력을 저하하기 때문에 익사와 관련이 있는 경우가 많다. 보트에서 발생하는 성인 사망 및 익사 사고의 20~30%는 음주로 인해 탑승자가 판단력이 떨어지거나 과속, 구명조끼 미착용, 무모하게 보트를 조작한 경우와 관련이 있다.
- 기저 질환 또는 외상. 기저 질환으로 인한 질병의 발병은 익사로 이어질 수 있다. 저혈당증, 심근경색, 부정맥, 우울증, 자살 충동, 실신은 익사 사고로 이어질 수 있다. 한 연구에 따르면 뇌전증 환자의 익사 위험은 일반인보다 15~19배 높다고 한다. 노인의 여러 가지 약물 복용으로 인해 65세 이상의 익사 비율이 증가했다. 목뼈 손상과 머리 외상은 보드 서퍼, 얕은 물에서 다이빙하는 피해자와 관련된 목격자가 없는 모든 사고와 손상에서 의심해야 한다. 긴척추고정판은 환자를 옮길 때나 이송하기 위해 사용할 수 있지만, 물 안팎에서 긴척추고정판을 오래 고정하는 것은 더 이상 권장하지 않는다(척추 보호에 대한 자세한 내용은 9장 척추 외상 참조).

- 아동학대. 특히 욕조에서 익사로 인한 사고가 아닌 외상 발생률이 높은 것으로 보고되고 있다. 1982~1992년 욕조에서 익사로 인해 사망한 아동을 대상으로 한 연구에 따르면 67%가 학대 또는 방임의 신체적 소견이 있는 것으로 나타났다. 따라서 욕조에 빠진 아동 익사 사고가 의심되는 경우 적절한 조사를 위해 관련 기관에 신고를 한다.
- 저체온증. 익사는 저체온증으로 이어지는 장기간의 침수로 인해 직접 발생할 수 있다(사고성 저체온증에 대한 자세한 내용은 제19장 환경 외상 I: 더위 및 추위 장의 한랭 관련 장애 부문을 참조). 저체온증은 중심체온이 35℃ 미만인 상태로 정의된다. 물에 잠기면 일반적으로 더 차가운 물로 체온이 빠르게 손실되어 저체온증이 발생하지만, 찬물에서 사망하는 대부분의 경우 저체온증으로 인한 이차적인 사망이 아닌 익사로 인한 직접적인 사망이 발생한다. 찬물에서 보트를 타거나 기타 수영 외 활동을 할 때 개인부양장치(PFD)를 준비해야 하며 물에 잠기거나 물에 잠길 수 있는 모든 작업 중에는 반드시 착용해야 한다.
- 흥미롭게도 수영 능력은 익사 사고의 일관된 위험 요소는 아니다. 이는 수영을 못하는 사람은 물을 피할 수 있지만, 수영 실력이 뛰어난 사람(서퍼나 정기적으로 수중 환경에 배치된 군인 등)은 더 높은 위험을 감수할 수 있기 때문일 수 있다. 백인 남성은 백인 여성보다 수영 능력이 더 뛰어나다고 알려졌지만, 익사 사고 발생률이 더 높다. 반면에 한 연구에 따르면 수영을 못하거나 초보자가 가정용 풀장에서 발생한 익사 사고의 73%를 차지하고 운하, 호수, 연못에서 발생한 익사 사고의 82%를 차지한다고 한다. 통계적으로 볼 때 수영 능력이 익사 위험 감소와 상관관계가 없을 수도 있지만, 그런데도 익사 예방 조치로 수영 교육을 권장하고 장려한다. 한 연구에 따르면 공식적인 수영 교육을 받은 1~4세 어린이는 그렇지 않은 대조군보다 익사로 인한 사망률이 8배 이상 낮다고 한다. 그러나 어린이들에게 수영 강습보다 훨씬 더 보호 효과가 큰 것은 어른들의 세심한 감독이다. 또한 서핑이나 급류가 아닌 비기술적인 물에 노출되는 경우 생존 능력은 수영이 아닌 물에 뜨는 능력과 관련이 있을 수 있으므로 개인부양장치(PFD) 또는 기타 부력 장치의 중요성을 강조하고 정확한 수영 기술보다는 생존 기술을 추구하는 사람들에게 교육 기회를 제공해야 한다.

손상 기전

머리가 물에 잠기거나 전신 익수 사고의 일반적인 시나리오는 공황 반응을 일으키는 상황에서 시작하여 숨을 참거나 공기 부족, 수면 위로 떠오르기 위해 신체 활동을 증가시키는 것으로 이어진다. 대부분의 목격자 진술에 따르면 물에 빠진 피해자가 수면 위로 떠오르기 위해 고군분투하면서 비명을 지르거나 손을 흔들며 도움을 요청하는 모습은 거의 보이지 않는다. 그보다는 수면 위에 떠 있거나 움직이지 않는 자세로 있거나 물속으로 잠수했다가 올라오지 못하는 모습을 볼 수 있다. 익사 과정이 진행됨에 따라 반사적인 흡기 노력으로 인두와 후두로 물이 유입되어 질식 반응을 일으킨다. 익사 전문가들은 후두연축은 매우 드물며 3% 이하에서 발생한다고 보고한다. 대부분은 의식을 잃게 되는 것은 물 흡인과 그에 따른 저산소혈증이다.

앞서 언급했듯이 익사의 병태생리학에 대한 구시대적이고 역사적인 논의는 현대 의학에서도 계속되고 있으며 주로 담수와 바닷물에서 익사한 경우와 폐로 물이 들어갔는지 아닌지에 대한 차이에 관한 것이다. 그런데도 최종적인 공통 경로는 뇌 무산소증이며 이러한 구분은 의학적으로 도움이 되지 않는다.

병원 전 처치 제공자에게 익사 사고의 공통 분모는 뇌 저산소증이다. 저산소혈증이 침수, 후두 경련 또는 흡인으로 인한 것인지 아니지는 환자 처치나 결과에 의미가 없다. 물에 잠기거나 물에 잠긴 후 저산소혈증, 무호흡, 의식 상실, 심정지, 맥박 없는 전기 활동, 무수축에 이르는 전체 익사 과정은 보통 몇 초에서 몇 분 안에 발생한다. 생존한 환자의 경우 물에 빠진 환자의 저산소혈증과 그에 따른 조직 저산소증(특히 뇌)을 신속하게 회복시켜 심정지 또는 뇌손상을 예방하는 데 환자 처치의 초점을 맞춰야 한다. 결과를 결정하는 가장 중요한 요소는 물에 잠긴 시간이다. 염분, 수온 또는 목격 여부는 결과를 예측하지 못한다.

찬물 침수 또는 수중에서 생존하는 방법

찬물에 잠기는 동안 신체의 반응과 사망 기전을 설명하는 4가지 단계가 있다. 이러한 단계는 1-10-1원칙과 관련이 있다.

1. 초기 침수 및 저온 쇼크 반응. 피해자는 1분 이내에 호흡 속도를 조절할 수 있다.
2. 단기 침수와 수행 능력 상실. 피해자는 물 밖으로 나오기 위해 10분 동안 의미 있는 움직임을 해야 한다.
3. 장기 침수와 저체온증 발병. 피해자는 저체온증으로 의식을 잃을 때까지 최대 1시간의 시간이 있다.
4. 구조 직전, 도중 또는 구조 직후 순환 붕괴. 피해자가 처음 3단계에서 살아남는 경우 최대 20%는 구조 중에 이러한 유형의 붕괴를 경험할 수 있다.

이러한 각 단계에서는 신체 크기, 수온, 신체가 물에 잠수되는 정도에 따라 개인 차이가 크게 나타난다. 각 단계에는 다양한 병태생리학적 기전에서 비롯되거나 영향을 받는 침수 피해자의 특정 생존 위험이 수반된다. 네 단계 모두에서 사망자가 발생했다.

드물게 장시간 물에 잠긴 경우(한 사례는 66분 동안 잠긴 경우)에는 심한 저체온증에 내원하여 부분적 또는 완전히 신경 기능을 회복한 환자들이 있었다. 이러한 침수 사고에서 생존자의 가장 낮은 체온은 성인 여성의 경우 중심체온이 13.7℃로 측정되었다. 또 다른 사례에서는 한 어린이가 얼음물에 40분간 잠긴 후 중심체온이 23.9℃로 측정되었고 완전히 정상적인 상태로 생존한 때도 있다. 소생술 1시간 후 자발 순환이 회복되었다. 이 사례는 예외적인 상황으로 주목할 만하지만, 이 생존자는 인구 기반 관점에서 결과를 예측할 수 있는 유일한 변수는 침수 시간(잠수 시간이 길수록 생존 가능성 낮아짐)이라는 것을 보여주었다.

이러한 경우에 대한 명확한 설명은 없다. 저체온증은 몇 분에서 몇 시간 동안 천천히 냉각되어 더 나쁜 결과를 초래할 수 있으며 보호 효과가 없다. 일부 어린이가 생존하는 이유를 설명할 수 있는 한 가지 요인은 포유류 잠수 반사이다(**Box 20-5**). 포유류 잠수 반사는 심박수를 늦추고 뇌로 가는 혈액을 차단한다. 최근의 증거에 따르면 다양한 포유류에 존재하는 잠수 반사는 인간 피험자의 15~30%에서만 활성화되므로 일부 어린이가 생존하는 이유에 대한 유일한 설명으로 간주할 수는 없지만, 여전히 이 현상의 일부를 설명할 수 있다. 자원을 수색 및 구조(SAR) 또는 복구에 투입할지 아니면 구조 후 소생술을 시작해야 하는지에 대한 많은 논의가 이루어진다. 앞서 언급했듯이 결과를 결정하는 유일한 검증된 요소는 침수 시간이다. 일부 자료에서는 구조 후 회복으로 전환하거나 소생술을 실시하지 않는 데 걸리는 잠수 시간을 60분으로 보고 있다. 이는 궁극적으로 현지의 인적, 정치적, 재정적 자원에 따라 개별 관할 구역에서 결정해야 하는 어려운 논의이다. 이 세 가지를 모두 무제한으로 이용할 수 있다면 복구로 전환할 필요 없이 각 수색 및 구조 작전을 무기한 계속할 수 있다. 이전에는 찬물에 장시간 잠겼을 때 생존한 사례 보고와 함께 "찬물 익사"에 대한 많은 관심을 기울여 왔다. 그러나 수온과 관계없이 물에 잠긴 시간만으로 결과를 예측할 수 있다. 인용된 검토에서는 장시간 물에 잠긴 후 생존한 예외적인 사례 보고를 제외했음을 인정한다. 팁턴과 골든은 제외된 이상값을 모두 포함할 수 있는 프로토콜을 결정하기 위해 검토를 수행했다. 이 작업은 영국 소방 구조서비스(UKFRS)의 프로토콜 개발에 영향을 미쳤다. UKFRS 지침에 따르면 0시에 동적 위험 평가(DRA)를 실시하고 30분이 지나면 수온이 6℃ 미만인 경우에만 수색을 계속하고 어린아이(즉, 12세 미만)인 경우에는 30분 더 수색을 진행해야 한다.

궁극적으로 소생술이 필요한 수색 및 구조 상태에서 소생술을 시도하지 않고 회복하는 단계로 전환하기 위한 일정 기간을 포함하는 프로토콜을 개발해야 한다. 이는 어려운 결정이며 문헌과 휴머니즘에 대한 균형 잡힌 해석이 있어야 한다. 핵심은 현지 의료책임자와 구조팀이 사고 발생 전에 이러한 논의를 거쳐 현지에서 사용 가능한 자원에 맞는 프로토콜을 개발하는 것이다.

수중 구조

많은 수상 안전 단체에서는 정기적으로 수중 구조 및 소생술 교육을 받은 고도로 숙련된 전문가를 활용할 것을 권장한다. 그러나 전문 수상 구조팀이 없는 경우 병원 전 처치 제공자는 수중 구조를 시도하기 전에 자신의 안전과 모든 구조대원의 안전을 고려한다. 물에서 조난자를 안전하게 구조하려면 다음 지침을 따르는 것이 좋다. 대부분의 수중 구조 시나리오에서 이 단계는 익사 과정을 잠재적으로 중단하고 추가 구조 개입을 계획할 시간을 벌기 위해 최우선으로 시도되는 초기 단계이다.

- 손을 뻗는다. 구조자가 육지나 보트에 머물 수 있도록 장대, 막대기, 노 등 도구를 이용하여 수상 구조를 시도한다. 실수로 물에 빠지지 않도록 주의한다.
- 던진다. 손을 뻗을 수 없을 때는 구명조끼나 밧줄과 같은 물건을 던져 피해자를 떠오를 수 있도록 한다.
- 끌기. 피해자에게 구조 줄이 있으면 피해자를 안전한 곳으로 견인한다.
- 노를 젓는다. 물에 들어가야 하는 경우 보트나 패들보드를 사용하여 피해자에게 접근하고 개인부유장치를 착용하는 것이 바람직하다.

- 가다(가지 않는다). 가장 위험한 기술은 구조대원을 배치하는 것이다. 일부 야생 EMS에서는 이 단계를 "가다(가지 않는다)"라고 명명하여 이 위험을 설명하는데 이는 적절한 훈련과 완전한 위험-이점 분석을 통해 이점이 위험을 초과하는 경우에만 "가기" 단계를 시작해야 함을 나타낸다. 구조대원은 물에 들어갈 때 개인부유장치를 착용해야 하며 급류 환경에서는 스스로 탈출할 수 있도록 가능한 한 빌레이 시스템에 줄을 묶는 것이 이상적이다.
- 헬기. 일부 지역에서는 홍수 또는 급류 구조에 헬기가 투입될 수 있다. 헬기 구조에 어느 정도의 복잡성과 위험을 수반하는 경향이 있고 추가적인 위험-이점 분석이 필요할 수 있으므로 헬기 구조는 신속하게 배치할 수 있는 경우가 드물며 일반적으로 즉각적인 익사 위험이 포함된 장기 구조 작업의 일부로 이루어진다.

병원 전 처치 제공자가 공황 상태에서 빠르게 폭력적으로 변해 잠재적인 이중 익사를 일으킬 수 있는 피해자를 관리할 수 있는 적절한 훈련을 받지 않은 한 수영 구조는 권장되지 않는다. 구조대원들이 자신의 안전을 우선시하지 않아 희생자가 되는 경우가 너무 많으며 일부 연구에 따르면 익사자의 5%가 구조자가 될 뻔한 사람이라고 한다. 수중 구조 시스템, 익수자 및 외상 환자를 위한 장비, 깊은 물속에서의 이동에 대한 몇 가지 방법은 **그림 20-3**을 참고한다.

생존의 예측 요인

다음은 익사자의 소생 결과를 예측하는 데 도움이 되는 중요한 요소이다.

1. 초기 BLS가 중요하다. 심정지 환자 또는 반응이 없는 익사 환자의 경우 지시에 따라 산소를 조기에 공급하고 구조 호흡 또는 심폐소생술을 실시하는 것이 결과에 매우 중요하다.
2. 물에 잠긴 시간이 길수록 퇴원 후 사망 또는 심각한 신경학적 장애가 발생할 위험이 커진다.

   - 0~5분 = 10%
   - 6~10분 = 56%
   - 11~25분 = 88%
   - 25분 이상 = 100%

4. 뇌간 손상의 징후는 사망 또는 심각한 신경학적 장애 및 결손을 예측한다.

평가

익사 환자에 대한 초기 우선순위는 다음과 같다.

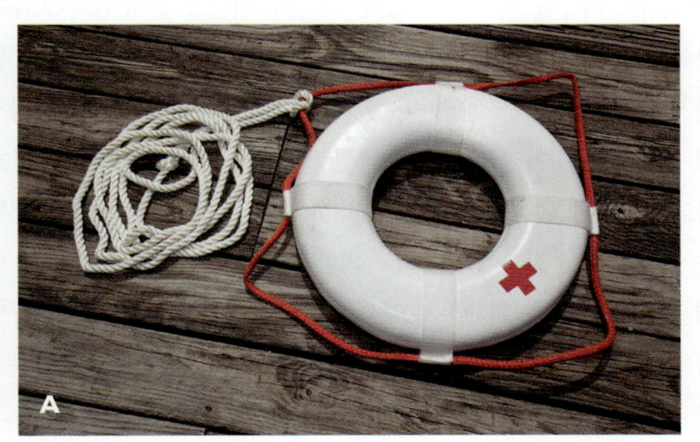

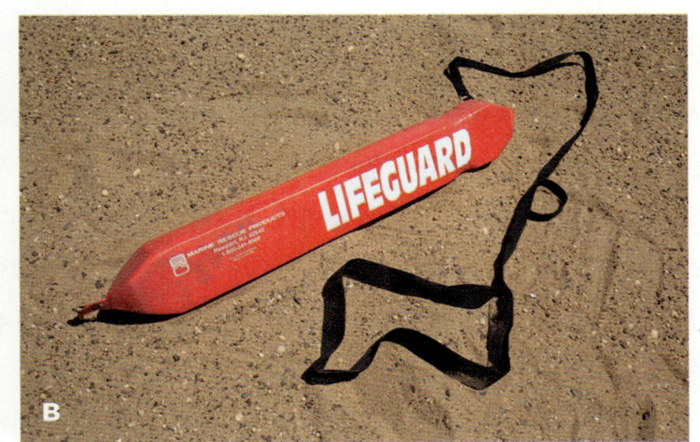

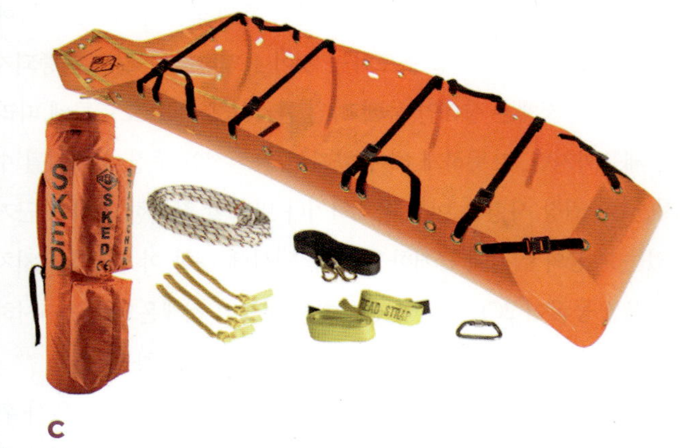

그림 20-3 수중 구조 장비 및 환자 고정 장비. **A.** 구조용 구명줄 **B.** 견인 장치 **C.** 수중 환자 고정 장비

A and B. Courtesy of Rick Brady; **C.** © National Association of Emergency Medical Technicians (NAEMT)

1. 환자와 구조대원의 손상을 방지하고 물에 있는 모든 사람이 부양 장치를 사용할 수 있도록 한다.

2. 물속에서 구조와 최소 BLS 수준의 EMS 처치, 응급실로의 신속한 이송을 위한 계획을 조기에 수립한다.

3. 안전한 수중 구조를 실시한다(다이빙 관련 원인 및 척추고정의 필요성을 고려한다). 이 방법을 훈련받으면 수중 소생술을 고려한다.

4. 저산소혈증으로 인해 CAB(순환, 기도, 호흡)가 아닌 기존 접근 방식을 사용하여 ABC(기도, 호흡, 순환)를 평가한다.

5. 처음에 5회의 구조 호흡으로 저산소혈증과 산혈증을 회복시킨 후 30회의 가슴 압박을 시행하고 이후에는 2회의 인공호흡을 계속한다(30:2). 구조 호흡 및 심폐소생술 중 가장 흔한 합병증인 역류가 발생하지 않도록 주의한다.

6. 익사한 사람에게는 가슴 압박만 시행하는 심폐소생술은 권장하지 않는다.

7. 심혈관계 안정성을 회복하거나 유지한다.

8. 저체온증 환자에게는 추가 체온 손실을 방지하고 재가온을 시작하며 구조 후 환자에게는 치료적 저체온 요법을 고려할 수 있음을 염두에 두어야 한다.

물에 빠진 환자는 달리 증명될 때까지 저산소혈증과 저체온증에 걸린 것으로 추정하는 것이 가장 안전하다. 따라서 익사로 인한 심정지는 주로 산소 부족으로 인해 발생하므로 수중 구조 중에 효과적인 호흡을 제공하기 위해 노력한다. 호흡이 정지된 익수 환자는 일반적으로 몇 번의 구조 호흡 후에 반응한다. 물속에서 가슴 압박을 시도하는 것은 효과가 없으므로 맥박이 있는지 확인하는 데 시간을 투자하는 것은 의미가 없으며 환자를 육지로 구출하는 것만 지연시킬 수 있다.

환자를 안전하게 물에서 구출한다. 육지에 도착한 환자는 머리와 몸통이 일직선이 되도록 바로누운자세를 취해야 하며 일반적으로 경사진 해변이나 제방에서는 해안과 평행한 높이에 놓아야 한다. 반응이 있는지 확인하고 필요에 따라 인공호흡을 계속 시행한다.

환자가 숨을 쉬고 있고 외상이 의심되지 않는 경우 환자를 회복 자세로 눕히고 호흡과 맥박이 효과적인지 모니터링한다. 외상이 의심되는 경우(예: 추락, 보트 사고, 수중 위험이 있는 물에 뛰어든 경우) 환자에게 다른 생명 위협이 없는지 신속하게 평가하고 머리와 목뼈 손상을 평가한다. 익사는 피해자가 물에 뛰어들었다는 사실이 알려지지 않는 한 외상성 손상의 가능성이 상대적으로 낮다. 호흡곤란, 수포음, 뻑뻑호흡음 등 다양한 폐 질환이 나타날 수 있으므로 활력징후를 평가하고 모든 폐 영역을 평가한다. 익사 환자는 초기에는 증상이 미미하다가 폐부종 징후와 함께 급격히 악화할 수 있다. 그러나 임상 검사에서 처음에는 증상이 전혀 없던 환자가 몇 시간 후 갑작스러운 후기 증상으로 사망한 사례는 의학 문헌에 발표된 적이 없다.

맥박산소측정기로 환자의 산소포화도를 평가하고 호기말이산화탄소 수치를 모니터링한다. 물에 잠긴 환자는 저산소증과 저체온증으로 인해 이차적으로 부정맥이 발생하는 경우가 많으므로 심장 리듬 장애가 있는지 평가한다. 많은 침수 환자가 지속적인 신경학적 손상을 입기 때문에 정신 상태와 모든 팔다리의 신경 기능에 변화가 있는지 평가한다. 저혈당이 침수 사고의 원인일 수 있으므로 환자의 혈당 수치를 확인한다. 기준이 되는 글래스고혼수척도(GCS) 점수를 측정하고 지속해서 평가한다. 항상 저체온증을 의심하고 추가 열 손실을 최소화한다. 젖은 옷을 모두 제거하고 체온을 측정(적절한 체온계가 있고 상황이 허락하는 경우)하여 저체온증 정도를 파악하고 추가 열 손실을 최소화하려는 조치를 한다(저체온증 처치에 대해서는 19장 환경 외상 I: 더위와 추위 참조).

처치

그림 20-4는 6등급 분류 체계에 따른 익사자 관리 도구와 각 등급에 따른 처치 지침을 제시한 것이다. 어떤 형태로든 익수 사고를 경험했지만, 일차평가 당시에는 아무런 증상이나 증후가 나타내지 않은 환자는 증상 발현이 지연될 가능성이 있으므로 현장에서 평가한 후 병원에서 후속 치료가 필요하다. 무증상 환자(2등급)의 대부분은 병원에서의 임상 소견에 따라 6~8시간 이내에 퇴원한다. 익사 사고를 경험한 수영 선수 52명을 대상으로 한 연구에서 사고 직후에는 모두 무증상이었지만, 21명(40%)이 4시간 이내에 저산소혈증으로 인한 호흡곤란 증상을 보였다. 일반적으로 모든 증상을 보이는 환자는 초기 임상 평가가 오해의 소지가 있을 수 있으므로 최소 24시간 동안 병원에 입원하여 지지적 처치와 관찰을 받아야 한다. 침수 시간 추정치와 과거 병력을 상세히 기록하는 등 사고에 대한 정확한 병력을 확보하는 것이 중요하다.

모든 익사 의심 환자는 초기 호흡 상태나 산소포화도와 관계없이, 특히 호흡곤란이 발생하는 경우 폐 손상 악화 우려에 따라 고유량 산소(15L/분)를 투여한다. 환자의 산소포화도를 모니터링하여 저산소증이 진행 중인지 확인한다. 특히 무맥성 전기 활동이나 무수축이 있는지 심전도를 적용하고 모니터링한다. 정맥 라인을 확보하고 환자가 저혈압이 아닌 경우 생리식염수 또는 락테이트링거액(LR)을 정맥 라인을 유지할 속도로 투여한다. 그런 다음 500mL의 수액을 볼루스로 주입하고 활력징후를 재평가한다.

모든 익사 환자를 응급실로 이송해서 평가받도록 한다. 익사 환자 중 상당수는 무증상이므로 일부는 즉각적인 주요호소 증상이 없다는 이유로 이송을 거부할 수 있다. 이 경우 시간을 들여 환자 교육을 잘하여 약간의 호흡곤란도 흡인의 징후일 수 있으며 향후 몇 시간 동안 악화할 수 있음을 설명한다. 환자가 이송에 동의하거나 추가 평가 및 관찰을 위해 가장 가까운 응급실로 이송하는 데 동의하도록 단호하고 끈질기게 설득해야 한다. 환자가 치료를 거부하는 경우 발생할 수 있는 결과를 환자에게 알리고 의학적 조언에 반하는 처치 거부 서명을 받아야 한다. 현재까지 익사 환자를 대상으로 한 가장 큰 규모의 연구에 따르면 초기 증상이 경미하거나 중간 정도에 불과한 환자의 사망률은 0.6~5%로 나타났다.

환자 소생술

익사한 심폐정지 환자에게 효과적인 BLS와 표준 ALS 절차를 신속하게 실시하는 것이 생존 확률을 높이는 것과 관련이 있다. 환자는 무수축, 무맥성 전기 활동, 무맥성 심실 빈맥, 심실세동을 보일 수 있다. 이러한 심장 리듬을 처치하려면 소아와 성인에 대한 미국 심장협회의 ALS와 ACLS에 대한 최신 지침을 따른다. 현재 심실세동으로 인한 심정지로 혼수상태에 있는 환자에게는 치료적 저체온요법을 사용할 것을 권장한다(이 주제는 19장 환경 외상 I: 더위와 추위에서 간략하게 설명한다). 다른 심정지 원인에도 똑같이 효과적일 수 있지만, 물에 빠진 환자에게 저체온증을 유도하는 것이 유익하다는 것은 입증되지 않았다. 이미 저체온 상태인 물에 빠진 환자의 경우 프로토콜에 따라 표준 체온까지만, 따뜻하게 해야 한다는 가설적인 주장이 제기될 수 있지만, 이 권장 사항은 이를 옹호하거나 반박할 강력한 과학적 근거가 없는 가상의 이점에 근거한 것이다. 익사에 대한 야생의학회 처치 지침(권장 등급이 2C)은 "익사 환자에서 치료적 저체온요법을 지시하거나 권장하지 않을 근거가 충분하지 않다."라고 명시하고 있다.

고통의 징후(예: 불안, 빠른 호흡, 호흡곤란, 기침)를 보이는 익사 환자에게는 산소를 공급하고 추가 평가를 위해 병원으로 이송해야 한다. 저산소혈증, 산혈증 및 저체온증을 교정하는 데 중점을 두어야 한다. 외상이 의심되는 모든 환자에게 척추 움직임 제한을 시행한다. 반응이 없는 환자의 경우 다량의 비심인성 폐부종(거품)이 있을 수 있다. 양압 환기 및 호기말양압은 이러한 거품을 관리하는 효과적인 방법이 될 수 있지만, 산소 공급과 환기를 희생하면서까지 흡인하는 것은 피해야 한다. 저산소혈증과 산혈증은 효과적인 환지 지원으로 교정할 수 있다. 무호흡 환자는 백마스크로 보조 환기를 시행한다. 익수 환자는 다량의 물을 삼키고 구토 및 위 내용물을 흡인할 위험이 있으므로 무호흡 또는 청색증이 있거나 정신 상태가 저하된 환자

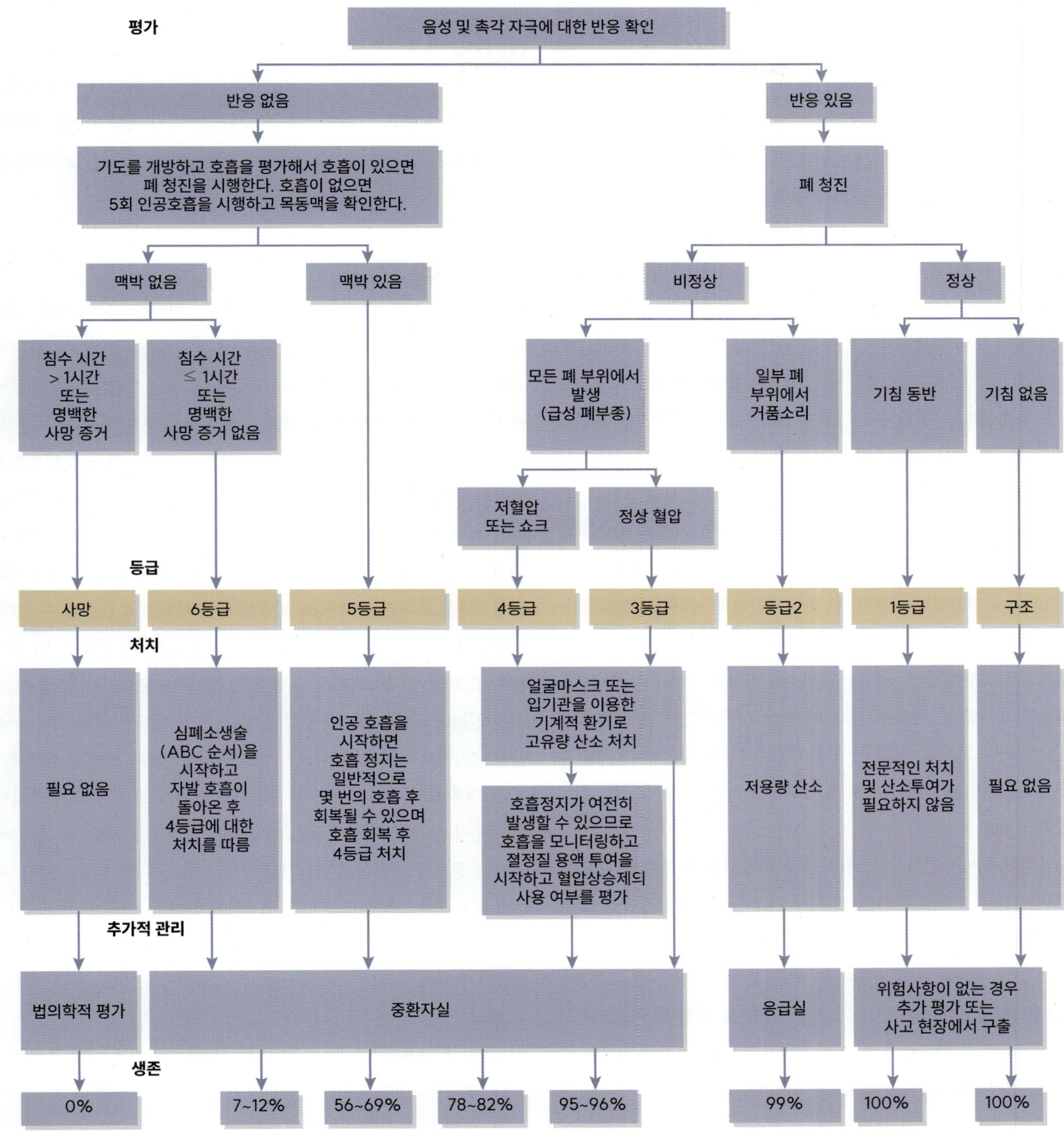

그림 20-4 6가지 중증도 등급에 따른 익사 환자 평가 및 처치.

의 기도를 보호하기 위해 기관내삽관을 조기에 고려한다. 환기에 문제가 있는 경우 환기가 쉽도록 적용되는 압력의 양을 조절해야 한다. 심전도를 모니터링하여 심박수 및 리듬 장애가 있는지 확인하고 침수 사고 전후에 심장 질환이 발생했을 수 있는지 조사한다. 비재호흡

마스크로 100% 산소(15L/분)를 공급하고 정맥 라인을 확보한 후 생리식염수 또는 락테이트링거액을 정맥 라인을 유지할 정도(KVO)로 투여하면서 의료기관으로 신속하게 이송한다.

물에 잠기게 된 원인(예: 다이빙, 워터슬라이드 사용, 손상 징후, 음

주)이 외상 가능성을 나타내지 않는 한 수중 구조 시 척추 고정에 대한 일반적인 주의는 필요하지 않다. 이러한 지표가 없으면 척추 손상의 가능성은 낮다. 수중 구조 시 일반적으로 시행하는 목뼈 고정 및 기타 척추 고정 수단은 기도 개방을 지연시켜 구조 호흡을 시작할 수 없게 할 수 있으므로 시행해서는 안 된다.

수중 구조를 시행하는 동안 가슴 압박은 여러 가지 이유로 권장되지 않는다. 첫째, 물속에서는 가슴 압박을 효과적으로 시행할 수 없다. 물 밖에서 효과적인 심폐소생술을 지연시키는 것 외에도 수중에서 심폐소생술을 시도하면 구조대원이 피로, 찬물, 파도, 해일 및 조류의 위험에 노출될 수 있다. 가능한 한 빨리 기도를 확보하고 무호흡 환자에게 구조 호흡을 제공하는 데 중점을 둔다. 수중 소생술은 환자가 물속에 있는 동안 구조 호흡을 제공하는 공인된 기술이다. 그러나 특정 상황에서 숙련된 병원 전 처치 제공자가 시행할 때만 효과가 있는 것으로 나타났으며 반드시 숙련된 의료진만 시행한다.

해변(또는 기타 장소)에서 경사진 지형에서 구조할 때는 기도를 확보하기 위해 환자를 엎드린 자세(또는 고개를 숙인 자세)로 눕히는 것은 더 이상 권장하지 않는다. 환자를 해안선과 평행하게 바닥에 누운자세에서 효과적인 인공호흡과 가슴압박을 실시할 때 소생술이 더 성공적으로 이루어지는 것으로 나타났다. 바닥에 똑바로 누운자세를 유지하면 고개를 든 자세에서 가슴압박을 시행하는 동안 전방 혈류가 감소하거나 고개를 숙인 자세에서 두개내압이 상승하는 것을 방지할 수 있다. 또한 특정 자세로 폐 배액이 효과적이라는 증거는 없으며 오히려 해로울 수 있다.

하임리히법은 이전에 익사 환자에게 사용하도록 제한된 적이 있다. 그러나 하임리히법은 기도 폐쇄 시 이물질을 제거하기 위해 고안된 것으로 기도나 폐에서 물을 제거하지 않는다. 오히려 익사 환자에게 구토를 유도하여 흡인 위험이 더 커질 수 있다. 현재 미국 심장협회, 야생의학회, 의학연구소는 기도가 이물질로 막힌 경우를 제외하고 하임리히법 처치를 하지 말 것을 권고하고 있다. 자발 호흡으로 회복된 피해자는 환자가 구토할 때 흡인 위험을 줄이기 위해 옆으로 누운 자세를 취해준다(19장, 환경 외상 I: 더위와 추위에서는 저체온 환자의 소생에 관한 ALS 절차를 설명한다. 이 지침은 추위에 노출된 원인과 관계없이 모든 저체온 환자에게 같이 적용된다.).

대부분의 익사 환자는 입에서 다량의 거품이 나오는데 이는 폐에 있는 계면활성제 및 기타 이물질과 물이 섞인 결과이다. 이 거품을 흡입하는 것은 아무런 이득이 없으며 실제로 기도에서 이물질을 제거하려고 노력하는 시간은 환자에게 산소 공급을 제공할 수 있는 시간을 낭비하는 것이다. 크고 단단한 이물질이 기도에서 제거된 후에는 거품을 다시 폐로 흡입할 수 있다.

심정지로 익사한 환자는 산소공급과 인공호흡이 매우 중요하므로 가능한 한 빨리 기관내삽관을 시행하는 것이 바람직하다. 성문위 기도기는 기도 저항이 높으므로 익사 환자에게 효과가 입증되지 않았다.

익사 예방

미국에서 익사 사고율을 낮추기 위한 예방 전략이 필수적이다. 전체 익사 사고의 85%는 감독, 수영 교육, 기술 규정 및 공공교육을 통해 예방할 수 있는 것으로 추정된다. 많은 교육 프로그램은 수영장 주변에 다양한 유형의 차단막(예: 격리 울타리, 수영장 덮개, 경보기)을 설치하고 구명조끼와 같은 개인부양장치를 사용하도를 권장함으로써 영유아의 의도치 않은 물놀이 사고를 줄이는 데 중점을 둔다. 또한, 병원 전 처치 제공자가 사고 현장에 도착하기 전에 목격자에 의해 시작된 심폐소생술은 환자의 예후 개선과 관련이 있으므로 지역 사회 심폐소생술 교육은 익사 사고 예방을 위한 개입으로 간주할 수 있다.

병원 전 처치 제공자는 이전에 파악한 위험 지역을 알리는 데 중점을 두고 해당 지역사회에서 수상 안전 및 교육 옹호자가 될 좋은 기회를 얻는다. 또한, 현장에 도착한 병원 전 처치 제공자 및 기타 공공 안전 요원에게 추가 익수 피해자가 발생하지 않도록 예방을 강조해야 한다. 당황하고 몸부림치는 익수자는 준비되지 않은 수중 구조자에게 위험할 수 있으며 잠재적으로 또 다른 익사를 초래할 수 있다. 구조자는 문제를 신속하게 평가하고 구경꾼이 물에 들어가지 못하도록 현장을 통제하고 자신의 안전을 확보해야 한다.

익수 사고에 관한 지역사회 교육에는 다음과 같은 권장 사항이 포함되어야 한다.

- 해변
  - 항상 인명구조요원 근처에서 수영한다.
  - 인명구조요원에게 안전한 수영 장소에 관해 물어본다.
  - 항상 다른 사람들과 함께 수영한다.
  - 자신의 수영 실력을 과대평가하지 않는다.
  - 항상 자녀를 지켜본다.
  - 교각, 바위 및 기둥에서 멀리 떨어져 수영한다.
  - 술을 마시지 않는다.
  - 수영하던 어린이가 보이지 않는 경우 가장 가까운 인명구조요원에게 도움을 요청한다.

- 바다에서 발생한 익사 사고의 대부분은 이안류에서 발생한다는 점에 유의한다.
- 물에 들어가기 전에 기상 상태를 파악한다.
- 자신이 무엇을 하고 있는지 모른 채 누군가를 구조하려고 시도해서는 안 된다. 많은 사람이 그러한 시도로 사망했다.
- 바위 위에서 낚시하는 경우 구명조끼를 착용한다.
- 얕은 물에는 항상 발부터 들어간다.
- 목뼈 손상이 발생할 수 있으므로 얕은 물에서 다이빙하지 않는다.
- 해양 동물에게 접근하지 않는다.
- 해안에 설치된 표지판과 깃발을 읽고 주의를 기울인다.
- 주거용 수영장 및 기타 수원
  - 성인이 어린이를 지속해 감독하도록 한다.
  - 물에서 안전을 위한 규칙을 정한다.
  - 수영장이나 욕조, 물통과 같은 수원 근처에 어린이를 혼자 두지 않는다.
  - 수영장 주변에 1.2m 이상의 4면 울타리를 설치하고 자동으로 닫히고 자동 잠금장치가 있는 문을 설치한다.
  - 어린이가 팔 부표나 기타 공기가 채워진 수영 보조기구를 사용하지 못하게 한다.
  - 승인된 구명조끼를 사용한다.
  - 수영장 주변에 어린이의 관심을 끄는 장난감을 두지 않는다.
  - 수영장을 사용할 때 9m 간격으로 배수구 2개와 머리카락 방지 덮개를 사용하거나 펌프 필터를 끈다.
  - 수영장 근처에서는 무선 전화기나 휴대전화를 사용하여 다른 곳에서 전화를 받기 위해 수영장을 떠나지 않도록 한다.
  - 구조 방비(예: 갈고리, 구명조끼)와 전화기를 수영장 옆에 비치한다.
  - 수중 수영 시간을 늘리기 위해 과다호흡을 시도하거나 허용하지 않는다.
  - 얕은 물에 다이빙하지 않는다.
  - 4세까지 모든 어린이에게 수영을 가르치되 될 수 있는 대로 만 1세까지 권장한다.
  - 어린이가 수영을 마친 후에는 수영장에 들어오지 못하도록 잠근다.
  - 모든 가족과 어린이를 보살피는 사람은 수상 안전, 응급처치 및 심폐소생술을 배워야 한다.

또한 지역사회는 홍수 시 운전의 위험성에 대해 대중에게 교육함으로써 익사를 예방할 수 있다. 홍수를 유발하는 폭풍우가 빈번해짐에 따라 이 메시지의 중요성이 점점 더 커지고 있다. 운전자가 물에 잠긴 차량에 갇히면 신속하고 안전하게 탈출하는 방법을 알아야 한다(**Box 20-6**)

Box 20-6 침수 차량에서 익사

연구에 따르면 익사 사고의 10%가 물에 잠기거나 물에 잠긴 차량에서 발생하며 재난 시 자동차 관련 사망 사고의 10%가 물에 잠긴 차량으로 인해 발생한다고 한다. 물이 가득 찬 차량에서 탈출하는 방법으로는 차에 물이 가득 찰 때까지 기다렸다가 문이 열리기를 기다리거나 갇힌 공기를 마시거나 앞 유리를 걷어차는 등 잘못된 방법이 언론을 통해 많이 알려졌다. 하지만 최근 이러한 방법들에 대한 철저한 조사 결과 위험하고 비효율적이라는 사실이 입증되어 침수 차량에서 탈출하기 위한 더욱 근거를 기반으로 한 지침이 마련되었다.

차량은 약 30초에서 120초 동안 떠 있다가 가라앉는다. 이 시간 동안 창문을 내리고 최대한 신속하게 차량에서 빠져나와야 한다. 연구에 따르면 성인 3명이 이 방법으로 차량에서 탈출하는 동시에 뒷좌석에 있는 어린이 마네킹도 51초 이내에 탈출할 수 있는 것으로 나타났다. 특히 신고자가 구급대원과 통화하는 동안 침수 차량으로 인한 익사 사망자가 다수 발생한 점을 고려할 때 병원 전 처치 제공자가 추가 조치를 취하기 전에 신고자에게 침수 차량에서 탈출하도록 조언하는 것을 알고 있어야 한다. 침수 차량 안에 있는 사람 또는 침수 차량 안에 있는 사람을 구조하려는 사람이 취해야 할 일련의 행동은 다음과 같다.

1. 안전띠를 푼다.
2. 창문을 연다.
3. 어린이가 있는 경우 안전띠를 풀고 탈출을 도와줄 수 있는 성인에게 가까이 온다.
4. 어린이를 먼저 창문 밖으로 밀어낸 다음 즉시 따라 나가야 한다.

© National Association of Emergency Mecical Technicians (NAEMT)

레크리에이션 스쿠버 관련 손상

수중 자가호흡기(SCUBA)를 사용하는 레크리에이션 다이빙은 다양한 연령대가 즐기는 흔한 활동이다. 이 활동의 인기는 계속 증가하여 매년 400,000명 이상의 신규 다이버가 자격증을 취득하고 있으며 현재 미국 내 레크리에이션 스쿠버 다이버는 총 400만 명에 육박하고 있다. 매년 증가하는 신규 다이버보다 손상이 발생하는 비율은 낮지만, 다이버의 다양성, 나이 증가, 체력 저하, 기저 질환 등으로 인해 다이빙을 위한 건강 상태에 대한 우려가 커지고 있다. 물은 문제가 발생하기 쉬운 환경이다. 현재 스쿠버 다이빙에 대한 상대적이고 일시적인 건강 위험과 절대적인 금기 사항을 나타내는 의료 지침이 있다.

다이버의 손상은 난파선, 산호초 등 다양한 수중 위험 요소나 위험한 해양생물을 취급으로 인해 발생한다. 그러나 병원 전 처치 제공자는 대부분의 심각한 다이빙 의학적 장애를 설명하는 감압증 또는 환경 압력 변화로 인한 스쿠버 관련 손상 및 사망에 대응하는 경우가 더 많다. 손상 기전은 다음 부문에서 자세히 설명하겠지만, 다양한 수심과 압력에서 압착 가스(예: 산소, 헬륨, 질소)를 호흡할 때 기체 법칙의 원리를 기반으로 한다.

다이빙 사망 사고와 관련된 원인은 최근 역사에서 크게 변하지 않았다. 가장 자주 언급되는 문제는 불충분한 기체(공기)나 가스 부족이다. 그 외의 일반적인 요인으로는 갇힘 또는 얽힘, 부력 조절 실패, 장비의 잘못된 사용, 거친 물살, 갑작스러운 상승 등이 있다. 주요 손상 또는 사망 원인으로는 물 흡입으로 인한 익사 또는 질식, 공기 색전증 및 심장 질환 등이 포함되어 있다. 나이가 많은 다이버일수록 심장 질환의 위험이 더 컸으며 65세까지 위험은 같았지만, 남성이 여성보다 손상의 위험이 더 컸다.

감압증으로 인한 대부분의 스쿠버 관련 손상은 수면 위로 떠오른 직후 또는 60분 이내에 징후(예: 하강시 귀 압박)와 증상이 나타나지만, 일부 증상은 다이빙 장소를 떠나 집으로 돌아온 후 최대 48시간까지 지연될 수 있다. 따라서 오늘날 미국, 카리브해 및 기타 외딴 지역의 인기 있는 다이빙 장소를 오가는 스쿠버 다이버들이 증가함에 따라 실제 다이빙 장소에서 멀리 떨어진 곳에서 다이빙과 관련 손상을 당할 가능성이 커지고 있다. 병원 전 처치 제공자는 이러한 스쿠버 관련 질환을 인지하고 초기 처치를 제공하며 가까운 응급실로 이송하거나 가장 가까운 재가압 챔버가 있는 기관에서 처치를 위한 계획을 조기에 시작해야 한다.

역학

다이버 경고 네트워크(DAN)는 북미 지역의 재가압 챔버에서 제공한 사상자 데이터를 근거로 광범위한 이환율과 사망률 데이터베이스를 수집한다. 다이빙 관련 사망률은 1970년대에 최고조에 달해 연간 150명에 달했지만, 그 이후에는 77~91명으로 훨씬 낮은 연간 사망률도 안정적으로 유지되고 있다. 다이버 경고 네트워크는 이러한 데이터를 웹사이트에서 확인할 수 있는 연례 보고서를 통해 발표한다. 다이버 경고 네트워크에 보고된 미국 내 사망자 수는 일반적으로 여름이 다가올수록 증가하여 7월경에 정점을 찍은 후 겨울이 다가올수록 감소한다. 북미에서 가장 많은 다이빙 사망자가 보고되고 있으며 유럽이 그 뒤를 잇고 있다. 남성이 여성보다 3~4배 더 많이 다이빙 중 손상을 입는다.

남성이 사망자의 81%를 차지하며 대부분의 사망은 40~59세 다이버에게서 발생한다. 익사가 가장 흔한 사망 원인이고 심혈관 질환은 두 번째로 흔한 사망 원인이며 장애를 남기는 가장 흔한 손상 원인이었다. 이 두 가지 원인은 세 번째로 흔한 질환인 동맥기체색전증(AGE)보다 사망 및 장애를 유발하는 원인으로 훨씬 더 흔했다. 익사가 사망의 주요 원인이긴 하지만, 심장 질환, 장비 문제, 공기 부족, 얽힘, 혼수, 공황, 방향 감각 상실, 저체온증, 동맥기체색전증 등 익사의 원인은 불분명하다. 스쿠버 다이빙 중 익사 사망자 중 일부는 동맥가스색전증으로 인해 사망한다.

압력의 기계적 영향

수중 환경의 압력 변화로 인해 발생하는 스쿠버 다이빙 관련 손상 또는 감압증은 1) 수중 환경의 압력 변화로 인해 신체 내 밀폐된 공기 공간(예: 귀, 부비동, 장, 폐)에 조직 손상이나 압력 손상이 발생하는 경우와 2) 감압병과 같이 높은 분압에서 압착된 기체를 호흡할 때 발생하는 문제로 구분할 수 있다.

스쿠버 다이빙과 관련된 압력 손상은 다이버에게 가해지는 공기와 물의 압력 효과와 직접적으로 관련이 있다. 해수면에 서 있을 때 대기압은 760토르(torr)이며 이는 기본적으로 760mmHg 또는 신체에 가해지는 14.7psi와 같다. 이 압력을 1기압이라고도 한다. 다이버가 더 깊은 수심으로 내려갈수록 절대 압력은 해수면에서 물속으로 10m 내려갈 때마다 1기압씩 증가한다. 따라서 수심 10m 깊이에서는 2기압(공기 1기압, 물 1기압)이 신체에 가하는 압력과 같다. **표 20-2**에는 수중 환경에서 일반적인 압력 단위를 나열한 것이다.

다이버가 물속으로 하강할 때 압력이 높아지면서 신체에 가해지는 힘의 영향은 조직 구획에 따라 달라진다. 단단한 조직에 가해지는 힘은 유체 매체와 비슷한 방식으로 작용하며 다이버는 일반적으로 압착력을 인식하지 못한다. 그러나 공기가 포함된 신체 공간에서는 다이버가 하강할 때 기체가 압착된다. 반대로 다이버가 수면으로 올라갈수록 이러한 가스는 팽창한다. 보일의 법칙과 헨리의 법칙은 수중에서 신체에 가해지는 압력의 영향을 설명한다.

보일의 법칙

보일의 법칙에 따르면 주어진 기체 질량의 부피는 해당 환경에서 발견되는 절대 압력에 반비례한다. 다시 말해, 다이버가 물속에서 더 깊은 수심으로 내려갈수록 압력이 증가하고 기체의 부피(예: 폐나 귀)

표 20-2 수중 환경에서 일반적인 압력 단위

깊이(FSW)	PSIA	대기압 (ATA)	Torr or mmHg (absolute)
해수면	14.7	1기압	760
10m	29.4	2기압	1,520
20m	44.1	3기압	2,280
30m	58.8	4기압	3,040
40m	73.5	5기압	3,800
50m	88.2	6기압	4,560
60m	102.9	7기압	5,320

Abbreviations: ATA, atmosphere absolute; FSW, feet seawater; mm Hg, millimeters of mercury; PSIA, pounds per square inch absolute.

© National Association of Emergency Medical Technicians (NAEMT)

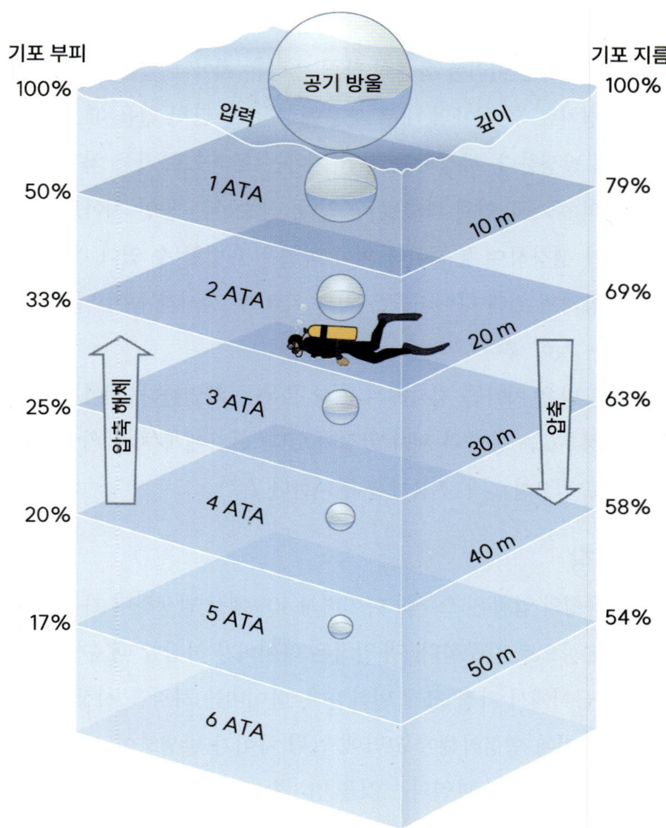

그림 20-5 코일의 법칙. 일정한 온도에서 주어진 양의 기체 부피는 압력에 반비례한다.

© National Association of Emergency Medical Technicians (NAEMT)

는 감소 한다. 그 반대도 마찬가지여서 다이버가 수면으로 올라갈 때 기체의 부피(예: 폐 또는 귀 안의 부피)는 증가한다. 이것이 바로 압력 손상과 동맥기체색전증이 신체에서 미치는 영향의 원리이다. **그림 20-5**는 기체 기포의 부피와 지름에 대한 압력의 영향을 보여준다.

헨리의 법칙

헨리의 법칙은 일정한 온도에서 액체에 용해되는 기체의 양은 액체 외부의 기체 부분압에 정비례한다는 법칙이다. 헨리의 법칙은 다이버가 물속으로 내려갈 때 압축 공기 실린더(스쿠버 탱크)의 기체가 체내에서 어떻게 작용하는지를 이해하는 데 기본이 된다. 예를 들어, 질소의 부분압이 증가하면 하강하는 동안 압력이 증가함에 따라 질소가 신체 조직의 체액에 용해된다. 수면으로 상승할 때 질소는 조직의 체액 용액에서 "기포"가 된다. 상승 속도가 느리면 질소가 거품을 형성하지 않고 소멸한다. 따라서 헨리의 법칙은 감압병이 발생하는 이유를 설명하는 원리를 설명한다.

압력 손상

압착이라고도 알려진 압력 손상은 스쿠버 다이빙과 관련된 가장 흔한 유형의 손상이다. 많은 유형의 압력 손상이 통증을 유발하지만, 대부분은 자연적으로 해결되며 병원 전 처치 제공자의 처치나 재가압 챔버 치료가 필요하지 않다. 그러나 일부 폐 과압 손상은 매우 심각하다. 스쿠버 다이빙 중 압력 손상은 비압착성 가스로 채워진 체강(예: 부비동) 내에서 발생한다. 다이빙 중 주변 압력이 증가함에 따

라 이러한 공간의 압력이 평형을 이루지 못하면 다이버가 하강할 때 기체 부피가 감소하여 혈관 충혈, 출혈 및 점막 부종이 발생하고 상승할 때 기체 부피가 증가하여 조직 파열이 발생한다. 다양한 유형의 압력 손상은 다음에 설명되어 있다.

하강에 의한 압력 손상

마스크 압착

이러한 유형의 압력 손상은 일반적으로 하강하는 동안 얼굴 마스크의 압력을 외부 수압과 같게 맞추지 못하는 미숙한 다이버에게서 발생한다. 환자의 눈 주위의 연부조직과 결막 조직에 모세혈관 파열이 있는지 검사한다. 마스크 압착의 징상과 징후로는 피부 반상출혈과 눈 주위 부종, 결막출혈 등이 있다. 마스크 압착은 자기 치료가 가능하며 조직 손상이 사라질 때까지 다이빙하지 않는 것이 좋다. 처치에는 눈에 냉찜질하고 환자가 휴식을 취하도록 권장하며 필요에 따라 진통제를 투여하는 것이 포함된다.

치아 압착

드물게 발견되는 이러한 유형의 압력 손상은 치아 보철물, 최근 발치 또는 신경치료 후 치아의 내부 부분에 가스가 갇혀 있을 때 다이버들에게서 발생한다. 하강하는 동안 치아는 혈액으로 가득 차거나 외부 압력의 증가로 인해 파열될 수 있다. 상승하는 동안 치아로 유입된 공기가 팽창하여 통증이나 치아 파열을 유발할 수 있다. 치아 압착을 예방하기 위해 다이버들은 치과 치료 후 24시간 동안 다이빙을 하지 않는 것이 좋다.

영향을 받은 치아를 검사해서 손상 유무를 확인한다. 치아 압착의 증상과 징후로는 통증과 치아 골절이 있다. 환자에게 치과 치료를 받도록 하고 필요한 경우 진통제를 투여한다.

중이 압착

이러한 유형의 압착은 스쿠버 다이버의 40%에서 발생하며 가장 흔한 다이빙 손상으로 간주한다. 귀 압착은 다이버가 하강할 때 수압 변화가 수면 근처에서 가장 크게 변화한다. 다이버는 하강을 시작하면서 중이를 조기에 평형화해야 고막에 압력 차이가 발생하여 심한 통증을 유발하고 고막이 파열되는 것을 방지할 수 있다. 고막이 파열되어 물이 중이로 들어가면 다이버는 현기증을 경험하게 된다. 상부 호흡기 감염이나 알레르기가 있는 다이버는 다이빙 중에 중이의 평형을 유지하는 데 어려움을 겪을 수 있다.

고막 파열로 인한 혈액이 있는지 이관을 검사한다. 중이 압착의 증상과 징후에는 통증, 현기증, 고막 파열로 인한 전도성 난청, 구토 등이 있다. 외이도 검사가 가능한 경우 고막의 발적이 종종 나타난다.

중이 압착이 있는 환자는 다이빙이나 비행과 같은 압력 변화가 발생할 수 있는 활동은 허용되지 않는다. 고막이 파열되지 않으면 유스타키오관을 열어 압력을 균등하게 하려고 충혈 완화제가 필요할 수 있다. 현기증이나 구토하는 환자는 프로클레페라진 또는 온단세트론과 같은 항구토제가 필요할 수 있다. 환자를 똑바로 세우거나 편안한 자세로 이송한다. 감염 예방을 위해 고막이 파열된 환자의 경우 항생제를 처방할 수 있다. 청력 손실 가능성을 평가하기 위해 환자에게 청력 평가를 받을 수 있도록 의료기관으로 이송한다.

부비동 압착(부비동 압력 손상)

일반적으로 부비동의 압력은 다이버가 하강 및 상승할 때 쉽게 균등해진다. 중이 압착과 같은 기전에 의해 압력이 발생하지만, 부비동 압착은 흔하지 않다. 다이버가 하강할 때 부비동의 압력을 유지할 수 없게 되고 부비동에 상대적인 진공 상태가 발생하여 부비동에 극심한 통증, 점막 벽 손상, 부비동에서 출혈을 유발할 수 있다. 이러한 부비동 압박은 충혈, 부비동염, 점막 비대(비대 또는 비후), 비염, 비강 폴립으로 인해 발생할 수 있다. 상승 중 역부비동 압착도 발생할 수 있다(뒷부분에서 설명하는 역 압착 참조).

환자의 코에 분비물이 있는지 검사한다. 부비동 압착의 증상과 징후로는 부비동 부위에 심한 통증이 있거나 부비동에서 피가 섞인 분비물이 나올 수 있다.

현장에서 특별한 처치는 필요하지 않다. 부비동 점막에서 출혈이 발생하므로 코뼈 바로 아래 콧구멍 끝부분을 꾹 눌러 코피를 지혈하는 것은 효과가 없을 수 있지만, 병원 전 유일한 처치 방법이다. 환자를 편안한 자세로 의료기관으로 이송한다.

역 압착

이러한 유형의 부비동 압착은 부비동 입구가 어떤 형태로든 막혀 팽창하는 가스가 빠져나가지 못할 때 상승 시 발생할 수 있다. 팽창하는 가스가 부비동 점막에 압력을 가하여 출혈과 함께 통증을 유발한다. 부비동 압력 손상은 상기도 감염이나 알레르기가 있는 다이버에게서 발생한다.

코에 분비물이 있는지 검사한다. 부비동 압력 손상의 증상과 징후로는 부비동 부위의 심한 통증과 피가 섞인 분비물이 나올 수 있다.

충혈 완화제는 점막 부종을 줄이고 부비동 배액을 촉진하는 데 도움이 될 수 있다. 광범위한 출혈이 관찰되지 않는 한 현장에서 다른 특별한 처치가 필요하지 않으며 이 경우 코뼈 바로 아래 콧구멍 끝부분을 꾹 눌러 코피를 지혈한다. 출혈이 코 앞부위의 정맥총이 아닌 부비동에서 발생한 것이므로 이 방법은 별 도움이 되지 않을 수 있으며 환자를 편안한 자세로 의료기관으로 이송한다.

내이의 압력 손상

중이 압착보다 훨씬 덜 흔하지만, 영구적인 난청으로 이어질 수 있으므로 가장 심각한 상태의 귀 압력 손상이다. 내이 압력 손상은 다이버가 하강하면서 중이의 압력 평형 시도에 실패했을 때 발생한다. 더 무리하게 시도하면 중이 압력이 크게 상승하여 달팽이창 구조가 파열될 수 있다.

이관에 분비물이 있는지 확인한다. 증상 및 증후에는 울리는 이명, 현기증, 청력 소실, 영향을 받은 귀의 꽉 찬 느낌 또는 막힌 느낌, 구역, 구토, 창백함, 발한, 방향 감각 상실, 운동 실조(근육 협응력 상실)가 포함된다.

환자는 두개내압을 높이는 활동, 격렬한 활동, 발살바법과 같은 동작, 튼 소음, 압력 변화가 없는 활동(예: 잠수 또는 비행)을 피해야 한다. 환자를 똑바로 선 자세로 이송한다. 환자가 내이 감압병을 겪고 있는지, 재가압 챔버 처치가 즉각적으로 필요한지 판단하기 어려울 수 있으므로 다이버 경고 네트워크 또는 응급의학과 전문의와 조기에 의료 상담을 받는 것이 좋다. 또한 환자는 이비인후과 전문의에게 신속하게 진료를 받아야 한다.

상승 시 압력 손상

압력 변화성 현기증

이것은 팽창하는 가스가 유스타키오관을 통해 이동하면서 발생하는 일종의 압력 손상으로 중이에 불균형한 압력이 발생하여 현기증을 유발할 수 있다. 증상은 짧지만, 현기증은 다이버에게 공황상태를 유발하여 수면으로 급격히 상승하여 다른 형태의 손상(예: 공기색전증, 익사)으로 이어질 수 있다.

이관에 분비물이 있는지 검사하고 청력 소실이 있는지 평가한다. 압력 변화성 현기증의 증상과 징후는 지속 시간이 짧으며 일시적인 현기증, 귀의 압력, 이명, 청력 소실이 발생한다.

환자가 다이빙 후 증상이 없고 이퀄라이징 문제가 발견되지 않는다면 특별한 처치가 필요하지 않다. 필요에 따라 EMS 시스템의 정책 및 절차에 따라 충혈 완화제를 제공한다. 증상이 신속하고 완전하게 해결되면 응급실로 이송할 필요가 없으며 환자는 주치의에게 후속 처치를 받을 수 있다. 증상이 지속되면 평가를 위해 의료기관으로 이송하는 것이 적절하다.

위장 압착

이러한 유형의 압력 손상은 다이버가 수면 위로 떠오를 때 장에서 팽창하는 가스가 빠져나가지 못할 때 발생한다. 위장관 압력 손상은 고개를 숙인 자세에서 발살바법을 자주하거나 호흡 중에 공기를 삼키거나 다이빙 전에 가스를 생성하는 음식을 섭취하는 다이버에게 발생하며 이로 인해 수심에서 위장의 공기량이 증가하여 상승 시 팽창하게 된다.

복부 사분면을 평가한다. 위장관 압박의 증상과 징후로는 복부 팽만감, 트림, 위장관가스참 등이 있다.

위장관 압착은 일반적으로 저절로 해결되며 처치가 필요한 경우는 거의 없다. 복통과 복부 팽만감이 해결되지 않으면 병원으로 이송하여 검사받는 것이 적절하다.

척수 감압병 등 수면 손상 후 복통의 다른 원인도 있다. 수면에서 해결되지 않는 복통은 응급실에서 즉시 처치를 받아야 한다.

폐 과도팽창 압력 손상

폐 과도팽창은 상승하는 동안 폐의 기체가 팽창하여 발생하는 심각한 유형의 압력 손상이다. 일반적으로 다이버는 수면으로 상승할 때 정상적인 날숨으로 팽창하는 가스를 제거한다. 팽창 가스가 빠져나가지 않으면 폐포가 파열된다. 이로 인해 폐 밖으로 빠져나가는 공기의 양과 최종 위치에 따라 여러 가지 형태의 손상이 발생할 수 있다. 일반적인 시나리오는 공기 부족, 공황 상태에 빠지거나 웨이트 벨트가 떨어지면서 다이버가 수면으로 빠르고 제어할 수 없을 정도로 상승하는 경우이다. 이러한 유형의 손상을 총칭하여 "폐 과도팽창증후군(POPS)" 또는 폐 파열이라고 한다. 재가압 요법은 동맥기체색전증을 제외한 모든 형태의 폐 과도팽창증후군에 금기이다.

다섯 가지 형태의 폐 과도팽창증후군은 다음과 같다.
1. 국소 손상을 동반한 과잉 확장
2. 세로칸기종
3. 피부밑기종
4. 기흉
5. 동맥기체색전증

국소 손상을 동반한 과잉확장

이는 폐 외 공기나 명백한 폐 손상 없이 발견되는 폐 압력 손상이다. 감소한 호흡을 평가하기 위해 폐 전체에서 호흡음을 청진한다. 가슴 통증이 있을 수도 있고 없을 수도 있다. 가래에 피가 보이면 응급실에서 즉시 처치를 받아야 한다.

환자가 편안한 자세로 쉬도록 하고 필요에 따라 환자의 증상을 처치한다. 환자의 활력징후와 산소포화도를 모니터링하고 100% 고농도의 산소를 공급하며 환자를 편안한 자세로 이송한다. 환자는 더 심각한 형태의 폐 과도팽창증후군을 배제하기 위해 추가 검사 필요하며 추가 압력 노출(예: 다이빙 또는 비행)을 피해야 한다.

세로칸기종

세로칸기종은 파열된 폐포에서 빠져나온 가스가 사이질 공간으로 들어가 세로칸으로 들어가서 발생하는 또 다른 형태의 폐 과도팽창증후군이다. 이 상태는 양성일 수 있다. 폐에서 호흡음이 감소하는지 평가한다. 쉰 소리, 목 충만감, 경미한 복장뼈 아래 가슴 통증, 호흡과 기침으로 악화하는 둔한 통증이나 압박감 등의 증상과 징후가 나타날 수 있다. 환자의 가슴과 목 부분에 피부밑기종이 있는지 검사한다. 심한 경우 다이버는 가슴 통증, 호흡곤란 및 삼킴 곤란을 호소한다.

환자가 편안한 자세로 휴식을 취할 수 있도록 한다. 환자의 활력징후와 산소포화도를 모니터링하고 고유량 산소를 공급한다. 일반적으로 세로칸기종은 특별한 처치가 필요하지 않다. 그러나 가슴 통증의 다른 원인과 더 심각한 형태의 폐 과도팽창증후군을 배제하기 위해 환자를 의학적으로 평가해야 할 수도 있다. 환자는 더 이상의 압력 노출(예: 다이빙 또는 비행)을 피해야 한다.

피부밑기종

피부밑기종이 있으면 파열된 폐포에서 빠져나온 공기가 목과 빗장뼈 부위로 계속 이동한다. 폐에서 호흡음이 감소했는지 평가한다. 피부밑기종의 증상과 징후로는 부기, 비빔소리, 쉰 목소리, 인후통 및 삼킴 곤란 등이 있다.

휴식 외에는 특별한 치료가 필요하지 않다. 환자의 활력징후와 산소포화도를 모니터링하고 고유량 산소를 공급한다. 환자는 더 심각한 형태의 폐 과도팽창증후군을 배제하기 위해 추가 의학적 평가가 필요하다. 환자를 바로누운자세로 이송한다. 환자는 더 이상의 압력 노출(예: 다이빙 또는 비행)을 피해야 한다.

기흉

기흉은 폐와 내장가슴막 사이의 사이질 공간을 통해 빠져나가는 공기보다 저항이 큰 폐 주변의 내장가슴막을 통해 빠져나가야 하므로 다른 형태의 폐 과도팽창증후군만큼 자주 나타나지 않는다. 폐 파열이 발생했을 때 다이버가 수심에 있는 경우 다이버가 수면으로 계속 올라갈 때 빠져나가는 가스의 양이 팽창하면서 긴장기흉이 발생할 수 있다. 폐에서 호흡음이 감소하는지 검사한다. 기흉의 크기에 따라 증상과 징후가 달라지며 날카로운 가슴 통증, 호흡음 감소, 호흡곤란, 피부밑기종 등이 나타날 수 있다.

호흡 또는 혈역학적 허탈의 증거와 같이 단순 기흉에서 긴장기흉으로 변화하는지를 모니터링하기 위해 지속해서 평가를 시행한다. 환자가 편안한 자세로 휴식을 취하게 한다. 환자의 활력징후와 산소포화도를 모니터링하고 비재호흡마스크로 100% 산소를 공급한다. 필요에 따라 길이가 8.5cm 이상인 14게이지 주삿바늘로 바늘감압을

시행한다. 환자를 편안한 자세로 이송한다. 환자는 더 심각한 형태의 폐 과도팽창증후군을 배제하기 위해 추가 의학적 평가가 필요하며 추가 압력 노출(예: 다이빙 또는 비행)을 피해야 한다.

동맥기체색전증(AGE)

이것은 가장 두려운 폐 가도팽창증후군 합병증이며 익사 다음으로 다이버의 주요 사망 원인이며 사망의 약 30%를 차지한다. 동맥기체색전증(AGE)은 앞서 언급한 네 가지 폐 과도팽창증후군 증상과 연관되어 발생하거나 공기가 빠져나와 공기색전증을 일으켜 단독으로 발생할 수 있다. 동맥기체색전증은 일반적으로 적절하게 숨을 내쉬지 않고 수면으로 상승하는 다이버에게서 발생하며 과잉 확장 폐 손상을 일으킨다. 그러나 기저 폐 질환 없이 천천히 수면 위로 올라온 다이버에게도 동맥기체색전증이 발생할 수 있다. 수면으로 상승하는 동안 폐 과잉 확장으로 폐포가 파열되면 공기가 폐정맥 모세혈관 순환으로 들어가고 기포는 좌심방과 좌심실로 들어간 다음 대동맥을 통해 심장을 빠져나와 대뇌, 관상동맥 및 기타 순환계로 분포된다. 기포가 관상동맥으로 들어가 폐색을 일으켜 부정맥, 심정지 또는 심근경색을 일으킬 수 있다. 기포가 뇌 순환계로 들어가면 다이버는 급성 뇌졸중과 유사한 증상과 징후를 보인다.

다이빙 후 몇 시간 후에 증상이 나타나는 감압병과 달리 동맥기체색전증의 증상은 수면에서 직시 나타나거나 일반적으로 10~15분 이내에 나타난다. 다이버가 수면으로 위로 떠오른 후 의식을 잃는다면 달리 증명될 때까지 동맥기체색전증으로 추정해야 한다. 동맥기체색전증에 대한 일차 처치는 재가압 챔버(고압산소) 요법이다.

과거에는 이 자세가 전신 혈관에서 기포가 순환하는 것을 방지하는 데 도움이 될 것이라는 믿음에 따라 동맥기체색전증 환자를 트렌델렌버그 자세로 이송할 것을 권장했다. 그러나 고개를 숙인 자세는 질소 기포의 전신 순환을 막지 못하고 환자에게 산소 공급을 더 어렵게 만들며 뇌부종을 악화시킬 수 있다는 증거가 있다. 현재 모든 동맥기체색전증 환자는 현장 및 이송 중에 바로누운자세를 취하는 것이 좋다. 비재호흡마스크로 고유량 100% 산소를 공급하면서 바로누운자세로 이송하면 다른 유익한 효과 외에도 질소 기포를 제거할 수 있다.

감압병

감압병(DCS)은 헨리의 법칙과 직접적인 관련이 있다. 스쿠버 다이버

가 산소(21%)와 질소(79%)가 포함된 압축 공기로 호흡할 때 액체에 용해되는 기체의 양은 액체와 접촉하는 기체의 부분압에 정비례한다. 산소는 용액 상태일 때 체내에서 조직 대사를 위해 사용되며 수심에서 상승하는 동안 기포를 형성하지 않는다.

다이버가 헬리옥스 탱크를 사용하는 경우 헬륨도 문제가 될 수 있지만, 신진대사에 사용되지 않는 불활성 가스인 질소가 감압병에서 가장 우려되는 주요 원인이다. 질소는 물보다 지방에 5배 더 잘 녹으며 주변 압력의 증가에 비례하여 조직에 용해된다. 따라서 다이버가 더 깊은 수중으로 들어가고 수심에 오래 머무를수록 조직에 용해되는 질소의 양은 더 많아진다. 다이버가 수면으로 상승할 때 흡수된 질소는 반드시 제거되어야 한다. 상승하는 동안 질소를 제거할 시간이 충분하지 않으면 질소가 혈관 내 기포의 형태로 조직의 용액에서 빠져나와 혈관 및 림프계를 폐쇄하고 조직 팽창을 유발하며 염증반응을 활성화한다.

대부분 다이버는 수면 위로 올라온 후 1시간 이내에 감압병을 경험하지만, 일부는 수면 위로 올라온 후 6~24시간까지 증상이 나타나기도 한다. 일반적으로 감압병의 증상은 피부, 림프계 및 근골격계와 관련된 경미한 형태인 제I형 또는 신경계 및 심폐계와 관련된 심각한 형태인 제II형으로 분류된다(**Box 20-7**). 감압병의 경미한 증상으로는 피로와 권태감이 있다. 그러나 경미한 증상은 무감각, 쇠약, 마비 등 더 심각한 증상과 징후의 전조 증상일 수 있다.

현재 연구에 따르면 임상적으로 감압병을 I형 또는 II형이 아닌 영향을 받은 신체 부위와 그 진행에 따라 설명하는 것이 더 중요하다. 이 제안은 경미한 감압병의 증상이 있는 환자라도 100% 산소를 제공하고 재가압 요법을 시행하기 위해 병원 전 처치 제공자는 조기에 환자를 신속하게 의료기관으로 이송한다. 경미한 형태의 감압병이 발생한 일부 다이버들은 의료 지원을 요청하지 않을 것이다. 다른 다이버들은 스쿠버 다이빙을 즐기는 사람들에서 감압병에 진료를 거부하는 것이 일반적이기 때문에 처치를 받는 것을 상당히 지연시킬 수 있다.

여러 가지 요인으로 인해 다이버가 감압병에 걸리기 쉽다. 일부 위험 요소는 하강 시 조직의 질소 흡수를 촉진하고 상승 시 질소 방출을 늦추는 것으로 알려져 있다. 특정 숙주 및 환경 요인, 부적절한 감압 및 공격적인 다이빙 관행은 감압병의 위험을 증가시킨다.

팔다리 통증(제I형 감압병)

이 형태의 감압병은 근골격계의 기포 형성으로 인해 발생하며 일반적으로 하나 이상의 관절에서 발생한다. 가장 흔하게 발생하는 관절은 어깨와 팔꿈치이며 무릎, 엉덩이 관절, 손목, 손, 발목 등이 그 뒤를 잇는다. 이 통증은 관절을 움직일 때 삐걱거리는 느낌을 동반하는 심한 힘줄염(관절 통증)으로 설명된다. 통증은 서서히 시작되어 경증에서 중증 강도의 깊고 둔한 통증으로 나타난다. 통증만 있는 형태의 감압병은 생명을 위협하지는 않지만, 더 심각한 형태의 감압병을 배제하기 위해 신경학적 평가와 시기적절한 치료가 필요하다.

피부 및 림프계(제I형 감압병)

피부 감압병은 흔하며 피부나 림프계에 영향을 미친다. 피부 굴곡은 일반적으로 심각한 증상이 아니며 경미한 감압병으로 분류되지만, 때때로 신경학적 증상과 연관될 수 있다. 때에 따라서는 다이빙 후 몇 분 후에 반점형성과 대리석 무늬가 생기는 징후는 심각한 감압병의 전조로 간주할 수 있다. 증상으로는 몸통과 팔다리 근위부 피부의 붉은 반점이나 푸르스름한 변색으로 진행되는 강렬한 발진이 있다. 림프관이 폐쇄되면 부기와 오렌지 껍질 모양을 유발할 수 있다. 모세혈관 누출 및 혈량저하 증후군과 관련될 수 있다. 활력징후, 신경학적 검사, 피부 변화를 사진으로 찍는다.

심폐(제II형 감압병)

이 심각한 유형의 감압병은 질식이라고 하며 정맥 기포가 폐 모세혈관 시스템을 압도할 때 발생한다. 저혈압은 폐에 대량의 정맥 공기색전증으로 인해 발생할 수 있다. 증상으로는 가래 없는 기침, 복장뼈 아래 가슴 통증, 청색증, 호흡곤란, 쇼크, 심폐정지 등이 있다. 이 질환은 급성 호흡곤란 증후군(ARDS)과 유사하다(자세한 내용은 7장 기도와 환기 참조).

척수(제II형 감압병)

척수의 백질은 기포 형성에 취약하며 질소는 척수 조직(수초)에 잘 용해된다. 이러한 유형의 감압병이 가장 흔하게 발생하는 부위는 하부 등뼈이고 허리뼈/엉치뼈 및 목뼈 부위가 그 뒤를 잇는다. 일반적인 증상과 징후로는 요통과 다리의 "무거움"이 이다. 이러한 유형의 감압병의 경우 환자는 종종 "이상한 감각" 또는 감각 이상을 설명하기

Box 20-7 감압병

감압병(DCI)이라는 용어는 제I형 및 제II형 감압병과 동맥기체색전증을 포함하기 위해 제안되었다.

위해 모호한 표현을 사용하며 이는 쇠약, 무감각 및 마비로 진행될 수 있다. 장 및 방광 기능 장애로 인한 요저류도 보고되었다.

동맥기체색전증과 감압병 평가

동맥기체색전증과 감압병 환자에 대한 표준화된 접근 방식이 제공되어 일관된 처치가 제공될 수 있도록 한다. 스쿠버 다이빙과 관련된 손상을 입은 모든 환자는 일차적이고 필수적인 처치는 재가압 요법이며 이를 위해서는 구체적인 계획과 물류가 필요하므로 동맥기체색전증 및 감압병의 증상과 징후가 있는지 검사할 것을 권장한다.

동맥기체색전증

모든 동맥기체색전증 환자의 약 5%에서 즉각적인 무호흡, 무의식 및 심정지 증상을 보인다. 다른 환자들은 의식상실, 무감각, 혼란, 반신불안전마비, 발작, 현기증, 시각 변화, 감각 변화, 두통 등을 동반한 급성 뇌졸중과 유사한 증상과 징후를 보인다.

감압병

제I형 감압병은 경미한 형태의 피부 가려움(심한 가려움)과 림프관 폐쇄(림프부종)를 포함한 관절의 심부 통증이 특징이다. 제II형 감압병은 쇠약 및 무감각에서 마비에 이르는 중추신경계와 관련된 증상이 특징이다.

　동료 다이버로부터 다이빙 관련 손상을 입게 된 사건에 관해 다음을 포함하여 다이빙 프로필과 병력을 확보한다.

- 증상 및 징후 시작 시간
- 호흡한 공기의 종류(예: 공기 또는 혼합 가스, 헬리옥스)
- 다이빙 프로필(다이빙 활동, 수심, 지속 시간, 다이빙 빈도, 수면 간격, 다이빙한 간격)
- 다이빙 장소 및 수질 조건
- 다이빙 위험 요인
- 상승 및 하강 시 수중 의료 및 장비 문제
- 다이버가 무감압 다이빙을 시도했는지 또는 감압 다이빙을 시도했는지 여부
- 상승 속도
- 감압 정지
- 다이빙 후 활동 수준
- 다이빙 후 항공기 여행 또는 고도 노출(유형 및 기간 포함)
- 과거 및 현재 병력(특히 이전 감압병 병력)

- 복용 중인 약물
- 현재 알코올이나 불법 약물 사용

처치

환자의 기도, 호흡, 순환을 평가하고 기도를 유지하며 필요에 따라서 BLS 또는 ALS 절차를 시작한다. 100% 산소를 분당 12~15L로 공급하고 생리식염수 또는 락테이터링거액(포도당 포함되지 않음)을 정맥 내로 투여(시간당 1~2mL/kg)한다. 환자의 활력징후, 산소포화도 및 심전도를 모니터링한다. 필요에 따라서 환자의 혈당 수치를 확인하고 처치하며 발작을 조절한다. 환자를 저체온증으로부터 보호하고 재가압 챔버가 있는 가장 가까운 의료기관이나 다이버 경고 네트워크에 문의한다. 다이버를 치료할 의사가 있는 재가압 챔버는 드물다(예: 플로리다주 전체에 4개). 즉 가장 가까운 적절한 시설로 신속하게 이송하기 위해서는 사고 발생 전 구체적인 계획이 필요하다. 다이버 경보 네트워크 연락처 정보는 **Box 20-8**을 참조한다. 미 해군 치료 표에 따라 100% 고압 산소를 사용한 재가압 요법이 제공된다. 환자를 바로누운자세로 이송한다. 스쿠버 다이빙 관련 손상의 경우 헬기나 기타 기압 유지 장치가 없는 항공기로 이송하는 경우 기포의 추가 팽창(보일의 법칙)과 감압 손상의 악화를 최소화하기 위해 가능한 한 안전하게 낮은 고도(예: 150 m)로 비행하며 300m를 넘지 않도록 하는 것이 좋다.

　동맥기체색전증 또는 감압병에 대한 결정적인 처치는 표준 프로토콜에 따라 재가압 챔버에서 대기압의 2~3에서 100% 산소를 투여하는 것이다. 스쿠버 관련 다이빙 손상에 대한 재가압 챔버 치료 방법에 대한 자세한 논의는 미 해군 다이빙 매뉴얼 또는 기타 출처를 참조한다. 보일의 법칙 원리에 따라 주변 압력을 높이고 형성되는 기포의 크기를 줄이며 조직의 산소 농도를 증가시킴으로써 환자는 즉각적인 효과를 얻을 수 있다. **Box 20-9**는 재가압 및 고압 산소요법의 이점에 관해 설명한 것이다.

　병원 전 이송 팀의 경우 환자를 수용할 수 있는 응급실 또는 기타 시설에서 동맥기체색전증과 감압병과 같은 다이빙 관련 상태가 진정한 응급 상황임을 인식하고 신경학적 검사를 포함한 자세한 검사를 신속하게 시행할 수 있도록 해야 한다는 사실을 인지하도록 하는 것이 중요하다. 팀 간의 의사소통 및 이러한 종류의 핸드오프를 최적화하는 기술을 설명하는 추가 읽기 자료가 있다. 환자 인계 절차에 대한 자세한 내용은 6장, 환자 평가 및 관리에서 확인할 수 있다.

표 20-3에는 압력 손상의 증상과 징후 및 그에 따른 처치법이 요약되어 있다. **표 20-4**에는 감압병의 증상과 징후 및 그에 따른 처치법이 요약되어 있다.

스쿠버 다이빙과 관련 손상 예방

공인 스쿠버 다이버는 스쿠버 다이빙 관련 손상을 예방하고 인식하기 위해 자주 보수교육을 받아야 한다. 인명구조요원, 소방관과 경찰관, 수색 및 구조대원, 해양경찰, 국방부 관련 직원 등 미국의 많은 스쿠버 전문가는 의료기관이나 재가압 챔버가 있는 기관으로 이송하기 위해 병원 전 처치 제공자에 의존하고 있다. 다이빙 훈련 중 의료 시나리오를 개발하기 위해 다이빙 팀과 지역 EMS 기관 간의 협력을 적극 권장한다. 여기에는 수중 수영자/다이버 구조 및 회복을 위해 안전하고 효과적으로 대응하는 데 가장 중요한 수중 구조 시나리오 및 초기 처치와 함께 다양한 수중 조건과 장소에서 빈번한 스쿠버 훈련이 포함되어야 한다. 의료 다이버 팀원들과 현지 병원 전 제공자 간의 스쿠버 훈련 조정은 효과적인 의사소통과 적절한 현장 처치의 연속성을 보장한다. 이 교육에는 지역 의료 통제 및 다이버 경고 네트워크와의 시나리오를 기반으로 하는 협의가 포함되어야 한다.

다이빙을 위한 건강 검진

병원 전 처치 제공자는 다이빙 적합성을 인증하지 않지만, 의사가 다이빙 적합성을 판단할 때 사용하는 요소를 알고 있어야 한다. 또한 다이빙 관련 사고에 대응하는 병원 전 처치 제공자는 모든 연령대의 다이버를 대상으로 잠수 사고와 관련된 주요 다이빙 장애(예: 감압병, 동맥기체색전증)뿐만 아니라 기저 질환(예: 심장질환, 폐 질환, 신경계 질환, 내분비계 질환, 정신과 질환 또는 의학적 장애와 압력 손상이 모두 있는 경우)에 대해서도 평가해야 한다. 모든 신규 다이버는 스쿠버 훈련을 시작하기 전에 의사의 진찰을 받는 것이 이상적이지만, 종 진찰받지 않는 경우가 있다. 다이빙 관련 문제가 발생할 위험이 높은 개인을 식별하기 위한 5가지 일반적인 건강 검진 권장 사항은 아래와 같다. 이러한 권장 사항은 의료 다이빙 전문가들의 합의를 기반

표 20-3　기압손상의 일반적인 증상 및 징후와 처치

유형	징후/증상	긴급	처치*
마스크 압축	각막 충혈, 결막출혈	비응급	자체 제한: 휴식, 냉찜질, 진통제
부비동 압착	통증, 혈액이 섞인 콧물 희귀한 후안와 폐기종 또는 기종	응급처치, 간단한 평가	진통제, 충혈제거제, 항히스타민제
중이 압착	통증, 현기증, 고막 파열, 청력 소실, 구토	응급처치, 간단한 평가	충혈제거제, 항히스타민제, 진통제, 항생제가 필요할 수 있으며 다이빙과 비행을 피함
내이 압력 손상	이명, 현기증, 실조, 난청	긴급	휴식, 머리를 올려줌, 소음을 피함, 대변 연화제, 격렬한 활동 피함, 몇 달 동안 다이빙 또는 비행 금지
외이 압력 손상	발살바 조작의 어려움, 귀통증, 피가 섞인 분비물, 고막 파열 가능성	응급처치, 간단한 평가	이관을 건조하게 유지, 감염에 필요한 경우 항생제 투여
치아 압착	다이빙 중 치아 통증	응급처치, 간단한 평가	자가 제한적, 진통제
기압변화성 현기증	압박감, 영향을 받은 귀의 통증, 현기증, 이명	응급처치, 간단한 평가	단기간, 충혈제거제, 정상 청력으로 회복될 때까지 다이빙 금지
폐 압력 손상	복장밑 통증, 목소리 변화, 호흡곤란, 피부밑기종	긴급	ABC 평가, 신경학적 기능 평가, 비재호흡마스크로 100% 산소를 분당 12~15L로 공급, 바로누운자세로 환자 이송, 동맥기체색전증을 배제하기 위한 검사
피부밑기종	빗장뼈 통증 및 비빔소리, 쉰 목소리, 목 부종, 호흡곤란, 혈성 가래	긴급	휴식, 다이빙과 비행 피하고 심한 경우 산소 공급 및 재가압 요법 시행
기흉	날카로운 가슴 통증, 호흡곤란, 호흡음 감소	응급	비재호흡마스크로 100% 산소를 분당 12~15L로 공급, 맥박산소측정기 모니터링, 편안한 자세로 환자 이송, 긴장기흉에 대한 평가
긴장기흉	청색증, 목정맥 팽창, 기관편위	응급	14 게이지 주삿바늘로 가슴막천자, 비재호흡마스크로 100% 산소를 분당 12~15L로 공급, 맥박산소측정기 모니터링
동맥기체색전증	무반응, 혼란, 두통, 시력장애, 발작	응급	ABC 평가, 신경학적 기능 평가, BLS 및 ALS 조기 시행, 발작 조절, 비재호흡마스크로 100% 산소를 분당 12~15L로 공급, 바로누운자세로 환자 이송, 정맥 내로 당분이 없는 수액 투여(1~2mL/kg/hr), 심전도 모니터링, 가장 가까운 재가압 챔버 설치 기관 확인

*경미한 기압손상은 자가 처치가 가능한 손상도 있고 의사의 평가가 필요한 손상도 있으며 주치의나 응급실에서 처치를 받아야 하는 손상도 있고 EMS 이송이 필요하지 않은 손상도 있으므로 현장에서 환자를 교육하는 것이 중요하다.

Abbreviations: ABCs, airway, breathing, circulation; AGE, arterial gas embolism; ALS, advanced life support; BLS, basic life support; DAN, Divers Alert Network; ECG, electrocardiogram.

Data from Clenney TL, Lassen LF: Recreational scuba diving injuries. *Am Fam Physician*. 1996;53(5):1761-1764; Salahuddin M, James LA, Bass ES. SCUBA medicine: A first-responder's guide to diving injuries. *Curr Sports Med Rep*. 2011;10(3):134-139; and Van Hoesen KB, Bird NH. Diving medicine. In: Auerbach PS, ed. *Wilderness Medicine*, 6th ed. Mosby Elsevier; 2012.

표 20-4 감압병의 일반적인 증상 및 증후와 처치

조건(상태)	징후/증상	처치
제 I 형 감압병		
피부 감압병	심한 가려움증, 어깨와 가슴 윗부분에 붉은 발진, 어깨와 몸통의 작열감과 및 가려움증이 먼저 나타날 수 있음, 국소적 청색증과 오목 부종	자가 제한적이며 저절로 해결됨, 감압병의 지연성 팔다리 통증 징후를 관찰, 신경학적 기능 평가 필수
감압병의 팔다리 통증	큰 관절 압통, 경증에서 중증의 관절이나 팔다리 통증, 통증은 일반적으로 환자의 75%에서 나타나고 욱신거림, 관절 운동 시 삐걱거리는 느낌, 움직임에 따라 악화, 제I형 감압병이 제 II 형 감압병으로 진행될 수 있음	경미한 통증만 있는 경우 저절로 호전되는 경우가 많으며 24시간 관찰, 중등도에서 중증의 통증이 있는 경우 비재호흡마스크로 100% 산소를 분당 12~15L로 공급하고 바로누운자세로 환자를 이송하며 정맥 내로 당분이 없는 수액을 1~2mL/kg/hr로 투여하고 가장 가까운 재가압 챔버가 설치되어 있는 기관 확인한다.
제 II 형 감압병		
심폐 질식	복장밑 통증, 경증의 기침, 호흡곤란, 효과 없는 기침, 청색증, 빠른호흡, 빈맥, 쇼크 및 심정지	ABCs, 비재호흡마스크로 100% 산소를 분당 12~15L로 공급, 필요한 경우 BLS 및 ALS 조기 시행, 정맥 내로 당분이 없는 수액을 1~2mL/kg/hr로 투여, 바로누운자세로 이송, 가장 가까운 재가압 챔버가 설치되어 있는 기관 확인한다.
신경계		
뇌	다양한 시각 변화, 두통, 혼란, 지남력 장애, 구역 및 구토	
척수	요통, 압박감, 쇠약, 무감각, 마비, 소변 정체, 변실금	
내이	현기증, 실조	

Abbreviations: ABCs, airway, breathing, circulation; ALS, advanced life support; BLS, basic life support; DAN, Divers Alert Network; DCS, decompression sickness; IV, intravenous.

Modified from Barratt DM, Harch PG, Van Meter K. Decompression illness in divers: A review of the literature. *Neurologist*. 2002;8:186-202; and Van Hoesen KB, Bird NH: Diving medicine. In: Auerbach PS, ed. *Wilderness Medicine*. 6th ed. Mosby/Elsevier; 2012.

으로 한다. 권당 사상은 다음과 같다.

- 신체 중 공기가 들어 있는 공간 중 하나 이상의 압력이 균일하지 않으면 압력 손상의 위험이 높아진다.
- 의학적 또는 정신적 상태는 수중이나 멀리 떨어진 다이빙 장소에서 나타날 수 있으며 상태 자체가 수중에서 발생하거나 적절한 의료 도움을 받을 수 없으므로 다이버의 생명을 위험에 빠뜨릴 수 있다.
- 조직 관류 장애 또는 불활성 기체의 확산은 감압병의 위험을 증가시킨다.
- 컨디션이 좋지 않으면 감압병이나 운동 관련 의학적 문제가 발생할 위험이 높아진다. 신체 컨디션을 저하하는 요인은 생리학적 또는 약리학적일 수 있다.
- 임신 중인 여성의 경우 태아의 압력 손상 위험이 높아질 수 있다.

수년 동안 당뇨병 환자들은 혈당 수치를 조절하고 있는 개인이 스쿠버 다이빙을 금기해야 하는가에 대해 다이빙 의학 전문가에게 질문해 왔다. 2005년 6월에 미국에서 해저고압의학회(UHMS)와 다이버 경고 네트워크가 공동으로 후원하는 국제 워크숍이 열렸다. 이 워크숍에서는 전 세계에서 50명이 넘는 의료 및 연구 전문가들이 모여 당뇨병을 앓고 있는 레크리에이션 다이버를 위한 지침을 개발했다. 이 패널은 당뇨병 치료를 위해 약물(경구 혈당강하제 또는 인슐린)을 사용하지만, 다른 방법으로 다이빙할 자격을 갖춘 다이버라면 여가생활을 위한 스쿠버 다이빙할 수 있다고 밝혔다. 그러나 그들은 다이빙하기 전에 엄격한 기준을 충족해야 한다고 말했다. 패널은 식이 조절을 하는 당뇨병 환자는 새로운 지침을 쉽게 충족할 수 있다는 데 동의했다. 합의된 지침(**Box 20-10**)은 다이빙 대상자 선정 및 감시, 다이빙 범위, 다이빙 당일 혈당 관리 등 19개 항목으로 구성되어 있다.

잠수 후 비행

다이빙은 미국 내 많은 유명한 다이빙 장소와 미국 외의 외딴 지역에서 이루어지기 때문에 비행 전날 다이빙을 할 수 있다. 보일의 법칙에

Box 20-10 당뇨병 환자의 레크리에이션 다이빙을 위한 지침

선택 및 감시

- 만 18세(특수 교육 프로그램 중 일부의 경우 16세 이상) 이상이어야 한다.
- 다음과 같은 약물 투여를 시작하거나 변경한 후에는 다이빙을 연기한다.
  - 경구 혈당강하제 복용 3개월 후
  - 인슐린 치료 시작 1년 후
- 최소 1년 이내에 제삼자의 처치가 필요한 저혈당 또는 고혈당 관련 사고가 없어야 한다.
- 저혈당으로 인한 의식소실 병력이 없어야 한다.
- 최초 평가 1개월 전과 매년 하는 검사에서 당화혈색소(HbA1c) 검사 결과가 9% 미만이어야 한다.
  - 9%를 초과하는 수치는 추가 평가 및 처치 방법 변경이 필요함을 나타낸다.
- 당뇨병으로 인한 심각한 이차 합병증이 없어야 한다.
- 내과 전문의/당뇨병 전문의가 매년 검토해야 하며 필요에 따라 다이빙 의학 전문가와 상의하여 다이버가 질병과 운동의 효과에 대해 잘 이해하고 있는지 확인해야 한다.
- 40세를 이상의 지원자는 무증상 심근허혈에 대해 평가를 실시해야 한다.
  - 초기 평가 후 당뇨병 환자의 평가에 대해 허용되는 지역/국가의 지침에 따라 주기적으로 무증상 심근허혈에 대한 감시를 실시할 수 있다.
- 지원자는 당뇨병이 있는 다이버를 위한 프로토콜을 따라 다이빙을 중단하고 당뇨병과 관련이 있을 수 있는 다이빙 중에 발생할 수 있는 부작용에 대해 의학적 검토를 하고 기록해야 한다.

다이빙 범위

- 다이빙은 다음을 피하도록 계획해야 한다.
  - 수심이 30m를 초과하는 바닷물

- 다이빙 지속시간이 60분을 초과하는 경우
- 강제 감압 중단
- 제한된 환경(예: 동굴, 난파선)
- 저혈당을 악화시킬 수 있는 상황(예: 장시간 춥고 힘든 잠수)
- 개인은 문제 발생 시 다이버 리더에게 알려야 한다.
  - 동료 다이버는 당뇨병이 없어야 한다.

다이빙 당일 혈당 관리

- 개인은 다이빙 적합성에 대한 일반적인 자체 평가를 해야 한다.
- 입수 전 혈당은 150mg/㎗ 이상으로 안정적이거나 상승해야 한다.
  - 최소 3회(60분 전, 30분 전, 다이빙 직전)의 혈당 검사를 시행하여 혈당 추이를 평가한다.
  - 다이빙 전날 저녁이나 당일에 경구 혈당강하제 또는 인슐린 용량을 변경하면 도움이 될 수 있다.
- 혈당이 다음과 같은 경우 다이빙을 연기한다.
  - 150mg/dL(8.3mmol/l) 미만인 경우
  - 300mg/dL(16.7mmol/l) 초과한 경우
- 구급 약물 고려 사항은 다음과 같다.
- 모든 다이빙 동안 쉽게 섭취할 수 있는 경구 포도당을 휴대한다.
  - 수면에서 비경구 글루카곤을 사용할 수 있도록 분비한다.
- 수중에서 저혈당이 발생하는 경우 다이버는 동료와 함께 수면으로 올라와서 부력을 확보하고 포도당을 섭취한 후 물 밖으로 나와야 한다.
- 다이빙 후 12~15시간 동안 혈당을 자주 확인한다.
- 다이빙 당일에는 충분한 수분을 섭취한다.
- 혈당 검사 결과 및 당뇨병 관리와 관련된 모든 정보를 포함하여 모든 다이빙을 기록한다.

의하면 다이빙 후 너무 빨리 비행하면 가압 또는 무가압 상용 항공기의 대기압 감소로 인해 비행 중 또는 목적지에 도착한 후 감압병의 위험이 높아질 수 있다. **Box 20-11**에는 다이빙 후 안전한 비행을 위해 다이버 경고 네트워크에서 권장하는 현재 지침이 나와 있다.

고소병

미국에서는 매년 4천만 명 이상의 사람들이 스노보드, 알파인 스키, 하이킹, 캠핑, 등산, 작업 등을 포함한 활동에 참여하기 위해 적응 없이 2,500m 이상의 고도를 여행한다. 따라서 많은 사람이 고지대에 도착한 후 몇 시간에서 며칠 이내에 발병할 수 있는 고산 관련 질환의 위험에 노출되어 있다. 병원 전 처치 제공자와 응급의학 전문의는 고지대 질환의 이환율과 사망률을 줄이기 위해 발병 요인, 증상 및 징후, 의학적 처치 방법, 교육 및 예방법을 숙지하고 있어야 한다.

Box 20-11 다이빙 후 안전한 비행을 위해 다이버 경보 네트워크에서 권장하는 현재 지침

다음 지침은 2002년 다이빙 후 비행을 위한 워크숍에 참석한 회원들의 합의에 따른 것이다. 이 지침은 감압병 증상이 없는 다이버가 다이빙한 후 610~2,440m의 기내 고도에서 비행할 때 적용된다. 권장되는 비행 전 휴식 시간은 감압병 예방을 보장하지 않는다. 휴식 시간을 더 길게 하면 감압병 발생 위험을 더 줄일 수 있다.

- 무감압 1회 다이빙의 경우 최소 12시간의 비행 전 휴식을 권장한다.
- 하루에 여러 번 또는 여러 날 다이빙을 한 경우 최소 18시간의 비행 전 휴식을 권장한다.

감압이 필요한 다이빙의 경우 권장 사항의 근거가 되는 증거가 거의 없으며 18시간보다 훨씬 긴 비행 전 휴식을 하는 것이 현명한 것으로 보인다.

이 부문에서는 고지대 환경으로 인해 직접적으로 발생하는 세 가지 의학적 질환을 소개하고 고지대 유발 저산소증(고도로 인해 악화

하는 기존 의학적 질환)으로 인해 악화하는 특정 기저 질환을 강조한다.

역학

고소병은 뇌 및 폐 증후군을 포괄하는 용어로 1) 급성 고산병(AMS), 2) 고지성 뇌부종(HACE), 고지성 폐부종(HAPE)이 있다. 급성 고산병과 고지성 뇌부종은 경증과 중증으로 나뉘지만, 고지성 폐부종은 별도의 과정을 거친다. 고소병에 걸릴 위험은 낮지만, 일단 발병하면 치명적일 수 있다.

급성 고산병은 경미한 형태의 고소병으로 2,000m 이하의 고도에서는 거의 발생하지 않지만, 고도가 2,060~2,440m로 높아지면 발생률은 1.4~25%까지 증가한다. 급성 고산병은 2,500m 이상에서는 20~25% 발생하고 4,270m 이상에서는 40~50% 발병한다. 이 급성 고산병의 발병률은 몇 시간에 4,270m까지 등반했을 때 발병률은 90% 이상이다. 또한, 일부 급성 고산병 환자(5~10%)는 경미한 증상에서 심각한 형태의 급성 고산병인 고지성 뇌부종으로 진행되기도 한다.

고지성 뇌부종은 고소병의 심각한 신경학적 형태이다. 해발 2,500m 이상의 고도에서는 일반 인구의 발병률(0.01%)이 낮지만, 신체 활동이 많은 사람에게서는 발병률이 1~2%까지 증가하고 급격한 상승이 이루어지는 해발 4,000m 이상에서는 발병률이 훨씬 더 높다.

고지성 폐부종은 일반적으로 특정 고산 작업 외에는 드물지만, 고산병으로 인한 사망의 대부분을 차지하며 조기에 발견하고 적절하게 처치하면 쉽게 회복할 수 있다. 고지성 폐부종은 일반적으로 고지대에 도착한 후 2~5일 이내에 나타난다. 해발 2,500m에서 일반 인구의 고지성 폐부종의 발생률은 0.01~0.1%이며 해발 4,000m의 등반가에게서는 2% 이상으로 증가한다.

저압 저산소증

고도는 세 가지 수준으로 정의된다. 고산병이 다른 지역보다 더 자주 보고되고 스키장이 유럽 알프스 같은 지역보다 일반적으로 높은 미국 동부 산댁에서 흔히 발생하는 높은 고도는 1,500~3,500m의 높이로 정의된다. 매우 높은 고도는 3,500~5,500m로 정의되며 심각한 형태의 고소병이 가장 흔하게 발생하는 고도이다. 극한 고도는 5,500m 이상의 고도로 정의되며 고도가 점진적으로 증가함에 따라 산소 가용성 감소어 적응하지 못한 사람에게는 환경이 매우 적대적으로 변하여 저압 저산소증이라는 질환이 발생할 수 있다. 그러나 저압 저산소증은 모든 고도에서 서로 다른 정도로 발생한다.

높은 고도는 호흡에 필요한 산소의 가용성이 감소하여 세포 저산소증을 유발하기 때문에 독특한 환경이다. 산소 농도는 모든 고도에서 21%로 유지되더라도 고도가 높을수록 대기압이 낮아져 산소분압(PO_2)이 감소한다. 예를 들어, 해수면(1기압)에서는 산소분압이 160mmHg이고 해발 5,500m(0.5 기압)에서 80mmHg이므로 호흡 시 사용할 수 있는 산소의 양이 줄어든다. **표 20-5**는 해수면에서 극한 고도로 고도가 높아질수록 기압, 동맥혈가스 및 동맥혈산소포화도

표 20-5 고도, 기압, 동맥혈 가스 및 산소포화도의 관계*				
고도(m)	기압(mmHg)	동맥혈산소분압 [PaO_2 (mmHg)]	산소포화도 [SaO_2 (%)]	동맥혈이산화탄소분압 [$PaCO_2$ (mmHg)]
해수면	760	100	98.0	40.0
1,646	630	73.0	95.1	35.6
2,810	543	60.0	91.0	33.9
3,660	489	47.6	84.5	29.5
4,700	429	44.6	78.0	27.1
5,340	401	43.1	76.2	25.7
6,140	356	35.0	65.6	22.0

*데이터는 20~40세 피험자의 평균값

Note: $PaCO_2$, arterial carbon dioxide partial pressure; PaO_2, arterial oxygen partial pressure; SaO_2, arterial oxygen saturation.

Modified from Hackett PH, Roach RC. High-altitude medicine. In: Auerbach PS, ed. *Wilderness Medicine*. 6th ed. Mosby/Elsevier; 2012.

(SaO_2)가 비례적으로 감소하는 것을 보여준다. 해발 2,800m 이상의 고도에 도달할 때까지 건강한 성인의 경우 평균적으로 산소포화도가 91% 이상을 유지한다는 사실에 주목할 필요가 있다.

고도 상승과 진행성 저산소증 사이의 이러한 관계는 환기 속도와 심박출량의 급성 생리학적 조절 및 생화학적인 변화의 기초를 형성한다. 결과적으로 고소병에 적응하지 못한 사람이 고소병에 걸리게 되는 것은 저압 저산소증과 저산소혈증이다.

고소병과 관련된 요인

고소병의 발병은 각 고산지대 노출에 따른 여러 요인에 따라 달라지지만, 주요 요인으로는 빠른 상승, 개인별 적응 속도, 고지에서의 신체 활동, 어린 나이, 이전 고소병 병력 등이 있다. 추가 요인으로는 다음과 같은 애용이 포함된다.

- 고도 및 상승 속도 증가: 고소병의 발생률과 중증도는 주로 상승 속도, 도달한 고도, 체류 시간(짧은 기간, 일정 시간이 지난 후 고도에 머무르는 시간이 길수록 위험도가 낮아짐)과 관련이 있는데 이는 이 세 가지 요인이 신체의 저산소성 스트레스를 증가시키기 때문이다.
- 고소병의 과거력: 고소병 과거력은 같은 고도에서 같은 속도로 등반할 때 고소병에 걸리기 쉬운 사람을 예측할 수 있는 중요한 지표이다. 고지성 폐부종(HAPE)의 병력이 있는 사람이 갑자기 4,560m로 올라갈 때 고지성 폐부종 발생률은 10%에서 60%까지 증가한다.
- 사전 적응: 해발 900m 이상의 고산지대에 거주하면 어느 정도 사전 적응이 가능하며 더 높은 고도로 올라갈 때 고소병의 발생률과 중증도가 낮아지는 것과 관련이 있다. 그러나 상승 속도가 빠르거나 극단적인 고도에 도달하는 경우 이러한 보호 기능은 제한적이다.
- 나이: 나이는 급성 고산병(AMS)에 영향을 미치는 요인으로 50세 이상에서는 발병률이 낮다. 고지성 폐부종은 어린이와 젊은 성인에서 더 자주 더 심각하게 발생하며 이 연령대에서는 남성과 여성은 같은 비율로 보고된다.
- 체력 및 운동: 고소병의 발병과 중증도는 체력과 무관하며 체력이 고도 적응을 가속하지 않는다. 체력이 높으면 개인이 더 많이 운동할 수 있지만, 고지대에 도착한 후 격렬한 운동은 저산소혈증을 더욱 악화시키고 고소병의 발병을 앞당긴다.
- 약물 및 중독 물질: 고지대에서 환기를 저하하고 수면 패턴을 방해하는 모든 물질은 고산증으로 인한 저산소혈증을 더욱 악화시킬 수 있으므로 피해야 한다. 이러한 물질에는 알코올, 바비투르산염 및 오피오이드가 포함된다.
- 추위: 추위는 폐동맥압을 높이기 때문에 차가운 주변 온도에 노출되면 고지성 폐부종의 위험이 높아진다.

기존 질환은 고소병과 관련된 또 다른 요인이다. 급성 고산병 및 고지성 폐부종에 효과적인 약물 용량을 결정하기 위한 임상 연구에는 일반적으로 기저 질환이 없는 건강한 사람만 참여한다는 점에 유의해야 한다. 그러나 오늘날 더 많은 고지대 여행객과 고지대로 거주지를 옮기는 사람들은 당뇨병, 고혈압, 심장병 또는 우울증과 같은 기저 질환을 앓고 있다. 고소병 처치를 위한 현재의 약물 권장 사항은 약물 상호작용의 가능성으로 인해 이러한 환자 및 신장 또는 간 기능부전 환자에게는 적절하지 않을 수 있다. 이러한 문제에 대한 논의는 건강한 사람을 위한 고소병(급성 고산병, 고지성 폐부종, 고지성 뇌부종) 예방 및 치료 약물과 기저 질환이 있는 환자를 위한 약물 선택 및 투약에 대한 검토 문서를 확인할 수 있다.

표 20-6에는 고소병 발병 우려를 높이는 질환이 나열되어 있다. 또한 고소병에 대한 취약성을 높이는 것으로 알려진 특정 의학적 질환은 다음과 같다.

- 심폐 선천성 이상: 폐동맥 결손, 원발성 폐고혈압, 선천성 심장 결함
- 목동맥 수술: 목동맥에 방사선 조사 또는 제거 수술

급성 고산병(AMS)

급성 고산병은 인플루엔자, 숙취, 탈진, 탈수 등의 일반적인 증상으로 인해 다른 여러 질환으로 쉽게 오인될 수 있는 자가 제한적이고 비특이적인 복합 증상이다. 최근 위원회에서 합의된 내용은 2,500m 이상의 고도에 도착한 적응되지 않은 사람이 한 가지 이상의 급성 고산병 증상을 보이는 경우 두통이 있는 것으로 급성 고산병을 정의했다. 그러나 급성 고산병은 2,000m의 낮은 고도에서도 발생할 수 있다. 고지성 뇌부종은 급성 고산병의 심각한 형태로 간주한다. 대부분의 급성 고산병 사례는 더 심각한 형태의 고소병으로 진행되지 않는다.

급성 고산병의 특징적인 증상은 저산소혈증에 의한 뇌혈관 확장으로 인해 발생하는 것으로 추정되는 경증에서 중증의 지속성 두통이다. 환자는 두통이 후두와 측두부에서 욱신거리고 밤이나 잠에서 깨어날 때 악화한다고 설명한다. 다른 증상으로는 구역, 구토, 불면증, 현기증, 무기력(피곤함), 피로, 수면 장애 등이 있다. 소변량 감소와 함께 불쾌감과 식욕부진이 나타날 수 있다. 예방 가능한 상태가 계속

표 20-6 고소병의 위험 범주	
위험 분류	설명
낮음	■ 고소병 병력이 없거나 2,800m 미만으로 등반한 경우 ■ 2,500~3,000m에 도착하는 데 2일 이상 걸리며 이후 하루에 500m 미만으로 상승하는 사람
보통	■ 급성 고산병의 병력이 있고 하루 동안 2,500~2,800m까지 등반한 경우 ■ 급성 고산병의 병력이 없으나 하루 동안 2,800m를 이상 등반한 경우 ■ 3,000m 이상의 고도에서 하루에 500m 이상 등반한 모든 경우
높음	■ 급성 고산병의 병력이 있고 하루 동안 2,800m 이상 등반한 경우 ■ 고지성 뇌부종 또는 고지성 폐부종의 병력이 있는 모든 경우 ■ 하루 동안 3,500m 이상을 등반한 모든 경우 ■ 3,500m 이상의 고도에서 하루에 500m 이상 등반한 모든 경우 ■ 매우 빠르게 등반한 경우

Abbreviations: AMS, acute mountain sickness; HACE, high-altitude cerebral edema; HAPE, high-altitude pulmonary edema.

Modified from Luk AM, McIntosh SE, Grissom, et al. Wilderness Medical Society consensus guidelines for the prevention and treatment of acute altitude illness. *Wilderness Environ Med*. 2010;21:146-155.

상승하여 심각한 형태의 고소성 뇌부종으로 진행되지 않도록 급성 고산병의 초기 증상을 인식하는 것이 중요하다.

급성 고산병의 증상 시작은 높은 고도에 도착한 후 빠르면 1시간 이내에 발생할 수 있지만, 일반적으로 6~10시간 노출 후에 발생한다. 증상은 보통 24~72시간 이내에 최고조에 달했다가 3~7일 이내에 가라앉는다. 증상이 고지대에 도착한 후 3일이 지나서 시작되고 두통이 동반되지 않고 산소 요법이 도움이 되지 않는다면 급성 고산병이 아닐 가능성이 높다.

낙뢰 및 익사 처치와 마찬가지로 야생 의학회에는 합의에 따라 도출된 급성 고산병 관련 실무 지침이 있다. 이러한 지침은 온라인으로 제공되며 실무자가 증거 기반의 최신 모범 사례를 결정하는 데 도움이 된다.

평가

환자가 의식이 있는 경우 증상의 시작과 중증도, 상승 속도, 노출 기간, 탈수를 유발할 수 있는 약물 사용, 음주 및 신체 활동 수준 등 병력을 잘 파악하는 것이 중요하다. 산소포화도를 포함한 활력징후를 측정한다. 또한 병력에 따라 기저 질환의 상태를 평가한다.

두통은 급성 고산병에서 가장 흔한 증상이므로 두통의 발생 위치와 질을 평가한다. 주기적인 호흡곤란은 약 3,000m 이상 고도에 오른 사람에게서 흔히 발견되는 증상이다. 신경학적 기능을 평가하고 특히 운동실조와 과도한 무기력증이 있는지 평가한다(이러한 증상은 고지성 뇌부종을 시사).

처치

해발 500~1,000m로 하강하면 증상이 가장 빨리 회복된다. 경증의 급성 고산병은 대개 저절로 해결되지만, 환자는 증상이 해결될 때까지 추가 등반 및 모든 활동을 피해야 한다. 프로토콜에 따라 구역질이 심한 경우 항구토제와 두통이 심한 경우 진통제를 제공해야 한다. 중등도의 증상이 나타나는 경우 낮은 고도로 하산한다. 맥박산소측정기를 이용하여 산소포화도가 90% 이상인지 평가한다. 산소포화도가 90% 미만이면 분당 1~2L의 산소를 제공한 후 재평가한다. 그러나 이는 고도와 관련이 있으며 해발 4,300m에서 정상적인 동맥혈 산소포화도는 80%대 중반이다. 예기치 않게 낮은 산소포화도는 고지성 뇌부종을 나타낼 수 있지만, 일반적으로 산소포화도 수치는 급성 고산병 진단에 큰 도움이 되지 않는다. 신경학적 증상이 있는 환자의 경우 고지성 뇌부종 처치를 참조한다. 고소병으로 인해 악화하는 기저 질환이 있는 환자는 일차 질환에 대한 의학적 평가와 고소병의 이차적 발병에 대한 의학적 평가를 위해 산소를 공급하며 이송해야 한다.

고소병의 증상과 징후, 처치 및 예방에 대한 요약은 **표 20-7**을 참조한다. 소아 급성 고산병 환자에 대한 투약 권장량은 **표 20-8**을 참조한다.

고지성 뇌부종(HACE)

고지성 뇌부종은 심각한 신경학적 증후군으로 급성 고산병 또는 고지성 폐부종을 앓고 있거나 다른 고소병과 무관하게 단독으로 발생할 수 있다. 해발 2,440m 이상의 고도에서는 저산소증으로 인한 혈관 확장으로 인해 뇌 혈류가 증가한다. 손상 기전은 지속적인 뇌혈관 확장, 혈액-뇌 장벽을 통과하는 모세혈관 투과성 증가, 과도한 뇌부종을 충분히 보상하지 못하는 것과 관련이 있는 것으로 보인다.

고지성 뇌부종은 해발 2,750m에 도착한 후에 3~5일 이내에 언제든지 발생할 수 있지만, 가장 흔하게는 해발 3,600m 이상에서 발생하며 몇 시간 이내에 증상이 시작된다. 급성 고산병의 일부 증상도 나타날 수 있지만, 고지성 뇌부종의 특징은 졸음, 혼미, 혼수상태로 진행되는 의식 수준 변화와 운동실조이다. 사망은 뇌탈출로 인해 발생한다.

평가

핵심은 증상의 시작과 중등도, 상승 속도, 노출 기간, 신체 활동 수준 등 정확한 병력을 파악하는 것이다. 이러한 정보는 환자의 동반자에게 질문하여 얻을 수 있으며 환자의 의식이 명료한 경우 환자에게 질문하여 얻을 수 있다. 산소포화도를 포함한 환자의 활력징후를 측정한다. 또한, 환자의 병력에 따라 기저질환의 상태를 평가한다. 고지성 뇌부종과 고지성 폐부종 사이에는 밀접한 연관성이 있으므로 환자의 폐음과 신경학적 기능 수준을 평가하는 것이 도움이 될 수 있다. 두 질환이 함께 발견되는 경우가 많지만, 고지성 폐부종은 휴식 시 호흡곤란, 기침 및 낮은 산소포화도를 나타내지만, 고지성 폐부종은 일반적으로 수포음 없이 발생한다.

처치

고지성 뇌부종의 첫 번째 증상이나 징후가 나타나면 처치 및 대피 계획을 지연시키지 않는다. 고지성 뇌부종이 있는 모든 환자의 최우선 순위는 비재호흡마스크로 고유량 산소(분당 15L)를 공급하고 산소포화도가 90% 이상으로 유지하는 것이다. 의식이 없는 환자는 기관내 삽관 및 기타 ALS 절차를 포함하여 뇌손상 환자와 같이 처치해야 한다(7장 기도와 환기, 8장 머리와 목 외상 참조). 덱사메타손을 투여해야 하며 보충 산소가 없거나 부족한 경우 휴대용 고압 챔버를 사용할 수 있다.

고지성 뇌부종의 증상과 징후, 처치 및 예방에 관한 요약은 **표 20-7**을 참조한다. 소아 고지성 뇌부종 환자에 대한 투약 권장량은 **표 20-11**을 참조한다.

고지성 폐부종(HAPE)

고지성 폐부종의 발병은 급성 고산병 및 고지성 뇌부종과 유사한 패턴을 보이며 높은 고도로 급격히 상승한 후 적응하지 못한 사람에게서 발생한다. 그러나 고소병은 저압 저산소증에 의해 유발되기 때문에 급성 고산병 및 고소성 뇌부종과는 다른 손상 기전을 가지고 있다. 고지성 폐부종은 폐고혈압 및 모세혈관 압력 상승과 관련된 비심인성 폐부종의 한 형태이다. 고지성 폐부종 환자의 50% 이상은 급성 고산병을 앓고 있으며 14%는 고지성 뇌부종을 앓고 있다. 증상과 징후는 대부분 둘째 날 밤(1~3일 사이에서 발병) 다음 날 아침에 나타나며 특정 고도에 도착한 후 4일이 지나면 거의 발생하지 않는다. 고지성 폐부종의 발병과 진행 속도는 추위에 노출되거나 격렬한 활동 및 지속적인 등반으로 가속화된다. 다른 두 가지 고소병과 비교했을 때 고지성 폐부종은 가장 많은 사망자 수를 차지한다.

평가

활력징후, 호흡음 및 병력 등을 포함한 환자 평가는 두 가지 이상의 증상(예: 휴식 시 호흡곤란, 기침, 쇠약감 또는 운동 능력 저하, 가슴 조임, 울혈)과 최소 두 가지 징후(예: 수포음 또는 쌕쌕거림, 중심 청색증, 낮은 산소포화도, 빠른 호흡, 빈맥)으로 정의되는 고지성 폐부종을 판단하는 데 필수적인 요소이다. 수포음은 일반적으로 오른쪽 겨드랑이 부위에서 시작하여 양측 폐에서 나타난다. 미열은 고지성 폐부종에서 나타날 수 있지만, 고열은 폐렴과 같은 다른 질환을 암시할 수 있다. 고지성 폐부종이 진행되면서 늦게 발견되는 증상은 휴식 시 빈맥, 빠른 호흡, 피가 섞인 가래이다. 처치가 이루어지지 않으면 몇 시간에서 며칠에 걸쳐 증상이 진행되어 목을 울리는 소리, 호흡곤란 및 결국 사망에 이를 수 있다.

처치

최소 500m~1,000m 낮은 고도로 하강하거나 대피하는 것이 가장 빠른 회복을 가져오지만, 초기에는 휴식과 산소 공급 또는 고압산소 요법으로 호전될 수 있다. 환자의 체온을 유지하고 무리하지 않도록 한다. 이러한 환자는 동맥 산소화를 개선해야 하므로 산소 공급을 분당 4~6L로 시작하거나 산소포화도를 90% 이상이 될 때까지 산소 공급을 조절한다. 동맥 산소화가 개선되면 빈맥과 빠른 호흡이 감소하므로 산소 공급을 시작한 후 환자의 활력징후를 재평가한다. 고지성 폐부종은 비심인성 형태의 폐부종이기 때문에 이뇨제는 도움이 되지 않는 것으로 나타났다. 증례 보고에 따르면 심각한 고지성 폐부종의 경우 지속기도양압(CPAP)을 사용하면 좋은 결과를 얻을 수 있으

표 20-7 고소병(급성 고산병, 고지성 뇌부종, 고지성 폐부종)의 증상 및 징후와 처치 및 예방

증상/징후	처치	예방
급성 고산병(AMS)		
경증: 처음 12시간 동안 두통, 구역, 어지럼 및 피로	코삽입관으로 분당 1~2L 산소 공공 및 500~1,000m로 하강하고 증상이 해결될 때까지 추가 상승을 피하고 아세타졸아마이드(250mg PO bid)를 투여하여 적응 속도를 높이며 필요에 따라 진통제 및 항구토제 투여	• 느린 속도로 오르고 중간 고도에서 하룻밤을 보내며 무리하지 말고 3,000m 이상 직접 이동하지 않음 • 아세타졸아마이드 250mg 하루 2번 등반 전날부터 시작하여 최고 고도에서 2일간 지속 투여하는 것을 고려 • 조기 급성 고산병 처치로 합병증을 예방할 수 있음
중등도: 중등도에서 중증의 두통, 현저한 구역, 구토, 식욕 감소, 어지럼, 불면증, 12시간 이상의 체액 정체	하산, 덱사메타손*(6시간마다 4mg PO/IM) 및 아세타졸아마이드(250mg PO bid) 투여를 고려, 하산할 수 없는 경우 상태 악화 여주를 주의 깊게 관찰, 가능한 경우 몇 시간 동안 산소를 분당 1~2L로 제공, 휴대용 고압 요법(2~4psi) 시행	경증 질환에서 나열한 것과 동일, 덱사메타손 2mg을 6시간마다 또는 12시간마다 4mg을 경구 투여, 등반 시작일부터 복용하고 최대 고도에서 2일 후 신중하게 중단하는 것을 고려할 수 있지만, 고위험 등반이고 아세타졸아마이드가 금기인 경우에만 사용해야 한다.
고지성 뇌부종(HACE)		
24시간 이상 지속되는 급성 고산병, 운동 실조, 혼란, 기이한 행동, 심각한 피로 일반적으로 급성 고산병의 증상은 고지성 뇌부종에도 나타남	즉시 1,000m로 하강하거나 대피, 산소를 분당 2~4L로 공급, 산소포화도를 90% 이상으로 유지, 덱사메타손(초기 8mg을 PO/IV/IM으로 투여, 이후 6시간마다 4mg 투여), 하강할 수 없는 경우 휴대용 고압 요법 시행	급성 고산병과 같음
고지성 폐부종(HAPE)		
안정 시 호흡곤란, 기침, 수포음, 심한 운동 제한, 청색증, 졸음, 빈맥, 빠른 호흡, 불포화화	분당 4~6L의 산소를 공급하여 산소포화도를 90% 이상으로 유지, 활동을 최소화하고 체온 유지, 500~1,000m로 하강하거나 대피, 고지성 폐부종이 없는 경우 니페디핀(12시간마다 서방형 30mg 경구 투여 또는 8시간마다 서방형 20mg 경구 투여)을 투여, 고위험 환자만 베타 흡입작용제(살메테롤 125mcg 또는 알부테롤을 12시간마다- 흡입)투여를 고려, 고지성 뇌부종이 발생한 경우에만 덱사메타손을 투여	느린 속도로 오르고, 과로를 방지, 반복적으로 고지성 폐부종이 발생하는 경우 니페디핀(12시간마다 서방형 30mg PO 또는 8시간마다 서방형 20mg PO) 투여를 고려, 등반 하루 전에 투여를 시작하여 최대 고도에서 2일간 지속 복용

Abbreviations: bid, twice daily; EPAP, expiratory positive airway pressure; IM, intramuscular; IV, intravascular; m, meter; mcg, microgram; mg, milligram; PO, by mouth; psi, pounds per square inch; SaO$_2$, arterial oxygen saturation.

*덱사메타손은 더 이상의 등반이 고려되지 않는 경우에만 사용해야 하며 어떤 운영상의 이유로 개인이 더 높이 등반해야 하는 경우 덱사메타손은 상대적으로 금기이다.

Data from Luks AM, Auerbach PS, Freer L, et al. Wilderness Medical Society consensus guidelines for the prevention and treatment of acute altitude illness: 2019 update. *Wilderness Environ Med*. 2019;30(4):S3-S18.

며 야생의학회에서는 이를 산소 보충의 보조 수단으로 고려할 수 있다고 제안하고 있다.

고지성 폐부종의 증상과 징후, 처치 및 예방에 관한 요약은 **표 20-7**을 참조한다. 고지성 폐부종이 있는 어린이에 대한 투약 권장량은 **표 20-8**을 참조한다.

예방

적응하지 않은 사람의 급성 고산병은 예방할 수 있다. 급성 고산병, 고지성 뇌부종 및 고지성 폐부종의 공통적인 발병 요인은 높은 고도로 상승 속도이다. 고소병은 항공기를 이용해 해발 2,100~4,500m 고도의 미국 도시에서 이른 아침 비행기를 타고 정오쯤 고지대에 도착

표 20-8 고산병이 있는 소아를 위한 약물 투여

2001년 국제 산악의학회(ISMM)는 성인 처치 알고리즘(급성 고산병, 고지성 뇌부종, 고지성 폐부종)에 따라 소아 약물 여량을 조정할 것을 권장하는 합의 성명을 발표했다.

급성 고산병	• 아세타졸아마이드 2.5mg/kg를 경구로 12시간마다(1회 최대 250mg) 투여
	• 덱사메타손 0.15 mg/kg을 경구로 6시간마다 최대 4mg 투여
고지성 뇌부종	• 아세타졸아마이드 2.5mg/kg를 경구로 12시간마다(1회 최대 250mg) 투여
	• 덱사메타손 0.3mg/kg 투여
고지성 폐부종	• 덱사메타손 0.15mg/kg를 경구로 6시간마다 최대 4mg 투여

Abbreviations: kg, kilogram; mg, milligram; PO, by mouth; q, every.

Data from Pollard AJ, Niermeyer S, Barry PB, et al. Children at high altitude: an international consensus statement by an ad hoc committee of the International Society for Mountain Medicine. *High Alt Med Biol*. 2001;2:389-401; and Luks AM, Auerbach PS, Freer L, et al. Wilderness Medical Society consensus guidelines for the prevention and treatment of acute altitude illness: 2019 update. *Wilderness Environ Med*. 2019;30(4):S3-S18.

한 후 이른 오후부터 스키를 타기 시작하는 스키어에게 발생할 수 있다. 고소병의 위험이 있는 또 다른 시나리오는 해발 1,000m 아래에 거주하는 다양한 공공 안전 요원에게 지원을 요청하는 것이다. 이들은 신속하게 집결한 후 2,750m 이상의 고도에 도착하여 실종된 등산객을 찾기 위해 더 높은 고도로 등반하는 수색 및 구조 자원봉사 팀을 지원한다. 환자를 다른 병원으로 이송하거나 오지에서 이송을 책임지는 지상 승무원이나 비행 승무원, 병원 전 저치 제공자는 자신과 동료의 안전을 위해 고소병 위험을 최소화할 수 있는 지식을 갖추고 있어야 한다(**Box 20-12**, **Box 20-13**).

고소병 예방을 위한 투약

모든 유형의 고소병을 예방하기 위해 모든 경우 완화를 위한 구체적인 전략(예: 높은 곳을 오르고 낮은 곳에서 잔다)과 함께 점진적인 등반을 권장한다.

급성 고산병/고지성 뇌부종의 약리학적 예방

해발 3,000m 이상의 고도를 하루 동안 여행하는 경우 또는 급성 고산병 병력이 있는 사람은 급성 고산병 및 고지성 뇌부종 예방을 위해 예방적 치료를 고려한다. 야생 의학회의 지침은 등반 계획과 과거

Box 20-12 고도 적응 절차

다음은 고지대 적응을 위한 핵심 사항이다.
■ 적응을 유도할 수 있을 정도로 높이 올라가되 고소병이 발생할 정도로 높지 않도록 한다.
■ 적응하지 않은 사람은 2,800m 이상에서는 천천히 조심스럽게 올라가야 한다.
■ 처음 3일간은 무리한 활동을 하지 않는다.
■ 물로 수분을 충분히 섭취한다.
■ 알코올, 수면제 및 기타 진정제를 복용하지 않는다.
■ 고탄수화물 음식을 섭취한다.
■ 과로하지 않는다.
■ 흡연하지 않는다.
■ 체력 훈련은 고산병 예방에 도움이 되지 않는다.

Box 20-13 고소병 황금 원칙

고산병의 "황금 원칙"은 다음과 같다.
1. 고산병에 걸렸다면 달리 증명되기 전까지 고산병으로 인한 증상으로 간주한다.
2. 고산병 증상이 나타나면 더 이상 올라가지 않는다.
3. 몸이 아프거나 악화하는 경우 또는 발뒤꿈치부터 발끝까지 일직선으로 걸을 수 없는 경우 즉시 하산한다.
4. 고산병 환자는 상상 하산이 필요한 경우 하산하거나 준비할 수 있는 책임 있는 동반자와 동행해야 한다.

병력에 따라 위험도와 그에 따른 예방 치료의 중요성을 구체화했다. 약리학적 예방이 바람직하다고 판단되면 경구용 아세타졸아마이드(125mg)를 1일 2회, 등반 1일 전부터 복용을 시작하여 최고 고도 또는 하산 시작 시까지 2일간 복용하는 것이 좋다. 대체 약물로는 덱사메타손 4mg을 6시간마다 경구 또는 근육 내로 투여하고 최고 고도에서 2일간 지속하는 방법이 있다(이 용량은 신체 활동을 통한 적극적인 등반을 가정한 것이다). 두 약물을 함께 복용하는 것이 단독으로 복용하는 것보다 더 효과적일 수 있지만, 야생 의학회 및 야생 EMS 전문가는 이 조합을 매우 빠른 속도로 등반해야 하는 응급 상황으로 제한할 것을 권장한다. 한 연구에서 아스피린(325mg)을 4시간마다 3회 복용하면 두통 발생률이 50%에서 7%로 감소했다.

두 연구에 따르면 이부프로펜 600mg을 해발 1,250~3,800m까지 등반하기 6시간 전부터 1일 3회 예방적으로 복용하면 위약 치료와 비교했을 때 이점이 있다고 한다. 립먼 등은 이부프로펜을 먹은 그룹

참가자의 43%가 급성 고산병이 발생했다고 보고했지만, 위약 그룹의 참가자는 69%가 발생했다고 보고했다. 또한 위약 그룹은 이부프로펜 그룹에서 보고된 것보다 급성 고산병의 중증도가 더 심했다고 보고했다. 이부프로펜 사용의 장점은 급성 고산병 예방을 위해 아세타졸아마이드를 사용하는 기존 방식에 비해 부작용이 없거나 적인 이차 선택 약물을 제공하고 등반 당일 복용할 수 있다는 점이다. 그러나 이부프로펜은 적응 속도가 빠르지 않다는 단점이 있다. 적어도 한 권의 야생 EMS 참고 교과서에서는 더 많은 데이터가 확보될 때까지 이부프로펜을 아세타졸아마이드보다 권장해서는 안 된다고 주장하고 있다. 또한, 아세타졸아마이드와 이부프로펜을 구체적으로 비교한 한 임상시험에서는 두 그룹에서 고산성 두통과 급성 고산병의 발생률이 같게 나타났다.

고지성 폐부종의 약리학적 예방

반복적인 사건의 병력이 있는 개인의 고지성 폐부종 예방을 위해 경구용 니페디핀 60mg을 매일 2~3회 복용(서방형 제제)으로 예방하는 것이 일차 처치로 권장된다. 살메테롤은 니페디핀의 보조제로 1일 2회 125mcg 흡입 용량을 고려할 수도 있지만, 재발 고지성 폐부종 병력이 명확한 고위험군에만 사용할 수 있다. 실데나필, 타다라필, 덱사메타손 등 잠재적인 가능성을 보이는 다른 고지성 폐부종 예방 약물도 연구 중이지만, 야생 EMS 목적으로 권장하기 위해서는 추가 연구가 필요하다.

현재 소아의 고소병 예방을 위한 예방적 처치는 임상 연구가 충분하지 않기 때문에 피해야 한다.

이송 지연

환경 외상은 종종 야생이나 구급차를 쉽게 이용할 수 없는 환경에서 발생하기 때문에 가장 가까운 적절한 외상센터로 환자를 이송하는 것이 지연될 수 있다. 병원 전 처치 제공자는 가장 가까운 병원으로 이송하거나 헬기 도착을 기다리는 동안 환자를 계속 처치해야 할 수 있다.

익사

증상이 경미한 환자는 장기 치료 상황에서 증상이 악화하기 4시간 전에 증상이 더 심해질 수 있다. 그러나 익사 환자가 처음에는 증상이 전혀 없다가 몇 시간 또는 며칠 후에 증상이 악화하거나 사망한 사례는 의학 문헌에 없다. 익사 환자에게 저산소혈증 교정을 시작하기 위해 CAB 방식이 아닌 일반적인 ABC 접근방법을 사용하여 5회 연속적인 호흡으로 심폐소생술을 실시한다. 산소 투여 전과 후에 맥박산소측정을 하고 비재호흡마스크로 분당 15L의 고유량 산소를 공급한다.

산소포화도가 92% 미만인 환자(특히 산소 투여 시작 후 이 수치를 보이는 환자), 의식 상태 변화, 무호흡 또는 혼수상태인 환자는 흡인으로부터 보호하기 위해 조기 침습적 기도 유지가 필요할 수 있다. 고유량 산소 투여 후에도 산소포화도 측정값이 92% 미만으로 저산소혈증이 지속되는 환자는 지속기도양압 또는 급속연속기관삽관을 시행해야 할 대상 환자이다. 기관내관을 통한 흡인은 분비물이 환기를 방해하는 경우 필요할 수 있지만, 산소 공급에 영향을 줄 수 있으므로 주의허야 한다. 가능한 경우 의료 지도 의사의 의료 지도를 받아 환자를 안정시키고 마비시켜(프로토콜에서 허용하는 경우) 성공적인 기관내삽관, 산소 공급 및 효과적인 환기를 보장한다.

효과적인 산소 공급과 환기를 보장하는 또 다른 효과적인 방법은 호흡을 보조하기 위해 호기말양압(PEEP)을 사용하는 것이다. 호기말양압은 허탈된 폐포를 보충하여 환기 관류 비율과 동맥혈 산소 공급을 개선한다.

환자의 글래스고혼수 척도를 평가하고 환자의 결과를 예측할 수 있으므로 주기적으로 재평가한다. 저체온증과 저혈당을 모니터링한다. 혼수상태인 환자는 혈당을 측정하거나 측정할 수 없는 경우 정맥내로 포도당을 투여한다. 기도가 확보된 후 침수 중에 삼킨 위 내용물과 물을 줄이기 위해 코위관을 삽입해야 할 수도 있다.

낙뢰 손상

낙뢰 피해자는 호흡정지, 심정지 또는 둘 다 발생할 수 있다. 순환, 기도, 호흡(CAB) 평가 후 신속하게 심폐소생술을 시작한다. 다수의 희생자가 발생한 상황에서는 역 분류법을 사용하여 사망한 것처럼 보이는 환자에게 먼저 소생술을 시행한다. 그러나 이러한 피해자에게 장시간 심폐소생술을 실시하면 환자의 예후가 좋지 않으며 20~30분 이상 지속하는 심폐소생술 또는 전문심장소생술의 이점은 거의 없다. 소생술을 중단하기 전에 저산소혈증, 저혈량증, 저체온증 및 산증을 교정하기 위해 환자를 안정화하는 모든 처치를 시도해야 한다.

환자의 뇌부종과 두개내압 증가 여부를 평가한다. 기준 글래스고혼수척도 점수를 설정하고 10분마다 환자를 재평가하여 진행성 뇌부종과 두개내압 상승을 지표로 삼는다(뇌부종에 대한 권장 사항에 따라 처치, 8장, 머리와 목 외상 부분 참조).

레크리에이션 스쿠버 관련 다이빙 손상

폐과도팽창증후군(예: 동맥기체색전증, 감압병)을 유발하는 스쿠버 관련 손상에 대한 표준 처치 프로토콜은 현장에서 고유량 산소(비재호흡마스크로 분당 15L)를 공급하고 고압산소 치료를 위해 환자를 가장 가까운 재가압 챔버가 있는 의료기관으로 이송하는 동안 산소 공급을 계속하는 것이다. 광범위한 신경학적 평가를 하고 증상과 징후의 진행을 확인하기 위해 자주 재평가해야 한다. 프로토콜에 따라 통증을 조절하기 위해 진통제를 사용한다. 또한 항 혈소판 작용을 위해 아스피린(325mg 또는 650mg)을 투여하는 것도 고려한다.

　가장 가까운 재가압 챔버가 있는 의료기관으로 이송하기 위해 다이빙 경보 네트워크(DAN)와 의료기관에 문의한다. 고압산소 치료를 위해 환자를 이송하기 전에 챔버 준비 상태가 예고 없이 변경될 수 있으므로 환자를 이송할 의료기관에 직접 연락한다. 항공으로 이송할 때는 비행 중에 해수면의 기압을 유지할 수 있는 항공기를 이용한다. 가압되지 않은 항공기는 재가압 챔버가 있는 의료기관으로 이송하는 동안 300m 이하의 고도를 유지해야 한다.

고소병

경증에서 중등도 정도의 급성 고산병은 코삽입관으로 분당 2~4L의 저용량 산소 공급으로 처치할 수 있으며 산소포화도가 90% 이상인 경우 분당 1~2L의 산소를 투여한 후 두통이 있는 경우 아스피린 650mg, 아세트아미노펜 650~1,000mg, 이부프로펜 600mg을 투여하고 메스꺼움이 있는 경우 프로클로로페라진(5~10mg IM) 또는 온단세트론(4mg 경구용해정 또는 IM)을 투여하거나 복용한다. 경증에서 중등도의 급성 고산병 처치에 사용되는 다른 약물로는 증상이 해소될 때까지 경구 아세타졸아마이드(1일 2회 250mg), 덱사메타손(6시간마다 4mg 경구 또는 IM)을 투여한다(단, 덱사메타손을 더 복용할 때 위험할 수 있음에 유의한다).

　고지성 뇌부종은 즉시 하강하고 코삽입관으로 산소를 공급하여 산소포화도를 90% 이상으로 유지(일반적으로 2~4L/분)하고 덱사메타손(처음에는 8mg을 PO, IV 또는 IM, 투여 후 6시간마다 4mg 투여)으로 처치한다. 하강이 장시간 지연되는 경우 경구용 아세타졸아마이드(1일 2회 250mg) 사용을 고려한다. 하강이 지연되는 경우 고압 챔버 사용을 고려한다. 중증 형태의 고지성 뇌부종이 발생하여 환자가 혼수상태면 뇌부종에 대한 권장 사항에 따라 처치한다(3장, 쇼크: 삶과 죽음의 병태 생리학 참조).

　고지성 폐부종의 장기간 처치는 주로 증상이 호전될 때까지 코삽입관으로 분당 4~6L 산소를 투여(산소포화도 90% 이상)한 다음 산소포화도를 유지하기 위해 분당 2~4L의 산소를 투여하거나 고압 챔버를 사용하는 것이다. 산소를 사용할 수 없는 경우 니페디핀(초기 10mg, 이후 12~24시간마다 30mg 서방형 용량)을 투여하고 지속성 기도양압을 고려한다. 환자가 고지성 뇌부종에 걸리면 덱사메타손(6시간마다 8mg을 PO 또는 IM)을 추가로 투여한다.

　휴대용 고압 챔버는 고소병을 처치하는 데 효과적이다. 이 가벼운 천으로 만들어진 압력 백은 보충 산소나 약물(예: 아세타졸아마이드, 덱사메타손, 니페디핀) 사용 여부와 관계없이 낮은 고도로 하강하는 것과 같은 효과를 나타낸다. 이 챔버는 수동 펌프로 최대 2psi까지 팽창시킬 수 있으며 이는 고지성 폐부종의 초기 고도 및 중증도에 따라 다양한 거리를 하강하는 것과 같은 효과가 있다. 이 챔버를 2~3시간 동안 사용하면 증상을 효과적으로 개선할 수 있다. 이는 최종적인 처치를 받을 수 있는 의료기관까지 이송되기를 기다리는 동안 이상적으로 사용할 수 있으며 때로는 환자의 증상이 호전되면 챔버 자체가 최종적 처치가 될 수도 있다.

요 약

- 병원 전 환경에서 신속한 평가와 처치가 이루어질 수 있도록 일반적인 환경 응급상황에 대한 기본 지식이 필요하다.

- 낙뢰
  - 낙뢰 손상은 경미한 표재성 손상에서 심각한 다발성 외상 및 사망에 이르기까지 다양하다.
  - 낙뢰로 인한 급사의 기전은 동시에 발생하는 심장 및 호흡 정지이다.
  - 낙뢰 피해자를 처치하기 위한 우선순위는 현장의 안전을 확보하고 XABCDE를 평가하여 심폐소생술과 제세동을 시행한다.
  - 낙뢰 다수의 사상자가 발생한 상황에서는 호흡 정지 또는 심정지 환자는 신속하게 처치하면 회복 가능성이 높으므로 역 분류법을 사용한다.

- 익사
  - 병원 전 처치 제공자는 익사의 병태생리학적 과정을 이해해야 한다. 익사 후 생존과 장기 기능의 주요 결정 요인은 중추신경계 손상 정도이다.
  - 익사 환자를 처치할 때 모든 환자에게 고유량 산소를 제공해야 한다. 일반으로 처치에는 정맥 라인 확보 및 수액 투여(생리식염수 또는 락테이트링거액), 평가를 위해 응급실로 이송한다.
  - 심폐정지 상태의 익사 환자에게 효과적인 BLS 및 표준 ALS 절차를 신속하게 실시하는 것이 생존 확률을 높이는 것과 관련이 있다.
  - 병원 전 처치 제공자가 지역 사회에서 권장할 수 있는 익사 예방 노력에는 수영장 주변에 차단막 설치, 물 근처에 있을 때 어린이 모니터링, 구명조끼와 같은 개인 부양 장치 사용,

  목격자에 의한 심폐소생술 시작, 수상 관련 활동에 참여할 때 음주와 같은 고위험 행동을 피하는 것이다.

- 레크리에이션 다이빙
  - 병원 전 처치 제공자가 가장 일반적으로 출동하는 여가 활동 관련 다이빙 손상 유형은 감압증(환경 압력 변화)으로 인한 스쿠버 관련 손상 또는 사망이다.
  - 압력 손상은 다양한 유형의 압력에 의한 손상을 초래할 수 있다. 하강 관련 손상의 예로는 마스크 압착, 치아 압착, 중이 압착(가장 흔함), 부비동 압착 및 내이 압력 손상 등이 있다. 상승 관련 손상에는 압력 변화성 현기증, 부비동 압력 손상 및 폐과도팽창증후군(POIS)이 포함된다. 병원 전 처치 제공자는 이러한 손상을 효과적으로 평가하고 처치할 수 있도록 준비가 되어 있어야 한다.
  - 다이빙 손상 처치에는 ABC를 평가하고 환자의 기도를 유지하며 BLS 또는 ALS 절차를 시작하는 것이 포함된다.

- 고소병
  - 고소병은 1) 급성 고산병(AMS), 2) 고지성 뇌부종(HACE), 3) 고지성 폐부종과 같은 뇌 및 폐 증후군을 포괄하는 용어이다.
  - 병원 전 처치 제공자와 응급실 직원은 고소병의 이환율과 사망률을 줄이기 위해 위험 요인, 증상 및 징후, 처치, 약물, 교육 및 예방 방법에 익숙해야 한다.
  - 이러한 질환에 대한 병원 전 처치에는 일반적으로 고지대에서 하강, 산소 투여 및 가능한 약리학적 처치가 포함된다.

- 환경 외상과 관련하여 이송 지연할 가능성이 있으므로 병원 전 처치 제공자는 구급차 내에서 지속해서 환자에게 처치를 제공할 준비가 되어 있어야 한다.

시나리오 재구성

어느 해안 마을에서 4인 가족이 쌀쌀한 겨울날 반려견과 함께 해변을 산책하고 있었다. 아들이 물가를 고무공을 던지자, 개가 쫓아갔다. 순식간에 해안을 거친 파도에 강아지가 휩쓸려 갔다. 17세의 아들은 개를 구하기 위해 가장 먼저 물로 뛰어들었지만, 물에 휩쓸려 버리고 말고 이 장면을 부모와 누나가 목격했다.

소년의 아버지와 어머니는 바닷가에 비치된 부력 장치를 잡고 소년을 따라 파도 속으로 들어가 도와주었다. 19세의 딸은 해변에 남아 휴대전화로 도움을 요청했다. 개는 결국 해안으로 돌아왔다. 부모는 아들이 차가운 물속에 잠긴 채 반응이 없는 것을 발견한 후 아들을 꺼냈다. 딸의 신고 후 7분 이내에 구급대가 현장에 도착했다.

구급차에서 내릴 때 의식을 잃은 10대 소년이 파도가 밀려오는 모래사장에 얼굴을 옆으로 돌린 채 반쯤 엎드린 채 누워 있는 것을 목격했다. 소년은 아직 파도가 밀려오는 지역에 있으며 파도에 휩쓸릴 수 있다. 당신은 현장에 도착한 119구조대와 함께 피해자에게 접근한다.

(다음 페이지에 계속)

시나리오 재구성 (이어서)

- 이 상황에서 환자에게 어떻게 접근해야 하는가?
- 환자의 맥박이나 호흡이 없는 경우 즉시 시행해야 할 처치는 무엇인가?
- 현장에서 해결해야 할 환자에 대한 다른 우려 사항은 무엇인가?

시나리오 해결책

여러분의 계획은 개인 부양 장치(PFD)를 착용한 소방관 한 명이 다가오는 파도의 위협을 감시하는 역할을 하도록 하고 당신과 동료 및 다른 소방관 두 명이 환자에게 접근하여 팔다리를 모두 잡고 밀려오는 파도로부터 신속하게 이동시키는 것이다. 물 근처에 있거나 물에 들어가는 모든 사람은 개인 부양 장치를 착용해야 한다.

병원 전 처치 제공자 팀의 리더로서 당신은 의식이 없는 환자를 머리와 몸통이 같은 높이로 위치할 수 있게 눕히도록 지시한 다음 즉시 반응 여부를 확인하도록 팀원에게 지시한다. 다른 동료들은 기도, 호흡, 순환을 평가하는 동안 환자 주변에 응급처치 장비를 배치한다. 이 상황에서 XABCDE 평가 순서가 부적절하다는 점을 기억한다. 환자는 무호흡 상태이므로 구조 호흡만 필요할 수도 있고 전체 심폐소생술이 필요할 수도 있다. 어떤 상황에서든 익사 시 처음에는 5회의 구조 호흡을 시행한 후 30회 가슴압박을 시행한 후 생명 징후가 나타나거나 소생술이 소용없다고 판단될 때까지 2회의 호흡과 30회의 가슴압박을 계속하는 것이 권장된다.

익사 피해자의 기도, 호흡, 순환에 대한 초기 접근은 저산소혈증을 해결하는 데 필수적이다. 백마스크 장비를 사용하여 고유량 산소를 제공한다. 정맥 라인을 확보한 후 결정질 용액을 투여한다. 이 경우 척추 손상을 의심할 만한 손상 기전이 없으므로 척추 고정은 필요하지 않다. 환자의 산소포화도가 92% 미만으로 악화 징후를 보이는 경우 조기 기관내삽관 또는 지속기도양압 환기와 같은 보조 기계 환기가 필요할 수 있다. 환자와 보호자를 병원으로 이송하여 지속해서 처치와 평가를 받도록 한다.

References

1. Curran EB, Holle RL, Lopez RE. Lightning fatalities, injuries and damage reports in the United States, 1959–1994. NOAA Tech Memo NWS SR-193; 1997.

2. Centers for Disease Control and Prevention. QuickStats: number of deaths from lightning among males and females—National Vital Statistics System, United States, 1968–2010. *Morb Mortal Wkly Rep*. Accessed January 18, 2022. https://www.cdc.gov/mmwr/preview/mmwrhtml/mm6228a6.htm

3. Gatewood MO, Zane RD. Lightning injuries. *Emerg Med Clin North Am*. 2004;22:369-403.

4. Huffines GR, Orville RE. Lightning ground flash density and thunderstorm duration in the continental United States: 1989–96. *J Appl Meteorol Climatol*. 1999;38(7):1013-1019.

5. Cummins KL, Krider EP, Malone MD. A combined TOA/MDF technology upgrade of the U.S. National Lightning Detection Network. *J Geophys Res*. 1998;103:9035-9044.

6. MacGorman, DR, Rust WD. Lightning strike density for the contiguous United States from thunderstorm duration records, Pub No NUREG/CR03759. Office of Nuclear Regulatory Research; 1984.

7. Hawkins SC, Simon RB, Beissinger JP, Simon D. *Vertical Aid: Essential Wilderness Medicine for Climbers, Trekkers, and Mountaineers*. The Countryman Press; 2017.

8. Cherington M, Walker J, Boyson M, Glancy R, Hedegaard H, Clark S. Closing the gap on the actual numbers of lightning casualties and deaths. 11th Conference on Applied Climatology. Dallas, TX: American Meteorological Society; 1999:379-380.

9. Dulcos PJ, Sanderson LM, Klontz KC. Lightning-related mortality and morbidity in Florida. *Pub Health Rep*. 1990;105:276-282.

10. Cooper MA, Andrews CJ, Holle RL, Blumenthal R, Aldana NN. Lightning-related injuries and safety. In: Auerbach PS, ed. *Auerbach's Wilderness Medicine*. 7th ed. Elsevier; 2017.

11. Nelson RD, McGinnis H. Lightning injuries and severe storms. In: Hawkins SC, ed. *Wilderness EMS*. Wolters Kluwer; 2018.

12. Jensenius JS. A detailed analysis of lightning deaths in the United States from 2006 through 2019. National Lightning Safety Council. Published February 2020. Accessed January 18, 2022. https://www.weather.gov/media/safety/Analysis06-19.pdf

13. Davis C, Engeln A, Johnson E, et al. Wilderness Medical Society practice guidelines for the prevention and treatment of lightning injuries: 2014 update. *Wilderness Environ Med.* 2014;25(4):S86-S95.

14. Cooper MA. Lightning injuries: prognostic signs of death. *Ann Emerg Med.* 1980;9:134-138.

15. Cooper MA, Edlich RF. Lightning injuries. Medscape. Updated September 17, 2021. Accessed October 25, 2021. http://emedicine.medscape.com/article/770642-overview

16. Andrews CJ, Darveniza M, Mackerras D. Lightning injury: a review of the clinical aspects, pathophysiology and treatment. *Adv Trauma.* 1989;4:241-287.

17. Ashish RP, Bartos JA, Cabañas JG, et al. 2020 American Heart Association guidelines for cardiopulmonary resuscitation and emergency cardiovascular care: cardiac arrest associated with electric shock and lightning strikes. *Circulation.* 2020;142(18):S366-S468.

18. Ritenour AE, Morton MJ, McManus JG, Barillo DJ, Cancio LC. Lightning injury: a review. *Burns.* 2008;34:585-594.

19. Beir M, Chen W, Bodnar E, Lee RC. Biophysical injury mechanisms associated with lightning injury. *Neurorehabilitation.* 2005;20(1):53-62.

20. Cooper MA. Electrical and lightning injuries. *Emerg Med Clin North Am.* 1984;2:489-501.

21. Casten JA, Kytilla J. Eye symptoms caused by lightning. *Acta Ophthalmol.* 1963;41:139-143.

22. Kleiner JP, Wilkin JH. Cardiac effects of lightning stroke. *JAMA.* 1978;240:2757-2759.

23. Taussig HB. Death from lightning and the possibility of living again. *Ann Intern Med.* 1968;68:1345-1353.

24. Hawkins SC, Williams J, Bennett BL, Islas A, Kayser DW, Quinn R. Wilderness Medical Society clinical practice guidelines for spinal cord protection. *Wilderness Environ Med.* 2019;30(4):S87-S99.

25. Zimmerman C, Cooper MA, Holle RL. Lightning safety guidelines. *Ann Emerg Med.* 2002;39:660-664.

26. National Lightning Safety Institute. Personal lightning safety. Accessed January 18, 2022. http://www.lightning-safety.com/nlsi_pls.html

27. National Weather Service. Lightning tips. Accessed January 18, 2022. https://www.weather.gov/safety/lightning-tips

28. Zafren K, Durrer B, Henry JP, Brugger H. Lightning injuries: prevention and on-site treatment in mountains and remote areas—official guidelines of the International Commission for Mountain Emergency Medicine and Medical Commission of the International Mountaineering and Climbing Federation (ICAR and UIAA MEDCOM). *Resuscitation.* 2005;65:369-372.

29. National Oceanic and Atmospheric Administration. Lightning myths. Accessed January 18, 2022. https://www.weather.gov/safety/lightning-myths

30. Sempsrott J, Schmidt AC, Hawkins SC, Cushing TA. Drowning and submersion injuries. In: Auerbach PS, ed. *Auerbach's Wilderness Medicine.* 7th ed. Elsevier; 2017.

31. Peden M, Oyegbite K, Ozanne-Smith J, et al., eds. World report on child injury prevention. World Health Organization; 2008.

32. Centers for Disease Control and Prevention. Nonfatal and fatal drowning in recreational water settings—United States, 2005–2009. *Morb Mortal Wkly Rep.* 2012;61(19):345.

33. Centers for Disease Control and Prevention. Drowning—United States, 2005–2009. *Morb Mortal Wkly Rep.* 2012;61(19);344-347.

34. Zuckerman GB, Conway EE Jr. Drowning and near-drowning. *Pediatr Ann.* 2000;29(6):360-366.

35. World Health Organization. Facts sheet: drowning. Updated April 27, 2021. Accessed October 25, 2021. https://www.who.int/news-room/fact-sheets/detail/drowning

36. Hawkins SC, Sempsrott J, Schmidt A. Drowning in a sea of misinformation: dry drowning and secondary drowning. *Emerg Med News.* 2017;39(8):1,39-40.

37. van Beeck EF, Branche CM, Szpilman D, et al. A new definition of drowning: towards documentation and prevention of a global public health program. *Bull World Health Organ.* 2005;83:853-856.

38. van Beeck EF, Branche CM, Szpilman D, et al. Definition of drowning. In: Bierens JJLM, ed. *Handbook on Drowning: Prevention, Rescue, Treatment.* Springer; 2006.

39. van Beek E, Branche C. Definition of drowning: a progress report. In: Bierens JJLM, ed. *Drowning: Prevention, Rescue, Treatment.* 2nd ed. Springer; 2014.

40. American College of Emergency Physicians. Death after swimming is extremely rare—and is NOT "dry drowning.' Published July 11, 2017. Accessed January 18, 2022. https://www.prnewswire.com/news-releases/death-after-swimming-is-extremely-rare--and-is-not-dry-drowning-300486302.html

41. Szpilman D, Bierens JJLM, Handley A, Orlowshi JP. Drowning. *N Engl J Med.* 2012;366:2102-2110.

42. World Health Organization. Global report on drowning: preventing a leading killer. Published November 17, 2014. Accessed October 25, 2021. https://www.who.int/publications/i/item/global-report-on-drowning-preventing-a-leading-killer

43. Schmidt AC, Sempsrott JR, Hawkins SC, Arastu AS, Cushing TA, Auerbach PS. Wilderness Medical Society practice guidelines for the prevention and treatment of drowning: 2019 update. *Wilderness Environ Med.* 2019;30(4):S70-S86.

44. Centers for Disease Control and Prevention. Injury Center: Drowning Prevention: Drowning Facts. Accessed January 18, 2022. https://www.cdc.gov/drowning/facts/index.html. Last reviewed June 17, 2021.

45. Centers for Disease Control and Prevention. Leading causes of injury and death. Accessed January 18, 2022. https://www.cdc.gov/injury/wisqars/index.html

46. Oshaker JS. Submersion. *Emerg Med Clin North Am.* 2004;22:357-367.

47. Moran K, Quan L, Franklin R, Bennett E. Where the evidence and expert opinion meet: a review of the open-water recreational safety messages. *Int J Aquatic Res Educ.* 2011;5:251-270.

48. Lavelle JM. Ten-year review of pediatric bathtub near-drownings: evaluation for child abuse and neglect. *Ann Emerg Med.* 1995;25:344-348.

49. Craig AB Jr. Underwater swimming and loss of consciousness. *JAMA.* 1961;176:255-258.

50. Dickinson P. Shallow water blackout. In: Bierens JJLM, ed. *Drowning: Prevention, Rescue, Treatment.* 2nd ed. Springer; 2014.

51. International Life Saving Federation. Medical Position Statement—MPS 16: shallow water blackout. International Life Saving Federation position statements. https://medical.ilsf.org/shallow-water-blackout/

52. Chimiak JM, Buzzacott P. Management of diving injuries. In: Hawkins SC, ed. *Wilderness EMS.* Wolters Kluwer; 2018.

53. United States Lifesaving Association. *Open Water Lifesaving: The United States Lifesaving Association Manual.* 3rd ed. Pearson; 2017.

54. Pearn JH, Franklin RC, Peden AE. Hypoxic blackout: diagnosis, risks, and prevention. *Int J Aquatic Res Educ.* 2015;9:342-347.

55. Royal Life Saving Australia. Hypoxic blackout. Accessed October 25, 2021. https://www.royallifesaving.com.au/stay-safe-active/risk-factors/hypoxic-blackout

56. Jensen LR, Williams SD, Thurman DJ, Keller PA. Submersion injuries in children younger than 5 years in urban Utah. *West J Med.* 1992;157(6):641-644.

57. Howland J, Hingson R, Mangione TW, Bell N, Bak S. Why are most drowning victims men? Sex differences, aquatic skills and behaviors. *Am J Public Health.* 1996;86:93-96.

58. Schuman SH, Rowe JR, Glazer HM, et al. The iceberg phenomenon of near-drowning. *Crit Care Med.* 1976;4:127-128.

59. Bell NS, Amoros PJ, Yore MM, et al. Alcohol and other risk factors for drowning among male active duty U.S. army soldiers. *Aviat Space Environ Med.* 2001;72(12):1086-1095.

60. DeNicola LK, Falk JL, Swanson ME, Kissoon N. Submersion injuries in children and adults. *Crit Care Clin.* 1997;13(3):477-502.

61. Howland J, Mangione T, Hingson R, et al. Alcohol as a risk factor for drowning and other aquatic injuries. In: Watson RR, ed. *Alcohol and Accidents: Drug and Alcohol Abuse Reviews.* Vol 7. Humana Press; 1995.

62. Howland J, Hingson R. Alcohol as a risk factor for drownings: a review of the literature (1950–1985). *Accid Anal Prev.* 1988;20(1):19-25.

63. Howland J, Smith GS, Mangione T, et al. Missing the boat on drinking and boating. *JAMA.* 1993;270:91-92.

64. Bell GS, Gaitatzis A, Bell CL, Johnson AL, Sander JW. Drowning in people with epilepsy. *Neurology.* 2008;71:578-582.

65. White J. *StarGuard: Best Practices for Lifeguards.* 5th ed. Human Kinetics; 2017.

66. Sempsrott J. Management of drowning. In: Hawkins SC, ed. *Wilderness EMS.* Wolters Kluwer; 2018.

67. Padgett J. Technical rescue interface: swiftwater rescue. In: Hawkins SC, ed. *Wilderness EMS.* Wolters Kluwer; 2018.

68. Smith B, Bledsoe B, Nicolazzo P. General management of trauma in the wilderness environment. In: Hawkins SC, ed. *Wilderness EMS.* Wolters Kluwer; 2018.

69. Smith W. Technical rescue interface introduction: principles of basic technical rescue, patient care integration, and packaging. In: Hawkins SC, ed. *Wilderness EMS.* Wolters Kluwer; 2018.

70. Rowe MI, Arango A, Allington G. Profile of pediatric drowning victims in a water-oriented society. *J Trauma.* 1977;17:587-591.

71. Brenner RA, Taneja GS, Haynie DL, et al. Association between swimming lessons and drowning in childhood: a case-control study. *Arch Pediatr Adolesc Med.* 2009;163:203-210.

72. Quan L, Mack CD, Schiff MA. Association of water temperature and submersion duration and drowning outcome. *Resuscitation.* 2014;85(6):790-794. doi: 10.1016/j.resuscitation.2014.02.024

73. Giesbrecht GG, Steinman AM. Immersion into cold water. In: Auerbach PS, ed. *Wilderness Medicine.* 6th ed. Mosby Elsevier; 2012.

74. Bolte RG, Black PG, Bowers RS. The use of extracorporeal rewarming in a child submerged for 66 minutes. *JAMA.* 1988;260:377-379.

75. Lloyd EL. Accidental hypothermia. *Resuscitation.* 1996;32:111-124. doi: 10.1016/0300-9572(96)00983-5

76. Gilbert M, Busund R, Skagseth A. Resuscitation from accidental hypothermia of 13.7°C with circulatory arrest. *Lancet.* 2000;355:375-376.

77. Siebke H, Breivik H, Rod T, et al. Survival after 40 minutes submersion without cerebral sequelae. *Lancet.* 1975;1:1275-1277.

78. Tipton MJ, Golden FSC. A proposed decision-making guide for the search, rescue and resuscitation of submersion (head under) victims based on expert opinion. *Resuscitation.* 2011;82(7)819-824. doi: 10.1016/j.resuscitation.2011.02.021

79. National Fire Chiefs Council. National Operational Guidance: Rescue from water. Accessed March 11, 2022. https://www.ukfrs.com/scenarios/rescue-water

80. Schmidt A, Sempsrott J, Abo B. Technical rescue interface: open water rescue. In: Hawkins SC, ed. *Wilderness EMS.* Wolters Kluwer; 2018.

81. James Cook University. Drowning researchers look for help. Media Release, July 12, 2017. Published July 12, 2017. Accessed October 25, 2021. https://www.jcu.edu.au/news/releases/2017/july/drowning-researchers-look-for-help

82. Zhu Y, Jiang X, Li H, et al. Mortality among drowning rescuers in China, 2013: a review of 225 rescue incidents from the press. *BMC Pub Health.* 2015;15:631. doi: 10.1186/s12889-015-2010-0

83. Hwang V, Frances S, Durbin D, et al. Prevalence of traumatic injuries in drowning and near-drowning in children and adolescents. *Arch Pediatr Adolesc Med.* 2003;157(1):50-53.

84. Pratt FD, Haynes BE. Incidence of "secondary drowning" after saltwater submersion. *Ann Emerg Med.* 1986;15(9):1084-1087.

85. Szpilman D. Near-drowning and drowning classification: a proposal to stratify mortality based on the analysis of 1,831 cases. *Chest.* 1997;112:660-665.

86. Kleinman ME, Brennan EE, Goldberger ZDD. Part 5: Adult Basic Life Support and Cardiopulmonary Resuscitation Quality. 2015 American Heart Association Guidelines Update for Cardiopulmonary Resuscitation and Emergency Cardiovascular Care. Accessed October 25, 2021. https://www.ahajournals.org/doi/full/10.1161/CIR.000000000000259

87. Rosen P, Stoto M, Harley J. The use of the Heimlich maneuver in near-drowning: Institute of Medicine report. *J Emerg Med.* 1995;13:397-405.

88. Moran K, Quan L, Franklin R, Bennett E. Where the evidence and expert opinion meet: a review of open-water recreational safety messages. *Int J Aquatic Res Educ.* 2011;5(3):251-270.

89. Baker PA, Webber JB. Failure to ventilate with supraglottic airways after drowning. *Anaesth Intensive Care.* 2011;39:675-677.

90. Smith T, ed. *Clinical Procedures and Guidelines: Comprehensive Edition, 2019-2022.* Guideline 11.1: Drowning. Accessed October 25, 2021. https://www.stjohn.org.nz/globalassets/documents/health-practitioners/clinical-procedures-and-guidelines---comprehensive-edition.pdf

91. Kyriacou DN, Arcinue EL, Peek C, Kraus JF. Effect of immediate resuscitation on children with submersion injury. *Pediatrics.* 1994;94:137-142.

92. Denny SA, Quan L, Gilchrist J, et al. American Academy of Pediatrics Policy Statement. Prevention of drowning prevention. *Pediatrics.* 2019;143(4):e20. Published May, 2019. Accessed October 25, 2021. https://pediatrics.aappublications.org/content/143/5/e20190850

93. Wintemute GJ, Kraus JF, Teret SP, Wright MA. Death resulting from motor vehicle immersions: the nature of the injuries, personal and environmental contributing factors, and potential interventions. *Am J Public Health.* 1990;80:1068-1070.

94. Hawkins SC. Submerged vehicles. *Wilderness Medicine Magazine.* Published February 26, 2015. Accessed October 25, 2021. www.wildernessmedicinemagazine.com/1137/drowning-submerged-vehicles

95. McDonald GK, Giesbrecht GG. Vehicle submersion: a review of the problem, associated risks, and survival information. *Aviat Space Environ Med.* 2013;84:498-510.

96. Hawkins SC. Setting the record straight to reduce fatalities in sinking vehicles. *Emerg Med News.* 2015;37:5B.

97. Melamed Y, Shupak A, Bitterman H. Medical problems associated with underwater diving. *N Engl J Med.* 1992;326:30-35.

98. Van Hoesen KB, Lang MA. Diving medicine. In: Auerbach PS, ed. *Auerbach's Wilderness Medicine.* 7th ed. Mosby Elsevier; 2017.

99. Salahuddin M, James LA, Bass ES. SCUBA medicine: a first-responder's guide to diving injuries. *Curr Sports Med Rep.* 2011;10(3):134-139.

100. Lynch JA, Bove AA. Diving medicine: a review of the current evidence. *J Am Board Fam Med.* 2009;22:399-407.

101. Strauss MB, Borer RC Jr. Diving medicine: contemporary topics and their controversies. *Am J Emerg Med.* 2001;19:232-238.

102. Morgan WP. Anxiety and panic in recreational scuba divers. *Sports Med.* 1995;20(6):398-421.

103. Della-Giustina D, Ingebretsen R. *Advanced Wilderness Life Support.* AdventureMed; 2013.

104. Divers Alert Network (DAN). Eleven-year trends (1987–1997) in diving activity: the DAN annual review of recreational SCUBA diving injuries and fatalities based on 2000 data. In: *Report on Decompression Illness, Diving Fatalities and Project Dive Exploration.* Divers Alert Network; 2000:17-29.

105. Divers Alert Network (DAN). *Report on Diving Fatalities: 2017 Edition.* Divers Alert Network; 2017.

106. Hardy KR. Diving-related emergencies. *Emerg Med Clin North Am.* 1997;15(1):223-240. doi: 10.1016/s0733-8627(05)70292-3

107. Green SM. Incidence and severity of middle-ear barotraumas in recreational scuba diving. *J Wilderness Med.* 1993;4:270-280.

108. Kizer KW. Dysbaric cerebral air embolism in Hawaii. *Ann Emerg Med.* 1987;16:535-541.

109. Cales RH, Humphreys N, Pilmanis AA, Heilig RW. Cardiac arrest from gas embolism in scuba diving. *Ann Emerg Med.* 1981;10(11):589-592.

110. Butler BD, Laine GA, Leiman BC, et al. Effect of Trendelenburg position on the distribution of arterial air emboli in dogs. *Ann Thorac Surg.* 1988;45(2):198-202.

111. Moon RE. Treatment of diving emergencies. *Crit Care Clin.* 1999;15:429-456.

112. Van Meter K. Medical field management of the injured diver. *Respir Care Clin North Am.* 1997;5(1):137-177.

113. Francis TJ, Dutka AJ, Hallenbeck JM. Pathophysiology of decompression sickness. In: Bove AA, Davis JC, eds. *Diving Medicine.* 2nd ed. Saunders; 1990.

114. Neuman TS. DCI/DCS: does it matter whether the emperor wears clothes? *Undersea Hyperb Med.* 1997;24(1):4-5.

115. Bove AA. Nomenclature of pressure disorders. *Undersea Hyperb Med.* 1997;24:1-2.

116. Spira A. Diving and marine medicine review: part II. diving diseases. *J Travel Med.* 1999;6:180-198.

117. Clenney TL, Lassen LF. Recreational scuba diving injuries. *Am Fam Physician.* 1996;53(5):1761-1774.

118. Kizer KW. Women and diving. *Physician Sportsmed.* 1981;9(2):84-92.

119. Lau AM, Johnston MJ, Rivard SC. Mottled, Blanching Skin Changes After Aggressive Diving. *J Spec Oper Med.* 2019;19(2):14-17. PMID: 31201746.

120. Estrada J, Meurer D, De Boer K, Huesgen K. Severe Decompression Illness: Case Report, Prehospital Recognition, and Regional Transport Considerations. *Case Rep Emerg Med.* 2017:2017:7203085. doi: 10.1155/2017/7203085. Epub 2017 Oct 4. PMID: 29109872; PMCID: PMC5646287.

121. Francis TJ, Dutka AJ, Hallenbeck JM. Pathophysiology of decompression sickness. In: Bove AA, Davis JC, eds. *Diving Medicine.* 2nd ed. Saunders; 1990.

122. Greer HD, Massey EW. Neurologic injury from undersea diving. *Neurol Clin.* 1992;10(4):1031-1045.

123. Kizer KW. Management of dysbaric diving casualties. *Emerg Med Clin North Am.* 1983;1:659-670.

124. Department of the Navy. *U.S. Navy Diving Manual.* Vol 1, Rev 4. U.S. Government Printing Office; 1999.

125. Davis JC. Hyperbaric medicine: critical care aspects. In: Shoemaker WC, ed. *Critical Care: State of the Art.* Society of Critical Care Medicine; 1984.

126. Pollock NW, Uguccioni DM, Dear GdeL, eds. Diabetes and recreational diving: guidelines for the future. Proceedings of the Undersea and Hyperbaric Medical Society/Divers Alert Network. June 19, 2005, Workshop. Divers Alert Network; 2005.

127. Gallagher SA, Hackett PH. High-altitude illness. *Emerg Med Clin North Am.* 2004;22:329-355.

128. Hackett PH, Roach RC. High-altitude illness. *N Engl J Med.* 2001;345(2):107-114. doi: 10.1056/NEJM200107123450206

129. Hackett PH, Luks AM, Lawley JS, Roach RC. High-altitude medicine and pathophysiology. In: Auerbach PS, ed. *Auerbach's Wilderness Medicine.* 7th ed. Mosby Elsevier; 2017.

130. Houston CS. High-altitude illness disease with protean manifestations. *JAMA.* 1976;236(19):2193-2195. doi:10.1001/jama.1976.03270200031025

131. Montgomery AB, Mills J, Luce JM. Incidence of acute mountain sickness at intermediate altitude. *JAMA.* 1989;261:732-734.

132. Gertsch JH, Seto TB, Mor J, Onopa J. Ginkgo biloba for the prevention of severe acute mountain sickness (AMS) starting day one before rapid ascent. *High Alt Med Biol.* 2002;3(1):29-37.

133. Honigman B, Theis MK, Koziol-McLain J, et al. Acute mountain sickness in a general tourist population at moderate altitudes. *Ann Intern Med.* 1993;118(8):587-592.

134. Zafren K, Honigman B. High-altitude medicine. *Emerg Clin North Am.* 1997;15(1):191-222.

135. Hultgren HN. *High-Altitude Medicine.* Hultgren Publications; 1997.

136. Luks AM, Auerbach PS, Freer LF, et al. Wilderness Medical Society consensus guidelines for the prevention and treatment of acute altitude illness: 2019 update. *Wilderness Environ Med.* 2019;30(4):S3-S18.

137. Schneider M, Bernasch D, Weymann J, et al. Acute mountain sickness: influence of susceptibility, pre-exposure, and ascent rate. *Med Sci Sports Exerc.* 2002;34(12):1886-1891.

138. Bartsch P. High-altitude pulmonary edema. *Med Sci Sports Exerc.* 1999;31(suppl 1):S23-S27.

139. Roach RC, Houston CS, Honigman B. How well do older persons tolerate moderate altitude? *West J Med.* 1995;162(1):32-36.

140. Roach RC, Maes D, Sandoval D, et al. Exercise exacerbates acute mountain sickness at simulated high altitude. *J Appl Physiol.* 2000;88(2):581-585.

141. Roeggla G, Roeggla H, Roeggla M, et al. Effect of alcohol on acute ventilation adaptation to mild hypoxia at moderate altitude. *Ann Intern Med.* 1995;122:925-927.

142. Reeves JWJ, Zafren K, Honigman B, Schoene R. Seasonal variation in barometric pressure and temperature in Summit County: effect on altitude illness. In: Sutton JHC, Coates

G, eds. *Hypoxia and Molecular Medicine*. Charles S. Houston; 1993:272-274.

143. Luks AM, Swenson ER. Medication and dosage considerations in the prophylaxis and treatment of high-altitude illness. *Chest*. 2008;133:744-755.

144. Roach RC, Bartcsh P, Oelz O, Hackett PH, Lake Louise Scoring Committee. The Lake Louise Acute Mountain Sickness Scoring System. In: Sutton JR, Houston CS, Coates G, eds. *Hypoxia and Molecular Medicine*. Charles S. Houston; 1993.

145. Muza SR, Lyons TP, Rock PB. Effect of altitude on exposure on brain volume and development of acute mountain sickness (AMS). In: Roach RC, Wagner PD, Hackett PH, eds. *Hypoxia: Into the Next Millennium: Advances in Experimental Medicine and Biology*. Vol 474. Kluwer-Academic/Plenum; 1999.

146. Hacket PH. High-altitude cerebral edema and acute mountain sickness: a pathological update. In: Roach RC, Wagner PD, Hackett PH, eds. *Hypoxia: Into the Next Millennium: Advances in Experimental Medicine and Biology*. Vol 474. Kluwer Academic/Plenum; 1999.

147. Sanchez del Rio M, Moskkowitz MA. High-altitude headache: lessons from aches at sea level. In: Roach RC, Wagner PD, Hackett PH, eds. *Hypoxia: Into the Next Millennium: Advances in Experimental Medicine and Biology*. Vol 474. Kluwer Academic/Plenum; 1999.

148. Hackett PH. The cerebral etiology of high-altitude cerebral edema and acute mountain sickness. *Wilderness Environ Med*. 1999;10(2):97-109.

149. Yarnell PR, Heit J, Hackett PH. High-altitude cerebral edema (HACE): the Denver/Front Range experience. *Semin Neurol*. 2000;20(2):209-217.

150. Hultgren HN, Honigman B, Theis K, Nicholas D. High-altitude pulmonary edema at ski resort. *West J Med*. 1996;164(3):222.

151. Stenmark KR, Frid M, Nemenoff R, et al. Hypoxia induces cell-specific changes in gene expression in vascular wall cells: implications for pulmonary hypertension. In: Roach RC, Wagner PD, Hackett PH, eds. *Hypoxia: Into the Next Millennium: Advances in Experimental Medicine and Biology*. Vol 474. Kluwer Academic/Plenum; 1999.

152. The Lake Louise consensus on the definition and quantification of altitude illness. In: Sutton JR, Coates G, Houston C, eds. *Hypoxia and Mountain Medicine*. Queen City Press; 1992.

153. Luks AM. Do we have a "best practice" for treating high-altitude pulmonary edema? *High Alt Med Biol*. 2008;9:111-114.

154. Koch RO, Burtscher M. Do we have a "best practice" for treating high-altitude pulmonary edema? [Letter to the Editor]. *High Alt Med Biol*. 2008;9:343-344.

155. Zafren K. Management of altitude illnesses. In: Hawkins SC, ed. *Wilderness EMS*. Wolters Kluwer; 2018.

156. Hackett PH, Rennie D, Levine HD. The incidence, importance, and prophylaxis of acute mountain sickness. *Lancet*. 1976;2:1149-1155.

157. Bartsch P, Maggiorini M, Mairbaurl H, et al. Pulmonary extravascular fluid accumulation in climbers. *Lancet*. 2002;360:571-572.

158. Singh I, Kapila CC, Khanna PK, et al. High-altitude pulmonary oedema. *Lancet*. 1965;191:229-234.

159. Lipman GS, Kanaan NC, Holck PS, et al. Ibuprofen prevents altitude illness: randomized controlled trial for prevention of altitude illness with nonsteroidal anti-inflammatories. *Ann Emerg Med*. 2012;59(6):484-490.

160. Gertsch JH, Corbett B, Holck PS, et al. Altitude sickness in climbers and efficacy of NSAIDs trial (ASCENT): randomized, controlled trial of ibuprofen versus placebo for prevention of altitude illness. *Wilderness Environ Med*. 2012;23:307-315.

161. Gertsch JH, Lipman GS, Holck PS, et al. Prospective, double-blind, randomized, placebo-controlled comparison of acetazolamide versus ibuprofen for prophylaxis against high altitude headache: the headache evaluation at altitude trial (HEAT). *Wilderness Environ Med*. 2010;21:236-243.

162. Pollard AJ, Niermeyer S, Barry PB, et al. Children at high altitude: an international consensus statement by an ad hoc committee of the International Society for Mountain Medicine. *High Alt Med Biol*. 2001;2(3):389-403.

Suggested Reading

Auerbach PS, ed. *Auerbach's Wilderness Medicine*. 7th ed. Mosby Elsevier; 2017.

Bechdel L, Ray S. *River Rescue: A Manual for Whitewater Safety*. 4th ed. CFS Press; 2009.

Bennett P, Elliott D. *Bennett and Elliots' Physiology and Medicine of Diving*. 5th ed. Saunders; 2003.

Bierens JJLM. *Drowning: Prevention, Rescue, Treatment*. 2nd ed. Springer; 2014.

Bove AA. *Bove and Davis' Diving Medicine*. 4th ed. Saunders; 2003.

Hawkins SC, ed. *Wilderness EMS*. Wolters Kluwer; 2018.

Hawkins SC, Simon RB, Beissinger JP, Simon D. *Vertical Aid: Essential Wilderness Medicine for Climbers, Trekkers, and Mountaineers*. The Countryman Press; 2017.

Rodway GW, Weber DC, McIntosh SE. *Mountain Medicine and Technical Rescue*. Carreg; 2016.

United States Lifesaving Association. *Open Water Lifesaving—The United States Lifesaving Association Manual*. 3rd ed. Pearson; 2017.

제**21**장

야생 외상 처치

Lead Editors
Will Smith, MD, Paramedic, FAEMS
John Trentini, MD, PhD, FAWM

학습 목표　이 장의 학습을 완료하면 다음과 같은 내용을 수행할 수 있다.

- 야생 EMS 운영 및 외상 처치에 대한 단순화된 접근 방식을 나타내는 LATE 약어의 네 가지 원칙에 관해 설명할 수 있다.
- 야생 EMS 처치 제공자의 수준과 손상 및 질병 발생 시점부터 의료 기관까지 표준 환자 처치를 어떻게 연속적으로 상호 작용해야 하지 파악할 수 있다.
- "모든 야생에서 발생한 환자는 다른 원인이 확인될 때까지 저체온증, 저혈당, 저혈량증 상태이다"라는 격언의 이유에 대해 논의할 수 있다.
- 야생에서 출혈을 지혈하는 단계별 방법, 어떤 상황에서 지혈대를 사용해야 하는지, 언제 지혈대 제거를 고려해야 하는지 설명할 수 있다.
- 야생에서 흔히 발생하는 물림과 쏘임의 증상과 징후 및 처치에 관해 설명할 수 있다.
- 야생에서 외성 처치 시 고려해야 할 몇 가지 운영상 구체적인(처치 범위 확대) 프로토콜에 관해 설명할 수 있다.

시나리오

당신은 지역 수색 및 구조팀 의료팀 리더이며 담당 지역의 유명한 계곡으로 출동하였다. 현재 가지고 있는 유일한 정보는 긴급 위성 통신을 통해 송출되는 조난 신호의 GPS 위치뿐이다. 현재 시각은 18시이고 기온은 23℃이다. 일기 예보에 따르면 저녁 내내 천둥 번개가 치고 밤새 최저기온이 2℃로 떨어질 것으로 예상된다. 팀은 LATE[위치(Location), 접근(Access), 처치(Treat), 구출(Excurrent)] 약어를 사용하여 대응 계획을 세우기 시작한다.

당신 팀은 수중 구조 키트, 고각 구조 키트, 개인보호장비 및 표준 의료키트 등 필요한 장비를 조립하고 해당 위치로 출동을 시작한다. 팀 리더인 당신은 사고지휘관과 연락하여 계곡 정상에서 사고지휘소까지 통신 중계가 가능하도록 단계별 팀원들과 통신 계획을 수립한다.

- 이러한 유형의 구조 시나리오에서 가장 심각하고 가능성이 높은 부상을 처리하기 위해 팀과 개인 의료 키트에 필수적인 항목은 무엇인가?
- 원격 및 장기간 현장에서 환자를 처치하기 위해 어떤 운영상 구체적인(업무 범위 확대) 프로토콜을 원하는가? 통신 방법이 제한적일 것으로 예상되므로 대기 명령이 있는가?
- 구조팀에 대한 어떤 안전 문제를 고려해야 하는가? 시간, 환자의 위치, 팀의 경험 및 훈련과 같은 상황적 요인이 안전에 어떤 영향을 미치는가?

(다음 페이지에 계속)

개요

야생의 혹독한 환경에서 병원 밖에서 의료서비스를 제공하는 것은 야생 EMS의 도전 과제이다. 여러 가지 의학적 상태는 야생과 기존 EMS 환경 모두에서 유사하게 발생할 수 있지만, 극한의 더위, 추위, 습기, 고도에 노출되는 등 야생 환경과 관련된 외상으로 인해 많은 질환이 악화할 수 있다. 또한 험난한 지형은 낙상 및 기타 손상의 위험을 증가시킨다. 야생 환경과 관련된 특정 문제는 아주 독특하고 복잡하여 하위 전문 자격 인증의 전체 영역이 야생 EMS에 전념하고 있다. 이러한 야생 환경에서 의료서비스를 제공하는 책임을 맡은 병원 전 처치 제공자는 직면할 수 있는 문제에 적절하게 대비한다.

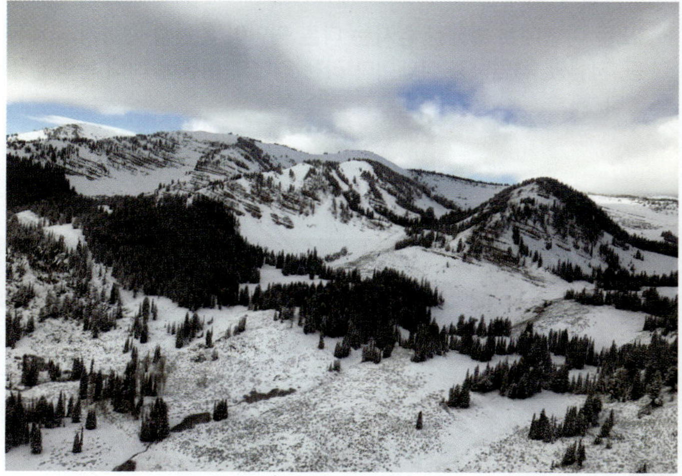

그림 21-1 야생은 전통적으로 문명에서 멀리 떨어진 지역으로 생각되지만, 재난이나 기타 자원이 제한된 사고(예: 다수 사상자 발생)가 발생하면 길거리의 EMS 환경에서도 유사한 상황이 발생할 수 있다.
Courtesy of Will Smith.

야생 EMS 정의

야생, 오지, 외딴 지역, 고립된 지역, 척박한 지역 등 문명에서 멀리 떨어진 지역을 설명하는 데 많은 용어가 사용된다(**그림 21-1**). EMS 요원은 이러한 용어를 "야생"이라는 범주로 묶어 사용하는 경향이 있다. 야생의 사전적 정의는 다음과 같다.

- 인간이 경작하지 않고 거주하지 않는 지역
- 자연적으로 발달한 생활 공동체와 함께 인간 활동으로 인해 본질적으로 방해받지 않는 지역

- 비어 있거나 길이 없는 지역

EMS는 환자 처치에 중점을 두기 때문에 야생 EMS의 정의는 앞서 정의한 야생 정의와 약간 다르다. 야생 EMS 정의는 실제로 야생에 있는 환자에게 의료서비스를 적용하는 것이다. 야생 외상 처치에 관한 이 장에서는 "언제 어디에서 야생 EMS를 접하게 되는가?"와 같은 질문에 대한 지침을 제공한다. 즉, "언제 우리는 최전선이나 길거리 EMS 환경에서 하는 방식과 다르게 생각하고 일해야 하는가?"와 같은 이 질문에 대한 지침을 제공한다. 이 질문에 대한 답은 단순한 지리적 위치를 넘어 다음과 같은 많은 고려 사항을 포함한다.

- 현장 접근
- 날씨
- 일조
- 지형 및 고도
- 특수 이송 및 이송 요구 사항
- 접근 및 이송 시간
- 가용 인원
- 통신
- 위험 요소
- 사용할 수 있는 의료 및 구조 장비
- 특정 환경에 대한 손상 패턴

야생 EMS에 대한 기존의 관점을 확장하는 수많은 사례가 존재한다. 예를 들어 다음을 고려한다.

- 지진이 발생한 후 도시에서는 부상자나 갇힌 사람들에게 접근하기 어렵고 이송을 위한 도로가 파괴되어 없을 수 있으며 지역 EMS 체계가 무력화되거나 과부하가 걸릴 수 있다. 이러한 상황에서는 환자가 상당한 시간 동안 해당 위치에 머물러 있을 가능성이 높다. 그들은 산에 넘어져 병원까지 몇 시간 또는 며칠이 걸리는 등산객과 같은 처치가 필요하다.
- 폭풍우가 몰아치는 늦은 저녁 교외의 넓은 공원에서 넘어진 환자는 야생과 같은 유형의 낙상 사고를 당한 환자와 같은 위험에 노출되어 있다. 환자는 저체온증, 고정 문제, 상처 관리 및 어려운 환자 구출과 같은 문제를 예상하고 관리할 수 있는 로프, 아이젠, 병원 전 처치 제공자로 포함된 구조팀이 필요할 수 있다.

야생 EMS와 기존 거리 EMS 비교

우리는 종종 야생 EMS가 기존의 거리 EMS와 무엇이 다른지에 대해 이야기하지만, 실제로는 EMS의 모든 측면이 스펙트럼에 존재한다. 스

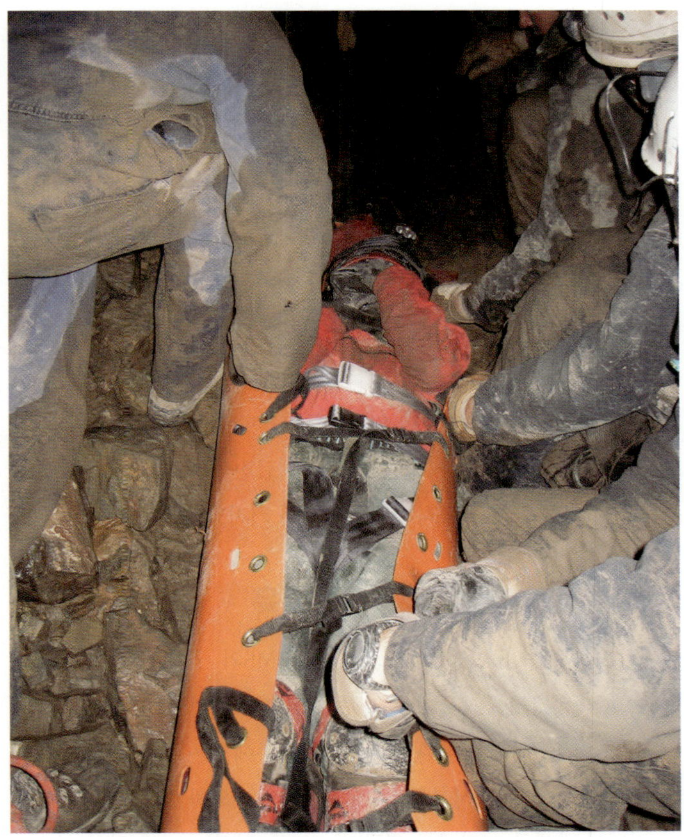

그림 21-2 동굴에서의 환자 처치는 의심할 여지없이 야생 EMS를 대표한다.
Courtesy of Will Smith

펙트럼의 한쪽 끝에는 Level I 외상센터에서 반 블록 떨어진 곳에서 발생한 사그가 있고 스펙트럼의 다른 쪽 끝에는 서부 와이오밍에 있는 윈드아이스 동굴 시스템의 가장 깊은 곳에서 발생한 사고가 있다 (**그림 21-2**). 야생 EMS는 시골과 국경 지역의 EMS 환경을 뛰어넘는다. 최종 분석에서 거리 EMS는 어디에서 끝나고 야생 EMS는 어디에서 시작되는가? 정답은 "상황에 따라 다르다"이다. 구급차에서 응급실까지의 거리, 날씨 및 지형에 따라 다르다. 사용할 수 있는 자원과 자원이 손상되지 않고 작동하는지에 따라 다르다. 더 중요한 것은 손상의 성격과 현장에 출동한 EMS 및 구조대원의 역량에 따라 달라진다.

이러한 상황별 EMS 변화를 인식할 때 손상을 입은 시점부터 외상센터에 제공되는 최종 처치, 재활 시설 또는 자택에서 환자가 기본 기능으로 돌아올 때까지 야생 EMS를 전체 의료시스템의 일부로 고려해야 한다는 것은 분명하다. 문서화, 품질 보증, 의료 감독, 프로토콜, 기술 검증 및 기타 요소는 기존 거리 EMS 시스템의 주축을 이루는 요소로 야생 EMS 시스템의 구성 요소이기도 하다.

야생 EMS 시스템

최적의 야생 환자 처치를 위해서는 몇 가지 문제가 중요하며 이는 일반 거리에서와 관리가 다른 일반적인 문제이다. 이 장에서는 야생의 의료 응급 상황과 관련된 여러 문제에 대한 개요를 제공한다. 야생 환경에서 활동하는 병원 전 처치 제공자는 공식적인 역할을 하는 병원 전 처치 제공자의 특정 교육을 받아야 한다(**Box 21-1**). 또한 지식이 풍부한 의사의 의료 지도는 야생 의료 활동의 필수 요소여야 한다. 미국의 많은 지역에서는 수색 및 구조팀(SAR)에 대한 의료 감독이 없다. 이는 차선책이긴 하지만, 의료 지도를 제공하는 모범 사례는 야생 및 기타 열악한 환경에서 활동하는 의료진을 포함하여 모든 병원 전 EMS 제공자에게 필수적이라는 인식이 커지고 있다.

야생 EMS 제공자를 위한 교육

야생 EMS 실무자는 전통적으로 기존 EMS와 구분됐다. 일부에서는 이들을 응급처치 제공자로 간주하여 EMS 규정의 적용을 받지 않는 것으로 간주하기도 했다. 심지어 일부 주에서는 스키 패트롤과 같은 특정 야생 EMS 종사자를 EMS 규정에서 제외하기도 했다. 손상이나 질병이 발생한 시점에서 제공되는 모든 처치는 전체 처치 시스템에 통합되어야 한다는 인식이 점차 확산하고 있다. 이러한 통합은 예방부터 시작해야 하며 손상 현장에서 기존의 응급 처치를 제공하는 대응자부터 기존 EMS 및 최종 병원 처치까지 모두 포함해야 한다. 일부 전통적인 야생 EMS 교육 프로그램 및 인증은 전통적인 길거리 EMS 모델과 직접적으로 일치하지 않지만, 야생의 특정 대응자는 일반적으로 지정된 수준의 교육을 받는다. 야생 지역에서 활동하는 병원 전 처치 제공자는 일반적으로 지정된 수준에서 훈련받지만, 일부 전통적인 야생 EMS 교육 프로그램 및 인증은 기존의 거리 EMS 모델과 직접적으로 일치하지 않는다. 미국 응급의학회(NAEMSP) 및 기타 조직은 이러한 병원 전 처치 제공자의 업무 범위를 표준화하여 훈련 및 환자 처치의 모범 사례를 보장하는 데 도움을 주시 시작했다.

일반적인 야생 EMS 인증에는 다음이 포함된다.

- 야생 응급의료 대응자(WFA). 기본 수준의 야생 응급처치 교육이고 일반적으로 16~20시간 과정이다.
- 야생 전문 응급처치(WAFA). 야생 응급처치 교육 과정을 기반으로 하는 교육이고 일반적으로 36~40시간 과정이다.
- 야생 응급의료 대응자(WEMR)/야생 최초반응자(WFR). 가장 일반적인 수준의 야생 응급의료종사자이다. 많은 수색 및 구조팀과 산악 및 기타 가이드 서비스에는 이 수준의 교육을 받은 개인이 있다. 일부 교육 모델에서는 국가가 인정하는 EMS 표준을 만들기 위해 응급의료 대응자(EMR) 인증을 충족하기 위해 NREMT 실무 범위와 결합하기도 한다. 이 과정은 일반적으로 70~80시간 과정이다. 일부 온라인 및 혼합 교육 프로그램도 개발 중이다. 이 과정은 원격 치료 환경에서 필요한 의학적 의사 결정, 중요한 술기 및 환자 처치, 대피 시기 및 안전한 작업 방법에 중점을 둔다.
- 야생 응급구조사(WEMT): 기존의 EMT 과정에 추가된 모듈로 구성된 과정으로 야생 응급의료 대응자/야생 최초반응자 의사결정, 술기 및 야생 프로토콜 등이 포함된다.
- 야생 응급처치(OEC): 국가 스키 패트롤 대원에게 일반적으로 가르치는 BLS 과정이 일반적으로 80~100시간으로 구성된다. 기존 EMT 및 WEMT 교육과 많은 유사점이 있지만, 몇 가지 차이점이 있다. 많은 환경에서 스키 패트롤 대원은 수색 및 구조팀과 협력하며 두 그룹 모두 야생 EMS 처치를 제공한다(**그림 21-3**).
- 파크메틱(ParkMedic): 일반적으로 많은 외딴 국립공원관리사무소(NPS)가 있는 지역에서 최적의 환자 처치를 위해 필요한 야생 응급의료 술기 세트를 갖춘 AEMT 수준의 과정이다. 국립공원 관리 사무소는 이 인증을 받기 위해 수년 동안 야생 EMS 제공자를 훈련시

<table>
<tr><td>

</td></tr>
</table>

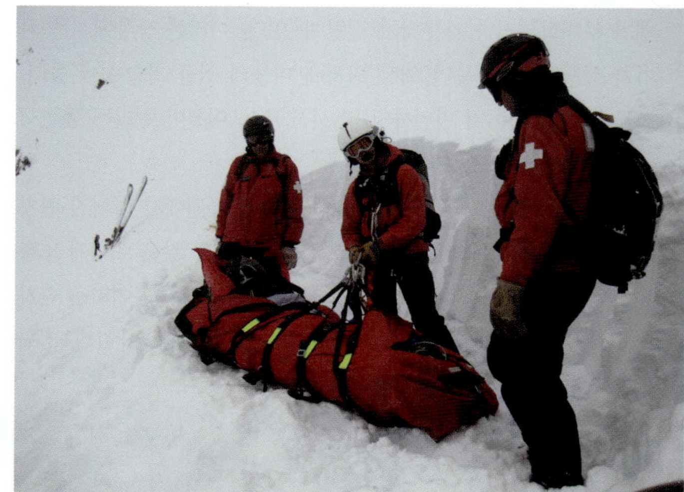

그림 21-3 스키 패트롤과 수색 및 구조대는 종종 최적의 환자 처치를 제공하기 위해 야생 EMS 환경에서 상호 작용한다.

Courtesy of Will Smith.

켜 왔다. 1970년대부터 캘리포니아 대학교 샌프란시스코 프레즈노 응급의학 프로그램에서 격년으로 1월에 교육을 실시해 왔다.

- 야생 고급 응급구조사(AEMT), 야생 파라메딕. 일반적으로 기존 EMS 프로그램과 유사한 교육을 받은 후 지역 및 전국 회의 및 교육 과정을 통해 ALS 제공자를 위한 증강 교육을 받는다.
- 야생 진료보조인력(PA), 야생 상급 전문 간호사(APRN): 야생 처치에 관여하거나 야생 EMS 시스템에서 공식적인 임무를 수행할 수 있는 사람들을 위해 제공되는 교육이다. 미국의 많은 지역, 특히 야생 지역이나 시골 지역에는 PA 또는 APRN이 배치되어 있다.
- 야생 의사: 일반적으로 1차 또는 하위 전문위원회 인증(예: 응급의학, 외과, 가정 의학 등)을 보유하고 있지만, 우연히 야생에서 환자를 돌보게 된 의사 또는 때에 따라서는 야생 응급의료 전담팀의 팀원이자 의료 책임자인 의사를 위한 교육이다. 이들은 팀이나 기관에 의료 지도를 제공할 뿐만 아니라 종종 직접 환자에게 처치를 제공하기도 한다. 다른 관련 의료 전문가(예: 수의사, 치과 의사)도 적절한 교육과 경험을 갖춘다면 야생 의료에 참여할 수 있다. 공식적인 학술 단체에서 다른 교육 프로그램에 이르기까지 의사에게 이러한 종류의 교육을 제공하는 여러 프로그램과 단체가 있다.

야생 EMS 의료 지도

이 장에서 전방 지역은 기존의 EMS가 출동할 수 있는 모든 지역을 의미하며 오지와 대조적으로 외딴곳, 종종 험준한 지역을 의미한다. 일부 국가의 EMS 체계에서 의료 지도를 받는 것처럼 야생 EMS 시스템도 의료 지도를 받아야 한다. 복잡한 의학적 의사결정과 장기간의 환자 처치는 사실상 모두 대기 명령이 필요하므로 어떤 측면에서는 더욱 중요하다. 이러한 의료 지도를 제공하는 의료 지도 의사는 이러한 환경에서 처치에 영향을 미치는 변수에 대해 잘 알고 있어야 한다. 또한 의료 지도 의사는 처치 제공자의 업무 범위와 한계도 이해해야 한다. 일부 환경에서는 의료 지도 의사가 현장에서 직접 의료 지도를 제공하고 때로는 환자를 직접 처치할 수도 있다. 의료 지도 의사가 현장에 투입되면 이러한 환경에서 안전하게 자신을 관리할 수 있도록 충분한 교육과 역량을 갖추어야 한다.

야생 EMS 기관

야생 EMS를 제공하는 기관이 많이 있다. 야생 EMS 기관의 예는 다음과 같다.

- 수색 및 구조팀
- 국립, 주립 및 지역 공원
- 스키 패트롤
- 원정 의료팀
- 특수 군사 팀

야생 EMS 상황

주요 야생 EMS/수색 및 구조 원칙: 위치 파악, 접근, 처치, 구출(LATE)

많은 수색 및 구조 작전의 공통 구성 요소인 야생 EMS에서는 몇 가지 핵심 원칙을 통해 전체 임무 또는 출동을 간소화할 수 있다. 첫 번째 시나리오에서 설명한 것처럼 LATE(위치 파악, 접근, 처치, 구출)는 대응을 구성하는 데 도움이 될 수 있다. 일반적으로 모든 야생 EMS 운영에는 각 단계의 일부 구성 요소가 포함된다(**Box 21-2**).

- 환자의 위치 파악은 모든 사건 또는 구조 요청의 첫 번째 단계이다. 환자를 찾아야 처치를 시작할 수 있다. 어떤 상황에서는 119에 신고해 정확한 위치를 알리고 있다면 이 과정이 쉬울 수 있다. 다른 상황에서는 이것이 더 어려울 수 있으며 광범위한 수색 작업을 수행해야 할 수도 있다.
- 접근은 기술적인 문제로 어려울 수 있다. 예를 들어, 환자가 발견되었지만, 거센 강물이 흐르는 반대편 기슭에 있을 수 있다. 이러한 유형의 상황은 기존의 길거리 EMS와 야생 EMS를 구별하는 요소이다.
- 처치는 종종 야생 EMS의 진정한 정의가 명확해지는 단계이다. 일부 처치는 길거리 EMS 환경에서 수행되는 것과 같을 수 있지만, 다

른 처치 개입은 언제 적용해야 하는지와 같은 의학적 의사결정은 중요한 방식에서 다를 수 있다. 이러한 결정에 따라 다음 단계의 구조 시간이 크게 달라질 수 있을 뿐만 아니라 환자와 구조자의 위험도 달라질 수 있다.

- 구출은 이러한 단순화된 구조 원칙의 마지막 단계이다. 이러한 원칙 중 일부는 중복될 수 있지만, 일부는 다른 원칙보다 우선시될 수 있다. 위험 물질이나 전술적 상황과 마찬가지로 정맥 라인을 확보하고 수액을 투여하는 것과 같은 표준 처치 방법보다 구조가 우선순위가 높을 수 있다.

전문적인 구조의 조화

야생 EMS 제공자는 적절한 처치를 제공해야 할 뿐만 아니라 험준한 지형에 있는 환자에게 안전하게 접근할 수 있어야 한다. 즉 전문적인 구조 방법을 탐색할 수 있어야 한다. 이러한 문제 또는 조화는 종종 야생 EMS 환경을 정의하는 데 도움이 된다. 구조대는 매우 다양할 수 있지만, 야생 EMS 제공 방식의 몇 가지 예는 다음과 같다.

- 자가 구조
- 동반자 구조
- 목격자 구조
- 조직된 소규모 그룹/스트라이크 팀 구조(예: 전문 수색 및 구조팀)
- 스키 패트롤
- 조직화한 대규모 그룹 구조
- 소방서 전문 구조대
- 산업 현장 구조팀
- 군대 시스템(예: 항공응급구조사)
- 복잡한 대응을 조율하는 다중 그룹/기관 간 구조

야생 EMS 영역

야생 EMS에는 많은 영역이 있다. 여기에는 몇 가지 잠재적인 시나리오가 나열되어 있으며 각 시나리오에는 특정 환자 처치 고려 사항, 환자 접근 제한 및 종종 완화하거나 극복해야 하는 기타 개별 요인이 있다.

- 공간
- 높은 각도(절벽/거의 수직)
- 가파른 각도(산길의 도로 측면)
- 낮은 각도
- 눈사태
- 동굴, 밀폐된 공간, 협곡(도보여행)

- 헬기 운영(장거리, 단거리)
- 잔잔한 물, 급류, 개방 수역
- 전지형 차량, 오프로드 차량, 스노모빌, 산악자전거
- 헬기를 이용한 구조
- 눈, 빙하, 크레바스 구조
- 등산, 암벽등반
- 높은 고도
- 다이빙

야생에서의 손상 유형

외상으로 인한 사망은 3단계 분포를 보인다. 자세한 내용은 1장 PHTLS: 과거, 현재 및 미래를 참조한다. 첫 번째 사망 단계는 손상 후 몇 초에서 몇 분 이내에 발생한다. 이 첫 번째 단계에서 발생하는 사망은 일반적으로 뇌, 뇌줄기, 위쪽 척수, 심장, 대동맥 또는 기타 큰 혈관의 손상으로 인해 발생하며 헬멧 착용과 같은 예방 조치로 가장 잘 관리할 수 있다. 이러한 환자 중 소수만을 살릴 수 있으며 일반적으로 신속한 이송이 가능한 대도시 지역에서만 생명을 구조할 수 있다.

두 번째 사망 단계는 손상 후 몇 분에서 몇 시간 이내에 발생합니다. 이 두 번째 단계의 외상 사망을 줄이기 위해 신속한 평가와 소생술이 시행된다. 이 단계에서 발생하는 사망은 일반적으로 경막밑혈종, 경막외혈종, 혈액기흉, 비장 파열, 간 열상, 골반 골절 또는 심각한 출혈과 관련된 다발성 손상으로 인해 발생한다. 이러한 환자에게는 외상 처치의 기본 원칙(지혈, 기도 관리, 균형 잡힌 수액 소생술 및 적절한 의료기관으로 이송)을 가장 잘 적용할 수 있다. 세 번째 사망 단계는 초기 손상 후 며칠 또는 몇 주 후에 발생하며 대부분 패혈증과 장기 부전으로 인해 발생한다.

병원 전 처치 제공자는 주로 두 번째 사망 단계에서 환자를 구하는 데 중점을 둔다. 야생에서 살아남아 구조되는 대부분 사람은 이미 첫 번째 사망 단계와 두 번째 단계를 통과했다. 그러나 수색 및 구조팀에 의료 교육을 받은 팀원이 있으면 두 번째 단계와 관련된 사망을 예방할 수 있다. 이러한 야생 응급처치는 종종 "환자가 사망하거나 나중에 심각한 합병증을 겪지 않도록 지금 무엇을 할 수 있을까?"에 초점을 맞추는 경우가 많다. 야생 EMS 제공자는 탈수로 인한 신부전, 굶주림으로 인한 저항력 저하로 인한 감염, 심각한 저체온증, 불필요한 고정으로 인한 욕창궤양으로 인한 피부 괴사 등의 문제가 발생하지 않도록 주의한다.

예방적 수색 및 구조 프로그램은 야생 EMS와 직면하는 것을 제한하고 줄이기 위해 중요한 초점이 되었다. 스키장의 헬멧과 기타 안전 장비의 사용으로 이용객의 이환율과 사망률을 감소시켰다. 와이오밍 주 잭슨에 있는 티턴 카운티 수색 및 구조팀과 협력하여 국립공원관리사무소(NPS) 및 Back Country Zero와 같은 기타 프로그램에서는 교육 및 예방을 촉진하는 광범위한 프로그램을 운영하고 있다.

안전

야생에서는 거리에서보다 훨씬 더 현장 안전이 중요한 고려 사항이다. 야생에서 다치거나 죽은 EMS 제공자는 환자의 처치에 집중하지 못하게 하고 성공적인 구조 임무의 가능성을 제한한다. 거리 현장의 안전 고려 사항은 야생에서도 적용된다. 특히 병원 전 처치 제공자가 주어진 환경에서 적절하게 훈련되지 않으면 현장의 위험이 거리보다 덜 분명할 수 있다.

야생 EMS 종사자와 환자는 환경과 날씨 변화에 노출된다. 예를 들어, 눈을 동반한 한랭 전선이 다가오면 구출 작업이 복잡해지거나 심지어 야생 의료 제공자와 환자가 다치거나 죽을 수도 있다. 구조가 몇 시간 또는 며칠 동안 지속되면 음식과 물 부족으로 쇠약해질 수 있다. 야생 지형은 종종 험준한 경우가 많으며 위험한 전문 기술이 필요한 지형 때문에 환자 처치와 구출을 복잡해질 수 있다(**그림 21-4**). 야생 EMS 제공자는 낙석, 눈사태 위험, 해수면 상승, 높은 고도 또는 고도 노출, 폭포 바닥의 소용돌이와 같은 환경 특유의 위험에 대해 알고 있어야 한다.

수색 및 구조팀의 각 구성원은 팀의 안전, 건강 및 복지를 종합적으로 보장하기 위해 적절한 준비와 예방 조처를 해야 한다. 모든 팀원은 작업할 특정 환경의 위험과 위험에 대해 교육을 받아야 한다. 또한 자신의 한계를 알고 손상 입은 환자를 구조하기 위해 자기 능력을 초과하지 않아야 한다. 수색 및 구조팀의 각 구성원은 환경 조건과 구조에 필요한 복장과 개인보호장비를 적절하게 준비한다. 마지막으로 수색 및 구조팀의 의학적 요구를 충족시키는 것은 대응 노력의 필수적인 요소여야 한다. 수색 및 구조팀 팀원의 잠재적인 질병이나 손상에 대처할 수 있는 적절한 물품과 작업-휴식 주기를 시행하면 수색 및 구조팀이 원활하게 활동하는 데 도움이 된다.

상황에 따른 적절한 처치

의학이 발전함에 따라 우리의 의학 지식, 이해 및 기술은 변화하지만, 기본 원칙 중 일부는 수년에 걸쳐 거의 변하지 않으며 환자의 위치와

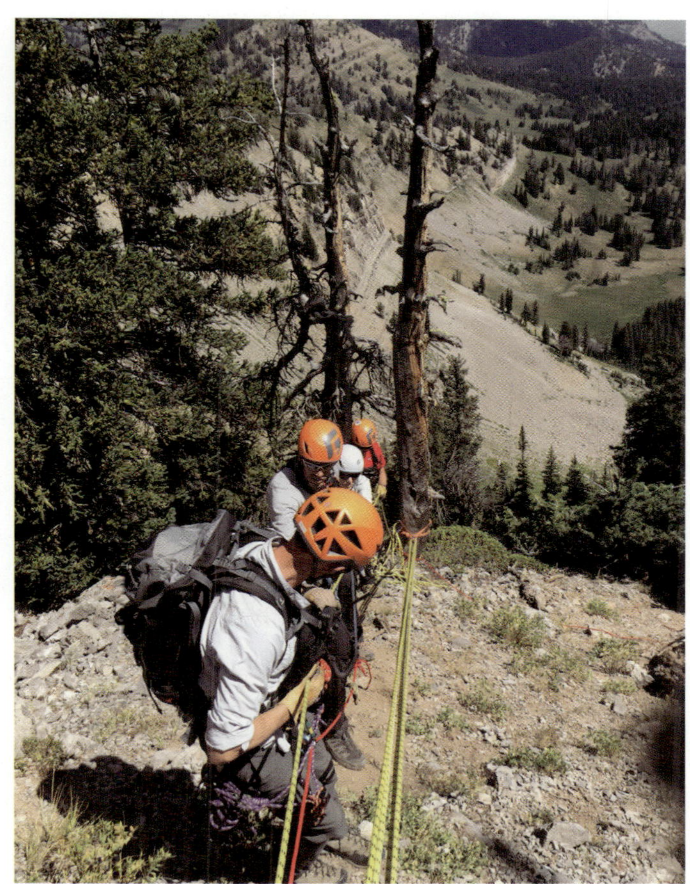

그림 21-4 가파른 경사면, 절벽, 낙석, 고르지 않은 지형은 야생 구조 시 위험하다.
Courtesy of Will Smith.

무관하다. PHTLS는 중상을 입은 환자를 가능한 한 빨리 적절한 의료기관으로 이송해야 한다고 오랫동안 주장해 왔으며 때로는 위급하지 않은 상태에 대한 자세한 신체검사 및 처치 없이도 이송할 수 있다. 그러나 적절한 처치는 상황에 따라 달라질 수 있다. 자세한 신체검사와 위급하지 않은 상태의 정의는 도시 거리에서와 깊은 산속에서 다를 수 있다(**그림 21-5**). 상황, 지식수준, 술기 능력, 현장 상황 및 이용할 수 있는 장비에 따라 외상 환자의 의학적 의사 결정 및 처치가 달라질 수 있다(이 개념은 2장, 황금 원칙, 선호도, 비판적 사고에 소개되어 있다).

이상적인 처치

야생 EMS에서는 복잡한 의료 결정이 "현실에 이상적인" 의료 개점을 기반으로 이루어져야 한다. 이러한 의사 결정 과정은 야생 EMS 제공자와 일반 거리 EMS 제공자와 야생 EMS 제공자를 구별하는 요소이다. 대부분의 야생 EMS 상황에서는 즉흥적으로 대처할 수 있는 능력

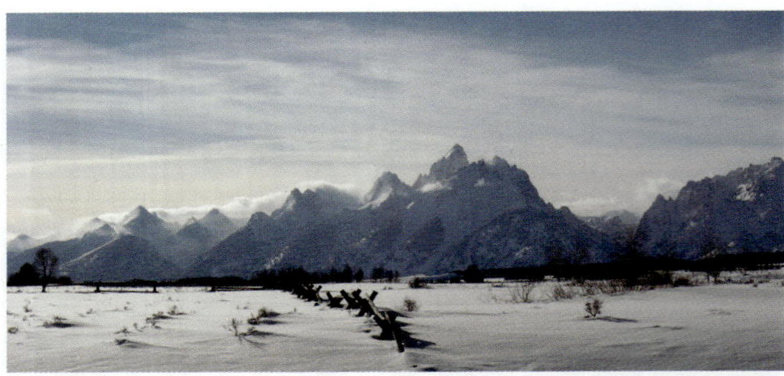

그림 21-5 야생 지형
Courtesy of Will Smith.

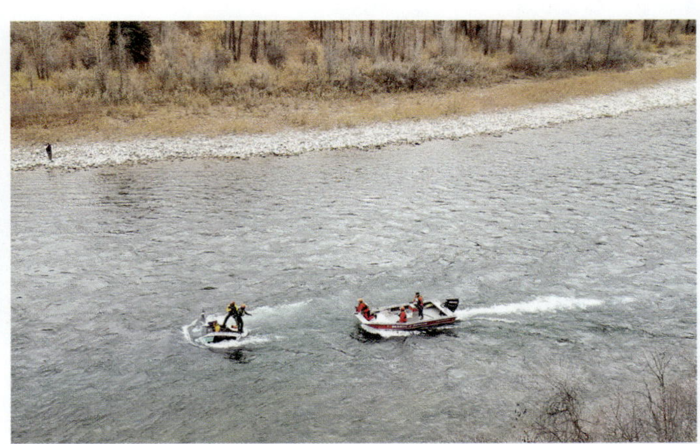

그림 21-6 자동차 충돌 후 흐르는 강 한가운데 차량에 갇힌 환자는 프로토콜을 변경하여 처치해야 할 수 있다. 야생에서의 외상 처치는 불리한 환경 조건, 물, 진흙, 덤불 및 밀폐된 공간으로 인해 종종 방해받는다.
Courtesy of Brian Coe.

이 거의 표준이며 EMS 제공자는 기존의 이상적인 처치 프로토콜이나 처치를 받아야 하며 자신이 처한 환경의 현실에 맞게 적용하거나 즉흥적으로 대처해야 한다.

복잡한 어깨 골절과 탈구가 있는 환자를 생각해 보면 수술실(OR)에서 적절한 처치는 무엇인가? 대부분은 개방정복 및 내부고정(ORIF)이 필요하다. 그러나 수술실에서 적절한 처치인 개방 정복을 시도하는 것이 응급실에서는 적절한 처치가 아닐 수 있다. 응급실에서는 골절과 탈구를 평가하기 위해 X-ray를 촬영하고 속효성 진통제를 투여하며 통증과 부종을 줄이고 뼈를 완전히 해부학적으로 재정렬하여 신경과 혈관에 가해지는 압력을 줄이기 위해 탈구 폐쇄 정복을 시행한다. 결정적인 개방정복 및 내부고정은 나중에 수술실에서 진행한다.

마찬가지로 응급실에서의 적절한 처치가 거리 EMS 환경에서는 적절한 처치가 아닐 수도 있다. 병원 전 처치 제공자는 평가를 수행하고 처치를 제공할 수 있는 넓고 따뜻하며 건조한 장소의 이점을 누리지 못할 수 있다. 빗속에서 환자가 찌그러진 차량 안에 거꾸로 매달려 있는 상황에서 구조대원이 절단기를 사용하여 금속을 절단하고 제거하여 환자에게 접근하기 위한 작업을 할 수도 있다. 구조대원이 환자를 구출하면 병원 전 처치 제공자는 환자의 다른 손상을 평가하고 팔의 원위부 신경 및 혈관 상태를 확인한 후 어깨를 고정하고 필요한 경우 진통제를 투여하며 환자를 응급실로 신속하게 이송한다. 마찬가지로 거리에서 골절과 탈구를 줄이기 위해 개방정복 및 내부고정을 시도하는 것이 적절한 처치가 아닐 수 있다(프로토콜에 근거).

마지막으로 거리에서의 적절한 처치가 야생에서는 적절한 처치가 아닐 수 있다. 자동차 충돌 후 흐르는 강 한가운데 있거나 물에 잠긴 자동차에 갇힌 환자를 위해 어떤 프로토콜을 수정해야 하는가(**그림**

21-6)? 이 경우 환자 처치 외에도 신속한 수중 구조 기술, 술기 및 변경된 우선순위를 수행해야 한다. 이와 같은 예가 바로 야생 EMS 프로토콜이 최상의 환자 처치를 위해 운영상 구체적인 처치 범위가 필요한 이유이다.

그러나 대부분 상황에서 적절한 처치는 수술실, 응급실, 거리 또는 야생에서 수행되는 경우에 상관없이 적절한 처치이다. 병원 전 처치 제공자는 풍부한 지식, 비판적 사고 능력, 교육, 주요 원칙에 대한 이해가 뒷받침된다면 현장에서 환자를 마주하게 될 다양한 상황을 반영하여 의학적 의사 결정을 내일 수 있다.

작지만 상당한 수의 상황에서 적절한 거리 EMS 처치와 적절한 야생 EMS 처치 사이에는 주목할 만한 차이가 존재한다. 이러한 상황에서는 다음과 같은 중요한 의문이 제기된다.

- 야생에서는 항상 거리 EMS 처치가 최선인가?
- 거리 EMS 처치가 최적의 처치가 아닌 경우 병원 전 처치 제공자는 최적의 처치가 무엇인지 어떻게 알 수 있는가? 이는 프로토콜에 명시되어 있는가?
- 병원 전 처치 제공자는 환자의 손상이 무엇인지 정확히 알 수 없을 때 현장에서 어떻게 대처하는가? 예를 들어, 동굴 깊숙한 곳에서 밧줄에 거꾸로 매달려 있는 환자를 평가할 때 야생 의료 제공자는 골절과 탈구가 있는지 어떻게 판단하는가?
- 병원 전 처치 제공자는 특정 상황 처한 특정 환자에게 거리 또는 야생 처치 중 어느 쪽이 더 적절한지 어떻게 결정하는가?
- 무엇이 상황을 야생이나 거리로 만드는가? 그 사이의 모든 사례는 어떻게 되는가?

이러한 모든 질문에 대한 명확한 답변을 제공하기는 쉽지 않다. 앞서 언급했듯이 "상황에 따라 다르다"라는 대답이 나오는 경우가 많다. 그러나 적어도 좋은 배경 정보는 제공될 수 있으므로 병원 전 처치 제공자는 특정 환자 처치 상황에서 필요에 따라 각자의 상황에 맞게 질문에 답할 수 있다. PHTLS의 철학은 항상 충분한 지식과 핵심 원칙이 제공되면 병원 전 처치 제공자가 환자 처치와 관련하여 합리적인 결정을 내릴 수 있다는 것이다. 결국 당면한 상황과 자원을 바탕으로 해당 환경의 표준이 되는 이상적인 처치를 기반으로 환자에게 진정한 처치를 제공하는 것이다.

야생 EMS 의사 결정: 위험과 이점의 균형

숙련된 의사, 간호사와 병원 전 처치 제공자는 기도 관리 및 상처 처치와 같은 절차가 의학에서 쉬운 부분이라는 것을 알고 있다. 어려운 부분은 언제 무엇을 해야 하는지 아는 것, 즉 비판적 사고이다. 거리에서 더 자주, 야생에서는 한 가지 위험을 다른 위험과 잠재적 비교하여 신중하게 검토해야 한다. 이 특정 환자의 경우 특별한 환경에서 특정 자원을 가지고 특정 시간에 이 특정 도움을 받을 가능성이 있는 경우 잠재적 위험은 무엇인가? 잠재적인 이점은 무엇인가? 야생 EMS는 각 환자에 대한 특정 위험과 이점의 균형을 맞추는 타협의 기술이다.

야생에서 외상 처치에 적용되는 TCCC 및 TECC 원칙

사건의 맥락을 고려하는 것의 중요성은 이라크와 아프가니스탄 분쟁의 전투 및 전술적 환경에서 분명하게 드러났다. TCCC 지침의 개발과 시행은 부상자 생존율 향상과 분명하게 연관되어 있다. 전투 환경에서 배운 많은 개념은 야생 상황에도 적용할 수 있다. 2016년 제7차 세계 야생 의학회에서 이 주제에 대한 전체 사전 회의가 열렸으며 그 결과 보고서가 발간되었다. 이 특별판에는 TCCC, 전장에서 배운 교훈을 다른 위험한 환경에서 적용하기이다. 위험의 원인은 같지 않을 수 있지만(예: 전투 중 입은 총상과 사냥 중 입은 손상 또는 급조 폭발물(IED)로 인한 손상과 눈사태로 인한 손상 등), 구조대와 환자 모두 같은 손상 패턴 및 처치 우선순위를 공유하는 경우가 많다.

TCCC에서 야생 환경으로 추정한 환자 처치 우선순위는 많은 조직에서 널리 채택되었다. 국립공원관리사무소는 매우 다양한 원거

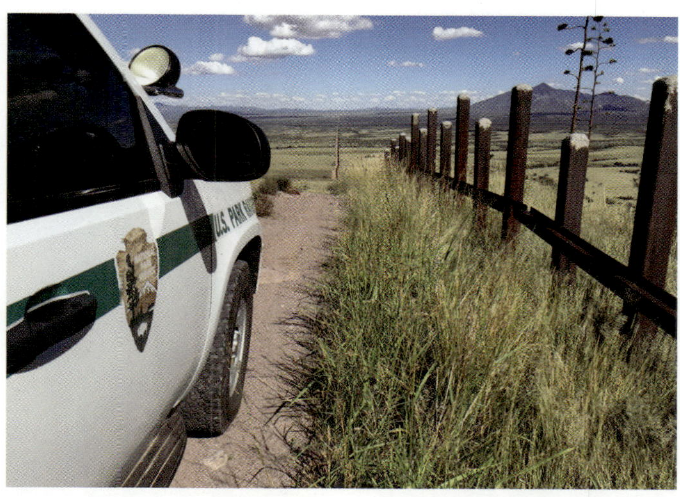

그림 21-7 외상 관련 손상의 가능성이 있는 야생 환경인 미국-멕시코 국경에서 순찰 중인 국립공원 관리사무소 직원
Courtesy of Will Smith.

리 환경에서 처치를 제공해야 하는 특별한 과제를 안고 있다(**그림 21-7**). 국립공원관리사무소의 레인저는 전술 및 야생 프로토콜을 모두 사용하여 외딴 야생 환경에서 환자를 처치한다.

TCCC 전술 지침은 TECC 위원회에서 민간과 정부 사용을 위해 수정 및 채택했다. TECC는 여러 모든 위험 지역(전술, 위험 물질 등)과 확대된 인구(어린이, 노인 등)에 대한 유사한 TCCC 개념을 적용한다. 많은 기관에서 TECC 지침에 따라 처치를 제공하기 시작했으며 구조 테스크포스 프로그램과 같은 공식화된 프로그램을 통해 이러한 처치를 전술 및 기타 위험한 상황(야생 및 원거리 외상 처치 포함)에 통합하고 있다. 전술적 환경에서의 TCCC, TECC 및 환자 처치 우선순위에 대한 자세한 내용은 22장 민간 전술응급의료지원(TEMS)을 참조한다.

환자 이송 원칙

궁극적으로 환자를 야생에서 구출하여 최종 처치를 받을 수 있는 의료기관으로 이송해야 하므로 이송은 야생 EMS에서 가장 중요한 문제가 된다. 때로는 단일 손상을 처치할 때 쉬운 일이 될 수 있다. 예를 들어, 팔의 손상은 부목으로 고정한 후 환자가 걸을 수 있거나 도움을 받아 걸을 수 있다. 그러나 다리 염좌나 골절과 같은 다른 경미한 손상은 환자를 이송해야 할 수도 있다. 더 치명적이거나 생명을 위협하는 손상은 항상 어느 정도의 환자 이송과 더 집중적인 구출이 필요하다. 전문적인 기술이 필요한 상황에서 보행할 수 없는 환자를 대피시키기 위해 다양한 구조 시스템을 사용할 수 있다. **그림 21-8**은

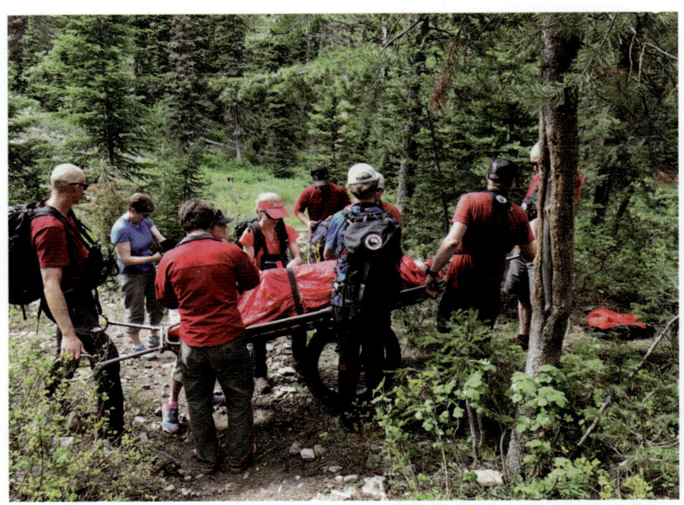

그림 21-8 산악자전거 사고 후 손상을 입은 환자를 이송하는 데 바퀴 달린 들것을 사용하고 있다. 보행할 수 없는 환자를 직접 이동하는 것보다 쉽지만, 여전히 여러 명의 도움이 필요하다.
Courtesy of Will Smith.

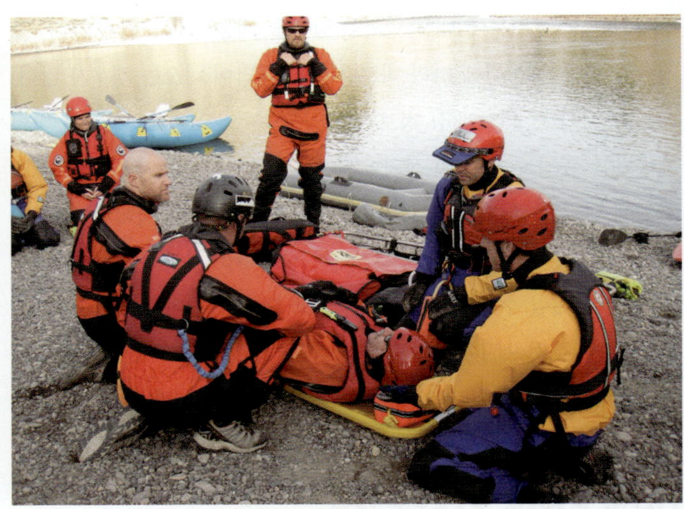

그림 21-9 개인부양장치는 환자를 물 위로 이송할 때마다 필수 이송 보조 장치이다.
Courtesy of Will Smith.

환자가 걸을 수 없을 때 이동시키는 데 사용되는 일반적인 구조 장비인 바퀴 달린 들것에 고정된 환자를 보여준다. 수중 구조작업에서는 구조 능력 외에도 환자에게 부양 장치(예: 개인 부양 장치)를 제공하도록 주의를 기울여야 한다(**그림 21-9**). 야생 EMS 상황에서 환자를 이송할 때는 이러한 모든 요소를 고려해야 한다. 구조가 장시간 지속되는 경우가 많으므로 환자를 이송할 때는 평소보다 더 많은 패딩을 사용해야 하며 환자에게 편안한 자세를 유지하기 위해 지속해 노력을 한다.

부목 적용

부목 적용은 야생뿐만 아니라 모든 EMS 환경에서 거의 모든 손상에 적용할 수 있는 개념이다. 부목은 손상 부위에 정상적인 생리적 기능적 자세로 정렬한 다음 그 위치에서 고정하거나 지지하는 것을 전제로 한다. 긴뼈 손상의 경우 위아래 뼈를 고정하는 것과 같은 개념이 통합되어 있다. 부목을 고정하기 전후에 순환, 감각 및 운동 기능 평가를 수행한 후 지속해서 재평가해야 한다.

야생에서 부목을 적용하려면 일반적으로 기존 EMS 현장보다 훨씬 더 많은 패딩이 필요하다. 이는 야생에서 환자를 이송하는 데 걸리는 시간이 길어지기 때문이다. 또한 환자 이송과 생리학적 부목이 처음에 올바르게 적용되었는지 확인하는 것도 중요하다. 패딩을 더 많이 적용하면 전반적으로 불편함을 줄일 뿐만 아니라 정상적인 신경 혈관 기능을 촉진하고 신속한 구조 작업을 가능하게 한다. 적절하게 부

목과 충분한 패딩을 적용하지 않고 서둘러 환자를 이송하는 경우 구조 작업이 지연될 수 있다.

전신 진공부목(**그림 21-10**)은 전신 고정(척추 움직임 제한/고정 포함)이 필요한 야생 EMS 환자를 위한 표준 처치가 되었다. 다른 특수 장비와 마찬가지로 구조 현장으로 가져가야 하지만, 도시에서 사용할 수 있는 장비보다 휴대성이 좋은 경우가 많다. 단일 팔다리 손상에 소형 진공부목을 사용할 수 있다. 그러나 대부분의 야생 EMS와 마찬가지로 이상적인 장비를 사용하지 못할 수도 있으며 동일한 환자 처치 목표를 달성하기 위해 즉흥적인 방법이 필요할 수도 있다. 이러한 상황은 앞서 설명한 것처럼 이상적인 처치와 실체 처치 개념의 또 다른 예이다.

기도 유지 고려 사항

기도 유지는 EMS 처치에서 최우선 순위이며 이는 오랫동안 ABC(기도, 호흡, 순환)로 이어져 왔다. 야생 EMS에서도 기도 유지를 고려해야 하지만, 때로는 더 높은 수준의 기도 유지가 필요하다. 움직이지 않는 환자를 구출하는 동안 특히 환자가 바로누운자세로 누워 있는 상태에서는 야생 EMS 제공자가 기도 유지를 모니터링하고 환자에게 접근하는 데 제한이 있을 수 있다. 구토 및 기도 손상 가능성이 있는 기도를 고려하는 것이 가장 중요하다. 전문 구조 및 대피 요소는 환자 이송 및 생리적 부목 고정과 균형을 이루어야 한다. 진공부목을 사용해서 환자를 측면으로 이송할 수 있다. 이 방법을 사용하면 중력에 따라 액체와 구토물이 기도에서 더 잘 배출될 수 있다(그

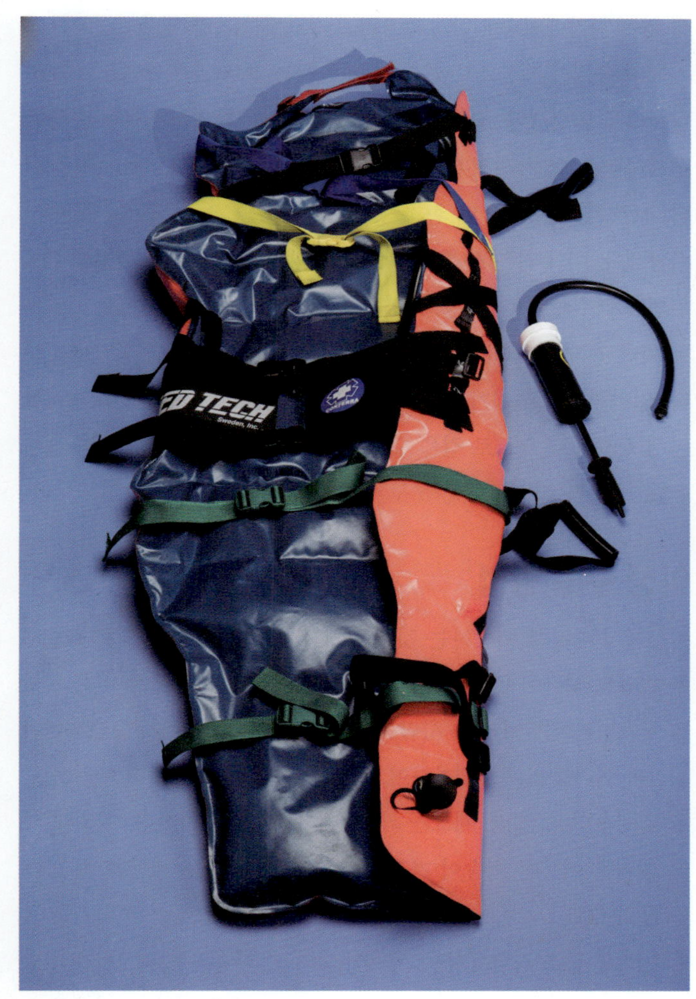

그림 21-10 전신형 진공부목

Courtesy of David Bowers.

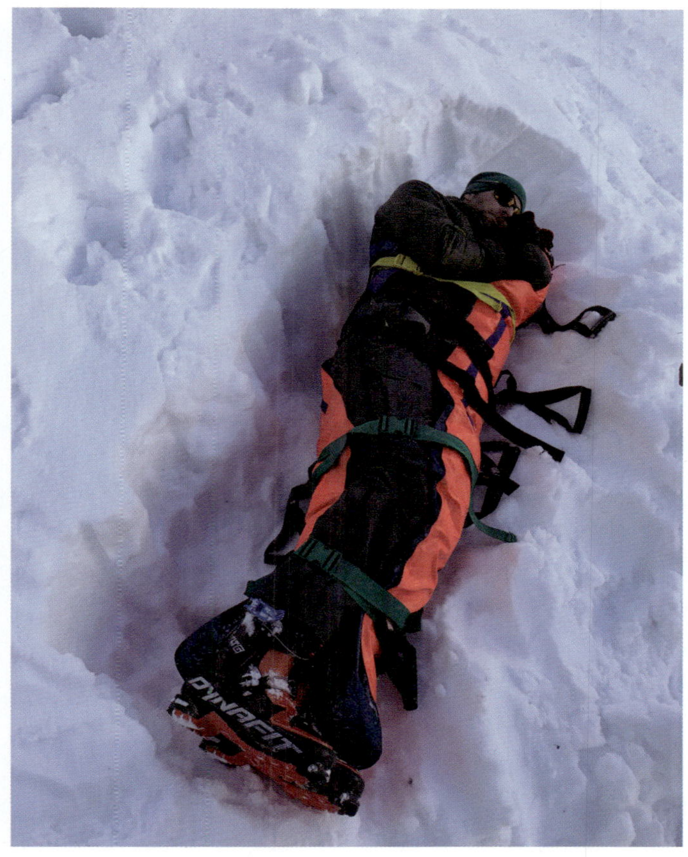

그림 21-11 환자를 진공부목에 옆으로 누운자세로 고정하면 기도를 유지하는 데 도움이 된다.

Courtesy of Will Smith.

림 21-11). 장기간 환자 처치 시 고려해야 할 다른 사항으로 구토가 우려되는 경우 환자에게 항구토제를 사전에 투여하는 등 잠재적인 문제를 예측하는 것이 있다. 쉽게 투여할 방법의 하나는 구강 용해성 정제인 온단세트론이다. 프로메타진과 같은 일반적인 항구토제와 다이펜히드라민과 같은 비정형 제제를 고려할 수 있으며 추가 효과가 있다. 항상 그렇듯이 약물은 적절한 업무 범위 내에서 EMS 제공자에 의해 관리되어야 하며 이에 대한 자세한 논의는 이 텍스트의 범위를 벗어난다.

척추 손상 및 척추 움직임 제한

실제 척추 손상과 의심되는 손상을 가장 잘 처치하는 방법에 대해 EMS가 탄생한 이래로 많은 논쟁이 있었다. 실제 척수 손상과 명백한 신경학적 결손이 있는 환자는 비교적 명확한 처치 방법이 있다. 이러한 환자들은 병원 전 단계에서 처치를 받을 때까지 척추 움직임을 제한해야 한다. 이송 시간이 길어지는 상황에서는 단단한 긴척추고정판보다는 척추 모양에 맞는 진공부목이나 기타 장비를 사용하는 것이 이상적이다.

야생 외상 처치에서 더 큰 딜레마는 명확한 신경학적 결손이 없지만, 척추 손상 가능성이 우려될 때 발생한다. 수년 동안 불안정한 손상이 실제 척수 손상과 장기적인 결손으로 이어질 수 있다는 예상 하에 손상 기전만을 근거하여 환자를 고정했다. 척추 손상 가능성에 대한 이러한 우려에 대한 처치가 EMS 훈련의 주축이 되었다. 척추 움직임 제한(척추 고정 또는 척추 안정화라고도 함)을 적용하는 것은 기존 EMS 처치의 특징적인 특징이었다. 수년 동안 많은 환자가 단단한 목뼈보호대와 함께 기존의 단단한 긴척추고정판을 사용하여 고정하였다.

지난 수십 년 동안 수많은 연구를 통해 "척추 손상 가능성"으로 인해 고정된 환자의 수를 제한하는 처치 방법이 수정되었다. 연구에 따르면 딱딱한 긴척추고정판과 목뼈보호대가 의도한 효과를 제공하지 않고 환자에게 해를 끼치는 경우가 있었다. 연구에 따르면 건강한 지원자라도 30분이 지나면 중간 정도의 통증이 있고 약 45분 정도 지나면 심한 통증을 느끼는 것으로 나타났다. 장시간 고정할 경우 기도 손상, 흡인 위험, 욕창 등 더 우려스러운 문제가 발생할 수 있다. 단단한 목뼈보호대는 부적절하게 적용하면 두개내압 증가, 뇌 유출 감소, 목뼈 떼어 당김과 같은 합병증이 발생할 수 있다. 이러한 합병증은 장시간의 처치 환경에서 발생하는 추가 요인으로 인해 더욱 악화한다. 이러한 이유로 야생 EMS 시스템과 의료진은 척추 움직임 제한을 조기에 시행했다.

야생 및 야생 환경에서의 척추 움직임 제한은 이송 결정, 전문적 구조 시 위험 및 기타 역학 관계에 큰 영향을 미친다. 환자와 구조자에 대한 이러한 위험 증가는 척추 손상 가능성의 작은 위험(많은 경우 정상 신경학적 검사에서 1% 미만)과 균형을 이루어야 한다. 야행 EMS 의사결정 과정을 설명하기 위해 다음 예를 고려한다.

건강한 22세의 여성이 강 협곡을 따라 암벽 등반을 하던 중 20m 아래로 추락했다. 절벽 틈새에 앵커를 설치한 후 하나씩 빠져나가면서 추락 속도를 약간 늦추었다. 하지만 결국 그녀는 땅에 부딪혔다. 헬멧을 쓰고 있던 그녀는 머리를 부딪치며 잠시 의식을 잃었다. 구급차로 최대한 접근할 수 있는 곳으로부터 강 협곡까지 1시간 동안 걸어서 야생 EMS 제공자가 환자에게 도착했다. 환자는 이제 의식이 돌아왔고 경미한 두통만 호소했으며 신경학적 검사와 신체검사 결과도 정상이었다. 친구들은 그녀에게 움직이지 말고 가만히 있으라고 권유했다. 늦가을이고 어두워지고 있으며 가장 가까운 헬기 착륙장까지 한 시간 거리에 있고 오늘 밤 눈보라가 시작될 것이라는 일기 예보가 있다. 환자가 척추 움직임 제한을 받아야 하는가? 가능한 경우 환자의 도움을 받아 걸어 나갈 수 있는가? 야생 EMS 제공자는 수레형 들것을 가지고 있는 수색 및 구조팀에게 지원을 요청하고 밤새도록 장시간 구조 작업을 진행해야 하는가? 이와 유사한 상황에서 환자를 평가하고 처치하기 위한 프로토콜이 있는가?

현재 많은 외상 전문가는 척수 손상이 의심되는 경우에도 야생 EMS 현장에서 단단한 긴척추고정판이 꼭 필요한 것은 아니라고 주장한다. 미국 외 지역에서 한동안 사용되어 온 진공부목은 척수 움직임 제한이 필요한 경우 표준 처치로 자리 잡고 있다. 이러한 장비는 척추에 맞게 유연성이 있으며 단단한 목뼈보호대가 없어도 머리의 움직임을 제한하는 데 사용할 수 있다.

고에너지 손상을 입은 후 눈에 띄는 결손은 없지만 심한 요통이 있는 환자는 잠재적으로 불안정한 척추 손상이 있을 수 있다. 일반적으로 야생 환경에서 환자가 걸을 수 있다면 걷는 것이 안전하다. 걸을

수 없는 환자에게 무리하게 걸으라고 강요해서는 안 된다.

척추 움직임 제한으로 인한 사망 사례는 2006년에 뉴햄프셔주 코니시에서 발생했다. 넘어져 발목을 다친 환자는 머리, 척추 손상을 우려하여 단단한 긴척추고정판에 고정한 후 구조 보트로 이송되었다. 보트가 침몰했을 때 환자는 경미한 손상이 아닌 구조 과정에서 사망했다. 이와 같은 사례는 야생 EMS 제공자에게 구조 결정의 실제 위험과 척추 손상 가능성 및 엄격한 프로토콜을 맹목적으로 따르는 데 따른 잠재적 위험을 균형 있게 고려해야 한다는 점을 상기시켜 준다. 일반적으로 환자가 최소한의 통증과 신경학적 증상 없이 위험한 야생 상황에서 스스로 걸을 수 있다면 가장 안전한 선택일 가능성이 높다.

야생 구출 방법

야생에서 환자를 이송하는 것은 환자와 이송하는 사람 모두에게 매우 어렵고 시간이 많이 소요되며 잠재적으로 위험한 활동이다. 수색 및 구조팀의 경험이 없는 사람들은 일반적으로 야생에서 구조까지의 시간과 어려움을 과소평가하며, 특히 동굴 구조와 같이 더 어려운 구조의 경우 최소 절반, 때로는 최대 5배까지 과소평가한다. 경우에 따라 헬기를 이용한 이송이 가장 적절한 이송 방법을 제공할 수 있다 (**그림 21-12**).

수색 및 구조 경험이 없는 사람이 "환자를 이송하는 데 2시간 정도 걸릴 것 같다"라고 말하는 경우 실제 소요 시간은 훨씬 더 길어질 수

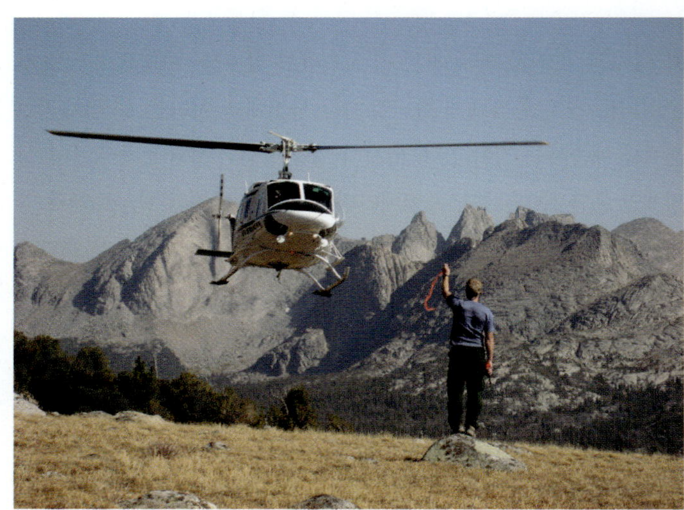

그림 21-12 헬기는 잠재적으로 위험이 더 높은 장비를 아주 짧은 시간 사용하여 많은 구조자가 장시간 험준한 지형에 노출되는 위험의 균형을 맞추는 데 사용될 수 있다. 이러한 위험의 균형은 모든 야생 구출에 대해 지속해서 평가를 한다.

있다. 환자가 동굴이나 기타 제한된 공간에 있는 경우 수색 및 구조 팀의 인력이 부족하거나 지형이 특히 어려운 경우 또는 날씨가 나쁜 경우 야생 EMS 제공자는 시간이 더 오래 걸릴 것으로 예상해야 한다. 특히 어둠이 다가오고 있거나 날씨가 악화할 때는 이 점을 기억하는 것이 중요하다.

여러 사람이 도와주더라도 환자를 걸어서 구출하는 것이 거의 항상 훨씬 빠르다. 수색 및 구조팀을 기다리지 않고 환자가 움직일 수 있고 지금 움직이기 시작하면 구출이 훨씬 더 빨라지고 일찍 완료할 수 있다. 발목 골절 등으로 환자가 걸을 수 없는 경우에 업거나 막대기와 밧줄을 이용해 즉석에서 들것을 만들어 사용할 수 있다.

기타 야생 EMS 환자 처치 고려 사항

환자 평가의 원칙

환자 평가가 야생 EMS 환경에서만 필요한 것은 아니지만, 병원 전 처치 제공자는 일반적으로 환자와 훨씬 더 오랜 시간 동안 함께 있다. 활력징후 경향은 특히 정신 상태의 변화는 장기간 환자를 처치하는 병원 전 처치 제공자에게 처치가 환자의 상태에 어떻게 영향을 미치는지 훨씬 더 잘 파악할 수 있는 통찰력을 제공한다. 정신 상태는 가장 중요한 활력징후로 간주하며 세 가지 주요 시스템(순환계, 호흡계, 신경계)이 제대로 작동하고 있는지 확인할 수 있다. 혈압과 같은 다른 전통적인 활력징후는 일부 야생 환경에서는 완전히 비실용적일 수 있다. 정상적인 정신 상태와 맥박의 속도 및 유무를 해석하는 훈련은 받으면 야생에서 환자 평가를 하는 데 필요한 모든 세부 정보를 얻을 수 있다.

MARCH PAWS

초기 환자 평가는 환경과 관계없이 같다. 우선순위는 손상 지점에서 즉시 완화할 수 있는 주요 생명 위협을 기반으로 한다. PHTLS에 따른 체계적인 접근 방법은 군대에서 개발한 MARCH PAWS 기억을 따를 수 있다. 이 접근 방법은 많은 군 의료 환경에서 인정받고 있다. 등반가 및 산악구조 전문가를 위한 MARCH PAWS에 대한 적응도 발표되었다.

- M(Massive hemorrhage) 대량출혈: 손상 발생 시 초치 처치의 우선순위는 대량출혈을 확인하고 지혈하는 것이다. 팔다리와 접합부 출혈 부위(겨드랑이 및 서혜부)의 초기 평가를 통해 이를 확인한

다. 그런 다음 골반이 불안정할 경우 골반고정대를 조기에 적용하는 것을 고려하여 골반 평가를 수행한다.

- A(Airway) 기도: 의식이 있는 환자의 기도 평가는 환자의 이름을 묻고 상황을 설명하는 것으로 간단히 평가할 수 있다. 의식이 없는 환자의 경우 간단하게 턱밀어올리기로 기도가 막힌 것을 완화할 수 있다. 코인두기도기는 가볍고 기도를 유지하기 위해 삽입할 수 있다. 심한 얼굴 손상이 있는 경우 코인두기도기 삽입은 피해야 한다. 때때로 일시적인 기도 확보를 위해 옆누운자세를 취하는 것이 필요할 수 있다. 급속연속마취유도를 시행하는 경우 숙련된 의료진이 수행해야 한다. 외과적 반지갑상연골절개는 적절한 교육을 받은 제공자가 시행할 수 있지만, 임상적으로 필수적이라고 판단되는 경우 조기에 시행한다.

- R(Respirations) 호흡: 호흡 평가는 청진기나 맥박산소측정기와 같은 장비를 사용하여 기존 거리 EMS 현장에서 시행할 수 있지만, 일부 야생 환경에서는 가슴 촉진과 같은 다른 환자 평가 술기가 필요할 수 있다. 갈비뼈 골절과 관련된 피부밑기종이나 비빔소리(마찰음)와 같은 이차적 소견은 기흉의 임상적 진단으로 이어질 수 있다.

- C(Circulation) 순환: 순환 평가의 주요 목표는 환자가 쇼크 징후를 보이는지 평가하는 것이다. 환자의 순환 상태에 대한 전반적인 평가는 정신 상태와 일반적인 외모를 바탕으로 결정해야 한다. 의식이 변하거나 혼란스러운 환자는 쇼크 징후가 있는 것으로 간주하고 그에 따라 처치해야 한다. 중심(목동맥, 넙적다리) 및 원위(노동맥, 뒤정강동맥, 발등동맥) 부위 맥박 유무를 평가하고 주의를 기울인다.

- H(Head/Hypothermia) 머리/저체온증: 환자의 의식 수준을 평가하기 위해 초기 신경학적 검사를 시행한다. 환자의 의식 상태는 AVPU를 이용해 명료, 언어에 반응, 통증에 반응 또는 무반응으로 분류할 수 있다. 중등도 또는 중증의 머리 손상이 의심되는 환자의 경우 처치의 우선순위는 저산소중, 저혈압 및 저혈당을 예방하는 것이다. 이 평가 단계에서는 환자를 노출해 전체적인 평가를 한다. 젖은 옷은 벗기고 환자를 따뜻하고 건조한 옷을 입히고 환자를 바닥어서 떨어뜨려 저체온증을 예방하도록 주의를 기울인다.

- P(Pain) 통증: MARCH 평가에서 초기 생명을 위협하는 처치를 완료한 후에는 환자의 통증을 관리한다. 깨어있고 의식이 명료한 환자에게는 초기에 아세트아미노펜을 투여하여 통증을 완화할 수 있다. 이부프로펜이나 나프록센과 같은 비스테로이드 항염증제(NSAID)는 항 혈소판 효과가 있으므로 출혈이 우려되는 경우 피해야 한다. 멜록시캄은 출혈 시간에 영향을 미치지 않으며 외상에 더 안전하게 사용할 수 있는 대체 지속성 비스테로이드 항염증제이다.

펜타닐이나 케타민과 같은 규제 약물을 휴대하고 있는 병원 전 처치 제공자는 투약 및 관리 지침에 대한 프로토콜을 준수한다.

- A(Antibiotics) 항생제: 외상성 손상 6시간 이내에 조기 항생제를 투여하는 것이 이상적이다. 외상성 손상을 일으킬 가능성이 가장 높은 병원체를 포괄하는 광범위한 항생제를 사용한다. 독시사이클린은 피부, 호흡기 및 위장 감염을 포함한 다양한 질환을 치료하는 데 사용할 수 있으므로 여행자가 휴대하기에 좋은 선택이다. 손상 부위 처치를 제공하는 Paramedic은 에르타페넴을 근육 또는 정맥 내로 투여할 수 있다. EMS 팀이 항생제를 하나만 휴대해야 하는 경우 일부 야생 EMS 현장에서 감염성 질환이 의심되는 경우 세프트리악손을 사용할 것을 권장한다. 병원 전 처치 제공자는 약물을 투여하기 전에 항상 알려진 약물 알레르기가 있는지 확인하여 아나필락시스를 유발하여 환자의 상태를 더욱 복잡하게 만들 수 있어 새로운 처치 문제를 일으킬 수 있는 위험을 줄인다.

- W(Wounds) 상처: 환자를 고정하고 이송하기 전에 평가 및 상처 처치를 완료한다. 일반적인 규칙은 마실 수 있는 물로 상처 부위를 깨끗하게 세척할 수 있다는 것이다. 오염을 완전히 제거하고 이물질을 제거한 다음 충분한 양의 물로 세척을 시행해야 하며 멸균 또는 깨끗한 드레싱을 상처에 적용한다.

- S(Splinting) 부목: 변형된 골절이나 심각한 연부조직 손상 부위에 부목을 적용하면 환자의 심한 통증을 완화효과를 제공할 수 있다. 어깨 탈구 시 가슴 부위에 손목을 위치시키고 삼각건이나 팔걸이로 고정하거나 발목 골절 시 등산용 지팡이를 사용하여 고정하는 것과 같은 간단한 고정만으로도 통증 조절을 개선하고 환자를 쉽게 이송할 수 있다.

장시간 환자 처치 시 고려 사항

앞서 언급했듯이 야생 EMS는 군대 및 기타 엄격한 환경과 유사할 수 있는 다양한 야생 환경에서 발생한다. 이라크와 파키스탄에서 전 세계의 다른 외딴 지역(예: 아프리카, 태평양)으로 군사 환경이 변경됨에 따라 몇 시간에서 며칠에 이르는 장기간의 환자 처치 환경에서 의료 및 외상 처치에 집중할 수 있도록 돕기 위해 장기간 현장 처치(PFC) 팀이 만들어졌다. 이 팀은 이러한 장기간 처치 환경에 대한 교육에 중점을 두고 10가지 필수 장기간 현장 처치 역량을 확인했다(**표 21-1**). 사실상 모든 환자 처치 교훈은 야생 EMS와 군 장기간 현장 처치 환경 사이에 연결될 수 있다.

배설(배뇨/배변) 욕구 충족

인기 있는 동화책 "누구나 똥을 싸다"에 묘사된 진실은 야생에 있는 환자에게도 적용된다. 도시 환경에서는 이송 시간이 비교적 짧으므로 대부분 환자는 대소변을 제거할 필요가 없다. 외상 환자는 병원 전이나 응급실에서 처치 중에 대소변을 보지 않는다. 그러나 하루 이상 야생에 머물렀던 환자를 돌보고 있고 환자에게 도착하는 데 몇 시간이 걸리는 경우 환자가 소변을 보거나 대변을 볼 수 있는 가능성이 훨씬 더 높다.

환자 밑에 깔 수 있는 패드가 포함된 환자 관리 용품, 위생 물티슈, 환자가 배변 또는 배뇨 후 교체할 수 있는 성인용 기저귀, 이동 중 환자가 소변 또는 배변할 수 있도록 잠시 멈추는 것도 모두 적절한 조치이다(**그림 21-13**). 전신 진공부목으로 고정 후 스토크스 들것(**그림 21-14**)에 고정된 상태에서도 소변을 볼 수 있다. 여성의 경우 도보여행을 할 때 여성들이 종종 휴대하는 작은 깔때기 장치가 필요할 수 있다. 일부 구조팀에서는 적절한 교육을 받으면 폴리 카테터를 사용할 수도 있다.

장시간 누워 있는 환자는 욕창성 궤양이 발생하는 경향이 있다. 이러한 궤양은 결국 수술이나 죽은조직제거가 필요할 수 있으며 이로 인해 입원 기간이 길어질 수 있다. 일부 환자는 감염 및 기타 합병증으로 사망할 수도 있다. 자신의 소변과 대변에 오랫동안(며칠이 아니라 몇 시간 동안) 누워 있으면 욕창성 궤양이 생길 가능성이 더 높아질 수 있다. 짧은 이송 중에 환자 처치가 몇 분 동안만 이루어지는 경우 소변과 대변은 큰 문제가 되지 않는다. 그러나 야생에서 병원 전 처치 제공자가 몇 시간 동안 환자를 처치하다가 대변에 누워 있는 상태로 응급실로 이송하는 경우 욕창성 궤양과 그로 인한 패혈증이 발생할 가능성이 훨씬 더 커진다.

식량과 물 필요량

모든 야생에 있는 환자는 춥고 배고프며 목마른 것으로 간주한다. 즉 환자는 저체온증, 굶주림 및 탈수로 간주하고 저체온증, 저혈당증 그리고 저혈량증을 고려한다. 굶주림은 단순한 저혈당 그 이상이며 모든 굶주린 환자가 심각한 저혈당 상태인 것은 아니다. 탈수는 혈관계 내의 혈관 내 용적만을 나타내는 혈량저하증 그 이상이다. 탈수 환자는 세포와 세포 사이의 사이질 공간에서도 수분이 손실된 상태이다.

거리에서는 일반적으로 환자에게 물과 음식을 제공하지 않는다.

표 21-1 위험한 환경에서 장기간 현장 처치(PFC)를 통해 확인된 10가지 핵심 기능

장기간 현장 처치 작업	최소	더 좋은	최고
1. 환자를 모니터링하여 유용한 활력징후를 확보한다.	혈압계, 청진기, 맥박산소측정기, 폴리카테터(소변량 측정), 정신상태 및 활력징후 해석에 대한 이해	호기말이산화탄소분압측정기 추가	일정한 간격으로 핸즈프리 활력징후 데이터를 모니터링
2. 결정질 또는 콜로이드 투여를 통한 환자 소생술을 시행한다.	현장에서 신선전혈(FWB) 수혈 키트	주요 화상 또는 폐쇄성 머리 손상 소생을 위해 준비된 결정질(젖산링거액 또는 플라즈마라이트 A 2~3개, 고장성식염수); 가능한 경우 동결건조혈장을 추가하는 것을 고려, 혈액 가온기	포장된 적혈구 및 신선한 동결 혈장 재고를 유지하고 즉각적인 신선전혈 확보를 위해 유형별 기증자를 확인
3. 환자에게 보조 환기를 시행하거나 산소를 공급한다.	백마스크를 이용한 호기말양압(PEEP)을 제공한다(호기말양압 환기를 시행하지 않으면 장기간 현장 처치에서 환자에게 환기를 시행할 수 없다. 환기를 시행할 수 없으면 환자가 급성 호흡곤란 증후군에 걸릴 위험이 있다.	산소통을 이용해 보충 산소 제공	보충 산소를 공급할 수 있는 휴대용 인공호흡기 사용
4. 기관에 팽창된 커프를 사용하여 환자의 기도를 확실하게 유지(환자를 편안하게 유지)	의사는 케타민을 투여하고 반지갑상연골절개 준비	장기간 진정제 투여 기능 추가	장기간 진정(흡인 및 마비 포함)을 제공하는 것 외에도 필요한 경우 추가로 빠른기관내삽관 시행
5. 진정/통증 조절을 사용하여 이전 처치를 시행한다.	아편제제를 정맥 내로 적정 투여	케타민 및 필요에 따라 미다졸람)으로 진정시키는 교육을 받음	정맥 내로 모르핀, 케타민, 미다졸람, 펜타닐 등을 투여하는 실습을 통해 술기 능력 유지
6. 신체검사 및 진단 검사사를 통해 잠재적인 문제를 파악한다.	전문적인 진단 없이 신체검사를 통해 눈에 보이지 않는 잠재적 손상(예: 복부출혈, 머리 손상)에 대한 인식 유지	초음파-, 휴대용 검사 등과 같은 고급 진단 장비를 사용할 수 있는 교육을 받음	두 가지 모두 경험
7. 간호, 위생 및 편의 조치를 제공한다.	환자가 깨끗하고 따뜻하며 건조하고 패딩을 적용하였는지 확인하고 기본적인 상처 처치를 제공	침상 거리 높이 조절, 상처 죽은조직제거, 상처 세척, 습식 및 건식 드레싱, 위 감압 시행	두 가지 모두 경험
8. 전문적인 외과적 처치를 시행한다.	가슴관, 반지갑상연골절개	근막 절제술, 상처 부위 죽은조직제거, 절단 등을 수행	두 가지 모두 경험
9. 원격 진료 상담을 수행한다.	신뢰할 수 있는 의사소통, 환자 상태 확인, 활력징후 전달	검사실 결과 및 초음파 이미지 추가	화상회의
10. 항공기를 이용한 환자 이송을 준비한다.	항공 이송 시 생리적 스트레스 요인에 대해 알고 있어야 함	중환자 이송에 대한 교육을 받음	중환자 이송 경험

Reproduced from Keenan S, Riesberg JC. Prolonged field care: beyond the "Golden Hour." *Wilderness Environ Med.* 2017;28(2S):S138.

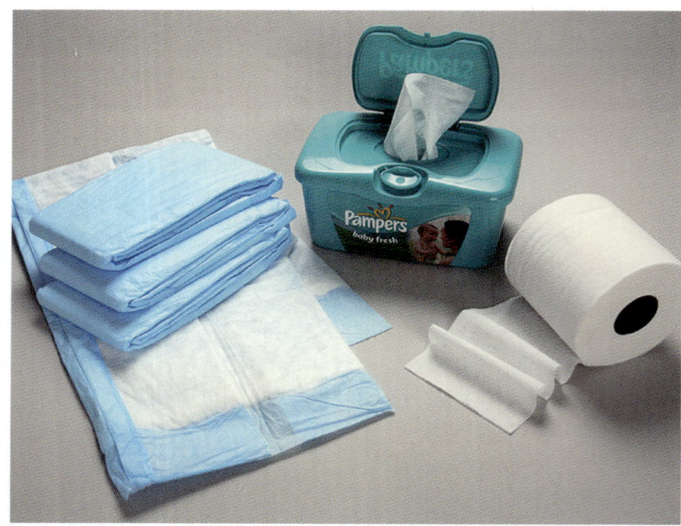

그림 21-13 소변 및 대변 제거에 필요한 용품
© National Association of Emergency Medical Technicians (NAEMT)

길거리 EMS 처치 중 환자에게 먹을 것을 주지 않는 데에는 여러 가지 이유가 있다. 환자가 수술을 받아야 하는 경우 위장에 음식이나 액체가 있으면 마취 유도 중 구토 또는 역류로 인한 흡인 가능성이 높아져 잠재적으로 해로울 수 있다. 또한 병원에 도착하는 시간 동안 환자가 굶거나 탈수되지 않는다.

야생에서는 구조된 환자가 수술이 필요한 경우 환자를 병원으로 이송하고 응급실에서 평가한 후 수술을 준비하는 데 시간이 걸린다. 야생에서 발생한 환자의 경우 일반적으로 이송 시간이 지연되기 때문에 환자가 칼로리 섭취와 수분 섭취를 유지할 수 있도록 하는 데 중점을 둔다. 마취 전 몇 시간 동안 금식하는 것이 이상적이기 때문에 야생에서 병원 전 처치 제공자는 안전하게 삼킬 수 있는 의식이 명료한 환자에게 음식과 물을 제공할 수 있다. 헬기를 이용해 환자를 구조 후 신속하게 이송할 수 있더라도 의료기관에서는 "위가 꽉 찬" 환자를 처치할 수 있다. 예를 들어 차량 충돌과 관련된 환자가 반드시 금식 상태인 것은 아니다.

구토와 흡인은 항상 위험하므로 환자의 기도 유지에 대한 세심한 주의가 항상 중요하다(예: 환자가 척추고정이 필요한 경우라도 이송 지연할 때는 옆으로 누운자세). 야생에서 EMS 제공자는 환자가 한두 번 구토하더라도 음식물과 물을 제공하려고 시도할 수 있다. 많은 환경에서 소량의 물을 자주 마시면 환자의 수분을 유지할 수 있다. 이 개념은 많은 소아 구토 처치의 주류를 이루던 정맥 내 수액 투여하던 것을 입으로 수분을 공급으로 대체하는 데 큰 변화를 가져왔다. 이는 야생 EMS 환자 처치에 희소식이다.

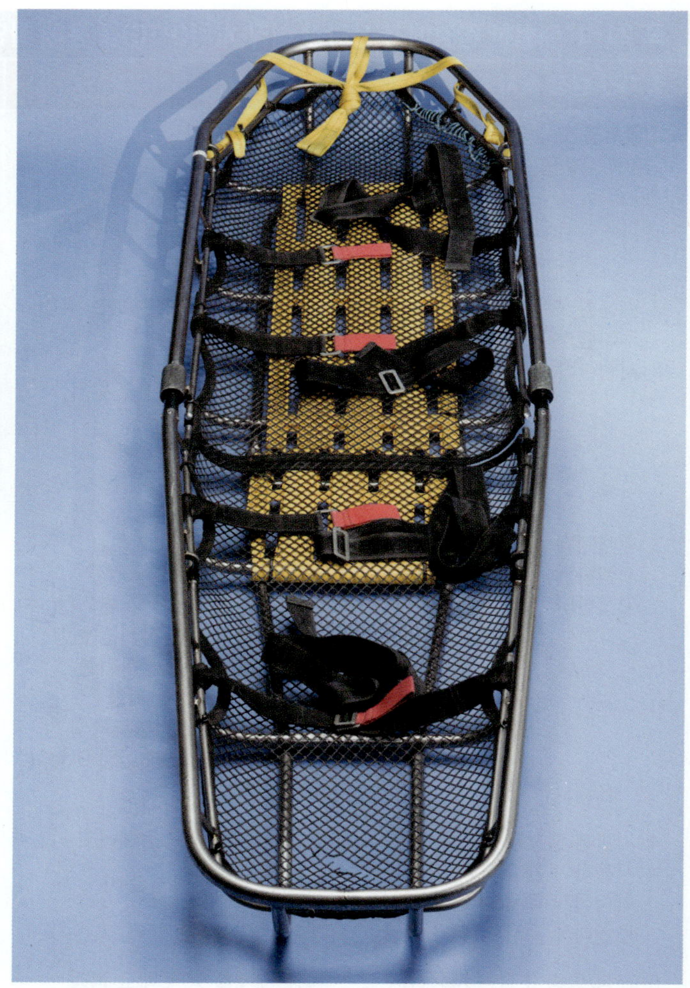

그림 21-14 스토크스 들것(Stokes litter). 일부 모델은 경량 운반을 위해 티타늄으로 제작되었으며 두 부분으로 나뉜다.
Courtesy of David Bowers.

의료 키트를 만들 때는 균형 잡힌 수분 공급을 위해 경구용 수분 보충제를 추가하는 것이 좋다. 또한 젤 형태의 고열량 저용량 간식도 고려한다. 당 함량이 높은 음식은 쉽게 흡수되어 이송 중 환자에게 상당한 양의 에너지를 공급할 수 있다.

서스펜션 증후군(현수 증후군)

서스펜션 증후군은 서스펜션 외상, 하네스로 인한 사망, 기립 불내성 및 하네스 행 증후군(HHS)을 포함하여 많은 이름으로 불려 왔다. 서스펜션 증후군은 직접적인 외상이 거의 없거나 전혀 없고 상태를 유발하는 데 하네스가 필요하지 않기 때문에 이러한 대체 용어보다 더 나은 용어로 확립되었다. 실제 병태생리학은 증후군과 관련된 일련의 사건으로 장시간 몸을 움직이지 않고 직립 상태로 유지되는 동안 다리에 혈액이 고여 쇼크 상태에 빠지는 것으로 마무리된다. 흔하지는 않지만, 야생 관련 활동에서 실제적인 우려 사항으로 남아 있다.

하네스를 착용하고 의존적인 자세로 다리를 움직일 수 없는 여러 유형의 여가 활동(예: 등산가, 동굴 탐험가)가가 이 증후군의 위험에 노출되기 쉽다. 직업 일부로 수직으로 매달릴 수 있는 산업근로자, 군인(낙하산부대), 서커스 공연자 및 스턴트 배우와 같은 다른 집단도 유사한 병태생리학에 노출될 수도 있다. 야생 EMS는 이러한 유형의 환자를 구출하고 처치하기 위해 고각 지형에 능숙해야 한다(**그림 21-15**).

서스펜션 증후군은 혈량저하증(예: 출혈, 탈수), 혈관 확장(예: 열, 감염) 또는 신체의 항상성 유지 능력을 변화시키는 기타 요인(예: 불법 또는 처방된 약물, 알코올)과 같은 다른 조건에 의해 악화할 수 있다. 주의해서 서 있는 병사들은 종아리 근육을 약간 구부리는 동작을 하도록 훈련받는다. 이 동작은 심장으로의 정맥혈복귀를 증가시키는 펌프 역할을 한다. 이러한 다리의 근육과 정맥의 한 방향 판막을 수축시킴으로써 혈액이 다시 중심 순환으로 돌아갈 수 있도록 돕는다. 이 정맥 펌프 기전이 없으면 서스펜션 증후군이 몇 분 만에 발생할 수 있으며 환자가 수직으로 매달린 채로 있는 경우 10분 이내에 사망할 수도 있다. 모티머가 2011년 야생 및 환경 의학 출판물은 서스펜션 증후군에 대한 최고의 사례 보고서 요약 중 하나를 제공한다.

환자가 수동적으로 매달려 있는 상황을 경험할 때마다 다리에는 혈액이 고이게 된다. 혈액 손실은 없지만, 상대적인 혈량저하 상태가 유도된다. 일부 학자들은 체내 혈액량의 최대 60%가 다리로 모일 수 있다고 추정한다. 이렇게 되면 심장의 전부하가 급격히 감소하여 후속 수축 시 충분한 양의 혈액을 펌핑할 수 없게 된다. 이렇게 혈류가 감소하면 뇌가 빠르게 영향을 받게 되고 환자는 의식을 잃게 된다. 이를 흔히 자세성 실신이라고 하며 대부분의 정상적이고 방해가 없는 환경에서는 환자가 바닥에 쓰러져 수평을 이루면서 뇌로 혈액 공급이 회복된다. 그러나 전문 기술이 필요한 구조 환경에서는 환자가 똑바로 매달려 있는 경우가 많고 신체의 보호 기전이 작동되지 않아 신속하게 반전시키지 않으면 사망에 이르는 경우가 많다.

정맥울혈과 심장 전부하 감소 외에도 추가적인 부적응 반응이 서스펜션 증후군의 혈류역학인 허탈에 기여하는 것으로 생각된다. 고칼륨혈증과 산혈증은 환자가 소생될 때 이환율과 사망률에 기여하는 것으로 생각된다. 저류 혈액은 상대적으로 저체온 상태가 되어 중심 순환계로 다시 유입될 때 전신 냉각을 유발할 수 있다. 특정 하네

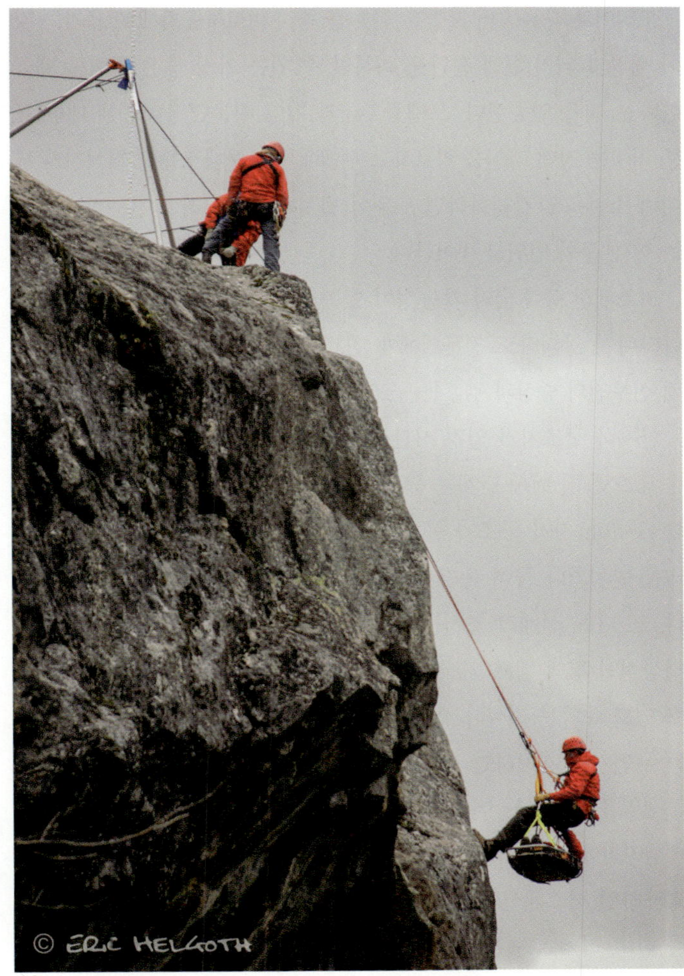

그림 21-15 고각 지형에 대한 기술적 숙련도는 야생 EMS 제공자에게 필수적이다. 이를 통해 구조대원에게 발생할 수 있는 서스펜션 증후군을 예방할 뿐만 아니라 잠재적인 서스펜션증후군이 있는 환자를 처치할 수 있다.
Courtesy of Eric He-goth.

스로 인한 질식 문제와 가슴 수축 또는 환자 위치 및 기도 손상이 겹치면 이러한 환자의 정신 상태 변화와 사망 가능성이 가속화될 수 있다는 추측도 있다. 이러한 추가 요인이 영향을 미칠 수 있지만, 아직 명확하게 밝혀지지 않은 병태생리학적 변수가 있다.

서스펜션 증후군에 대한 처치 권장 사상은 가능한 한 빨리 환자를 바로누운자세로 구출하는 데 중점을 둔다. 이 중요한 단계 후 야생 EMS 제공자는 전통적인 BLS 및 ALS 처치를 시작하고 환자를 최종 처치를 받을 수 있는 의료기관으로 신속하게 이송할 수 있다. 환자가 장기간의 정지 상태에서 구출된 직후 심정지를 겪은 "구조 사망" 사례 연구에 대한 우려가 제기되었다. 이전 권장 사항에서는 구조가 지연되고 하네스를 천천히 제거하면 이환율과 사망률이 낮아질 수 있다고 제안했지만, 더 이상 권장되지 않는다.

모티머와 다른 연구자들은 환자를 즉시 바로누운자세로 옮기는 것이 심장과 뇌의 혈액 순환을 회복할 수 있는 가장 좋은 기회를 제공한다는 것을 입증했다. 으깸증후군과 기타 횡문근융해증에 대한 표준 처치는 정맥 라인을 확보하고 수액에 중탄산나트륨을 희석시켜 투여해 소변을 알칼리화하면 도움이 될 수 있다. 이러한 전문적인 논의는 이 본문의 범위를 벗어난다.

서스펜션 증후군의 가능성이 있는 환자는 겉으로 뚜렷한 증상이 나타나지 않더라도 전문의에게 진료를 받아야 한다. 횡문근융해증 및 신부전의 증상과 징후는 구조 중 또는 나중에 발생할 수 있다.

환자나 구조자가 일정 시간 동안 수직으로 매달린 자세로 움직일 수 없으면 첫 번째 단계는 즉시 도움을 요청하고 자가 구조를 시도하는 것이다. 자가 구조가 불가능하거나 희생자가 탈진한 상태라면 다리를 받치거나 들어 올리거나 움직여 혈액이 고이는 것을 줄여야 한다. 또 다른 선제적 조치는 종아리와 다리 근육을 수축시켜 신체의 정상적인 정맥 펌프 기전을 작동시켜 혈액을 중앙 순환계로 되돌릴 수 있도록 하는 것이다. 암벽을 밀거나 로프 끈을 사용하여 밀 수 있는 무언가를 제공하면 서스펜션 증후군의 진행을 지연시킬 수 있다.

생명을 위협하는 이 질환은 문헌에 보고된 바 있지만, 최근에야 병태생리학에 대해 이해가 높아지고 처치 권장 사항이 업데이트되었다. 요약하면 서스펜션 증후군에 대한 최선의 처치 방법은 환자를 가능한 한 빨리 바로누운자세로 구출하고 중요한 장기로 혈류를 회복시킨 다음 표준 소생술 프로토콜을 계속해서 시행하는 것이다.

눈과 머리 보호

구조하는 동안 환자를 의인성 손상으로부터 보호하고 모든 구조대원이 상황에 적합한 개인보호장비(예: 헬멧, 보호안경)를 착용하고 있는지 세심한 주의를 기울인다. 환자가 구출되는 동안 미끄러져 넘어지거나 바위에 머리를 부딪쳐 이차 충격을 받으면 경미한 반복되는 머리 손상도 뇌진탕으로 악화할 수 있다. 수풀과 나무 사이로 환자를 옮기거나 눈에 띄지 않는 파편이 환자에게 떨어지면 눈 손상으로 이어질 수 있다. 따라서 환자의 눈을 보호할 수 있도록 고글이나 보호안경이 달린 헬멧을 착용시킨다. 수레형 들것에는 때때로 얼굴과 머리 보호막이 포함된 예도 있다.

자외선 차단

햇빛은 인체의 비타민 D 합성에 필수적이며 기분에도 유익한 영향을 미친다. 그러나 태양의 자외선(UV)은 피부를 손상할 수 있다. 급성 손상에는 일부 심각한 노출 사례에서 볼 수 있는 표재성, 부분층 및 전층 햇빛 화상이 포함될 수 있다. 극단적이면 햇빛 화상은 특히 다른 동반 질환이나 외상이 있는 경우 쇼크나 사망으로 이어질 수도 있다. 특히 태양의 자외선이 가장 강한 10:00~15:00시 사이에 직사광선에 노출되는 것을 피하면 햇빛 화상 및 장기적인 손상(광노화 및 피부암)의 위험이 감소하지만, 완전히 제거되지는 않는다.

국소 자외선 차단제는 일반적으로 다양한 파장의 자외선을 흡수하는 유기 화합 물질 및 무기물 필터의 조합을 포함한다. 산화아연과 이산화티타늄은 인위적인 필터의 일반적인 예이다. 두 가지 유형의 자외선 차단제는 모두 두 가지 특정 주파수인 A와 B(UVA와 UVB)에서 자외선 노출을 차단하는 것을 목표로 한다. UVA는 한때 해가 없는 것으로 여겨졌지만, 이제는 UVB와 시너지 효과를 일으켜 햇빛 화상을 유발한다는 사실이 밝혀졌다. 햇빛 화상에 의한 홍반(발적) 대부분은 UVB가 원인이다. UVA는 광 독성 및 광노화의 발생과 관련이 있다. 따라서 자외선 차단제나 선크림은 UVA와 UVB를 모두 차단해야 효과적이다. 제품 라벨에서 광범위 자외선 차단 지수(SPF)라는 용어를 찾아 UVA나 UVB를 모두 차단하는지 확인한다.

SPF는 옷이나 크림이 피부를 붉게 만드는 최소 자외선량을 얼마나 증가시키는지를 수치로 나타낸 것이다(**그림 21-16**). 예를 들어, 자외선 차단 지수 45등급의 자외선 차단제를 사용하면 자외선 차단제는 바르지 않았을 때보다 약 45배 더 오랫동안 햇빛 화상으로부터 피부를 보호한다. 자외선 차단 지수 10은 UVB를 90%를 차단하고 자외선 차단 지수 15는 93%, 30이면 97%, 50이면 98%를 차단한다. 2012년부터 FDA는 자외선 차단 제품의 추가 차단 효과가 제한적이라는 이유로 SPF 50으로 제한했지만, 2019년에는 SPF 60+로 상한선을 제시하면서 최대 SPF 80의 제품 판매를 허용했다. UVA에 대한 차단

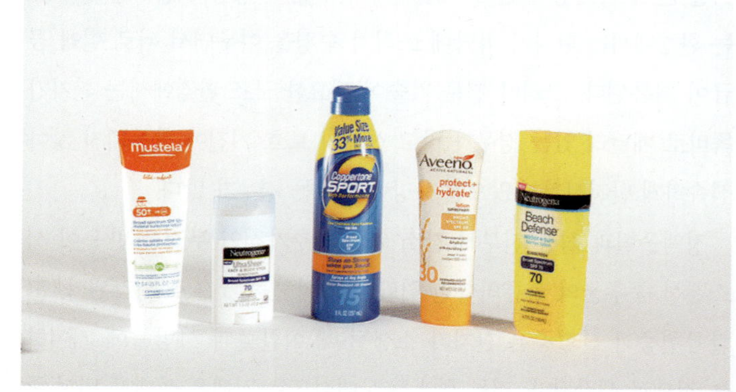

그림 21-16 선크림
© Jones & Bartlett Learning. Photographed by Darren Stahlman.

Box 21-3 자외선 차단 지수 효과를 감소시키는 요인

바람, 더위, 습도 및 고도는 모두 자외선 차단제의 유효 자외선 차단 지수 (SPF)를 감소시킬 수 있다. DEET(N, N-dietyl-meta-toluamide)가 함유된 자외선 차단제와 방충제를 함께 사용하면 자외선 차단 지수 효과가 감소한다.

Data from Prevention and treatment of sunburn. Med Lett Drugs Ther. 2004;46:45.

Box 21-4 자외선 차단제로 인한 알레르기 반응

로션에 파라아미노벤조산(PABA)이 함유된 경우 일부 환자는 급성 알레르기 반응을 일으킬 수 있으므로 PABA가 없는 제품을 사용하는 것이 좋다.

© National Association of Emergency Medical Technicians (NAEMT)

정도는 정량화하기 어렵고 일반적으로 UVB에 대한 차단보다 훨씬 적다.

챙이 넓은 모자, 바지, 긴팔 셔츠와 같은 보호 의류를 착용하고 노출된 피부에는 자외선 차단제를 바르는 것이 좋다. 의류의 여러 요소가 자외선 차단지수(UPF)에 영향을 미치며 현재 많은 아웃도어 의류 브랜드에서 자외선 차단 지수 등급을 제공하고 있다. 원단의 자외선 차단 지수 등급에 미치는 요소는 다음과 같다.

- 실의 구성(예: 면, 폴리에스테르)
- 직조 또는 니트의 조임(조일수록 등급이 향상되며 직조의 조임은 다른 요인보다 의복의 자외선 차단 지수에 더 많은 영향을 미친다.)
- 색상(일반적으로 어두운 색상이 더 좋음)
- 신축성(신축성이 높을수록 등급이 낮아짐)
- 수분(많은 원단은 젖었을 때 등급이 낮음)
- 상태(낡고 색이 바랜 의류는 등급이 낮을 수 있음)
- 마감 처리(일부 원단은 자외선 흡수 소재로 처리됨)

햇빛 노출로 인한 잠재적인 손상을 최소화하기 위해 노출된 피부에는 최소 SPF 15의 보호 로션을 발라야 한다. 장기간 구조 및 이송할 경우 SPF 30의 로션을 사용해야 하지만, 90분마다 다시 바르지 않는 한 SPF 30만으로는 거의 효과를 기대할 수 없다. 자외선 차단제는 햇볕에 노출되기 15~30분 전에 바르는 것이 가장 이상적이다. 대부분 사람은 표시된 SPF를 달성할 만큼 아주 두껍게 바르지 않는다. 해변에서 보통 성인의 경우 노출되는 부위에 최소 30mL를 사용해야 한다. 땀을 많이 흘리거나 물에 담글 때는 제품 라벨에 따라 자외선 차단제를 자주 덧발라야 한다. 일반적으로 방수 자외선 차단제는 제품 설명에 따라 최대 40~80분 동안 효과가 지속된다. 자외선 차단제 도포에 관한 추가 고려 사항은 **Box 21-3** 및 **Box 21-4**에 포함되어 있다.

햇빛 화상은 다른 화상과 마찬가지로 취급되며 처치는 야생에서나 길거리에서나 본질적으로 같다(**Box 21-5**). 유일한 주요 차이점은 야생에서 병원 전 처치 제공자는 지연성 감염, 체액 손실, 탈수 또는 쇼

Box 21-5 햇빛 화상 처치

예방
자외선차단 의복을 착용하고 SPF >30의 자외선 차단제를 바르는 것이 가장 좋다.

통증 완화
비스테로이드성 항염증제(NSAID)(예: 이부프로펜, 나프록센, 아스피린, 인도메타신)
진통제: 아세트아미노펜

면역조절제
코르티코스테로이드: 국소 또는 전신(프리드니손)

피부 관리
물 또는 아세트산 알루미늄 용액에 적진 냉찜질(Burrow 용액)
알로에 베라
국소 마취제
필요에 따라 수액 소생술(입안 또는 드물게 정맥 내)

© National Association of Emergency Medical Technicians (NAEMT)

크의 가능성을 인지하고 처치해야 하며 햇빛 화상 환자는 저체온증에 걸릴 위험이 높다는 점을 인식한다.

야생 EMS의 특성

이 부문에서는 적절한 야생 외상 처치가 길거리에서의 처치와 다른 가장 중요한 몇 가지 상황을 검토한다. 운영상 특정(업무 범위 확대)한 프로토콜이 도움이 될 수 있는 분야에는 상처 관리, 관절 탈구, 심정지 및 물림 및 쏘임 등이 포함된다.

상처 관리

상처 관리에는 다음이 포함된다.

- 지혈
- 소득(감염 예방)
- 기능 회복(피부를 보호 기능으로 되돌리고 팔다리 또는 기타 신체

부위를 정상 기능으로 회복)

- 성형

야생에서는 감염 예방과 기능 회복이 매우 중요합니다.

지혈

출혈을 지혈하는 것은 일차평가의 일부이며 길거리에서는 동맥 출혈로 사망할 수 있다. 야생에서는 정맥 출혈도 충분한 시간 동안 지속되면 사망할 수 있다. 모든 적혈구가 중요하다는 것을 기억한다. 직접 압박 같은 표준 처치를 포함한 지혈은 특히 야생에서 더 중요하다. 의료진이 실제 손상이 발생한 그룹에 속해 있지 않는 한 지혈되지 않은 심각한 출혈은 수색 및 구조팀이 도착하기 전에 환자가 사망하는 결과를 초래할 수 있다(**Box 21-6**).

야생 환경으로 여행을 떠나는 사람들을 위한 교육 프로그램에서는 이러한 인명 구조 기술을 다루어야 한다.

- 생명을 위협하는 심각한 출혈에는 지혈대를 먼저 사용해야 한다. 야생의 일부 상황(예: 다수 사상자 발생 현장)에서는 환자가 많고 자원이 제한되어 있어 상처에 직접 압박을 가하는 것이 어렵거나 불가능하다. 구조가 다음 중요한 단계이고 직접 압박을 유지하는 것이 불가능한 구조 상황(예: 절벽 측면)에서도 비슷한 어려운 문제가 존재한다. 일부 상황에서는 더 이상 생명을 위협하는 출혈이 없고 다른 수단으로 출혈을 조절할 수 있는 경우 6시간 미만 동안 적용한 지혈대를 압박붕대로 교체(즉, 지혈대를 제거하고 다른 지혈 방법으로 교체)할 수 있다. 이러한 유형의 환경에서 환자를 처치하는 병원 전 처치 제공자를 위한 구체적인 프로토콜을 마련해야 한다.
- 출혈 부위에 직접 10~15분 동안 직접 압박을 가한 다음 압박 붕대를 감아야 한다.
- 지혈제는 야생에서 심각한 출혈을 조절하는 데 유용할 수 있다. 야생 병원 전 처치 제공자는 다른 사람이 이미 지혈제를 사용한 손상

을 입은 환자를 만날 수 있다. 이러한 제품 중 일부는 일반인에게 판매되고 있지만, 효과적으로 사용하는 방법에 대한 교육은 여전히 권장된다. 지혈제를 사용하더라도 상처에 직접 압박을 가하는 것은 처치 과정에서 여전히 중요한 부분이라는 점을 기억하는 것이 중요하다.

장시간(2시간 이상) 지혈대를 사용할 것으로 예상되는 야생 상황에서는 지혈대를 상처 위쪽에 적용하지만, 가능한 한 상처에 가깝게 적용해야 한다(**Box 21-7**). 그 이유는 지혈대로 인해 허혈이 발생한 조직의 양(사망의 위험이 있고 절단이 필요한 경우)이 가능한 한 근위부에 지혈대를 적용했을 때보다 이론적으로 적기 때문이다(지혈제, 지혈대 및 기타 출혈 조절 원칙과 선호도에 대한 자세한 내용은 3장 쇼크: 삶과 죽음의 병태생리학을 참조한다).

즉석에서 만든 지혈대

많은 야생 상황에서 병원 전 처치 제공자는 처치를 제공하기 위해 사용하는 도구를 즉석에서 만들어 사용할 수 있다. 벨트나 옷가지 등 주변에서 구할 수 있는 제품을 사용하여 즉석에서 지혈대를 만드는 것은 야생 환경에서 매우 중요한 기술이다. 일반적으로 상용화된 지혈대가 더 빨리 사용할 수 있고 더 빠르고 안정적으로 지혈을 할 수 있지만, 야생 외상 처치에서 항상 상용화된 지혈대를 사용할 수 있는 것은 아니다.

Box 21-6 업데이트된 출혈 조절 원칙

2015년 AHA가 소집한 국제 컨센서스 패널은 출혈 조절 원칙을 포함한 응급처치 기술을 발표했다. 여기에는 손으로 직접 압박하고 거즈와 압박 드레싱, 지혈제, 지혈대를 사용하여 심한 출혈을 조절할 것을 권장했다. 선택적 동맥 압박점 및 팔다리 거상법은 과거에 사용되었던 방법일 뿐이며 그 효과를 뒷받침하는 증거가 부족하여 권장되지 않는다.

Data from Singletary EM, Charlton NP, Epstein JL, et al. Part 15: first aid: 2015 American Heart Association and American Red Cross guidelines update for first aid. Circulation. 2015;132(Suppl 2):S574-S589.

Box 21-7 지혈대 사용 시 피해야 할 실수

- 손상으로 인해 지혈대를 사용해야 할 때 사용하지 않는 경우(생명을 위협하거나 출혈이 조절되지 않는 경우)
- 지혈대를 적용하기까지 너무 오래 기다리는 경우(생명을 위협하는 출혈이 명백한 경우 지혈대를 먼저 적용)
- 환자가 쇼크 상태이거나 병원으로 이송 시간이 짧을 때(1~2시간 미만) 지혈대를 제거
- 지혈대 적용 시간이 6시간 미만인 경우 의료 지도에 따라 제거하지 않는 경우(즉, 다른 지혈 방법으로 전환하지 않는 경우)
- 충분히 꽉 조이지 않음(지혈대 적용 후 원위부 맥박이 촉지되지 않아야 함)
- 필요한 경우 두 번째 지혈대를 사용하지 않음(첫 번째 지혈대와 바로 옆)
- 손상된 팔다리에 혈류가 흐를 수 있도록 주기적으로 지혈대를 느슨하게 함
- 출혈을 최소화하기 위해 지혈대 사용(직접 압박이나 압박 붕대로 지혈할 수 있는 경우)

Modified from Department Defense Lessons Learned from the Committee on Tactical Combat Casualty Care. See Chapter 27 in the 8th edition of *PHTLS: Prehospital Trauma Life Support, Military Edition.*

미 육군 외과 연구소는 이라크 및 아프가니스탄 분쟁에서 지혈대를 평가할 때 성공적인 지혈대의 주요 특징을 확인했다. 이러한 기능은 EMS 기관의 의료 키트에 지혈대가 포함되어야 하며 즉석에서 만들어 사용할 수 있는 지혈대의 기본이 되어야 한다.

- 폭이 최소 2.5cm(예: 등산용 웨빙 또는 벨트)
- 밴드를 조일 수 있는 조임 막대
- 조임을 고정할 수 있는 능력
- 간단한 적용(자가 적용 시 60초 미만 소요)
- 조절 가능
- 미끄럼 방지

감염 예방

야생에서 손상을 입은 후 응급실에서 상처를 결정적으로 처치하기까지 오랜 시간이 걸릴 수 있다. 응급실에서의 일상적인 상처 처치에는 감염을 예방하기 위한 적절한 세척이 포함된다. 먼지로 오염되거나 더러운 물체가 관통하여 생긴 상처는 고압으로 세척하고 오염되지 않은 상처는 저압으로 세척한다.

고압으로 세척하면 상처가 부어오를 수 있지만, 이물질과 세균으로 가득 한 오염된 상처의 경우 세균 제거의 이점이 상처가 붓는 위험보다 더 크다. 감염이 빠르게 진행될 수 있다. 상처가 발생하고 약 8시간 동안 개방되어 있으면 세균이 피부에서 상처 깊숙이 퍼져나가기 때문에 상처를 봉합하면 심부 상처 감염으로 이어질 가능성이 높아진다. 심부 상처 감염은 감염에 대한 신체의 정상적인 방어 기전인 백혈구를 차단하는 압력을 발생시킨다.

환자가 응급실에 도착할 때까지 몇 분간 상처 세척을 미루는 것이 환자의 상처를 세척하고 평가하는 데 더 적합하므로 길거리 EMS에서의 일상적인 상처 처치에는 상처 세척이 포함되지 않는다. 응급실에 도착하는 데 몇 시간이 걸리는 경우 상처를 깨끗이 세척해야 한다. 극도로 외딴 지역에서는 환자가 며칠 후 응급실에 도착하기 전에 상처가 감염될 수도 있다.

연구에 따르면 조기 세척은 세균을 제거하고 상처 감염을 줄이는 데 필수적인 것으로 나타났다. 상처 세척을 위해 멸균 용액을 휴대할 필요도 없고 실용적이지 않다. 물에 소독제를 첨가할 필요는 없으며 마실 수 있을 정도의 물이면 상처를 세척하기에 충분하다. 시냇물이나 눈 녹은 물은 야생에서 식수로 사용할 수도 있고 상처를 세척하는 데 사용할 수 있다.

상처가 오염되면 세균을 제거할 수 있을 만큼 충분한 압력으로 세척해야 한다. 기존 연구에 따르면 18 게이지 바늘이 달린 35mL 주사기가 적절한 압력(5~15psi)을 제공하는 것으로 나타났다. 상처 전체에 고압으로 물을 분사한다. 생수병이나 카멜 백에서 깨끗한 물을 분출하는 것도 효과가 있다. 그러나 이 방법은 구조자에게 주요 혈액매개 병원체 위험을 초래하므로 세척 시 가운이나 깨끗한 쓰레기봉투 또는 비옷으로 혈액이 튀지 않도록 보호한다. 이 환자를 처치할 때 보호안경과 글러브가 필수이다.

때때로 상처에 묻은 이물질을 제거해야 하는 경우가 있다. 거즈 패드나 깨끗한 천, 겸자/핀셋 또는 글러브를 낀 손가락을 사용하여 가능한 한 상처 부위에 추가 손상을 주지 않으면서 죽은 조직을 제거한다. 상처를 세척하기 전에 환자의 통증을 먼저 조절해야 할 수도 있다. 리도카인을 상처에 국소적으로 바르거나 국소 마취를 위해 피하 주사하면 대부분의 경우 통증을 완화할 수 있다. 반대로 마약성 진통제는 환자의 보행 능력을 손상해 이송이나 구조가 지연될 수 있다. 세척이 완료되면 상처 부위에 드레싱을 적용하고 붕대를 감는다. 붕대가 젖거나 더러워지면 적어도 매일 또는 더 자주 깨끗하게 드레싱을 다시 시행한다.

상처가 벌어져 있는 경우 젖은 드레싱을 사용하면 건조로 인한 조직 손상을 방지할 수 있으므로 하루에 여러 번 깨끗한 드레싱으로 갈아주거나 깨끗한 물로 최소한 다시 적셔야 한다.

심각한 외상을 입은 환자에게 응급실 도착하자마자 항생제를 조기에 투여하는 것이 일반적이다. 도시 환경에서는 이송 시간이 짧기 때문에 대부분의 병원 전 EMS에서는 항생제를 투여하지 않는다. 야생 환경에서는 이동 거리가 길고 험준한 지형에서 구조를 고려해야 하므로 결정적인 처치가 지연될 수 있으며 이러한 환경에서는 조기 항생제 사용이 적절할 수 있다.

손상 후 조기에 항생제를 투여하면 상처 감염을 예방하는 데 더 효과적이다. 돼지 상처 감염 모델에서 손상 후 1시간 이내에 근육 내로 벤질페니실린 투여를 시작하면 연쇄상구균 감염을 예방하는 데 효과적인 것으로 나타났다. 손상 후 6시간까지 투여가 지연된 경우 약물의 투여 효과가 없었다.

전장에서의 항생제 사용에 대한 최근 군의 검토에 따르면 의료시설에 도착하는 데 3시간 이상 걸릴 것으로 예상되는 경우 항생제를 사용할 것을 권장했다. 미 국방성의 TCCC 과정은 손상 지점에서 개방성 상처에 대해 항생제를 조기에 투여할 것을 권장한다. TCCC는 군인들이 전장에서 항생제를 투여받았을 때 상처 감염이 발생하지 않았다는 여러 사례 연구를 인용한다. TCCC는 또한 부상자가 삼킬 수 있는 경우 하루에 한 번 경구 항생제를 투여할 것을 권장한다. 민간 환경에서 이와 유사한 연구가 수행되지 않았지만, 이러한 권장 사항은 의료 지도의사의 지시가 있다면 야생 환경에서도 적용하는 것이 합리적이다.

기능 회복 및 성형: 야생에서 상처의 지연된 봉합

밝은 조명, 적절하고 깨끗한 멸균 용품, 따뜻하고 건조한 처치장소가 부족하므로 대부분 야생에서는 상처를 최종적으로 봉합하는 것은 적절하지 않다. 상처를 깨끗이 세척한 후 드레싱을 시행하고 일상적인 상처 관리를 지속한 다음 적절한 의료진이 지연된 1차 봉합을 시행하는 것이 바람직하다. 상처가 감염되지 않았다면 며칠 후 방금 발생한 것처럼 상처를 봉합해도 안전하다. 손상 직후에는 세균이 상처로 이동하지만, 결국에는 백혈구 등 신체의 방어 기능이 상처에 들어가 상처를 안전하게 봉합할 수 있다. 의사나 상처 봉합 경험이 있는 사람이 있다면 현장에서 상처를 봉합할 수 있다. 그러나 상처를 간단히 세척하고 드레싱을 시행한 후 나중에 봉합하는 것이 좋다. 대부분 상황에서 야생 환경에서 상처를 봉합하는 것이 뚜렷한 이점이 없으며 그렇게 하면 이송 노력이 상당히 길어지는 경우가 많다.

어떤 방법으로도 출혈을 조절할 수 없는 야생의 상황에서는 상처를 봉합하는 것이 중요할 수 있다. 이러한 상황은 드물고 일반적으로 두피 열상을 수반한다. 이러한 이유로 야생에서 처치 제공자는 일회용 수술 스테이플러를 사용하여 두피 상처를 봉합할 수 있도록 교육을 받는다. 그러나 상처 봉합은 복잡하며 충분한 훈련과 경험 없이 시도해서는 안 된다.

통증 관리

야생 EMS에서 적절한 통증 관리는 구조 및 구출에 대한 환자의 내성을 극적으로 변화시킬 수 있다. 이상적인 목표는 환자가 정상 또는 거의 정상에 가까운 생리적 기능을 유지하면서 통증과 때때로 함께 나타나는 불안을 견딜 수 있는 수준으로 줄이는 것이다. 케타민과 펜타닐과 같은 다른 단기 작용 마약성 진통제를 사용하는 대체 통증 조절 전략이 등장하고 있다.

새로운 전달 전략이 유용해지고 있으며 야생 EMS 환경에서 사용하기 위해 사용하고 있다. 펜타닐의 입안 점막을 통한 투여는 이러한 환경(예: 군대, 스키 패트롤, 수색 및 구조)에서 큰 성공을 거두었습니다. 코 안 투여(케타민, 펜타닐)는 구조 중에 진통제를 투여하는 경로로 훨씬 더 빈번하게 사용한다. 아세트아미노펜뿐만 아니라 이부프로펜과 같은 비스테로이드성 항염증제(NSAID)는 부작용이 거의 없이 적절한 통증 관리를 제공할 수 있는 훌륭한 비마약성 약물이다. 일부 손상에는 더 광범위한 통증 조절 방법이 필요하며 이러한 경우 마약성 진통제 및 기타 진통제[(예: 케타민, 아산화질소, 메톡시플루란(펜트란)]를 투여할 수 있다. 복합적인 통증 조절 전략은 필요한 마약성 약물의 총량을 줄일 수 있을 뿐만 아니라 투여 용량과 관련된 부작용도 줄일 수 있다. 예를 들어, 케타민 50mg과 펜타닐 50mcg을 코안으로 투여하면 두 약물을 고용량으로 단독 투여하는 것보다 더 나은 진통 효과를 얻을 수 있다. 다른 약물과 마찬가지로 야생 EMS 제공자는 다중약물 요법 방법을 통해 선택한 단일 약물의 위험과 이점의 균형을 맞춰야 한다. 많은 구조 환경에서는 환자를 자세히 모니터링하기가 어려울 수 있다. 휴대용 산소포화도측기가 사용할 수 있는 유일한 모니터링 장비일 수 있지만, 적절한 교육을 받으면 충분한 데이터를 제공할 수 있다. **그림 21-17**은 야생 구조에서 넓적다리뼈 골절 환자를 처치하는 데 사용하는 야생 EMS 처치 키트이다. 환자를 모니터링하기가 종종 어려울 수 있으므로 일반적인 알고리즘을 사용하지 않고 특정 환자에 대한 개별화된 통증 조절 계획을 선택하는 것이 중요하다. 병원에서 시행하는 전문적인 통증 조절은 야생에서 시행하기가 어렵다. 이러한 많은 전문적인 약물을 투여하려면 다른 전문적인 처치 관행과 마찬가지로 적절한 교육이 필수적이다.

그러나 통증 조절은 야생 EMS 제공자가 제공할 수 있는 특정 약물에만 국한되지 않고 훨씬 더 넓은 의미에서 접근해야 한다. 여기에

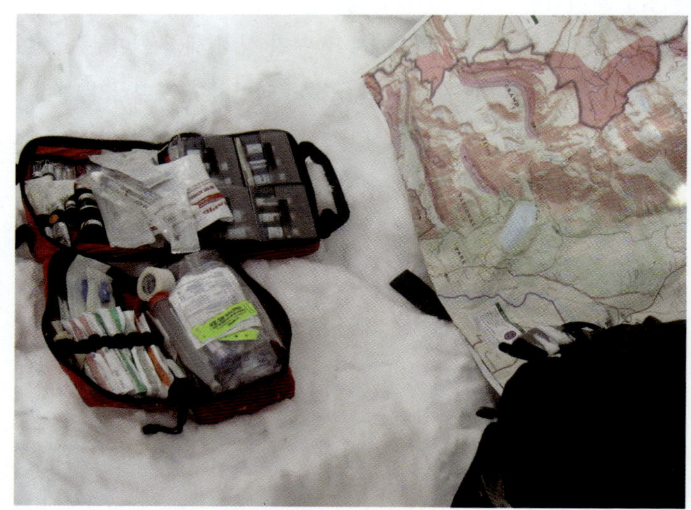

그림 21-17 넓적다리뼈 골절 환자를 야생에서 구조하는 데 사용되는 전문 생명 유지 의료키트. 통증 조절 방법은 열악한 환경에서 환자를 처치하는 데 매우 중요하다.
Courtesy of Will Smith.

는 심리적 안정, 부목 고정 그리고 약물 투여를 포함하여 훨씬 더 많은 것이 포함된다. 심리적 응급처치는 확장된 개념이며 모든 통증 조절 전략에서 유용한 전술이 될 수 있다. 야생 EMS 제공자는 최적의 환자 처치를 제공하기 위해 이러한 모든 방법과 균형을 유지해야 한다. 오지 환경에서 급성 통증을 조절하기 위한 야생 의학회의 처치 지침은 편안한 처치와 PRICE(보호, 휴식, 냉찜질, 압박, 거상) 방법으로 처치를 시작하여 정맥 및 골내 약물 투여에 이르는 전문적인 처치 방법에 대한 좋은 요약본을 제공한다.

탈구

건강한 20세 남성이 급류를 따라 카약을 타던 중 카약 패들 윗부분이 처진 나뭇가지에 부딪혀 오른쪽 어깨에 간접적인 외상을 입었다. 그의 오른쪽 어깨는 변형되고 통증이 심해졌다. 그는 오른팔을 가슴에 대거나 팔꿈치를 옆구리로 움직일 수 없다. 원위부 맥박, 모세혈관 재충전, 감각 및 운동 기능은 정상이었다. 구급차에서 내린 구급대원은 숲을 가로질러 약 2km 정도 걸어 계곡에 도착했다. 그들은 발견된 자세 그대로 부목을 적용해야 하는가? 아니면 전방 어깨 탈구처럼 보이는 것을 줄이려고 노력해야 하는가?

길거리에서 골절과 탈구에 대한 일반적인 처치는 그대로 누운 상태에서 부목을 고정하고 최종 처치를 시행할 수 있는 의료기관으로 신속하게 이송하는 것이다. 유일한 예외는 환자의 손상된 원위부 맥박이 촉지되지 않는 경우 혈액 순환을 회복하기 위해 손상된 팔다리를 해부학적 자세로 재정렬한다.

길거리에서는 "발견된 자세 그대로 부목을 고정한다"가 일반적인 규칙이지만, 야생에서 발생한 환자에게는 부목을 해부학적 자세를 위해 부목으로 고정해 정상적으로 보이게 하는 것이 더 나은 일반적 규칙이다. 이 방법은 이송이 지연될 때 골절과 탈구 모두에 확실히 적절하지만, 병원 전 처치 제공자의 업무 범위도 고려해야 한다. 일부 지역에서는 EMS 프로토콜에서 탈구에 대해 교정술을 허용하기 시작했다.

손가락, 발가락, 어깨, 무릎뼈, 무릎, 팔꿈치, 엉덩관절, 발목, 턱 등 다양한 유형의 탈구가 있으며 야생에서 성공적으로 재정렬할 수 있는 탈구도 있었으며 일부는 다른 탈구보다 더 쉽게 재정렬되었다. 발목(대부분 골절-탈구 동반), 무릎뼈, 발가락, 손가락의 탈구는 일부 둘째손가락의 가락뼈사이관절(PIP)을 제외하고는 일반적으로 쉽게 재정렬할 수 있다. 팔꿈치, 무릎, 엉덩관절의 탈구는 일반적으로 상당히 어렵다. 모든 것은 교육과 연습을 통해 훨씬 쉬워진다. 특히, 단

순방사선 촬영 없이도 관절이 탈구될 가능성이 있는 부위를 파악하고 정렬을 시도하려면 교육이나 많은 경험이 필요하다.

기존의 거리 EMS 교육 과정에서는 탈구 정복에 대한 교육을 거의 제공하지 않았다. 그러나 야생에서 탈구가 매우 흔하게 발생하므로 거의 모든 야생 EMS 교육이나 야생의학회의 정형외과 워크숍에서 손가락, 무릎뼈 또는 어깨 탈구 교정을 교육한다. 야생에서 EMS를 제공할 가능성이 있거나 정기적으로 오지를 여행하는 사람은 이러한 과정 중 하나를 수강하는 것이 좋다. 그러나 교육받았더라도 다른 환자 처치와 마찬가지로 이러한 술기를 수행할 수 있는 인증과 자격을 받아야 한다. 또한, 업무 범위를 고려할 때 탈구 정복은 현장 팀의 일원으로 배치된 EMS 의사가 특히 도움이 될 수 있는 상황 중 하나이다.

야생에서의 심폐소생술

길거리에서 외상성 심정지가 발생하면 Level I 외상센터까지 몇 분 이내에 도착하더라도 예후가 좋지 않다. 외상성 심정지 후 심폐소생술을 시행하더라도 몇 분 이상 생존하는 사람은 없다. 이러한 현실은 많은 길거리 EMS 프로토콜에서 인정되고 있다. 외상성 심정지의 경우 다음과 같은 상황에서 심폐소생술 시행하는 것을 고려한다.

- EMS 종사자가 있는 곳에서 심정지가 발생한 경우
- 관통 손상을 입은 환자가 EMS 종사자가 도착한 후 15분 이내에 생명의 징후를 보인 경우

야생에서 발생한 외상성 심정지

다음 징후는 일률적으로 생존 가능성이 없는 것과 동일시할 수 있다.

- 참수
- 몸통 절단
- 환자가 너무 단단하게 얼어서 환자의 가슴을 압박할 수 없는 경우
- 환자의 직장 체온이 매우 낮거나 주변 환경과 같은 경우
- 부패가 진행된 경우

다음과 같은 사망을 추정할 수 있는 징후는 야생에서 병원 전 처치 제공자에게 유용할 수 있지만, 그 자체로 신뢰할 수 있는 징후는 없다.

- 사후강축: 사후경축은 잘 알려졌지만, 항상 나타나는 것은 아니며 저체온증 환자 중에서도 유사한 경직이 종종 관찰된다.
- 시반: 이러한 소견은 시체에서 흔히 볼 수 있지만, 압력 괴사 및 동상과 함께 장시간 외부에 노출된 일부 환자 중에서도 발견될 수

있다.

- 부패: 이 징후는 일반적으로 자명하다.
- 생존을 추정할 수 있는 징후 부족: 저체온증은 맥박이 촉지되지 않거나 호흡이 감지되지 않을 수 있으며 동공이 확장되고 의식이 없으며 반응하지 않을 수 있으므로 사망한 것처럼 보일 수 있다. 그러나 심한 저체온증 환자도 간혹 소생하여 신경학적으로 완전히 회복되는 경우가 있다.

따라서 야생 상황에서 대부분의 외상성 심정지 환자에게 심폐소생술을 시행하는 것은 부적절하다. 야생 의학 전문의와 수색 및 구조팀원은 환자를 평가한 후 동료에게 피해자가 사망했으며 소생술을 시작하거나 계속할 이유가 없다고 부드럽지만 단호하게 말하는 것이 적절하다. 사망이라는 단어를 사용하기 어려운 경우가 많지만, 완곡한 표현은 종종 실제로 말하는 내용에 대한 오해와 오해를 불러일으킬 수 있다.

야생에서 내과적 심정지

내과적 심정지란 기저 질환이 있거나 급성 질환(예: 가슴 통증, 호흡 곤란, 당뇨병)을 앓고 있다가 심정지가 발생한 환자에게 적용되는 용어이다. 다시 말하지만, 야생 환경에서는 환자에게 심폐소생술 또는 제세동 시행 후 몇 분 이상 지나면 생존 가능성이 작거나 아예 없다. 수색 및 구조팀원은 환자 또는 팀원의 갑작스러운 심정지에 대응해야 할 수도 있다. 현재 경량 제세동기를 사용할 수 있으며 일부 수색 및 구조팀은 제세동기를 휴대하거나 최소한 사고지휘소 또는 현장응급 의료소에 비치하고 있다. 모든 의료 및 기타 장비와 마찬가지로 무게 대비 사용 비율을 자세히 검토해야 한다.

저체온증으로 인한 심실세동 심정지 또는 폐색전증으로 인한 심정지 등 야생에서는 다양한 원인으로 심정지가 발생할 수 있다. 이러한 심정지의 경우 심근경색으로 인한 이차 심정지보다 생존 가능성이 훨씬 낮다. 그러나 다음과 같은 상황에서는 비외상성 심정지가 야생에서 발생하면 생존할 수 있다.

- 저체온증
- 찬물에 익수
- 낙뢰
- 감전
- 약물 과다 복용
- 눈사태로 매몰

이 모든 경우에서 환자는 심정지 상태인 것처럼 보이지만, 기본 심폐소생술로 소생할 수 있다. 특히 저체온증의 경우 "환자는 따뜻해져서 죽을 때까지 죽은 것이 아니다."라는 말이 있다(19장, 환경 외상 I: 더위와 추위 참조). 이러한 기전으로 인해 죽은 것처럼 보이는 사람 중 상당수는 소생할 수 있다. 이러한 각각의 상황에 대해 특별한 고려 사항이 있다. 예를 들어 감전되었지만, 여전히 전선에 닿아 있는 환자의 현장 안전이나 저체온증 환자에게 외부 가슴압박이 심실세동으로 인한 심정지를 유발할 수 있다. 야생 EMS 과정에서는 적절하지만, 이러한 주제에 대한 자세한 논의는 이장의 범위를 벗어난다(19장 환경 외상 I: 더위 및 추위, 20장 환경 외상 II: 낙뢰, 익사, 다이빙 및 고도를 참조).

두 가지 간단한 표준 야생에서의 심폐소생술 권장 사항은 다음과 같다.

- 환자가 외상 이외 원인으로 심정지가 발생한 것 같으면 15~30분 동안 심폐소생술을 시행하고 이 시간이 지나도 소생되지 않으면 심폐소생술을 중단하고 환자가 사망한 것으로 간주한다.
- 햇빛, 지형, 날씨 및 근처에 대피소가 있는지 등을 고려하여 구조자를 위험에 빠뜨리고 현장에서 안전하게 빠져나올 기회를 감소시킬 수 있는 경우 심폐소생술을 시작하지 않는다.

NAEMSP 웹사이트에서 확인할 수 있는 미국 응급의학회의 "비외상성 심폐소생술의 종료"는 심정지 소생술 중단을 고려해야 하는 시기에 대한 지침을 제공한다.

물림 및 쏘임

물리거나 쏘이는 것은 야생에서 흔히 발생하는 문제이다. 야생 지역에서 발생할 수 있는 물림이나 쏘임의 정확한 유형은 특정 지역에 따라 다르다. 이러한 환자를 처치하는 데 도움이 되는 현지 지식과 자원이 중요하지만, 일상적인 환자 처치 지침도 여전히 필요하다.

곤충 물림 및 쏘임

북미의 야생 환경에서는 많은 곤충(예: 무는 파리, 모기)이 골칫거리가 될 수 있지만, 질병을 옮기지는 않는다. 곤충에게 물리거나 쏘인 대부분 사람은 경미한 국소 반응만 나타난다. 통증이 있고 일반적으로 상당한 불안감을 동반하지만, 일반적으로 생명을 위협하는 문제는 없다. 그러나 웨스트 나일 바이러스, 지카 바이러스와 같은 모기 매개 질병은 최근 큰 우려를 불러일으키고 있다. 또한 열대 지역을 여행하는 사람들은 말라리아, 뎅기열 등 다른 매개체로 전염 질병에 대해 알고 있어야 한다.

알레르기 반응은 국소적인 증상과 징후부터 생명을 위협하는 아나필락시스까지 다양한 범위에서 발행한다. 쏘인 후 심각한 증상이 나타나기까지 걸리는 시간은 다양할 수 있지만, 보통 쏘인 후 1시간 이내에 가장 심각한 증상이 나타난다. 더 심각한 전신 반응은 48시간 후에 최고조에 달할 수 있으며 일부 지연형 과민증에서는 더 오래 지속될 수도 있다. 아나필락시스는 쏘인 사람의 0.3~8%에서 보고된다. 미국에서는 매년 최소 40명의 사망자가 보고되고 있다.

야생 EMS 제공자는 종종 사고와 관련된 불안감으로부터 반응의 심각성을 파악할 수 있어야 한다. 이전에 심각한 알레르기 반응을 보인 적이 있는 모든 환자가 두 번째 노출 시 똑같이 심각한 반응을 보이는 것은 아니지만, 그럴 수도 있고 더 심할 수도 있다. 이러한 이유로 누가 덜 심각한 반응을 보일지 예측하기는 매우 어려울 수 있으며 병원 전 처치 제공자는 처치와 조기 이송을 신중하게 시행한다.

쏘인 일부 사람 중 일부는 몇 분 안에 전신 알레르기 반응으로 진행된다. 이 반응은 두드러기에서 아나필락시스 반응에 이르기까지 다양하다. 전신 알레르기 반응의 정확한 범위는 주입된 독소의 함량(벌과 말벌의 종에 따라 다름)과 환자의 알레르기 병력에 따라 다르지만, 일반적으로 다음 중 하나 이상의 증상이 나타난다.

- 두드러기(**그림 21-18**)
- 입술 및 얼굴 부기
- 쉰 목소리 또는 협착음
- 쌕쌕거림 및 호흡곤란
- 복부 경련, 구토 또는 설사
- 빈맥 또는 서맥
- 저혈압
- 실신 및 정신 상태 변화

벌에 쏘인 후 경미하거나 국소적으로 두드러기가 발생한 환자는 아마도 상태가 좋아질 것이다. 그러나 물리거나 쏘인 후 두드러기가 발생한 환자가 실제 아나필락시스로 진행되면 쉰 목소리와 저혈압이 가장 흔한 초기 징후이다. 벌에 쏘여 알레르기 반응 후 사망의 주요 원인은 기도 부종으로 인한 기도 폐쇄이며 쉰 목소리는 일반적으로 기도 부기의 첫 징후이다. 벌레 물림이나 쏘임에 대한 전신 반응을 보이는 환자는 즉시 처치를 받아야 한다.

꿀벌 침은 가시가 있으므로 쏘고 날아갈 때 보통 피부에 남아 있다. 침을 제거하지 않으면 침과 독주머니에서 나온 독이 45~60초 동

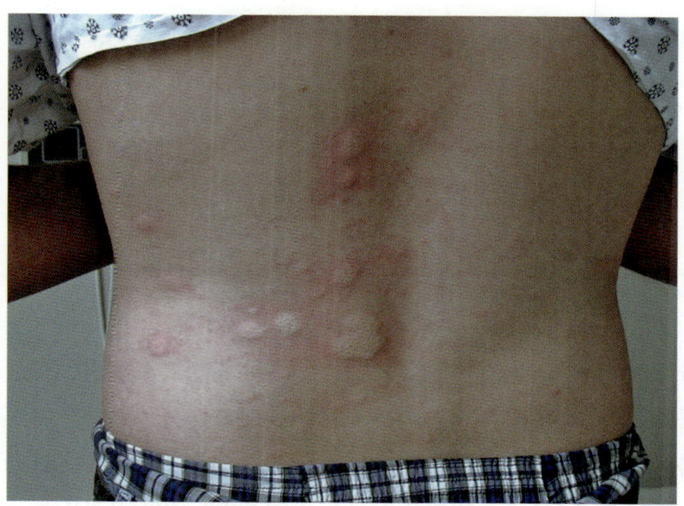

그림 21-18 알레르기성 두드러기
© Chuck Stewart, MD, EMDM, MPH

안 피부에 계속 주입되므로 침을 빨리 제거하는 것이 중요하다. 벌침을 제거하는 올바른 방법에 대한 많은 논의가 있었지만, 최근 정보에 따르면 가능한 한 빨리 제거하기만 하면 벌침을 제거하는 방법은 크게 중요하지 않다고 한다. 손톱, 칼날 가장자리 또는 신용카드는 박힌 벌침을 제거하는 데 효과적인 도구이다. 쏘인 후 15초 이내에 침을 제거하면 쏘임의 심각성이 감소한다. 말벌과 같은 다른 곤충은 알레르기 반응을 일으킬 수 있으며 침을 삽입하지 않고도 환자에게 여러 번 침을 쏠 수 있다.

기본소생술 처치는 일반적으로 환자를 편안한 자세로 유지하고 기도 유지를 시행하며 산소를 공급하는 것이 포함된다.

벌레에게 물리거나 쏘인 경우 나타나는 알레르기 반응을 처치하는 데 사용하는 주요 약물은 다음과 같다.

1. 에피네프린(아드레날린). 에피네프린은 몇 분 동안만 작용하지만, 생명을 구할 수 있다. 심하면 반복 투여가 필요할 수 있다.
2. 항히스타민제. 히스타민-1(예: 디이펜하이드라민과 히스타민-2(예: 파모티딘) 차단제가 모두 사용된다. 벌침 알레르기로 인해 에피네프린 투여가 필요한 사람은 항히스타민제를 투여한다.
3. 스테로이드(예: 프레드니손, 덱사메타손). 에피네프린이 필요한 대부분의 사람은 장기간의 알레르기 반응을 억제하기 위해 스테로이드를 투여한다.

가장 중요한 약물은 에피네프린으로 급성 반응을 빠르게 역전시키는 작용을 한다. 에피네프린은 펜 크기의 자가 주사기로 사용할 수 있으며 벌침에 대한 전신 알레르기가 있는 환자에게 처방되는 경우

가 많다(**Box 21-8**). 이러한 자가 주사기는 많은 야생 EMS 처치 키트에 들어 있다. 야생의학회는 야생에서의 에피네프린 사용에 관한 지침을 발표했다. 이 지침은 급성 아나필락시스를 인지하고 에피네프린을 투여할 수 있도록 교육받은 야생 EMS 제공자가 에피네프린을 투여할 것을 권장한다.

일부 야생 수색 및 구조팀의 구급 가방에 알레르기 반응에 대한 약물을 휴대하고 있으며 야생 EMS 제공자는 약물 사용에 대한 특별 교육을 받았다. 심한 알레르기 병력이 있는 사람은 개인 구급상자에 이러한 약물을 가지고 다니는 경우가 많다.

이 장에서는 벌레 물림과 쏘임을 포함할 수 있는 야생 외상 처치에 초점을 맞추고 있지만, 병원 전 처치 제공자는 환자가 다른 노출 및 음식으로 인해 심각한 알레르기가 발생할 수 있으며 같은 환자 평가와 처치가 적용될 수 있음을 명심해야 한다.

뱀에게 물린 상처

약 3,000종의 뱀이 있으며 그 중 약 600종이 독을 가지고 있지만, 의학적으로 중요한 독을 가진 뱀은 200종에 불과하다. 북반구에서는 거의 발견되지 않는다. 대부분은 열대 지역에 자연적으로 서식하며 많은 뱀에 독샘을 가지고 있지만, 북미에 서식하는 토종 뱀 중 인간에게 경미한 자극 이상을 일으킬 정도로 강한 독을 가진 뱀은 두 종류뿐이다. 모든 뱀에게 물린 상처는 감염 및 기타 국소 조직 손상을 일으킬 가능성이 있으므로 다른 찔린 상처와 마찬가지로 처치를 한다.

산호 뱀은 북아메리카 남부에서 발견되는 작은 뱀이다(**그림 21-19**). 이 뱀은 신경독성이 있고 마비를 일으키는 독을 가지고 있다. 이 뱀은 몸집이 작고 독니가 작으며 큰 뱀에 비해 입을 크게 벌릴 수 없고 다른 살무사에 비해 소심하여서 심각한 독이 주입되는 경우는 흔하지 않다. 북아메리카 산호 뱀 중에서 동부 또는 플로리다에 서식하는 산호 뱀이 가장 독성이 강한 독을 가지고 있다. 색깔이 있는 띠를 기준으로 산호 뱀을 식별하는 데 사용하는 방법은 특정 북

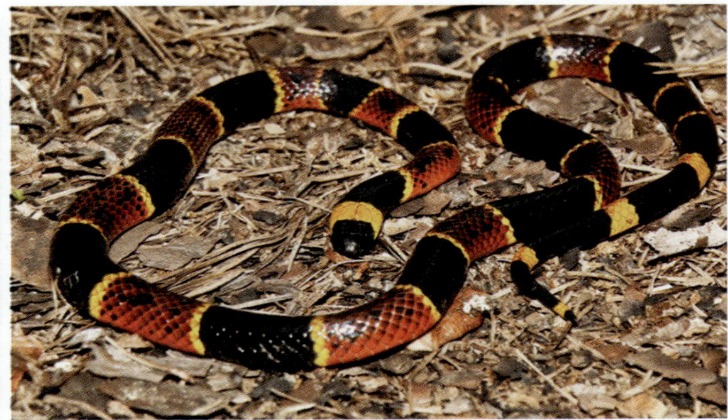

그림 21-19 산호 뱀
© JasonOndreicka/iStock/Getty Images

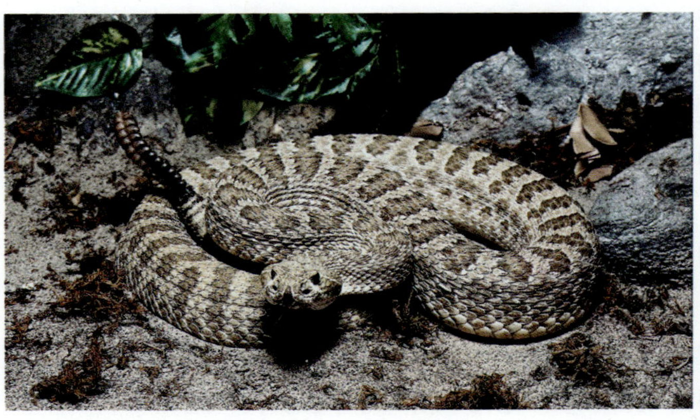

그림 21-20 방울뱀
© Jason Ondreicka/Thinkstock

아메리카 종에만 적용되며 뱀을 구별하는 데 의존해서는 안 된다. 독에 중독되면 최대 15시간까지 증상이 지연될 수 있으며 빠르게 나타나고 중추 마비(눈꺼풀 처짐, 복시, 안구의 부동화, 입안 분비물 관리 곤란)로 시작된다.

흔히 살무사라고 불리는 살무사아과 독사는 북아메리카 전역에서 발견되며 다양한 종류의 방울뱀(**그림 21-20**), 아메리카 살무사(**그림 21-21**), 물뱀 또는 늪살무사를 포함한다(**그림 21-22**). 대부분의 살무사아과 독사에게 물리는 사고는 야생이 아닌 시골, 교외, 심지어 도시 지역에서 발생한다. 대표적인 예는 술에 취한 남자가 애완용 방울뱀과 뽀뽀하다가 입술이나 혀를 물린 경우이다. 신체의 다른 부위, 특히 팔다리에 물리는 경우도 흔하다(**그림 21-23**).

뱀에게 물리는 것은 생각만큼 드문 일이 아니다. 미국에서는 매년 약 10,000명의 환자가 뱀에게 물려 치료를 받고 약 5명이 사망한다. 세계적으로 매년 약 421,000건의 뱀에게 물려 20,000명이 사망하는

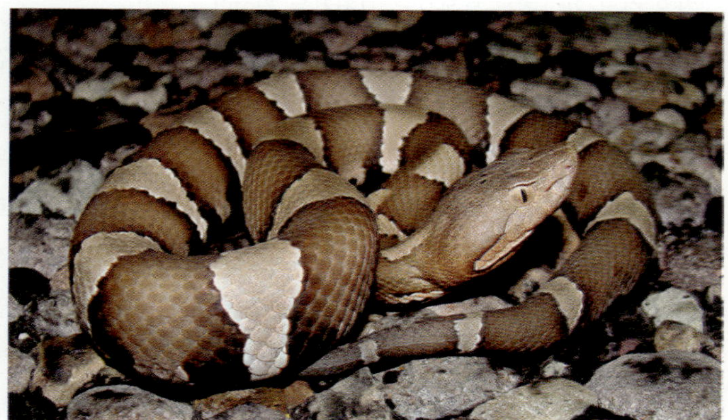

그림 21-21 아메리카 살무사
© Matt Jeppson/Shutterstock

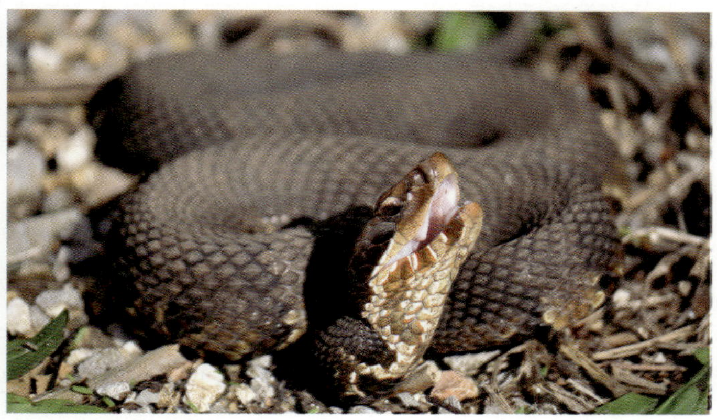

그림 21-22 늪살모사
© James DeBoer/Shutterstock

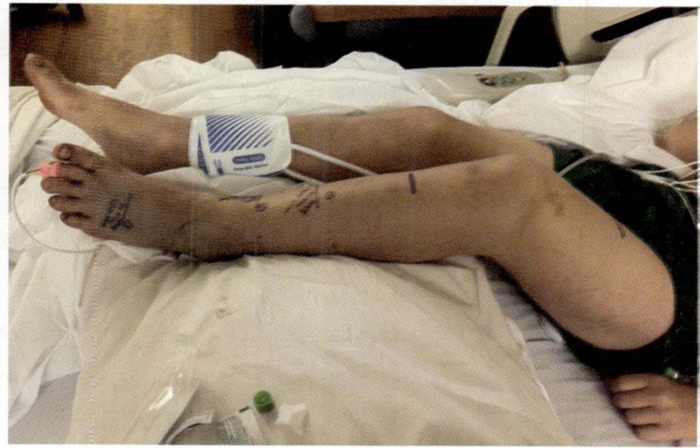

그림 21-23 늪살모사에 왼쪽 다리 아래 부위를 물린 상처로 진행성 부종과 반상출혈에 유의한다.
Courtesy of Ben Abo.

과 같다.

- 심한 국소 발적, 부기, 멍 및 통증
- 물린 부위의 심한 통증 및 압통(예: 발에 물린 경우 서혜부 또는 무릎까지 통증이나 압통이 있는 경우)
- 물린 부위에서 무시할 수 있는 출혈이 지속되는 경우
- 손가락과 발가락의 감각 이상(감각 이상은 일반적으로 신경 손상이나 생화학적 이상으로 인해 발생하는 비정상적인 감각으로 "핀과 바늘로 찌르는 듯한 느낌"이 일반적인 감각 이상)
- 입안의 금속성 맛
- 심한 불안감
- 구역, 구토 및 복통

것으로 추정되지만, 많은 국가에서 사망에 대한 기록이 부실하므로 실제로는 이보다 훨씬 더 많을 수 있다.

역사적으로 환자, 목격자 또는 EMS 제공자가 다양한 병원 전 처치를 시도해 왔다. 독사에게 물렸을 때 효과가 있는 것으로 알려진 유일한 처치법은 해독제인 데 이 해독제는 매우 비싸므로 구급 가방에 일상적으로 갖춰져 있지 않다. 도움이 되는 것으로 입증된 유일한 길거리 EMS 처치는 지지요법과 신속하게 병원으로 이송하는 것이다.

뱀에게 물렸을 때 처치의 첫 번째 단계는 독의 징후를 관찰하는 것이다(즉, 독이 주입되었는지 확인). 살무사아과 독사에 물린 부위 중 일부만 실제로 독이 주입되며(20~25%는 독이 없음) 독 주입의 징후는 상당히 뚜렷하다. 독사에게 물렸을 때 나타나는 증상과 징후는 보통 몇 분 안에 나타나지만, 6~8시간 또는 그 이상 지연되는 경우는 드물지 않으므로 독사에게 물린 것으로 의심되면 환자를 병원으로 이송하는 것이 적절하다. 독사에게 물렸을 때 나타나는 징후는 다음

살무사아과 독사에게 물려 독액 주입이 의심되는 경우 병원 전 처치

독 주입이 의심되는 환자를 처치할 때 초기 처치는 다른 중증 내과 질환이나 중증 손상 환자와 유사하다. 기도, 호흡, 순환을 유지하고 적절한 산소포화도를 유지하기 위해 산소 공급, 심장 모니터링, 정맥 라인 확보, 환자의 활력징후를 모니터링한다.

물린 부위에 홍반, 부기, 반상출혈, 압통, 수포 또는 연부조직 괴사 발생, 통증 및 압통이 얼마나 방사되는지 등 독에 중독된 징후가 있는지 평가한다. 장신구나 몸에 꽉 끼는 옷은 모두 제거한다.

15분마다 부기의 앞쪽 가장자리를 검은색 펜으로 표시하여 부기의 심각성과 진행 속도를 확인한다. 마찬가지로 통증과 압통이 방사되는 앞쪽 가장자리를 표시한다. 해당 팔다리를 고정하고 심장 높이와 비슷하게 위치시켜야 한다(심장보다 높아지거나 의존적으로 유지하

지 않아야 함). 팔꿈치와 같은 주요 관절은 상대적인 신전 상태(45도 미만으로 굴곡)를 유지한다. 부기가 발생하면 부목이나 의복이 순환 장애를 일으키지 않는지 지속해서 고려한다.

환자에게 통증 완화가 필요한 경우 일부 독 주입과 관련된 출혈 위험과 비스테로이드성 항염증제(NSAID) 사용 시 혈소판 효과 때문에 통증 완화에는 비스테로이드성 항염증제(NSAID)보다 아편제가 선호된다.

뱀을 죽이려고 시도하지 않는다. 죽이거나 목이 잘린 뱀은 여전히 EMS 제공자에게 독을 주입할 위험이 있다. 상황이 허락하는 경우 안전한 거리에서 뱀의 사진을 찍는다. 이 시나리오에서 안전은 아무리 강조해도 지나치지 않는다.

환자를 구조하는 것이 바람직하지만, 필요한 경우 환자를 천천히 걸어서 대피시킬 수 있으며 자주 휴식을 취하고 안심시켜 침착하게 이송할 수 있다. 환자를 적절한 의료기관으로 신속하게 이송을 시작하고 이송할 의료기관에 상황을 보고하여 처치할 준비를 할 수 있도록 한다.

팔다리 고정

호주에서는 코브라과(코브라, 맘바, 북미 산호) 뱀에게 물렸을 때 현장에서 압박 고정이 효과적으로 사용되었다(**그림 21-24**). 이 술기는 뱀에게 물린 팔다리 전체를 탄력이 있는 랩이나 붕대로 즉시 단단히 감은 다음 팔다리를 부목으로 고정하는 것이다.

북아메리카 이외의 지역에서 환자가 병원 처치를 받기까지 2시간 이상 걸리고 팔다리를 물린 경우 압박 고정을 시행하는 것이 합리적일 수 있다. 물린 부위에 5×5cm 패드로 덮고 그런 다음 물린 부위 양쪽에서 최소 10~15cm의 여유를 두고 패드로 덮은 물린 부위 바로 위에 탄력 붕대로 단단히 감는다. 손가락과 발가락의 혈액 순환이 잘 되는지(정상 맥박, 감각, 색) 주의 깊게 확인한다. 또 다른 방법은 압박 붕대로 팔다리 전체를 뱀처럼 단단히 감싸는 것이다. 붕대는 압박된 조직과 팔다리 표면 근처의 미세한 혈액 및 림프관 내에 독을 넣어 독이 일반 순환계로 흡수되는 것을 지연시키기 위한 것이다. 마지막으로 팔다리의 움직임을 방지하기 위해 부목으로 고정한다. 손이나 팔에 물린 경우 슬링을 적용한다. 일부 전문가들은 독이 한 부위에 국한되면 국소 조직 손상 가능성이 높아질 수 있다고 생각하기 때문에 이 권장 사상은 논란의 여지가 있다는 점에 유의한다.

역사적으로 다음과 같은 치료법이 권장되었지만, 문헌에 의해 뒷받침되지는 않는다.

1. 휴식을 취한다. 일부 권장 사항은 뱀에게 물린 사람은 항상 무리한 활동을 피해야 한다고 주장한다. 북아메리카에서 뱀에게 물려 사망하는 경우는 매우 드물며 야생 지역에서 무리한 하이킹으로 인해 뱀에게 물린다고 해서 훨씬 더 통증이 증가할 가능

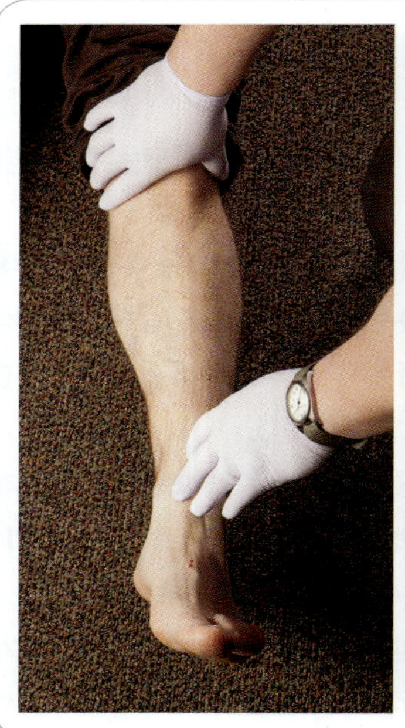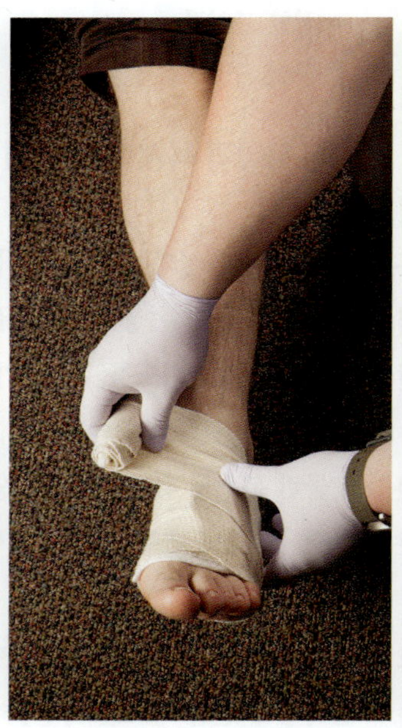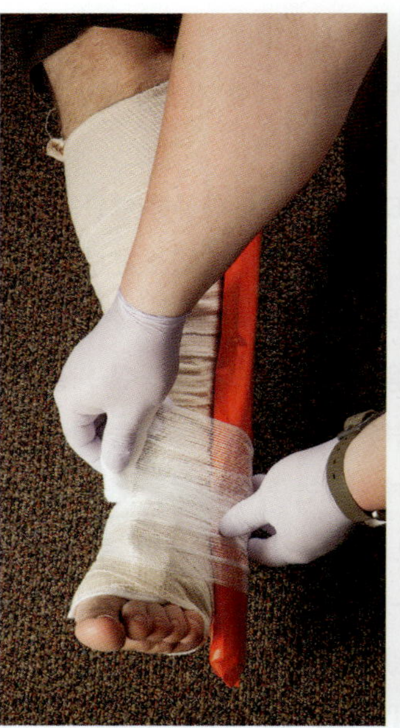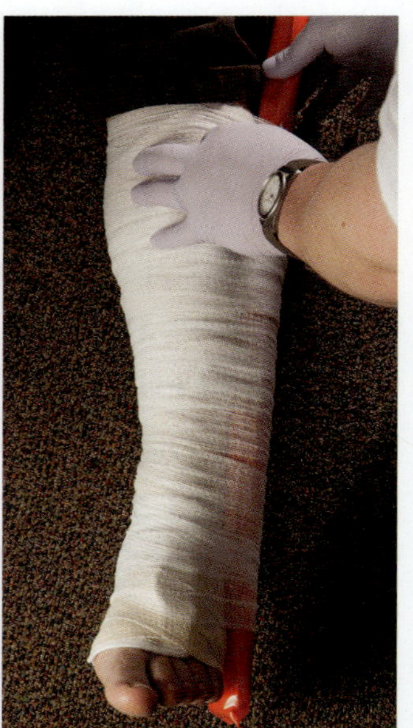

그림 21-24 압박 고정 기술

성은 거의 없다. 피해자가 걸을 수 있다면 가장 이상적이다. 그러나 이송을 기다리는 것이 환자를 병원으로 이송하는 것을 지연시키는 경우 환자는 가능한 모든 도움을 받아 걸어서 이동을 할 수 있다.

2. 뱀을 잡아 병원으로 가지고 간다. 독사로 의심되는 뱀을 잡으려다 물린 목격자에 대한 신고가 많이 접수되고 있다. 미국에서는 모든 살무사아과 독사의 독에 대해 단일해독제가 사용하며 처치는 이전의 증상과 징후에 따라 임상적 독 주입 정도에 따라 이루어진다. 따라서 뱀을 식별하는 것은 뱀을 잡으려는 시도의 위험성에 비해 중요도가 낮다. 뱀 사진이 유용할 수 있지만, 추가 물림의 위험을 무릅쓰고 뱀을 확인하는 것은 가치가 없다.

3. 흡인 또는 절개. 독사에게 물렸을 때 절개 여부와 관계없이 흡인은 필요가 없는 것으로 밝혀졌다. 구급 가방에 흡인기가 있는 경우를 제외하고는 뱀에게 물린 상처에 흡인을 시행하지 않는다.

4. 전기 충격. 뱀에게 물린 부위에 전기 충격을 가하는 것은 전혀 효과가 없는 것으로 밝혀졌으므로 절대로 사용하지 않는다.

5. 얼음찜질. 북아메리카 살무사아과 독사에게 물렸을 때 조직 손상을 증가시키는 것으로 밝혀졌으므로 사용하지 않는다.

6. 부목 고정. 동맥 또는 정맥 지혈대, 림프 수축기 또는 탄력 붕대 등은 권장되지만, 이러한 처치 방법 중 어느 것도 효과가 입증되지 않았으며 물린 부위의 국소 손상을 악화시킬 수 있다.

야생의 EMS 상황 재조명

이 장의 시작 부분에서 우리는 다음과 같이 질문했다. "언제 야생 EMS에 대해 생각해야 하는가? 즉, 언제 거리에서 하는 일과 다르게 생각하고 일해야 하는가?"라고 질문했다. 짧은 대답은 "상황에 따라 다르다."

시간, 거리, 날씨, 지형 등이 모두 결정에 영향을 미친다. 특정 상황에서 특정 손상을 입은 특정 환자에게 길거리에서의 처치가 아닌 야생 처치가 필요하다는 결정은 환자를 직접 처치하는 병원 전 처치 제공자가 내리는 것이 가장 좋은 의학적 결정이다. 현장에 있는 병원 전 처치 제공자가 의료 지도 의사에게 연락할 수 있다면 특히 의료 지도 의사가 야생 EMS 상황에 대해 잘 알고 있다면 의료 지도를 받을 가치가 있다. 궁극적으로 결정은 업무 범위, 자율성에 관한 프로토콜, 의료 지도에 따라 현장의 병원 전 처치 제공자에게 달려 있다.

PHTLS는 자율적 의료 의사 결정 및 야생 의료에 대한 의료 지도 의사의 충분한 지식, 핵심 원칙, 교육이 충분하다면 병원 전 처치 제공자가 야생 환경에서 환자 처치와 관련하여 가장 절절한 결정을 내릴 수 있다고 믿는다.

요 약

- 야생 EMS의 많은 원칙은 거리 EMS와 같지만, 특수한 상황으로 인해 선호도와 관행이 변경될 수 있다. 이러한 요소의 균형을 맞추는 것은 야생 EMS 제공자의 전문 분야가 된다.

- 지식이 풍부한 의료 지도 의사의 의료 지시와 야생 EMS 상황에 직면할 가능성이 있는 병원 전 처치 제공자를 위한 전문 교육은 야생 EMS의 필수 구성 요소이다.

- LATE라는 약어는 수색 및 구조팀, 기타 야생 EMS 작업의 단순화된 원칙을 나타낸다.

- 야생 EMS는 특별한 환자 고정 및 이송 고려 사항, 특수 장비, 표준 절차 및 프로토콜의 수정, 환자와 병원 전 처치 제공자 모두를 위한 상황별 안전 고려사항이 필요한 다양한 환경과 상황을 제시한다.

- 초기 환자 평가는 환경과 관계없이 같다. 우선순위는 손상이 발생한 지점에서 즉시 완화할 수 있는 주요 생명을 위협하는 것을 기준으로 한다.

- 많은 야생 상황에서 병원 전 처치 제공자는 처치를 제공하는 데 사용하는 장비와 방법을 즉석에서 만들어 사용할 수 있다. 즉석에서 만든 지혈대 사용에 능숙해야 하며 항생제 투여, 통증 관리, 심폐소생술 및 제세동과 같은 표준 처치 방법을 야생 환경에 가장 잘 적용하는 방법을 이해한다.

- 야생에서 환자를 처치할 때 야생 EMS 제공자는 음식과 물 요구량과 배설물 제거 필요성도 고려한다.

- 야생 처치의 기본 원칙은 달리 입증될 때까지 모든 환자에게 저체온증, 저혈당 및 혈량저하 상태라는 것이다.

- 물림과 쏘임은 야생에서 흔히 발생하는 문제이다. 이러한 환자를 처치하는 데는 현지 지식과 자원이 중요하지만, 일상적인 환자 처치 지침도 필요하다.

시나리오 재구성

당신은 지역 수색 및 구조팀 의료팀 리더이며 담당 지역의 유명한 계곡으로 출동하였다. 현재 가지고 있는 유일한 정보는 긴급 위성 통신을 통해 송출되는 조난 신호의 GPS 위치뿐이다. 현재 시각은 18시이고 기온은 23℃이다. 일기 예보에 따르면 저녁 내내 천둥 번개가 치고 밤새 최저기온이 2℃로 떨어질 것으로 예상된다. 팀은 LATE[위치(Location), 접근(Access), 처치(Treat), 구출(Excurrent)] 약어를 사용하여 대응 계획을 세우기 시작한다.

당신 팀은 수중 구조 키트, 고각 구조 키트, 개인보호장비 및 표준 의료키트 등 필요한 장비를 조립하고 해당 위치로 출동을 시작한다. 팀 리더인 당신은 사고지휘관과 연락하여 계곡 정상에서 사고지휘소까지 통신 중계가 가능하도록 단계별 팀원들과 통신 계획을 수립한다.

- 이러한 유형의 구조 시나리오에서 가장 심각하고 가능성이 높은 부상을 처리하기 위해 팀과 개인 의료 키트에 필수적인 항목은 무엇인가?
- 원격 및 장기간 현장에서 환자를 처치하기 위해 어떤 운영상 구체적인(업무 범위 확대) 프로토콜을 원하는가? 통신 방법이 제한적일 것으로 예상되므로 대기 명령이 있는가?
- 구조팀에 대한 어떤 안전 문제를 고려해야 하는가? 시간, 환자의 위치, 팀의 경험 및 훈련과 같은 상황적 요인이 안전에 어떤 영향을 미치는가?

당신은 GPS 위치를 찾아 30m 레펠이 3개가 설치되어 있을 계곡을 발견한다. 소리를 지르며 연락을 시도하지만, 아무런 응답이 없었다. 호루라기를 불면 희미한 호루라기 소리가 들린다. 당신 팀은 안전하게 해당 위치로 이동한다. 두 번째 레펠의 정상에서 비상 신호를 울린 두 명을 발견한다. 그들은 팀원 중 한 명이 13시에 계속에서 15m 아래로 추락했다고 말한다. 그들은 비상 신호등을 이용해 신호를 보내기 위해 그 위치에서 다시 올라가야 했다. 다른 친구는 피해자를 평가하기 위해 하강했고 손상 부위에 대량출혈과 변형된 개방성 넓적다리뼈 골절이 보이고 환자가 혼란스러워 보인다고 말했다. 환자는 의식을 잃거나 다른 머리 외상 징후를 보이지 않았으며 그는 헬멧을 쓰고 있었다. 그 친구는 출혈이 계속되는 상태에서 출혈 부위에 직접 압박을 가하고 있었다.

당신은 레펠을 내려가면서 환자를 돌보는 친구와 구두로 의사소통한다. 출혈이 계속되는 상처 근위부에, 즉석에서 지혈대를 적용하는 방법을 설명하고 지혈대를 적용하라고 지시한다. 환자의 친구가 출혈이 조절되었다고 이야기했다.

(다음 페이지에 계속)

시나리오 재구성 (이어서)

추가 장비가 지원되면 환자에 접근하기 위한 마지막 레펠을 시작한다. 환자에게 도착했을 때 25세의 건강한 남성이 깨어 있었고 오른쪽 넓적다리뼈 개방성 골절이 변형된 것을 발견할 수 있었다. 친구는 여분의 옷을 입히려고 했지만, 환자는 얕은 차가운 물웅덩이에 있었고 옷이 젖어 떨고 있었다. 당신은 처치를 어떻게 시행할지 계획하고 시작하지만, 날이 어두워지고 있어 환자를 구출하려면 아침까지 기다려야 한다.

- 야생 환경에서 다른 사람에게 처치를 제공하도록 지시할 수 있는가? 119 신고 시 구급 및 구조대원이 도착하기 전에 지침을 지원하기 위해 출동 방법을 잘 알고 있으며 다른 사람에게 원격으로 초기 처치를 제공하도록 지시할 수 있는가? 환자에게 도착하는 데 시간이 더 지연되는 경우 친구에게 어떤 조치를 하도록 지시하겠는가?
- 평가 및 처치에 있어 우선순위는 무엇인가? 장기간에 걸친 환자 처치 시 고려해야 할 사항은 무엇인가?
- 환자의 체온을 유지하고 구출하기 위한 계획은 무엇인가?

시나리오 해결책

현장에 가장 먼저 도착하면 헤드램프를 켜고 신속하게 주변을 파악하여 자신과 부상자 및 동료의 안전을 확보한다. 협곡 정상에 있는 통신 중계기를 통해 구조 진행 상황을 사고지휘관에게 보고했다. 구름이 거의 없고 뇌우가 발생하지 않는 날씨가 유지되는 것 같으며 밤새 이 위치에 머물러야 한다고 결정한다. 이 지역에는 야간 작전을 수행할 수 있는 헬기가 없으며 오늘 밤에는 환자를 이 위치에서 안전하고 효율적으로 이동할 수 없다. 현재 위치에서 약 100m 정도 떨어진 협곡의 입구에서 환자를 인양하기 위해 동이 트면 대기 중인 구조 헬기가 출동할 수 있도록 요청한다.

환자가 있는 위치에는 공간이 제한되어 있지만, 환자를 옆으로 이동할 수 있으므로 다른 구조대원이 내려올 때 직접적인 경로를 벗어나지 않고 환자를 건조한 장소와 단열 패드 위로 조심스럽게 옮길 수 있다.

MARCH PAWS 알고리즘에 따라 환자 평가가 진행된다. 이미 원격으로 대량 출혈을 확인하고 지혈했으며 환자의 동료가 적용한 지혈대를 확인한다. 지혈대는 적당히 효과적인 것으로 보이므로 첫 번째 지혈대 바로 옆에 두 번째 지혈대를 적용하고 시간을 기록했다. 두 번째 적용한 지혈대로 추가 출혈이 완전히 멈췄고 더 이상 원위부 맥박이 촉지되지 않는 것을 확인했다. 대량 출혈의 다른 징후를 발견하지 못했다. 그러나 환자의 골반을 평가하니 불안정하고 통증이 심해 골반고정대를 적용한다.

환자는 기도 손상의 징후 없이 깨어 있고 말을 한다. 가슴벽에 손을 대고 호흡곤란이나 가슴벽 외상의 징후 없이 양쪽 가슴이 대칭적으로 움직이는 것을 평가한다. 원위부 맥박을 평가하여 혈액 순환을 확인하고 노동맥의 맥박수가 분당 120회로 빠른 것을 확인한다. 환자의 피부는 차갑고 약간 발한이 있다. 환자의 젖은 옷을 제거하고 건조하고 따뜻한 옷을 입혀 저체온증을 처치한다. 당신은 팀원에게 추가 핫팩이 있는 침낭을 준비하도록 지시한다. 머리를 평가한 결과 머리나 목 및 허리 손상의 명백한 징후는 보이지 않지만, 심각한 낙상으로 손상을 입었을 가능성이 있으므로 척추 손상의 가능성을 고려하여 전신 진공부목을 사용하여 척추 움직임 제한을 시행한다. 환자는 의식이 있고 지남력이 있으며 신경학적 검사 결과도 정상이다. 그는 약간의 메스꺼움은 있지만, 구토는 하지 않았으며 온단세트론 4mg을 경구 붕해 정제로 투여한다. 통증을 조절하기 위해 경구 아세트아미노펜 1g을 투여하고 코안으로 케타민 100mg의 해리성 용량을 투여한다. 이렇게 하면 10점 만점에 10점이던 통증이 10점 만점에 2점으로 낮아지고 평가와 부목 고정 및 처치를 쉽게 한다.

개방 골절에 대한 기존 항생제 처방 프로토콜에 따라 다른 모든 생명을 위협하는 문제가 해결되었으므로 정맥 라인을 확보하고 항생제에 대한 알레르기가 없는지 확인한 후 세파졸린 2g을 투여한다. 환자의 머리부터 발끝까지 다른 상처나 손상이 있는지 재평가하고 주의가 필요한 유일한 부위는 개방성 넓적다리뼈 골절을 확인한다. 개방성 골절 부위를 생수로 조심스럽게 세척한다. 이제 구출 시간이 길어졌다는 것을 알고 지혈대를 다른 형태의 지혈 방법으로 전환하려고 시도한다. 지혈대에서 압박 드레싱으로 안전하게 전환하여 출혈을 조절할 수 있다. 당신은 압박 드레싱 부위를 자주 재평가하고 지혈이 유지되는지 확인한다. 원위부 맥박과 감각이 회복되었다.

마지막으로 적절한 부목으로 환자를 고정하고 이송할 준비를 완료한다. 개방성 넓적다리뼈 골절의 경우 도수 견인으로 다리를 해부학적 자세를 취한 후 그 상태를 유지하면서 진공부목을 적용한다. 이제 진공부목은 과도한 압력 부위 없이 목, 등, 골반 및 넓적다리뼈 골절을 포함한 전신을 고정할 수 있다. 우선순위가 높은 손상을 처치한 후 가장 심각한 손상이 아닌 오른쪽 손목 골절이 의심되는 환자를

(다음 페이지에 계속)

References

1. Wilderness. In: *Merriam-Webster's Collegiate Dictionary*. 11th ed. Merriam-Webster; 2014:1432.

2. McGinnis KK. *Rural and Frontier Emergency Medical Services*. National Rural Health Association; 2004.

3. Liffrig JR, Tarter SL, Schimelpfenig T, et al. Wilderness medicine education. In: Auerbach PS, ed. *Auerbach's Wilderness Medicine*. 7th ed. Elsevier; 2017:2440-2471.

4. Winstead C, Hawkins SC. Wilderness EMS education. In: Hawkins SC, ed. *Wilderness EMS*. Wolters Kluwer; 2018:61-81.

5. Bennett BL. A time has come for wilderness emergency medical service: a new direction. *Wilderness Environ Med*. 2012;23(1):5-6.

6. Warden CR, Millin MG, Hawkins SC, et al. Medical direction of wilderness and other operational emergency services programs. *Wilderness Environ Med*. 2012;23(1):37-43.

7. Millin M. Wilderness EMS medical oversight. In: Hawkins SC, ed. *Wilderness EMS*. Wolters Kluwer; 2018:101-110.

8. Russell K, Weber D, Scheele B, et al. Search and rescue in the intermountain west states. *Wilderness Environ Med*. 2013;24:429-433.

9. National Highway Traffic Safety Administration. *The National EMS Scope of Practice Model*. Department of Transportation/ National Highway Traffic Safety Administration; 2005.

10. Millin MG, Johnson DE, Schimelpfenig T, et al. Medical oversight, educational core content, and proposed scopes of practice of wilderness EMS providers: a joint project developed by wilderness EMS educators, medical directors, and regulators using a Delphi approach. *Prehosp Emerg Care*. 2017;21(6):673-681.

11. Smith W. Medical professionals role in search and rescue. In: Rodway G, Weber DC, McIntosh SE, eds. *Mountain Medicine and Technical Rescue*. Carreg; 2016:207-223.

12. Hawkins SC, Millin MC, Smith W. Wilderness emergency medical services and response systems. In: Auerbach P, ed. *Auerbach's Wilderness Medicine*. 7th ed. Elsevier; 2017:1200-1213.

13. Johnson DE, Schimelpfenig T, Hubbel F. Minimum guidelines and scope of practice for wilderness first aid. *Wilderness Environ Med*. 2013;24(4):456-462.

14. Tilton B. *Wilderness First Responder*. Falcon Guides (Globe Pequot Press); 2010.

15. American Society for Testing and Materials. *Standard Guide for Training First Responders Who Practice in Wilderness, Delayed, or Prolonged Transport Settings*. American Society for Testing and Materials; 1995:F1616-F1695.

16. Wilderness Medical Society Curriculum Committee. Wilderness first responder: recommended minimum course topics. *Wilderness Environ Med*. 1999;10:13-19.

17. McNamara EC, Johe DH, Endly DA, eds. *Outdoor Emergency Care*. 5th ed. National Ski Patrol. Brady (Pearson); 2012.

18. Hawkins SC. The relationship between ski patrols and emergency medical services systems. *Wilderness Environ Med*. 2012;23:106-111.

19. Constance BB, Auerbach PS, Johe DH. Prehospital medical care and the National Ski Patrol: how does outdoor emergency care compare to traditional EMS training? *Wilderness Environ Med*. 2012;23:177-189.

20. Spano SJ. National Park Service medicine. In: Auerbach P, ed. *Auerbach's Wilderness Medicine*. 7th ed. Elsevier; 2017: 2487-2497.

21. Smith WR. Integration of tactical EMS in the National Park Service. *Wilderness Environ Med*. 2017;28(2S):S146-S153.

22. Lipman GS, Weichenthal L, Harris NS, et al. Core content for Wilderness Medicine fellowship training of emergency medicine graduates. *Acad Emerg Med*. 2014;21(2):204-207.

23. Hawkins S, Millin M, Smith W. Care in the wilderness. In: Cone D, Brice JH, Delbridge TR, Myers JB, eds. *Emergency Medical Services: Clinical Practice and System Oversight*. 2nd ed. Vol 2: Medical Oversight of EMS. John Wiley & Sons; 2015:377-391.

24. Vines T, Hudson S. Medical considerations in technical rescue. In: *High-Angle Rope Rescue Techniques: Levels I and II*. 4th ed. Jones & Bartlett Learning; 2016:224-245.

25. Smith WR. Principles of basic technical rescue, packaging, and patient care integration. In: Hawkins SC, ed. *Wilderness EMS*. Wolters Kluwer; 2018:101-110.

26. Hawkins SC. WEMS systems. In: Hawkins SC, ed. *Wilderness EMS*. Wolters Kluwer; 2018:21-59.

27. Zafren K, McCurley L, Shimanski C, et al. Technical rescue. In: Auerbach PS, ed. *Auerbach's Wilderness Medicine*. 7th ed. Elsevier; 2017:1242-1280.

28. Goodman T, Iserson KV, Strich H. Wilderness mortalities: a 13-year experience. *Ann Emerg Med*. 2001;37:279-283.

29. Gentile DA, Morris JA, Schimelpfenig T, Bass SM, Auerbach PS. Wilderness injuries and illnesses. *Ann Emerg Med.* 1992;21:853-861.

30. Singletary EM, Markenson DS. Injury prevention: decision making, safety, and accident avoidance. In: Auerbach PS, ed. *Auerbach's Wilderness Medicine.* 7th ed. Elsevier; 2017:593-616.

31. Isaac JE, Johnson DE. *Wilderness and Rescue Medicine.* 6th ed. Jones & Bartlett Learning; 2013.

32. Hawkins SC. Setting the record straight to reduce fatalities in sinking vehicles. *Emerg Med News.* 2015;37(8):28-29.

33. Butler FK, Blackbourne LH. Battlefield trauma care then and now: a decade of tactical combat casualty care. *J Trauma Acute Care Surg.* 2012;73:S395-S402.

34. Holcomb JB, Stansbury LG, Champion HR, Wade C, Bellamy RF. Understanding combat casualty care statistics. *J Trauma Acute Care Surg.* 2006;60:397-401.

35. Kelly J, Ritenour AE, McLaughlin DF, et al. Injury severity and causes of death from Operation Iraqi Freedom and Operation Enduring Freedom: 2003–2004 versus 2006. *J Trauma.* 2008;6:S21-S27.

36. Eastridge BJ, Mabry RL, Seguin P, et al. Death on the battlefield (2001–2011): implications for the future of combat casualty care. *J Trauma Acute Care Surg.* 2012;73: S431-S437.

37. Kotwal RS, Montgomery HR, Mabry RL, et al. Eliminating preventable death on the battlefield. *Arch Surg.* 2011;146:1350-1358.

38. Bennett BL, Butler FK, Wedmore I, eds. Tactical combat casualty care: transitioning battlefield lessons learned to other austere environments. *Wilderness Environ Med.* 2017;28(2S):S1-S154.

39. Smith B, Bledsoe BE, Nicolazzo P. General management of trauma in the wilderness. In: Hawkins SC, ed. *Wilderness EMS.* Wolters Kluwer; 2018:371-392.

40. Smith W. Episode 3: medical direction with Will Smith, MD [podcast]. RAW Medicine website. Published February 1, 2018. Accessed March 1, 2022. https://rawmedicine.libsyn.com/episode-3-medical-direction-with-will-smith-md

41. What is C-TECC? Committee for Tactical Emergency Casualty Care website. Accessed March 1, 2022. https://www.c-tecc.org/about-us/what-is-ctecc

42. Smith W, Grange K. Mission success: how a rural EMS agency implemented a tactical EMS program. *JEMS.* 2018;43(1):24-30.

43. Chan D, Goldberg R, Tascone A, et al. The effect of spinal immobilization on healthy volunteers. *Ann Emerg Med.* 1994;23(1):48-51.

44. Kwan I, Bunn F, Roberts IG. Spinal immobilisation for trauma patients. *Cochrane Database Syst Rev.* 2001(2): CD002803.

45. Ben-Galim P, Dreiangel N, Mattox KL, et al. Extrication collars can result in abnormal separation between vertebrae in the presence of dissociative injury. *J Trauma.* 2010;69:447-450.

46. Hauswald M, Ong G, Tandeberg D, et al. Out-of-hospital spinal immobilization: its effect on neurologic injury. *Acad Emerg Med.* 1998;5:214-219.

47. Oto B, Corey DJ II, Oswald J, Sifford D, Walsh B. Early secondary neurological deterioration after blunt spinal trauma: a review of the literature. *Acad Emerg Med.* 2015;22:1200-1212.

48. Senz K. New Hampshire rescue squad denies fault in woman's drowning. EMS World website. Published September 10, 2007. Accessed March 1, 2022. https://www.hmpgloballearningnetwork.com/site/emsworld/news/10408685/new-hampshire-rescue-squad-denies-fault-womans-drowning

49. Scheele BM. Technical rescue interface: off-road vehicle and helicopter WEMS response. In: Hawkins SC, ed. *Wilderness EMS.* Wolters Kluwer; 2018:503-518.

50. Kosecuat J, Rush SC, Simonsen I, et al. Efficacy of the mnemonic device "MARCH PAWS" as a checklist for pararescuemen during tactical field care and tactical evacuation. *J Spec Operations Med.* 2017;4:80-84.

51. Hawkins SC, Simon RB, Beissinger JP, Simon D. *Vertical Aid: Essential Wilderness Medicine for Climbers, Trekkers, and Mountaineers.* The Countryman Press; 2017.

52. Davis C. Part 2: management of infectious diseases: general infectious diseases in the wilderness environment. In: Hawkins SC, ed. *Wilderness EMS.* Wolters Kluwer; 2018:355-370.

53. Keenan S, Riesberg JC. Prolonged field care: beyond the "Golden Hour." *Wilderness Environ Med.* 2017;28(2S): S135-S139.

54. Gomi T. *Everyone Poops.* Kane/Miller Book Publishers; 1993.

55. Wing-Gaia SL, Askew W. Nutrition, malnutrition and starvation. In: Auerbach PS, ed. *Auerbach's Wilderness Medicine.* 7th ed. Elsevier; 2017:1964-1985.

56. Kenefick RW, Cheuvront SN, Leon LR, Obrien K. Dehydration and rehydration. In: Auerbach PS, ed. *Wilderness Medicine.* 7th ed. Elsevier; 2017:2031-2044.

57. Madsen P, Svendsen LB, Jorgenesen LG, et al. Tolerance to head-up tilt and suspension with elevated legs. *Aviat Space Environ Med.* 1998;69:781-784.

58. Mortimer RB. Risks and management of prolonged suspension in an Alpine harness. *Wilderness Environ Med.* 2011;22:77-86.

59. Seddon P. *Harness Suspension: Review and Evaluation on Existing Information.* Health Safety Executive Books; 2002:CRR 451/2002.

60. Kolb JJ, Smith EL. Redefining the diagnosis and treatment of suspension trauma. *JEMS.* Published June 9, 2015. Accessed March 1, 2022. https://www.jems.com/operations/rescue-vehicle-extrication/redefining-the-diagnosis-and-treatment-of-suspension-trauma/

61. Prevention and treatment of sunburn. *Med Lett Drugs Ther.* 2004;46:45.

62. Department of Health and Human Services. Food and Drug Administration. 21 CFR Parts 201, 310, 347, and 352. Sunscreen drug products for over-the-counter human use. *Federal Register.* Vol 84. No 38. February 26, 2019/Proposed Rules. Accessed April 20, 2022. https://www.govinfo.gov/content/pkg/FR-2019-02-26/pdf/2019-03019.pdf

63. Krakowski AC, Goldenberg A. Exposure to radiation from the sun. In: Auerbach PS, ed. *Auerbach's Wilderness Medicine.* 7th ed. Elsevier; 2017:335-353.

64. Stern RS. Clinical practice: treatment of photoaging. *N Engl J Med.* 2004;350:1526-1534.

65. Richardson SD. Environmental mass spectrometry: emerging contaminants and current issues. *Anal Chem.* 2012;84:747-778.

66. Gies P. Photoprotection by clothing. *Photodermal Photimmunol Photomed.* 2007;23:264-274.

67. Singletary EM, Charlton NP, Epstein JL, et al. Part 15: first aid: 2015 American Heart Association and American Red Cross guidelines update for first aid. *Circulation.* 2015;132(Suppl 2): S574-S589.

68. Kragh JF, Walters TJ, Baer DG, et al. Practical use of emergency tourniquets to stop bleeding in major limb trauma. *J Trauma.* 2008;64(Suppl 2):38-50.

69. Drew B, Bird D, Matteucci M, Keenan S. Tourniquet conversion: a recommended approach in the prolonged field care setting. *J Spec Operations Med.* 2015;15(3):81-85.

70. Kragh JF, Dubick MA. Bleeding control with limb tourniquet use in the wilderness setting: review of science. *Wilderness Environ Med.* 2017;28(Suppl 2):S25-S32.

71. Edlich RF, Rodeheaver GT, Morgan RF, et al. Principles of emergency wound management. *Ann Emerg Med.* 1988;17(12):1284-1302.

72. Edlich RF, Thacker JG, Buchanan L, Rodeheaver GT. Modern concepts of treatment of traumatic wounds. *Adv Surg.* 1979;13:169-197.

73. Bhandari M, Thompson K, Adili A, Shaughnessy SG. High and low pressure irrigation in contaminated wounds with exposed bone. *Int J Surg Invest.* 2000;2(3):179-182.

74. Bhandari M, Adili A, Lachowski RJ. High pressure pulsatile lavage of contaminated human tibiae: an in vitro study. *J Orthop Trauma.* 1998;12(7):479-484.

75. Bhandari M, Schemitsch EH, Adili A, et al. High and low pressure pulsatile lavage of contaminated tibial fractures: an in vitro study of bacterial adherence and bone damage. *J Orthop Trauma.* 1999;13(8):526-533.

76. Anglen JO. Wound irrigation in musculoskeletal injury. *J Am Acad Orthop Surg.* 2001;9(4):219-226.

77. Valente JH, Forti RJ, Freundlich LF, et al. Wound irrigation in children: saline solution or tap water? *Ann Emerg Med.* 2003;41(5):609-616.

78. Backer HD. Field water disinfection. In: Auerbach PS, ed. *Auerbach's Wilderness Medicine.* 7th ed. Elsevier; 2017: 1985-2030.

79. Griffiths RD, Fernandez RS, Ussia CA. Is tap water a safe alternative to normal saline for wound irrigation in the community setting? *J Wound Care.* 2001;10(10):407-411.

80. Moscati R, Mayrose J, Fincher L, Jehle D. Comparison of normal saline with tap water for wound irrigation. *Am J Emerg Med.* 1998;16(4):379-381.

81. Moscati RM, Reardon RF, Lerner EB, Mayrose J. Wound irrigation with tap water. *Acad Emerg Med.* 1998;5(11):1076-1080.

82. Rodeheaver GT, Pettry D, Thacker JG, et al. Wound cleansing by high pressure irrigation. *Surg Gynecol Obstet.* 1975;141(3):357-362.

83. Edlich RF, Reddy VR. Revolutionary advances in wound repair in emergency medicine during the last three decades: a view toward the new millennium. 5th Annual David R. Boyd, MD, Lecture. *J Emerg Med.* 2001;20(2):167-193.

84. Singer AJ, Hollander JE, Subramanian S, et al. Pressure dynamics of various irrigation techniques commonly used in the emergency department. *Ann Emerg Med.* 1994;24(1):36-40.

85. Luck JB, Campagne D, Falcon Bachs R, et al. Pressures of wilderness improvised wound irrigation techniques: how do they compare? *Wilderness Environ Med.* 2016;27(4):476-481.

86. Mellor SG, Cooper GJ, Bowyer GW. Efficacy of delayed administration of benzylpenicillin in the control of infection in penetrating soft tissue injuries in war. *J Trauma.* 1996;40(Suppl 3):S128-S134.

87. Hospenthal DR, Murray CK, Andersen RC, et al. Guidelines for the prevention of infection after combat-related injuries. *J Trauma.* 2008;64(Suppl 3):S211-S220.

88. Jamshidi R. Wound management. In: Auerbach PS, ed. *Wilderness Medicine.* 7th ed. Elsevier; 2017: 440-450.

89. Russell KW, Scaife CL, Weber DC, et al. Wilderness Medical Society practice guidelines for the treatment of acute pain in remote environments: 2014 update. *Wilderness Environ Med.* 2014;25:S96-S104.

90. McGladrey L. Psychological first aid and stress injuries. In: Hawkins SC, ed. *Wilderness EMS.* Wolters Kluwer; 2018:189-202.

91. Switzer JA, Bovard RS, Quinn RH. Wilderness orthopedics. In: Auerbach PS, ed. *Auerbach's Wilderness Medicine.* 7th ed. Elsevier; 2017:450-492.

92. Kranc DA, Jones AW, Nackenson J, et al. Use of ultrasound for joint dislocation reduction in an austere wilderness setting: a case report. *Prehosp Emerg Care.* 2018;23(2):1-14.

93. Fulton RL, Voigt WJ, Hilakos AS. Confusion surrounding the treatment of traumatic cardiac arrest. *J Am Coll Surg.* 1995;181:209-214.

94. Pasquale MD, Rhodes M, Cipolle MD, et al. Defining "dead on arrival": impact on a level I trauma center. *J Trauma.* 1996;41:726-730.

95. Mattox KL, Feliciano DV. Role of external cardiac compression in truncal trauma. *J Trauma.* 1982;22:934-936.

96. Shimazu S, Shatney CH. Outcomes of trauma patients with no vital signs on admission. *J Trauma.* 1983;23(3):213-216.

97. Forgey WW, Wilderness Medical Society. *Practice Guidelines for Wilderness Emergency Care.* 5th ed. Globe Pequot Press; 2006.

98. Goth P, Garnett G, Rural Affairs Committee, National Association of EMS Physicians. Clinical guidelines for delayed/prolonged transport. I. Cardiorespiratory arrest. *Prehosp Disaster Med.* 1991;6(3):335.

99. Eisenberg MS, Bergner L, Hallstrom AP. Cardiac resuscitation in the community: importance of rapid provision and implications of program planning. *JAMA.* 1979;241:1905-1907.

100. Kellermann AL, Hackman BB, Somes G. Predicting the outcome of unsuccessful prehospital advanced cardiac life support. *JAMA.* 1993;270(12):1433-1436.

101. Bonnin MJ, Pepe PE, Kimball KT, Clark PS. Distinct criteria for termination of resuscitation in the out-of-hospital setting. *JAMA.* 1993;270(12):1457-1462.

102. Millin MG, Khandker SR, Malki A. Termination of resuscitation of nontraumatic cardiopulmonary arrest: resource document for the National Association of EMS Physicians position statement. *Prehosp Emerg Care.* 2011;15(4):547-554.

103. Leavitt M, Podgorny G. Prehospital CPR and the pulseless hypothermic patient. *Ann Emerg Med.* 1984;13:492.

104. Zafren K, Giesbrecht G, Danzl D, et al. Wilderness Medical Society practice guidelines for the out-of-hospital evaluation and treatment of accidental hypothermia: 2014 update. *Wilderness Environ Med.* 2014;25:S66-S85.

105. Keatinge WR. Accidental immersion hypothermia and drowning. *Practitioner.* 1977;219:183-187.

106. Olshaker JS. Near drowning. *Emerg Med Clin North Am.* 1992;10(2):339-350.

107. Bolte RG, Black PG, Bowers RS, et al. The use of extracorporeal rewarming in a child submerged for 66 minutes. *JAMA.* 1988;260(3):377-379.

108. Orlowski JP. Drowning, near-drowning, and ice-water drowning. *JAMA.* 1988;260(3):390-391.

109. Cooper MA, Andrews CJ, Holle RL, et al. Lightning-related injuries and safety. In: Auerbach PS, ed. *Auerbach's Wilderness Medicine.* 7th ed. Elsevier; 2017:71-117.

110. Davis C, Engeln A, Johnson E, McIntosh S, et al. Wilderness Medical Society practice guidelines for the prevention and treatment of lightning injuries: 2014 update. *Wilderness Environ Med.* 2014;25:S86-S95.

111. Durrer B, Brugger H. Recent advances in avalanche survival. Presented at the Second World Congress on Wilderness Medicine. Aspen, CO; 1995.

112. Van Tilburg C, Grissom CK, Zafren K, et al. Wilderness Medical Society practice guidelines for prevention and

management of avalanche and nonavalanche snow burial accidents. *Wilderness Environ Med.* 2017;25(28):23-42.

113. Steinman AM. Cardiopulmonary resuscitation and hypothermia. *Circulation.* 1986;74(6, pt 2):29-32.

114. Zell SC. Epidemiology of wilderness-acquired diarrhea: implications for prevention and treatment. *J Wild Med.* 1992;3(3):241-249.

115. Lloyd EL. *Hypothermia and Cold Stress.* Aspen Systems; 1986.

116. Maningas PA, DeGuzman LR, Hollenbach SJ, et al. Regional blood flow during hypothermic arrest. *Ann Emerg Med.* 1986;15(4):390-396.

117. Groves LJ, Cushing TA. General management of medical conditions in the wilderness. In: Hawkins SC, ed. *Wilderness EMS.* Wolters Kluwer; 2018:393-412.

118. Sampson HA, Muñoz-Furlong A, Campbell RL, et al. Second symposium on the definition and management of anaphylaxis: summary report—Second National Institute of Allergy and Infectious Disease/Food Allergy and Anaphylaxis Network symposium. *J Allergy Clin Immunol.* 2006;117:391-397.

119. Graif Y, Romano-Zelekha O, Livne I, et al. Allergic reactions to insect stings: results from a national survey of 10,000 junior high school children in Israel. *J Allergy Clin Immunol.* 2006;117:1435-1439.

120. Golden DB. Insect sting anaphylaxis. *Immunol Allergy Clin North Am.* 2007;27:261-272.

121. Bilò BM, Bonifazi F. Epidemiology of insect-venom anaphylaxis. *Curr Opin Allergy Clin Immunol.* 2008;8:330-337.

122. Graft DF. Insect sting allergy. *Med Clin North Am.* 2006;90:211-232.

123. Valentine MD, Schuberth KC, Kagey-Sobotka A, et al. The value of immunotherapy with venom in children with allergy to insect stings. *N Engl J Med.* 1990;323:1601-1603.

124. Barnard JH. Studies of 400 *Hymenoptera* sting deaths in the United States. *J Allergy Clin Immunol.* 1973;52:259-264.

125. Gaudio F, Lemery J, Johnson D. Wilderness Medical Society practice guidelines for the use of epinephrine in outdoor education and wilderness settings: 2014 update. *Wilderness Environ Med.* 2014;25:S15-S18.

126. Hawkins S, Weil C, Fitzpatrick D. Letter to the editor: epinephrine autoinjector warning. *Wilderness Environ Med.* 2012;23:371-378.

127. Snakes. *National Geographic.* Accessed March 1, 2022. https://www.nationalgeographic.com/animals/reptiles/facts/snakes-1

128. Kasturiratne A, Wickremasinghe AR, de Silva N, et al. The global burden of snakebite: a literature analysis and modelling based on regional estimates of envenoming and deaths. *PLoS Med.* 2008;5(11):e218. doi: 10.1371/journal.pmed.0050218

129. Abo B. Management of animal bites and envenomation. Hawkins SC, ed. *Wilderness EMS.* Wolters Kluwer; 2018:333-346.

130. O'Neil ME, Mack KA, Gilchrist J, Wozniak EJ. Snakebite injuries treated in United States emergency departments, 2001–2004. *Wilderness Environ Med.* 2007;18(4):281-287.

131. Lavonas EJ, Ruha AM, Banner W, et al. Unified treatment algorithm for the management of crotaline snakebite in the United States: results of an evidence-informed consensus workshop. *BMC Emerg Med.* 2011;11:2. doi: 10.1186/1471-227X-11-2

132. Norris RL, Bush SP, Cardwell MD. Bites by venomous reptiles in Canada, the United States, and Mexico. In: Auerbach PS, ed. *Auerbach's Wilderness Medicine.* 7th ed. Elsevier; 2017:729-760.

133. Warrell DA. Bites by venomous and nonvenomous reptiles worldwide. In: Auerbach PS, ed. *Auerbach's Wilderness Medicine.* 7th ed. Elsevier; 2017:760-828.

134. Kanaan NC, Ray J, Stewart M, et al. Wilderness Medical Society practice guidelines for the treatment of pit viper envenomations in the United States and Canada. *Wilderness Environ Med.* 2015;26:472-487.

135. Curry SC, Kunkel DB. Death from a rattlesnake bite. *Am J Emerg Med.* 1985;3(3):227-235.

136. Bush SP. Snakebite suction devices don't remove venom: they just suck. *Ann Emerg Med.* 2004;43(2):187-188.

137. Alberts MB, Shalit M, LoGalbo F. Suction for venomous snakebite: a study of "mock venom" extraction in a human model. *Ann Emerg Med.* 2004;43(2):181-186.

138. Davis D, Branch K, Egen NB, et al. The effect of an electrical current on snake venom toxicity. *J Wild Med.* 1992;3(1):48-53.

139. Howe NR, Meisenheimer JL Jr. Electric shock does not save snakebitten rats. *Ann Emerg Med.* 1988;17(3):254-256.

140. Gill KA Jr. The evaluation of cryotherapy in the treatment of snake envenomation. *South Med J.* 1968;63:552-556.

141. Norris RL. A call for snakebite research. *Wilderness Environ Med.* 2000;11(3):149-151.

Suggested Reading

Auerbach PS, ed. *Auerbach's Wilderness Medicine.* 7th ed. Elsevier; 2017.

Hawkins SC, ed. *Wilderness EMS.* Wolters Kluwer; 2018.

Rodway G, McIntosh S, Weber D, eds. *Mountain Medicine and Technical Rescue: A Manual of the Diploma in Mountain Medicine.* Carreg; 2016.

민간 전술적 응급의료지원 (TEMS)

Lead Editors
Faroukh Mehkri, DO
Alexander L. Eastman, MD, MPH, FACS, FAEMS

학습 목표 이 장의 학습을 완료하면 다음과 같은 내용을 수행할 수 있다.

- 전술적 응급의료지원(TEMS)의 구성 요소에 관해 설명할 수 있다.
- 전술적 응급의료지원의 운영 및 지원 기능을 이해할 수 있다.
- 전술적 응급의료지원 프로그램의 이점을 설명할 수 있다.
- 전술적 응급의료지원의 세 가지 처치 단계에서 응급의료가 무엇이 다른지어 대해 논의할 수 있다.
- 전술적 임무에서 원격 평가 방법(RAM)이 어떻게 사용될 수 있는지 설명할 수 있다.
- 대테러 작전에 대한 의료 지원의 역할에 관해 설명할 수 있다.

시나리오

당신이 속한 EMS 기관은 지역 경찰특공대(SWAT)팀을 지원하고 현지 경찰과 함께 엄격한 통합 훈련 프로그램을 갖추고 있다. TEMS 팀은 해가 진 직후 오래된 이동식 주택에 총기 난사범이 숨어있다는 신고를 받고 출동한다. 진입을 준비하고 있을 때 두 명의 SWAT 대원이 용의자의 마당을 가로질러 집에 접근하여 문을 부수기 위해 준비한다. 앞쪽 창문에서 총성이 울려 퍼지고 SWAT 대원이 손상을 입었다. SWAT 대원 한 명이 용의자의 집 출입구에 쓰러졌고 다른 한 명은 낡은 픽업트럭 근처에 쓰러졌다. 근처에 서 있던 경찰관이 "우리가 구하러 가자!"라고 외친다. 당신은 경찰관의 팔을 잡고 SWAT 지휘관을 바라본다.

- 당신은 어떻게 행동해야 하는가?
- 현장의 위험성을 고려할 때때 쓰러진 SWAT 대원을 어떻게 평가하고 처치해야 하는가?

개요

전술적 응급의료지원은 특수 작전 법 집행 임무의 성공을 높이고 임무의 의료 책임과 위험을 줄이며 공공 안전을 증진하기 위한 병원 외 처치 시스템이다. TEMS은 군진 의학, 야생 의학, 재난 대응, 도시 수색 및 구조, 기존 EMS의 원칙을 기반으로 하여 법 집행 임무를 지원하고 자원이 부족하고 이송 지연이 필요한 환경에서 사상자의 임상 결과를 극대화하는 동시에 병원 전 처치 제공자에 대한 위협을 최소화하는 치료 시스템을 구축한다.

이 장에서는 TEMS에 대한 개요를 설명한다. TEMS에 참여하고 전술적 사상자 처치(TCC)를 제공하려면 다른 특수 작전 상황과 마찬가지로 특정 훈련과 전문 지식이 필요하다. TEMS에 대한 자세한 개요를 위해 NAEMT에서 TEMS개념에 대한 16시간 교육 과정인 전술적 응급사상자처치(TECC)를 제공한다.

전술적 응급의료지원의 역사와 발전

최초의 SWAT 팀은 1968년 로스앤젤레스에서 창설되었다. 얼마 지나지 않아 SWAT 팀에 "의료"라는 개념이 발전했는데, 이는 전투 의료진을 팀에 배치하는 군대 모델과 유사하다. 오늘날 TEMS는 고위험 전술 환경에서 작동하도록 구조와 기능이 수정된 광범위한 의료서비스를 포함한다. 현재 경찰과 의료계 모두에서 TEMS에 대한 광범위한 지지가 존재한다.

30여 년 전에 마약 및 테러 작전 의료지원(CONTOMS) 과정이 개발되었다. 이 프로그램은 숙련된 응급의료 제공자를 선발하여 56시간 동안 전술적 환경에서 의료서비스를 제공하는 데 몰입할 수 있도록 하는 증거 기반 TEMS 교육 과정으로 개발되었다. 마약 및 테러 작전 의료지원을 통해 손상 데이터베이스를 개발하여 전술 의료의 효능을 뒷받침하는 데 필요한 연구 자료를 제공했다.

그 이후로 마약 및 테러 작전 의료지원과 유사한 많은 과정이 개발되었다. TCCC 과정은 미국 국방성 국방보건위원회(DHB) 산하 CoTCCC에서 개발했다. 이 과정은 특정 전술 상황에 따라 달라지는 전술 환경에서 필요한 필수 의료 개입을 가르친다. 최초 TCCC 프로젝트는 1993년부터 1996년까지 특수 작전 의료진과 사관학교의 공동 노력으로 진행되었다. 4년에 걸친 이 연구 노력은 1996년 최초의 TCCC 논문이 발표되면서 절정에 달했다.

TCCC 지침은 현재 미국 특수작전사령부가 2001년에 설립하여 현재 국방부 합동 외상시스템(JTS)의 한 구성 요소인 TCCC 위원회(CoTCCC)에서 관리하고 있다. TCCC 지침은 다음을 기반으로 업데이트된다. 1) 발표된 민간 및 군 병원 전 외상 문헌에 대한 지속적인 검토, 2) 군 전투 사상자 처치 연구 실험실과의 지속적인 상호 작용, 3) 숙련된 전투 부대원, 의무병 및 항공응급구조사(PJ)의 직접적인 의견, 4) 군 의료 교육 센터의 의견, 5) 주간 합동 현장 외상시스템(JTTS) 프로세스 개선 화상 회의에서 논의된 사례 보고서, 6) JTS-군 의료 검시관 시스템(AFMES) 회의에서 수집한 전투 사상자의 사망 원인에 대한 관찰, 7) 군 및 민간 외상 전문가들의 전문가 의견 등을 기반으로 한다.

이제 의료 및 비의료 등 다양한 범주의 전투 요원을 위한 세 가지 TCCC 과정이 제공된다. TCCC-ASM은 7시간 과정으로 모든 군인을 대상으로 한다. TCCC 전투 인명 구조자(TCCC-CLS)는 전투 작전 지원을 위해 배치되는 비의료 군인을 위한 40시간 과정이다. 의료 요원을 위한 TCCC-MP는 전투 작전 지원을 위해 배치되는 의무병, 군의관, 응급구조사 등 군 의료 요원을 위한 16시간 과정이다. TCCC 과정 중 어느 것도 전술적 사고의 구성 요소를 가르치는 과정은 없다. 전술적 이동과 계획에 대한 지식은 완벽하고 잘 개발된 TEMS 프로그램을 위해 필요하다. 전술 환경에서의 응급의료 문제를 해결하기 위해 모든 TEMS 교육 프로그램에는 TCCC-MP 프로그램과 그 의료 목표가 포함되어야 한다.

2013년에는 27명의 경찰관이 중범죄 사건 중 직무 수행 중에 발생한 손상으로 사망했다. 2020년에는 70% 증가한 46명이 사망했다. 이러한 증가는 전국적으로 총기 난사 사건/적대적 사건(ASHE)의 발생률이 계속 증가하는 것과 맞물려 TEMS의 필요성을 더욱 강화했다. 미국 전술 경관 협회(NTOA)는 1994년 최초 입장 발표를 시작으로 TEMS를 지지해 왔으며 전술 의료진을 위한 표준 운영 절차이자 "전술적 법 집행의 중요한 요소"라고 계속 주장하고 있다. 2001년 9월 11일 테러 이후 미국 응급의료 지도 의사협의회(NAEMSP)와 미국 응급의학회(ACEP)는 모두 법 집행 특수 작전에 EMS 기능을 통합하는 것을 공식적으로 승인했다.

CoTCCC는 군 병원 전 의료에 대한 글로벌 표준으로 인정받는 지침을 제정했다. 미국 외과학회 외상위원회(ACS-COT)와 NAEMT는 모두 TCCC 지침을 승인했다. NAEMT는 전 세계 교육 센터 네트워크를 통해 국방보건위원회 합동 외상시스템(DHA-JTS)에서 지정한 TCCC 과정을 제공한다. 군과 법 집행 기관의 특수 작전은 독특하지만, 전술적 의료 측면에서는 유사점이 존재한다. NTOA가 승인한 TCCC 지침은 TEMS 프로토콜의 표준화를 위한 강력한 기반을 제공했다.

전술적 의료가 중요한 문제라는 인식이 확산하고 군 TCCC 교육 프로그램을 개발하기 위한 CoTCCC의 활동이 활발해지면서 군사 정보를 민간 환경에 적용하기 위한 노력이 진행 중이다. 민간 CoTCCC의 대응 기관인 전술적 응급사상자처치위원회(C-TECC)는 민간 법 집행 기관의 병원 전 고위험 요구 사항을 해결하기 위해 맞춤화된 일련의 TECC 지침을 개발했다. 이 지침은 이후 FBI, 미국 연방 재난관리청(FEMA), 국가 테러센터가 사용하는 국가 합동 테러 인식 워크숍에 통합되었다. NAEMT는 민간 병원 전 처치 제공자를 위한 TECC 과정을 개발했다.

TCCC 교육 프로그램과 TECC 과정은 유사한 원칙을 기반으로 하지만, TCCC와 TECC가 항상 같은 권장 사항을 제시하는 것은 아니다. 각 그룹에는 제안된 지침 변경 사항을 평가하는 자체 주제 전문가와 자체 프로세스가 포함되어 있다. 두 과정의 차이점은 각각 군사 전투 환경과 민간 전술 환경 간의 관련성 높은 차이점과 CoTCCC 및 C-TECC 구성원의 주제별 전문성을 반영한다.

민간 전술적 응급의료지원의 실습 구성 요소

민간 전술적 응급의료지원은 기존의 EMS와 몇 가지 차이점이 있다. 기존 EMS와는 달리 포괄적인 TEMS 프로그램에는 건강 유지, 예방의학(예: 면역, 적절한 수면 습관 및 신체 단련), 의료 위협 평가, 다양한 지역 의료 자원을 이용한 처치 조정이 포함된다. 운영 관점에서 TEMS 의료진은 처치 및 퇴원 결정에 자주 직면하게 된다. 이러한 상황은 탈수 증세를 보이는 TEMS 팀원부터 전술 작전 중 손상을 입은 화난 포로에 이르기까지 다양하다. 두 상황 모두 고유한 문제가 있다.

일부 주에서 EMS 프로토콜에 TEMS 실무에 관한 특정 부록을 포함하고 있다. 전술적 환경에서 운영할 때와 잠재적인 고급 술기를 인증할 때 TEMS 제공자와 의료 책임자는 해당 프로토콜을 숙지해야 한다.

TEMS의 의료 술기 능력은 기존 EMS와 일치하며 종종 확장되기도 한다. 술기가 유사할 수 있지만, TEMS에서는 이러한 술기의 적용이 전술적 상황과 임무에 의해 크게 영향을 받는 경우가 많다. 예를 들어, LMA의 사용은 정상적인 작전 상황에서는 부상자에게 임상적으로 적합할 수 있지만, 부상자를 위험한 지역을 가로질러 구출하거나 거친 지형을 넘어야 하는 경우 LMA는 안전한 기도유지 장비가 아니므로 적절하지 않을 수 있다.

기존 EMS 이용의 장애 요인

법 집행 기관의 특수 작전 현장에서는 기존 EMS 접근에 다양한 장애 요인이 존재한다. 일반적으로 지리적 경계가 설정되어 있다. 이 경계선 내에서 EMS가 통과하거나 의료 활동 수행하기에 안전한 구역이 어디인지 명확히 할 수 있는 경우는 드물다. 의료 구성 요소가 SWAT 팀의 임무 수행에 방해가 돼서는 안 된다. 이미 부족한 경찰 자원을 의료 지원 임무에 투입할 필요가 없어야 한다.

EMS가 현장에 도착하여 환자와 접촉할 때까지의 시간 간격은 기존 EMS 운영에서 병원 처치 시작을 지연시키는 중요한 원인이 될 수 있다. 이러한 유형의 지연은 전술적 임무 중에는 훨씬 더 길어질 수 있다. 통합 TEMS 프로그램은 TEMS 처치 제공자가 전술 팀의 중요한 일부로서 경계 내에서 일상적으로 활동하는 경찰관이 손상을 당한 첫 순간에 상처 치료를 시작할 수 있으므로 지연을 최소화한다.

일부 소방서장 및 구조 책임자와 EMS 관리자는 전술 의학이 너무 위험하다고 인식하여 소속 대원들이 전술 의료를 시행하는 것을 반대할 수 있다. 자신의 지휘를 받는 소방관이 왜 불타는 건물에 들어가는지(명백히 위험한 상황) 묻는 말에 소방관들은 화재 위협에 대해 잘 훈련되고 적절한 장비를 갖추고 있으므로 소방은 법 집행 기관의 작전과 다르다고 대답하는 경우가 많다. TEMS도 마찬가지이다(**Box 22-1**).

안전이 확보되지 않은 경찰 경계 구역에 들어가기 위해 해당 임무에 대한 교육이나 장비가 미흡한 EMS 대원을 투입하는 것은 기본적인 현장 안전 원칙을 위반하는 행위이다. 그런데도 단순히 경계선 밖으로 환자가 이송되기를 기다리는 것은 효과적인 방법이 아니라는 것을 알고 있다. TEMS 의료진의 부재로 인한 지연은 불필요한 생명 또는 기능 손실을 초래지만, 군대 내 원거리(손상 지점에 최대한 근접) 의료 서비스는 사망률과 이환율을 모두 낮추는 것으로 나타났다. 황금 기간은 각 손상과 사람마다 다르며 몇 시간이 걸리는 경우도 있고 몇 초밖에 걸리지 않는 예도 있으므로 가능한 한 빨리 손상

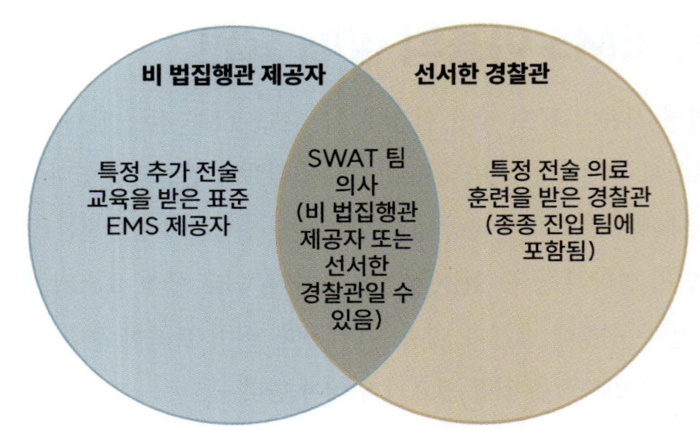

그림 22-1 TEMS 모델(안전한 작전 경계 내에서 운영).
© National Association of Emergency Medical Technicians (NAEMT)

표 22-1 처치 단계

전술적 상황	TCCC	TECC
즉각적이거나 능동적인 위협 (HOT ZONE)	교전 중 처치(CUF)/ 위협 상황에서의 처치	교전 중 처치(CUF)/ 위협 상황에서의 처치
위협이 차단되었으나 재개될 수 있음 (WARM ZONE)	전술적 현장 처치 (TFC)	전술적 현장 처치 (TFC)
위협 없음 (COLD ZONE)	전술적 후송 처치 (TEC)	전술적 후송 처치 (TEC)

© National Association of Emergency Medical Technicians (NAEMT)

을 처치하기 위해 모든 노력을 기울여야 한다. 확실한 해결책은 법 집행 특수 작전의 의료 지원은 안전한 작전지역 내에서 안전하게 작전을 수행할 수 있는 잘 훈련되고 적절한 장비를 갖춘 TEMS 의료진이 수생하는 것이다. 전진 운용 TEMS 요원에는 여러 모델이 있다. 민간인 자원봉사자, 선서한 경찰관, 전술 의료 훈련을 받은 경찰관, 의사 또는 여러 인력이 혼합된 모델로 구성할 수 있다(**그림 22-1**). 일부 모델은 진입 팀 내에 TEMS 요원을 포함한다. 다른 곳에서는 TEMS 요원을 안전한 경계선 내에 배치하지만, 직접 사선에 있지 않고 일반적으로 수송 차량 근처에 배치한다.

작전 지역

전술 임무 시행 시 전술 법 집행 팀의 작전 개념은 목표 지역을 작전 구역으로 나눈다. 팀은 지리적 경계로 내부 경계와 외부 경계를 설정하여 안전지역(safe zone/위협이 존재해서는 안 되는 외부 경계 외부), 전방통제 지역(warm zone/위협의 위험이 존재할 수 있는 외부 경계와 내부 경계 사이), 위험지역(kill zone/즉각적인 위험을 초래하거나 대응자가 명확한 표적이 될 수 있는 지역)으로 나눈다. 이 개념은 위험물질 사고의 운영 구역과 유사하다. 통제되지 않은 사건과 마찬가지로 이러한 구역은 정적인 것이 아니라 본질적으로 동적이며 상황에 따라 다양한 구역의 지리적 경계가 급변할 수 있다는 점을 인식하는 것이 중요하다. TEMS 의료진은 자신과 환자에 대한 위험을 최소화하기 위해 항상 상황 인식을 유지해야 한다.

처치 단계

TCCC 또는 TECC에서 처치가 제공되는 시점의 전술적 전투 사상자

(TCC) 지침은 전술적 상황과 관련 위협에 따라 응급의료 제공을 처치 단계로 구분한다(**표 22-1**).

TCCC 또는 TECC 지침을 사용하든 각 단계에서 제공되는 처치는 기본적으로 같다. 처치 단계는 더 역동적이며 분 단위 위험 평가의 영향을 받으며 동심원이거나 연속적일 필요가 없고 전술적 환경에서 위험 수준은 급변한다. 따라서 처치 단계가 항상 작전 지역과 일치하지 않을 수도 있다. TEMS 요원은 전술 환경에서 규율에 따라 효과적으로 기능하기 위해 두 패러다임의 관계를 이해해야 한다(**Box 22-2**).

교전 중 처치(CUF)/위협 상황에서의 처치(직접 위협 관리)

교전 중 처치 및 위협 상황에서의 처치(CUFT) 중에는 위협이 직접적이고 즉각적이다. 사상자와 구조대원에게는 제한된 보호가 제공된다. 이 구역 내에서의 작전은 매우 위험하므로 정찰 및 전술팀 요원으로 제한해야 한다. CUFT 중 위험지역 내에서 안전하게 작전을 수행하려면 적절한 개인보호장비(예: 헬멧, 고글, 조끼, 방패, 전투화)와 전술적 이동법(예: 조명/소음 억제, 은폐/엄폐 사용)을 사용한다. 거실에 은신한 총격범이 창문으로 총을 쏘는 집 앞마당에 경찰관이 쓰러져 있는 장면은 전형적인 CUFT 시나리오의 예시이다.

이 단계에서 부상자 처치는 막대한 위험이 수반되며 기존 EMS의 원칙에서 크게 벗어난다. 즉각적인 조치에는 위협을 진압하고 사상자를 대피시켜 은폐와 엄폐하는 것이 포함된다. 위협이 빨리 무력화될수록 부상자를 치료하기 위한 모든 의료 자원이 더 빨리 투입될 수 있다. 그전까지는 부상자를 보호하는 것이 필수적이다. 반응이 있고 움직일 수 있는 부상자는 엄폐물로 이동하도록 지시해야 한다. 부상

자가 움직일 수 없는 경우 조 계획을 고려할 수 있다. 이 단계에서 의학적 처치는 부상자의 추가 손상을 줄이고 구조대원의 부상을 방지하며 위협을 제압하고 생명을 위협하는 팔다리 출혈을 조절하는 데 중점을 둔다. 관통성 목 손상에서 목뼈 고정, 기도관리 또는 심폐소생술과 같은 기타 "영웅적" 처치를 시행하기 위해서 시간을 소모하지 않는다.

자가 처치와 동료에 의한 처치는 CUFT의 중요한 구성요소다. 경찰관이 입은 대부분의 치명적이지 않은 관통상은 일반적으로 완전히 무능력 화되지 않으며 반드시 경찰관이 작전에서 완전히 배제되는 것은 아니다. 베트남, 이라크, 아프가니스탄에서의 군사 작전에서 얻은 자료에 따르면 자가 처치와 동료에 의한 처치를 훈련한 결과 사망률이 현저히 감소한 것으로 나타났다. 실제로 조기 지혈대 사용을 시작한 후 팔다리 출혈로 인한 사망률이 67% 감소한 것으로 나타났다. 예를 들어, 생명을 위협하는 팔다리 관통상에 지혈대를 스스로 적용하면 자신을 구할 수 있을 뿐만 아니라 추가 부상을 최소화하며 TEMS 요원이 적의 총격에 불필요하게 노출되는 것을 방지할 수 있다.

많은 CUFT 전술 환경에서 직접 압박 및 압박 드레싱을 적용하는 것은 비현실적이며 불필요한 출혈을 초래하고 부상자를 대피시키는 데 지연을 초래할 수 있다. 팔다리 출혈을 조절하기 위한 지혈대 사용은 CUFT 단계의 처치 표준이며 지혈대 사용과 관련된 낮은 위험보다 출혈을 멈출 수 있는 이점이 훨씬 더 크다. 지혈대는 가능한 한 팔다리의 출혈 부위보다 위쪽에 단단하게 적용한다. CUFT 상황에서는 지혈대를 옷 위에 적용한다. 동맥 혈류가 차단되었는지 확인하는 것이 중요하다. 이 단계에서는 팔다리 및 접합부 상처를 처치하기 어렵다. 부상자를 신속하게 엄폐할 수 있는 위치로 이동시키고 전술적 현장 처치 단계로 전환하면서 이러한 상처에 직접 압박을 시행해야 한다.

전술적 현장 처치(간접적 위협 관리)

전술적 현장 처치(TFC) 단계에서는 위협이 계속 존재할 수 있지만, 직접적이거나 즉각적이지 않을 수 있다. 예를 들어, SWAT 대원이 앞마당에 쓰러진 경우 부상자가 적절한 엄폐물이나 은폐물 뒤로 이동하거나(예: 무장 괴한의 시야에서 벗어나 두꺼운 벽돌 벽) 위협이 진압된 후에는 전술적 현장 처치 원칙이 적용된다(**그림 22-2**). 엄폐와 은폐는 공격 및 방어 전술의 핵심 요소이므로 엄폐와 은폐의 차이점을 이해하는 것이 중요하다. 엄폐는 날아오는 발사체(예: 총알)를 막거나 굴절시켜 보호하는 벽을 말한다. 엄폐물의 예로는 벽돌, 바위, 강철 또는 차량 엔진 블록 등이 있지만, 필요한 엄폐물의 유형은 가해자가 사용하는 무기와 탄약에 따라 달라진다. 은폐는 발사체로부터 보호하는 것이 아니라 가해자의 시야에서 벗어난 지역이나 물체를 제공하는 것이다. 은폐는 덤불, 내려진 블라인드 또는 건식 벽체 뒤, 심지어 연기 속에서도 찾을 수 있다. 자연 지형은 엄폐물 또는 은폐물을 제공한다.

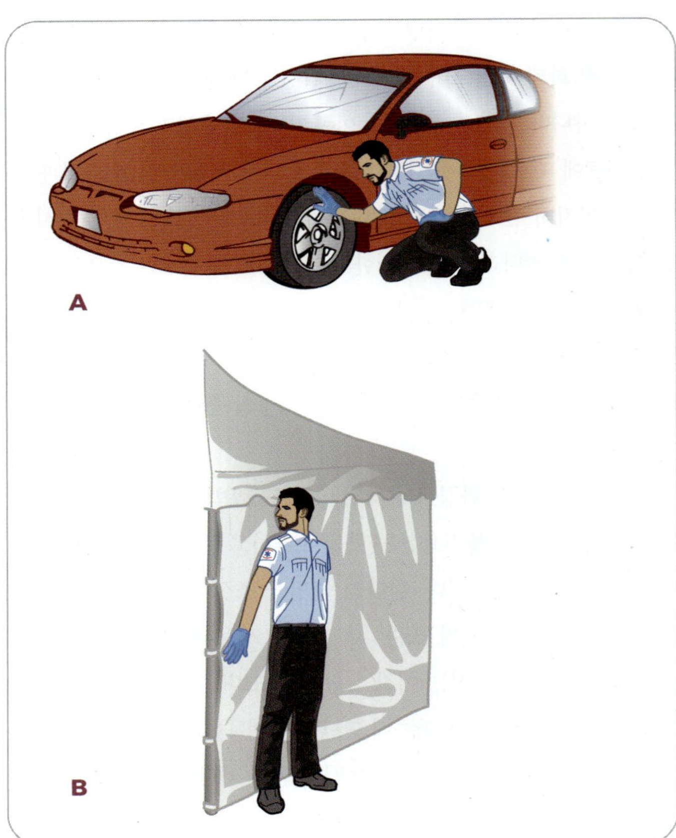

그림 22-2 **A.** 엄폐, **B.** 은폐.
© National Association of Emergency Medical Technicians (NAEMT)

이 단계에서는 위협 수준이 크게 달라지므로 유연하고 유동적인 의료 대응이 필요하다. TEMS 의료진은 동적 요인을 분석하고 데이터를 신속하게 수집하며 자신과 부상자에 대한 위험 측면에서 모든 의료 결정을 신속하게 평가할 수 있어야 한다. TEMS 시나리오에서 상대적으로 안전한 환경이 언제든지 CUFT 상황으로 돌아갈 수 있다. TEMS 의료진은 현장에서 의학적 의사 결정과 처치에 신중해야 한다.

전술적 현장 처치 시 전술적으로 적절하다면 모든 손상 부위를 노출하고 신속한 외상 평가를 시행해야 한다. 처치는 전술적 환경에서 예방할 수 있는 외상 사망의 주요 원인인 박동성 출혈, 긴장기흉, 단순 기도 손상, 저체온증을 신속하게 안정시키는 데 중점을 두어야 한다. MARCH 알고리즘은 전술적 현장 처치 초기에 신속하게 적용하여 즉각적인 TEMS 문제를 해결하고 중증도에 따라 부상자를 분류해야 한다.

지혈

전술적 현장 처치 중 직접 압박으로 외부출혈을 지혈하는 것이 매우 중요하다. 압박으로 중증 외부출혈은 일반적으로 신속하게 지혈할 수 있으므로 최우선으로 시행해야 한다. 지혈대는 잠재적으로 생명을 위협할 수 있는 팔다리 출혈을 지혈하기 위해 언제 어디서나 적용할 수 있는 일차 처치법이다. 출혈이 생명을 위협하는 경우 지혈대는 손상 부위 위쪽 서혜부, 겨드랑이에 옷을 제거하고 피부 위에 단단하게 적용한다. 조임막대를 돌리기 전에 조임끈을 최대한 당겨 벨크로에 붙인다. 지혈대의 본체가 변형되는 것을 방지하기 위해 윈들러스를 3회(540도) 이상 돌리지 않는다. 하나의 지혈대로 출혈이 조절되지 않으면 적용한 지혈대 위쪽에 추가 지혈대를 나란히 적용하는 것이 적극 권장된다. CUFT 단계에서 팔다리에 사용한 모든 지혈대는 재평가를 통해 계속 적용해야 하는지 결정해야 한다. 부상으로 인한 출혈이 생명을 위협하지 않는다고 판단되면 지혈대를 적절한 압박 드레싱으로 전환할 수 있다. 의심스러운 경우 특히 상황에 따라 추가 이동이 필요하거나 위험한 상황이 완전히 끝나지 않으면 조심하는 편히 좋으며 지혈대를 계속 착용하는 것이 좋다.

현재 TCCC 지침에서는 지혈대 사용이 불가능한 부위의 출혈에 대한 대안으로 Combat Gauze, Celox Gauze 및 ChitoGauze 등의 지혈거즈를 이용한 드레싱을 권장한다. 이러한 드레싱을 적용한 후에는 3분간 직접 압박을 시행해야 한다. 오래된 분말 또는 과립형 제제는 열화상, 이물질에 의한 색전, 내피(혈관 내층) 독성을 유발할 수 있으므로 사용하지 않는다. 대신 목, 겨드랑이, 서혜부와 같은 접합 부위에는 지혈 성분이 함유된 지혈 거즈를 사용한다. 모든 지혈제 및 기타 새로운 상처 패킹 수단의 사용은 해당 부대 의료 책임자의 승인을 받아야 한다.

기도 관리

이 단계의 기도 관리는 부상자가 임박한 기도 폐쇄 또는 심혈관 허탈의 징후를 보이는 경우 적절하다. 부상자가 의식이 있고 정상적인 구역반사가 있는 경우 자기의 기도 유지를 위해 편안하게 않아서 앞으로 기대는 자세로 앉도록 하는 것이다. 의식이 없는 환자의 경우 기도 손상의 징후 유무와 관계없이 외상 턱밀어올리기를 시행한 후 즉시 코인두기도기를 삽입하는 것이 일차적인 방법으로 권장된다. 코인두기도기 삽입한 후 부상자를 회복자세로 유지하여 기도를 개방하고 분비물이 흡인되는 것을 방지한다(**그림 22-3**). 코인두기도기를 삽입한 후에도 기도 폐쇄가 발생하거나 지속하는 경우 적절한 교육을 받은 TEMS 제공자는 전술적 상황에 따라 기관내삽관 또는 성문위기도기 삽입을 고려할 수 있다. 이러한 장치는 부상자가 의식이 저하된

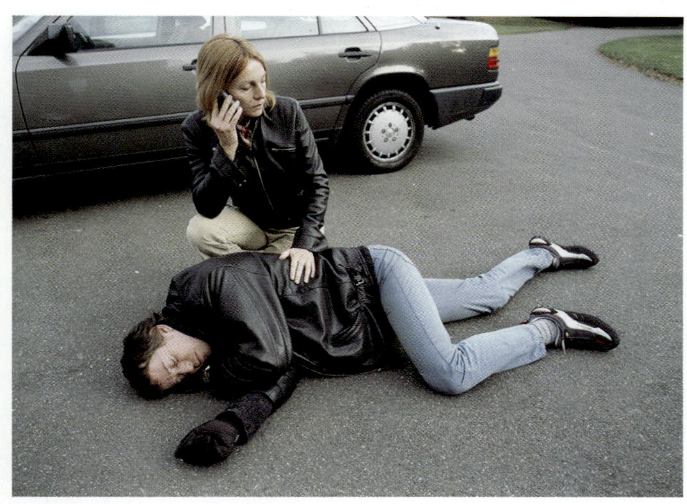

그림 22-3 회복 자세를 취한 환자
© Cordelia Molloy/Science Photo Library/Science Source

경우가 아니라면 잘 견디지 못한다.

때에 따라 외과적 반지갑상연골절개술이 필요할 수 있다. 위턱 얼굴 손상이나 흡입 화상으로 인해 기도가 손상된 부상자의 반지 갑상연골절개술을 일차 기도 유지 방법으로 선택해야 할 수 있다. CricKey 장치는 TCCC 지침에 따라 반지갑상연골절개술에 선호되는 방법이며 데이터에 따르면 이 절차를 수행하도록 훈련받은 전투 의무병이 시체를 이용한 실습에서 100%의 성공률을 보였다. 이 독특한 장치에 대한 교육용 비디오를 온라인에서 확인할 수 있다. 반지갑 상연골절개술은 고도의 기술이 필요하고 거의 시행하지 않는 술기이며 성공하기 위해서는 훈련이 절대적으로 중요하다. 이 술기를 시행하고, 교육하고 승인하는 것은 TEMS 의료 책임자의 몫이며 일부 실무자 그룹(주로 교육을 많이 받은 Paramedic 또는 EMT)의 정상적인 업무 범위 내에서 이 시술을 시행할 수 있다.

호흡 관리

무딘 손상 및 가슴 관통상의 처치는 TEMS 제공자에게 특히 중요하다. 특히 TEMS 제공자는 가슴 관통상과 긴장기흉 처치에 익숙해야 한다. 목 아래에서 배꼽까지 몸통의 모든 개방성 또는 흡입성 관통상은 피부에 폐쇄드레싱을 시행하며 즉석에서 사용할 수 있는 다양한 재료와 접착력이 뛰어난 상업적으로 제작된 체스트 씰(chest seals)을 사용할 수 있다. 흡입성 가슴 관통상 부위에서 긴장기흉이 발생할 위험을 최소화하기 위해 체스트 씰을 사용하는 것을 권장한다. TEMS 제공자에게 적용 직전에 피부 표면을 빠르게 닦아 재료의 밀

착력을 향상하도록 교육하는 것이 중요하다.

관통성 가슴 상처와 진행성 호흡곤란이 있는 부상자의 경우 긴장 기흉이 있는 것으로 추정하고 관통상을 입은 쪽에 바늘감압(NDC)을 하여 환자를 안정시키는 것이 타당하다. 기관 편위나 목정맥 팽창과 같은 소견은 초기 긴장기흉에서 나타나는 것은 아니며 전술적 환경에서는 발견하기 어려울 수 있으므로 이러한 소견에 의존해서는 안 된다. 많은 전술적 환경에서는 호흡음이 없는 것을 판단하는 것조차 불가능할 수 있으며 관통성 가슴 외상이 있는 경우 호흡곤란이 증가하거나 혈역학적 허탈의 증거가 있으면 바늘감압을 시행할 만한 충분한 근거가 된다(**Box 22-3**).

14 게이지 또는 그 이상, 길이가 8cm인 카테터가 있는 바늘을 부상자의 앞겨드랑선과 네 번째 또는 다섯 번째 갈비 사이 공간에 삽입하거나 빗장중앙선과 두 번째 갈비 사이가 만나는 지점에서 젖꼭지 바깥쪽으로 바늘을 삽입하여 긴장기흉을 처치한다. 가슴 관통 손상을 입은 부상자는 긴장기흉이 존재하지 않더라도 일반적으로 일차 손상의 결과로 어느 정도의 기흉이나 혈흉이 발생한다. 바늘감압으로 인한 추가 손상은 긴장기흉이 없는 경우 부상자의 상태를 악화시키지 않는다. 성공적인 바늘감압은 부상자의 호흡 상태가 개선되고 여건이 허락되는 경우 가슴 내부의 압력이 완화될 때 감압 바늘을 통해 공기가 밀려 나오는 소리를 들음으로써 확인할 수 있다.

14 게이지(또는 그 이상) 길이가 8cm인 주삿바늘로 부상자의 앞겨드랑선과 다섯 번째 갈비사이 공간에 삽입하여 긴장기흉을 처치한다. 또는 빗장중간선과 두 번째 갈비사이 공간에 바늘감압을 시행할 수 있다. 관통성 가슴 손상을 입은 부상자는 긴장기흉이 없더라도 일반적으로 일차 상처로 인해 어느 정도의 기흉이나 혈흉이 있을 수 있다. 바늘감압으로 인한 추가 외상은 긴장기흉이 없는 상태에서 부상자의 상태를 악화시키지 않는다. 성공적인 바늘감압은 부상자의 호흡 상태가 개선되고 조건이 허락하는 경우 흉부 내 압력이 완화되면서 바늘감압을 통해 공기가 빠져나오는 소리를 들으면서 확인할수 있다.

14게이지 길이가 8cm 주삿바늘을 사용하고 카테터를 부상자의 가슴에 삽입한 채로 고정하는 것이 TCCC 권장 사항이다. TEMS 제공자는 시술 후 부상자를 모니터링하여 카테터가 빠지거나 혈액으로 막히지 않았는지, 호흡곤란 증상이 재발하지 않았는지 확인하기 확인해야 한다. 호흡 곤란 증상이 재발하거나 카테터가 막히거나 빠진 경우 첫 번째 바늘감압을 시행한 인접한 부위에 두 번째 바늘감압을 한다. 바늘감압을 시행한 후에는 부상자에게 가슴관 삽입 또는 추가 처치가 필요할 수 있으므로 부상자에 대해 시술 적응증을 기록하는 것이 중요하다. 마지막으로 한 가지 권장 사항은 몸통 외상이나 다발성 외상을 입은 부상자가 병원 전 심정지가 발생하면 소생술을 중단하기 전에 가슴 양쪽에 바늘감압을 해야 한다는 것이다. 의료 지시 권한이 있는 의사, TEMS 제공자 또는 상위 레벨 시술자의 경우 손가락 가슴관삽입이 불가능하거나 초기 바늘감압 시도가 실패한 경우 손가락 가슴관삽입로 바늘감압을 대체할 수 있다.

혈관 확보 및 병원 전 수액 처치

많은 연구에서 외상 환자에게 저혈압("균형 잡힌") 소생술의 이점을 보여준다(자세한 내용은 3장 쇼크: 삶과 죽음의 병태생리학 참조). 따라서 특정 전술 시나리오에서는 이송이 지연된 정맥 라인 확보를 시행할 수 있다. 전술적 현장 처치 단계에서 의료 지도를 받은 경우에만 정맥 라인 확보를 시행한다. 전통적인 외상 교육에서는 정맥 라인을 확보하는 것을 가르치지만, 전술적 환경에서는 18게이지 카테터를 사용하는 것이 적절하며 의료진은 특히 전술적 환경에서 해를 끼치지 않고 지연을 최소화하기 위한 노력을 먼저 한다. 18게이지 카테터는 수액과 약물을 신속하게 투여할 수 있어 적합하고 삽입하기 쉬우며 응급처치 가방에 휴대해야 하는 소모품을 줄일 수 있다. 정맥 라인을 확보하려는 부위에 심각한 상처가 있는 팔다리 부위에 정맥 라인 확보를 시도해서는 안 된다. 부상자를 일반 EMS로 이송하기 전에 먼 거리로 이송해야 하는 경우 카테터가 빠지지 않도록 정맥 라인을 고정하는 것이 좋다.

부상자가 수액 소생술이나 정맥 내 약물 투여가 필요하지만, 정맥 라인을 확보할 수 없는 경우 골내 경로(IO)가 효과적이고 효율적인 대안이 될 수 있다. 선택한 부위에 심각한 손상이 없는 경우 복장뼈나 팔다리에 골내 경로 확보를 시행할 수 있다. 대부분 전문적인 처치와 마찬가지로 이 시술에는 TEMS 제공자에게 자신감과 역량을 심어주기 위해 엄격한 교육 프로그램이 필요하다.

민간인 TEMS 손상 유형은 군인 손상 유형보다 더 빈번하게 팔과 다리 모두에서 골내 라인을 확보하는 것이 적절할 수 있다. 가 가능하다. 따라서 골내 경로를 확보하기 위해 정강뼈에 라인을 확보하는 것이 적절할 수 있다. 몸쪽 위팔뼈에 골내 경로를 확보할 수 있지만, 전술적 환경에서 부상자를 이동하는 중에 위팔뼈 부분에 골내 경로를 확보하면 의도치 않게 쉽게 골내로 주입된 바늘이 빠질 수 있다는 점에 주의한다.

현재 인정되는 저혈압 소생술 프로토콜과 손상 관리 소생술에 따르면 머리 손상 없고 노동맥이 약하거나 촉지되지 않는 정신 상태 변화를 보이는 경우 출혈성 쇼크라고 인지하고 부상자에게 수액을 투여해야 한다(**Box 22-4**). 이러한 소견은 상당한 출혈과 쇼크의 진행된 단계를 나타내며 혈액제제를 사용할 수 없는 경우 수액 투여가 필요하다는 것을 의미한다.

전술 현장 처치 및 TEMS는 지난 몇 년 동안 수액 처치 영역에서 많은 변화를 겪었다. 소생술 수액의 선택은 대부분 프로토콜과 선호도에 따라 달라진다. 제한적인 결정질 용액과 허용적 저혈압으로 개선된 결과가 입증됨에 따라 광범위한 결정질 수액 투여에 대한 이전의 권장 사항은 삭제되었다.

가능하면 전혈을 수혈하는 것이 TCCC의 출혈 관리에서 권장되는 수혈 전략이다. 출혈성 쇼크에 빠진 부상자에게는 냉장 보관된 저역가 O형 전혈(CS-LTOWB)이 가장 선호되는 소생술 수액이다. 사전 선별된 기증자 풀에서 얻은 신선한 전혈 사용은 차선책이다. 그런 다음 TCCC는 단위마다 부상자를 재평가하고 노동맥이 촉지되거나 정신 상태가 개선되거나 수축기 혈압이 100mmHg가 될 때까지 수액 소생술을 계속 시행할 것을 권장한다. 혈액 제제를 수혈하는 경우 이제 TCCC 지침에서는 첫 번째 수혈 후 칼슘 1g을 정맥 내/골내로 투여할 것을 권장한다. 외상성 뇌손상이 의심되고 정신 상태에 변화가 있는 부상자의 노동맥이 약하거나 촉지되지 않는 경우 지점에서는 정상 노동맥박을 회복하고 유지하는 데 필요하면 수액 소생술을 실시할 것을 권장한다. 이러한 환자에게 혈압 모니터링이 가능한 경우 목표 수축기 혈압을 100~110mmHg로 설정한다. 특히 TCCC는 더 이상 군 전투 환경에서 수액 소생술에 결정질 용액 사용을 권장하지 않는다. 민간 전술 시나리오에서 혈액 제제의 가용성이 훨씬 제한되어 있으므로 결정질 및 기타 비혈액량 확장제에서 벗어나 전혈 사용으로 완전히 전환하는 것은 아직 대부분의 민간 전술 프로토콜에 도달하지 못했다.

저체온증

외상 환자의 저체온증은 사망률의 독립적인 예측 인자이다. 외상 환자는 주변 온도와 관계없이 저체온증이 발생할 위험이 높다. 특히 습한 환경에서 처치 및 대피 중에 환자가 환경에 더 오래 노출될수록 저체온증에 걸릴 가능성이 높아진다. TEMS 제공자는 부상자가 외부 환경에 노출되는 것을 최소화한다. 가능하면 젖거나 피가 묻은 옷을 갈아입거나 벗기고 마른 담요, 재킷, 침낭과 같이 사용할 수 있는 모든 방법을 이용하여 부상자를 따뜻하게 유지한다. 가능하다면 손상을 처치한 후에도 부상자에게 모든 보호 장비를 착용시킨다. 이 보호 장비는 다시 교전이 발생하는 경우 부상자를 보호할 수 있다. 매우 추운 환경에서 장시간 병원 전 단계에 있을 가능성이 있는 군 전투 시나리오의 경우 TCCC 지침은 부상자의 앞쪽 몸통과 겨드랑이의 팔 아래에 발열 담요를 덮을 것을 권장한다. 화상을 예방하기 위해 열원을 피부에 직접 대거나 몸통을 완전히 감싸서는 안 된다. 가능한 한 빨리 후드가 달린 침낭이나 기타 쉽게 구할 수 있는 단열재를 사용하여 저체온증을 예방한다. 이러한 전투 환경에서는 정맥 내 수액을 투여하는 경우 배터리로 작동하는 가온 장치를 사용하는 것도 저체온증을 해결하는 데 도움이 될 수 있다.

사상자 구출 및 대피

구출은 사상자를 위험 지역에서 전방통제 지역(내부 경계선 내)으로 이동하는 것이고 대피는 외부 경계선(전방통제 지역)내 지역에서 안전지역으로 사상자를 옮기는 것이다. 사상자 구출은 육체적으로 힘든 과정으로 임무 흐름이 중단되고 전술팀이 사상자를 구출하는 취약한 상황에서 적의 공격에 노출되어 위험에 처할 가능성이 있다.

사상자를 구출하기 전에 TEMS 제공자는 이송 위험과 부상자 생존 가능성을 분석한다. 이는 팀장과의 공동 결정이며 궁극적으로 전체 임무를 담당하는 팀장의 결정이며 손상 위치, 총기 손상, 손상 시간 등에 영향을 받는다. 부상자를 안전지역으로 이동하는 데 필요한

시간은 부상자의 지원 능력, 이동 거리, 부상자의 장비 무게, 해당 지역의 상대적 위협 수준 및 팀의 체력 등에 따라 영향을 받는다. 일부 상황에서 시작 시나리오에서와 같이 가해자가 현장을 장악하고 있어 안전하지 않은 넓은 지역을 만들 수도 있다. 많은 민간 전술 작전에서 임무의 목표는 상대적으로 제한된 장소에 있는 한 두 명의 가해자일 수 있다. 이러한 유형의 임무에는 위험이 높은 영장 집행, 마약 단속, 고위급 인사 경호 등이 포함된다. 이러한 임무는 가해자를 체포하거나 제압하여 신속하게 완료하는 경향이 있다. 이러면 일단 해당 지역을 확보하던 전술적 현장 처치로 신속하게 전환한 다음 "정상적이고 일반적인" EMS 처치로 전환한다.

이송 위험의 두 번째 요소는 이동 경로다. 교전 지역(Zones of fire)은 불규칙한 형태의 비연속적인 지리적 영역으로 위험 수준이 유동적이다. 구출을 위해서는 선형 위험 지역을 가로질러야 할 수 있으며 이 경우 제자리에서 처치하는 것의 가치와 즉각적인 전문 인명 소생술 처치의 필요성을 비교 검토해야 한다. 지휘관은 구조 임무를 시작하기 전에 사용할 수 있는 자원을 고려한다. 이러한 고위험 구조에는 여러 가지 요인이 작용하며 역사적으로 비효과적이고 비현실적인 방법이 사용되어 궁극적으로 불필요한 손상과 사망의 위험을 증가시켜 왔다. 비대칭 구에는 구출 작전을 시작하기 전에 여러 명의 인력, 특수 장비(예: 휴대용 들것, 하네스, 드래그 스트랩) 및 적극적인 보호 자세가 필요하다(**그림 22-4**).

마지막으로 TEMS 제공자는 이송 중 처치를 제공할 수 있는 능력을 고려한다. 예를 들어, 실제 교전 지역에서 빠르게 들것을 이용해 이동하는 동안 TEMS 제공자는 외상 환자에게 턱 밀어올리기를 유지하지 못할 수 있다. 이 경우 이동하기 전에 보조기도기를 삽입하는 것이 현명할 수 있다. 이동 위험 또는 잠재적 교전 지역을 통해 부상자를 이동하는 위험은 해당 지역을 통과하는 데 걸리는 시간 및 이동 경로와 관련된 위험과 이동 중 필수적인 처치 제공으로 인해 발생하는 위험과 관련이 있다. 전술적 환경에서 대부분의 의사 결정과 마찬가지로 경험과 판단이 중요하다.

신속한 원격 평가 방법(RAM)

신속한 원격 평가 방법(RAM)은 미국 국방성 의과대학인 보건과학대학의 CONTOOMS 프로그램에서 개발했다. 이 평가 알고리즘의 주요 목적은 구조 가능한 사상자를 구조하고 처치할 기회를 극대화하는 동시에 불필요한 구출 시도로 인한 TEMS 제공자의 위험을 최소화하는 것이다. 이 알고리즘은 전술적 사상자 처치(TCC)의 CUFT 단계

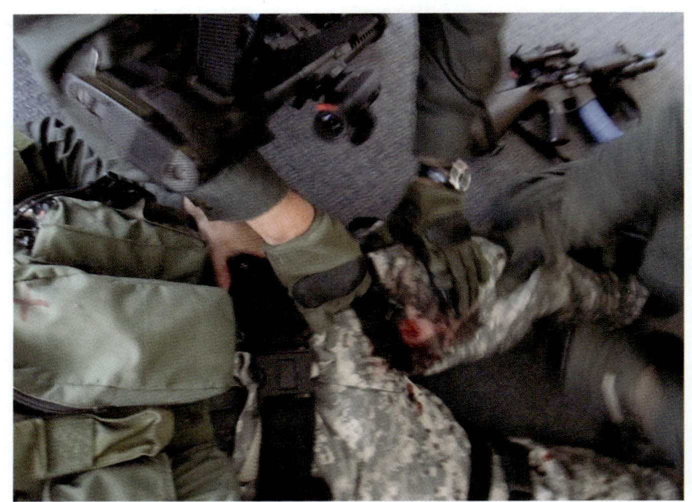

그림 22-4 교전 중 처치/ 위협 상황에서의 처치 및 구출
Courtesy of Commander Al Davis, Ventura Police Department.

에 가장 적합하다(**그림 22-5**). 불필요한 구조는 부상자가 스스로 탈출할 수 있는 경우와 이미 사망한 경우(시신 수습이라고 부르는 것이 더 적절함)의 두 가지 범주로 나뉜다. 신속한 원격 평가 방법은 지휘관에게 구조 시도를 권장하기 전에 보호된 위치에서 전체 상황을 평가할 수 있는 체계적인 접근 방법을 제공한다.

신속한 원격 평가 방법을 실시하는 첫 번째 단계는 해당 지역이 안전한지 확인하는 것이다. 안전하다면 부상자가 TEMS 제공자에게 해를 끼칠 수 없는지 확인한 후 표준 EMS 처치를 하는 것이 적절하다. 해당 지역이 안전하지 않으면 사용할 수 있는 정보를 활용하여 사상자가 가해자인지 아니면 다른 위협을 나타내는지 판단한다. 이러한 상황에서 위협이 통제될 때까지 추가적인 의료 개입을 하지 않는다. 그렇지 않으면 전술 요원, TEMS 요원 및 무고한 부대원의 안전이 위태로워질 수 있다. 사상자가 가해자로 간주하지 않으면 신속하게 원격 평가를 시작하여 손상의 본질과 사상자 상태의 안정성을 평가한다.

원격 관찰은 TEMS 제공자가 적대 세력에게 자신의 위치나 의도를 드러내지 않고 정보를 수집할 수 있으므로 원격 평가 시 가장 먼저 사용되는 기술이다. SWAT 팀이 사용할 수 있는 기술은 이 평가의 신뢰성을 향상할 수 있다. 예를 들어, 쌍안경이나 야간 투시경을 잘 사용하면 부상자가 숨을 쉬고 있는지, 호흡 속도와 호흡의 질, 생명을 위협하는 출혈이 있는지, 생명에 지장이 없는 명백한 상처가 있는지 확인

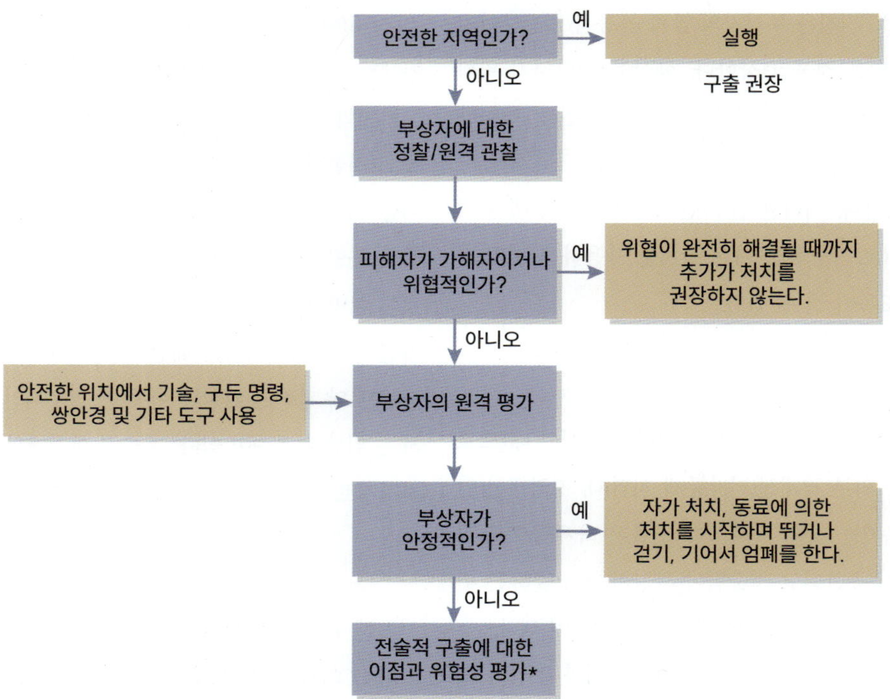

그림 22-5 신속 및 원격 평가 방법(RAM) 흐름도
© National Association of Emergency Medical Technicians (NAEMT)

하는 데 도움이 될 수 있다. 전술팀 사이에서 무인 항공 시스템(UAS)과 항공 드론이 점점 더 보편화되고 있으며 TEMS 제공자의 업무에 지장을 주지 않으면서도 신속한 원격 평가에 도움을 줄 수 있다. 추운 날씨에 부상자가 숨을 쉬고 있으면 부상자의 입에서 입김을 흔히 볼 수 있다. 가능한 경우 음향 감시 장비를 사용하여 음성, 신음, 심지어 호흡음까지 감지할 수 있다. 열화상 기술은 최근 몇 년 동안 향상 개선되었으며 신속한 원격 평가에 적용하는 것을 고려할 수 있다.

부상자가 안정적으로 보이면 가능한 한 부상자에게 자가 처치를 지시하고 안위를 도모해야 하며 전술적 상황이 개선될 때까지 구출을 기다려야 한다. 지휘관은 언제든지 부상자를 전술적으로 구출하는 것이 최선이라고 판단할 수 있지만, 이 결정에는 부상자의 의학적 안정성이 아닌 상황을 먼저 고려해야 한다. 부상자의 상태가 불안정한 경우 구출의 위험과 즉각적인 처치의 이점을 비교 검토해야 한다. 이는 지휘관의 결정이지만, 지휘관은 환자의 상태와 즉각적인 구출의 필요성에 대한 TEMS 제공자의 평가에 의존할 것이다. 이익이 위험성보다 매우 높으면 구출이 진행할 수 있다.

이 알고리즘은 논리적으로 보이지만 감정이 이성을 압도하여 불필요한 구출이 이루어지기 전에 올바른 판단을 내릴 수 있는 의사 결정 구조를 갖추는 것이 중요하다. 군대에서는 시신을 수습하기 위해 발생한 사상자와 결국 도움 없이 일어서서 엄호하러 달려온 사상자를 구조하려는 시도가 실패한 수많은 사례가 있다.

추가 고려 사항

일부 일반적인 기존 EMS 개입은 전술적 상황에서 부적절할 수 있다. 예를 들어, 심폐소생술은 외상성 심정지 환자에게는 거의 도움이 되지 않으며 EMS 제공자의 위험 노출을 증가시킨다. 따라서 심폐소생술은 전술적 의료 대응에서 매우 제한적인 역할을 하며 익사, 감전, 저체온증 및 일부 독성 물질에 노출된 피해자에게만, 고려한다. CUFT와 전술적 현장 처치(TFC)의 두 단계 모두에서 심폐소생술, 정맥 라인 확보 및 수액 처치에 대한 강조가 줄어든 것은 TEMS와 기존 EMS 사이의 몇 가지 차이점을 보여준다. 이러한 예시는 TEMS 제공자의 임상적 판단을 대체할 수 없다.

진통제 고려 사항

간단히 고려해야 할 한 가지 영역은 TEMS 통증 관리이다. 초기 TEMS 제공자들은 처음에는 모르핀을 사용했으며 필요에 따라 병원 전 임무 중 사용 빈도와 용량을 조절했다. 그러나 경구용 점막 펜타닐의 잠재적인 효과를 발견한 후 이 약물은 기도 또는 정신 상태에 문제가 없는 부상자의 경증에서 중등도 통증에 대한 TCCC 지침에 추가되었다. 케타민은 사용 범위가 넓고 금기 사항이 제한적인 또 다른 예외적인 약물로 2012년 TCCC 지침에 추가되었다. 케타민은 혈류역학, 호흡수 및 기도 반사를 보존하며 의식이 없거나 의식을 잃은 환자에게 사용할 수 있다. 진통, 해리성 기억 상실 및 처치를 시행하기 전에 진정이 필요한 대부분 부상자는 적절한 모니터링과 의료 지도 의사의 의료 지도를 받아 케타민을 사용하면 효과를 볼 수 있다.

2014년 TCCC는 민간 영역에서도 권장할 수 있는 세 가지 선택 통증 관리 방법을 개발했다. 처음에는 경미한 통증에 대해 경구용 약물(예: NSAIDs, 아세트아미노펜)을 지속해 복용하는 것이 권장된다. 중등도 통증이 있지만, 쇼크나 악화 위험이 없는 경우 경구용 점막 펜타닐(또는 설하 수펜타닐)이 권장된다. 마지막으로 부상자가 심한 통증을 느끼며 쇼크 또는 폐 손상의 위험이 있거나 경험하고 있는 경우 정맥 내 펜타닐 투여와 함께 케타민을 추가 방법으로 선택할 수 있다. 권장 사항은 가용성, 선호도 및 TEMS 의료 책임자의 재량에 따라 달라진다.

전술적 후송 처치(후송 중 처치)

전술적 후송 처치(TEC)는 외부 경계선을 지나 작전상 안전 지역에서 이루어지며 상대적으로 위험이 낮은 구역이다. 외부 경계는 사고 현장을 격리하고 일반적으로 현장 통제, 사건 격리 및 일반 공공 안전을 주요 임무로 하는 기존의 경찰관이 담당한다. 전술적 후송 처치 단계에서 적절한 의료기관으로 이송하는 동안 처치는 계속된다. 외상 환자에 대한 기존의 EMS 처치와 유사하게 여기에는 부상자를 구급차로 이송하거나 장갑차와 같은 대체 응급 차량을 사용하는 것이 포함될 수 있다(**그림 22-6**). 이 단계에서의 처치는 상황과 부상에 따라 다르며 팀 표준 운영 절차와 사고 지휘관의 결정에 따라 이루어진다. 사고 지휘관의 재량과 필요에 따라 가해자가 사용하는 무기가 손이 닿지 않는 곳에 의료 통제 구역을 설정할 수 있으며 이 구역에 추가 EMS 의료 자원을 배치할 수 있다.

부상자 이송에 대체 응급 차량을 사용하는 경우 의료 교육을 받았거나 받지 않은 팀원의 역할을 포함하도록 표준 운영 절차를 심도 있게 연습해야 한다. 이러한 차량에는 추가 의료 장비를 준비해야 하며 모든 팀원은 지혈대, 코인두기도기, 체스트 씰, 저체온증 예방과 같은

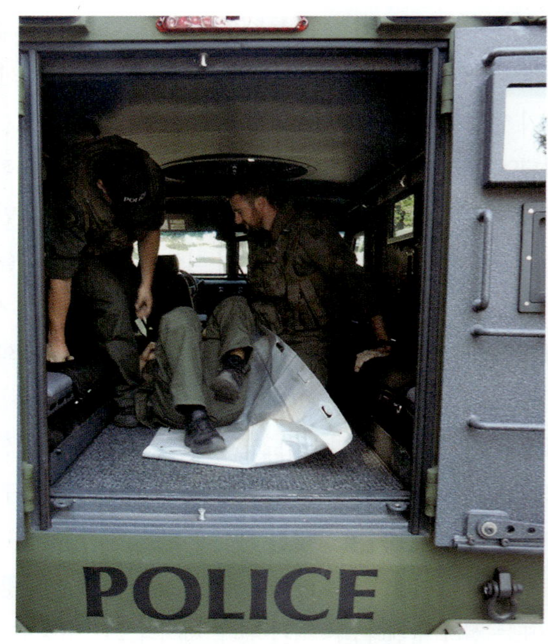

그림 22-6 비표준 전술 후송 차량.
Courtesy of Commander Al Davis, Ventura Police Department.

인명구조 처치를 시행하여 예방할 수 있는 4가지 사망 원인(출혈, 기도 폐쇄, 기흉, 저체온증)을 처치하는 교차 훈련을 받아야 한다.

안전하다고 판단되는 지역이라도 모든 구급대원은 경계를 늦추지 말아야 한다. 전술 작전은 복잡하고 역동적이다. 1999년 콜럼바인 고등학교 총기 난사 사건 당시 범인들은 파이프 폭탄과 사제 폭발물을 설치하여 구급대원을 표적으로 삼았다. 다행히도 기술적 오류로 인해 이러한 장치는 폭발하지 않았다. 이와 유사하게 2012년 콜로라도주 오로라 영화관 총격 사건의 범인은 폭발물을 준비하여 자기 아파트에 설치했다. 이 장치에는 현장에 출동한 경찰관을 살해 사고 건물을 파괴할 수 있는 인화성 물질이 든 트립 와이어와 부비트랩이 포함되어 있었다. 이 모든 장치는 숙련된 폭발물 처리팀에 의해 처리되었다.

FBI는 경찰관을 의도적으로 매복한 사건을 여러 차례 보고했으며 이러한 사건의 빈도는 점점 더 증가하고 있다. 또한 바리케이드를 친 용의자를 이용해 경찰관을 현장으로 유인하여 매복하는 작전을 명시적으로 자세히 설명하는 테러 훈련 매뉴얼도 발간되었다. 근면함과 상황 인식은 대응하는 경찰관과 TEMS 제공자의 안전한 작전을 위한 초석이다. 최근 몇 년 동안 화재부터 차량, 유기화합물 용액에 이르기까지 모든 것을 활용한 민간인과 경찰관에 대한 공격이 발생하고 있다. 기민한 TEMS 제공자는 작전 중 예상치 못한 부상 패턴을 고려해야 한다.

다수 사상자 사고

총기 난사범이 연루된 다수 사상자 사건(MCI)은 점점 더 빈번하고 위험해지고 있으며 복잡한 기관 간 협업 과제를 안고 있다. 플로리다주 올랜도에서 발생한 펄스 나이트클럽 총격 사건과 라스베이거스 루트 91번 국도 하베스트 컨트리 뮤직 페스티벌 총격 사건은 비극적인 사례로 꼽힌다. TEMS 제공자는 다수 사상자 사고에서 고유한 임무를 수행한다. 첫째 TEMS 팀은 경찰과 소상서 및 전술적 EMS 시스템을 연결하는 역할을 한다. 둘째 TEMS 제공자는 혼란스럽고 위험하며 자원이 부족한 환경에서 일하도록 훈련받았다. 셋째 TEMS 제공자는 다양한 통신 매체 활용, 즉각적인 조치 훈련. 임무 계획에 대한 폭넓은 경험이 있다. TEMS 제공자는 잘 조율된 다수 사상자 사고 대응을 계획하고 실행하는 과정을 수행할 때 고려해야 할 귀중한 자원이다.

의료 정보 및 의료 지침

TEMS 제공자의 역할 중 하나는 의료 정보를 사전 계획, 수집하여 유지하는 것이다. 지역 및 지역팀에서 TEMS 제공자는 지역 EMS 및 외상 시스템에 대한 심층적인 지식을 갖추고 있어야 한다. 이러한 지식은 임무 수행 중 사상자가 발생할 때 TEMS 제공자가 처치와 환자를 이송할 의료기관과 관련하여 적절한 결정을 내릴 수 있게 해준다. 야생 지역과 같이 알려지지 않은 지역에서 원격으로 활동하는 TEMS 팀은 실행할 수 있는 이송 계획과 연장된 처치 계획을 개발하기 위해 훨씬 더 심층적인 의료 계획을 수행한다.

TEMS에서 항공 의무 후송 플랫폼의 역할은 매우 유용할 수 있지만, TEMS 제공자는 항공 의무 후송 자산의 가용성을 지속해서 모니터링 또한, 전술적 상황에 대한 항공 후송 플랫폼의 대응에는 항공 의료 부대가 적의 공격을 받지 않도록 적절한 안전 예방 조치가 포함되어야 한다.

마지막으로 민간 TEMS의 확산을 고려할 때 각 팀의 의료 지도 책임자를 팀의 일원으로 파악하고 포함하는 것이 필수적이다. 전술 EMS는 본질적으로 EMS의 하위 전문 분야이므로 이와 같이 취급해야 한다. 전술 의학에 관심이 있는 EMS 의사를 찾아서 확보해야 팀원의 안전과 팀 성과를 개선하는 데 도움을 주어야 한다. EMS 의사는 자료수집, 증거 기반 의학, 우수한 품질 관리 및 임상 교육 프로그램의 과학적 원칙을 준수한다. 이와 같은 원칙을 경찰과 SWAT 팀에도 적용하여 가능한 최고 품질의 시스템을 구축한다.

요 약

- 일반적으로 전술 환경에서 의료 원칙은 병원 전 처치 제공자에게 익숙한 원칙과 같다.
- 작전 환경의 긴박성과 위험성 때문에 모든 처치의 이점과 해당 처치를 제공하는 데 내재한 위험을 비교 검토해야 한다. 이러한 결정에는 고유한 의사결정 기술이 필요하다.
- TEMS 제공자는 특정 처치의 이점과 이러한 환경에서 처치를 수행할 때 내재한 특수한 위험 사이의 균형을 지속해서 유지한다.
- 전술적 상황에서 세 가지 단계의 처치로 구성된다.
  - 교전 중 처치/위협 상황에서의 처치(직접적인 위협이 있는 상황에서 처치): 적의 공격 또는 적극적인 위험 상황(오염지역)에서 제공되는 처치
  - 전술적 현장 처치(간접적인 위협이 있는 상황에서 처치): 즉각적인 위험이 진압되거나 통제된 후 제공되는 처치로 상황이 교전 중 처치로 돌아갈 수 있음을 알고 제공하는 처치
  - 전술적 후송 처치(후송 중 처치): 상황이 안전하다고 판단되면 제공되는 처치로 일반적인 민간 EMS에 도움을 요청하는 것과 유사하다.
- 의료 정보 수집을 통해 TEMS 제공자는 전술 작전이 수행될 지역의 환경, 지리 및 이용할 수 있는 자원을 파악할 수 있다.

시나리오 재구성

당신이 속한 EMS 기관은 지역 경찰특공대(SWAT)팀을 지원하고 현지 경찰과 함께 엄격한 통합 훈련 프로그램을 갖추고 있다. TEMS 팀은 해가 진 직후 오래된 이동식 주택에 총기 난사범이 숨어있다는 신고를 받고 출동한다. 진입을 준비하고 있을 때 두 명의 SWAT 대원이 용의자의 마당을 가로질러 집에 접근하여 문을 부수기 위해 준비한다. 앞쪽 창문에서 총성이 울려 퍼지고 SWAT 대원이 손상을 입었다. SWAT 대원 한 명이 용의자의 집 출입구에 쓰러졌고 다른 한 명은 낡은 픽업트럭 근처에 쓰러졌다. 근처에 서 있던 경찰관이 "우리가 구하러 가자!"라고 외친다. 당신은 경찰관의 팔을 잡고 SWAT 지휘관을 바라본다.

- 당신은 어떻게 행동해야 하는가?
- 현장의 위험성을 고려할 때때 쓰러진 SWAT 대원을 어떻게 평가하고 처치해야 하는가?

시나리오 해결책

SWAT 지휘관이 신속한 원격 평가 방법(RAM)을 사용하여 구조 활동의 유용성을 판단하라고 명령한다. SWAT 팀은 쌍안경과 음향 장치를 사용하여 쓰러진 두 명의 팀원을 확인한다. 총격범의 이동식 주택 출입문 앞에 누워 있는 첫 번째 대원의 가슴벽 움직임이나 호흡하는 것이 보이지 않는다. 팀원의 호출에도 불구하고 음향 장치에서 어떤 소리 반응도 감지할 수 없다.

두 번째 경찰관은 낡은 픽업트럭의 보닛 부분으로 이동했다. 허벅지 아랫부분에서 출혈이 보인다. 다행히도 당신은 대원들을 위해 광범위한 전술 의료 훈련을 시행했다. 당신은 팀 보안 무전기를 통해 그와 교신하고 출혈 부위보다 위쪽 서혜부에 지혈대를 단단히 적용하도록 지시한다. 그는 지혈대를 확실하게 적용하고 더 이상의 부상은 없다고 말한다.

당신의 추천과 위협 평가에 따라 SWAT 지휘관은 생명의 징후가 보이지 않는 대원에 대한 고위험 구출을 수행하지 않기로 한다. 협상 전문가가 용의자에게 항복하도록 설득하는 동안 두 번째 손상을 입은 대원과 연락을 유지한다. 그리고 지역 외상센터에 연락하여 부상자의 잠재적인 손상 관련 정보를 알려준다. 30분 후 용의자가 항복하고 체포되었다. 당신 팀은 부상자를 지역 외상센터로 이송하였고 혈관 재건술을 통해 다리와 생명을 구하였다.

References

1. Rinnert KJ, Hall WL. Tactical emergency medical support. *Emerg Med Clin N Am.* 2002;20:929-952.
2. Butler FK, Hagmann J, Butler EG. Tactical combat casualty care in Special Operations. *Milit Med.* 1996;161(Suppl):1–16.
3. Federal Bureau of Investigation. Crime data explorer. Accessed January 17, 2022. https://crime-data-explorer.app.cloud.gov/pages/home
4. Federal Bureau of Investigation. Uniform crime reports. Accessed October 6, 2021. https://ucr.fbi.gov/leoka
5. National Tactical Officers Association. Position statement on the inclusion of physicians in tactical law enforcement operations. Accessed January 17, 2022. https://www.ntoa.org/sections/tems/tems-position-statement/
6. Heck JJ, Pierluisi G. Law enforcement special operations and medical support. *Prehosp Emerg Care.* 2001;5:403-406.
7. American College of Emergency Physicians. Policy statement on tactical emergency medical support. *Ann Emerg Med.* 2005;45:108.
8. National Association of Emergency Medical Technicians. Pollak AN, ed. *Prehospital Trauma Life Support.* 9th ed. Jones & Bartlett Learning; 2018.
9. Callaway DW, Reed S, Shapiro G, et al. The Committee for Tactical Emergency Care (C-TECC): evolution and application of TCCC guidelines to civilian high threat medicine. *J Special Operations Med.* 2011;11:2.
10. Smith ER, Shapiro G, Sarani B. Fatal wounding pattern and causes of potentially preventable death following the Pulse Night Club shooting event. *Prehosp Emerg Care.* 2018;22(6):662-668.
11. Kanable R. Peak performance: well-trained tactical medics can help the team perform at its best. *Law Enforcement Tech.* August 1999.
12. Cooke, MC. How much to do at the accident scene? *BMJ.* 1999;319:1105-1106. doi: 10.1136/bmj.320.7240.1005/
13. Jagoda A, Pietrzek M, Hazen S, Vayer J. Prehospital care and the military. *Mil Med.* 1992;157(1):11-15. doi: 10.1093/milmed/157.1.11
14. Bellamy RF. The causes of death in conventional land warfare: implications for combat casualty care research. *Mil Med.* 1984;149:55-62.
15. Callaway DW. Tactical emergency services. In: Hogan DE, Burstein JL, eds. *Disaster Medicine.* 2nd ed. Lippincott, Williams and Wilkins; 2007.
16. Gerold KB, Gibbons M, McKay S. The relevance of Tactical Combat Casualty Care (TCCC) guidelines to civilian law enforcement operations. National Tactical Officers TEMS Overview. Updated November 1, 2009. Accessed March 18, 2022. https://www.east.org/content/documents/MilitaryResources/TCCC/TCCC.pdf
17. Parsons, DL, Mott JC. *Tactical Combat Casualty Care Handbook: Observations, Insights, and Lessons.* Center for Army Lessons Learned; 2012.
18. Kragh JF, Walters TJ, Baer DG, et al. Survival with emergency tourniquet use to stop bleeding in major limb trauma. *Ann Surg.* 2009;249(1):1-7.
19. Thunholm P, Henåker L. A tentative model on effective army combat tactics. *Comparative Strategy.* 2020;39(5):490-504. doi: 10.1080/01495933.2020.1803713
20. Kragh JF, O'Neill ML, Walters TJ, et al. The military emergency tourniquet program's lessons learned with devices and designs. *Mil Med.* 2011;176:10, 1144.
21. Butler FK, Giebner SD, McSwain N, et al., eds. *Prehospital Trauma Life Support.* Military 8th ed. Jones & Bartlett Learning; 2014.
22. Bennett BL, Littlejohn LF, Kheirabadi BS, et al. Management of external hemorrhage in Tactical Combat Casualty Care: chitosan-based hemostatic gauze dressings. *J Spec Oper Med.* 2014;14:12-29.
23. Bennett BL, Littlejohn L. Review of new topical hemostatic dressings for combat casualty care. *Mil Med.* 2014;179:497-514.
24. Littlejohn L, Bennett B, Drew B. Application of current hemorrhage control techniques for backcountry care: part 2: hemostatic dressings and other adjuncts. *Wilderness Environ Med.* 2015;26:246-254.
25. Drew B, Bennett B, Littlejohn L. Application of current hemorrhage control techniques for backcountry care. Part 1: tourniquets and hemorrhage control adjuncts. *Wilderness Environ Med.* 2015;26:236-245.
26. Kheirabadi BS, Edens JW, Terrazas IB, et al. Comparison of new hemostatic granules/powders with currently deployed hemostatic products in a lethal model of extremity arterial hemorrhage in swine. *J Trauma.* 2009;66:316-326.
27. Kheirabadi BS, Mace JE, Terrazas IB, et al. Safety evaluation of new hemostatic agents, smectite granules, and kaolin-coated gauze in a vascular injury wound model in swine. *J Trauma.* 2010;68:269-278.
28. Kheirabadi BS, Edens JW, Terrazas IB, et al. Comparison of new hemostatic granules/powders with currently deployed hemostatic products in a lethal model of extremity arterial hemorrhage in swine. *J Trauma.* 2009;66(2):316-326; discussion 327-328.
29. Butler FK Jr, Hagmann J, Butler EG. Tactical combat casualty care in special operations. *Mil Med.* 1996;161(suppl):3-16.
30. Mabry R, Frankfurt A, Kharod C, et al. Emergency cricothyroidotomy in Tactical Combat Casualty Care. *J Spec Oper Med.* 2015;15:11-19.
31. Hessert MJ, Bennett BL. Optimizing emergent surgical cricothyrotomy for use in austere environments. *Wilderness Environ Med.* 2013;24:53-66.
32. Mabry R, Nichols M, Shiner D, et al. A comparison of two open surgical cricothyroidotomy techniques by military medics using a cadaver model. *Ann Emerg Med.* 2014;63:1-5.
33. Tien HC, Jung V, Riool SB, et al. An evaluation of tactical combat casualty care interventions in a combat environment. *J Am Coll Surg.* 2008;207(2):174-178.
34. Hacked HT, Parse LA, Levy AD, et al. Chest wall thickness in military personnel: implications for needle thoracentesis in tension pneumothorax. *Mil Med.* 2008;172:1260-1263.
35. Zengerink I, Brink PR, Laupland KB, et al. Needle thoracostomy in the treatment of tension pneumothorax in trauma patients: what size needle? *J Trauma.* 2008;64:111-114.
36. Givens ML, Ayotte K, Manifold C. Needle thoracostomy: implications of computed tomography chest wall thickness. *Acad Emerg Med.* 2004;11:211-213.
37. Revell M, Greaves I, Porter K. Endpoints for fluid resuscitation in hemorrhagic shock. *J Trauma.* 2003;54(suppl 5):S63-S67.
38. Morrison CA, Carrick MM, Norman MA, et al. Hypotensive resuscitation strategy reduces transfusion requirements and severe postoperative coagulopathy in trauma patients with hemorrhagic shock: preliminary results of a randomized controlled trial. *J Trauma.* 2011;70(3):652-663.

39. Benson G. Intraosseous access to the circulatory system: an under-appreciated option for rapid access. *J Perioper Pract.* 2015;25:140-143.

40. Byars DV, Tsuchitani SN, Erwin E, et al. Evaluation of success rate and access time for an adult sternal intraosseous device deployed in the prehospital setting. *Prehosp Disaster Med.* 2011;26:127-129.

41. Lewis P, Wright C. Saving the critically injured trauma patient: a retrospective analysis of 1000 uses of intraosseous access. *Emerg Med J.* 2015;32:463-467.

42. Ley E, Clond M, Srour M, et al. Emergency department crystalloid resuscitation of 1.5 L or more is associated with increased mortality in elderly and non-elderly trauma patients. *J Trauma.* 2011;70:398-400.

43. Duke MD, Guidry C, Guice J, et al. Restrictive fluid resuscitation in combination with damage control resuscitation: time for adaptation. *J Trauma.* 2012;73:674-678.

44. Spinella P, Pidcoke H, Strandenes G, et al. Whole blood transfusion for hemostatic resuscitation of major bleeding. *Transfusion.* 2016;56:S190-S202.

45. Cap A, Pidcoke H, DePasquale M, et al. Blood far forward: time to get moving! *J Trauma.* 2015;78:S2-S6.

46. Stubbs J, Zielinski M, Jenkins D. The state of the science of whole blood: lessons learned at Mayo Clinic. *Transfusion.* 2016;56:S173-S881.

47. Spinella PC, Perkins JG, Grathwohl KW, et al. Warm fresh whole blood is independently associated with improved survival for patients with combat-related traumatic injuries. *J Trauma.* 2009;66:S69-S76.

48. Montgomery HR, Drew BG, Torrisi J, et al. TCCC Guidelines Comprehensive Review and Edits 2020: TCCC Guidelines Change 20-05 01 November 2020. *J Spec Oper Med.* 2021;21(2):122-127.

49. Zafren K, Giesbrecht GG, Danzl DF, et al. Wilderness Medical Society practice guidelines for the out-of-hospital evaluation and treatment of accidental hypothermia: 2014 update. *Wilderness Environ Med.* 2014;25(suppl):S66-S85.

50. McKeague AL. Evaluation of patient active warming systems. Military Health System Research Symposium, Tactical Combat Casualty Care breakout session. Ft. Lauderdale, FL. August 2012.

51. Allen PB, Salyer SW, Dubick MA, et al. Preventing hypothermia: comparison of current devices used by the U.S. Army in an in vitro warmed fluid model. *J Trauma.* 2010;69(suppl 1):S154-S161.

52. McKay S, Hoyne S. High threat immediate extraction: the Immediate Reaction Team (IRT) model. *Tactical Edge.* Spring 2007 50-54.

53. Callaway DW. Emergency medical services in disasters. Hogan DE, Burstein JL, eds. *Disaster Medicine.* 2nd ed. Philadelphia, PA: Lippincott, Williams and Wilkins; 2007:127-139.

54. Cloonan C. *Proceedings of the Third International Conference on Tactical Emergency Medical Support.* Bethesda, MD: Uniformed Services University of the Health Sciences; 1999.

55. Rosemary AS, Norris PA, Olson SM, et al. Prehospital traumatic cardiac arrest: the cost of futility. *J Trauma.* 1998;38:468-474.

56. Butler FK, Kotwal RS, Buckenmaier CC III, et al. A triple-option analgesia plan for Tactical Combat Casualty Care. *J Spec Oper Med.* 2014;14:13-25.

57. Kotwal R, O'Connor K, Johnson T, et al. A novel pain management strategy for combat casualty care. *Ann Emerg Med.* 2004;44:121-127.

58. Dickey N, Jenkins D, Butler F. Prehospital use of ketamine in battlefield analgesia. Defense Health Board Memorandum. Published March 8, 2012. Accessed January 17, 2022. https://health.mil/Reference-Center/Reports/2012/03/08/Prehospital-Use-of-Ketamine-in-Battlefield-Analgesia

Suggested Reading

National Association of Emergency Medical Technicians. *PHTLS: Prehospital Trauma Life Support.* Military 9th ed. Jones & Bartlett Learning; 2019.

특수 술기

정맥 라인 고정

원리: 외상 환자를 원거리로 이동, 움직이거나 직접 이송해야 할 때 정맥 라인을 확보하고 고정한다.

외상 환자가 움직이거나 원거리도 이동, 움직이거나 직접 이송해야 하는 경우 환자에게 확보한 정맥 라인이 이 과정에서 빠지는 경우가 종종 있다. 미군은 정맥 라인이 빠지지 않고 이러한 이동을 가능하게 하는 정맥 라인을 고정하는 방법을 개발했다. 여기서 시연하는 술기는 군에서 사용하는 방법을 민간에서 사용할 수 있도록 수정한 것이다.

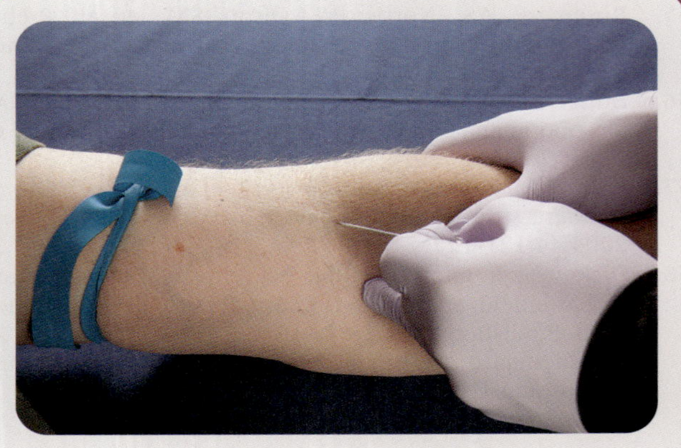

1 TEMS 제공자는 18 또는 16게이지 IV 카테터를 사용하여 일반적인 절차에 따라 정맥 라인을 확보한다.

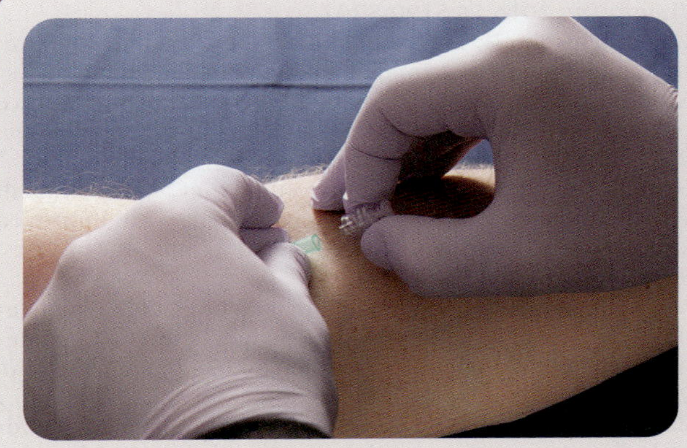

2 TEMS 제공자는 IV 카테터에 식염수 잠금 장치를 부착한다.

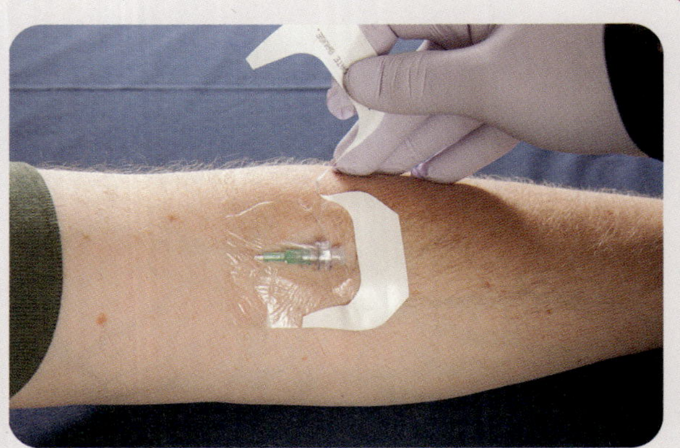

3 TEMS 제공자는 IV 카테터와 식염수 잠금장치를 투영한 상처 드레싱 필름(예: 테가덤)으로 완전히 덮는다.

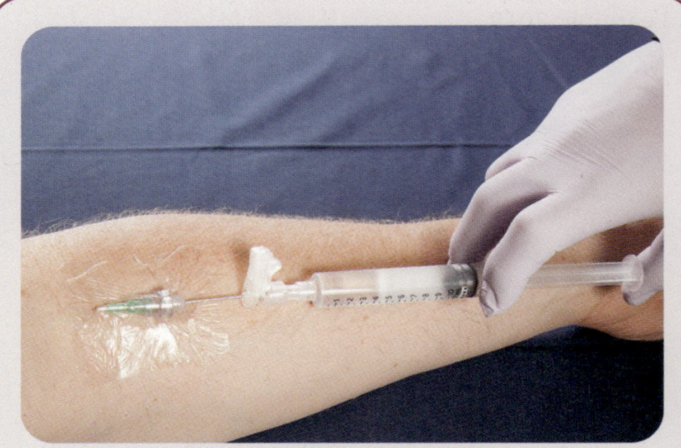

4 TEMS 제공자는 식염수 잠금장치의 드레싱 필름과 고무마개에 직접 구멍을 뚫어 식염수 잠금장치를 5mL의 생리식염수를 플러시한다.

(다음 페이지에 계속)

정맥 라인 고정 (이어서)

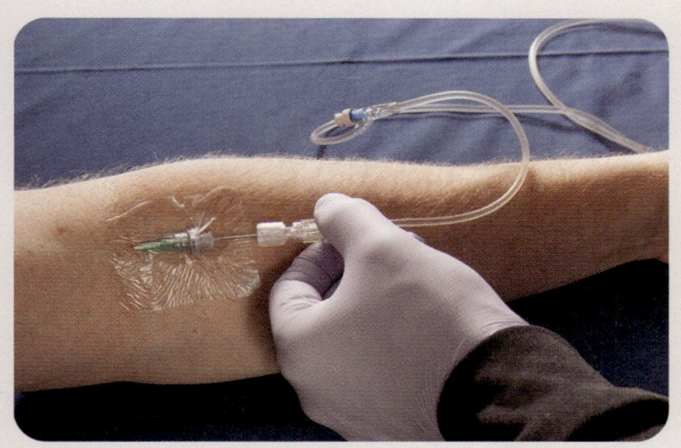

5　TEMS 제공자는 식염수 잠금장치의 드레싱 필름과 고무마개를 통해 두 번째 IV 카테터(18게이지)를 직접 삽입하고 이 카테터를 통해 수액과 약물을 투여한다.

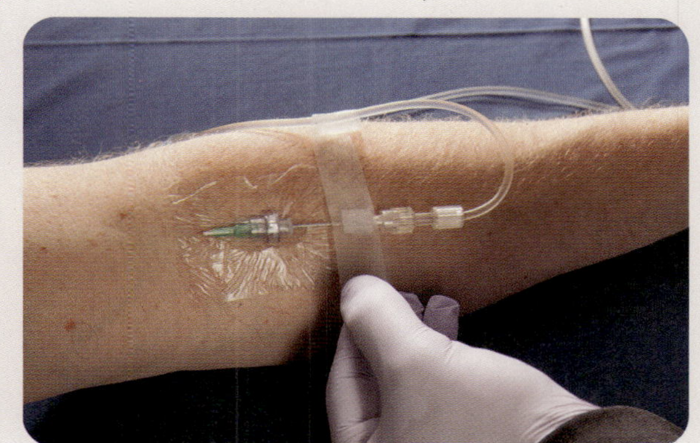

6　TEMS 제공자는 두 번째 카테터를 고정하고 벨크로 고정 장치 또는 테이프로 정맥 라인을 팔에 부착한다.

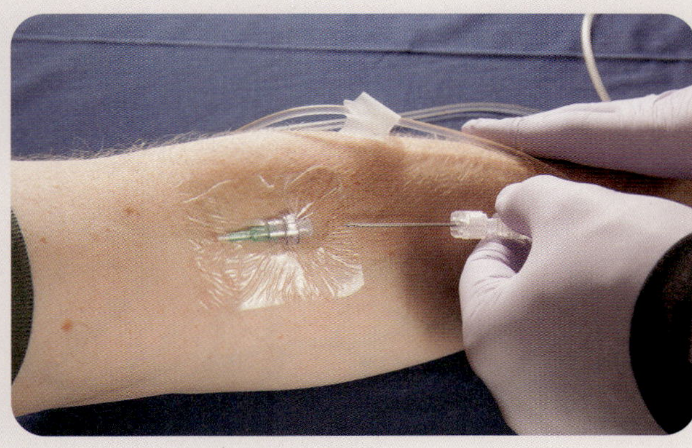

7　외상 환자를 이동해야 하는 경우 고정 장치 또는 테이프, 정맥 라인 보조 카테터를 제거한다. 기본 카테터와 식염수 잠금장치는 그대로 유지되므로 환자가 이동한 후에도 신속하게 정맥 라인을 확보할 수 있다.

용어 해설

Abbreviated Injury Scale (AIS; 간이 손상 척도): 손상을 1에서 6 사이의 값을 부여하는 손상 분류 시스템으로 1) 경미함, 2) 보통, 3) 심각함, 4) 중증, 5) 치명적임, 6) 생존 불가능으로 분류한다.

acetylcholine (아세틸콜린): 신경 자극을 전달하기 위해 신경세포 말단에서 분비되는 신경전달 물질로 작용하는 화학물질이다.

acid (산): pH 7 미만이며 알칼리를 중화시키는 화학 물질

active strategy (적극적 전략 손상): 예방과 관련하여 개인의 적극적인 참여가 필요한 예방 조치(예: 헬멧 착용)를 말한다.

acute mountain sickness (급성 고산병): 고지대(보통 24,000m 이상) 여행으로 인해 발생하는 일련의 증상

acute respiratory distress syndrome (ARDS; 급성 호흡곤란 증후군): 폐의 모세혈관과 폐포 내벽이 손상되어 간질 공간과 폐포로 체액이 누출되어 발생하는 호흡부전이다.

acute tubular necrosis (ATN; 급성 요세관 괴사): 일반적으로 쇼크와 관련된 허혈로 인해 발생하는 신세뇨관의 급성 손상

aerosol (에어로졸): 공기 중에 부유하는 고체 입자 및 액체 입자

afterload (후부하): 좌심실이 심장박동마다 혈액을 펌프질해야 하는 압력

air density (공기 밀도): 이 본문에서 사용되는 것으로 폐 조직과 같이 공기와 거의 같은 무게와 밀도를 가진 기관의 특성이다.

air-purifying respirator (APR; 공기 정화기): 필터, 여과장치, 카트리지를 사용하여 공기 정화 부품을 통과하는 주변 공기에서 오염 물질을 제거하고 호흡하기 안전한 공기를 만드는 장치이다.

alpha particle (α 입자): 방사성 물질이 붕괴할 때 방출되는 입자로 양성자 2개와 중성자 2개로 구성되며 양전하를 띠는 입자이다.

alveoli (폐포): 호흡기와 순환계가 만나 가스 교환이 일어나는 호흡기의 말단 공기주머니

anastomosis (문합): 두 개의 혈관 또는 인접한 장과 같은 두 구조물 사이의 연결

anhidrosis (무한증): 땀이 나지 않음

anisocoria (동공부등): 동공 크기가 서로 다름

anterior cord syndrome (전방 척수 증후군): 일반적으로 뼛조각이나 척추 동맥 압박으로 인해 척수 앞부분에 손상된 상태이다.

apnea (무호흡): 호흡이 없는 상태

appendicular skeleton (팔다리 뼈대): 팔다리 뼈대(어깨와 팔, 골반과 다리를 포함하는 골격 부위)

arachnoid mater (거미막): 경막과 연막 사이에 있는 거미줄 모양의 투명한 막으로 뇌를 둘러싸고 있는 세 개의 수막 막 중 중간막이다.

aspiration pneumonitis (흡인성 폐렴): 구토물이나 위 내용물을 흡입하여 발생하는 염증 및 폐렴

assist control (A/C) ventilation (보조 제어 환기): 기계 호흡의 한 형태로 환자가 적절하게 숨을 들이마시려고 시도하여 장치를 작동시키면 인공호흡기가 호흡을 보즈하거나

환자가 숨을 쉬지 않으면 자동으로 호흡이 이루어질 수 있다.

ataxic breathing (무호흡): 호흡량과 무호흡 주기가 불규칙하고 조정되지 않는 불규칙한 호흡 패턴이다.

atelectasis (무기폐): 폐포 또는 폐의 일부가 허탈된다.

atherosclerosis (죽상경화증): 혈관이 좁아지고 동맥벽의 안쪽 층이 두꺼워지면서 동맥 내에 지방 침전물이 쌓이는 상태이다.

atlas (고리뼈): 첫 번째 목뼈로 두개골이 그 위에 자리 잡고 있다.

atropine (아트로핀): 부교감신경 말단에서 아세틸콜린의 효과를 경쟁적으로 막는 화학 물질로 항콜린성 약물, 신경작용제 중독의 피해자를 처치하는 데 사용된다.

austere environment (통제된 환경): 자원, 소모품, 장비, 인력, 교통 및 물리적, 정치적, 사회적, 경제적 여건의 기타 측면이 극도로 제한된 환경

autonomic nervous system (자율신경계): 신체의 불수의적 기능을 지지하고 제어하는 중추신경계의 일부이다.

autonomy (자율성): 간섭이나 부당한 영향에서 벗어나 자신의 건강관리를 지시할 수 있는 성인 환자의 권리

autoregulation (자동조절): 시스템 내에서 변화를 감지하고 그 변화에 맞게 적응하도록 하는 생물학적 과정으로 순환계에서는 혈압의 변화에 따라 일정한 혈류를 유지하는 과정이다.

axial loading (축 부하): 물체의 장축에 작용

하거나 장축에 가해지는 힘이다. 일반적으로 머리에서 아래쪽으로 척추에 가해지는 힘을 말하며 높은 곳에서 넘어져 발로 착지할 때와 같이 몸의 무게가 척추 아래쪽 부분에 가해지는 때도 발생할 수 있다.

axis (중쇠뼈): 그 모양은 머리의 가능한 넓은 범위의 회전을 허용한다. 또한 몸의 중심을 통과하는 가상의 선이다.

baroreceptor (압력수용기): 혈압 변화로 자극받는 감각 신경 말단으로 압력수용기는 심장의 심방, 대정맥, 대동맥활, 목동맥팽대의 벽에서 발견된다.

barotrauma (압력 손상): 기압의 변화로 인해 발생하는 공기가 함유된 기관의 손상

basal level (기저 수준): 기준선 또는 최소 수준

basal metabolic rate (기초대사율): 인체가 휴식 중에 연소하여 신진대사의 부산물로 열이 생성되는 열량의 수이다.

base (염기): 물에 용해되면 수산화 이온을 방출하거나 수소 이온을 수용하여 조직의 액화 괴사를 일으키는 pH 7보다 높은 화학물질

basilar skull fracture (두개골 기저골절): 두개골 기저부의 골절

behavioral regulation (행동 조절): 환경의 열 변화에 대한 개인의 의식적인 반응과 따뜻하게 하거나 시원하게 유지하기 위해 취하는 신체적 행동

beneficence (선행): "선을 행한다"라는 뜻의 윤리적 용어로 병원 전 처치 제공자가 환자에게 이익을 극대화하고 위험을 최소화하는 방식으로 행동해야 한다.

biologic agent (생물학적 작용제): 대량살상무기로 사용될 수 있는 박테리아, 바이러스 또는 독소

blast lung injury (BLI; 폭발성 폐 손상): 높은 폭발성 과압파에 노출되어 발생하는 폐 손상으로 폐 손상은 점상출혈에서 타박상 및 폐출혈에 이르기까지 다양하다.

blast overpressure (폭발 과압): 고성능 폭발물 폭발로 인해 의해 발생하는 일반 대기압을 초과하는 압력

blast wave (폭발파): 폭발 중심에서 바깥쪽으로 퍼져나가는 증가한 압력의 파형

blast wind (폭발풍): 폭발로 인해 발생하는 공기 갑자기 이동한 결과이다.

blind nasotracheal intubation (맹목적 코 기관내삽관): 후두와 성대를 눈으로 보지 않고 기관내관을 콧구멍을 통해 기관으로 삽입하는 술기이다.

blister agent (수포제): 화상 같은 손상을 유발하는 화학물로 대량살상용무기로 사용된다.

blunt trauma (무딘 외상): 빠르게 움직이는 물체가 신체에 충격을 가하여 발생하는 비관통성 외상

bradypnea (느린 호흡): 비정상적으로 느린 호흡 속도를 말하며 일반적으로 분당 12회 미만의 호흡

brain stem (뇌줄기): 대뇌 반구와 척수를 연결하는 뇌의 줄기 같은 부분

bronchioles (세기관지): 공기가 폐포로 전달되는 기관지의 작은 부분

Brown-Sequard syndrome (브라운세카르증후군): 척수의 반절단을 수반하는 관통성 손상으로 인해 발생하며 척수의 한쪽만 관련된다.

capillary (모세혈관): 가장 작은 유형의 혈관. 이 미세 혈관은 폭이 세포 하나에 불과하여 모세혈관벽을 통해 산소와 영양분의 확산과 삼투를 허용한다.

capnography (호기말이산화탄소분압측정): 가스 샘플에서 이산화탄소의 분압을 측정하고 모니터링하는 방법이다. 동맥과 관련이 있을 수 있다.

capnometry (호기말이산화탄소분압측정): 호흡기 가스의 이산화탄소측정(분석만), 연속적인 기록이나 파형 없이 호흡 가스의 이산화탄소를 측정한다.

cardiac output (심박출량): 심장이 펌프질하는 혈액의 양(L/분)

cardiac tamponade (심장눌림증): 심장을 둘러싸고 있는 심낭에 액체가 축적되어 심장이 압박을 받는 상태이다. 외상의 경우에는 체액은 보통 혈액이며 체액이 축적되면 심장을 압박하여 정상적인 혈액이 심장으로 돌아가는 것을 방해하여 혈액 순환에 장애가 발생한다.

care under fire/threat (CUFT): 적의 사격 또는 위협이 계속되는 상황에서 현장에 도착한 최초 구조자 또는 전투원이 제공하는 처치이다.

casualty collection point (사상자 수집 장소): 다수 사상자가 발생한 사고에서 사상자를 수집, 분류, 처치 및 대피시키는 데 사용되는 장소이다.

cataract (백내장): 수정체가 점차 불투명해져 눈에 들어오는 빛을 차단하고 왜곡하여 시야를 흐리게 하는 눈의 상태이다.

catecholamine (카테콜아민): 중요한 신경전달로 작용하는 신체에서 생성되는 화학물질 그룹이다. 신체에서 생성되는 주요 카테콜아민에는 도파민, 에피네프린(아드레날린), 노르에피네프린이다. 이는 우리 몸의 교감방

어 기전의 일부이다.

caudad (꼬리 쪽으로): 꼬리 쪽으로(꼬리뼈)

cavitation (공동화): 신체 조직을 정상 위치에서 강제로 밀어내어 일시적 또는 영구적인 공동을 발생시키는 행위(예: 신체가 총알에 맞았을 때 조직 입자가 총알에서 멀어지는 가속으로 인해 큰 일시적 공동이 발생하는 손상 부위가 생긴다).

cellular respiration (세포 호흡): 세포가 에너지를 생산하기 위해 산소를 사용하는 것이다.

central chemoreceptor (중추 화학수용체): 이산화탄소 또는 pH의 뇌 분압 변화에 민감하며 혈류에 이산화탄소가 축적되거나 대사성 산증에 의해 유발되는 호흡 자극에 기여하는 세포이다.

central cord syndrome (중심척수증후군): 일반적으로 목뼈 부위의 과신전으로 발생하는 척수 중심부의 손상으로 팔은 약화하거나 마비되지만, 다리는 마비되지 않는 것이 특징이다.

central neurogenic hyperventilation (중심 신경성 과다환기): 머리 손상과 두개내압 증가와 관련된 병리학적으로 빠르고 얕은 환기 패턴이다.

cerebellum (소뇌): 대뇌의 아래쪽과 연수 뒤쪽에 위치하며 운동 조정과 관련된 뇌 일부분이다.

cerebral perfusion pressure (CPP; 뇌관류압): 뇌 혈류를 유지하는 데 필요한 압력으로 평균 동맥압(MAP)에서 두개내압(ICP)의 차이로 계산한다.

cerebrospinal fluid (뇌척수액): 거미막밑공간과 경막집에서 발견되는 액체로 충격 흡수제 역할을 하여 뇌와 척수를 외부 충격으로부터 보호한다.

cerebrum (대뇌): 뇌에서 가장 큰 부분으로 지능, 감각, 운동기능의 조절을 담당한다.

chemosis (결막부종): 눈을 덮고 있는 결막이 부어오르는 증상이다.

Cheyne-Stokes ventilation (체인-스톡스 호흡): 환자의 호흡이 무호흡과 과다호흡 사이에서 진동하는 주기적 호흡(즉, 폐와 화학 수용체가 잘 조정되지 않음)이다.

chilblains (동창): 가렵고 통증이 있으며 특히 기저 순환이 좋지 않은 환자에서 추위에 노출된 후 나타나는 피부의 붉은색 또는 보라색 피부 병변을 말한다.

choke (쵸크): 사격 후 총알이 퍼져 나가는 것을 줄이기 위해 산탄총의 배럴을 수축시키는 장치

cilia (섬모): 기관지에서 이물질과 점액을 밀어내는 털 모양의 진동 세포이다.

circuferential burn (둘레 화상): 팔, 다리 또는 가슴 같은 부위 전체를 포함하는 화상이다.

classic heatstroke (전형적인 열사병): 높은 습도와 고온에 노출되어 발생하는 장애로 체온이 40℃ 이상으로 상승하고 신경학적 이상(정신 상태 변화)이 특징이다.

closed fracture (폐쇄골절): 상부 피부가 손상되지 않는 뼈의 골절을 말한다.

coagulative necrosis (응고성 괴사): 산성에 노출되어 발생하는 조직 손상 유형으로 손상된 조직은 산의 더 깊은 침투를 막는 장벽을 형성한다.

coagulopathy (응고병): 정상적인 혈액 응고 능력의 손상

cold-induced diuresis (한랭 유발 이뇨): 추위에 노출되면 혈관 수축으로 인해 소변 생산량이 증가한다.

cold-induced vasodilation (CIVD; 한랭 유도 혈관 확장): 추위로부터 어느 정도 보호하기 위해 팔다리가 10℃로 냉각된 후 발생하는 생리적 반응

command (지휘부): 모든 사고 감독과 관리를 담당하는 사고지휘체계의 첫 번째 구성요소이다. 사고지휘체계에서 항상 인력이 배치되어야 하는 유일한 직책이다.

command staff (지휘부 직원): 공보 책임자, 안전 책임자, 연락 책임자이며 현장지휘관에 직접 보고한다.

commission (위원회): 의도적인 행위

commotio cordis (심장진탕): 가슴 앞쪽이나 복장뼈에 타격을 받아 발생하는 갑작스러운 심장 부정맥으로 종종 치명적일 수 있다.

compartment syndrome (구획증후군): 혈관 손상으로 발생할 수 있는 허혈 및 순환 장애로 인해 팔다리 구획의 근육에 저산소증을 유발하여 나타나는 임상 소견이다. 세포 부종으로 인해 폐쇄된 근막 또는 뼈 구획의 압력이 증가한다.

competence (능력): 1) 스스로 올바른 결정을 내릴 수 있는 개인의 일반적인 능력, 2) 어떤 일을 성공적으로 수행할 수 있는 능력, 기술, 지식 및 자격을 지칭하는 법적 용어이다.

complete cord transection (척수 완전 절단): 척수의 완전한 손상 및 절단으로 모든 척수가 끊어지고 해당 부위 원위부의 모든 정상적인 신경 기능이 상실된 상태이다.

comprehensive emergency management(포괄적 응급처치): 사고를 관리하는 데 필요한 완화, 준비, 대응, 회복 등 네 가지 구성 요소로 구성된다.

compressibility (압축성): 에너지 전달로 변형될 수 있는 능력

compression (압박): 두 개 이상의 물체 또는 신체 부위 사이에 조직, 장기 또는 기타 신체 일부가 눌리는 충격과 관련된 힘의 유형이다.

compression injur (압박 손상): 심한 압박 및 눌림으로 인해 발생하는 손상으로 신체의 외부 구조 또는 내부 장기에 발생할 수 있다.

conduction (전도): 서로 직접 접촉하는 두 물체 사이에 열이 전달되는 현상

confidentiality (비밀성): 환자와 의료제공자 관계에서 환자에게 공개된 환자 정보를 환자가 승인한 사람, 환자 처치에 관여한 다른 의료 전문가 또는 의무화한 보고를 처리할 책임이 있는 기관 이외의 다른 사람에게 공유하지 않아야 하는 의료서비스 제공자의 의무이다.

conjunctiva (결막): 공막(눈의 흰자위 부분)을 덮고 눈꺼풀을 감싸고 있는 투명한 점막이다.

contact wound (접촉 상처): 탄환이 발사될 때 총구가 환자에게 닿았을 때 발생하는 상처의 유형으로 종종 문에 보이는 화상, 그을음 또는 총구의 자국과 관련된 원형 입구 상처가 생긴다.

convection (대류): 신체와 접촉한 물이나 공기의 가열, 바람 등에 의해 해당 공기 또는 물이 제거된 후 남은 것을 대체하는 새로운 공기 또는 물을 가열하는 것과 같이 기체 또는 액체의 이동 또는 순환에서 열이 전달되는 현상이다.

cord compression (척수압박): 부기, 뼛조각 또는 혈종으로 인해 척수에 압력이 가해져 조직 허혈이 발생할 수 있으며 때에 따라 영구적인 기능 상실을 방지하기 위해 감압이 필요할 수 있다.

cord concussion (척수진탕): 척수 손상 부위 원위부의 척수 기능에 일시적인 장애가 발생한 경우이다.

cord contusion (척수타박상): 척수 조직에 타박상이나 출혈이 발생하여 손상 부위 원위부의 척수 기능이 일시적으로 상실될 수 있다.

cord laceration (척수열상): 척수 조직이 찢어지거나 절단될 때 발생하는 손상이다.

core temperature (중심체온): 1) 중요 장기가 유지되고 가장 잘 기능하는 온도, 2) 인체의 깊은 구조와 기관의 측정된 온도

cornea (각막): 동공과 색이 있는 홍채를 덮고 있는 돔 모양의 투영한 눈 바깥 부분

corneal abrasion (각막 찰과상): 각막에 경미한 상처나 긁힘을 특징으로 하는 일반적인 유형의 눈 손상이다.

coup-contrecoup injury (충격-맞충격 손상): 머리가 고정된 물체에 부딪힐 때 발생하는 뇌손상으로 충격 부위에 손상이 발생하고 반대쪽에 손상이 발생하여 뇌가 두개골의 반대쪽과 충돌하는 손상이 발생할 수 있다.

cranial vault (머리덮개뼈): 두개골 또는 두개골 내의 공간

crepitus (비빔소리): 뼈끝이 서로 부딪혀서 나는 딱딱거리는 소리

critical incident stress management (CISM; 위기 상황 스트레스 관리): 사건 발생 후 스트레스를 예방하고 관리하는 데 사용되는 중재적 전략 그룹이다.

Cushing reflex (쿠싱 반사): 두개 내 고혈압이 특징이다.

cyanosis (청색증): 피부, 점막 도는 손톱 바닥의 푸른색 착색으로 헤모글로빈이 산소화되지 않았고 혈액 내 적절한 산소 수준이 부족함을 나타내며 일반적으로 부적절한 환기 또는 관류 감소로 인해 이차적으로 발생한다.

dead space (사강): 가스 교환에 참여하지 않는 환기된 공기의 양으로 전도성 기도에 남아 있거나 관류가 되지 않거나 관류가 잘 되지 않는 폐포에 도달한다.

debridement (죽은조직제거): 일반적으로 외과적으로 죽은 조직이나 손상된 조직을 제거한다.

decerebrate posturing (대뇌제거자세): 통증 자극이 가해졌을 때 나타나는 특징적인 자세로 팔다리가 신전되고 머리는 뒤로 당겨진다. 일반적으로 두개내압 증가와 관련된 병적 자세의 형태 중 하나이다.

decomposition (분해): 부패 또는 썩은 상태

decompression sickness (감압병): 다이버의 체내 기체에 가해지는 압력 증가의 영향으로 인해 발생하는 질환으로 몸에 있는 기체의 증가한 압력에 의해 발생하는 장애 그룹이다.

decontamination (오염제거): 해로운 화학물질, 생물학적 또는 방사성 물질의 감소 또는 제거

decorticate posturing (피질제거자세): 두개내압이 증가한 환자의 특징적인 병리학적 자세로 통증 자극이 가해지면 환자는 팔을 구부리고 주먹을 쥔 채 등과 다리를 뻗은 채 경직된 자세를 취한다.

deep frostbite (심부 동상): 피부, 근육, 뼈에 영향을 미치는 조직이 얼어붙은 상태

delayed primary closure (지연 일차 봉

합): 부기가 가라앉고 감염 징후가 없는지 확인하기 위해 48~72시간 동안 상처 봉합을 지연하는 것이다.

delayed-sequence intubation (DSI; 지연 연속기관삽관): 삽관 중 CPAP를 통한 사전 산소화 및 무호흡 산소화를 강조하는 약물 보조 삽관 방법이다.

delirium (섬망): 급성 질환으로 인해 이차적으로 발생하는 정신 상태의 갑작스러운 변화이며 일반적으로 근본적인 급성 과정이 교정되면 가역적이다.

dementia (치매): 일상생활에 지장을 초래하는 인지 능력의 저하를 총칭하는 용어이다.

denuded (벗겨진): 덮개 또는 표면층이 제거됨

dependent lividity (시반): 사망한 시신의 가장 아래쪽에 누워 있는 부분에 혈액이 고이거나 고여 있는 상태

dermatome (피부 분절): 신경근이 담당하는 신체의 감각 영역. 총체적으로 척추 수준별로 신체 부위를 매핑하고 척수 손상의 위치를 찾는 데 도움이 된다.

dermis (진피): 피부. 혈관, 신경 말단, 피부 기름샘, 땀샘을 포함하는 결합조직의 골격으로 구성된 표피 바로 아래의 피부층이다.

designated incident facility (지정된 사고 시설): 특정 사고 지휘 체계 기능이 수행되는 지정된 장소이며 예를 들어 현장 지휘는 현장지휘소에서 이루어진다.

devitalized (죽음): 생명이 없거나 죽은 상태

diaphragm (가로막): 가슴과 복부를 나누는 호흡 과정의 일부로 기능하는 돔 모양의 근육

diastole (확장기): 심실 이완

distraction (떼어 당김): 두 구조물을 분리하는 것으로 예를 들면 뼈의 고정된 구성 요소나 척추 일부가 분리되는 것을 말한다.

distributive shock (분포성 쇼크): 수분량의 비례적 증가 없이 혈관 내 물질이 증가할 때 발생하는 쇼크

diverter (전환기): 산탄총의 장치로 발사할 때 펠릿을 더 넓은 수평 경로로 퍼뜨리는 역할을 한다.

dorsal root (뒤 뿌리): 감각 자극을 담당하는 척추 신경 뿌리

DUMBELS (DUMBELS 암기법): 신경작용제 독성의 무스카린 효과와 관련된 증상(설사, 배뇨, 축동, 서맥, 기관지루, 기관지연축, 구토, 눈물, 타액 분비, 발한)을 나타내는 암기법이다.

dura mater (경막): 뇌와 척수를 덮고 있는 바깥쪽의 단단한 막으로 세 개의 수막층 중 가장 바깥쪽에 있다. 말 그대로 강인한 어머니를 의미한다.

dynamic pressure (동압): 방향성이 있는 폭발 바람으로 느껴지는 폭발의 구성 요소

dysarthria (구음장애): 말하기의 어려움

dysbarism (감압증): 주변 환경 압력의 변화로 인해 생리학적으로 발생하는 변화

ecchymosis (반상출혈): 피부 아래 출혈로 인해 발생하는 푸르스름하거나 자주색으로 불규칙하게 형성된 반점 또는 부위

eclampsia (자간증): 고혈압, 말초부종 및 발작을 포함하는 임신부의 증후군으로 임신 중독증이라고도 한다.

edema (부종): 신체 조직에 과도한 양의 체액이 포함된 국소적 또는 전신적 상태이며 일반적으로 조직의 부종을 포함한다.

edentulism (무치아): 치아가 없는 상태

effective ventilation (유효 환기량): 총 분당 환기량에서 사강 환기량을 뺀 값이다.

elasticity (탄성): 늘어나는 능력

endotracheal tube (기관내관): 기도를 개방하기 위해 기관에 삽입하여 환자의 호흡을 돕는 데 사용되는 플라스틱 튜브이다.

environmental temperature (환경 온도): 개인을 둘러싼 공기의 온도

epidermis (표피): 혈관 없이 죽은 상피세포로만 구성된 피부의 가장 바깥층이다.

epidural hematoma (경질외혈종): 두개골과 경막 사이에 모이는 동맥 출혈

epidural space (경막외 공간): 뇌와 두개골을 둘러싸고 있는 경막 사이의 잠재적인 공간으로 뇌 수막 동맥을 포함한다.

epiglottis (후두덮개): 게이트 또는 플랩퍼 밸브 역할을 하며 공기는 기관으로 액체와 고체는 식도로 보내는 나뭇잎 모양의 구조물

epinephrine (에피네프린): 부신에서 분비되는 화학물질로 심장을 자극하여 수축의 강도와 속도를 증가시켜 심박출량을 증가시킨다.

eschar (가피): 죽은 조직의 두꺼운 딱지로 종종 화상으로 인해 발생한다.

escharotomy (가피절개): 심한 화상으로 인해 생긴 질기고 가죽 같은 손상된 피부의 기저 조직이 부풀어 오르면서 팽창할 수 있도록 에스카로 절개하는 수술이다.

esophagus (식도): 입과 위를 연결하는 근육 관이다.

eucapnic state (정상 이산화탄소): 혈중 이산화탄소 수치가 정상 범위 내에 있는 상태

evaporation (증발): 액체에서 기체로의 변화

event phase (사건단계): 실제 외상이 발생한 순간과 관련된 외상 처치 단계

evisceration (내장적출): 장 또는 기타 복부 장기의 일부가 개방성 상처를 통해 복강 외부로 튀어나오는 상태이다.

exercise-associated hyponatremia (EAH; 운동 관련 저나트륨혈증): 장시간 활동 시 과도한 수분 섭취(시간당 1.4L)로 인해 혈중 나트륨 농도가 현저하게 낮아져 생명을 위협하는 질환이다.

exercise-associated hyponatremic encephalopathy (EAHE; 운동 관련 저나트륨성 뇌병증): 장시간 활동 중 과도한 수분 섭취(시간당 1.4L 이상)로 인해 혈중 나트륨 농도가 낮아져 생명을 위협할 수 있는 뇌부종 상태이다.

exertional heatstroke (EHS; 운동성 열사병): 고온 다습한 환경에서 일하거나 운동하는 남성에게 주로 나타나는 체온 상승 상태로 창백하고 땀에 젖은 피부, 체온 상승, 정신 상태 변화 등이 특징이다.

exsanguination (실혈): 혈액량의 총손실로 사망에 이르는 상태

extracellular fluid (세포외액): 세포 내에 포함되지 않은 모든 체액

extramural (extraluminal) pressure (혈관외 압력): 혈관을 둘러싸고 있는 조직의 압력

extreme altitude (극한 고도): 5,500m 이상의 높은 고도

eyelid laceration (눈꺼풀열상): 눈꺼풀에 상처를 입는 것으로 얼굴 외상의 중요한 하위 집합을 구성하며 안와 골절, 누액 배출 시스템 장애, 이물질, 각막 찰과상 또는 안구 개방을 포함한 다른 안구 손상을 동반하는 경우가 많다.

face-to-face intubation (대면 삽관): 환자의 머리 위쪽에서 일반적으로 시행하는 것이 아니라 환자의 얼굴을 마주 보고 구조자가 기관내삽관을 시행하는 술기이다.

fascia (근막): 여러 층을 분리하는 평평한 조직의 띠로 근육을 감싸고 있는 섬유질 조직 띠이다.

field exercise (현장 훈련): 지역사회 재난 대응 계획을 실제 실행 및 수행과 관련된 훈련이다.

finance/administration section (재정/행정 부문): 사고의 모든 비용 및 재정 조치를 담당하는 부서

first-degree frostbit (1도 동상): 찬 공기나 금속에 잠깐 접촉한 피부에 국한된 표피 손상으로 관련된 피부가 흰색 또는 노란 판처럼 보이고 물집이나 조직 손실이 없으며 피부가 빨리 녹고, 감각이 없으며, 주위 부종과 함께 붉게 보이며 7~10일 이내에 치유된다.

first phase of death (사망의 첫 번째 단계): 손상 후 몇 초에서 몇 분 이내에 발생하는 외상성 손상으로 인한 사망

flail chest (동요가슴): 여러 갈비뼈가 두 군데 이상 골절되거나 복장뼈 골절로 인해 불안정한 부분이 생긴 흉부

flail sternum (동요 복장뼈): 흉골 양쪽의 갈비뼈가 골절되어 흉골이 자유롭게 떠다니는 동요 가슴의 변형이다.

fontanelle (숫구멍): 영아의 두개골에서 융합되지 않은 뼈 사이에 있는 부드러운 막질의 공간

foramen magnum (큰 구멍): 수질이 통과하는 두개골 기저부의 구멍을 말한다.

fourth-degree frostbite (4도 동상): 피부, 기저 조직, 근육 및 뼈를 포함하는 동상이다.

fragmentation (조각남): 여러 부분이나 파편을 생성하기 위해 물체가 부서지는 것

frostbite (동상): 동결 또는 영하의 온도에 노출되어 신체 조직이 얼어붙는 현상이다.

full-thickness (third-degree) burn (전층 화상): 표피와 진피가 모두 포함된 화상

galea aponeurotica (머리덮개널힘줄): 두피 아래 두개골을 덮고 있는 거칠고 두꺼운 조직층

gamma ray (감마선): 방사성 물질 붕괴의 결과로 방출되는 고에너지 전자기 방사선의 광선

group training (그룹 훈련): 특별 대응 그룹을 대상으로 하는 재난 대응 훈련

Haddon matrix (해든 매트릭스): 사건에서 숙주, 병인, 환경 요인의 상호 작용을 보여주는 표이다.

heat stress index (열 스트레스 지수): 주위 온도와 상대습도의 조합

heat syncope (열 실신): 더운 환경에 장시간 서 있다가 실신하거나 어지러움, 다리에 정맥이 확장되고 정맥혈이 고임으로 인해 저혈압이 발생하는 경우이다.

hemiparesis (반신불완전마비): 신체 한쪽에 국한된 쇠약감

hemiplegia (반신마비): 신체 한쪽의 마비

hemothorax (혈흉): 가슴막 안에 혈액이 차는 것

high altitude (고지대): 1,500~3,500m 이상의 고도

high-altitude cerebral edema (HACE; 고지대 뇌부종): 고지대(2,400m 이상)로의 여행으로 인해 뇌가 부어 생명을 위협하는 합병증이다.

high-altitude pulmonary edema (HAPE; 고지대 폐부종): 고지대(2,400m 이상)로의 여행으로 인해 폐에 체액이 축적되어 생명을 위협하는 합병증이다.

high explosive (고성능 폭약): 매우 빠르게 폭발하여 에너지를 방출하도록 설계된 폭발물의 일종으로 충격파 또는 과압 현상을 일으켜 일차 폭발 손상을 초래할 수 있다.

homeostasis (항상성): 일정하고 안정적인 내부 환경, 건강을 생명 과정을 유지하는 데 필요한 균형

homeotherm (온혈동물): 온혈 동물

hot zone (오염 지역): 위험 물질이 있는 지역 또는 위험하다고 간주하는 지역을 말한다.

hydrofluoric acid (불산): 산의 일종으로 소량이라도 노출되면 생명을 위협하는 혈중칼슘 수치 저하와 부정맥을 유발할 수 있다.

hypercarbia (고이산화탄소혈증): 체내 이산화탄소 수치가 증가한다.

hyperchloremic acidosis (고염소혈증 산증): 혈중 애 염화 이온의 양 증가와 관련된 대사성 산증(혈중 pH 감소)의 일종으로 다량의 생리식염수 투여로 인해 발생할 수 있다.

hyperextension (과신전): 관절이 극단적으로 또는 비정상적으로 확장된 상태, 최대로 확장된 위치. 목의 과산전은 머리가 중립 위치보다 후방으로 확장될 때 발생하며 척추가 불안정한 환자의 경우 척추의 골절이나 탈구 또는 척수 손상을 초래할 수 있다.

hyperflexion (과굴곡): 관절의 극단적이거나 비정상적인 굴곡. 최대 굴곡의 위치. 목의 굴곡이 증가하면 척추가 불안정한 환자의 경우 척추 골절이나 탈구 또는 척수 손상을 초래할 수 있다.

hyperkalemia (고칼륨혈증): 혈중 칼륨 수치 상승을 나타내는 의학용어이다.

hyper-rotation (과회전): 과도한 회전

hypertension (고혈압): 정상 범우의 상한을 포함하는 혈압으로 일반적으로 환자의 수축기 혈압이 140mmHg 이상인 경우 고혈압이 있는 것으로 간주한다.

hypertonic saline (고장식염수): 체액과 같은 0.9% 염화나트륨인 생리식염수보다 염화나트륨 농도가 높은 물에 담긴 염화나트륨 용액이다.

hyphema (앞방출혈): 투명한 Z-막과 홍채 사이의 눈 앞방에 혈액이 고여 있는 상태이다.

hypobaric hypoxia (저압 저산소증): 점점 더 높은 고도에서 대기압과 산소 분압의 감소로 인해 발생하는 저산소증

hypochlorite solution (차아염소산염): 화학식이 CIO-인 염소와 산소로 구성된 음이온. 용액 가정용 표백제, 공업용 세제제로 쓰이는 용액

hypoperfusion: 관류저하 산소가 공급된 혈액이 세포로 불충분하게 흐르는 것

hypopharynx (후인두): 앞쪽은 후두로 뒤쪽은 식도로 연결된 인두의 아랫부분

hypothalamus (시상하부): 체온 조절 및 호르몬을 조절하는 뇌의 체온 조절 중추

hypothermia (저체온증): 중심체온이 정상 범위보다 낮은 상태(보통 26~32℃)를 말한다.

hypoxemia (저산소혈증): 혈중 산소 농도가 정상 이하인 상태를 발한다.

hypoxia (저산소증): 신체 또는 신체 부위에 조직 수준에서 충분한 산소가 공급되지 않는 상태

ICS general staff (사고지휘체계의 임원): 운영, 계획, 물류, 재정/행정 등 사고지휘체계의 네 가지 주요 부서의 각 책임자

immersion foot (침수발): 차갑고 습한 물에 다리를 장시간 담가서 발생하는 비동결성 저온 노출 손상으로 참호족이라고도 한다.

impact phase (충격 단계): 실제 사고나 재난과 관련된 재난 주기의 단계이다.

incident action plan (IAP;사고 대응 계획): 사고지휘체계(ICS)의 현장지휘관이나 명령체계 담당자가 개발한 전반적인 전략, 전술 및 위험 관리 계획에 대해 지속해 업데이트되는 개요이다.

incident commander (IC; 재난지휘관): 사고 목표 개발, 모든 사고 운영 관리, 우선순위 설정, 특정 대응을 위한 사고 지휘 시스템 조직 정의 등 사고 대응의 모든 측면을 책임지는 개인으로 재난지휘관 직책은 항상 채워져 있다.

incident command post (지휘본부): 사고 지휘 기능이 수행되는 위치

incident command system (ICS; 사고지휘체계): 재난 발생 시 대응하는 다양한 자원의 지휘 체계와 조직을 정의하는 시스템이다.

incomplete cord transection (불완전 척수 절단): 척수의 일부 기관과 운동/감각 기능은 그대로 유지되는 척수의 부분 절단

independent learning (독립 학습): 스스로 공부하는 것

inferior vena cava (아래대정맥): 하반신에서 탈산호화된 혈액을 다시 심장으로 운반하는 주요 정맥

inhalation (흡입): 공기를 폐로 끌어들이는 과정

injury (손상): 특정 형태의 물리적 에너지가

방출되거나 정상적인 에너지 흐름에 장애가 발생하여 발생하는 해로운 사건

injury process (손상 과정): 질병과 유사하게 숙주, 병인(외상의 경우 병인은 에너지), 숙주와 병인이 상호 작용할 수 있는 환경 또는 상황과 관련된 과정이다.

Injury Severity Score (ISS; 손상 중증도 점수): 손상을 해부학적으로 구분되는 6개의 신체 부위로 분류하는 손상분류시스템으로 1) 머리와 목, 2) 얼굴, 3) 가슴, 4) 복부이다.

inner perimeter (내부 경계): 가장 위험하고 잠재적 치사율이 높은 지역을 둘러싼 위험 사고의 지리적 경계

insensible loss (불감성 손실): 내쉬는 공기, 피부, 점막에서 측정할 수 없는 수분 및 열 손실

integrated communications (통합통신시스템): 사고 현장의 모든 대응자가 상사 및 부하 직원과 소통할 수 있는 통신 시스템

intentional injury (의도적 손상): 대인 관계 또는 자기 주도적 폭력 행위와 관련된 손상

intercostal muscles (늑간근): 갈비뼈와 갈비뼈 사이에 있는 근육으로 갈비뼈와 갈비뼈를 서로 연결하고 호흡을 돕는 근육이다.

interdisaster period (재난 간 기간): 재난 또는 다수 사상자 발생 사이에 위험 평가 및 완화 활동이 수행되고 발생 가능성이 있는 사건에 대한 대응 계획이 개발, 테스트 및 실행되는 기간이다.

intermediate-range wound (중거리 상처): 약 1.8~5.5m 거리에서 발생한 관통성 총상을 말한다.

intermittent mandatory ventilation (IMV; 간헐적 강제 환기): 환자에게 정해진 속도와 일회호흡량을 제공하는 기계식 호흡의 한 형태이다.

interstitial fluid (사이질액): 모세혈관벽과 세포벽 사이에 있는 세포외액이다.

intervertebral foramen (추간공): 척추의 아래쪽 측면에 신경이 지나가는 홈.

intracellular fluid (세포내액): 세포 내의 체액

intracranial pressure (ICP; 두개내압): 뇌조직, 혈액 및 뇌척수액이 두개골 내부에 가하는 압력이며 일반적으로 성인의 경우 15mmHg 미만, 소아에서는 3~7mmHg이다.

intramural (intraluminal) pressure (혈관 내 압력): 혈관 내 체액 및 혈액 압력 사이클로 혈관 벽 내부에 가해지는 압력

involuntary guarding (불수의적 보호): 복막염에 반응하는 복벽 근육의 긴장과 연축

ionization (이온화): 전자를 얻거나 잃음으로써 분자가 전하를 띠게 되는 과정

iris (홍채): 동공의 조절 가능한 개구부를 포함하는 눈의 색깔 부분

justice (정의): 공평하거나 공정한 것, 의학에서는 일반적으로 의료서비스와 관련하여 의료 자원이 분배되는 방식을 말한다.

kinetic energy (KE; 운동에너지): 움직임에서 사용할 수 있는 에너지. 물체의 무게와 속도의 함수: 운동에너지=1/2 질량 x 속도의 제곱

kyphosis (척주후만증): 일반적으로 노화 과정과 관련된 척추의 앞쪽으로 굽은 휘어짐. 척추 후만증은 척추의 노화, 구루병 또는 결핵으로 인해 발생할 수 있다.

lactated Ringer's (LR; 젖산 링거 용액): 혈액과 등장성이며 순환량과 전해질을 보충하는 데 사용되는 정맥 내 결정성 용액으로 물, 나트륨, 염화물, 칼슘, 칼륨, 젖산염이 함유되어 있다.

laryngeal mask airway (후두마스크 기도기): 기도 관리 장치로 환자의 입에 삽입되는 원위부 끝이 타원형 마스크 모양으로 성문위 구조를 덮고 기관을 분리하여 공기가 통과할 수 있도록 한다.

laryngeal tube airway (LTA; 후두튜브기도기): 폐의 기계적 인공호흡에 사용되며 후두마스크기도기, 마스크 인공호흡, 기관내삽관과 같은 기도 관리 기술의 대안이다.

larynx (후두): 기관의 바로 위에 있는 구조물로 성대와 성대를 움직이게 하는 근육이 있다.

Lewisite (루이사이트): 화상과 같은 물집을 생성하는 화학 무기로 사용되는 유성 액체로 수포제라고도 한다.

liaison officer (연락관): 여러 기관을 지원하거나 조정하는 지취 참모로 사고 지휘관과 외부 기관 간의 중개자 역할을 한다.

Lichetenberg's figure (리히텐베르그 모양): 낙뢰에 맞았을 때 생기는 통증이 없는 가지 모양 또는 고사리 모양의 붉은 피부 자국이다.

ligament (인대): 뼈와 뼈를 서로 연결하여 관절에 안정성과 강도를 제공하는 섬유질 결합조직

liquefaction necrosis (액화 괴사): 알칼리성 물질이 인체 조직을 손상할 때 발생하는 조직 손상 유형으로 염기가 조직을 액화시켜 화학 물질이 더 깊이 침투할 수 있게 한다.

logistics section (물류 관리): 사고에 대한 모든 서비스, 장비와 시설 제공을 담당하는 부서이다.

logistics section chief (물류 관리 위임장): 사건 지휘관을 위해 물류 기능을 지휘하는

직책이다.

long-range wound (장거리 상처): 5.5m 이상의 거리에서 발생하는 관통상

low explosive (저성능 화약): 고체나 액체에서 기체 상태로 비교적 느리게 변화하는 (폭발보다는 연소 작용이 더 특징적인) 폭발물의 일종으로 에너지를 훨씬 더 느리게 방출하기 때문에 저성능 화약은 폭발 과압을 일으키지 않는다.

lung sliding sign (폐 슬라이딩 징후): 호흡 중에 발생하는 두 개의 가슴막층 사이의 움직임(두 개의 가슴막층이 서로 붙어 있고 호흡과 함께 미끄러짐

maceration (짓무름): 지속적인 수분 노출로 인한 피부 연화, 피부가 하얗게 변하고 부서지며 쉽게 감염될 수 있다.

maculopapular rash (반구진 발진): 작고 융기된 돌기와 함께 붉은색으로 변색한 부위가 특징인 피부 발진이다.

magnesium (마그네슘): 소이탄을 만드는 데 사용되는 인화성이 높은 화학 원소이며 인체 생리학에서 필수적인 전해질이기도 하다.

mammalian diving reflex (포유류 잠수 반사): 차가운 물(21℃ 미만)에 잠길 때 발생하는 반사로 신체의 신진대사가 급격히 느려지고 후두 경련, 말초에서 심장과 뇌로 혈액이 이동하며 심박수 및 호흡수가 현저하게 감소한다.

mass-casualty incident (MCI; 다수 사상자 사고): 비행기 추락, 건물 붕괴, 화재 등 하나의 기전으로 한 장소에서 동시에 다수의 희생자를 발생시키는 사고

mass-casualty incident (MCI) response(다수 사상자 사고 대응): 사고로 인한 피해, 이환율, 사망률을 최소화하기 취하는 사건 후 조치

mean arterial pressure (MAP; 평균 동맥압): 맥박 압력의 1/3을 이완기 압력에 더하여 추정되는 혈관계의 평균 압력이다.

mediastinum (세로칸): 심장, 대혈관, 기관, 주기관지 및 식도를 포함하는 가슴안의 중앙

meninges (수막): 뇌 조직과 척수를 덮고 있는 세 개의 막(경막, 지주막, 연막)

minute ventilation (V̇; 분당환기량): 매분 교환되는 공기의 양으로 일회호흡량에 분당 호흡 횟수를 곱하여 계산한다.

minute volume (분당 호흡량): 매분 교환되는 공기의 양의로 분당 호흡수에 일회호흡량을 곱하여 계산한다.

mitigation (완화): 응급의학에서 재난의 영향을 줄여 인명 및 재산 손실을 줄이는 것을 말한다.

Monro-Kellie doctrine (먼로-켈리 법칙): 뇌 조직, 혈액 및 뇌척수액의 부피의 합은 온전한 두개골 내에서 일정하게 유지되어야 한다.

MTWHF (MTWHF 기억법): 일반적으로 신경 작용제에 노출된 후 나타나는 니코틴 수용체의 자극과 관련된 일련의 증상을 나타내는 기억방법으로 동공확대(mydriasis, 드물게 나타남), 빈맥(tachycardia), 쇠약(weakness), 고혈압(hypertension), 고혈당(hyperglycemia), 근섬유 다발수축(fasciculation)의 약자이다.

mucocutaneous (점막): 피부와 점막으로 구성되거나 피부와 관련된 것이다.

multisystem trauma patient (다발성 외상 환자): 둘 이상의 신체 계통에 손상을 입은 환자

muscarinic site (무스카린): 수용체 민무늬근육과 샘에서 주로 발견되는 아세틸콜린 수용체

myocardial hypertrophy (심근비대): 심장의 근육량과 크기가 증가하는 현상

myoglobin (미오글로빈): 근육에서 발견되는 단백질로 근육에 특징적인 붉은색을 부여하는 역할을 한다.

nasopharyngeal airway (코인두기도기): 콧구멍으로 삽입하여 코인두 뒤에 위치시켜 혀를 들어 올리는 기도기이다. 이 기도기는 일반적으로 구역반사가 있는 환자에게 삽입할 수 있다.

nasopharynx (코인두): 연구개 위에 있는 기도의 윗부분

neural arches (신경활): 척추뼈의 구부러진 두 측면

neutral position (중립 자세): 최대한 움직일 수 있는 관절의 위치로 구부러지거나 펴지지 않은 상태이다.

Newton's first law of motion (뉴턴의 운동 제1 법칙): 물체는 외부의 힘이 작용하지 않는 한 정지한 물체는 정지한 상태를 유지하고 운동 중인 물체는 운동 상태를 유지한다는 물리학의 기본 법칙이다.

Newton's second law of motion (뉴턴의 운동 제2 법칙): 물체에의 가속도는 가해진 힘의 크기에 정비례하며 가해진 힘과 같은 방향이며 물체의 질량에 반비례한다는 물리학의 기본 법칙이다.

Newton's third law of motion (뉴턴의 운동 제3 법칙): 모든 작용에는 크기가 같고 방향이 반대인 반작용이 있다는 물리학의 기본 법칙이다.

nicotinic site (니코틴 수용체): 주로 골격근

에서 발견되는 아세틸콜린 수용체

nitrogen mustard (질소머스터드): 화상 같은 물집을 생성하는 화학 무기로 사용되는 기름 같은 화학 물질로 호흡기, 위장관 및 골수를 손상할 수 있으며 물집 제거제, 수포제, 항암제로 사용된다.

nonfreezing cold injury (NFCI; 비동결 한랭 손상): 습한/추위에 장시간(수 시간에서 수일) 노출되어 말초 조직이 손상되어 발생하는 증후군으로 침수발 또는 참호발이라고도 한다.

nonmaleficence (무해성): 의료제공자가 환자에게 해를 끼치거나 환자를 빠뜨릴 수 있는 조치를 하지 않아야 하는 윤리적 원칙

norepinephrine (노르에피네프린): 교감신경계에서 분비되는 화학물질로 혈관 수축을 유발하여 혈관 용기의 크기를 줄이고 남은 체액의 부피에 더 밀접하게 비례하게 한다.

normal saline (생리식염수): 0.9% 농도의 물과 염화나트륨으로 구성된 정맥 내 결정질 용액이다.

obtunded (둔화): 환자의 정신 능력이 둔해지거나 저하된 상태, 감각 지각이 손상된 경증에서 중등도의 의식 수준 저하를 말한다.

oculomotor nerve (눈돌림신경): 3번 뇌신경으로 동공 수축과 특정 안구 운동을 조절한다.

omentum (그물망): 위장과 다른 복부 장기를 덮고 연결하는 복막의 주름

omission (누락): 행동하지 않음

oncotic pressure (삼투압): 혈관 내의 체액량을 조절하는 압력

open fracture (개방골절): 피부의 손상을 동반한 골절

open globe (개방성 눈): 관통성 눈의 손상으로 각막 또는 공막의 전층을 포함하는 안구 손상

open pneumothorax (개방성 기흉): 가슴에 관통상을 입어 가슴벽에 개방성 상처가 발생하고 외부 환경에서 가슴안으로 공기가 이동하는 우선적인 통로가 생기는 경우

operations section (작전 부서): 사건 발생 시 모든 전술 작전을 담당하는 부서

operations section chief (작전 참모/부서장): 현장 지휘체계에서 모든 작전 활동을 관리하는 책임을 맡은 직위

oropharyngeal airway (입인두기도기): 혀보다 위쪽 입인두에 위치하여 혀를 앞으로 잡아주어 기도를 개방하고 유지하는 데 도움이 되는 기도기로 구역반사가 없는 환자에게만 사용한다.

oropharynx (입인두): 연구개와 후두개 상부 사이에 있는 인두의 중앙 부분이다운데 부분

orotracheal intubation (입기관삽관): 기관 내관을 입을 통해 기관으로 삽입하여 기도 개방을 확보하는 방법이다.

osmosis (삼투): 저장성 영역에서 고장성 영역으로 막을 통과하여 물이 이동하는 현상이다.

osteoarthritis (OA; 골관절염): 관절에 영향을 미치는 퇴행성 질환으로 관절 운동에 매끄러운 표면을 제공하는 관절의 연골이 손상되는 질환이다.

osteophytosis (골증식증): 일반적으로 관절, 특히 척추를 따라 뼈가 자라는 현상으로 골극이라고도 한다.

osteoporosis (골다공증): 뼈조직이 얇아지고 뼈에 작은 구멍이 생기면서 정상적인 골밀도가 감소하는 질환이다. 이 질환은 통증, 잦은 골절, 키 감소 및 다양한 신체 여러 부위의 형성 불량을 일으킬 수 있다. 일반적으로 정상적인 노화 과정의 일부이다.

outer perimeter (외부 경계): 위험한 사건에서 위협이 존재하지 않아야 하는 안전 구역을 정의하는 지리적 경계

overpressure phenomenon (과다압력 현상): 고성능 폭발물에 근접하여 발생하는 개기압 또는 충격파의 갑작스러운 증가

oxygenation (산소공급): 산소를 공급, 처리 또는 농축하는 과정

paradoxical pulse (모순맥박): 일반적으로 긴장기흉이나 심장눌림증으로 인한 가슴안의 압력 상승으로 인해 매 흡기 시 환자의 수축기 혈압이 10~15mmHg 이상 떨어지는 상태이다.

parasympathetic nervous system (부교감신경계): 정상적인 신체 기능을 유지하는 신경계의 한 부분

parietal pleura (벽가슴막): 가슴안의 안쪽을 감싸고 있는 얇은 막이다.

partial-thickness burn (부분층 화상): 표피와 진피층 일부를 포함하는 화상

passive strategy (수동적 전략): 손상 예방에서 개인의 조치가 필요하지 않은 예방 방법 (예: 차량 에어백)

patent (개방): 개방적이고 명확한

patient care report (PCR; 환자 처치 기록지): 환자에게 제공된 병원 전 처치를 기록한 서면 보고서로 병력, 평가, 병원 전 처치, 재평가 및 처치에 대한 환자 반응을 포함한다.

peak overpressure value (최대 과압 값): 고성능 폭발물의 폭발파가 해당 위치에 도달하는 순간 특정 위치에서 경험하는 압력의 최대값이다.

Pediatric Assessment Triangle (PAT; 소아 평가 삼각구도): 첫 번째 접촉 지점에서 사용되는 소아 환자의 신속한 평가 도구로 병원 전 처치 제공자가 환자의 외모, 호흡, 피부 순환을 평가한다.

pelvic ring (골반 고리): 골반을 구성하는 둥근 모양으로 엉덩뼈, 궁둥뼈, 두덩뼈, 엉치뼈, 꼬리뼈로 구성되며 골반띠라고도 한다.

penetrating trauma (관통성 외상): 물체가 피부를 관통하여 기저 구조물에 손상을 입힐 때 발생하는 외상이다. 일반적으로 영구적 및 일시적 공동을 생성한다.

percutaneous (경피): 피부를 통해 발생하는 경우(예: 주삿바늘)

pericardial effusion (심낭삼출): 심장을 둘러싸고 있는 주머니, 즉 심낭 사이에 과도한 체액이 비정상적으로 축적되는 것을 말한다.

pericardiocentesis (심장막천자): 심낭 공간에 바늘을 삽입하여 축적된 혈액이나 체액을 제거하는 시술

peripheral chemoreceptors (말초 화학수용체): 동맥혈 산소의 변화를 감지하고 저산소혈증 동안 항상성을 유지하는 데 중요한 반사를 시작하는 목동맥 및 대동맥소체

peritoneal space (복막강): 앞쪽 복막강으로 장, 비장, 간, 위, 담낭을 포함한 공간이고 복막 공간은 복막으로 덮여있다.

peritonitis (복막염): 복막의 염증

pharynx (인두): 목구멍으로 호흡기와 소화관이 지나가는 관 모양의 구조이다. 입인두-입 뒤쪽 인두 부위, 코인두-코 뒤쪽 콧구멍 넘어 인두 부위

physiologic reserve (생리적 예비): 장기 또는 기관 시스템의 초과 기능 용량

physiologic thermoregulation (생리학적 체온 조절): 체온이 조절되는 과정으로 체온을 제거하거나 보존하는 데 도움이 되는 혈관의 확장 및 수축을 포함한다.

pia mater (연막): 뇌와 척수 및 신경의 근위부에 밀착된 얇은 혈관 막으로 뇌를 덮고 있는 세 개의 수막 중 가장 안쪽에 있는 막이다.

planning section (계획 부서): 사고와 관련된 정보의 수집 및 평가를 탐상하는 ICS 부서

planning section chief (계획 부서 임원): 정보 수집 및 평가를 담당하고 현장지휘관과 함께 계획을 지원하는 ICS 직책이다.

pneumothorax (기흉): 가슴막 안에 공기가 차는 손상이며 일반적으로 폐허탈 증상이 나타난다. 기흉은 가슴벽을 통해 외부로 구멍이 뚫린 개방성 기흉일 수 있고 둔기에 의한 외상이나 자연적인 허탈로 인해 발생한 폐쇄성 기흉일 수도 있다.

polypharmacy (다중약물요법): 5가지 이상의 약물을 복용하는 환자를 설명하는 데 사용되는 용어이다.

positive end-expiratory pressure (PEEP; 호기말양압): 호기말에 대기압보다 높은 폐의 압력으로 호기말에 폐에 더 많은 압력을 가하여 폐에 남아있는 공기의 양을 늘리고 가스 교환을 강화하는 보조 환기 기술을 말한다.

post event phase (사건 후 단계): 외상 사건의 결과와 관련된 외상 처치 단계이다.

posttraumatic endophthalmitis (외상 후 눈속염): 일반적으로 눈에 관통하는 외상으로 인해 안구 내 내용물이 감염되는 질환이다.

posttraumatic stress disorder (PTSD; 외상 후 스트레스 장애): 끔찍하거나 무서운 사건에 노출되어 그 사건에 대한 회상, 악몽, 불안, 통제할 수 없는 사고에 관한 생각으로 이어지는 정신 건강 상태이다.

powered air-purifying respirator (PAPR; 전동식 공기정화 호흡기): 필터 정화통을 통해 주변 공기를 흡입하여 양압으로 얼굴 마스크나 후드에 전달하는 호흡 보조기 장치이다.

preference (선호): 주어진 시간과 병원 전 처치 단계에서 처치 원칙을 달성하는 방식

pre-event phase (사건 발생 전 단계): 손상으로 이어지는 상황과 관련된 외상 처치 단계이다.

preload (전부하): 전신 순환계에서 심장으로 들어오는 혈액의 양과 압력(정맥혈복귀)

preparedness (대비): 사고 발생 전에 필요한 특정 물품, 장비, 인력을 파악하는 포괄적인 응급 관리 단계로 구체적인 실행 계획이 포함된다. 구체적인 실행 계획을 파악하는 종합적인 응급 관리 단계이다.

presbycusis (노년난청): 점진적인 청력 감소를 특징으로 하는 상태

primary contamination (1차 오염): 방출 지점에서 유해 물질에 노출되는 경우

primary hypothermia (1차 저체온증): 건강한 사람이 과도한 급성 또는 만성 추위에 노출될 준비가 되어 있지 않을 때 발생하는 체온의 감소

principle (원리): 환자의 생존과 결과를 최적화하기 위해 의료제공자가 반드시 갖추어야 하거나 달성하고 보장해야 하는 요소로 자율성, 비해악성, 선행, 정의의 네 가지 윤리적 개념을 의미한다.

principlism (원칙주의): 자율성, 비해악성,

선행, 정의의 네 가지 윤리적 개념을 사용하여 특정 환자를 처치할 때 얻을 수 있는 득과 실을 비교하고 균형을 맞춰 환자에게 가장 이익이 되는 일을 할 수 있는 틀을 제공한다.

privacy (프라이버시): 환자가 개인 건강 정보에 접근할 수 있는 사람을 통제할 수 있는 권리

prodrome/predisaster (전조/재난 전 단계): 재난 지역에서 특정 이벤트가 필연적으로 발생할 것으로 확인되고 후속 이벤트의 영향을 완화하기 위해 특정 조치를 할 수 있는 단계이다.

profile (프로필): 관통하는 물체의 초기 크기와 충격 시 발생하는 크기 변화 정도

public information officer (PIO; 공공 정보 책임자): 대중과 미디어와 소통하고 정보를 배포하는 ICS 지휘 참모 책임자

pulmonary contusion (폐 타박상): 폐의 타박상, 무딘 손상에 의한 이차적일 수 있음

pulseless electrical activity (무맥성 전기 활동): 맥박이 촉지되지 않으며 심장 모니터링에서 조직화한 전기 활동을 특징으로 하는 상태

pulse oximeter (맥박산소포화도측정기): 동맥 산소 헤모글로빈 포화도를 측정하는 장치이다. 이 값은 조직을 통과한 적색광과 적외선의 흡수 비율을 측정하여 결정된다.

pulse pressure (맥압): 1) 심장이 수축할 때마다 새로운 혈액이 좌심실을 떠날 때마다 발생하는 압력의 증가, 2) 수축기 혈압과 이완기 혈압의 차이(수축기 혈압에서 이완기 혈압을 뺀 값은 맥압과 같음)

radiation (복사): 적외선에 의해 따뜻한 물체에서 차가운 물체로 에너지가 직접 전달되는 것을 말한다.

radiation dispersion device (RDD; 방사선 분산 장치): 이 장치는 핵폭발 없이 방사성 물질을 분산시키기 위해 재래식 폭발을 사용한다.

Rapid and Remote Assessment Methodology (RAM; 신속 및 원적 평가 방법): 전술적 EMS 제공자의 위험을 최소화하면서 구조 가능한 사상자를 구출하고 처치할 기회를 극대화하기 위해 활용되는 평가 알고리즘이다.

rapid-sequence intubation (RSI; 급속연속기관삽관): 진정제와 속효성 마비제를 사용하여 환자의 의식을 잃고 반응이 없는 상태로 만들어 흡인 위험 기간을 최소화하는 약물 보조 삽관 방법이다.

rebound tenderness (반동압통): 복부를 깊숙이 눌렀다가 빠르게 압력을 풀면 발생하는 신체검사 소견으로 복압이 갑자기 풀리면 더 심한 통증을 유발한다.

recovery or reconstruction phase (복구 또는 재건 단계): 의료, 공중보건, 지역사회 인프라(물리적, 정치적)의 조율된 노력을 통해 재난의 영향을 견디고, 극복하고, 재건하기 위한 지역 사회의 자원을 다루는 재난 주기 동안의 기간으로 지역사회가 완전히 회복되기까지 가장 길고 수개월에서 수년간 지속되는 기간이다.

remote assessment (원격 평가): 전술 운영자와 제공자가 적대 세력에게 자신의 위치나 의도를 드러내지 않고 정보를 수집하는 과정으로 쌍안경을 이용한 원격 관찰, 원격 음향 감시, 열화상 촬영 등이 포함된다.

rescue, emergency or relief phase (구조, 응급 또는 구호 단계): 재난 발생 직후의 재난 주기 중 대응이 이루어지고 적절한 처치로 생명을 구할 수 있는 기간이다.

resouce managememt (자원 관리): 대규모 사고 발생 시 지자체, 중앙정부가 하나의 지휘체계 아래에 협력할 수 있도록 하는 계약 및 절차

respiration (호흡): 외부 공기와 인체 세포 간에 산소와 이산화탄소를 교환하는 데 관여하는 전체 환기 및 순환 과정. 의학에서는 호흡과 환기의 단계를 의미하는 것으로 제한되기도 한다.

reticular activating system (그물체활성계): 의식과 각성 수준을 유지하는 중추신경계 제어 센터의 일부

retroperitoneal space (복막 뒤 공간): 신장, 요관, 방광, 생식 기관, 아래대정맥, 복부 대동맥, 췌장, 십이지장, 결장과 직장 일부가 있는 복막 뒤 공간이다.

rhabdomyolysis (횡문근융해): 세포 내 근육 성분이 순환계로 방출되면서 근육 조직이 분해되는 질환이다. 근육 조직이 파괴되어 근육의 세포 성분이 유리되는 손상

rheumatoid arthritis (RA; 류마티스관절염): 자가 면역 반응으로 인한 염증성 질환으로 관절이 붓고 기형이 생길 수 있다.

rifling (강선): 총신 안쪽의 홈으로 하나의 탄환을 목표물을 향해 안정되게 날아가면서 회전시키는 역할을 한다.

rigor mortis (사후경축): 사망 후 발생하는 근육과 관절의 일시적인 경직 및 강직으로 사망 후 2~4시간 이내에서 시작하여 약 36~48시간 지속된다.

riot control agent (폭동 진압제): 피부, 점막, 폐, 눈 등에 자극을 유발하여 노출된 사람을 빠르고 짧게 무력화시키는 데 사용되는 화학물질이다.

sacrum (엉치뼈): 허리뼈 아래 척추의 일부로 움직이지 않는 관절로 연결되어 엉치뼈를 형성하는 5개의 엉치뼈를 포함한다. 엉치뼈는 척추의 체중을 지탱하는 기저부이며 다리 이음뼈 일부이기도 하다.

safety officer (안전 책임자): 응급 요원의 안전을 모니터링, 평가 및 보장할 책임이 있는 ISC 지휘 참모 책임자

SAMPLE history (SAMPLE 병력): 병력의 구성 요소를 기억하기 위한 암기법으로 증상(symptoms), 알레르기(allergies), 복용 중인 약물(medication), 과거력과 및 수술력(past medical and surgical history), 마지막 식사(last meal), 손상을 초래한 사건(events leading up to the injury) 등을 나타낸다.

secondary contamination (이차 오염): 피해자, 구조자 또는 장비 때문에 유해 물질이 발생 지점에서 이동한 후 유해 물질에 노출되는 경우

secondary hypothermia (이차성 저체온증): 갑상샘저하증, 부신저하증, 외상, 종양, 패혈증 등 환자의 전신 장래로 인한 체온저하

second-degree frostbite (2도 동상): 표피와 진피를 포함하는 추위 노출로 인한 동상, 처음에는 1도 손상과 비슷하게 보이지만, 동결된 조직이 더 깊고 해동 후 홍반과 부종으로 둘러싸인 표피성 피부 물집이 생기고 조직의 영구적인 손실은 없으며 3~4주 이내에 치유된다.

second phase of death (두 번째 사망 단계): 손상 후 몇 분에서 몇 시간 이내에 발생하는 외상성 손상으로 인한 사망

self-aid/buddy aid (SA/BA; 자가 응급처치/동료 응급처치): 자신을 구하거나 동료의 생명을 구하기 위해 사용하는 응급처치 절자. 예를 들어, 생명을 위협하는 손상에 지혈대를 스스로 적용하는 것이다.

self-contained breathing apparatus (SCBA; 자가 호흡 장치): 산소가 부족하거나 유독성 흡입 위험이 있는 환경에서 사용하는 마스크와 휴대용 공기 공급 장치로 구성된 개인보호장비이다.

self-contained underwater breathing apparatus (SCUBA; 수중 자가 호흡 장치): 압축 공기 탱크에 연결된 튜브가 있는 마스크로 구성된 수중 휴대용 자가 호흡 장치이다.

senescence (노화): 노화의 과정

sepsis (패혈증): 전신으로 퍼진 감염

sequelae (후유증): 질병이나 손상의 후유증 또는 합병증

shear (전단): 신체 부위가 절단되거나 찢어지는 속도 변화의 힘

shear force (전단력): 인접한 부분이 다른 방향으로 움직이거나 제자리에 고정되는 동안 장기나 신체 일부를 한 방향으로 움직이게 하는 경향을 가진 신체에 가해지는 에너지

shock wave (비틀림파): 전단력을 참조한다.

shock front (충격파의 전면): 고성능 폭발로 생성되는 폭발 과압파와 정상 대기압 사이의 경계

shock wave (충격파): 충격파의 전면을 참조한다.

shock index (SI; 쇼트 지수): 심박수와 수축기 혈압 사이의 비율이다.

short bone: 짧은 뼈 손허리뼈, 발허리뼈, 손가락뼈

simple pneumothorax: 단순 공기가슴증 가슴막 안에 공기가 존재하는 것

simulation (시뮬레이션): 사고 또는 환자 처치를 구두 또는 모형을 통해 모방, 재정 또는 표현하는 훈련의 한 형태이다.

single command (단일 명령): 한 개인이 사고 발생 시 모든 전략적 목표를 책임지는 명령 구조이다. 일반적으로 사고가 단일 관할권 내에 있고 단일 분야에 의해 관리될 때 사용한다.

single-system trauma patient (단일 계통 외상 환자): 하나의 신체 계통에만 손상을 입은 외상을 경험한 환자를 말한다.

sniffing position (냄새 맡는 자세): 기관내 삽관 시 시야와 환기를 최적화하기 위해 머리와 목의 약간 앞쪽에 위치.

solar keratitis (일광 각막염): 자외선에 노출되어 눈의 각막에 화상을 입는 것으로 눈에 반사되어 발생하며 설맹이라고도 한다.

solid density (고체 밀도): 뼈와 일치하는 조직 밀도

span of control (통제 범위): 현장 지휘체계에서 대응 조직 내 모든 수준에서 한 명의 상급자에게 보고하는 부하 직원의 수. 대부분은 한 사람이 3~7명의 사람 또는 자원만 효과적으로 감독할 수 있다.

spinal shock (척수 쇼크): 감각 및 운동 기능의 일시적 상실을 초래하는 척수 손상

spinal stenosis (척추관협착증): 척주관이 좁아진 상태

spinous process (가시돌기): 척추의 뒤쪽에 있는 꼬리 모양의 구조물

sprain (염좌): 관절에 스트레스를 가하는 손상으로 인해 관절을 지지하는 인대가 과도하게 늘어나거나 파열되어 발생하는 관절 내

인대의 급성 연부조직 손상이다.

spray (스프레이): 산탄총에서 발사된 총알의 분산 패턴

spread (확산): 스프레이를 참조한다.

staging area (집결 지역): 자원, 장비 및 인력을 안전하게 배치하고 배치 준비를 마칠 수 있는 미리 정해진 구역

START triage algorithm (START 분류 알고리즘): 다중사상자 발생 시 환자를 평가하고 처치 및 이송 우선순위를 지정하는 방법으로 환자의 호흡 상태, 순환 상태, 정신 상태를 평가하는 것이 포함된다.

status epilepticus (뇌전증 지속상태): 발작이 5분 이상 지속되거나 그사이에 깨어나는 시간 없이 2회 이상의 발작이 발생하는 생명을 위협하는 상태

steady-state metabolism: 안정 시 대사 안정된 상태의 세포, 장기 및 신체 기능의 상태

stellate wound (별 모양 상처): 별 모양 상처

stipple (반점): 총상으로 인한 화약으로 생긴 여러 개의 작은 점

stopping distance (정지거리): 움직이는 물체가 정지하는 거리로 에너지가 얼마나 빨리 소멸하거나 전달되는지를 나태는 척도이다.

stress wave (응력파): 1) 작고 빠른 비틀림으로 높은 국부적 힘을 생성하고, 2) 미세혈관 손상을 일으키며, 3) 조직 표면에서 강화 및 반사되어 특히 폐, 귀, 장과 같이 가스로 채워진 기관에서 손상 가능성을 높이는 초음속 종방향 압력파이다.

stroke volume (일회박출량): 왼심실이 수축 시마다 나오는 혈액의 양이다.

subarachnoid hemorrhage (SAH; 거미막밑 혈종): 거미막 아래 뇌척수액으로 채워진 공간에 혈액이 모여 있는 것을 말한다.

subconjunctival hemorrhage (결막밑 출혈): 눈을 덮고 있는 투명한 결막과 흰 공막 사이에서 발견되는 출혈

subcutaneous emphysema (피부밑기종): 신체의 연부조직에 공기가 축적된 상태

subdermal burn (피하 화상): 피부의 모든 층과 기저 지방, 근육, 뼈 또는 내부 장기를 포함하는 화상이다.

subdural hematoma (경막밑 혈종): 경막과 거미막 사이에 혈액이 고이는 것을 말한다.

sublimation (승화): 고체가 액체 상태를 우회하여 증기를 방출하는 과정

subluxation (불완전 탈구): 부분적 또는 불완전한 탈구

submersion: 익수 몸의 전체가 완전히 물속으로 빠진 상황

sulfur mustard (황화 머스타드): 폭탄 폭발이나 분무기로 에러로졸화할 수 있는 기름지고 투명하거나 황갈색 액체, 대량살상무기로 사용되는 소포제 또는 발포제이다.

superficial burn (표재성 화상): 표피에만 화상을 입은 경우로 붉고 염증이 생기며 통증이 있는 피부

superficial frostbite (표재성 동상): 추위에 노출되어 피부와 피하 조직에 영향을 미치는 동결 손상으로 다시 따뜻하게 하면 투명한 물집이 생긴다.

superior vena cana (위대정맥): 신체 상부에서 탈산소화된 혈액을 심장으로 다시 운반하는 주요 정맥이다.

supplied air respirator (SAR; 공기공급 호흡 장치): 마스크와 구조자가 휴대하지 않는 공기 공급원으로 구성된 개인보호장비로 산소가 부족하거나 독성 흡입 위험이 있는 환경에서 사용된다.

supraglottic airway (SGA; 성문위기도기): 입과 인두로 맹목적으로 삽입하는 기도 장치로 기관과 식도를 분리하도록 설계되어 있으며 어떤 장치고 기관을 완전히 밀봉하지 못하므로 흡인 위험을 낮추지만, 완전히 예방할 수는 없다.

surgical cricothyrotomy (외과적 반지갑상연골절개): 목의 반지갑상막을 절개하여 기도를 기관으로 열어 환자의 기도를 개방하는 시술이다.

surveillance (감시): 일반적으로 전염병에 대해 지역 사회 내에서 자료를 수집하는 과정이다.

suspension syndrome (현수 증후군): 장기간 몸을 움직이지 않고 똑바로 서 있는 동안 의지하는 다리에 혈액이 고여 쇼크 상태에 빠지게 되는 일련의 사건

sympathetic nervous system (교감신경계): 투쟁 또는 도피 반응을 일으키는 신경계의 교감신경계 분열

systemic vascular resistance (전신 혈관 저항): 혈관을 통한 혈액의 흐름에 대한 저항의 양이다. 혈관이 수축함에 따라 증가한다. 내강 지름이나 혈관 탄성의 변화는 저항의 양에 영향을 미칠 수 있다.

systolic (수축기): 혈액이 다시 채워진 후 심장 근육의 일부 방이 수축하는 동안 율동적으로 반복되는 심장 수축이다.

tachypnea (빠른호흡): 증가한 호흡수

tactical casualty care (TCC; 전술적 사상자 처치): 위험하거나 전술적인 상황에서의 제공되는 응급의료 서비스이다.

tactical emergency medical support

(TEMS; 전술 응급의료 지원): 특수 작전 법률 집행 임무의 성공 가능성을 높이고 임무의 의료 책임과 위험을 줄이며 공공 안전을 증진하기 위한 병원 외 처치 시스템이다.

tactical evacuation care (전술적 대피 처치): 기존의 EMS 상황과 유사하게 위협이나 위험이 완전히 해결된 후 의료 서비스를 제공하는 전술적 사상자 처치의 치료 단계로 대피 처치라고도 한다.

tactical field care (전술적 현장 처치): 위협이나 위험이 억제되었지만, 재개될 수 있을 때 의료 서비스를 제공하는 전술적 사상자 처치의 치료 단계로 간접 위협 처치라고도 한다.

tamponade (눌림증): 상처나 혈관의 폐쇄 또는 막힘, 심낭에 혈액 또는 체액이 축적되어 심장이 압박되는 상태이다.

tendon (힘줄): 근육과 뼈를 연결하는 질기고 비탄력적이며 섬유질 조직으로 이루어진 띠이다.

tension pneumothorax (긴장기흉): 가슴막 공간의 기압이 외부 대기압을 초과하여 빠져나가지 못하고 영향을 받는 쪽이 과팽창되어 관련 쪽의 폐를 압박하고 세로칸을 반대쪽으로 이동시켜 다른 쪽 폐를 부분적으로 허탈된 상태로 대개 진행성이며 생명을 위협하는 상태이다.

tentorium cerebelli (소뇌천막): 소뇌를 덮고 있는 경막을 덮고 있는 경막의 주름이다. 천막은 뇌 바로 아래 두개골 상부 바닥의 일부이다.

thermal equilibrium (열평형): 따뜻한 물체에서 차가운 물체로 열을 전달하여 두 물체 사이의 온도를 같게 만드는 현상

thermal gradient (열 경사도): 두 물체 사이의 온도 차이를 말한다.

thermite (테르밋): 1,982℃에서 맹렬하게 연소하고 녹은 철을 흩뿌리는 분말 알루미늄과 산화철로 구성된 소이화 화합물이다.

thermoregulatory center (체온조절 중추): 체온을 조절하는 뇌의 영역이다.

third-degree frostbite (3도 동상): 표피와 진피층을 포함하는 추위 노출로 인한 동상, 피부가 얼어붙어 움직임이 제한되그, 조직이 해동된 후 피부가 부풀어 오르고 피가 찬 물집(출혈성 수포)이 발생하여 심부 조직에 혈관 외상이 있음을 나타내며 피부 손실이 천천히 일어나 미라화되고 벗겨지며 치유가 느리다.

tidal volume (Vt; 일회호흡량): 환기할 때마다 정상적으로 교환되는 공기량이다. 건강한 성인이 휴식 중일 때 숨을 쉴 때마다 폐와 대기 사이에서 약 500mL의 공기가 교환된다.

total lung capacity (TLC; 총 폐용량): 강제 흡입 후 폐에 들어온 공기의 총량

toxidrome (중독증후군): 특정 종류의 화학물질 또는 독소에 노출되었음을 시사하는 임상 징후 및 증상의 모음

tracheal shift (기관편위): 가슴안 내 불균등한 가슴안 내 압력으로 인해 기관의 위치가 정순선의 정상 위치에서 한쪽으로 멀어지는 변화를 나타내는 임상 징후이다.

transesophageal echocardiography (경식도 심초음파): 식도에 삽입한 초음파 탐색자를 사용하여 심장 초음파를 수행하는 기술이다.

transmission-based PPE (전파 기본 개인보호장비): 표준 예방조치 외에 질병 전염을 방지하기 위해 사용하는 개인보호장비로 에어로졸, 접촉 및 비말 예방 조치가 포함된다.

transmural preesure (전층 압력): 혈관 벽을 가로지르는 압력 차는 림프 내 및 림프 외 힘의 영향을 받는다.

transverse process (가로돌기): 척추의 양쪽 측면 가장자리 부근에 있는 돌기

trauma chin lift (외상 턱 들기): 자발 호흡을 하는 환자의 다양한 해부학적 기도 폐쇄를 완화하는 데 사용되는 술기로 턱과 아래 앞니를 잡은 다음 들어 올려 아래턱뼈를 앞으로 당겨서 수행한다.

trauma jaw thrust (외상 턱 밀어올리기): 머리와 목뼈의 움직임이 거의 또는 전혀 없이 기도를 개방할 수 있는 술기로 엄지손가락을 양쪽 광대활에 대고 양쪽 두 번째, 세 번째 손가락을 아래턱뼈에 같은 각도로 위치시켜 아래턱뼈를 앞으로 밀면서 올리는 술기이다.

traumatic asphyxia (외상 질식): 혈관 내 압력이 현저하게 증가하여 모세혈관이 파열되는 가슴과 복부에 무딘 손상이나 으깸손상을 입어 발생한다. 상반신과 얼굴의 피부가 자줏빛으로 변색하고 피부의 점상출혈이 특징이다.

trench foot (참호발): 차갑고 축축한 곳에 발이 장시간 침수되어 발생하는 동결되지 않은 한랭 노출 손상이다. 침수발이라고도 한다.

triage (분류): '분류한다.'라는 뜻의 프랑스어 단어로 환자 처치의 우선순위에 따라 그룹별로 분류하는 과정이다. 여러 명의 환자만 관련되면 분류에는 각 환자를 평가하고 우선순위가 가장 높은 모든 환자의 요구 사항을 먼저 충족한 다음 우선순위가 낮은 항목으로 이동하는 것이 포함된다. 다수의 환자가 관

련된 다수 사상자 사고의 경우 긴급성과 생존 가능성을 모두 판단하여 분류를 수행한다.

triage officer (분류 책임자): 손상에 따른 분류와 치료와 이송의 우선순위를 결정하는 과정을 관리, 감독하도록 훈련받은 개인

tumble (텀블): 끝에서 끝까지 움직이는 동작이다. 탄환은 일반적으로 총알의 앞쪽 가장자리에서 저항에 부딪히면 텀블한다.

unified command (통합 지휘 사건): 대응하는 모든 다양한 기관의 사고 지휘관이 함께 협력하여 사건을 관리하는 ICS 지휘 구조이다.

unintentional injury (비의도적 손상): 계획되지 않았고 해를 입히려는 의도와 관련이 없는 손상이다.

units(단위): 단일하고 완전한 것으로 간주하지만, 전체 또는 그룹 일부이기도 한 개별 사물 또는 사람

unity of command (단일 지휘): 각 대응자에게 한 명의 직속상관만 있는 사고 지휘 시스템 관리 개념이다.

vapor (증기): 기체 상태의 고체 또는 액체로 미세한 구름이나 안개로 보인다.

vertebral foramen (척추뼈 구멍): 혈관과 신경이 통과하는 척추뼈의 뼈 구조에 있는 구멍 또는 개구부

very high altitude (매우 높은 고도): 3,500m~5,500m 사이의 고도

vesicant (수포제): 대량살상무기로 사용되는 황화 머스타드 및 루이사이트와 같은 화학 작용제로 시각적으로 화상과 유사한 손상을 입히기 때문에 수포 작용제라고도 한다.

vestibular folds (안뜰주름): 성대를 통해 공기의 흐름을 유도하는 가짜 성대

vestibular nuclei (안뜰핵): 균형 감각을 담당하는 전정신경이 발생하는 뇌 영역이다.

viral hemorrhagic fever (VHF; 바이러스성 출혈열): 여러 가지 바이러스로 인해 발생하는 임상 증후군으로 발열, 불쾌감, 출혈성 증상이 임상적으로 나타나는 것이 특징이다.

viscera (내장): 신체의 내부 장기

visceral pleura (내장가슴막): 각 폐의 외부 표면을 덮고 있는 얇은 막

volatility (휘발성): 고체나 액체가 실온에서 기체 형태로 기화할 가능성

voluntary guarding (수의적 보호): 의사가 복부의 압통 부위를 촉진할 때 환자가 복근을 긴장시키는 평가 소견

warning phase (경고 단계): 재난 또는 응급 상황의 혼돈과 혼란이 발생하기 전에 사람들에게 전달되는 마지막 지침, 통지 및 알림

water density (수분 밀도): 물과 유사한 조직 밀도를 가진 장기(예: 간, 비장, 근육)

weapon of mass destruction (대량살상무기): 심각한 피해와 다수의 사상자를 발생시키도록 고안된 화학적, 생물학적, 방사능, 폭발성 제제이다.

white blood cell (WBC; 백혈구): 침입한 미생물에 대응하는 순환계의 거의 무색에 가까운 혈액 세포

white phosphorus (백린): 군수품 생산에 사용되는 소이탄

work of breathing (호흡 작업): 숨을 쉬기 위해 가슴벽과 횡격막을 움직일 때 수행되는 신체적 작업 또는 노력

years of potential life lost (YPLL; 잠재적 수명 손실 연수): 검사 대상 그룹의 고정 연령(일반적으로 65세 또는 70세) 또는 그룹의 기대 수명에서 사망 연령을 빼서 계산한 손상의 영향 추정치이다.

zone of coagulation (응고구역): 전층 화상 시 조직 파괴가 가장 심한 영역으로 이 영역의 조직은 괴사하여 조직 복구가 불가능하다.

zone of hyperemia (충혈구역): 전층 화상의 가장 바깥쪽 영역으로 세포 손상이 적고 화상 손상으로 인한 염증 반응으로 인해 이차적으로 혈류가 증가하는 것이 특징이다.

zone of stasis (정체구역): 응고구역 옆의 영역으로 이 영역으로의 혈류가 정체되어 있으며 이 영역의 세포가 손상되었지만, 돌이킬 수 없을 정도로 손상되지는 않았다. 이후 산소나 혈류가 공급되지 않으면 생존할 수 있는 세포가 죽어 괴사하게 된다. 시기적절하고 적절한 화상 처치는 이러한 손상된 세포에 혈류와 산소 공급을 보존한다.

찾아보기

ㄱ

가락뼈사이관절 _ 695
가로막 _ 215
가로막신경 _ 208
가로막 파열 _ 366, 367
가슴관 _ 357
가슴관삽입 _ 357
가슴막 감압 _ 356
가슴막안 _ 353
가슴안 _ 61
가슴우리 _ 233
가시성 _ 150
가피 _ 426
가피절개 _ 429
각막 찰과상 _ 286
각 충돌 _ 120
간편 손상척도 _ 191
간헐필수 환기 _ 237
갈고리이랑탈출 _ 273, 274
갈비뼈 _ 344
갈비뼈 골절 _ 188, 350
갈비사이공간 _ 215, 356
갈비사이근 _ 303, 344
갈비척추관절 _ 300
감각기능 _ 400
감압병 _ 652
감압증 _ 648
갑상연골 _ 288
개방골절 _ 404
개방 기흉 _ 236, 353
개인보호장비 _ 155
개인부양장치 _ 640
거리 EMS _ 675
거미막밑출혈 _ 271
거미막밑혈종 _ 266
견인부목 _ 40, 406
결막밑출혈 _ 286
결정질 용액 _ 39
경구 수액제 _ 442
경막밑혈종 _ 270
경막외혈종 _ 269
경막정맥동 _ 285
경막하혈종 _ 266

경성 부목 _ 406
경증 _ 166
고리뼈 _ 299
고막 파열 _ 650
고산소증 _ 276
고성능 폭약 _ 554
고소병 _ 659
고에너지 무기 _ 132
고에너지 손상 _ 684
고이산화탄소혈증 _ 278
고지성 뇌부종 _ 659, 661, 666
고지성 폐부종 _ 659, 662
고형장기 _ 136, 378
골관절염 _ 485
골내 _ 77, 182
골반 고리 골절 _ 403
골반 고정대 _ 75, 385
골반 골절 _ 320, 379, 402
골증식증 _ 485
공간형성 _ 107
공공 정보 책임자 _ 532
공기색전증 _ 348
공기 정화기 _ 577
공기호흡기 _ 550
공막 열상 _ 286
과거 병력 및 수술 이력 _ 186
과공명음 _ 355
과불화탄소 _ 80
과산소화 _ 217
과소 분류 _ 190
과잉 분류 _ 190
관류압 _ 228
관통상 _ 66, 347
교감신경계 _ 55, 56
교류 _ 436
교전 중 처치 _ 712
교전 지역 _ 717
구강 건조증 _ 482
구역반사 _ 220, 456
구획증후군 _ 402, 408, 436
국가 사고관리체계 _ 528
그레이–터너 징후 _ 382
근거리 상처 _ 138
근골격 외상 _ 38

근육마비제 _ 226
글래스고혼수척도 _ 75, 459
급성 고산병 _ 660
급성세관괴사 _ 84
급성 호흡곤란 증후군 _ 85, 564, 653
급속연속기관삽관 _ 226, 280
급속연속마취유도 _ 685
기관기관지 파열 _ 363
기관내관 _ 226, 356
기관내삽관 _ 222, 352, 428, 456
기관편위 _ 62, 355
기능잔기용량 _ 206
기도 _ 63
기밀 유지 _ 32
기본소생술 _ 195
기술자 _ 154
기초대사율 _ 587
긴장기흉 _ 62, 356
긴장혈흉 _ 357

ㄴ

낙뢰 손상 _ 633
낙상 _ 486
내과적 심정지 _ 194
내부고정 _ 680
내부출혈 _ 62, 401
내장탈출 _ 387
내층 _ 113
냄새 맡는 자세 _ 456
넓적다리뼈 골절 _ 404
노인 학대 _ 487
노화 과정 _ 480
농축 적혈구 _ 58
뇌 관류압 _ 267
뇌내출혈 _ 272
뇌부종 _ 275
뇌정맥 배액 _ 268, 290
뇌줄기 _ 266
뇌진탕 _ 269
뇌척수액 _ 55, 266
뇌타박상 _ 272
뇌탈출 징후 _ 467
뇌 혈류량 _ 268
눈꺼풀 열상 _ 286

눈돌림신경 _ 274
뉴턴의 운동 제1 법칙 _ 104
느린 호흡 _ 176
능동적 재가온 _ 623

ㄷ

다기관 외상 _ 408
다발성 장기 기능장애 증후군 _ 85
다수 사상자 _ 165
다수 사상자 사고 _ 527
다중약물 요법 _ 694
단순 기흉 _ 224, 352
대기 _ 166
대뇌제거자세 _ 180, 274
대동맥 내 풍선폐쇄술 _ 385
대동맥 파열 _ 128, 362
대동맥 협착 _ 362
대동맥활 _ 127, 362
대량살상무기 _ 155, 524
대량 출혈 _ 63
대류 _ 588
대면 삽관 _ 226
덩이 효과 _ 275
도뇨관 _ 198
도수 조작 _ 35
동결건조 혈장 _ 78
동공부등 _ 189
동맥기체색전증 _ 555, 652, 654
동맥이산화탄소분압 _ 345
동맥 출혈 _ 177
동맥 포화도 _ 233
동맥혈가스 _ 281
동맥혈산소분압 _ 236
동맥혈이산화탄소분압 _ 64, 74, 234
동상 _ 605
동요가슴 _ 351
동의 _ 32
동적 위험 평가 _ 642
동창 _ 606
두개골 골절 _ 285
두개골 바닥 골절 _ 285
두개내 덩이 효과 _ 272
두개내압 _ 267
두개내압 증가 _ 237, 467
두개내출혈 _ 269, 273
두덩결합 _ 188
두창 _ 569
두피 _ 284, 285
두피 타박상 _ 125

둘레 화상 _ 428, 429
뒤당김 _ 215
뒤뿌리 _ 303
뒤뿌리신경절 _ 299
뒤척수동맥 _ 302
들숨 _ 209
등세모근 _ 303
떨림 _ 587
떼어당김 _ 305

ㄹ

룬드-브로더 _ 431
류마티스관절염 _ 485
리히텐베르크 도형 _ 636

ㅁ

마그네슘 _ 558
만성폐쇄폐질환 _ 231, 345, 482
맘대로근육 _ 397
망상 진피 _ 423
맥박산소측정기 _ 64, 181
맹목적 코기관삽관 _ 225, 280
머리/저체온증 _ 63
먼로-켈리 법칙 _ 273
메트헤모글로빈 _ 439
모세혈관 재충전 시간 _ 66
모세혈관 출혈 _ 177
모순맥박 _ 361
모순운동 _ 351
목동맥 _ 288
목뼈보호대 _ 275
목정맥구멍패임 _ 464
목정맥패임구멍 _ 364
목정맥 팽대 _ 356
몸통뼈대 _ 396
무딘 손상 _ 62, 195, 450
무딘 심장 파열 _ 359
무딘 외상 _ 109
무산소대사 _ 48
무산소증 _ 276
무인 항공 시스템 _ 719
무작위 대조 실험 _ 41
무해성 _ 31
무호흡 _ 176
물리학 _ 35
미국 응급구조사협회 _ 6
미만성 축삭 손상 _ 125
민간 전술적 응급의료지원 _ 28, 711

ㅂ

바늘감압 _ 356, 715
바로누운자세 _ 321
바빈스키 반사 _ 274
바이러스성 출혈열 _ 571
박힌 물체 _ 386
반신마비 _ 284
반신불안전마비 _ 270
반신불완전마비 _ 284
반지갑상연골절개 _ 232
반지갑상연골절개술 _ 715
발열 담요 _ 717
방사능 분산 장치 _ 573
방사선 재난 _ 574
방사선 피폭 _ 442
방사선 화상 _ 441
방임 _ 494
백린 _ 445, 558
백질 _ 302
베타 차단제 _ 489
병원 전 외상 소생술 _ 3
보상 예비 측정 _ 68
보일의 법칙 _ 648
보조 제어 _ 237
보충 산소 _ 467
보툴리눔 독소 _ 572
보폭전압 _ 633
보행자 충돌 _ 121
복강 _ 376
복막 _ 380
복막뒤공간 _ 376
복막뒤 출혈 _ 367
복막염 _ 379, 383
복부 검사 _ 461
복사 _ 588
복장뼈파임 _ 215
부교감신경계 _ 56
부목 고정 _ 405
부분층 화상 _ 425
부비동 압착 _ 650
부유 복장뼈 _ 359
분당 호흡량 _ 211
분당 환기량 _ 347
분류 _ 164
분포 _ 52
분포 쇼크 _ 59
불완전(생나무)골절 _ 469
브라운-시쿼드증후군 _ 306

브룩 공식 _ 434
비말 _ 566
비보상성 쇼크 _ 356
비보상성 저혈량 쇼크 _ 59
비보상 쇼크 _ 453
비색이산화탄소 감지기 _ 231
비스테로이드성 소염제 _ 69
비스테로이드성소염진통제 _ 196
비어스 기준 _ 490
비재호흡마스크 _ 235
비통기성 체스트 씰 _ 354
비틀림파 _ 555
비판적 사고 _ 28, 29
빈맥 _ 57, 453
빈혈 _ 277
빗장중간선 _ 356, 464
빠른 호흡 _ 37, 176
뼘 _ 412

ㅅ

사강 _ 210, 347
사고 단계 _ 12, 103
사고성 저체온증 _ 612
사고 전 단계 _ 11, 102
사고 지휘관 _ 150
사고 후 단계 _ 13, 103
사구체여과율 _ 484
사람면역결핍바이러스 _ 161
사망 _ 166
사망 징후 _ 194
사이안화물 _ 439, 561
사이질액 _ 54
사이토카인 _ 423
사제폭발물 _ 73, 554
사후경축 _ 695
산소운반체 _ 80
산소 전달 _ 212
산소 흡입량 _ 209
산탄총 _ 136
삼차 손상 _ 140
삼투 _ 55
삽관형 후두마스크기도기 _ 221
상기도 _ 206, 213
상행신경로 _ 302
상향경로 _ 112
상향 방전 _ 633
생리식염수 _ 78
생명윤리 _ 31
생명의 별 _ 6

생물학적 작용제 _ 564
서맥 _ 228
서스펜션 증후군 _ 688
선 골절 _ 285
선행 _ 31
선호 _ 25
설맹 _ 606
섬락 전류 _ 633
섬망 _ 484
성문위기도기 _ 219, 220
성형 부목 _ 406
세로칸 _ 62
세로칸기종 _ 651
세포 _ 49
세포 관류 _ 52
세포 내 공간 _ 55
세포 내액 _ 54
세포 대사 _ 49
세포 사멸 _ 34, 50
소뇌 _ 266
소뇌편도탈출 _ 274
소생 테이프 _ 461
소아 외상센터 _ 466
소아 평가 삼각구도 _ 455, 458
소이제 _ 558
속목정맥 _ 288
속빈장기 _ 136
손바닥 법칙 _ 430, 470
손상 중증도 점수 _ 191
쇼크 _ 48, 49
쇼크 지수 _ 53, 57
수색 및 구조 _ 534, 641
수액 소생술 _ 412
수축기 혈압 _ 52
수포음 _ 662
수포 작용제 _ 564
수포제 _ 445
순환 _ 63
스탈링의 법칙 _ 53
습구흑구온도지수 _ 600
시반 _ 695
시상하부 _ 587
시안화물 중독 _ 213
식도괄약근 _ 482
식도 밀폐 _ 220
신경성 쇼크 _ 59, 323
신경성 저혈압 _ 59
신경세포 _ 278
신경작용제 _ 561

신경학적 결손 _ 298
신경학적 기능 _ 400
신경활 _ 299
신속한 원격 평가 방법 _ 717
신체적 학대 _ 494
심낭 _ 61
심박출량 _ 50, 53
심부 동상 _ 609
심부전 _ 483
심부정맥혈전증 _ 389
심장근육 _ 59
심장눌림증 _ 360
심장막 _ 360
심장막천자 _ 361
심장성 _ 52
심장성 쇼크 _ 59
심장 진탕 _ 361
심장 타박상 _ 359
심장 탈출 _ 359

ㅇ

아데노신삼인산 _ 34, 48
아동 학대 _ 472
아래대정맥 _ 322, 355
아래턱 골절 _ 288
아세타졸아마이드 _ 664
안구내염 _ 287
안와 손상 _ 286
안전띠 _ 117
안전띠 징후 _ 188, 382
안전지대 _ 155
안전지역 _ 552, 712
안전 책임자 _ 532
알레르기 반응 _ 697
압력손상 _ 140, 344, 649
압박 골절 _ 305
압박 드레싱 _ 71
압착 _ 649
앞겨드랑선 _ 356
앞방출혈 _ 286
앞뿌리 _ 303
앞척수동맥 _ 302
야생 고급 응급구조사 _ 677
야생 응급구조사 _ 676
야생 응급의료 대응자 _ 676
야생 응급처치 _ 676
야생 전문 응급처치 _ 676
야생 진료보조인력 _ 677
야생 최초반응자 _ 676

야생 EMS _ 675
약물 보조 삽관 _ 226
양압 환기 _ 219, 352
얼굴 골절 _ 286
얼굴중간 골절 _ 287
엄폐 _ 713
에너지 보존 법칙 _ 104
에어백 _ 118
역트렌델렌버그 _ 317
역학적 3요소 _ 503
연결정맥 _ 266, 270
연부조직 손상 _ 400
열 발진 _ 591
열 부종 _ 591
열사병 _ 594
열 생산 _ 587
열 손실 방지 자세 _ 612
열 순응 _ 602
열 스트레스 지수 _ 600
열 실신 _ 592
열전도율 _ 422
열탈진 _ 593
열탕 화상 _ 471
영구적 공동 _ 108
예방산소투여 _ 217, 228
예방적 과다환기 _ 278, 291
예상 도착 시간 _ 193
오른아래사부역 _ 378
오른위사분역 _ 378
오름대동맥 _ 127
오염 제거 _ 157, 539, 553
오염지역 _ 155, 552
외과적 반지갑상연골절개 _ 457
외부 재가온 _ 623
외부출혈 _ 64, 289, 402
외상성 뇌손상 _ 59, 264, 453, 487
외상성 대동맥 파열 _ 362
외상성 심정지 _ 194
외상성 질식 _ 364
외상성 척추 손상 _ 298
외상 초음파 검사를 통한 확장된 집중 평가 _ 62
외상 턱들기 _ 216
외상 턱밀어올리기 _ 216
외호흡 _ 211
왼아래사분역 _ 378
왼위사분역 _ 378
요추전만증 _ 305
운동 관련 근육 경련 _ 591

운동 관련 저나트륨혈증 _ 597
운동 관련 저나트륨혈증 뇌병증 _ 597
운동기능 _ 400
운동성 열사병 _ 595
운동성 열탈진 _ 594
운동실조성 호흡 _ 274
운동에너지 _ 105, 129
운영 _ 154
움켜쥐는 반사 _ 180
원시 _ 484
원칙 _ 24
원형 사입구 _ 138
위기 상황 스트레스 관리 _ 540
위장관 _ 198
위장관 탄저병 _ 567
위험지역 _ 712
유두 진피 _ 423
유산소대사 _ 48
유스타키오관 _ 651
유해 물질 _ 154
윤곽 _ 129
윤리 _ 31
윤리적 원칙 _ 31
으깸 손상 _ 436
으깸증후군 _ 411
은폐 _ 713
응고 괴사 _ 442
응고구역 _ 424
응고병증 _ 85, 277
응고연쇄반응 _ 84
응급의료반응자 _ 205
응력파 _ 555
의도적 손상 _ 505
의사소통 장애 _ 311
의식 수준 _ 59, 453
이산화탄소의 분압 _ 234
이완기 혈압 _ 52
이차 뇌손상 _ 272
이차 폭발물 _ 158
익사 _ 638
익사 과정 _ 639
인식 _ 154
일산화탄소 _ 438
일산화탄소 중독 _ 240
일산화헤모글로빈 _ 438
일시적 공동 _ 108
일차 뇌손상 _ 269
일차평가 _ 173
일차 폭발 손상 _ 140

일회호흡량 _ 74, 233, 347
임신 중독증 _ 389
입구 상처 _ 134
입기관삽관 _ 225
입인두기도기 _ 217, 218

ㅈ

자동호기말양압 _ 74
자외선 차단 지수 _ 690
자율성 _ 31
자율신경계 _ 55
잠복성 출혈 _ 488
잠재 수명 손실 기간 _ 507
장거리 상처 _ 139
장기간 현장 처치 _ 686
재가압 챔버 _ 652
재난 대응계획 _ 161
재난 분류표 _ 535
재난 의료지원팀 _ 538
재난 주기 _ 525
재난지휘체계 _ 158
저나트륨혈증 _ 598
저산소 구동 _ 346
저산소증 _ 48, 224, 280, 452
저산소혈증 _ 48, 213
저성능 폭약 _ 555
저에너지 무기 _ 130
저온 두드러기 _ 605
저온 손상 _ 606
저이산화탄소혈증 _ 278, 281
저체온증 _ 586
저칼슘혈증 _ 444
저혈당 _ 278
저혈량 _ 52
저혈량 쇼크 _ 56
저혈압 소생술 _ 75
적대적 사건 _ 710
적혈구 _ 48
전기 손상 _ 436
전기 화상 _ 436
전단 _ 125
전단파 _ 555
전도 _ 588
전두골 _ 264
전리방사선 _ 573
전문가 _ 154
전문소생술 _ 195
전방충돌 _ 111
전방통제지역 _ 155, 552, 712

전복 _ 116
전복벽 _ 128
전부하 _ 52
전술적 응급사상자처치위원회 _ 711
전술적 전투 사상자 _ 712
전술적 전투 사상자 처치 _ 4
전술적 전투 사상자 처치 위원회 _ 7
전술적 현장 처치 _ 713, 719
전술적 후송 처치 _ 719
전신성 저혈압 _ 275
전신 순환 _ 54
전신 피폭량 _ 574
전척수증후군 _ 306
전층 압력 _ 70
전층 화상 _ 426
전혈 _ 58
절단 _ 409
접촉 상처 _ 138
접촉 화상 _ 440, 471
접합부 지혈대 _ 73
접합부 출혈 _ 175
정맥 라인 _ 182
정맥울혈 _ 689
정맥 출혈 _ 177
정맥 폐쇄 _ 275
정맥혈복귀 _ 62, 229
정서적 학대 _ 494
정신 상태 _ 65
정신 상태 변화 _ 311
정체구역 _ 424
제 I 형 감압병 _ 654
종이 봉지 효과 _ 126
좌심실 _ 54
죽상경화증 _ 483
중간수막동맥 _ 269, 279
중거리 상처 _ 138
중성자 _ 441, 574
중쇠뼈 _ 299
중심척수증후군 _ 306
중심탈출 _ 274
중에너지 무기 _ 132
중이 압착 _ 650
중증 급성 호흡기 증후군 _ 567
중증외상 환자 _ 39
중증 출혈 _ 177
중추신경계 _ 62, 454
중추 청색증 _ 457
즉시 _ 166
증발 _ 588

지갑상연골절개술 _ 279
지속기도양압 _ 228, 665
지속적기도양압기 _ 352
지속적양압환기기 _ 367
지속적인 의료 교육 _ 27
지속적 품질 개선 _ 240
지연 _ 166
지연성 손상 _ 424
지연연속기관삽관 _ 226
지혈대 _ 71, 178, 402
지혈제 _ 73
직접 압박 _ 71, 177, 462
진공부목 _ 312
진정제 _ 199
진통제 _ 197
진피 돌기 _ 423
질식 중독 증후군 _ 560

ㅊ

차량 충돌 _ 103
참호발 _ 607
척수 _ 302
척수 관류압 _ 307
척수 손상 _ 298, 323
척수 쇼크 _ 307
척수 절단 _ 306
척주후만증 _ 492
척추 고정 _ 38, 312
척추고정판 _ 317
척추공 _ 299
척추뼈 _ 299
척추뼈 몸통 _ 299
척추 손상 _ 323
척추 움직임 _ 38
척추 움직임 제한 _ 214, 308, 684
청력 저하 _ 484
청진 _ 349
체수분 _ 55
체스트 씰 _ 715
체인-스톡스 _ 274
체질량 지수 _ 356
체판 _ 187
체표면적 _ 423
촉진 _ 349
총상 _ 132, 380
총체액량 _ 590
총 폐용량 _ 347
최대 날숨 _ 377
추간공 _ 299

추락 _ 123
출구 상처 _ 134
출혈 _ 64
출혈쇼크 _ 59
충격-맞충격 _ 279
충격파 _ 555
충혈구역 _ 424
측면 섬광 _ 633
측면충돌 _ 114
치매 _ 483
치아염소산나트륨 _ 553
침수 저체온증 _ 612
침수 화상 _ 440

ㅋ

칼슘 채널 차단제 _ 490
코기관삽관 _ 225
코뼈 골절 _ 287
코삽입관 _ 235, 666
코 안 투여 _ 694
코인두기도기 _ 218, 714
콜레스골절 _ 485
콜린성 중독 _ 560
쿠싱 반사 _ 289
쿨렌징후 _ 382
큰구멍 _ 302

ㅌ

타진 _ 349
탄산수소염 _ 210
탄저 _ 567
탈구 _ 407
탈수 _ 590
탈출증 _ 273, 281
탈출증후군 _ 273
태반조기박리 _ 387
텀블 _ 130
테러 _ 538
테러 작전 의료지원 _ 710
테르밋 _ 558
토혈 _ 224
통기성 체스트 씰 _ 354
통증 완화 _ 40
통합지휘체계 _ 159
퇴행관절염 _ 492
투과성 _ 55
투쟁-도피 반응 _ 56
튜브 가슴관삽입 _ 357
트라넥삼산 _ 58, 84, 465

트라이카복실산 회로 _ 212
트렌델렌버그 자세 _ 76

ㅍ

파종혈관내응고 _ 389
파크랜드 공식 _ 434
파크메틱 _ 676
파편 _ 130
파형 호기말이산화탄소분압측정 _ 350
판막 손상 _ 61
판막 파열 _ 359
팔다리뼈대 _ 396
팔오금 _ 465
펜타닐 _ 466
편향 징후 _ 284
평균 동맥압 _ 53, 75, 267
폐 과도팽창 _ 651
폐 독성 물질 _ 563
폐렴흑사병 _ 569
폐부종 _ 662
폐 손상 _ 135
폐쇄골절 _ 404
폐쇄드레싱 _ 353
폐쇄 함몰두개골 골절 _ 285
폐 타박상 _ 348
폐포 _ 206
포도당 용액 _ 78
폭발파 _ 139, 140
폭발풍 _ 555
폭풍파 _ 555
표재성 동상 _ 609
표재 화상 _ 425
풍속냉각지수 _ 620
플래티넘 10분 _ 39
피라미드형 골절 _ 287
피부밑기종 _ 364, 652
피부밑조직 _ 424
피부밑 화상 _ 426
피부 분절 _ 303
피질제거자세 _ 180, 274
피크의 원리 _ 50, 51

ㅎ

하기도 _ 206
하네스 행 증후군 _ 688
하이드록소코발라민 _ 561
하임리히법 _ 646
하행대동맥 _ 362
하행신경로 _ 303

하향 경로 _ 112
학대 _ 197
함몰두개골 골절 _ 268, 285
합동 외상시스템 _ 710
항공 이송 _ 193
항균 코팅 드레싱 _ 432
항상성 _ 589
항이뇨호르몬 _ 56
해든 매트릭스 _ 503
햇빛 화상 _ 690
헐떡임 반사 _ 614
헤타스타치 _ 80
헨리의 법칙 _ 649
현장 지휘관 _ 532
현장 지휘소 _ 532
현장 평가 _ 148
혈관 내액 _ 54
혈관 용적 _ 54
혈당강하제 _ 490
혈압 _ 67
혈흉 _ 357
협착 _ 483
형질막 _ 424
형평성 _ 512
호기말양압 _ 237, 665
호기말양압환기 _ 367
호기말이산화탄소 _ 234
호기말이산화탄소분압 _ 64, 234, 456
호기말이산화탄소분압측정기 _ 182
호흡 _ 63
호흡곤란 _ 349, 457
호흡근 _ 345
호흡 노력 _ 347
호흡부전 _ 482
화상 손상 _ 427
화상 쇼크 _ 422
화학 물질 _ 549
화학 작용제 _ 442
화학 화상 _ 442
확산 이상 _ 213
환기 _ 345
환기 속도 _ 66
환자 분류 _ 536, 552
환자처치기록지 _ 40
황금 기간 _ 14, 33, 172
황금 시간 _ 33
황색포도상구균 _ 566
회복자세 _ 714
회색질 _ 302

회전충돌 _ 116
횡문근융해증 _ 411
후두 골절 _ 288
후두마스크기도기 _ 219
후두튜브기도기 _ 219, 221
후방 추돌 _ 113
후부하 _ 52
후천면역결핍증후군 _ 161
흉복부 _ 376
흉추후만증 _ 305
흑사병 _ 569
흡인 _ 216
흡인 가슴 상처 _ 353
흡입 손상 _ 437
흡입 화상 _ 435

A

AEMT _ 677
AVPU _ 179, 685

B

Beck의 3 징후 _ 360

C

C-A-T 지혈대 _ 71
CBRNE _ 548
CONTOOMS _ 717
CS-LTOWB _ 716
CUFT _ 712

D

DUMBELS _ 562

E

eFAST _ 385

F

FACES _ 473
FAST _ 383

I

i-gel _ 221
IO _ 77, 182
IV _ 182

J

JumpStart _ 535

L

LATE _ 677

Level A 개인보호장비 _ 569
Lund−Browder _ 431

M

MARCH _ 63
MARCH PAWS _ 685
MARH _ 620
MASS _ 535, 553
MTWHF _ 562

N

N95 마스크 _ 570

O

OEC _ 676

P

PA _ 677
ParkMedic _ 676
PRICE _ 695

S

SALT _ 166, 535, 553
SAMPLE _ 186
SAMPLER 병력 _ 39
SCIWORA _ 468
SOFT−W 지혈대 _ 71
START _ 166, 535, 553

T

TCA _ 212
TNE _ 473

U

UKFRS 지침 _ 642

W

WAFA _ 676
WEMR _ 676
WEMT _ 676
WFA _ 676
WFR _ 676

기타

1단계 출혈 _ 57
1도 동상 _ 608
1차 폭발 손상 _ 555
2단계 출혈 _ 57
2도 동상 _ 609
2차 폭발 손상 _ 556
3단계 출혈 _ 57
3도 동상 _ 609
3차 폭발 손상 _ 557
4단계 출혈 _ 58
4도 동상 _ 609
9의 법칙 _ 430
10의 법칙 _ 430, 435